CONTENTS IN BRIEF

SECTION I Children, Their Families and the Nurse

1 Perspectives of Paediatric Nursing, 1
2 Social, Cultural, Religious and Family Influences on Child Health Promotion, 11
3 Hereditary Influences on Health Promotion of the Child and Family, 25

SECTION II Childhood and Family Assessment

4 Communication, Physical and Developmental Assessment of the Child and Family, 50
5 Pain Assessment and Management in Children, 97
6 Childhood Communicable and Infectious Diseases, 121

SECTION III Family-centred Care of the Newborn

7 Health Promotion of the Newborn and Family, 137
8 Health Problems of the Newborn, 168
9 The High-risk Newborn and Family, 196

SECTION IV Family-centred Care of the Infant

10 Health Promotion of the Infant and Family, 241
11 Health Problems of the Infant, 272

SECTION V Family-centred Care of the Toddler and Preschooler

12 Health Promotion of the Toddler and Family, 290
13 Health Promotion of the Preschooler and Family, 310
14 Health Problems of Early Childhood, 324

SECTION VI Family-centred Care of the School-age Child

15 Health Promotion of the School-age Child and Family, 337
16 Health Problems of the School-age Child, 360

SECTION VII Family-centred Care of the Adolescent

17 Health Promotion of the Adolescent and Family, 381
18 Health Problems of the Adolescent, 400

SECTION VIII Family-centred Care of the Child with Special Needs

19 Impact of Chronic Illness, Disability or End-of-life Care for the Child and Family, 423
20 Impact of Cognitive or Sensory Loss on the Child and Family, 448

SECTION IX The Child Who is Hospitalised

21 Family-centred Care of the Child During Illness and Hospitalisation, 467
22 Paediatric Nursing Interventions and Skills, 481

SECTION X Childhood Nutrition and Elimination Problems

23 The Child with Fluid and Electrolyte Imbalance, 520
24 The Child with Renal Dysfunction, 556
25 The Child with Gastrointestinal Dysfunction, 592

SECTION XI Childhood Oxygenation Problems

26 The Child with Respiratory Dysfunction, 637

SECTION XII Childhood Blood Production and Circulation Problems

27 The Child with Cardiovascular Dysfunction, 701
28 The Child with Haematological or Immunological Dysfunction, 752

SECTION XIII Childhood Regulatory Problems

29 The Child with Cancer, 783
30 The Child with Cerebral Dysfunction, 819
31 The Child with Endocrine Dysfunction, 865

SECTION XIV Childhood Physical Mobility Problems

32 The Child with Integumentary Dysfunction, 891
33 The Child with Musculoskeletal or Articular Dysfunction, 911
34 The Child with Neuromuscular or Muscular Dysfunction, 960

WONG'S Nursing Care of Infants and Children

AUSTRALIA AND NEW ZEALAND EDITION—FOR PROFESSIONALS

Australian adaptation edited by:

Lisa Speedie, RN Div 1, BN, Grad Dip Women's Health, MNS

Senior Fellow, Higher Education Academy (United Kingdom)
Lecturer, School of Nursing, Paramedicine and Healthcare Sciences, Charles Sturt University
Higher Education Research and Development Society of Australasia member
Australian College of Nursing member

Andrea Middleton, RN, BN (Hons), MCN (Paediatrics)

Clinical Nurse Educator (Paediatrics), Centre for Education and Research, Royal Hobart Hospital
Tasmanian Health Service—South
Lecturer, School of Nursing, College of Health and Medicine, University of Tasmania

US editors:

Marilyn J. Hockenberry, PhD, RN, PPCPNP-BC, FAAN

Professor of Pediatrics
Baylor College of Medicine
Director, Global HOPE Nursing
Texas Children's Hospital
Houston, Texas
Bessie Baker Professor Emerita of Nursing
Chair, Duke Institutional Review Board
Duke University
Durham, North Carolina

David Wilson, MS, RN, C(INC), (deceased)

Staff
Children's Hospital at Saint Francis
Tulsa, Oklahoma

Cheryl C. Rodgers, PhD, RN, CPNP, CPON (deceased)

Associate Professor
Chair, Duke Institutional Review Board
Duke University School of Nursing
Durham, North Carolina

ELSEVIER

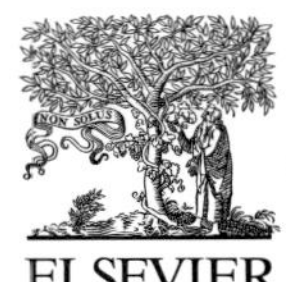

ELSEVIER

Elsevier Australia, ACN 001 002 357
(a division of Reed International Books Australia Pty Ltd)
Tower 1, 475 Victoria Avenue, Chatswood, NSW 2067

Wong's Nursing Care of Infants and Children

ISBN: 978-0-323-54939-4

This adaptation of Wong's Nursing Care of Infants and Children, 11e by Marilyn J. Hockenberry, David Wilson and Cheryl C. Rodgers, was undertaken by Elsevier Australia and is published by arrangement with Elsevier Inc.

Wong's Nursing Care of Infants and Children - For Professionals

ISBN: 978-0-7295-4366-8

National Library of Australia Cataloguing-in-Publication Data

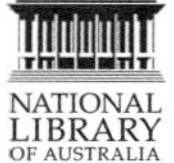

A catalogue record for this book is available from the National Library of Australia

Senior Content Strategist: Natalie Hunt
Content Project Manager: Shruti Raj
Edited by Leanne Peters
Proofread by Tim Learner
Cover by Georgette Hall
Index by SPi Global
Typeset by GW Tech India
Printed in Singapore by KHL Printing Co Pte Ltd

Dedication

To April and Tiffany

'The future belongs to those who believe in the beauty of their dreams.' (Eleanor Roosevelt)

To Benjamin, Samuel and Jacob

'The more that you read, the more things you will know. The more that you learn, the more places you'll go.' (Dr Seuss)

AUSTRALIAN AND NEW ZEALAND CONTRIBUTORS

Lauren Kendrick, RN, BN, MN, GradCert (Neonatal Intensive Care)
Senior Academic Staff Member and Neonatal Paper Coordinator
School of Nursing
Auckland University of Technology
Auckland
Neonatal Intensive Care Unit
Starship Child Health
Auckland District Health Board
New Zealand

Elyce Kenny, RN, BN, GradCert (Nurs Ed), GradDip (Paed, Child and Yth Hlth Nursing)
Lecturer
Adelaide Nursing School
The University of Adelaide
Adelaide, South Australia
Australia

Christine Taylor, RN, BAppSc (Adv Nsg), BSc (Hons), MHScEd, PhD, MACN
Senior Lecturer
School of Nursing and Midwifery
Western Sydney University
Parramatta, New South Wales
Australia

Lynne Staff, RN, RM, MMid (Hons)
Lecturer in Nursing and Midwifery
School of Nursing
University of Tasmania
Launceston, Hobart
Australia

Amy Vaccaro, RN, RM, BN, MMid, GradCert (Acute Care)
Clinical Support Nurse/Midwife
Albury–Wodonga Health and Sessional Lecturer
School of Nursing, Paramedicine and Healthcare Science
Charles Sturt University
Albury, New South Wales
Australia

Emma Collins, RN, BEd, MN, DipTchng, PGCert (Higher Ed), FHEA
Professional Practice Fellow
Women's and Children's Health
University of Otago
Dunedin
New Zealand

Tameeka Mulquiney, RN, RM, MMid (Dist)
Lecturer
School of Nursing, Paramedicine and Healthcare Science
Charles Sturt University
Albury, New South Wales
Australia

Deb Surman, RN, DipNsg, BN, GradCert (Emerg Nsg), MN
Senior Academic Staff Member
School of Nursing
Waikato Institute of Technology (Wintec)
Hamilton
New Zealand

Patience Moyo, RN, M (AdNursPrac), GradCert (LTHE), GradCert (Acute Care Nurs), MACN
Lecturer in Nursing
School of Nursing, Paramedicine and Healthcare Science
Charles Sturt University
Dubbo, New South Wales
Australia

Kylie Smith, RN, DipHlthSci (Nursing)
eClinician
Clinical eHealth Project team
Health ICT
Dubbo, New South Wales
Australia

Felicity Radford, RN, BNurs
Paediatric Registered Nurse
Paediatric Unit
Dubbo Health Service
Dubbo, New South Wales
Australia

Julia Laing, RCompN, MHSc
Clinical Nurse Specialist
Waikids—Waikato Child and Youth Health
Waikato District Health Board
Waikato
New Zealand

Jane Mateer, NSC, RN, Cert Emergency, GD Nurse Specialisation (NP), MPH, FCENA
Clinical Nurse Educator
Monash Children's Hospital
Melbourne, New South Wales
Australia

Maryanne Podham, RN, BHlthSci, MN (Clinical Education), MACN,
Lecturer in Nursing
School of Nursing, Paramedicine and Healthcare Science
Charles Sturt University
Dubbo, New South Wales
Australia

Ibi Patane, RN, BN, GCPCYHN, GradDip (EBP), MNsg, CCN, FHEA
Clinical Lecturer
School of Nursing
Queensland University of Technology
Brisbane, Queensland
Australia

Sarah Dechert, RN, BN, PostGradCert (Neonatal Intensive Care)
Associate Nurse Unit Manager
Special Care Nursery
Albury Wodonga Health
Wodonga, Victoria
Australia

CONTRIBUTORS TO US EDITION

Caroline E. Anderson, RN, MSN, CPHON
Clinical Practice and Advanced Education Specialist
Cook Children's Medical Center
Fort Worth, Texas

Annette L. Baker, RN, BSN, MSN, CPNP
Pediatric Nurse Practitioner
Department of Cardiology
Boston Children's Hospital
Boston, Massachusetts

Rose Ann Urdiales Baker, PhD, PMHCNS, RN
Associate Instructor
School of Nursing
College of Health Professions
University of Akron
Akron, Ohio

Raymond C. Barfield, MD, PhD
Professor of Pediatrics and Christian Philosophy; Director, Medical Humanities
Pediatrics, and Trent Center for Bioethics, Humanities, and History of Medicine
Duke University
Durham, North Carolina

Amy Barry, MSN, RN, PNP-BC
Pediatric Nurse Practitioner
Children's Healthcare of Atlanta
Atlanta, Georgia

Heather Bastardi, RN, cPNP, CCTC
Pediatric Nurse Practitioner
Advanced Cardiac Therapies
Boston Children's Hospital
Boston, Massachusetts

Debra Brandon, PhD, RN, CNS, FAAN
Associate Professor
School of Nursing
Duke University
Associate Professor
Department of Pediatrics, School of Medicine
Duke University
Neonatal CNS
Duke Intensive Care Nursery
Durham, North Carolina

Rosalind Bryant, PhD, RN-CS, PNP
Clinical Instructor
Baylor College of Medicine
Houston, Texas

Cynthia J. Camille, MSN, RN, CPNP, FNP-BC
Pediatric Nurse Practitioner
Pediatric Urology
Duke University Health System
Durham, North Carolina

Brigit M. Carter, PhD, RN, CCRN
Director
Accelerated BSN Program
Duke University School of Nursing
Durham, North Carolina

Lisa M. Cleveland, PhD, RN, PNP-BC, IBCLC, NTMNC
Assistant Professor
School of Nursing
UT Health San Antonio
San Antonio, Texas

Patricia Conlon, MS, APRN, CNS, CNP
Pediatric Clinical Nurse Specialist
Assistant Professor of Nursing
Mayo Clinic Children's Center
Rochester, Minnesota

Erin Connelly, APRN, CPNP, CPON
Developmental Therapeutics Nurse Practitioner
Department of Hematology
Children's Healthcare of Atlanta
Clinical Manager of Advance Practice
Department of Oncology
Aflac Cancer and Blood Disorders Center
Atlanta, Georgia

Anne Derouin, DNP, APRN, CPNP, FAANP
Associate Professor, Faculty Lead, MSN/PNP-PC and Pediatric Behavioral Mental Health Specialty
School of Nursing
Duke University
Durham, North Carolina

Sharron L. Docherty, PhD, PNP-BC, FAAN
Associate Professor
Department of Pediatrics
Duke University
Durham, North Carolina

Angela Drummond, MS, APRN, CPNP
Pediatric Nurse Practitioner–Orthopedics
Gillette Children's Specialty Healthcare
St Paul, Minnesota

Elizabeth A. Duffy, DNP, RN, CPNP
Clinical Assistant Professor
Health Behavior and Biological Sciences
The University of Michigan School of Nursing
Ann Arbor, Michigan

Kimberley Fisher, PhD, FNP-BC
Research Director
Neonatal Perinatal Research Unit
Division of Neonatology
Duke University
Durham, North Carolina

Jan M. Foote, DNP, CPNP, ARNP, FAANP
Pediatric Nurse Practitioner
Blank Children's Hospital
Des Moines, Iowa
Adjunct Clinical Associate Professor
University of Iowa College of Nursing
Iowa City, Iowa

Quinn Franklin, MS, CCLS
Assistant Director
Psychosocial Division
Cancer and Hematology Centers
Texas Children's Hospital
Houston, Texas

Ruth Anne Herring, MSN, RN, CPNP-AC/PC, CPHON
Pediatric Nurse Practitioner
Center for Cancer and Blood Disorders
Children's Health
Dallas, Texas

Mystii Kidd, MSN, RN, CPNP
Pediatric Nurse Practitioner
TLC Pediatrics, PA
Allen, Texas

Teri A. Huddleston Lavenbarg, MSN, APRN, PPCNP-BC, FNP-BC, CDE
Nurse Practitioner
Medical Center
University of Kansas
Kansas City, Kansas

Shirley D. Martin, PhD, RN, CPN
Outpatient Surgery
Cook Children's Medical Center
Fort Worth, Texas

Maggie Maxtin, RN, BSN, CPN
Hematology/Oncology RN
Cook Children's Medical Center
Fort Worth, Texas

Patricia Barry McElfresh, MN, RN, PNP
Clinical Program Manager—Advanced Practice Providers
Hematology Oncology-Bone Marrow Failure
Aflac Cancer & Blood Disorders Center
Atlanta, Georgia

Tara Merck, MSN, APRN, CPNP
Director of Advanced Practice Providers
Children's Specialty Group
Medical College of Wisconsin
Milwaukee, Wisconsin

Mary A. Mondozzi, MSN, BSN, WCC
Burn Center Education/Outreach Coordinator
The Paul and Carol David Foundation Burn Institute
Akron Children's Hospital
Akron, Ohio

Rebecca A. Monroe, MSN, RN, CPNP
Pediatric Nurse Practitioner
Collin County Pediatrics
Frisco, Texas

Kim Mooney-Doyle, PhD, CPNP-AC, RN
Assistant Professor
School of Nursing
University of Maryland
Baltimore, Maryland

Patricia O'Brien, CPNP-AC
Nurse Practitioner
Cardiology
Boston Children's Hospital
Boston, Massachusetts

Sue Park, APN, CPNP-PC
Pediatric Nurse Practitioner
Pediatric Anesthesia
Ann and Robert H. Lurie Children's Hospital of Chicago
Chicago, Illinois

Katherine Soss Prihoda, DNP, RN, PPCNP-BC
Assistant Professor
School of Nursing
Rutgers University, Camden
Camden, New Jersey

Cynthia A. Prows, MSN, APRN, FAAN
Clinical Nurse Specialist
Human Genetics and Patient Services
Cincinnati Children's Hospital Medical Center
Cincinnati, Ohio

Patricia A. Ring, MSN, RN, CPNP
Pediatric Nephrology
Children's Hospital of Wisconsin
Milwaukee, Wisconsin

Kathleen S. Ruccione, PhD, RN, MPH, CPON, FAAN
Associate Professor and Chair
Department of Doctoral Programs
Azusa Pacific University
Azusa, California

Margaret L. Schroeder, MSN, RN, PPCNP-BC
Pediatric Nurse Practitioner
Cardiovascular Surgery
Boston Children's Hospital
Boston, Massachusetts

Maureen Sheehan, CPNP
Child Neurology, Epilepsy, and Ketogenic Diet Nurse Practitioner
Child Neurology and Advanced Practice
Stanford Children's Health
Palo Alto, California

Katherine Smalling, RN, BSN, CPON
Nurse Case Manager
Children's Medical Center Dallas
Center for Cancer and Blood Disorders
Dallas, Texas

Anne Feierabend Stanton, APRN, PCNS, BC
Pediatric Clinical Nurse Specialist
University of Kansas Medical Center
Kansas City, Kansas

Alexandra Kathleen Superdock, MD
Pediatric Resident
University of Pittsburgh Medical Center
Pittsburgh, Pennsylvania

Barbara J. Wheeler, RN, MN, IBCLC
Neonatal Clinical Nurse Specialist
St Boniface General Hospital
Winnipeg, Canada

Kristina D. Wilson, PhD, CCC-SLP
Senior Speech Pathologist and Clinical Research
Division of Speech, Language, and Learning
Texas Children's Hospital
Houston, Texas

AUSTRALIAN AND NEW ZEALAND REVIEWERS

Kelly Grant, RN, BN, MCN (Paediatrics)
Clinical Nurse Consultant
Children's and Adolescent Ward
Royal Hobart Hospital
Hobart, Tasmania
Australia

Gracie Patten, RN, BN (ClinHons), GradCertN (Paediatrics)
Children's and Adolescent Ward
Royal Hobart Hospital
Hobart, Tasmania
Australia

Leah Campbell, RN, BN, GradCertN (Paediatrics)
Children's and Adolescent Ward
The Royal Children's Hospital
Royal Hobart Hospital
Hobart, Tasmania
Australia

Grace Shallard, RN, BN, MPhil (Nursing)
Nurse Specialist, Child Protection
Te Puaruruhau, Starship Children's Hospital
Auckland
New Zealand

Lola Bishop, RN, BNsg, CCHNS (CAFHN), Cert IV TAELLN, M (Professional Education &Training)
Lecturer
Flinders University
Adelaide, South Australia
Australia

Deaane Terlich, RN, RM, EM
Albury Wodonga Health
Wodonga, Victoria
Australia

PREFACE

The first edition of *Wong's Nursing Care of Infants and Children* adaptation for Australia and New Zealand was a huge undertaking especially when the decision was made to edit two versions, Student and Professional. As co-editors we began the challenge of sourcing contributors from both Australia and New Zealand and, due to the two versions, sourced both academics and clinical experts.

In a rapidly changing environment, supporting the educational needs of nurses working with infants, children and young people and their families is essential. At a time where nurse recruitment and retention is at the forefront of healthcare in both Australia and New Zealand, nurses need to be supported to provide safe and fulfilling care across many clinical contexts, such as tertiary centres, paediatric units within adult-focused hospitals, emergency departments, theatres, rural centres and outpatient clinics, just to name a few. We hope that Wong's Nursing Care of Infants and Children finds a place in supporting both students new to paediatric nursing and nurses who have found their niche in caring for infants, children, young people and their families and want to enhance their expertise in the care they provide.

We would like to take a moment to reflect on the legacy of this textbook. The first edition of Whaley and Wong's *Nursing Care of Infants and Children*, published by Elsevier in 1979, was the first of its kind to integrate important principles from the biological, physical and behavioural sciences into a paediatric nursing textbook. With the first United States (US) edition, the principles and concepts of nursing practice were conceptualised to give both nursing students and experienced nurses an opportunity to expand and refine nursing care; this proves true with the 11th US edition. This, the first Australian and New Zealand (ANZ) edition, has divided the US text, providing the student with a more streamlined text suited to their beginner needs. The professional text contains more in-depth content and appropriate research cues for nurses practising paediatric nursing. Neither text has come without its challenges for both ourselves as editors and for the contributors. Asking such passionate and knowledgeable contributors to split the content was difficult.

The first ANZ edition clearly reflects 21st-century changes in paediatric nursing and demonstrates how scientific evidence has had a significant impact on the specialty in the ANZ environment. It continues to be about providing best practice care to children their families, and it emphasises the philosophy of family-centred care. This book has retained the theme that Donna Wong so passionately advocated: providing care that minimises the psychological and physical stress that health promotion and illness can inflict. The first edition's preface stated, 'This book truly embodies the concept of [family-centred] care.' We are proud to note that with this new edition, this foundation remains true. Features such as Family-centred Care, Community Focus and Nursing Care Considerations boxes bring these philosophies to life throughout the text. We believe strongly that children and families need consistent caregivers. Establishing therapeutic relationships with the child and family is explored as the essential foundation for providing quality nursing care.

This first ANZ edition has been revised to keep pace with new innovations in paediatric nursing care, particularly in Australia and New Zealand. We feel a unique accountability and responsibility to continue to strive to provide students and professionals with the latest information they need to become competent critical thinkers and to attain the sensitivity necessary to become caring paediatric nurses. As editors for the first ANZ Wong textbooks, we have developed an expert panel of more than 20 nurses and multidisciplinary specialists who assisted in reviewing, revising, rewriting and authoring portions of the text on areas undergoing rapid and complex change, such as immunisations, genetics, high-risk newborn care, adolescent health issues, numerous diseases and care specific to Aboriginal and Torres Strait Islander and Māori children and families. We have carefully preserved aspects of the book that have met with such universal acceptance—its state-of-the-art evidence-based information; strong, integrated focus on the family and community; logical and user-friendly organisation; and easy reading style. We have placed additional emphasis on research with concise reviews of important evidence in Research Focus boxes within the Professional edition. With this first ANZ edition we emphasised the importance of care evaluation and have added Nursing Care Consideration boxes throughout the book to demonstrate how quality of care can be assessed among the paediatric population. This feature allows students and professionals to review new evidence and quality indicators on important topics in a concise way.

Pathophysiology review figures throughout the text provide a concise evaluation of major healthcare diseases in children. With an understanding of the pathophysiological process, the nurse is better prepared to develop evidence-based nursing interventions for patient care. In addition, more than 130 figures are colour enhanced to focus on the importance on visual learning. This provides the visual learner with a tangible connection to the content of the text for application to clinical practice.

Within the Student edition we have tried to meet the increasing demands of faculty and students to teach and to learn in an environment characterised by rapid change, enormous amounts of information, fewer traditional clinical facilities and less time to teach. To help students quickly locate essential information, most of the features used in the US edition have been retained. Within the Professional edition we continue to use Evidence-Based Practice boxes incorporating the PICOT approach and GRADE evidence quality assessment criteria. Most importantly, this text continues to encourage professionals to *think critically*.

These two texts serve as reference manuals for the practising student nurse and professional. The latest recommendations have been included from authoritative organisations such as the Royal Children's Hospital Melbourne, Sydney Children's Hospital, Australian Institute of Health and Welfare, Ministry of Health New Zealand, Wellington Children's Hospital and Starship Children's Hospital, Auckland. To expand the universe of available information, websites have been included for many of organisations and other educational resources used and referenced throughout the two texts.

ORGANISATION OF THE BOOK

The same general approach to the presentation of content has been preserved from previous US editions, although much content has been added, condensed and rearranged within this framework to improve flow, minimise duplication, emphasise healthcare trends (such as home and community care) and ensure the relevance to Australia and New Zealand. The two books continue to be divided into two broad parts. The first part of the book, sometimes called the 'age and stage' approach, considers infancy, childhood and adolescence from a developmental context. It emphasises the importance of the nurse's role in health promotion and maintenance and in considering the family as the focus of care. From a developmental perspective, the care of common health problems is presented, giving readers a sense of what normal problems can be expected in otherwise healthy children and demonstrating when during childhood these problems are most likely to occur. The second part of the book presents the more serious health problems not specific to any particular age group but that frequently require hospitalisation or major medical and nursing interventions. Both books also take into consideration cultural needs and a rural and remote aspect addressing the needs of ANZ children and families.

Unit I (Chapters 1 to 3) provides an overview of the multitude of influences on a child who is developing as a member of a family unit and maturing within a culture, community and society. Chapter 1 includes a discussion of morbidity and mortality in infancy and childhood and examines child healthcare from a historical perspective. Because unintentional injury is one of the leading causes of death in children, an overview of this topic is included. The chapter presents the nursing process with an emphasis on nursing diagnosis and outcomes and the Professional edition focuses on the importance of developing critical thinking skills. The critical components of evidence-based practice provide the template for exploring the latest paediatric nursing research and practice guidelines throughout the Professional edition. Discussion of nursing care considerations and their importance in evaluating the quality of nursing care has been added in several sections of the Student edition.

Chapter 2 in both books provides the opportunity to expand the discussion of social, cultural, religious, rural/regional and family influences on child development and health promotion, including socioeconomic factors, customs and health beliefs and practices. The content clearly describes the role of the nurse, with such information as guidelines for culturally sensitive interactions and nursing consideration discussions.

Unit II (Chapters 4 to 6) is concerned with the principles of critical nursing assessment by keeping pace with the newest evaluation strategies in nursing. Chapter 4 contains guidelines for communicating with children, adolescents and their families; telephone triage; and a detailed description of a health assessment, including an extensive discussion of family assessment and nutritional assessment. This chapter provides a comprehensive approach to physical examination and developmental assessment, using the latest literature.

In this edition, an important chapter with new contributors is devoted to critical assessment and management of pain in children. Although the literature on pain assessment and management in children has grown considerably, this knowledge has not been widely applied in practice. Chapter 5 addresses this concern by presenting detailed pain assessment and management strategies, including discussion of common pain states in children. Chapter 6 was a newly developed chapter for the 11th US edition focusing on the various infectious diseases encountered in childhood, and has been adapted to include ANZ infectious requirements. In addition, it details hospital-acquired infections, childhood communicable diseases and childhood immunisations within both books.

Unit III (Chapters 7 to 9) in both books stresses the importance of the neonatal period, the time of greatest risk to a child's survival, and discusses several health concerns encountered in the vulnerable first month of life. Chapter 7 has been updated and revised to include the latest information on the benefits of breastfeeding. Nursing consideration sections have been revised to include the latest evidence-based recommendations for pain management in newborns. Newborn screening guidelines have also been extensively updated. Chapter 8 has also been revised and updated. The latest guidelines for the management of hyperbilirubinaemia in late-preterm and term newborns and for follow-up and management of hyperbilirubinaemia in the breastfeeding pair are included in this edition. Updated management protocols for neonatal hypoglycaemia are also included. Nursing considerations of the newborn remains an important concept in these chapters. Evidence-based practice and critical thinking exercises have also been updated in the Professional book. Chapter 9 contains information regarding maternal conditions that may adversely affect the fetus and newborn, including maternal viruses, maternal diabetes, fetal alcohol and tobacco exposure, and neonatal drug exposure.

Units IV through VII (Chapters 10 to 18) in both books present the major developmental stages in childhood, expanded to provide a broader concept of the stages and the health problems most often associated with each age group. Special emphasis is placed on the preventive aspects of care. The health promotion chapters follow a standard approach that is used consistently for each age group.

The chapters on health problems primarily reflect typical and age-related concerns. The information on many disorders has been revised to reflect recent changes, particularly within Australia and New Zealand. Examples include the latest information on food sensitivity, attention-deficit/hyperactivity disorder, contraception, teenage pregnancy, substance abuse, self-harm and eating disorders such as anorexia nervosa and childhood obesity. The section on sudden infant death syndrome (SIDS) has been extensively updated to include the latest ANZ considerations for recognised SIDS protective and risk factors. A common theme in these chapters is the recognition of the impact of accidental childhood injury on childhood morbidity and mortality and efforts for prevention of such injuries.

Childhood obesity information is now located in the school-age child chapter to emphasise the need for earlier assessment and intervention of this health problem. Sections on male and female reproductive health conditions, sexual orientation and gender identity and support have been revised and updated.

Unit VIII (Chapters 19 and 20) in both books deals with children who have the same developmental needs as growing children but who, because of congenital or acquired physical, cognitive or sensory impairment, require alternative interventions to facilitate development. Chapter 19 combines discussions of chronic illness, disability and end-of-life care for the child and family. It reflects the latest trends in the care of families and children with chronic illness or disability, such as home care, normalising children's lives, focusing on developmental needs, enabling and empowering families and providing early intervention. The content in Chapter 20 on cognitive, sensory and communication impairment includes the latest information on cognitive impairment and learning disorders.

Unit IX (Chapters 21 and 22) is concerned with the impact of hospitalisation on the child and the family and presents a comprehensive overview of the stressors imposed by hospitalisation and nursing interventions available to prevent or eliminate these stressors. Chapter 21 discusses the care of the hospitalised child and family with consideration for increasing care in ambulatory centres. Chapter 22 explores safe implementation of procedures in children, including emphasis on the use of therapeutic holding. The Professional edition also includes numerous boxes that are designed to provide rationales for the interventions discussed in this edition. Recommendations for practice are based on the evidence and are concisely presented in boxes throughout the chapter.

Units X through XIV (Chapters 23 to 34) in both books consider serious health problems of infants and children primarily from a biological system orientation, which has the practical organisational value of permitting healthcare problems and nursing considerations to relate to specific pathophysiological disturbances. Important additions and revisions include discussion of blood disorders, acute respiratory distress syndrome and the latest classification for asthma, seizures, chemotherapy, diabetes mellitus and burns. Examples of the updates and revisions for these units include Chapter 27 on the child with cardiovascular dysfunction, which has major revisions to the latest guidelines for assessment and management of the most common heart disorders in children, and Chapter 34, which includes updates on Guillain-Barré syndrome, cerebral palsy and respiratory management of neuromuscular conditions such as spinal muscular atrophy and muscular dystrophy.

UNIFYING PRINCIPLES

Several unifying principles have guided the organisational structure of the US book since its inception and we have continued this in the ANZ 1st edition. These principles continue to strengthen the book with each revision to maintain a consistent approach throughout each chapter and we felt it was important to maintain this approach in the ANZ edition.

The Family as the Unit of Care

The child is an essential member of the family unit. Nursing care is most effective when it is delivered with the belief that *the family is the patient.* This belief permeates the book. The family is seen as a myriad of structures; each has the potential to provide a caring, supportive environment in which the child can grow, mature and maximise his or her human potential. In addition to family-centred care being integrated into every chapter, an entire chapter is devoted to understanding the family as the core focus in children's lives. Another chapter discusses the social, cultural and religious influences on family beliefs. Separate sections in yet another chapter deal in depth with family communication and family assessment. The impact of illness, hospitalisation and the death of a child are covered extensively in three additional chapters.

An Integrated Approach to Development

Children are not small adults but are special individuals with unique minds, bodies and needs. No book on paediatric nursing is complete without extensive coverage of communication, nutrition, play, safety, dental care, sexuality, sleep, self-esteem and, of course, parenting. Nurses promote the healthy expression of development and need to understand how this is observed in children at different ages and stages. Effective parenting depends on the parents' knowledge of development, and it is often the nurse's responsibility to provide parents with a developmental awareness of their children's needs. For these reasons, coverage of the many dimensions of childhood is integrated within each developmental-stage chapter, rather than being presented in a separate chapter. Safety concerns, for instance, are very different for a toddler to those of an adolescent. Sleep needs change with age, as do nutritional needs. As a result, the units on each stage of childhood contain complete information on all these subjects as they relate to the specific age. Using the integrated approach, students and professionals gain an appreciation for the unique characteristics and needs of children at every age and stage of development.

Focus on Wellness and Illness: Child, Family and Community

In a paediatric nursing text, a focus on illness is expected. Children become ill, and nurses typically are involved in helping children get well. However, it is not sufficient to prepare students to care primarily for sick children. First, health is more than the absence of disease. Being healthy is being whole in mind, body and spirit; therefore, the majority of the first half of the book is devoted to discussions that promote physical, psychosocial, mental and spiritual wellness. Much emphasis is placed on anticipatory guidance of parents to prevent injury or illness in the child. Second, more than ever, healthcare is prevention focused. Competent nursing care flows from this knowledge and is enhanced by an awareness of childhood development, family dynamics and communication skills. The books are enhanced further with Critical Thinking Case Study boxes within the Student edition and Research Focus boxes in the Professional edition.

Nursing Care

Although both books incorporate information from numerous disciplines (e.g. medicine, pathophysiology, pharmacology, nutrition, psychology, sociology), its primary purpose is to provide information on the nursing care of children and families. Discussions of disorders conclude with a section on Nursing Care Management. Although many aspects of the nursing care of children and families have changed significantly over the last few decades, the focus must continue to be on the quality of care. For the quality of care to be maintained, paediatric nurses must be proactive in staying informed about the strength of evidence that supports specific nursing practices. The Nursing Care Considerations sections are designed to provide the latest evidence for the implementation of evidence-based nursing practice.

Critical Role of Research and Evidence-based Practice

This first ANZ edition is the product of an extensive review of the literature published within the 11th US edition and from ANZ contributors. In addition, Research Focus boxes provide the professional with a concise discussion of the latest research on a given topic. So that information is accurate and current, most citations are less than 5 years old, and almost every chapter has entries within 1 year of publication. Examples of current cutting-edge information include recommendations from the appropriate ANZ paediatric providers and government sites.

• • •

Just as children and their families bring with them a value system and unique background that affect their role within the healthcare system, so too must each nurse bring to each child and family an individual set of characteristics and values that will affect their relationship. Although we have attempted to present a total picture of the child in each age group, both in wellness and in illness, no one child, family or nurse will be found in these books. We hope that each page, chapter and unit builds a foundation on which the nurse can begin to construct an ideal of comprehensive, atraumatic and individualised nursing care for infants, children, adolescents and their families.

SPECIAL FEATURES

Much effort has been directed towards making this book easy to teach from and, more importantly, easy to learn from. In this edition, the following features have been included to benefit educators, students and practitioners/professionals.

APPLYING EVIDENCE TO PRACTICE

Applying Evidence to Practice boxes are new specialty boxes throughout the Professional edition outlining up-to-date procedures to show best practice and focus on applying evidence.

 NURSING CARE CONSIDERATIONS

Nursing Care Considerations boxes highlight important factors to enhance critical thinking. These could be to identify signs or triggers for deterioration and the importance of providing competent care without creating undue physical and psychological distress.

LEARNING OUTCOMES

Learning Outcomes have been added to the beginning of each chapter to focus the attention of students and professionals on the unique principles found in each chapter, as well as to aid students and professionals in using concept-based curricula, system-focused curricula or a hybrid approach.

 CRITICAL THINKING CASE STUDY

Critical Thinking Case Study boxes have been revised in this Student edition to describe brief scenarios of the child-family-nurse interaction that depict real-life clinical situations. From the synthesis of the topical content and a critical analysis of possible options, the reader builds on their knowledge of intervention and learns to make clinical judgments.

 CULTURAL CONSIDERATIONS

Cultural Considerations boxes integrate concepts of culturally sensitive care throughout both texts. Their emphasis is on the clinical application of the information.

 DRUG ALERT

Drug Alert boxes highlight critical drug safety concerns for better therapeutic management.

 FAMILY-CENTRED CARE

Family-centred Care boxes present issues of special significance to families who have a child with a particular disorder. This feature is another method of highlighting the needs or concerns of families that should be addressed when family-centred care is provided.

 NURSING CARE GUIDELINES

Nursing Care Guidelines boxes summarise important nursing interventions for a variety of situations and conditions.

QUALITY PATIENT OUTCOMES

Quality Patient Outcomes boxes are added throughout the text to provide a framework for measuring nursing care performance. Nursing-sensitive outcome measures are integrated into the outcome indicators used throughout the book.

 RESEARCH FOCUS

Research Focus boxes review new evidence on important topics in a concise way.

TRANSLATING EVIDENCE INTO PRACTICE

Translating Evidence into Practice boxes have been completely revised in this edition to focus the reader's attention on application of both research and critical thought processes to support and guide the outcomes of nursing care and to provide measurable outcomes that nurses can use to validate their unique role in the healthcare system.

Numerous pedagogic devices that enhance student learning have been retained from previous editions.

- More than 100 **COLOUR PHOTOGRAPHS** are included in this edition to reflect the latest in nursing care. Anatomical drawings are easy to follow, with appropriate use of colour to illustrate important aspects, such as saturated and desaturated blood. New figures reflecting a **PATHOPHYSIOLOGY REVIEW** of various disorders have been added throughout the book. For example, the full-colour heart illustrations in Chapter 27 clearly depict congenital cardiac defects and associated haemodynamic changes.
- A functional and attractive **FULL-COLOUR DESIGN** visually enhances the organisation of each chapter, as well as the special features.
- An **INDEX**, detailed and cross-referenced, allows readers to quickly access discussions.
- **KEY TERMS** are highlighted throughout each chapter to reinforce student learning.
- **BLOOD PRESSURE LEVELS** on the inside back cover provide information nurses refer to often.
- Hundreds of **TABLES** and **BOXES** highlight key concepts and nursing interventions.

ACKNOWLEDGMENTS

This first edition of the Australia and New Zealand *Wong's Nursing Care of Infants and Children* brings with it not only two new co-editors but numerous new contributors from both countries. We have continued the excellence in nursing education and knowledge by seeking contributors from diverse backgrounds, bringing a wealth of expertise to the ANZ edition and to paediatric education and nursing. We are grateful for their time and contribution to this new project and to the commitment and many hours that they have provided during a very difficult time due to COVID-19. We are thankful and appreciative of the many hours reviewers have also given to provide constructive feedback to assist with this challenging project. The books would never have been completed without the enormous task undertaken by these professionals in both the academic and the clinical environment, and we thank them for their ongoing commitment.

These books would not have been a reality without the dedication and perseverance of the editorial staff. It would be impossible to list all involved at Elsevier that have made the Student and Professional editions possible, but to all we thank you. To Sukanthi and Shruti and the endless emails, we thank you. To Leanne Peters for her patience and exceptional input throughout the project to assist with producing an outstanding result, we are especially grateful. Leanne on many occasions was able to provide feedback and assistance that has enhanced the content of both editions. To Natalie Hunt, we thank you for your belief that both of us could achieve this and for your ongoing support through some very difficult times, personal loss and a forever-changing environment with COVID-19.

Finally, we would like to thank our families—Glenn, April and Tiffany Monte and Pete, Ben, Sam and Jacob Middleton—who have been there to support and encourage us from the beginning. They have allowed us to spend many hours of family time on this project, and our love and thanks is endless for this.

Lisa Speedie
Andrea Middleton

CONTENTS

SECTION I Children, Their Families and the Nurse

1 Perspectives of Paediatric Nursing, 1
Lynne Staff and Lisa Speedie
Healthcare for children, 1
Australia's Health System, 2
New Zealand's Health System, 2
Infant, child and adolescent health promotion, 3
Development, 3
Nutrition, 3
Oral Health, 4
Childhood health problems, 4
Obesity and Type 2 Diabetes, 4
Childhood Injuries, 4
Mental Health Problems, 6
Infant Mortality, 6
The art of paediatric nursing, 7
Philosophy of Care, 7
Role of the Paediatric Nurse, 8
Research and Evidence-based Practice, 8
Quality Outcome Measures, 9

2 Social, Cultural, Religious and Family Influences on Child Health Promotion, 11
Julia Laing and Lisa Speedie
General concepts, 11
Definition of Family, 11
Family Theories, 11
Family Nursing Interventions, 13
Family Strengths and Functioning Style, 13
Family roles and relationships, 13
Parental Roles, 14
Role Learning, 14
Parenting, 14
Parenting Styles, 14
Limit Setting and Discipline, 14
Special parenting situations, 15
Parenting the Adopted Child, 15
Parenting and Relationship Breakdown, 15
Single Parenting, 16
Parenting in Reconstituted Families, 17
Parenting in Dual-earner Families, 17
Foster Parenting, 18
Sociocultural influences on children and families, 18
Cultural safety in nursing practice, 18
Influences in the surrounding environment, 18
School Communities: School Health and School Connectedness, 18
Schools, 19
Peer Cultures, 19
Community, 19
Broader influences on child health, 19
Social Media and Mass Media, 19
Race and Ethnicity, 20
Poverty, 20
Land of Origin, Refugee and Immigration, 22
Religion/Spiritual Identity, 22

3 Hereditary Influences on Health Promotion of the Child and Family, 25
Lisa Speedie
Genetic/genomic nursing competencies, 25
Genetics and Genomics, 25
Congenital Anomalies, 27
Genetic Disorders, 28
Single-gene Disorders, 33
Variable Patterns of Gene Expression and Inheritance, 38
Mitochondrial Disorders, 39
Hereditary Cancer Predisposition Genes, 40
Inborn errors of metabolism, 41
Phenylketonuria, 42
Galactosaemia, 43
Cytogenetic Diagnostic Techniques, 44
Molecular Diagnostic Techniques, 44
Predisposition Genetic Testing, 45
Therapeutic Management of Genetic Disease, 45
Impact of hereditary disorders on the family, 45
Genetic Testing, 45
Prenatal Testing, 46
Genetic Evaluation and Counselling, 47
Role of Nurses, 47

SECTION II Childhood and Family Assessment

4 Communication, Physical and Developmental Assessment of the Child and Family, 50
Andrea Middleton
Guidelines for communication and interviewing, 50
Establishing a Setting for Communication, 50
Computer Privacy and Applications in Nursing, 50
Telephone Triage, Telehealth and Counselling, 50
Communicating with families, 51
Communicating with Parents, 51
Communicating with Children, 53
Communication Techniques, 55
History taking, 57
Performing a Health History, 57
Nutritional assessment, 63
Dietary Intake, 63
Clinical Examination of Nutrition, 63
Evaluation of Nutritional Assessment, 64
General approaches towards examining the child, 64
Sequence of the Examination, 64
Preparation of the Child, 64
Physical examination, 68
Growth Measurements, 68
Physiological Measurements, 71
General Appearance, 72
Skin, 74
Lymph Nodes, 76
Head and Neck, 76
Eyes, 76
Ears, 79

Nose, 81
Mouth and Throat, 82
Chest, 83
Lungs, 84
Heart, 86
Abdomen, 88
Genitalia, 89
Anus, 91
Back and Extremities, 91
Neurological Assessment, 92
Developmental Assessment, 93

5 Pain Assessment and Management in Children, 97
Maryanne Podham and Patience Moyo
Fundamentals of pain, 97
What is pain and how does it occur?, 97
What does pain do besides hurt?, 98
Common acute pain conditions in children, 98
Needlestick Pain, 100
Postoperative Pain, 100
Common chronic pain conditions in children, 100
Headaches, 101
Abdominal Pain, 101
Musculoskeletal Pain, 101
Neuropathic Pain Syndromes, 101
Common mixed-pain conditions in children, 101
Burn Pain, 101
Cancer Pain, 102
Sickle Cell Pain, 102
Measuring pain in children, 103
Observational Pain Measures, 103
Special Populations, 104
Self-report Pain Rating Scales, 104
Chronic and recurrent pain assessment, 105
Multidimensional Measures, 105
Prevention and treatment of pain in children, 108
Biobehavioural Interventions, 108
Pharmacological Management of Pain, 109

6 Childhood Communicable and Infectious Diseases, 121
Andrea Middleton
Infection control, 121
Immunisations, 122
Communicable diseases, 128
Nursing Care Management, 128
Conjunctivitis, 134
Stomatitis, 134
Intestinal parasitic diseases, 135
General Nursing Care Management, 135

SECTION III Family-centred Care of the Newborn

7 Health Promotion of the Newborn and Family, 137
Tameeka Mulquiney and Amy Vaccaro
Adjustment to extrauterine life, 137
Immediate Adjustments, 137
Physiological Status of Other Systems, 138
Nursing and midwifery care of the newborn and family, 140
Assessment, 140
Maintain a Patent Airway, 155
Maintain a Stable Body Temperature, 156
Protect from Infection and Injury, 156
Promote Parent–Infant Bonding (Attachment), 162
Prepare for Discharge and Home Care, 165

8 Health Problems of the Newborn, 168
Tameeka Mulquiney and Sarah Dechert
Birth injuries, 168
Soft Tissue Injury, 168
Head Injury, 168
Fractures, 170
Nerve Injuries, 171
Cranial deformities, 172
Microcephaly, 173
Craniosynostosis, 173
Craniofacial Abnormalities, 174
Pierre Robin Sequence, 174
Cleft Lip and Cleft Palate, 174
Dermatological problems in the newborn, 178
Erythema Toxicum Neonatorum, 178
Candidiasis, 178
Oral Candidiasis, 178
Herpes Simplex Virus, 178
Bullous Impetigo, 179
Birthmarks, 179
Problems Related to Physiological Factors, 180
Hyperbilirubinaemia, 180
Haemolytic Disease of the Newborn, 185
Hypoglycaemia, 188
Hyperglycaemia (Transient), 190
Hypocalcaemia, 191
Haemorrhagic Disease of the Newborn, 192
Problems caused by perinatal environmental factors, 192
Chemical Agents, 192
Radiation, 193

9 The High-risk Newborn and Family, 196
Sarah Dechert, Tameeka Mulquiney & Lisa Speedie
General management of high-risk newborns, 196
Identification of High-risk Newborns, 196
Intensive Care Facilities, 197
Nursing care of high-risk newborns, 198
Assessment, 198
Monitoring Physiological Data, 199
High-risk conditions related to dysmaturity, 210
Premature Infants, 210
Postterm Infants, 211
High risk related to disturbed respiratory function, 211
Apnoea of Prematurity, 211
Respiratory Distress Syndrome, 212
Meconium Aspiration Syndrome, 217
Air Leak Syndromes, 218
Persistent Pulmonary Hypertension of the Newborn, 218
Chronic Lung Disease, 219
High risk related to infectious processes, 220
Sepsis, 220
Necrotising Enterocolitis, 222
High risk related to cardiovascular and haematological complications, 223
Patent Ductus Arteriosus, 223
Anaemia, 224
Polycythaemia, 224
Retinopathy of Prematurity, 224

High risk related to neurological disturbance, 225
Perinatal Hypoxic-ischaemic Brain Injury, 225
Intraventricular Haemorrhage, 226
Intracranial Haemorrhage, 227
Neonatal/perinatal Stroke, 228
Neonatal Seizures, 228
High risk related to maternal conditions, 229
Infants of Diabetic Mothers, 229
Drug-exposed Infants, 230
Maternal Infections, 234

SECTION IV Family-centred Care of the Infant

10 Health Promotion of the Infant and Family, 241
Christine Taylor and Jane Mateer
Promoting optimum growth and development, 241
Biological Development, 241
Psychosocial Development, 247
Cognitive Development, 249
Development of Body Image, 250
Development of Gender Identity, 251
Social Development, 251
Temperament, 253
Coping with Concerns related to Normal Growth and Development, 253
Promoting optimum health during infancy, 261
Nutrition, 261
Sleep and Activity, 263
Dental Health, 264
Safety Promotion and Injury Prevention, 264
Anticipatory Guidance—Care of Families, 269
11 Health Problems of the Infant, 272
Jane Mateer and Christine Taylor
Nutrition in children, 272
Obesity, 272
Nutritional imbalances, 273
Vitamin Imbalances, 273
Mineral Imbalances, 274
Health problems related to nutrition, 274
Severe Acute Malnutrition (Protein–energy Malnutrition), 274
Food Sensitivity, 276
Faltering Growth, 279
Special health problems, 281
Colic (Paroxysmal Abdominal Pain), 281
Sudden Infant Death Syndrome, 282
Positional Plagiocephaly, 286
Brief Resolved Unexplained Event, 287

SECTION V Family-centred Care of the Toddler and Preschooler

12 Health Promotion of the Toddler and Family, 290
Julia Laing
Promoting optimum growth and development, 290
Biological Development, 290
Cognitive Development, 292
Moral Development: Preconventional or Premoral Level, 295
Spiritual Development, 295
Development of Body Image, 295
Development of Gender Identity, 296
Social Development, 296
Temperament, 298
Coping with concerns related to normal growth and development, 298
Toilet Training, 298
Temper Tantrums, 301
Stress, 302
Regression, 302
Promoting optimum health during toddlerhood, 302
Nutrition, 302
Sleep and Activity, 303
Dental Health, 304
Safety Promotion and Injury Prevention, 304
Anticipatory Guidance—Care of Families, 308
13 Health Promotion of the Preschooler and Family, 310
Emma Collins
Promoting optimum growth and development, 310
Biological Development, 310
Psychosocial Development, 311
Cognitive Development, 312
Moral Development (Kohlberg), 312
Spiritual Development, 312
Development of Body Image, 313
Development of Sexuality, 313
Social Development, 313
Temperament, 317
Coping with Concerns Related to Normal Growth and Development, 317
Promoting optimum health during the preschool years, 320
Nutrition, 320
Sleep and Activity, 320
Oral Healthcare, 322
Injury Prevention, 322
Anticipatory Guidance—Care of Families, 322
14 Health Problems of Early Childhood, 324
Emma Collins
Sleep problems, 324
Poisoning, 324
Principles of Emergency Treatment, 325
Child maltreatment, 328
Child Neglect, 329
Physical Abuse, 329
Sexual Abuse, 330
Nursing Care of the Maltreated Child, 331

SECTION VI Family-centred Care of the School-age Child

15 Health Promotion of the School-age Child and Family, 337
Andrea Middleton
Promoting optimum growth and development, 337
Biological Development, 337
Cognitive Development (Piaget), 340
Moral Development (Kohlberg), 341
Language Development, 342
Social Development, 342
Play, 344
Development of Self-concept, 345
Development of Sexuality, 347

Coping with concerns related to normal growth and development, 348
Discipline, 348
Coping with Stress, 349
Promoting optimum health during the school years, 350
Health Behaviours, 350
Nutrition, 351
Sleep and Rest, 352
Physical Activity, 353
Dental Health, 354
Injury Prevention, 355
Anticipatory Guidance—Care of Families, 358

16 Health Problems of the School-age Child, 360
Andrea Middleton
Obesity: complications, treatment and prevention, 360
Obesity, 360
Dental disorders, 365
Dental Decay, 365
Trauma, 366
Disorders of continence, 366
Enuresis, 366
Encopresis, 368
Disorders with behavioural components, 369
Attention Deficit/Hyperactivity Disorder, 369
Learning Disability, 372
Tic Disorders, 372
Gilles de la Tourette's Syndrome, 372
Posttraumatic Stress Disorder, 373
School Phobia, 374
Functional Abdominal Pain, 375
Childhood Depression, 376
Childhood Schizophrenia, 377
Anxiety Disorders, 377
Conduct Disorders, 378

SECTION VII Family-centred Care of the Adolescent

17 Health Promotion of the Adolescent and Family, 381
Lisa Speedie
Promoting optimum growth and development, 381
Biological Development, 382
Cognitive Development, 386
Development of Value Autonomy, 387
Psychosocial Development, 388
Social Environments, 390
Promoting optimum health during adolescence, 391
Health Concerns of Adolescence, 392
Health Promotion among Special Groups of Adolescents, 396
Nursing Care Management, 397

18 Health Problems of the Adolescent, 400
Lisa Speedie
Health conditions of the male reproductive system, 400
Penile Conditions, 400
Varicocele, 400
Epididymitis, 400
Testicular Torsion, 401
Gynaecomastia, 401
Health conditions of the female reproductive system, 401
Gynaecological Examination, 401
Menstrual Disorders, 401
Endometriosis, 402
Premenstrual Syndrome, 403
Abnormal Uterine Bleeding, 403
Vulvar Pain, 405
Vaginal Infections, 405
Sexually Transmitted Infections, 405
Sexually Transmitted Protozoa Infections, 406
Sexually Transmitted Bacterial Infections, 406
Sexually Transmitted Viral Infections, 408
Health conditions related to reproduction, 409
Adolescent Pregnancy, 409
Adolescent Abortion, 410
Contraception, 411
Sexual Assault (Rape), 411
Health conditions with a behavioural component, 413
Anorexia Nervosa and Bulimia Nervosa, 413
Substance abuse, 416
Motivation, 416
Types of Drugs Abused, 416
Tobacco, 417
Alcohol, 417
Cocaine, 417
Narcotics, 417
Central Nervous System Depressants, 417
Central Nervous System Stimulants, 418
Mind-altering Drugs, 418
Nursing Care Management, 418
Self-harm, 418
Aetiology, 418
Diagnostic Evaluation, 418
Therapeutic Management, 418
Suicide, 418
Aetiology, 419
Methods, 419
Nursing Care Management, 419

SECTION VIII Family-centred Care of the Child with Special Needs

19 Impact of Chronic Illness, Disability or End-of-life Care for the Child and Family, 423
Lisa Speedie
Perspectives on the care of children and families living with or dying from chronic or complex diseases, 423
Scope of the Problem, 423
Trends in Care, 424
The family of the child with a chronic or complex condition, 425
Impact of the Child's Chronic Illness, 425
Coping with Ongoing Stress and Periodic Crises, 426
Assisting Family Members in Managing their Feelings, 427
Establishing a Support System, 427
The child with a chronic or complex condition, 428
Developmental Aspects, 428
Coping Mechanisms, 428

Nursing care of the family and child with a chronic or complex condition, 428
Assessment, 428
Provide Support at the Time of Diagnosis, 428
Support the Family's Coping Methods, 428
Educate about the Disorder and General Healthcare, 431
Promote Normal Development, 431
Establish Realistic Future Goals, 431
Palliative care in childhood terminal illness, 432
Scope of the Problem, 432
Principles of Palliative Care, 432
Goals of Care, 432
Awareness of Dying in Children with Life-threatening Illness, 433
Children's Understanding of and Reactions to Dying, 434
Delivery of Palliative Care Services, 436
Nursing care of the child and family at the end of life, 437
Management of Pain and Suffering, 437
Parents' and Siblings' Need for Education and Support through the Caregiving Process, 437
Care at the Time of Death, 438
Care of the Family Experiencing Unexpected Childhood Death, 439
Special decisions at the time of dying and death, 440
Advance Care Planning, 440
Viewing of the Body, 441
Organ or Tissue Donation and Autopsy, 441
Siblings' Attendance at Funeral Services, 441
Care of the grieving family, 441
Grief, 442
Mourning, 444
The nurse and the child with life-threatening illness, 444
Nurses' Reactions to Caring for Children with Life-threatening Illnesses, 444
Coping with Stress, 445

20 Impact of Cognitive or Sensory Loss on the Child and Family, 448
Andrea Middleton
Cognitive disability, 448
General Concepts, 448
Nursing care of children with impaired cognitive function, 449
Educate Child and Family, 449
Down Syndrome, 452
Fragile X Syndrome, 454
Sensory loss, 455
Deafness and Hard of Hearing, 455
Blindness and Low Vision, 458
Hearing Loss and Low Vision, 462
Communication difficulties, 462
Autism Spectrum Disorders, 462

SECTION IX The Child Who is Hospitalised

21 Family-centred Care of the Child During Illness and Hospitalisation, 467
Deb Surman and Julia Laing
Stressors of hospitalisation and children's reactions, 467
Separation Anxiety, 467
Loss of Control, 469
Effects of Hospitalisation on the Child, 469
Stressors and reactions of the family of the child who is hospitalised, 469
Parental Reactions, 469
Sibling Reactions, 470
Nursing care of the child who is hospitalised, 470
Preparation for Hospitalisation, 470
Nursing Interventions, 472
Supporting Family Members, 475
Providing Information, 476
Encouraging Parent Participation, 476
Preparing for Discharge and Home Care, 476
Care of the child and family in special hospital situations, 477
Ambulatory or Outpatient Setting, 477
Isolation, 477
Emergency Admission, 478
Intensive Care Unit, 479

22 Paediatric Nursing Interventions and Skills, 481
Deb Surman
General concepts related to paediatric procedures, 481
Informed Consent, 481
Preparation for Diagnostic and Therapeutic Procedures, 482
Surgical Procedures, 484
Compliance, 487
Skin care and general hygiene, 488
Maintaining Healthy Skin, 488
Bathing, 489
Oral Hygiene, 489
Hair Care, 489
Feeding the sick child, 489
Controlling elevated temperatures, 490
Therapeutic Management, 490
Family Teaching and Home Care, 491
Safety, 491
Environmental Factors, 492
Infection Control, 493
Transporting Infants and Children, 493
Restraining Methods, 494
Positioning for procedures, 494
Femoral Venepuncture, 494
Extremity Venepuncture or Injection, 494
Lumbar Puncture, 495
Bone Marrow Aspiration or Biopsy, 496
Collection of specimens, 496
Urine Specimens, 496
Stool Specimens, 498
Blood Specimens, 498
Respiratory Secretion Specimens, 500
Administration of medication, 500
Determination of Drug Dosage, 500
Oral Administration, 501
Intramuscular Administration, 502
Subcutaneous and Intradermal Administration, 505
Intravenous Administration, 505
Maintaining fluid balance, 507
Measurement of Intake and Output, 507
Parenteral Fluid Therapy, 507
Securement of a Peripheral Intravenous Line, 508
Safety Catheters and Needleless Systems, 509

Infusion Pumps, 509
Maintenance, 510
Complications, 510
Removal of a Peripheral Intravenous Line, 510
Rectal Administration, 510
Optic, Otic and Nasal Administration, 511
Aerosol Therapy, 511
Family Teaching and Home Care, 511
Nasogastric, Orogastric and Gastrostomy Administration, 511
Alternative feeding techniques, 511
Gavage Feeding, 512
Gastrostomy Feeding, 514
Nasoduodenal and Nasojejunal Tubes, 515
Total Parenteral Nutrition, 515
Family Teaching and Home Care, 516
Procedures related to elimination, 516
Enema, 516
Ostomies, 516
Family Teaching and Home Care, 516

SECTION X Childhood Nutrition and Elimination Problems

23 The Child with Fluid and Electrolyte Imbalance, 520
Patience Mayo
Introduction, 520
Distribution of body fluids, 520
Water Balance, 520
Disturbances of fluid and electrolyte balance, 523
Dehydration, 523
Water Intoxication, 529
Oedema, 529
Nursing responsibilities in fluid and electrolyte disturbances, 530
Assessment, 530
Shock, 531
Septic Shock, 535
Anaphylaxis, 536
Toxic Shock Syndrome, 538
Burns, 538
Overview, 538
Burn Wound Characteristics, 539
Pathophysiology, 541
Therapeutic Management, 545
Nursing Care Management, 550
Future Research Needs, 553

24 The Child with Renal Dysfunction, 556
Lisa Speedie
Renal structure and function, 556
Renal Physiology, 556
Renal Pelvis and Ureters: Structure and Function, 558
Urethrovesical Unit: Structure and Function, 558
Genitourinary tract disorders, 563
Urinary Tract Infection, 563
Vesicoureteral Reflux, 566
Glomerular disease, 567
Acute Glomerulonephritis, 567
Chronic or Progressive Glomerulonephritis, 570
Nephrotic Syndrome, 570
Renal tubular disorders, 573
Tubular Function, 573
Renal Tubular Acidosis, 573
Nephrogenic Diabetes Insipidus, 574
Miscellaneous renal disorders, 574
Familial Nephritis (Alport's Syndrome), 574
Unexplained Proteinuria, 574
Renal Trauma, 575
Renal Failure, 575
Acute Kidney Injury, 575
Chronic Kidney Disease, 578
Renal replacement therapy, 581
Haemodialysis, 581
Peritoneal Dialysis, 582
Continuous Venovenous Haemofiltration, 583
Transplantation, 583
Defects of the genitourinary tract, 584
Phimosis, 584
Hydrocele, 584
Cryptorchidism, 585
Hypospadias, 586
Epispadias and Exstrophy Complex, 586
Disorders of sex development, 587
Pathophysiology, 587
Therapeutic Management, 588
Family Support, 588
Obstructive Uropathy, 588

25 The Child with Gastrointestinal Dysfunction, 592
Lisa Speedie
Gastrointestinal structure and function, 592
Development of the Gastrointestinal Tract, 592
Digestion, 592
Absorption, 593
Assessment of Gastrointestinal Function, 594
Gastrointestinal disorders, 594
Diarrhoea, 594
Constipation, 602
Vomiting, 603
Ingestion of foreign substances, 605
Pica, 605
Foreign Bodies, 605
Disorders of motility, 606
Hirschsprung's Disease (Congenital Aganglionic Megacolon), 606
Gastro-oesophageal Reflux, 607
Irritable Bowel Syndrome, 608
Inflammatory conditions, 609
Acute Appendicitis, 609
Meckel's Diverticulum, 610
Inflammatory Bowel Disease, 611
Peptic Ulcer Disease, 614
Obstructive disorders, 616
Hypertrophic Pyloric Stenosis, 616
Intussusception, 617
Malrotation and Volvulus, 618
Malabsorption syndromes, 618
Coeliac Disease (Gluten-sensitive Enteropathy), 619
Short Bowel Syndrome, 620
Gastrointestinal Bleeding, 620
Hepatic disorders, 622
Acute Hepatitis, 622

Biliary Atresia, 624
Cirrhosis, 626
Structural defects, 627
Oesophageal Atresia and Tracheo-oesophageal Fistula, 627
Abdominal Wall Defects, 629
Hernias, 631
Umbilical Hernia, 631
Inguinal Hernia, 631
Femoral Hernia, 632
Anorectal Malformations, 633

SECTION XI Childhood Oxygenation Problems

26 The Child with Respiratory Dysfunction, 637
Kylie Smith and Felicity Radford
Introduction, 637
Respiratory tract structure, 637
Respiratory Function, 638
Defences of the respiratory tract, 638
Assessment of respiratory function, 639
Physical Assessment, 639
Diagnostic Procedures, 639
General aspects of respiratory tract infections, 641
Aetiology and Characteristics, 641
Clinical Manifestations, 641
Nursing Care of the Child with a Respiratory Tract Infection, 641
Upper respiratory tract infections (URTI), 644
Acute Viral Nasopharyngitis, 644
Acute Streptococcal Pharyngitis, 645
Tonsillitis, 646
Glandular Fever (Infectious Mononucleosis), 648
Influenza, 649
Coronavirus (COVID-19), 650
Otitis Media, 650
Acute Otitis Externa, 653
Croup syndromes, 653
Acute Epiglottitis, 653
Acute Laryngitis, 655
Acute Laryngotracheobronchitis (Croup), 655
Acute Spasmodic Laryngitis, 656
Bacterial Tracheitis, 657
Infections of the lower airways, 657
Bronchitis, 657
Respiratory Syncytial Virus (RSV) and Bronchiolitis, 657
Pneumonia, 659
Viral Pneumonia, 660
Primary Atypical Pneumonia, 660
Bacterial Pneumonia, 660
Neonatal Pneumonia, 662
Other infections of the respiratory tract, 663
Pertussis (Whooping Cough), 663
Tuberculosis, 663
Respiratory disturbance caused by non-infectious irritants, 666
Foreign Body Ingestion and Aspiration, 666
Foreign Body in the Nose, 668
Aspiration Pneumonia, 668
Pulmonary Oedema, 669
Acute Respiratory Distress Syndrome and Acute Lung Injury, 670
Smoke Inhalation Injury, 672
Environmental Tobacco Exposure, 673
Structural defects, 673
Congenital Diaphragmatic Hernia, 673
Pierre Robin Sequence, 675
Choanal Atresia, 675
Long-term respiratory dysfunction, 675
Allergic Rhinitis, 675
Asthma, 677
Cystic Fibrosis, 687
Obstructive Sleep Apnoea, 696
Respiratory emergency, 697
Respiratory Failure, 697
Nursing Care Management, 697

SECTION XII Childhood Blood Production and Circulation Problems

27 The Child with Cardiovascular Dysfunction, 701
Lauren Kendrick
Cardiac structure and function, 701
Cardiac Development and Function, 701
Assessment of Cardiac Function, 704
Tests of Cardiac Function, 705
Cardiac catheterisation, 706
Congenital Heart Disease, 708
Altered Haemodynamics, 708
Clinical Consequences of Congenital Heart Disease, 708
Congestive Heart Failure, 709
Classification of Congenital Heart Defects, 723
Nursing Care of the Child with Congenital Heart Disease and Their Family, 724
Acquired cardiovascular disorders, 730
Infective Endocarditis, 730
Acute Rheumatic Fever and Rheumatic Heart Disease, 731
Cultural Considerations, 734
Kawasaki Disease, 734
Systemic Hypertension, 737
Dyslipidaemia (Abnormal Lipid Metabolism), 740
Cardiac Dysrhythmias, 743
Pulmonary Hypertension, 745
Cardiomyopathy, 747
Advanced Heart Failure, 747
Heart Transplantation, 748
28 The Child with Haematological or Immunological Dysfunction, 752
Julia Laing
The haematological system and its function, 752
Origin of Formed Elements, 752
Assessment of Haematological Function, 756
Red blood cell disorders, 756
Anaemia, 756
Blood Transfusion Therapy, 759
Anaemia caused by nutritional deficiencies, 760
Iron Deficiency Anaemia (IDA), 760
Anaemias caused by increased destruction of red blood cells, 763

Hereditary Spherocytosis, 763
Sickle Cell Anaemia, 763
Beta-thalassaemia (β-thalassaemia or Cooley's Anaemia), 768
Anaemias caused by impaired or decreased production of red blood cells, 771
Aplastic Anaemia, 771
Defects in Haemostasis, 771
Mechanisms Involved in Normal Haemostasis, 771
Haemophilia, 772
Von Willebrand Disease, 775
Immune Thrombocytopenia (Idiopathic Thrombocytopenic Purpura), 775
Other haematological disorders, 776
Neutropenia, 776
Henoch-Schönlein Purpura, 776
Immunological deficiency disorders, 777
Mechanisms Involved in Immunity, 777
Human Immunodeficiency Virus Infection and Acquired Immunodeficiency Syndrome, 778

SECTION XIII Childhood Regulatory Problems

29 The Child with Cancer, 783
Elyce Kenny
Cancer in children, 783
Epidemiology, 783
Aetiology, 784
Diagnostic Evaluation, 784
Clinical Trials, 786
Treatment Modalities, 787
Complications of Therapy, 791
Nursing care management, 792
Signs and Symptoms of Cancer in Children, 792
Managing Side Effects of Treatment, 793
Nursing Care during Haematopoietic Stem Cell Transplantation, 796
Preparation for Procedures, 796
Pain Management, 796
Health Promotion, 797
Family Education, 797
Completion of Therapy, 797
Cancers of blood and lymph systems, 798
Acute Leukaemias, 798
Lymphomas, 801
Nervous system tumours, 803
Brain Tumours, 803
Neuroblastoma, 808
Bone tumours, 809
General Considerations, 809
Osteosarcoma, 809
Ewing's Sarcoma (Primitive Neuroectodermal Tumour of the Bone), 810
Other solid tumours, 811
Wilms Tumour, 811
Rhabdomyosarcoma, 812
Retinoblastoma, 813
Germ Cell Tumours, 815
Liver Tumours, 815
The childhood cancer survivor, 815

30 The Child with Cerebral Dysfunction, 819
Emma Collins
Cerebral structure and function, 819
Development of the Neurological System, 819
Central Nervous System, 819
Increased Intracranial Pressure, 821
Evaluation of neurological status, 822
Assessment: General Aspects, 822
Altered States of Consciousness, 823
Neurological Examination, 825
Special Diagnostic Procedures, 826
The child with cerebral compromise, 827
Nursing Care of the Unconscious Child, 827
Head Injury, 833
Submersion Injury, 839
The child with cerebral malformation, 841
Hydrocephalus, 841
Intracranial infections, 845
Bacterial Meningitis, 845
Non-bacterial (Aseptic) Meningitis, 848
Brain Abscess, 849
Encephalitis, 849
Seizures and epilepsy, 850
Epilepsy, 850
Headache, 860
Assessment, 860
Migraine Headache, 861

31 The Child with Endocrine Dysfunction, 865
Lisa Speedie
The endocrine system, 865
Hormones, 865
Neuroendocrine Interrelationships, 865
Disorders of pituitary function, 866
Hypopituitarism, 866
Pituitary Hyperfunction, 870
Precocious Puberty, 870
Diabetes Insipidus, 871
Syndrome of Inappropriate Antidiuretic Hormone, 872
Disorders of thyroid function, 872
Juvenile Hypothyroidism, 872
Goitre, 873
Chronic Lymphocytic Thyroiditis, 873
Hyperthyroidism, 874
Disorders of parathyroid function, 875
Hypoparathyroidism, 875
Hyperparathyroidism, 876
Disorders of adrenal function, 876
Adrenal Hormones, 876
Acute Adrenocortical Insufficiency, 877
Chronic Adrenocortical Insufficiency (Addison's Disease), 878
Cushing's Syndrome, 879
Congenital Adrenal Hyperplasia, 880
Hyperaldosteronism, 881
Phaeochromocytoma, 882
Disorders of pancreatic hormone secretion, 882
Diabetes Mellitus, 882

SECTION XIV Childhood Physical Mobility Problems

32 The Child with Integumentary Dysfunction, 891
Ibi Patane
Integumentary dysfunction, 891
Skin Lesions, 891
Wounds, 892
Infections of the skin, 894
Bacterial Infections, 894
Viral Infections, 896
Dermatophytoses (Fungal Infections), 896
Systemic Mycotic (Fungal) Infections, 897
Skin disorders related to chemical or physical contacts, 897
Contact Dermatitis, 897
Allergic Contact Dermatitis to Plants, 899
Drug Reactions, 899
Skin disorders related to animal contacts, 900
Arthropod Bites and Stings, 900
Scabies, 900
Pediculosis Capitis, 902
Rickettsial Diseases, 903
Animal Bites, 903
Human Bites, 904
Cat-scratch Disease, 904
Flying Fox (Bat) Bites, 904
Miscellaneous skin disorders, 904
Skin disorders associated with specific age groups, 904
Nappy Rash, 904
Atopic Dermatitis (Eczema), 906
Seborrhoeic Dermatitis, 908
Acne, 908
Cold injury, 909

33 The Child with Musculoskeletal or Articular Dysfunction, 911
Patience Moyo
The child and trauma, 911
Trauma Management, 911
The immobilised child, 914
Immobilisation, 914
The Child in a Cast, 921
The Child in Traction, 922
Distraction, 924
Amputation, 925
Mobilisation Devices, 925
The child with a fracture, 928
Fracture Complications, 932
Injuries and health problems related to sports participation, 934
Preparation for Sports, 934
Types of Injury, 934
Contusions, 935
Dislocations, 935
Sprains and Strains, 936
Overuse Injury, 937
Exercise-induced Heat Stress, 937
Health Concerns Associated with Sports, 937
Nurse's Role in Children's Sports, 940
Musculoskeletal dysfunction, 940
Torticollis, 940
Kyphosis and Lordosis, 940
Idiopathic Scoliosis, 941
Skeletal Limb Deficiency, 943
Developmental Dysplasia of the Hip, 944
Legg-Calvé-Perthes Disease, 946
Slipped Capital Femoral Epiphysis, 947
Metatarsus Adductus, 948
Congenital Talipes Equinovarus (Clubfoot), 948
Nursing Care Management, 949
Orthopaedic infections, 949
Osteomyelitis, 949
Septic Arthritis, 950
Skeletal Tuberculosis, 950
Skeletal and articular dysfunction, 951
Osteogenesis Imperfecta, 951
Juvenile Idiopathic Arthritis, 952
Systemic Lupus Erythematosus, 955

34 The Child with Neuromuscular or Muscular Dysfunction, 960
Andrea Middleton
Neuromuscular dysfunction, 960
Classification and Diagnosis, 960
Cerebral Palsy, 961
Defects of neural tube closure, 969
Aetiology, 969
Anencephaly, 970
Spina Bifida and Myelodysplasia, 971
Myelomeningocele (Meningomyelocele), 971
Hypotonia, 977
Spinal Muscular Atrophy Type 1 (Werdnig-Hoffmann Disease), 978
Juvenile Spinal Muscular Atrophy (Kugelberg-Welander Disease), 979
Guillain-Barré Syndrome, 979
Spinal Cord Injuries, 981
Muscular dysfunction, 991
Muscular Dystrophies, 991
Duchenne's Muscular Dystrophy, 992

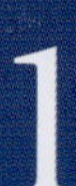

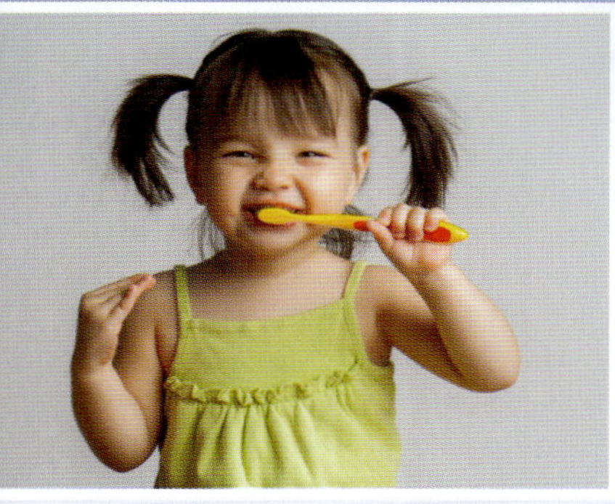

Perspectives of Paediatric Nursing

Lynne Staff and Lisa Speedie

LEARNING OBJECTIVES

- Begin to understand family-centred care
- Understand clinical reasoning and critical thinking in paediatric nursing
- Be able to show strength-based approaches and assessments
- Understand the nursing process and role of the nurse

HEALTHCARE FOR CHILDREN

The major goal for paediatric nursing is to enable children's wellbeing by providing access to quality healthcare for children and their families. While childhood is a time of rapid growth and development where health behaviours are established, it is also a time of vulnerability. Many health problems experienced by adults originate in infancy and childhood, and early intervention can prevent later illnesses. Key indicators known to influence a person's long-term wellbeing are healthcare availability, access and uptake, where a child lives, their family's culture and social circumstances, lifestyle, community and environment.

To begin to appreciate the concept of infant, child and adolescent health and wellbeing, a brief examination of some background data is warranted. In 2017, Australia's population was 23.5 million people, with children making up just over 19% of the population, or 4.7 million (Australian Bureau of Statistics 2018). In New Zealand, the total population according to the 2013 Census data was 4.475 million people. Of these, 25%, or 1.12 million, were children under the age of 18 years (Office of the Children's Commissioner 2016).

Understanding the determinants of health and the healthcare needs of this proportion of the population is fundamental in terms of planning, infrastructure and provision of current and future health services. For example, in Australia, immunisation rates for all children have increased. In 2019, 94.2% of 1-year-old, 91.4% of 2-year-old and 94.8% of 5-year-old Australian children were fully immunised (Australian Government Department of Health 2020). However, in New Zealand, the 2019 immunisation rates for 1-, 2- and 5-year-old children have decreased by 92%, 91% and 88% respectively (Ministry of Health 2019b). The percentage of women smoking in the first 20 weeks of pregnancy in Australia has decreased from 13% in 2011 to 11% in 2015 (Australian Institute for Health and Welfare [AIHW] 2020) and in New Zealand, 13% of pregnant women smoked in 2017, compared to 16% in 2008 (Ministry of Health 2014, Smokefree Aotearoa 2025 2017). Similarly, the infant death rate in Australia has reduced from 5.0 to 3.3 per 1000 live births between 1997 and 2017 (AIHW 2020), and in New Zealand, reduced from 5 per 1000 live births in 2008 to 3.8 per 1000 live births in 2018 (Ministry of Health 2019a).

Despite these positive advances in infant health, reports in Australia and New Zealand (see, for example, *Australia's children: in brief* [AIHW 2019] and the Annual Update of Key Results 2019/20: New Zealand Health Survey [Ministry of Health 2020d]) identified a number of areas for improvement. For example, 1 in 4 Australian children aged 5 to 14 years are classified as overweight or obese, and obesity among children in New Zealand varied by ethnicity as follows: Pacific (29.1%), Māori (13.2%), Asian (3.4%) and European/Other (7.2%). Accidental injury remains a frequent cause of hospitalisation, and 1 in 5 Australian 9-year-old children reported experiencing bullying on a weekly basis in 2015 (AIHW 2019). This report also highlighted that the majority of 12- to 13-year-old children (97%) had someone they could talk to if they had a problem with poor health, and this was identified by children aged 9 to 13 years as important, second to family, for having a good life. Similarly, in 2019 the Education Review Office in New Zealand reported that 46% of primary school students and 31% of secondary school students reported that they had experienced bullying.

In Australia, the AIHW collects, collates, regularly updates and presents statistical health and welfare data. Relevant to infant health and wellbeing are the Children's Headline Indicators (CHIs) outlined in Box 1.1. In 2008 the CHIs were endorsed at the Australian Health Ministers' Conference, the Community and Disability Services Ministers' Conference and the Australian Education, Early Childhood Development and Youth Affairs Senior Officials Committee in 2008. First reported in 2009, the CHIs are 19 high-level measurable indicators that identify the fundamental effect of immediate environment as a key influence on children's health, development and wellbeing. The CHIs are assembled into three general topic areas: health; early learning and care; and family and community.

BOX 1.1 Australian Institute of Health and Welfare Children's Headline Indicator list

Health	Smoking and drug use during pregnancy
	Infant mortality
	Low birthweight
	Breastfeeding
	Immunisation
	Overweight and obesity
	Dental health
	Injury deaths
	Teenage births
Early learning and care	Early childhood education
	Transition to primary school
	Attendance at primary school
	Literacy
	Numeracy
Family and community	Family social network
	Family economic situation
	Child abuse and neglect
	Social and Emotional wellbeing
	Shelter

RESEARCH FOCUS

Australia's Children

Take some time to look at the reports highlighted in this section. They provide excellent background to children's health and wellbeing in the Australia and New Zealand contexts.

The AIHW highlights that reporting on national data informs an understanding of how Australian children are faring over time. It also enables comparisons across different groups and internationally, and these comparisons support more local-level reporting. *Australia's children: in brief* provides an inclusive overview of the wellbeing of children living in Australia. Building on previous AIHW reporting, it provides a comprehensive overview of the latest available Australian data on a wide range of topics relevant to infant, child and adolescent health and wellbeing. The *Australia's children* reports aim to:

- collate and contextualise vital national statistics on child wellbeing and present these data in one place
- provide updated data not published under other AIHW child reporting frameworks
- provide a more comprehensive understanding of related data gaps.

Each topic area in the report profiles the importance of that particular issue to infant, child and adolescent health and wellbeing, and longitudinal data is presented on established measures and, wherever possible, for specific priority population groups. International comparisons are also provided where available. The report discusses limitations in current national reporting and suggests opportunities for development and refinement. Additionally, the report provides information regarding further sources of information. Where established measures are not yet obtainable for particular topics, the use of available national data sources or subnational data sources provide some insight on the topic.

New Zealand also has a comprehensive reporting system on the health and wellbeing of its youngest citizens, with health outcomes data readily available. Examples of these include:

- *Children and young people living well and staying well: New Zealand childhood obesity programme baseline report 2016/2017* (2017)
- *Te ohonga ake: the health status of Māori children and young people in Aotearoa/New Zealand* (2017)
- *Te ohonga ake: the determinants of health for Māori children and young people in New Zealand* (2015).

The structure of the health systems in Australia and New Zealand is also worthy to note for those involved in paediatric nursing, as this is relevant to the availability of, access to and affordability of services, and how health services are organised, offered and provided.

Australia's Health System

Australia's health system has been described as an intricate arrangement of public and private providers, settings, services and support mechanisms (AIHW 2020). Australia's public health system, Medicare, is funded by Australian taxpayers and is made up of the Medicare Benefits Schedule (MBS) which covers health services and hospital care, and the Pharmaceutical Benefits Scheme (PBS) which covers prescribed medications. Those who may access Medicare services include Australian citizens and residents, and individuals from a country which has a reciprocal health service agreement with Australia (e.g. the United Kingdom). The MBS provides full or partial cover for medical services provided to healthcare users who are registered with the system and who hold a Medicare card. These include general practitioner (GP) billing costs, hospitalisation costs and some diagnostic and screening costs. While the PBS reduces the cost of many medications for the public, many more medications are not listed on the PBS and incur significant out-of-pocket expenses for the healthcare user. Similarly, patients who require ongoing screening, tests and treatments may also incur significant healthcare expenses. To help address this, the Medicare Safety Net was established to support people with health issues that incur high and ongoing health and pharmaceutical expenses.

Patients may be bulk billed (where the cost is covered by Medicare) or privately billed (where they are charged a fee that is usually more than the Medicare rebate). Mixed billing is the term used when the patient is charged for and pays the entire fee upfront but a rebate from Medicare can be claimed at a later date.

Because Medicare does not cover all medical services, many people take out private healthcare insurance; however, the number of people taking out private health insurance is decreasing. In December 2019, 40% of Australian citizens held private health insurance compared to 47.3% in December 2014 (Australian Prudential Regulation Authority [APRA] 2020). The demographics of the person who holds private health insurance is also changing with fewer people having insurance, but their use of services is increasing (APRA 2020). Many Australian children are covered by their parents' private health insurance, and some paediatric services/procedures may only be covered by a private specialist.

There are two types of private health insurance cover:

1. hospital cover (taken out for in-hospital treatment)
2. ancillary or 'extras' cover (taken out for ambulance, optometry, dental, physiotherapy and other ancillary services).

Private health insurance may cover full or partial costs of certain treatments for private patients, and privately insured patients may choose to be cared for in private or public hospitals, with a medical practitioner of their choice. Private health insurance may also cover some additional services that Medicare does not; for example, dental, optical, physiotherapy and chiropractic care costs.

New Zealand's Health System

Similar to Australia, New Zealand's health and disability services are also provided by a complex network of organisations and people who work together across the system to attain better health for New Zealanders, and public and private health services are available.

The public health system is funded by taxpayers as well as the Accident Compensation Corporation (ACC) and several government agencies. Essential healthcare services are available at no cost for all New Zealand citizens and also to people on a work permit valid for 2 years or longer. Overseas visitors from countries with respective reciprocal health agreements (e.g. Australia and the United Kingdom) can also access some services. The public system uses a community-focused model, comprising three key sectors. These are the district health boards (DHBs), primary health care and primary health organisations (PHOs). DHBs are government funded and overarch PHOs. They provide and fund health and disability services in their district whereas PHOs coordinate local collaborative primary health services. Primary health care includes first-level services (e.g. GP services) and mobile nursing and community health services. The public healthcare system in New Zealand gives permanent residents access to free or heavily subsidised hospital care, as well as emergency treatment.

The ACC is another element of the system. ACC is the New Zealand Government's personal injury organisation which assists medical and treatment fees payment, and rehabilitation and residential care costs caused by an accident or injury.

Private healthcare services, including private hospitals or clinics, are not funded by the government and are based on a user-pays scheme. Private healthcare services offer non-urgent and elective treatments, and private accident, emergency and medical clinics provide out-of-hours services outside of the public system. Specialists often work across private and public services, and there are also privately owned screening and diagnostic services. As in Australia, patients with private health insurance are able to utilise public or private hospital care and are able to choose their medical care provider.

The two types of private healthcare policies are:

1. 'comprehensive cover' that cover all medical costs, including GP visits and prescriptions
2. those that cover combinations of specialist care and elective (non-urgent) surgery.

The Pharmaceutical Management Agency (PHARMAC) was established by the New Zealand Government in 1983. This agency makes subsidised medications available and negotiates low medication prices.

INFANT, CHILD AND ADOLESCENT HEALTH PROMOTION

Child health promotion provides opportunities to reduce differences in current health status among members of different groups and to ensure equal opportunities and resources to enable all children to achieve their fullest health potential. Health indicators provide a background by identifying essential components to enable child health promotion programs to be designed to prevent future health problems in children in Australia and New Zealand. According to Aotearoa's Te Hiringa Hauora/Health Promotion Agency, health promotion initiatives encompass:

- *promotion of health and wellbeing and encouragement of healthy lifestyles*
- *prevention of disease, illness and injury*
- *enabling environments that support health, wellbeing and healthy lifestyles*
- *reduction of personal, social and economic harm.*

(Aotearoa Te Hiringa Hauora/Health Promotion Agency 2018)

The *National Action Plan for the Health of Children and Young People 2020-2030* was developed by the Australian Government's Department of Health in 2020 as a foundation for the formulation and enactment of a series of policies, interventions and approaches with the purpose of improving health outcomes for children and young people. Five priority areas were identified as essential to drive change and improve outcomes so that the health of Australia's children and young people is maximised. The five priority areas in the action plan are to:

1. improve health equity across populations
2. empower parents and caregivers to maximise healthy development
3. tackle mental health and risky behaviours
4. address chronic conditions and preventive health
5. strengthen the workforce.

Healthy Kids and Go4Fun are examples of Australian child health promotion initiatives with an overarching goal to improve the health of Australia's children. Major themes of these initiatives are promoting family support, child development, mental health and healthy nutrition. These support the development of healthy weight, physical activity, oral health, healthy sexual development and sexual identity, safety and injury prevention, and an understanding of the importance of community relationships and resources. Developmentally appropriate health promotion strategies are discussed throughout this book. Key examples of child health promotion themes that are essential for all age groups include promoting development, nutrition and oral health. Recommendations for preventive health and primary healthcare during infancy, early childhood and adolescence are found in Chapters 7, 10, 12, 13, 15 and 17.

Development

Health promotion recognises the physical, psychological and emotional changes that occur in human beings in the period before birth until the end of adolescence. Developmental processes are unique to each stage of development, and continuous screening and assessment are adjuncts to enable early intervention when problems are found. The most dramatic times of physical, motor, cognitive, emotional and social development occur before birth and during infancy. Interactions between the parent and infant are central to promoting optimal developmental outcomes and are a key component of infant assessment. During early childhood, early identification of developmental delays is critical for establishing early interventions. Health promotion accompanied by the provision of timely and age- and family-appropriate education can help to ensure that parents are aware of the specific needs of each developmental stage of their child. Ongoing observation and screening during middle childhood provides opportunities to positively develop and strengthen cognitive and emotional attributes, communication skills, self-esteem and independence. Recognition that adolescents differ greatly in their physical, social and emotional maturity is an important consideration for health professionals when caring for them throughout this developmental period. Investment in the early years of a person's life, coupled with the benefits of early intervention (should it be required), demonstrate a positive cumulative effect on health in the long term (Australian Health Minister's Advisory Council 2015).

An important example for health promotion during early child development is to be aware of changing recommendations that address the fast-changing world of technology in our society. An important example is the changes in recommendations on screen viewing by infants and children. For infants less than 18 months of age, no screen time is recommended except for video calling with a grandparent or loved one, yet Tooth et al (2019) found in their study of Australian children that infants up to 12 months of age were having 50 and 58 minutes of screen time on weekdays and weekend days respectively. Parents should be advised to use technology sparingly before 5 years of age and to always participate during screen time viewing.

Nutrition

Nutrition is an essential component for healthy growth and development. Human milk is the preferred form of nutrition for all infants and exclusive breastfeeding is recommended for all infants at least up to 6 months of age (Council of Australian Governments [COAG]

Health Council 2019). Breastfeeding provides the infant with micronutrients, immunological properties and several enzymes that enhance digestion and absorption of these nutrients. A recent resurgence in breastfeeding has occurred as a result of the education of parents regarding its benefits and increased social support for breastfeeding women. However, there are still many infants who are never breastfed, or breastfed for a very limited time, and whose health suffers because of this. The significance of breastfeeding to the overall health of the infant and child and the ongoing benefits to health throughout the lifespan, because of having been breastfed as an infant, are still being discovered.

Children establish lifelong eating habits during the first 3 years of life, and the nurse is ideally positioned to support and educate parents on the importance of nutrition. Most eating preferences and attitudes related to food develop from family influences and culture. During adolescence, parental influence diminishes and the adolescent makes food choices related to independent decision-making, peer acceptability and sociability. Many food choices can be detrimental to adolescents who have chronic illnesses including, but not limited to, diabetes, obesity, anorexia nervosa, binge eating disorder, chronic lung disease, hypertension, cardiovascular risk factors and renal disease. The importance of good nutrition balanced with regular exercise cannot be underscored enough.

Families that struggle with lower incomes, who live in remote and very remote communities, who experience homelessness or overcrowding, and who have migrant status may lack the resources and knowledge to provide their children with adequate and nutritious foods including fresh fruits and vegetables, and appropriate protein foods (Lee et al 2018). The result can be nutritional deficiencies with subsequent growth and developmental delays, depression and behaviour problems.

Oral Health

Oral health is an essential component of overall health, and should be a key feature of health promotion throughout infancy, childhood and adolescence. Preventing dental caries and developing healthy oral hygiene habits must occur early in childhood. Dental caries have been recognised for decades as a significant yet preventable health problem for children (Clark et al 2015). Children in racial or cultural minority groups experience disparities in oral healthcare and are much more likely to have dental disease. Australian Indigenous children aged 2 to 8 years are twice as likely to experience any dental caries in primary teeth compared with non-Indigenous children (Baker et al 2018).

Preschoolers of low-income families are twice as likely to develop tooth decay and only half as likely to visit the dentist as other children (Baker & Edlund 2018). Early childhood caries is a preventable disease, and nurses play an essential role in health promotion and health education in relation to practising dental hygiene (beginning with the first tooth eruption), drinking fluoridated water and instituting early dental preventive care. Oral healthcare practices established during the early years of development prevent destructive periodontal disease and dental decay.

CHILDHOOD HEALTH PROBLEMS

Changes in modern society, including pandemics, advancing medical knowledge and technology, the proliferation of information systems, economically troubled times, and various changes and disruptive influences on the family, are leading to significant medical problems that affect the health of children. Problems that can negatively affect a child's development include poverty, violence, aggression, non-compliance, school failure and adjustment to parental separation and divorce. In addition, mental health issues cause challenges in childhood and adolescence. Recent concern has focused on groups of children who are at highest risk, such as children born preterm or with a very low birth weight (VLBW) or low birth weight (LBW), children attending childcare centres, children who live in poverty or are homeless and children with chronic medical issues and disabilities. In addition, these children and their families face multiple barriers to adequate health, dental and mental healthcare. A perspective of several health problems facing children and the major challenges for paediatric nurses is discussed in the following sections.

Obesity and Type 2 diabetes

Childhood obesity, the most common nutritional problem among children in Australia and New Zealand, is increasing in epidemic proportions (AIHW 2020). *Obesity* in children and adolescents is defined as a body mass index (BMI) at or greater than the 95th percentile for youth of the same age and gender. *Overweight* is defined as a BMI at or above the 85th percentile and below the 95th percentile for children and teens of the same age and sex.

Increasing evidence associates maternal obesity as a major influence on offspring health during childhood and in adult life (Godfrey et al 2017). An optimal nutritional and microbial environment during pregnancy may reduce the risk of infants being obese or overweight during early life (Haszard et al 2019).

Lack of physical activity related to limited resources, unsafe environments and inconvenient play and exercise facilities, combined with easy access to television and video games, increases the incidence of obesity among children from low-income backgrounds and minority groups (AIHW 2020). Overweight youth have increased risk for cardiometabolic changes (a cluster of cardiovascular factors that include hypertension, altered glucose metabolism, dyslipidaemia and abdominal obesity) in the future (Weiss et al 2013, AIHW 2020) (Fig 1.1).

Children aged 5 to 14 years and living in the rural and remote environments are more likely to be overweight or obese than those living in metropolitan cities (AIHW 2020) (Fig 1.2). It is recommended that nurses begin with prevention strategies focusing on reducing the incidence of overweight as early as possible, educating about nutrition and obesity in infancy (AIHW 2020).

Childhood Injuries

Injuries are the most common cause of death and disability to children in Australia (AIHW 2020). For New Zealand it was transport and assault (Ministry of Health 2019c, 2020c).

In Australia and New Zealand, injury is a major cause of death and hospitalisation. Children are vulnerable to certain types of injuries depending on their age, and this is reflected by their stage of development. Very young children are more vulnerable to injury where they are not yet able to assess the potential dangers. Injuries among older children are increasingly influenced by risk-taking behaviour and peers (AIHW: Pointer 2014).

The child's developmental stage partially determines the types of injuries that are most likely to occur at a specific age and helps provide clues to preventive measures. For example, small infants are helpless in any environment. When they begin to roll over or propel themselves, they can fall from unprotected surfaces. The crawling infant, who has a natural tendency to place objects in the mouth, is at risk for aspiration or poisoning. The mobile toddler, with the instinct to explore and investigate and the ability to run and climb, may experience falls, burns or collisions with objects. As children grow older, their absorption with play makes them oblivious to environmental hazards such as street

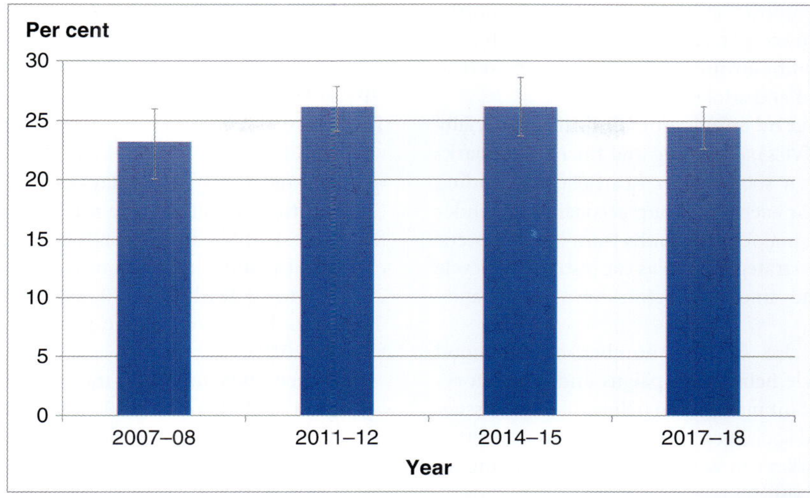

Fig 1.1 Overweight or obese children aged 5–14, Australia, 2007–08 to 2017–18. (Source: Australian Institute of Health and Welfare (AIHW). 2020. Australia's children. 3 April. AIHW, Canberra. https://www.aihw.gov.au/reports/children-youth/australias-children/contents/health/health-australias-children. Data from: Australian Bureau of Statistics (ABS) 2019. Microdata: National Health Survey, 2017–18. ABS cat. no. 4324.0.55.001. Canberra: ABS. Customised data report; AIHW 2017. A picture of overweight and obesity in Australia 2017. Cat. no. PHE 216. AIHW, Canberra.)

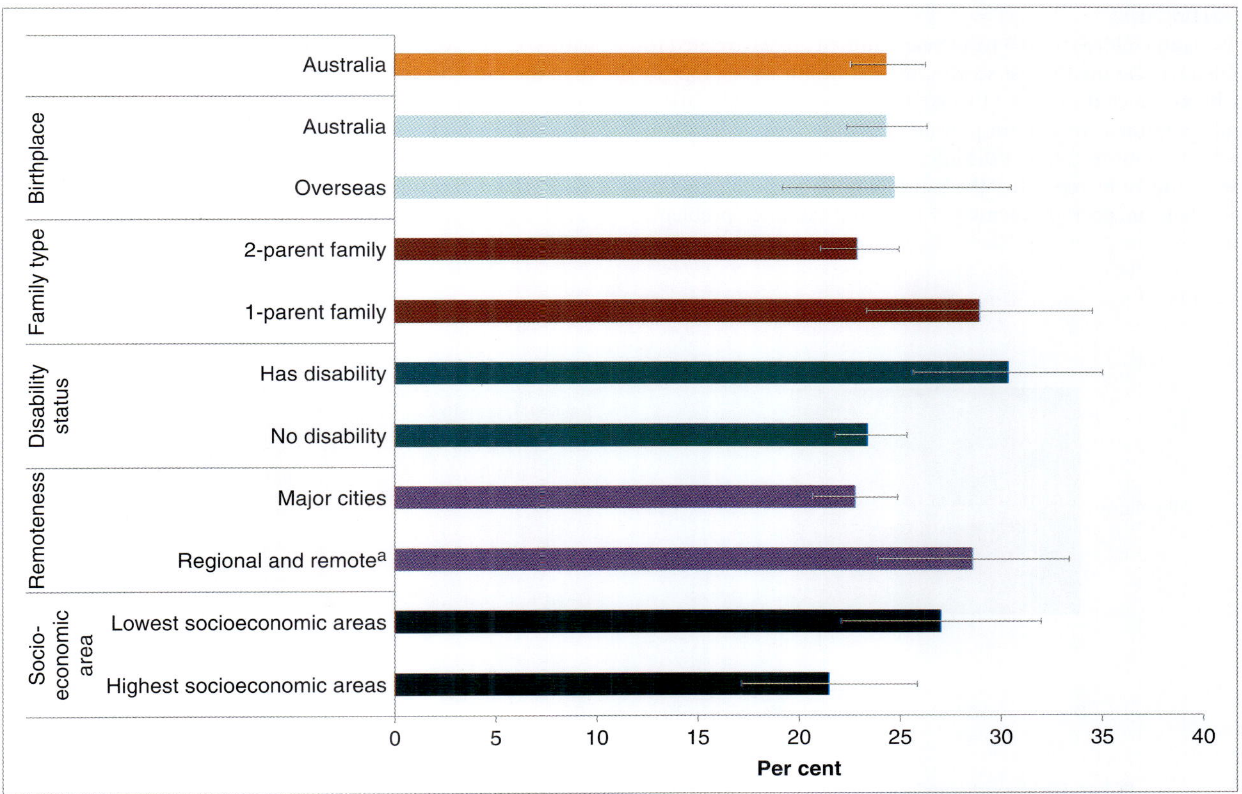

Fig 1.2 Proportion (%) of children aged 5–14 who were overweight or obese, by priority population groups, Australia, 2017–18. (a) Regional and remote includes *Inner regional, Outer regional* and *Remote* areas. *Very remote* areas were excluded from the survey. (Source: Australian Institute of Health and Welfare (AIHW). 2020. Australia's children. 3 April. AIHW, Canberra. https://www.aihw.gov.au/reports/children-youth/australias-children/contents/health/health-australias-children. Data from ABS 2019.)

traffic or water. The need to conform and gain acceptance compels older children and adolescents to accept challenges and dares. Although the rate of injuries is high in children younger than 9 years, most fatal injuries occur in later childhood and adolescence.

The pattern of deaths caused by unintentional injuries, especially from motor vehicle crashes (MVCs), drowning and burns, is remarkably consistent in most Western societies. In Australia, the leading causes of death from injuries for each age group according to gender are presented in Figure 1.3. The majority of deaths from injuries occur in boys. Fortunately, prevention strategies such as car restraints, bicycle helmets, sleeping positions and smoke detectors have significantly decreased fatalities for children.

Bicycle-associated injuries also cause a number of childhood deaths. Community-wide bicycle helmet campaigns and mandatory-use laws have resulted in significant increases in helmet use. Still, issues such as stylishness, comfort and social acceptability remain important factors in non-compliance. Nurses can educate children and families about pedestrian and bicycle safety.

Mental Health Problems

In Australia in 2013–14, an estimated 314,000 children aged 4 to 11 years (almost 14%) experienced a mental disorder. Boys were more commonly affected than girls (17% compared with 11%). Attention deficit hyperactivity disorder (ADHD) was the most common disorder for children (8.2%). It was also the most common disorder among boys (11%). Anxiety disorders were the second most common disorders among all children (6.9%), and the most common among girls (6.1%) (AIHW 2019).

New Zealand children aged 3 to 14 years showed anxiety related to peer problems to be the highest scoring mental health issue (13.7%) followed by conduct disorders (10.3%) (Ministry of Health 2018). Emotional symptoms were more prevalent in older age groups and boys experienced more conduct disorders than girls. For Māori children it was similar in reporting the same issues and problems but higher numbers in peer problems (17.8%) and conduct problems (16.7%), and again, higher in boys than girls (Ministry of Health 2018).

Infant Mortality

The infant mortality rate is the number of deaths during the first year of life per 1000 live births. It may be further divided into neonatal mortality (< 28 days of life) and post-neonatal mortality (28 days to 11 months). The infant death rate in Australia decreased from a peak of 5.7 deaths per 1000 babies in 1999 to 3.3 in 2017. The child death rate for children aged 1–14 halved between 1998 and 2017 (20 to 10 deaths per 100,000 children); however, since 2011, the death rate has stayed in the range of 10 to 12 deaths per 100,000 (AIHW 2020).

Between 2008 and 2017, the total number of births has decreased by 7%. In 2017 there were 390 fetal deaths and 284 infant deaths registered. Infant death rates in 2017 for the Pacific and Māori peoples were the highest (8.7 and 5.9 per 1000 live births, respectively) compared to European or Other and Asian ethnic groups (3.4 and 3.7 per 1000 live births, respectively). This has been the pattern for the previous 5 years (Ministry of Health 2020c).

In 2015–17, the leading causes of child (aged 1–14) deaths in Australia were injuries, cancer and diseases of the nervous system (AIHW 2019). Halving the gap between Australian Indigenous and non-Indigenous child deaths (ages 0 to 4 years) by 2018 was a key priority of the Closing the Gap framework established by COAG in 2008.

In New Zealand, one major factor leading to high rates of infant death is sudden unexpected death in infancy (SUDI). Rates for babies in the Māori and Pacific peoples ethnic groups were higher than the rates for babies in the Asian and European or Other ethnic groups. For mothers 25 years of age or less, the rates for SUDI were significantly higher again. The SUDI rate for babies born in the most deprived areas (quintile 5, low socioeconomic areas and multiple low social determinants of health) was significantly higher than the rate for all other deprivation quintiles (Ministry of Health 2020c).

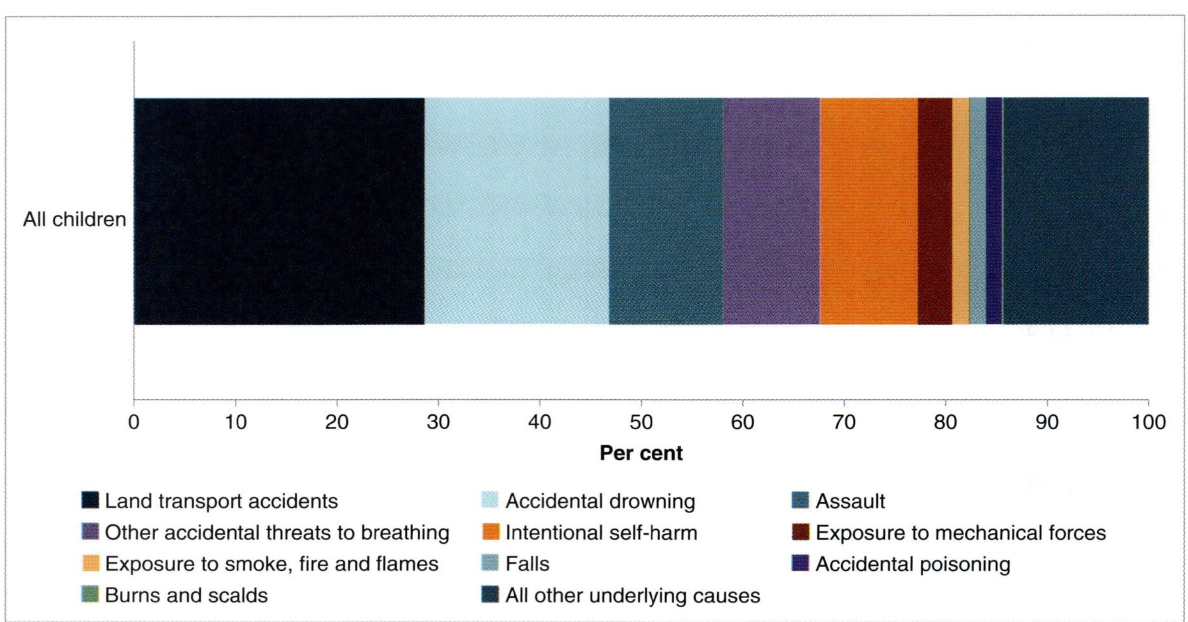

Fig 1.3 Leading causes of injury deaths among children aged 0–14, Australia, 2015–17. (Source: AIHW 2019 Australia's children: in brief. 17 December. AIHW, Canberra. https://www.aihw.gov.au/reports/children-youth/australias-children-in-brief/contents/table-of-contents. Data from: AIHW analysis of AIHW National Mortality Database.)

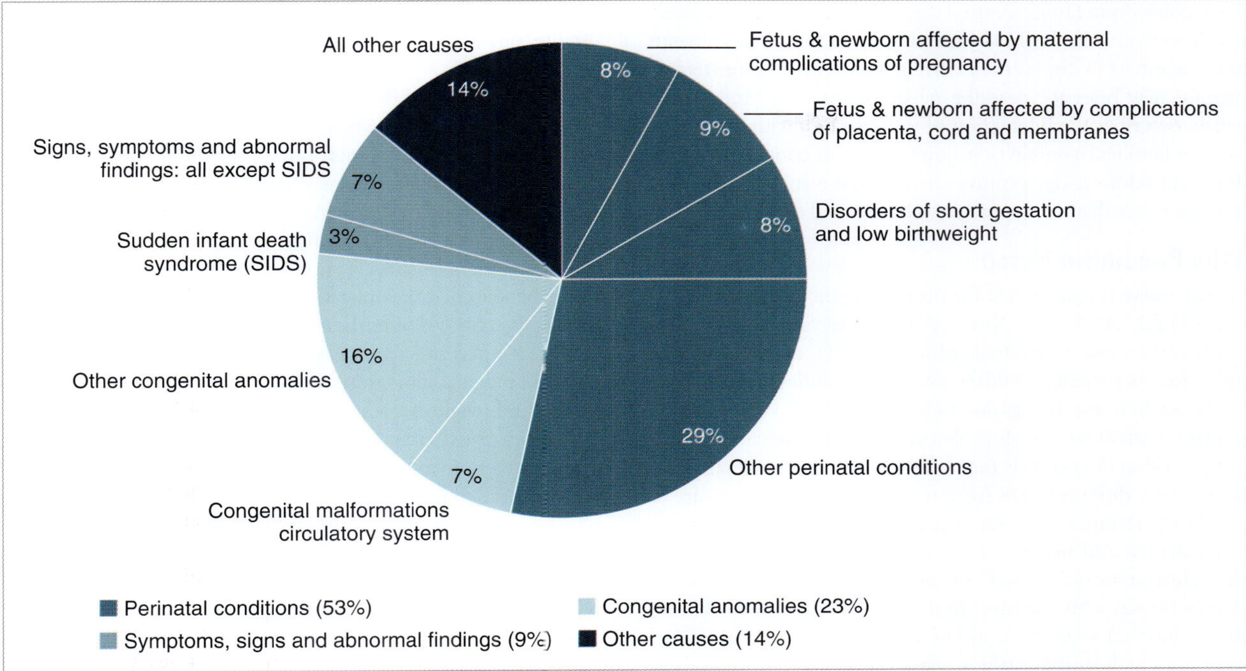

Fig 1.4 Leading causes of infant death, Australia, 2017. (Note: Due to rounding the proportions do not sum to 100. Source: Australian Institute of Health and Welfare (AIHW). 2020. Australia's children. 3 April. AIHW, Canberra. https://www.aihw.gov.au/reports/children-youth/australias-children/contents/health/health-australias-children)

As Figure 1.4 demonstrates, many of the leading causes of death during infancy continue to occur during the perinatal period. In 2015–17, 3 leading causes of infant deaths accounted for the majority (86%) of deaths: perinatal conditions (53%), congenital anomalies (23%), and symptoms, signs and abnormal findings including sudden infant death syndrome (SIDS) (a subtype of SUDI) (9.3%).

Childhood Mortality

In Australia, death rates for children older than 1 year of age have always been lower than those for infants. Children ages 5 to 14 years have the lowest rate of death. However, a sharp rise occurs during later adolescence, primarily from injuries, homicide and suicide. In 2017, 453 children aged 1–14 died—a rate of 10 per 100,000 children (12 per 100,000 for boys and 9.3 for girls). Boys accounted for 57% of child deaths (AIHW 2020). The death rate for children aged 1 to 4 years (15 per 100,000 children) was almost twice the rate for children aged 5 to 9 years (7.8) and 1.5 times as high as the rate for children aged 10 to 14 years (9.5). In 2015–17, the leading causes of child deaths were injuries (33%), cancer (19%) and diseases of the nervous system (10%)—rates of 3.5, 2.1 and 1.0 per 100,000 children, respectively. Children aged 1 to 4 years had the highest rates of death due to injury and diseases of the nervous system. Children aged 5 to 9 years had the highest rates of cancer (AIHW 2020).

THE ART OF PAEDIATRIC NURSING

Philosophy of Care

> *Childhood is an important time for healthy development, learning and establishing the foundations for future wellbeing. Most Australian children are healthy, safe and doing well. However, childhood is also a time of vulnerability and a child's growth and development can vary depending on where they live and their family's circumstances.*
>
> *(AIHW 2019)*

Health is influenced by social determinants such as individual and psychological make-up, lifestyle, environment, education, cultural influences, socioeconomic conditions and access to quality healthcare programs and services (WHO 2020). The WHO defines health as a multidimensional construct that incorporates physical, mental and social wellbeing and so is more than just the absence of disease or infirmity (WHO 1946).

While the WHO's definition of health is widely accepted, there can be variation across cultures. Aboriginal and Torres Strait Islander peoples take a broader perspective of health and view it not just as the physical wellbeing of the individual, but as the social, emotional and cultural wellbeing of the whole community (AIHW 2020). The He Korowai Oranga aim is whānau ora, whereby Māori families support each other to achieve their full potential for health and wellbeing. Whānau (kuia, koroua, pakeke, rangatahi and tamariki) is identified as the foundation of Māori society and is the central role in assisting families to reach their full potential for health and wellbeing (Ministry of Health 2002).

Child and family health nursing is family centred, and assessments must include both the family and the individual's data when planning care. The child's community must also be considered when planning care. The community has the ability to influence the type of care and support that will be available for a child and the family.

Family-centred Care

The philosophy of family-centred care recognises the family as the constant in a child's life. Family-centred care is an approach to the planning, delivery and evaluation of healthcare that is grounded in mutually beneficial partnerships among healthcare providers, patients and families (Institute for Patient- and Family-Centered Care 2014). Nurses support families in their natural caregiving and decision-making roles by building on their unique strengths and acknowledging their expertise in caring for their child both within and outside the hospital setting. The nurse considers the needs of all family members in relation to the care of the child.

Two basic concepts in family-centred care are enabling and empowerment. Professionals enable families by creating opportunities and means for all family members to display their current abilities and competencies and to acquire new ones to meet the needs of the child and family. *Empowerment* describes the interaction of professionals with families in such a way that families maintain or acquire a sense of control over their family's lives and acknowledge positive changes that result from helping behaviours that foster their own strengths, abilities and actions.

Role of the Paediatric Nurse

The paediatric nurse is responsible for promoting the health and wellbeing of the child and family. Nursing functions vary according to regional job structures, individual education and experience, and demography. Just as patients (children and their families) have unique backgrounds, each nurse brings an individual set of variables that affect the nurse–patient relationship. No matter where paediatric nurses practise, their primary concern is the welfare of the child and family.

There are many different roles for nurses specialising in the care of children and their families. For example, a paediatric nurse can pursue an advanced degree and become a clinical nurse specialist (CNS) in paediatrics, clinical nurse consult or nurse practitioner. CNSs are master-degree nurses who function in a variety of settings in both a direct and an indirect role. They model expert direct family-centred patient care. As our hospital settings change, so does the role of the paediatric nurse. The Australian Health Practitioner Regulation Agency (AHPRA) can provide further information on legislation, regulation and registration. In New Zealand, the National Framework for Nursing Professional Development and the Nursing Council of New Zealand provide information on legislation, regulation and registration.

Therapeutic Relationship

The establishment of a therapeutic relationship is the essential foundation for providing high-quality nursing care. Paediatric nurses need to have meaningful relationships with children and their families and yet remain separate enough to distinguish their own feelings and needs. In a therapeutic relationship, caring, well-defined boundaries separate the nurse from the child and family. These boundaries are positive and professional and promote the family's control over the child's healthcare. Both the nurse and the family are empowered and maintain open communication. In a non-therapeutic relationship, these boundaries are blurred, and many of the nurse's actions may serve personal needs, such as a need to feel wanted and involved, rather than the family's needs. Exploring whether relationships with patients are therapeutic or non-therapeutic helps nurses identify problem areas early in their interactions with children and families.

Coordination and Collaboration

The nurse, as a member of the healthcare team, collaborates and coordinates nursing care with the care activities of other professionals and works within a multidisciplinary team approach. A nurse working in isolation rarely serves the child's best interests. The concept of holistic care can be realised through a unified, interdisciplinary approach by being aware of individual contributions and limitations and collaborating with other specialists to provide high-quality health services. Failure to recognise limitations can be non-therapeutic at best and destructive at worst. For example, the nurse who feels competent in counselling but who is really inadequate in this area may not only prevent the child from dealing with a crisis but also impede future success with a qualified professional. Nursing should be seen as a major contributor to ensuring that the healthcare team focuses on high-quality, safe care.

Ethical Decision-making

Ethical dilemmas arise when competing moral considerations underlie various alternatives. Parents, nurses, medical practitioners and other healthcare team members may reach different but morally defensible decisions by assigning different weights to competing moral values. These competing moral values may include: autonomy, the patient's right to be self-governing; non-maleficence, the obligation to minimise or prevent harm; beneficence, the obligation to promote the patient's wellbeing; and justice, the concept of fairness. Nurses must determine the most beneficial or least harmful action within the framework of societal mores, professional practice standards, the law, institutional rules, the family's value system and religious traditions, and the nurse's personal values.

Nurses must prepare themselves systematically for collaborative ethical decision-making. They can accomplish this through formal coursework, continuing education, contemporary literature and work to establish an environment conducive to ethical discourse.

The nurse also uses the professional code of ethics for guidance and as a means for professional self-regulation. Nurses may face ethical issues regarding patient care, such as the use of lifesaving measures for VLBW newborns or the terminally ill child's right to refuse treatment. Ethical arguments are presented to help nurses clarify their value judgments when confronted with sensitive issues.

Research and Evidence-based Practice

Nurses should contribute to research because they are the individuals observing human responses to health and illness. The current emphasis on measurable outcomes to determine the efficacy of interventions (often in relation to cost) demands that nurses know whether clinical interventions result in positive outcomes for their patients. This demand has influenced the current trend towards evidence-based practice (EBP), which implies questioning why something is effective and whether a better approach exists. The concept of EBP also involves analysing and translating published clinical research into the everyday practice of nursing. When nurses base their clinical practice on science and research and document their clinical outcomes, they will be able to validate their contributions to health, wellness and cure not only to their patients, third-party payers and institutions but also to the nursing profession. Evaluation is essential to the nursing process, and research is one of the best ways to accomplish this.

EBP is the collection, interpretation and integration of valid, important and applicable patient-reported, nurse-observed and research-derived information. Using the population/patient problem, intervention, comparison, outcome and time (PICOT) question format to clearly define the problem of interest, nurses are able to obtain the best evidence to improve care. Evidence-based nursing practice combines knowledge with clinical experience and intuition. It provides a rational approach to decision-making that facilitates best practice (Murphy 2019). EBP is an important tool that complements the nursing process by using critical thinking skills to make decisions based on existing knowledge. The traditional nursing process approach to patient care can be used to conceptualise the essential components of EBP in nursing. During the assessment and diagnostic phases of the nursing process, the nurse establishes important clinical questions and completes a critical review of existing knowledge. EBP also begins with identification of the problem. The nurse asks clinical questions in a concise, organised way that allows for clear answers. Once the specific questions are identified, extensive searching for the best information to answer the question begins. The nurse evaluates clinically relevant research, analyses findings from the history and physical examination and reviews the specific pathophysiology of the defined problem. The third step in the nursing process is to develop a care plan. In evidence-based nursing practice, the care plan is established on completion of a critical appraisal of what is known and not known about the defined problem. Next, in the traditional nursing process, the nurse implements the care plan. By integrating evidence with clinical expertise, the nurse focuses care on the patient's unique needs. The final step in EBP is consistent with the final phase of the nursing process—to evaluate the effectiveness of the care plan.

Searching for evidence in this modern era of technology can be overwhelming. For nurses to implement EBP, they must have access to appropriate, recent resources such as online search engines and journals. In many institutions, computer terminals are available on patient care units, with the internet and online journals easily accessible. Another important resource for the implementation of EBP is time. The nursing shortage and ongoing changes in many institutions have compounded the issue of nursing time allocation for patient care, education and training. In some institutions, nurses are given paid time away from performing patient care to participate in activities that promote EBP. This requires an organisational environment that values EBP and its potential impact on patient care. As knowledge is generated regarding the significant impact of EBP on patient care outcomes, it is hoped that the organisational culture will change to support the staff nurse's participation in EBP. As the amount of available evidence increases, so does our need to critically evaluate the evidence.

Quality Outcome Measures

National Health Strategies for Children

A key objective of the National Healthcare Agreement from the Council of Australian Governments (COAG) is that Australians are born healthy and remain healthy. This is also the vision of the *Healthy, Safe and Thriving*: National Strategic Framework for Child and Youth Health (the framework). Even though a new National Federation Reform Council (NFRC) was announced, which is to replace the COAG meetings, the National Cabinet is to remain at the centre of the NFRC and the focus is to remain as above: that Australians are born health and remain healthy. At present the National Cabinet will focus specifically on responding to the COVID-19 pandemic.

The framework was endorsed by the Australian Health Ministers' Advisory Council (AHMAC) in 2015 and provides a 10-year overarching vision and set of priorities for child and youth health, on which other targeted health policies at the national and/or state and territory level can build. The framework's priorities are to:

- equip children and young people with the foundations for a healthy life
- support children and young people to become strong and resilient adults
- support children and young people to live in healthy and safe homes, communities and environments
- ensure children and young people have equitable access to healthcare services and equitable health outcomes
- improve systems to optimise the health outcomes of children and young people.

Improvement of child health and wellbeing outcomes is also the goal of the Australian Government's *National Action Plan for the Health of Children and Young People: 2020–2030* (the action plan).

This plan builds on the framework. It has these five key priority areas:

- improve health equity across populations
- empower parents and caregivers to maximise healthy development
- tackle mental health and risky behaviours
- address chronic conditions and preventive health
- strengthen the workforce.

Improving Child Wellbeing

Making New Zealand the best place in the world to be a child is a top priority for the New Zealand Government. The health system is well-placed to contribute to achieving this, by providing services that keep children healthy and identifying and addressing issues at an early stage. This gives all children the foundation upon which to thrive socially, emotionally and developmentally.

Universal healthcare for children in New Zealand is delivered by the Well Child/Tamariki Ora program. This service is the main provider of the government's child wellbeing programs. The aim is to ensure that Well Child/Tamariki Ora is well resourced and achieves its outcomes. This program will be reviewed to strengthen Well Child/Tamariki Ora by:

1. improving sustainability and performance of the Well Child/Tamariki Ora service
2. driving equitable health and development outcomes for children
3. enabling Well Child/Tamariki Ora to more effectively contribute to wider child wellbeing
4. ensuring value for money.

The main aim of the review is to assess how Well Child/Tamariki Ora can improve in meeting the needs of children, caregivers and wider communities and enable children to be empowered to thrive and achieve (Ministry of Health 2020a).

REFERENCES

Aotearoa Te Hiringa/Health Promotion Agency. (2018). T m tou whakat nga. Our role. https://www.hpa.org.nz/about/our-role

Australia's National Research Organisation for Women's Safety (ANROWS). (2018). Research summary: the impacts of domestic and family violence on children. ANROWS, Sydney. https://www.anrows.org.au/publication/research-summary-the-impacts-of-domestic-and-family-violence-on-children/ Accessed 22 May 2019.

Australian Bureau of Statistics (ABS). (2018). Immunisation coverage rates for all children. Canberra: ABS. https://www.abs.gov.au/AUSSTATS/abs@.nsf/Lookup/3235.0Main+Features12017?OpenDocument=

ABS. (2019). Microdata: National Health Survey, 2017–18. ABS cat. no. 4324.0.55.001. Canberra: ABS. Customised data report.

Australian Government Department of Health. (2020). National action plan for the health of children and young people 2020-2030. https://www1.health.gov.au/internet/main/publishing.nsf/Content/4815673E283EC1B6CA2584000082EA7D/$File/FINAL%20National%20Action%20Plan%20for%20the%20Health%20of%20Children%20and%20Young%20People%202020-2030.pdf Accessed 5 March 2020.

Australian Health Minister's Advisory Council. (2015). Healthy, safe and thriving: National strategic framework for child and youth health, COAG Health Council. http://www.coaghealthcouncil.gov.au/Publications/Reports Accessed 5 March 2020.

AIHW. (2019). Australia's children: in brief. 17 December. AIHW: Canberra. https://www.aihw.gov.au/reports/children-youth/australias-children-in-brief/contents/table-of-contents

AIHW. (2020). Australia's children. 3 April. AIHW: Canberra. https://www.aihw.gov.au/reports/children-youth/australias-children/contents/health/health-australias-children

Australian Institute of Health and Welfare (AIHW). (2017). A picture of overweight and obesity in Australia 2017. Cat. no. PHE 216. AIHW: Canberra.

AIHW: Pointer S. (2014). Hospitalised injury in children and young people 2011–12. Injury research and statistics series no. 91. Cat. no. INJCAT 167. AIHW: Canberra.

Australian Prudential Regulation Authority (APRA). (2020). Statistics. Quarterly private health insurance statistics – highlights. September 2020 (released 17 November 2020). https://www.apra.gov.au/sites/default/files/2020-11/Quarterly%20private%20health%20insurance%20statistics%20highlights%20September%202020_0.pdf

Baker S R, Foster Page L, Thomson W M et al. (2018). Structural determinants and children's oral health: a cross-national study. Journal of Dental Research, Sep, 97(10), 1129–1136.

Baker, J. L. & Edlund, A. (2018). Exploiting the oral microbiome to prevent tooth decay: has evolution already provided the best tools? Switzerland: Frontiers Research Foundation Frontiers in microbiology, 9, p.3323.

Campo, M. (2015). Children's exposure to domestic and family violence: key issues and responses. CFCA paper no. 36. Melbourne: Child Family Community Australia information exchange, Australian Institute of Family Studies. Viewed 22 May 2019.

Clark, C. A., Kent, K. A., & Jackson, R. D. (2015). Open mouth, open mind: expanding the role of primary care nurse practitioners. Journal of Pediatric Health Care, 30(5), 480–488.

COAG Health Council. (2019). Australian national breastfeeding strategy 2019 and beyond. Council of Australian Governments. www.coaghealthcouncil.gov.au/Publications/Reports Accessed 5 March 2020.

Education Review Office New Zealand. (2019). Bullying Prevention and Response in New Zealand Schools May 2019. https://www.ero.govt.nz/publications/bullying-prevention-and-response-in-new-zealand-schools-may-2019/introduction/

Finkelhor, D., Turner, H., Ormrod, R., et al. (2009). Violence, abuse and crime exposure in a national sample of children and youth. Paediatrics, 124, 1411–1423.

Godfrey, K. M., Reynolds, R. M., Prescott, S. L., et al. (2017). Influence of maternal obesity on the long-term health of offspring. The Lancet. Diabetes & Endocrinology, 5(1), 53–64.

Haszard, J. J., Russell, C. G., Byrne, R. A., et al. (2019). Early maternal feeding practices: associations with overweight later in childhood. Appetite , 1 January, 132(1), 96.

Holt, S., Buckley, H., & Whelan, S. (2008).' The impact of exposure to domestic violence on children and young people: a review of the literature. Child Abuse and Neglect, 32, 797–810.

Institute for Patient- and Family-Centered Care. (2014). What is patient- and family-centered health care? http://www.ipfcc.org

Jaffe, P., Wolfe, D., & Campbell, M. (2012). Growing up with domestic violence: assessment, intervention, and prevention strategies for children and adolescents. Hogrefe Publishing, Cambridge.

Knight, C. (2015). Trauma-informed social work practice: practice considerations and challenges. Clinical Journal of Social Work, 43, 25–37.

Lee, H., Hall, A., Reilly, K. L., et al. (2018). Mechanisms of implementing public health interventions: a pooled causal mediation analysis of randomised trial. Implementation Science Open Access, 13(42), 1–11.

Lewis, T., Kotch, J., Thompson, R., et al. (2010). Witnessed violence and youth behavior problems: a multi-informant study. American Journal of Orthopsychiatry, 80(4), 443–450.

Ministry of Health. (2002). He Korowai Oranga: Māori Health Strategy. November. Wellington: Ministry of Health.

Ministry of Health. (2014). Tobacco use 2012/13. NZ Health Survey. Wellington: Ministry of Health.

Ministry of Health. (2018). Social, emotional and behavioural difficulties in New Zealand children: Summary of findings. Wellington: Ministry of Health.

Ministry of Health. (2019a). Report on Maternity 2017. 11 April. Wellington: Ministry of Health. https://www.health.govt.nz/publication/report-maternity-2018

Ministry of Health. (2019b). Tatau Kahukura: Māori health statistics. Immunisation. 23 September. Wellington: Ministry of Health. https://www.health.govt.nz/our-work/populations/maori-health/tatau-kahukura-maori-health-statistics/nga-mana-hauora-tutohu-health-status-indicators/immunisation

Ministry of Health. (2019c). Mortality 2017 data tables, Summary. Wellington: Ministry of Health. https://www.health.govt.nz/publication/mortality-2017-data-tables

Ministry of Health 2020a. Well Child Tamariki Ora Review, Improving child wellbeing. 21 January. Wellington: Ministry of Health. https://www.health.govt.nz/our-work/life-stages/child-health/well-child-tamariki-ora-services/well-child-tamariki-ora-review

Ministry of Health. (2020a). Health Statistics. Child obesity statistics. 19 November. Wellington: Ministry of Health. https://www.health.govt.nz/nz-health-statistics/health-statistics-and-data-sets/obesity-statistics?mega=Health%20statistics&title=Obesity

Ministry of Health. (2020c). Fetal and infant deaths web tool. 19 November. Wellington: Ministry of Health. https://www.health.govt.nz/publication/fetal-and-infant-deaths-web-tool

Ministry of Health. (2020d). Annual Data Explorer 2019/20: New Zealand Health Survey [Data File]. 19 November. Wellington: Ministry of Health. https://minhealthnz.shinyapps.io/nz-health-survey-2019-20-annual-data-explorer/

Mitchell, K., Hamby, S., Turner, H., et al. (2015). Weapon involvement in the victimization of children. Pediatrics 136(1):10–17.

Office of the Children's Commissioner. (2016). Stats on Kids. Our Work. https://www.occ.org.nz/our-work/statsonkids/

Smokefree Aotearoa 2025. (2017). Smokefree Aotearoa 2025 Progress Report 2017. Wellington, New Zealand, August 2017. https://aspire2025.files.wordpress.com/2017/08/asap-progress-report-for-web.pdf

Tooth, L., Moss, K., Hockey, R., et al. (2019). Adherence to screen time recommendations for Australian children aged 0–12 years. Medical Journal of Australia, 211(4), 181–182. doi: 10.5694/mja2.50286

Weiss, R., Bremer, A. A., & Lustig, R. H. (2013). What is metabolic syndrome, and why are children getting it? Annals of the New York Academy of Sciences, 1281, 123–140.

World Health Organization (WHO). (1946). Constitution of the World Health Organization. Geneva: WHO.

WHO. (2016). Violence against children fact sheet. Geneva: WHO. https://www.who.int/news-room/fact-sheets/detail/violence-against-children Accessed 1 May 2019.

WHO. (2020). Health promotion. Focus. Geneva: WHO. https://www.who.int/health-topics/health-promotion#tab=tab_3

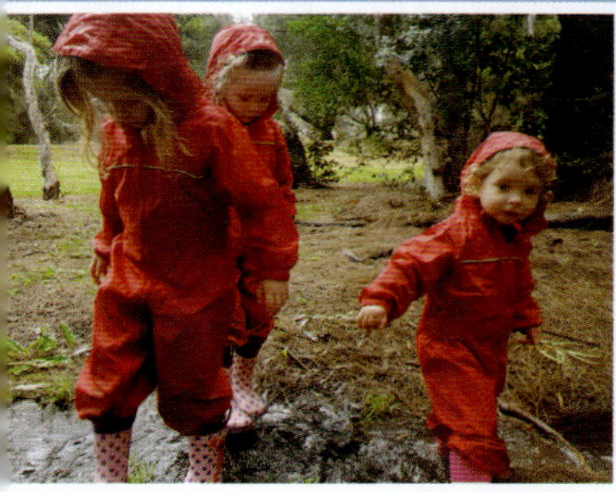

2

Social, Cultural, Religious and Family Influences on Child Health Promotion

Julia Laing and Lisa Speedie

LEARNING OUTCOMES

- Begin to understand the effect of family and family dynamics on a child's health and wellbeing
- Understand the impact of culture on health and the child and family's experience of healthcare

GENERAL CONCEPTS

Definition of Family

The term ***family*** has been defined in many different ways according to the individual's own frame of reference, values or discipline. There is no universal definition of family; a family is what an individual considers it to be. Biology describes the family as fulfilling the biological function of perpetuation of the species. Psychology emphasises the interpersonal aspects of the family and its responsibility for personality development. Economics views the family as a productive unit providing for material needs. Sociology depicts the family as a social unit interacting with the larger society, creating the context within which cultural values and identity are formed. Others define family in terms of the relationships of the persons who make up the family unit. The most common types of relationships are **consanguineous** (blood relationships), **affinal** (marital relationships) and **family of origin** (family unit a person is born into).

Earlier definitions of family emphasised that family members were related by legal ties or genetic relationships and lived in the same household with specific roles. Later definitions have been broadened to reflect both structural and functional changes. A family can be defined as an institution in which individuals, related through biology or enduring commitments and representing similar or different generations and genders, participate in roles involving mutual socialisation, nurturance and emotional commitment (Kaakinen & Coehlo 2015).

To accommodate these and other varieties of family styles, the descriptive term ***household*** is frequently used.

Family Theories

A **family theory** can be used to describe families and how the family unit responds to events both within and outside the family. Each family theory makes assumptions about the family and has inherent strengths and limitations (Kaakinen & Coehlo 2015). Most nurses use a combination of theories in their work with children and families. Commonly used theories are family systems theory, family stress theory and developmental theory (Table 2.1).

Family Systems Theory

Family systems theory is derived from general systems theory, a science of 'wholeness' that is characterised by interaction among the components of the system and between the system and the environment (Bomar 2004, Papero 1990). **General systems theory** expanded scientific thought from a simplistic view of direct cause and effect (*A* causes *B*) to a more complex and interrelated theory (*A* influences *B*, but *B* also affects *A*). In family systems theory, the family is viewed as a system that continually interacts with its members and the environment. The emphasis is on the interaction between the members; a change in one family member creates a change in other members, which in turn results in a new change in the original member.

The family is viewed as a whole that is different from the sum of the individual members. For example, a household of parents and one child consists of not only three individuals but also four interactive units. These units include three dyads (the parental relationship and the relationship the child has with each parent) and a triangle (the parent–parent–child relationship). In this ecological model, the family system functions within a larger system, with the family dyads in the centre of a circle surrounded by the extended family, the subculture and the culture, with the larger society at the periphery.

Bowen's family systems theory (Kaakinen & Coehlo 2015, Papero 1990) emphasises that the key to healthy family function is the members' ability to distinguish themselves from one another both emotionally and intellectually. The family unit has a high level of **adaptability**. When problems arise within the family, change occurs by altering the interaction or feedback messages that perpetuate disruptive behaviour. **Feedback** refers to processes in the family that help identify strengths and needs and determine how well goals are accomplished. Positive feedback initiates change; negative feedback resists change (Goldenberg & Goldenberg 2012). When the family system is disrupted, such as when a child is unwell or requiring healthcare, change can occur at any point in the system.

A major factor that influences a family's adaptability is its **boundary**, an imaginary line that exists between the family and its environment (Kaakinen & Coehlo 2015). Families have varying degrees of openness and closure in these boundaries. For example, one family has the capacity to reach out for help, whereas another considers help threatening. Knowledge of boundaries is critical when teaching or counselling families. Families with open boundaries may demonstrate a greater receptivity to interventions, whereas families demonstrating closed boundaries often require increased sensitivity and skill on the part of the nurse to gain their trust and acceptance. The nurse who uses family systems theory should assess the family's ability to accept new ideas, information, resources and opportunities and to plan strategies.

TABLE 2.1 Summary of Family Theories and Application

Assumptions	Strengths	Limitations	Applications
FAMILY SYSTEMS THEORY			
A change in any one part of a family system affects all other parts of the family system (circular causality). Family systems are characterised by periods of rapid growth and change and periods of relative stability. Both too little change and too much change are dysfunctional for the family system; therefore, a balance between morphogenesis (change) and morphostasis (no change) is necessary. Family systems can initiate change, as well as react to it.	Applicable for family in normal everyday life, as well as for family dysfunction and pathology. Useful for families of varying structure and various stages of life cycle.	More difficult to determine cause-and-effect relationships because of circular causality.	Mate selection, courtship processes, family communication, boundary maintenance, power and control within family, parent–child relationships, adolescent pregnancy and parenthood.
FAMILY STRESS THEORY			
Stress is an inevitable part of family life, and any event, even if positive, can be stressful for family. Family encounters both normative expected stressors and unexpected situational stressors over the life cycle. Stress has a cumulative effect on family. Families cope with and respond to stressors with a wide range of responses and effectiveness.	Potential to explain and predict family behaviour in response to stressors and to develop effective interventions to promote family adaptation. Focuses on positive contribution of resources, coping and social support to adaptive outcomes. Can be used by many disciplines in healthcare field.	Relationships between all variables in framework not yet adequately described. Not yet known if certain combinations of resources and coping strategies are applicable to all stressful events.	Transition to parenthood and other normative transitions, single-parent families, families experiencing work-related stressors (dual-earner family, unemployment), acute or chronic childhood illness or disability, infertility, death of a child, divorce, teenage pregnancy and parenthood.
DEVELOPMENTAL THEORY			
Families develop and change over time in similar and consistent ways. Family and its members must perform certain time-specific tasks set by themselves and by persons in the broader society. Family role performance at one stage of family life cycle influences family's behavioural options at next stage. Family tends to be in stage of disequilibrium when entering a new life cycle stage and strives towards homeostasis within stages.	Provides a dynamic, rather than static, view of family. Addresses both changes within family and changes in family as a social system over its life history. Anticipates potential stressors that normally accompany transitions to various stages and when problems may peak because of lack of resources.	Traditional model more easily applied to two-parent families with children. Use of age of oldest child and marital duration as marker of stage transition sometimes problematic (e.g. in stepfamilies, single-parent families).	Anticipatory guidance, educational strategies and developing or strengthening family resources for management of transition to parenthood; family adjustment to children entering school, becoming adolescents, leaving home; management of 'empty nest' years and retirement.

Family Stress Theory

Family stress theory explains how families react to stressful events and suggests factors that promote adaptation to stress (Kaakinen & Coehlo 2015). Families encounter **stressors** (events that cause stress and have the potential to effect a change in the family social system), including those that are predictable (e.g. parenthood) and those that are unpredictable (e.g. illness, unemployment). These stressors are cumulative, involving simultaneous demands from work, family and community life. Too many stressful events occurring within a relatively short period (usually 1 year) can overwhelm the family's ability to cope and place it at risk for breakdown or physical and emotional health problems among its members. When the family experiences too many stressors for it to cope adequately, a state of crisis ensues. For adaptation to occur, a change in family structure or interaction is necessary.

The **resiliency model of family stress, adjustment and adaptation** emphasises that the stressful situation is not necessarily pathological or detrimental to the family but demonstrates that the family needs to make fundamental structural or systemic changes to adapt to the situation (McCubbin & McCubbin 1994).

Developmental Theory

Developmental theory is an outgrowth of several theories of development. Duvall (1977) described eight developmental tasks of the family throughout its life span (Box 2.1). The family is described as a small group, a semiclosed system of personalities that interacts with the larger cultural social system. As an interrelated system, the family does not have changes in one part without a series of changes in other parts.

Developmental theory addresses family change over time, using Duvall's family life cycle stages. This theory is based on the predictable changes in the family's structure, function and roles, with the age of the oldest child as the marker for stage transition. The arrival of the first child marks the transition from stage I to stage II. As the first child grows and develops, the family enters subsequent stages. In every stage the family faces certain developmental tasks. At the same time, each

BOX 2.1 Duvall's Developmental Stages of the Family

Stage I—Marriage and An Independent Home: The Joining of Families
- Re-establish couple identity.
- Realign relationships with extended family.
- Make decisions regarding parenthood.

Stage II—Families with Infants
- Integrate infants into the family unit.
- Accommodate to new parenting and grandparenting roles.
- Maintain marital bond.

Stage III—Families with Preschoolers
- Socialise children.
- Parents and children adjust to separation.

Stage IV—Families with Schoolchildren
- Children develop peer relations.
- Parents adjust to their children's peer and school influences.

Stage V—Families with Teenagers
- Adolescents develop increasing autonomy.
- Parents refocus on midlife marital and career issues.
- Parents begin a shift towards concern for the older generation.

Stage VI—Families as Launching Centres
- Parents and young adults establish independent identities.
- Parents renegotiate marital relationship.

Stage VII—Middle-aged Families
- Reinvest in couple identity with concurrent development of independent interests.
- Realign relationships to include in-laws and grandchildren.
- Deal with disabilities and death of older generation.

Stage VIII—Ageing Families
- Shift from work role to leisure and semiretirement or full retirement.
- Maintain couple and individual functioning while adapting to the ageing process.
- Prepare for own death and dealing with the loss of spouse and/or siblings and other peers.

Source: Modified from Wright L M, Leahey M 1984. *Nurses and families: A guide to family assessment and intervention.* Philadelphia, PA: Davis.

family member must achieve individual developmental tasks as part of each family life cycle stage.

Developmental theory can be applied to nursing practice. For example, the nurse can assess how well new parents are accomplishing the individual and family developmental tasks associated with transition to parenthood. New applications should emerge as more is learned about developmental stages for non-nuclear and non-traditional families.

Family Nursing Interventions

In working with children, the nurse must include family members in their care plan. Research confirms parents' desire and expectation to participate in their child's care (Power & Franck 2008). To discover family dynamics, strengths and weaknesses, a thorough family assessment is necessary (see Chapter 4).

BOX 2.2 Qualities of Strong Families

- A belief and sense of **commitment** towards promoting the wellbeing and growth of individual family members, as well as the family unit
- **Appreciation** for the small and large things that individual family members do well and **encouragement** to do better
- Concentrated effort to spend **time** and do things together, no matter how formal or informal the activity or event
- A sense of **purpose** that permeates the reasons and basis for 'going on' in both bad and good times
- A sense of **congruence** among family members regarding the value and importance of assigning time and energy to meet needs
- The ability to **communicate** with one another in a way that emphasises positive interactions
- A clear set of **family rules, values and beliefs** that establishes expectations about acceptable and desired behaviour
- A varied repertoire of **coping strategies** that promote positive functioning in dealing with both normative and non-normative life events
- The ability to engage in **problem-solving** activities designed to evaluate options for meeting needs and procuring resources
- The ability to be **positive** and see the positive in almost all aspects of their lives, including the ability to see crisis and problems as an opportunity to learn and grow
- **Flexibility** and **adaptability** in the roles necessary to procure resources to meet needs
- A **balance** between the use of internal and external family resources for coping and adapting to life events and planning for the future

Source: Dunst C, Trivette C, Deal A 1988. *Enabling and empowering families: Principles and guidelines for practice.* Cambridge, MA: Brookline Books.

Family Strengths and Functioning Style

Family function refers to the interactions of family members, especially the quality of those relationships and interactions (Bomar 2004). Researchers are interested in family characteristics that help families function effectively. Knowledge of these factors guides the nurse throughout the nursing process and helps the nurse predict ways that families may cope and respond to a stressful event, to provide individualised support that builds on family strengths and unique functioning style, and to assist family members in obtaining resources.

Family strengths and unique functioning styles (Box 2.2) are significant resources that nurses can use to meet family needs. Building on qualities that make a family work well and strengthening family resources make the family unit even stronger. All families have strengths as well as vulnerabilities.

FAMILY ROLES AND RELATIONSHIPS

Each individual has a position, or status, in the family structure and plays culturally and socially defined roles in interactions within the family. Each family also has its own traditions and values and sets its own standards for interaction within and outside the group. Each determines the experiences the children should have, those they are to be shielded from and how each of these experiences meets the needs of family members. When family ties are strong, social control is highly effective and most members conform to their roles willingly and with commitment. Conflicts arise when people do not fulfil their roles in ways that meet other family members' expectations, either because they are unaware of the expectations or because they choose not to meet them.

Parental Roles

Historically, in family groups the socially recognised status of father and mother existed within socially sanctioned roles that prescribed appropriate sexual behaviour and childrearing responsibilities. The guides for behaviour in these roles served to control sexual conflict in society and provide for prolonged care of children. The degree to which parents were committed and the way they played their roles were influenced by a number of variables and by the parents' unique socialisation experience.

Parental role definitions have changed as a result of changes in society. Currently, parental and family roles are as individual as the family structure. Each family assigns roles to members which work best for the family as a whole and meet the needs of family members, achieving the goals of the family unit. In order to build a strong partnership between the family and nurse, gaining an understanding of the way a family functions and the roles of its members is a key part of the family assessment, thus creating a platform to build on the strengths of the family in the planning and delivery of care.

Role Learning

Roles are learned through the socialisation process. During all stages of development, children learn and practise, through interaction with others and in their play, a set of social roles and the characteristics of other roles. They behave in patterned and more or less predictable ways because they learn roles that define mutual expectations in typical social relationships. Although role definitions are changing, the basic determinants of parenting remain the same. Several determinants of parenting infants and young children are parental personality and mental wellbeing, systems of support and child characteristics. These determinants have been used as consistent measurements to determine a person's success in fulfilling the parental role.

Parents, peers, authority figures and other socialising agents who use positive and negative sanctions to ensure conformity to their norms transmit role conceptions. Role behaviours positively reinforced by rewards such as love, affection, friendship and honours are strengthened. Negative reinforcement takes the form of ridicule, withdrawal of love, expressions of disapproval or banishment.

In some cultures, the role behaviour expected of children conflicts with desirable adult behaviour. One of the family's responsibilities is to develop culturally appropriate role behaviour in children. Children learn to perform in expected ways consistent with their position in the family and culture. The observed behaviour of each child is a single manifestation—a combination of social influences and individual psychological processes. In this way the uniting of the child's intrapersonal system (the self) with the interpersonal system (the family) is simultaneously understood as the child's conduct.

PARENTING

Parenting Styles

Children respond to their environment in a variety of ways. A child's temperament heavily influences his or her response (see Chapter 10), but styles of parenting have also been shown to affect a child and lead to particular behavioural responses. There are many different parenting styles and more evolve over time. Some common parenting styles are outlined here. Parenting styles are often classified as authoritarian, permissive or authoritative (Baumrind 1971, 1996). **Authoritarian** parents try to control their children's behaviour and attitudes through unquestioned mandates. They establish rules and regulations or standards of conduct that they expect to be followed rigidly and unquestioningly. The message is: 'Do it because I say so'. Punishment need not be corporal but may be stern withdrawal of love and approval. Careful training often results in rigidly conforming behaviour in the children, who tend to be sensitive, shy, self-conscious, retiring and submissive. They are more likely to be courteous, loyal, honest and dependable, but docile. These behaviours are more typically observed when close supervision and affection accompany parental authority. If not, this style of parenting may be associated with both defiant and antisocial behaviours.

Permissive parents exert little or no control over their children's actions. They avoid imposing their own standards of conduct and allow their children to regulate their own activity as much as possible. These parents consider themselves to be resources for the children, not role models. If rules do exist, the parents explain the underlying reason, elicit the children's opinions and consult them in decision-making processes. They employ lax, inconsistent discipline; do not set sensible limits; and do not prevent the children from upsetting the home routine. These parents rarely punish the children.

Authoritative parents combine practices from both of the previously described parenting styles. They direct their children's behaviour and attitudes by emphasising the reason for rules and negatively reinforcing deviations. They respect the individuality of each child and allow the child to voice objections to family standards or regulations. Parental control is firm and consistent but tempered with encouragement, understanding and security. Control is focused on the issue, not on withdrawal of love or the fear of punishment. These parents foster 'inner-directedness', a conscience that regulates behaviour based on feelings of guilt or shame for wrongdoing, not on fear of being caught or punished. Parents' realistic standards and reasonable expectations produce children with high self-esteem who are self-reliant, assertive, inquisitive, content and highly interactive with other children.

There are differing philosophies in regard to parenting. Childrearing is a culturally bound phenomenon, and children are socialised to behave in ways that are important to their family. When working with individual families, nurses should give these differing styles equal respect.

Limit Setting and Discipline

In its broadest sense, **discipline** means 'to teach' or refers to a set of rules governing conduct. In a narrower sense, it refers to the action taken to enforce the rules after non-compliance. **Limit setting** refers to establishing the rules or guidelines for behaviour. For example, parents can place limits on the amount of time children spend watching television or chatting online. The clearer the limits that are set and the more consistently they are enforced, the less need there is for disciplinary action.

Nurses can help parents establish realistic and concrete 'rules'. Limit setting and discipline are positive, necessary components of childrearing and serve several useful functions as they help children:

- test their limits of control
- achieve in areas appropriate for mastery at their level
- channel undesirable feelings into constructive activity
- protect themselves from danger
- learn socially acceptable behaviour.

Children want and need limits. Unrestricted freedom is a threat to their security and safety. By testing the limits imposed on them, children learn the extent to which they can manipulate their environment and gain reassurance from knowing that others are there to protect them from potential harm.

Challenging Behaviour

The reasons for misbehaviour may include attention, power, defiance and a display of inadequacy (e.g. the child misses classes because of a fear that he or she is unable to do the work). Children may also misbehave because the rules are not clear or consistently applied. Acting-out behaviour, such as a temper tantrum, may represent uncontrolled frustration, anger, depression or pain. There are numerous books available about different ways to manage challenging behaviours in children of various ages. Many of these books focus on particular parenting styles and management of specific concerns, addressing contemporary societal issues. The range of topics and differing approaches to management of challenging behaviour is too large and out of the scope of this nursing care text; however, having an understanding of contemporary parenting issues and a healthy interest in further research on those issues and their management is helpful in child health nursing.

SPECIAL PARENTING SITUATIONS

Parenting is a demanding task under ideal circumstances, but when parents and children face situations that deviate from 'the norm', the potential for family disruption is increased. For many parents, managing the challenging behaviours of their child in public can be difficult as the parent may feel that they are being watched or judged by those around them. In addition, as our communities become more culturally diverse many immigrants are making the transition to parenthood and a new country, culture and language simultaneously. Other situations that create unique parenting challenges are parental addiction, poverty, homelessness and incarceration. Although these topics are not addressed here, the reader may wish to investigate them further.

Parenting the Adopted Child

Adoption establishes a legal relationship between a child and parents who are not related by birth but who have the same rights and obligations that exist between children and their biological parents. Unlike biological parents, who prepare for their child's birth with prenatal classes and the support of friends and relatives, adoptive parents have fewer sources of support and preparation for the new addition to their family. Nurses can provide the information, support and reassurance needed to reduce parental anxiety regarding the adoptive process and refer adoptive parents to parental support groups.

For the child, difficulties in forming an attachment depend on the amount of time he or she has spent with caregivers early in life, as well as the number of caregivers (e.g. the birth mother, nurse, adoption agency personnel).

Siblings (adopted or biological) who are old enough to understand should be included in discussions regarding the commitment to adopt, with reassurance that they are not being replaced.

Issues of Origin

The task of telling children that they are adopted can be a cause of deep concern and anxiety. There are no clear-cut guidelines for parents to follow in determining when and at what age children are ready for the information. Parents are naturally reluctant to present such potentially unsettling news. However, it is important that parents not withhold the adoption from the child because it is an essential component of the child's identity.

The timing arises naturally as parents become aware of the child's readiness. Most authorities believe that children should be informed at an age young enough so that, as they grow older, they do not remember a time when they did not know they were adopted. The time is highly individual, but it must be right for both the parents and the child. It may be when children ask where babies come from, at which time children can also be told the facts of their adoption. It is wise for parents who have not previously discussed adoption to tell children that they are adopted before the children enter school to avoid having them learn it from third parties. Complete honesty between parents and children strengthens the relationship.

Parents should anticipate behaviour changes after the disclosure, especially in older children. Children who are struggling with the revelation that they are adopted may benefit from individual and family counselling.

Adolescence may be an especially trying time for parents of adopted children. The normal confrontations of adolescents and parents assume more painful aspects in adoptive families. Adolescents may use their adoption to defy parental authority or as a justification for aberrant behaviour. As they attempt to master the task of identity formation, they may begin to have feelings of abandonment by their biological parents.

Adopted children fantasise about their biological parents and may feel the need to discover their parents' identity to define themselves and their own identity. It is important for parents to keep the lines of communication open and to reassure their child that they understand the need to search for their identity.

Cross-racial and International Adoption

Adoption of children from racial backgrounds that are different from that of the family is commonplace. In addition to the problems faced by adopted children in general, children of a cross-racial adoption must deal with physical and sometimes cultural differences. It is advised that parents who adopt children with different ethnic backgrounds work to support the adopted children's racial heritage.

In international adoptions the medical information the parents receive may be incomplete or sketchy; weight, height and head circumference are often the only objective information present in the child's medical record. Many internationally adopted children were born prematurely, and common health problems such as infant diarrhoea and malnutrition delay growth and development. Some children have serious or multiple health problems that can be a source of stress for the parents.

Parenting and Relationship Breakdown

Since the mid-1960s, a marked change in the stability of families has been reflected in increased rates of divorce, single parenthood and remarriage. Although almost half of all divorcing couples are childless, it is estimated that more than 1 million children experience divorce each year.

Quality time is essential with the child during family separations and divorce; this also includes time spent with grandparents (Fig 2.1).

During a relationship breakdown, parents' coping abilities may be compromised. The parents may be overwhelmed with their own feelings, needs and life changes and have limited energy to support their children. The child/children are likely to experience a change in usual arrangements and childcare during the separation and while new households and routines are established. Newly employed parents, often mothers, are likely to leave children with new caregivers, in unfamiliar settings or alone after school. Sometimes, however, the adult feels frightened and alone and begins to depend on the child as a substitute for the absent parent. This dependence places an enormous burden on the child.

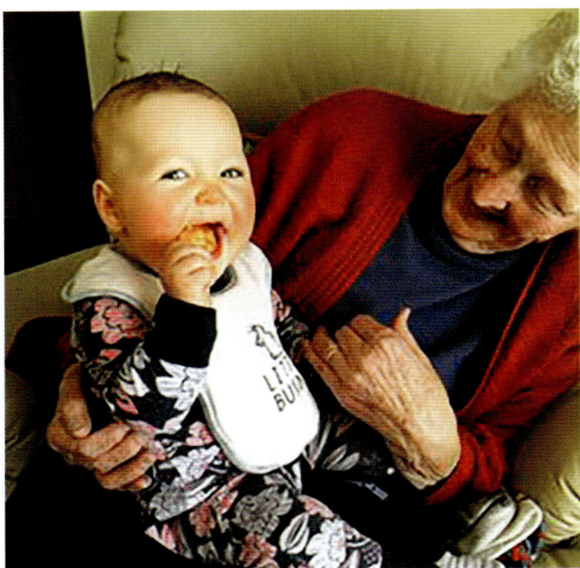

Fig 2.1 Quality time spent with a child during a divorce is essential to a family's health and wellbeing.

Impact of Relationship Breakdown on Children

Parental relationship breakdown or divorce is an additional childhood adversity that contributes to poor mental health outcomes. Even when a divorce is amicable and open, children recall parental separation with the same emotions felt by victims of a natural disaster: loss, grief and vulnerability to forces beyond their control.

The impact of divorce on children depends on several factors, including the age and sex of the children, the outcome of the divorce and the quality of the parent–child relationship and parental care during the years following the divorce. Family characteristics are more crucial to the child's wellbeing than specific child characteristics, such as age or sex. High levels of ongoing family conflict are related to problems of social development, emotional stability and cognitive skills for the child (see Research Focus box).

A major problem occurs when children are 'caught in the middle' between the separating parents. They become the message bearer between the parents, are often quizzed about the other parent's activities and have to listen to one parent criticise the other. A nurse may be able to help the child get out of the middle by stating 'I-messages' based on the formula of 'I feel (state the feeling) when you (state the source). I would like it if you ...' An example of an 'I-message' is: 'I do not feel comfortable when you ask me questions about Mum; maybe you could ask her yourself'. This approach enables the child to feel in control.

Feelings of children towards divorce vary with age (Box 2.3). Previously, researchers believed that divorce had a greater impact on younger children, but recent observations indicate that divorce constitutes a major disruption for children of all ages. The feelings and behaviours of children may be different for various ages and gender, but all children suffer stress second only to the stress produced by the death of a parent. Although considerable research has looked at sex differences in children's adjustments to divorce, the findings are not conclusive.

Some children may feel a sense of shame and embarrassment concerning the family situation if they don't know others from similar situations. Depending on the developmental stage of the child they may see themselves as different, inferior or unworthy of love, especially if they feel responsible for the family dissolution. Although the social stigma attached to divorce no longer produces the emotions it did in the past, such feelings may still exist in small towns or in some cultural groups and can reinforce children's negative self-image. The lasting effects of divorce depend on the children's and the parents' adjustment to the transition from their original family to a new family dynamic.

Although most studies have concentrated on the negative effects of divorce on youngsters, some positive outcomes of divorce have been reported. A successful post-separation family, either a single-parent or a reconstituted family, can improve the quality of life for both adults and children. If conflict is resolved, a better relationship with one or both parents may result. Greater stability in the home setting and the removal of arguing parents can be a positive outcome for the child's long-term wellbeing.

RESEARCH FOCUS

Impact of Divorce

Children who reported that their divorced parents were cooperative had better relationships with their parents, grandparents, step-parents, and siblings (Ahrons 2007). Complications associated with divorce include efforts on the part of one parent to subvert the child's loyalties to the other, abandonment to other caregivers and adjustment to a step-parent.

Parenting Children After Separation

Changes in the parenting partnership after relationship breakdown need to promote and focus on the ongoing wellbeing of the children, supporting each child to maintain a healthy relationship with each parent. Changes in family dynamics may also affect wider family connections and relationships. The amount of time children spend with people with whom they have a significant relationship may change and cause the child sadness or distress.

Co-parenting offers substantial benefits for the family: children can be close to both parents and life with each parent can be more relaxed. To be successful, parents in these arrangements must be highly committed to providing normal parenting and to separate their marital conflicts from their parenting roles. No matter what type of custody arrangement is awarded, the primary consideration is the welfare of the children.

Parents may find themselves separated and caring for their children under parenting orders. In **joint physical custody**, the parents alternate the physical care of the children on an agreed-on basis while maintaining shared parenting responsibilities legally. This custody arrangement works well for families who live close to each other and whose occupations permit an active role in the care and raising of the children. In **joint legal custody**, the children reside with one parent, but both parents are the children's legal guardians, and both participate in childrearing.

Single Parenting

An individual may acquire single-parent status as a result of divorce, separation, death of a spouse or birth or adoption of a child. Managing shortages of money, time and energy is often a concern for single parents. Studies repeatedly confirm the financial difficulties of single-parent families, particularly single mothers. These families are often forced by their financial status to live in communities with inadequate housing and personal safety concerns. Single parents often feel guilty about the time spent away from their children. Many single parents have challenges relating to childcare, particularly for a sick child.

Social supports and community resources needed by single-parent families include healthcare services that are open on evenings and

BOX 2.3 Feelings and Behaviours of Children Related to Divorce

Infancy
- Effects of reduced mothering or lack of mothering
- Increased irritability
- Disturbance in eating, sleeping and elimination
- Interference with attachment process

Early Preschool Children (Ages 2 to 3 Years)
- Frightened and confused
- Blame themselves for the divorce
- Fear of abandonment
- Increased irritability, whining, tantrums
- Regressive behaviours (e.g. thumb sucking, loss of elimination control)
- Separation anxiety

Later Preschool Children (Ages 3 to 5 Years)
- Fear of abandonment
- Blame themselves for the divorce; decreased self-esteem
- Bewilderment regarding all human relationships
- Become more aggressive in relationships with others (e.g. siblings, peers)
- Engage in fantasy to seek understanding of the divorce

Early School-age Children (Ages 5 to 6 Years)
- Depression and immature behaviour
- Loss of appetite and sleep disorders
- May be able to verbalise some feelings and understand some divorce-related changes
- Increased anxiety and aggression
- Feelings of abandonment by departing parent

Middle School-age Children (Ages 6 to 8 Years)
- Panic reactions
- Feelings of deprivation—loss of parent, attention, money and secure future
- Profound sadness, depression, fear and insecurity
- Feelings of abandonment and rejection
- Fear regarding the future
- Difficulty expressing anger at parents
- Intense desire for reconciliation of parents
- Impaired capacity to play and enjoy outside activities
- Decline in school performance
- Altered peer relationships—become bossy, irritable, demanding and manipulative
- Frequent crying, loss of appetite, sleep disorders
- Disturbed routine, forgetfulness

Later School-age Children (Ages 9 to 12 Years)
- More realistic understanding of divorce
- Intense anger directed at one or both parents
- Divided loyalties
- Ability to express feelings of anger
- Ashamed of parental behaviour
- Desire for revenge; may wish to punish the parent they hold responsible
- Feelings of loneliness, rejection and abandonment
- Altered peer relationships
- Decline in school performance
- May develop somatic complaints
- May engage in aberrant behaviour such as lying, stealing
- Temper tantrums
- Dictatorial attitude

Adolescents (Ages 12 to 18 Years)
- Able to disengage themselves from parental conflict
- Feelings of a profound sense of loss—of family, childhood
- Feelings of anxiety
- Worry about themselves, parents, siblings
- Expression of anger, sadness, shame, embarrassment
- May withdraw from family and friends
- Disturbed concept of sexuality
- May engage in acting-out behaviours

weekends, high-quality childcare and support from family and friends to offer respite childcare to relieve parental exhaustion and prevent burnout. Single parents need social contacts separate from their children for their own emotional growth and that of their children.

Parenting in Reconstituted Families

The entry of a step-parent into a family requires adjustments for all family members. Some obstacles to the role adjustments and family problem-solving include disruption of previous lifestyles and interaction patterns, complexity in the formation of new ones and lack of social supports.

Cooperative parenting relationships can allow more time for each set of parents to be alone to establish their own relationship with the children. Under ideal circumstances, power conflicts between the two households can be reduced, and tension and anxiety can be lessened for all family members. Flexibility, mutual support and open communication are critical in successful relationships in stepfamilies and step-parenting situations.

Parenting in Dual-earner Families

Many families are dual-earner families, whether to meet basic family needs or to increase the resources available to enhance the family's life and lifestyle. This can result in the family being subject to considerable stress as members attempt to meet often competing demands of occupational needs and family life.

Role definitions are frequently altered to arrange a more equitable division of time and labour, as well as to resolve conflict, especially conflict related to traditional cultural norms. Overload is a common source of stress in a dual-earner family, and social activities could be significantly curtailed. Time demands and scheduling are major challenges for all individuals who work. When the individuals are parents, the demands can be even more intense. Dual-earner couples may increase the strain on themselves to avoid creating stress for their children. Although there is no evidence to indicate that the dual-earner lifestyle is stressful to children, the stress experienced by the parents may affect the children indirectly.

The quality of childcare is a persistent concern for all working parents. Determinants of childcare quality are based on health and safety requirements, responsive and warm interaction between staff and children, developmentally appropriate activities, trained staff, limited group size, age-appropriate caregivers, adequate staff-to-child ratios and adequate indoor and outdoor space.

Kinship Care

Kinship care refers to the placement of a child in the care of a grandparent or other relative. There are a number of cultural models of kinship care among different ethnicities and Indigenous groups. Among Māori, kinship care is not uncommon. The Māori term for kinship care is whāngai and is often adoption within the wider family/whānau. The whole family/whānau is involved in the decision and the child is aware that they are whāngai and who their birth parents are. This arrangement may be confirmed under law or agreed within the wider family/whānau and tribe/iwi. This practice keeps the child within the family and tribe and the child is raised in these customs and traditions as they would be if they were kept by their birth parents.

Foster Parenting

The term ***foster care*** is the temporary placement of a child in an approved living situation away from the birth parents. The living situation may be an approved foster home, possibly with other children, or a pre-adoptive home. Each country has its own legal requirements for approving and monitoring foster homes to ensure the child is placed in an environment which supports the child's growth and wellbeing.

Foster homes include both kinship and non-relative placements. Since the 1980s, the proportion of children in out-of-home care placed with relatives has increased rapidly and has been accompanied by a decrease in the number of foster families. As with their non-foster counterparts, much of the child's adjustment depends on the family's stability and available resources. Even though foster homes are designed to provide short-term care, it is not unusual for children to stay for many years.

Foster children are often at risk because of their previous caretaking environment. Nurses should strive to implement strategies to improve the healthcare for this group of children. In particular, assessment and case management skills are required to involve other disciplines in meeting their needs.

SOCIOCULTURAL INFLUENCES ON CHILDREN AND FAMILIES

A child and his or her immediate family are nested within a local community of school, peers and extended family and within a larger community that may be bound by common geography, background, traditions and an even broader community that incorporates the social, political and economic elements that influence many aspects of family life. These layers of influence are often multifactorial: parents, extended family and community exert influence most directly when thinking about any aspect of the culture of the family. These elements do come into play when we think about children moving into the wider world, such as their interactions with other children at school or potential biases a child/adolescent might face because of cultural identity. Thus, the sociopolitical context, though an outer layer of a social ecological model, can exert significant influence on a child's daily life, opportunities and outcomes. Equally important to child and family health outcomes, the sociopolitical context draws our attention to factors and health policies at the local, regional, state or federal government levels that can serve as barriers to health equity. This is also made evident through research on the social determinants of health. This section of the chapter will now delve into a deeper discussion of such factors.

The social ecological model (Kazak 2001, Kazak et al 2010), rooted in Bronfenbrenner's ecological model (Bronfenbrenner 1979, 2005), offers a perspective of viewing children and their families within the context of various circles of influence, called an ecological framework.

Promoting the health of children requires a nurse to understand social, cultural and religious influences on children and their families as populations are constantly evolving. Patients experience negative health outcomes when social, cultural and religious factors are not considered as influencing their healthcare (Chavez 2012, Williams 2012). Educating healthcare providers is one way to reduce disparities in healthcare.

CULTURAL SAFETY IN NURSING PRACTICE

The nursing regulatory authorities in both Australia (Nursing and Midwifery Board of Australia) and New Zealand (Nursing Council of New Zealand) provide professional guidelines and codes which aim to ensure that the nursing care provided is culturally safe. As with any professional guideline, these are regularly reviewed to ensure reflection of society and current health issues. Therefore, ensuring nurses maintain an awareness of current health concerns and the latest professional information is essential to support the health and wellbeing of all people. Of particular focus for both countries is addressing the impact of social determinants of health on the Indigenous peoples of each country. Statistics have shown over a long period of time the lack of equity in healthcare outcomes for both Aboriginal and Torres Strait Islander and Māori and Pasifika peoples. Both countries have government health strategies to improve the health outcomes in this area of their communities; however, nurses can work in partnership with healthcare consumers to ensure that the care they are receiving is culturally appropriate and acceptable.

Along with ensuring that care given is culturally safe, the Nursing Council of New Zealand requires all nurses to engage in cultural safety education which includes reflection on the individual nurse's own culture and the impact this might have on their practice (Nursing Council of New Zealand 2011). This critical consciousness leads the nurse to step back and examine his or her own beliefs, cultures and positions in the world, as well as assumptions, biases and values, and it is viewed as an ongoing process. Through this teaching and coaching, the aim is to be more engaged in understanding the social determinants of health, their impacts and their roots, and how to counteract their negative effects.

An individual's culture is not a single identity; rather, it is a complex intersection of various aspects of the person. Consider the notion that culture is not just ethnicity or race, but age, gender, sexual orientation and many other things, including the culture of being a child, being a student and/or being a parent. That culture is unique to the individual and healthcare needs to support and respect the culture of the health consumer. For example, when we gather demographic data about those in our care, they might indicate that they are a specific religion or ethnicity but they may not have any strong links to the religion or cultural traditions because of their experience, distance, estrangement or lack of interest in that aspect of their culture. Therefore, to assume that they need some specific care due to this information would not be culturally safe in that you are making an assumption about them from limited information.

Culture can influence the ways children, youth and their families interact with healthcare providers and engage with the healthcare system. Gaining an understanding of the culture of the child and family is essential to ensure culturally safe care. Questions to start this conversation can begin with the following: 'Is there anything you would like me to know about your child or your family so that I can take the best possible care of you all?'

INFLUENCES IN THE SURROUNDING ENVIRONMENT

School Communities: School Health and School Connectedness

Environments differentially support learning through the kinds of opportunities and support provided. Learning and development are cumulative and synergistic; one supports the other. High-quality early childhood education is especially beneficial to set children up for success in later grades.

Within communities, schools are important sites for health promotion. Initiatives can emphasise and build on this critical connection between youth academic performance and health by addressing important elements of children's and adolescents' lives that cut across domains.

An important concept when considering schools as a site of health promotion is connectedness (Centers for Disease Control and Prevention [CDC] 2009). Feeling connected at school has important health benefits. Children and youth who feel more connected are more likely to engage in healthy behaviours and do well academically. School connectedness has been found particularly protective against substance abuse, early sexual debut and violence in both boys and girls. In addition, school connectedness was second only to family connectedness in protection against emotional distress, disordered eating and suicidal ideation and attempts. Finally, it also promotes academic outcomes in addition to health outcomes, including improved grades, decreased absence and delayed dropout.

Schools

When children enter school, their radius of relationships extends to include a wider variety of peers and a new source of authority. Although parents continue to exert the major influence on children, in the school environment teachers have the most significant psychological impact on children's development and socialisation. In addition to academic and cognitive progress, teachers are concerned with the emotional and social development of the children in their care. Both parents and teachers act to model, shape and promote positive behaviour, constrain negative behaviour and reinforce standards of conduct. Ideally, parents and teachers work together for the benefit of the children in their care.

Schools serve as a major source of socialisation for children. Next to the family, schools exert a major force in providing continuity. This, in turn, prepares children to carry out the social roles they are expected to assume as they develop into adults. School is the centre of **cultural diffusion** wherein the cultural standards of the larger group are disseminated into the community. It governs what is taught and, to a great extent, how it is taught. School rules and regulations regarding attendance, authority relationships and the system of rewards and penalties based on achievement transmit to children the expectations of the adult world of employment and relationships. School is an important institution in which children systematically learn about the negative consequences of behaviour that departs from social expectations. School also serves as an avenue for children to participate in the larger society in rewarding ways, to promote social mobility and to connect the family with new knowledge and services. Like parents, teachers are responsible for transmitting knowledge and culture (i.e. values on which there is a broad consensus) to the children in their care. Teachers are also expected to stimulate and guide children's intellectual development and creative problem-solving.

Peer Cultures

Peer groups also have an impact on the socialisation of children (Fig 2.2). Peer relationships become increasingly important and influential as children proceed through school. In school, children have what can be regarded as a culture of their own. This is even more apparent in unsupervised playgroups because the culture in school is partly produced by adults.

During their lives, children are subjected to many influential factors, such as family and religious community. In peer-group interactions, they confront a variety of these sets of values. The values imposed by the peer group are especially compelling because children must accept and conform to them to be accepted as members of the group. When the peer values are not too different from those of family and teachers, the mild conflict created by these small differences serves to separate children from the adults in their lives and to strengthen the feeling of belonging to the peer group.

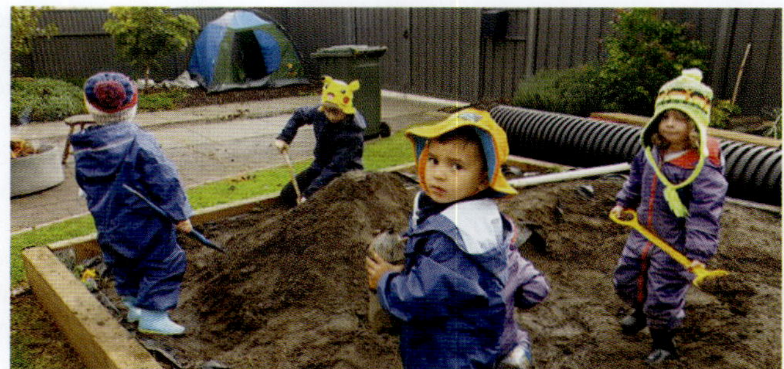

Fig 2.2 Children from different cultural backgrounds interact within the larger culture.

Community

Families and communities are often interwoven in their impact on child health. Although both are essential to socioemotional growth and improved learning outcomes in children, their influence on children is synergistic. When families live in areas of concentrated poverty, residents experience risk at population and individual levels. Children and families living in areas of concentrated poverty are at risk for negative health outcomes and experience higher rates of crime and violence. In addition, it is more likely that these challenges affect education provision in affected communities. If parents have grown up in the area or a similar area, they have also experienced unfavourable effects on their health or educational outcomes. As a result, they may not be able to secure employment that provides greater resources for them to invest in their child or that provides economic stability for the family. Financial stressors in parents contribute to their stress and depression, which can inhibit effective parenting. Thus, we see an important need for two-generation programs or strategies to both build on family and community strengths and diminish their stressors. Community-level factors are especially important as we consider the life, safety and causes of death in older adolescents.

BROADER INFLUENCES ON CHILD HEALTH

Social Media and Mass Media

Digital technologies that serve as an avenue to mass and social media are pervasive in most parts of society. Technology has a role in the lives of children more than ever before. This frequent use carries risks for increased rates of obesity, disrupted sleep and delays in cognitive, social and language development, potentially related to diminished parent–child interaction in preschoolers. Research has demonstrated that there is limited benefit of digital technology for children younger than 2 years. Benefits related to digital technology use are related to the type of content viewed and used. For example, high-quality programming, such as programs and apps that encourage cognitive and social development, can bolster cognitive and social outcomes in preschool-age children, and applications from educational organisations can promote literacy skills. Unfortunately, many programs and applications targeted to children and their parents or caregivers are not created under the direction of educators or developmental experts and may not prove as beneficial to child social and cognitive outcomes. Despite technological advances, play, social interactions with peers and parent–child interactions remain vital to young children's development of the skills needed to succeed in school, including persistence, emotional regulation and creative thinking (Australian Institute of Health and Welfare [AIHW] 2020).

The digital landscape for older children and adolescents seems to change and grow on a daily basis and is woven into daily life for many youth. Most adolescents have a smartphone or mobile device (AIHW 2020). While using these mobile devices, most adolescents are engaging in social media, with nearly three-quarters engaging in multiple social media sites and cultivating a portfolio (Reid Chassiakos et al 2016). This immersion poses both benefits and risks to these youth. In terms of the benefits, youth have an unprecedented chance to learn and gather information and consider new perspectives; connect with other youth, which is especially important for youth who may feel marginalised or isolated; and maintain connections with family and friends who live at a distance.

On the other hand, navigating this landscape includes potential risks to physical and mental health, such as obesity, disrupted sleep, addictive behaviour, negative impact on academics, bullying and sexual exploitation and normalisation of maladaptive behaviour (e.g. sites that promote disordered eating or self-harm). Similar to traditional forms of media (e.g. television), research has demonstrated that social media postings can influence perceptions of alcohol and drug use and younger age of initiating sexual activity as normal in the eyes of adolescents (AIHW 2020). Finally, communication among adolescents has shifted and become more pervasive through texting, messaging through gaming systems and messaging on social media sites. This continual access and inlet to the lives of peers can serve as both a source of support and a source of stress. Thus, it is essential for nurses and other healthcare providers to talk with older children and adolescents about the frequency, content and nature of their digital and social media use and how they maintain their privacy and safety. Equally important, nurses can help families devise strategies and personalised plans for safe and healthy technology use (AIHW 2020) (Box 2.4 and Table 2.2).

Race and Ethnicity

Race and ethnicity are socially constructed terms used to group people who share similar characteristics, traditions or historical experience. **Race** is a term that groups together people by their outward physical appearance. **Ethnicity** is a classification aimed at grouping 'individuals who consider themselves, or are considered by others, to share common characteristics that differentiate them from the other collectivities in a society, and from which they develop their distinctive cultural behaviour' (Scott & Marshall 2009). Ethnicities may be differentiated from one another by customs and language and may influence family structure, food preferences and expressions of emotion. The composition and definition of ethnic groups can be fluid in response to changes in geography (i.e. moving from one country to another). Race and ethnicity influence a family's health when they are used as criteria by which a child or family is discriminated against.

Racism remains an important social determinant of health. According to Williams (2012), for minority or other groups who experience stigmatisation, 'inequalities in health are created by larger inequalities in society', meaning that prevailing social conditions and obstacles to equal opportunities for all influences the health of all individuals.

BOX 2.4 Actions to Promote Positive Media

Parents

- For children aged 2 to 4 years who are not in school, the recommended guidelines are no more than 60 minutes a day of screen-based activity. For children aged 5 to 12 and 13 to 17 years, the recommended guidelines are no more than 2 hours a day of screen-based activity (AIHW 2020).
- Establish clear guidelines for internet use and provide direct supervision. Have frank discussions about what young people may encounter in viewing media. Be mindful of own media use in the home.
- Encourage unstructured play in the home and plan to help children readjust to this change in family dynamic. Consider planned, deliberate use of media to experience the benefits (e.g. watching a television show together to bond or start a sensitive discussion).

Nurses/Healthcare Providers

- Dedicate a few minutes of each visit to provide media screening and counselling.
- Discourage presence of electronic devices in children's rooms.
- Be sensitive to the challenges that parents face in carrying this out.

Schools

- Offer timely, accurate sexuality and drug education.
- Promote resilience.
- Develop programs to educate children and adolescents on wise use of technology.
- Develop and implement policies on dealing with cyberbullying and sexting.

Addressing race and ethnicity in nursing practice should reflect the aspects of cultural safety discussed previously in this chapter.

Poverty

Our health starts in the environment where we live, work and play. Opportunities to promote this health or risks to this health often begin in our families, schools, where we live and places of employment. Thus, to fully promote child health and diminish risks to it, we need to understand how the surrounding context and environments are influential. Children are nested within layers of family, peers, school and community; we can consider the direct impact of these outside systems interacting with the child and family. Equally important, however, is the influence of factors within the sociopolitical landscape at local/state/regional/national and international levels. These factors affect the creation of health and social policies that may perpetuate health disparities or make health equity possible.

Economy and Poverty

Poverty affects children and their families across all geographical areas, including urban, suburban and rural. Several social factors associated with poverty that can negatively affect child health are family disruption, parental depression, substance use, other mental illnesses, unsafe homes or areas, housing instability, homelessness, decreased educational opportunities and low parent educational levels and health literacy (Fierman et al 2016).

Poverty influences these social determinants of health, the circumstances and environments in which people are born, live, work, learn and play. In turn, these social determinants shape child health in major and lasting ways. Poverty itself is a major cause of acute and chronic stress for adults and children. The daily stressors associated with poverty are overwhelming, and other circumstances, such as trauma or violence, can add to the stress experienced by parents and children. This overwhelming stress can undermine skills in dealing with

TABLE 2.2 Media Effects on Children and Adolescents

Media Effect	Potential Consequences
Violence	Government, medical and public health data show that exposure to media violence is one factor in violent and aggressive behaviour. Both adults and children become desensitised by violence witnessed through various media, including television (including children's programming), movies (including G rated), music and video games. In addition, cyberbullying and harassment via text messages are a growing concern among primary school and high school students.
Sex	A significant body of research shows that sexual content in the media can contribute to beliefs and attitudes about sex, sexual behaviour and initiation of intercourse. Teens access sexual content through a variety of media: television, movies, music, magazines, the internet, social media and mobile devices. Current issues receiving attention for the role they play in teen sexual behaviour include: sending of sexual images via mobile devices (i.e. sexting); impact of violent media on youth views of women and forced sex/rape; cyberbullying lesbian, gay, bisexual, transgender, intersex, queer/questioning (LGBTIQ+) youth. Media can also serve as a positive source of sexual information (i.e. information, apps, social media about sexually transmitted infections, teen pregnancy and promoting acceptance and support of LGBTIQ+ youth).
Substance use and abuse	Although the causes of teen substance use and abuse are numerous, media play a significant role. Alcohol and tobacco are still heavily marketed to adolescents/young adults. Television and movies featuring the use of these substances can influence initiation of use. Media also show substance used to be pervasive and without consequences. Finally, content shared over social networking sites can serve as a form of peer pressure and can influence likelihood of use.
Obesity	Highly prevalent public health issue among children of all ages and increasing rates around the world. A number of studies have demonstrated a link between the amount of screen time and obesity. Advertising of unhealthy food to children is a long-standing marketing practice, which may increase snacking in the face of decreased activity. In addition, both increased screen time and unhealthy eating may also be related to unhealthy sleep.
Body image	Media may play a significant role in the development of body image awareness, expectations and body dissatisfaction among young and older adolescents. Their beliefs may be influenced by images on television, movies and magazines. New media also contribute to this through internet images, social networking sites and websites that encourage disordered eating (Strasburger et al 2012).

challenging situations. The stressors associated with poverty can be psychologically and emotionally depleting, yet supports to deal with this depletion may not be available, such as adequate mental health services, high-quality and affordable childcare or social supports (Center on the Developing Child at Harvard University 2016).

Considering the impact of poverty on children, an important place to look is the brain. Children's brains are dynamic and plastic (adaptable) and change according to what they experience. This impact is greatest in young children and adolescents because their brains go through such rapid development. Even as early as the prenatal period, children are affected by the stressors of their surrounding environments, and poverty carries multiple important stressors with it that affect health, such as housing instability, poor or compromised nutrition and unsafe living conditions. Additionally, parents and caregivers who are overwhelmed by the stressors associated with poverty or trauma may be less able to participate in reciprocal communication with an infant or young child. Affected caregivers may not respond to infant crying or cues as needed or may become irritable, which then propels the infant towards a dysregulated state. Parent and infant are caught in a stressful cycle, and it may then be harder for the parent to prevent a harsh response in this challenging situation. Serious, early, adverse events can affect development of the prefrontal cortex, influencing later self-regulation, emotional responsiveness and reactivity. Severe, chronic adversity early in life can trigger toxic stress responses that affect brain development and response and diminish mental health. Early exposure to stressful events is associated with challenges to working memory, attention, emotional regulation skills and perception of new situations as potential threats that require quick action. Thus 'the ways in which we have experienced the world fundamentally frame how we perceive our environment and the choices made in this environment' (Center on the Developing Child at Harvard University 2016, p. 7).

Poverty and the link between poverty and poor environments impacts on the healthy development and education of children and adolescents. Poor nutrition affects growth and development from intrauterine development to adolescence, and the effects of this impact on lifelong health and wellness. High costs of quality food and healthcare affect access to these resources and compromise other aspects of family life such as the cost of bills, school trips or needed clothing. Access to healthcare can include an inability to get to medical centres due to a remote or rural situation, a lack of transport to seek healthcare, attendance to medical centres that don't bulk bill which adds additional cost that many families are unable to afford. The additional financial stress for families with children who have significant or complex needs adds to the difficulty and challenges of managing and caring for the child.

Parental Education

Parent level of education is another important consideration when we consider economic influences on child health. Child economic status is directly tied to parental earnings. Parental earnings from employment and health literacy are affected by parental level of education.

The high incidence and pervasive nature of child poverty demands that paediatric nurses and other healthcare providers incorporate screening for poverty or financial hardship into everyday practice. Paediatric nurses, despite geographical context, are likely to care for children and families encountering poverty. Context influences the experience of poverty and how healthcare providers address it. Nurses can screen in various ways and connect children and families with the right services, including those local to the communities in which the families live.

Often the paediatric nurse is best placed to assess and support families to access supports. Performing a 'Healthy Kids Check' (Australia) or 'Well Child Tamariki Ora' check (New Zealand) in the home enables assessment and discussion about their needs in the privacy of the family's home. Barriers to completing those assessments and accessing support include: not recognising the impact of poverty or the measurable outcomes associated with it; lack of time; limited and insufficient training in assessment and limited familiarity with assessment tools; and limited knowledge about available community resources. Paediatric nurses and healthcare providers can initiate surveillance and screening to elicit and address parent concerns, identify risk and protective factors, screen for specific issues and refer the child and family to the right place with the right services. To address the social determinants of health, screening can be tailored to the most sensitive or sustained issues in the community, to the parents' sources of concern and to the child's developmental stage.

Land of Origin, Refugee and Immigration

Cultural factors are woven into social, economic and political influences on child health, including the misconception that children are oblivious to or not deeply affected by the world around them. This perception of children can colour the work that governments and policymaking bodies do on behalf of children and families.

The demographics of countries are changing, yet race and ethnicity remain important social determinants of health for many children. Aboriginal, Torres Strait Islander, Māori and Pasifika children are disproportionately represented in impoverished communities and schools. This demonstrates one way in which a child's chances for thriving depend not only on child, family and community characteristics, but also on the region in which the child lives because of variations in access to health and social services available. Policy choices and investments can have a significant impact on child health (Annie E. Casey Foundation 2014, 2017).

Considering the broader context of where children and families live, work and play is complex when we care for children and families who are considered refugees or immigrants. For these children and families, we must consider not only where they are within the country and in our particular sight for care, but also where they have been and where they have left. Nearly half of the world's displaced people are children (Murray 2015), amounting to over 20 million children. Within this group are both children and families who have fled their home countries and those who are internally displaced within their home country. Nonetheless, these children and their families often experience mental and physical trauma; they may have experienced danger and violence in both staying in their homes and fleeing. For children and families who journey to a new destination, there are dangers along the journey.

Religion/Spiritual Identity

Religion and spirituality are important aspects in the lives of individuals, families and communities. Spirituality and religion are significant principles around which families organise their responses to illness experiences and life transitions. Indeed, nearly 80% of people report that religion is fairly important to them. The terms, however, are often conflated. Religion and spirituality, although frequently grouped together, denote different entities. Religion is a specific set of beliefs enacted through a practice (religiosity) (Taylor et al 2015). Spirituality is described as a unique awareness, belief, practice and experience starting in childhood and is rooted over time. Religion and spirituality are important avenues through which children participate in meaning-making around important life events, such as illness in themselves or loved ones (Lima et al 2013), and are shaped by the developmental stage of the child (Taylor et al 2015). Further, spiritual assessment is necessary to provide family-centred care that is aligned with spiritual and religious needs. Finally, many regulatory bodies that guide practice call for assessment of and intervention for spiritual concerns, including the International Council of Nurses.

When individuals become parents, they may connect to their religion as a guide in raising their children, to enhance their wellbeing and to provide a moral and social context for their childrearing (Fig 2.3). Although parents may employ an approach to parenting that is informed by their religion and spirituality, how this is enacted or operationalised varies dramatically because of variability in beliefs about parenting goals and roles, the parent–child relationship and child discipline (Holden & Williamson 2014).

Additionally, parents' spirituality, religious practices and beliefs are a guiding force on their children. Thus, considering the 'family-based spirituality care', comprehensive, collaborative, spiritual care is important in addressing the spiritual needs of children who are ill and acknowledges the interrelated relationships of child, parent and family spirituality (Box 2.5). In the context of paediatric illness, this is also important as children and families are often isolated from their faith communities and experience crises for which they have no prior experience to draw on or that cause existential questioning and meaning-seeking. Children and families receiving a new or life-threatening diagnosis often experience fear and anxiety and may benefit from healthcare providers helping them connect to those spiritual and religious practices that are important to them. For example, nurses can help families find a suitable place to pray and asking families which of their healthcare practices may be most helpful in addressing their spiritual needs.

Children who experience major life transitions, such as being diagnosed with a life-threatening illness or the death of a loved one, often experience spirituality as a source of hope and comfort that promotes their resilience and helps them discern the meaning of the life transition for them. Yet there is a paucity of research on children's spiritual development in a contemporary context (Taylor et al 2015). Children, adolescents and young adults have unique spiritual needs related to their developmental stage. Providing space in the physical environment for children to participate in their spirituality in ways that bring them comfort and provide for meaning-making opportunities is essential as it can provide a glimpse into their spiritual distress and sources of hope. For example, the provider can elicit an adolescent's narrative of his or her illness situation or life event and invite parents

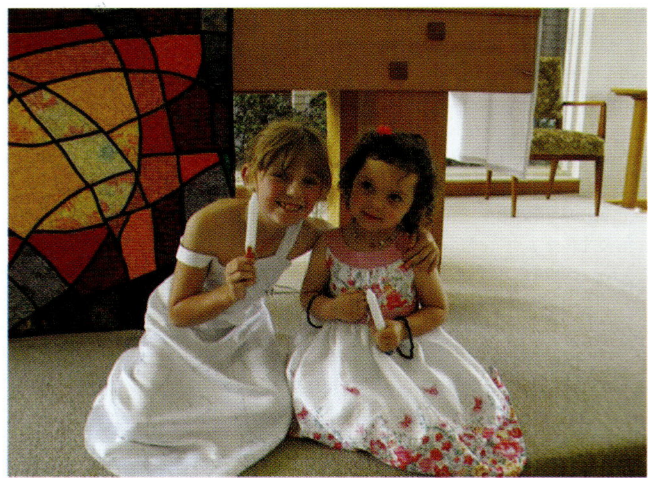

Fig 2.3 Many families have special religious ceremonies.

BOX 2.5 Guidelines for Integrating Spiritual Care into Paediatric Nursing Practice

- Respect the child's and family's religious beliefs and practices.
- Consider the child's development when talking about spiritual concerns.
- Contact the institution's chaplaincy department for patients and families who have symptoms of spiritual distress or ask for specific religious rituals.
- Become knowledgeable about the religious worldviews of cultural groups found in the patients you care for.
- Encourage visitation with family members, members of the patient's spiritual community and spiritual leaders.
- Allow children and families to teach you about the specifics of their religious beliefs.
- Develop awareness of your own spiritual perspective.
- Listen for understanding rather than agreement or disagreement.

Source: Data from Brooks, B. (2004). Spirituality. In N. Kline (Ed.) *Essentials of pediatric oncology nursing: A core curriculum* (2nd ed.). Glenview, IL: Association of Pediatric Oncology Nurses; Barnes, L. L., Plotnikoff, G. A., Fox, K., et al. (2000). Spirituality, religion, and pediatrics: Intersecting worlds of healing. Pediatrics, 106(4 suppl), 899–908.

or caregivers to listen and share their reaction to promote family connection and communication.

Religion can affect children across multiple domains, including physical health, healthy behaviours, mental and emotional health, participation in risky behaviours or demonstrating externalising problems, and academic/cognitive functioning.

Regarding physical health, religion has demonstrated mixed effects, with positive effects resulting from the emphasis on healthy behaviours and respect for others. Conversely, deleterious effects may be associated with some religions that are more authoritarian and prohibit healthcare interventions, such as cases of religiously motivated declining of treatment, when a child suffers injury or dies because parents did not seek treatment for a particular ailment or when immunisations or screenings are declined. Additionally, adolescents who identified as highly religious were less likely to use contraception at sexual debut, despite being older than non-religious adolescents, putting them at risk for unplanned pregnancy or sexually transmitted infections. Considering mental and emotional health, connection to religion or spirituality has been associated with less adolescent depression, anxiety and suicidality, as well as lower rates of criminal or delinquent behaviour. However, religion or spirituality can contribute to psychological distress if youth are subjected to negative relationships or experiences that are imbued with a requirement to adhere to strict rules and criticism. Thus, the social context in which the religion is practised may be more important than the religion itself (Holden & Williamson 2014). Parents weave religion and spirituality into their family life generally because it was an important part of their lives and because they believe it will promote their child's wellbeing. Religion and spirituality can help parents cope with the demands of parenting and help parents find meaning in the role.

However, conflicts can arise between religion and healthcare, and parental religious objections have been a major focus of literature on family spirituality versus other forms of engagement. Although parents' refusal of medical care for their children falls under the scope of parental authority, the child's best interest is priority. Failure to provide essential healthcare is increasingly viewed as a form of neglect. Religions and spiritual traditions vary in the depth and nature of treatment they refuse, from refusal of all treatment to refusal of select interventions or therapeutics, such as blood products. These arguments and considerations become murky when the conditions are not life-threatening or when the proposed treatment has significant adverse effects, or the efficacy is limited. Negative psychological effects must also be considered (AIHW 2020).

REFERENCES

Ahrons, C. R. (2007). Family ties after divorce: Long-term implications for children. Family Process, 46(1), 53–65.

Annie E. Casey Foundation. (2014). African American, American Indian and Latino Children have the most barriers. Retrieved from http://www.aecf.org/blog/african-american-american-indian-and-latino-children-have-the-most-barriers.

Annie E. Casey Foundation. (2017). 2017 kids count data book: State profiles of child well-being. Retrieved from http://www.aecf.org/resources/2017-kids-count-data-book/.

Australian Institute of Health and Welfare (AIHW). 2020. Australia's children. 3 April. AIHW, Canberra. https://www.aihw.gov.au/reports/children-youth/australias-children/contents/health/health-australias-children

Baumrind, D. (1971). Harmonious parents and their preschool children. Developmental Psychology, 41, 92–102.

Baumrind, D. (1996). The discipline controversy revisited. Family Relations, 45, 405–414.

Bomar, P. J. (2004). Promoting health in families (3rd ed.). Philadelphia: Saunders.

Bronfenbrenner, U. (1979). The ecology of human development: Experiments by nature and design. Cambridge, MA: Harvard University Press.

Bronfenbrenner, U. (2005). Making human beings human: Bioecological perspectives on human development. Thousand Oaks, CA: Sage Publications.

Center on the Developing Child at Harvard University. (2016). Building core capabilities for life: The science behind the skills adults need to succeed in parenting and in the workplace. http://www.developingchild.harvard.edu.

Centers for Disease Control and Prevention (CDC). (2009). School connectedness: Strategies for increasing protective factors among youth. Atlanta, GA: US Department of Health and Human Services.

Chavez, V. (2012). Cultural humility: People, principles and practices - Part 1 of 4 (documentary film). Retrieved from https://www.youtube.com/watch?v=_Mbu8bvKb_U

Duvall, E. R. (1977). Family development (5th ed.). Philadelphia: Lippincott.

Fierman, A. H., Beck, A. F., Chung, E. K., et al. (2016). Redesigning healthcare practices to address childhood poverty. Academic Pediatrics, 16, S136–S146.

Goldenberg, I., Goldenberg, H. (2012). Family therapy: An overview (8th ed.). Pacific Grove, CA: Brooks-Cole Cengage Learning.

Holden, G. W., Williamson, P. A. (2014). Religion and child well-being. In B.-A. Asher, F. Casas, I. Frones, et al. (Eds.), Handbook of child well-being. Dordrecht: Springer.

Kaakinen, J. R., Coehlo, D. P. (2015). Family health care nursing (5th ed.). Philadelphia: Davis.

Kazak, A. E. (2001). Comprehensive care for children with cancer and their families: A social ecological framework guiding research, practice, and policy. Children's Services: Social Policy, Research, and Practice, 4(4), 217–233.

Kazak, A. E., Rourke, M. T., Navasaria, N. (2010). Families and other systems in pediatric psychology. In M. C. Roberts & R. G. Steele (Eds.), Handbook of pediatric psychology. Guilford Press.

Lima, N. N., do Nascimento, V. B., de Carvalho, S. M., et al. (2013). Spirituality in childhood cancer care. Neuropsychiatric Disease and Treatment, 9, 1539–1544.

McCubbin, M. A., McCubbin, H. I. (1994). Families coping with illness: The resiliency model of family stress, adjustment, and adaptation. In C. B. Danielson, B. H. Bissell, & P. Winstead-Fry (Eds.), Families, health, and illness. St Louis, MO: Mosby.

Murray, J. S. (2015). Displaced and forgotten child refugees: A humanitarian crisis. Journal for Specialists in Pediatric Nursing, 21, 29–36.
Nursing Council of New Zealand (2011). Guidelines for Cultural Safety, the Treaty of Waitangi and Māori Health in Nursing Education and Practice. Nursing Council of New Zealand, Wellington.
Papero, D. V. (1990). Bowen family systems theory. Boston, MA: Pearson.
Power, N., Franck, L. (2008). Parent participation in the care of hospitalized children: A systematic review. Journal of Advanced Nursing, 62(6), 622–641.
Reid Chassiakos, Y. L., Radesky, J., Christakis, D., et al. (2016). Children and adolescents and digital media. Pediatrics, 138(5), e20162593.
Scott, J., & Marshall, G. (2009). Ethnicity, Oxford Dictionary of Sociology. Oxford: Oxford University Press.
Strasburger, V., Jordan, A., & Donnerstein, E. (2012). Children, adolescents, and the media: Health effects. Pediatric Clinics of North America, 59, 533–587.
Taylor, E. J., Petersen, C., Oyedele, O., et al. (2015). Spiritualty and spiritual care of adolescents and young adults with cancer. Seminars in Oncology Nursing, 31(3), 227–241.
Williams, D. R. (2012). Miles to go before we sleep: Racial inequities in health. Journal of Health and Social Behavior, 53, 279–296.

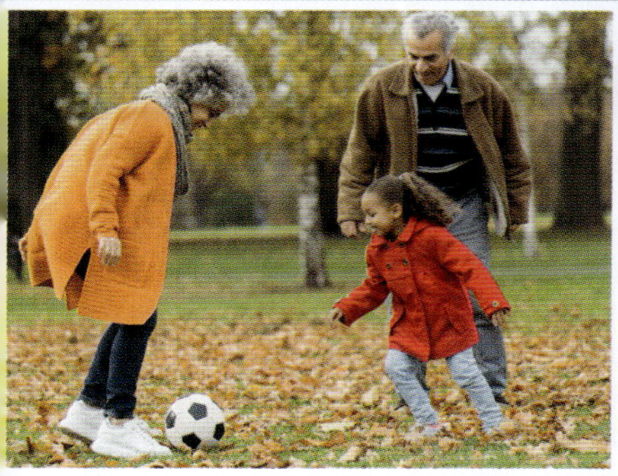

3

Hereditary Influences on Health Promotion of the Child and Family

Lisa Speedie

LEARNING OBJECTIVES

- Ensure genetic assessments and education are family centred
- Be able to discuss expected outcomes and make sure they meet the family and child's needs
- Achieve effectiveness of care by ensuring nursing care plans are discussed and family centred

GENETIC/GENOMIC NURSING COMPETENCIES

Nurses and midwives are increasingly faced with incorporating genetic and genomic information into their practice. To assist with providing information to both professionals and the public, the Genetics Society of AustralAsia was formed to provide up-to-date research in this area (https://genetics.org.au/). Genetics and genomics are strong forces influencing the role of nurses in patient care. This chapter provides foundational information to help nurses begin using genetics and genomics information and technology when caring for children and families. (See Box 3.1 for definitions of relevant terms.)

Genetics and Genomics

A human genome consists of 22 nuclear autosome chromosomes and a sex chromosome (either an X or a Y), as well as a single circular molecule of DNA within the mitochondria. Every cell in the human body, except the egg or the sperm, contains a maternally inherited and a paternally inherited copy of the genome in its nucleus, as well as the maternally inherited mitochondrial DNA. The ovum contains a single nuclear genome (22 autosomes and the X chromosome), as well as the circular DNA strand within the mitochondria. The sperm head contains a single nuclear genome (22 autosomes and either the X or the Y chromosome) but does not contain mitochondria. **Genes** are segments of DNA that code for structural or functional proteins. Areas of

BOX 3.1 Key Genetic Terms

AFP—Abbreviation of alpha-fetoprotein, a protein produced by the developing fetus. Alterations in AFP can be used as a marker suggestive of neural tube defect (increased AFP) and Down syndrome (decreased AFP).

Allele—One version of a gene at a given location (locus) along a chromosome. The most common version of a gene in a population is called the **wild-type allele**.

Amniocentesis—Prenatal diagnostic procedure that consists of transabdominally withdrawing a small sample of amniotic fluid for genetic analysis of embryonic cells. Biochemical analysis and chromosome studies can be performed in such cells. This procedure is usually performed between 14 and 20 weeks' gestation.

Aneuploidy—An abnormal chromosome pattern in which the total number of chromosomes is not a multiple of the haploid number ($n = 23$) (e.g. persons with 45 or 47 chromosomes, as in Turner or Down syndrome, respectively). Such monosomies and trisomies are examples of aneuploidy.

Association—Non-random cluster of malformations, the cause of which varies from person to person (e.g. VATERL).

Autosomes—The 22 pairs of chromosomes in somatic cells that do not greatly influence sex determination at conception. This does not include the sex chromosomes, X and Y.

Carrier—A clinically normal (asymptomatic) person who possesses a genetic alteration, in the form of either a gene or a chromosome change. A carrier has the potential of transmitting that abnormality to an offspring who will then express the abnormal phenotype. Examples of carrier states include a sickle cell disease carrier ('trait') and a balanced carrier of a chromosome translocation.

Centromere—Chromosomal region that separates the chromosome arms and unites the chromatids. Centromeres attach to spindle fibres during cell division, ensuring through disjunction an equal distribution of chromosomes or chromatids.

Chromosome—Filament-like nuclear structure that consists of chromatin, stores genetic information as base sequences in DNA and has a constant number for each species. Chromosomes are found in pairs in somatic cells (homologous chromosomes) and in single copies in germ cells. One member of a homologous pair is of paternal origin, the other of maternal origin. Homologous chromosomes have identical number and arrangement of genes.

Chromosome aberrations—Genetic disorders that result from variation in number or structure of chromosomes.

Chromosomes, acrocentric—Chromosomes in which the centromere is distally placed. Human chromosomes in groups D and G are acrocentric.

Chromosomes, metacentric—Chromosomes in which the centromere is located approximately in the midpoint of the chromosome, resulting in arms of approximately equal length. Human chromosomes A(1), A(3) and E(16) are metacentric.

Chromosomes, submetacentric—Chromosomes in which the centromere is located closer to one telomere than to the other. Human B group chromosomes are submetacentric.

Continued

BOX 3.1 Key Genetic Terms–cont'd

Concordant—A condition in which two individuals have the same genetic trait; usually applied to monozygotic twin concordance studies.

Congenital—Present at birth. A congenital disease may or may not be genetic. Likewise, a genetic disease may or may not be congenital, although the causative genes are present at birth.

Crossing-over—The genetic event that results in exchange of genetic material between homologous chromosomes during prophase I of meiosis.

CVS—Abbreviation of chorionic villi sampling, a prenatal diagnostic procedure in which a small amount of chorionic villi material (embryonic tissue) is aspirated for genetic analysis of the developing embryo. This procedure is usually performed during the first trimester of pregnancy.

Cytogenetics—Study of chromosomes, with special focus on chromosome abnormalities.

Deformation—Fetal abnormality caused by extrinsic factors (e.g. uterine position).

Diploid—A cell that contains two copies of each chromosome. The term is often extended to include an individual carrying such cells. The diploid number ($2n$) in humans is 46.

Deletion—The loss of chromosomal material. An example of a terminal deletion is found in cri-du-chat (cat's cry) syndrome, in which there is loss of a portion of the short arm of chromosome B(5). Deleted fragments may attach to another chromosome (see Translocation).

DNA—Abbreviation of deoxyribonucleic acid, a double-helix molecule consisting of an assembly of nucleotides (phosphate–sugar [deoxyribose]–nitrogenous base). DNA bases (cytosine, guanine, thymine, adenine) encode genetic information, which is *transcribed* into messenger RNA and further *translated* into proteins.

DNA, mitochondrial (mtDNA)—DNA located in the mitochondria of cells. Inheritance of mtDNA is independent of paternal genetics.

DNA, nuclear (nDNA)—DNA located in the nucleus of cells.

Dominant—An allele that is phenotypically expressed in single copy (heterozygote) and in double copy (homozygote). Example: polydactyly.

FISH analysis—Fluorescent in situ hybridisation, a process by which chromosomes or portions of chromosomes are 'painted' with fluorescent molecules. This technique is useful for identifying chromosomal microdeletions.

Gamete (germ cell)—A mature reproductive cell containing the haploid number of chromosomes ($n = 23$); in males, the spermatozoon; in females, the ovum. The union of gametes in sexual reproduction initiates the development of a new individual.

Gametogenesis—A series of mitotic and meiotic cell divisions occurring in the gonads that lead to the production of gametes; in males, spermatogenesis; in females, oogenesis. Reduction in the number of chromosomes ($2n \rightarrow n$) during gametogenesis occurs in the first meiotic division (meiosis I).

Gene—A segment of nucleic acid that contains genetic information necessary to control a certain function, such as the synthesis of a polypeptide (structural gene). This segment is often referred to as a site, or locus, on a chromosome.

Genetic counselling—The process by which genetic information is given to patients and their families. Information about a genetic disease may include its natural history, recurrence risk and management.

Genetics—Study of individual genes and their impact on relatively rare single-gene disorders.

Genome—Complete genetic information of an organism, usually described as total number of base pairs. The human genome contains approximately 3 billion base pairs.

Genomics—Study of all the genes in the human genome together, including their interactions with each other and the environment, and the influence of other psychosocial and cultural factors.

Genotype—Genetic constitution that determines the physical and chemical characteristics of an individual.

Haploid—The number of chromosomes present in a gamete. Also, a cell that contains one copy of each chromosome. The haploid number (n) in humans is 23. The diploid number of chromosomes (46) is reconstituted in the zygote on fertilisation of two haploid gametes.

Hemizygote—A condition in which an allele is present in a single copy. Males are hemizygous for all markers (genes) located on the X chromosome.

Heterozygote—An individual who has two different alleles at a given locus on a pair of homologous chromosomes; for example, in the case of the *HexA* gene, Hh (or +/−).

Homologous—Referring to chromosomes with matching genes, or to those genes individually.

Homozygote—An individual possessing a pair of identical alleles at a given locus; for example, in the case of the *HexA* gene, above, HH (or +/+) and hh (or −/−).

Human Genome Project—International research project to map each human gene and sequence the human genome.

Imprinting—Phenomenon in which an allele at a given locus is altered or inactivated, depending on whether it is inherited from the mother or father; implies a functional difference in genes inherited from the two parents and explains some variation in expression.

Karyotype—The chromosome constitution of an individual represented by a laboratory-made display in which chromosomes are arranged by size and centromere position.

Locus—The chromosome location of a specific gene (or site). Plural: loci.

Malformation—A primary morphological defect occurring as a result of abnormal morphogenesis.

Malformation, major—Structural abnormality with serious medical, surgical or cosmetic consequences.

Malformation, minor—Structural abnormality that has no serious consequences or is a normal variation (e.g. extra nipple or umbilical hernia).

Meiosis—A reductional type of cell division, in which the chromosome number is halved. In humans, meiosis is one of the processes that lead to the formation of haploid gametes ($n = 23$).

Mendelian inheritance—The mode of inheritance of single-gene traits. The term is derived from Gregor Mendel, the pioneer of genetics.

Microdeletion—Chromosome deletion too small to be detected by standard cytogenetic techniques; can be detected by FISH analysis, which is a molecular cytogenetic technique.

Mitochondrion—Cellular organelle responsible for converting nutrients into energy and for many other specialised tasks. Mitochondria are the only part of the body known to have their own separate and unique DNA; mitochondrial DNA (mtDNA) is inherited exclusively from the mother. Plural: mitochondria.

Mitosis—Type of equational cell division in which the resulting daughter cells have the same number of chromosomes as each other and the mother cell.

Monosomy—The aneuploid condition of having a chromosome represented by a single copy in a somatic cell, that is, the absence of a chromosome from a given pair. Generally, monosomies are not compatible with life, except in the case of a missing X chromosome in Turner syndrome (45,XO).

Mosaicism—Condition in which an individual harbours two or more genetically distinct cell lines. Generally, one cell line is normal and one is abnormal; it results from mitotic non-disjunction, a postzygotic event.

Multifactorial—Complex interaction of both genetic and environmental factors that produces an effect on an individual. Disease processes resulting from multifactorial inheritance are referred to as *complex diseases.*

Mutation—Structural or chemical alteration in genetic material that persists and is transmitted to future generations. Mutations can occur naturally (spontaneous) or can be induced by a variety of physical (temperature, radiation), chemical (various substances such as nitrogen mustard) or biological (certain viruses) mutagens.

BOX 3.1 Key Genetic Terms–cont'd

Non-disjunction—Failure of homologous chromosomes or chromatids to separate properly during anaphase meiosis I and II, or mitosis, resulting in daughter cells with unequal chromosome numbers. Meiotic non-disjunction may result in gametes with an abnormal chromosome number, which on fertilisation may produce aneuploidy. Mitotic non-disjunction in a developing embryo may result in mosaicism.

Oncogene—A gene or group of genes, usually involved in cell division, whose malfunction (e.g. a mutation) will result in malignant transformation.

Pedigree chart (family tree, genogram)—A diagram that describes family relationships, gender, disease status or other relevant information about a family, illustrating the genetic variation within a family.

Penetrance—Frequency with which a heritable trait is manifested in individuals possessing the gene.

Phenotype—Any observable or measurable expression of gene function in an individual. For instance, eye colour and haemoglobin type are phenotypical expressions of specific genes. Phenotypes may result from interaction of genotype and environment.

Polygenic—Inheritance involving many genes at separate loci whose combined additive effects produce a given phenotype.

Polyploidy—Chromosome condition in which the diploid chromosome number of a cell varies by increments of 23. For example, a triploid cell or individual would have 69 chromosomes (46 + 23); a tetraploid, 92 (46 + 23 + 23).

Proband (index case)—The clinically identified person who displays the characteristics of features of the disease in question; also referred to as propositus (feminine: proposita).

Recessive—Refers to an allele whose phenotypical expression occurs in homozygous or hemizygous conditions. In heterozygosity, a recessive allele is masked by its dominant homologous counterpart. Example: cystic fibrosis.

Recombination—The occurrence among the offspring of new combinations of alleles as a result of genetic material exchange following crossovers during parental gametogenesis.

RNA—Abbreviation of ribonucleic acid, a single-stranded molecule consisting of an assembly of nucleotides (phosphate–sugar [ribose]–nitrogenous base). RNA bases (cytosine, guanine, uracil, adenine) encode genetic information, which is *translated* into proteins.

Sex-linked—The transmission of a trait whose causative gene is located on a sex chromosome (X or Y). Most sex-linked genes in humans are located on the X chromosome (X-linked).

Somatic cell—Body tissue cells with diploid complement of 46 chromosomes.

Sporadic—A descriptor for birth defects or disorders occurring as a new case in a family and not inherited.

Syndrome—A collection of multiple primary malformations or defects all due to a single underlying cause. Examples: Down syndrome (chromosome abnormality), Marfan syndrome (single-gene disorder).

Telomere—The distal portion of a chromosome.

Teratogen—An environmental agent capable of producing a congenital anomaly.

Transcription—The process by which genetic information is copied from DNA to RNA.

Translation—The step in protein synthesis during which an amino acid sequence is assembled according to the genetic information contained in messenger RNA (mRNA).

Translocation—Transfer of all or part of a chromosome to a different chromosome after chromosome breakage; can be balanced, producing no phenotypical effects, or unbalanced, producing severe or lethal effects.

Trisomy—An aneuploid condition caused by the presence of an extra chromosome, which is added to a given chromosome pair and results in a total number of 47 chromosomes per cell. Down syndrome is the most common human autosomal trisomy.

X inactivation (lyonisation)—The process by which, in a normal female, most of the genes on one of the X chromosomes are inactivated during early embryonic development, so that alleles on active chromosomes are allowed full expression.

X-linked inheritance—Transmission of a trait whose causative gene is located on the X chromosome.

Zygote—Cell resulting from the fusion of male and female gametes.

DNA that do not code for proteins still have essential regulatory functions that are beginning to be better understood. The locations of genes or non-coding regulatory elements are often referred to as *sites*, or *loci*, indicating a physical or 'geographic' location on a chromosome. Each gene is made up of exons and introns. Exons are the portions of a gene that contain the code for a specific protein. Introns may have important regulatory elements or function as spacers between exons to improve the efficiency of the cellular molecules that transcribe the gene (make a copy in the form of messenger RNA [mRNA]). Although the entire gene is transcribed, the intron portions of the mRNA are removed so that only the exonic codes remain in the mature mRNA that leaves the nucleus and enters the cytoplasm where it is translated into an eventual protein. Mutations in genes may have significant qualitative and quantitative effects on the synthesis of the corresponding protein, with potential clinical consequences. Proteins can be classified as structural (or constitutive) proteins, and functional, those that affect the metabolism of other molecules or substrates (enzymes). Table 3.1 summarises the effects of protein disorders on selected genetic diseases. Such alterations in an individual genome may have been inherited from a parent or may represent an event that is new to that person and may be the first case in that family (**new mutation**). It is therefore erroneous to consider all genetic disorders as having a positive family history.

Evidence is growing that genes play an important role in human susceptibility and resistance to infection even in cases with a clear environmental cause of the infectious disease. Evidence for this genetic element in resistance gained heightened recognition during the first decade of the acquired immunodeficiency syndrome (AIDS) epidemic.

Variations in the genes predispose a person to experiencing unintended effects from normal doses of certain medications. Unintended effects include absent or reduced therapeutic effect resulting from subtherapeutic levels of the active drug or adverse drug reactions caused by toxicity from abnormally high levels of the active drug after being given a normal dose. In this way, pharmacogenomics is another example of the interplay of genes and environmental factors.

Congenital Anomalies

Embryogenesis and fetal development are an intricate and precisely timed series of events in which all parts must be properly integrated to ensure a coordinated whole. Insults during development or abnormalities in differentiation or in the proper timing of organogenesis may result in a variety of congenital anomalies. **Congenital anomalies**, or birth defects, occur in 2% to 4% of all live-born children and are often classified as deformations, disruptions, dysplasias or malformations.

TABLE 3.1 **Selected Proteins Involved in Genetic Disease**

Protein Involved	Altered Mechanism of Action Due to Mutations	Resulting Disorder
	CONSTITUTIVE PROTEINS	
Globins	Altered oxygen transport	Haemoglobinopathies: • Sickle cell disease • thalassaemias
Dystrophin	Muscle cell defect	Muscular dystrophies
Coagulation factors VIII and IX	Abnormal clotting activity	Haemophilia A and B
	ENZYMES	
Phenylalanine hydroxylase	Interrupted metabolism of phenylalanine and accumulation of toxic precursors (phenylalanine and phenylketones)	Phenylketonuria
Hexosaminidase A (*HexA*)	Interrupted metabolism and accumulation of precursors (GM_2 ganglioside)	Tay-Sachs disease
Hypoxanthine-guanine phosphoribosyltransferase (HGPRT)	Disruption of metabolic feedback mechanism and accumulation of end product (uric acid)	Lesch-Nyhan syndrome
3-Hydroxy-3-methylglutaryl coenzyme A (HMG-CoA) reductase	Disruption of metabolic feedback mechanism and accumulation of end product (cholesterol)	Familial hypercholesterolaemia

Deformations are often caused by extrinsic mechanical forces on normally developing tissue. Club foot is an example of a deformation often caused by uterine constraint. **Disruptions** result from the breakdown of previously normal tissue. Congenital amputations caused by amniotic bands (fibrous strands of amnion that wrap around different body parts during development) are examples of disruption anomalies (Passias et al 2019).

Dysplasias result from abnormal organisation of cells into a particular tissue type. Congenital abnormalities of the teeth, hair, nails or sweat glands may be manifestations of one of the more than 100 different ectodermal dysplasia syndromes. **Malformations** are abnormal formations of organs or body parts resulting from an abnormal developmental process. Most malformations occur before 12 weeks' gestation. Cleft lip, an example of a malformation, occurs at approximately 5 weeks' gestation when the developing embryo naturally has two clefts in the area. Normally between 5 and 7 weeks, cells rapidly divide and migrate to fill in those clefts. If there is an abnormality in this developmental process, the embryo is left with either a unilateral or bilateral cleft lip that may also involve the palate.

The types of anomalies that can result from genetic or prenatal environmental agents can be major structural abnormalities with serious medical, surgical or quality-of-life consequences, or they can be minor anomalies or normal variants with no serious consequences, such as a sacral dimple, an extra nipple or a café-au-lait spot. Congenital anomalies can occur in isolation, such as congenital heart defect, or multiple anomalies may be present. A recognised pattern of anomalies resulting from a single specific cause is called a **syndrome** (e.g. Down syndrome or fetal alcohol syndrome). A non-random pattern of malformations for which a cause has not been determined is called an **association** (e.g. VACTERL [vertebral defects, anal atresia, cardiac defect, tracheo-oesophageal fistula, and renal and limb defects] association). When a single anomaly leads to a cascade of additional anomalies, the pattern of defects is referred to as a **sequence**. Pierre Robin sequence begins with the abnormal development of the mandible, resulting in abnormal placement of the tongue during development. The normal developmental process for the palate is prevented because the tongue obstructs the migration of the palatal shelves towards the midline, and a cleft palate remains. Consequently, infants born with Pierre Robin sequence have a recessed mandible and an abnormally placed tongue and are at risk for obstructive apnoea. NTDs, cleft lip and palate, deafness, congenital heart defects and cognitive impairment are examples of congenital malformations that can occur in isolation or as part of a syndrome, association or sequence and can have different causes, such as single-gene or chromosome abnormalities, prenatal exposures or multifactorial causes.

Genetic Disorders

Genetic disorders can be caused by: chromosome abnormalities as seen in Turner's syndrome, Down syndrome or velocardiofacial syndrome (VCFS); single-gene mutations as seen in sickle cell anaemia, neurofibromatosis or Duchenne's muscular dystrophy; a combination of genetic and environmental factors as seen in NTDs or maturity-onset diabetes in the young; and mitochondrial DNA (mtDNA) mutations as seen in non-syndromic deafness susceptibility due to aminoglycoside sensitivity. Whereas numerical or structural chromosome aberrations automatically involve large groups of genes, a small gene mutation does not alter chromosome structure and number. Alterations in single genes (**single-gene disorders**) or in many genes (**polygenic disorders**) may represent a lesion too small to cause an identifiable alteration in chromosomal structure. Human nucleated somatic cells contain approximately 25,000 genes distributed across 46 chromosomes. Because human chromosomes vary in size, the larger the chromosome, the greater the number of genes carried.

Both numerical and structural abnormalities of **autosomes** (all chromosomes except the X and Y chromosomes) account for a variety of syndromes usually characterised by cognitive deficiencies. A few are associated with a group of characteristics that clearly indicate the precise chromosome anomaly. Nurses often note dysmorphic facial features, behavioural characteristics such as an unusual cry and poor feeding behaviour, and other neurological manifestations such as hypotonia or abnormal reflex responses, which may alert them to these and other chromosome abnormalities.

Numerical Chromosome Abnormalities

With the exception of brief periods of gametogenesis, human beings are diploid individuals, and human somatic cells are **diploid** (a cell that contains two copies of each chromosome). A diploid chromosome number in humans is represented by the notation $2n = 46$. A **haploid** chromosome constitution ($n = 23$) is found in **germ cells**, the male and female **gametes** (sperm and ova). Somatic cells contain 44 autosomes (the 22 pairs of chromosomes that do not greatly influence sex determination at conception) and 2 sex chromosomes: XX in females and XY in males. For the purpose of cytogenetic studies, chromosomes are usually displayed in a **karyotype**, the laboratory-made arrangement of specially prepared chromosomes according to their size, banding patterns and centromere position. The location of the centromere allows the classification of human chromosomes as **acrocentric**, **submetacentric** and **metacentric** chromosomes.

Numerical chromosome abnormalities occur whenever entire chromosomes are added or deleted. The addition of one or more chromosomes to each pair (increments of the haploid number, 23) will result in triploid cells with 69 chromosomes (46 + 23), or tetraploid cells with 92 chromosomes (46 + 23 + 23), and so on. The product of this uniform addition of chromosomes to all the original pairs is termed ***euploidy***, a euploid cell being one whose chromosome number is a multiple of 23.

Individuals who are triploid ($3n = 69$) have a genetic imbalance of such magnitude that the few who are carried to term have severe multiple abnormalities that limit their life span to a few hours or days. On the other hand, one chromosome may be added to or lost from one of the pairs, creating a condition of **aneuploidy**. When one chromosome is added to a pair, the embryo, fetus or child is described as having a **trisomy**, and the total chromosome number is 47. Most fetuses that have an autosomal trisomy are not live-born. Fetuses with trisomy 21, trisomy 18 and trisomy 13 may be live-born. When one chromosome is lost from the pair, the fetus is described as having a **monosomy**, and the total chromosome number in somatic cells is 45. The loss of a chromosome and its related complement of genes is overall more detrimental than the addition of a chromosome. The only monosomy compatible with life is monosomy X (Turner's syndrome), yet most 45,X pregnancies spontaneously miscarry (The Royal Children's Hospital [RCH] 2020, Scherdel et al 2018).

The most common cause of alteration in the number of chromosomes is a misdistribution of chromosomes during mitosis or meiosis. As somatic cells multiply by mitosis, each daughter cell receives the same chromosome number as the mother cell. This equitable chromosome sharing in anaphase is due to a phenomenon termed ***disjunction***, by which chromatids of each chromosome separate and migrate to opposite poles of the cell. Disruption of this orderly chromosome distribution occurs in ***non-disjunction***, which can occur during both mitosis and meiosis. In mitosis, failure of chromatids to separate properly during anaphase will result in daughter cells with different chromosome numbers (e.g. 45 and 47, instead of 46 and 46). Of those, the 45-chromosome monosomic cells will tend to degenerate and die, but those with the extra chromosome (trisomic) may continue to divide and generate a complete line of trisomic cells.

When **mitotic non-disjunction** occurs during embryonic development (Fig 3.1), the trisomic cell line proliferates concomitantly with the normal cell line and results in an individual with **mosaicism** for that particular chromosome. Mosaicism therefore results in an individual (mosaic) with two or more genetically different cell populations. The chromosomal notation for a male with mosaic type of Down syndrome, for example, is 46,XY/47,XY,+21. The slash (/) indicates a dual cell population in which one has the normal chromosomal constitution (46,XY), whereas the other carries an extra chromosome 21 and has a total chromosome number of 47 (RCH n.d., Peng et al 2019). The percentage, or level, of mosaicism depends on the stage of embryonic development in which the cell division error occurs. If it occurs at the first cell division after fertilisation, the level of mosaicism may be as high as 50%. If the cell division error occurs in later development, the abnormal cells may be localised to one cell type, such as the brain tissue or germ cell line (ovaries or testes). The extent of clinical manifestations

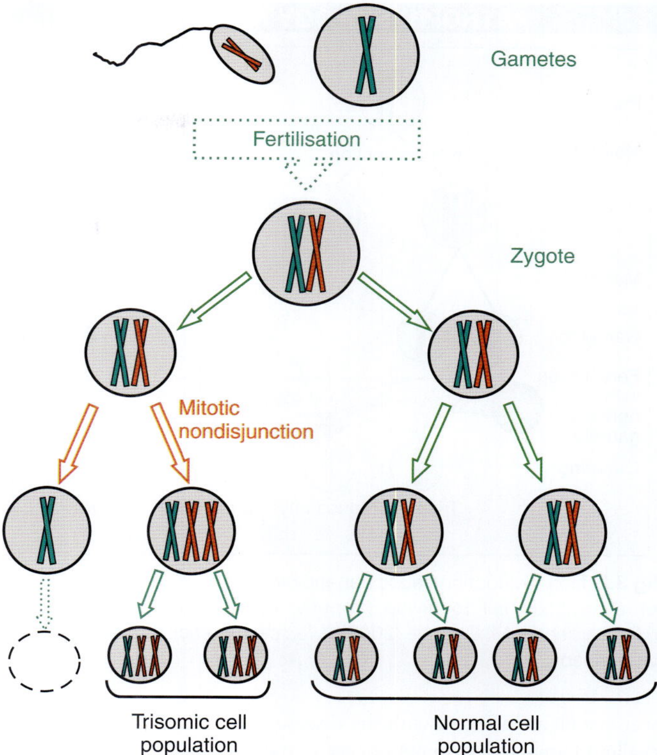

Fig 3.1 Mitotic non-disjunction resulting in an individual with different cell populations (mosaicism). This event occurs during embryonic development, after the normal zygote was formed by fertilisation of two normal gametes. Only one chromosome pair is represented. As represented here, mitotic non-disjunction and uneven chromosome distribution result in some cell populations with the extra chromosome, whereas other cell lines have the normal chromosome complement.

is determined by the type of tissues that contain cells with abnormal chromosome numbers and the percentage of affected cells, and may vary from near normal to a fully manifested syndrome.

Meiotic non-disjunction (Fig 3.2) is a major cause of aneuploidy, an abnormal chromosome pattern in which the total number of chromosomes is not a multiple of the haploid number, 23. Non-disjunction can occur during meiosis I and II, during both oogenesis and spermatogenesis, resulting in gametes with an aneuploid chromosome number (e.g. 22 or 24, instead of 23). As in the case of somatic cells, gametes lacking a chromosome are not likely to survive, but gametes with an extra chromosome are more often viable. Fertilisation of an aneuploid gamete with a normal gamete will produce an aneuploid zygote. The most common aneuploidies in humans are trisomies.

Autosome Aneuploidies

Examples of numerical alterations affecting the autosomes include some of the most common trisomies found in humans: trisomy 21 (Down syndrome), trisomy 18 (Edwards' syndrome) and trisomy 13 (Patau's syndrome) (Table 3.2).

Trisomy 21. Down syndrome affects 1 in 800 to 1 in 1000 live births and is the most common aneuploidy compatible with life expectancy into adulthood. Physical and cognitive abnormalities vary (Down Syndrome Australia 2020). Intelligence quotient (IQ) range is typically mild to moderate impairment. In spite of modern medical developments, life expectancy is still shortened, with 20% dying in the first decade and 50% by age 60 years. Adults with Down syndrome are also more likely to develop Alzheimer's disease; more than 75% of those

PATHOPHYSIOLOGY REVIEW

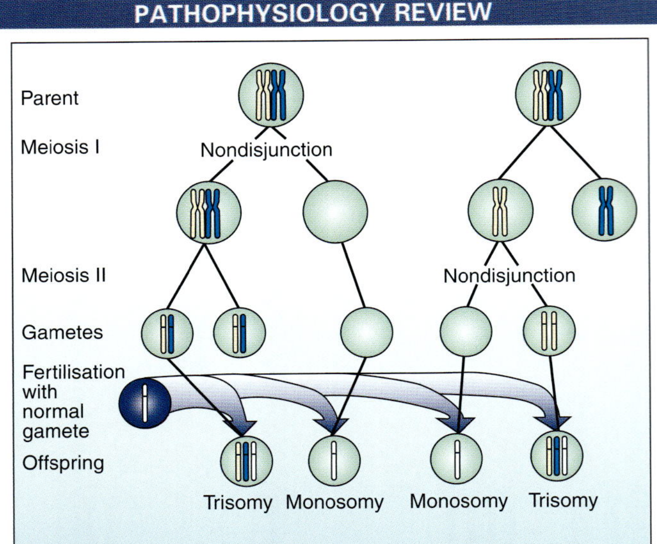

Fig 3.2 Non-disjunction causes aneuploidy when chromosomes or sister chromatids fail to divide properly. (Source: Jorde, L. B., Carey, J. C., Bamshad, M. J., et al. (2003). *Medical genetics* (3rd ed.). St Louis, MO: Mosby.)

over age 60 are affected with the disease (Waisman Center 2016, New Zealand Down Syndrome Association n.d.).

The chromosomal constitution of Down syndrome is variable, with three possible configurations.

1. **Trisomy**—The nomenclature for a female with trisomy is 47,XX,+21 and for a male with trisomy is 47,XY,+21. Trisomy encompasses 92% of all cases of Down syndrome. The extra chromosome 21 is unattached and segregates freely during meiosis. The risk for this type of Down syndrome increases linearly with increasing maternal age (Peng et al 2019); however, because young women have more babies, about 75% of babies with trisomy 21 are born to younger mothers.
2. **Translocation Down syndrome**—The accepted nomenclature for a male with Down syndrome due to robertsonian translocation between acrocentric chromosomes 14 and 21 is 46,XY,t(14;21). Translocation (discussed later) accounts for approximately 4% of all male and female Down syndrome cases. The majority of cases are sporadic (without family history), but about 25% have one balanced translocation carrier parent. When one such carrier and a partner with normal chromosomes reproduce, their theoretical chances of producing a live-born child with Down syndrome are 33%, but the actual observed risk is approximately 15% if the mother is the carrier and less than 10% if the father is the carrier. The observed chance of producing a live-born child who is a balanced translocation carrier approaches 50%. Because chromosome 21 is an acrocentric chromosome, it is possible for the translocation to be with both chromosome 21s. A carrier mother [45,XX,t(21;21)] or father [45,XY,t(21;21)] of the translocation would have a 100% chance of producing a pregnancy with Down syndrome because the other parent normally would contribute one chromosome 21. This latter situation is one of the rare examples in genetics where an abnormality is passed on to *all* living progeny.
3. **Mosaic Down syndrome**—The nomenclature for a female with mosaic Down syndrome is 46,XX/47,XX,+21. This rarer type of Down syndrome can occur in males and females. It results from mitotic non-disjunction during early embryonic development of a normal zygote. Children with this type have mixed cell populations, some with the normal karyotype, others with the extra chromosome. Contrary to what one might expect, children with mosaic

TABLE 3.2 Partial List of Chromosomal Genetic Disorders

Disorder	Genetic Aetiology	Possible Periods of Recognition	Major Findings
Angelman's syndrome	Chr—deletion, uniparental disomy or abnormal methylation of chromosome 15	Prenatal to early childhood	Significant motor, cognitive and speech delays; microcephaly; ataxia
Beckwith-Wiedemann syndrome	AD or Chr—abnormal methylation of chromosome 11, uniparental disomy of paternal chromosome 11 or structural abnormality in critical region	Prenatal to newborn	Overgrowth syndrome; often recognised in newborn period due to abnormally large tongue; abdominal wall defects; hypoglycaemia in infancy
Cri-du-chat syndrome	Chr—46,XX,del(5p) or 46,XY,del(5p)	Prenatal to newborn	Microcephaly; high-pitched, catlike cry; significant motor and cognitive delays
Down syndrome (trisomy 21)	Chr—47,XX,+21 or 47,XY,+21	Prenatal to newborn	Mild to moderate cognitive impairment, characteristic facial features, hypotonia
Edwards' syndrome (trisomy 18)	Chr—47,XX,+18 or 47,XY,+18	Prenatal to newborn	Multiple congenital anomalies; significantly shortened life span; if survival beyond 1 year, severe cognitive impairment
Klinefelter's syndrome	Chr—47,XXY	Prenatal; adolescence to adulthood	Gynaecomastia, small testes, normal sex drive and function but infertility common
Patau's syndrome (trisomy 13)	Chr—47,XX,+13 or 47,XY,+13	Prenatal to newborn	Multiple congenital anomalies; significantly shortened life span; if survival beyond 1 year, severe cognitive impairment
Prader-Willi syndrome	Chr—absence of paternally derived region of chromosome 15 or abnormally methylated critical region of chromosome 15	Prenatal; infancy to early childhood	Severe hypotonia, failure to thrive in early infancy; after 1–2 years of age, excessive eating—including non-food items; morbid obesity; cognitive impairment; distinctive behavioural problems; hypogonadism
Turner's syndrome	Chr—45,XO	Prenatal to adolescence	Lymphoedema at birth, coarctation, short stature, ovarian dysgenesis, lack of secondary sex characteristics during adolescence

AD, Autosomal dominant; *Chr,* chromosomal.

Down syndrome do not necessarily have a better developmental outcome than those with free trisomy type. The proportion of trisomic cells in various tissues and organs plays a role in the child's developmental potential and syndrome-associated potential health problems.

Trisomy 18. Edwards' syndrome is a fairly common trisomy in fetuses. Those who are live-born have severe cognitive impairment and physical abnormalities that contribute to a limited life span.

Trisomy 13. Patau's syndrome carries more severe malformations than the previous two trisomies discussed, consistent with the increased size of the extra chromosome and greater gene imbalance. Life span is significantly shortened.

Sex Chromosome Aneuploidies

Alterations in number may also involve the sex chromosomes. The possible mechanisms by which sex chromosome abnormalities may occur are the same as those previously described (i.e. pre-fertilisation non-disjunction during one of the meiotic divisions of gametogenesis in either parent or in the early post-fertilisation divisions of the zygote). An alteration in the number of sex chromosomes usually does not produce the profound effects that are associated with the autosomal trisomies. Intelligence may be normal or low normal, or the child may have some learning disabilities, but moderate or severe cognitive impairment is less common. Some of the most common genetic disorders caused by sex chromosome aneuploidies are Klinefelter's, XYY, triple X female and Turner's syndromes.

47,XXY. Klinefelter's syndrome is the most common of all sex chromosome aneuploidies. Physical abnormalities include: elements of decreased masculinisation, such as gynaecomastia; hypogonadism (with sterility resulting from degeneration of seminiferous tubules); and increased pubis-to-sole length, reflecting elongated lower limbs (Fig 3.3). Mental development is normal in most cases, with a mean full-scale IQ between 85 and 90. Cognitive difficulties tend to be in expressive language, auditory processing and auditory memory. Chromosome mosaicism (46,XY/47,XXY) rarely occurs and results in individuals with milder manifestations than their trisomic counterparts. Overall, the phenotype of Klinefelter's syndrome is highly variable, making it difficult, in the absence of chromosome studies, to make a prepubertal clinical diagnosis.

47,XYY. This genotype was reported in the early 1960s by Patricia Jacobs, a Scottish cytogeneticist who detected an increased frequency of double-Y men among inmates of penal institutions in Great Britain. This and subsequent early studies that linked this karyotype with criminal behaviour were significantly flawed by selection bias. Males with XYY may be at increased risk for autism spectrum disorder (Peng et al 2019). The extra Y is paternally derived. Although XYY fathers have an increased risk for offspring with abnormal Y chromosome complement, the majority of live births have a normal number of sex chromosomes.

45,XO. Turner's syndrome, originally described clinically as ovarian dysgenesis (with gonads consisting of streaks of connective tissue and devoid of germ cells), is an example of a monosomy that is compatible with life. Clinical manifestations are variable in expression. Intellectually, verbal IQ exceeds performance IQ. There is no prepubertal growth spurt, and girls with Turner's syndrome are generally infertile. It is common practice to administer female hormones around the time that puberty would occur to provide the girl with Turner's syndrome some secondary sex characteristics; however, the female hormones may further stunt growth and must be used judiciously. The child's growth is usually normal until 3 years of age and then slows, gradually drifting away from the normal growth curve. Treatment for the decreased growth velocity includes growth hormone and anabolic steroids. Mosaicism also occurs in Turner's syndrome (e.g. 46,XX/45,XO), resulting in milder expression of the phenotype. Girls with Turner's syndrome may have difficulty with peer relationships and with understanding social cues. They may exhibit behavioural problems, especially immature, socially isolated behaviour. Most, however, lead productive lives and function as independent adults.

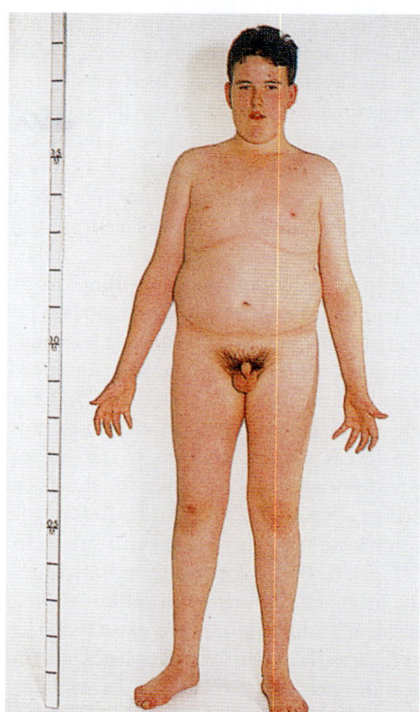

Fig 3.3 Klinefelter's syndrome. This young man exhibits many characteristics of Klinefelter's syndrome: small testes, some development of the breasts, sparse body hair and long limbs. This syndrome results from the presence of two or more X chromosomes with one Y chromosome (genotypes XXY or XXXY, for example). (Source: Patton, K. T. (2019). *Anatomy and physiology* (10th ed.). St Louis, MO: Elsevier.)

47,XXX. A relatively common condition (1:1000 live female births), females with triple X display a normal phenotype, with an increased risk of learning disabilities compared with their euploid sisters. Gynaecological complications include delayed menarche and premature menopause. As with XYY men, the offspring of XXX women is largely normal, indicative of a selective advantage of euploid gametes.

Structural Chromosome Abnormalities

Chromosomes are subject to structural alterations resulting from breakage and rearrangement. Chromosome **breakage** has long been recognised as a significant source of genetic abnormalities. Many **clastogens** (chromosome-breaking agents) have been identified, including physical (e.g. ionising radiation), chemical (e.g. chlorpromazine) and biological (e.g. viral infections) agents. Chromosome breakage can also result from many non-specific causes, such as influenza. These breaks are usually restricted to somatic cells and are temporary. Chromosome breakage becomes significant when it is permanent (or long lasting) and when these permanent changes, in addition to appearing in somatic cells, are also present in germ cells and thus have the potential of being transmitted to the offspring.

A chromosome **deletion** occurs when chromosome breakage results in loss of the broken fragment at a chromosome's terminal end or within the chromosome. Chromosome deletions often have significant clinical impact, as in a chromosome 5 terminal deletion that results in cri-du-chat syndrome. Chromosome breakage can create unstable end points ('sticky ends'), which predispose the chromosomes to a variety of rearrangements of the fragments. A relatively rare structural abnormality that can occur as a result of chromosomal 'sticky ends' is a ring chromosome. If a break occurs in the terminal end of both arms of a chromosome, the ends may fuse together, forming a circle. Like any structural alteration of a chromosome, the clinical manifestations depend on which genes are lost.

A more common rearrangement resulting from chromosome breakage is a **translocation**, which occurs when a chromosomal fragment reunites with another, non-homologous chromosome. Two types of translocations have clinical significance: reciprocal translocations and robertsonian translocations. In a **reciprocal translocation**, breaks occur in two different chromosomes and the fragments are mutually exchanged, resulting in derivative chromosomes. **Robertsonian translocations** occur when the short arms of two acrocentric chromosomes (pairs 13 to 15 and pairs 21 and 22) break off and the remaining long arms fuse at the centromere, forming a 'single chromosome' (Fig 3.4). Both types result in individuals who have the correct amount of genetic information (although 'rearranged'), and therefore no clinical manifestations are expected. These persons are termed ***balanced translocation carriers***. These asymptomatic, balanced translocation carriers (either male or female) may pass the translocation to their offspring in a balanced or unbalanced form, depending on how the chromosomes segregate to the gametes. If it is passed in the unbalanced form, the combination is often lethal, and an early spontaneous abortion occurs. The chance of having a liveborn child with birth defects associated with the unbalanced translocation depends on the quantity and role of the missing or additional genetic material. Approximately 5% of cases of repeated spontaneous abortion (two or more) can be attributed to a balanced translocation carrier parent.

Some structural chromosome abnormalities are too small to reliably visualise under a light microscope but are still clinically relevant. Fragile, or weak, sites associated with expanded triplet repeats (described later in the chapter) have been identified on both the autosomes and the X chromosome. A classic example is fragile X syndrome. **Contiguous gene syndromes** are disorders characterised by a microdeletion or microduplication of smaller chromosome segments, which may require special analysis techniques or molecular testing to detect.

46,XX,del(5p) or 46,XY,del(5p). Cri-du-chat, or cat's cry, syndrome is a rare (1:50,000 live births) (Jorde et al 2016, Peng et al 2019) chromosome deletion syndrome resulting from loss of the small arm of chromosome 5. In early infancy this syndrome manifests with a typical but non-distinctive facial appearance, often a 'moon-shaped' face with wide-spaced eyes (hypertelorism) (Fig 3.5). As the child grows, this feature is progressively diluted, and by age 2 years the child is indistinguishable from age-matched controls. Profound cognitive impairment persists throughout their short life; many die in infancy. Typical of this disease is a crying pattern that is abnormal and catlike. At times it sounds like an angry cat, and at others like a soft mewing sound. This is a result of a laryngeal atrophy that improves with age. By age 3 years the crying pattern is still abnormal, but it acquires a normal pitch and loses its catlike quality.

Fragile X Syndrome. Fragile X syndrome acquired its name from the fact that, in special cell culture conditions, the affected X chromosome may display a gap in its terminal portion. However, it is an X-linked condition caused by an unstable expansion (described later in the chapter). Fragile X is the most common cause of inherited cognitive impairment. Common clinical features include: a typical facial appearance, with an elongated face and large ears; macroorchidism in

PATHOPHYSIOLOGY REVIEW

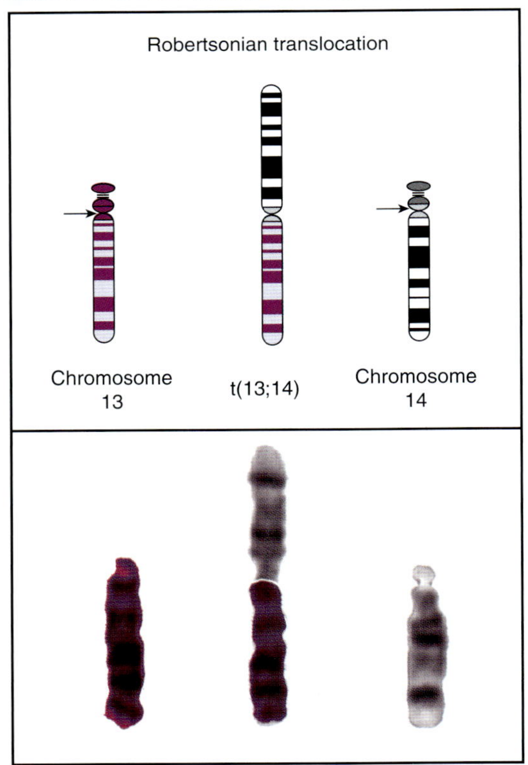

Fig 3.4 Translocation. In a robertsonian translocation, the long arms of two acrocentric chromosomes (13 and 14) fuse, forming a single chromosome. (Source: Jorde, L. B., Carey, J. C., Bamshad, M. J., et al (2003). *Medical genetics* (3rd ed.). St Louis, MO: Mosby.)

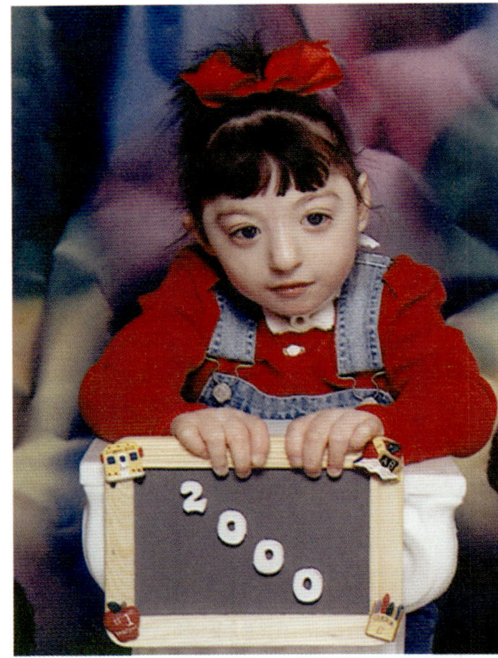

Fig 3.5 Eight-year-old child with cri-du-chat (cat's cry) syndrome. Notice the wide-spaced eyes (hypertelorism) and 'moon face'.

adolescent males; connective tissue dysplasia; and behavioural problems, including autism spectrum disorder (Committee on Genetics 2011).

Velocardiofacial Syndrome. Velocardiofacial syndrome (VCFS), sometimes called DiGeorge's syndrome or CATCH22, is a common (1:4000) microdeletion syndrome. It is caused by a specific microdeletion within the long arm of chromosome 22 (22q11.2 deletion) (McDonald-McGinn et al 1999, updated 2013). Manifestations of this condition are variable, with nearly 200 different possible clinical features described. Although no one feature is found in every patient, cognitive impairment is common and can range from full-scale measured IQ in the borderline low-normal range with characteristic learning disabilities to mild cognitive impairment (Antshel et al 2008). Although most patients' deletion is caused by a sporadic event, those with the condition can transmit the microdeletion in an autosomal dominant manner. Therefore, their chances of producing a child with VCFS are 50% with each pregnancy.

Chromosome Instability Syndromes. **Chromosome instability syndromes** are a heterogeneous group of genetic disorders characterised by a high frequency of chromosome breakage observed in vitro. They include ataxia telangiectasia, Fanconi's anaemia and xeroderma pigmentosum. These syndromes are associated with decreased immune function and an increased incidence of cancer.

Single-gene Disorders

Chromosome anomalies typically affect large numbers of genes; however, a **single-gene disorder** is caused by an abnormality within a gene or in a gene's regulatory region. Single-gene disorders can affect all body systems and may have mild to severe expression. These disorders display a mendelian pattern of dominant or recessive inheritance that was first delineated in the mid-19th century by Gregor Mendel's experiments with plants. Single-gene disorders cannot be detected by chromosome analysis and demand specific and sophisticated molecular detection methods, such as DNA-based techniques.

Mendelian inheritance laws allow for risk prediction in single-gene disorders; however, phenotypical expression may be altered by incomplete penetrance or variable expressivity of the responsible **allele**. An allele is said to have **reduced** or **incomplete penetrance** in a population when a proportion of persons who possess that allele do not express the phenotype. An allele is said to have **variable expressivity** when individuals possessing that allele display the features of the syndrome in various degrees, from mild to severe. If a person expresses even the mildest possible phenotype, the allele is penetrant in that individual.

Autosomal Inheritance Patterns

Autosomal Dominant Inheritance. A clear understanding of transmission of autosomal inheritance patterns requires the understanding of a few basic facts. First, most genetic diseases are rare. The probability that two affected persons will mate is very low for most genetic disorders (with the exception of societal selection, as in the case of achondroplasia). Second, depending on the disease, if one parent is affected, he or she is much more likely to be heterozygous (have one mutant allele) than homozygous (have two mutant alleles). Usually, an individual with two dominant mutant alleles will experience physical or cognitive abnormalities at a much more severe level.

Those assumptions being accepted, two questions remain: What are the chances of transmitting the mutant allele to the offspring? And what are the risks of the offspring being affected? If a gene has only two alleles, one normal and one mutant, three possible allele combinations exist: normal/normal, normal/mutant and mutant/mutant. In autosomal dominant conditions, only persons with normal/normal combination will be disease-free, assuming that the mutant allele is 100% penetrant. Figure 3.6 shows the relationships between genotypes and phenotypes for an autosomal dominant trait. Considering that genetic diseases are rare and that persons who are homozygous for the mutated allele are more severely affected, it is most likely that an affected individual who is heterozygous for the mutant allele will mate with a genotypically normal partner (Fig 3.7A). The outcomes of these matings are best expressed by the use of **Punnett squares.** Also depicted (Fig 3.7B) is the mating of a homozygote for the mutated gene with a genotypically normal partner. The result of these matings is one of the few instances in medical genetics in which *all* progeny have a 100% chance of being affected, assuming that the mutant allele they receive is 100% penetrant. These matings, however, are extremely rare.

Many children diagnosed with an autosomal dominant disorder have a positive family history of the disease. In other instances, that child may represent the first occurrence of that condition in the family. In the latter case, the event may be due to a new mutation (**de novo**

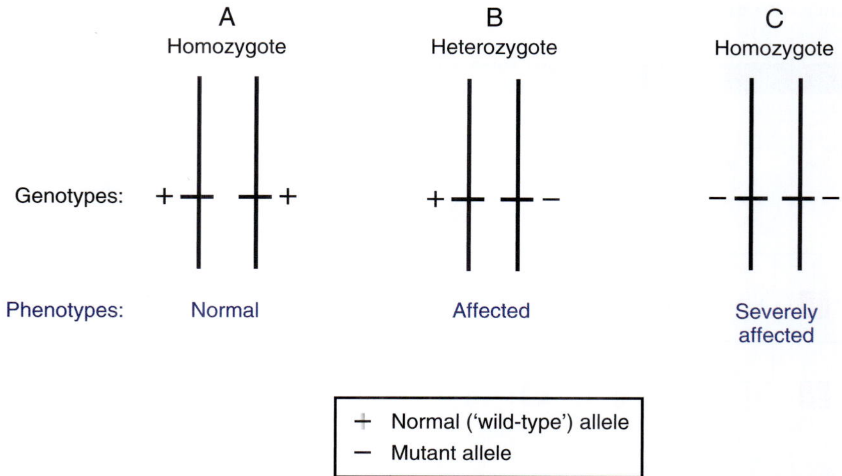

Fig 3.6 Dominant inheritance pattern. Schematic representation of the three possible allelic arrangements of a gene with two alleles. Depicted here are genotypes and possible phenotypes for a trait transmitted by a dominant gene. The presence of a single copy of the mutant allele in heterozygous person (**B**) is sufficient to express the phenotype in question. Double dose of the mutated allele, in homozygous person (**C**), results in more severe expression of the phenotype.

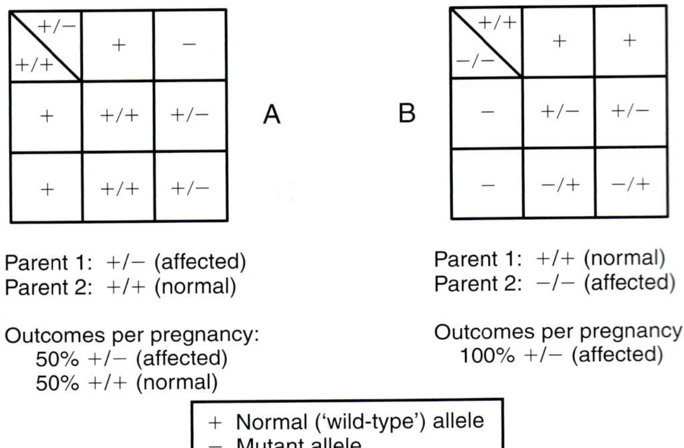

Fig 3.7 Determination of mating outcomes in autosomal dominant inheritance obtained with Punnett squares. (*A*) Possible outcomes of the mating of an affected heterozygous individual (+/−) with a normal partner (+/+). (*B*) Mating of an affected homozygous individual (−/−) and a normal partner (+/+).

mutation) in that child or to the presence of the mutation only in a subset of the germ cells of a healthy parent. The birth of other affected children indicates the second possibility. The range of expression of autosomal dominant gene mutations is highly variable, from minor manifestations (e.g. polydactyly), to severe, debilitating and life-threatening disease (e.g. neurofibromatosis). Depending on the degree of disability the condition imposes on the individual and the ability to procreate, the mutated gene will either be eliminated or continue to be passed on through several generations. In addition, in diseases that have a late age of onset (e.g. Huntington's disease), a person with a disease-associated mutation may be healthy and asymptomatic during childbearing years and be unaware of the risk of passing on the mutant allele to offspring. Consequently, the mutant allele continues to be passed on through several generations.

Other examples of autosomal dominant disorders include achondroplasia, neurofibromatosis and Marfan's syndrome. An idealised pedigree for autosomal dominant inheritance is found in Figure 3.8. The gene mutation associated with achondroplasia is considered 100% penetrant. The pedigree in the figure demonstrates that although an affected parent has a 50% chance with each pregnancy of transmitting the gene mutation associated with achondroplasia, 50% of offspring do not necessarily inherit the gene mutation. Selected examples of autosomal dominant disorders are found in Table 3.3.

Autosomal Recessive Inheritance. Children who display an autosomal recessive disorder are always homozygous for that trait (both the maternally and the paternally inherited alleles contain disease-associated mutations). This is due to the fact that a recessive allele is one whose phenotypical expression occurs only when both genes have disease-associated mutations. Although this makes the alleles homozygous because both alleles are recessive, the disease-associated mutation may be different in each allele. When this is the case, the pair of alleles is more accurately referred to as **compound heterozygous** for the recessive trait. In the heterozygote, a recessive allele is 'masked' by the wild-type (normal) allele, which is dominant. Whereas the possible pregnancy outcomes in autosomal dominant pattern are children who are either affected (if the gene mutation is fully penetrant) or unaffected when completely free of the gene mutation, in autosomal recessive inheritance a third possibility arises: that of a **heterozygous carrier**. These are individuals who are clinically normal (or nearly normal) but who are at risk of having offspring who are affected.

Identification of such carriers is of paramount importance for genetic counselling. In the case of an unaffected couple who produce a child with a recessive disease, identification is straightforward, assuming lack of misattributed paternity; because they each must contribute a mutant allele, they are considered obligate carriers, even in the absence of specific carrier testing for that gene.

Other examples of autosomal recessive disorders include the thalassaemias, congenital adrenal hyperplasia and galactosaemia. Figure 3.9 illustrates two situations involving autosomal recessive traits. Figure 3.9A depicts the most common occurrence in autosomal recessive disorders: the mating of two carrier parents, with each pregnancy carrying a 25% chance of producing an affected child. Figure 3.9B reflects the mating of an affected parent with a genotypically normal partner, in which 100% of the offspring will be carriers. An idealised pedigree representing the mating of two heterozygous (asymptomatic) carriers and its possible outcomes in each and every pregnancy is shown in Figure 3.10. Selected examples of autosomal recessive disorders are found in Table 3.3.

Sex-linked Inheritance Patterns

The transmission of genes located on one of the sex chromosomes (either X or Y) is termed ***sex-linked inheritance***. However, few genes

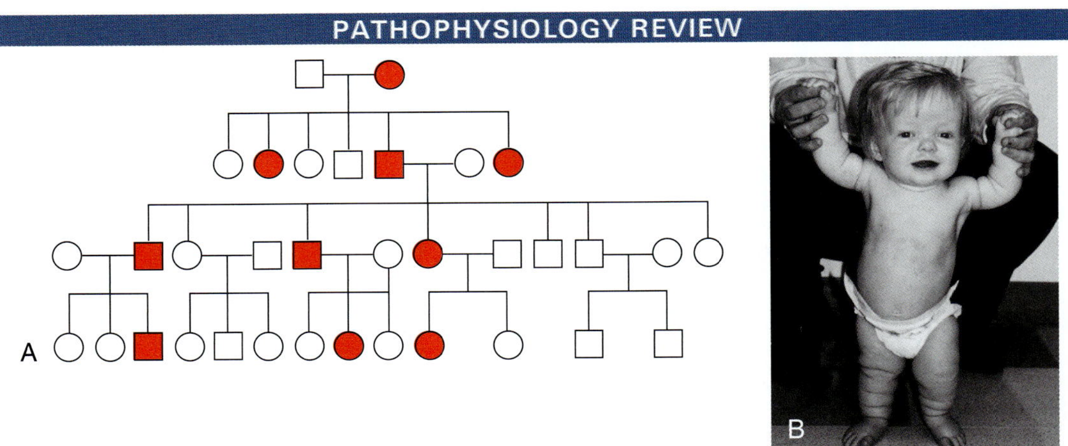

Fig 3.8 Pedigree for achondroplasia. (*A*) Pedigree showing the transmission of an autosomal dominant disease. (*B*) Achondroplasia. This girl has short limbs relative to trunk length. She also has a prominent forehead, low nasal root and redundant skin folds in the arms and legs. (Source: *B,* from Jorde, L. B., Carey, J. C., Bamshad, M. J., et al. (2003). *Medical genetics* (3rd ed.). St Louis, MO: Mosby.)

TABLE 3.3 Partial List of Mendelian-inherited Genetic Disorders

Disorder	Genetic Aetiology	Possible Periods of Recognition	Major Findings
Achondroplasia	AD	Prenatal to newborn	Dwarfism with legs and arms significantly shorter than torso; characteristic facial features
Adenosine deaminase deficiency	AR	Prenatal*; infant period most common; onset can be delayed until adulthood	Enzyme deficiency that results in severe combined immunodeficiency
Ataxia telangiectasia	AR	Prenatal* to early childhood	Immunodeficiency, neurodegenerative, acute sensitivity to ionising radiation that increases risk for cancer
Beckwith-Wiedemann syndrome	AD or Chr—Abnormal methylation of chromosome 11, uniparental disomy of paternal chromosome 11, or structural abnormality in critical region	Prenatal to newborn	Overgrowth syndrome; often recognised in newborn period due to abnormally large tongue; abdominal wall defects; hypoglycaemia in infancy
Bloom's syndrome	AR	Prenatal* to early childhood	Prenatal and postnatal growth retardation; chromosome instability leading to sun sensitivity, high cancer risk, immunodeficiency
Congenital adrenal hyperplasia	AR	Prenatal* to newborn	Ambiguous genitalia—virilisation of female external genitalia due to elevated androgen levels; salt loss in some due to inability to reabsorb sodium
Cystic fibrosis	AR	Prenatal* to toddler	Meconium ileus at birth; pancreatic insufficiency and malabsorption; chronic pulmonary inflammation and infection
Duchenne's muscular dystrophy	XL recessive	Prenatal* to early childhood	Delayed milestones, progressive skeletal muscle disease, dilated cardiomyopathy
Familial adenomatous polyposis (Gardner's syndrome, Turcot's syndrome)	AD—Mutation in APC gene	Childhood to adulthood	Hundreds to thousands of adenomatous polyps in the distal portion of colon; colon cancer; extra colonic polyps and tumours
Fanconi's anaemia	Most forms AR; at least one form XL	Prenatal* to childhood	Multiple malformations, progressive bone marrow failure, chromosome breakage in cell culture
Fragile X syndrome	XL—Expanded triplet repeat	Prenatal; childhood to adolescent	Moderate cognitive impairment in males, mild cognitive impairment in females
Friedreich's ataxia	AR (most have expanded triplet repeat in one or both genes)	Prenatal* to childhood, sometimes not until adulthood	Slowly progressive ataxia, cardiomyopathy
Galactosaemia	AR	Prenatal* to neonatal	Failure to thrive, hepatocellular damage, sepsis, bleeding, cognitive impairment, death if untreated
Gaucher's disease	AR	Prenatal* to adulthood	Three major types: • Type 1 most common; hepatosplenomegaly, bone disease, sometimes lung disease • Type 2 neurodegenerative, lethal by 4 years • Type 3 neurodegenerative disease, can live to adulthood
Glucose-6-phosphate dehydrogenase (G6PD) deficiency	XL recessive	Infant to adulthood	Haemolytic anaemia; expression dependent on exposure to environmental triggers (eating fava beans, certain infections and certain drugs)
Haemophilia A, haemophilia B	XL recessive	Prenatal* to adulthood depending on extent of deficient clotting activity	Haemophilia A—Factor VIII deficiency; haemophilia B—Factor IX deficiency Both diagnosed in infancy period in those with severe deficiency; brought to attention by spontaneous joint or deep muscle bleeds
Hunter's syndrome	XL recessive	Prenatal* to childhood	Progressive multisystem disorder due to glycosaminoglycans accumulation; CNS deterioration common in severe form but not attenuated form
Huntington's disease	AD expanded triplet repeat	Prenatal for couples with family history; most often diagnosed in adulthood	Progressive neurodegenerative disease with mean age of onset in third to fourth decade of life; death typically within 20 years of symptom onset
Hurler's syndrome	AR	Prenatal*; infant to childhood	Progressive lysosomal storage disease; death by 10 years of age in severely affected; mildly affected can live into adulthood

Continued

TABLE 3.3 **Partial List of Mendelian-inherited Genetic Disorders–cont'd**

Disorder	Genetic Aetiology	Possible Periods of Recognition	Major Findings
Hypophosphataemic vitamin D–resistant rickets	XL dominant	Infant to adulthood	Kidney abnormality resulting in overexcretion of phosphate in urine; secondary bone defects result
Incontinentia pigmenti	XL dominant	Prenatal*; newborn to infant	Often prenatally lethal in males; those who survive should have chromosome testing; a de novo mutation is the cause in most affected individuals; blistering of skin, later linear hypopigmentation of skin; small, missing teeth; sparse, wiry hair; vascular retinal abnormalities
Li-Fraumeni cancer syndrome	AD	Prenatal*; 50% have first cancer by age 40	Predisposition to multiple primary cancers at various body sites
Malignant hyperthermia	AD	Prenatal* or before drug exposure (if family history and family mutation known)	Susceptibility to uncontrolled skeletal muscle hypermetabolism when exposed to certain anaesthetics and succinylcholine; first symptoms tachycardia, tachypnoea, then progressive symptoms and death if not quickly treated
Marfan's syndrome	AD	Prenatal*; neonatal to adulthood depending on number and severity of features and presence or absence of family history	Connective tissue disorder primarily affecting cardiovascular, skeletal and ocular systems
Myotonic dystrophy	AD expansion mutation; *DMPK* for type 1; *CNBP* for type 2	Prenatal if gene expansion mutation identified in affected parent Type 1—Birth in congenital form; child to adulthood for other forms Type 2—Onset typically in third decade	Variable presentation Classic type 1—Affects skeletal and smooth muscle characterised by muscle weakness, wasting, myotonia, cardiac conduction abnormalities Type 2—Muscle weakness, myotonia, posterior subcapsular cataracts, insulin insensitivity (increasingly common with age)
Neurofibromatosis	AD	Type 1—Childhood to adulthood Type 2— Adolescence to adulthood	Type 1—Six or more café-au-lait spots, axillary and inguinal freckling, neurofibromas, iris Lisch nodules; learning disabilities common Type 2—Vestibular schwannomas
Oculocutaneous albinism type 1	AR	Prenatal*; birth to childhood	Hypopigmentation of skin and hair due to reduced melanin production; nystagmus, iris translucency; significant vision impairment
Phenylketonuria	AR	Prenatal*; newborn	Minimal or absent phenylalanine hydroxylase activity resulting in profound cognitive impairment if not treated early with dietary restriction of phenylalanine
Pompe's disease (glycogen storage disease type II)	AR	Prenatal*; newborn to infant	Hypotonia, cardiomegaly and hypertrophic cardiomyopathy, failure to thrive; death within first year of life; early enzyme therapy may prevent or delay symptoms
Porphyria, acute intermittent	AD (low penetrance)	Adolescence to adulthood	Acute attacks include abdominal pain; peripheral neuropathy; neuropsychiatric symptoms
Sickle cell disorder (sickle cell anaemia; sickle-haemoglobin C disease; sickle β-thalassaemia)	AR	Prenatal to newborn; if missed on newborn screen, childhood	Severe pain at site of vascular occlusion leading to tissue ischaemia; organ dysfunction possible at site of vascular occlusion
Tay-Sachs disease (hexosaminidase A deficiency)	AR	Prenatal to infant	Neurodegenerative disease Acute type—Progressive weakness, loss of motor skills, seizures, blindness, spasticity, death by about 4 years Subacute type—May have onset in childhood or adulthood with variable progressive neurological findings
Beta-thalassaemia	AR	Prenatal*; newborn screening; by 2 years of age if missed on screen	Microcytic hypochromic anaemia, absent or reduced haemoglobin A; severe anaemia and secondary hepatosplenomegaly
Velocardiofacial syndrome	AD and Chr—46,XX,del(22.11.2) or 46,XY,del(22.11.2)	Prenatal to adulthood	Extremely variable condition; nearly 200 possible features described; most common are cognitive impairment, palatal structural or functional abnormalities, conotruncal heart defects, mild immunodeficiencies

TABLE 3.3 Partial List of Mendelian-inherited Genetic Disorders–cont'd

Disorder	Genetic Aetiology	Possible Periods of Recognition	Major Findings
Xeroderma pigmentosum	AR (abnormalities in genes responsible for DNA repair)	Prenatal* to 2 years	Acute sun sensitivity (severe sunburns and blistering with minimal exposure) and over 1000-fold increased risk of cutaneous and ocular neoplasms; in some cases, sensitivity to x-rays

*Mutation(s) in affected family member or in carrier parents need to be known before prenatal testing can be informative.
AD, autosomal dominant; *AR*, autosomal recessive; *Chr*, chromosomal; *CNS*, central nervous system; *DNA*, deoxyribonucleic acid; *XL*, X-linked.

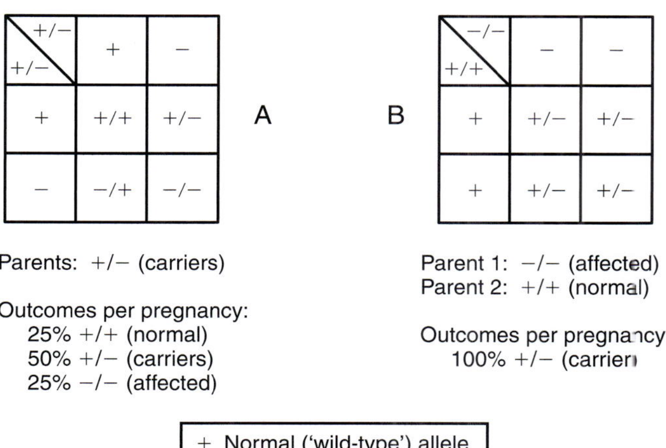

Fig 3.9 Autosomal recessive inheritance: Punnett squares. **A** Possible outcomes of mating of two heterozygous carriers (+/−). **B** Mating of affected homozygous individual (−/−) and normal partner (+/+). Percentages shown refer to outcome possibilities in each pregnancy.

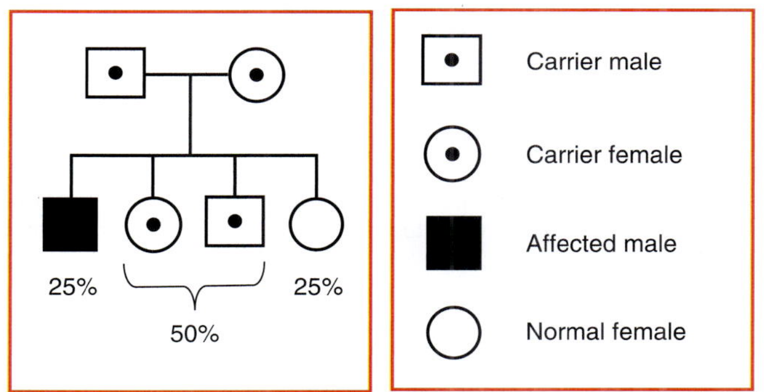

Fig 3.10 Autosomal recessive inheritance: typical pedigree. The idealised pedigree on the left represents possible outcomes of the mating of two heterozygous carriers (+/−). Percentages express risks for each pregnancy resulting from this mating.

have been found on the Y chromosome, so frequently the terms *sex-linked* and *X-linked* are interchangeably (and incorrectly) used. The testicular organising region of the Y chromosome determines the formation of testes and the development of male sexual structures during embryonic growth. A gene for hairy ears, with high prevalence in southern Asia, has also been located on the Y chromosome. Inheritance of Y-linked genes follows a father-to-son, or male-to-male, pattern. It is important to remember that men give their X chromosomes to their daughters (and their Y to their sons), so in analysing a family pedigree, male-to-male transmission of a gene rules out X-linked inheritance.

Sex-linked Traits. Women have two X chromosomes; therefore, inheritance of genes located on the X chromosome (X-linked inheritance) follows the same pattern as that for autosomal genes. However, in the case of males, the X and Y chromosomes have small areas of homology and therefore do not pair side-by-side during meiosis. Because of this, men are hemizygous for all genes on the X chromosome that do not have a homologous site on the Y chromosome, and their alleles are represented as single copies. Therefore, in the inheritance of an X-linked gene, the single-copy presence of its normal, or its mutant, allele will result in the expression of the normal or mutant phenotype, respectively. This is true for both dominant and recessive X-linked diseases in males (Fig 3.11).

X-linked Recessive Inheritance. In females the alleles of an X-linked recessive gene behave as the alleles of any autosomal recessive gene: the effect of the abnormal allele is 'hidden' by the normal (dominant) allele. Therefore, females who have a disease-associated mutation in both members of the gene pair will express the phenotype. Although it is rare for females to express the phenotype if only one member of the gene pair carries a disease-associated mutation, it is possible due to X inactivation.

Soon after fertilisation, it is normal for one X chromosome in females to be inactivated through a natural process called **methylation.** This occurs in each cell in the early blastocyst stage, and whether the paternal or maternally inherited X is inactivated is random in each cell. At the time this occurs, the X that has been inactivated will remain so through all subsequent cell divisions. Females who express a phenotype may have a greater proportion of X chromosome with the normal allele inactivated within the tissues or organs associated with the disorder. Examples of X-linked recessive disorders include haemophilia types A and B and Duchenne's muscular dystrophy. Figure 3.12 illustrates the outcomes of each pregnancy between an affected man and a normal woman (Fig 3.12A) and between a normal man and a carrier woman (Fig 3.12B). An idealised pedigree depicting the mating between a genetically normal man and a carrier woman, and its possible outcomes per pregnancy, is shown in Figure 3.13.

X-linked Dominant Inheritance. X-linked dominant inheritance (see Fig 3.11) is rare. The main characteristics of X-linked dominant inheritance are: (1) both males and females can be affected, but females, because of the random nature of X inactivation, are usually less severely affected than males; (2) affected men do not transmit the mutant allele to their sons; and (3) all daughters of an affected man are affected and have a 50% chance of passing on the mutant allele to their sons and daughters. Examples of X-linked dominant disorders are hypophosphataemic vitamin D–resistant rickets and incontinentia pigmenti. Figure 3.14 illustrates the outcomes of each pregnancy between an affected man and an unaffected woman (Fig 3.14A) and between an unaffected man and an affected woman (Fig 3.14B). An idealised pedigree representing the mating of an affected man with an unaffected woman is shown in Figure 3.15.

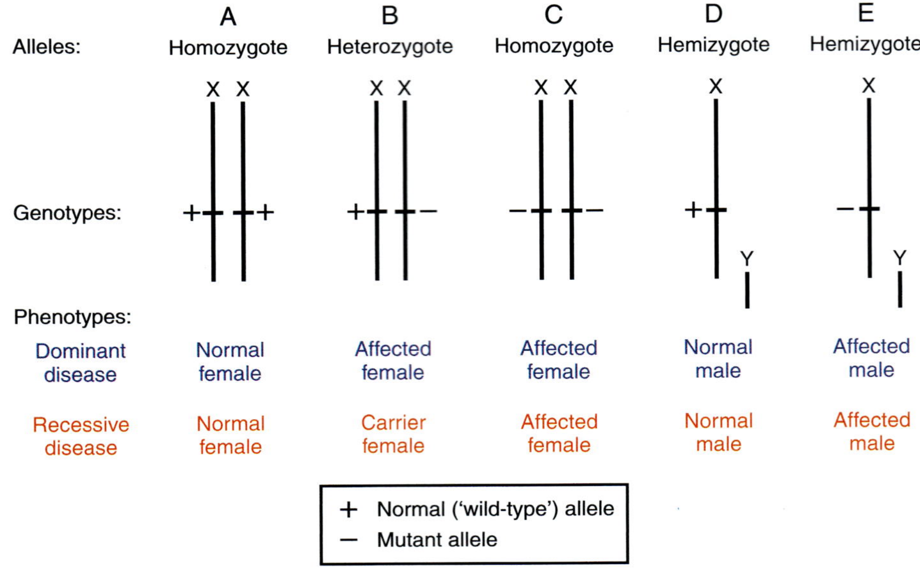

Fig 3.11 X-linked inheritance pattern. (*A*) to (*C*) Possible allelic arrangements of an X-linked gene in females. Note that phenotypical expression of an X-linked gene in women is typically similar to that of an autosomal gene. However, unequal X inactivation could result in more active X chromosomes with the mutation and could result in symptoms. (*D*) and (*E*) Uneven pairing of X and Y chromosomes in males, and its phenotypical expressions. Note that there are no carrier males because the phenotype is determined solely by the characteristic of X-linked allele. Hemizygous males are either normal or affected.

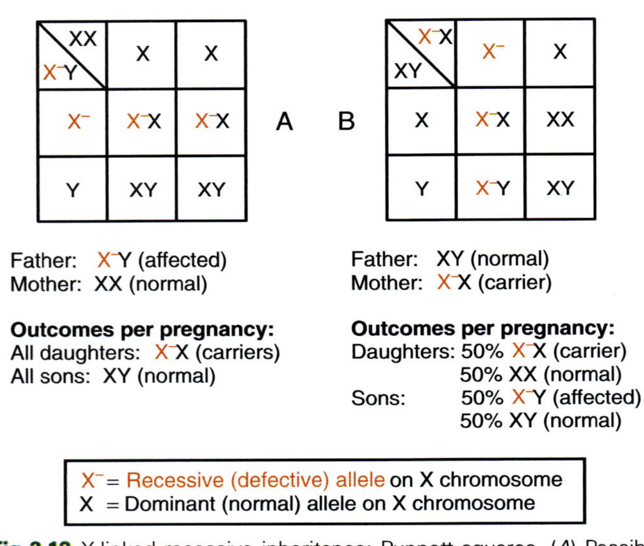

Fig 3.12 X-linked recessive inheritance: Punnett squares. (*A*) Possible outcomes of mating of affected male with normal female. (*B*) Mating of normal male and carrier female. Percentages refer to outcome possibilities in each pregnancy.

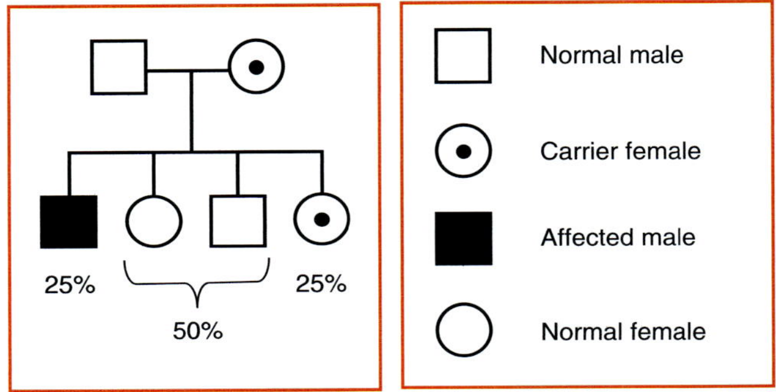

Fig 3.13 X-linked recessive inheritance: typical pedigree. The idealised pedigree on the left represents possible outcomes of mating of normal male and carrier female. Percentages express risks for each pregnancy resulting from this mating.

Variable Patterns of Gene Expression and Inheritance

A number of variables have been observed that explain or modify basic inheritance patterns and the effects of chromosome abnormalities. Some of these variations have been recognised for some time; others are newly discovered phenomena that explain some apparent contradictions in the established patterns of inheritance. Also, some disorders have been reported to follow more than one inheritance pattern in different families (e.g. a classically recessive disorder occasionally may be reported to be following a dominant or X-linked pattern in other families). This phenomenon is known as **locus heterogeneity** (Jorde et al 2016).

The most notable of these gene variations is mutation. As discussed earlier, mutations are heritable changes in the DNA sequence of a gene. Mutations can result from a substitution of bases (**point mutations**) or the insertion or deletion of bases. Some genes have a high mutation rate, and various forms of the resulting disease may have varying expression. One example is the *CFTR* gene, in which more than 1000 different cystic fibrosis (CF) associated mutations have been identified (the vast majority being point mutations or small deletions). Mutation rates are not constant for all genes, so some diseases may occur with much greater frequency than others.

Variable expression is an important concept that describes differences in the extent, severity and onset of phenotype. There is a continuum of expression for any affected person from very mild to severe clinical manifestations. For those with very mild manifestations, it may take an expert clinician to identify the condition. For example, a parent of a child with classic neurofibromatosis may exhibit only a few 'birthmarks' that a medical geneticist, genetics advanced practice nurse or

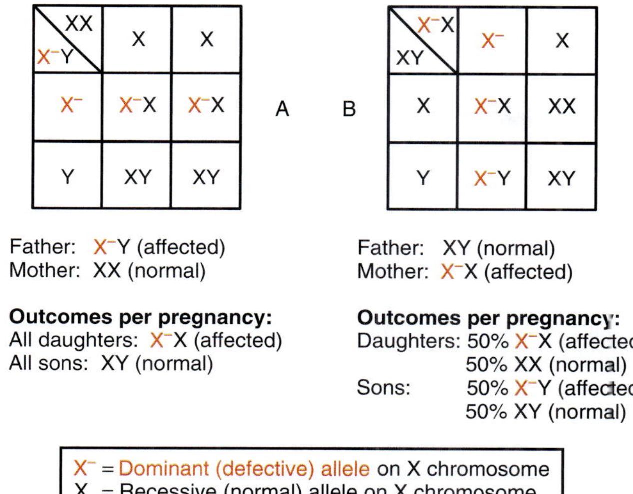

Fig 3.14 X-linked dominant inheritance: Punnett squares. (*A*) Possible outcomes of mating of affected male with normal female. (*B*) Mating of normal male and affected female. Percentages shown refer to outcome possibilities in each pregnancy.

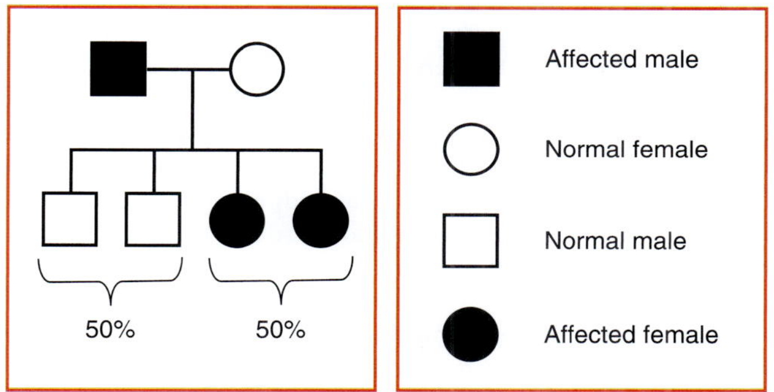

Fig 3.15 X-linked dominant inheritance: typical pedigree. The idealised pedigree on the left represents possible outcomes of mating of affected male and normal female. Percentages depicted express risks for each pregnancy resulting from this mating. Because the mutant allele is carried in the X chromosome, an affected male will transfer it to 100% of his daughters.

genetic counsellor would recognise as café-au-lait spots, one of the manifestations of neurofibromatosis.

Some genetic disorders are caused by an abnormal expansion of a short DNA sequence that naturally repeats. The size of an **expansion mutation** can influence the age of onset and severity of the disorder. For example, the *FMR1* gene on the X chromosome usually has about 5 to 40 repeats of three nucleotides: cytosine, guanine and guanine (CGG). When *FMR1* has 59 to 200 CGG repeats, that area of the gene can become unstable and gain further repeats during meiosis. Females who have this number of repeats are considered carriers of a **premutation** for fragile X syndrome. A person with fragile X has a full mutation allele with hundreds to thousands of repeats. Because fragile X syndrome is an X-linked disorder, females are less likely to be affected because of the presence of a normal allele on the homologous X chromosome. These expanding repeats have also been found to occur in autosomal dominant disorders such as myotonic dystrophy and in autosomal recessive disorders such as Friedreich's ataxia. Expansion mutations that have a tendency to further expand when transmitted from one generation to the next can display phenotypical anticipation. Pedigrees display anticipation when individuals in successive generations develop the disorder at an earlier age and/or with more severe manifestations.

Genomic imprinting and uniparental disomy are two genetic phenomena that consider the parental origin of genetic information (i.e. maternally or paternally derived). The concept of **genomic imprinting** refers to modification, in some instances, of genetic material. Methyl groups are naturally added to (and in some cases removed from) certain regions of the genome to control the expression of select genes. Methylation patterns can be specific to parent of origin. For example, during sperm formation, methyl groups are removed from the father's chromosomes that were inherited from his mother and methyl groups added to areas of those chromosomes to ensure that genes that should be turned on or off in paternally inherited chromosomes are transmitted to future offspring. Genomic imprinting is exhibited during pregnancy, when paternally derived chromosomes seem to positively influence placental development and maternally derived chromosomes seem to positively influence fetal development. This phenomenon also occurs in some genetic disorders, such as Prader-Willi and Angelman's syndromes. In both these disorders about two-thirds of affected individuals have a deletion of the same segment of chromosome 15 that is normally methylated. However, the clinical manifestations of Prader-Willi and Angelman's syndromes are markedly different. If the deletion occurs on the paternally derived chromosome 15 so only the mother's genes are expressed, the child exhibits Prader-Willi syndrome; if the deletion occurs on the maternally derived chromosome 15 so that only the father's genes are expressed, the child manifests Angelman's syndrome (Jorde et al 2016). Prader-Willi syndrome is characterised by failure to thrive and central hypotonia in the newborn and infancy period with later insatiable hunger that can lead to morbid obesity during childhood. Children with Prader-Willi syndrome also have cognitive dysfunction, typical dysmorphic features, behavioural disturbances, hypothalamic hypogonadism and short stature. In contrast, Angelman's syndrome includes severe cognitive impairment, characteristic facies, abnormal (puppet-like) gait, and paroxysms of inappropriate laughter. Children with Angelman's syndrome are usually non-verbal.

In some cases both copies of a chromosome pair are discovered to have come from one parent, either the mother or the father, instead of one from each; this phenomenon is called **uniparental disomy**. An example of uniparental disomy was reported with CF, in which both chromosomes, each with a mutant recessive gene, came from the carrier mother; the father was not a carrier. In cases that appear to be misattributed paternity, uniparental disomy may be a factor. One of several theories about uniparental disomy is that the chromosome pair was originally a trisomy and the father's chromosome was randomly eliminated, leaving two copies of the mother's chromosome. Because the chromosomes appear as a normal 'pair', diagnosis of this situation is only possible with molecular (DNA) techniques. Uniparental disomy has also been reported with Beckwith-Wiedemann syndrome, which is characterised by overgrowth and hypoglycaemia at birth (see Table 3.2).

Mitochondrial Disorders

Mitochondrial disorders can be caused by mutations in the nuclear genes and exhibit mendelian inheritance. However, mitochondrial disorders can also be caused by DNA found in a cytoplasmic cellular organelle, the **mitochondrion**, whose primary function in cellular metabolism is the production of energy. Mutations in mtDNA also account for non-mendelian inheritance patterns. Inheritance of traits contained in mtDNA is exclusively maternal because only the mitochondria from the ovum are transmitted to the zygote. Mitochondria are not contained within the sperm head.

An additional complexity in mitochondrial inheritance results from the fact that, during mitosis, mitochondria are randomly distributed among the daughter cells, so both normal and mutated mitochondria may be found in the same cell, a phenomenon known as **heteroplasmy**. This leads to variable dosages of mutated mtDNA between tissues and organs. This variation in mutation load leads to a highly variable spectrum of clinical manifestations, and individuals with the same mtDNA mutation may range from symptom free, to mildly affected, to severely impaired. Symptoms may include seizures, pancreatitis and metabolic disease. Different manifestations may be seen in different members of the same family. Heteroplasmy complicates the use of prenatal diagnosis. Once the mtDNA mutation is identified in the mother, her pregnancies can be tested for the same mutation. However, the mutation load identified in sampled fetal tissue (chorionic villi or amniocytes) may not correspond to other fetal tissues, the mutational load of which will continue to change during development due to random mitotic segregation of cytoplasmic organelles. Consequently, it is not possible to predict the unborn child's phenotype based on prenatal test results.

mtDNA mutations are responsible for various childhood diseases (Table 3.4), such as Leigh syndrome (movement disorder, respiratory dyskinesia, regression, hypotonia, seizures and failure to thrive). Because mitochondrial disorders have such variability of expression, determining the diagnosis can be confusing. However, when a child has an unexplained constellation of abnormal findings in tissue or organs that require high energy (e.g. heart, skeletal muscle, eyes), a mitochondrial disorder should be considered.

Hereditary Cancer Predisposition Genes

The process of carcinogenesis implies permanent changes in the DNA of the targeted cell. Early observations recognised genetic influences in cancer: (1) certain types of cancer occur more frequently within certain families (breast, colon, ovarian, some leukaemias); (2) some well-defined genetic disorders show a predisposition to various malignancies (familial adenomatous polyposis and colon cancer, Bloom's syndrome, and lymphomas); (3) chromosome abnormalities occur frequently with malignancies (Philadelphia chromosome in chronic myelogenous leukaemia); and (4) certain chromosome aneuploidies predispose the person to cancer (Down syndrome and acute leukaemias).

The discovery of **oncogenes** in the early 1970s marked the beginning of a new era in the field of cancer genetics. Initially thought to be carried exclusively by retroviruses, oncogenes were later identified as natural genes that existed in all mammals. Early investigations suggested that oncogenes were found in inactive form (i.e. no correlation with cancer could be identified in this state). In reality, oncogenes are normally involved in cell growth and division. A mutation in an oncogene can disrupt this normal process and transform a normal cell into one that has uncontrolled cell growth or division, predisposing the cell to further mutations that eventually transform the cell into one that is malignant.

Since the discovery of oncogenes, two other classes of genes associated with cancer development have been identified: tumour suppressor genes and mismatch repair genes. **Tumour suppressor genes** normally inhibit cell growth and division. A mutation in these genes can interfere with this normal function and lead to uninhibited cell growth and division. Among this group is *p53* (sometimes called *TP53*), whose germ cell (or hereditary) mutations are associated with Li-Fraumeni cancer syndrome and whose somatic cell mutations (sporadic) result in various malignancies, such as bladder cancer. Li-Fraumeni cancer syndrome is inherited as an autosomal dominant trait that predisposes children and young adults to the development of various tumours, including: osteosarcoma; soft tissue sarcomas; breast, brain and adrenocortical carcinomas; and leukaemia (Schneider et al 1999, updated 2013).

Mismatch repair genes normally function by recognising and repairing DNA errors that occur during replication or mutations that

TABLE 3.4 Partial List of Mitochondrial Genetic Disorders

Disorder	Genetic Aetiology	Possible Periods of Recognition	Major Findings
Kearns-Sayre syndrome	Mit—maternal inheritance but affected women only have approximately 1 in 24 risk of having affected offspring; maternal transmission to more than one child has not been reported	Infancy; before 20 years of age	Three overlapping phenotypes that can be seen in the same family and used to be distinguished as three different diseases; multisystem disease primarily affecting CNS, endocrine system, skeletal muscles, heart, retina
Leigh syndrome; NARP (neurogenic muscle weakness, ataxia, retinitis pigmentosa)	Mit—many different mitochondrial genes implicated	Leigh—infancy NARP—childhood	Symptoms depend on mutation load and tissue distribution of disease causing mtDNA mutation; progressive, neurodegenerative disorder Leigh onset typically after viral infection; 75% die by 3 years of age NARP onset typically in childhood; ataxia, learning difficulties, episodic deterioration possible following viral infections
MELAS (mitochondrial encephalomyopathy, lactic acidosis and stroke-like episodes)	Mit	Early childhood	Encephalopathy, seizures, recurrent vomiting, recurrent headaches, exercise intolerance, stroke-like episodes
MERRF (myoclonic epilepsy associated with ragged red fibres)	Mit	Childhood	Myoclonus, generalised epilepsy, ataxia, dementia

CNS, central nervous system; *Mit*, mitochondrial; *mtDNA*, mitochondrial deoxyribonucleic acid.

are caused by external agents such as ultraviolet light or chemical exposure. Xeroderma pigmentosum is a classic example of inherited predisposition to cancers caused by a germline mutation in one of several possible mismatch repair genes. Infants and children with xeroderma pigmentosum are at considerable risk for skin cancers triggered by sun and ultraviolet light exposure.

INBORN ERRORS OF METABOLISM

Inborn errors of metabolism (IEMs) include a large number of inherited diseases caused by interruptions in the various pathways involved in the metabolism of protein, carbohydrates or lipids. Figure 3.16 is a conceptual model representing the multiple interactions in a metabolic pathway in health and disease. **Metabolic pathways** are series of biochemical reactions by which substrates are sequentially converted into other by-products, aiming at a final end-product that can be successfully used or eliminated by the body. Each of these transformations is mediated by an enzyme, which is under the control of a specific structural gene. Figure 3.16A represents the normal metabolic conversion of substance **A** into end-product **K**, via by-products **B**, **C**, **D** and so on. Enzymes **b** and **c**, whose synthesis is controlled by genes β and δ, catalyse steps **B** → **C** and **C** → **D**, respectively. A feedback loop ensures physiological levels of **K**. A gene mutation may result in qualitative or quantitative changes in the enzyme, resulting in a different (and therefore ineffective) enzyme, or in the decreased synthesis of the enzyme, including its total absence. This ineffective (or missing) enzyme will interrupt the pathway, resulting in accumulation of the by-product that immediately precedes the blockage, as well as lack of the by-products beyond the blockage. IEMs can occur as a result of such accumulations or absences of an essential byproduct.

In Figure 3.16B, a mutation in gene β prevents normal synthesis of enzyme **b**, creating an interruption of the pathway between **B** and **C**. Assuming a continuous uptake of **A**, two outcomes ensue: accumulation of **B** and depletion of all products beyond the block (**C, D, ... K**). An example of this situation is Tay-Sachs disease (or GM_2 gangliosidosis). In this disease, a mutation in the *HexA* gene (here exemplified by β) causes the lack of the enzyme hexosaminidase A (*HexA*), represented by **b**. Absence of **b** creates an accumulation of ganglioside GM_2 (**B**)—lipids, in nerve cells, resulting in the clinical manifestations of this progressive neurological disorder because the lipids are not broken down by the cellular liposomes.

Figure 3.16C depicts a mutation in gene δ, which causes depletion of enzyme **c** and interrupts the metabolic conversion of **C** into **D**. In this instance an alternative pathway **C** → **E** → **F** is opened. This event may have two outcomes: product **F** may eventually be converted into **K**, with no significant clinical consequences, or **F** may represent the endpoint to the alternative pathway. If accumulation of **F** reaches toxic levels, a disease process may occur. Such is the case with PKU, an IEM that creates an intolerance to the amino acid phenylalanine. The missing enzyme (**c**, in this case), which results from mutation in the phenylalanine hydroxylase (PAH) gene (δ), is phenylalanine hydroxylase. The alternative pathway leads to the formation and accumulation of phenylketones (**F**). In combination with phenylalanine deficiency, an excessive amount of phenylketones contributes to the postnatal completion of myelination of nerves, resulting in profound cognitive impairment.

Figure 3.16D represents a genetic alteration of the enzyme **d**, which is involved in the feedback control of synthesis of **K**. As a result, **K** may accumulate to toxic levels. The prototype genetic disease here is

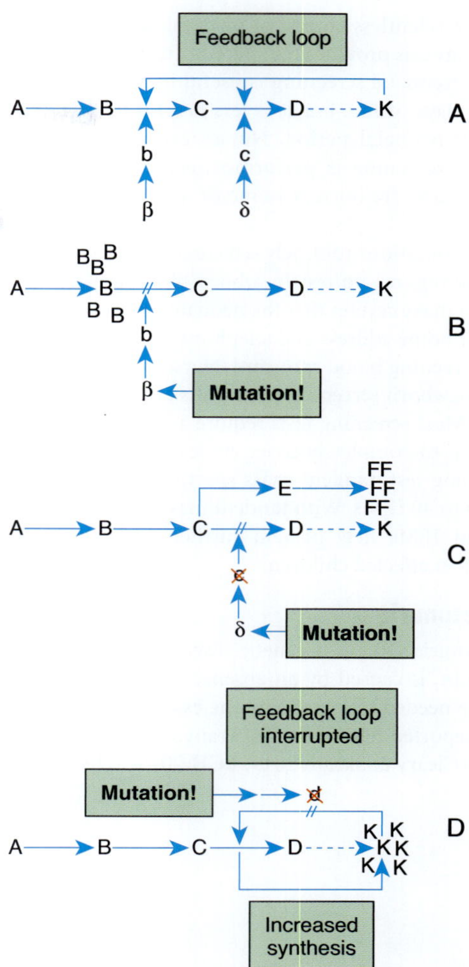

Fig 3.16 Metabolic pathway. (**A**) Normal metabolic pathway. (**B**) Mutation of gene β. (**C**) Mutation of gene δ. (**D**) Genetic alteration of enzyme d. A, substance; B–F, by-products; K, end-product; b, c and d, enzymes; β and δ, genes. (Source: Adapted from da Cunha, M. F. (2000). Genetic basis of human disease. In B. A. Bullock & R. L. Henze (Eds.), *Focus on physiology.* Philadelphia, Pennsylvania: Lippincott.)

Lesch-Nyhan syndrome, in which **d** is the enzyme hypoxanthine-guanine phosphoribosyltransferase (HGPRT) and **K** is uric acid. A deficiency in HGPRT and accumulation of uric acid to extremely high levels will result in the development of cognitive impairment and self-mutilation tendency.

The mode of inheritance in IEMs is almost always autosomal recessive. The heterozygote has one gene with a normal effect and is still able to produce the enzyme in sufficient amounts to carry out the metabolic function under normal circumstances. Therefore, the heterozygote does not exhibit symptoms of the disorder. The homozygote, who inherits a defective gene from both parents, has no functioning enzyme and thus is clinically affected.

Individually, different IEMs are rare; collectively they account for a significant proportion of health problems in children. It is becoming possible to detect and screen for an increasing number of IEMs—to detect the disease in the heterozygote, the newborn and the fetus and to identify heterozygotes at risk for having a child with an IEM. With most IEMs, early diagnosis and prompt treatment are essential to prevent a relentless course of physical and mental deterioration. Prenatal diagnosis provides for special care of the infant immediately after birth. Neonatal screening is useful in detecting many disorders after a few days of life, but it is less helpful in detecting symptoms early in the neonatal period. Nurses caring for neonates must be certain that screening is performed, especially in infants who are discharged early, are born at home or are in neonatal intensive care units.

A list of conditions routinely screened in each state can be found at https://www.vcgs.org.au/tests/newborn-bloodspot-screening. Nurses also need to make certain that the neonate has a primary care provider and current home address and telephone number documented on the newborn screening blood spot card. Nurses should instruct parents to ask about newborn screening test results at their newborn's first well-child visit. Most screening tests require a heel puncture to obtain sufficient blood to completely cover circles on special blotting paper. A new screening test, tandem mass spectrometry, has the potential to identify up to 40 IEMs. With tandem mass spectrometry, earlier identification of IEMs may prevent further developmental delays and morbidities in affected children.

Phenylketonuria

Phenylketonuria (PKU), a genetic disease inherited as an autosomal recessive trait, is caused by an absence of the enzyme phenylalanine hydroxylase needed to metabolise the essential amino acid phenylalanine. The reported figures for PKU range from 1 per 10,000 to 15,000 live births (Cleary & Skeath 2019, RCH 2019). The disease has a wide variation of incidence by ethnic groups. The disease is most prevalent among individuals of Northern European ancestry, American Indians and Alaskan Natives, whereas African American, Hispanic, Jewish and Asian individuals account for the lowest frequencies.

Pathophysiology

In PKU the hepatic enzyme phenylalanine hydroxylase, which controls the conversion of phenylalanine to tyrosine, is absent. This results in the accumulation of phenylalanine in the bloodstream and urinary excretion of abnormal amounts of its metabolites, the phenyl acids (Fig 3.17). One of these phenyl ketones, phenylpyruvic acid, gives urine the characteristic musty odour associated with this disease and is responsible for the term *phenylketonuria.*

Amino acids produced by the metabolism of phenylalanine are absent in PKU. One of these, tyrosine, is needed to form the pigment melanin and the hormones adrenaline and thyroxine. Decreased melanin production results in similar phenotypes of most children with PKU: blond hair, blue eyes and fair skin that is particularly susceptible to eczema and other dermatological problems. Children with a genetically darker skin colour may be red haired or brunette.

Severe hyperphenylalaninaemia (>360 to 600 mmol/L) causes progressive damage to the developing brain with severe consequences: defective myelination, cystic degeneration of the grey and white matter and disturbances in cortical lamination. Cognitive impairment occurs before the metabolites are detected in the urine and will progress if ingested phenylalanine levels are not lowered.

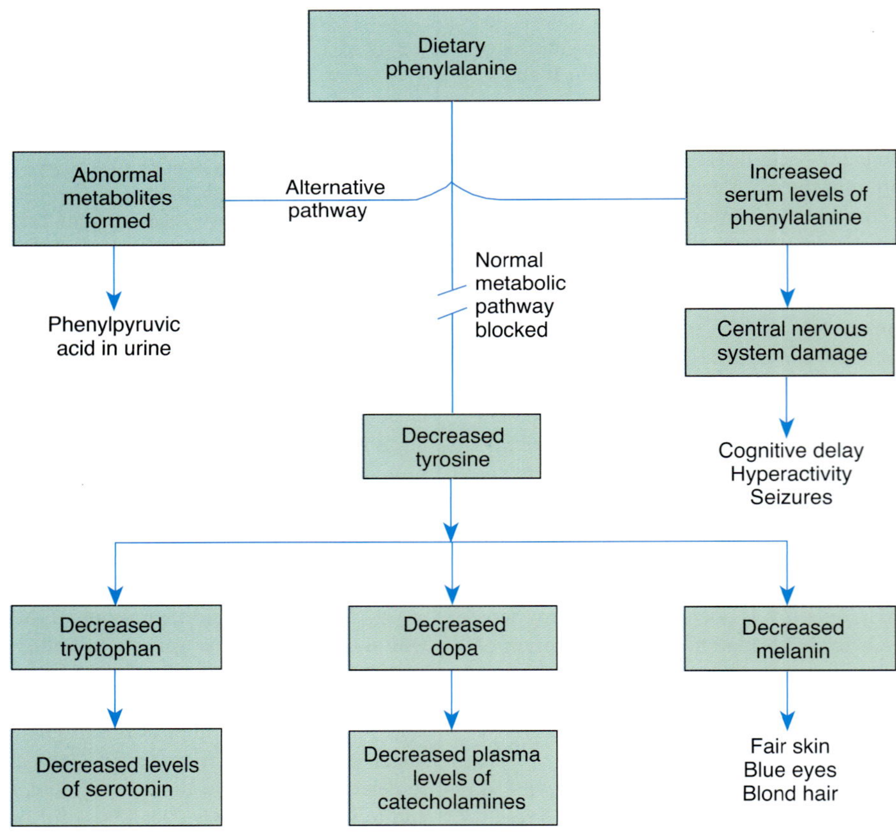

Fig 3.17 Metabolic errors and consequences in phenylketonuria.

Clinical Manifestations

Clinical manifestations of PKU include: growth failure (failure to thrive); frequent vomiting; irritability; hyperactivity; and unpredictable, erratic behaviour. Older children commonly display bizarre or schizoid behaviour patterns such as fright reactions, screaming episodes, head banging, arm biting, disorientation, failure to respond to strong stimuli and spasticity or catatonia-like positions. Many of the severely cognitively impaired children have seizures, and approximately 80% of untreated persons with PKU demonstrate abnormal electroencephalographs, regardless of whether overt seizures occur.

Diagnostic Evaluation

The objective in diagnosing or treating the disorder is to prevent cognitive impairment. The most commonly used test for screening newborns is Guthrie's bacterial inhibition assay for phenylalanine in the blood. *Bacillus subtilis,* present in the culture medium, grows if the blood contains an excessive amount of phenylalanine. The normal range of blood phenylalanine concentration in newborns is 0.5 to 1 mg/dL. The Guthrie test detects serum phenylalanine levels greater than 4 mg/dL (normal value is 1.6 mg/dL). Only fresh heel blood, not cord blood, can be used for the test.

Newborn screening tests are mandatory in Australia and New Zealand. In New Zealand, the newborn screening tests are attended by the midwives or nurse within the first 48 hours where possible, or as close to this time as possible (Ministry of Health 2019). The midwife or nurse collects a small amount of blood from the baby's heel onto the spot card, which is then sent for testing. In Australia and New Zealand, regardless of the gestational age of the newborn, the baby is screened where possible in the first 48 hours. If needed, collection can be repeated if the infant is receiving multiple transfusing or complex care and treatment, but if possible do not delay too long. Guidelines to assist with when to repeat are as follows.

- Birth weight < 1000 g: repeat sample no later than 6 weeks of age
- Birth weight 1000–1500 g: repeat sample no later than 4 weeks of age

If recollection has been missed, collect the sample as soon as this is recognised.

Therapeutic Management

Treatment of PKU involves the restriction of dietary protein. As with most genetic disorders, because the genetic enzyme is intracellular, systemic administration of phenylalanine hydroxylase is of no value. Phenylalanine cannot be totally eliminated because it is an essential amino acid in tissue growth. Therefore, dietary management must meet two criteria: fulfil the child's nutritional need for optimum growth and maintain phenylalanine levels within a safe range.

Treatment for infants with sustained blood phenylalanine levels greater than 360 micromol/L is recommended. Although the threshold for adverse effects of elevated blood phenylalanine is not known, treatment of phenylalanine levels between 120 and 360 micromol/L is not recommended, but close follow-up for the first few years of life is important (Vockley et al 2014). A lifetime reduction of phenylalanine intake is necessary to prevent neuropsychological and cognitive deficits. To evaluate the effectiveness of dietary treatment, frequent monitoring of blood phenylalanine and tyrosine levels is necessary. The blood **phenylalanine** concentration in newborns is normally 0.5 to 1 mg/dL (30 to 60 micromol/L).

Phenylalanine levels should be carefully monitored throughout the first 12 years of age and, once stable, monthly assessments are still recommended.

A low-phenylalanine diet begins as soon as possible after birth and continues throughout life. Adherence to this diet can be especially challenging in adolescence and adulthood. To evaluate the effectiveness of dietary treatment, frequent monitoring of blood phenylalanine and tyrosine levels is necessary. Because phenylalanine levels greater than or equal to 20 mg/dL in mothers with PKU affect the normal embryonic development of the fetus, women with PKU who are not on a lifelong diet must resume a low-phenylalanine diet before pregnancy.

Prognosis. Although many individuals with treated PKU manifest no cognitive and behavioural deficits, many comparisons of individuals with PKU to controls show lower performance on IQ tests, with larger differences in other cognitive domains. However, their performance is still in the average range. Evidence for differences in behavioural adjustment is inconsistent despite anecdotal reports suggesting greater risk for internalising psychopathology and attention disorders. In addition, there are insufficient data on the effects of phenylalanine restriction over many decades of life (Vockley et al 2014). Total bone mineral density is considerably lower in children who are on a low-phenylalanine diet, even though calcium, phosphorus and magnesium intakes are higher than normal.

Nursing Care Management

The principal nursing considerations involve educating the family regarding the dietary restrictions. Although the treatment may sound simple, the task of maintaining such a strict dietary regimen is demanding, especially for older children and adolescents. Foods with low phenylalanine levels (e.g. some vegetables [except legumes]; fruits; juices; and some cereals, breads and starches) must be measured to provide the prescribed amount of phenylalanine. Most high-protein foods, such as meat and dairy products, are either eliminated or restricted to small amounts.

Maintaining the diet during infancy presents few problems. Parents can introduce solid foods such as cereal, fruits and vegetables as usual to the infant. Difficulties arise as the child gets older. A decreased appetite and refusal to eat may reduce intake of the calculated phenylalanine requirement. The child's increasing independence may inhibit absolute control of what he or she eats. Either factor can result in decreased or increased phenylalanine levels. During the school years, peer pressure becomes a major force in deterring the child from eating the prescribed foods or abstaining from high-protein foods such as milkshakes or ice cream. Adolescence is a particularly difficult period, and limiting foods containing phenylalanine in adolescents with PKU is challenging.

Parents need a basic understanding of the disorder and practical suggestions regarding food selection and preparation; therefore, the assistance of a dietitian is highly recommended. For rural and remote regions, this may not be possible so telehealth or connecting with the Children's Hospitals for support may be needed.

Galactosaemia

Galactosaemia transferase deficiency is caused by galactose-1-phosphate uridyl. The birth incidence is 1:40,000 in 2018 in most Western countries (Sydney Children's Hospitals Network n.d.). The disorder presents itself through an accumulation in the blood of one of the sugars (galactose) in milk. If left untreated babies can become extremely unwell and die.

Clinical Features

In its most severe form, galactosaemia is due to an almost complete deficiency of galactose-1-phosphate uridyl transferase (Gal-1-PUT) enzyme activity occurring in all cells within the body. Early clinical presentation includes neonatal hypoglycaemia, jaundice, vomiting and (if left untreated) liver failure and death if gram-negative sepsis presents within 1 to 2 weeks of birth. If the infant can survive until past the neonatal period, there are long-term impacts such as failure to thrive, cirrhosis, kidney disease (proximal renal tubular acidosis), cataracts and possible intellectual delay.

Mild Bariants

Galactosaemia can present with several genetic variants while only demonstrating partial enzyme deficiency. The Duarte variant, where babies are asymptomatic and no treatment is required, is one presentation. Mild elevation of galactose metabolites due to reduced activity in the Gal-1-PUT enzyme may be the only indicator in the first 3 months of life to demonstrate galactosaemia.

Galactokinase Deficiency

This is a rare defect which is associated with the development of cataracts within infancy and has a possible link to delayed intellectual development. Life-threatening symptoms do not present in this instance.

Laboratory Tests

The use of manual fluormetic assay for galactose and/or galactose-1-phosphate are preferred to detect elevated galactose metabolites, usually indicating an elevation of 1 mmol/L in normal neonates. When this is detected, a follow-up test is required to further separate the sugars, which allows for determination of the levels of galactose or galactose-1-phosphate. Upon completion of this follow-up test, the metabolite increase demonstrates the enzyme defect leading to galactosaemia. Urgent testing of the elevated galactose metabolites is carried out for Gal-1-PUT activity.

Treatment

Exclusion of all galactose within the diet is the primary treatment for galactosaemia syndromes. Other treatments if galactosaemia is suspected are the implementation of supportive treatment of the baby and family, ongoing monitoring for hypoglycaemia, liver failure, bleeding disorders and in particular *Escherichia coli* sepsis (Sydney Children's Hospitals Network n.d.).

Prognosis

Studies following the children's treatment from birth or within the first 2 months of life after the presentation of symptoms have demonstrated several long-term complications. Ovarian dysfunction, cataracts, abnormal speech, growth restrictions, cognitive impairment and delayed motor development have all been reported (Coelho et al 2017). These findings also demonstrated that the elimination of the sources of galactose has no significant impact on improving the outcome. Ongoing research with new therapeutic interventions such as replacing depleted metabolites, enhancing residual transferase activity and the use of gene replacement therapy are all being explored to improve the outcome and prognosis for children with galactosaemia.

Screening Considerations

In severe (classical) galactosaemia, the Gal-1-PUT assay should present abnormal in all cases, regardless of whether the specimen has been obtained before lactose is ingested. The only time this may not be the case is if the infant has had an exchange transfusion prior to specimen collection. Due to galactosaemia being fatal, it should always be considered in an infant with non-glucose-reducing substances in the urine. Regardless of this not being a reliable test, it must be considered along with aminoacidopathies other than PKU.

Nursing Care Management

When considering nursing interventions, dietary restrictions are a priority and much easier to maintain in this instance because compared to other IEMs, more foods are allowed. Encourage families to read food labels carefully to monitor for the presence of all forms of lactose, particularly in dairy products. Educate families to check for lactose in medications and in syrups and liquids in particular. Many oral liquid antibiotics contain high levels of lactose within the mixture and are often unlabelled. Encourage families to always ask the pharmacist about galactose content within all products and medications, prescription and over the counter.

Cytogenetic Diagnostic Techniques

Chromosomes have traditionally been studied under light microscopy. After a significant number of cells are prepared so the chromosomes can be visualised during mitotic metaphase under a light microscope and imaged through a computer, their chromosomes are displayed in a karyotype, arranged according to their size, position of their centromeres and banding patterns. The most common human cells used for chromosome studies are peripheral blood leucocytes obtained by venepuncture and cells obtained by biopsy from a variety of tissues, such as skin (including fetal skin cells), chorionic villi and bone marrow. Robotic cell harvesters and computerised imaging systems have drastically cut down on manual labour; however, expert technicians and cytogeneticists are still necessary to analyse and interpret karyotypes.

Although karyotypes still have an important role in identifying large chromosomal rearrangements such as translocations, they have been replaced by chromosomal microarray testing as the preferred tool for evaluating children with congenital malformations and intellectual or global developmental delays and for whom a clinical diagnosis is uncertain (Rosenfeld & Patel 2017).

When clinical examination, health history and developmental history are strongly suggestive of a known condition, a less expensive targeted test can be used to identify the specific microdeletion, microduplication or fragile site.

Molecular Diagnostic Techniques

Identification of single-gene mutations responsible for a growing number of genetic disorders is now possible with a variety of molecular tests. In some conditions, such as CF, sickle cell disease, myotonic dystrophy and fragile X syndrome, the specific gene is known and tests are available that target many of the known disease-associated mutations or that sequence the coding portions of the gene associated with the specific condition. Gene panels for some disorders have become available as technology improves to make it easier and less expensive to analyse a number of genes at one time. Finally, technology has made it possible to target sequencing of exons within a group of genes or the entire genome (Korf & Rehm 2013). When exons in the entire genome are sequenced, it is called *whole exome sequencing*. When all accessible DNA within a genome is sequenced, it is called *whole genome sequencing*. Whole exome or whole genome sequencing is used to diagnose rare disorders for which specific testing is not available or when a clinically diagnosed condition can be caused by a mutation in one of many possible genes. The use of whole exome or whole genome sequencing in healthy newborns is being studied (Ceyhan-Birsoy et al 2017).

Predisposition Genetic Testing

Molecular diagnostic techniques have enabled **predisposition testing**, which is the identification of gene mutations associated with genetic disorders in asymptomatic individuals. Depending on the penetrance of the allele(s), these may be considered presymptomatic or susceptibility tests.

Familial adenomatous polyposis is one of several overlapping conditions associated with mutations in the *APC* gene. These mutations are considered virtually 100% penetrant, resulting in hundreds to thousands of adenomatous polyps and eventual colon cancer. Once the *APC* mutation has been identified in an affected family member, at-risk family members can be tested for the same mutation. Because of the high penetrance, such testing in asymptomatic individuals would be considered presymptomatic testing. *APC* mutation testing in at-risk children is done to identify those who need colon screening and to identify polyp formation early so cancer-preventive surgical decisions can be made (Hegde et al 2014).

Therapeutic Management of Genetic Disease

Therapy for genetic disease is currently aimed at correcting the phenotypical expression of a variant gene; therefore, the major goal of therapy is modification of the internal or external environment to correct or minimise the effects of the variant gene or pair of variant genes. However, genomic advances have opened doors to genotype intervention, and clinical applications of gene manipulation techniques are currently being tested.

Phenotype Modification

Examples of currently used intervention aimed at modifying the phenotypical expression of genetic disorders follow.

Surgical Management. Surgical repair of structural defects has made it possible to prolong life in a number of multifactorial disorders, such as congenital heart disease and NTDs. Numerous facial and limb deformities can be corrected by plastic and reconstructive techniques.

Diet Modification. For disorders in which an enzyme deficiency causes a toxic accumulation of a substance or its by-products, restricting the intake of foods containing that substance may prevent irreversible damage from the improper metabolism of these compounds. This dietary control is lifelong and requires a high level of adherence.

Metabolic Manipulation. In some deficiency diseases, supplying the missing product that cannot be synthesised prevents undesirable effects. For example, thyroid hormone is prescribed to prevent the damaging effects of hypothyroidism, and providing the missing blood factors prevents life-threatening and debilitating haemorrhages in persons with different types of haemophilia. Other examples are insulin for diabetes mellitus, growth hormone for growth hormone deficiency and corticosteroids for adrenogenital syndrome.

Removal of toxic substances that accumulate in vital tissues as a result of a hereditary disease can prevent disabling complications. Some of the deleterious effects of haemochromatosis, a hereditary disorder characterised by an excess accumulation of iron in the liver, heart and pancreas, can be reduced with the removal of iron by periodic therapeutic phlebotomies or administration of chelating agents.

Avoidance of Drugs or Other Harmful Substances. In drug-induced disease, such as glucose-6-phosphate dehydrogenase (G6PD) deficiency and the porphyrias, avoidance of the drugs that precipitate a reaction is a simple preventive measure. These include aspirin and quinine-based antimalarial medications in the case of G6PD deficiency, and ethanol, barbiturates, anticonvulsants, sulfonamides and oral contraceptives in the case of acute intermittent porphyria (Valle et al 2014). Some anaesthetic agents may precipitate symptoms of malignant hyperthermia.

Immunological Prevention. The administration of immunoglobulin to Rh-negative mothers after the birth of an Rh-positive infant is effective in preventing Rh-antibody formation, which causes haemolytic disease of the newborn in subsequent births.

Transplantation. Better control of tissue incompatibility problems is improving the survival of children undergoing replacement of nonfunctioning organs with normal organs. Transplanted organs include the kidneys in hereditary polycystic kidneys, the heart in severe cardiac myopathy, the liver in hepatic atresia and stem cell transplant for Fanconi's anaemia.

Gene Product Replacement. Recombinant DNA technology makes it possible to produce large quantities of certain gene products. Such technology avoids the infectious contamination risk that accompanied extraction of gene products from mass quantities of human blood or tissue.

The administration of gene products is especially applicable when the missing product is a circulatory peptide or protein, as in coagulation factor VIII or IX in haemophilia type A and type B, respectively (Saenko & Pipe 2006). If the gene product is membrane bound, as is the case for enzymes deficient in various lysosomal storage diseases, the natural enzyme product may need to be purposely altered so that it can enter the cell through a naturally occurring cell receptor.

Environmental Modification

Inherited diseases or defects with no therapeutic modality can be modified to enhance the quality of life for the affected individual. Some examples of environmental manipulation include hearing aids for children with congenital hearing loss, glasses or vision enhancers such as books in enlarged print or braille for the visually impaired, mobilising devices such as braces and wheelchairs for persons with muscle and bone impairment, prosthetic devices for those with limb deficiencies and infant stimulation programs to maximise the potential of children who are developmentally delayed. Environmental manipulation also includes protection from the damaging effects of the environment, such as exposure to sunlight, which can cause skin fragility and blistering in persons with porphyrias and increases the risk of skin cancers in patients with xeroderma pigmentosum and oculocutaneous albinism.

IMPACT OF HEREDITARY DISORDERS ON THE FAMILY

Genetic Testing

Genetic testing can be broadly divided into two categories: diagnostic testing and screening. Tests to detect a disease-associated gene mutation or chromosome abnormality in symptomatic individuals are rapidly assuming greater importance in management of genetic disorders as more genes and mutations are identified and techniques are developed for easy application of the tests.

With improved technology, mass screening for numerous genetic disorders will probably become routine. However, to be truly effective, screening programs depend on thorough education of both health professionals and the public regarding these programs and the limitations and implications of testing. The religious, moral, ethical and legal issues revolving around screening and prenatal diagnosis are extensive and change over time.

Purposes of Screening

Genetic screening is presumptive identification of an unrecognised genetic predisposition for future disease in individuals or their progeny for which preventive or disease course–altering interventions exist. In general, genetic screening targets populations, whereas genetic diagnostic testing targets individuals. The first corollaries of any genetic screening intervention must be *voluntary participation, equal access to all* and *confidentiality* (both in conducting the tests and in handling records and results). In addition, education and counselling about tests and procedures must be an integral part of any screening program. Attention must be paid to quality control of all aspects of testing and laboratory procedures.

Genetic screening has three purposes: (1) to provide for early recognition of a disease, before signs and symptoms occur, for which effective intervention and therapy exist (e.g. PKU); (2) to identify carriers of a genetic disease for the purpose of maximising parenthood planning options (e.g. Tay-Sachs disease); and (3) to obtain population data on frequency, spectrum and natural history of genetic variations not currently known to be associated with disease.

Screening for genetic disorders can occur during various times in a person's life: (1) preconception screening of selected populations for heterozygous carriers (e.g. Ashkenazi Jewish carrier screening panel); (2) screening of relatives of known carrier or affected individuals within a family, for the purpose of reproductive decision-making; (3) postconceptional (prenatal) screening (e.g. maternal serum screen for identifying risks for NTDs and chromosome abnormalities); and (4) newborn screening.

Screening for Reproductive Information. Screening for heterozygotes (carriers) can detect unaffected persons with certain variant genes who, when they mate with an individual who carries a mutation in the same gene, are at high risk of producing an affected offspring. These individuals are thus provided with the information they need for making decisions about family planning. Carriers of a number of diseases can be detected by laboratory tests, but, because of the rarity of these diseases, mass screening is not feasible except in persons or populations known to be at risk. Persons at risk include close relatives of those with an inborn error of metabolism or other detectable disorder and certain ethnic populations known to have a high incidence of a specific disease, such as sickle cell anaemia in African Americans, Tay-Sachs disease in Ashkenazi Jews and thalassaemia in persons of Mediterranean ancestry (Holtkamp et al 2017).

Newborn screening tests reveal carrier status for certain conditions such as CF and sickle cell disease. Careful counselling is necessary with carrier screening to ensure that individuals understand the limitations of testing and the implications of results. Even with careful counselling, there may be significant misunderstanding or misuse of information.

Screening for Epidemiological Information. Public health officials may use screening as a method for monitoring the incidence of diseases or malformations in a population to detect environmental or other causes that might significantly influence the incidence of the disorders. For example, geographical and socioeconomic variations in the incidence of NTDs eventually led to research that determined that folic acid supplementation of 0.4 mg/day in women of childbearing age reduces NTD occurrence within the population.

Significance of Screening to Families

Mass screening programs have received mixed acceptance from health professionals and the general public. Potential benefits of carrier screening include facilitating genetic counselling and reproductive planning and providing useful information to other at-risk family members.

Prenatal Testing

Paediatric nurses may encounter couples who had prenatal testing and are preparing for the anticipated care of their unborn child. Such couples may be making primary care arrangements; meeting professionals in the newborn intensive care unit; meeting with surgeons to learn about the surgeries their newborn will need in the first few days, weeks or months of life; and talking with other parents who have children with the same condition. Thus it is important that paediatric nurses have a general understanding of the capabilities, limitations and risks of prenatal testing.

Prenatal Screening Tests

Non-invasive screening uses maternal blood or ultrasound to assess fetal risk for certain congenital malformations or chromosome abnormalities. Maternal age has been the longest-standing screening measure to detect women at increased risk for having a child with a chromosome abnormality. The most common laboratory screening method is to analyse maternal serum for abnormal levels of pregnancy-related chemical markers (such as free human chorionic gonadotropin [hCG], unconjugated oestriol and pregnancy-associated plasma protein A).

Prenatal Diagnostic Procedures

Recommendations for diagnostic testing may be triggered by preexisting risks (e.g. previous child with a genetic disorder), personal characteristics (e.g. member of subpopulation at risk for certain genetic diseases) or a newly identified risk following prenatal screening for the current pregnancy (see Box 3.2). Specific risk factors are usually identified in the family history, previous pregnancy outcomes or the mother's medical history. Ethnic risk factors are based on a higher

BOX 3.2 Indications for Prenatal Testing

General Risk Factors

- Maternal age of at least 35 years at time of delivery or at least 31 years if twin gestation
- Elevated or low trisomy profile screen results

Specific Risk Factors

- Previous child with a structural defect or chromosome abnormality
- Previous stillbirth or neonatal death
- Structural abnormality in mother or father
- Balanced translocation in mother or father
- Inherited disorders—cystic fibrosis, metabolic disorders, sex-linked recessive disorders
- Medical disease in mother—diabetes mellitus, phenylketonuria
- Exposure to a teratogen—ionising radiation, anticonvulsant medicines, lithium, isotretinoin, alcohol
- Infection—rubella, toxoplasmosis, cytomegalovirus
- Abnormal ultrasound findings

Ethnic Risk Factors

- Disorder—ethnic or racial group
- Tay-Sachs disease—Ashkenazi Jewish, French Canadian
- Sickle cell anaemia—Black African, Mediterranean, Arab, Indian, Pakistani
- α- and β-thalassaemia—Mediterranean, Southern and Southeast Asian, Chinese

carrier frequency for certain genetic diseases in selected populations. Indications for prenatal diagnosis when any of these risk factors is present are based on a greater than general population risk that a congenital anomaly or genetic disorder will occur in the pregnancy. The specific risk is, of course, different for each situation.

A few additional diagnostic tests are infrequently used. Fetal biopsy is sometimes used to diagnose certain genetic skin disorders and metabolic disorders when DNA studies are unavailable or are uninformative. Fetal echocardiography may be performed for further diagnosis when a cardiac defect is noted on ultrasound or if prior prenatal procedures reveal the fetus has a genetic disorder in which cardiac malformations may occur.

Genetic Evaluation and Counselling

The expanded recognition of genetic diseases and disorders and an increasingly well-informed public are creating a justified demand for genetic evaluation, diagnosis, information regarding risks to present and future generations, and access to available therapies. Unfortunately, however, persons who need expert genetic counselling often make uninformed decisions on their own or are the victims of well-meaning but equally uninformed relatives, acquaintances or paraprofessionals. Nurses involved in infant and child care continually encounter families that have a risk of transmitting a disorder to an offspring, as well as children who may have an undiagnosed genetic disorder that needs expert evaluation.

More often, persons who inquire about the possibility of recurrence of a disease or disorder have a child with a genetic disease or disorder or had a child who died of the disease. They are concerned about the likelihood of having another similarly affected child and may want to know what reproductive choices are available.

Genetic Services

Comprehensive genetic services consist of a group of specialists, which may include clinical geneticists, advanced practice nurses in genetics, genetic counsellors, psychologists, biochemical geneticists, cytogeneticists, nurses, social workers and other allied health professionals.

Genetic counselling is a communication process that deals with the human problems associated with the occurrence, or risk of occurrence, of a genetic disorder in a family. This process involves an attempt by one or more appropriately trained persons to help the individual or family:

- comprehend the medical facts, including the diagnosis, the probable course of the disorder and the available management
- appreciate the way heredity contributes to the disorder and the risk of recurrence in specified relatives
- understand the options for dealing with the risk of recurrence
- choose the course of action that seems appropriate to them in view of their risk and family goals and act in accordance with that decision
- make the best possible adjustment to the disorder in an affected family member and to the risk of recurrence of that disorder.

Estimation of Risks

Risks for occurrence or recurrence of a genetic disorder are estimated from a thorough family history and any known genetic screening information. A careful, detailed family history not only provides a picture of the **proband** (the affected person, or index case) in relation to other family members, but also may identify others who are similarly affected or who might be presymptomatic or at risk of producing affected children. Analysing the pattern of affected family members can assist in confirming a tentative diagnosis or in determining the level of risk in multifactorial inheritance.

An accurate diagnosis is essential to provide specific risk figures. There are more than 10,000 known inherited disorders, many of which have similar clinical manifestations but different modes of inheritance. For example, symptoms in the early stages of severe X-linked muscular dystrophy appear much like those of the milder autosomal recessive and autosomal dominant varieties, autosomal recessive neurogenic muscular atrophies and non-genetic poliomyelitis. The significance of the risks related to each type of disorder is readily apparent. For disorders with an unknown or multifactorial cause, recurrence risks are termed *empiric,* meaning they are based on observations of recurrence in similar situations, rather than *theoretic,* meaning they are based on mendelian inheritance patterns.

Communicating Risks

Genetic professionals do not attempt to make recommendations or decisions for patients when discussing reproductive risks. Instead, they discuss comprehensive and current information about the nature of the disorder, the extent of risk, the probable consequences and alternative solutions. The goal of this communication process is to enable patients to make their own decisions about whether to pursue preconception or prenatal testing and what to do in response to test results. However, genetics professionals recognise that recommendations do have a place when genetic testing is used to identify risk for diseases or disorders that have available treatments that can prevent, delay or improve symptoms.

Role of Nurses

All nurses need to be prepared to use genetic and genomic information and technology when providing care. The professional practice domains include applying/integrating genetic knowledge into nursing assessment; identifying and referring clients who may benefit from genetic information or services; identifying genetics resources and services to meet clients' needs; and providing care and support before, during and after providing genetic information and/or services. Often a nurse is the first one to recognise the need for genetic evaluation by identifying an inherited disorder in a family history or by noting physical, cognitive or behavioural abnormalities when performing a nursing assessment (Box 3.3).

Genetic counsellors support people through genetic testing including:

- assisting with decision-making about whether to have a test and what test(s) to have
- waiting for the results, understanding the meaning of the results and adjusting to the results
- providing supportive counselling to families
- arranging referrals to other health professionals
- linking families with community support services.

Nursing Assessment: Applying and Integrating Genetic and Genomic Knowledge

Family health history is an important tool to identify individuals and families at increased risk for disease, risk factors for disease (such as obesity) and inheritance patterns of diseases. Because of its importance, all nurses need to be able to elicit family history information and, when feasible, document the collected information in pedigree format.

Identification and Referral

It is a nurse's responsibility to learn basic genetic principles, to be alert to situations in which families could benefit from genetic evaluation and counselling, to know about special services that can help manage and support affected children and to be familiar with facilities in their

BOX 3.3 Assessment Clues to Genetic Disorders*

Major or minor birth defects (anomalies) and dysmorphic features—Cardiac defect, ear or eye abnormalities, micrognathia, forehead prominence, hairline low set on forehead or nape of neck, wide-set eyes (hypertelorism), epicanthal folds, low-set or abnormal ears.

Growth abnormalities—Short stature, overgrowth, asymmetrical growth, intrauterine growth retardation

Skeletal abnormalities—Limb abnormalities, asymmetry, scoliosis, hyperextensible joints, hypotonic or hypertonic muscle tone, pectus excavatum, finger or joint abnormalities

Visual or hearing problems—Coloboma of the iris, hearing loss, congenital or early-onset cataracts

Metabolic disorders—Unusual odour of breath, urine or stool

Sexual development abnormalities—Ambiguous genitalia, micropenis, delayed onset of puberty, primary amenorrhoea, precocious sexual development, large testicles

Skin disorders—Unusual pigmentation patterns (e.g. café-au-lait spots, vitiligo), dry and scaly skin, skin tumours, hyperextensible skin

Recurrent infection or immunodeficiency—Ear infection, pneumonia, poor healing of umbilicus

Development and Speech Delays or Loss of Developmental Milestones

Cognitive delays—Learning disabilities, mild to severe cognitive impairment

Behavioural disorders—Attention-deficit disorders with or without hyperactivity, autistic behaviour, aggressive behaviour

*Increased concern for genetic aetiology if two or more findings are present.

areas where these services are available. In this way, nurses will be able to direct individuals and families to needed services and be active participants in the genetic evaluation and counselling process.

Early identification of a genetic disorder allows anticipation of associated conditions and implementation of available preventive measures and therapy to avoid potential complications and to enhance the child's health. It may also prevent the unexpected birth of another affected child in the immediate or extended family.

Providing Education, Care and Support

Maintaining contact with the family or making a referral to a healthcare practice or an agency that can provide a sustained relationship is critical. It is becoming more common for genetics healthcare professionals to provide regular follow-up and management, particularly for children with rare genetic disorders. However, some families choose not to have follow-up visits with genetic experts.

Nurses must assess for and address parents' feelings of guilt about carrying 'bad genes' or having 'made my child sick'. Depending on the type of cytogenetic disorder, the nurse may be able to absolve the parents of guilt by explaining the random nature of segregation during both gamete formation and fertilisation and that those errors in cell division unique to the pregnancy in question are not likely to happen again and are not inherited. If the condition is a mendelian-inherited or mitochondrial disorder, it is important to assess parents' understanding of recurrence risk, help them understand the chances that a subsequent pregnancy will not be affected and ensure that they have been given information about their options for future children (preimplantation diagnosis, use of donor egg or sperm, prenatal diagnosis or adoption). Families often try to reason that some unrelated event caused the abnormality (e.g. a fall, a urinary tract infection or 'one glass of wine') before the mother was aware that she was pregnant. These misconceptions need to be assessed and dispelled.

After a genetics visit, and sometimes before the visit, parents often use the internet to find answers to their questions. During the initial genetics evaluation, a diagnosis may not be possible. Instead, findings in medical, developmental and family histories lead the professional to order genetic tests and other diagnostic procedures. Diagnoses under consideration are discussed briefly with the parents. Some parents are satisfied with the brief information and do not care to find out more until the actual diagnosis is established. Other parents go home and seek as much information as they can about the diagnoses under consideration. The information they find can be terrifying and overwhelming and inaccurate or misleading. Nurses can play an important role in helping parents identify reliable, accurate resources for information at whatever time they desire it. It is also important to stress that everything that is described for a genetic condition may not be relevant to their child. Before the follow-up genetics visit when test and procedure results are discussed, nurses can help parents identify and write down the questions and concerns they need addressed before leaving the clinic.

Initial and ongoing assessment of the family's coping abilities, resources and support systems is vital to determine their need for additional assistance and support. As with any family who has a child with chronic healthcare needs, nurses must teach the family to become the child's advocate. Nurses can help families locate agencies and clinics specialising in a specific disorder or its consequences that can provide services (e.g. equipment, medication and rehabilitation), educational programs and parent support groups. Referral to local and national support groups or contact with a local family that has a child with the same condition can be helpful for new parents. Privacy and confidentiality are imperative, and both families must give permission before their contact information is given. Nurses can also be instrumental in helping parents evaluate disease-specific social media groups and blogs or starting a local support group when none is available.

Parental attachment and adjustment to the baby can be supported and facilitated by nursing interventions. Assessing the parents' understanding of the child's disorder and providing simple and truthful explanations can help them begin to understand their child's health issues. Guiding the parents in recognising their child's cues, responses and strengths can be helpful even for experienced parents. A caring attitude conveys the value of their child and, by extension, their value as parents. The nurse can help the parents identify their strengths as a family and identify support that is available to them.

Some families do struggle after learning their child has a genetic disorder. Families may feel ashamed of a hereditary disorder and seek to blame their partner for transmitting a faulty gene or chromosome. Intrafamilial strife, hostility and marital or couple disharmony, sometimes to the point of family disintegration, can occur. Nurses should be alert for evidence of risk factors that indicate poor adjustment (e.g. child abuse, divorce or other maladaptive behaviours). Referral to psychosocial professionals for crisis intervention may be necessary.

REFERENCES

Antshel, K. M., Fremont, W., Kates, W. R., et al. (2008). The neurocognitive phenotype in velo-cardio-facial syndrome: A developmental perspective. Developmental Disabilities Research Reviews, 14(1), 43–51.

Bennett, R. L., French, K. S., Resta, R. G., et al. (2008). Standardized human pedigree nomenclature: Update and assessment of the recommendations of the National Society of Genetic Counselors. Journal of Genetic Counseling, 17, 424–433.

Ceyhan-Birsoy, O., Machini, K., Lebo, M. S., et al. (2017). A curated gene list for reporting results of newborn genomic sequencing. Genetics in Medicine, 19(7), 809–818.

Cleary, M. A., & Skeath, R. (2019). Phenylketonuria. Paediatrics and child health, 29(3), 111–115.

Coelho, A. I., Rubio-Gozalbo, M. E., Vicente, J. B., et al. (2017). Sweet and sour: An update on classic galactosemia. Journal of Inherited Metabolic Disease, 40(3), 325–342.

Committee on Genetics. (2011). Health supervision for children with fragile X syndrome. Pediatrics, 127, 994–1006.

Down Syndrome Australia. (2020). Resources. About Down syndrome. What is Down syndrome? https://www.downsyndrome.org.au/about-down-syndrome/what-is-down-syndrome/

Hegde, M., Ferber, M., Mao, R., et al. (2014). ACMG technical standards and guidelines for genetic testing for inherited colorectal cancer (Lynch syndrome, familial adenomatous polyposis, and MYH-associated polyposis). Genetics in Medicine, 16(1), 101–116.

Holtkamp, K. C., Mathijssen, I. B., Lakeman, P., et al. (2017). Factors for successful implementation of population-based expanded carrier screening: Learning from existing initiatives. European Journal of Public Health, 27(2), 372–377.

Jorde, L. B., Carey, J. C., Bamshad, M. J., et al. (2016). Medical genetics (5th ed.). Philadelphia: Elsevier.

Korf, B. R., & Rehm, H. L. (2013). New approaches to molecular diagnosis. JAMA: The Journal of the American Medical Association, 309(14), 1511–1521.

McDonald-McGinn, D. M., Emanuel, B. S., & Zackai, E. H. (1999). 22q11.2 Deletion syndrome. In R. A. Pagon, T. D. Bird, C. R. Dolan, et al. (Eds.), GeneReviews™ [Internet]. Seattle, Washington. http://www.ncbi.nlm.nih.gov/books/NBK1523/. Updated 2013 Feb 28.

Ministry of Health. (2019). Your Health. Pregnancy and kids. Newborn metabolic screening. https://www.health.govt.nz/your-health/pregnancy-and-kids/first-year/first-6-weeks/health-checks-first-6-weeks/newborn-screening-tests/newborn-metabolic-screening

New Zealand Down Syndrome Association. (n.d.). Support and information. Health. https://nzdsa.org.nz/support/health/

Passias, P., Poorman, G., Jalai, C. et al (2019) Incidence of congenital spinal abnormalities among pediatric patients and their association with scoliosis and systemic anomalies. Journal of Pediatric Orthopedics, 39(8), 608–613. ISSN: 0271-6798 PMID: NLM31393300

Peng, R., Zheng, J., Xie, H. N., et al. (2019). Genetic anomalies in fetuses with tetralogy of Fallot by using high-definition chromosomal microarray analysis. Cardiovascular Ultrasound, 17(1), 8.

Prows, C. A., Hopkin, R. J., Barnoy, S., et al. (2013). An update of childhood genetic disorders. Journal of Nursing Scholarship, 45(1), 34–42.

Rosenfeld, J. A., & Patel, A. (2017). Chromosomal microarrays: Understanding genetics of neurodevelopmental disorders and congenital anomalies. Journal of Pediatric Genetics, 6(1), 42–50.

Saenko, E. L., & Pipe, S. W. (2006). Strategies towards a longer acting factor VIII. Haemophilia: The Official Journal of the World Federation of Hemophilia, 12(Suppl. 3), 42–51.

Scherdel, P., Matczak, S., Léger, J., et al. (2018). Algorithms to define abnormal growth in children: external validation and head-to-head comparison. Journal of Clinical Endocrinology & Metabolism, 104(2), 241–249.

Schneider, K., Zelley, K., Nichols, K. E., et al. (1999). Li-Fraumeni syndrome. In R. A. Pagon, M. P. Adam, T. D. Bird, et al. (Eds.), GeneReviews™ [Internet]. University of Washington, Seattle, Washington. http://www.ncbi.nlm.nih.gov/books/NBK1311/. [Updated 2013 Apr 11].

Sydney Children's Hospitals Network. (n.d.). Laboratory services. https://www.schn.health.nsw.gov.au/find-a-service/laboratory-services/nsw-newborn-screening/disorders

The Royal Children's Hospital (RCH). (2019). Newborn bloodspot screening. RCH, Parkville.

The Royal Children's Hospital (RCH). (2020). Endocrinology and diabetes. Turner's syndrome. RCH, Parkville. https://www.rch.org.au/endo/Conditions/turner-syndrome

The Royal Children's Hospital. Division of Medicine. Department of General Medicine. Screening for children with Down syndrome. (n.d.). RCH, Parkville. https://www.rch.org.au/genmed/clinical_resources/Screening_for_children_with_Down_Syndrome/

Valle, D., Beaudet, A. L., Vogelstein, B., et al. (Eds.) (2014). The online metabolic and molecular bases of inherited disease. New York: McGraw-Hill. http://ommbid.mhmedical.com/content.aspx?bookid=971§ionid=62632315

Vockley, J., Andersson, H. C., Antshel, K. M., et al. (2014). Phenylalanine hydroxylase deficiency: Diagnosis and management guideline. Genetics in Medicine, 16(2), 188–200.

Waisman Center. (2016). Waisman Center DWTE DS 2016 - Christian [video], *Waisman Center*. 18 March. YouTube. https://www.youtube.com/watch?v=aqhaC3R3tP4&feature=youtu.be

INTERNET RESOURCES

GeneReviews—https://www.ncbi.nlm.nih.gov/books/NBK1116/ (expert-written, peer-reviewed, regularly updated resource of comprehensive descriptions of genetic conditions that include diagnosis, management and genetic counselling for patients and their families)

Australian Institute of Family Studies—https://aifs.gov.au/publications/family-matters/issue-96/ethical-research-involving-children (Graham, A., Powell, M. A., & Taylor, N. [2015]. Ethical research involving children: Putting the evidence into practice. *Family Matters*, 96, 23–28.)

International Society of Nurses in Genetics—http://www.isong.org/ (provides information about various education resources, conferences targeting nurses)

National Human Genome Research Institute—http://www.genome.gov (information on genome research and its ethical, legal and social implications)

National Organization for Rare Disorders—https://rarediseases.org/ (a federation of voluntary health organisations dedicated to helping people with rare 'orphan' diseases)

United Mitochondrial Disease Foundation—http://www.umdf.org/ (provides information about mitochondrial defects, including professional and lay materials)

4

Communication, Physical and Developmental Assessment of the Child and Family

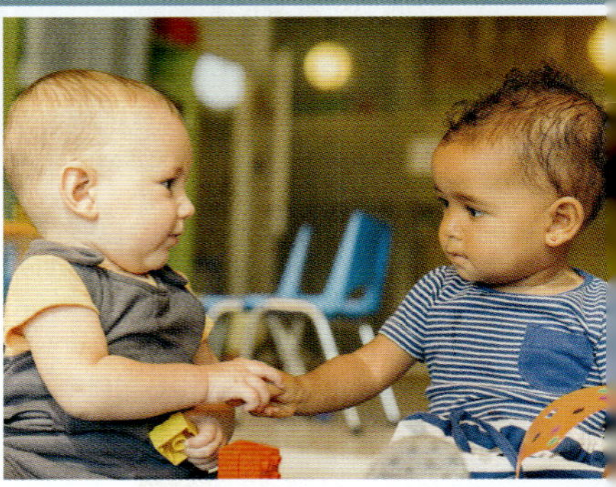

Andrea Middleton

LEARNING OUTCOMES

- Understand the complexities in physical and developmental assessment of infants, children and adolescents
- Understand the importance of family centred care and building therapeutic relationships with patients and their families/caregiver
- Explore communication and distraction techniques

GUIDELINES FOR COMMUNICATION AND INTERVIEWING

The most widely used method of communicating with parents on a professional basis is the interview process. Unlike social conversation, **interviewing** is a specific form of goal-directed communication. As nurses converse with children and adults, they focus on the individuals to determine the kind of persons they are, their usual mode of handling problems, whether they need help and the way they react to counselling. Developing interviewing skills requires time and practice, but following some guiding principles can facilitate this process. An organised approach is most effective when using interviewing skills in patient teaching.

Establishing a Setting for Communication

Appropriate Introduction

Introduce yourself and ask the name of each family member who is present and their preferred name, ensuring to document this on the medical record and other spaces as appropriate such as beside the child's bed.

At the beginning of the interview, include children in the interaction by asking them their name, preferred name, age and other information. Nurses often direct all questions to adults even when children are old enough to speak for themselves. This only terminates one extremely valuable source of information—the patient. When including the child, follow the general rules for communicating with children given in the Nursing Care Considerations box later in the chapter.

Assurance of Privacy and Confidentiality

The place where the nurse conducts the interview is almost as important as the interview itself. The physical environment should allow for as much privacy as possible, with distractions (such as interruptions, noise or other visible activity) kept to a minimum. At times, it is necessary to turn off a television, radio or mobile phone. The environment should also have some play provision for young children to keep them occupied during the parent–nurse interview (Fig 4.1). Parents who are constantly interrupted by their children are unable to concentrate fully and tend to give brief answers to finish the interview as quickly as possible.

Confidentiality is another essential component of the initial phase of the interview. Because the interview is usually shared with other members of the healthcare team or the teacher (in the case of students), be certain to inform the family of the limits regarding confidentiality. If confidentiality is a concern in a particular situation, such as when talking to a parent suspected of child abuse or a teenager contemplating suicide, deal with this directly and inform the person that in such instances, confidentiality cannot be assured. However, the nurse judiciously protects information of a confidential nature.

Computer Privacy and Applications in Nursing

The use of computer technology to store and retrieve health information has become widespread; most institutions now maintain electronic health records for patients. The healthcare community is increasingly concerned about the privacy and security of this health information and all nurses are engaged in protecting confidentiality of healthcare records. Any person accessing confidential health information is charged with managing safeguards for disclosure, including password protection to prevent violation of patient privacy and confidentiality.

Telephone Triage, Telehealth and Counselling

Telephone triage care management and telehealth have increased access to high-quality healthcare services and empowered parents to participate in their child's healthcare. It has the potential to engage hard-to-reach populations; for example, socially isolated families living in regional areas, families of low socioeconomic status, families with English as a second language and families with a parent with

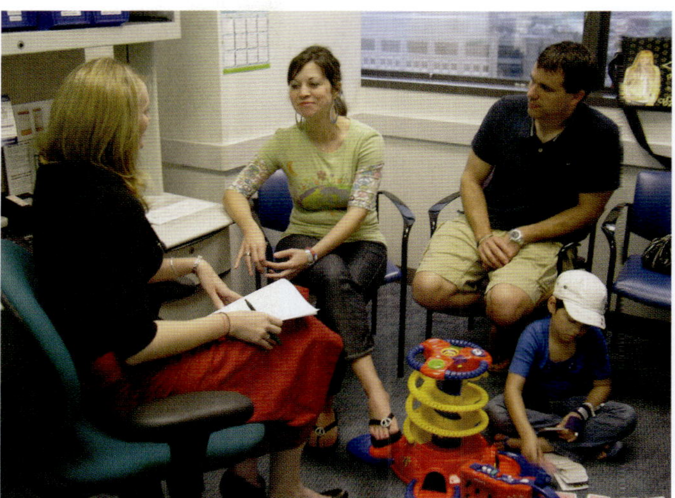

Fig 4.1 Child plays while the nurse interviews parent.

mental health issues (Campbell et al 2019, Smith et al 2020). Consequently, patient satisfaction has significantly improved.

Telephone triage is more than 'just a phone call' because a child's life is a high price to pay for poorly managed or incompetent telephone assessment skills. Typically, guidelines for telephone triage include asking screening questions, determining when to immediately refer to emergency medical services (dial 000 in Australia, 111 in New Zealand) or the emergency department, and determining when to refer to same-day appointments, appointments in 24 to 72 hours, appointments in 4 days or more or home care (Box 4.1). Telehealth could include a pre-arranged phone appointment with a nurse, medical specialist or allied health professional. Successful outcomes are based on the consistency and accuracy of the information provided. Telehealth professionals require advanced communication skills, in part to compensate for lack of visual cues (Campbell et al 2019) and to decipher information given from patients, parents or caregivers.

A systematic review of 49 studies where nurses triaged calls found that the appropriateness of a decision and subsequent compliance often varied (Blank et al 2012). A meta-analysis of 13 studies provided further insight and found that patient compliance with triage recommendations were influenced by the quality of provider communication (Purc-Stephenson & Thrasher 2012). The importance of nurse–patient communication is reinforced as an essential aspect of telephone triage training. Training of communication skills that are patient and family centred and specifically address active listening and advising skills offers the greatest opportunity for success. Assessment skills used in direct nurse-to-patient interactions are not directly transferable to the telephone and provide further support for training in decision-making skills for phone triage (Purc-Stephenson & Thrasher 2010). Evidence-based clinical protocols for telephone triage can provide a structured method for assessment (Stacey et al 2013).

BOX 4.1 Telephone Triage Guidelines

- Date and time
- Background:
  - name, age, sex, contact information
  - chronic illness
  - allergies, current medications, treatments or recent immunisations
- Chief complaint
- General symptoms:
  - severity
  - duration
  - other symptoms
  - pain
- Systems review
- Steps taken:
  - advised to call emergency medical services (000 in Australia, 111 in NZ)
  - advised to go to emergency department
  - advised to see practitioner (today, tomorrow or later appointment)
  - advised regarding home care
  - advised to call back if symptoms worsen or fail to improve

COMMUNICATING WITH FAMILIES

Communicating with Parents

Although the parent and the child are separate and distinct individuals, the nurse's relationship with the child is frequently mediated by the parent, particularly with younger children. For the most part, nurses acquire information about the child by direct observation or through communication with the parents. Usually it can be assumed that because of the close contact with the child, the parent gives reliable information. Assessing the child requires input from the child (verbal and non-verbal), information from the parent and the nurse's own observations of the child and interpretation of the relationship between the child and the parent. When children are old enough to be active participants in their own healthcare, the parent becomes a collaborator.

Encouraging the Parents to Talk

Interviewing parents offers not only the opportunity to determine the child's health and developmental status but also information about factors that influence the child's life. Whatever the parent sees as a problem should be a concern of the nurse. These problems are not always easy to identify. Nurses need to be alert for clues and signals by which a parent communicates worries and anxieties. Careful phrasing with broad, open-ended questions (such as 'What is Ari eating now?') provides more information than several single-answer questions (such as 'Is Ari eating what the rest of the family eats?').

Sometimes the parent will take the lead without prompting. At other times, it may be necessary to direct another question on the basis of an observation, such as 'Yindi seems unhappy today', or 'How do you feel when Yindi cries?' If the parent appears to be tired or distraught, consider asking, 'What do you do to relax?' or 'What help do you have with the children?' A comment such as 'You handle Kirra very well. What kind of experience have you had with babies?' to new parents who appear comfortable with their first child gives positive reinforcement and provides an opening for questions they might have on the infant's care. Often all that is required to keep parents talking is a nod or saying 'yes' or 'uh-huh'.

Directing the Focus

Directing the focus of the interview while allowing maximum freedom of expression is one of the most difficult goals in effective communication. One approach is the use of open-ended or broad questions, followed by guiding statements. For example, if the parent proceeds to list the other children by name, say, 'Tell me their ages, too'. If the parent continues to describe each child in depth, which is not the purpose of the interview, redirect the focus by stating, 'Let's talk about the other children later. You were beginning to tell me about Kai's activities at school'. This approach conveys interest in the other children but focuses the assessment on the patient.

Listening and Cultural Awareness

Listening is the most important component of effective communication. When the purpose of listening is to understand the person being interviewed, it is an active process that requires concentration and attention to all aspects of the conversation—verbal, non-verbal and abstract. Major blocks to listening are environmental distraction and premature judgment.

Although it is necessary to make some preliminary judgments, listen with as much objectivity as possible by clarifying meanings and attempting to see the situation from the parent's point of view. Effective interviewers consciously control their reactions and responses and the techniques they use. (See Cultural Considerations box.)

CULTURAL CONSIDERATIONS

Interviewing without Judgment

It is easy to inject one's own attitudes and feelings into an interview. Often nurses' own prejudices and assumptions, which may include racial, religious and cultural stereotypes, influence their perceptions of a parent's behaviour. What the nurse may interpret as a parent's passive hostility or lack of interest may be shyness or an expression of anxiety. For example, in Western cultures, eye contact and directness are signs of paying attention. However, in many non-Western cultures, including that of some Indigenous Australians, directness (e.g. looking someone in the eye) can be viewed as being rude, disrespectful or even aggressive (Queensland Health 2015). Children are taught to avert their gaze and to look down when being addressed by an adult, especially one with authority (Ball et al 2014). Therefore, nurses must make judgments about 'listening', as well as verbal interactions, with an appreciation of cultural differences.

Careful listening relies on the use of clues, verbal leads or signals from the interviewee to move the interview along. Frequent references to an area of concern, repetition of certain key words or a special emphasis on something or someone serve as cues to the interviewer for the direction of inquiry. Concerns and anxieties are often mentioned in a casual, offhand manner. Even though they are casual, they are important and deserve scrutiny to identify problem areas. For example, a parent who is concerned about a child's habit of bedwetting may casually mention that the child's bed was 'wet this morning'.

Using Silence

Silence as a response is often one of the most difficult interviewing techniques to learn. The interviewer requires a sense of confidence and comfort to allow the interviewee space in which to think without interruptions. Silence permits the interviewee to sort out thoughts and feelings and search for responses to questions. Silence can also be a cue for the interviewer to go more slowly, re-examine the approach and not push too hard (Ball et al 2014).

Sometimes it is necessary to break the silence and reopen communication. Do this in a way that encourages the person to continue talking about what is considered important. Breaking a silence by introducing a new topic or by prolonged talking essentially terminates the interviewee's opportunity to use the silence. Suggestions for breaking the silence include statements such as the following.

- 'Is there anything else you wish to say?'
- 'I see you find it difficult to continue; how may I help?'
- 'I don't know what this silence means. Perhaps there is something you would like to put into words but find difficult to say.'

Being Empathic

Empathy is the capacity to understand what another person is experiencing from within that person's frame of reference; it is often described as the ability to put oneself in another's shoes. The essence of empathic interaction is accurate understanding of another's feelings. Empathy differs from **sympathy**, which is having feelings or emotions similar to those of another person, rather than understanding those feelings.

Providing Anticipatory Guidance

The ideal way to handle a situation is to deal with it before it becomes a problem. The best preventive measure is anticipatory guidance. Traditionally, **anticipatory guidance** focused on providing families information on normal growth and development and nurturing childrearing practices. For example, one of the most significant areas in paediatrics is injury prevention. Beginning prenatally, parents need specific instructions on home safety. Because of the child's maturing developmental skills, parents must implement home safety changes early to minimise risks to the child.

Unprepared parents can be disturbed by many normal developmental changes, such as a toddler's diminished appetite, negativism, altered sleeping patterns and anxiety towards strangers. The chapters on health promotion provide nurses with information for counselling parents. However, anticipatory guidance should extend beyond giving general information to empowering families to use the information as a means of building competence in their parenting abilities (Dosman & Andrews 2012). To achieve this level of anticipatory guidance, the nurse should do the following:

- base interventions on needs identified by the family, not by the professional
- view the family as competent or as having the ability to be competent
- provide opportunities for the family to achieve competence.

Avoiding Blocks to Communication

A number of blocks to communication can adversely affect the quality of the helping relationship. The interviewer introduces many of these blocks, such as giving unrestricted advice or forming prejudged conclusions. Another type of block occurs primarily with the interviewees and concerns **information overload**. When individuals receive too much information or information that is overwhelming, they often demonstrate signs of increasing anxiety or decreasing attention. Such signals should alert the interviewer to give less information or to clarify what has been said. Box 4.2 lists some of the more common blocks to communication, including signs of information overload.

The nurse can correct communication blocks by careful analysis of the interview process. One of the best methods for improving interviewing skills is audiotape or videotape feedback. With supervision and guidance, the interviewer can recognise the blocks and consciously avoid them.

Communicating with Families Through an Interpreter

Sometimes communication is impossible because two people speak different languages. In this case it is necessary to obtain information through a third party: the interpreter. When using an interpreter, the nurse follows the same interviewing guidelines. Specific guidelines for using an adult interpreter are given in the Nursing Care Considerations box.

BOX 4.2 Blocks to Communication

Communication Barriers (Nurse)
- Socialising
- Giving unrestricted and sometimes unsought advice
- Offering premature or inappropriate reassurance
- Giving overready encouragement
- Defending a situation or opinion
- Using stereotyped comments or clichés
- Limiting expression of emotion by asking directed, closed-ended questions
- Interrupting and finishing the person's sentence
- Talking more than the interviewee
- Forming prejudged conclusions
- Deliberately changing the focus

Signs of Information Overload (Patient)
- Long periods of silence
- Wide eyes and fixed facial expression
- Constant fidgeting or attempting to move away
- Nervous habits (e.g. tapping, playing with hair)
- Sudden interruptions (e.g. asking to go to the bathroom)
- Looking around
- Yawning, eyes drooping
- Frequently looking at a watch or clock
- Attempting to change the topic of discussion

NURSING CARE CONSIDERATIONS

Using an Interpreter

- Explain to the interpreter the reason for the interview and the type of questions that will be asked.
- Clarify whether a detailed or brief answer is required and whether the translated response can be general or literal.
- Introduce the interpreter to the family, and allow some time before the interview for them to become acquainted.
- Communicate directly with family members when asking questions to reinforce interest in them and to observe non-verbal expressions, but do not ignore the interpreter.
- Pose questions to elicit only one answer at a time, such as 'Do you have pain?' rather than 'Do you have any pain, tiredness or loss of appetite?'
- Refrain from interrupting family members and the interpreter while they are conversing.
- Avoid commenting to the interpreter about family members because they may understand some English.
- Be aware that some medical words, such as *allergy,* may have no similar word in another language; avoid medical jargon whenever possible.
- Be aware that cultural differences may exist regarding views on sex, marriage or pregnancy.
- Allow time after the interview for the interpreter to share something that he or she thought could not be said earlier; ask about the interpreter's impression of non-verbal clues to communication and family members' reliability or ease in revealing information.
- Arrange for the family to speak with the same interpreter on subsequent visits whenever possible.

Communicating with families through an interpreter requires sensitivity to cultural, legal and ethical considerations (see Cultural Considerations box). In some cultures, class differences between the interpreter and the family may cause the family to feel intimidated and less inclined to offer information. Therefore, it is important to choose the interpreter carefully and provide time for the interpreter and family to establish rapport.

CULTURAL CONSIDERATIONS

Using Children as Interpreters

When no one else is available to interpret, there may be temptation to use a bilingual child within the family as an interpreter. However, the use of children in healthcare interpreting is strongly discouraged because they are often not mature enough to understand healthcare questions, answers or messages. Children may inadvertently commit interpretive errors, such as inaccuracies, omissions or substitutions. In addition, children can be adversely affected by serious or sensitive information that may be discussed. In some cultures, using a child as an interpreter is considered an insult to an adult because children are expected to show respect by not questioning their elders. Note that some institutions prohibit the use of children as interpreters; check institutional policy for compliance. If a trained on-site or community-based interpreter is not available, a *language line* using a telephonic interpreter may be an option.

In obtaining informed consent through an interpreter, the nurse should fully inform the family of all aspects of the particular procedure to which they are consenting. Issues of confidentiality may arise when family members related to another patient are asked to interpret for the family, thus revealing sensitive information that may be shared with other families on the unit. With increased sensitivity towards patient rights and confidentiality, many institutions now require consent forms translated in the patient's primary language.

Communicating with Children

Although the greatest amount of verbal communication is usually carried out with the parent, do not exclude the child during the interview. Pay attention to infants and younger children through play or by occasionally directing questions or remarks to them. Include older children as active participants so that they can share their own experiences and perspectives.

In communication with children of all ages, the non-verbal components of the communication process convey the most significant messages. It is difficult to disguise feelings, attitudes and anxiety when relating to children. They are alert to surroundings and attach meaning to every gesture and move that is made; this is particularly true of very young children.

Active attempts to make friends with children before they have had an opportunity to evaluate an unfamiliar person tend to increase their anxiety. Continue to talk to the child and parent but go about activities that do not involve the child directly, thus allowing the child to observe from a safe position. If the child has a special toy or doll, 'talk' to the doll first. Ask simple questions such as 'Does your teddy bear have a name?' to ease the child into conversation. Other guidelines for communicating with children are in the Nursing Care Considerations box. Specific guidelines for preparing children for procedures are provided in Chapter 22.

Communication Related to Development of Thought Processes

The normal development of language and thought offers a frame of reference for communicating with children. Thought processes progress from sensorimotor to perceptual to concrete and finally to abstract, formal operations. An understanding of the typical characteristics of these stages provides the nurse with a framework to facilitate social communication.

Infancy. Because they are unable to use words, infants primarily use and understand non-verbal communication. Infants communicate their needs and feelings through non-verbal behaviours and vocalisations that can be

NURSING CARE CONSIDERATIONS

Communicating with Children

- Allow children time to feel comfortable.
- Avoid sudden or rapid advances, broad smiles, extended eye contact or other gestures that may be seen as threatening.
- Talk to the parent if the child is initially shy.
- Communicate through transition objects (such as dolls, puppets and stuffed animals) before questioning a young child directly.
- Give older children the opportunity to talk without the parents present.
- Assume a position that is at the same level as the child (Fig 4.2).
- Speak in a quiet, unhurried and confident voice.
- Speak clearly, be specific and use simple words and short sentences.
- State directions and suggestions positively.
- Offer a choice only when one exists.
- Be honest with children.
- Allow children to express their concerns and fears.
- Use a variety of communication techniques.

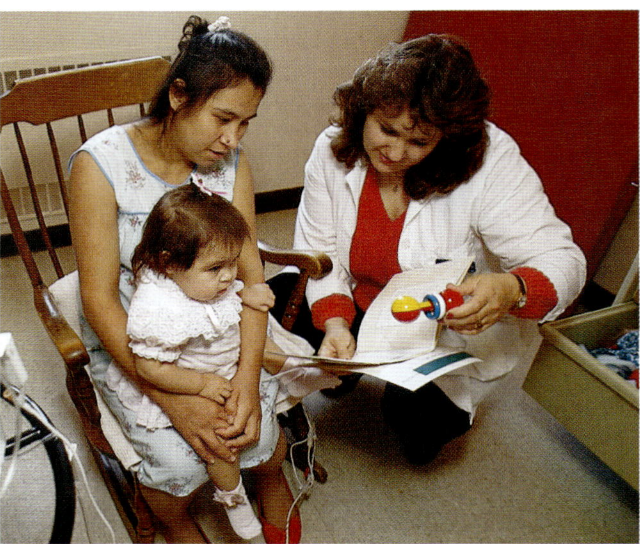

Fig 4.2 Nurse assumes position at the child's level.

interpreted by someone who is around them for a sufficient time. Infants smile and coo when content and cry when distressed. Crying is provoked by unpleasant stimuli from inside or outside, such as hunger, pain, body restraint or loneliness. Adults interpret this to mean that an infant needs something and consequently try to alleviate the discomfort by meeting their physical needs, speaking softly and communicating through touch.

Infants respond to adults' non-verbal behaviours. They become quiet when they are cuddled, rocked or receive other forms of gentle physical contact. They receive comfort from the sound of a soft voice even though they do not understand the words that are spoken. Until infants reach the age at which they experience stranger anxiety, they readily respond to any firm, gentle handling and quiet, calm speech. Loud, harsh sounds and sudden movements are frightening.

Early Childhood. Children younger than 5 years of age are **egocentric**. They see things only in relation to themselves and from their point of view. Therefore, focus communication on them. Tell them what they can do or how they will feel. Experiences of others are of no interest to them. It is futile to use another child's experience in an attempt to gain the cooperation of small children. Allow them to touch and examine articles they will come in contact with. A stethoscope bell will feel cold; palpating a neck might tickle. Although they have not yet acquired sufficient language skills to express their feelings and wants, toddlers can effectively use their hands to communicate ideas without words. They push an unwanted object away, pull another person to show them something, point and cover the mouth that is saying something they do not wish to hear.

Everything is direct and concrete to small children. They are unable to work with abstractions and interpret words literally. Analogies escape them because they are unable to separate reality from fantasy. For example, they attach literal meaning to such common phrases as 'two-faced', 'sticky fingers' or 'coughing your head off'. Children who are told they will get 'a little stick in the arm' may not be able to envision an injection (Fig 4.3). Therefore use simple, direct language rather than phrases that might be misinterpreted by a small child.

School-age Years. Younger school-age children rely less on what they see and more on what they know when faced with new problems. They want explanations and reasons for everything but require no verification beyond that. They are interested in the functional aspect of all procedures, objects and activities. They want to know why an object exists, why it is used, how it works and the intent and purpose of its user. They need to know what is going to take place and why it is being done to them specifically. For example, to explain a procedure such as taking blood pressure, show the child how squeezing the bulb pushes air into the cuff and makes the 'arrow' move. Let the child operate the bulb. An explanation for the procedure might be as simple as, 'I want to see how far the arrow moves when the cuff squeezes your arm'. Consequently, the child becomes an enthusiastic participant.

School-age children have a heightened concern about body integrity. Because of the special importance they place on their body, they are sensitive to anything that constitutes a threat or suggestion of injury to it. This concern extends to their possessions, so they may appear to overreact to loss or threatened loss of treasured objects. Encouraging children to communicate their needs and voice their concerns enables the nurse to provide reassurance, to dispel myths and fears and to implement activities that reduce their anxiety. For example, if a shy child dislikes being the centre of attention, ignore that particular child by talking and relating to other children in the family or group. When children feel more comfortable, they will usually interject personal ideas, feelings and interpretations of events.

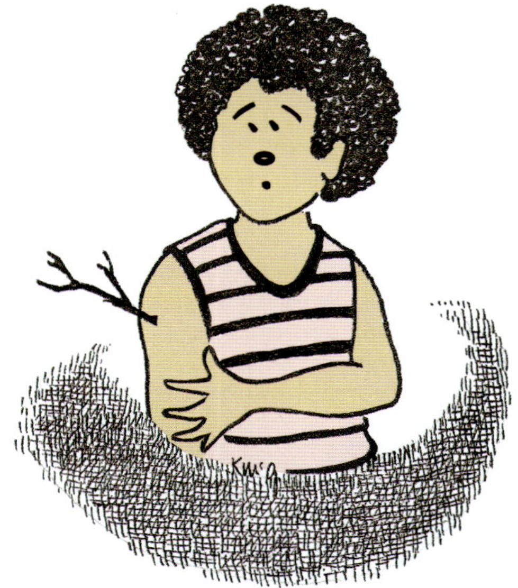

Fig 4.3 A young child may take the expression 'a little stick in the arm' literally.

Adolescence. As children move into adolescence, they fluctuate between child and adult thinking and behaviour. They are riding a current that is moving them rapidly towards a maturity that may be beyond their coping ability. Therefore when tensions rise, they may seek the security of the more familiar and comfortable expectations of childhood. Anticipating these shifts in identity allows the nurse to adjust the course of interaction to meet the needs of the moment. No single approach can be relied on consistently, and encountering cooperation, hostility, anger, bravado and a variety of other behaviours and attitudes is common. It is as much a mistake to regard an adolescent as an adult with an adult's wisdom and control as it is to assume that the teenager has the concerns and expectations of a child.

Interviewing the adolescent presents some special issues. The first may be whether to talk with the adolescent alone or with the adolescent and parents together. If the parents and teenager are together, talking with the adolescent first has the advantage of immediately identifying with the young person, thus fostering the interpersonal relationship. However, talking with the parents initially may provide insight into the family relationship. In either case, give both parties an opportunity to be included in the interview. If time is limited (such as during history taking), clarify this at the onset to avoid appearing to 'take sides' by talking more with one person than with the other.

Privacy and confidentiality are of great importance when interviewing adolescents because it is consistent with developmental maturity and autonomy. Explain to parents and teenagers the legal and ethical protections and limits of confidentiality. Nurses need to know and understand the consent, mandatory reporting and confidentiality laws pertaining to adolescent circumstances, such as suspected abuse, alcohol or other drug use, suicidal or homicidal ideation, contraceptive care, pregnancy, sexually transmitted infections and sexual assault (Child Family Community Australia [CFCA] 2020). Another dilemma in interviewing adolescents is that two views of a problem frequently exist: the teenager's and the parents'. Clarification of the problem is a major task. However, providing both parties an opportunity to discuss their perceptions in an open and unbiased atmosphere can, by itself, be therapeutic. Demonstrating positive communication skills can help families with adolescents to communicate more effectively (see Nursing Care Considerations box).

NURSING CARE CONSIDERATIONS

Communicating with Adolescents

Build a Foundation

- Spend time together.
- Encourage expression of ideas and feelings.
- Respect their views.
- Tolerate differences.
- Praise good points.
- Respect their privacy.
- Set a good example.

Communicate Effectively

- Give undivided attention.
- Listen, listen, listen.
- Be courteous, calm, honest and open minded.
- Try not to overreact. If you do, take a break.
- Avoid judging or criticising.
- Avoid the 'third degree' of continuous questioning.
- Choose important issues when taking a stand.
- After taking a stand:
  - think through all options
  - make expectations clear.

Communication Techniques

Nurses use a variety of verbal techniques to encourage communication. Some of these techniques are useful to pose questions or explore concerns in a less threatening manner. Others can be presented as word games, which are often well received by children. However, for many children and adults, talking about feelings is difficult, and verbal communication may be more stressful than supportive. In such instances, use several non-verbal techniques to encourage communication.

Box 4.3 describes both verbal and non-verbal techniques. Because of the importance of play in communicating with children, play is discussed more extensively in the section. Any of the verbal or non-verbal techniques can give rise to strong feelings that surface unexpectedly. Be prepared to handle them or to recognise when issues go beyond your ability to deal with them. At that point, consider an appropriate referral.

Play

Play is a universal language of children. It is one of the most important forms of communication and can be an effective technique in relating to them. The nurse can often pick up on clues about physical, intellectual and social developmental progress from the form and complexity of a child's play behaviours. Play requires minimum equipment or none at all. Many providers use therapeutic play to reduce the trauma of illness and hospitalisation (see Chapter 21) and to prepare children for therapeutic procedures (see Chapter 22).

Because their ability to perceive precedes their ability to transmit, infants respond to activities that register on their physical senses. Patting, stroking and other skin play convey messages. Repetitive actions, such as stretching infants' arms out to the side while they are lying on their backs and then folding the arms across the chest or raising and revolving the legs in a bicycling motion, will elicit pleasurable sounds. Colourful items to catch the eye or interesting sounds, such as a ticking clock, chimes, bells or singing, can be used to attract infants' attention.

Older infants respond to simple games. The old game of peek-a-boo is an excellent means of initiating communication with infants while maintaining a 'safe', non-threatening distance. After this intermittent eye contact, the nurse is no longer viewed as a stranger but as a friend. This can be followed by touch games. Clapping an infant's hands together for pat-a-cake or wiggling the toes for 'this little piggy' delights an infant or small child. Talking to a foot or other part of the child's body is another effective tactic. Much of the nursing assessment can be carried out with the use of games and simple play equipment while the infant remains in the safety of the parent's arms or lap.

The nurse can capitalise on the natural curiosity of small children by playing games such as 'Which hand do you take?' and 'Guess what I have in my hand', or by manipulating items such as a torch or stethoscope. Finger games are useful. More elaborate materials, such as puppets and replicas of familiar or unfamiliar items, serve as excellent means of communicating with small children. The variety and extent are limited only by the nurse's imagination.

Through play, children reveal their perceptions of interpersonal relationships with their family, friends or healthcare personnel. Children may also reveal the wide scope of knowledge they have acquired from listening to others around them. For example, through needle play, children may reveal how carefully they have watched each procedure by precisely duplicating the technical skills. They may also reveal how well they remember those who performed procedures. In one example, a child painstakingly re-enacted every detail of a tedious medical procedure, including the role of the physician who had repeatedly shouted

BOX 4.3 Creative Communication Techniques with Children

Verbal Techniques

'I' Messages

- Relate a feeling about a behaviour in terms of 'I'.
- Describe effect behaviour had on the person.
- Avoid use of 'you'.
- 'You' messages are judgmental and provoke defensiveness.

Example: 'You' message: 'You are being uncooperative about doing your treatments'.

Example: 'I' message: 'I am concerned about how the treatments are going because I want to see you get better'.

Third-person Technique

- Express a feeling in terms of a third person ('he', 'she', 'they'). This is less threatening than directly asking children how they feel because it gives them an opportunity to agree or disagree without being defensive.

Example: 'Sometimes when a person is sick a lot, he feels angry and sad because he cannot do what others can.' Either wait silently for a response or encourage a reply with a statement, such as 'Did you ever feel that way?'

- This approach allows children three choices: (1) to agree and, one hopes, express how they feel; (2) to disagree; or (3) to remain silent, which means they probably have such feelings but are unable to express them at this time.

Facilitative Response

- Listen carefully and reflect back to patients the feelings and content of their statements.
- Responses are empathic and non-judgmental and legitimise the person's feelings.
- Formula for facilitative responses: 'You feel _________ because _________'.

Example: If the child states, 'I hate coming to the hospital and getting needles', a facilitative response is, 'You feel unhappy because of all the things that are done to you'.

Storytelling

- Use the language of children to probe into areas of their thinking while bypassing conscious inhibitions or fears.
- The simplest technique is asking children to relate a story about an event, such as 'being in the hospital'.
- Other approaches:
  - show children a picture of a particular event, such as a child in a hospital with other people in the room, and ask them to describe the scene
  - cut out comic strips, remove words and have the child add statements for scenes.

Mutual Storytelling

- Reveal the child's thinking and attempt to change their perceptions or fears by retelling a somewhat different story (more therapeutic approach than storytelling).
- Begin by asking the child to tell a story about something; then tell another story that is similar to the child's tale but with differences that help the child in problem areas.

Example: The child's story is about going to the hospital and never seeing their parents again. The nurse's story is also about a child (using different names but similar circumstances) in a hospital whose parents visit every day, but in the evening after work, until the child is better and goes home with them.

Bibliotherapy

- Use books in a therapeutic and supportive process.
- Provide children with an opportunity to explore an event that is similar to their own but sufficiently different to allow them to distance themselves from it and remain in control.
- General guidelines for using bibliotherapy.
  1. Assess the child's emotional and cognitive development in terms of readiness to understand the book's message.
  2. Be familiar with the book's content (intended message or purpose) and the age for which it is written.
  3. Read the book to the child if the child is unable to read.
  4. Explore the meaning of the book with the child by having the child:
     - retell the story
     - read a special section with the nurse or parent
     - draw a picture related to the story and discuss the drawing
     - talk about the characters
     - summarise the moral or meaning of the story.

Dreams

- Dreams often reveal unconscious and repressed thoughts and feelings.
- Ask the child to talk about a dream or nightmare.
- Explore with the child what meaning the dream could have.

'What If' Questions

- Encourage the child to explore potential situations and to consider different problem-solving options.

Example: 'What if you got sick and had to go the hospital?' Children's responses reveal what they know already and what they are curious about, providing an opportunity for them to learn coping skills, especially in potentially dangerous situations.

Three Wishes

- Ask, 'If you could have any three things in the world, what would they be?'
- If the child answers, 'That all my wishes come true', ask the child for specific wishes.

Rating Game

- Use some type of rating scale (numbers, sad to happy faces) to have the child rate an event or feeling.

Example: Instead of asking youngsters how they feel, ask how their day has been 'on a scale of 1 to 10, with 10 being the best'.

Word Association Game

- State key words and ask children to say the first word they think of when they hear the word.
- Start with neutral words and then introduce more anxiety-producing words, such as 'illness', 'needles', 'hospitals' and 'operation'.
- Select key words that relate to some relevant event in the child's life.

Sentence Completion

- Present a partial statement and have the child complete it. Some sample statements include the following:
  - The thing I like best (least) about school is _________.
  - The best (worst) age to be is _________.
  - The most (least) fun thing I ever did was _________.
  - The thing I like most (least) about my parents is _________.
  - The one thing I would change about my family is _________.
  - If I could be anything I wanted, I would be _________.
  - The thing I like most (least) about myself is _________.

Pros and Cons

- Select a topic, such as 'being in the hospital', and have the child list 'five good things and five bad things' about it.
- This is an exceptionally valuable technique when applied to relationships, such as things family members like and dislike about each other.

BOX 4.3 **Creative Communication Techniques with Children—cont'd**

Non-verbal Techniques

Writing

- Writing is an alternative communication approach for older children and adults.
- Specific suggestions include the following:
  - keep a journal or diary
  - write down feelings or thoughts that are difficult to express
  - write 'letters' that are never mailed (a variation is making up a 'pen pal' to write to).
- Keep an account of the child's progress from both a physical and an emotional viewpoint.

Drawing

- Drawing is one of the most valuable forms of communication—both non-verbal (from looking at the drawing) and verbal (from the child's story of the picture).
- Children's drawings tell a great deal about them because they are projections of their inner selves.
- Spontaneous drawing involves giving the child a variety of art supplies and providing the opportunity to draw.
- Directed drawing involves a more specific direction, such as 'draw a person' or the 'three themes' approach (state three things about the child and ask the child to choose one and draw a picture).

Guidelines for Evaluating Drawings

- Use spontaneous drawings and evaluate more than one drawing whenever possible.
- Interpret the drawings in light of other available information about the child and their family, including the child's age and stage of development.
- Interpret the drawings as a whole rather than focusing on specific details of the drawings.
- Consider individual elements of the drawings that may be significant.
  - Sex of figure drawn first—Usually relates to the child's perception of his or her own sex role
  - Size of individual figures—Expresses importance, power or authority
  - Order in which figures are drawn—Expresses priority in terms of importance
  - The child's position in relation to other family members—Expresses feelings of status or alliance
  - Exclusion of a member—May denote feeling of not belonging or desire to eliminate
  - Accentuated parts—Usually express concern for areas of special importance (e.g. large hands may be a sign of aggression)
  - Absence of or rudimentary arms and hands—Suggest timidity, passivity or intellectual immaturity; tiny, unstable feet may express insecurity, and hidden hands may mean guilt feelings
  - Placement of drawing on the page and type of stroke—Free use of paper and firm, continuous strokes express security, whereas drawings restricted to a small area and lightly drawn in broken or wavering lines may be signs of insecurity
  - Erasures, shading or cross-hatching—Expresses ambivalence, concern or anxiety with a particular area

Magic

- Use simple magic tricks to help establish rapport with the child, encourage compliance with health interventions and provide effective distraction during painful procedures.
- Although the 'magician' talks, no verbal response from the child is required.

Play

- Play is the universal language and 'work' of children.
- It tells a great deal about children because they project their inner selves through the activity.
- Spontaneous play involves giving the child a variety of play materials and providing the opportunity to play.
- Directed play involves a more specific direction, such as providing medical equipment or a dollhouse for focused reasons, such as exploring the child's fear of injections or exploring family relationships.

at her to be still for the long ordeal. Her anger at him was most evident during the play session and revealed the cause for her abrupt withdrawal and passive hostility towards the medical and nursing staff after the test.

HISTORY TAKING

Performing a Health History

The format used for history taking may be: (1) **direct**, in which the nurse asks for information via direct interview with the informant; or (2) **indirect**, in which the informant supplies the information by completing some type of questionnaire. The direct method is superior to the indirect approach or a combination of both. However, because time is limited, the direct approach is not always practical. If the nurse cannot use the direct approach, he or she should review parents' written responses and question them regarding any unusual answers. The categories listed in Box 4.4 encompass children's current and past health status and information about their psychosocial environment.

Identifying Information

Much of the identifying information may already be available from other recorded sources. However, if the parent and child seem anxious, use this opportunity to ask about such information to help them feel more comfortable.

Informant. One of the important elements of identifying information is the **informant**, the person(s) who furnishes the information. Record: (1) who the person is (child, parent or other); (2) an impression of reliability and willingness to communicate; and (3) any special circumstances such as the use of an interpreter or conflicting answers by more than one person.

Chief Complaint

The **chief complaint** is the specific reason for the child's visit to the clinic, office or hospital. It may be the theme, with the present illness viewed as the description of the problem. Elicit the chief complaint by asking open-ended, neutral questions (e.g. 'What seems to be the matter?', 'How may I help you?' or 'Why did you come here today?'). Avoid labelling-type questions (e.g. 'How are you sick?' or 'What is the problem?'). It is possible that the reason for the visit is not an illness or problem.

Occasionally, it is difficult to isolate one symptom or problem as the chief complaint because the parent may identify many. In this situation, be as specific as possible when asking questions. For example, asking informants to state which one problem or symptom prompted them to seek help now may help them focus on the most immediate concern.

BOX 4.4 Outline of a Paediatric Health History

Identifying Information
1. Name
2. Address
3. Telephone
4. Birth date and place
5. Race or ethnic group
6. Sex
7. Religion
8. Date of interview
9. Informant

Chief complaint (CC): To establish the major specific reason for the child's and parents' seeking of healthcare

Present illness (PI): To obtain all details related to the chief complaint

Past history (PH): To elicit a profile of the child's previous illnesses, injuries or surgeries
1. Birth history (pregnancy, labour and delivery, perinatal history)
2. Previous illnesses, injuries or surgeries
3. Allergies
4. Current medications
5. Immunisations
6. Growth and development
7. Habits

Review of systems (ROS): To elicit information concerning any potential health problem
1. General appearance
2. Integument
3. Eyes
4. Ears
5. Nose
6. Mouth
7. Throat
8. Neck
9. Chest
10. Respiratory
11. Cardiovascular
12. Gastrointestinal
13. Genitourinary
14. Gynaecological
15. Musculoskeletal
16. Neurological
17. Endocrine
18. Haematological/lymphatic
19. Allergic/immunological
20. Psychiatric

Family medical history: To identify genetic traits or diseases that have familial tendencies and to assess exposure to a communicable disease in a family member and family habits that may affect the child's health, such as smoking and chemical use

Psychosocial history: To elicit information about the child's self-concept

Sexual history: To elicit information concerning the child's sexual concerns or activities and any pertinent data regarding adults' sexual activity that influences the child

Family history: To develop an understanding of the child as an individual and as a member of a family and a community
1. Family composition
2. Home and community environment
3. Occupation and education of family members
4. Cultural and religious traditions
5. Family function and relationships

Nutritional assessment: To elicit information on the adequacy of the child's nutritional intake and needs
1. Dietary intake
2. Clinical examination

Present Illness

The history of the present illness* is a narrative of the chief complaint from its earliest onset through its progression to the present. Its four major components are the details of onset, a complete interval history, the present status and the reason for seeking help now. The focus of the present illness is on all factors relevant to the main problem, even if they have disappeared or changed during the onset, interval and present.

Analysing a Symptom. Because pain is often the most characteristic symptom denoting the onset of a physical problem, it is used as an example for analysis of a symptom. Assessment includes type, location, severity, duration and influencing factors (see Nursing Care Considerations).

History

The history contains information relating to all previous aspects of the child's health status and concentrates on several areas that are ordinarily passed over in the history of an adult, such as birth history, detailed feeding history, immunisations, and growth and development. Because this section includes a great deal of information, use a combination of open-ended and fact-finding questions. For example, begin interviewing for each section with an open-ended statement (such as 'Tell me about your child's birth') to provide the informants the opportunity to relate what they think is most important. Ask fact-finding questions related to specific details whenever necessary to focus the interview on certain topics.

Birth History. The **birth history** includes all data concerning: (1) the mother's health during pregnancy; (2) the labour and delivery; and (3) the infant's condition immediately after birth. Because prenatal influences have significant effects on a child's physical and emotional development, a thorough investigation of the birth history is essential. Because parents may question what relevance pregnancy and birth have on the child's present condition, particularly if the child is past infancy, explain why such questions are included. An appropriate statement may be 'I will be asking you some questions about your pregnancy and ____'s [refer to child by name] birth. Your answers will give me a more complete picture of his [or her] overall health'.

Because emotional factors also affect the outcome of pregnancy and the subsequent parent–child relationship, investigate concurrent crises during pregnancy and prenatal attitudes towards the fetus. It is best to approach the topic of parental acceptance of pregnancy through indirect questioning. Asking the parents if the pregnancy was planned is a leading statement because they may respond affirmatively for fear of criticism if the pregnancy was unexpected. Rather, encourage parents to state their true reactions by referring to specific facts relating to the pregnancy, such as the spacing between offspring, an extended or short interval between marriage and conception, or a pregnancy during adolescence. The parent can choose to explore such statements with further explanations or, for the moment, may not be

*The term *illness* is used in its broadest sense to denote any problem of a physical, emotional, or psychosocial nature. It is actually a history of the chief complaint.

NURSING CARE CONSIDERATIONS

Analysing the Symptom: Pain

Type

Be as specific as possible. With young children, asking the parents how they know the child is in pain may help describe its type, location and severity. For example, a parent may state, 'My child must have a severe earache because she pulls at her ears, rolls her head on the floor and screams. Nothing seems to help'. Help older children describe the 'hurt' by asking them if it is sharp, throbbing, dull or stabbing. Record whatever words they use in quotes.

Location

Be specific. 'Stomach pains' is too general a description. Children can better localise the pain if they are asked to 'point with one finger to where it hurts' or to 'point to where mummy or daddy would put a Band-Aid'. Determine whether the pain radiates by asking, 'Does the pain stay there or move? Show me with your finger where the pain goes'.

Severity

Severity is best determined by finding out how it affects the child's usual behaviour. Pain that prevents a child from playing, interacting with others, sleeping and eating is most often severe. Assess pain intensity using a rating scale, such as a numeric or Wong-Baker FACES Pain Rating Scale (see Chapter 5).

Duration

Include the duration, onset and frequency. Describe this in terms of activity and behaviour, such as 'pain reported to last all night; child refused to sleep and cried intermittently'.

Influencing Factors

Include anything that causes a change in the type, location, severity or duration of the pain: (1) precipitating events (those that cause or increase the pain); (2) relieving events (those that lessen the pain, such as medications); (3) temporal events (times when the pain is relieved or increased); (4) positional events (standing, sitting, lying down); and (5) associated events (meals, stress, coughing).

able to reveal such feelings. If the parent remains silent, return to this topic later in the interview.

Dietary History. Because parental concerns are common and nursing interventions are important in ensuring optimum nutrition, the dietary history is discussed in detail under the Nutritional Assessment section of this chapter.

Previous Illnesses, Injuries and Surgeries. When inquiring about past illnesses, begin with a general statement (e.g. 'What other illnesses has your child had?'). Because parents are most likely to recall serious health problems, ask specifically about colds, earaches and childhood diseases such as gastroenteritis, chickenpox, pertussis (whooping cough), recurrent ear infections, gastro-oesophageal reflux or allergic manifestations.

In addition to illnesses, ask about injuries that required medical intervention, surgeries, procedures and hospitalisations, including the dates of each incident. Focus on injuries (e.g. accidental falls, poisoning, choking, concussion, fracture or burns) because these may be potential areas for parental guidance.

Allergies. Ask about commonly known allergic disorders, such as hay fever and asthma; unusual reactions to drugs, food or latex products; and reactions to other contact agents such as poisonous plants, animals, household products or fabrics. If asked appropriate questions, most people can give reliable information about drug reactions.

Current Medications. Inquire about current medications, including vitamins, antipyretics (especially aspirin), antibiotics, antihistamines, decongestants, nutritional supplements, herbs, essential oils and homeopathic medications. List all medications, including name, dose, route, schedule, duration and reasons for use. Often parents are unaware of a medication's actual name. Whenever possible, ask the parents to bring the containers with them to the next visit or ask for the name of the pharmacy and call for a list of all the child's recent prescription medications. However, this list will not include over-the-counter medications, which are important to know.

Immunisations. A record of all immunisations is essential. As many parents are unaware of the exact name and date of each immunisation, sources of information include Australian Immunisation Register (Australian Government Department of Health [AGDH] 2020) and National Immunisation Register (Ministry of Health 2020). All immunisations and 'boosters' are listed, stating: (1) the name of the specific disease; (2) the number of injections; (3) the dosage (sometimes lesser amounts are given if a reaction is anticipated); (4) the date when administered; and (5) the occurrence of any reaction following the immunisation. Children should be screened for contraindications and precautions before every vaccine is administered (see Immunisations, Chapter 6).

Growth and Development. Review the child's growth, including the following:

- measurements of weight, length and head circumference at birth
- patterns of growth on the growth chart and any significant deviations from previous percentiles
- concerns about growth from the family or child.

Developmental milestones include the following:

- age of holding up head steadily
- age of sitting alone without support
- age of walking without assistance
- age of saying first words with meaning
- age of achieving bladder and bowel control
- present year in school
- school performance
- if the child has a best friend
- interactions with other children, peers and adults.

Use specific and detailed questions when inquiring about each developmental milestone. For example, 'sitting up' can mean many different activities, such as sitting propped up, sitting in someone's lap, sitting with support, sitting up alone but in a hyperflexed position for assisted balance or sitting up unsupported with the back slightly rounded. A clue to misunderstanding of the requested activity may be an unusually early age of achievement (see Developmental Assessment at the end of this chapter).

Habits. Habits are an important area to explore (Box 4.5). Parents frequently express concerns during this part of the history. Encourage their input by saying, 'Please tell me any concerns you have about your child's habits, activities or development'. Investigate further any concerns that parents express.

BOX 4.5 Habits to Explore During a Health Interview

- Behaviour patterns, such as nail biting, thumb sucking, pica (habitual ingestion of non-food substances), rituals ('security' blanket or toy) and unusual movements (head banging, rocking, overt masturbation, walking on toes)
- Activities of daily living, such as hours of sleep and arising, duration of night-time sleep and naps, type and duration of exercise, regularity of stools and urination, age of toilet training, and daytime or night-time bedwetting
- Unusual disposition; response to frustration
- Use or abuse of alcohol, drugs, caffeine or tobacco

One of the most common concerns relates to sleep. Many children develop a normal sleep pattern, and all that is required during the assessment is a general overview of night-time sleep and nap schedules. However, a number of children develop sleep problems (see Sleep Problems, Chapters 11 and 14).

Habits related to the use of chemicals apply primarily to older children and adolescents. If a youngster admits to smoking, drinking or using drugs, ask about the quantity and frequency. Questions such as 'Many kids your age are experimenting with drugs and alcohol; have you ever had any drugs or alcohol?' may give more reliable data than questions such as 'How much do you drink?' or 'How often do you drink or take drugs?' Clarify that 'drinking' includes all types of alcohol, including beer and wine. When quantities such as a 'glass' of wine or a 'can' of beer are given, ask about the size of the container.

If older children deny use of chemical substances, inquire about past experimentation. Asking 'You mean you never tried to smoke or drink?' implies that the nurse expects some such activity, and the youngster may be more inclined to answer truthfully. Be aware of the confidential nature of such questioning, the adverse effect that the parents' presence may have on the adolescent's willingness to answer and the fact that self-reporting may not be an accurate account of chemical abuse.

Sexual History

The sexual history is an essential component of adolescents' health assessment. The history uncovers areas of concern related to sexual activity, alerts the nurse to circumstances that may indicate need for screening for sexually transmitted infections or testing for pregnancy, and provides information related to the need for sexual health counselling, such as safer sex practices. Box 4.6 gives guidelines for anticipatory guidance topics for parents and adolescents.

One approach to initiating a conversation about sexual concerns is to begin with a history of peer interactions. Open-ended statements (e.g. 'Tell me about your social life' or 'Who are your closest friends?') generally lead into a discussion of dating and sexual issues. To probe further, include questions about the adolescent's attitudes on such topics as sex education, 'going steady', 'living together' and premarital sex. Phrase questions to reflect concern rather than judgment or criticism of sexual practices.

In any conversation regarding sexual history, be aware of the language that is used in either eliciting or conveying sexual information. For example, avoid asking whether the adolescent is 'sexually active' because this term is broadly defined. 'Are you having sex with anyone?' is probably the most direct and best understood question. Because same-sex experimentation may occur, refer to all sexual contacts in non-gender terms, such as 'partners', rather than 'girlfriends' or 'boyfriends'.

BOX 4.6 Anticipatory Guidance—Sexuality

Ages 12 to 14 Years

- Have the adolescent identify a supportive adult with whom to discuss sexuality issues and concerns.
- Discuss the advantages of delaying sexual activity.
- Discuss making responsible decisions regarding normal sexual feelings.
- Allow space to discuss a variety of gender and sexual attraction possibilities.
- Discuss the roles of gender, peer pressure and the media in sexual decision-making.
- Discuss contraceptive options (advantages and disadvantages).
- Provide education regarding sexually transmitted infections (STIs), including human immunodeficiency virus (HIV) infection; clarify risks and discuss condoms.
- Discuss abuse prevention, including avoiding dangerous situations, the role of drugs and alcohol, and the use of self-defence.
- Have the adolescent clarify his or her values, needs and ability to be assertive.
- If the adolescent is sexually active, discuss limiting partners, use of condoms and contraceptive options.
- Have a confidential interview with the adolescent (including a sexual history).
- Discuss the evolution of sexual identity and expression.
- Discuss breast examination or testicular examination.

Ages 15 to 18 Years

- Support delaying sexual activity.
- Discuss alternatives to intercourse.
- Discuss 'When are you ready for sex?'
- Clarify values; encourage responsible decision-making.
- Discuss consequences of unprotected sex: early pregnancy and STIs, including HIV infection.
- Discuss negotiating with partner and barriers to safer sex.
- If the adolescent is sexually active, discuss limiting partners, use of condoms and contraceptive options.
- Emphasise that sex should be safe and pleasurable for both partners.
- Have a confidential interview with the adolescent.
- Discuss concerns about sexual expression and identity.

Source: Data from Wright, K. (1997). Anticipatory guidance: Developing a healthy sexuality. *Pediatr Ann, 26*(2 suppl), S142–S144, C3; Fonseca, H., & Greydanus, D. (2007). Sexuality in the child, teen and young adult: Concepts for the clinician. *Prim Care Clin Office Pract, 34,* 275–292.

Family Health History

The family health history is used primarily to discover any genetic or chronic diseases in the child's family members. Assess for the presence or absence of consanguinity (if anyone in the family is related to their spouse's/partner's family). Family health history is generally confined to **first-degree relatives** (parents, siblings, grandparents and immediate aunts and uncles). Information includes age, marital status, health status, cause of death if deceased and any evidence of conditions, such as early heart disease, stroke, sudden death from unknown cause, hypertension, cancer, diabetes mellitus, obesity, congenital anomalies, allergies, asthma, seizures, cognitive impairment, hearing or visual deficits and psychiatric disorders (e.g. depression or psychosis, and emotional problems). Confirm the accuracy of the reported disorders by inquiring about the symptoms, course, treatment and sequelae of each diagnosis.

Geographic Location. One of the important areas to explore when assessing the family health history is geographic location, including the birthplace and travel to different areas in or outside of the country, for identification of possible exposure to endemic diseases. Include current and past housing, whether they rent or own, reside in an urban or rural location, the age of the home and whether there are significant threats such as moulds or pests within the housing structure. Children are especially susceptible to parasitic infestation in areas of poor sanitary conditions.

Family Structure

Assessment of the family, both its structure and function, is an important component of the history-taking process. Because the quality of the functional relationship between the child and family members is a major factor in emotional and physical health, family assessment is discussed separately and in greater detail apart from the more traditional health history.

Family assessment is the collection of data about the composition of the family and the relationships among its members. In its broadest sense, **family** refers to all those individuals who are considered by the family member to be significant to the nuclear unit, including relatives, friends and social groups (e.g. the school and church). Although family assessment is not family therapy, it can and frequently is therapeutic. Involving family members in discussing family characteristics and activities can provide insight into family dynamics and relationships.

Because of the time involved in performing an in-depth family assessment as presented here, be selective in deciding when knowledge of family function may facilitate nursing care. During brief contacts with families, a full assessment is not appropriate, and screening with one or two questions from each category may reflect the health of the family system or the need for additional assessment.

The most common method of eliciting information on the family structure is to interview family members. The principal areas of concern are family composition, home and community environment, occupation and education of family members, and cultural and religious traditions (Box 4.7).

Psychosocial History

The traditional medical history includes a personal and social section that concentrates on children's personal status, such as school adjustment and any unusual habits, and the family and home environment. Because several personal aspects are covered under development and habits, only those issues related to children's ability to cope and their self-concept are presented here.

Through observation, obtain a general idea of how children handle themselves in terms of confidence in dealing with others, answering questions and coping with new situations. Observe the parent–child relationship for the types of messages sent to children about their coping skills and self-worth. Do the parents treat the child with respect, focusing on strengths, or is the interaction one of constant reprimands, with emphasis on weaknesses and faults? Do the parents help the child learn new coping strategies or support the ones the child uses?

Parent–child interactions also convey messages about body image. Do the parents label the child and body parts (e.g. 'bad boy', 'skinny legs' or 'ugly scar')? Do the parents handle the child gently, using soothing touch to calm an anxious child, or do they treat the child roughly, using slaps or restraint to make the child obey? If the child

BOX 4.7 Family Assessment Interview

General Guidelines

- Schedule the interview with the family at a time that is most convenient for all parties; include as many family members as possible; clearly state the purpose of the interview.
- Begin the interview by asking each person's name and their relationship to one another.
- Restate the purpose of the interview and the objective.
- Keep the initial conversation general to put members at ease and to learn the 'big picture' of the family.
- Identify major concerns and reflect these back to the family to be certain that all parties receive the same message.
- Terminate the interview with a summary of what was discussed and a plan for additional sessions if needed.

Structural Assessment Areas

Family Composition

- Immediate members of the household (names, ages and relationships)
- Significant extended family members
- Previous marriages, separations, death of spouses or divorces

Home and Community Environment

- Type of dwelling, number of rooms, occupants
- Sleeping arrangements
- Number of floors, accessibility of stairs and lifts
- Adequacy of utilities
- Safety features (fire and smoke alarm, guardrails on windows, use of car restraint)
- Environmental hazards (e.g. chipped paint, poor sanitation, pollution, heavy street traffic)
- Availability and location of healthcare facilities, schools, play areas
- Relationship with neighbours
- Recent crises or changes in home
- Child's reaction and adjustment to recent stresses

Occupation and Education of Family Members

- Types of employment
- Work schedules
- Work satisfaction
- Exposure to environmental or industrial hazards
- Sources of income and adequacy
- Effect of illness on financial status
- Highest degree or year-level attained

Cultural and Religious Traditions

- Religious beliefs and practices
- Cultural and ethnic beliefs and practices
- Language spoken in home
- Assessment questions include the following:
  - Does the family identify with a particular religious or ethnic group? Are both parents from that group?
  - How is religious or ethnic background part of family life?
  - What special religious or cultural traditions are practised in the home (e.g. food choices and preparation)?
  - Where were family members born, and how long have they lived in this country?
  - What language does the family speak most frequently?
  - Do they speak and understand English?
  - What do they believe causes health or illness?
  - What religious or ethnic beliefs influence the family's perception of illness and its treatment?
  - What methods are used to prevent or treat illness?
  - How does the family know when a health problem needs medical attention?
  - Who does the family contact when a member is ill?
  - Does the family rely on cultural or religious healers or remedies? If so, ask them to describe the type of healer or remedy.
  - Who does the family go to for support (clergy, medical healer, relatives)?
  - Does the family experience discrimination because of their race, beliefs or practices? Ask them to describe.

Continued

BOX 4.7 Family Assessment Interview—cont'd

Functional Assessment Areas

Family Interactions and Roles

- *Interactions* refer to ways family members relate to each other. The chief concern is the amount of intimacy and closeness among the members, especially spouses.
- *Roles* refer to behaviours of people as they assume a different status or position.
- Observations include the following:
  - family members' responses to each other (cordial, hostile, cool, loving, patient, short-tempered)
  - obvious roles of leadership versus submission
  - support and attention shown to various members.
- Assessment questions include the following:
  - What activities does the family perform together?
  - Who do family members talk to when something is bothering them?
  - What are family members' household chores?
  - Who usually oversees what is happening with the children, such as at school or healthcare?
  - How easy or difficult is it for the family to change or accept new responsibilities for household tasks?

Power, Decision-making and Problem-solving

- *Power* refers to individual family members' control over others in the family; it is manifested through family decision-making and problem-solving.
- Chief concern is clarity of boundaries of power between parents and children.
- One method of assessment involves offering a hypothetical conflict or problem, such as a child failing school, and asking family how they would handle this situation.
- Assessment questions include the following:
  - Who usually makes the decisions in the family?
  - If one parent makes a decision, can the child appeal to the other parent to change it?
  - What input do children have in making decisions or discussing rules?
  - Who makes and enforces the rules?
  - What happens when a rule is broken?

Communication

- Communication is concerned with clarity and directness of communication patterns.
- Further assessment includes periodically asking family members if they understood what was just said and to repeat the message.
- Observations include the following:
  - who speaks to whom
  - if one person speaks for another or interrupts
  - if members appear uninterested when certain individuals speak
  - if there is agreement between verbal and non-verbal messages.
- Assessment questions include the following:
  - How often do family members wait until others are through talking before 'having their say'?
  - Do parents or older siblings tend to lecture and preach?
  - Do parents tend to 'talk down' to the children?

Expression of Feelings and Individuality

- Expressions are concerned with personal space and freedom to grow, with limits and structure needed for guidance.
- Observing patterns of communication offers clues to how freely feelings are expressed.
- Assessment questions include the following:
  - Is it OK for family members to get angry or sad?
  - Who gets angry most of the time? What do they do?
  - If someone is upset, how do other family members try to comfort this person?
  - Who comforts specific family members?
  - When someone wants to do something, such as try out for a new sport or get a job, what is the family's response (offer assistance, discouragement or no advice)?

touches certain parts of the body, such as the genitalia, do the parents make comments that suggest a negative connotation?

With older children, many of the communication strategies discussed earlier in this chapter are useful in eliciting more definitive information about their coping and self-concept. Children can write down five things they like and dislike about themselves. The nurse can use sentence completion statements, such as 'The thing I like best (or worst) about myself is ____________'; 'If I could change one thing about myself, it would be ____________'; or 'When I am scared, I ____________'.

Review of Systems

The review of systems is a specific review of each body system, following an order similar to that of the physical examination (see Nursing Care Considerations box). Often the history of the present illness provides a complete review of the system involved in the chief complaint. Because asking questions about other body systems may appear irrelevant to the parents or child, precede the questioning with an explanation of why the data are necessary (similar to the explanation concerning the relevance of the birth history) and reassure the parents that the child's main problem has not been forgotten.

NURSING CARE CONSIDERATIONS

Review of Systems

General health—Overall state of health, fatigue, recent or unexplained weight gain or loss (period of time for either), contributing factors (change of diet, illness, altered appetite), exercise tolerance, fevers (time of day), chills, night sweats (unrelated to climatic conditions), general ability to carry out activities of daily living

Integument—Pruritus, pigment or other colour changes (including birthmarks), acne, eruptions, rashes (location), bruises, petechiae, excessive dryness, general texture, tattoos or piercings, disorders or deformities of nails, hair growth or loss, hair colour change

Eyes—Visual problems (behaviours indicative of blurred vision, such as bumping into objects, clumsiness, sitting close to television, holding a book close to face, writing with head near desk, squinting, rubbing the eyes, bending head in an awkward position), crossed eyes or lazy eye (strabismus), eye infections, oedema of lids, excessive tearing, use of glasses or contact lenses, date of last vision examination

Ears—Earaches, ear discharge, evidence of hearing loss (ask about behaviours, such as the need to repeat requests, loud speech, lack of response to noises, inattentive behaviour), results of any previous auditory testing

NURSING CARE CONSIDERATIONS

Review of Systems—cont'd

Nose—Nosebleeds (epistaxis), constant or frequent runny or stuffy nose, nasal obstruction (difficulty breathing), alteration or loss of sense of smell

Mouth—Mouth breathing, gum bleeding, number of teeth and pattern of eruption/loss, toothaches, tooth brushing, use of fluoride, difficulty with teething (symptoms), last visit to dentist (especially if temporary dentition is complete)

Throat—Sore throats, difficulty swallowing, choking, hoarseness or other voice irregularities

Neck—Pain, limitation of movement, stiffness, difficulty holding head straight (torticollis), thyroid enlargement, enlarged lymph nodes or other masses

Chest—Breast enlargement, discharge, masses; for adolescent girls, ask about breast self-examination

Respiratory—Chronic cough, wheezing, shortness of breath at rest or on exertion, difficulty breathing, snoring, sputum production, infections (pneumonia, tuberculosis), skin reaction from tuberculin testing

Cardiovascular—Cyanosis or fatigue on exertion, history of heart murmur or rheumatic fever, tachycardia, syncope, oedema

Gastrointestinal—Appetite, nausea, vomiting (not associated with eating; may be indicative of brain tumour or increased intracranial pressure), abdominal pain, jaundice or yellowing skin or sclera, belching, flatulence, distension, diarrhoea, constipation, recent change in bowel habits, blood in stools

Genitourinary—Pain on urination, frequency, hesitancy, urgency, haematuria, nocturia, polyuria, enuresis (daytime and/or nocturnal), unpleasant odour to urine, force of stream, discharge, change in size of scrotum, date and result of last urinalysis; for adolescents, sexually transmitted infection and type of treatment; for adolescent boys, ask about testicular self-examination

Gynaecological—Menarche, date of last menstrual period, regularity or problems with menstruation, vaginal discharge, pruritus; if sexually active, type of contraception, sexually transmitted infection and type of treatment; if sexually active with weakened immune system or if 21 years old and older, date and result of last Papanicolaou (Pap) smear; obstetric history (as discussed under birth history, when applicable)

Musculoskeletal—Weakness, clumsiness, lack of coordination, unusual movements, scoliosis, back pain, joint pain or swelling, muscle pains or cramps, abnormal gait, deformity, fractures, serious sprains, activity level

Neurological—Headaches, seizures, tremors, tics, dizziness, head injury (specific details), loss of consciousness episodes, loss of memory, developmental delays or concerns

Endocrine—Intolerance to heat or cold, excessive thirst or urination, excessive sweating, salt craving, rapid or slow growth, signs of puberty (regardless of age)

Haematological/lymphatic—Easy bruising or bleeding, anaemia, date and result of last blood count, blood transfusions, swollen or painful lymph nodes (cervical, axillary, inguinal)

Allergic/immunological—Allergic responses, anaphylaxis, eczema, rhinitis, unusual sneezing, autoimmunity, recurrent infections, infections associated with unusual complications

Psychiatric—General affect, anxiety, depression, mood changes, hallucinations, attention span, tantrums, behaviour problems, suicidal ideation, substance abuse

Begin the review of a specific system with a broad statement (e.g. 'How has your child's general health been?' or 'Has your child had any problems with his eyes?') If the parent states that the child has had problems with some body function, pursue this with an encouraging statement such as 'Tell me more about that'. If the parent denies any problems, query for specific symptoms (e.g. 'No headaches, bumping into objects or squinting?'). If the parent reconfirms the absence of such symptoms, record positive statements in the history, such as 'Mother denies headaches, bumping into objects or squinting'. In this way, anyone who reviews the health history is aware of exactly what symptoms were investigated.

NUTRITIONAL ASSESSMENT

Dietary Intake

Knowledge of the child's dietary intake is an essential component of a nutritional assessment. However, it is also one of the most difficult factors to assess. Individuals' recall of food consumption, especially amounts eaten, is frequently unreliable. The food intake history of children and adolescents is prone to reporting error, mostly in the form of underreporting. People from different cultures may have difficulty adequately describing the types of food they eat. Despite these obstacles, a dietary evaluation is an important component of the child's assessment. Specific questions used to conduct a nutritional assessment are given in Box 4.8. Every nutritional assessment should begin with a **dietary history**. The exact questions used to elicit a dietary history vary with the child's age. In general, the younger the child, the more specific and detailed the history should be. The overview elicited from the dietary history can be helpful in evaluating food frequency records. The history is also concerned with financial and cultural factors that influence food selection and preparation.

The most common and probably easiest method of assessing daily intake is the **24-hour recall**. The child or parent recalls every item eaten and drunk in the past 24 hours and the approximate amounts. The 24-hour recall is most beneficial when it represents a typical day's intake. Some of the difficulties with a daily recall are the family's inability to remember exactly what was eaten and inaccurate estimation of portion size. To increase accuracy of reporting portion sizes, the use of food models and additional questions are recommended. In general, this method is most useful in providing qualitative information about the child's diet.

To improve the reliability of the daily recall, the family can complete a **food diary** by recording every food and liquid consumed for a certain number of days. A 3-day record consisting of 2 weekdays and 1 weekend day is representative for most people. Providing specific charts to record intake can improve compliance. The family should record items immediately after eating.

Clinical Examination of Nutrition

A significant amount of information regarding nutritional deficiencies comes from a clinical examination, especially from assessing the skin, hair, teeth, gums, lips, tongue and eyes. Hair, skin and mouth are vulnerable because of the rapid turnover of epithelial and mucosal tissue. Table 4.1 summarises clinical signs of possible nutritional deficiency or excess. Few are diagnostic for a specific nutrient, and if suspicious signs are found, they must be confirmed with dietary and biochemical data. Faltering growth is discussed in Chapter 11. Obesity and eating disorders are discussed in Chapter 18.

Anthropometry, an essential parameter of nutritional status, is the measurement of height (length), weight, head circumference, proportions, skinfold thickness and arm circumference in children. Height and head circumference reflect past nutrition, whereas weight, skinfold thickness and arm circumference reflect present nutritional status, especially of protein and fat reserves. Skinfold thickness is a measurement

BOX 4.8 Assessment of Nutritional Intake

Dietary History

- What are the family's usual mealtimes?
- Do family members eat together or at separate times?
- Who does the family grocery shopping and meal preparation?
- How much money is spent to buy food each week?
- How are most foods prepared—baked, broiled, fried, other?
- How often does the family or your child eat out?
  - What kinds of restaurants do you go to?
  - What kinds of food does your child typically eat at restaurants?
- Does your child eat breakfast regularly?
- Where does your child eat lunch?
- What are your child's favourite foods, beverages and snacks?
  - What are the average amounts eaten per day?
  - What foods are artificially sweetened?
  - What are your child's snacking habits?
  - When are sweet foods usually eaten?
  - What are your child's tooth brushing habits?
- What special cultural practices are followed? What ethnic foods are eaten?
- What foods and beverages does your child dislike?
- How would you describe your child's usual appetite (hearty eater, picky eater)?
- What are your child's feeding habits (breast, bottle, cup, spoon, eats by self, needs assistance, any special devices)?
- Does your child take vitamins or other supplements? Do they contain iron or fluoride?
- Does your child have any known or suspected food allergies? Is your child on a special diet?
- Has your child lost or gained weight recently?
- Are there any feeding problems (excessive fussiness, spitting up, colic, difficulty sucking or swallowing)? Are there any dental problems or appliances, such as braces, that affect eating?
- What types of exercise does your child do regularly?
- Is there a family history of cancer, diabetes, heart disease, high blood pressure or obesity?

Additional Questions for Infants

- What was the infant's birth weight? When did it double? Triple?
- Was the infant premature?
- Are you breastfeeding or have you breastfed your infant? For how long?
- If you use a formula, what is the brand?
  - How long has the infant been taking it?
  - How many millilitres (mL) does the infant drink a day?
- Are you giving the infant cow's milk (whole, low fat, skim)?
  - When did you start?
  - How many millilitres (mL) does the infant drink a day?
- Do you give your infant extra fluids (water, juice)?
- If the infant takes a bottle to bed at nap or night-time, what is in the bottle?
- At what age did the child start on cereal, vegetables, meat or other protein sources, fruit or juice, finger food and table food?
- Do you make your own baby food or use commercial foods, such as infant cereal?
- Does the infant take a vitamin or mineral supplement? If so, what type?
- Has the infant had an allergic reaction to any food(s)? If so, list the foods and describe the reaction.
- Does the infant spit up frequently; have unusually loose stools; or have hard, dry stools? If so, how often?
- How often do you feed your infant?
- How would you describe your infant's appetite?

Source: Modified from Murphy, S. P., & Poos, M. I. (2002). Dietary reference intakes: Summary of applications in dietary assessment. *Pub Health Nutr, 5*(Suppl 6A), 843–849.

of the body's fat content because approximately half the body's total fat stores are directly beneath the skin. The upper arm muscle circumference is correlated with measurements of total muscle mass. Because muscle serves as the body's major protein reserve, this measurement is considered an index of the body's protein stores. Ideally, growth measurements are recorded over time, and comparisons are made regarding the velocity of growth based on previous and present values.

Numerous **biochemical tests** are available for assessing nutritional status. The most common laboratory studies to assess for undernutrition are haemoglobin, red blood cell indices and serum albumin or prealbumin. For obese children, fasting serum glucose, lipids and liver function studies may be performed to assess for complications.

Evaluation of Nutritional Assessment

After collecting the data needed for a thorough nutritional assessment, evaluate the findings to plan appropriate counselling. From the data, assess whether the child is malnourished, at risk for becoming malnourished, well-nourished with adequate reserves or overweight or obese.

GENERAL APPROACHES TOWARDS EXAMINING THE CHILD

Sequence of the Examination

Ordinarily, the sequence for examining patients follows a head-to-toe direction. The main function of such a systematic approach is to provide a general guideline for assessment of each body area to avoid omitting segments of the examination. The standard recording of data also facilitates exchange of information among different professionals. In examining children, this orderly sequence is frequently altered to accommodate the child's developmental needs, although the examination is recorded following the head-to-toe model. Using developmental and chronological age as the main criteria for assessing each body system accomplishes several goals:

- minimises stress and anxiety associated with assessment of various body parts
- fosters a trusting nurse–child–parent relationship
- allows for maximum preparation of the child
- preserves the essential security of the parent–child relationship, especially with young children
- maximises the accuracy and reliability of assessment findings.

Preparation of the Child

Although the physical examination consists of painless procedures, for some children the use of a tight arm cuff, probes in the ears and mouth, pressure on the abdomen or a cold piece of metal to listen to the chest is stressful. Therefore, the nurse should use the same considerations discussed in Chapter 22 for preparing children for procedures. In addition to that discussion, general guidelines related to the examining process are given in the Nursing Care Considerations box.

TABLE 4.1 Clinical Assessment of Nutritional Status

Evidence of Adequate Nutrition	Evidence of Deficient or Excess Nutrition	Deficiency or Excess*
General Growth		
Between 5th and 95th percentiles for height, weight and head circumference	< 5th or > 95th percentile for growth	Protein, calories, fats and other essential nutrients, especially vitamin A, pyridoxine, niacin, calcium, iodine, manganese, zinc
Steady gain with expected growth spurts during infancy and adolescence	Absence of or delayed growth spurts; poor weight gain	
Sexual development appropriate for age	Delayed sexual development	Excess vitamins A, D
Skin		
Smooth, slightly dry to touch Elastic and firm Absence of lesions Colour appropriate to genetic background	Hardening and scaling	Vitamin A
	Seborrhoeic dermatitis	Excess niacin
	Dry, rough, petechiae	Riboflavin
	Delayed wound healing	Vitamin C
	Scaly dermatitis on exposed surfaces	Riboflavin, vitamin C, zinc
	Wrinkled, flabby	Niacin
	Crusted lesions around orifices, especially nares	Protein, calories, zinc
	Pruritus	Excess vitamin A, riboflavin, niacin
	Poor turgor	Water, sodium
	Oedema	Protein, thiamine Excess sodium
	Yellow tinge (jaundice)	Vitamin B_{12} Excess vitamin A, niacin
	Depigmentation	Protein, calories
	Pallor (anaemia)	Pyridoxine, folic acid, vitamins B_{12}, C, E (in premature infants), iron Excess vitamin C, zinc
	Paraesthesia	Excess riboflavin
Hair		
Lustrous, silky, strong, elastic	Stringy, friable, dull, dry, thin	Protein, calories
	Alopecia	Protein, calories, zinc
	Depigmentation	Protein, calories, copper
	Raised areas around hair follicles	Vitamin C
Head		
Even moulding, occipital prominence, symmetrical facial features	Softening of cranial bones, prominence of frontal bones, skull flat and depressed towards middle	Vitamin D
Fused sutures after 18 months	Delayed fusion of sutures	Vitamin D
	Hard, tender lumps in occiput	Excess vitamin A
	Headache	Excess thiamine
Neck		
Thyroid not visible, palpable in midline	Thyroid enlarged, may be grossly visible	Iodine
Eyes		
Clear, bright	Hardening and scaling of cornea and conjunctiva	Vitamin A
Good night vision	Night blindness	Vitamin A
Conjunctiva—pink, glossy	Burning, itching, photophobia, cataracts, corneal vascularisation	Riboflavin
Ears		
Tympanic membrane—pliable	Calcified (hearing loss)	Excess vitamin D
Nose		
Smooth, intact nasal angle	Irritation and cracks at nasal angle	Riboflavin Excess vitamin A

Continued

TABLE 4.1 Clinical Assessment of Nutritional Status—cont'd

Evidence of Adequate Nutrition	Evidence of Deficient or Excess Nutrition	Deficiency or Excess*
Mouth		
Lips—smooth, moist, darker colour than skin	Fissures and inflammation at corners	Riboflavin Excess vitamin A
Gums—firm, coral pink, stippled	Spongy, friable, swollen, bluish red or black, bleed easily	Vitamin C
Mucous membranes—bright pink, smooth, moist	Stomatitis	Niacin
Tongue—rough texture, no lesions, taste sensation	Glossitis	Niacin, riboflavin, folic acid
	Diminished taste sensation	Zinc
Teeth—uniform white colour, smooth, intact	Brown mottling, pits, fissures	Excess fluoride
	Defective enamel	Vitamins A, C, D, calcium, phosphorus
	Caries	Excess carbohydrates
Chest		
In infants, shape almost circular	Depressed lower portion of rib cage	Vitamin D
In children, lateral diameter increased in proportion to anteroposterior diameter	Sharp protrusion of sternum	Vitamin D
Smooth costochondral junctions	Enlarged costochondral junctions	Vitamins C, D
Breast development—normal for age	Delayed development	See under General Growth; especially zinc
Cardiovascular System		
Pulse and BP within normal limits	Palpitations	Thiamine
	Rapid pulse	Potassium Excess thiamine
	Arrhythmias	Magnesium, potassium Excess niacin, potassium
	Increased BP	Excess sodium
	Decreased BP	Thiamine Excess niacin
Abdomen		
In young children, cylindrical and prominent	Distended, flabby, poor musculature	Protein, calories
	Prominent, large	Excess calories
In older children, flat	Potbelly, constipation	Vitamin D
Normal bowel habits	Diarrhoea	Niacin Excess vitamin C
	Constipation	Excess calcium, potassium
Musculoskeletal System		
Muscles—firm, well-developed, equal strength bilaterally	Flabby, weak, generalised wasting	Protein, calories
	Weakness, pain, cramps	Thiamine, sodium, chloride, potassium, phosphorus, magnesium Excess thiamine
	Muscle twitching, tremors	Magnesium
	Muscular paralysis	Excess potassium
Spine—cervical and lumbar curves (double S curve)	Kyphosis, lordosis, scoliosis	Vitamin D
Extremities—symmetrical; legs straight with minimum bowing	Bowing of extremities, knock-knees	Vitamin D, calcium, phosphorus
	Epiphyseal enlargement	Vitamins A, D
	Bleeding into joints and muscles, joint swelling, pain	Vitamin C
Joints—flexible, full range of motion, no pain or stiffness	Thickening of cortex of long bones with pain and fragility, hard tender lumps in extremities	Excess vitamin A
	Osteoporosis of long bones	Calcium Excess vitamin D
Neurological System		
Behaviour—alert, responsive, emotionally stable	Listless, irritable, lethargic, apathetic (sometimes apprehensive, anxious, drowsy, mentally slow, confused)	Thiamine, niacin, pyridoxine, vitamin C, potassium, magnesium, iron, protein, calories Excess vitamins A, D, thiamine, folic acid, calcium

TABLE 4.1 Clinical Assessment of Nutritional Status—cont'd

Evidence of Adequate Nutrition	Evidence of Deficient or Excess Nutrition	Deficiency or Excess*
Absence of tetany, convulsions	Masklike facial expression, blurred speech, involuntary laughing	Excess manganese
	Convulsions	Thiamine, pyridoxine, vitamin D, calcium, magnesium Excess phosphorus (in relation to calcium)
Intact peripheral nervous system	Peripheral nervous system toxicity (unsteady gait, numb feet and hands, fine motor clumsiness)	Excess pyridoxine
Intact reflexes	Diminished or absent tendon reflexes	Thiamine, vitamin E

*Nutrients listed are deficient unless specified as excess.

NURSING CARE CONSIDERATIONS

Performing a Paediatric Physical Examination

Perform the examination in an appropriate, non-threatening area.

- Have the room well-lit and decorated with neutral colours.
- Have the room temperature comfortably warm.
- Place all strange and potentially frightening equipment out of sight.
- Have some toys and games available for the child.
- If possible, have rooms decorated and equipped for different-age children.
- Provide privacy, especially for school-age children and adolescents.
- Provide time for play and becoming acquainted.

Observe behaviours that signal child's readiness to cooperate:

- talking to the nurse
- making eye contact
- accepting the offered equipment
- allowing physical touching
- choosing to sit on the examining table rather than the parent's lap.

If signs of readiness are not observed, use the following techniques.

- Talk to the parent while essentially 'ignoring' the child; gradually focus on the child or a favourite object, such as a doll.
- Make complimentary remarks about the child, such as about his or her appearance, dress or a favourite object.
- Tell a funny story or play a simple magic trick.
- Have a non-threatening 'friend' available, such as a hand puppet to 'talk' to the child for the nurse (see Fig 4.24A later in this chapter).

If child refuses to cooperate, use the following techniques.

- Assess the reason for uncooperative behaviour; consider that a child who is unduly afraid may have had a traumatic experience.
- Try to involve the child and parent in the process.
- Avoid prolonged explanations about examining procedure.
- Use a firm, direct approach regarding expected behaviour.
- Perform examination as quickly as possible.
- Minimise any disruptions or stimulation.
- Limit the number of people in the room.
- Use an isolated room.
- Use a quiet, calm, confident voice.

Begin examination in a non-threatening manner for young children or children who are fearful.

- Use approaches such as Simon Says to encourage child to make a face, squeeze a hand, stand on one foot and so on.
- Use the paper-doll technique.
  1. Lay the child supine on an examining table or floor that is covered with a large sheet of paper.
  2. Trace around the child's body outline.
  3. Use the body outline to demonstrate what will be examined, such as drawing a heart and listening with a stethoscope before performing the activity on the child.

If several children in the family will be examined, begin with the most cooperative child to model desired behaviour.

Involve the child in the examination process.

- Provide choices, such as sitting on the table or in the parent's lap.
- Allow the child to handle or hold equipment.
- Encourage the child to use equipment on a doll, family member or examiner.
- Explain each step of the procedure in simple language.

Examine the child in a comfortable and secure position:

- sitting on parent's lap
- sitting upright if in respiratory distress.

Proceed to examine the body in an organised sequence (usually head to toe) with the following exceptions.

- Alter the sequence to accommodate the needs of different-age children (see Table 4.2).
- Examine painful areas last.
- In an emergency SITUATION, examine vital functions (airway, breathing and circulation) and injured area first.

Reassure the child throughout the examination, especially about bodily concerns that arise during puberty.

Discuss findings with the family at the end of the examination.

Praise the child for cooperation during the examination; give a reward such as a small toy or sticker.

The physical examination should be as pleasant as possible, as well as educational. The paper-doll technique is a useful approach to teaching children about the body part that is being examined (Fig 4.4). At the conclusion of the visit, the child can take home the paper doll as a memento.

Table 4.2 summarises guidelines for positioning, preparing and examining children at various ages. Because the child may not fit precisely into one age category, it may be necessary to vary the approach after a preliminary assessment of the child's developmental achievements and needs. Even with the best approach, many toddlers are uncooperative and inconsolable for much of the physical examination. However, some seem intrigued by the new surroundings and unusual equipment and respond more like preschoolers than toddlers. Likewise, some early preschoolers may require more of the 'security measures' employed with younger children, such as continued parent–child contact, and less of the preparatory measures used with preschoolers, such as playing with the equipment before and during the actual examination (Fig 4.5).

TABLE 4.2 Age-specific Approaches to Physical Examination During Childhood

Position	Sequence	Preparation
	INFANT	
Before able to sit alone—supine or prone, preferably in parent's lap; before 4–6 months, can place on examining table After able to sit alone—sitting in parent's lap whenever possible; if on table, place with parent in full view	If quiet, auscultate heart, lungs, abdomen. Record heart and respiratory rates. Palpate and percuss same areas. Proceed in usual head-to-toe direction. Perform traumatic procedures last (eyes, ears, mouth [while crying]). Elicit reflexes as body part is examined. Elicit Moro reflex last.	Completely undress if room temperature permits. Leave nappy on male infant. Gain cooperation with distraction, bright objects, rattles, talking. Smile at infant; use soft, gentle voice. Use pacifier (if used) or bottle with feeding (if bottle feeding). Enlist parent's aid for restraining to examine ears, mouth. Avoid abrupt, jerky movements.
	TODDLER	
Sitting or standing on or by parent Prone or supine in parent's lap	Inspect body area through play: 'Count fingers', 'tickle toes'. Use minimum physical contact initially. Introduce equipment slowly. Auscultate, percuss, palpate whenever quiet. Perform traumatic procedures last (same as for infant).	Have parent remove child's outer clothing. Remove underwear as body part is examined. Allow toddler to inspect equipment; demonstrating use of equipment is usually ineffective. If uncooperative, perform procedures quickly. Use restraint when appropriate; request parent's assistance. Talk about examination if cooperative; use short phrases. Praise for cooperative behaviour.
	PRESCHOOL CHILD	
Prefer standing or sitting Usually cooperative prone or supine Prefer parent's closeness	If cooperative, proceed in head-to-toe direction. If uncooperative, proceed as with toddler.	Request self-undressing. Allow to wear underpants if shy. Offer equipment for inspection; briefly demonstrate use. Make up story about procedure (e.g. 'I'm seeing how strong your muscles are' [blood pressure]). Use paper-doll technique. Give choices when possible. Expect cooperation; use positive statements (e.g. 'Open your mouth').
	SCHOOL-AGE CHILD	
Prefer sitting Cooperative in most positions Younger child prefers parent's presence Older child may prefer privacy	Proceed in head-to-toe direction. May examine genitalia last in older child.	Respect need for privacy. Request self-undressing. Allow to wear underpants. Give gown to wear. Explain purpose of equipment and significance of procedure, such as otoscope to see eardrum, which is necessary for hearing. Teach about body function and care.
	ADOLESCENT	
Same as for school-age child Offer option of parent's presence	Same as older school-age child. May examine genitalia last.	Allow to undress in private. Give gown. Expose only area to be examined. Respect need for privacy. Explain findings during examination (e.g. 'Your muscles are firm and strong'). Matter-of-factly comment about sexual development (e.g. 'Your breasts are developing as they should be'). Emphasise normalcy of development. Examine genitalia as any other body part; may leave to end.

PHYSICAL EXAMINATION

Although the approach to and sequence of the physical examination differ according to the child's age and development, the following discussion outlines the traditional model for physical assessment. The focus includes all paediatric age groups (see Chapter 7 for a detailed discussion of a newborn assessment).

Growth Measurements

Measurement of physical growth in children is a key element in evaluating their health status. Physical growth parameters include weight, height (length), skinfold thickness, arm circumference and head circumference. Values for these growth parameters are plotted on percentile charts, and the child's measurements in percentiles are compared with those of the general population.

Growth Charts

Growth charts use a series of percentile curves to demonstrate the distribution of body measurements in children. The Australasian Paediatric Endocrine Group (APEG) (2020) recommends that the World Health Organization (WHO) growth standards be used to

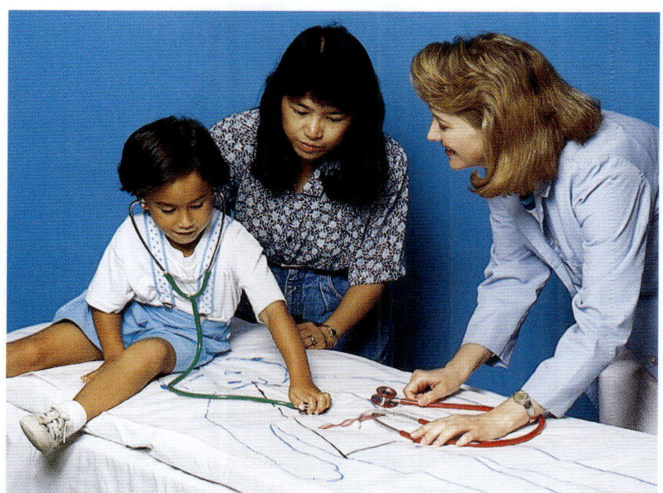

Fig 4.4 Using the paper-doll technique to prepare a child for physical examination.

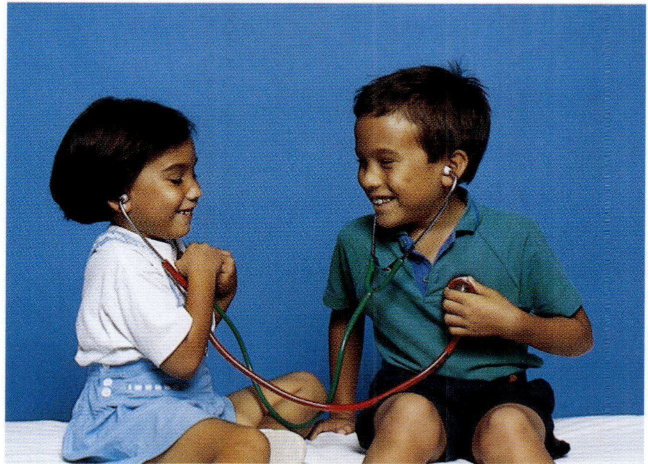

Fig 4.5 Preparing children for physical examination.

monitor growth for infants and children between the ages of 0 and 2 years old in Australia and New Zealand. Because breastfeeding is the recommended standard for infant feeding, the WHO growth charts are used; they reflect growth patterns among children who were predominantly breastfed for at least 4 months and are still breastfeeding at 12 months old. For children and adolescents aged 2 to 18 years APEG (2020) recommends using their endorsed growth charts or CDC clinical growth charts (Centres for Disease Control and Prevention [CDC] 2017).

Children whose growth may be questionable include the following:

- children whose height and weight percentiles are widely disparate (e.g. height in the 10th percentile and weight in the 90th percentile, especially with above-average skinfold thickness)
- children who fail to follow the expected growth velocity in height and weight
- children who show a sudden increase (except during normal puberty) or decrease in a previously steady growth pattern (i.e. crossing two major percentile lines after 3 years old)
- children who are short in the absence of short parents.

Because growth is a continuous but uneven process, the most reliable evaluation lies in comparing growth measurements over time because they reflect change. It is important to remember that same-age children (whether short, average or tall in stature) should grow at similar rates (Fig 4.6).

Length

The term ***length*** refers to measurements taken when children are supine (also referred to as **recumbent length**). Until children are 24 months old (or 36 months if using the chart for birth to 36 months), measure recumbent length using a length board (see Fig 4.7A). Because of the normally flexed position during infancy, fully extend the body by: (1) holding the head in midline; (2) grasping the knees together gently; and (3) pushing down on the knees until the legs are fully extended and flat against the table. When using a length board, place the head firmly at the top of the board and the heels of the feet firmly against the footboard. A tape measure should not be used to measure the length of infants and children because the methods are inaccurate and unreliable (Foote et al 2009).

Height

The term ***height*** (or ***stature***) refers to the measurement taken when a child is standing upright. Wall charts and flip-up horizontal bars (floppy-arm devices) mounted to weighing scales should not be used to measure the height of children (Foote et al 2009). These devices are not steady and do not maintain a right angle to the vertical ruler, preventing an accurate and reliable height. Measure height by having the child, with shoes removed, stand as tall and straight as possible with the head in midline and the line of vision parallel to the ceiling and floor. Be certain the child's back is to the wall or other vertical flat surface, with the head, shoulder blades, buttocks and heels touching

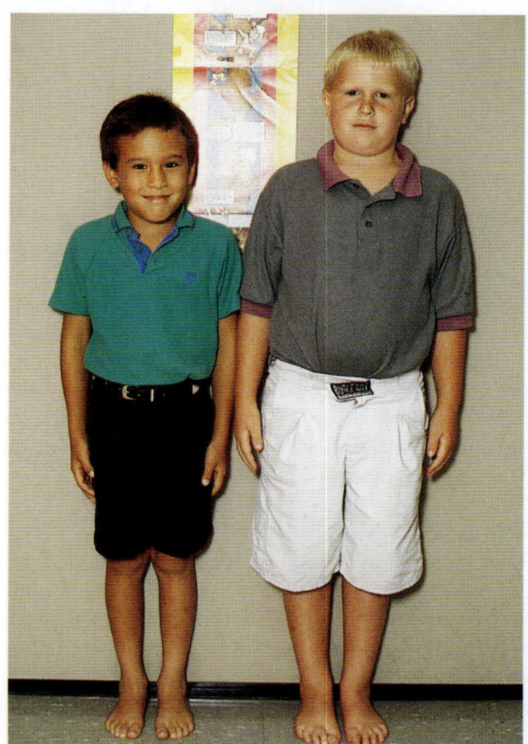

Fig 4.6 These children of identical age (8 years) are markedly different in size. The child on the left, of Asian descent, is at the 5th percentile for height and weight. The child on the right is above the 95th percentile for height and weight. However, both children demonstrate normal growth patterns because they are growing and gaining weight at normal rates.

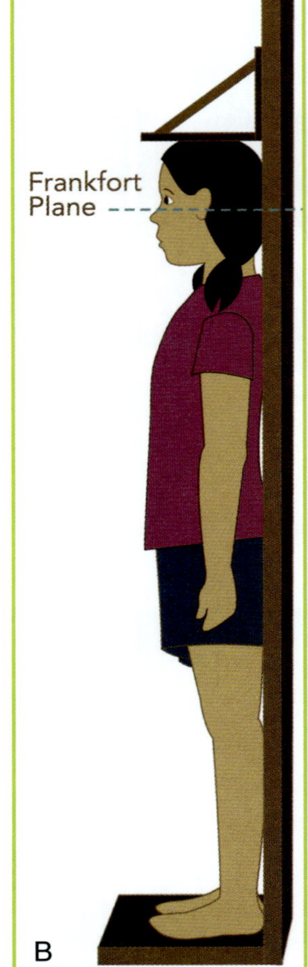

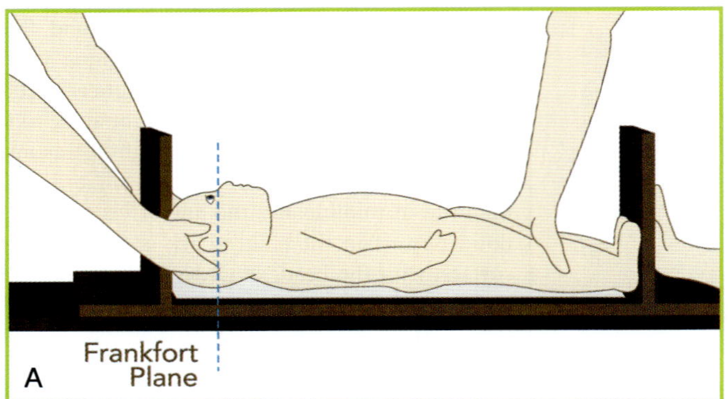

Fig 4.7 Measurement of linear growth. **A** Infant length. **B** Child height. (Source: Courtesy Jan M. Foote, Blank Children's Hospital, Des Moines, IA.)

the wall and the medial malleoli touching if possible (Fig 4.7B). Check for and correct slumping of the shoulders, positional lordosis, bending of the knees or raising of the heels.

For the most accurate measurement, use a wall-mounted unit (**stadiometer**; see Fig 4.7B). To improvise a flat, vertical surface for measuring height, attach a paper or metal tape or yardstick to the wall, position the child adjacent to the tape and place a three-dimensional object, such as a thick book or box, on top of the head. Rest the side of the object firmly against the wall to form a right angle. Measure height or stature to the last completed millimetre.

Weight

Weight is measured with an appropriately sized electronic or balance beam scale, which measures weight to the nearest 10 g for infants and 100 g for children. Before weighing the child, balance the scale by setting it at 0 and noting if the balance registers at exactly 0 or in the middle of the mark. If the end of the balance beam rises to the top or bottom of the mark, more or less weight, respectively, is needed. Some scales are designed to self-correct, but others need to be recalibrated according to the manufacturer's instructions. Take measurements in a comfortably warm room. When birth-to-2-year or birth-to-36-month growth charts are used, children should be weighed nude. Older children are usually weighed while wearing their underpants, a gown or light clothing, depending on the setting. However, always respect the privacy of all children. If the child must be weighed wearing some type of special device, such as a prosthesis or an arm board for an intravenous device, note this when recording the weight. Children who are measured for recumbent length are usually weighed on an infant scale and placed in a lying or sitting position. When weighing a child, place your hand slightly above the infant to prevent him or her from accidentally falling off the scale (Fig 4.8A) or stand close to the toddler, ready to prevent a fall (Fig 4.8B). For maximum asepsis, clean the scale and cover the scale with a clean sheet of paper between each child's weight measurement.

Nurses need to be familiar with determining body mass index (BMI), which requires accurate information about the child's weight and height.

$$\text{BMI} = \text{Weight in kilograms} \div [\text{Height in metres}]^2$$

With the increasing number of overweight children in Australia and New Zealand, BMI charts are a critical component of children's physical assessment. BMI-for-age and gender is used to identify children and adolescents who are underweight (<5th percentile), healthy weight (5th to <85th percentile), overweight (≥85th percentile and <95th percentile) or obese (≥95th percentile).

Skinfold Thickness and Arm Circumference

Measures of relative weight and stature cannot distinguish between adipose (fat) tissue and muscle. One convenient measure of body fat is **skinfold thickness**, which is increasingly recommended as a routine

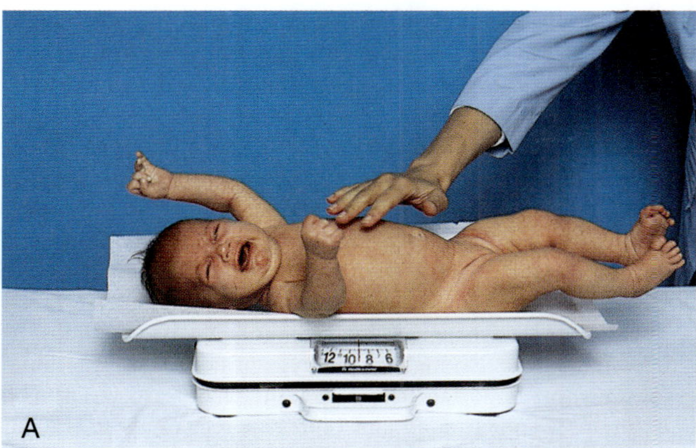

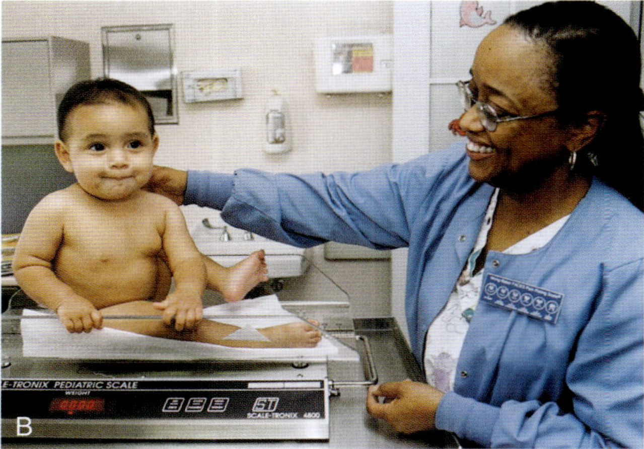

Fig 4.8 **A** Infant on scale. **B** Toddler on scale. Note the presence of nurse to prevent falls. (Source: *B*, Courtesy Paul Vincent Kuntz, Texas Children's Hospital, Houston, TX.)

measurement. Measure skinfold thickness with special callipers, such as the Lange callipers. The most common sites for measuring skinfold thickness are the triceps (most practical for routine clinical use), subscapular, suprailiac, abdomen and upper thigh. For greatest reliability, follow the exact procedure for measurement and record the average of at least two measurements of one site.

Arm circumference is an indirect measure of muscle mass. Measurement of arm circumference follows the same procedure as for skinfold thickness except the midpoint is measured with a paper, non-stretchable plastic or steel tape. Place the tape vertically along the posterior aspect of the upper arm from the acromial process to the olecranon process; half the measured length is the midpoint. WHO growth curves are available for triceps skinfold and arm circumference measurements.

Head Circumference

Head circumference is a reflection of brain growth. Measure head circumference in children up to 36 months of age and in any child whose head size is questionable. Measure the head at its greatest fronto-occipital circumference, usually slightly above the eyebrows and pinna of the ears and around the occipital prominence at the back of the skull (Fig 4.9). Use a paper or non-stretchable tape, or insert-a-tape, marked in millimetre increments because a cloth tape can stretch and give a falsely small measurement. Because head shape can affect the location of the maximum circumference, more than one

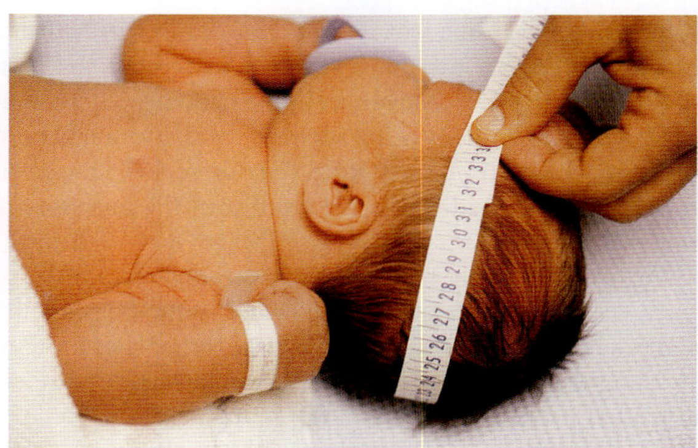

Fig 4.9 Measurement of head circumference. (Source: Seidel, H. M., Ball, J. W., Dains, J. E., et al. (1999). *Mosby's guide to physical examination* (4th ed.). St Louis, MO: Mosby.)

measurement is necessary to obtain the most accurate measure. Measure head circumference to the last completed millimetre.

Plot the head size on the appropriate growth chart for head circumference. Generally, head and chest circumferences are equal at about 1 to 2 years of age. During childhood, chest circumference exceeds head size by about 5 to 7 cm. For newborns, see Chapter 7.

Physiological Measurements

Physiological measurements, key elements in evaluating physical status of vital functions, include temperature, pulse, respiration and blood pressure. Compare each physiological recording with normal values for that age group. In addition, compare the values taken on preceding health visits with present recordings. For example, a falsely elevated blood pressure reading may not indicate hypertension if previous recent readings have been within normal limits. The isolated recording may indicate some stressful event in the child's life.

As in most procedures carried out with children, treat older children and adolescents much the same as adults. However, give special consideration to preschool children (see Nursing Care Considerations box). For best results in taking vital signs of infants, count respirations first (before the infant is disturbed), take the pulse next and measure temperature last. If vital signs cannot be taken without disturbing the child, record the child's behaviour (e.g. crying) along with the measurement.

> **NURSING CARE CONSIDERATIONS**
>
> ***Reducing Young Children's Fears***
>
> Young children, especially preschoolers, fear intrusive procedures because of their poorly defined body boundaries. Therefore avoid invasive procedures, such as measuring rectal temperature, whenever possible. Also, avoid using the word 'take' when measuring vital signs because young children interpret words literally and may think that their temperature or other function will be taken away. Instead, say, 'I want to know how warm you are'.

Temperature

Temperature is the measure of heat content within an individual's body. The **core temperature** most closely reflects the temperature of the blood flow through the carotid arteries to the hypothalamus. Core temperature is relatively constant despite wide fluctuations in the external environment. When a child's temperature is altered, receptors in the skin, spinal cord and brain respond in an attempt to achieve **normothermia**, a normal temperature state. In paediatrics, there is a lack of consensus regarding what temperature constitutes normothermia for every child. For neonates, a core body temperature between 36.5° and 37.6° C is a desirable range. In the neonate, obtain temperature measurements for monitoring adequacy of thermoregulation, not just for fever; therefore, temperature measurements in each infant should be carefully considered in the context of the purpose and the environment.

The nurse can measure temperature in healthy children at several body sites via oral, rectal, axillary, ear canal (tympanic membrane), temporal artery or skin route. For the ill child, other sites for temperature measurement have been investigated. Skin temperature sensors are most often used for neonates and infants placed in radiant heat warmers or incubators. The pulmonary artery is the closest to the hypothalamus and best reflects the core temperature (Batra et al 2012). Tympanic membrane thermometry for children older than 2 years of age and temporal artery thermometry in all age groups are taking precedence over other methods (Batra & Goyal 2013, Batra et al 2012). One of the most important influences on the accuracy of temperature is improper temperature-taking technique. Detailed discussion of temperature-taking methods and visual examples of proper techniques are given in Table 4.3.

The most frequently used temperature measurement devices in infants and children include the following.

- **Electronic intermittent thermometers** measure the patient's temperature at oral, rectal and axillary sites and are used as primary diagnostic indicators.
- **Infrared thermometers** measure the patient's temperature by collecting emitted thermal radiation from a particular site (e.g. ear canal).
- **Electronic continuous thermometers** measure the patient's temperature during the administration of general anaesthesia, treatment of hypothermia or hyperthermia and other situations that require continuous monitoring.

Pulse

A satisfactory pulse can be taken radially in children older than 2 years of age. However, in infants and young children, the **apical impulse** (heard through a stethoscope held to the chest at the apex of the heart) is more reliable (see Fig 4.31 later in this chapter for location of pulses). Count the pulse for 1 full minute in infants and young children because of possible irregularities in rhythm. However, when frequent apical rates are necessary, use shorter counting times (e.g. 15- or 30-second intervals). For greater accuracy, measure the apical rate while the child is asleep; record the child's behaviour along with the rate. Grade pulses according to the criteria in Table 4.4. Compare radial and femoral pulses at least once during infancy to detect the presence of circulatory impairment, such as coarctation of the aorta.

Respiration

Count the respiratory rate in children in the same manner as for adult patients. However, in infants, observe abdominal movements because respirations are primarily diaphragmatic. Because the movements are irregular, count them for 1 full minute for accuracy (see also the Chest section later in this chapter).

Blood Pressure

Auscultation remains the recommended method of blood pressure (BP) measurement in children, under most circumstances. Use of the automated devices is preferred for BP measurement in newborns and young infants, in whom auscultation is difficult and in the intensive care setting, where frequent BP measurement is needed.

Oscillometric devices measure mean arterial BP and then calculate systolic and diastolic values. The algorithms used by companies are proprietary and differ from company to company and device to device. These devices can yield results that vary widely when one is compared with another, and they do not always closely match BP values obtained by auscultation. An elevated BP reading obtained with an oscillometric device should be repeated using auscultation.

BP readings using oscillometry, such as Dinamap, are generally higher (10 mmHg higher) than measurements using auscultation (Park et al 2005). Differences between Dinamap and auscultatory readings prevent the interchange of the readings by the two methods.

Selection of Cuff. No matter what type of non-invasive technique is used, the most important factor in accurately measuring BP is the use of an appropriately sized cuff (**cuff size** refers only to the inner inflatable bladder, not the cloth covering). A technique to establish an appropriate cuff size is to choose a cuff with a **bladder width** that is approximately 40% of the arm circumference midway between the olecranon and the acromion. This will usually be a cuff **bladder length** that covers 80% to 100% of the circumference of the arm (Fig 4.10). Cuffs that are either too narrow or too wide affect the accuracy of BP measurements. If the cuff size is too small, the reading on the device is falsely high. If the cuff size is too large, the reading is falsely low. Similarly, sites for assessing BP are important. Generally, the upper arm is used (Fig 4.11). When using a site other than the arm, BP measurements using non-invasive techniques may differ. A systolic BP in the lower extremities (thigh or calf) is greater than that in the upper extremities, and systolic BP in the calf is higher than that in the thigh (Schell et al 2011).

Orthostatic Hypotension. **Orthostatic hypotension (OH)**, also called *postural hypotension* or *orthostatic intolerance,* often manifests as **syncope** (fainting), **vertigo** (dizziness) or light-headedness and is caused by decreased blood flow to the brain (**cerebral hypoperfusion**). Normally blood flow to the brain is maintained at a constant level by several compensating mechanisms that regulate systemic BP. When one assumes a sitting or standing position from a supine or recumbent position, peripheral capillary vasoconstriction occurs and blood that was pooling in the lower vasculature is returned to the heart for redistribution to the head and remainder of the body. When this mechanism fails or is slow to respond, the person may experience vertigo or syncope. One of the most common causes of OH is hypovolaemia, which may be induced by medications such as diuretics, vasodilator medications and prolonged immobility or bed rest. Other causes of OH include dehydration, diarrhoea, emesis, fluid loss from sweating and exertion, alcohol intake, dysrhythmias, diabetes mellitus, sepsis and haemorrhage.

BP measurements taken with the child first supine and then standing (at least 2 minutes in each position) may demonstrate variability and assist in the diagnosis of OH. The child with a sustained drop in systolic pressure of more than 20 mmHg or in diastolic pressure of more than 10 mmHg after standing for 2 minutes without an increase in heart rate of more than 15 beats/min most likely has an autonomic deficit. Non-neurogenic causes of OH have a compensatory increase in pulse of more than 15 beats/min, as well as a drop in BP, as noted previously. For children or adolescents with vertigo, light-headedness, nausea, syncope, diaphoresis and pallor, it is important to monitor BP and heart rate to determine the original cause. BP is an important diagnostic measurement in children and adolescents and must be a part of the routine monitoring of vital signs.

General Appearance

The child's general appearance is a cumulative, subjective impression of the child's physical appearance, state of nutrition, behaviour, personality,

TABLE 4.3 Temperature Measurement Locations for Infants and Children

Temperature Site

Oral

Place tip under tongue in right or left posterior sublingual pocket, not in front of tongue. Have child keep mouth closed, without biting on thermometer.

Pacifier thermometers measure intraoral or supralingual temperature and are available but lack support in the literature.

Several factors affect mouth temperature: Eating and mastication, hot or cold beverages, open-mouth breathing and ambient temperature.

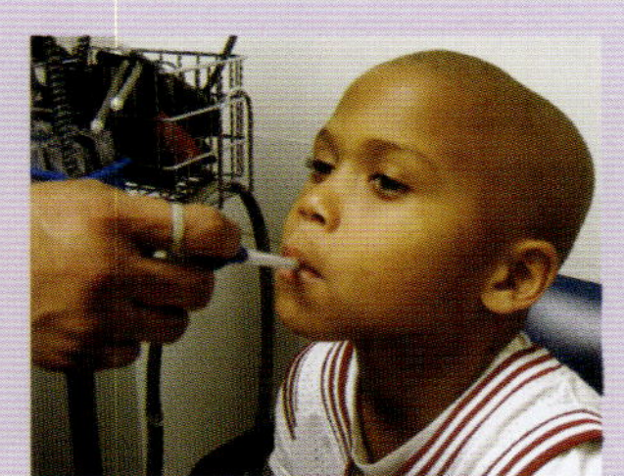

Axillary

Place tip under arm in centre of axilla and keep close to skin, not clothing. Hold child's arm firmly against side. Temperature may be affected by poor peripheral perfusion (results in lower value); clothing or swaddling, use of radiant warmer or amount of brown fat in cold-stressed neonate (results in higher value).

Advantage: Avoids intrusive procedure and eliminates risk of rectal perforation.

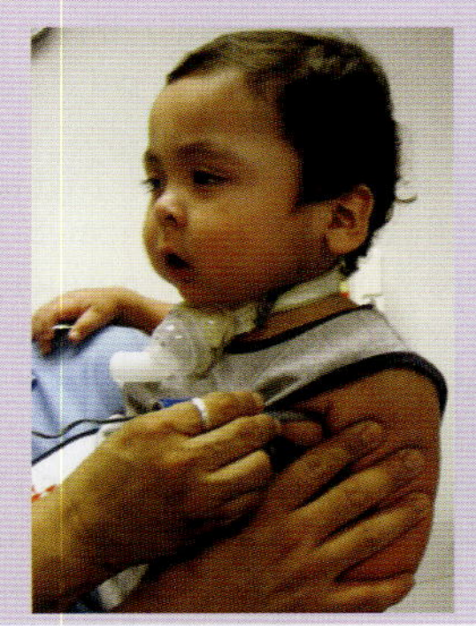

Ear Based (Aural)

Insert small infrared probe deeply into canal to allow sensor to obtain measurement from tympanic membrane. Size of probe (most are 8 mm) may influence accuracy of result. In young children, this may be a problem because of small diameter of canal.

Proper placement of ear is controversial related to whether the pinna should be pulled in a manner similar to that used during otoscopy.

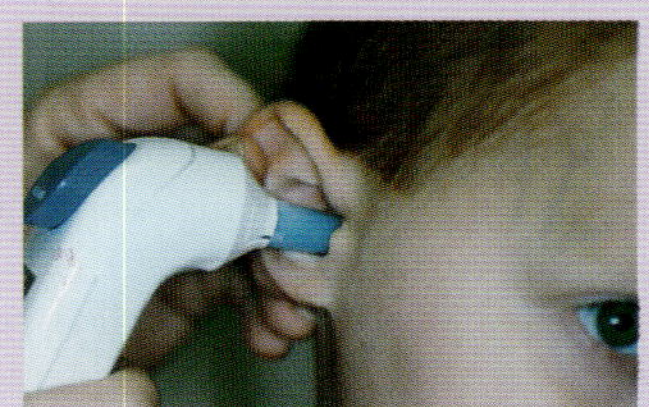

Rectal

Place well-lubricated tip at maximum 2.5 cm into rectum for children and 1.5 cm for infants; securely hold thermometer close to anus.

Child may be placed in side-lying, supine or prone position (i.e. supine with knees flexed towards abdomen); cover penis because procedure may stimulate urination. A small child may be placed prone across parent's lap.

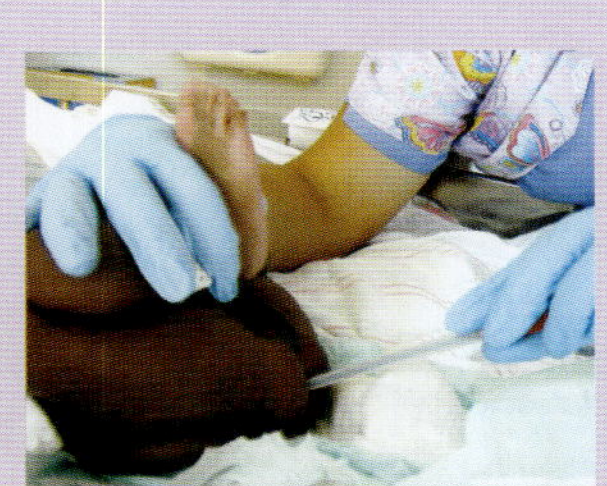

Temporal Artery

An infrared sensor probe scans across forehead, capturing heat from arterial blood flow.Temporal artery is only artery close enough to skin's surface to provide access for accurate temperature measurement.

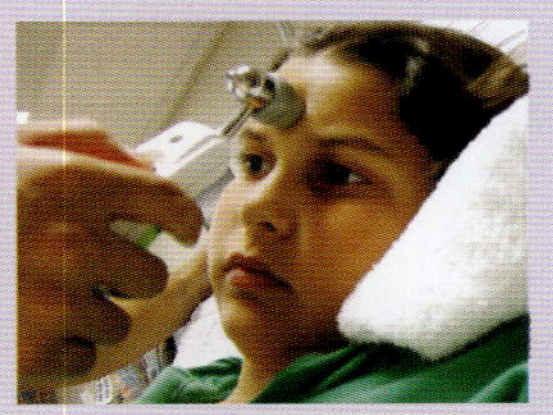

Source: Data from Martin, S. A., & Kline, A. M. (2004). Can there be a standard for temperature measurement in the pediatric intensive care unit? *AACN Clinical Issues, 15*(2), 254–266; Falzon, A., Grech, V., Caruana, B., et al. (2003). How reliable is axillary temperature measurement? *Acta Paediatrica, 92*(3), 309–313. Oral, axillary, rectal, and temporal artery images courtesy Paul Vincent Kuntz, Texas Children's Hospital, Houston, TX.

TABLE 4.4 Grading of Pulses

Grade	Description
0	Not palpable
+1	Difficult to palpate, thready, weak, easily obliterated with pressure
+2	Difficult to palpate, may be obliterated with pressure
+3	Easy to palpate, not easily obliterated with pressure (normal)
+4	Strong, bounding, not obliterated with pressure

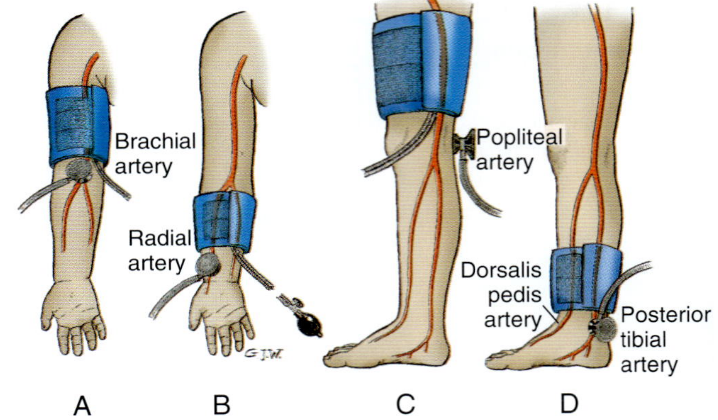

Fig 4.11 Sites for measuring BP. **A** Upper arm. **B** Lower arm or forearm. **C** Thigh. **D** Calf or ankle.

interactions with parents and nurse (also siblings if present), posture, development and speech. Although the nurse records general appearance at the beginning of the physical examination, it encompasses all the observations of the child during the interview and physical assessment.

Note the **facies**, the child's facial expression and appearance. For example, the facies may give clues to children who are in pain; have difficulty breathing; feel frightened, discontented or unhappy; are mentally delayed; or are acutely ill.

Observe the posture, position and types of body movement. A child with hearing or vision loss may characteristically tilt the head in an awkward position to hear or see better. A child in pain may favour a body part. A child with low self-esteem or a feeling of rejection may assume a slumped, careless and apathetic pose. Likewise, a child with confidence, a feeling of self-worth and a sense of security usually demonstrates a tall, straight, well-balanced posture. While observing such body language, do not interpret too freely but rather record objectively.

Note the child's hygiene in terms of cleanliness; unusual body odour; the condition of the hair, neck, nails, teeth and feet; and the condition of the clothing. Such observations are excellent clues to possible instances of neglect, inadequate financial resources, housing difficulties (e.g. no running water) or lack of knowledge concerning children's needs.

Behaviour includes the child's personality, activity level, reaction to stress, requests, frustration, interactions with others (primarily the parent and nurse), degree of alertness and response to stimuli. Some mental questions that serve as reminders for observing behaviour include the following.

- What is the child's overall personality?
- Does the child have a long attention span, or is he or she easily distracted?
- Can the child follow two or three commands in succession without the need for repetition?
- What is the child's response to delayed gratification or frustration?
- Does the child use eye contact during conversation?
- What is the child's reaction to the nurse and family members?
- Is the child quick or slow to grasp explanations?

Skin

Assess skin for colour, texture, temperature, moisture, turgor, lesions and rashes. Examination of the skin and its accessory organs primarily involves inspection and palpation. Touch allows the nurse to assess the texture, turgor and temperature of the skin. The normal colour in

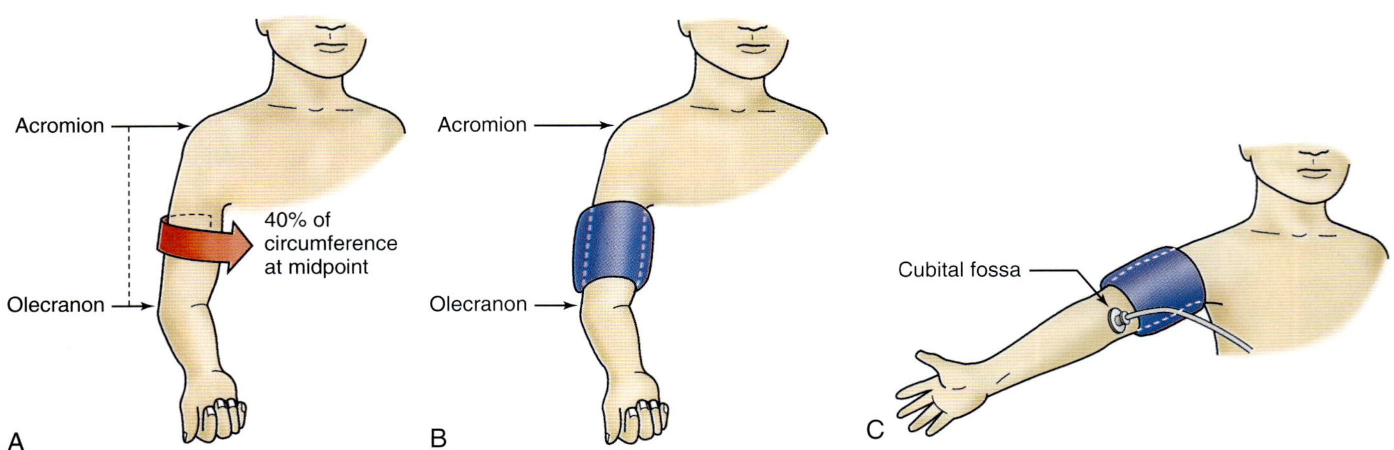

Fig 4.10 Determination of proper cuff size. **A** Cuff bladder width should be approximately 40% of circumference of arm measured at a point midway between olecranon and acromion. **B** Cuff bladder length should cover 80% to 100% of circumference of arm. **C** BP should be measured with the cubital fossa at the level of the heart. The arm should be supported. The stethoscope bell is placed over the brachial artery pulse proximal and medial to the cubital fossa and below the bottom edge of the cuff. (Source: National Institutes of Health, National Heart, Lung, and Blood Institute. (2005). *The fourth report on the diagnosis, evaluation, and treatment of high blood pressure in children and adolescents.* May. NIH Pub No 05-5267, originally printed 1996 (96-3790). Bethesda, MD: Author.)

light-skinned children varies from a milky white and rose to a deeply hued pink. Dark-skinned children, such as Aboriginal and Torres Strait Islanders or those of Māori decent, may have inherited various brown, red, yellow, olive green and bluish tones in their skin. Persons of Asian descent have skin that is normally of a yellow tone. Several variations in skin colour can occur, some of which warrant further investigation. The types of colour change and their appearance in children are summarised in Table 4.5.

Normally the skin texture of young children is smooth, slightly dry and not oily or clammy. Evaluate skin temperature by symmetrically feeling each part of the body and comparing upper areas with lower ones. Note any difference in temperature.

Determine **tissue turgor**, or elasticity in the skin, by grasping the skin on the abdomen between the thumb and index finger, pulling it taut and quickly releasing it. Elastic tissue immediately resumes its normal position without residual marks or creases. In children with poor skin turgor, the skin remains suspended or tented for a few seconds before slowly falling back on the abdomen. Skin turgor is one of the best estimates of adequate hydration and nutrition.

Accessory Structures

Inspection of the accessory structures of the skin may be performed while examining the skin, scalp or extremities. Inspect the hair for colour, texture, quality, distribution and elasticity. Children's scalp hair is usually lustrous, silky, strong and elastic. Genetic factors affect the appearance of hair. For example, the hair of Māori and Aboriginal or Torres Strait Islander children is usually curlier and coarser than that of Caucasian children. Hair that is stringy, dull, brittle, dry, friable and depigmented may suggest poor nutrition. Record any bald or thinning spots. Loss of hair in infants may indicate lying in the same position and may be a cue to counsel parents concerning the child's stimulation needs.

Inspect the hair and scalp for general cleanliness. Persons in some ethnic groups condition their hair with oils or lubricants that, if not thoroughly washed from the scalp, clog the sebaceous glands, causing scalp infections. Examine the scalp for lesions, scaliness, evidence of infestation (e.g. lice or ticks) and signs of trauma (e.g. ecchymosis, masses or scars).

In children who are approaching puberty, look for growth of secondary hair as a sign of normally progressing pubertal changes. Note precocious or delayed appearance of hair growth because, although not always suggestive of hormonal dysfunction, it may be of great concern to the early-maturing child or late-maturing adolescent.

Inspect the nails for colour, shape, texture and quality. Normally the nails are pink, convex, smooth and hard but flexible (not brittle). The edges, which are usually white, should extend over the fingers. Dark-skinned individuals may have more deeply pigmented nail beds. Short, ragged nails are typical of habitual biting. Uncut, dirty nails are a sign of poor hygiene.

The palm normally shows three flexion creases (Fig 4.12A). In some conditions, such as Down syndrome, the two distal horizontal creases may be fused to form a single horizontal crease (the single palmar crease, or transpalmar crease) (Fig 4.12B). If grossly abnormal lines or folds are observed, sketch a picture to describe them and refer the finding to a specialist for further investigation.

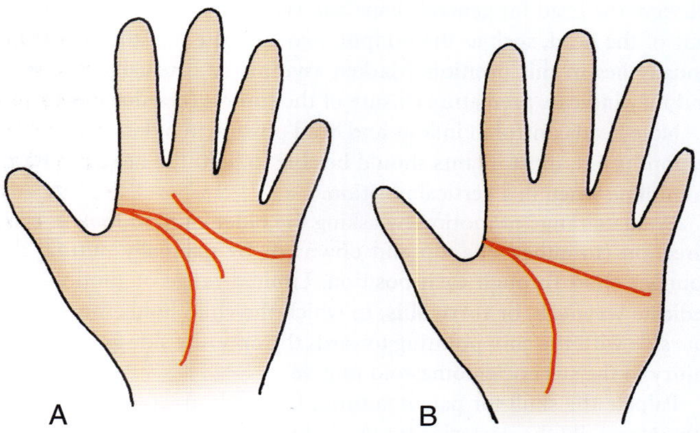

Fig 4.12 Examples of flexion creases on palm. **A** Normal. **B** Single palmar crease (transpalmar crease).

TABLE 4.5 Differences in Colour Changes of Light and Dark Skin

Description	Appearance in Light Skin	Appearance in Dark Skin
Cyanosis—bluish tone through skin; reflects reduced (deoxygenated) haemoglobin	Bluish tinge, especially in palpebral conjunctiva (lower eyelid), nail beds, earlobes, lips, oral membranes, soles and palms	Ashen grey lips and tongue
Pallor—paleness; may be sign of anaemia, chronic disease, oedema or shock	Loss of rosy glow in skin, especially face	Ashen grey appearance in black skin More yellowish brown colour in brown skin
Erythema—redness; may be result of increased blood flow from climatic conditions, local inflammation, infection, skin irritation, allergy or other dermatoses, or may be caused by increased numbers of red blood cells as compensatory response to chronic hypoxia	Redness easily seen anywhere on body	Much more difficult to assess; rely on palpation for warmth or oedema
Ecchymosis—large, diffuse areas, usually black and blue, caused by haemorrhage of blood into skin; typically result of injuries	Purplish to yellow-green areas; may be seen anywhere on skin	Very difficult to see unless in mouth or conjunctiva
Petechiae—same as ecchymosis except for size: small, distinct, pinpoint haemorrhages ≤ 2 mm in size; can denote some type of blood disorder, such as leukaemia	Purplish pinpoints most easily seen on buttocks, abdomen and inner surfaces of arms or legs	Usually invisible except in oral mucosa, conjunctiva of eyelids and conjunctiva covering eyeball
Jaundice—yellow staining of skin usually caused by bile pigments	Yellow staining seen in sclerae of eyes, skin, fingernails, soles, palms and oral mucosa	Most reliably assessed in sclerae, hard palate, palms and soles

Lymph Nodes

Lymph nodes are usually assessed during examination of the part of the body in which they are located. The body's lymphatic drainage system is extensive. Fig 4.13 shows the usual sites for palpating accessible lymph nodes.

Palpate nodes using the distal portion of the fingers and gently but firmly pressing in a circular motion along the regions where nodes are normally present. During assessment of the nodes in the head and neck, tilt the child's head upwards slightly but without tensing the sternocleidomastoid or trapezius muscles. This position facilitates palpation of the **submental**, **submandibular**, **tonsillar** and **cervical nodes.** Palpate the **axillary nodes** with the child's arms relaxed at the sides but slightly abducted. Assess the **inguinal nodes** with the child in the supine position. Note size, mobility, temperature and tenderness, as well as reports by the parents regarding any visible change of enlarged nodes. In children, small, non-tender, movable nodes are usually normal. Tender, enlarged, warm, erythematous lymph nodes generally indicate infection or inflammation close to their location. Report such findings for further investigation.

Head and Neck

Observe the head for general shape and symmetry. A flattening of one part of the head, such as the occiput, may indicate that the child continually lies in this position. Marked asymmetry is usually abnormal and may indicate premature closure of the sutures (**craniosynostosis**).

Note head control in infants and head posture in older children. By 4 months old, most infants should be able to hold the head erect and in midline when in a vertical position.

Evaluate range of motion by asking the older child to look in each direction (to either side, up and down) or by manually putting the younger child through each position. Limited range of motion may indicate **wryneck**, or **torticollis**, in which the child holds the head to one side with the chin pointing towards the opposite side as a result of injury to the sternocleidomastoid muscle.

Palpate the skull for patent sutures, fontanels, fractures and swellings. Normally the posterior fontanel closes by 2 months old, and the anterior fontanel fuses between 12 and 18 months. Early or late closure is noted because either may be a sign of a pathological condition.

While examining the head, observe the face for symmetry, movement and general appearance. Ask the child to 'make a face' to assess symmetrical movement and disclose any degree of paralysis. Note any unusual facial proportion, such as an unusually high or low forehead; wide- or close-set eyes; or a small, receding chin.

In addition to assessment of the head and neck for movement, inspect the neck for size and palpate its associated structures. The neck is normally short, with skinfolds between the head and shoulders during infancy; however, it lengthens during the next 3 to 4 years.

Eyes

Inspection of External Structures

Inspect the lids for proper placement on the eye. When the eye is open, the upper lid should fall near the upper iris. When the eyes are closed, the lids should completely cover the cornea and sclera (Fig 4.14).

Determine the general slant of the **palpebral fissures** or lids by drawing an imaginary line through the two points of the medial canthus and across the outer orbit of the eyes and aligning each eye on the line. Usually the palpebral fissures lie horizontally. However, in Asians, the slant is normally upwards.

Inspect the inside lining of the lids, the **palpebral conjunctivae.** To examine the lower conjunctival sac, pull the lid down while the patient looks up. To evert the upper lid, hold the upper lashes and gently pull down and forwards as the child looks down. Normally the conjunctiva appears pink and glossy. Vertical yellow striations along the edge are the **meibomian glands**, or **sebaceous glands**, near the hair follicle. Located in the inner or medial canthus and situated on the inner edge of the upper and lower lids is a tiny opening, the **lacrimal punctum.** Note any excessive tearing, discharge or inflammation of the lacrimal apparatus.

The **bulbar conjunctiva**, which covers the eye up to the limbus, or junction of the cornea and sclera, should be transparent. The **sclera** should be white, contrasting with the coloured iris. Tiny black marks in the sclera of heavily pigmented individuals are normal.

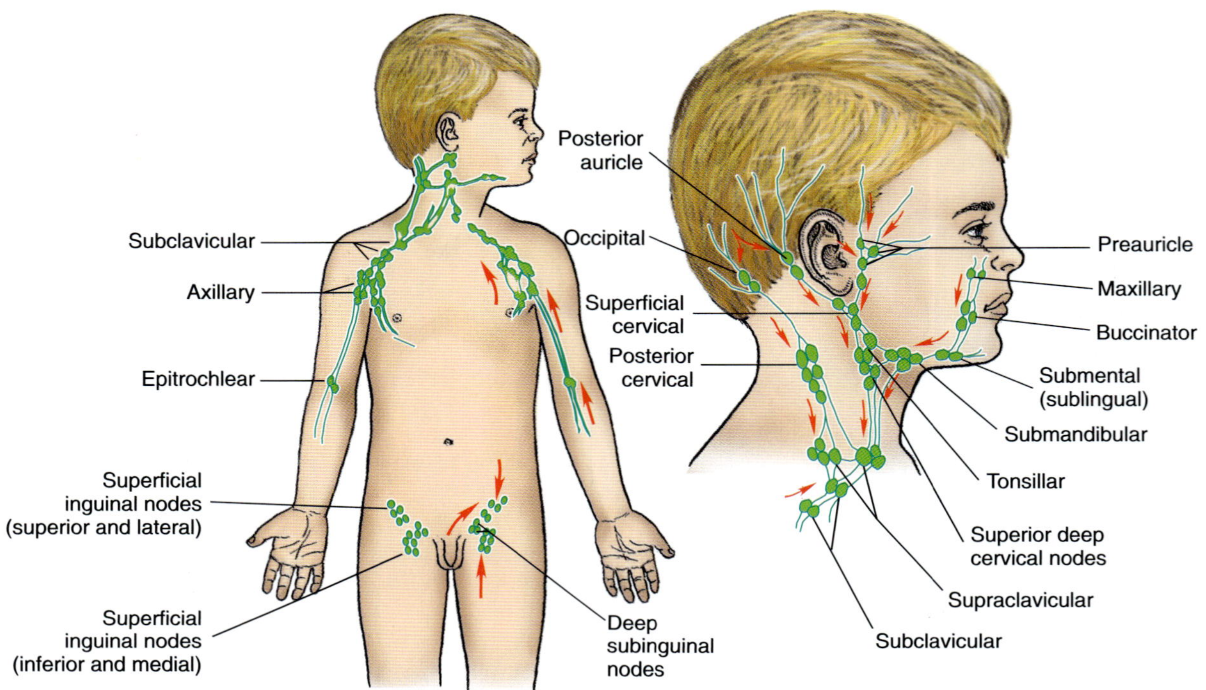

Fig 4.13 Location of superficial lymph nodes. Arrows indicate directional flow of lymph.

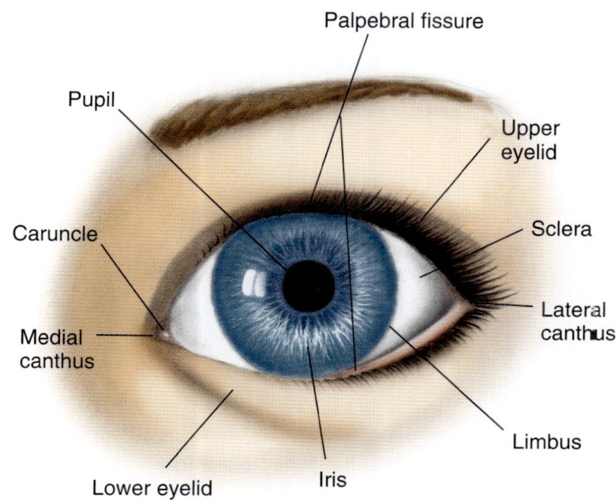

Fig 4.14 External structures of the eye.

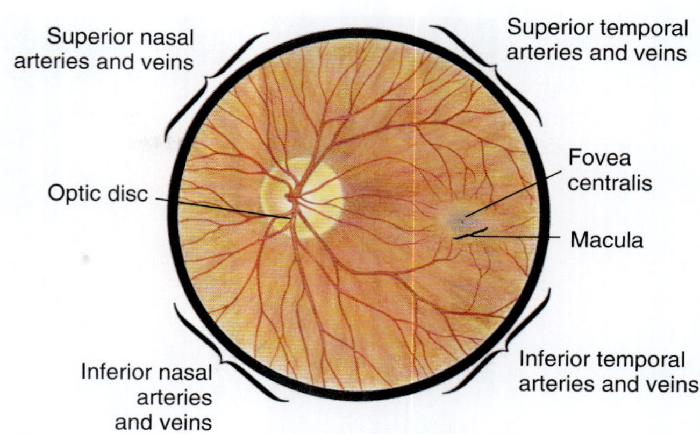

Fig 4.15 Structures of fundus. (Source: Ball, J. W., Dains, J. E., Flynn, J. A., et al. (2014). *Seidel's guide to physical examination* (8th ed.). St Louis, MO: Elsevier.)

The **cornea**, or covering of the iris and pupil, should be clear and transparent. Record opacities because they can be signs of scarring or ulceration, which can interfere with vision. The best way to test for opacities is to illuminate the eyeball by shining a light at an angle (**obliquely**) towards the cornea.

Compare the pupils for size, shape and movement. They should be round, clear and equal. Test their reaction to light by quickly shining a light towards the eye and removing it. As the light approaches, the pupils should constrict; as the light fades, the pupils should dilate. Test the pupil for any response of **accommodation** by having the child look at a bright, shiny object at a distance and quickly moving the object towards the face. The pupils should constrict as the object is brought near the eye. Record normal findings on examination of the pupils as **PERRLA**, which stands for 'Pupils Equal, Round, React to Light and Accommodation'.

Inspect the iris and pupil for colour, size, shape and clarity. Permanent eye colour is usually established by 6 to 12 months of age. While inspecting the iris and pupil, look for the lens. Normally the lens is not visible through the pupil.

Inspection of Internal Structures

The ophthalmoscope permits visualisation of the interior of the eyeball with a system of lenses and a high-intensity light. The lenses permit clear visualisation of eye structures at different distances from the nurse's eye and correct visual acuity differences in the examiner and child. Use of the ophthalmoscope requires practice to know which lens setting produces the clearest image.

Preparing the Child. The nurse can prepare the child for the ophthalmoscopic examination by showing the child the instrument, demonstrating the light source and how it shines, and explaining the reason for darkening the room. For infants and young children who do not respond to such explanations, it is best to use distraction to encourage them to keep their eyes open. Forcibly parting the eyelids results in an uncooperative, watery-eyed child and a frustrated nurse. Usually, with some practice, the nurse can elicit a red reflex almost instantly while approaching the child and may also gain a momentary inspection of the blood vessels, macula or optic disc.

Funduscopic Examination. Figure 4.15 shows the structures of the back of the eyeball, or the **fundus**. The fundus is immediately apparent as the **red reflex**. The intensity of the colour increases in darkly pigmented individuals.

As the ophthalmoscope is brought closer to the eye, the most conspicuous feature of the fundus is the **optic disc**, the area where the blood vessels and optic nerve fibres enter and exit the eye. The disc is orange to creamy pink with a pale centre and lighter in colour than the surrounding fundus. Normally, it is round or vertically oval.

After locating the optic disc, inspect the area for blood vessels. The central retinal artery and vein appear in the depths of the disc and emanate outwards with visible branching. The veins are darker and about 25% larger than the arteries. Normally, the branches of the arteries and veins cross one another.

Other structures that are common are the **macula**, the area of the fundus with the greatest concentration of visual receptors and in the centre of the macula, a minute glistening spot of reflected light called the **fovea centralis**; this is the area of most perfect vision.

Vision Testing

Vision screening is recommended for the presence of amblyopia and its risk factors for all children 3 to 5 years of age. Several tests are available for assessing vision. This discussion focuses on ocular alignment, visual acuity, peripheral vision and colour vision. Chapter 20 discusses behavioural and physical signs of visual impairment. Nurses can provide accurate vision screening with appropriate training (Mathers et al 2010).

Ocular Alignment. Normally, by the age of 3 to 4 months, children are able to fixate on one visual field with both eyes simultaneously (binocularity). In **strabismus**, or cross-eye, one eye deviates from the point of fixation. If the misalignment is constant, the weak eye becomes 'lazy' and the brain eventually suppresses the image produced by that eye. If strabismus is not detected and corrected by 4 to 6 years old, blindness from disuse, known as **amblyopia**, may result.

Tests commonly used to detect misalignment are the corneal light reflex and the cover tests. To perform the **corneal light reflex test**, or **Hirschberg test**, shine a torch or the light of the ophthalmoscope directly into the patient's eyes from a distance of about 40.5 cm. If the eyes are **orthophoric**, or normal, the light falls symmetrically within each pupil (Fig 4.16A). If the light falls off-centre in one eye, the eyes are misaligned. **Epicanthal folds**, excess folds of skin that extend from the roof of the nose to the inner termination of the eyebrow and that partially or completely overlap the inner canthus of the eye, may give a false impression of misalignment (**pseudostrabismus**) (Fig 4.16B). Epicanthal folds are often found in Asian children.

In the **cover test**, one eye is covered and the movement of the uncovered eye is observed while the child looks at a near (33 cm away) or distant (6 m away) object. If the uncovered eye does not move, it is aligned. If the uncovered eye moves, a misalignment is present because

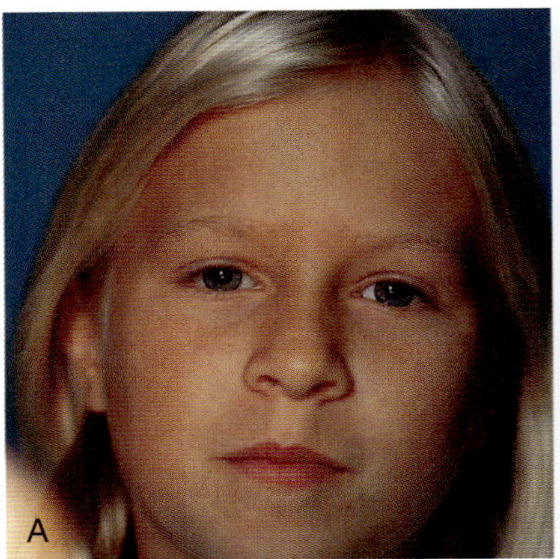

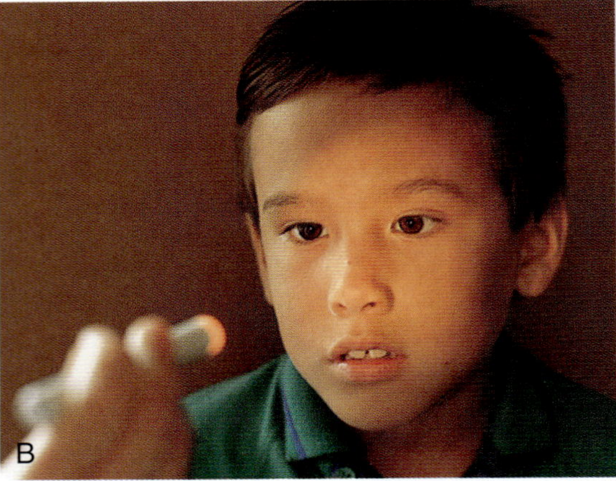

Fig 4.16 **A** Corneal light reflex test demonstrating orthophoric eyes. **B** Pseudostrabismus. Inner epicanthal folds cause the eyes to appear misaligned; however, the corneal light reflexes fall perfectly symmetrically.

when the stronger eye is temporarily covered, the misaligned eye attempts to fixate on the object.

In the **alternate cover test**, occlusion shifts back and forth from one eye to the other, and movement of the eye that was covered is observed as soon as the occluder is removed while the child focuses on a certain point (Fig 4.17). If normal alignment is present, shifting the cover from one eye to the other will not cause the eye to move. If misalignment is present, eye movement will occur when the cover is moved. This test takes more practice than the other cover test because the occluder must be moved back and forth quickly and accurately to see the eye move. Because deviations can occur at different ranges, it is important to perform the cover tests at both close and far distances.

Visual Acuity Testing in Children. The most common test for measuring visual acuity is the **Snellen letter chart**, which consists of lines of letters of decreasing size. The child stands with his or her heels at a line 3 metres away from the chart. When screening for visual acuity in children, the nurse tests the child's right eye first by covering the left. Children who wear glasses should be screened with them on. Tell the child to keep both eyes open during the examination. If the child fails to read the current line, move up the chart to the next larger line. Continue up the chart until the child is able to read the line. Then begin moving down the chart again until the child fails to read the line. To pass each line, the child must correctly identify four of six symbols on the line. Repeat the procedure, covering the right eye.

For children unable to read letters and numbers, the **tumbling E** or **HOTV** test is useful. The tumbling E test uses the capital letter **E** pointing in four different directions. The child is asked to point in the direction the **E** is facing. The HOTV test consists of a wall chart composed of the letters **H, O, T** and **V**. The child is given a board containing a large **H, O, T** and **V**. The examiner points to a letter on the wall chart, and the child matches the correct letter on the board held in his or her hand. The tumbling E and HOTV are excellent tests for preschool-age children.

Visual Acuity Testing in Infants and Difficult-to-test Children. In newborns, vision is tested mainly by checking for **light perception** by shining a light into the eyes and noting responses, such as pupillary constriction, blinking, following the light to midline, increased alertness or refusal to open the eyes after exposure to the light. Although the simple manoeuvre of checking light perception and eliciting the pupillary light reflex indicates that the anterior half of the visual apparatus is intact, it does not confirm that the infant can see. In other words, this test does not assess whether the brain receives the visual message and interprets the signals.

Another test of visual acuity is the infant's ability to fix on and follow a target. Although any brightly coloured or patterned object can be used, the human face is excellent. Hold the infant upright while moving your face slowly from side to side. Signs that may indicate visual loss or other serious eye problems include fixed pupils, strabismus, constant nystagmus, the setting-sun sign and slow lateral movements. Unfortunately, it is difficult to test each eye separately; the presence of such signs in one eye could indicate unilateral blindness.

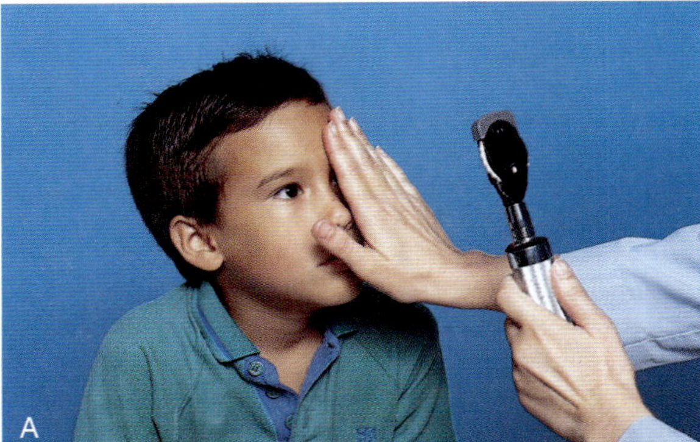

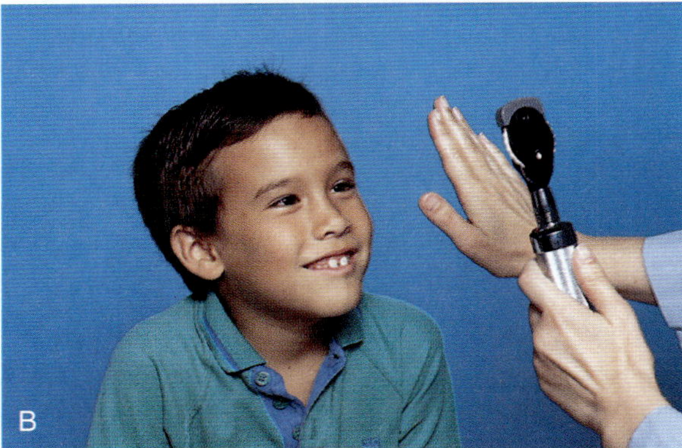

Fig 4.17 Alternate cover test to detect amblyopia in a patient with strabismus. **A** The eye is occluded, and the child is fixating on light source. **B** If the eye does not move when uncovered, the eyes are aligned.

Special tests are available for testing infants and other difficult-to-test children to assess acuity or confirm blindness. For example, in **visually evoked potentials**, the eyes are stimulated with a bright light or pattern, and electrical activity to the visual cortex is recorded through scalp electrodes.

Peripheral Vision. In children who are old enough to cooperate, estimate **peripheral vision** or the visual field of each eye, by having the children fixate on a specific point directly in front of them while an object, such as a finger or a pencil, is moved from beyond the field of vision into the range of peripheral vision. As soon as children see the object, have them say 'Stop'. At that point measure the angle from the anteroposterior axis of the eye (straight line of vision) to the peripheral axis (point at which the object is first seen). Check each eye separately and for each quadrant of vision. Normally children see about 50 degrees upwards, 70 degrees downwards, 60 degrees nasalwards and 90 degrees temporally. Limitations in peripheral vision may indicate blindness from damage to structures within the eye or to any of the visual pathways.

Colour Vision. The tests available for colour vision include the Ishihara test and the Hardy-Rand-Rittler test. Each consists of a series of cards (pseudoisochromatic) containing a colour field composed of spots of a certain 'confusion' colour. Against the field is a number or symbol similarly printed in dots but of a colour likely to be confused with the field colour by a person with a colour vision deficit. As a result, the figure or letter is invisible to an affected individual but is clearly seen by a person with normal vision.

Ears

Inspection of External Structures

The outer portion of the ear is called the pinna, or auricle; one is located on each side of the head. Measure the height alignment of the pinna by drawing an imaginary line from the outer orbit of the eye to the occiput, or most prominent protuberance of the skull. The top of the pinna should meet or cross this line. Low-set ears are commonly associated with renal anomalies or cognitive impairment. Measure the angle of the pinna by drawing a perpendicular line from the imaginary horizontal line and aligning the pinna next to this mark. Normally the pinna lies within a 10-degree angle of the vertical line (Fig 4.18). If it falls outside this area, record the deviation and look for other anomalies.

Normally the pinna extends slightly outwards from the skull. Except in newborn infants, ears that are flat against the head or protruding away from the scalp may indicate problems. Flattened ears in an infant may suggest a frequent side-lying position and, just as with isolated areas of hair loss, may be a clue to investigate parents' understanding of the child's stimulation needs.

Inspect the skin surface around the ear for small openings, extra tags of skin, sinuses or earlobe creases. If a sinus is found, note this because it may represent a fistula that drains into some area of the neck or ear. Note an earlobe crease, if found, because it may be associated with a rare syndrome. However, having one small abnormality is not uncommon and is often not associated with a serious condition. Cutaneous tags represent no pathological process but may cause parents' concern in terms of the child's appearance.

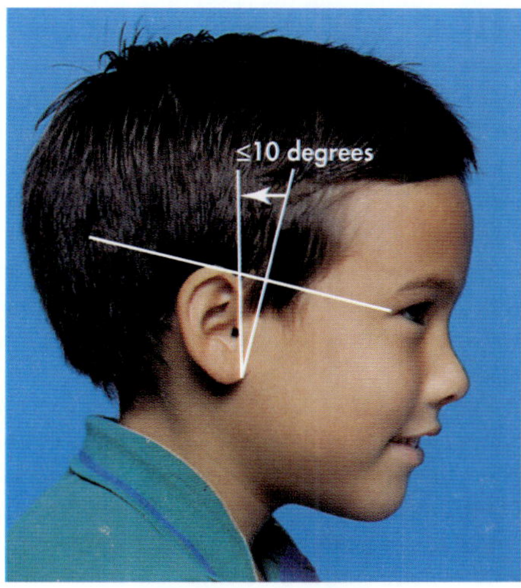

Fig 4.18 Ear alignment.

Assess the ear for hygiene. An otoscope is not necessary for looking into the external canal to note the presence of **cerumen**, a waxy substance produced by the ceruminous glands in the outer portion of the canal. Cerumen is usually yellow-brown and soft. If an otoscope is used and any discharge is visible, note its colour and odour. Avoid transmitting potentially infectious material to the other ear or to another child through hand washing and using disposable specula or sterilising reusable specula between each examination.

Inspection of Internal Structures

The head of the otoscope permits visualisation of the tympanic membrane by use of a bright light, a magnifying glass and a speculum. Some otoscopes have an attachment for a pneumonic device to insert air into the canal to determine membrane compliance (movement). The speculum, which is inserted into the external canal, comes in a variety of sizes to accommodate different canal widths. The largest speculum that fits comfortably into the ear is used to achieve the greatest area of visualisation. The lens, or magnifying glass, is movable, allowing the examiner to insert an object, such as a curette, into the ear canal through the speculum while still viewing the structures through the lens.

Positioning the Child. Before beginning the otoscopic examination, position the child properly and gently restrain him or her (child sits on a parent's lap and the parent holds their body and head) if necessary. Older children usually cooperate and do not need restraint. However, prepare them for the procedure by allowing them to play with the instrument, demonstrating how it works and stressing the importance of remaining still. A helpful suggestion is to let them observe you examining the parent's ear. Restraint is needed for younger children because the ear examination upsets them (see Nursing Care Considerations box).

> **NURSING CARE CONSIDERATIONS**
>
> ***Reducing Distress from Otoscopy in Young Children***
>
> Make examining the ear a game by explaining that you are looking for a 'big elephant' in the ear. This kind of make-believe is an absorbing distraction and usually elicits cooperation. After examining the ear, clarify that 'looking for elephants' was only pretend and thank the child for letting you look in his or her ear. Another great distraction technique is asking the child to put a finger on the opposite ear to keep the light from getting out.

As you insert the speculum into the meatus, move it around the outer rim to accustom the child to the feel of something entering the ear. If examining a painful ear, examine the unaffected ear, then return to the painful ear and touch a non-painful part of the affected ear first. By this time, the child is usually less fearful of anything causing discomfort to the ear and will cooperate more.

For their protection and safety, restrain infants and toddlers for the otoscopic examination. There are two general positions of restraint. In one, the child is seated sideways in the parent's lap with one arm hugging the parent and the other arm at the side. The ear to be examined is towards the nurse. With one arm the parent holds the child's head firmly against his or her chest and hugs the child with the other arm, thereby securing the child's free arm (Fig 4.19A). Examine the ear using the same procedure for holding the otoscope as described later.

The other position involves placing the child on the side, back or abdomen with the arms at the side and the head turned so that the ear to be examined points towards the ceiling. Lean over the child, use the upper part of the body to restrain the arms and upper trunk movements, and use the examining hand to stabilise the head. This position is practical for young infants or for older children who need minimum

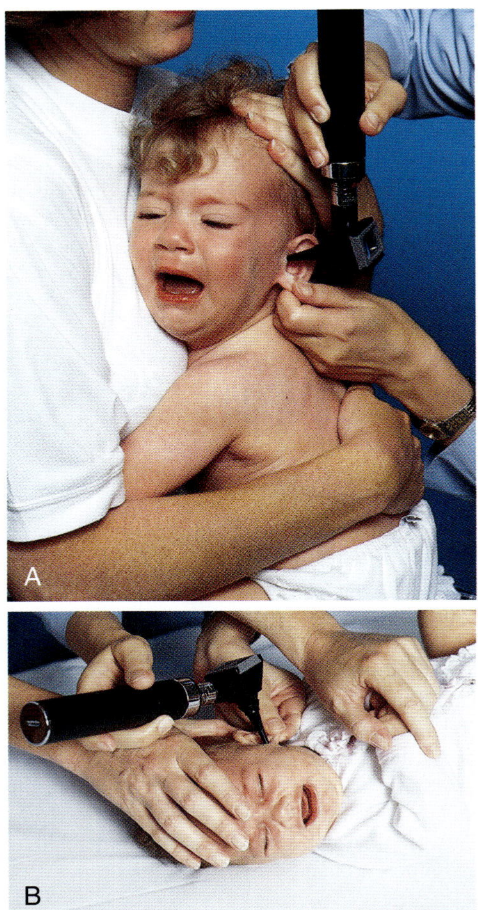

Fig 4.19 Position for restraining a child (**A**) and an infant (**B**) during otoscopic examination.

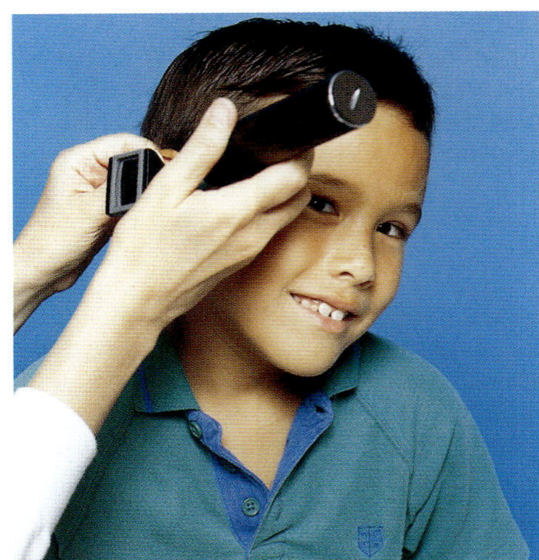

Fig 4.20 Positioning the head by tilting it towards the opposite shoulder for full view of the tympanic membrane.

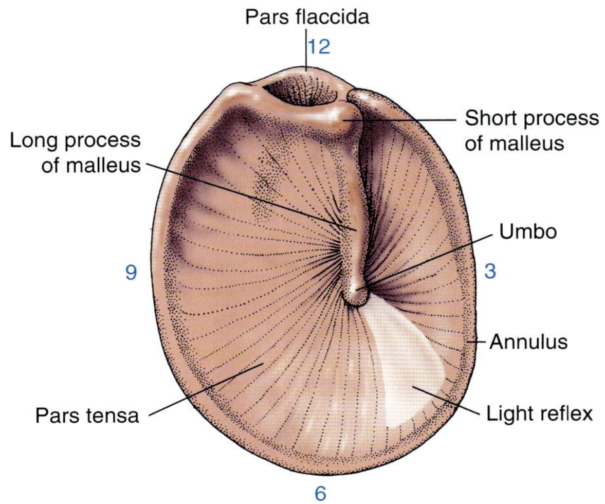

Fig 4.21 Landmarks of the tympanic membrane. (Source: Ignatavicius, D. D., & Workman, M. L. (2013). *Medical-surgical nursing: Patient-centred collaborative care* (7th ed.). St Louis, MO: Saunders.)

restraint, but it may not be feasible for other children who protest vigorously. For safety, enlist the parent's or an assistant's help in immobilising the head by firmly placing one hand above the ear and the other on the child's side, abdomen or back (Fig 4.19B).

With cooperative children, examine the ear with the child in a side-lying, sitting or standing position. One disadvantage to standing is that the child may 'walk away' as the otoscope enters the canal. If the child is standing or sitting, tilt the head slightly towards the child's opposite shoulder to achieve a better view of the drum (Fig 4.20).

With the thumb and forefinger of the free hand, grasp the auricle. For the two positions of restraint, hold the otoscope upside down at the junction of its head and handle with the thumb and index finger. Place the other fingers against the skull to allow the otoscope to move with the child in case of sudden movement. In examining a cooperative child, hold the handle with the otic head upright or upside down. Use the dominant hand to examine both ears or reverse hands for each ear, whichever is more comfortable.

Before using the otoscope, visualise the external ear and the tympanic membrane as being superimposed on a clock (Fig 4.21). The numbers are important geographic landmarks. Introduce the speculum into the meatus between the 3 and 9 o'clock positions in a downward and forward position. Because the canal is curved, the speculum does not permit a panoramic view of the tympanic membrane unless the canal is straightened. In infants, the canal curves upwards. Therefore, pull the pinna down and back to the 6 to 9 o'clock range to straighten the canal (Fig 4.22A). With older children, usually those older than 3 years of age, the canal curves 'downwards' and forwards. Therefore, pull the pinna up and back towards a 10 o'clock position (Fig 4.22B). If you have difficulty visualising the membrane, try repositioning the head, introducing the speculum at a different angle and pulling the pinna in a slightly different direction. Do not insert the speculum past the cartilaginous (outermost) portion of the canal, usually a distance of 0.6 to 1.25 cm in older children. Insertion of the speculum into the posterior or bony portion of the canal causes pain.

In neonates and young infants, the walls of the canal are pliable and floppy because of the underdeveloped cartilaginous and bony structures. Therefore, the very small 2-mm speculum usually needs to be inserted deeper into the canal than in older children. Exercise great care not to damage the walls or drum. For this reason, only an experienced examiner should insert an otoscope into the ears of very young infants.

Otoscopic Examination. As you introduce the speculum into the external canal, inspect the walls of the canal, the colour of the tympanic membrane, the light reflex and the usual landmarks of the bony prominences of the middle ear. The walls of the external auditory canal are pink, although they are more pigmented in dark-skinned children. Minute hairs are evident in the outermost portion, where cerumen is produced. Note signs of irritation, foreign bodies or infection.

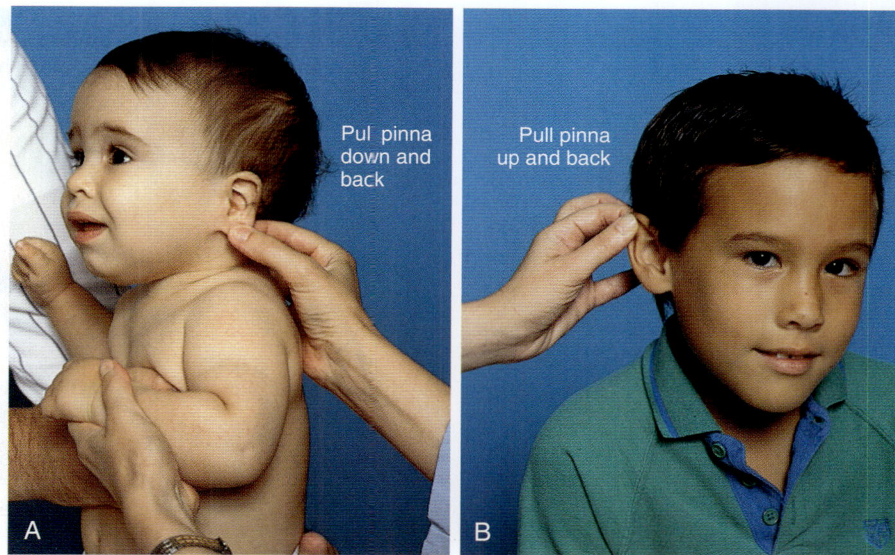

Fig 4.22 Positioning for visualising the eardrum in an infant (**A**) and in a child older than 3 years old (**B**).

Foreign bodies in the ear are common in children and range from erasers to beans. Symptoms may include pain, discharge and affected hearing. Remove soft objects, such as paper or insects, with forceps. Remove small, hard objects, such as pebbles, with a suction tip, a hook or irrigation. However, irrigation is contraindicated if the object is vegetative matter, such as beans or pasta, which swells when in contact with fluid.

The **tympanic membrane** is a translucent, light pearly pink or grey. Note marked erythema (which may indicate suppurative otitis media); a dull, non-transparent, greyish colour (sometimes suggestive of serous otitis media); or ashen grey areas (signs of scarring from a previous perforation). A black area usually suggests a perforation of the membrane that has not healed.

The characteristic tenseness and slope of the tympanic membrane cause the light of the otoscope to reflect at about the 5 or 7 o'clock position. The **light reflex** is a fairly well-defined, cone-shaped reflection, which normally points away from the face.

The **bony landmarks** of the drum are formed by the **umbo**, or tip of the malleus. It appears as a small, round, opaque, concave spot near the centre of the drum. The **manubrium** (long process or handle) of the malleus appears to be a whitish line extending from the umbo upwards to the margin of the membrane. At the upper end of the long process near the 1 o'clock position (in the right ear) is a sharp, knoblike protuberance, representing the **short process** of the malleus. Note the absence or distortion of the light reflex or loss or abnormal prominence of any of these landmarks.

Auditory Testing

Several types of hearing tests are available and recommended for screening in infants and children (Table 4.6). The nurse must operate under a high index of suspicion for those children who may have conditions associated with hearing loss, whose parents are concerned about hearing loss and who may have developed behaviours that indicate auditory impairment. Chapter 20 discusses types of hearing loss, causes, clinical manifestations and appropriate treatment.

Nose

Inspection of External Structures

Compare the placement and alignment of the nose by drawing an imaginary vertical line from the centre point between the eyes down

TABLE 4.6 Auditory Tests for Infants and Children

Age	Auditory Test	Type of Measurement	Procedure
Newborns	Auditory brainstem response (ABR)	Electrophysiological measurement of activity in auditory nerve and brainstem pathways	Placement of electrodes on child's head detects auditory stimuli presented through earphones one ear at a time.
Infants	Behavioural audiometry	Used to observe their behaviour in response to certain sounds heard through speakers or earphones	The child's responses to the sounds heard are observed.
Toddlers	Play audiometry	Uses an audiometer to transmit sounds at different volumes and pitches	The toddler is asked to do something with a toy (i.e. touch a toy, move a toy) every time the sound is heard.
Children and adolescents	Pure tone audiometry	Uses an audiometer that produces sounds at different volumes and pitches in the child's ears	The child is asked to respond in some way when the tone is heard in the earphone.
	Tympanometry (also called *impedance* or *admittance*)	Determines how the middle ear is functioning and detects any changes in pressure in the middle ear	A soft plastic tip is placed over the ear canal and the tympanometer measures eardrum movement when the pressure changes.
All ages	Evoked otoacoustic emissions (EOAE)	Physiological test specifically measuring cochlear (outer hair cell) response to presentation of stimulus	Small probe containing sensitive microphone is placed in ear canal for stimulus delivery and response detection.

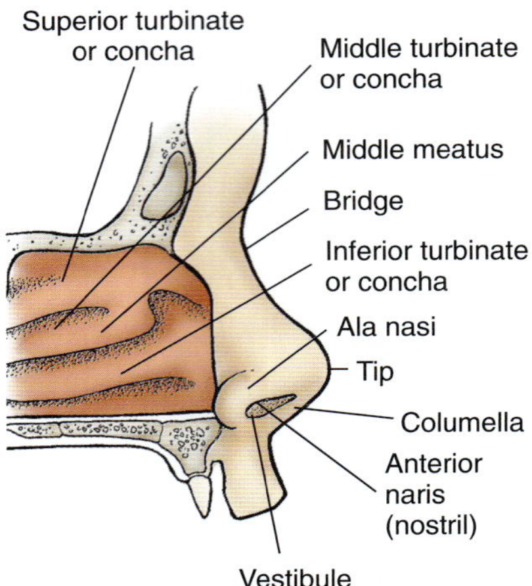

Fig 4.23 External landmarks and internal structures of the nose.

to the notch of the upper lip. The nose should lie in the middle of the face, with each side exactly symmetrical on both sides of the imaginary line. Note its location, any deviation to one side and asymmetry in overall size and in diameter of the nares (nostrils). The bridge of the nose is sometimes flat in Asian children. Observe the **alae nasi** for any sign of flaring, which indicates respiratory difficulty. Always report any flaring of the alae nasi. Fig 4.23 illustrates the landmarks used in describing the external landmarks and internal structures of the nose.

Inspection of Internal Structures

Inspect the **anterior vestibule** of the nose by pushing the tip upwards, tilting the head backwards and illuminating the cavity with a torch or otoscope without the attached ear speculum. Note the colour of the **mucosal lining**, which is normally redder than the oral membranes, as well as any swelling, discharge, dryness or bleeding. There should be no discharge from the nose.

On looking deeper into the nose, inspect the **turbinates** or **concha**, plates of bone that jut into the nasal cavity and are enveloped by mucous membrane. The turbinates greatly increase the surface area of the nasal cavity as air is inhaled. The spaces or channels between the turbinates are called the **meatus** and correspond to each of the three turbinates. Normally the front end of the inferior and middle turbinate and the middle meatus are seen. They should be the same colour as the lining of the vestibule.

Inspect the **septum**, which should divide the vestibules equally. Note any deviation, especially if it causes an occlusion of one side of the nose. A perforation may be evident within the septum. If this is suspected, shine the light of the otoscope into one naris and look for admittance of light to the other. Because olfaction is an important function of the nose, testing for smell may be done at this point or as part of cranial nerve assessment (see Table 4.10 later in this chapter).

Mouth and Throat

With a cooperative child, the nurse can accomplish almost the entire examination of the mouth and throat without the use of a tongue blade. Ask the child to open the mouth wide; to move the tongue in different directions for full visualisation; and to say 'ahh', which depresses the tongue for full view of the back of the mouth (tonsils, uvula and oropharynx). For a closer look at the **buccal mucosa**, or lining of the cheeks, ask children to use their fingers to move the outer lip and cheek to one side (see Nursing Care Considerations box).

NURSING CARE CONSIDERATIONS

Encouraging Opening the Mouth for Examination

- Perform the examination in front of a mirror.
- Let the child first examine someone else's mouth, such as the parent, the nurse or a puppet (Fig 4.24A), and then examine the child's mouth.
- Instruct the child to tilt the head back slightly, breathe deeply through the mouth and hold the breath; this action lowers the tongue to the floor of the mouth without the use of a tongue blade.
- Lightly brushing the palate with a cotton swab also may open the mouth for assessment.

Infants and toddlers usually resist attempts to keep the mouth open. Because inspecting the mouth is upsetting, leave it for the end of the physical examination (along with examination of the ears) or do it during episodes of crying. However, the use of a tongue blade (preferably flavoured) to depress the tongue may be needed. Place the tongue blade along the side of the tongue, not in the centre back area where the gag reflex is elicited. Fig 4.24B, illustrates proper positioning of the child for the oral examination.

The major structure of the exterior of the mouth is the lips. The lips should be moist, soft, smooth and pink, or a deeper hue than the surrounding skin. The lips should be symmetrical when relaxed or tensed. Assess symmetry when the child talks or cries.

Inspection of Internal Structures

The major structures that are visible within the oral cavity and oropharynx are the mucosal lining of the lips and cheeks, gums (or

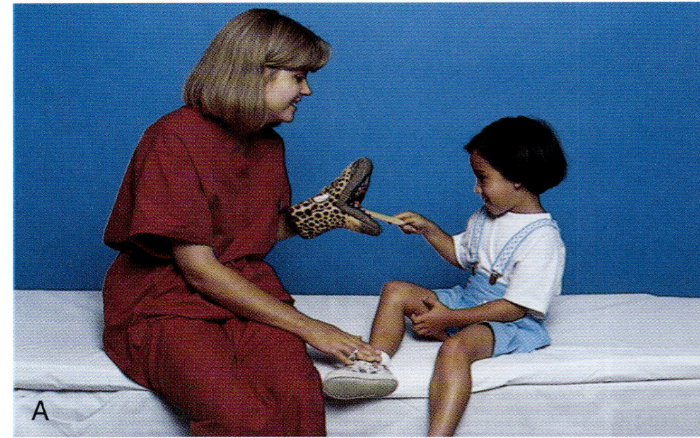

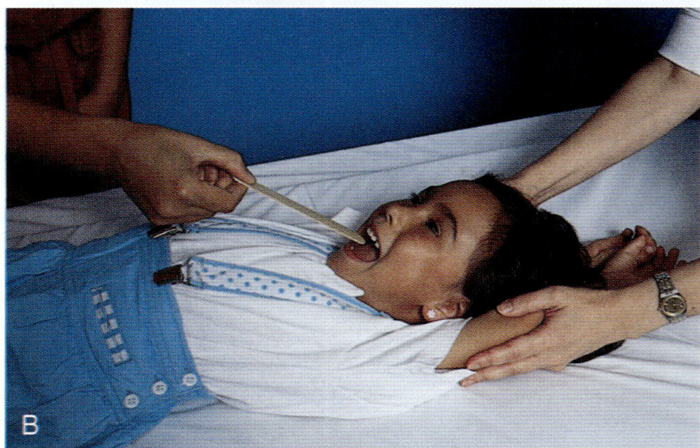

Fig 4.24 **A** Encouraging a child to cooperate. **B** Positioning a child for examination of the mouth.

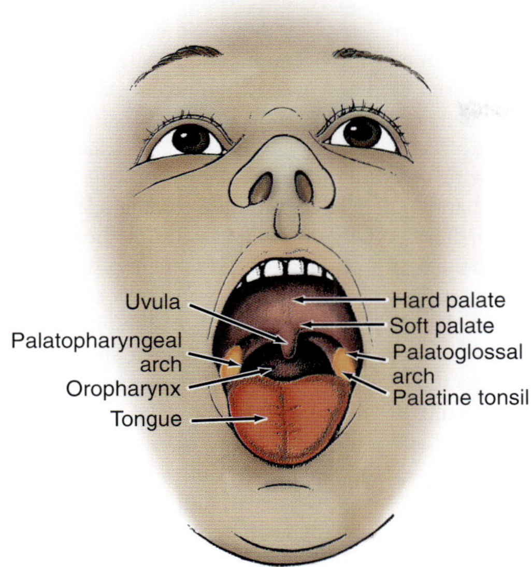

Fig 4.25 Interior structures of the mouth.

gingiva), teeth, tongue, palate, uvula, tonsils and posterior oropharynx (Fig 4.25). Inspect all areas lined with **mucous membranes** (inside the lips and cheeks, gingiva, underside of the tongue, palate and back of the pharynx) for colour, any areas of white patches or ulceration, petechiae, bleeding, sensitivity and moisture. The membranes should be bright pink, smooth, glistening, uniform and moist.

Inspect the teeth for number (deciduous, permanent or mixed dentition) in each dental arch, for hygiene and for occlusion or bite (see also Teething, Chapter 10). Discolouration of tooth enamel with obvious **plaque** (whitish coating on the surface of the teeth) is a sign of poor dental hygiene and indicates a need for counselling. Brown spots in the crevices of the crown of the tooth or between the teeth may be **caries** (cavities). Chalky white to yellow or brown areas on the enamel may indicate **fluorosis** (excessive fluoride ingestion). Teeth that appear greenish black may be stained temporarily from ingestion of supplemental iron.

Examine the gums (**gingiva**) surrounding the teeth. The colour is normally coral pink and the surface texture is stippled, similar to the appearance of an orange peel. In dark-skinned children, the gums are more deeply coloured and a brownish area is often observed along the gum line.

Inspect the tongue for papillae, small projections that contain taste buds and give the tongue its characteristic rough appearance. Note the size and mobility of the tongue. Normally the tip of the tongue should extend to the lips or beyond.

The roof of the mouth consists of the **hard palate**, which is located near the front of the oral cavity, and the **soft palate**, which is located towards the back of the pharynx and has a small midline protrusion called the **uvula**. Carefully inspect the palates to ensure they are intact. The arch of the palate should be dome shaped. A narrow, flat roof or a high, arched palate affects the placement of the tongue and can cause feeding and speech problems. Test movement of the uvula by eliciting a gag reflex. It should move upwards to close off the nasopharynx from the oropharynx.

Examine the oropharynx and note the size and colour of the **palatine tonsils**. They are normally the same colour as the surrounding mucosa; glandular, rather than smooth in appearance; and barely visible over the edge of the palatoglossal arches. The size of the tonsils varies considerably during childhood. However, report any swelling, redness or white areas on the tonsils.

Chest

Inspect the chest for size, shape, symmetry, movement, breast development and the bony landmarks formed by the ribs and sternum. The **rib cage** consists of 12 ribs on each side and the sternum, or breastbone, located in the midline of the trunk (Fig 4.26). The **sternum** is composed of three main parts. The **manubrium**, the uppermost portion,

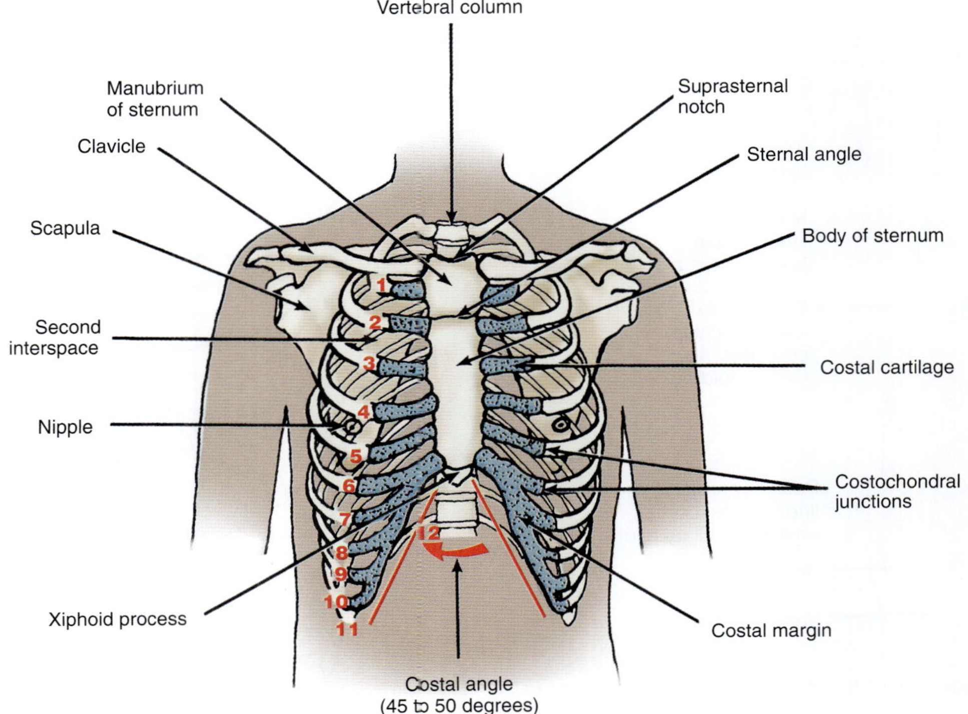

Fig 4.26 The rib cage.

can be felt at the base of the neck at the **suprasternal notch**. The largest segment of the sternum is the **body**, which forms the **sternal angle (angle of Louis)** as it articulates with the manubrium. At the end of the body is a small, movable process called the **xiphoid**. The angle of the costal margin as it attaches to the sternum is called the **costal angle** and is normally about 45 to 50 degrees. These bony structures are important landmarks in the location of ribs and **intercostal spaces (ICSs)**, which are the spaces between the ribs. They are numbered according to the rib directly above the space. For example, the space immediately below the second rib is the second ICS.

The **thoracic cavity** is also divided into segments by drawing imaginary lines on the chest and back. Fig 4.27 illustrates the anterior, lateral and posterior divisions.

Measure the size of the chest by placing the measuring tape around the rib cage at the nipple line. For greatest accuracy, take two measurements—one during inspiration and the other during expiration—and record the average. Always report marked disproportions because most are caused by abnormal head growth, although some may be a result of altered chest shape, such as **barrel chest** (chest is round), **pectus excavatum** (sternum is depressed) or **pectus carinatum** (sternum protrudes outwards).

During infancy, the chest's shape is almost circular, with the anteroposterior (front-to-back) diameter equalling the transverse, or lateral (side-to-side), diameter. As the child grows, the chest normally increases in the transverse direction, causing the anteroposterior diameter to be less than the lateral diameter. Note the angle made by the lower costal margin and the sternum, and palpate the junction of the ribs with the costal cartilage (costochondral junction) and sternum, which should be fairly smooth.

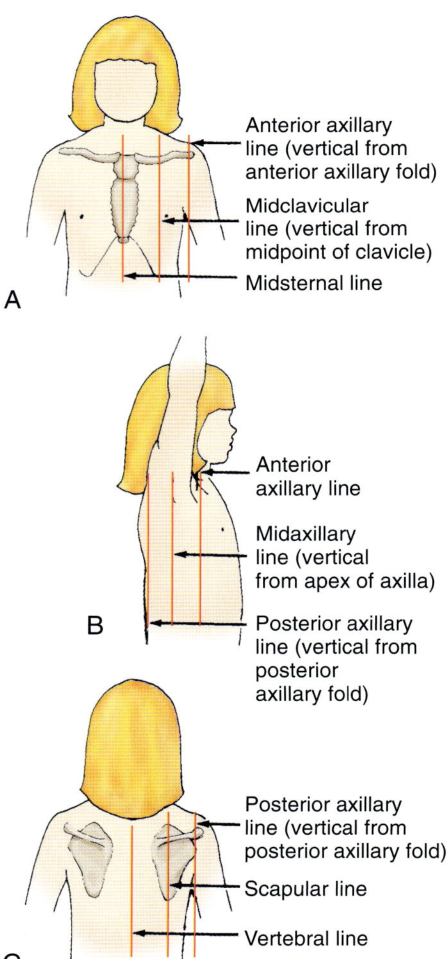

Fig 4.27 Imaginary landmarks of the chest. **A** Anterior. **B** Right lateral. **C** Posterior.

Movement of the chest wall should be symmetrical bilaterally and coordinated with breathing. During inspiration, the chest rises and expands, the diaphragm descends and the costal angle increases. During expiration, the chest falls and decreases in size, the diaphragm rises and the costal angle narrows (Fig 4.28). In children younger than 6 or 7 years of age, respiratory movement is principally abdominal or diaphragmatic. In older children, particularly girls, respirations are chiefly thoracic. In either case, the chest and abdomen should rise and fall together. Always report any asymmetry of movement.

While inspecting the skin surface of the chest, observe the position of the nipples and any evidence of breast development. Normally the nipples are located slightly lateral to the midclavicular line between the fourth and fifth ribs. Note symmetry of nipple placement and normal configuration of a darker pigmented areola surrounding a flat nipple in the prepubertal child.

Pubertal breast development usually begins in girls between 8 and 12 years of age (see Chapter 17). Record early (precocious) or delayed breast development, as well as evidence of any other secondary sexual characteristics. In males, breast enlargement (**gynaecomastia**) may be caused by hormonal or systemic disorders but more commonly is a result of adipose tissue from obesity or a transitory body change during early puberty. In either situation, investigate the child's feelings regarding breast enlargement.

In adolescent girls who have achieved sexual maturity, palpate the breasts for evidence of any masses or hard nodules. Use this opportunity to discuss the importance of routine breast self-examination. Emphasise that most palpable masses are benign to decrease any fear or concern that results when a mass is felt.

Lungs

The lungs are situated inside the thoracic cavity, with one lung on each side of the sternum. Each lung is divided into an **apex**, which is slightly

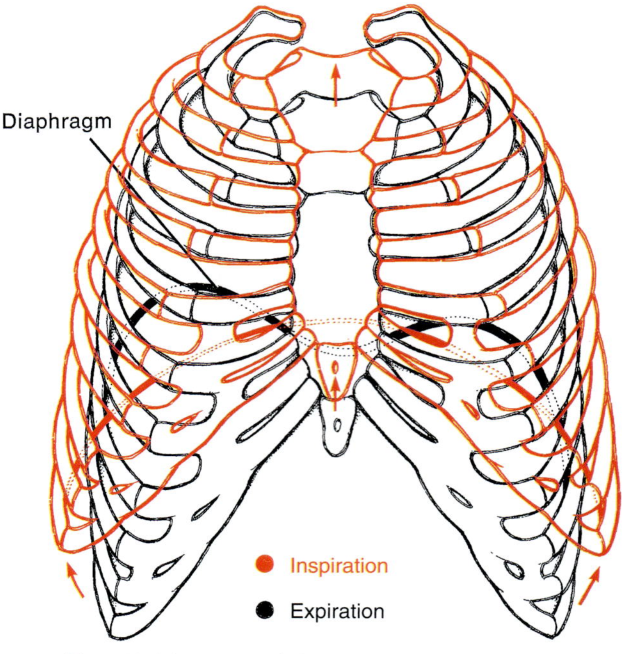

Fig 4.28 Movement of the chest during respiration.

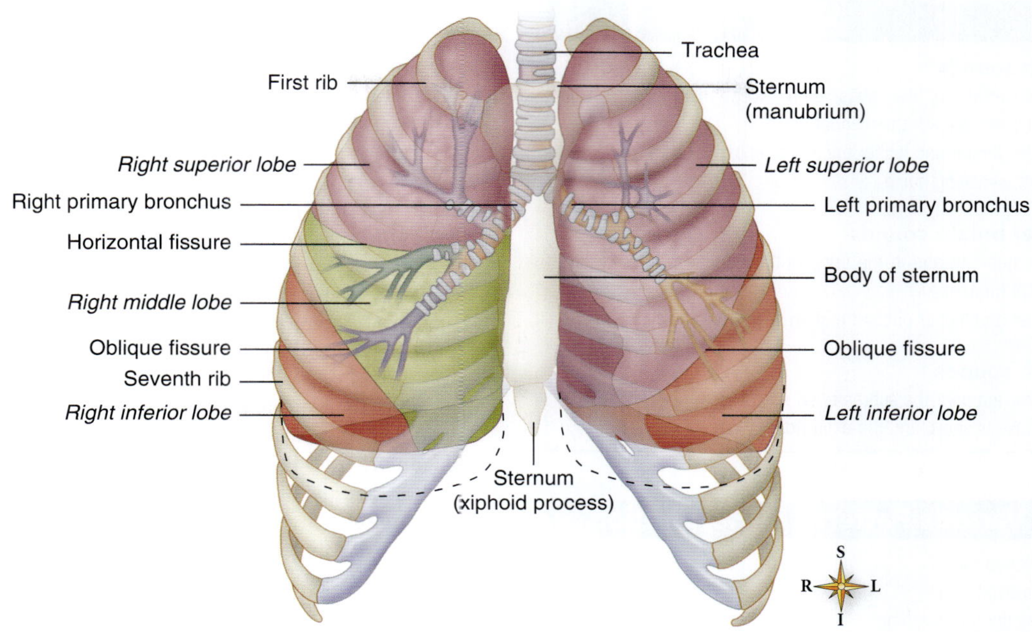

Fig 4.29 Location of the lobes of the lungs within the thoracic cavity. (Source: Patton, K. T., & Thibodeau, G. A. (2013). *Anatomy and physiology* (8th ed.). St Louis, MO: Mosby.)

pointed and rises above the first rib; a **base**, which is wide and concave and rides on the dome-shaped diaphragm; and a **body**, which is divided into lobes. The right lung has three lobes: the right superior (upper) lobe, right middle lobe and right inferior (lower) lobe. The left lung has only two lobes, the left superior (upper) and left inferior (lower) lobes because of the space occupied by the heart (Fig 4.29).

Inspection of the lungs primarily involves observation of respiratory movements. Evaluate respirations for: (1) rate (number per minute); (2) rhythm (regular, irregular or periodic); (3) depth (deep or shallow); and (4) quality (effortless, automatic, difficult or laboured). Note the character of breath sounds, such as noisy, grunting, snoring or heavy.

Evaluate respiratory movements by placing each hand flat against the back or chest with the thumbs in midline along the lower costal margin of the lungs. The child should be sitting during this procedure and, if cooperative, should take several deep breaths. During respiration, your hands will move with the chest wall. Assess the amount and speed of respiratory excursion and note any asymmetry of movement.

Experienced examiners may percuss the lungs. Percuss the anterior lung from apex to base, usually with the child in the supine or sitting position. Percuss each side of the chest in sequence to compare the sounds. When percussing the posterior lung, the procedure and sequence are the same, although the child should be sitting. Resonance is heard over all the lobes of the lungs that are not adjacent to other organs. Record and report any deviation from the expected sound.

Auscultation

Auscultation involves using the stethoscope to evaluate breath sounds; these are best heard if the child inspires deeply (see Nursing Care Considerations box). In the lungs breath sounds are classified as vesicular, bronchovesicular or bronchial (Box 4.9).

NURSING CARE CONSIDERATIONS

Effective Auscultation

- Make certain the child is relaxed and not crying, talking or laughing. Record if child is crying.
- Check that room is comfortable and quiet.
- Warm stethoscope before placing it against skin.
- Apply firm pressure on chest piece but not enough to prevent vibrations and transmission of sound.
- Avoid placing stethoscope over hair or clothing, moving it against skin, breathing on tubing or sliding fingers over chest piece, which may cause sounds that falsely resemble pathological findings.
- Use a symmetrical and orderly approach to compare sounds.

Encouraging Deep Breaths

- Ask the child to 'blow out' the light on an otoscope or pocket torch; discreetly turn off the light on the last try so that the child feels successful.
- Place a cotton ball in the child's palm; ask the child to blow the ball into the air and have the parent catch it.
- Hold a tissue in front of the child and ask them to blow the tissue in the air.
- Have the child blow a pinwheel, a party horn or bubbles.

Absent or diminished breath sounds are always an abnormal finding warranting investigation. Fluid, air or solid masses in the pleural space all interfere with the conduction of breath sounds. Diminished breath sounds in certain segments of the lung can alert the nurse to pulmonary areas that may benefit from chest physiotherapy. Increased breath sounds after pulmonary therapy indicates improved passage of air through the respiratory tract. Box 4.10 lists terms used to describe various respiration patterns.

BOX 4.9 Classification of Normal Breath Sounds

Vesicular Breath sounds
- Heard over entire surface of the lungs, with exception of upper intrascapular area and area beneath the manubrium.
- Inspiration is louder, longer and higher pitched than expiration.
- The sound is a soft, swishing noise.

Bronchovesicular breath sounds
- Heard over the manubrium and in the upper intrascapular regions where trachea and bronchi bifurcate.
- Inspiration is louder and higher pitched than in vesicular breathing.

Bronchial breath sounds
- Heard only over trachea near the suprasternal notch.
- The inspiratory phase is short, and the expiratory phase is long.

BOX 4.10 Various Patterns of Respiration

Tachypnoea—Increased rate
Bradypnoea—Decreased rate
Dyspnoea—Distress during breathing
Apnoea—Cessation of breathing
Hyperpnoea—Increased depth
Hypoventilation—Decreased depth (shallow) and irregular rhythm
Hyperventilation—Increased rate and depth
Kussmaul respiration—Hyperventilation, gasping and laboured respiration; usually seen in diabetic coma or other states of respiratory acidosis
Cheyne-Stokes respiration—Gradually increasing rate and depth with periods of apnoea
Seesaw (paradoxical) respirations—Chest falls on inspiration and rises on expiration

Various pulmonary abnormalities produce **adventitious sounds** that are not normally heard over the chest. These sounds occur in addition to normal or abnormal breath sounds. They are classified into two main groups: (1) **crackles**, which result from the passage of air through fluid or moisture; and (2) **wheezes**, which are produced as air passes through narrowed passageways, regardless of the cause, such as exudate, inflammation, spasm or tumour. Considerable practice with an experienced tutor is necessary to differentiate the various types of lung sounds. Often it is best to describe the type of sound heard in the lungs rather than trying to label it. Always report any abnormal sounds for further evaluation.

Heart

The heart is situated in the thoracic cavity between the lungs in the mediastinum and above the diaphragm (Fig 4.30). About two-thirds of the heart lies within the left side of the rib cage, with the other third on the right side as it crosses the sternum. The heart is positioned in the thorax like a trapezoid:

- **vertically** along the right sternal border (RSB) from the second to the fifth rib
- **horizontally** (long side) from the lower right sternum to the fifth rib at the left midclavicular line (LMCL)
- **diagonally** from the left sternal border (LSB) at the second rib to the LMCL at the fifth rib
- **horizontally** (short side) from the RSB and LSB at the second ICS—base of the heart.

Inspection is easiest when the child is sitting in a semi-Fowler's position. Look at the anterior chest wall from an angle, comparing both sides of the rib cage with each other. Normally they should be symmetrical. In children with thin chest walls, a pulsation may be visible. Because comprehensive evaluation of cardiac function is not limited to the heart, also consider other findings such as the presence of all pulses (especially the femoral pulses) (Fig 4.31), distended neck veins, clubbing of the fingers, peripheral cyanosis, oedema, BP and respiratory status.

Use palpation to determine the location of the **apical impulse (AI)**, the most lateral cardiac impulse that may correspond to the apex. The AI is found at the:

- fifth ICS and LMCL in children older than 7 years of age
- fourth ICS and just lateral to the LMCL in children younger than 7 years of age.

Although the AI gives a general idea of the size of the heart (with enlargement, the apex is lower and more lateral), its normal location is variable, making it an unreliable indicator of heart size.

The **point of maximum intensity (PMI)**, as the name implies, is the area of most intense pulsation. Usually the PMI is located at the

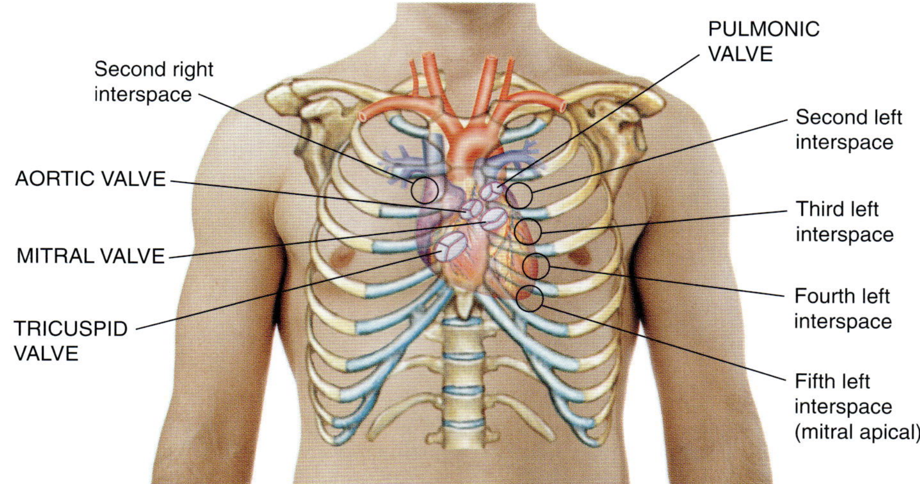

Fig 4.30 Position of the heart within the thorax. (Source: Ball, J. W., Dains, J. E., Flynn, J. A., et al. (2014). *Seidel's guide to physical examination* (8th ed.). St Louis, MO: Elsevier.)

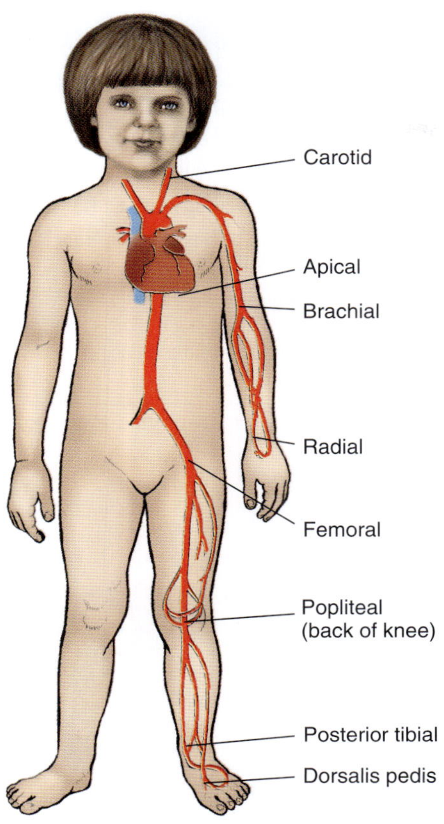

Fig 4.31 Location of pulses.

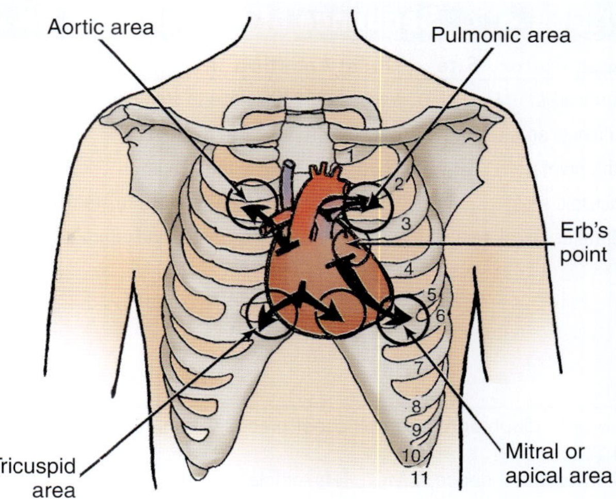

Fig 4.32 Direction of heart sounds for anatomical valve sites and areas *(circled)* for auscultation.

same site as the AI, but it can occur elsewhere. For this reason, the two terms should not be used synonymously.

Assess **capillary refill time**, an important test for circulation, by pressing the skin lightly on a central site, such as the forehead, or a peripheral site, such as the nail beds, to produce a slight blanching. The time it takes for the blanched area to return to its original colour is the capillary refill time.

Auscultation

Origin of Heart Sounds. The heart sounds are produced by the opening and closing of the valves and the vibration of blood against the walls of the heart and vessels. Normally two sounds—S_1 and S_2—are heard, which correspond, respectively, to the familiar 'lub dub' often used to describe the sounds. S_1 is caused by closure of the **tricuspid** and **mitral valves** (sometimes called the **atrioventricular valves**). S_2 is the result of closure of the **pulmonic** and **aortic valves** (sometimes called **semilunar valves**). Normally the split of the two sounds in S_2 is distinguishable and widens during inspiration. **Physiological splitting** is a significant normal finding.

Two other heart sounds, S_3 and S_4, may be produced. S_3 is normally heard in some children. S_4 is rarely heard as a normal heart sound; it usually indicates the need for further cardiac evaluation.

Differentiating Normal Heart Sounds. Figure 4.32 illustrates the approximate anatomical position of the valves within the heart chambers. Note that the anatomical location of valves does not correspond to the area where the sounds are heard best. The auscultatory sites are located in the direction of the blood flow through the valves.

Normally S_1 is louder at the apex of the heart in the mitral and tricuspid area, and S_2 is louder near the base of the heart in the pulmonic and aortic area (Table 4.7). Listen to each sound by inching down the chest. Auscultate the following areas for sounds, such as murmurs, which may radiate to these sites: sternoclavicular area above the clavicles and manubrium, area along the sternal border, area along the left midaxillary line and area below the scapulae.

Auscultate the heart with the child in at least two positions: sitting and reclining. If adventitious sounds are detected, further evaluate them with the child standing, sitting and leaning forwards, and lying on the left side. For example, atrial sounds such as S_4 are heard best with the person in a recumbent position and usually fade if the person sits or stands.

Evaluate heart sounds for: (1) quality (they should be clear and distinct, not muffled, diffuse or distant); (2) intensity, especially in relation to the location or auscultatory site (they should not be weak or pounding); (3) rate (they should have the same rate as the radial pulse); and (4) rhythm (they should be regular and even). A particular arrhythmia that occurs normally in many children is **sinus arrhythmia**, in which the heart rate increases with inspiration and decreases with expiration. Differentiate this rhythm from a truly abnormal arrhythmia by having children hold their breath. In sinus arrhythmia, cessation of breathing causes the heart rate to remain steady.

Heart Murmurs. Another important category of the heart sounds is **murmurs**, which are produced by vibrations within the heart chambers or in the major arteries from the back-and-forth flow of blood. (For a more detailed discussion, see Assessment of Cardiac Function, Chapter 27). Murmurs are classified as follows.

- **Innocent**—No anatomical or physiological abnormality exists.
- **Functional**—No anatomical cardiac defect exists, but a physiological abnormality (e.g. anaemia) is present.
- **Organic**—A cardiac defect with or without a physiological abnormality exists.

The description and classification of murmurs are skills that require considerable practice and training. In general, recognise murmurs as distinct swishing sounds that occur in addition to the normal heart sounds and record the: (1) location, or the area of the heart in which the murmur is heard best; (2) time of the occurrence of the murmur within the S_1–S_2 cycle; (3) intensity (evaluate in relationship to the child's position); and (4) loudness. Table 4.8 lists the usual subjective method of grading the loudness or intensity of a murmur.

TABLE 4.7 Sequence of Auscultating Heart Sounds*

Auscultatory Site	Chest Location	Characteristics of Heart Sounds
Aortic area	Second right ICS close to sternum	S_2 heard louder than S_1; aortic closure heard loudest
Pulmonic area	Second left ICS close to sternum	Splitting of S_2 heard best, normally widens on inspiration; pulmonic closure heard best
Erb's point	Third left ICS close to sternum	Frequent site of innocent murmurs and those of aortic or pulmonic origin
Tricuspid area	Fourth right and left ICSs close to sternum	S_1 heard as louder sound preceding S_2 (S_1 synchronous with carotid pulse)
Mitral or apical area	Fifth ICS, LMCL (fourth ICS and lateral to LMCL in infants)	S_1 heard loudest; splitting of S_1 may be audible because mitral closure is louder than tricuspid closure S_3 heard best at beginning of expiration with child in recumbent or left side-lying position; occurs immediately after S_2 S_4 heard best during expiration with child in recumbent position (left side-lying position decreases sound); occurs immediately before S_1

*Use both diaphragm and bell chest pieces when auscultating heart sounds. Bell chest piece is necessary for low-pitched sounds of murmurs, S_3 and S_4.
ICS, Intercostal space; *LMCL*, left midclavicular line.

TABLE 4.8 Grading the Intensity of Heart Murmurs

Grade	Description
I	Very faint; often not heard if child sits up
II	Usually readily heard; slightly louder than grade I; audible in all positions
III	Loud, but not accompanied by a thrill
IV	Loud, accompanied by a thrill
V	Loud enough to be heard with a stethoscope barely touching the chest; accompanied by a thrill
VI	Loud enough to be heard with the stethoscope not touching the chest; often heard with the human ear close to the chest; accompanied by a thrill

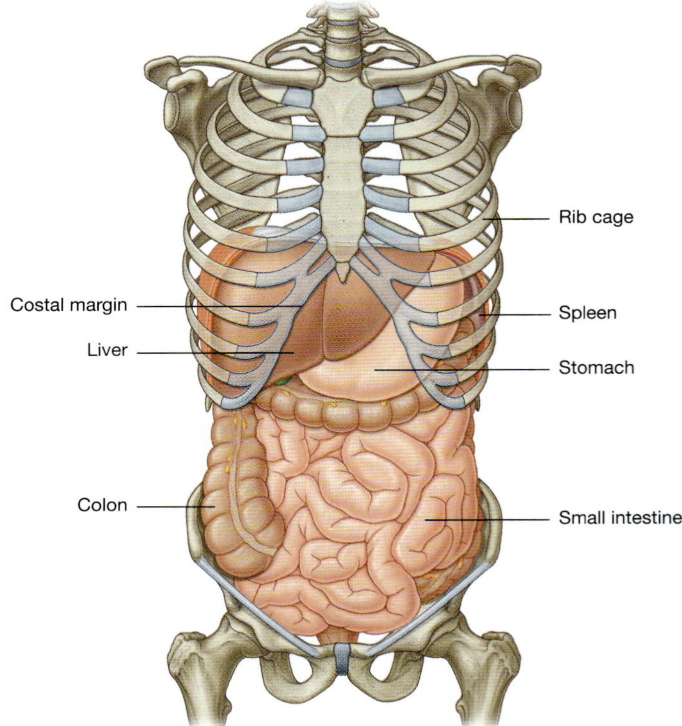

Fig 4.33 Location of structures in the abdomen. (Source: Drake, R. L., Vogl, W., & Mitchell, A. W. M. (2015). *Gray's anatomy for students* (3rd ed.). New York: Churchill Livingstone.)

Abdomen

Examination of the abdomen involves inspection, followed by auscultation and then palpation. Experienced examiners may also percuss the abdomen to assess for organomegaly, masses, fluid and flatus. Perform palpation last because it may distort the normal abdominal sounds. Knowledge of the anatomical placement of the abdominal organs is essential to differentiate normal, expected findings from abnormal ones (Fig 4.33).

For descriptive purposes, the abdominal cavity is divided into four quadrants by drawing a vertical line midway from the sternum to the symphysis pubis and a horizontal line across the abdomen through the umbilicus. The sections are named as follows:

- left upper quadrant
- left lower quadrant
- right upper quadrant
- right lower quadrant.

Inspection

Inspect the contour of the abdomen with the child erect and supine. Normally the abdomen of infants and young children is cylindrical and, in the erect position, fairly prominent because of the physiological lordosis of the spine. In the supine position the abdomen appears flat. A midline protrusion from the xiphoid to the umbilicus or symphysis pubis is usually **diastasis recti**, or failure of the rectus abdominis muscles to join in utero. In a healthy child, a midline protrusion is usually a variation of normal muscular development.

The skin covering the abdomen should be uniformly taut, without wrinkles or creases. Sometimes silvery, whitish striae ('stretch marks') are seen, especially if the skin has been stretched as in obesity. Superficial veins are usually visible in light-skinned, thin infants, but distended veins are an abnormal finding.

Observe movement of the abdomen. Normally chest and abdominal movements are synchronous. In infants and thin children **peristaltic waves** may be visible through the abdominal wall; they are best observed by standing at eye level to and across from the abdomen. Always report this finding.

Examine the umbilicus for size, hygiene and evidence of any abnormalities, such as hernias. The umbilicus should be flat or only

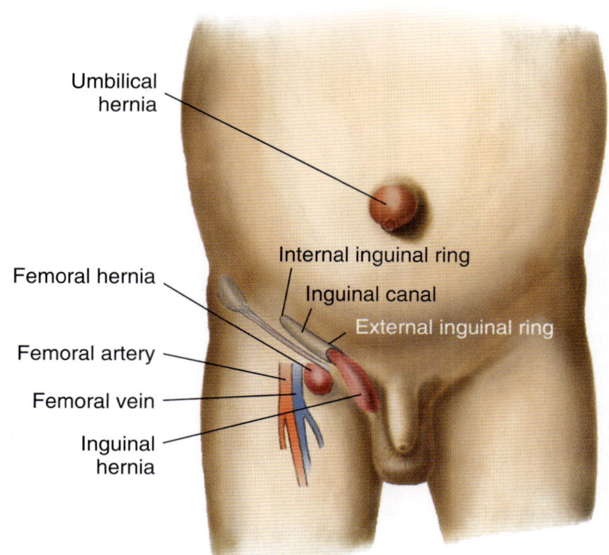

Fig 4.34 Location of hernias.

slightly protruding. If a herniation is present, palpate the sac for abdominal contents and estimate the approximate size of the opening. **Umbilical hernias** are common in infants, especially in African American children.

Hernias may exist elsewhere on the abdominal wall (Fig 4.34). An **inguinal hernia** is a protrusion of peritoneum through the abdominal wall in the inguinal canal. It occurs mostly in males, is frequently bilateral and may be visible as a mass in the scrotum. To locate a hernia, slide the little finger into the external inguinal ring at the base of the scrotum and ask the child to cough. If a hernia is present, it will hit the tip of the finger.

A **femoral hernia**, which occurs more frequently in girls, is felt or seen as a small mass on the anterior surface of the thigh just below the inguinal ligament in the femoral canal (a potential space medial to the femoral artery). Feel for a hernia by placing the index finger of your right hand on the child's right femoral pulse (left hand for left pulse) and the middle finger flat against the skin towards the midline. The ring finger lies over the femoral canal, where the herniation occurs. Palpation of hernias in the pelvic region is often part of the genital examination.

Auscultation

The most important finding to listen for is **peristalsis**, or **bowel sounds**, which sound like short metallic clicks and gurgles. Record their frequency per minute (e.g. 5 sounds/min). Listen for up to 5 minutes before determining that bowel sounds are absent. Stimulate bowel sounds by stroking the abdominal surface with a fingernail. Report absence of bowel sounds or hyperperistalsis because either usually denotes an abdominal disorder.

Palpation

There are two types of palpation: superficial and deep. For **superficial palpation**, lightly place your hand against the skin and feel each quadrant, noting any areas of tenderness, muscle tone and superficial lesions such as cysts. Because superficial palpation is often perceived as tickling, use several techniques to minimise this sensation and relax the child (see Nursing Care Considerations box). Admonishing the child to stop laughing only draws attention to the sensation and decreases cooperation.

NURSING CARE CONSIDERATIONS

Promoting Relaxation During Abdominal Palpation

- Position the child comfortably, such as in a semireclining position in the parent's lap, with knees flexed.
- Warm your hands before touching the skin.
- Use distraction, such as telling stories or talking to the child.
- Teach the child to use deep breathing and to concentrate on an object.
- Give an infant a bottle or soother (dummy).
- Begin with light, superficial palpation and gradually progress to deeper palpation.
- Palpate any tender or painful areas last.
- Have the child hold the parent's hand and squeeze it if palpation is uncomfortable.
- Use the non-palpating hand to comfort the child, such as placing the free hand on the child's shoulder while palpating the abdomen.

To minimise sensation of tickling during palpation:

- have children 'help' with palpation by placing a hand over the palpating hand
- have them place a hand on the abdomen with the fingers spread wide apart, and palpate between their fingers.

Deep palpation is for palpating organs and large blood vessels and for detecting masses and tenderness that were not discovered during superficial palpation. Palpation usually begins in the lower quadrants and proceeds upwards to avoid missing the edge of an enlarged liver or spleen. Except for palpating the liver, successful identification of other organs (e.g. the spleen, kidney and part of the colon) requires considerable practice with tutored supervision. Report any questionable mass. The lower edge of the liver is sometimes felt in infants and young children as a superficial mass 1 to 2 cm below the right costal margin (the distance is sometimes measured in fingerbreadths). Normally the liver descends during inspiration as the diaphragm moves downwards. Do not mistake this downward displacement as a sign of liver enlargement.

Palpate the **femoral pulses** by placing the tips of two or three fingers (index, middle or ring) along the inguinal ligament about midway between the iliac crest and symphysis pubis. Feel both pulses simultaneously to make certain that they are equal and strong (Fig 4.35).

Genitalia

Examination of genitalia conveniently follows assessment of the abdomen while the child is still supine. In adolescents, inspection of

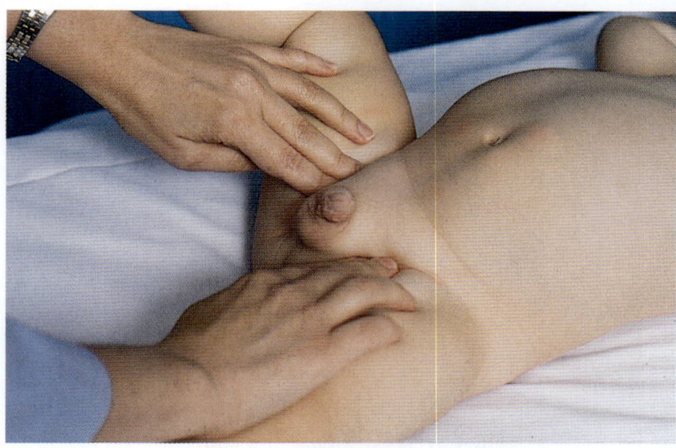

Fig 4.35 Palpating for femoral pulses.

the genitalia may be left to the end of the examination. The best approach is to examine the genitalia matter-of-factly, placing no more emphasis on this part of the assessment than on any other segment. It helps relieve children's and parents' anxiety by telling them the results of the findings; for example, the nurse might say, 'Everything looks fine here'.

If it is necessary to ask questions, such as about discharge or difficulty urinating, respect the child's privacy by covering the lower abdomen with the gown or underpants. To prevent embarrassing interruptions, keep the door or curtain closed and post a 'do not disturb' sign. Have a drape ready to cover the genitalia if someone enters the room.

In examining the genitalia, wear gloves when touching the child. It might be helpful for the adolescent to know that wearing gloves also prevents skin-to-skin contact.

The genital examination is an excellent time for eliciting questions or concerns about body function or sexual activity. Use this opportunity to increase or reinforce the child's knowledge of sexual anatomy by naming each body part and explaining its function. This part of the health assessment is an opportune time to teach testicular self-examination to boys.

Male Genitalia

Note the external appearance of the glans and shaft of the penis, the prepuce, the urethral meatus and the scrotum (Fig 4.36). The penis is generally small in infants and young boys until puberty, when it begins to increase in both length and width. In an obese child, the penis often looks abnormally small because of the folds of skin partially covering it at the base. Be familiar with normal pubertal growth of the external male genitalia to compare the findings with the expected sequence of maturation (see Chapter 17).

Examine the **glans** (head of the penis) and **shaft** (portion between the perineum and prepuce) for signs of swelling, skin lesions, inflammation or other irregularities. Any of these signs may indicate underlying disorders, especially sexually transmitted infections.

Carefully inspect the **urethral meatus** for location and evidence of discharge. Normally it is centred at the tip of the glans. Note the hair distribution. Normally, before puberty, no pubic hair is present. Soft, downy hair at the base of the penis is an early sign of pubertal maturation. In older adolescents, hair distribution is diamond shaped from the umbilicus to the anus.

Note the location and size of the **scrotum**. The scrota hang freely from the perineum behind the penis, and the left scrotum normally hangs lower than the right. In infants, the scrota appear large in relation to the rest of the genitalia. The skin of the scrotum is loose and highly rugated (wrinkled). During early adolescence, the skin normally becomes redder and coarser. In dark-skinned children, the scrota are usually more deeply pigmented.

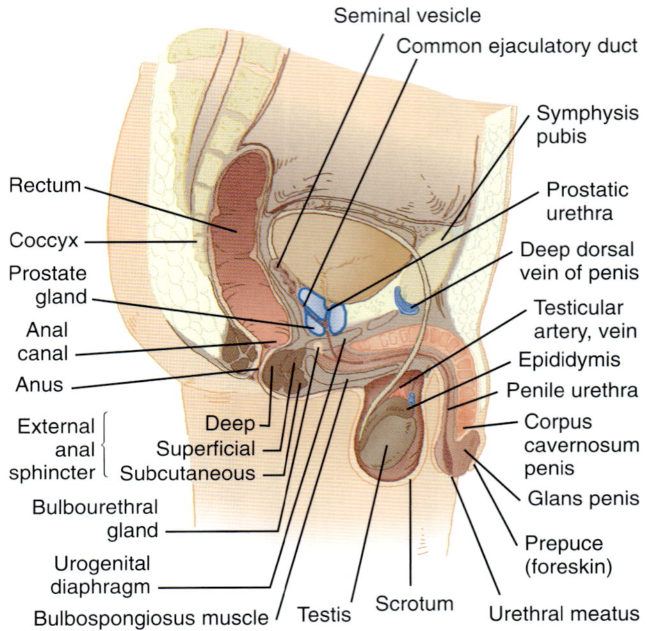

Fig 4.36 Major structures of genitalia in an uncircumcised postpubertal male. (Source: Douglas, G., Nicol, F., & Robertson, C. (2013). *Macleod's clinical examination* (13th ed.). Philadelphia, PA: Elsevier.)

Palpation of the scrota includes identification of the testes, epididymis and, if present, inguinal hernias. In the prepubertal child, the two **testes** are felt as small, ovoid bodies about 1.5 to 2 cm long (1 to 3 mL in volume)—one in each scrotal sac. They do not enlarge until puberty (see Chapter 17). Pubertal testicular development normally begins in boys between 9 and 13 years old. Record early (precocious) or delayed pubertal development, as well as evidence of any other secondary sexual characteristics.

When palpating for the presence of the testes, avoid stimulating the **cremasteric reflex**, which is stimulated by cold, touch, emotional excitement or exercise. This reflex pulls the testes higher into the pelvic cavity. Several measures are useful in preventing the cremasteric reflex during palpation of the scrotum. First, warm the hands. Second, if the child is old enough, examine him in a tailor or 'Indian' position, which stretches the muscle, preventing its contraction (Fig 4.37A). Third, block the normal pathway of ascent of the testes by placing the

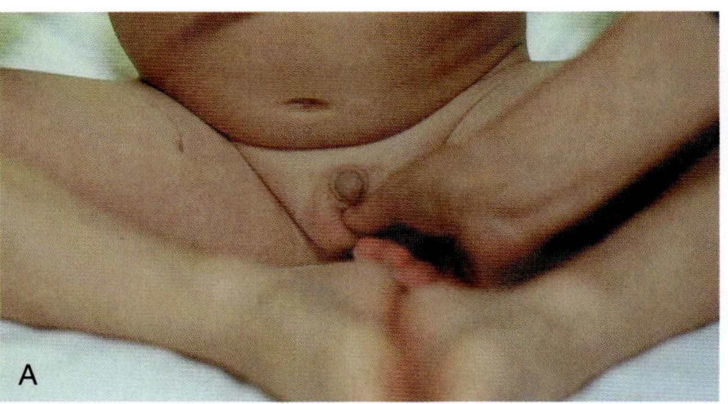

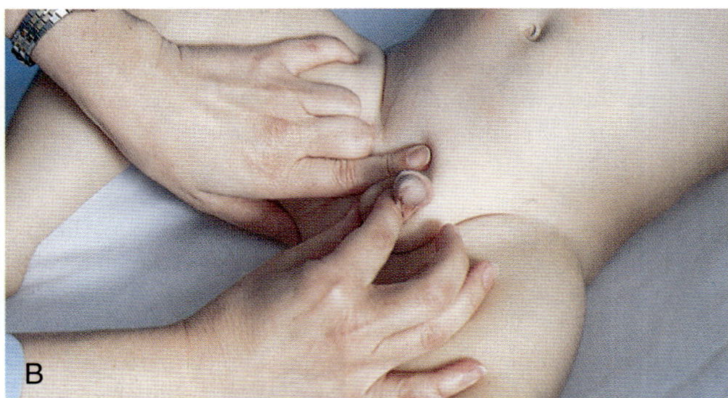

Fig 4.37 **A** Preventing the cremasteric reflex by having the child sit in the tailor position. **B** Blocking the inguinal canal during palpation of the scrotum for descended testes.

thumb and index finger over the upper part of the scrotal sac along the inguinal canal (Fig 4.37B). If there is any question concerning the existence of two testes, place the index and middle fingers in a scissors fashion to separate the right and left scrota. If, after using these techniques, you have not palpated the testes, feel along the inguinal canal and perineum to locate masses that may be undescended testes. Report any failure to palpate the testes for further evaluation.

Female Genitalia

The examination of female genitalia is limited to inspection and palpation of external structures. If a vaginal examination is required, the nurse should make an appropriate referral unless he or she is qualified to perform the procedure.

A convenient position for examination of the genitalia involves placing the young child supine on the examining table or in a semi-reclining position on the parent's lap with the feet supported on your knees as you sit facing the child. Divert the child's attention from the examination by instructing her to try to keep the soles of her feet pressed against each other. Separate the labia majora with the thumb and index finger and retract outwards to expose the labia minora, urethral meatus and vaginal orifice.

Examine the female genitalia for size and location of the structures of the **vulva**, or **pudendum** (Fig 4.38). The **mons pubis** is a pad of adipose tissue over the symphysis pubis. At puberty, the mons is covered with hair, which extends along the labia. The usual pattern of female hair distribution is an inverted triangle. The appearance of soft, downy hair along the labia majora is an early sign of sexual maturation. Note the size and location of the **clitoris**, a small, erectile organ located at the anterior end of the labia minora. It is covered by a small flap of skin, the **prepuce**.

The **labia majora** are two thick folds of skin running posteriorly from the mons to the posterior commissure of the vagina. Internal to the labia majora are two folds of skin called the **labia minora**. Although the labia minora are usually prominent in the newborn, they gradually atrophy, which makes them almost invisible until their enlargement during puberty. The inner surface of the labia should be pink and moist. Note the size of the labia and any evidence of fusion, which may suggest male scrota. Normally, no masses are palpable within the labia.

The **urethral meatus** is located posterior to the clitoris and is surrounded by the Skene glands and ducts. Although not a prominent structure, the meatus appears as a small V-shaped slit. Note its location, especially if it opens from the clitoris or inside the vagina. Gently palpate the glands, which are common sites of cysts and sexually transmitted lesions.

The **vaginal orifice** is located posterior to the urethral meatus. Its appearance varies depending on individual anatomy and sexual activity. Ordinarily, examination of the vagina is limited to inspection. In virgins, a thin crescent-shaped or circular membrane, called the **hymen**, may cover part of the vaginal opening. In some instances, it completely occludes the orifice. After rupture, small rounded pieces of tissue called **caruncles** remain. Although an imperforate hymen denotes lack of penile intercourse, a perforate one does not necessarily indicate sexual activity.

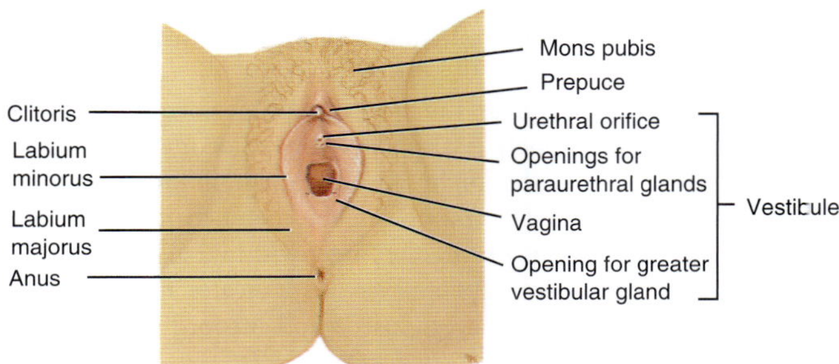

Fig 4.38 External structures of the genitalia in a postpubertal female. The labia are spread to reveal deeper structures. (Source: Paulsen, F., & Waschke, J. (2013). *Sobotta atlas of human anatomy* (2nd vol., 15th ed.). Munich, Germany: Elsevier.)

Surrounding the vaginal opening are **Bartholin's glands**, which secrete a clear, mucoid fluid into the vagina for lubrication during intercourse. Palpate the ducts for cysts. Note the discharge from the vagina, which is usually clear or white.

Anus

After examination of the genitalia, it is easy to identify the anal area, although the child should be placed on the abdomen. Note the general firmness of the buttocks and symmetry of the **gluteal folds**. Assess the tone of the anal sphincter by eliciting the **anal reflex** (**anal wink**). Gently scratching the anal area results in an obvious quick contraction of the external anal sphincter.

Back and Extremities

Spine

Note the general **curvature** of the spine. Normally the back of a newborn is rounded or C shaped from the thoracic and pelvic curves. The development of the cervical and lumbar curves approximates development of various motor skills, such as cervical curvature with head control, and gives the older child the typical double S curve.

Marked curvatures in posture are abnormal. **Scoliosis**, lateral curvature of the spine, is an important childhood problem, especially in girls. Although scoliosis may be identified by observing and palpating the spine and noting a sideways displacement, more objective tests include the following.

- With the child standing erect, clothed only in underpants (and bra if older girl), observe from behind, noting asymmetry of the shoulders and hips.
- With the child bending forwards so that the back is parallel to the floor, observe from the front and side, noting asymmetry or prominence of the rib cage.
- A slight limp, a crooked hemline, asymmetrical heights of shoulders or hips, or complaints of a sore back are other signs and symptoms of scoliosis.

Inspect the back, especially along the spine, for any tufts of hair, dimples or discolouration. Mobility of the vertebral column is easy to assess in most children because of their tendency to be in constant motion during the examination. However, you can test mobility by asking the child to sit up from a prone position or to do a modified sit-up exercise.

Movement of the cervical spine is an important diagnostic sign of neurological problems, such as meningitis. Normally movement of the head in all directions is effortless.

Extremities

Inspect each extremity for symmetry of length and size; refer any deviation for orthopaedic evaluation. Count the fingers and toes to be certain of the normal number. This is so often taken for granted that an extra digit (**polydactyly**) or fusion of digits (**syndactyly**) may go unnoticed.

Inspect the arms and legs for temperature and colour, which should be equal in each extremity, although the feet may normally be colder than the hands.

Assess the shape of bones. There are several variations of bone shape in children. Although many of them cause parents concern,

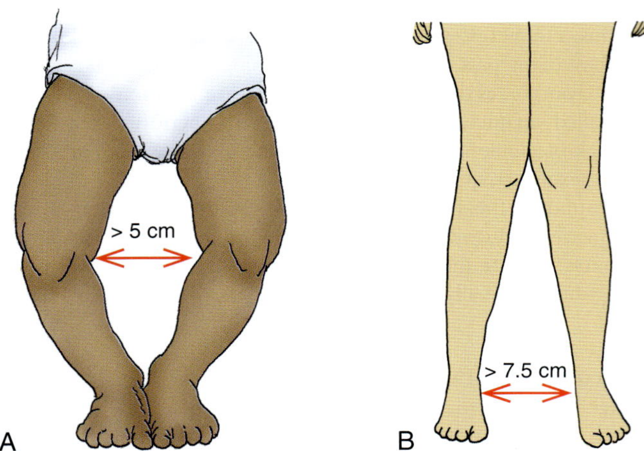

Fig 4.39 A Genu varum. **B** Genu valgum.

most are benign and require no treatment. **Bowleg**, or **genu varum**, is lateral bowing of the tibia. It is clinically present when the child stands with an outward bowing of the legs, giving the appearance of a bow. Usually there is an outward curvature of both femur and tibia (Fig 4.39A). Toddlers are usually bowlegged after beginning to walk until all their lower back and leg muscles are well developed. Unilateral or asymmetrical bowlegs that are present beyond 2 to 3 years old, particularly in African American children, may represent pathological conditions requiring further investigation.

Knock-knee, or **genu valgum**, appears as the opposite of bowleg, in that the knees are close together but the feet are spread apart. It is determined clinically by using the same method as for genu varum but by measuring the distance between the malleoli, which normally should be less than 7.5 cm (see Fig 4.39B). Knock-knee is normally present in children from about 2 to 7 years of age. Knock-knee that is excessive, asymmetrical, accompanied by short stature or evident in a child nearing puberty requires further evaluation.

Next inspect the feet. Infants' and toddlers' feet appear flat because the foot is normally wide and the arch is covered by a fat pad. Development of the arch occurs naturally from the action of walking. Normally at birth the feet are held in a valgus (outward) or varus (inward) position. To determine whether a foot deformity at birth is a result of intrauterine position or development, scratch the outer, then inner, side of the sole. If the foot position is self-correctable, it will assume a right angle to the leg. As the child begins to walk, the feet turn outwards less than 30 degrees and inwards less than 10 degrees.

Toddlers have a 'toddling' or broad-based gait, which facilitates walking by lowering the centre of gravity. As the child reaches preschool age, the legs are brought closer together. By school age, the walking posture is much more graceful and balanced.

The most common gait problem in young children is **pigeon toe**, or **toeing in**, which usually results from torsional deformities, such as internal tibial torsion (abnormal rotation or bowing of the tibia). Tests for tibial torsion include measuring the thigh-foot angle, which requires considerable practice for accuracy.

Elicit the **plantar** or **grasp reflex** by exerting firm but gentle pressure with the tip of the thumb against the lateral sole of the foot from the heel upwards to the little toe and then across to the big toe. The normal response in children who are walking is flexion of the toes. **Babinski's sign**, dorsiflexion of the big toe and fanning of the other toes, is normal during infancy but abnormal after about 1 year old or when locomotion begins (see Fig 7.10).

Joints

Evaluate the joints for range of motion. Normally this requires no specific testing if you have observed the child's movements during the examination. However, routinely investigate the hips in infants for congenital dislocation by checking for subluxation of the hip (see Chapter 33). Report any evidence of joint immobility or hyperflexibility. Palpate the joints for heat, tenderness and swelling. These signs, as well as redness over the joint, warrant further investigation.

Muscles

Note symmetry and quality of muscle development, tone and strength. Observe development by looking at the shape and contour of the body in both a relaxed and a tensed state. Estimate tone by grasping the muscle and feeling its firmness when it is relaxed and contracted. A common site for testing tone is the biceps muscle of the arm. Children are usually willing to 'make a muscle' by clenching their fist.

Estimate strength by having the child use an extremity to push or pull against resistance, as in the following examples.

- **Arm strength**—Child holds the arms outstretched in front of the body and tries to raise the arms while downward pressure is applied.
- **Hand strength**—Child shakes hands with nurse and squeezes one or two fingers of the nurse's hand.
- **Leg strength**—Child sits on a table or chair with the legs dangling and tries to raise the legs while downward pressure is applied.

Note symmetry of strength in the extremities, hands and fingers, and report evidence of **paresis**, or weakness.

Neurological Assessment

The assessment of the nervous system is the broadest and most diverse part of the examination process because every human function, both physical and emotional, is controlled by neurological impulses. Much of the neurological examination has already been discussed, such as assessment of behaviour, sensory testing and motor function. The following focuses on a general appraisal of cerebellar function, deep tendon reflexes and the cranial nerves.

Cerebellar Function

The cerebellum controls balance and coordination. Much of the assessment of cerebellar function is included in observing the child's posture, body movements, gait and development of fine and gross motor skills. Tests (e.g. balancing on one foot and the heel-to-toe walk) assess balance. Test coordination by asking the child to reach for a toy, button clothes, tie shoes or draw a straight line on a piece of paper (provided the child is old enough to do these activities). Coordination can also be tested by any sequence of rapid, successive movements, such as quickly touching each finger with the thumb of the same hand.

Several tests for cerebellar function can be performed as games (Box 4.11). When a Romberg test is done, stay beside the child if there is a possibility that he or she might fall. School-age children should be able to perform these tests, although in the finger-to-nose test, preschoolers normally can only bring the finger within 5 to 7.5 cm of the nose. Difficulty in performing these exercises indicates a poor sense of position (especially with the eyes closed) and incoordination (especially with the eyes opened).

Reflexes

Testing reflexes is an important part of the neurological examination. Persistence of primitive reflexes (see Chapter 7), loss of reflexes or

BOX 4.11 Tests for Cerebellar Function

Finger-to-nose test—With the child's arm extended, ask the child to touch the nose with the index finger with eyes open and then closed.

Heel-to-shin test—Have the child stand and run the heel of one foot down the shin or anterior aspect of the tibia of the other leg, both with the eyes opened and then with the eyes closed.

Romberg test—Have the child stand with the eyes closed and heels together; falling or leaning to one side is abnormal and is called the Romberg sign.

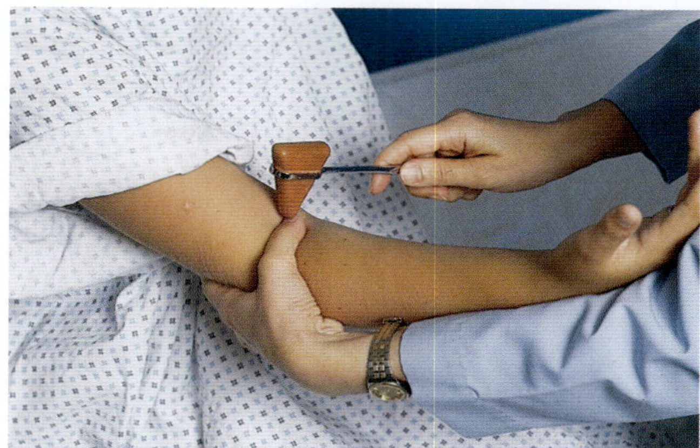

Fig 4.41 Testing for the biceps reflex. The child's arm is held by placing the partially flexed elbow in the examiner's hand with the thumb over the antecubital space. The examiner's thumbnail is struck with a hammer. Normal response is partial flexion of the forearm.

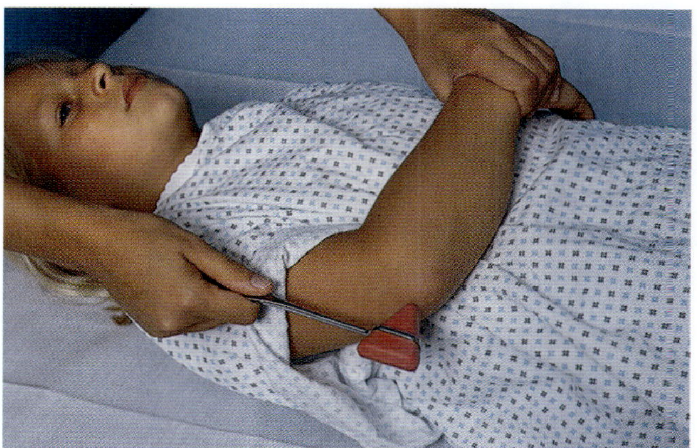

Fig 4.40 Testing for the triceps reflex. Child is placed supine, with the forearm resting over the chest, and the triceps tendon is struck. *Alternative procedure:* The child's arm is abducted, with the upper arm supported and the forearm allowed to hang freely. The triceps tendon is struck. Normal response is partial extension of the forearm.

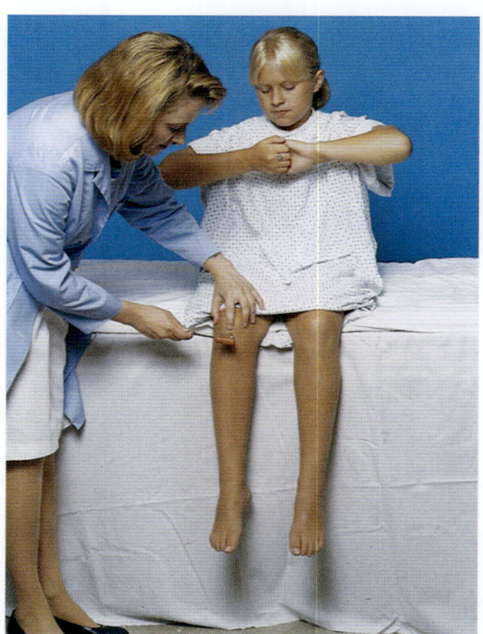

Fig 4.42 Testing for the patellar, or knee-jerk, reflex, using distraction. The child sits on the edge of the examining table (or on the parent's lap) with the lower legs flexed at the knee and dangling freely. The patellar tendon is tapped just below the kneecap. Normal response is partial extension of the lower leg.

hyperactivity of deep tendon reflexes is usually a result of a cerebral insult.

Elicit reflexes by using the rubber head of the reflex hammer, flat of the finger or side of the hand. If the child is easily frightened by equipment, use your hand or finger. Although testing reflexes is a simple procedure, the child may inhibit the reflex by unconsciously tensing the muscle. To avoid tensing, distract younger children with toys or talk to them. Older children can concentrate on the exercise of grasping their two hands in front of them and trying to pull them apart. This diverts their attention from the testing and causes involuntary relaxation of the muscles.

Deep tendon reflexes are stretch reflexes of a muscle. The most common deep tendon reflex is the **knee-jerk reflex**, or **patellar reflex** (sometimes called the **quadriceps reflex**). Figs. 4.40 to 4.43 illustrate the reflexes normally elicited. Report any diminished or hyperreflexive response for further evaluation.

Cranial Nerves

Assessment of the cranial nerves is an important area of neurological assessment (Fig 4.44; Table 4. 9). With young children, present the tests as games to foster trust and security at the beginning of the examination. Include the cranial nerve test when examining each system, such as tongue movement and strength, gag reflex, swallowing, cardinal positions of gaze (Fig 4.45) and position of the uvula during examination of the mouth.

Developmental Assessment

One of the most essential components of a complete health appraisal is assessment of developmental function. **Screening** procedures are designed to identify quickly and reliably children whose developmental level is below normal for their age and who therefore require further evaluation. The earlier that developmental problems are identified and treated, the more likely the child can reach his or her potential. Developmental screening also provides a means of recording objective measurements of present developmental function for future reference.

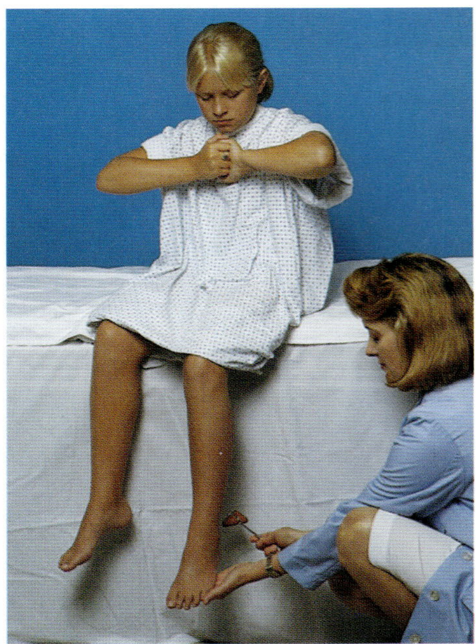

Fig 4.43 Testing for the Achilles reflex. The child should be in the same position as for the knee-jerk reflex. The foot is supported lightly in the examiner's hand, and the Achilles tendon is struck. Normal response is plantar flexion of the foot (the foot pointing downwards).

PATHOPHYSIOLOGY REVIEW

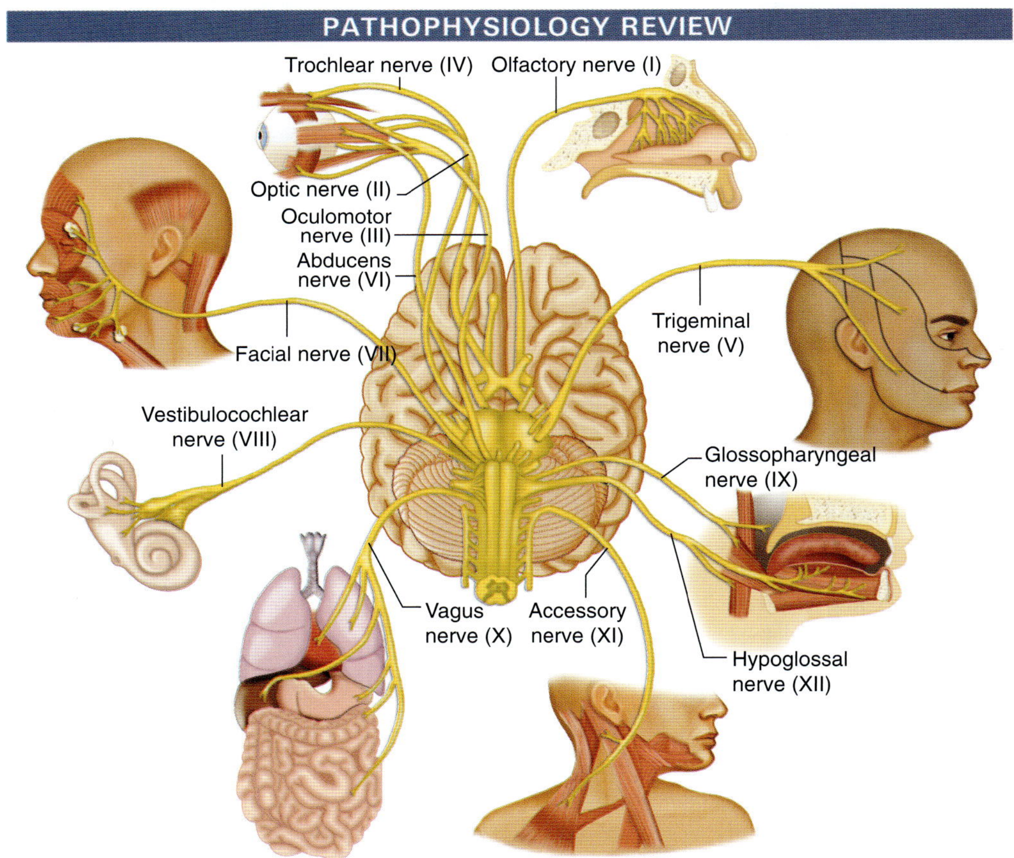

Fig 4.44 Cranial nerves. (Source: Patton, K. T., & Thibodeau, G. A. (2013). *Anatomy and physiology* (8th ed.). St Louis, MO: Mosby.)

TABLE 4.9 Assessment of Cranial Nerves

Description and Function	Tests
I—Olfactory Nerve	
Olfactory mucosa of nasal cavity Smell	With eyes closed, have child identify odours such as coffee, alcohol from a swab or other smells; test each nostril separately.
II—Optic Nerve	
Rods and cones of retina, optic nerve Vision	Check for perception of light, visual acuity, peripheral vision, colour vision and normal optic disc.
III—Oculomotor Nerve	
Extraocular muscles of eye: • Superior rectus—moves eyeball up and in • Inferior rectus—moves eyeball down and in • Medial rectus—moves eyeball nasally • Inferior oblique—moves eyeball up and out	Have child follow an object (toy) or light in six cardinal positions of gaze (see).Fig 4.45
Pupil constriction and accommodation	Perform PERRLA (Pupils Equal, Round, React to Light and Accommodation).
Eyelid closing	Check for proper placement of lid.
IV—Trochlear Nerve	
Superior oblique muscle (SO)—moves eye down and out	Have child look down and in (see .Fig 4.45)
V—Trigeminal Nerve	
Muscles of mastication	Have child bite down hard and open jaw; test symmetry and strength.
Sensory—face, scalp, nasal and buccal mucosa	With child's eyes closed, see if child can detect light touch in mandibular and maxillary regions. Test corneal and blink reflex by touching cornea lightly with a whisk of cotton ball twisted into a point (approach from side so that child does not blink before cornea is touched).
VI—Abducens Nerve	
Lateral rectus (LR) muscle—moves eye temporally	Have child look towards temporal side (see).Fig 4.45
VII—Facial Nerve	
Muscles for facial expression	Have child smile, make funny face or show teeth to see symmetry of expression.
Anterior two-thirds of tongue (sensory)	Have child identify sweet or salty solution; place each taste on anterior section and sides of protruding tongue; if child retracts tongue, solution will dissolve towards posterior part of tongue.
VIII—Auditory, Acoustic or Vestibulocochlear Nerve	
Internal ear Hearing and balance	Test hearing; note any loss of equilibrium or presence of vertigo.
IX—Glossopharyngeal Nerve	
Pharynx, tongue	Stimulate posterior pharynx with a tongue blade; child should gag.
Posterior third of tongue Sensory	Test sense of sour or bitter taste on posterior segment of tongue.
X—Vagus Nerve	
Muscles of larynx, pharynx, some organs of gastrointestinal system, sensory fibres of root of tongue, heart and lung	Note hoarseness of voice, gag reflex and ability to swallow. Check that uvula is in midline; when stimulated with tongue blade, it should deviate upwards and to stimulated side.
XI—Accessory Nerve	
Sternocleidomastoid and trapezius muscles of shoulder	Have child shrug shoulders while applying mild pressure; with examiner's hands placed on shoulders, have child turn head against opposing pressure on either side; note symmetry and strength.
XII—Hypoglossal Nerve	
Muscles of tongue	Have child move tongue in all directions; have child protrude tongue as far as possible; note any midline deviation. Test strength by placing tongue blade on one side of tongue and having child move it away.

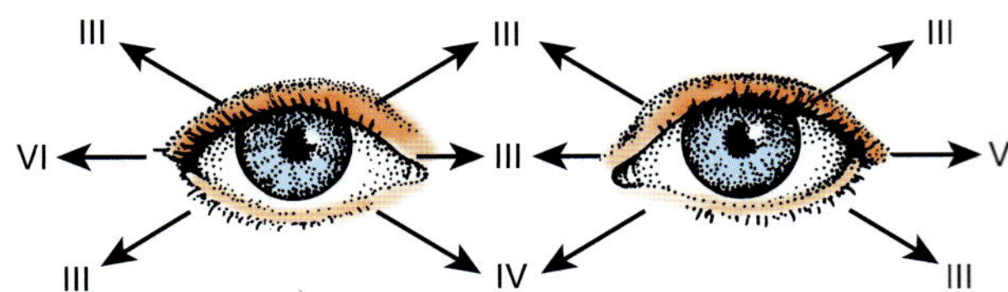

Fig 4.45 Checking extraocular movements in the six cardinal positions indicates the functioning of cranial nerves III, IV and VI. (Source: Ignatavicius, D. D., & Workman, L. M. (2016). *Medical-surgical nursing: Patient-centered collaborative care* (8th ed.). St Louis, MO: Elsevier.)

REFERENCES

Australian Government Department of Health (AGDH). (2020). Australian Immunisation Register. https://www.servicesaustralia.gov.au/individuals/services/medicare/australian-immunisation-register

Australasian Paediatric Endocrine Group (APEG). (2020). Growth and Growth Charts. https://apeg.org.au/clinical-resources-links/growth-growth-charts/

Ball, J. W., Dains, J. E., Flynn, J. A., et al. (2014). Seidel's guide to physical examination (8th ed.). St Louis, MO: Elsevier.

Batra, P., Faridi, M. M., & Saha, A. (2012). Thermometry in children. Journal of Emergencies, Trauma, and Shock, 5(3), 246–249.

Batra, P., & Goyal, S. (2013). Comparison of rectal, axillary, tympanic, and temporal artery thermometry in the pediatric emergency room. Pediatric Emergency Care, 29(1), 63–66.

Blank, L., Coster, J., O'Cathain, A., et al. (2012). The appropriateness of, and compliance with, telephone triage decisions: A systematic review and narrative synthesis. Journal of Advanced Nursing, 68(12), 2610–2621.

Campbell, J., Theodoros , D., Russell, T., et al. (2019) Client, provider and community referrer perceptions of telehealth for the delivery of rural paediatric allied health services. Australian Journal of Rural Health, 27(5), 419–426.

Centers for Disease Control and Prevention (CDC). (2017). Clinical Growth Charts. https://www.cdc.gov/growthcharts/clinical_charts.htm

Child Family Community Australia (CFCA). (2020). Mandatory Reporting of Child Abuse and Neglect. https://aifs.gov.au/cfca/sites/default/files/publication-documents/2006_mandatory_reporting_of_child_abuse_and_neglect.pdf

Dosman, C., & Andrews, D. (2012). Anticipatory guidance for cognitive and social-emotional development: Birth to five years. Paediatrics & Child Health, 17(2), 75–80.

Foote, J. M., Brady, L. H., Burke, A. L., et al. (2009). Evidence-based clinical practice guideline on linear growth measurement of children. http://www.blankchildrens.org/linear-growth-measurement.aspx.

Mathers, M., Keyes, M., & Wright, M. (2010). A review of the evidence on the effectiveness of children's vision screening. Child: Care, Health and Development, 36(6), 754–780.

Ministry of Health. (2015). National Immunisation Register. https://www.health.govt.nz/our-work/preventative-health-wellness/immunisation/national-immunisation-register

Park, M. K., Menard, S. W., & Schoolfield, J. (2005). Oscillometric blood pressure standards for children. Pediatric Cardiology, 26(5), 601–607.

Purc-Stephenson, R. J., & Thrasher, C. (2012). Patient compliance with telephone triage recommendations: A meta-analytic review. Patient Education and Counseling, 87, 135–142.

Queensland Health. (2015). Communicating effectively with Aboriginal and Torres Strait Islander people. https://www.health.qld.gov.au/__data/assets/pdf_file/0021/151923/communicating.pdf

Schell, K., Briening, E., Lebet, R., et al. (2011). Comparison of arm and calf automatic non-invasive blood pressures in pediatric intensive care patients. Journal of Pediatric Nursing, 26, 3–12.

Smith, W., Taki, S., & Wen, L. (2020). The role of telehealth in supporting mothers and children during the COVID-19 pandemic. Australian Journal of Advanced Nursing, 37(3). doi: 10.37464/2020.373.168.

Stacey, D., Macartney, G., Carley, M., et al. (2013). Development and evaluation of evidence-informed clinical nursing protocols for remote assessment, triage and support of cancer treatment-induced symptoms. Nursing Research and Practice, 2013, 171872.

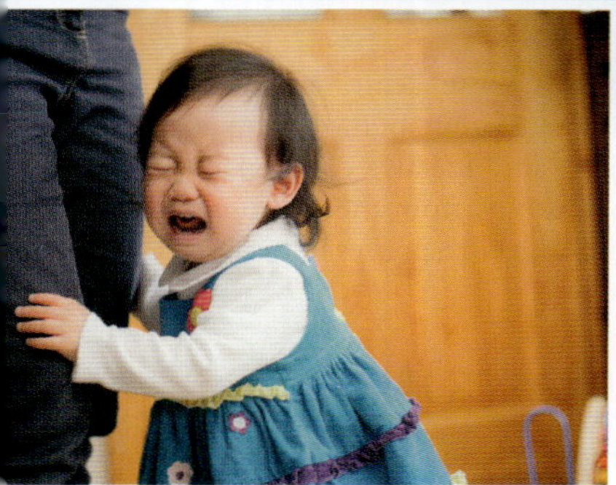

5

Pain Assessment and Management in Children

Maryanne Podham and Patience Moyo

LEARNING OBJECTIVES

- Discuss the fundamentals of pain.
- Describe the various types of pain.
- Identify various types of pain.
- Describe the factors which influence the pain response.
- Identify acute and chronic conditions which contribute to pain in children.
- Explain the methods used to assess pain in children.
- Establish nursing care interventions related to the management of pain in children through pharmacological and non-pharmacological strategies.

FUNDAMENTALS OF PAIN

Pain is a very complex phenomenon which is highly individualised involving multiple factors. The prevalence of persistent pain (pain extending beyond the expected healing timeframe) in childhood is estimated to range from 11% to 54% (Pate et al 2019). Pain is noted to be one of the sources of distress not only in children but also in the children's families. Children may not be able to accurately describe pain and often their families, carers and even healthcare providers have misconceptions about pain experienced by children. If pain is poorly managed, this can lead to serious long-lasting health and emotional consequences thereby impacting on one's quality of life and health journey. It is crucial for pain to be anticipated and appropriately managed. It should be noted that access to pain management is considered to be a fundamental right and as such healthcare professionals have a mandate to ensure that they alleviate pain and suffering for the children they care for (Australian and New Zealand College of Anaesthetists [ANZCA] 2010, Brennan & Gwyther 2019). This chapter will therefore describe the mechanisms of pain in children, differentiate the types of pain, explain the various pain assessment tools and also outline the various pharmacological and non-pharmacological strategies used to manage pain.

Pain is a significant problem for children of all ages in all healthcare settings. Pain experience is subjective and as such this necessitates that health professionals need to be considerate of the patient's self-report of pain. Needle procedures are one of the most painful and fear-inducing procedures for children (McMurtry, Noel et al 2015). Exposure to needle procedures is highest in preterm infants in neonatal intensive care units, but neonates experience from 1 to 10 or more painful procedures during each day of hospitalisation (Courtois et al 2016, Johnston et al 2011). Up to 86% of hospitalised children experience acute pain (Kozlowski et al 2014, Solodiuk et al 2014, Walther-Larsen et al 2016) from their disease or injury, treatment and invasive procedures, including surgery, and more than 5% of children will have persistent postsurgical pain for 2 months or longer (Fortier et al 2011, Kristensen et al 2012, Sieberg et al 2013). Uncontrolled acute pain has been recognised as a significant risk factor for the development of chronic pain (Chapman & Vierck 2017). Reported prevalence rates of chronic pain in children in Australia vary from 25% to 35% (Australian Institute of Health and Welfare [AIHW] 2020), and 5% of children are reported to commonly experience moderate to severe pain from headaches, limb pain, abdominal pain and complex regional pain syndrome (Bennett 2017). Differences in chronic pain prevalence rates are found by gender, age, ethnicity and geographical region.

Paediatric nurses play a pivotal role in preventing, advocating for and managing children's pain. Unfortunately, evidence suggests that paediatric nurses are not translating pain prevention, assessment and treatment knowledge into their routine care of managing children's pain (Manworren 2017). Pain occurs in children of all ages and may manifest as acute, recurrent, chronic, or a mixture of acute and chronic pain. Nurses with a foundational understanding of pain, developmental differences in pain expression and developmental implications of pain can prevent, assess, treat and advocate for optimal paediatric pain reduction and relief.

WHAT IS PAIN AND HOW DOES IT OCCUR?

Pain is a complex biopsychosocial phenomenon with multiple components. According to the International Association for the Study of Pain (IASP) (2012) pain is defined as 'an unpleasant sensory and emotional experience associated with actual or potential tissue damage, or described in terms of such damage' (Schug et al 2015, p. 1). Processes involved in the experience of pain include the peripheral and central nervous systems' reactions that are characteristic of acute pain. At the same time, responses and interactions within the neuronal matrix are evolving and influence both acute and chronic pain experiences (Table 5.1).

Figure 5.1 depicts these processes and indicates areas where interventions can influence or modulate pain signalling. When a tissue injury is sustained (e.g. to the finger from a blood test), peripheral sensory neurons synapse onto interneurons in the spinal cord that then transmit information within a spinal segment and into ascending pathways for processing by the brain. Positron emission tomography studies confirm that painful stimulation activates somatosensory and limbic cortices of the brain. These areas have projections to the frontal cortex, an area implicated in many of our most complex human behaviours (e.g. attention, emotional regulation, mood).

A painful stimulus also activates the periaqueductal grey matter (PAG). Stimulation of the PAG with opiate administration or electrical stimulation results in significant analgesia (Tryon & Mizumori 2018). The PAG sends projections to the raphe nucleus magnus in the rostroventral medulla, which projects to the dorsal horn of the spinal cord. These descending projections inhibit further activation in ascending pathways, thereby modulating the amount of pain information transmitted up from the spinal cord to the brain (Ossipov et al 2014, Tryon & Mizumori 2018). Additionally, there are direct connections to the PAG from the prefrontal cortex, amygdala and hypothalamus, and these connections are capable of eliciting analgesia (Tryon & Mizumori 2018).

The neural network, or **brain neuromatrix** (Huether & Rodway 2019), is a series of connected neural cells with cognitive, sensory and affective pathways combined in a feedback loop unique to each individual. Therefore, the brain neuromatrix is able to assign meaning to the stimulus and modulate the perceptual experience and response through the descending pathway, which both inhibits and facilitates pain. In addition, the connections between emotional and cognitive processing areas and these descending pathways offer other paths by which pain is modulated and by which prior painful experience may affect modulatory processes. Often the effect of descending inhibition is to increase threshold or decrease pain sensitivity during times of stress.

Prior experiences may alter the modulatory tone of this pathway, setting up circumstances where the system is perpetually sensitised and eliciting disproportionate responses to incoming painful stimuli without temporal tissue damage. Once these pain tracks are created in the brain, it is possible for pain to exist purely in the brain. This pain, however, is real and it feels the way the child says it feels—regardless of the location of origin, whether the message is coming straight from the brain or as a result of body tissue damage.

The neuromatrix is involved in both acute and chronic stress responses that contribute to pain perception. In the case of acute stress responses, each sensory, cognitive and affective component provides input to the brain about pain. Outputs from the brain neuromatrix influence the neural web and also trigger responses in the body that are perceived as the pain experience.

WHAT DOES PAIN DO BESIDES HURT?

In addition to being uncomfortable, pain is harmful. Stress regulation includes hormonal responses and immune system activity. Pain triggers a number of physiological stress responses in the body, and these may lead to negative consequences involving multiple systems. Long-term amplification of the sympathetic nervous system hinders healing. Unrelieved pain, whether from trauma, surgery or disease, may prolong stress response and adversely affect a child's recovery. Box 5.1 provides a list of numerous complications of untreated pain in preterm neonates.

Poorly controlled acute pain also predisposes patients to chronic pain syndromes (Chapman & Vierck 2017). When pain is unrelieved, sensory input from injured tissues causes recruitment of peripheral and spinal cord neurons to amplify pain responses even to non-painful stimuli. Severe and sustained pain is more difficult to control. Nurses who care for infants and children need to consider the potential acute and long-term effects of pain on their young patients and be advocates in preventing and treating pain.

COMMON ACUTE PAIN CONDITIONS IN CHILDREN

Children experience numerous **acute pain** episodes during childhood, but certain children are at higher risk than others. Children may sustain acute pain from immunisations, minor injuries (e.g. knee abrasion), illnesses or medical and surgical procedures during hospitalisation. Nurses may find it easy to overlook certain painful experiences as part of normal care and perform invasive procedures without any

TABLE 5.1 What is Pain? Pain Definitions

Pain	'Pain is an unpleasant sensory and emotional experience associated with actual or potential tissue damage, or described in terms of such damage' (IASP 2012). Pain has sensory, emotional, cognitive and social components (Williams & Craig 2016).
Acute pain	Pain (as described) felt acutely for a short period of time. Acute pain may occur in response to illness, stress or injury.
Chronic pain	Persistent or recurrent pain lasting longer than 3 months.
Chronic primary pain	Pain in one or more anatomical regions that persists or recurs for longer than 3 months and is associated with significant emotional distress or significant functional disability (interference with activities of daily life and participation in social roles) and that cannot be better explained by another chronic pain condition.
Chronic cancer pain	Pain caused by the cancer itself (the primary tumour or metastases) and pain that is caused by the cancer treatment (surgical, chemotherapy, radiotherapy and others). Cancer-related pain will be subdivided based on location into visceral, bony (or musculoskeletal) and somatosensory (neuropathic). It will be described as either continuous (background pain) or intermittent (episodic pain) if associated with physical movement or clinical procedures.
Chronic postsurgical or posttraumatic pain	Pain that develops after a surgical procedure or a tissue injury (involving any trauma, including burns) and persists at least 3 months after surgery or tissue trauma. This is a definition of exclusion, as all other causes of pain (infection, recurring malignancy) as well as pain from a preexisting pain problem need to be excluded.
Chronic neuropathic pain	Pain caused by a lesion or disease of the somatosensory nervous system.
Chronic headache or chronic orofacial pain	Pain defined as headaches or orofacial pains that occur on at least 50% of the days during at least 3 months.
Chronic visceral pain	Persistent or recurrent pain that originates from the internal organs of the head and neck region and the thoracic, abdominal and pelvic cavities.
Chronic musculoskeletal pain	Persistent or recurrent pain that arises as part of a disease process directly affecting bone(s), joint(s), muscle(s) or related soft tissue(s).

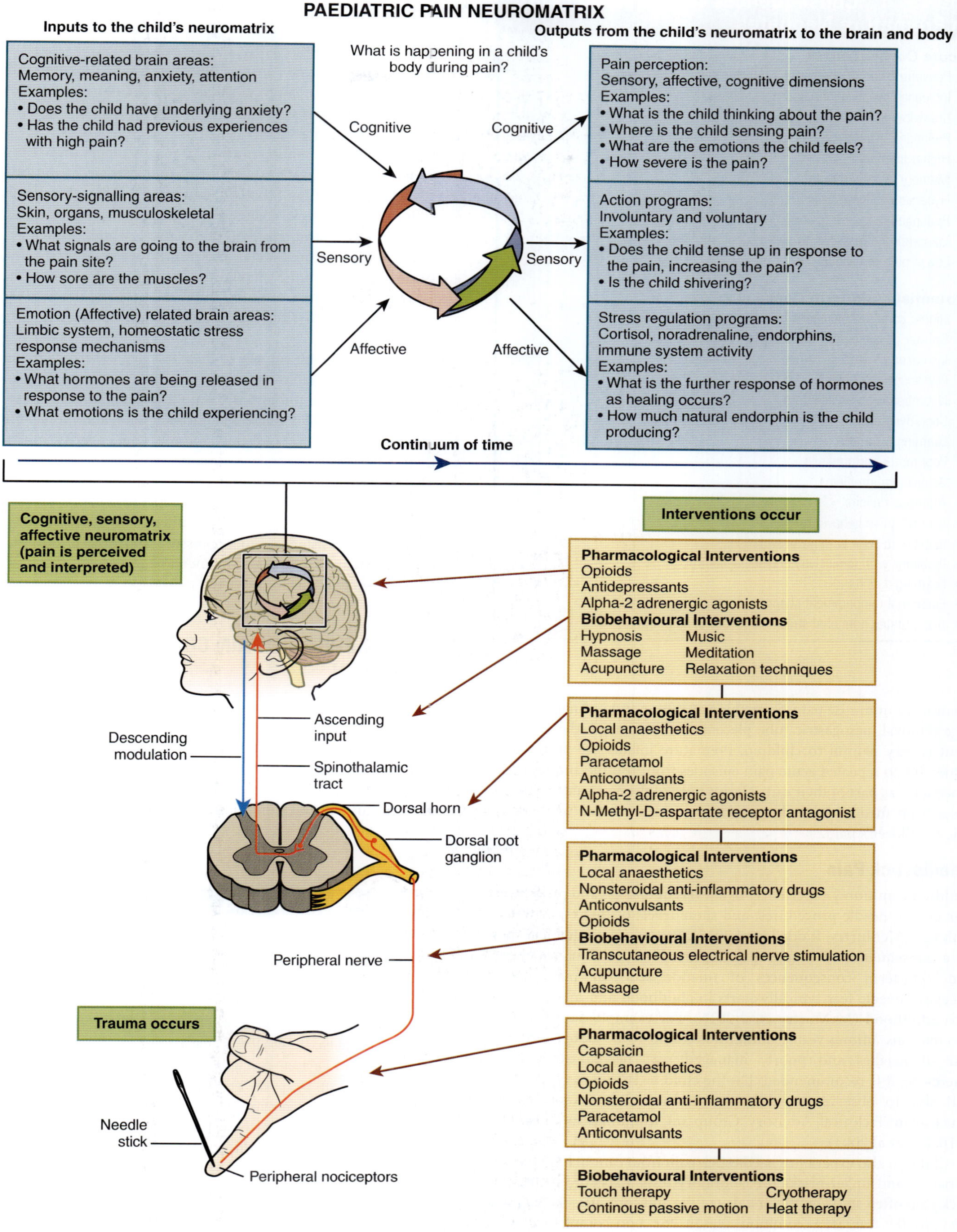

PAEDIATRIC PAIN NEUROMATRIX

Inputs to the child's neuromatrix

Cognitive-related brain areas:
Memory, meaning, anxiety, attention
Examples:
- Does the child have underlying anxiety?
- Has the child had previous experiences with high pain?

Sensory-signalling areas:
Skin, organs, musculoskeletal
Examples:
- What signals are going to the brain from the pain site?
- How sore are the muscles?

Emotion (Affective) related brain areas:
Limbic system, homeostatic stress response mechanisms
Examples:
- What hormones are being released in response to the pain?
- What emotions is the child experiencing?

What is happening in a child's body during pain?

Cognitive
Sensory
Affective

Cognitive
Sensory
Affective

Outputs from the child's neuromatrix to the brain and body

Pain perception:
Sensory, affective, cognitive dimensions
Examples:
- What is the child thinking about the pain?
- Where is the child sensing pain?
- What are the emotions the child feels?
- How severe is the pain?

Action programs:
Involuntary and voluntary
Examples:
- Does the child tense up in response to the pain, increasing the pain?
- Is the child shivering?

Stress regulation programs:
Cortisol, noradrenaline, endorphins, immune system activity
Examples:
- What is the further response of hormones as healing occurs?
- How much natural endorphin is the child producing?

Continuum of time

Cognitive, sensory, affective neuromatrix (pain is perceived and interpreted)

Descending modulation
Ascending input
Spinothalamic tract
Dorsal horn
Dorsal root ganglion
Peripheral nerve

Trauma occurs

Needle stick
Peripheral nociceptors

Interventions occur

Pharmacological Interventions
Opioids
Antidepressants
Alpha-2 adrenergic agonists
Biobehavioural Interventions
Hypnosis
Music
Massage
Meditation
Acupuncture
Relaxation techniques

Pharmacological Interventions
Local anaesthetics
Opioids
Paracetamol
Anticonvulsants
Alpha-2 adrenergic agonists
N-Methyl-D-aspartate receptor antagonist

Pharmacological Interventions
Local anaesthetics
Nonsteroidal anti-inflammatory drugs
Anticonvulsants
Opioids
Biobehavioural Interventions
Transcutaneous electrical nerve stimulation
Acupuncture
Massage

Pharmacological Interventions
Capsaicin
Local anaesthetics
Opioids
Nonsteroidal anti-inflammatory drugs
Paracetamol
Anticonvulsants

Biobehavioural Interventions
Touch therapy
Cryotherapy
Continous passive motion
Heat therapy

Fig 5.1 Pain model.

BOX 5.1 Consequences of Untreated Pain in Premature Neonates

Acute Consequences
- Periventricular-intraventricular haemorrhage
- Increased chemical and hormone release
- Breakdown of fat and carbohydrate stores
- Prolonged hyperglycaemia
- Higher morbidity
- Memory of painful events
- Hypersensitivity to pain
- Prolonged response to pain
- Inappropriate response to non-noxious stimuli
- Lower pain threshold

Potential Long-term Consequences
- Higher somatic complaints of unknown origin
- Greater physiological and behavioural responses to pain
- Increased prevalence of neurological deficits
- Psychosocial problems
- Neurobehavioural disorders
- Cognitive deficits
- Learning disorders
- Poor motor performance
- Behavioural problems
- Attention deficits
- Poor adaptive behaviour
- Inability to cope with novel situations
- Problems with impulsivity and social control
- Learning deficits
- Emotional temperament changes in infancy or childhood
- Accentuated hormonal stress responses in adult life

attempts to minimise pain. Something as minor and ordinary as bandage removal, nasogastric tube placement or urinary catheter placement is very painful to children. Premature infants are particularly vulnerable to repeated acute pain episodes from routine and frequent procedures as part of their care. Nurses need to prevent painful experiences from medical procedures and use evidence-based methods to relieve children's pain.

Needlestick Pain

Children commonly experience high levels of distress and procedural fear during needle procedures, and these levels of distress correlate with age (McMurtry, Riddell et al 2015). Procedure-related fear may be a consequence of inappropriate procedural pain management, and long-term consequences of unaddressed fear may follow. Excessive needle fear typically starts in childhood and may progress into adulthood (McMurtry et al 2016). For example, fainting with vaccinations among young adults was found to be associated with fear of needles and poorly managed past needle experiences. Therefore, it is recommended that the child be sitting or lying down and also to observe the child for 15 minutes post vaccination (Australian Technical Advisory Group on Immunisation [ATAGI] 2018, Nir et al 2003).

Children also experience needlestick pain from cannulation or heel puncture and finger-pricks for laboratory tests. Exposure to needlestick pain often starts on the first day of life and continues throughout life. Needle fear is a common reason for non-compliance with immunisations and also avoidance of seeking healthcare services (McMurtry, Noel et al 2015, Taddio et al 2012).

Postoperative Pain

Nurses and parents often consider postoperative pain an unavoidable painful consequence of surgery. At least 60% of children who undergo surgery are likely to report moderate to severe pain the first day after surgery (Kozlowski et al 2014).

Surgery and traumatic injuries (fractures, lacerations, burns) generate a catabolic state as a result of increased secretion of hormones (e.g. adrenaline, cortisol, glucagon). This then leads to alterations in blood flow, coagulation, fibrinolysis, substrate metabolism and water and electrolyte balance, which increases the demands on the cardiovascular and respiratory systems. The major endocrine and metabolic changes occur during the first 48 hours after surgery or trauma. Opioids and local anaesthetic nerve blocks are routinely used to alter the physiological responses to surgical injury.

Pain associated with surgery to the chest (e.g. repair of congenital heart defects, chest wall or spinal deformities) or abdomen (e.g. colectomy) may result in pulmonary complications. Pain leads to splinting and guarding. This decreased thoracic and abdominal muscle movement leads to decreased tidal volume, vital capacity, functional residual capacity and alveolar ventilation. The patient is unable to cough and clear secretions, and the risk for complications (e.g. atelectasis and pneumonia) is high. Severe postoperative pain also results in sympathetic overactivity, which is manifested by increases in heart rate, peripheral resistance, blood pressure and cardiac output. The patient eventually experiences an increase in cardiac demand and myocardial oxygen consumption and a decrease in oxygen delivery to the tissues.

COMMON CHRONIC PAIN CONDITIONS IN CHILDREN

Pain that persists for 3 months or more is defined as **chronic pain**. The three most common sites for chronic pain in paediatrics are headaches (up to 83%), abdominal pain (up to 53%) and musculoskeletal pain (up to 36%) (Friedrichsdorf et al 2016). Chronic pain may also be episodic with recurrent bouts of pain at least every 3 months (see Research Focus box and Community Focus box).

RESEARCH FOCUS

Pain in School-age Children

Friedrichsdorf et al (2016) reported that 44% of school-age children have at least one recurrent pain (headaches, stomach pains, facial pain and back pain) and at least 12% have persistent pain, mostly seen in females.

Chronic or recurrent pain adversely affects the psychosocial and physical wellbeing of children. The domains for the assessment of chronic or recurrent pain are the same for acute pain (pain intensity, global judgment of satisfaction with treatment, symptoms and adverse events, physical functioning, emotional functioning, economic factors), plus two additional domains: role functioning and sleep. Because the time course of chronic or recurrent pain is different from that of acute pain, measures used to assess chronic pain often evaluate the symptom over time.

A systematic review of treatment for functional abdominal pain disorders found no evidence to support pharmacological therapy (Korterink et al 2015).

COMMUNITY FOCUS

Chronic Pain and School Absenteeism in Children

Children with chronic pain may experience a problematic cycle of school absenteeism that progresses from absences to poor performance and school refusal. Children miss school because of pain exacerbations and healthcare appointments. Missed days may translate into lowered academic performance and an inability to deal with the complexities of the school environment (Logan 2017). Children with various chronic pain sources have reported missing an average of 13.5 days of school in a 3-month period (Logan et al 2012). Absence from school may require special accommodations and a modified school plan. Children with frequent or long-term absences may need a comprehensive and coordinated plan for a return to school. A team approach among healthcare clinicians, parents, teachers and school staff can help improve reintegration of children into school (Miro et al 2017, Jones et al 2014). As part of this team approach, cognitive-behavioural counsellors/psychologists may provide strategies to help children work through self-esteem and peer perception issues. Nurses, medical practitioners and therapists can educate parents about the importance of school attendance, set boundaries for compliance with attendance policies and teach parents to avoid reinforcement of negative behaviours.

Headaches

Almost every child reports having had a headache in the last 3 months. Most children with recurrent headaches have a family history of headaches. Headache prevalence also increases with age. Prevalence for boys and girls is similar before 12 years of age; after 12 years, prevalence for girls is triple that of boys.

Primary headaches, as classified by the International Headache Society, do not have an identified cause. Primary headaches common in children include migraines and tension-type headaches. Secondary headaches are associated with a cause, such as head or neck trauma, intracranial pressure, inflammatory disorders, infection, medication overuse or substance use and withdrawal, and tumour. The aetiology of the headache should dictate the treatment plan. Therefore, the goal of treating migraines and other headaches without known cause is pain relief or reduction to minimise associated functional disability.

Migraines are theorised to be a sensory processing disorder of dysfunctional modulation of the nociceptive system. There may be a migraine generator in the dorsal midbrain and pons. Children typically describe migraines as throbbing, unilateral or bilateral, frontotemporal and of moderate to severe intensity. The term *migraine* is often misused to describe an intensely painful headache; however, there are specific diagnostic criteria of migraines in children. To meet these diagnostic criteria, migraine headaches must also have at least one of these characteristics: (1) aggravated by physical activity; (2) associated with nausea or vomiting; (3) photophobia; (4) phonophobia (ligyrophobia); (5) behavioural interference; or (6) lack of identified cause of recurrent headache. Children rarely report an aura with migraines.

Abdominal Pain

The Rome criteria for a diagnosis of functional abdominal pain includes episodic or continuous abdominal pain for greater than 3 months without identified pathology on physical examination and a negative stool for occult blood. Functional abdominal pain is described as non-radiating pain that lasts 1 to 3 hours and is typically located around the umbilicus. Accompanying symptoms may include altered bowel pattern, pallor, diaphoresis, nausea, vomiting, sleep disturbances and changes in oral intake. In at least 25% of cases, patients also have some loss of daily function and other somatic symptoms, such as headache or limb pain. Other terms that have erroneously been used interchangeably with functional abdominal pain are non-organic abdominal pain, psychogenic abdominal pain and recurrent abdominal pain. Other common chronic abdominal pain conditions include functional dyspepsia, irritable bowel syndrome and abdominal migraine. (See Chapter 16.)

Musculoskeletal Pain

Chronic musculoskeletal pain can be categorised into three subtypes: injury-related, illness-related or primary musculoskeletal pain. Pain can be localised to specific joints or muscle groups, such as ankle injuries or back pain, or may occur in multiple joints or muscle groups, as occurs with arthritis.

Musculoskeletal pain may also be diffuse as with fibromyalgia. Sometimes musculoskeletal pain appears as both diffuse and idiopathic in nature, making the pain difficult to characterise. Diffuse types of musculoskeletal pain have a high comorbidity with depressive symptoms (Kashikar-Zuck & Ting 2014, Vinall et al 2016). Researchers believe the stress adaptation response is altered in children with fibromyalgia, possibly due to immune-mediated processes (Kashikar-Zuck & Ting 2014, Vinall et al 2016).

Neuropathic Pain Syndromes

Neuropathic pain results from injury or dysfunction of the somatosensory system. Neuropathic pain is thought to be less common in children, but there are no current epidemiological studies (Howard et al 2014). Children experience neuropathic pain from nerve injury as a result of surgery or trauma (e.g. phantom limb pain or complex regional pain syndrome [CRPS]), autoimmune or degenerative neuropathies (e.g. Guillain-Barré syndrome or Charcot-Marie-Tooth disease) and neuropathies related to cancer or cancer treatment.

CRPS manifests as severe localised pain with allodynia, swelling and colour and temperature changes. CRPS typically affects a single extremity. A minor to severe injury, trauma, infection or stressful event precipitates the syndrome. A precipitating event to any extremity can also cause CRPS to recur (Howard et al 2014, Weissmann & Uziel 2016).

COMMON MIXED-PAIN CONDITIONS IN CHILDREN

Burn Pain

Burn pain is challenging to control because of multiple pain triggers, manipulations over injured sites during care and the changing patterns of pain across time (Griggs et al 2017). Pain perception is mediated by the degree of the burn, sensory input and individual child factors such as underlying anxiety (Gamst-Jensen et al 2014, Griggs et al 2017). Symptoms such as anxiety, depression and insomnia modulate the chronicity of burn pain (McIntyre et al 2016). Long-term posttraumatic stress symptoms vary inversely with early opiate dosing in children recovering from serious burns (Sheridan et al 2014).

Subtypes of burn pain have been categorised as background pain, breakthrough pain, procedural pain and postoperative pain (Gamst-Jensen et al 2014). Burns often result in constant background pain that is felt at the wound sites and surrounding areas. This background pain is often described as a throbbing or burning sensation (McIntyre et al 2016). Burn sites may trigger breakthrough pain during movements, such as position changes, walking or even breathing. Procedures that cause pain include wound debridement, dressing changes, physical therapy, baths and removal of skin graft staples (McIntyre et al 2016). Postoperative pain includes both the area of the burn and the donor sites for skin grafts. Pain is commonly experienced with intense tingling or itching sensations in skin graft sites. The healing process and side effects (itch, tingling, cold sensations) may last for months to years (Van Loey et al 2016). Researchers have explored mechanisms of itch to develop treatments for both itch and neuropathic pain.

Cancer Pain

Children with cancer experience pain from different causes at different points throughout their cancer experience. Pain may be a symptom of cancer and therefore children may be in pain when diagnosed with cancer (Table 5.2). Cancer treatment may also relieve cancer pain; however, treatment-related pain is also common. Survivors of childhood cancer may experience chronic pain from their cancer treatment; for example, from phantom limb pain, graft-versus-host disease or post herpetic neuralgia.

Mucositis, inflammation of mucosal lining, is a common source of treatment-related pain. Inflammation may occur in the mouth, oesophagus, stomach, intestine, rectal and vaginal areas after patients undergo chemotherapy, radiotherapy or bone marrow transplantation. Mucositis appears at different time intervals based on the type and duration of chemotherapy/radiology a patient receives, generally sooner after chemotherapy than after radiotherapy. Its maximum expression occurs 7 to 10 days after chemotherapy, and erythema progresses towards ulceration. Mucositis gradually subsides over a period of 2 to 3 weeks after the patient's cytotoxic treatment (Chaveli-López & Bagán-Sebastián 2016). Mucositis after bone marrow transplantation may be prolonged and continuously intense. Mucositis pain is exacerbated by mouth care and function (swallowing, drinking, eating and talking). There are no effective treatments to adequately relieve mucositis pain; this is an area of active research for prevention and better treatment options. Children at risk of mucositis should have regular oral assessments and bowel charts completed.

The types of treatment-related pain experienced by children with cancer vary with progression of the disease and the type of treatment protocol. Other treatment-related pain includes: (1) abdominal pain after allogeneic bone marrow transplantation, which may be associated with acute graft-versus-host disease; (2) abdominal pain associated with typhlitis (infection of the caecum), which occurs when the patient is immunocompromised; (3) phantom sensations and phantom limb pain after an amputation; (4) peripheral neuropathy after administration of vincristine; (5) medullary bone pain, which may be associated with administration of granulocyte colony–stimulating factor; and (6) pain associated with immunotherapy.

Sickle Cell Pain

Pain is a hallmark symptom of sickle cell disease (SCD) (see Chapter 28). The pain is severe, acute and episodic. **Vaso-occlusive crisis** (VOC) pain begins in infants as young as 6 months and continues throughout life. Chronic pain can also develop from repeated tissue

TABLE 5.2 Cancer Pain in Children

Type	Clinical Presentation	Causes
Bone		
Skull Vertebrae Pelvis and femur	Aching to sharp, severe pain generally more pronounced with movement; point tenderness common Skull—headaches, blurred vision Spine—tenderness over spinous process Extremities—pain associated with movement or lifting Pelvis and femur—pain associated with movement; pain with weight bearing and walking	Infiltration of bone Skeletal metastases—irritation and stretching of pain receptors in periosteum and endosteum Prostaglandins released from bone destruction Aches from biological agents and immunotherapy Bone marrow pain from immature blood cell proliferation
Neuropathic		
Peripheral Plexus Epidural Cord compression	Complaints of pain without any detectable tissue damage Abnormal or unpleasant sensations, generally described as tingling, burning or stabbing Often a delay in onset Brief, shooting pain Increased intensity of pain with receptive stimuli	Nerve injury caused by tumour infiltration; nerve injury from treatment (e.g. vincristine toxicity) Infiltration or compression of peripheral nerves Surgical interruption of nerves (phantom pain after amputation)
Visceral		
Soft tissue Tumours of bowel Retroperitoneum	Poorly localised Varies in intensity Pressure, deep or aching	Obstruction—bowel, urinary tract, biliary tract Metabolic alteration Nociceptor activation, generally from distension or inflammation of visceral organs
Treatment Related		
Mucositis Infection typhlitis Radiation dermatitis Postsurgical Post lumbar puncture headaches	Difficulty swallowing, pain from lesions in oropharynx; may extend throughout entire gastrointestinal tract Infection may be localised pain from focused infection or generalised (i.e. tissue infection versus septicaemia) Severe headache after lumbar puncture Skin inflammation causing redness and breakdown Pain related to tissue trauma secondary to surgery	Direct side effects of treatment for cancer: • chemotherapy • radiation • surgery • tumour removal • central line placement/removal • diagnostic procedures venipuncture • lumbar puncture • bone marrow biopsy • other biopsies

damage or avascular joint necrosis. There are preventive treatments, but the only cure for SCD is a bone marrow transplant.

VOC pain in infants and toddlers is typically characterised by dactylitis—visible painful swelling of fingers, hands, toes or feet or extremity pain. As children get older, headaches, low back pain and bone pain are common. Children with SCD may also have increased frequency of surgical procedures (e.g. splenectomy following splenic sequestration or cholecystectomy for gallbladder sludging). VOC, however, is the most frequent reason for emergency department visits and hospital admissions among children with SCD (Fosdal 2015).

Sickle cell pain has been described as stronger than surgical, arthritis and childbirth pain (Fosdal 2015). Children may experience this pain from a very young age, and changes in level of activity, guarding certain body parts and fussiness may provide hints that the child is experiencing a pain crisis. Parents of children with SCD may notice that pain crises coincide with weather changes or acute illnesses such as respiratory viral infections or other bacterial infections.

MEASURING PAIN IN CHILDREN

Nurses may fail to recognise, treat and prevent acute and chronic pain without a strategic plan in place to assess pain at key times during care delivery. It is important to use a pain assessment tool appropriate for the child's developmental level and condition. Pain assessment should commence with a comprehensive pain history utilising the PQRST mnemonic (provoking/palliative factors, quality, region [location] and radiation, severity and temporal pattern [onset, duration, pattern]) and also evaluate the psychosocial factors such as pain beliefs, mood, coping strategies, social interactions and the impacts of pain on the level of functioning and quality of life (Chisengantambu & McDonald 2018). Pain assessment tools are available as observational pain measures, self-report rating scales and multidimensional pain assessment tools. Pain assessment should be more thorough than merely obtaining a pain rating. Understanding the location, frequency and duration and the precipitating, aggravating and alleviating factors of the pain experienced by the child is also essential for effective pain management. Nurses should assess other symptoms, including pain's effect on sleep, emotional function (mood, anxiety, depression), physical recovery (acute pain) or physical functioning, disability (chronic pain), role functioning (chronic pain) and satisfaction with pain treatment (Eccleston et al 2014, Swift 2015).

Consistent use of the same measurement tools is necessary to standardise communication related to pain and evaluate the effectiveness of pain management strategies. The current trend is to choose pain assessment tools with a common metric for measurement of pain. A common metric would make pain scores easier to read, interpret and integrate into research and practice (Gregory 2019). Most instruments consist of 0 for no pain to a range of 4 to 160 for the top anchors in pain measures. A pain score of 5 may mean a lot of pain (if a 0 to 5 scale is used) or very little (if a 0 to 100 scale is used), and it may not be clearly specified which score corresponds to which scale. Tools based on a 0 to 10 scale have been reported as the metric most commonly preferred by healthcare professionals, but not by patients (Gregory 2019). The goal of interpreting all pain scores based on a common metric is flawed because pain assessment tools measure different pain expressions; for example, self-report measures patients' perceived pain intensity, whereas observational pain measures are used to quantify patients' behavioural and physiological responses to pain.

Observational Pain Measures

Observational measures of pain are generally used for children from infancy until they are able to provide a self-report of pain and distinguish increments of pain intensity, typically around 3 to 4 years of age (Table 5.3). Observational pain measurement tools require a trained observer to watch and record children's behaviours, such as vocalisation, facial expression and body movements, that are associated with painful stimulus. Facial expression is the most consistent and specific indicator of pain in infants. Scales are available to systematically evaluate facial features, such as eye squeeze, brow bulge, open mouth and taut tongue (Figs 5.2 and 5.3). Understanding which behaviours are associated with pain helps nurses assess pain in infants and small children who are unable to provide self-report. However, discriminating between pain behaviours and reactions to other sources of distress, such as hunger, anxiety or other types of discomfort, is not always easy. Observational pain measures are most reliable when used to measure short, sharp procedural pain, such as pain due to heel puncture or

TABLE 5.3 Examples of Commonly used Behavioural Observational Pain Assessment Scales for Children

	FLACC (Malviya et al 2006, Merkel et al 1997, Voepel-Lewis et al 2010)	COMFORT-B (Harris et al 2016, Ista et al 2005, van Dijk et al 2000)
Age range	0–3 2 months to 7 years in PACU* 0–19 years in ICU* 0–19 years with cognitive impairment (use revised descriptors)*	0–18 years
Type of pain	Acute pain including postoperative pain, pain in children with cognitive impairment (revised descriptors) and critically ill	Acute pain in critically ill, ventilated children
Variables assessed	Face (0–2) Legs (0–2) Activity (0–2) Cry (0–2) Consolability (0–2)	Alertness Calmness/agitation Respiratory response or crying Physical movement Muscle tone Facial tension
Score range	0–10	6–30 Consider pain > 17

*Crellin et al (2015)
ICU, Intensive care unit; *PACU,* postanaesthesia care unit.

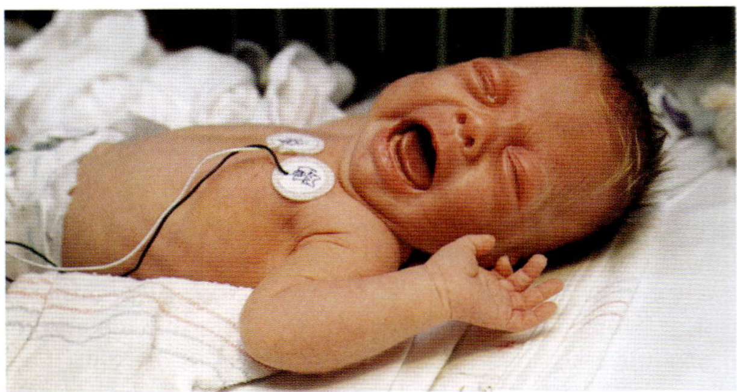

Fig 5.2 Full, robust crying of preterm infant after heel puncture. (Source: Courtesy of Halbouty Premature Nursery, Texas Children's Hospital, Houston, TX; photo by Paul Vincent Kuntz.)

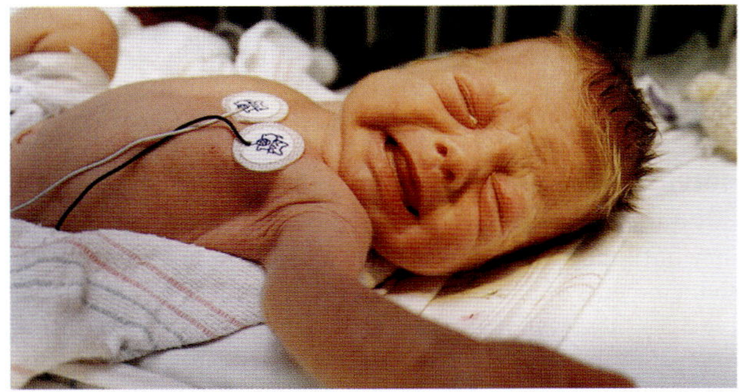

Fig 5.3 The face of pain after heel puncture. Note eye squeeze, brow bulge, nasolabial furrow and wide-spread mouth. (Source: Courtesy of Halbouty Premature Nursery, Texas Children's Hospital, Houston, TX; photo by Paul Vincent Kuntz.)

injections. They are less reliable when measuring acute pain and not reliable or valid for assessing chronic pain or pain in older children. Pain scores on observational measures do not correlate with children's own reports of pain intensity.

One commonly used clinical observational tool is the FLACC Pain Assessment Tool. It is an interval scale that includes the five categories of behaviour: **F**acial expression, **L**eg movement, **A**ctivity, **C**ry and **C**onsolability (Freund & Bolick 2019, Haley 2016, Howard et al 2012, Merkel et al 1997, The Royal Children's Hospital Melbourne 2019). Observers rate each category of behaviour on a 0 to 2 scale, for total scores ranging from 0 (no pain behaviours) to 10. This procedure of rating each category and then summing them for a score is common to the observational pain assessment tools.

Special Populations

Preterm Infants

Early pain experiences greatly influence the developing nervous system with persistent long-term effects. Nurses must consider the infant's maturity, behavioural state, energy resources available to respond to pain and risk factors for pain. Evaluation of pain in preterm infants is complex and based on gestational age, state, condition, previous response to pain, physiological changes and validated observational tools (Hatfield & Ely 2015). Several pain assessment tools for neonates have been validated in preterm infants (Table 5.4).

Preterm infants in awake or alert states demonstrate a more robust reaction to painful stimuli than infants in sleep states. Preterm infants' responses to pain may be behaviourally blunted or absent. Also, an infant receiving a muscle-paralysing agent (vecuronium) is incapable of a behavioural or visible pain response; however, there is ample evidence that such infants are neurologically capable of feeling pain. In preterm infants with diminished ability to respond robustly to pain, it is imperative to presume that pain exists in all situations that are usually considered painful for adults and children, even in the absence of behavioural or physiological signs.

Cognitively Impaired Children

Cognitively impaired children may not be able to express pain through behaviours or self-report methods validated for developmentally similar peers. Children who are cognitively impaired often have their levels of pain underestimated by both health professionals and parents. The most frequent pain behaviours reported by parents of children with cognitive impairment were: crying; being less active; seeking comfort; moaning; not cooperating; being irritable; being stiff, spastic, tense or rigid; sleeping less; being difficult to satisfy or pacify; flinching or moving the body part away; and being agitated or fidgety. Parents also reported that some daily living activities were painful, such as assisted stretching and walking, independent standing, toileting, putting on splints, occupational therapy, range of motion and physical therapy. There are three tools that have been found reliable and valid for this population: Revised Faces Legs Activity Cry Consolability Scale (r-FLACC), Non-communicating Children's Pain Checklist–Revised (NCCPC-r) and Paediatric Pain Profile (PPP) (Chen-Lim et al 2012, Hunt et al 2003, Malviya et al 2006, Quinn et al 2015). When using the r-FLACC, nurses must include parent-reported pain behaviours to customise the tool to use with individual children.

Children Post Anaesthesia

Pain assessment can be challenging in children recovering from anaesthesia. For this reason, nurses often use observational pain assessment tools and then transition to self-report tools when the child is more alert. The only tool found reliable and valid for pain assessment of children 2 months to 7 years of age recovering in the post anaesthesia care unit is the FLACC tool (Merkel et al 1997).

Children in the Paediatric Intensive Care Unit

It is challenging to differentiate a child's pain from distress, anxiety and agitation due to physiological compromise when a child is in the paediatric intensive care unit. Sedating pain medications (opioids) and other sedatives are used to treat these complex patients. One of the most commonly used pain scales to assess critically ill ventilated children who are non-verbal due to sedation or their condition is the COMFORT behaviour scale (COMFORT-B). There are six COMFORT scales: COMFORT, COMFORT plus crying, COMFORT behaviour, COMFORT-modified, COMFORT-adapted and COMFORTneo. Each scale has been developed and studied as measures of several different comfort concepts (pain, stress, distress and sedation) with different patient populations. See Tables 5.3 and 5.4 for examples of COMFORT-B and COMFORTneo compared with other scales. The COMFORT-B scale is able to detect specific changes in pain or distress intensity in critically ill children (Boerlage et al 2015, Freund & Bolick 2019) and is particularly helpful in children who are mechanically ventilated.

Self-report Pain Rating Scales

Self-report is the single most reliable indicator of pain and must be accepted and respected by nurses as the most important pain assessment data available. Self-report measures are most often used for children older than 3 to 4 years, but even 2 year olds can report pain. Several cognitive skills, such as measurement, classification and seriation (the ability to accurately place items in rank order), become apparent between 7 and 10 years of age. Therefore, most school-age

TABLE 5.4 Summary of Pain Assessment Scales for Infants

	PIPP-revised (Stevens et al 2014)	NIPS (Lawrence et al 1993)	N-PASS (Hummel et al 2008)	COMFORTneo (van Dijk et al 2009)	CRIES (Krechel & Bildner 1995)
Age range	25–40 weeks	26–40 weeks	23–40 weeks	24–42 weeks	32–40 weeks
Type of pain	Procedural and postoperative		Procedural and prolonged	Prolonged pain	Postoperative pain
Variables assessed	Scored at (0–3) each Heart rate Oxygen saturation Brow bulge Eye squeeze Nasolabial furrow Behavioural state	Breathing (0–1) Face (0–1) Arms (0–1) Legs (0–1) Cry (0–2) Arousal (0–1)	Scored at (0–2) each Vital signs Crying/irritability Facial expressions Behavioural state Extremities/tone	Scored at (1–5) each Alertness Calmness/agitation Respiratory response or crying Body movement Muscle tone Facial tension	Scored at (0–2) each Crying Oxygen requirement Changes to vital signs Facial expressions Sleeplessness
Score range	0–21	0–7	Pain: 0–10	6–30	0–10
Adjusted for gestational age	Yes Scored at (0–3)	No	Yes	No	No

Source: Adapted from Harris et al (2016). Clinical recommendations for pain, sedation, withdrawal and delirium assessment in critically ill infants and children: An ESPNIC position statement for healthcare professionals. *Intensive Care Medicine, 42*, 972–986.

children have the cognitive ability required to use a numeric rating scale. Many self-report pain rating scales exist, but not all have well-established psychometric properties. It is necessary to have multiple tools available because validity and reliability of each tool varies across age groups and types of pain (Manworren & Stinson 2016).

There are many different 'faces' scales for the measurement of pain intensity. Although children at 3 or 4 years of age are able to self-report pain, they do not have the cognitive ability to understand rank order. Self-report measures with 'faces' provide a pictorial representation of pain intensity. The ability to discriminate degrees of pain in facial expressions appears to be reasonably established by 3 years old. However, cognitive characteristics of the preoperational stage influence their ability to separate feelings of pain and mood. It has been suggested that smiling faces on pain assessment scales may lead younger children to rate the affective domain of pain; or, in other words, rate their feelings about having pain rather than report the intensity of their physical pain (Freund & Bolick 2019, Quinn et al 2014). Simple, concrete anchor words, such as the script originally used to validate the tool, should be used (Table 5.5). The faces are appealing and valid for use with children of all ages (even adults); patients can simply point to the face that represents their pain intensity to report pain.

For children 8 years old and older, there are a number of numeric rating scales. The numeric rating scales (NRSs), such as the 0 to 10 scale, are the most widely used in clinical practice because they are easy to use. The NRS is also called the verbal numeric scale (VNS) (Bailey et al 2010). In contrast, the visual analog scale (VAS) is classically a 10-centimetre line with or without anchors from 0 to 10 or 0 to 100, sometimes anchored with the words *no pain* and *worst pain*. Word-graphic scales use descriptors along a line that provides a highly subjective evaluation of a pain or other symptom. All have established reliability and validity.

Pain assessment in the patient who can provide self-report should not be limited to pain intensity. Other dimensions (such as pain quality, location and spatial distribution) may change without a change in pain intensity. Valid pain charts, diagrams or drawings may be used to help children over 8 years of age describe the location of their pain (Freund & Bolick 2019, von Baeyer et al 2011).

Cultural Considerations

Expression of pain can be greatly affected by communication barriers (Azize et al 2011, Givler & Maani-Fogelman 2019). Culture also exerts a profound influence on pain expression. Some cultures train children to withhold pain expression whereas others encourage pain expression (Bisogni et al 2014). In addition, underlying genetic and biological factors contribute to ethnic and gender differences in pain expression and pain perceptions (Kozlowski et al 2014).

Children with Autism Spectrum Disorder. Children with autism may be unable to engage in the social interactions required to both verbally and non-verbally communicate pain. Because there is a wide range of cognitive abilities among individuals with autism spectrum disorder (ASD), self-report measures should be used whenever possible. Ask the verbal child with ASD where the pain is located and to describe how it feels (Ely et al 2016). Individuals with ASD who are non-verbal may have an escalation of repeated self-stimulating activities (i.e. rocking or hand flapping) when in pain. Consulting with the child's caregiver is essential in providing patient-centred care, assessing pain and providing appropriate pain relief.

CHRONIC AND RECURRENT PAIN ASSESSMENT

Tools that measure acute pain intensity may not be sensitive to the subtle changes and slow resolution characteristic of chronic and recurrent pain because pain expression becomes more complex. Specialised assessment tools are used to assess the domains of pain experienced by children with chronic or recurrent pain and the accompanying functional disability.

Multidimensional Measures

The Pediatric Pain Questionnaire (PPQ) is a multidimensional pain instrument to assess patients' perceptions of their pain experience in a manner appropriate for the cognitive-developmental level of the child (Lootens & Rapoff 2011, Manworren & Stinson 2016). The PPQ consists of eight areas of inquiry: pain history, pain language, the colours the child associates with pain, emotions the child experiences, the worst pain experiences, the way the child copes with pain, the positive aspects of pain and the location of the current pain. The three

TABLE 5.5 Pain Rating Scales for Children

Pain Scale, Description	Instructions	Recommended Age, Comments
	WONG-BAKER FACES PAIN RATING SCALE*	
Consists of six cartoon faces ranging from smiling face for 'no pain' to tearful face for 'worst pain'	*Original instructions:* Explain to child that each face is for a person who feels happy because there is no pain (hurt) or sad because there is some or a lot of pain. FACE 0 is very happy because there is no hurt. FACE 1 hurts just a little bit. FACE 2 hurts a little more. FACE 3 hurts even more. FACE 4 hurts a whole lot, but FACE 5 hurts as much as you can imagine, although you don't have to be crying to feel this bad. Ask child to choose face that best describes own pain. Record number under chosen face on pain assessment record. *Brief word instructions:* Point to each face using the words to describe the pain intensity. Ask child to choose face that best describes own pain, and record appropriate number.	For children as young as 3 years old. Using original instructions without affect words, such as happy or sad, or brief words resulted in same range of pain rating, probably reflecting child's rating of pain intensity. For coding purposes, numbers 0, 2, 4, 6, 8 and 10 can be substituted for 0–5 system to accommodate 0–10 system. The Wong-Baker FACES Pain Rating Scale provides three scales in one: facial expressions, numbers and words. Research supports cultural sensitivity of FACES for Caucasian, African American, Hispanic, Thai, Chinese and Japanese children.
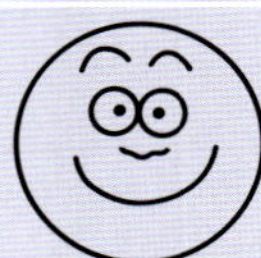 0 No hurt 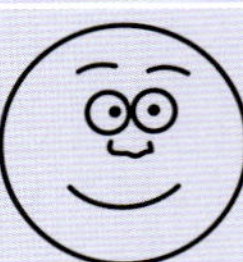 1 or 2 Hurts little bit	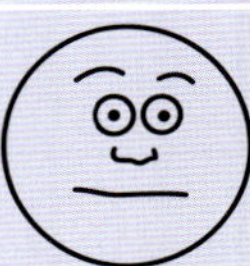 2 or 4 Hurts little more 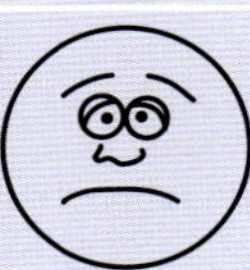 3 or 6 Hurts even more	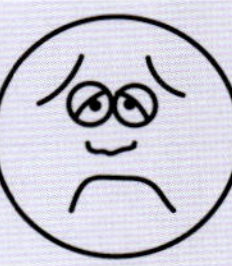 4 or 8 Hurts whole lot 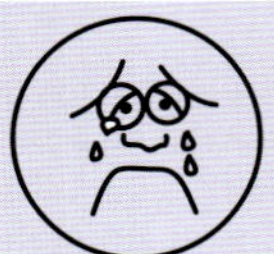 5 or 10 Hurts worst
	FACES PAIN SCALE–REVISED (FPS-R) (HICKS ET AL 2001)	
Consists of six cartoon faces ranging from neutral face for 'no pain' to grimacing face 'worst possible pain' The child is asked to select the picture of a face that best represents their pain intensity For children 5–17		
	WORD-GRAPHIC RATING SCALE[†] (TESLER ET AL 1991)	
Uses descriptive words (may vary in other scales) to denote varying intensities of pain	Explain to child, 'This is a line with words to describe how much pain you may have. This side of the line means no pain, and over here the line means worst possible pain'. (Point with your finger where 'no pain' is, and run your finger along the line to 'worst possible pain', as you say it.) 'If you have no pain, you would mark like this.' (Show example.) 'If you have some pain, you would mark somewhere along the line, depending on how much pain you have.' (Show example.) 'The more pain you have, the closer to worst pain you would mark. The worst pain possible is marked like this.' (Show example.) 'Show me how much pain you have right now by marking with a straight, up-and-down line anywhere along the line to show how much pain you have right now.' With millimetre rule, measure from the 'no pain' end to mark and record this measurement as pain score.	For children 8–17 years old.
No pain	Little pain · Medium pain · Large pain	Worst possible pain
	THE OUCHER PAIN SCALE (BEYER ET AL 1992)	
Consists of six photographs of a white child's face r epresenting 'no hurt' to 'biggest hurt you could ever have'; also includes vertical scale with numbers from 0–100; scales for African American and Hispanic children have been developed	*Numeric scale:* Point to each section of scale to explain variations in pain intensity: '0 means no hurt.' 'This means little hurts' (pointing to lower part of scale, 1–29). 'This means middle hurts' (pointing to middle part of scale, 30–69). 'This means big hurts' (pointing to upper part of scale, 70–99). '100 means the biggest hurt you could ever have.' Score is actual number stated by child.	For children 3–17 years old. Use numeric scale if child can count off any two numbers or by 10s Determine whether child has cognitive ability to use photographic scale; child should be able to rate six geometric shapes from largest to smallest. Determine which ethnic version of Oucher to use; allow child to select version of Oucher or use version that most closely matches physical characteristics of child.

TABLE 5.5 **Pain Rating Scales for Children–cont'd**

Pain Scale, Description	Instructions	Recommended Age, Comments
	Photographic scale: Point to each photograph and explain variations in pain intensity using following language: First picture from the bottom is 'no hurt', second is 'a little hurt', third is 'a little more hurt', fourth is 'even more hurt than that', fifth is 'pretty much or a lot of hurt', and sixth is 'biggest hurt you could ever have'. Score pictures from 0–5, with bottom picture scored as 0. *General:* Practice using Oucher by recalling and rating previous pain experiences (e.g. falling off bike). Child points to number or photograph that describes pain intensity associated with experience. Obtain current pain score from child by asking, 'How much hurt do you have right now?'	*Note:* Ethnically similar scale may not be preferred by child when given choice of ethnically neutral cartoon scale (Luffy & Grove 2003).
NUMERIC RATING SCALE		
Verbal scale or may have a line If a line is used, it may be oriented horizontally or vertically.	Explain to child that is 0 is no pain (hurt), and 5 or 10, is the worst pain. Ask child to choose number that best describes own pain.	For children as young as 8 years old, as long as they can count and have some concept of numbers and their values in relation to other numbers.
No pain 0 1 2 3 4 5 6 7 8 9 10 Worst pain		
VISUAL ANALOG SCALE (VAS) (CLINE ET AL 1992)		
Defined as vertical or horizontal line that is drawn to certain length, such as 10 cm, and anchored by items that represent extremes of the subjective phenomenon being measured, such as pain	Ask child to place mark on line that best describes amount of own pain. With centimetre ruler, measure from 'no pain' end to the mark, and record this measurement as the pain score.	For children as young as 8 years old. Vertical or horizontal scale may be used. Research shows that children ages 3–18 years old least prefer VAS compared with other scales (Luffy & Grove 2003, Wong & Baker 1988).
No pain — Worst pain		

*Copyright 1983, Wong-Baker FACES Foundation, http://www.WongBakerFACES.org. Used with permission. Originally published in *Whaley & Wong's Nursing Care of Infants and Children.* ©Elsevier Inc.

†Word-Graphic Rating Scale is part of the Adolescent Pediatric Pain Tool and is available from Pediatric Pain Study, University of California, School of Nursing, Department of Family Health Care Nursing, San Francisco, CA 94143-0606; 415-476-4040.

components of the PPQ are (1) VASs; (2) colour-coded rating scales; and (3) verbal descriptors to provide information about the sensory, affective and evaluative dimensions of chronic pain. There is also information about the child's and family's pain history, symptoms, pain relief interventions and socioenvironmental situations that may influence pain. The child, parent and medical practitioner each complete the form separately to report their individual perceptions of the child's pain experiences.

For the child with chronic pain, a measure such as the Functional Disability Inventory (FDI) (Walker & Greene 1991) provides a more comprehensive evaluation of the influence of pain on physical functioning. The FDI assesses the child's ability to perform everyday physical activities and has established psychometric properties with different populations (Claar & Walker 2006, Kashikar-Zuck et al 2011). For the child younger than 7 years old, the Pediatric Quality of Life Scale (PedsQL) is a multidimensional scale with both parent and child versions. It is recommended for assessing physical, emotional, social and academic functioning as they relate to the child's pain (Varni et al 1999). The PedsQL and the PedMIDAS (Gold et al 2009, Hershey et al 2001, 2004) have been validated for measurement of role functioning in the child with chronic or recurrent pain. The PedMIDAS is specifically designed to evaluate pain caused by migraines.

Pain diaries are commonly used to assess pain triggers, symptoms, peaks and troughs and response to treatment in children and adolescents with recurrent or chronic pain (Fortier et al 2014, Chisengatambu & McDonald 2018, Stinson et al 2008). Diary studies have included children as young as 6 years old. Conventional paper-and-pencil measures have been associated with several limitations, such as poor compliance, missing data, hoarding of responses and back-and-forward filling. Electronic diaries to assess paediatric chronic pain have been developed to address these limitations. Refinement continues and holds promise for efficient clinical translation.

Chronic and recurrent types of pain often occur with some level of depression and anxiety in children (Fisher et al 2015). Among the many validated tools to measure anxiety and depression in children are the Children's Depression Inventory (CDI) (Kovacs 1981) and the Revised Child Anxiety and Depression Scale (Chorpita et al 2000, Kösters et al 2015). These two validated scales may be used together to better measure negative affect (Manworren & Stinson 2016).

Sleep disruption is also common in children with chronic or recurrent pain (Valrie et al 2013, Allen et al 2016). A sleep diary can be useful in keeping a record of activities surrounding sleep, including bedtime, time to fall asleep, number of night awakenings, waking in the morning and especially any pain or other circumstance that interfered with sleeping. Sleep diaries have been validated using actigraphy in healthy adolescents (Gaina et al 2004, Allen et al 2016). The Sleep Habits Questionnaire, which is useful for assessing sleep behaviours in school-age children with chronic or recurrent pain, has also been evaluated for use in preschool and toddlers using parent proxy (Sneddon et al 2013).

PREVENTION AND TREATMENT OF PAIN IN CHILDREN

Nurses' knowledge, unfortunately, does not always translate into improved pain outcomes for children. Nurses and other clinicians may hold onto outdated or incorrect beliefs and attitudes about pain or may work in a culture that does not support good pain management practices. Improving pain prevention and management requires a multifaceted approach of education, institutional support, attitude shifts and change leadership. (See Nursing Care Guidelines box.)

NURSING CARE GUIDELINES

Goals of a Pain Treatment Program

A multidisciplinary approach helps provide the most comprehensive treatment of acute, chronic and mixed types of pain. The primary care provider must first rule out and/or treat any systemic disease. When children experience chronic pain, intensive physical therapy, occupational therapy and psychological support for parents and children can be especially helpful. The ultimate goal in the experience of any pain is to improve function, improve quality of life and facilitate a return to daily activities. Clinicians may emphasise the importance of participation in normal activities, including daily school attendance, sports or physical activities, social life and adequate sleep (see Community Focus: Chronic Pain and School Absenteeism in Children).

Biobehavioural interventions and adequate analgesics are essential for effective pain prevention and treatment. Biobehavioural interventions are also known as non-pharmacological interventions. The term *biobehavioural intervention* is preferred over *non-pharmacological* because it is a term that reflects the mechanism of action. The term *non-pharmacological* reflects the lack of pharmaceutical treatment as though medications are the gold standard of treatment. Sometimes biobehavioural interventions are as effective as, or even more effective than, pharmacological interventions. The type of intervention(s) needed to prevent and treat a child's pain depends on the situation and specific needs of the child. Multimodal, also known as combinations of analgesic and biobehavioural therapies, is the preferred pain treatment plan. By targeting different mechanisms of pain, medications combined with biobehavioural interventions are more effective at relieving pain.

Biobehavioural Interventions

Pain is often associated with fear, anxiety and stress. Most **biobehavioural interventions** prevent and treat pain by interrupting the pain, fear, anxiety and stress cycle. A number of biobehavioural techniques such as distraction, relaxation, guided imagery, hypnosis, cognitive behaviour therapy, massage, heat, cold and transcutaneous electrical nerve stimulation (TENS) can help with pain control. Some techniques have combined targets of action. For example, music therapy is used for both distraction and relaxation. Coping strategies can help reduce pain perception, make pain more tolerable, decrease anxiety and enhance the effectiveness of analgesics or reduce the dosage required. Biobehavioural interventions are accompanied by few if any side effects and at the same time may have crossover benefits in unintended areas. For example, use of regular relaxation and deep breathing practice to reduce chronic headaches could also improve a child's sleep.

It is helpful to think of biobehavioural pain prevention and treatment strategies as a box of available tools for acute, chronic or recurrent pain. Nurses may consider the individual child's needs when deciding on a strategy or series of strategies to use in prevention and treatment of pain. What helps one child may not be as effective for another. The child's developmental age and cognitive abilities are important considerations when choosing biobehavioural strategies.

If the child cannot identify a familiar coping technique, the nurse can describe several strategies (e.g. distraction, breathing, guided imagery) and let the child select the most appealing one (see Research Focus box). Experimentation with several strategies that are suitable to the child's developmental abilities is often necessary to determine the most effective approach. Parents should be involved in the selection process; they may be familiar with the child's usual coping style and can help identify potentially successful strategies. Involving parents also encourages their participation in learning the skill with the child and acting as coach. If the parent cannot assist the child, other appropriate persons may include a grandparent, older sibling, nurse or play specialist.

RESEARCH FOCUS

Biobehavioural Methods of Pain Management—Preterm and Newborn Infants

Sucrose is safe and effective in reducing pain during needlesticks in neonates (Gray et al 2015, Pillai et al 2015). In a randomised controlled trial of 71 infants comparing oral sucrose, facilitated tucking and a combination of both interventions, sucrose with and without facilitated tucking had pain-relieving effects (Cignacco et al 2012) (see Fig 5.4). Significant differences were found in pain responses during heel puncture between infants who were held skin-to-skin and those who were not. Infant responses to pain during heel-puncture procedures were studied using skin-to-skin care, with the neonate held upright at a 60-degree angle between the mother's breasts for maximal skin-to-skin contact (Wilson-Smith 2011). A blanket was placed over the neonate's back and the mother's clothes were wrapped around the neonate for 30 minutes before the lancing procedure, during and at least 30 minutes after the heel puncture. Another group remained in the isolette in a prone position, swaddled with a blanket and the heel accessible, for 30 minutes before the heel-puncture procedure. Pain scores were significantly lower in skin-to-skin–held infants.

Although there is lack of evidence on the effectiveness of sweet-tasting solutions in reducing injection pain in infants and children 1 to 12 months old, the data are promising (Kassab et al 2012). One randomised controlled trial found that sucrose reduced 16- to 19-month-old infant distress during immunisations (Yilmaz et al 2014), while another found that sucrose and warmth are more effective in reducing pain in healthy newborns than sucrose alone (Gray et al 2015). Breastfeeding, but not breast milk, is as effective as sucrose and skin-to-skin care (Johnston et al 2017).

Children should learn to use a specific strategy before pain occurs or before it becomes severe. Instructions for a strategy, such as distraction or relaxation, can be recorded and played during a period of comfort. However, even after they have learned an intervention, children often need help using it during a painful procedure. The intervention can also be used after the procedure. This gives the child a chance to recover, feel mastery and cope more effectively.

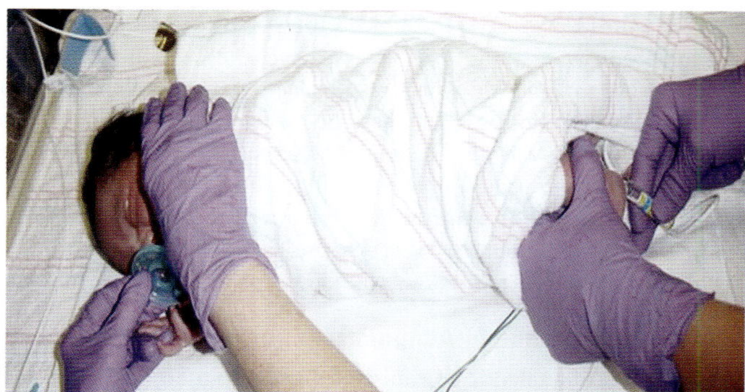

Fig 5.4 Sucking following oral sucrose can enhance analgesia before a heel puncture in a preterm infant.

Biobehavioural interventions used to treat certain disease-specific pain syndromes may be helpful in prevention and treatment of other types of pain. Researchers have found good effect sizes and significant results using virtual reality, various mind-body techniques, creative arts therapy, listening to music, massage and hypnosis in treatment of pain and anxiety in children with cancer (Thrane 2013). Creative arts therapy incorporates any of the following into a program to reduce pain and anxiety: dance, movement, music, art, theatre, yoga and/or poetry (Poder & Lemieux 2014).

Pharmacological Management of Pain

The World Health Organization (WHO) (2012) states that the principles for pharmacological pain management should include the following:

- using a two-step strategy
- dosing at regular intervals
- using the appropriate route of administration
- adapting treatment to the individual child.

The traditional WHO stepladder has been replaced with a two-step approach for use with children. For children older than 3 months of age the first step is to administer a non-opioid analgesic. Opioids are started when pain is severe or unrelieved by non-opioids. Morphine is the medicine of choice for the second step, although other opioids may be considered (WHO 2012). The following sections discuss the most common pain medications used in children in the non-opioid and opioid categories.

Non-opioids

Non-opioids include medications such as paracetamol and non-steroidal anti-inflammatory drugs (NSAIDs). NSAIDs are known for their antipyretic, anti-inflammatory and analgesic actions. Paracetamol has antipyretic and analgesic actions, but no anti-inflammatory action. Non-opioids are usually the first analgesics for pain related to tissue injury, also known as *nociceptive pain*. Non-opioid analgesics can provide safe and effective pain relief when dosed at appropriate levels with adequate frequency.

Opioids

Opioids are indicated for nociceptive pain that is severe or unrelieved by non-opioids. Morphine remains the standard agent used for comparison to other opioids. Opioids are titrated to safely achieve optimal analgesia.

Genetic Variants of Drug Metabolism. Genetic background influences how children and adults metabolise medications, placing certain children at particular risk. Codeine was once a commonly used opioid in children. Children with *CYP2D6* allele combinations associated with poor metabolism of codeine may get no analgesia, whereas children with combinations associated with ultrarapid metabolism are at risk of morphine toxicity and death (Isaacson 2014, Manworren et al 2016). Over 400 variations of the *CYP2D6* gene are known (Baugh et al 2011, Isaacson 2013, Khetani et al 2012, Lauder & Emmott 2014). For this reason, in 2018 the new Therapeutic Goods Administration (TGA) guideline stipulated that all codeine-containing products need to be prescription only so as to minimise harm from codeine (TGA 2018). Genetic differences in metabolism, however, may explain differences in opioid analgesic effectiveness and adverse reactions to an estimated 50% of currently available medications, including opioids, NSAIDs and co-analgesics (Trescot 2014).

Co-analgesic Drugs

Several drugs, known as co-analgesics or adjuvants, may be used alone or with non-opioids and opioids to control pain and associated symptoms, including opioid side effects. Benzodiazepines are frequently used to treat anxiety; however, these drugs do not provide analgesia and should not be used as a substitute for analgesics. The concomitant use of opioids and sedatives, such as diazepam, is associated with increased risk of death. Tricyclic antidepressants (e.g. amitriptyline, imipramine), antiepileptics (e.g. gabapentin, pregabalin), steroids, α_2-agonists, ketamine and intravenous (IV) lidocaine (lignocaine) are being used to treat chronic pain; these co-analgesics are also being used with increased frequency to treat acute pain (American Pain Society 2016). Other medications commonly prescribed to address opioid-related side effects include peristaltics for constipation, antiemetics for nausea and vomiting, opioid antagonists for itching and stimulants for sedation.

Choosing the Pain Medication Dose

Children's dosages are usually calculated according to body weight, with two exceptions. First, children achieve adult capabilities of cytochrome P450 metabolism (CYP2D6) by 1 year of age and over 50% by 6 months of age. Therefore, doses of opioids for infants less than 6 months of age should be a quarter to a third of the starting dose recommended for children over 6 months of age. The infant receiving opioid analgesics should be monitored closely for signs of pain relief and respiratory depression (see Nursing Care Guidelines). Doses of other analgesics are also adjusted to account for this age difference in drug metabolism. Second, most adult analgesic doses are based on a weight of 50 to 60 kg. Children with a weight greater than 50 kg should be prescribed the average adult dose (see Pain Management in Obese and Overweight Children later in this chapter). The child's comorbidities should also be considered for safe opioid dosing (Schug et al 2015).

NURSING CARE GUIDELINES

Managing Opioid-induced Respiratory Depression

- Assess sedation level.
- If sedated, stimulate patient (squeeze the shoulder gently, call by name, ask to breathe).
- Stop or reduce opioid.
- Monitor closely for pain and progressive sedation and respiratory depression.
- If patient cannot be aroused and respirations are depressed or patient is apnoeic:
  - Activate the Clinical Emergency Response System (Medical Emergency Team/Rapid Response System).
  - Stop or reduce opioid.

NURSING CARE GUIDELINES

Managing Opioid-induced Respiratory Depression—cont'd

- Initiate resuscitation efforts as appropriate.
- Administer oxygen.
- Support respirations.
- Administer naloxone (Narcan).
  - IM and IV 0.1 mg/kg/dose – given stat. Withdraw ordered dose. No dilution required.
  - IV infusion 0.01 mg/kg/hr – titrated to response since its action is shorter than most opioids. Withdraw ordered dose and make up to ordered volume of infusion fluid. Either Sodium Chloride 0.9% or Glucose 5%
- Closely monitor patient. Naloxone's duration of antagonist action may be shorter than that of the opioid, requiring repeated doses of naloxone after 2 to 3 minutes.

Note: Respiratory depression caused by benzodiazepines (e.g. diazepam or midazolam) can be reversed with flumazenil. Paediatric dosing experience suggests 0.01 mg/kg given IV over 15 seconds (maximum dose 0.2mg); if no (or inadequate) response after 1 to 2 minutes, administer same dose and repeat as needed at 60-second intervals for maximum dose of 1 mg. Flumazenil is contraindicated in intentional overdose (it can precipitate seizures in withdrawal or mixed overdoses).

A major difference between opioids and non-opioids is that non-opioids have a ceiling effect. This means that doses higher than the recommended dose will not produce greater pain relief. Opioids do not have a ceiling effect other than that imposed by side effects. Therefore, recommended initial opioid dosages are titrated to effect. If the patient experiences pain relief and opioid side effects, the dosage should be titrated downwards. However, if pain relief is inadequate, the dosage is increased to provide greater analgesic effect. Decreasing the interval between doses may also provide more continuous pain relief. Because tolerance to opioids can develop, large doses may be needed for continued or increasing pain.

Parenteral and oral dosages of opioids are not the same. Because of the first-pass effect, an oral opioid is absorbed from the gastrointestinal tract and is partially metabolised in the liver before reaching the central circulation. Therefore, oral dosages must be larger to compensate for the partial loss of analgesic potency to achieve an equal analgesic effect. Conversion factors for selected opioids should be used when a change is made from the IV to the oral route.

NURSING CARE CONSIDERATIONS

The optimum dosage of an opioid analgesic is one that controls pain without causing undesirable side effects. This usually requires titration, the gradual adjustment of drug dosage (usually by increasing the dose) until optimum pain relief without excessive sedation is achieved. Dosages must be checked in an appropriate dosing guide such as the *Australian Medication Handboook (AMH) Children's Dosing Companion*. Monitoring is required to determine safe and optimal dose for each patient.

Choosing the Timing of Analgesia

The right timing for administering analgesics depends on the type of pain and the drug-specific duration of analgesia. For continuous pain control, such as for postoperative or VOC pain, medications should be administered around the clock (ATC). The ATC schedule achieves steady-state analgesia. If analgesics are administered only when the patient has pain or requests pain medications (a typical use of the PRN, or 'as needed', order), the child is then being required to endure pain to demonstrate a need for pain treatment. Pain is then not controlled. Uncontrolled pain is less responsive to pain medications and thus requires more and higher doses of medications. This places the child at greater risk for adverse analgesic effects. This cycle of erratic pain control also promotes 'clock watching', which may be erroneously equated with addiction. Nurses can effectively use PRN orders by giving the drug at regular intervals because 'as needed' should be interpreted 'as needed to prevent and treat pain', not 'as little as possible'.

Choosing the Method of Administration

Several routes of analgesic administration can be used (Box 5.2), and the most effective and least traumatic route of administration should be selected. The intramuscular route is never appropriate. Continuous analgesia is not always appropriate because not all pain is continuous. Frequently, temporary pain control or sedation is needed to provide analgesia for medical procedures. When pain can be predicted, the drug's peak effect should be timed to coincide with the painful event. For example, with opioids the onset of effect is usually 5 to 10 minutes after administration and peak effect is approximately 30 minutes for the IV route. Analgesics given by the oral route typically have onset of action by 30 minutes and the peak effect occurs about 60 minutes after administration. Time of onset and peak effect is dependent on drug metabolism and therefore varies by drug, route and patient. For extended pain control with fewer administration times, drugs that provide longer duration of action (e.g. some NSAIDs, time-released morphine or oxycodone, methadone) can be used.

Patient-controlled Analgesia

A significant advance in the administration of IV or epidural analgesics is the use of **patient-controlled analgesia** (PCA). As the name implies, the patient controls the frequency of analgesic administration, which is typically delivered through a special infusion device. Children who are physically able to activate the device and who can understand the concept of cause and effect (usually by 7 to 8 years of age) can use PCA. Nurses can also efficiently use the infusion device to administer analgesics and this is known as nurse-controlled analgesia (NSW Health Agency for Clinical Innovation 2016). The pump is typically locked, programmed and verified to deliver a specific dose, making the infusion device an efficient alternative to witnessing and preparing each dose every time it is needed.

PCA infusion devices typically allow for three modes of drug administration.

- Patient-administered boluses that can be infused at a preset dose and lockout interval (time between doses). More frequent attempts at self-administration may mean the patient needs the dose and time adjusted for better pain control.
- Nurse-administered boluses are typically used to give an initial loading dose to increase analgesia rapidly and to relieve breakthrough pain (pain not relieved with the usual programmed dose).
- Continuous infusion that delivers a constant analgesic amount. This mode has been shown to increase sedation from opioids without providing improved analgesia, but may be appropriate in critical care settings.

PCA is typically used for controlling pain from surgery, sickle cell crisis, trauma and cancer. If more than one dose of an IV opioid is needed, it is more cost-effective to administer intermittent doses by infusion pump or PCA. With any type of analgesic management plan, continued assessment of the child is essential for the greatest benefit from PCA. Pain and sedation observations must be recorded hourly on the PCA chart and all other vital observations recorded on the appropriate paediatric chart every hour (NSW Health Agency

BOX 5.2 Routes and Methods of Analgesic Drug Administration

Oral

- Oral route preferred because of convenience, cost and relatively steady blood levels
- Higher dosages of oral form of opioids required for equivalent parenteral analgesia
- Peak drug effect occurring after 1 hour for most analgesics
- Delay in onset a disadvantage when rapid control of severe or fluctuating pain is desired

Sublingual, Buccal or Transmucosal

- Tablet or liquid placed between cheek and gum (buccal) or under tongue (sublingual)
- Highly desirable because more rapid onset than oral route
- Produces less first-pass effect through liver than oral route, which normally reduces analgesia from oral opioids (unless sublingual or buccal form is swallowed, which occurs often in children)
- Few drugs commercially available in this form
- Many drugs can be compounded into sublingual troche or lozenge
- Actiq: Oral **transmucosal** fentanyl citrate in hard confection base on a plastic holder; indicated only for management of breakthrough cancer pain in patients with malignancies who are already receiving and are tolerant to opioid therapy

Intravenous (Bolus)

- Preferred for rapid control of severe pain
- First-choice alternative when oral route not available
- Provides most rapid onset of effect, usually in about 5 minutes
- Advantage for acute pain, procedural pain and breakthrough pain
- Needs to be repeated for continuous pain control

Intravenous (Continuous)

- Preferred for sedation
- Easy to titrate dosage
- Need to provide boluses for analgesia

Subcutaneous (Continuous)

- Used when oral and intravenous (IV) routes not available
- Provides equivalent blood levels to continuous IV infusion
- Total 24-hour dose usually requires concentrated opioid solution to minimise infused volume; use smallest gauge needle that accommodates infusion rate

Patient-controlled Analgesia

- Generally refers to self-administration of drugs, regardless of route
- Typically uses programmable infusion pump (IV, epidural, subcutaneous [SC]) that permits self-administration of boluses of medication at preset dose and time interval (lockout interval is time between doses)
- Patient-controlled analgesia (PCA) bolus administration often combined with initial bolus may be combined with continuous (basal or background) infusion of opioid, but not recommended in opioid-naïve patients or unless sedation is desired
- Optimum lockout interval not known but must be at least as long as time needed for onset of drug
- Should effectively control pain during movement or procedures

Nurse-activated Analgesia

- Child's primary nurse designated as primary pain manager and is only person who presses PCA button during that nurse's shift
- Guidelines for selecting primary pain manager for family-controlled analgesia also applicable to nurse-activated analgesia
- Because nurse is not with patient at all times, dose is typically higher than PCA but lower than traditional boluses and lockout is longer
- May be used in addition to basal rate to treat breakthrough pain with bolus doses; patient assessed every 30 minutes for need for bolus dose
- May be used without a basal rate as a means of maintaining analgesia with around-the-clock bolus doses

Intramuscular

Note: Not recommended for pain control; not current standard of care

- Painful administration (hated by children)
- Tissue and nerve damage caused by some drugs
- Wide fluctuation in absorption of drug from muscle
- Time consuming for staff and unnecessary delay for child

Intranasal

- Short acting
- Beneficial for procedural sedation/analgesia
- Should not be used in patients receiving morphine-like drugs

Intradermal

- Used primarily for skin anaesthesia (e.g. before lumbar puncture, bone marrow aspiration, arterial puncture, skin biopsy)
- Local anaesthetics (e.g. lidocaine [lignocaine]) cause stinging, burning sensation:

Topical or Transdermal (Zempsky 2014)

- EMLA (eutectic mixture of local anaesthetics [lidocaine (lignocaine) and prilocaine]) cream:
  - eliminates or reduces pain from most procedures involving skin puncture
  - must be placed on intact skin over puncture site and covered by occlusive dressing for 30 minutes or more before procedure
- Local AnGel (tetracaine [amethocaine] gel 4%):
  - apply for 20 to 30 minutes
  - do not apply to broken skin
- Transdermal fentanyl (Duragesic):
  - available as patch for continuous pain control
  - safety and efficacy not established in children younger than 12 years old
  - not appropriate for initial relief of acute pain because of long interval to peak effect (24–72 hours); for rapid onset of pain relief, give an immediate-release opioid
  - orders for 'rescue doses' of an immediate-release opioid recommended for breakthrough pain, a flare of severe pain that breaks through the medication being administered at regular intervals for persistent pain
  - has duration of up to 72 hours for prolonged pain relief
  - if respiratory depression occurs, possible need for several doses of naloxone

Regional Nerve Block

- Use of long-acting local anaesthetic (bupivacaine or ropivacaine) injected to block nerve transmission of pain
- Provides up to 8 hours of analgesia postoperatively, such as after inguinal herniorrhaphy
- May be used to provide local anaesthesia for surgery, such as dorsal penile nerve block for circumcision, or for reduction of fractures

Inhalation

- Use of anaesthetics, such as nitrous oxide, to produce partial or complete analgesia for painful procedures
- Side effects (e.g. headache) possible from occupational exposure to high levels of nitrous oxide

Continued

BOX 5.2 Routes and Methods of Analgesic Drug Administration–cont'd

Epidural or Intrathecal

- Involves catheter placed into epidural, caudal or intrathecal space for continuous infusion or single or intermittent administration of opioid with or without a long-acting local anaesthetic (e.g. bupivacaine, ropivacaine)
- Analgesia primarily from drug's direct effect on opioid receptors in spinal cord
- Respiratory depression rare but may have slow and delayed onset; can be prevented by checking level of sedation and respiratory rate and depth hourly for initial 24 hours and decreasing dose when excessive sedation is detected
- Nausea, pruritus and urinary retention are common dose-related side effects from the epidural opioid
- Hypotension, urinary retention, pruritus and temporary motor or sensory deficits common unwanted effects of epidural local anaesthetic
- Catheter for urinary retention inserted during surgery to decrease trauma to child; if inserted when child is awake, anaesthetise urethra with lidocaine (lignocaine)

American Pain Society. (2016). *Principles of analgesic use* (7th ed.). Chicago, IL.
Data from Pasero, C., & McCaffrey, M. (2011). *Pain assessment and pharmacologic management*. St Louis, MO: Elsevier.

for Clinical Innovation 2016). The child is to be maintained on oxygen therapy to maintain oxygen saturation above 95% and continuous pulse oximetry should be used (NSW Health Agency for Clinical Innovation 2016). Unless specifically ordered by the acute pain service or paediatric medical officer, no other opioids or sedatives must be administered (NSW Health Agency for Clinical Innovation 2016).

Epidural Analgesia

Epidural analgesia is recommended to manage postoperative pain in children hospitalised for pain control from surgeries below the neck (Chou et al 2016). Although an epidural catheter can be inserted at any vertebral level, it is usually placed into the epidural space at the lumbar or caudal level (Suresh et al 2012). The thoracic level is usually reserved for older children or adolescents who have had an upper abdominal or thoracic procedure, such as a cardiac or chest surgery. A local anaesthetic (which is often combined with a preservative-free opioid such as fentanyl, hydromorphone or morphine) is instilled by continuous infusion, with or without patient-controlled epidural analgesia. Careful monitoring of sedation level and respiratory status is critical to prevent opioid-induced respiratory depression. Assessments of pain and motor function are also critical to promptly identify epidural haematoma and avoid paralysis.

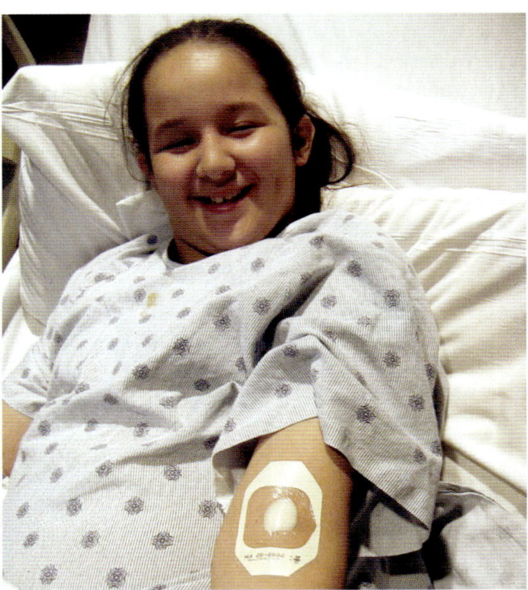

Fig 5.5 Topical anaesthetics are effective before intravenous (IV) insertion or blood draw.

Transmucosal and Transdermal Analgesia

One of the most significant improvements in the ability to provide atraumatic care to children undergoing procedures is the development of anaesthetic creams. EMLA (eutectic mixture of local anaesthetics: lidocaine [lignocaine] 2.5% and prilocaine 2.5%) is one well-studied topical anaesthetic found to be effective in children when applied to intact skin, but must be administered at least an hour before the painful intervention (Olsen & Weinberg 2017). EMLA and other topical anaesthetic creams should be used with caution in neonates (Watterberg et al 2016) (Fig 5.5). Topical anaesthetics can reduce pain of immunisation when allowed sufficient time for action (Shah 2015).

The intradermal route is sometimes used to inject a local anaesthetic, typically lidocaine (lignocaine), into the skin to reduce the pain from a lumbar puncture, bone marrow aspiration or venous or arterial access. One problem with the use of lidocaine (lignocaine) is the stinging and burning that initially occurs. Needleless injection systems (i.e. J-tip) can be used to numb the skin for needle procedures.

Local anaesthetics are lipophilic and have been successfully manipulated to penetrate intact skin. Fentanyl is also lipophilic. Fentanyl is available as a **transdermal** patch for continuous administration through intact skin for 72 hours per patch.

Monitoring Side Effects

All analgesics have side effects and risk of adverse effects. Respiratory depression is rare, but is the most serious adverse effect from analgesics. Respiratory depression from opioids progresses in a predictable pattern. The patient first becomes sedated and unarousable. Then depth of respirations decreases and rate of respirations increases. End-tidal CO_2 increases, oxygen saturation decreases and respiratory rate decreases and then ceases. Sedation from opioids is to be avoided and nurses must increase their monitoring vigilance while patients sleep. Early recognition of respiratory compromise and prompt intervention is critical. (See Nursing Care Guidelines box and Box 5.3 for further discussion of opioid side effects.)

BOX 5.3 Side Effects of Opioids

General
- Nausea and vomiting
- Miosis (may be sign of toxicity)
- Constipation (possibly severe)
- Sedation
- Euphoria
- Agitation
- Mental clouding
- Hallucinations
- Pruritus
- Orthostatic hypotension
- Respiratory depression
- Anaphylaxis (rare)

Signs of Tolerance
- Decreasing pain relief
- Decreasing duration of pain relief

Signs of Withdrawal Syndrome in Patients with Physical Dependence

Initial Signs of Withdrawal
- Rhinorrhoea
- Yawning
- Sweating
- Restlessness

Later Signs of Withdrawal
- Irritability
- Tremors
- Anorexia
- Dilated pupils
- Piloerection
- Nausea, vomiting
- Abdominal cramping, diarrhoea
- Seizure

NURSING CARE GUIDELINES

Biobehavioural Strategies for Pain Management

General Strategies
- Form a trusting relationship with child and family.
- Express concern regarding their reports of pain and intervene appropriately.
- Take an active role in seeking effective pain management strategies.
- If available, consult a child-life or play specialist.
- Use biobehavioural interventions to supplement, not replace, pharmacological interventions.
- Use general guidelines to prepare child for procedure.
- Prepare child before potentially painful procedures. Honestly describe procedure.
  - For example, instead of saying, 'This doesn't hurt', say, 'Sometimes this feels like pushing, sticking or pinching, and sometimes it hurts and sometimes it doesn't bother people. Tell me what it feels like to you'.
  - Use descriptors when possible (e.g. 'It feels like heat' rather than 'It's a burning pain'). This allows for variation in sensory perception and gives the child control in describing reactions.
  - Avoid evaluative statements or descriptions (e.g. 'This is a terrible procedure' or 'It really will hurt a lot').
- Ensure one person takes the lead in biobehavioural strategies for the child.
- Stay with the child during a painful procedure.
- Allow parents to stay with the child if the child and parent desire; encourage parent to talk softly to child and to remain near child's head.
- Involve parents in learning specific biobehavioural strategies and in coaching child in their use.
- Educate child about the pain, especially when explanation may lessen anxiety (e.g. that pain may occur after surgery and does not indicate something is wrong); reassure the child that he or she is not responsible for the pain.
- Educate the child in a developmentally appropriate manner, for example, offer the child a doll, which represents 'the patient', and allow child to do everything to the doll that is done to the child; emphasise pain control through the doll by stating, 'Dolly feels better after the medicine'.
- Allow the child to de-brief after the procedure.
- Teach procedures to child and family for later use.

Specific Strategies

Distraction
- Involve parent and child in identifying strong distractors.
- Involve child in play; use radio, CD player, computer game or smart phone; have child sing or use rhythmic breathing.
- Have child take a deep breath and blow it out until told to stop.
- Have child blow bubbles to 'blow the hurt away'.
- Have child concentrate on yelling or saying 'ouch', with instructions to 'yell as loud or soft as you feel it hurt; that way I know what's happening'.
- Have child look through kaleidoscope (type with glitter suspended in fluid-filled tube) and encourage him or her to concentrate by asking, 'Do you see the different designs?'
- Use humour, such as watching cartoons, telling jokes or funny stories or acting sillily with child.
- Have child read, play games or visit with friends.

Relaxation
- With an infant or young child:
  - Hold in a comfortable, well-supported position, such as vertically against the chest and shoulder.
  - Rock in a wide, rhythmic arc in a rocking chair or sway back and forth, rather than bouncing child.
  - Repeat one or two words softly, such as 'Mummy's here'.
- With a slightly older child:
  - Ask child to take a deep breath and 'go limp as a rag doll' while exhaling slowly; then ask child to yawn (demonstrate if needed).
  - Help child assume a comfortable position (e.g. pillow under neck and knees).
  - Begin progressive relaxation: starting with the toes, systematically instruct child to let each body part 'go limp' or 'feel heavy'. If child has difficulty relaxing, instruct child to tense or tighten each body part and then relax it.
  - Allow child to keep eyes open because children may respond better if eyes are open rather than closed during relaxation.

Guided Imagery
- Have child identify some highly pleasurable real or imaginary experience.
- Have child describe details of the event, including as many senses as possible (e.g. 'feel the cool breezes', 'see the beautiful colours', 'hear the pleasant music').
- Have child write down or record script.

Continued

NURSING CARE GUIDELINES

Biobehavioural Strategies for Pain Management—cont'd

- Encourage child to concentrate only on the pleasurable event during the painful time; enhance the image by recalling specific details by reading the script or playing the recording.
- Combine with relaxation and rhythmic breathing.

Positive Self-talk

- Teach child positive statements to say when in pain (e.g. 'I will be feeling better soon', or 'When I go home, I will feel better, and we will eat ice cream').

Thought Stopping

- Identify positive facts about the painful event (e.g. 'It does not last long').
- Identify reassuring information (e.g. 'If I think about something else, it does not hurt as much').
- Condense positive and reassuring facts into a set of brief statements and have child memorise them (e.g. 'Short procedure, good veins, little hurt, nice nurse, go home').
- Have child repeat the memorised statements whenever thinking about or experiencing the painful event.

Behavioural Contracting

- Informal: May be used with children as young as 4 or 5 years old:
  - Use stars, tokens or cartoon character stickers as rewards.
  - Give a child who is uncooperative or procrastinating during a procedure a limited time (measured by a visible timer) to complete the procedure.
  - Proceed as needed if child is unable to comply.
  - Reinforce cooperation with a reward if the procedure is accomplished within specified time.
- Formal: Use written contract, which includes the following:
  - Realistic (seems possible) goal or desired behaviour
  - Measurable behaviour (e.g. agrees not to hit anyone during procedures)
  - Contract written, dated and signed by all persons involved in any of the agreements
  - Identified rewards or consequences that are reinforcing
  - Goals that can be evaluated
  - Commitment and compromise requirements for both parties (e.g. while timer is used, nurse will not nag or prod child to complete procedure)

Although respiratory depression is the most dangerous side effect, nausea is the most common side effect of analgesics. Non-sedating antiemetics should be given to prevent nausea, such as ondansetron. Sedating antiemetics such as lorazepam may be tried in the vomiting child, but the patient must be monitored for sedation. Constipation is also a common side effect of opioids due to a decrease in gastric peristalsis. Prevention of constipation with peristaltic agents and laxatives is more effective than treatment once constipation occurs. Dietary treatment, such as increased fibre and the use of stool softeners, is usually not sufficient to promote regular bowel evacuation. However, increased fluid intake and physical activity, such as rocking and walking, should be encouraged. Gum chewing has also been used to effectively increase peristalsis. Pruritus from epidural or IV opioid infusions is treated with low-dose opioid agonists such as naloxone. Diphenhydramine is often erroneously used to treat opioid-related pruritus; however, appreciable relief is the result of sedation rather than the antihistamine effect. Nausea, vomiting, pruritus and sedation usually subside after 2 days of regular opioid administration.

Both tolerance and physical dependence can occur with prolonged use of opioids. Tolerance occurs when the dose of an opioid needs to be increased to achieve the same analgesic effects to that which was previously achieved at a lower dose. Treatment of tolerance involves increasing the dose or decreasing the duration between doses.

Physical dependence to opioids is a normal, natural, physiological state of 'neuroadaptation'. When opioids are abruptly discontinued in physically dependent patients without weaning, withdrawal symptoms occur. Symptoms of withdrawal include signs of neurological excitability (irritability, tremors, increased motor tone, insomnia, seizures), gastrointestinal dysfunction (nausea, vomiting, diarrhoea, abdominal cramps) and autonomic dysfunction (sweating, fever, chills, tachypnoea, nasal congestion, rhinitis). Withdrawal symptoms can be anticipated and prevented by weaning patients from opioids that were administered for more than 5 days. In children (7 months to 10 years old) the Withdrawal Assessment Tool–1 may be used to assess and monitor withdrawal symptoms in paediatric critically ill children who are exposed to opioids and benzodiazepines for prolonged periods (Franck et al 2008).

Opioids are rarely indicated for long-term management of chronic pain in children due to the risk of efficacy and safety compromise associated with long-term use (IASP 2018, Palermo et al 2013) but may be indicated for short-term treatment. Parents and older children may fear addiction when opioids are prescribed. The nurse should address these concerns (see Community Focus box). Infants may be at risk for physical tolerance and physical dependence but not psychological dependence or addiction when using opioids for short-term pain management. The use of opioid analgesics early in life has not been demonstrated to increase the risk for addiction later in life. However, there is new evidence of increased risk of prescription opioid misuse in young adults who were treated with opioids as adolescents (Miech et al 2015). Nurses need to explain to parents the differences between tolerance, physical dependence and addiction and allow patients and parents to express concerns about the use and duration of opioid use. Nurses must counsel parents to secure opioids used to treat pain and promptly dispose of opioids that are no longer needed for pain treatment (Manworren & Gilson 2015).

COMMUNITY FOCUS

*Prescription Drug Abuse**

Prescription opioid diversion, misuse and addiction are at epidemic levels. In 2018, deaths from opioid misuse were estimated to be slightly over 3 per day (Australian Bureau of Statistics 2019). Prescription drug misuse is defined as use other than prescribed, including use of another person's prescription or use only for the feeling the drug causes (Hasin et al 2013).

Opioids are appropriate for treating severe acute pain. Opioids are prescribed at greater than 5% of adolescents' primary care and emergency department visits (Fortuna et al 2010). Previous prescriptions for acute pain are a commonly identified source of opioids for misuse (Boyd et al 2009). This association is strongest among young adults who reported little to no previous history of drug use and disapproval of illegal drug use as adolescents.

Nurses should counsel families to monitor home opioid use and to secure opioids in locked medication safes or other locked cabinets to protect their children and children who visit (Manworren & Gilson 2015). Nurses should also inform families of methods to dispose of opioids when they are no longer needed for the reason they are prescribed.

*Box created by Renee C. B. Manworren.

BOX 5.4 Evidence-based Strategies to Reduce Needlestick Pain

Vaccination Specific	
Injection technique	Avoid aspiration, use rapid injection technique
Vaccination order and sequencing	Administer the least painful vaccine first when administering multiple vaccines in one visit (e.g. Priorix before MMR-II)
	Consider simultaneous vaccine administration if possible
General Needlestick Pain Prevention Strategies	
Positioning	Avoid supine position if possible
	Use position of comfort in all ages; use breastfeeding for small infants or at least skin-to-skin care
Type of soothing	Caregivers and nurses should *avoid* verbal reassurance, empathy and apology
	Caregivers can be encouraged to use physical soothing and coaching
Topical agents/numbing agents/sucrose	Topical numbing recommended in appropriate age groups
	Sucrose recommended in children under 6 months of age
Other	Consider age-appropriate distraction

BOX 5.5 Levels of Sedation

Minimal Sedation (Anxiolysis)
- Patient responds to verbal commands.
- Cognitive function may be impaired.
- Respiratory and cardiovascular systems are unaffected.

Moderate Sedation
- Patient responds to verbal commands but may not respond to light tactile stimulation.
- Cognitive function is impaired.
- Respiratory function is adequate; cardiovascular system is unaffected.

Deep Sedation
- Patient cannot be easily aroused except with repeated or painful stimuli.
- Ability to maintain airway may be impaired.
- Spontaneous ventilation may be impaired; cardiovascular function is maintained.

General Anaesthesia
- Loss of consciousness, patient cannot be aroused with painful stimuli.
- Airway cannot be maintained adequately and ventilation is impaired.
- Cardiovascular function may be impaired.

From Meredith et al (2008).

Specific Strategies for Special Populations

Pain Prevention for Needlestick. A number of interventions have been studied for prevention of needlestick pain in children. The most effective biobehavioural intervention to reduce needlestick pain in infants is breastfeeding (Benoit et al 2017). Other effective methods to reduce needlestick distress include: the use of 24% sucrose or glucose and skin-to-skin care in infants; comfort holds for toddlers and small children; and deep breathing, distraction, hypnosis and virtual reality for children and adolescents (Stevens & Marvicsin 2016). There is strong evidence that these strategies are effective interventions to manage distress and help children and adolescents cope with needle pain, but there is no evidence these interventions prevent, reduce or relieve needle pain (Birnie et al 2014, Jones et al 2016). Local anaesthetics are the most effective pharmacological agents for preventing and reducing needlestick pain. Best practice to manage needlestick pain requires a team approach with clinicians and families. Box 5.4 highlights evidence-based strategies to reduce needlestick pain.

Care during Painful and Invasive Procedures. Combining pharmacological and biobehavioural interventions provides the best approach for reducing pain from invasive procedures. Severe pain associated with invasive procedures and anxiety associated with diagnostic imaging may require sedation and analgesia.

Procedural sedation and analgesia. Sedation involves a wide range of levels of consciousness (Box 5.5). A thorough patient assessment including the child's history is essential before procedural sedation. Key components of the patient's history include the following.

- Past medical history—Major illnesses, such as asthma, psychiatric disorders, cardiac disease, hepatic or renal impairment; previous hospitalisations or surgeries; history of previous anaesthesia or sedation
- Allergies—Opiates, benzodiazepines, barbiturates, local anaesthetics or other drug allergies and side effects
- Current medications—Cardiovascular medications, central nervous system depressants; use caution with chronic benzodiazepine and opiate users; administration of reversal agents may induce withdrawal or seizures
- Drug use—Opiates, benzodiazepines, barbiturates, cocaine, tobacco, marijuana and alcohol
- Last oral intake—For non-emergent cases, some guidelines recommend more than 4 hours for solid food and 2 hours for clear liquid
- Hydration status—Vomiting, diarrhoea, fluid restriction, urinary output, making tears
- Baseline observations—Heart rate, respiratory rate, SpO_2, blood pressure, temperature and pain score

To provide a safe environment for procedural sedation and analgesia, equipment should be readily available to prevent or manage adverse events and complications (Box 5.6). If nitrous oxide alone is not appropriate, the patient should have IV access for titration of sedatives and analgesics and for administration of antagonists and fluids, if needed. A trained healthcare provider whose sole responsibility is to monitor the patient (rather than performing or assisting with the procedure) should be present to monitor for level of pain, sedation and adverse events and complications.

Biobehavioural Interventions with Postsurgical Pain. A number of biobehavioural interventions have been studied to manage children's postoperative pain. Parental presence has been associated with significantly lower pain scores after surgery (Scalford et al 2013). Therapeutic

BOX 5.6 Procedural Sedation and Analgesia Equipment Needs

- High-flow oxygen and delivery method
- Airway management materials: endotracheal tubes, bag valve masks and laryngoscopes
- Pulse oximetry, blood pressure monitor, electrocardiography,* capnography*
- Suction and large-bore catheters
- Vascular access supplies
- Resuscitation drugs, intravenous fluids
- Reversal agents, including flumazenil and naloxone

*May be optional devices.

suggestion under anaesthesia, a script of positively worded suggestions (no mention of pain or nausea) for promoting a sense of calm and healing delivered to a child while emerging from anaesthesia, significantly lowered pain in children after tonsillectomy (Martin et al 2014) (see Research Focus box). Music therapy (Van der Heijden et al 2015) has also been successfully used to reduce postoperative pain in conjunction with pharmacological management. However, there is limited and conflicting research support for these interventions.

RESEARCH FOCUS

Therapeutic Suggestions

Therapeutic suggestions (TSs) delivered to children while emerging from anaesthesia may be a potential tool to lower pain and reduce opioid use in children after painful surgery. TSs are positively worded statements with suggestions for feeling comfortable. TSs do not include references to pain or nausea. Martin and colleagues (2014) found that children aged 4 to 8 who had TS in the postanaesthesia care unit (PACU) after tonsillectomy had significantly lowered pain scores 30 minutes after extubation compared with children who heard PACU noises only. The children who received TSs also had 70% lower risk of receiving higher opioid doses. Further research is necessary to determine generalisability to other age groups.

Pain Management in Obese and Overweight Children. Little evidence exists on proper dosing of pharmaceuticals in children, including obese and overweight (OB/OW) children. Paediatric medication doses are calculated based on measures of height and weight. Children with excess body fat may have altered metabolism of medications compared with normal-weight peers (Ross et al 2015). There is some evidence that OB/OW children may be at risk for prolonged episodes of acute pain after painful surgery (Martin 2016). There are no current practice guidelines across all settings for OB/OW children requiring dosing of analgesics. Ross and colleagues (2015) produced a support tool to guide medication use in critically ill OB children. This tool includes some of the commonly used analgesic medications and contains instructions to adjust medications based on calculations of ideal body weight (IBW) and adjusted body weight (ABW). When medications are calculated using the ABW calculation, the ABW has been multiplied by a medication-specific cofactor. Controlled trials of this support tool, use of adult dose limits, IBW and ABW are needed to provide evidence for safety and effectiveness.

Adjusted weight calculations for obese and overweight children. Calculate IBW:

$$(50\%\ \text{BMI for age})/[\text{height (in metres)}]^2$$

Calculate ABW doses:

$$\text{IBW} + (\text{total body weight} - \text{IBW}) \times \text{specific cofactor}$$

Treatment for Chronic Pain. Management of chronic pain is highly individualised to reflect the causes of the pain and the psychosocial needs of the child and family. A clear understanding of the child's characteristics (anxiety, physical health, temperament, coping skills, experience, learned response, depression), child's disability (school attendance, activities with family, social interactions, pain behaviours), environmental factors (family attitudes and behavioural patterns, school environment, community, friendships) and the pain stimulus (disease, injury, stress) is important in planning management strategies (Oakes 2011).

Before any workup of chronic pain, the nurse informs the family that chronic pain is common in children and only 10% of children with chronic pain have an identifiable and treatable organic cause for their pain symptom. Medical workup is dictated by the child's symptoms in combination with knowledge about common organic causes of chronic pain. Even if no organic cause is found, the nurse needs to communicate to the child and family acceptance of the pain and the belief that the pain is real.

The management plan includes regular follow-up at 3- to 4-month intervals, a list of symptoms that call for earlier contact and biobehavioural pain management techniques. Cognitive behaviour therapy (CBT) may be required. The goal is to minimise the impact of the pain on the child's activities and the family's quality of life.

The use of CBT has been documented to reduce or eliminate pain in children with chronic pain. Parent involvement is a necessary supportive component. Case reports have demonstrated the effectiveness of implementing a time-out procedure, token systems and positive reinforcement based on operant theory treatment modalities. Parent training in how to avoid positive reinforcement of sick behaviours and focus on rewarding healthy behaviours is important. Stress management strategies may be taught as part of the training. Over the course of several sessions, parents are educated about the chronic pain syndrome, how to distinguish between sick and well behaviours, how to implement a reward system for well behaviours and how to reinforce relaxation and coping skills taught to children for pain management. Treatment may consist of a varying number of sessions over 1 to 6 months and may include various components, such as monitoring symptoms, limiting parent attention, relaxation training and requiring school attendance. No negative side effects of symptom substitution occurred with the interventions (see the Research Focus box).

RESEARCH FOCUS

What is Cognitive Behaviour Therapy?

Cognitive behaviour therapy (CBT) is an evidence-based psychological approach for managing paediatric pain. Environmental and psychological factors exert a powerful influence on children's pain perceptions. CBT uses strategies that focus on thoughts and behaviours to modify negative beliefs and enhance the child's ability to solve pain-related problems that result in better pain management.

Pain with Paediatric Cancer. Sedation or general anaesthesia may be required to prevent the significant pain of procedures performed to diagnose and treat cancer. The pain related to bone marrow aspiration is due to the insertion of a large needle into the posterior iliac space and the unpleasant sensation experienced at the time of marrow aspiration. Lumbar puncture (LP) for administration of chemotherapy (e.g. cytarabine, methotrexate) and collection of cerebrospinal fluid may lead to a leak at the puncture site and low intracranial pressure. Some children may experience post–dural puncture headache after LP, which may be treated by administering non-opioid analgesics and placing the patient in the supine position. Rarely, post–dural puncture pain that persists may require a blood patch. Adequate pain control during immunotherapy infusions may minimise other side effects such as bronchospasm (Parsons 2013).

The most common clinical syndrome of cancer-related neuropathic pain is painful peripheral neuropathy caused by chemotherapeutic agents, particularly vincristine and cisplatin, and rarely cytarabine (Edwards et al 2019, Hickman 2014). After withdrawal of the chemotherapy, the neuropathy may resolve over weeks to months, or it may persist. Neuropathic pain is associated with at least one of the following: (1) pain that is described as a tingling, pins-and-needles, electric or shock-like, stabbing, allodynia, burning or numbness; (2) signs of neurological involvement (paralysis, neuralgia) other than those associated with the progression of the tumour; or (3) the location of the solid organ cancer consistent with neurological damage that could give rise to neuropathic pain. Tricyclic antidepressants (amitriptyline, desipramine) and anticonvulsants (gabapentin, pregabalin) have demonstrated effectiveness in neuropathic cancer pain (Rastogi & Campbell 2014) (see Research Focus box).

RESEARCH FOCUS

Tricyclic Antidepressants to Treat Neuropathic Pain

Although there is limited evidence for the use of antidepressants for the management of pain in children, there is clinical use of amitriptyline for pain management in children (WHO 2012). A study of 90 children with irritable bowel syndrome, functional abdominal pain or functional dyspepsia randomised participants to 4 weeks of placebo or amitriptyline (Saps et al 2009). Both amitriptyline and placebo were associated with excellent therapeutic response. There was no significant difference between amitriptyline and placebo after 4 weeks of treatment. Patients with mild to moderate intensity of pain responded better to treatment.

If the patient has neutropenia (absolute neutrophil count less than 500/mm^3), the antipyretic action of paracetamol may mask a fever. Therefore, paracetamol (acetaminophen) should only be administered as needed and with timed temperature monitoring. NSAIDs are contraindicated in patients with thrombocytopenia (platelet count less than 50,000/mm^3) who may be at risk for bleeding. Trilisate and COX-2 inhibitors do not affect platelet function and may be used to treat pain in patients with thrombocytopenia.

Pain Prevention and Treatment for Children with SCD. A multidisciplinary approach combining pharmacological and biobehavioural modalities is useful in treating the pain of SCD (sickle cell disease) (Williams & Tanabe 2016). The main treatment goal of the acute episode is to make the pain tolerable because complete pain relief is usually impossible even with the use of high-dose opioids. Other goals include patient participation in activities of daily living and a return to baseline physical function (Oakes 2011).

SCD pain has both acute and chronic pain components; clinicians should not rely on typical physiological response (outward distress, guarding) during assessment to determine level of pain. There is evidence that clinicians have undervalued patient-reported pain due to mismatch of observed and expected behaviours in relation to the severity of self-reported pain intensity (Schiavenato & Alvarez 2013). Nurses should ask patients to rate their pain, and believe the patient's response, even if the patient's appearance does not match the nurses' expectations. The nurse should expect and not promote functional disability with reports of severe pain.

At home, most patients with SCD have treatment protocols that include escalation of opioids to prevent hospitalisation. For example, patients may be given a regimen where they attempt to control pain and prevent hospitalisation. Therefore, patients coming to an emergency department for acute painful episodes usually have exhausted all home management options or outpatient therapy. Nurses should be aware that patients may be on long-term opioid therapy at home and may have developed some degree of tolerance (Han et al 2016). It is important to collect accurate information on the patient's current doses and home treatment for pain control so that hospital dosing may be adequate during times of crisis.

Patients may require inpatient management of severe pain if adequate relief is not achieved in the emergency department. For severe pain, IV administration with bolus dosing and continuous infusion using a PCA device may be necessary. Rapid treatment is needed to prevent chest syndrome and further patient deterioration. VOC (vaso-occlusive crisis) lasts an average 7 to 10 days, but hospitalisation is typically less than half this time. The goal while inpatient is to provide adequate pain control and transition from IV pain medication to oral so that the patient may be discharged home. Rehospitalisation is common after a rapid return to home. Dehydration can trigger and prolong the sickle cell pain crisis. Close attention should be given to the patient's fluid status to ensure adequate hydration. IV fluids may be necessary to achieve optimal intake. In addition to opioids (oral or IV), the patient may also be on oral or IV NSAIDs such as ibuprofen or ketorolac. Patients with localised pain can benefit from heat applied to the affected area. Use of cold therapy should be avoided because cold is known to precipitate VOC. Other treatments that may be effective for pain from SCD include massage therapy, physical therapy, distraction, music therapy, art therapy and CBT.

Pain Treatment during End-of-Life Care. Many patients at the end of life require doses of opioids to treat the pain of their disease as their disease progresses (e.g. cancer, human immunodeficiency virus, cystic fibrosis, neurodegenerative diseases). Patients achieve comfort with a combination of opioids and adjuvant analgesics in most situations. Parents need reassurance that the opioids are treating pain but not causing the child's death and that the child's advancing disease is the cause of death.

A small group of patients have intolerable side effects or inadequate analgesia despite extremely aggressive use of medications to relieve pain and side effects. Continuous sedation may be a means of relieving suffering when there is no feasible or acceptable means of providing analgesia that preserves alertness. A continuing high-dose infusion of opioids along with sedation is prescribed to reduce the possibility that a child might experience unrelieved pain but be too sedated to report it. Sedation in these situations is widely regarded as providing comfort, not euthanasia. Clinicians and ethicists have a range of views regarding assisted suicide and euthanasia, but they all agree that no child or parent should choose death because of inadequate efforts to relieve pain and suffering.

REFERENCES

Allen, J. M., Graef, D. M., Ehrentraut, J. H., et al. (2016). CNS Neuroscience & Therapeutics, 22(11), 880–893. doi: 10.1111/cns.12583

American Pain Society. (2016). Principles of Analgesic Use, 7th Ed. Chicago, IL: APS.

Australian and New Zealand College of Anaesthetists (ANZCA). (2010). Faculty of Pain Medicine: Statement on Patients' Rights to Pain Management and Associated Responsibilities. http://www.anzca.edu.au/documents/ps45-2010-statement-on-patients-rights-to-pain-man.pdf

Australian Bureau of Statistics. (2019). Opioid-induced deaths in Australia. 25 September. https://www.abs.gov.au/articles/opioid-induced-deaths-australia

Australian Institute of Health and Welfare (AIHW). (2020). Australia's Children. AIHW, Canberra. https://immunisationhandbook.health.gov.au/vaccination-procedures/after-vaccination

Australian Technical Advisory Group on Immunisation (ATAGI). (2018). Australian Immunisation Handbook. Australian Government Department of Health, Canberra.

Azize, P. M., Humphreys, A., & Cattani, A. (2011). The impact of language on the expression and assessment of pain in children. Intensive & Critical Care Nursing, 27(5), 235–243.

Bailey, B., Daoust, R., Doyon-Trottier, S., et al. (2010). Validation and properties of the verbal numeric scale in children with acute pain. Pain, 149, 216–221.

Baugh, R. F., Archer, S. M., Mitchell, R. B., et al. (2011). Clinical practice guideline. Otolaryngology–Head and Neck Surgery, 144(1 Suppl.), S1–S30.

Bennett, C. (2017). Power through knowledge: patient education and self-management keys to successfully managing chronic pain. https://ahha.asn.au/sites/default/files/docs/policy-issue/evidence_brief_17_power_through_knowledge_patient_education_and_self-management_keys_to_successfully_managing_chronic_pain_0.pdf

Beyer, J. E., Denyes, M. J., Villarruel, A. M. (1992). The creation, validation, and continuing development of the Oucher: a measure of pain intensity in children. J Pediatr Nurs, 7(5), 335–346.

Benoit, B., Martin-Misener, R., Newman, A., et al. (2017). Neurophysiological assessment of acute pain in infants: A scoping review of research methods. Acta Paediatrica, 106(7), 1053–1066.

Birnie, K. A., Noel, M., Parker, J. A., et al. (2014). Systematic review and meta-analysis of distraction and hypnosis for needle-related pain and distress in children and adolescents. Journal of Pediatric Psychology, 39(8), 783–808.

Bisogni, S., Calzolai, M., Olivini, N., et al. (2014). Cross-sectional study on differences in pain perception and behavioral distress during venipuncture between Italian and Chinese children. Pediatric Reports, 6(3), 56–60'

Boerlage, A. A., Ista, E., Duivenvoorden, H. J., et al. (2015). The COMFORT behavior scale detects clinically meaningful effects of analgesic and sedative treatment. European Journal of Pain, 19(4), 473–479.

Boyd, C. J., Young, A., Grey, M., et al. (2009). Teens' nonmedical use of prescription medications and other problem behaviors. The Journal of Adolescent Health, 45(6), 543–550.

Brennan, F., & Gwyther, L. (2019). Access to Pain Management as a Human Right. American Journal of Public Health: Pain Management, 109, 61–65. doi: 10.2105/AJPH.2018.304743

Carter, B., Arnott, J., Simons, J., et al. (2017). Developing a Sense of Knowing and Acquiring the Skills to Manage Pain in Children with Profound Cognitive Impairments: Mothers' Perspectives. Pain Research & Management, 2017, 2514920. https://doi.org/10.1155/2017/2514920

Chapman, C. R., & Vierck, C. J. (2017). The transition of acute postoperative pain to chronic pain: An integrative overview of research on mechanisms. The Journal of Pain, 18(4), 359.e1–359.e38.

Chaveli-López, B., & Bagán-Sebastián, J. V. (2016). Treatment of oral mucositis due to chemotherapy. Journal of Clinical and Experimental Dentistry, 8(2), e201.

Chen-Lim, M. L., Zarnowsky, C., Green, R., et al. (2012). Optimizing the assessment of pain in children who are cognitively impaired through the quality improvement process. Journal of Pediatric Nursing, 27(6), 750–759.

Chisengantambu, C., & McDonald, P. (2018). Management of chronic pain. In Chang & Johnson (2018). Living with chronic illness and disability, (3rd ed.). Chatswood: Australia.

Chorpita, B. F., Yim, L., Moffitt, C., et al. (2000). Assessment of symptoms of DSM-IV anxiety and depression in children: A revised child anxiety and depression scale. Behaviour Research and Therapy, 38(8), 835–855.

Chou, R., Gordon, D. B., de Leon-Casasola, O. A., et al. (2016). Management of postoperative pain: A clinical practice guideline from the American Pain Society, the American Society of Regional Anesthesia and Pain Medicine, and the American Society of Anesthesiologists' committee on regional anesthesia, executive committee, and administrative council. The Journal of Pain, 17(2), 131–157.

Cignacco, E. L., Sellam, G., Stoffel, L., et al. (2012). Oral sucrose and 'facilitated tucking' for repeated pain relief in preterms: A randomized controlled trial. Pediatrics, 129(2), 299–308.

Claar, R. L., & Walker, L. S. (2006). Functional assessment of pediatric pain patients: Psychometric properties of the functional disability inventory. Pain, 121(1–2), 77–84.

Courtois, E., Droutman, S., Magny, J. F., et al. (2016). Epidemiology and neonatal pain management of heelsticks in intensive care units: EPIPPAIN 2, a prospective observational study. International Journal of Nursing Studies, 59, 79–88.

Eccleston, C., Palermo, T. M., Williams, A. C. D., et al. (2014). Psychological therapies for the management of chronic and recurrent pain in children and adolescents. The Cochrane Library, CD003968.

Edwards, L., Mulvey, M., & Bennett, M. (2019). Cancer-Related Neuropathic Pain. Cancers, 11(373), 1–8.

Ely, E., Chen-Lim, M. L., Carpenter, K. M., et al. (2016). Pain assessment of children with autism spectrum disorders. Journal of Developmental and Behavioral Pediatrics, 37(1), 53–61.

Fisher, E., Law, E., Palermo, T. M., et al. (2015). Psychological therapies (remotely delivered) for the management of chronic and recurrent pain in children and adolescents. The Cochrane Database of Systematic Reviews, (3), CD011118.

Fortier, M. A., Chou, J., Maurer, E. L., et al. (2011). Acute to chronic postoperative pain in children: Preliminary findings. Journal of Pediatric Surgery, 46, 1700–1705.

Fortier, M. A., Wahi, A., Bruce, C., et al. (2014). Pain management at home in children with cancer: A daily diary study. Pediatric Blood & Cancer, 61(6), 1029–1033.

Fortuna, R. J., Robbins, B. W., Caiola, E., et al. (2010). Prescribing of controlled medications to teens and young adults in the United States. Pediatrics, 126(6), 1108–1116.

Fosdal, M. B. (2015). Perception of pain among pediatric patients with sickle cell pain crisis. Journal of Pediatric Oncology Nursing, 32(1), 5–20.

Franck, L. S., Harris, S. K., Soetenga, D. J., et al. (2008). The Withdrawal Assessment Tool–1 (WAT-1): An assessment instrument for monitoring opioid and benzodiazepine withdrawal symptoms in pediatric patients. Pediatric Critical Care Medicine: A Journal of the Society of Critical Care Medicine and the World Federation of Pediatric Intensive and Critical Care Societies, 9(6), 573–580.

Freund, D., & Bolick, B.N. (2019). Assessing a Child's Pain. American Journal of Nursing, 119(5), 34–41. doi: 10.1097/01.NAJ.0000557888.65961.c6.

Friedrichsdorf, S. J., Giordano, J., Desai Dakoji, K., et al. (2016). Chronic pain in children and adolescents: Diagnosis and treatment of primary pain disorders in head, abdomen, muscles and joints. Children, 3(4), 42.

Gaina, A., Sekine, M., Chen, X., et al. (2004). Validity of child sleep diary questionnaire among junior high school children. Journal of Epidemiology, 14(1), 1–4.

Gamst-Jensen, H., Vedel, P. N., Lindberg-Larsen, V. O., et al. (2014). Acute pain management in burn patients: Appraisal and thematic analysis of four clinical guidelines. Burns: Journal of the International Society for Burn Injuries, 40(8), 1463.

Givler, A., Maani-Fogelman, P. A. (2019). The Importance of Cultural Competence in Pain and Palliative Care. Retrieved from StatPearls website: https://www.ncbi.nlm.nih.gov/books/NBK493154/

Gold, J. I., Mahrer, N. E., Yee, J., et al. (2009). Pain, fatigue and health-related quality of life in children and adolescents with chronic pain. The Clinical Journal of Pain, 25(5), 407.

Gray, L., Garza, E., Zageris, D., et al. (2015). Sucrose and Warmth for Analgesia in Healthy Newborns: An RCT. Pediatrics: Academy of Pediatrics, 135(3), e607–e614. doi: 10.1542/peds.2014-1073

Gregory, J. (2019). Use of pain scales and observational pain assessment tools in hospital settings. Nursing Standard. doi: 10.7748/ns.2019.e11308

Griggs, C., Goverman, J., Bittner, E., et al. (2017). Sedation and pain management in burns patients. Clinical Plastic Surgery, 44(3), 535–540.

Haley, C. (2016). Pillitteri's Child and family health nursing in Australia and New Zealand, (2nd ed.). Philadelphia: Lippincott Williams and Wilkins.

Han, J., Saraf, S. L., Zhang, X., et al. (2016). Patterns of opioid use in sickle cell disease. American Journal of Hematology, 91(11), 1102–1106.

Hasin, D. S., O'Brien, C. P., Auriacombe, M., et al. (2013). DSM-5 criteria for substance use disorders: Recommendations and rationale. The American Journal of Psychiatry, 170(8), 834–851.

Hatfield, L. A., & Ely, E. A. (2015). Measurement of acute pain in infants: A review of behavioural and physiological variables. Biological Research for Nursing, 17(1), 100–111.

Hershey, A. D., Powers, S. W., Vockell, A. L., et al. (2001). PedMIDAS development of a questionnaire to assess disability of migraines in children. Neurology, 57(11), 2034–2039.

Hershey, A. D., Powers, S. W., Vockell, A. L., et al. (2004). Development of a patient-based grading scale for PedMIDAS. Cephalalgia: An International Journal of Headache, 24(10), 844–849.

Hickman, J., Varadarajan, J., Weisman, S. J., et al. (2014). Paediatric cancer pain. In P. C. McGrath, B. J. Stevens, & S. M. Walker (Eds.), Oxford Textbook of Paediatric Pain. Oxford: Oxford University Press.

Hicks, C. L., von Baeyer, C. L., Spafford, P. A., et al. (2001). The faces pain scale–revised: Toward a common metric in pediatric pain measurement. Pain, 93(2), 173–183.

Howard, R., Carter, B., Curry, J., et al. (2012). Good practice in postoperative and procedural pain management. Paediatric Anaesthesia, 22(July Suppl. 1), 1–79.

Howard, R. F., Wiener, S., & Walker, S. M. (2014). Neuropathic pain in children. Archives of Disease in Childhood, 99(1), 84–89.

Hummel, P., Puchalski, M., Creech, S. D., et al. (2008). Clinical reliability and validity of the N-PASS: Neonatal pain, agitation and sedation scale with prolonged pain. Journal of Perinatology, 28(1), 55–60.

Huether, S. E., & Rodway, G. W. (2019). Pain, temperature regulation, sleep, and sensory function. In McCance, K.L. & Huether, S.E. (2019). Pathophysiology: The Biologic Basis for Disease in Adults and Children, (8th ed.). Missouri: Elsevier.

Hunt, A., Goldman, A., Seers, K., et al. (2003). Clinical validation of the Paediatric Pain Profile. Developmental Medicine and Child Neurology, 46(1), 9–18.

International Association for the Study of Pain (IASP). (2012 May). Pain Terms, IASP Taxonomy. IASP: Washington. http://s3.amazonaws.com/rdcms-iasp/files/production/public/Content/ContentFolders/Publications2/ClassificationofChronicPain/Part_III-PainTerms.pdf

International Association for the Study of Pain. (2018). IASP Statement on Opioids. IASP: Washington. https://www.iasp-pain.org/Advocacy/Content.aspx?ItemNumber=7194

Isaacson, G. (2013). Further concerns regarding opioids after tonsillectomy in children. Otolaryngology–Head and Neck Surgery, 148, 892.

Isaacson, G. (2014). Pediatric tonsillectomy: An evidence-based approach. Otolaryngologic Clinics of North America, 47, 673–690.

Ista, E., van Dijk, M., Tibboel, D., et al. (2005). Assessment of sedation levels in pediatric intensive care patients can be improved by using the COMFORT 'behavior' scale. Pediatric Critical Care Medicine: A Journal of the Society of Critical Care Medicine and the World Federation of Pediatric Intensive and Critical Care Societies, 6(1), 58–63.

Johnston, C., Barrington, K. J., Taddio, A., et al. (2011). Pain in Canadian NICUs: Have we improved over the past 12 years? The Clinical Journal of Pain, 27(3), 225–232.

Johnston, C., Campbell-Yeo, M., Disher, T., et al. (2017). Skin-to-skin care for procedural pain in neonates. The Cochrane Database of Systematic Reviews, CD008435.

Johnston, C. C., Stevens, B., Pinelli, J., et al. (2003). Kangaroo care is effective in diminishing pain response in preterm neonates. Archives of Pediatrics and Adolescent Medicine, 157(11), 1084–1088.

Jones, K. M., King, S., & MacLaren Chorney, J. E. (2014). Supporting children with chronic pain in their return to school. Pediatric Pain Letter, 16(1–2), 8–14. http://www.childpain.org/ppl.

Jones, T., Moore, T., & Choo, J. (2016). The impact of virtual reality on chronic pain. PLoS ONE, 11(12), e0167523.

Kashikar-Zuck, S., Flowers, S. R., Claar, R. L., et al. (2011). Clinical utility and validity of the Functional Disability Inventory among a multicenter sample of youth with chronic pain. Pain, 152(7), 1600–1607.

Kashikar-Zuck, S., & Ting, T. V. (2014). Juvenile fibromyalgia: Current status of research and future developments. Nature Reviews. Rheumatology, 10(2), 89–96.

Kassab, M., Foster, J. P., Foureur, M., et al. (2012). Sweet-tasting solutions for needle-related procedural pain in infants one month to one year of age. The Cochrane Database of Systematic Reviews, (12), CD008411.

Khetani, J. D., Madadi, P., Sommer, D. D., et al. (2012). Apnea and oxygen desaturations in children treated with opioids after adenotonsillectomy for obstructive sleep apnea syndrome. Paediatric Drugs, 14, 411–415.

Korterink, J. J., Rutten, J. M., Venmans, L., et al. (2015). Pharmacologic treatment in pediatric functional abdominal pain disorders: A systematic review. The Journal of Pediatrics, 166(2), 424–431.

Kösters, M.P., Chinapaw, M.J.M., Zwaanswijk, M. et al. (2015). Structure, reliability, and validity of the revised child anxiety and depression scale (RCADS) in a multi-ethnic urban sample of Dutch children. BMC Psychiatry 15, 132. https://doi.org/10.1186/s12888-015-0509-7

Kovacs, M. (1981). Rating scales to assess depression in school-aged children. Acta Paedopsychiatrica, 46(5–6), 305–315.

Kozlowski, L. J., Kost-Byerly, S., Colantuoni, E., et al. (2014). Pain prevalence, intensity, assessment and management in a hospitalized pediatric population. Pain Management Nursing, 15, 22–35.

Krechel, S. W., & Bildner, J. (1995). CRIES: A new neonatal postoperative pain measurement score. Initial testing of validity and reliability. Paediatric Anaesthesia, 5, 53–61.

Kristensen, A. D., Ahlburg, P., Lauridsen, M. C., et al. (2012). Chronic pain after inguinal hernia repair in children. British Journal of Anaesthesia, 109(4), 603–608.

Lauder, G., & Emmott, A. (2014). Confronting the challenges of effective pain management in children following tonsillectomy. International Journal of Pediatric Otorhinolaryngology, 78, 1813–1827.

Lawrence, J., Alcock, D., McGrath, P., et al. (1993). The development of a tool to assess neonatal pain. Neonatal Network: NN, 12(6), 59–66.

Logan, D. E., Simons, L. E., & Carpino, E. (2012). Too sick for school? Parent influences on school functioning among children with chronic pain. Pain, 153(2), 437–443.

Logan, D, Gray, L., Iversen, C., et al. (2017). School self-concept in adolescents with chronic pain. Journal of Pediatric Psychology, 42(8), 892–901.

Lootens, C. C., & Rapoff, M. A. (2011). Measures of pediatric pain: 21-numbered circle visual analog scale (VAS), E-Ouch electronic pain diary, Oucher, pain behavior observation method, pediatric pain assessment tool (PPAT), and Pediatric Pain Questionnaire (PPQ). Arthritis Care and Research, 63(Suppl. 11), S253–S262.

Luffy, R., & Grove, S. K. (2003). Examining the validity, reliability, and preference of three pediatric pain measurement tools in African-American children. Pediatric Nursing, 29(1), 54–60.

Malviya, S., Voepel-Lewis, T., Burke, C., et al. (2006). The revised FLACC observational pain tool: Improved reliability and validity for pain assessment in children with cognitive impairment. Paediatric Anesthesia, 16(3), 258–265.

Manworren, R. C. B. (2017). We do still hurt babies. Journal of Perinatal & Neonatal Nursing, 31(2), 89–90.

Manworren, R. C. B., & Gilson, A. M. (2015). Nurses' role in preventing prescription opioid diversion. The American Journal of Nursing, 115(8), 34–40. http://journals.lww.com/ajnonline/Abstract/2015/08000/CE___Nurses__Role_in_Preventing_Prescription.21.aspx.

Manworren, R. C. B., Jeffries, L., Pantaleao, A., et al. (2016). Pharmacogenetic testing for analgesic adverse effects: Pediatric case series. The Clinical Journal of Pain, 32(2), 109–115.

Manworren, R. C. B., & Stinson, J. (2016). Pediatric pain measurement, assessment, and evaluation. Seminars in Pediatric Neurology, 23(3), 189–200.

Martin, S. (2016). Associations between weight status and post-tonsillectomy pain experiences in children: A retrospective study (Order No. 10585181), available from Dissertations & Theses @ University of Texas–Arlington; ProQuest Dissertations & Theses Global.

Martin, S., Smith, A. B., Newcomb, P., et al. (2014). Effects of therapeutic suggestion under anesthesia on outcomes in children post tonsillectomy. Journal of Perianesthesia Nursing, 29(2), 94–106.

McIntyre, M. K., Clifford, J. L., Maani, C. V., et al. (2016). Progress of clinical practice on the management of burn-associated pain: Lessons from animal models. Burns: Journal of the International Society for Burn Injuries, 42(6), 1161–1172.

McMurtry, C. M., Noel, M., Taddio, A., et al. (2015). The Clinical Journal of Pain, 31, (Suppl 10), S109–S123. doi: 10.1097/AJP.0000000000000273

McMurtry, C. M., Riddell, R. P., Taddio, A., et al. (2015). Far from 'Just a Poke': Common painful needle procedures and the development of needle fear. The Clinical Journal of Pain, 31, S3–S11.

McMurtry, C. M., Taddio, A., Noel, M., et al. (2016). Exposure-based interventions for the management of individuals with high levels of needle fear across the lifespan: A clinical practice guideline and call for further research. Cognitive Behaviour Therapy, 45(3), 217–235.

Merkel, S. I., Voepel-Lewis, T., Shayevitz, J. R., et al. (1997). The FLACC: A behavioral scale for scoring postoperative pain in young children. Pediatric Nursing, 23(3), 293–297.

Miech, R., Johnston, L., O'Malley, P. M., et al. (2015). Prescription opioids in adolescence and future opioid misuse. Pediatrics, 136(5), e1169–e1177.

Miro, J., McGrath, P. J., Finley, G. A., et al. (2017). Pediatric chronic pain programs: current and ideal practice. Pain Reports, 2(5), e613. doi: 10.1097/PR9.0000000000000613

NSW Health Agency for Clinical Innovation. (2016). Paediatric PCA (patient-controlled analgesia) / NCA (nurse controlled analgesia) chart. https://www.health.nsw.gov.au/kidsfamilies/paediatric/Documents/paeds-pca-chart-educational.pdf

Nir, Y., Paz, A., Sabo, E., et al. (2003). Fear of injections in your adults: Prevalence and associations. The American Journal of Tropical Medicine and Hygiene, 68(3), 341–344.

Oakes, L. L. (2011). Infant and child pain management. New York: Springer Publishing.

Olsen, K., & Weinberg, E. (2017). Pain-less practice: Techniques to reduce procedural pain and anxiety in pediatric acute care. Clinical Pediatric Emergency Medicine, 18(1), 32–41.

Ossipov, M. H., Morimura, K., & Porreca, F. (2014). Descending pain modulation and chronification of pain. Current Opinion in Supportive and Palliative Care, 8(2), 143–151.

Palermo, T., Eccleston, C., Goldschneider, K., et al. (2013). Assessment and management of children with chronic pain: A position statement from the American Pain Society. http://americanpainsociety.org/uploads/get-involved/pediatric-chronic-pain-statement.pdf.

Parsons, K., Bernhardt, B., & Strickland, B. (2013). Targeted immunotherapy for high-risk Neuroblastoma—The role of monoclonal antibodies. The Annals of Pharmacotherapy, 47(2), 210–218.

Pasero, C., & McCaffrey, M. (2011). Pain assessment and pharmacologic management. St Louis, MO: Elsevier.
Pate, J. W., Noblet, T., Hush, J. M., et al. (2019). Exploring the concept of pain of Australian children with and without pain: qualitative study. BMJ Open, 9:e033199, 1–12. doi:10.1136/ bmjopen-2019-033199
Pillai Riddell, R. R., Racine, N. M., Gennis, H. G., et al. (2015). Non-pharmacological management of infant and young child procedural pain. The Cochrane Database of Systematic Reviews, CD006275.
Poder, T. G., & Lemieux, R. (2014). How effective are spiritual care and body manipulation therapies in pediatric oncology? A systematic review of the literature. Global Journal of Health Science, 6(2), 112.
Quinn, B. L., Sheldon, L. K., & Cooley, M. E. (2014). Pediatric pain assessment by drawn faces scales: A review. Pain Management Nursing, 15(4), 909–918.
Quinn, B. L., Seibold, E., & Hayman, L. (2015). Pain assessment in children with special needs: A review of the literature. Exceptional Children, 82(1), 44–57.
Rastogi, S., & Campbell, F. (2014). Drugs for neuropathic pain. In P. C. McGrath, B. J. Stevens, S. M. Walker, et al. (Eds.), Oxford Textbook of Paediatric Pain. Oxford: Oxford University Press.
Ross, E. L., Heizer, J., Mixon, M. A., et al. (2015). Development of recommendations for dosing of commonly prescribed medications in critically ill obese children. American Journal of Health-System Pharmacy, 72(7), 542–556.
Saps, M., Youssef, N., Miranda, A., et al. (2009). Multicenter, randomized, placebo-controlled trial of amitriptyline in children with functional gastrointestinal disorders. Gastroenterology, 137(4), 1261–1269.
Scalford, D., Flynn-Roth, R., Howard, D., et al. (2013). Pain management of children aged 5 to 10 years after adenotonsillectomy. Journal of Perianesthesia Nursing, 28(6), 353–360.
Schiavenato, M., & Alvarez, O. (2013). Pain assessment during a vaso-occlusive crisis in the pediatric and adolescent patient: Rethinking practice. Journal of Pediatric Oncology Nursing, 30(5), 242–248.
Schug, S. A., Palmer, G. M., Scott, D. A., et al. (2015). Acute Pain Management: Scientific Evidence (4th ed.) Australian and New Zealand College of Anaesthetists and Faculty of Pain Medicine: Melbourne. http://fpm.anzca.edu.au/documents/apmse4_2015_final
Shah, V., Taddio, A., McMurtry, C. M., et al. (2015). Pharmacological and combined interventions to reduce vaccine injection pain in children and adults: Systematic review and meta-analysis. The Clinical Journal of Pain, 31(Suppl. 10), S38–S63.
Sheridan, R. L., Stoddard, F. J., Kazis, L. E., et al. (2014). Long-term posttraumatic stress symptoms vary inversely with early opiate dosing in children recovering from serious burns. The Journal of Trauma and Acute Care Surgery, 76(3), 828–832.
Sieberg, C. B., Simons, L. E., Edelstein, M. R., et al. (2013). Pain prevalence and trajectories following pediatric spinal fusion surgery. The Journal of Pain, 14(12), 1694–1702.
Sneddon, P., Peacock, G. G., & Crowley, S. L. (2013). Assessment of sleep problems in preschool aged children: An adaptation of the children's sleep habits questionnaire. Behavioral Sleep Medicine, 11(4), 283–296.
Solodiuk, J. C., Brighton, H., McHale, J., et al. (2014). Documented electronic medical record-based pain intensity scores at a tertiary pediatric medical center: A cohort analysis. Journal of Pain and Symptom Management, 48(5), 924–933.
Stevens, B. J., Gibbins, S., Yamada, J., et al. (2014). The premature infant pain profile-revised (PIPP-R): Initial validation and feasibility. The Clinical Journal of Pain, 30, 238–243.
Stevens, K., & Marvicsin, D. (2016). Evidence-based recommendations for reducing pediatric distress during vaccination. Pediatric Nursing, 432(6), 267.
Stinson, J. N., Stevens, B. J., Feldman, B. M., et al. (2008). Construct validity of a multidimensional electronic pain diary for adolescents with arthritis. Pain, 136(3), 281–292.
Suresh, S., Birmingham, P. K., & Kozlowski, R. J. (2012). Pediatric pain management. Anesthesiology Clinics, 30(1), 101–117.
Swift, A. (2015). Pain management 3: the importance of assessing pain in adults. Nursing Times; 11(41), 12–17. https://www.nursingtimes.net/clinical-archive/pain-management/pain-management-3-the-importance-of-assessing-pain-in-adults-05-10-2015/
Taddio, A., Ipp, M., Thivakaran, S., et al. (2012). Survey of the prevalence of immunization non-compliance due to needle fears in children and adults. Vaccine, 30(32), 4807–4812.
Tesler, M. D., Savedra, M. C., Holzemer, W. L., et al. (1991). The word-graphic rating scale as a measure of children's and adolescents' pain intensity. Research in Nursing and Health, 14(5), 361–371.
The Royal Children's Hospital Melbourne. (2019). Pain assessment and measurement. https://www.rch.org.au/rchcpg/hospital_clinical_guideline_index/Pain_assessment_and_measurement/
Therapeutic Goods Administration (TGA). (2018). Codeine information hub. 10 April. Australian Government Department of Health. https://www.tga.gov.au/codeine-info-hub
Thrane, S. (2013). Effectiveness of integrative modalities for pain and anxiety in children and adolescents with cancer. Journal of Pediatric Oncology Nursing, 30(6), 320–332.
Trescot, A. M. (2014). Genetics and implications in perioperative analgesia. Best Practice & Research Clinical Anaesthesiology, 28(2), 153–166.
Tryon, V. L. & Mizumori, S. J. Y. (2018). A Novel Role for the Periaqueductal Gray in Consummatory Behavior. Frontiers in Behavioral Neuroscience, 12(178), 1–15. https://doi.org/10.3389/fnbeh.2018.00178
Valrie, C. R., Bromberg, M. H., Palermo, T., et al. (2013). A systematic review of sleep in pediatric pain populations. Journal of Developmental and Behavioral Pediatrics, 34(2), 120–128.
Van der Heijden, M. J. E., Oliai Araghi, S., van Dijk, M., et al. (2015). The effects of perioperative music interventions in pediatric surgery: A systematic review and meta-analysis of randomized controlled trials. PLoS ONE, 10(8).
van Dijk, M., de Boer, J., & Koot, H. (2000). The reliability and validity of the COMFORT scale as a postoperative pain instrument in 0 to 3-year-old infants. Pain, 84(2–3), 367–377.
van Dijk, M., Roofthooft, D. W. E., Anand, K. J. S., et al. (2009). Taking up the challenge of measuring prolonged pain in (premature) neonates: The COMFORTneo scale seems promising. The Clinical Journal of Pain, 25(7), 607–616.
Van Loey, N. E., Hofland, H. W., Hendrickx, H., et al. (2016). Validation of the burns itch questionnaire. Burns: Journal of the International Society for Burn Injuries, 42(3), 526–534.
Varni, J. W., Seid, M., & Rode, C. A. (1999). The PedsQL: Measurement model for the pediatric quality of life inventory. Medical Care, 37(2), 126–139.
Vinall, J., Pavlova, M., Asmundson, G. J. G., et al. (2016). Multidisciplinary Digital Publishing Institute: Children, 3(4), 1–31. doi: 10.3390/children3040040
Voepel-Lewis, T., Zanotti, J., Dammeyer, J. A., et al. (2010). Reliability and validity of the face, legs, activity, cry, consolability behavioral tool in assessing acute pain in critically ill patients. American Journal of Critical Care, 19(1), 55–61.
von Baeyer, C., Lin V., Seidman L., et al. (2011). Pain charts (body maps or manikins) in assessment of the location of pediatric pain. Pain Management, 1(1), 61–68.
Walker, L. S., & Greene, J. W. (1991). The functional disability inventory: Measuring a neglected dimension of child health status. Journal of Pediatric Psychology, 16(1), 39–58.
Walther-Larsen, S., Pedersen, M. T., Friis, S. M., et al. (2016). Pain prevalence in hospitalized children. Acta Anaesthesiologica Scandinavica, 61(3), 328–337.
Watterberg, K. L., Cummings, J. J., Benitz, W. E., et al. (2016). Prevention and management of procedural pain in the neonate. Pediatrics, 137(2), e20154271.
Weissmann, R. & Uziel, Y. (2016). Pediatric complex regional pain syndrome: a review. Pediatr Rheumatol, 14(29), 1–10. https://doi.org/10.1186/s12969-016-0090-8
Williams, A. C. C., & Craig, K. D. (2016). Updating the definition of pain. Pain, 157(11), 2420–2423.
Williams, H., & Tanabe, P. (2016). Sickle cell disease: A review of nonpharmacological approaches for pain. Journal of Pain and Symptom Management, 51(2), 163–177.
Wong, D. L., & Baker, C. M. (1988). Pain in children: Comparison of assessment scales. Pediatric Nursing, 14(1), 9–17.
World Health Organization. (2012). WHO guidelines on the pharmacological treatment of persisting pain in children with medical illnesses. Geneva: World Health Organization.
Yilmaz, G., Cavlan, N., Oguz, M., et al. (2014). Oral sucrose administration to reduce pain response during immunization in 16-19-month infants: A randomized, placebo-controlled trial. European Journal of Pediatrics, 173(11), 1527–1532.
Zempsky, W. T. (2014). Topical anesthetics and analgesics. In P. C. McGrath, B. J. Stevens, S. M. Walker, et al. (Eds.), Oxford Textbook of Paediatric Pain. Oxford: Oxford University Press.

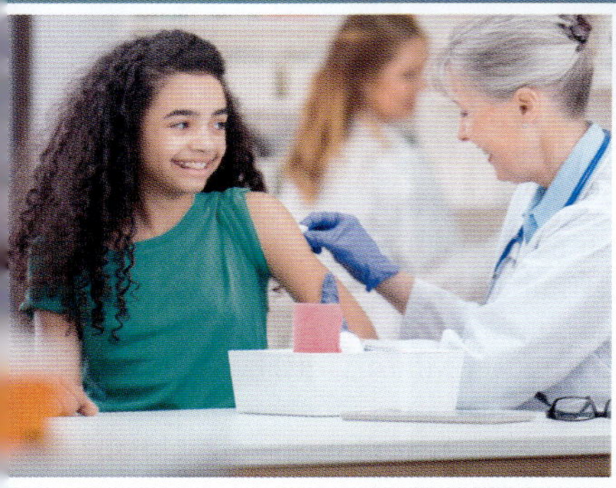

6

Childhood Communicable and Infectious Diseases

Andrea Middleton

LEARNING OUTCOMES

- Outline nursing care, infection control measures, safety concerns and preventive actions to take in caring for children with common communicable and infectious diseases
- Build an understanding of immunity and safety concerns with administering vaccinations
- Outline of vaccines listed in the Australian and New Zealand immunisation schedules

INFECTION CONTROL

Healthcare-associated infections (HAIs) are a safety risk to patients in the hospital setting. Infections to the blood stream, respiratory system and gastroenterological system remain high with approximately 165,000 HAIs occurring each year in Australia (Mitchell et al 2017). These infections occur when there is interaction among patients, healthcare professionals, equipment and bacteria. HAIs are preventable and effective infection control is central to providing high-quality healthcare for patients and a safe working environment for healthcare workers (NHMRC 2019).

Standard precautions synthesise the major features of universal (i.e. blood and body fluid) precautions (designed to reduce the risk of transmission of blood-borne pathogens) and body substance isolation (designed to reduce the risk of transmission of pathogens from moist body substances). Standard precautions involve the use of barrier protection (personal protective equipment [PPE]), such as gloves, goggles, gowns and masks, to prevent contamination from: blood; all body fluids, secretions and excretions, except sweat, regardless of whether they contain visible blood; non-intact skin; and mucous membranes. Standard precautions are designed for the care of all patients to reduce the risk of transmission of microorganisms from both recognised and unrecognised sources of infection.

Hand hygiene continues to be the single most important practice to reduce the transmission of infectious diseases in healthcare settings (Bolon 2016). Hand hygiene includes handwashing with soap and water, as well as the use of alcohol-based products for hand disinfection.

Transmission-based precautions are designed for patients with documented or suspected infection or colonisation (i.e. presence of microorganisms in or on patient but without clinical signs and symptoms of infection) with highly transmissible or epidemiologically important pathogens for which additional precautions beyond standard precautions are needed to interrupt transmission in hospitals. The three types of transmission-based precautions are: (1) airborne precautions; (2) droplet precautions; and (3) contact precautions. They may be combined for diseases that have multiple routes of transmission. They are to be used in addition to standard precautions.

Airborne precautions reduce the risk of airborne transmission of infectious agents. Airborne transmission occurs by dissemination of either airborne droplet nuclei (i.e. small-particle residue [≤ 5 mm] of evaporated droplets that may remain suspended in the air for long periods) or dust particles containing the infectious agent. Microorganisms carried in this manner can be dispersed widely by air currents and may become inhaled by or deposited on a susceptible host within the same room or over a longer distance from the source patient, depending on environmental factors. Special air handling and ventilation are required to prevent airborne transmission. The term *airborne infection isolation room* (AIIR) has replaced *negative pressure isolation room*; this room is used to isolate persons with a suspected or confirmed airborne infectious disease transmitted by the airborne route such as measles, varicella and tuberculosis.

Droplet precautions reduce the risk of droplet transmission of infectious agents. Droplet transmission involves contact of the conjunctivae or the mucous membranes of the nose or mouth of a susceptible person with large-particle droplets (> 5 mm) containing microorganisms generated from a person who has a clinical disease or who is a carrier of the microorganism. Droplets are generated from the source person primarily during coughing, sneezing or talking and during procedures such as suctioning and bronchoscopy. Transmission requires close contact between source and recipient persons because droplets do not remain suspended in the air and generally travel only short distances, usually 1 metre or less, through the air. Because droplets do not remain suspended in the air, special air handling and ventilation are not required to prevent droplet transmission. Droplet precautions apply to any patient with known or suspected infection with pathogens that can be transmitted by infectious droplets.

Contact precautions reduce the risk of transmission of microorganisms by direct or indirect contact. Direct-contact transmission involves skin-to-skin contact and physical transfer of microorganisms to a susceptible host from an infected or colonised person, such as occurs when turning or bathing patients. Direct-contact transmission also can occur between two patients (e.g. by hand contact). Indirect contact transmission involves contact of a susceptible host with a contaminated intermediate object, usually inanimate, in the patient's environment. Contact precautions apply to specified patients known or suspected to be infected or colonised with microorganisms that can be transmitted by direct or indirect contact.

NURSING CARE CONSIDERATIONS

The most common piece of medical equipment, the stethoscope, can be a potent source of harmful microorganisms and nosocomial infections. Consider also the keyboard and desktop as potential sources.

Nurses caring for young children are frequently in contact with body substances, especially urine, faeces and vomitus. Nurses need to exercise judgment concerning those situations when gloves, gowns or masks are necessary. For example, wear gloves and possibly gowns for changing nappies when there are loose or explosive stools. Otherwise, the plastic lining of disposable nappies provides a sufficient barrier between the hands and body substances and gloves are adequate.

Antimicrobial-resistant organisms are causing increasing numbers of HAIs. In hospitals, patients are the most significant sources of methicillin-resistant *Staphylococcus aureus* (MRSA), and the main mode of transmission is patient-to-patient transmission via the hands of a healthcare provider. Handwashing is the most critical infection control practice.

During feedings, wear gowns if the child is likely to vomit or spit up, which often occurs during burping. When wearing gloves, wash the hands thoroughly after removing the gloves because gloves fail to provide complete protection. The absence of visible leaks does not indicate that gloves are intact.

Another essential practice of infection control is that all needles (uncapped and unbroken) are disposed of in a rigid, puncture-resistant container located near the site of use. Consequently, these containers are installed in each patient's room. Because children are naturally curious, extra attention is needed in selecting a suitable type of container and a location that prevents access to the discarded needles. The use of needleless systems allows secure syringe or intravenous (IV) tubing attachment to vascular access devices without the risk of needle stick injury to the child or nurse.

Immunisations

One of the most dramatic advances in paediatrics has been the decline of infectious diseases during the 20th century because of the widespread use of immunisation for preventable diseases. This trend has continued into the 21st century with the development of newer vaccines. Although many of the immunisations can be given to individuals of any age, the recommended primary schedule begins during infancy and, with the exception of boosters and human papillomavirus (HPV) vaccines, is completed during early childhood. This section includes a discussion of childhood immunisations for diphtheria, tetanus and acellular pertussis (DTaP); poliovirus; measles, mumps and rubella (MMR); *Haemophilus influenzae* type b (Hib); hepatitis B virus (HBV); hepatitis A virus (HAV); meningococcal; pneumococcal conjugate vaccine (PCV); influenza; varicella-zoster virus (VZV; chickenpox); rotavirus; human papilloma virus (HPV); and COVID-19. Selected vaccines generally reserved for children considered at high risk for the disease are discussed here and as appropriate throughout the text.

To facilitate an understanding of immunisations, key terms are listed in Box 6.1. Although in this discussion the terms *vaccination* and *immunisation* are used interchangeably in reference to active immunisation, they are not synonymous because the administration of a vaccine cannot automatically be equated with the development of adequate immunity.

Schedule for Immunisations

Australia and New Zealand each have a national immunisation program which consists of a series of immunisations scheduled to be given at specific times throughout your life (Australian Technical Advisory Group on Immunisation [ATAGI] 2018, Ministry of Health 2020a). There is a different schedule for Indigenous and non-Indigenous people. The immunisations range from birth through to adulthood and all vaccines listed in the schedule are free.

Nurses need to be knowledgeable about the program and keep informed of the latest advances and changes in the schedule.

- The Australian National Immunisation Program Schedule is available at https://www.health.gov.au/health-topics/immunisation/immunisation-throughout-life/national-immunisation-program-schedule#national-immunisation-program-schedule-from-1-july-2020.
- The New Zealand Immunisation Schedule is available at https://www.health.govt.nz/our-work/preventative-health-wellness/immunisation/new-zealand-immunisation-schedule.

The recommended age for beginning primary immunisations of infants is at birth or within 2 weeks of birth. Children born preterm should receive the full dose of each vaccine at the appropriate chronological age. A recommended catch-up schedule for Australian children under 10 years not immunised during infancy is available in the Australian Immunisation Handbook (ATAGI 2018) and for New Zealand children is in the Immunisation Handbook 2020 (Ministry of Health 2020b).

Recommendations for Routine Immunisations

Because of constant changes in the pharmaceutical industry, trade names of single and combination vaccines may differ from those currently available. Check the Australian Register of Therapeutic Goods (https://www.tga.gov.au/australian-register-therapeutic-goods or the New Zealand Ministry of Health's therapeutic products regulatory regime (https://www.health.govt.nz/our-work/regulation-health-and-disability-system/therapeutic-products-regulatory-regime).

Hepatitis B Virus. Hepatitis B virus (HBV) is a significant paediatric disease because HBV infections that occur during childhood and adolescence can lead to fatal consequences from cirrhosis or liver cancer during adulthood. It is recommended that newborns receive a monovalent vaccine of Hepatitis B (HepB) before hospital discharge if the mother is hepatitis B surface antigen (HBsAg) negative. Monovalent HepB should be given as the birth dose, whereas a combination vaccine containing HepB may be given for subsequent doses in the series. Both full-term and preterm infants born to mothers whose HBsAg status is positive or unknown should receive HepB and hepatitis B immune globulin (HBIg) 0.5 mL within 12 hours of birth at two different injection sites. Because the immune response to HepB is not optimum in newborns weighing less than 2 kg, the first HepB dose should be given to such infants at a chronological age of 1 month, as long as the mother's HBsAg status is negative (ATAGI 2018).

The vaccine is given intramuscularly in the vastus lateralis in newborns or in the deltoid for older infants and children. Regardless of age, avoid the dorsogluteal site because it has been associated with low antibody seroconversion rates, indicating a reduced immune response. No data exist regarding the seroconversion when the ventrogluteal site is used. The vaccine can be safely administered simultaneously at a separate site with DTaP, MMR and Hib vaccines.

BOX 6.1 Key Immunisation Terms

Acquired immunity—Immunity from exposure to the invading agent, either bacteria, virus or toxin

Active immunity—A state where immune bodies are actively formed against specific antigens, either naturally by having had the disease clinically or subclinically or artificially by introducing the antigen into the individual

Antibody—A protein, found mostly in serum, that is formed in response to exposure to a specific antigen

Antigen—A variety of foreign substances, including bacteria, viruses, toxins and foreign proteins, that stimulate the formation of antibodies

Antitoxin—A solution of antibodies (e.g. diphtheria antitoxin, botulinum antitoxin) derived from the serum of animals immunised with specific antigens and used to confer passive immunity and for treatment

Attenuate—Reduce the virulence (infectiousness) of a pathogenic microorganism by such measures as treating it with heat or chemicals or cultivating it on a certain medium

Cocooning—Strategy of protecting infants from pertussis by vaccinating all persons who come in close contact with the infant, including the parents, grandparents and healthcare care workers.

Combination vaccine—Combination of multiple vaccines into one parenteral form

Conjugate vaccine—A carrier protein with proven immunological potential combined with a less antigenic polysaccharide antigen to enhance the type and magnitude of the immune response (e.g. *Haemophilus influenzae* type b [Hib])

Herd immunity—A condition in which the majority of the population is vaccinated and the spread of certain diseases is stopped because the population that has been vaccinated protects those in the same population who are unvaccinated

Immunisation—Inclusive term denoting the process of inducing or providing active or passive immunity artificially by administering a vaccine

Immunity—An inherited or acquired state in which an individual is resistant to the occurrence or the effects of a specific disease, particularly an infectious agent

Immunoglobulin (Ig) or intravenous immunoglobulin (IVIg)—A sterile solution containing antibodies from large pools of human blood plasma; primarily indicated for routine maintenance of immunity of certain immunodeficient persons and for passive immunisation against measles and hepatitis A

Monovalent vaccine—Vaccine designed to vaccinate against a single antigen or organism

Natural immunity—Innate immunity or resistance to infection or toxicity

Passive immunity—Temporary immunity obtained by transfusing immunoglobulins or antitoxins either artificially from another human or an animal that has been actively immunised against an antigen or naturally from the mother to the fetus via the placenta

Polyvalent vaccine—Vaccine designed to vaccinate against two or more antigens or organisms (e.g. inactivated poliovirus vaccine [IPV])

Specific immunoglobulins—Special preparations obtained from blood plasma from donor pools preselected for a high antibody content against a specific antigen (e.g. hepatitis B immunoglobulin, varicella-zoster immunoglobulin, tetanus immunoglobulin and cytomegalovirus immunoglobulin); as with Ig and IVIg, do not transmit hepatitis B virus, human immunodeficiency virus or other infectious diseases

Toxoid—A modified bacterial toxin that has been made non-toxic but retains the ability to stimulate the formation of antitoxin

Vaccination—Originally referred to inoculation with vaccinia smallpox virus to make a person immune to smallpox; currently denotes physical act of administering any vaccine or toxoid

Vaccine—A suspension of live (usually attenuated) or inactivated microorganisms (e.g. bacteria, viruses or rickettsiae) or fractions of the microorganism administered to induce immunity and prevent infectious disease or its sequelae

Hepatitis A virus. Hepatitis A virus (HAV) has been recognised as a significant child health problem, particularly in Aboriginal and Torres Strait Islander communities in Queensland, the Northern Territory, South Australia and Western Australia, experiencing unusually high infection rates. HAV is spread by the faecal-oral route and from person-to-person contact, by ingestion of contaminated food or water and, rarely, by blood transfusion. The illness has an abrupt onset, with fever, malaise, anorexia, nausea, abdominal discomfort, dark urine and jaundice being the most common clinical signs of infection. In children under 6 years of age, who represent approximately one-third of all cases of hepatitis A, the disease may be asymptomatic, and jaundice is rarely evident.

Hepatitis A vaccine is not recommended on the National Immunisation Schedule in New Zealand or for non-Indigenous children in Australia. For Aboriginal and Torres Strait Islander children living in Queensland, the Northern Territory, South Australia or Western Australia it is recommended for all children beginning at age 18 months. The recommendation for the second dose in the two-dose series is at 4 years. Since the implementation of widespread childhood hepatitis A vaccination, infection rates among children ages 5 to 14 years have declined significantly.

Tetanus. Tetanus is rare in Australia and New Zealand. It is caused by a bacterium found in soil. The bacteria can enter wounds and produce a neurotoxin that acts on the central nervous system to cause muscle rigidity with painful spasms.

Tetanus-containing vaccines are only available in Australia and New Zealand as combination vaccines that include other antigens such as pertussis and diphtheria. These are: diphtheria and tetanus (dT); or diphtheria, tetanus and acellular pertussis (DTPa); or a combination DTPa.

Tetanus-containing vaccines are recommended as a 5-dose schedule for children at 2, 4, 6 and 18 months and at 4 years of age. The first dose can be administered from 6 weeks (ATAGI 2018). Adolescents require a booster dose of tetanus-containing vaccine between 11 and 13 years of age to extend the protective level of immunity into adulthood.

If a child <10 years old obtains a tetanus-prone wound, they may require a booster of a tetanus-containing vaccine if it is 5 years since their last administration of a DTPa or DTPa-containing vaccine. For children over 10 years, tetanus immunisation may be accomplished by administering dT. A resource table can be found at https://immunisationhandbook.health.gov.au/resources/handbook-tables/table-guide-to-tetanus-prophylaxis-in-wound-management.

Diphtheria. Although cases of diphtheria are rare in Australia and New Zealand, the disease can result in significant morbidity. Respiratory manifestations include respiratory nasopharyngitis or obstructive laryngotracheitis with upper airway obstruction. Diphtheria-containing vaccines are only available in Australia as combination vaccines that include other antigens such as pertussis and tetanus. Diphtheria-containing vaccines are recommended for children at 2, 4, 6 and 18 months and at 4 years of age, and adolescents between 11 and 13 years of age (ATAGI 2018).

Although the diphtheria vaccine does not produce absolute immunity, protective antitoxin persists for 10 years or more when given according to the recommended schedule, and boosters are given every 10 years for life.

Pertussis. Pertussis-containing vaccine is recommended for all children in a 5-dose schedule at 2, 4, 6 and 18 months and at 4 years of age. Infants can have their first dose from 6 weeks old. Concerns over outbreaks of the disease in the past decade have prompted discussion about vaccinating infants and adults. Many cases of pertussis have occurred in children less than 6 months or persons over 7 years, with both groups falling in the category for which pertussis immunisation previously was not recommended. Pertussis vaccine is only available in Australia in combination with diphtheria and tetanus. Vaccines may also include inactivated poliovirus, hepatitis B and *Haemophilus influenzae* type b. The acronym DTPa, using capital letters, signifies a child formulation of diphtheria, tetanus and acellular pertussis-containing vaccine. The acronym dTpa signifies a formulation that contains substantially less diphtheria toxoid and pertussis antigens than the child formulation. dTpa is recommended between ages 11 and 13 years for persons who have completed the DTPa childhood schedule. The dTpa is also recommended for adolescents 13 to 18 years old who have not received a tetanus booster (dT) or dTpa dose and have completed the childhood DTPa schedule. When the dTpa is used as a booster dose, it may be administered regardless of the interval from the previous tetanus, diphtheria and pertussis-containing vaccine. Children aged 7 through 10 years who are not fully vaccinated for pertussis (i.e. did not receive five doses of DTPa or four doses of DTPa with the fourth dose being administered on or after the fourth birthday) should receive a dose of dTpa (ATAGI 2018).

The Australian Immunisation Handbook (ATAGI 2018) recommends women, including adolescents, receive the dTpa vaccine during each pregnancy, including pregnancies that are closely spaced, optimally between 20 and 32 weeks' gestation or postpartum before discharge from the hospital. Breastfeeding is not a contraindication to dTpa vaccination. The concept of cocooning is promoted to reduce the spread of pertussis to vulnerable infants. Cocooning involves the strategy of vaccinating pregnant women during or after pregnancy, as well as all persons who will have close contact with the infants (including healthcare workers, fathers and adults [especially those aged 65 years and older]) (Rowe et al 2018). Cocooning can prevent pertussis in vulnerable infants; however, actual implantation of the cocooning strategy among all family members is difficult (Rowe et al 2018).

Healthcare workers who may be susceptible to pertussis as a result of waning immunity and who have potential exposure to children or adults with pertussis should receive a single dose of dTpa (if not previously vaccinated with same) and take the necessary protective precautions against droplet contamination (i.e. wear procedural or surgical masks and practise handwashing). The diagnosis of pertussis may be missed or delayed in unvaccinated infants, who often are seen with respiratory distress and apnoea without the typical cough.

Pertussis (both suspected and confirmed) is a notifiable disease in all states and territories in Australia and New Zealand (Communicable Disease Network Australia [CDNA] 2020, Ministry of Health 2020c). National guidelines are available with details about the management of pertussis cases and contacts.

Polio. Inactivated poliovirus (IPV)–containing vaccine is recommended for infants and children in a four-dose schedule at 2, 4 and 6 months and at 4 years of age. Infants can have their first dose of IPV-containing vaccine as early as 6 weeks of age. Infants and children receive IPV vaccines in combination with DTPa-HepB and Hib (*Haemophilus influenzae* type b) in one injection (ATAGI 2018). The use of combination vaccines provides equivalent immunogenicity and decreases the number of injections an infant receives. However, it is important that they be given to the appropriate-age child.

Measles, Mumps and Rubella. Measles, mumps and rubella are highly infectious viral illnesses that are transmitted by respiratory aerosols. It is recommended that children have the MMR (measles, mumps and rubella) vaccine at 12 months of age, and then at 18 months of age the MMRV (measles, mumps, rubella and varicella) vaccine (ATAGI 2018). During the course of measles outbreaks, the MMR vaccine can be given at 6 to 11 months of age, followed by a second inoculation after 12 months of age. The MMRV vaccine is an attenuated live virus vaccine and may be given to children at 18 months of age.

People who receive the MMR vaccine may develop a fever 7 to 10 days (range 5 to 12 days) after vaccination. This can last 2 to 3 days. The fever may be associated with malaise and/or a non-infectious rash. Up to 15% of MMR vaccine recipients develop a high fever (> 39.4°C) (Strebel et al 2018). An increased risk of febrile seizures of about one case per 3000 to 4000 doses occurs in the same time period. The risks and benefits of administering the MMRV vaccine should be fully explained to the parent or caregiver including how to manage the symptoms, such as using paracetamol for fever.

Rubella is a relatively mild infection in children, but in a pregnant woman the actual infection presents serious risks to the developing fetus. Therefore, the aim of rubella immunisation is actually protection of the unborn child rather than the recipient of the immunisation.

Increased emphasis should also be placed on vaccinating all unimmunised prepubertal children and susceptible adolescents and adult women in the childbearing age group. Postpubertal females without evidence of rubella immunity should be immunised unless they are pregnant; they should be counselled not to become pregnant for 28 days after receiving the rubella-containing vaccine (ATAGI 2018). Because the live attenuated virus may cross the placenta and theoretically present a risk to the developing fetus, rubella vaccine is currently not given to any pregnant woman.

Varicella.A varicella-containing vaccine is recommended for all children aged 12 months to < 14 years (ATAGI, 2019) According to the schedule for immunisations in Australia and New Zealand, infants receive the MMRV (measles-mumps-rubella-varicella) vaccine at 18 months of age. A second dose of varicella-containing vaccine can provide extra protection and minimise the chance of breakthrough varicella in children <14 years of age; however, is it not included in the schedule. Adolescents (≥14 years of age) and adults need to receive 2 doses of varicella vaccine to achieve adequate protection from varicella. The 2 doses should be given at least 4 weeks apart (ATAGI, 2018). This can be administered as a monovalent varicella vaccine. Varicellacontaining vaccine may also be given simultaneously with DTaP, IPV, HepB or Hib (ATAGI, 2019). The vaccine is administered subcutaneously.

Haemophilus Influenzae Type B. Hib conjugate vaccines protect against a number of serious infections caused by *H. influenzae* type b, especially bacterial meningitis, epiglottitis, bacterial pneumonia, septic arthritis and sepsis. (Hib is not associated with the viruses that cause influenza, or 'flu'). It is recommended that infants and children receive Hib-containing vaccine at 2, 4, 6 and 18 months of age. Infants can receive their first dose from 6 weeks (ATAGI 2018). All Hib-containing vaccines are administered by intramuscular injection using a separate syringe and at a site separate from any concurrent vaccinations.

Pneumococcal Disease. *Streptococcus pneumoniae* is responsible for a number of bacterial infections in children under 2 years, which may cause serious morbidity and mortality. Among these are generalised infections, such as septicaemia and meningitis, or localised infections, such as otitis media, sinusitis and pneumonia. These illnesses are particularly problematic in children who attend day care facilities (the incidence in day care children is two or three times higher than in children not attending out-of-home day care) and in those who are immunocompromised. A 13-valent pneumococcal vaccine (13vPCV [Prevenar 13]) is currently recommended as the standard pneumococcal vaccine for children aged 6 weeks to 24 months old. The 13vPCV vaccine is administered at 2, 4 and 12 months of age. Infants can receive their first dose of pneumococcal conjugate vaccine as early as 6 weeks of age. If the first dose is given at the age of 6 weeks, infants should still receive their next scheduled dose at 4 months of age.

In addition to the three doses for all children < 5 years of age, it is recommended that Aboriginal and Torres Strait Islander children living in the Northern Territory, Queensland, South Australia and Western Australia receive an additional dose of 13vPCV at 6 months of age (ATAGI 2018). This is because of the higher risk of pneumococcal disease in these children (Naidu et al 2013). It is also recommended that these children receive two doses of 23vPPV, one dose at 4 years of age and a second dose at least 5 years later. This is because a considerable proportion of pneumococcal disease in these children is caused by serotypes that are present in 23vPPV but not in 13vPCV. The 13vPCV and 23vPPV vaccine may be administered in conjunction with all other immunisations in a separate syringe and at a separate intramuscular site.

Influenza. The annual influenza vaccine is recommended annually for everyone > 6 months of age, particularly children aged > 6 months to < 5 years and Aboriginal and Torres Strait Islander people. The vaccine is not funded by Australia's National Immunisation Program. The vaccine is administered in early autumn before the flu season begins and is repeated yearly for ongoing protection. The intramuscular vaccine is administered as two separate doses 4 weeks apart in first-time recipients younger than 9 years old (ATAGI, 2021). The vaccine may be given simultaneously with other vaccines but in a separate syringe and at a separate site. The vaccine is administered yearly because different strains of influenza are used each year in the manufacture of the vaccine.

The Australian Immunisation Handbook (ATAGI 2018) recommends an assessment of the egg allergenic reaction—mild (such as hives alone) versus severe (such as an anaphylactic reaction)—before making a decision about the vaccine administration to children who have a history of egg allergy. Several options for administering the influenza vaccine are described in the literature, and individuals should discuss the risks and benefits with a knowledgeable healthcare practitioner.

The pandemic of H1N1 in 2009–2010 caused significant morbidity and mortality worldwide, but particularly in Mexico and the United States. **Antigenic shift** occurs when influenza viruses undergo significant changes that result in new infection subtypes; such is the case in the 2009 pandemic. The signs and symptoms of H1N1 flu are the same as those mentioned for influenza.

Meningococcal Disease. Meningococcal disease is caused by the bacterium *Neisseria meningitidis*. There are 13 known meningococcal serogroups, distinguished by differences in surface polysaccharides of the bacterium's outer membrane capsule. Globally, serogroups A, B, C, W-135 and Y most commonly cause disease (ATAGI 2018).

Invasive meningococcal disease is a rare but serious condition, often presenting as septicaemia and/or meningitis (ATAGI 2018). Infants younger than 1 year of age are particularly susceptible, yet the highest fatalities occur in adolescents and young adults. Meningococcal infections are also responsible for significant morbidities, including limb or digit amputation, skin scarring, hearing loss and neurological disabilities.

Infants can receive MenACWY and MenB vaccines from as early as 6 weeks of age. Dose schedules are dependent on vaccine brand used and age of child when first dose administered. Nurses must consult an Australian or New Zealand Immunisation Handbook for confirmation.

MenB vaccination is included in the Australian NIPS for Aboriginal and Torres Strait Islander infants and children at 6 weeks, 2 months, 4 months, 6 months and 12 months. MenACWY is on the Australian NIPS for both Indigenous and non-Indigenous children at 12 months and again between 14 and 16 years (ATAGI 2018).

Rotavirus. Rotavirus is one of the leading causes of severe diarrhoea in infants and young children and is transmitted by the faecal-oral route. The incidence of rotavirus has decreased dramatically since rotavirus vaccines became available in 2006. Infants in Australia and New Zealand are routinely immunised with either three doses of RotaTeq at 2, 4 and 6 months of age or two doses of Rotarix at 2 and 4 months of age. RotaTeq is licensed for administration to infants at 6 to 14 weeks of age, with two additional doses administered at 4- to 10-week intervals but not after 32 weeks of age (ATAGI 2018). Rotarix (1 mL) may be administered beginning at 6 weeks of age, with a second dose at least 4 weeks after the first dose but before 24 (AM) weeks of age (ATAGI 2018). Both vaccines are administered orally. Infants who contract rotavirus infection before completing the vaccine series should complete the vaccinations following the standard intervals (ATAGI 2018).

Human Papillomavirus. Human papillomaviruses (HPVs) are a large family of viruses that consist of cutaneous (i.e. skin wart) and genital (i.e. mucosal) types. Genital HPVs can be classified as low risk and high risk according to their association with cancers. Three human papillomavirus (HPV) vaccines have been licensed for use in adolescents but Gardasil 9 is the only HPV vaccine available in Australia and New Zealand. The vaccine is administered intramuscularly, preferably in the deltoid muscle, in three separate doses; the first dose in the series is commonly administered at 11 to 12 years of age; the second dose is given 2 months after the first; and the third dose is given 6 months after the first dose (ATAGI 2018). The vaccine is recommended for both boys and girls at a minimum age of 9 years and a maximum age of 26 years (ATAGI 2018). Women who receive the HPV vaccines must continue to have regular cervical screening tests (ATAGI 2018).

COVID-19. COVID-19 (SARS-CoV-2) is a coronavirus belonging to the β-coronavirus cluster (Sun et al 2020). Coronaviruses cause a wide range of illness, ranging from the common cold to severe, fatal illness. Since the World Health Organization (WHO) declared coronavirus disease 2019 (COVID-19, the disease caused by SARS-CoV-2) a pandemic health emergency in 2020 (WHO 2020) scientists have worked tirelessly to develop a vaccine.

All COVID-19 vaccines used in Australia and New Zealand require approval by the Therapeutic Goods Administration (TGA) in Australia or Medsafe in New Zealand which both have a rigorous process to ensure the safety, quality and efficacy of vaccines (AGDH 2021, Ministry of Health 2021). The TGA has approved two vaccines for use in Australia: BNT162b2 (BioNTech/Pfizer) and ChAdOx1 nCoV-19/AZD1222 (AstraZeneca) (AGDH 2021). Medsafe has approved BNT162b2 (BioNTech/Pfizer) for use in New Zealand (Ministry of Health 2021). Rollout has begun in both countries but neither vaccine is approved for children at the time of writing.

Ensuring public confidence in both the safety and the effectiveness of COVID-19 vaccines will be critical to achieving high vaccine uptake among target populations during vaccine rollout in Australia and New Zealand. As COVID-19 vaccines become available for use in children, nurses can take early steps to prepare for vaccine introduction, such as ensuring connectivity to the Australian Immunisation Register and engagement with other systems such as adverse events following immunisation reporting (McIntyre et al 2021). In the meantime protective measures, including improving personal hygiene, wearing medical masks and keeping rooms well ventilated, can effectively prevent COVID-19 (Sun et al 2020). Nurses must be aware of and adhere to COVID-19 policies and protocols and COVID-19 safety plans within their workplace.

Reactions

Vaccines for routine immunisations are among the safest and most reliable drugs available. However, minor side effects do occur after many of the immunisations and, rarely, a serious reaction may result from the vaccine. A number of inactive components are incorporated in vaccines to enhance their effectiveness and safety. Some of these components include preservatives, stabilisers, adjuvants, antibiotics (e.g. neomycin) and purified culture medium proteins (e.g. egg) to enhance effectiveness. A child may react to the preservative in the vaccine rather than the vaccine component; an example of this is the hepatitis B vaccine, which is prepared from yeast cultures. Therefore, yeast hypersensitivity would preclude one from receiving that particular vaccine without consulting an allergist. Trace amounts of neomycin are used to decrease bacterial growth within certain vaccine preparations, and persons with documented anaphylactic reactions to neomycin should avoid those vaccines.

Most vaccine preparations now contain vial stoppers with a synthetic rubber to prevent latex allergy reactions, but healthcare personnel administering vaccines should make sure that the package insert specifies there is no latex in the stopper. In the event that an individual has a severe reaction to a vaccine and subsequent immunisations are required, an allergist should be consulted to determine the best course of action. Although influenza vaccines contain small amounts of egg protein, recent evidence shows no risk of an anaphylactic reaction with the inactivated influenza vaccine among children with an egg allergy and these children should receive the influenza vaccine (ATAGI 2018). Some vaccines contain a preservative, thimerosal, which contains ethyl mercury. Concerns regarding possible mercury poisoning in the 1990s prompted many to put off vaccination of infants and small children for fear of childhood developmental problems, such as autism. A number of manufacturers have since stopped producing vaccines containing thimerosal. No local hypersensitivity reactions to thimerosal have been recorded, and studies on thimerosal and the potential link to autism or any other pervasive developmental disorder failed to establish a causal relationship between the two (DeStefano et al 2013, Yoshimasu et al 2014). The Institute of Medicine (2004), following an in-depth 3-year study, concluded that there was no link between autism and the MMR vaccine or vaccines containing the preservative thimerosal.

With inactivated antigens, such as DTPa, side effects are most likely to occur within a few hours or days of administration and are usually limited to: local tenderness, erythema and swelling at the injection site; low-grade fever; and behavioural changes (e.g. drowsiness, eating less, prolonged or unusual cry). Local reactions tend to be less severe when a needle of sufficient length to deposit the vaccine in the muscle is used (see Nursing Care Considerations box). Rarely, more severe reactions may occur. If adrenaline is administered, observe for adverse reactions such as tachycardia, hypertension, irritability, headaches, nausea and tremors.

NURSING CARE CONSIDERATIONS

Immunisations

Needle length and injection techniques are important factors and must be considered for each individual child. Fewer reactions to immunisations are observed when the vaccine is given deep into the muscle rather than into subcutaneous tissue. The dorsogluteal site is not recommended as an injection site for children because of the potential for sciatic nerve damage (Rishovd 2014). In addition, aspiration for blood is no longer recommended for an intramuscular injection because large blood vessels are not present at recommended injection sites and slow aspiration causes more pain than injection without aspiration (Rishovd 2014).

To ensure appropriate needle size for vaccine administration (Rishovd 2014):

- newborns (0–28 days old)—recommended needle size is 16 mm, 22 to 25 gauge, recommended injection site: vastus lateralis
- infant/toddler (1 month to 2 years)—recommended needle size/site is 25 mm, 22 to 25 gauge for vastus lateralis or 16 to 25 mm, 22 to 25 gauge in the deltoid only if muscle mass is adequately developed
- child/adolescent (3 to 18 years)—less than 60 kg: 16 to 25 mm, 22 to 25 gauge in deltoid; greater than 60 kg: 25 to 38 mm, 22 to 25 gauge in deltoid.

Use one or more of the following techniques to minimise pain (Rishovd 2014, World Health Organization 2015).

- Apply topical anaesthetic EMLA (lidocaine [lignocaine]-prilocaine) to the injection site and cover with an occlusive dressing for at least 1 hour.
- Ensure comfort positioning of the patient: being held by a parent or caregiver for infants and young children, and sitting upright for older children and adolescents.
- Encourage breastfeeding during or before the immunisations.
- For children less than 6 years old, use distraction, such as asking the child to blow bubbles or telling the child to 'take a deep breath and blow and blow and blow until I tell you to stop'. Evidence does not show any benefit in using distraction during injections with adolescents.
- Nurses administering the injections should remain calm and use neutral words such as 'here I go' instead of 'here comes the sting'.

Do not manually stimulate (i.e. rubbing or applying pressure) the injection site.

MEDICATION SAFETY

Emergency Management of Anaphylaxis

EpiPen Jr (150mcg; or 0.01mg/kg of 1:1000) intramuscularly (IM) for child weighing 7.5 kg to 20 kg

EpiPen (300mcg; 0.01mg/kg of 1:1000 up to 0.5mg per dose) IM for child weighing 20 kg or more

Source: Australian Society of Clinical Immunology and Allergy (ASCIA). (2019). ASCIA Guidelines. https://www.allergy.org.au/hp/anaphylaxis/adrenaline-autoinjector-prescription

Contraindications and Precautions

Nurses need to be aware of the reasons for withholding immunisations—both for the child's safety in terms of avoiding reactions and for the child's maximum benefit from receiving the vaccine. Unfounded fears and lack of knowledge regarding contraindications can needlessly prevent a child from having protection from life-threatening diseases. Issues that have surfaced regarding vaccines include the misconception that administering combination vaccines may overload the child's immune system; the combined vaccines have undergone rigorous study in relation to side effects and immunogenicity rates following administration. Others may express concern that vaccines are not a part of the individual's natural immunity and that administering too many vaccines may decrease the child's immunity to such diseases. A recent evaluation of parents' vaccination concerns identified through posts on social media found that parents were concerned about adverse reactions, such as autism, pain, compromised immunity and death associated with vaccinations (Tangherlini et al 2016).

A *contraindication* is considered as a condition in an individual that increases the risk for a serious adverse reaction (e.g. not administering a live virus vaccine to a severely immuno-compromised child). Thus one would not administer a vaccine when a contraindication is present. A *precaution* is a condition in a recipient that might increase the risk for a serious adverse reaction or that might compromise the ability of the vaccine to produce immunity. If conditions are such that the benefit of receiving the vaccine would outweigh the risk of an adverse event or incomplete response, a precaution would not prevent vaccine administration (ATAGI 2018).

The general contraindication for all immunisations is a severe febrile illness. This precaution avoids adding the risk of adverse side effects from the vaccine to an already ill child or mistakenly identifying a symptom of the disease as having been caused by the vaccine. The presence of minor illnesses, such as the common cold, is not a contraindication. Live virus vaccines are generally not administered to anyone with an altered immune system because multiplication of the virus may be enhanced, causing a severe vaccine-induced illness.

In general, live virus vaccines should not be administered to persons who are severely immunocompromised or among persons whose immune function is not known (ATAGI 2018). Another contraindication to live virus vaccines (e.g. MMR, varicella and rotavirus) is the presence of recently acquired passive immunity through blood transfusions, immunoglobulin or maternal antibodies. Administration of MMR and varicella should be postponed for a minimum of 3 months after passive immunisation with immunoglobulins and blood transfusions (except washed red blood cells, which do not interfere with the immune response). Suggested intervals between administration of immunoglobulin preparations and MMR and varicella depend on the type of immune product and dosage. If the vaccine and immunoglobulin are given simultaneously because of imminent exposure to disease, the two preparations are injected at sites far from each other. Vaccination should be repeated after the suggested intervals unless there is serological evidence of antibody production.

A final contraindication is a known allergic response to a previously administered vaccine or a substance in the vaccine. An anaphylactic reaction to a vaccine or its component is a true contraindication. MMR vaccines contain minute amounts of neomycin; measles and mumps vaccines, which are grown on chick embryo tissue cultures, are not believed to contain significant amounts of egg cross-reacting proteins. Therefore, only a history of anaphylactic reaction to neomycin, gelatine or the vaccine itself is considered a contraindication to their use.

Pregnancy is a contraindication to MMR vaccines, although the risk of fetal damage is primarily theoretic. Breastfeeding is not a contraindication for any vaccine. The only vaccine virus that has been isolated in human milk is rubella, and there is no indication that this is harmful to infants; rubella infection in an infant as a result of exposure to rubella virus in human milk would likely be well tolerated because the vaccine is attenuated (ATAGI 2018).

To identify the rare child who may not be able to receive the vaccines, take a careful allergy history. If the child has a history of anaphylaxis, report this to the practitioner before administering the vaccine. Contact dermatitis in reaction to neomycin is not considered a contraindication to immunisation. Evidence indicates that children who are egg sensitive are not at increased risk for untoward reactions to MMR vaccine. Furthermore, skin testing of egg-allergic children with vaccine has failed to predict immediate hypersensitivity reactions (ATAGI 2018). A family history of seizures, or adverse events following vaccination, penicillin allergy, allergies to duck meat or duck feathers and a family history of sudden unexpected death in infancy (SUDI) are not considered contraindications to receiving childhood vaccines (ATAGI 2018).

Nurses are at the forefront in providing parents with appropriate information regarding childhood immunisation benefits, contraindications and side effects and the effects of non-vaccine and their interaction with patients and parents is a critical factor shaping parental attitudes to vaccination (Leask et al 2012). Nurses often administer vaccines, and thus they may have the responsibility for obtaining valid informed consent by adequately informing parents of: the nature, prevalence and risks of the disease; the type of immunisation product to be used; the expected benefits and risks of side effects of the vaccine; and the need for accurate immunisation records.

Some suggestions for communicating with parents about the benefits of immunisations in childhood and obtaining consent prior to administration is to include the following (ATAGI 2018, Leask et al 2012).

- Provide accurate and user-friendly information on vaccines (the necessity for each one, the disease each prevents, potential adverse effects).
- Acknowledge the parent's concerns in a genuine, empathetic manner.
- Tailor the discussion to the needs of the parent; avoid judgmental or threatening language.
- Be knowledgeable about the benefits of individual vaccines, the common adverse effects and how to minimise those effects.
- Help the parent make an informed decision regarding the administration of each vaccine.
- Communicate risk effectively. Give information about common but minor side effects, and rare but serious ones.
- Use written materials, web links or decision aids that can be given prior to, or used during, the consultation.
- Be flexible and provide options to parents regarding the administration of multiple vaccines, especially in infants, who must receive multiple injections at 2, 4 and 6 months (i.e. allow parents to space the vaccinations at different visits to decrease the total number of injections at each visit; make provisions for office visits for immunisation purposes 'only,' (not necessary to mention 'fee' in ANZ contexts) provided the child is healthy).
- Involve the parent in minimising the potential adverse effects of the vaccine (e.g. administering an appropriate dose of paracetamol 45 minutes before administering the vaccine [as warranted], following up to check on the child if untoward reactions have occurred in the past or parent is especially anxious about the child's wellbeing).
- Respect the parent's ultimate wishes.

Although immunisation rates have increased significantly, health professionals should use every opportunity to encourage complete immunisation of all.

Administration

The principal precautions in administering immunisations include proper storage of the vaccine to protect its potency and institution of recommended procedures for injection. The nurse must be familiar with the manufacturer's directions for storage and reconstitution of the vaccine. For example, if the vaccine is to be refrigerated, it should be stored in a dedicated vaccine fridge on a centre shelf, not in the door, where frequent temperature increases from opening the refrigerator can alter the vaccine's potency.

The DTPa vaccines contain an adjuvant to retain the antigen at the injection site and prolong the stimulatory effect. Because subcutaneous or intracutaneous injection of the adjuvant can cause local irritation, inflammation or abscess formation, excellent intramuscular injection technique must be used (see Nursing Care Considerations: Immunisation box earlier in this chapter).

The total series requires several injections, and every attempt is made to rotate the sites and administer the injections as painlessly as possible. (See discussion on intramuscular injections, Chapter 22.) When two or more injections are given at separate sites, the order of injections is arbitrary. Some practitioners suggest injecting the less painful one first. Some believe this is DTP (or DTaP), whereas others suggest the MMR or Hib vaccine. Still others advocate injecting at two sites simultaneously (requires two operators) (see Research Focus box).

RESEARCH FOCUS

Order of Injections

Ipp and colleagues (2009) evaluated the administration order of the diphtheria-tetanus, acellular pertussis and *Haemophilus influenzae* type b (DTPa-Hib) vaccine and pneumococcal conjugate vaccine (13vPCV) and pain perception in 120 infants 2 to 6 months of age. The infants who were given the primary DTPa-Hib vaccine before the 13vPCV vaccine had significantly lower pain scores than those who received the 13vPCV vaccine first. Fallah and colleagues (2016) evaluated the best order for immunisations: intramuscular injection (diphtheria, pertussis and tetanus) versus subcutaneous injection (measles, mumps and rubella) among 70 children. Pain was significantly lower when the subcutaneous injection was administered before the intramuscular injection.

One of the most important features of injecting vaccines is adequate penetration of the muscle for deposition of the drug intramuscularly and not subcutaneously (depending on the manufacturer's recommendation for administration). The use of appropriate needle length is an essential component of administering vaccines. A recent systematic review reported the appropriate needle size to be 16 mm for infants less than 28 days old; 25 mm for infants 1 month to 2 years; and 16 mm if the skin is stretched tightly and not bunched to 25 mm for children 3 to 18 years (Beirne et al 2015). In two studies, the use of longer needles significantly decreased the incidence of localised oedema and tenderness when vaccines were administered to a group of infants (Diggle & Deeks 2000, Diggle et al 2006). Similar findings have been recorded for children 4 to 6 years of age receiving the fifth DTPa vaccine (Jackson et al 2011).

Another important nursing responsibility is accurate documentation. Each child should have an immunisation record for parents to keep, especially for families who move frequently. In Australia all people, of all ages and who are enrolled in Medicare are included in the Australian Immunisation Register (AIR), a national register that records all vaccines given to all people in Australia. Prompt and correct submission of data to the AIR is essential. It provides a central record of the vaccination history of every Medicare-registered Australian and AIR data is used to determine a family's entitlement to government family assistance payments (ATAGI 2018). In New Zealand, immunisations are recorded on the National Immunisation Register (NIR) (Ministry of Health 2015).

On the patient's medical record, document the following information: day, month and year of administration; manufacturer and lot number of vaccine; and name, address and title of the person administering the vaccine. Additional data to record are the site and route of administration and evidence that the parent or legal guardian gave informed consent before the immunisation was administered. Report any adverse reactions after the administration of a vaccine to the state or territory authorities or directly to the Therapeutic Goods Administration (TGA) Australian Adverse Drug Reaction Reporting System https://www.ebs.tga.gov.au/ebs/ADRS/ADRSRepo.nsf?OpenDatabase.

COMMUNICABLE DISEASES

The incidence of childhood communicable diseases has declined significantly since the advent of immunisations. The use of antibiotics and antitoxins has further reduced serious complications resulting from such infections. However, infectious diseases do occur, and nurses must be familiar with the infectious agent to recognise the disease and to institute appropriate preventive and supportive interventions (Table 6.1 and Figs 6.1 to 6.6).

Nursing Care Management

Table 6.1 describes the more common communicable diseases of childhood, their therapeutic management and specific nursing care. The following is a general discussion of nursing care management for communicable diseases.

Identification of the infectious agent is of primary importance to prevent exposure to susceptible individuals. Nurses in ambulatory care settings, childcare centres and schools are often the first persons to see signs of a communicable disease, such as a rash or sore throat. The nurse must operate under a high index of suspicion for common childhood diseases to identify potentially infectious cases and to recognise diseases that require medical intervention.

When the nurse suspects a communicable disease, it is important to assess the following:

- recent exposure to a known case
- **prodromal symptoms** (symptoms that occur between early manifestations of the disease and its overt clinical syndrome) or evidence of constitutional symptoms, such as a fever or rash (see Table 6.1)
- immunisation history
- history of having the disease.

Immunisations are available for many diseases, and infection usually confers lifelong immunity; therefore, the possibility of many infectious agents can be eliminated based on these two criteria.

Prevent Spread

Prevention consists of two components: prevention of the disease; and control of its spread to others. **Primary prevention** rests almost exclusively on immunisation.

Control measures to prevent spread of disease should include techniques to reduce risk of cross-transmission of infectious organisms between patients and to protect healthcare workers from organisms harboured by patients. If the child is hospitalised, follow the facility's policies for infection control. The most important procedure is handwashing. Persons directly caring for the child or handling contaminated articles must wash their hands and practise effective standard precautions in the care of their patients.

Instruct the child to practise good handwashing technique after toileting and before eating. For those diseases spread by droplets, instruct the parents in measures to reduce airborne transmission. The child who is old enough should use a tissue to cover the face during coughing or sneezing; otherwise the parent should cover the child's mouth with a tissue and then discard it in the bin. Stress the usual hygiene measures of not sharing eating and drinking utensils to the family.

TABLE 6.1 Communicable Diseases of Childhood

Disease	Clinical Manifestations	Therapeutic Management and Complications	Nursing Care Management
CHICKENPOX (VARICELLA) (FIG 6.1)			
Agents—Varicella-zoster virus (VZV) **Source**—Primary secretions of respiratory tract of infected persons; to a lesser degree, skin lesions (scabs not infectious) **Transmissions**—Direct contact, droplet (airborne) spread and contaminated objects **Incubation period**—2–3 weeks, usually 14–16 days **Period of communicability**—Probably 1 day before eruption of lesions (prodromal period) to 6 days after first crop of vesicles when crusts have formed	**Prodromal stage**—Slight fever, malaise and anorexia for first 24 hours; rash highly pruritic; begins as macule, rapidly progresses to papule and then vesicle (surrounded by erythematous base; becomes umbilicated and cloudy; breaks easily and forms crusts); all three stages (papule, vesicle, crust) present in varying degrees at one time **Distribution**—Centripetal, spreading to face and proximal extremities but sparse on distal limbs and less on areas not exposed to heat (i.e. from clothing or sun) **Constitutional signs and symptoms**—Elevated temperature from lymphadenopathy, irritability from pruritus	**Specific**—Antiviral agent aciclovir (Zovirax); varicella-zoster immune globulin or intravenous immune globulin (IVIg) after exposure in high-risk children **Supportive**—Diphenhydramine hydrochloride or antihistamines to relieve itching; skin care to prevent secondary bacterial infection **Complications**—Secondary bacterial infections (abscesses, cellulitis, necrotising fasciitis, pneumonia, sepsis) Encephalitis Varicella pneumonia (rare in healthy children) Haemorrhagic varicella (tiny haemorrhages in vesicles and numerous petechiae in skin) Chronic or transient thrombocytopenia **Preventive**—Childhood immunisation	Maintain standard, airborne and contact precautions if hospitalised until all lesions are crusted; for immunised child with mild breakthrough varicella, isolate until no new lesions are seen. Keep child in home away from susceptible individuals until vesicles have dried (usually 1 week after onset of disease), and isolate high-risk children from infected children. Administer skin care: give bath and change clothes and linens daily; administer topical calamine lotion; keep child's fingernails short and clean; apply mittens if child scratches. Keep child cool (may decrease number of lesions). Lessen pruritus; keep child occupied. Remove loose crusts that rub and irritate skin. Teach child to apply pressure to pruritic area rather than scratching it. Avoid use of aspirin (possible association with Reye's syndrome).
ERYTHEMA INFECTIOSUM (FIFTH DISEASE) (FIG 6.2)			
Agent—Human parvovirus B19 **Source**—Infected persons, mainly school-age children **Transmission**—Respiratory secretions and blood, blood products **Incubation period**—4–14 days; may be as long as 21 days **Period of communicability**—Uncertain but before on-set of symptoms in children with aplastic crisis	Rash appears in three stages: **I**—Erythema on face, chiefly on cheeks ('slapped face' appearance); disappears by 1–4 days **II**—About 1 day after rash appears on face, maculopapular red spots appear, symmetrically distributed on upper and lower extremities; rash progresses from proximal to distal surfaces and may last ≥1 week **III**—Rash subsides but reappears if skin is irritated or traumatised (sun, heat, cold, friction) In children with aplastic crisis, rash usually absent and prodromal illness includes fever, myalgia, lethargy, nausea, vomiting and abdominal pain Child with sickle cell disease may have concurrent vaso-occlusive crisis	**Symptomatic and supportive**—Antipyretics, analgesics, anti-inflammatory drugs Possible blood transfusion for transient aplastic anaemia **Complications**—Self-limited arthritis and arthralgia (arthritis may become chronic); more common in adult women May result in serious complications (anaemia, hydrops) or fetal death if mother infected during pregnancy (primarily second trimester) Aplastic crisis in children with haemolytic disease or immunodeficiency Myocarditis (rare)	Isolation of child is not necessary, except hospitalised child (immunosuppressed or with aplastic crises) suspected of parvovirus infection is placed on droplet precautions and standard precautions. Pregnant women need not be excluded from workplace where parvovirus infection is present; they should not care for patients with aplastic crises. Explain low risk of fetal death to those in contact with affected children; assist with routine fetal ultrasound for detection of fetal hydrops.
EXANTHEM SUBITUM (ROSEOLA INFANTUM) (FIG 6.3)			
Agent—Human herpesvirus type 6 (HHV-6; rarely HHV-7) **Source**—Possibly acquired from saliva of healthy adult person; entry via nasal, buccal or conjunctival mucosa	Persistent high fever > 39.5°C for 3–7 days in child who appears well Precipitous drop in fever to normal with appearance of rash Bulging fontanel	Non-specific Antipyretics to control fever **Complications**—Recurrent febrile seizures (possibly from latent infection of central nervous system that is reactivated by fever)	Use standard precautions. Teach parents measures for lowering temperature (antipyretic drugs); ensure adequate parental understanding of specific antipyretic dosage to prevent accidental overdose.

Continued

TABLE 6.1 Communicable Diseases of Childhood—cont'd

Disease	Clinical Manifestations	Therapeutic Management and Complications	Nursing Care Management
Transmission—Year round; no reported contact with infected individual in most cases (virtually limited to children < 3 years but peak age is 6–15 months old) **Incubation period**—Usually 5–15 days **Period of communicability**—Unknown	Rash—Discrete rose-pink macules or maculopapules appearing first on trunk, then spreading to neck, face and extremities; non-pruritic; fades on pressure; lasts 1–2 days **Associated signs and symptoms**—Cervical and postauricular lymphadenopathy, inflamed pharynx, cough, coryza	Encephalitis Hepatitis (rare)	If child is prone to seizures, discuss appropriate precautions and possibility of recurrent febrile seizures.
MEASLES (RUBEOLA) (FIG 6.4)			
Agent—Virus **Source**—Respiratory tract secretions, blood and urine of infected person **Transmission**—Usually by direct contact with droplets of infected person; primarily in the winter **Incubation period**—10–20 days **Period of communicability**—From 4 days before to 5 days after rash appears, but mainly during prodromal (catarrhal) stage	**Prodromal (catarrhal) stage**—Fever and malaise, followed in 24 hours by coryza, cough, conjunctivitis, Koplik's spots (small, irregular red spots with a minute, bluish-white centre first seen on buccal mucosa opposite molars 2 days before rash); symptoms gradually increasing in severity until second day after rash appears, when they begin to subside Rash—Appears 3–4 days after onset of prodromal stage; begins as erythematous maculopapular eruption on face and gradually spreads downwards; more severe in earlier sites (appears confluent) and less intense in later sites (appears discrete); after 3–4 days assumes brownish appearance, and fine desquamation occurs over area of extensive involvement **Constitutional signs and symptoms**—Anorexia, abdominal pain, malaise, generalised lymphadenopathy	**Preventive**—Childhood immunisation **Supportive**—Bed rest during febrile period; antipyretics Antibiotics to prevent secondary bacterial infection in high-risk children **Complications**—Otitis media Pneumonia (bacterial) Obstructive laryngitis and laryngotracheitis Encephalitis (rare but has high mortality) **Treatment**—Administer vitamin A (World Health Organization recommendation) for children with acute illness: 200,000 international units for children 12 months and older; 100,000 international units for children 6 through 11 months old; 50,000 international units for infants younger than 6 months	Maintain isolation until fifth day of rash; if child is hospitalised, institute airborne precautions. Encourage rest during prodromal stage; provide quiet activity. Fever—Instruct parents to administer antipyretics; avoid chilling; if child is prone to seizures, institute appropriate precautions. Eye care—Dim lights if photophobia present; clean eyelids with warm saline solution to remove secretions or crusts; keep child from rubbing eyes. Coryza, cough—Use cool-mist vaporiser; protect skin around nares with layer of petrolatum; encourage fluids and soft, bland foods. Skin care—Keep skin clean; use tepid baths as necessary.
PERTUSSIS (WHOOPING COUGH)			
Agent—Bordetella pertussis **Source**—Discharge from respiratory tract of infected persons **Transmission**—Direct contact or droplet spread from infected person; indirect contact with freshly contaminated articles **Incubation period**—6–20 days; usually 7–10 days **Period of communicability**—Greatest during catarrhal stage before onset of paroxysms	**Catarrhal stage**—Begins with symptoms of upper respiratory tract infection, such as coryza, sneezing, lacrimation, cough and low-grade fever; symptoms continue for 1–2 weeks, when dry, hacking cough becomes more severe **Paroxysmal stage**—Cough most common at night, consists of short, rapid coughs followed by sudden inspiration associated with a high-pitched crowing sound or 'whoop'; during paroxysms, cheeks become flushed or cyanotic, eyes bulge and tongue protrudes; paroxysm may continue until thick mucus plug is dislodged; vomiting frequently follows attack; stage generally lasts 4–6 weeks, followed by convalescent stage Infants < 6 months old may not have characteristic whoop cough, but have difficulty maintaining adequate oxygenation with amount of secretions, frequent vomiting of mucus and formula or breast milk	**Preventive**—Immunisation; current belief is that childhood immunisations for pertussis do not confer lifelong immunity to adolescents and adults, so a pertussis booster is recommended for adolescents (see Immunisations section in this chapter) Antimicrobial therapy (e.g. erythromycin, clarithromycin, azithromycin) **Supportive**—Hospitalisation sometimes required for infants, children who are dehydrated or those who have complications Increased oxygen intake and humidity Adequate fluids Intensive care and mechanical ventilation if needed for infants < 6 months old **Complications**—Pneumonia (usual cause of death in younger children)	Maintain isolation during catarrhal stage; if child is hospitalised, institute standard and droplet precautions. Obtain nasopharyngeal culture for diagnosis. Encourage oral fluids; offer small amount of fluids frequently. Ensure adequate oxygenation during paroxysms; position infant on side to decrease chance of aspiration with vomiting. Provide humidified oxygen; suction as needed to prevent choking on secretions. Observe for signs of airway obstruction (e.g. increased restlessness, apprehension, retractions, cyanosis). Encourage compliance with antibiotic therapy for household contacts.

TABLE 6.1 Communicable Diseases of Childhood—cont'd

Disease	Clinical Manifestations	Therapeutic Management and Complications	Nursing Care Management
	Pertussis may occur in adolescents and adults with varying manifestations; cough and whoop may be absent; however, as many as 50% of adolescents may have a cough for up to 10 weeks Additional symptoms in adolescents include difficulty breathing and posttussive vomiting (See also Immunisations, for discussion of pertussis immunisat on schedule.)	Atelectasis Otitis media Seizures Haemorrhage (scleral, conjunctival, epistaxis; pulmonary haemorrhage in neonate) Weight loss and dehydration Hernias (umbilical and inguinal) Prolapsed rectum Complications reported among adolescents include syncope, sleep disturbance, rib fractures, incontinence and pneumonia	Encourage adolescents to obtain pertussis booster (Tdap) (see I mmunisations section in this chapter). Use standard precautions and droplet precautions in healthcare workers exposed to children with persistent cough and high suspicion of pertussis. Observe for respiratory paralysis (e.g. difficulty talking, ineffective cough, inability to hold breath, shallow and rapid respirations); report such signs and symptoms to practitioner.

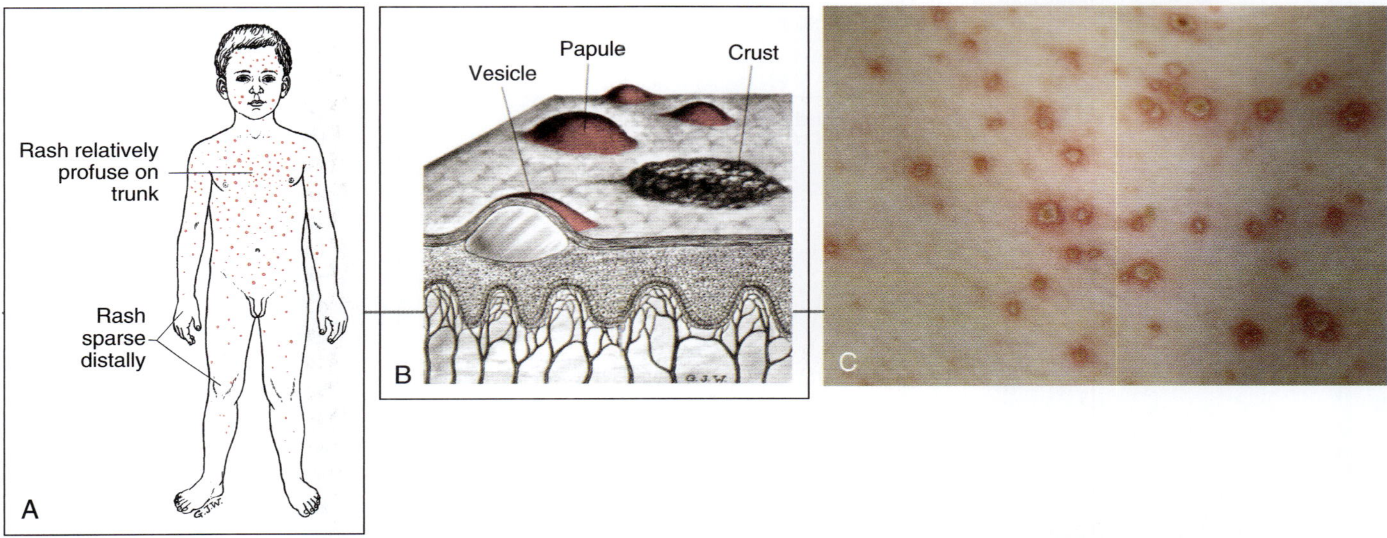

Fig 6.1 Chickenpox (varicella). (**A**) Progression of disease. (**B**) Simultaneous stages of lesions. (**C**) Clinical view. (Source: *C*, Habif, T. P. (2016). *Clinical dermatology: A color guide to diagnosis and therapy* (6th ed.). St Louis, MO: Mosby.)

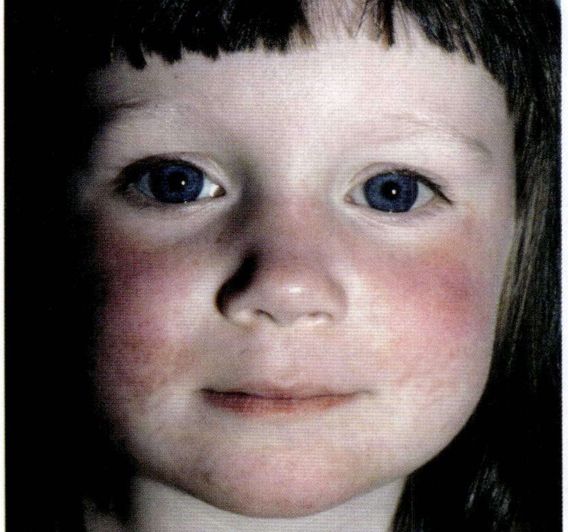

Fig 6.2 Erythema infectiosum (fifth disease). (Source: Habif, T. P. (2016). *Clinical dermatology: A color guide to diagnosis and therapy* (6th ed.). St Louis, MO: Mosby.)

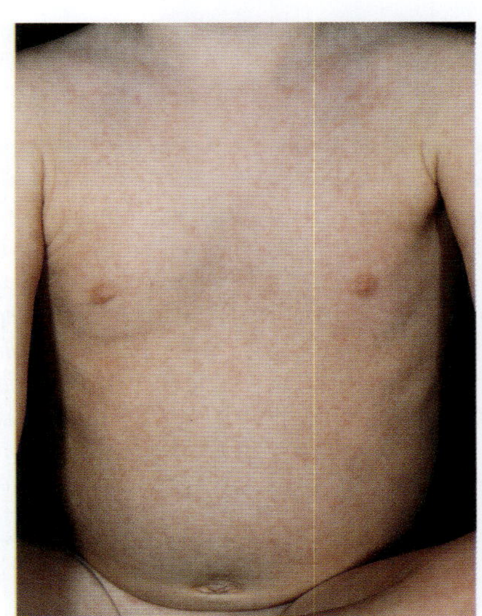

Fig 6.3 Exanthem subitum (roseola infantum). (Source: Habif, T. P. (2016). *Clinical dermatology: A color guide to diagnosis and therapy* (6th ed.). St Louis, MO: Mosby.)

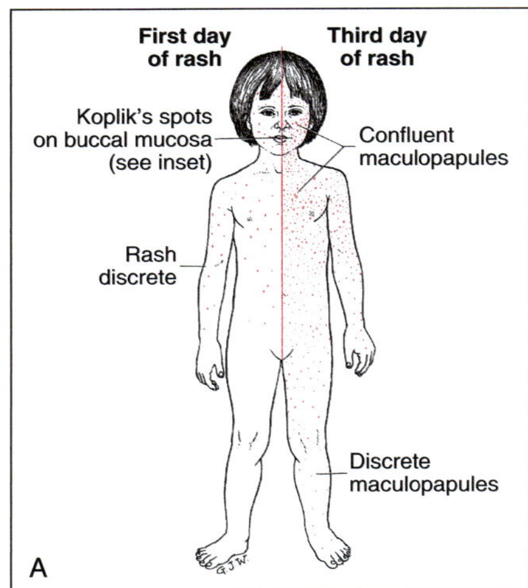

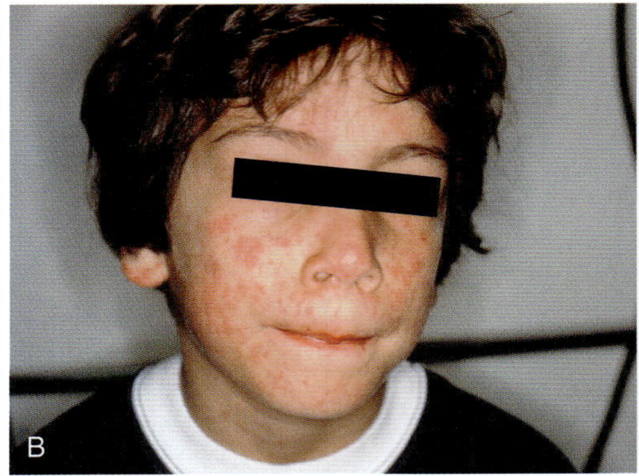

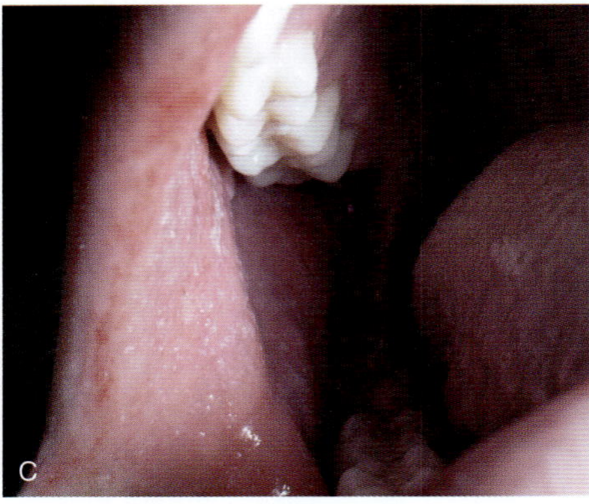

Fig 6.4 Measles (rubeola). (**A**) Progression of disease. (**B**) Clinical view. (**C**) Koplik's spots. (Source: B, Paller, S. A., & Mancini, A. J. (2011). Hurwitz clinical pediatric dermatology (4th ed.). St Louis, MO: Saunders; C, Habif, T. P. (2016). Clinical dermatology: A color guide to diagnosis and therapy (6th ed.). St Louis, MO: Mosby.)

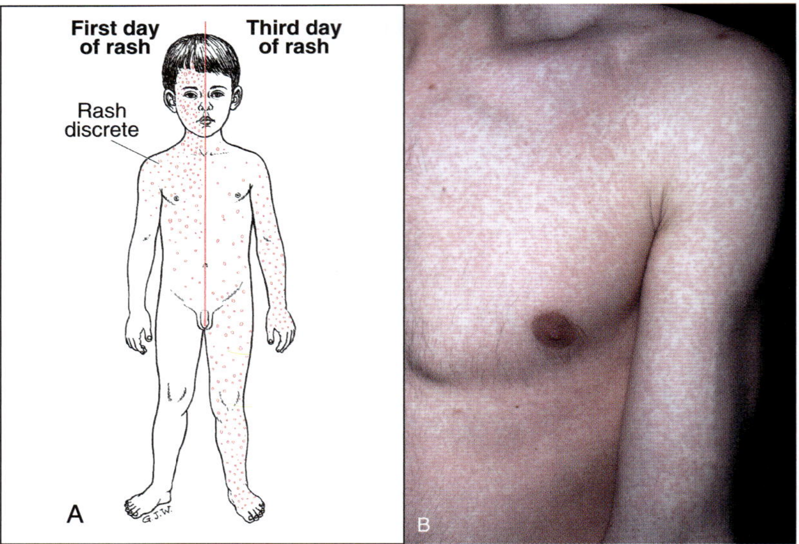

Fig 6.5 Rubella (German measles). (**A**) Progression of rash. (**B**) Clinical view. (Source: B, Zitelli, B. J., & Davis, H. W. (2007). Atlas of pediatric physical diagnosis (5th ed.). St Louis, MO: Mosby; courtesy Dr. Michael Sherlock, Lutherville, Md.)

NURSING CARE CONSIDERATIONS

If a child is admitted to the hospital with an undiagnosed skin eruption or rash (exanthema), institute strict transmission-based precautions (contact, airborne and droplet) and standard precautions until a diagnosis is confirmed. Childhood communicable diseases requiring these precautions include diphtheria, VZV (chickenpox), measles, tuberculosis, adenovirus, *Haemophilus influenzae* type b (Hib), influenza, mumps, *Neisseria meningitides, Mycoplasma pneumoniae* infection, pertussis, plague, rhinovirus, group A streptococcal pharyngitis, severe acute respiratory syndrome, pneumonia or scarlet fever (National Health and Medical Research Council, Australian Commission on Safety and Quality in Healthcare 2019).

Prevent Complications

Although most children recover without difficulty, certain groups are at risk for serious, even fatal, complications from communicable diseases, especially the viral diseases chickenpox and erythema infectiosum (fifth disease) caused by **human parvovirus B19**.

Children with immunodeficiency—those receiving steroid or other immunosuppressive therapy, those with a generalised malignancy such as leukaemia or lymphoma or those with an immunological disorder—are at risk for viraemia from replication of the **varicella-zoster virus** in the blood. VZV is so named because it causes two distinct diseases: **varicella** (**chickenpox**) and **zoster** (**herpes zoster** or **shingles**). Varicella occurs primarily in children younger than 15 years of age. However, it leaves the threat of herpes zoster, an intensely painful varicella that is localised to a single **dermatome** (body area innervated by a particular segment of the spinal cord). Immunocompromised patients and healthy infants younger than 1 year of age (who also have reduced immunity) are at a higher risk for reactivation of VZV causing herpes zoster, probably as a result of a deficiency in cellular immunity (ATAGI 2018). Complications of herpes zoster virus in children

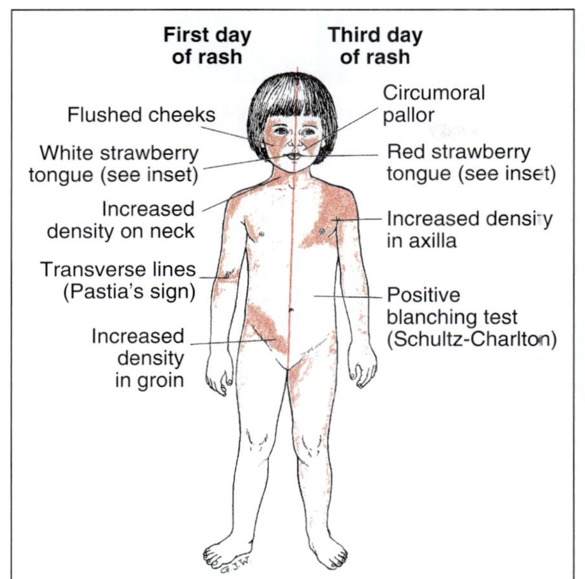

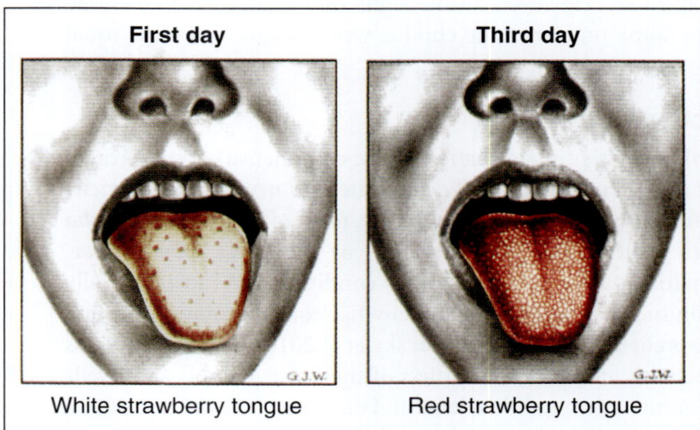

Fig 6.6 Scarlet fever.

include secondary bacterial infection, depigmentation and scarring. Postherpetic neuralgia in children is uncommon (ATAGI 2018).

The use of varicella-zoster immune globulin (VariZIG) or intravenous immune globulin (IVIg) is recommended for children who are immunocompromised, who have no previous history of varicella and who are likely to contract the disease and have complications as a result (ATAGI 2018). The antiviral agent aciclovir (Zovirax) or valaciclovir may be used to treat varicella infections in susceptible immunocompromised persons. It is effective in decreasing the number of lesions; shortening the duration of fever; and decreasing itching, lethargy and anorexia.

Children with haemolytic disease, such as sickle cell disease, are at risk for aplastic anaemia from erythema infectiosum. Human parvovirus B19 infects and lyses red blood cell precursors, thus interrupting the production of red blood cells. Therefore, the virus may precipitate a severe aplastic crisis in patients who need increased red blood cell production to maintain normal red blood cell volumes. Thrombocytopenia and neutropenia may also occur as a result of human parvovirus B19 infection. The fetus has a relatively high rate of red blood cell production and an immature immune system; it may develop severe anaemia and hydrops as a result of maternal human parvovirus infection. Fetal death rates as a result of human parvovirus B19 have been estimated to be between 2% and 6%, with the greatest risk appearing to be in the first 20 weeks (Koch 2016).

Since about 2010 the incidence of pertussis has increased, particularly in infants less than 6 months old and in children 10 to 14 years of age. Early clinical manifestations of pertussis in infants may include gagging and gasping, followed by posttussive emesis, apnoea and cyanosis; the typical 'whoop' associated with the disease is absent (Long 2016). In older children the disease may manifest as a common cold, but a prolonged cough (at least 21 days) is common in adolescents (Long 2016) (see Table 6.1). There is now a recommendation that children ages 11 to 12 receive a booster pertussis vaccine (dTpa) to prevent the disease. Because pertussis is contagious, especially among close household members, identify pertussis early and initiate treatment for the child and those who have been exposed. Azithromycin (for infants younger than 1 month old) and erythromycin, clarithromycin or azithromycin are administered to infants and children with pertussis.

Prevention of complications from diseases such as diphtheria, pertussis and scarlet fever requires compliance with antibiotic therapy. With oral preparations, educate the importance to complete the entire course of therapy. (See Compliance, Chapter 22.)

Provide Comfort

Many communicable diseases cause skin manifestations that are bothersome to the child. The chief discomfort from most rashes is itching, and measures such as cool baths (usually without soap) and lotions (e.g. calamine) are helpful. Cooling the lotion in the refrigerator beforehand often makes it more soothing on the skin than at room temperature.

To avoid overheating, which increases itching, children should wear lightweight, loose, non-irritating clothing and keep out of the sun. If the child persists in scratching, keep the nails short and smooth or use mittens and clothes with long sleeves or legs. For severe itching, antipruritic medication, such as diphenhydramine (Benadryl), may be required, especially when the child has trouble sleeping because of itching. Loratadine or cetirizine do not cause drowsiness and may be preferred for urticaria during the day.

An elevated temperature is common, and both antipyretic medicine (paracetamol or ibuprofen) and environmental manipulation are implemented. (See Controlling Elevated Temperatures, Chapter 22.) Paracetamol is effective in lowering the fever but does not significantly reduce the symptoms of itching, anorexia, abdominal pain, fussiness or vomiting.

A sore throat, another frequent symptom, is managed with lozenges, saline rinses (if the child is old enough to cooperate) and analgesics. Because most children are anorectic during an illness, bland foods and increased liquids are usually preferred. During the early stages of the disease, children voluntarily curtail their activity, and although bed rest is beneficial, it should not be imposed unless specifically indicated. During periods of irritability, quiet activity (e.g. reading, music, television, video games, puzzles, colouring) helps distract children from the discomfort.

Support Child and Family

Most communicable diseases are benign but may produce considerable concern and anxiety for parents. Often the occurrence of a disease, such as chickenpox, is the first time the child is acutely uncomfortable. Parents need assistance to cope with manifestations of the illness, such as intense itching. The family and child need reassurance that recovery is generally rapid. However, visible signs of the dermatosis may be present for some time after the child is well enough to resume usual activities.

Conjunctivitis

Acute **conjunctivitis** (inflammation of the conjunctiva) occurs from a variety of causes that are typically age related. In newborns conjunctivitis can occur from infection during birth, most often from *Chlamydia trachomatis* (inclusion conjunctivitis) or *Neisseria gonorrhoeae.* Conjunctivitis in a neonate is a serious condition and can potentially lead to blindness; all signs of conjunctivitis require prompt reporting and a comprehensive evaluation (Olitsky et al 2016). The clinical signs of conjunctivitis are similar regardless of the cause: redness and swelling of the conjunctiva, eyelid oedema and discharge (Olitsky et al 2016). In infants, recurrent conjunctivitis may be a sign of nasolacrimal (tear) duct obstruction or dacryocystitis, an infection of the lacrimal sac. Timing of the infection may provide signs of the cause. A chemical conjunctivitis may occur within 24 hours of instillation of neonatal ophthalmic prophylaxis; *N. gonorrhoeae* usually occurs within 2 to 5 days after birth, and *C. trachomatis* occurs 5 to 14 days after birth (Olitsky et al 2016). In children the usual causes of conjunctivitis are viral, bacterial, allergic or related to a foreign body. Bacterial infection accounts for most instances of acute conjunctivitis in children. Diagnosis is made primarily from the clinical manifestations (Box 6.2), although cultures of purulent drainage may be needed to identify the specific cause.

BOX 6.2 Clinical Manifestations of Conjunctivitis

Bacterial conjunctivitis ('pink eye')

- Purulent drainage
- Crusting of eyelids, especially on awakening
- Inflamed conjunctiva
- Swollen eyelids

Viral conjunctivitis

- Usually occurs with upper respiratory tract infection
- Serous (watery) drainage
- Inflamed conjunctiva
- Swollen eyelids

Allergic conjunctivitis

- Itching
- Watery to thick, stringy discharge
- Inflamed conjunctiva
- Swollen eyelids

Conjunctivitis caused by foreign body

- Tearing
- Pain
- Inflamed conjunctiva
- Usually only one eye affected

Therapeutic Management

Treatment of conjunctivitis depends on the cause. Viral conjunctivitis is self-limiting, and treatment is limited to removal of the accumulated secretions. Bacterial conjunctivitis has traditionally been treated with topical antibiotics such as chloramphenicol. Infants with bacterial conjunctivitis may require systemic antibiotics (Olitsky et al 2016). For children 1 year and older, fluoroquinolones and aminoglycosides are commonly used ophthalmic antimicrobial agents. Fourth-generation fluoroquinolones such as moxifloxacin provide broad-spectrum coverage, are bactericidal and are generally well tolerated (Alter et al 2011). Drops may be used during the day and an ointment at bedtime because the ointment preparation remains in the eye longer but blurs the vision. Corticosteroids are avoided because they reduce ocular resistance to bacteria.

Nursing Care Management

Nursing care includes keeping the eye clean and properly administering ophthalmic medication. Remove accumulated secretions by wiping from the inner canthus downwards and outwards, away from the opposite eye. Warm, moist compresses, such as a clean washcloth wrung out with hot tap water, are helpful in removing the crusts. Compresses are *not* kept on the eye because an occlusive covering promotes bacterial growth. Instil medication immediately after the eyes have been cleaned and according to correct procedure. (See Chapter 22.)

Prevention of infection in other family members is an important consideration with bacterial conjunctivitis. Keep the child's washcloth and towel separate from those used by others. Discard tissues used to clean the eye. Instruct the child to refrain from rubbing the eye and to use good handwashing technique.

NURSING CARE CONSIDERATIONS

Signs of serious conjunctivitis include reduction or loss of vision, ocular pain, photophobia, exophthalmos (bulging eyeball), decreased ocular mobility, corneal ulceration and unusual patterns of inflammation (e.g. the perilimbal flush associated with iritis or localised inflammation associated with scleritis). If a patient has any of these signs, refer him or her immediately to an ophthalmologist.

Stomatitis

Stomatitis is inflammation of the oral mucosa, which may include the buccal (cheek) and labial (lip) mucosa, tongue, gingiva, palate and floor of the mouth. It may be infectious or non-infectious and may be caused by local or systemic factors. In children, aphthous stomatitis and herpetic stomatitis are typically seen. Children with immunosuppression and those receiving chemotherapy or head and neck radiotherapy are at high risk for developing mucosal ulceration and herpetic stomatitis.

Aphthous stomatitis (aphthous ulcer, mouth ulcer) is a benign but painful condition whose cause is unknown. Its onset is usually associated with mild traumatic injury (e.g. biting the cheek, hitting the mucosa with a toothbrush or a mouth appliance rubbing on the mucosa), allergy or emotional stress. The lesions are painful, small, whitish ulcerations surrounded by a red border. They are distinguished from other types of stomatitis by healthy adjacent tissues, absence of vesicles and no systemic illness. The ulcers persist for 4 to 12 days and heal uneventfully.

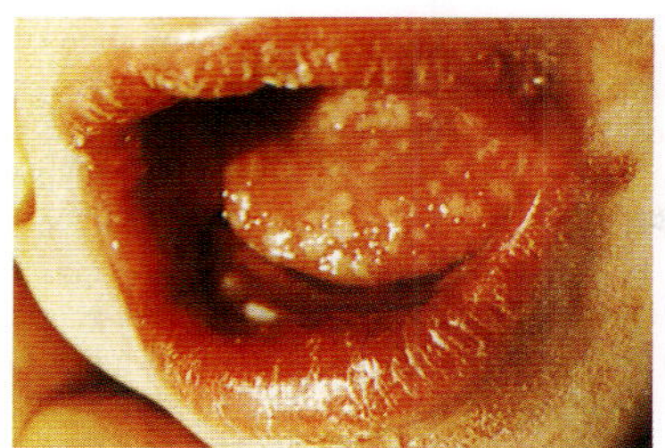

Fig 6.7 Primary gingivostomatitis. (Source: Thompson, J. M., McFarland, G. M., Hirsch, J. E., et al. (2002). Mosby's clinical nursing (5th ed.). St Louis, MO: Mosby.)

Herpetic gingivostomatitis (HGS) is caused by herpes simplex virus (HSV), most often type 1, and may occur as a primary infection or recur in a less severe form known as **recurrent herpes labialis** (commonly called *cold sores* or *fever blisters*). The primary infection usually begins with a fever; the pharynx becomes oedematous and erythematous; and vesicles erupt on the mucosa, causing severe pain (Fig 6.7). Cervical lymphadenitis often occurs, and the breath has a distinctly foul odour. In the recurrent form, the vesicles appear on the lips, either singly or in groups. The precipitating factors for the cold sores include emotional stress, trauma (often related to dental procedures), immunosuppression or exposure to excessive sunlight. The disease can last 5 to 14 days, with varying degrees of severity.

Stomatitis may occur as a manifestation of hand-foot-and-mouth disease (HFMD) and herpangina; both manifest with scattered vesicles on the buccal mucosa and are commonly caused by the non-polio enteroviruses (primarily coxsackieviruses). Children with either HFMD or herpangina often have poor intake as a result of the mouth sores; infants may refuse to nurse or take a bottle or may pull away and cry after a few seconds of nursing.

Therapeutic Management

Treatment for all types of stomatitis is aimed at relief of symptoms, primarily pain. Paracetamol and ibuprofen are usually sufficient for mild cases, but with more severe HGS, stronger analgesics such as codeine may be needed. Topical anaesthetics are helpful and include over-the-counter preparations such as Orabase. Lignocaine gel 2% or Xylocaine viscous can be prescribed for the child who can keep 1 tsp of the solution in the mouth for 2 to 3 minutes and then expectorate the drug. Treatment for children with severe cases of HGS includes the use of antiviral agents such as aciclovir (Tinanoff 2016).

Nursing Care Management

The chief nursing goals for children with stomatitis are relief of pain and prevention of spread of the herpes virus. Analgesics and topical anaesthetics are used as needed to provide relief, especially before meals to encourage food and fluid intake. Educating parents regarding the use of these medications is important to maintain adequate hydration in the child whose mouth is too sore to take liquids. Drinking bland fluids through a straw is helpful in avoiding the painful lesions. Encourage mouth care; the use of a very soft bristle toothbrush or disposable foam-tipped toothbrush provides gentle cleaning near ulcerated areas.

Careful handwashing is essential when caring for children with HGS. Because the infection is autoinoculable, children should keep their fingers out of the mouth; contaminated hands can infect other body parts. Very young children may require elbow restraints to ensure compliance. Articles placed in the mouth are cleaned thoroughly. Newborns and individuals with immunosuppression should not be exposed to infected children.

> **NURSING CARE CONSIDERATIONS**
>
> When examining herpetic lesions, wear gloves. The virus easily enters breaks in the skin and can cause herpetic whitlow of the fingers.

Because herpes infection is often associated with sexual transmission, explain to parents and older children that HGS is usually caused by type 1 HSV, the type not associated with sexual activity.

INTESTINAL PARASITIC DISEASES

Intestinal parasitic diseases, including helminths (worms) and protozoa, constitute the most frequent infections in the world. Young children are especially at risk because of typical hand-to-mouth activity and uncontrolled faecal activity.

Various infecting organisms cause intestinal parasitic diseases in humans. This discussion is limited to threadworm (also called pinworm), a type of roundworm that is commonly found in preschool and school-aged children; however, the whole family can become infected.

General Nursing Care Management

Nursing responsibilities related to intestinal parasitic infections involve assistance with identification of the parasite, treatment of the infection and prevention of initial infection or reinfection. Clinical manifestations are identified in Box 6.3. Laboratory examination of substances containing the worm, its larvae or ova can identify the organism. Most are identified by examining faecal smears from the stools of persons suspected of harbouring the parasite. Fresh specimens are best for revealing parasites or larvae; therefore, take collected specimens directly to the laboratory for examination. If this is not possible, place the specimen in a container with a preservative. Parents need clear instructions on obtaining an adequate sample and the number of samples required (see Stool Specimens, Chapter 22). In most parasitic infections, other family members, especially children, may be examined to identify those who are similarly affected.

After the diagnosis is confirmed and appropriate treatment is planned, parents need further explanation and reinforcement. Compliance in terms of drug therapy and other measures, such as thorough handwashing, is essential for eradication of the parasite. The family needs to understand the nature of transmission and that in some cases the medication must be repeated in 2 weeks to 1 month to kill organisms hatched since initial treatment.

The nurse's most important function is preventive education of children and families regarding hygiene and health habits. Thorough handwashing before eating or handling food and after using the toilet is the most important precautionary method. The Family-Centred Care box lists other preventive practices.

> **BOX 6.3 Clinical Manifestations of Threadworm**
>
> Intense perianal itching is the principal symptom. Evidence of itching in young children includes the following:
> - general irritability
> - restlessness
> - poor sleep
> - bed-wetting
> - distractibility
> - short attention span
> - perianal dermatitis and excoriation secondary to itching
> - if worms migrate, possible vaginal (vulvovaginitis) and urethral infection.

FAMILY-CENTRED CARE

Preventing Intestinal Parasitic Disease

- Always wash hands and fingernails with soap and water before eating and handling food and after toileting.
- Avoid placing fingers in mouth and biting nails.
- Discourage children from scratching bare anal area.
- Use superabsorbent disposable nappies to prevent leakage.
- Change nappies as soon as soiled and dispose of nappies in closed receptacle out of children's reach.
- Do not rinse cloth or disposable nappies in toilet.
- Disinfect toilet seats and nappy-changing areas; use dilute household bleach (10% solution) or ammonia (Lysol) and wipe clean with paper towels.
- Drink only treated water or bottled water, especially if camping.
- Wash all raw fruits and vegetables and food that have fallen on the floor.
- Avoid growing foods in soil fertilised with human or untreated animal excreta.
- Teach children to defecate only in a toilet, not on the ground.
- Keep dogs and cats away from playgrounds and sandpits.
- Avoid swimming in pools frequented by children in swimmer nappies.
- Wear shoes outside.

REFERENCES

Alter, S. J., Vidwan, N. K., Sobande, P. O., et al. (2011). Common childhood bacterial infections. Current Problems in Pediatric and Adolescent Healthcare, 41(10), 256–283.

Australian Government Department of Health (AGDH). (2021). COVID 19 vaccines. https://www.health.gov.au/initiatives-and-programs/covid-19-vaccines

Australian Technical Advisory Group on Immunisation (ATAGI). (2018). Australian Immunisation Handbook, Australian Government Department of Health, Canberra. http://immunisationhandbook.health.gov.au.

Australian Technical Advisory Group on Immunisation (ATAGI). Australian Immunisation Handbook, Australian Government Department of Health, Canberra, 2021, "https://immunisationhandbook.health.gov.au/vaccine-preventable-diseases/influenza-flu" Influenza (flu) | The Australian Immunisation Handbook (health.gov.au)

Beirne, P. V., Hennessy, S., Cadogan, S. L., et al. (2015). Needle size for vaccination procedures in children and adolescents. Cochrane Database of Systematic Reviews, (6), CD010720.

Bolon, M. K. (2016). Hand hygiene: An update. Infectious Disease Clinics of North America, 30, 591–607.

Communicable Disease Network Australia (CDNA). (2020). Australian national notifiable diseases and case definitions. https://www1.health.gov.au/internet/main/publishing.nsf/Content/cdna-casedefinitions.htm

DeStefano, F., Price, C. S., & Weintraub, E. S. (2013). Increasing exposure to antibody-stimulating proteins and polysaccharides in vaccines is not associated with risk of autism. The Journal of Pediatrics, 163(2), 561–567.

Diggle, L., & Deeks, J. (2000). Effect of needle length on incidence of local reactions to routine immunizations in infants aged 4 months: Randomized controlled trial. BMJ (Clinical Research Ed.), 321(7266), 931–993.

Diggle, L., Deeks, J. J., & Pollard, A. J. (2006). Effect of needle size and immunogenicity and reactogenicity of vaccines in infants: A randomized controlled trial. BMJ (Clinical Research Ed.), 333(7568), 571.

Fallah, R., Gholami, H., Ferdosian, F., et al. (2016). Evaluation of vaccines injection order on pain score of intramuscular injection of diphtheria, whole cell pertussis and tetanus vaccine. Indian Journal of Pediatrics, 83, 1405–1409.

Institute of Medicine. (2004). Immunization safety review: Vaccines and autism. Washington, DC: National Academies Press.

Ipp, M., Parkin, P. C., Lear, N., et al. (2009). Order of vaccine injection and infant pain response. Archives of Pediatrics and Adolescent Medicine, 163(5), 469–472.

Jackson, L. A., Yu, O., Nelson, J. C., et al. (2011). Injection site and risk of medically attended local reactions to acellular pertussis vaccine. Pediatrics, 127(3), e681–e687.

Koch, W. C. (2016). Parvoviruses. In R. M. Kliegman, B. F. Stanton, J. W. St Geme, et al. (Eds.), Nelson textbook of pediatrics (20th ed.). Philadelphia: Saunders/Elsevier.

Leask J., Kinnersly, P., Jackson, C., et al. (2012). Communicating with parents about vaccination: a framework for health professionals. BMC Pediatrics, 12, 154. http://www.biomedcentral.com/1471-2431/12/154

Long, S. S. (2016). Pertussis. In R. M. Kliegman, B. F. Stanton, J. W. St Geme, et al. (Eds.), Nelson textbook of pediatrics (20th ed.). Philadelphia: Saunders.

McIntyre, P., Ye, J. J., Chiu, C., et al. (2021) COVID 19 Vaccines—Are we there yet? Australian Prescriber, 44(1), 19–25.

Ministry of Health. (2021). COVID-19: Vaccine safety and approval. https://www.health.govt.nz/our-work/diseases-and-conditions/covid-19-novel-coronavirus/covid-19-vaccines/covid-19-vaccine-safety-and-approval

Ministry of Health. (2020a). Immunisation Handbook. Wellington: Ministry of Health. https://www.health.govt.nz/our-work/immunisation-handbook-2020/

Ministry of Health. (2020b). Appendix 2: Planning immunisation catch-ups. Immunisation Handbook. Wellington: Ministry of Health. https://www.health.govt.nz/our-work/immunisation-handbook-2020/appendix-2-planning-immunisation-catch-ups

Ministry of Health. (2020c). Notifiable Diseases. https://www.health.govt.nz/our-work/diseases-and-conditions/notifiable-diseases

Ministry of Health. (2015). National Immunisation Register, https://www.health.govt.nz/our-work/preventative-health-wellness/immunisation/national-immunisation-register

Mitchell, B., Shaban, R., MacBeth, D., et al. (2017). The burden of healthcare-associated infection in Australian hospitals: A systematic review of the literature. Infection, Disease & Health, 22, 117–128.

National Health and Medical Research Council, Australian Commission on Safety and Quality in Healthcare. (2019). Australian Guidelines for the Prevention and Control of Infection in Healthcare. https://www.nhmrc.gov.au/about-us/publications/australian-guidelines-prevention-and-control-infection-healthcare-2019

Olitsky, S. E., Hug, D., Plummer, L. S., et al. (2016). Disorders of the conjunctiva. In R. M. Kliegman, B. F. Stanton, J. W. St Geme, et al. (Eds.), Nelson textbook of pediatrics (20th ed.). Philadelphia: Saunders.

Rishovd, A. (2014). Pediatric intramuscular injections: Guidelines for best practice. The American Journal of Maternal Child Nursing, 39, 107–112.

Rowe, S. L., Tay, E. L., Franklin, L. J., et al. (2018). Effectiveness of parental cocooning as a vaccination strategy to prevent pertussis infection in infants: A case-control study. , Vaccine, 36(15), 2012–2019.

Strebel, P. M., Papania, M. J., Dastañaduy, P. A., et al. (2018). Measles vaccines. In: Plotkin SA, Orenstein WA, Offit PA, Edwards KM, eds. Plotkin's vaccines. 7th ed. Philadelphia, PA: Elsevier.

Sun, P., Lu, X., Xu, C., et al. (2020). Understanding of COVID-19 based on current evidence. Journal of Medical Virology. 5 March. https://www.ncbi.nlm.nih.gov/pmc/articles/PMC7228250/

Tangherlini, T. R., Roychowdhury, V., Glenn, B., et al. (2016). 'Mommy blogs' and the vaccination exemption narrative: Results from a machine-learning approach for story aggregation on parenting social media sites. JMIR Public Health and Surveillance, 2, 1–15.

Tinanoff, N. (2016). Common lesions of the oral soft tissues. In R. M. Kliegman, B. F. Stanton, J. W. St Geme, et al. (Eds.), Nelson textbook of pediatrics (20th ed.). Philadelphia: Saunders.

World Health Organization (WHO). (2020). WHO Director-General's opening remarks at the media briefing on COVID-19: 11 March 2020. https://www.who.int/dg/speeches/detail/who-director-general-s-opening-remarks-at-the-media-briefing-on-covid-19---11-march-2020

World Health Organization (WHO). (2015). Reducing pain at the time of vaccination: WHO position paper – September 2015. World Health Organization Weekly Epidemiological Record, 39, 505–516.

Yoshimasu, K., Kiyohara, C., Takemura, S., et al. (2014). A meta-analysis of the evidence on the impact of prenatal and early infancy exposures to mercury on autism and attention deficit/hyperactivity disorder in the childhood. Neurotoxicology, 44, 121–131.

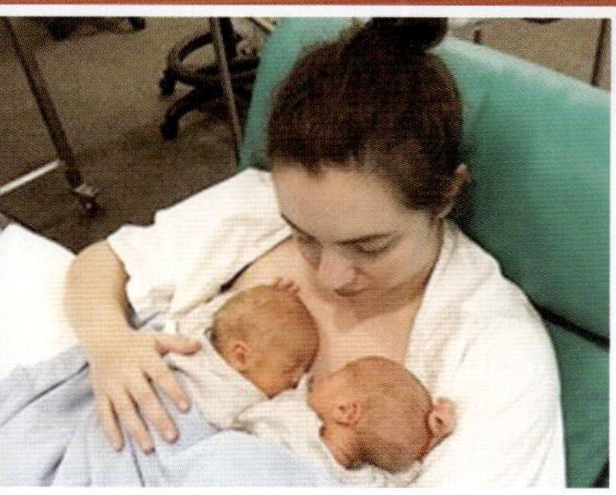

7 Health Promotion of the Newborn and Family

Tameeka Mulquiney and Amy Vaccaro

LEARNING OBJECTIVES

- Be able to recognise and demonstrate the normal adjustment to extrauterine life for full-term newborn
- Be able to discuss and document the initial assessment of the newborn
- Demonstrate and document the nursing care of the newborn and family
- Be able to discuss and implement daily care needs of the newborn

ADJUSTMENT TO EXTRAUTERINE LIFE

The most profound physiological change required of the newborn is transition from fetal or placental circulation to independent respiration. The loss of the placental connection means the loss of complete metabolic support, particularly the supply of oxygen and the removal of carbon dioxide. The normal stresses of labour and birth cause alterations in placental gas exchange patterns, acid–base balance in the blood and cardiovascular activity in the neonate. Factors that interfere with normal transition or that interfere with fetal oxygenation (including conditions such as hypoxaemia, hypercapnia and acidosis) will affect the fetus's adjustment to extrauterine life.

Immediate Adjustments

Respiratory System

The most critical and immediate physiological change required of the newborn is the onset of breathing. The stimuli that help initiate respiration are primarily chemical and thermal. Chemical factors in the blood (low oxygen, high carbon dioxide and low pH) initiate impulses that excite the respiratory centre in the medulla. The primary thermal stimulus is the sudden chilling of the infant, who leaves a warm environment and enters a relatively cooler atmosphere. This abrupt change in temperature excites sensory impulses in the skin that are transmitted to the respiratory centre. Tactile stimulation may assist in initiating respiration. Descent through the birth canal and normal handling during birth, such as drying the skin, help stimulate respiration in uncompromised infants. Acceptable methods of tactile stimulation include drying with a soft towel or rubbing the newborn's back, trunk or extremities with a soft towel (Victorian Agency for Health Information [VAHI] & Safer Care Victoria [SCV] 2020a).

The initial entry of air into the lungs is opposed by the surface tension of the fluid that filled the fetal lungs and alveoli. Some fetal lung fluid is removed during the normal forces of labour and birth. As the chest emerges from the birth canal, fluid is squeezed from the lungs through the nose and mouth. After complete emergence of the neonate's chest, a brisk recoil of the thorax occurs. Air enters the upper airway to replace the lost fluid. In caesarean birth the chest is not compressed, and the newborn may need additional respiratory support or monitoring until remaining fetal lung fluid is absorbed by the pulmonary capillaries and lymphatic vessels.

In the alveoli the fluid's surface tension is reduced by **surfactant**, a substance produced by the alveolar epithelium that coats the alveolar surface. Chapter 9 discusses the effect of surfactant in facilitating breathing in relation to respiratory distress syndrome.

Circulatory System

As important as the initiation of respiration are the circulatory changes that allow blood to flow through the lungs. These changes occur more gradually and are the result of pressure changes in the lungs, heart and major vessels. The transition from fetal circulation to postnatal circulation involves the functional closure of the **fetal shunts:** the foramen ovale, the ductus arteriosus and eventually the ductus venosus. (For a brief review of fetal circulation, see Chapter 27.)

Once the lungs are expanded, the inspired oxygen dilates the pulmonary vessels, which decreases pulmonary vascular resistance and consequently increases pulmonary blood flow. As the lungs receive blood, the pressure in the right atrium, right ventricle and pulmonary arteries decreases. At the same time, there is a progressive rise in systemic vascular resistance and an increased volume of blood as a result of cord clamping. This increases the pressure in the left side of the heart. Because blood flows from an area of high pressure to one of low pressure, the circulation of blood through the fetal shunts is reversed (see Fig 27.2).

The most important factor controlling ductal closure is the increased oxygen concentration of the blood. Secondary factors are the fall in endogenous prostaglandins and acidosis. The foramen ovale closes functionally at or soon after birth from compression of the two portions of the atrial septum. The ductus arteriosus is closed functionally by the fourth day in well neonates, but closure may be delayed in ill or preterm infants. Anatomical closure from deposition of fibrin and cell products takes considerably longer. Because of the reversible flow of blood through the ductus arteriosus during the early neonatal period, a functional murmur is occasionally heard.

Physiological Status of Other Systems

Thermoregulation

Next to establishing respiration, heat regulation is most critical to the newborn's survival. Although the newborn's capacity for heat production is adequate, several factors predispose the newborn to excessive heat loss. First, the newborn's large surface area relative to his or her weight facilitates heat loss to the environment. The newborn's large body surface is partially compensated for by a usual position of flexion, which decreases the amount of surface area exposed to the environment.

The second factor that contributes to loss of body heat is the newborn's thin layer of subcutaneous fat. Because core body temperature is approximately 0.5°C higher than surface body temperature, this temperature gradient (difference) causes a heat transfer from a higher to lower temperature.

A third factor is the newborn's mechanism for producing heat. Unlike the child or adult, who can increase heat production through shivering, the chilled neonate cannot shiver but produces heat through **non-shivering thermogenesis (NST)**. NST (or chemical thermogenesis) is produced by stimulating cellular respiration, resulting in increased need for oxygen and glucose (see Thermoregulation, Chapter 9). A thermogenic source, once believed to be unique to the full-term newborn, is **brown adipose tissue (BAT)**, or brown fat, which owes its name to its larger content of mitochondrial cytochromes. BAT has a greater capacity for heat production through intensified metabolic activity than does ordinary adipose tissue. Heat generated in the brown fat is distributed to other parts of the body by the blood, which is warmed as it flows through the layers of this tissue. Superficial deposits of brown fat are located between the scapulae, around the neck, in the axillae and behind the sternum. Deeper layers surround the kidneys, trachea, oesophagus, some major arteries and adrenals. The location of the brown fat may explain why the nape of the neck often feels warmer than the rest of the body.

Because of these factors predisposing infants to loss of body heat, it is essential that a newly born infant is quickly dried and either placed skin-to-skin with the mother after birth and covered with a blanket, or, if that is not possible, wrapped with warm, dry blankets. Although concern is usually for newborns' ability to conserve heat, they may also have difficulty dissipating heat in an overheated environment, increasing the risk of hyperthermia.

Haematopoietic System

The blood volume of the newborn depends largely on the amount of blood transferred via the placenta before clamping the cord. The blood volume of the full-term infant is about 80 to 85 mL/kg of body weight. Immediately after birth, the total blood volume averages 300 mL, but, depending on how long cord clamping is delayed, or if cord is milked, as much as 100 mL may be added to the blood volume (Rabe et al 2019).

Fluid and Electrolyte Balance

Changes occur in the total body water volume, extracellular fluid volume and intracellular fluid volume during the transition from fetal to postnatal life. The fetus is composed almost entirely of water early in gestation and at term is 73% fluid, compared with 58% in the adult. The fetus has more extracellular fluid than intracellular fluid, but this shifts progressively throughout postnatal life, probably because of the growth of cells at the expense of extracellular fluid.

An important aspect of fluid balance is its relationship to other systems. The infant's rate of metabolism is twice that of an adult in relation to body weight. As a result, more acid is formed, leading to more rapid development of acidaemia. In addition, the immature kidneys cannot sufficiently concentrate urine to conserve body water. These three factors make the infant more prone to dehydration, acidosis and overhydration.

Gastrointestinal System

The newborn's ability to digest, absorb and metabolise food is adequate but limited in certain functions. Enzymes are available to catalyse proteins and simple carbohydrates (monosaccharides and disaccharides), but deficient production of pancreatic amylase impairs utilisation of complex carbohydrates (polysaccharides). A deficiency of pancreatic lipase limits the absorption of fats, especially with ingestion of foods that have high saturated fatty acid content, such as cow's milk. Human milk, despite its high fat content, is easy to digest and absorb because it contains enzymes such as lipase, which assist in digestion.

The liver is the most immature of the gastrointestinal organs. The activity of the enzyme glucuronyl transferase is reduced, affecting the conjugation of bilirubin with glucuronic acid, which contributes to physiological jaundice of the newborn. The liver is also deficient in forming plasma proteins, which is likely to play a role in the oedema usually seen at birth. Prothrombin and other coagulation factors are also low. The liver stores less glycogen at birth than later in life. Consequently, the newborn is prone to hypoglycaemia, which may be prevented by early and effective feeding, ideally breastfeeding.

Some salivary glands are functioning at birth, but the majority do not begin to secrete saliva until about age 2 to 3 months, when drooling is common. Newborn stomach capacity is difficult to determine; however, Bergman (2013) reviewed six published studies exploring this, concluding that stomach capacity is about 20 mL at birth, thus the infant requires frequent small feedings. Newborns who breastfeed usually have more frequent feedings and more frequent stools than infants who receive formula.

The infant's intestine is longer in relation to body size than that in the adult. Therefore, it has a proportionately larger number of secretory glands and a larger surface area for absorption compared with the adult's intestine. Rapid peristaltic waves and simultaneous non-peristaltic waves occur along the entire intestine. These waves, called the **migrating motor complex (MMC)**, propel nutrients forwards. The relative immaturity of the MMC, combined with decreased lower oesophageal sphincter (LES) pressure, inappropriate relaxation of the LES and delayed gastric emptying, makes regurgitation a common occurrence. Progressive changes in the stooling pattern indicate a properly functioning gastrointestinal tract (Box 7.1).

Renal System

All structural components are present in the renal system, but the kidney has a functional deficiency in its ability to concentrate urine and to cope with fluid and electrolyte fluctuations, such as dehydration or a concentrated solute load.

Total volume of urinary output per 24 hours is about 200 to 300 mL by the end of the first week. The bladder involuntarily empties when stretched by a volume of 15 mL, resulting in as many as 20 voidings per day. It can be much less in early stages after birth: day 1 = 1, day 2 = 2, day 3 = 3, and so on (Australian Breastfeeding Association 2017). The first voiding should occur within 24 hours. The urine is colourless and odourless and has a specific gravity of approximately 1.020.

BOX 7.1 Change in Stooling Patterns of Newborns

Meconium

- This is the infant's first stool, composed of amniotic fluid and its constituents, intestinal secretions, shed mucosal cells and possibly blood (ingested maternal blood or minor bleeding of alimentary tract vessels).
- Passage of meconium occurs within the first 24 hours for the vast majority of newborns, although it is delayed in premature infants.

Transitional Stools

- These usually appear by the third day after initiation of feeding.
- They are greenish brown to yellowish-brown, thin and less sticky than meconium and may contain some milk curds.

Milk Stools

- These usually appear by the fourth day.
- In breastfed infants stools are yellow to golden, are pasty in consistency and have an odour similar to that of sour milk.
- In formula-fed infants stools are pale yellow to light brown, are firmer in consistency and have a more offensive odour.

Integumentary System

At birth all the structures within the skin are present, but many of the functions of the integument are immature. The two layers of the skin, the epidermis and dermis, are loosely bound to each other and are very thin. Rete pegs, which later in life anchor the epidermis to the dermis, are not developed. Slight friction across the epidermis, such as from rapid removal of tape, can cause separation of these layers and blister formation or loss of the epidermis. In full-term infants the transitional zone between the cornified and living layers of the epidermis is effective in preventing fluid from reaching the skin surface.

The sebaceous glands are active late in fetal life and in early infancy because of high levels of maternal androgens. They are most densely located on the scalp, face and genitalia and produce the greyish-white, greasy **vernix caseosa** that covers the infant at birth. Plugging of the sebaceous glands causes **milia**.

The eccrine glands, which produce sweat in response to heat or emotional stimuli, are functional at birth, and by 3 weeks of age palmar sweating on crying reaches levels equivalent to those of anxious adults. The eccrine glands produce sweat in response to higher temperatures than those required in adults, and the retention of sweat may result in milia. The apocrine glands, sweat glands that develop as attachments to hair follicles, remain small and non-functional until puberty.

The growth phases of hair follicles usually occur simultaneously at birth. During the first few months, the synchrony between hair loss and regrowth is disrupted, and there may be overgrowth of hair or temporary alopecia.

Because the amount of melanin is low at birth, newborns are lighter skinned than they will be as children. Consequently, infants are more susceptible to the harmful effects of ultraviolet light such as sunlight.

Musculoskeletal System

At birth the skeletal system contains more cartilage than ossified bone, although the process of ossification is fairly rapid during the first year. The nose, for example, is predominantly cartilage at birth and is frequently flattened by the force of the birthing process. The six skull bones are relatively soft and not yet joined. The sinuses are incompletely formed as well.

Unlike the skeletal system, the muscular system is almost completely formed at birth. Hypertrophy, rather than hyperplasia, of cells causes the growth in the size of muscular tissue.

Defences Against Infection

The infant is born with several defences against infection. The first line of defence is the skin and mucous membranes, which protect the body from invading organisms. The second line of defence is the cellular elements of the immunological system, which produces several types of cells capable of attacking a pathogen. The neutrophils and monocytes are **phagocytes**, cells that engulf, ingest and destroy foreign agents. Eosinophils also probably have a phagocytic property because in the presence of foreign protein they increase in number. The **lymphocytes** (T and B cells) are capable of being converted to other cell types, such as monocytes and antibodies. Although the phagocytic properties of the blood are present in the infant, the tissues' inflammatory response to localise an infection is immature.

The third line of defence is the formation of specific antibodies to an antigen. This process requires exposure to various foreign agents for antibody production to occur. Infants are generally not capable of producing their own immunoglobulins until the beginning of the second month of life, but they receive considerable passive immunity in the form of immunoglobulin G (IgG) from the maternal circulation and from human milk. They are protected against most major childhood diseases, including diphtheria, measles, poliomyelitis and rubella, for about 3 months, provided that the mother has developed antibodies to these illnesses.

Endocrine System

Ordinarily, the newborn's endocrine system is adequately developed, but its functions are immature. For example, the posterior lobe of the pituitary gland produces limited quantities of antidiuretic hormone, or vasopressin, thus risk of diuresis is increased. This renders the newborn highly susceptible to dehydration.

The effect of maternal sex hormones is particularly evident in the newborn. The labia are hypertrophied, and the breasts in both sexes may be engorged and secrete milk during the first few days of life to as long as 2 months of age. Female newborns may have pseudomenstruation (more often seen as a milky secretion rather than actual blood) from a sudden drop in progesterone and oestrogen levels.

Neurological System

At birth the nervous system is incompletely integrated but sufficiently developed to sustain extrauterine life. Most neurological functions are primitive reflexes. The autonomic nervous system is crucial during transition because it stimulates initial respirations, helps maintain acid–base balance and partially regulates temperature control.

Myelination of the nervous system follows the **cephalocaudal-proximodistal** (head-to-toe–centre-to-periphery) laws of development and is closely related to the observed mastery of fine and gross motor skills. Myelin is necessary for rapid and efficient transmission of some, but not all, nerve impulses along the neural pathway. Tracts that develop myelin earliest are the sensory, cerebellar and extrapyramidal. This accounts for the acute senses of taste, smell and hearing and the perception of pain in the newborn. All cranial nerves are myelinated except the optic and olfactory nerves.

Sensory Functions

The newborn's sensory functions are remarkably well developed and have a significant effect on growth and development, including the attachment process.

Vision. At birth the eye is structurally incomplete. The fovea centralis is not yet completely differentiated from the macula. The ciliary muscles are also immature, limiting the eyes' ability to accommodate and fixate on an object for any length of time. The pupils react to light, the blink reflex is responsive to minimum stimulus and the corneal reflex is activated by a light touch. Tear glands usually do not begin to function until 2 to 4 weeks of age.

The newborn has the ability to momentarily fixate on a bright or moving object that is within 20 cm and in the midline of the visual field. The infant's ability to fixate or coordinate movement is greater during the first hour of life than during the succeeding several days. Visual acuity is reported to be between 20/100 and 20/400, depending on the vision measurement techniques (see Chapter 4).

The infant also demonstrates visual preferences: medium colours (yellow, green, pink) over dim or bright colours (red, orange, blue); black-and-white contrasting patterns, especially geometric shapes and checkerboards; large objects with medium complexity rather than small, complex objects; and reflecting objects over dull ones.

Hearing. Once the amniotic fluid has drained from the ears, the infant probably has auditory acuity similar to that of an adult. The newborn is able to detect a loud sound of about 90 dB and reacts with a startle (**Moro**) reflex. The newborn's response to sounds of low frequency and high frequency differs; the former, such as a heartbeat, metronome or lullaby, tends to decrease an infant's motor activity and crying, whereas the latter elicits an alerting reaction.

Infants have an early sensitivity to the sound of human voices and to specific speech sounds. For example, infants younger than 3 days of age can distinguish their mother's voice from that of other females. As early as 5 days, newborns can differentiate between stories read by their mother's voice (in utero) versus stories read by another woman's voice after birth.

The internal and middle ear structures are large at birth, but the external canal is small. The mastoid process and the bony part of the external canal have not yet developed. Consequently, the tympanic membrane and facial nerve are close to the surface and can be easily damaged.

Smell. Newborns react to strong odours such as alcohol or vinegar by turning their heads away. Breastfed infants are able to smell breast milk and will cry for their mothers when the breasts are leaking. Infants are also able to differentiate their mother's breast milk from that of other women by scent alone. Many believe maternal odours influence the attachment process and successful breastfeeding. Unnecessary routine washing of the breasts may interfere with establishment of early breastfeeding. It is preferable to avoid washing newborns within the first 24 hours, to assist with scent and attachment and also temperature regulation.

Taste. The newborn can distinguish between tastes, and various types of solutions elicit differing facial reflexes. A tasteless solution elicits no facial expression; a sweet solution elicits an eager suck and a look of satisfaction; a sour solution causes the usual puckering of the lips; and a bitter liquid produces an angry, upset expression.

Touch. The newborn perceives tactile sensation in any part of the body, although the face (especially the mouth), hands and soles of the feet seem to be the most sensitive. Sufficient evidence now shows that touch and motion are essential components in the attachment process and in normal growth and development. Gentle patting of the back or rubbing of the abdomen usually elicits a calming response from the infant.

NURSING AND MIDWIFERY CARE OF THE NEWBORN AND FAMILY

Assessment

The newborn requires thorough, skilled observation to ensure a satisfactory adjustment to extrauterine life. Physical assessment after birth is divided into four phases: (1) the initial assessment, which includes the Apgar scoring system; (2) transitional assessment during periods of reactivity; (3) assessment of gestational age; and (4) a comprehensive, systematic physical examination. In addition, the nurse/midwife must be aware of those behaviours that signal successful attachment between the infant and parents. Awareness of the expected normal findings during each assessment process helps the nurse/midwife recognise any deviation that may prevent the infant from progressing uneventfully through the early postnatal period. With shorter hospital stays, accomplishing a thorough newborn assessment and comprehensive parent teaching requires focused nursing/midwifery observations and interventions with every parent and newborn encounter.

Initial Assessment: Apgar Scoring

The most frequently used method to assess the newborn's immediate adjustment to extrauterine life is the **Apgar scoring system.** The score is based on observation of heart rate, respiratory effort, muscle tone, reflex irritability and colour (Table 7.1). Each item is given a score of 0, 1 or 2. Evaluations of all five categories are made 1 and 5 minutes after birth and are repeated every 5 minutes until the infant's condition stabilises. Total scores of 0 to 3 represent severe distress, scores of 4 to 6 signify moderate difficulty and scores of 7 to 10 indicate absence of difficulty in adjusting to extrauterine life. Many healthy newborns do not achieve a score of 10 because the body is not completely pink. The degree of physiological immaturity affects the Apgar score. For example, a healthy preterm infant may receive a low score due to low tone and reduced reflex irritability. Infection, congenital anomalies, maternal sedation or analgesia, hypovolaemia and neuromuscular disorders also affect the Apgar score.

The Apgar score reflects the infant's general condition at 1, 5 and 10 minutes based on the five parameters described previously. The Apgar score is not a tool, however, that stands on its own to interpret past events, determine need for newborn resuscitation or predict future events linked to the infant's neurological or physical status (AIHW 2020).

TABLE 7.1 Infant Evaluation at Birth: Apgar Scoring System

Sign	0	1	2
Heart rate	Absent	Slow, $<$ 100 beats/min	$>$ 100 beats/min
Respiratory effort	Absent	Irregular, slow, weak cry	Good, strong cry
Muscle tone	Limp	Some flexion of extremities	Well flexed
Reflex irritability	No response	Grimace	Cry, sneeze
Colour	Blue, pale	Body pink, extremities blue	Completely pink

Transitional Assessment: Periods of Reactivity

The newborn exhibits behavioural and physiological characteristics that can at first appear to be signs of stress. During a newborn's initial 24 hours, changes in heart rate, respiration, motor activity, colour, mucus production and bowel activity occur in an orderly, predictable sequence, which is normal and indicates lack of stress. Distressed infants also progress through these stages but at a slower rate.

For 6 to 8 hours after birth the newborn is in the **first period of reactivity**. During the first 30 minutes the infant is alert, cries vigorously, may suck his or her fingers or fist and appears interested in the environment. At this time the neonate's eyes are usually open; thus, this is an excellent opportunity for mother, father and child to see one another. Because the healthy, full-term newborn has a vigorous suck reflex, this is an opportune time to begin breastfeeding. The newborn usually grasps the nipple quickly, satisfying both mother and child. This is important to remember because it is likely that after this initial highly active state, the infant may be sleepy and uninterested in sucking. Physiologically, the respiratory rate can be as high as 80 breaths/min, crackles may be heard, heart rate may reach 180 beats/min, bowel sounds are active, mucus secretions are increased and temperature may decrease slightly. Maintaining appropriate temperature for the newborn is best accomplished by practising skin-to-skin care, whereby only a nappy is worn, to allow the majority of the skin surface to be in contact with the mother's skin. A light blanket is used to cover the mother and newborn. Research has shown that skin-to-skin care is effective in ensuring the newborn remains normothermic (Widström et al 2019). Being in skin-to-skin contact with the mother after birth elicits the newborn infant's internal process to go through what could be called *nine instinctive stages*: birth cry, relaxation, awakening, activity, rest, crawling, familiarisation, suckling and sleeping (Table 7.2).

After this initial stage of alertness and activity, the infant enters the second stage of the first reactive period, which generally lasts 2 to 4 hours. Heart and respiratory rates decrease, temperature continues to fall,

TABLE 7.2 Nine Instinctive Stages

Stages	Behaviours
1. Birth cry	Intense cry just after birth, transition to breathing air.
2. Relaxation stage	Infant rests. No activity of mouth, head, arms, legs or body.
3. Awakening stage	Infant begins to show signs of activity. Small thrusts of head: up, down, from side-to-side. Small movements of limbs and shoulders.
4. Active stage	Infant moves limbs and head, more determined movements. Rooting activity, 'pushing' with limbs without shifting body.
5. Resting stage*	Infant rests, with some activity, such as mouth activity, sucks on hand.
7. Familiarisation	Infant has reached areola/nipple with mouth positioned to brush and lick areola/nipple.
8. Suckling stage	Infant has taken nipple in mouth and commences suckling.
9. Sleeping stage	Infant closes eyes and falls asleep.

*The Resting Stage could be interspersed with all the stages.
Source: Widström, A., Brimdyr, K., Svensson, K., et al. (2019). Skin-to-skin contact the first hour after birth, underlying implications and clinical practice. Acta Paediatrica, 108(7), 1192–1204. https://doi.org/10.1111/apa.14754

mucus production decreases and urine or stool is usually not passed. The infant is in a state of sleep and relative calm. Any attempt at stimulation usually elicits a minimal response. Because of the decrease in body temperature, avoid undressing or bathing the infant during this time.

The **second period of reactivity** begins when the infant wakes from this deep sleep; it lasts about 2 to 5 hours and provides another excellent opportunity for child and parents to interact. The infant is again alert and responsive, heart and respiratory rates increase, the gag reflex is active, gastric and respiratory secretions are increased and passage of meconium commonly occurs. This period is usually over when the amount of respiratory mucus has decreased. After this stage is a period of stabilisation of physiological systems and a vacillating pattern of sleep and activity.

Behavioural Assessment

An important area of assessment is observation of behaviour. Infants' behaviour helps shape their environment, and their ability to react to various stimuli affects how others relate to them. The principal areas of behaviour for newborns are sleep, wakefulness and activity such as crying.

One method of systematically assessing the infant's behaviour is use of the Newborn Behavioural Observations (NBO) assessment (The Royal Women's Hospital n.d.). It is generally used as a research or diagnostic tool and requires special training.

The scale may be used to assess and support parent–child relationships, guiding parents to focus on their infant's individuality and develop a deeper attachment. Studies have demonstrated that exposure to the NBO results in increased maternal confidence and improved parent–infant interaction and developmental outcome (Nugent 2013).

The NBO system is a structured set of observations designed to help the clinician and parent together, to observe the infant's behavioural capacities and identify the kind of support the infant needs for his successful growth and development. There has been renewed interest in the NBO recently, and it is being used by nurses and midwives, doctors, home visitors and others to optimise parent–infant relationships (VAHI & SCV 2020b).

Patterns of Sleep and Activity. Infants have six distinct sleep-wake states, which represent a particular form of neural control (Table 7.3). As gestational and postconceptional maturity increases, each state becomes more precisely defined according to the behaviours observed. **State** is defined as a 'group of characteristics that regularly occur together' (Davies & Baddock 2019); these include body activity, eye and facial movements, respiratory pattern and response to internal and external stimuli. The six **sleep-wake states** are quiet (deep) sleep, active (light) sleep, drowsy, awake (quiet), active alert and crying. Infants respond to internal and external environmental factors by controlling sensory input and regulating the sleep-wake states; the ability to make smooth transitions between states is called **state modulation**. The ability to regulate sleep-wake states is essential in the infant's neurobehavioral development. The more immature the infant, the less he or she is able to cope with factors, external or internal, that affect the sleep-wake patterns.

Newborns typically spend as much as 16 to 18 hours a day sleeping and do not necessarily follow a pattern of light-dark diurnal rhythm. With increasing age, sleep-wake states change, with increasing amounts of time spent in awake alert states and decreasing amounts in sleep time. Approximately 50% of total sleep time is spent in irregular or rapid eye movement sleep.

Cry. Variations in the initial cry can indicate underlying abnormalities. A weak, groaning cry or grunting during expiration usually indicates a respiratory disturbance. Absent, weak or constant

TABLE 7.3 **States of Sleep and Activity**

State and Behaviour	Implications for Parents
DEEP SLEEP (QUIET)	
Closed eyes Regular breathing No movement except for occasional sudden bodily twitch No eye movement	Continue usual household noises because external stimuli do not arouse infant. Leave infant alone if sudden loud noise awakens infant and child cries. Do not attempt to feed.
LIGHT SLEEP (ACTIVE)	
Closed eyes Irregular breathing Slight muscular twitching of body Rapid eye movements under closed eyelids May smile	External stimuli that did not arouse infant during regular sleep may minimally arouse child. Periodic groaning or crying is usual; do not interpret as indication of pain or discomfort.
DROWSY	
Eyes may be open Irregular breathing Active body movement variable, with occasional mild startles	Most stimuli arouse infant, but infant may return to sleep state. Pick infant up during this time rather than leaving in cot. Provide mild stimulus to awaken. Infant may enjoy non-nutritive sucking.
QUIET ALERT	
Eyes wide open and bright Responds to environment by active body movement and staring at close-range objects Minimum body activity Regular breathing Focuses attention on stimuli	Satisfy infant's needs such as hunger or non-nutritive sucking. Place infant in area of home where activity is continuous. Place toys in cot or playpen. Place objects within 17.5–20 cm of infant's view. Intervene to console.
ACTIVE ALERT	
May begin with whimpering and slight body movement Eyes open Irregular breathing	Remove intense internal or external stimuli because of increased sensitivity to stimuli.
CRYING	
Progresses to strong, angry crying and uncoordinated thrashing of extremities Eyes open or tightly closed Grimaces Irregular breathing	Comforting measures that were effective during alert state are usually ineffective. Rock and swaddle to decrease crying. Intervene to reduce fatigue, hunger or discomfort.

Source: Portions adapted from Blackburn, S., & Loper, D. L. (2007). *Maternal, fetal, and neonatal physiology: A clinical perspective.* Philadelphia, PA: Saunders.

crying requires further investigation for possible drug withdrawal or a neurological problem. Crying status alone, however, is not a diagnostic tool.

Assessment of Attachment Behaviours

One of the most important areas of assessment is careful observation of those behaviours thought to indicate the formation of emotional bonds between the newborn and family, especially the mother. Although **bonding** and **attachment** are sometimes referred to as separate phenomena, with bonding representing the development of emotional ties from parent to infant and attachment representing the emotional ties from infant to parent, in this discussion the terms are used interchangeably to denote both processes.

Unlike physical assessment of the neonate, which follows concrete guidelines, assessment of parent–child attachment requires much more skill in terms of observation and interviewing. The assessment process is even more challenging with short hospital stays for mothers and their newborn infants. Rooming-in of mother and infant and visits by partner, siblings and grandparents facilitate recognition of behaviours that demonstrate positive or negative attachment. Guidelines for assessment of bonding behaviours are in the Nursing Care Guidelines box.

NURSING CARE GUIDELINES

Assessing Attachment Behaviour

- When you bring the infant to the parents, do they reach out for the child and call the child by name?
- Do the parents speak about the child in terms of identification (e.g. whom the infant looks like; what appears special about their child compared with other infants)?
- When parents are holding the infant, what kind of body contact is there? Do parents feel at ease in changing the infant's position; are fingertips or whole hands used; are there parts of the body they avoid touching or parts of the body they investigate and scrutinise?
- When the infant is awake, what kinds of stimulation do the parents provide? Do they talk to the infant, to each other or to no one? How do they look at the infant—direct visual contact, avoidance of eye contact or looking at other people or objects?
- How comfortable do the parents appear in terms of caring for the infant? Do they express any concern regarding their ability or disgust for certain activities, such as changing nappies?
- What type of affection do they demonstrate to the newborn, such as smiling, stroking, kissing or rocking?
- If the infant is fussy, what kinds of comforting techniques do the parents use, such as rocking, swaddling, talking or stroking?

Clinical Assessment of Gestational Age

Assessment of gestational age is important because perinatal morbidity and mortality are related to gestational age and birth weight. A frequently used method is the **Ballard Scale (BS)** by Ballard and colleagues (1991) (Fig 7.1A). The BS, an abbreviated version of the Dubowitz scale (Dubowitz & Dubowitz 1977), assesses six external physical and six neuromuscular signs. Each sign has a number score, and the cumulative score correlates with a maturity rating of 20 to 44 weeks of gestation.

The New Ballard Scale (NBS) can be used with newborns as young as 20 weeks of gestation, as it includes scores that reflect signs of extremely premature infants such as: fused eyelids; imperceptible breast tissue; sticky, friable, transparent skin; no lanugo; and square-window (flexion of wrist) angle of greater than 90 degrees (see Fig 7.1A and a description of the tests in Box 7.2). For infants with a gestational age of at least 26 weeks, the examination may be performed up to 96 hours after birth, but it is recommended that the initial examination be performed within the first 48 hours of life. In a study of preterm infants ranging from 29 to 35 weeks at birth, Ballard scores completed 7 days after birth were found to either overestimate or underestimate gestational age by up to 2 weeks (Sasidharan et al 2009).

Weight Related to Gestational Age. The infant's weight at birth also correlates with the incidence of perinatal morbidity and mortality. Birth weight alone, however, is a poor indicator of gestational age and fetal maturity. Maturity implies functional capacity—the degree to which the neonate's organ systems are able to adapt to the requirements of extrauterine life. Therefore, gestational age is more closely related to fetal maturity than is birth weight. Because heredity influences size at birth, it is important to note the sizes of other family members as part of the assessment process.

Classification of infants at birth by both **birth weight** and **gestational age** provides a more satisfactory method for predicting mortality risks and providing guidelines for management of the neonate than estimating gestational age or birth weight alone. The infant's birth weight, length and head circumference are plotted on standardised graphs that identify normal values for gestational age. The infant whose weight is **appropriate for gestational age (AGA)** (between the 10th and 90th percentiles) can be presumed to have grown at a normal rate regardless of the length of gestation—preterm, term or postterm. The infant who is **large for gestational age (LGA)** (> 90th percentile) can be presumed to have grown at an accelerated rate during fetal life; the **small-for-gestational-age (SGA)** infant (< 10th percentile) can be presumed to have grown at a restricted rate during intrauterine life. When gestational age is determined according to the NBS, the newborn will fall into one of the following nine possible categories for birth weight and gestational age: AGA—term, preterm, postterm; SGA—term, preterm, postterm; or LGA—term, preterm, postterm. Figure 7.2 illustrates the disparity between birth weights of three preterm infants of the same gestational age. Birth weight influences mortality rate: the lower the birth weight, the higher the mortality rate. The same is true for gestational age: the lower the gestational age, the higher the mortality rate.

Physical Assessment

The discussion of physical examination focuses on normal findings, variations from the norm that require little or no intervention, and specific potential danger signs that require more careful observation. General guidelines for conducting a physical examination are in the Nursing Care Guidelines box. Table 7.4 summarises the physical examination of the newborn. (See Chapter 4 for further discussion of examination techniques.)

NURSING CARE GUIDELINES

Physical Examination of the Newborn

- Provide a normothermic and non-stimulating examination area.
- Check that equipment and supplies are working properly and are accessible.
- Proceed quickly to avoid stressing infant.
- Undress only body area examined to prevent heat loss.
- Proceed in an orderly sequence (usually head to toe) with the following exceptions:
  - perform all procedures that require quiet first, such as auscultating the lungs, heart and abdomen
  - perform disturbing procedures, such as testing reflexes, last
  - measure head, crown-to-rump and head-to-heel length at same time to compare results.
- Comfort infant during and after examination; involve parent in the following:
  - talking softly
  - holding the infant's hands against the chest
  - swaddling and holding
  - giving a soother or gloved finger to suck.

General Measurements. Several measurements of the newborn are significant compared with each other, as well as when recorded over time on a graph. For the full-term infant, average head circumference is between 33 and 35 cm. Head circumference may be somewhat less than that immediately after birth because of the moulding process that occurs during vaginal birth. Usually by the second or third day the normal size and contour of the skull will have replaced the moulded one. In a mature newborn, the head circumference is approximately 34 to 36 cm; if the circumference is outside these measurements, the newborn will need to be assessed for neurological concerns.

Head-to-heel length is also measured. It is important to extend the legs completely when measuring total body length (Fig 7.3). The average length of the newborn is 48 to 53 cm.

Abdominal circumference need not be routinely measured in the newborn but should be done in the event of abdominal distension to determine changes in girth over time. Abdominal circumference is measured just above the level of the umbilicus. Because the umbilical cord is still attached, measurements across the umbilicus are too variable in newborns. Measuring the abdominal circumference below the umbilical region is also unsuitable because bladder status may affect the reading.

Measure body weight soon after birth because weight loss occurs fairly rapidly. Normally the newborn loses up to 10% of the birth weight by 3 to 4 days of age because of loss of excessive extracellular fluid and meconium, as well as limited food intake, especially in breastfed infants. The birth weight is usually regained by the 10th to 14th day of life, depending on the method of feeding. Most newborns weigh 2700 to 4000 g, with the average weight being about 3400 g. Accurate birth weights and lengths are important because they provide a baseline for assessment of risk status and future growth.

Vital Signs. Another category of measurements is vital signs. Core (internal) body temperature varies according to the period of reactivity but is normally 36.5°C to 37.6°C.

In addition to axilla temperature measurements, several other techniques may be used for newborns; however, the single best and most accurate method for determining the newborn infant's temperature is unclear when considering published research.

ESTIMATION OF GESTATIONAL AGE BY MATURITY RATING

NEUROMUSCULAR MATURITY

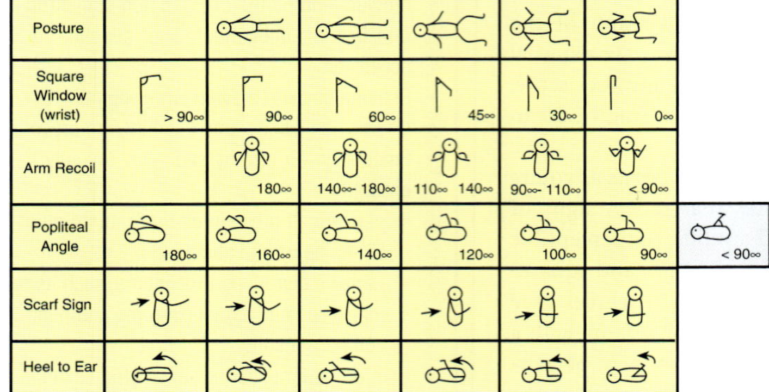

PHYSICAL MATURITY

	-1	0	1	2	3	4	5
Skin	sticky friable transparent	gelatinous red, translucent	smooth pink, visible veins	superficial peeling &/or rash, few veins	cracking pale areas rare veins	parchment deep cracking no vessels	leathery cracked wrinkled
Lanugo	none	sparse	abundant	thinning	bald areas	mostly bald	
Plantar Surface	heel-toe 40-50 mm: -1 <40 mm: -2	>50 mm no crease	faint red marks	anterior transverse crease only	creases ant. 2/3	creases over entire sole	
Breast	imperceptible	barely perceptible	flat areola no bud	stippled areola 1-2 mm bud	raised areola 3-4 mm bud	full areola 5-10 mm bud	
Eye/Ear	lids fused loosely: -1 tightly: -2	lids open pinna flat stays folded	slightly curved pinna; soft; slow recoil	well-curved pinna; soft but ready recoil	formed & firm instant recoil	thick cartilage ear stiff	
Genitals (male)	scrotum flat, smooth	scrotum empty faint rugae	testes in upper canal rare rugae	testes descending few rugae	testes down good rugae	testes pendulous deep rugae	
Genitals (female)	clitoris prominent labia flat	prominent clitoris small labia minora	prominent clitoris enlarging minora	majora & minora equally prominent	majora large minora small	majora cover clitoris & minora	

MATURITY RATING

score	weeks
-10	20
-5	22
0	24
5	26
10	28
15	30
20	32
25	34
30	36
35	38
40	40
45	42
50	44

A

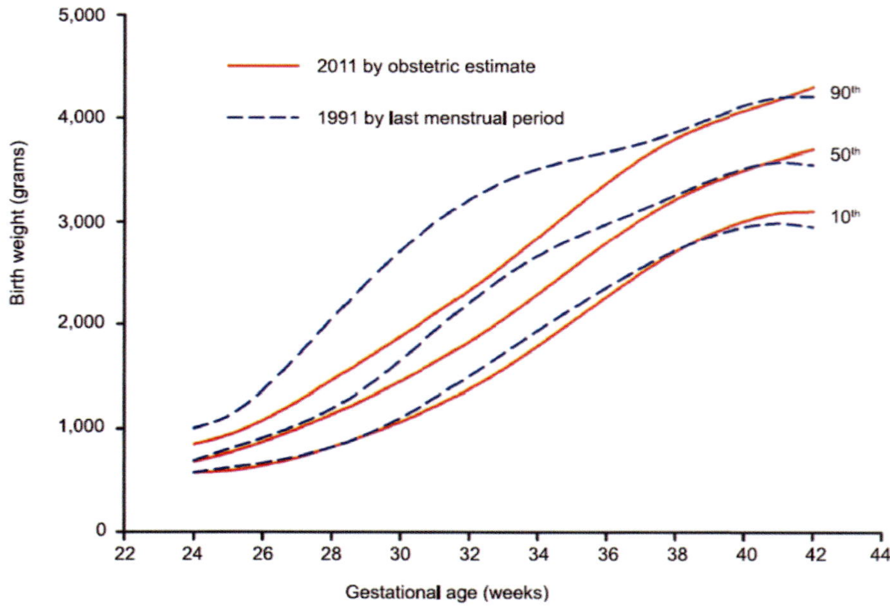

Fig 7.1 (**A**) Ballard Scale for newborn maturity rating. Expanded scale includes extremely premature infants and has been refined to improve accuracy in more mature infants. (Source: *A,* Ballard, J. L., Khoury, J. C., Wedig, K., et al. (1991). New Ballard score expanded to include extremely premature infants. The Journal of Pediatrics, 119 417.) (**B**) Intrauterine growth: Birth weight curves for 1991 neonates dated by last menstrual period compared with 2011 neonates dated by obstetrics estimate. (Source: *B,* Duryea, E. L., Hawkins, J. S., McIntire, D. D., et al. (2014). A revised birth weight reference for the United States. Obstetrics & Gynecology, 124(1), 16–22.)

BOX 7.2 Tests Used in Assessing Gestational Age

See Fig 7.1A for score categories and manoeuvres.

- **Posture**—With infant quiet and in a supine position, observe degree of flexion in arms and legs. Muscle tone and degree of flexion increase with maturity. *Score:* Full flexion of the arms and legs = 4.
- **Square window**—With thumb supporting back of arm below wrist, apply gentle pressure with index and third fingers on dorsum of hand without rotating infant's wrist. Measure angle between base of thumb and forearm. *Score:* Full flexion (hand lies flat on ventral surface of forearm) = 4.
- **Arm recoil**—With infant supine, fully flex both forearms on upper arms, hold for 5 seconds; pull down on hands to fully extend and rapidly release arms. Observe rapidity and intensity of recoil to a state of flexion. *Score:* A brisk return to full flexion = 4.
- **Popliteal angle**—With infant supine and pelvis flat on a firm surface, flex lower leg on thigh and then flex thigh on abdomen. While holding knee with thumb and index finger, extend lower leg with index finger of other hand. Measure degree of angle behind knee (popliteal angle). *Score:* An angle of less than 90 degrees = 5.
- **Scarf sign**—With infant supine, support head in midline with one hand; use other hand to pull infant's arm across the shoulder so that infant's hand touches shoulder. Determine location of elbow in relation to midline. *Score:* Elbow does not reach midline = 4.
- **Heel to ear**—With infant supine and pelvis flat on a firm surface, pull foot as far as possible up towards ear on same side. Measure distance of foot from ear and degree of knee flexion (same as popliteal angle). *Score:* Knees flexed with a popliteal angle of less than 10 degrees = 4.

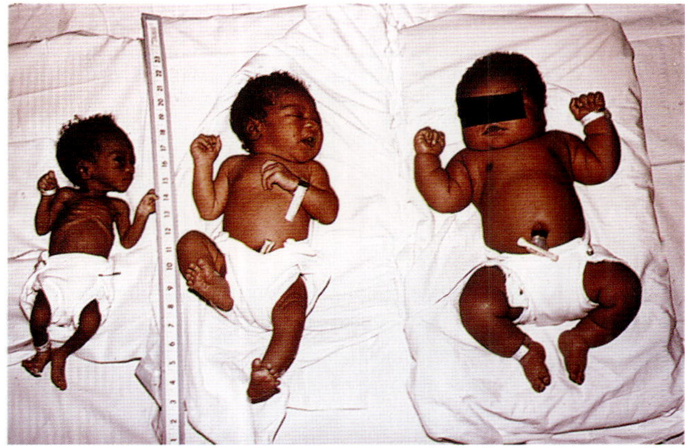

Fig 7.2 Three infants, same gestational age, weighing 600, 1400 and 2750 g, respectively, from left to right. (Source: *Perinatal assessment of maturation,* National Audiovisual Center, Washington, DC.)

Despite their usefulness in older children and adults, the accuracy of tympanic membrane thermometers has been problematic in infants. A comprehensive review of the literature exploring methods and devices for temperature measurement in the newborn resulted in the authors concluding that the accuracy of the tympanic route in the neonate is controversial (Smith 2014, Smith et al 2013). The Canadian Paediatric Society (CPS) (2015) has outlined concerns regarding safety and accuracy of tympanic temperature measurement in newborns because of the size of a newborn's external ear canal relative to the size of the thermometer probe. To ensure accuracy, the probe, which may be up to 8 mm in diameter, must be deeply inserted into the ear canal to allow orientation of the sensor near or against the tympanic membrane. At birth, the average diameter of the canal is just 4 mm; at 2 years of age it is just 5 mm. The CPS concludes that current infrared tympanic thermometry lacks sufficient safety and precision to meet clinical needs for use in newborn infants and children under 2 years of age.

Temporal artery thermometers (TATs), in which a battery-powered instrument is gently slid across the newborn's forehead, are available for use in the general paediatric population, and parents often report ease of use and increased comfort with such methods. Beginning research in the neonatal population suggests that TAT may be a reasonable method for newborn temperature measurement in healthy full-term newborns. Haddad and colleagues (2012), in a study of healthy newborns in a mother and baby unit, compared TAT with axillary temperature measurement. Although a slightly statistically significant difference was found between TAT and axillary temperatures, the difference was deemed clinically insignificant, and the unit has adopted TAT as their standard of care for healthy newborns. Similarly, Sim and colleagues (2016) report, after a prospective comparative study, that TAT and axillary temperatures did not differ significantly for newborns nursed in room air. They recommend that TAT measurements are a reasonable alternative to axillary temperatures for stable, afebrile infants nursed in room air. The use of TAT for infants under phototherapy or those in incubators or under radiant warmers was deemed inappropriate in this study, as there was poor correlation between TAT and axillary temperatures in those newborns.

Infrared axillary and digital thermometers are used in many neonatal units because they give rapid readings and are easy to clean. An extensive review by Smith and colleagues (2013) of the literature on temperature measurement in term and preterm infants reported that the axillary route is the most common one used in newborns.

A suggested schedule for monitoring heart and respiratory rates and temperature for healthy full-term newborns is within the first hour of life, once every 30 minutes until the newborn has been stable for 2 hours, and then once every 8 hours until discharge. This schedule may vary according to institutional policy. Any change in the infant's colour, breathing, muscle tone or behaviour necessitates more frequent monitoring.

Measurement of blood pressure (BP) provides baseline data and may indicate cardiovascular problems. BP is affected by gestational age and birth weight. For infants with **murmurs**, suspicion of congenital heart disease or any concerns regarding tissue perfusion or fluid volume, BP is most easily and accurately assessed using oscillometry (DINAMAP) (Fig 7.5). Oscillometric BP is more accurate when the newborn is in a quiet or sleep state and an appropriate cuff width–to–arm or calf ratio of 0.45 to 0.70 is used. It is recommended that two or three BP measurements be taken in sick infants and that the mean BP be used because there is less error than when using systolic and diastolic readings. For healthy full-term infants, the average oscillometric systolic/diastolic BP is 65/45 mmHg on day 1 of life, changing to 69.5/44.5 by day 3 (Casey 2018). Compare BP in the upper and lower extremities, which should be equal.

Although uncommon, neonatal hypertension may be a sign of a significant underlying problem such as a renal, cardiac or thromboembolic pathological condition, or it may be associated with a

TABLE 7.4 Summary of Physical Assessment of the Newborn

Usual Findings	Common Variations, Minor Abnormalities	Potential Signs of Distress, Major Abnormalities
GENERAL MEASUREMENTS		
Head circumference—33–35 cm; equal or up to 2 cm larger than crown-to-rump length	Moulding after birth altering head circumference	Head circumference < 10th or > 90th percentile
Crown-to-rump length—31–35 cm; approximately equal to head circumference Head-to-heel length—48–53 cm		
Birth weight—2700–4000 g	Loss of 10% of birth weight in first week; regained in 10–14 days, depending on feeding method	Birth weight < 10th or > 90th percentile Loss of > 10% of birth weight in first week
VITAL SIGNS		
Temperature, axillary—36.5–37°C	Crying increasing body temperature slightly Radiant warmer falsely increasing axillary temperature	Hypothermia Hyperthermia
Heart rate, apical—120–140 beats/min	Crying increasing heart rate; sleep decreasing heart rate During 1st period of reactivity (6–8 hours), rate ≤ 180 beats/min	Bradycardia—resting rate < 80–100 beats/min Tachycardia—rate > 160–180 beats/min Irregular rhythm
Respirations—30–60 breaths/min	Crying increasing respiratory rate; sleep decreasing respiratory rate During 1st period of reactivity (6–8 hours), rate up to 80 breaths/min	Tachypnoea—rate > 60 breaths/min Apnoea—cessation of respirations for 20 seconds or more
Blood pressure (BP), oscillometric—65/41 mmHg in arm and calf	Crying and activity increasing BP	Oscillometric systolic pressure in calf 6–9 mmHg less than in upper extremity (possible sign of coarctation of aorta) Systolic pressure > 90 mmHg is considered hypertension
GENERAL APPEARANCE		
Posture—flexion of head and extremities, which rest on chest and abdomen	Frank breech—extended legs, abducted and fully rotated thighs, flattened occiput, extended neck	Limp posture—extension of extremities
SKIN		
At birth, bright red, puffy, smooth 2nd–3rd day, pink, flaky, dry Vernix caseosa Lanugo Oedema around eyes, face, legs, dorsa of hands, feet and scrotum or labia Acrocyanosis—cyanosis of hands and feet Cutis marmorata—transient mottling when infant is exposed to decreased temperature	Neonatal jaundice after first 24 hours Ecchymoses or petechiae caused by birth trauma Milia—distended sebaceous glands that appear as tiny white papules on cheeks, chin and nose Miliaria or sudamina—distended sweat (eccrine) glands that appear as minute vesicles, especially on face Erythema toxicum—pink papular rash with vesicles superimposed on thorax, back, buttocks and abdomen; may appear in 24–48 hours and resolve after several days Harlequin colour change—clearly outlined colour change as infant lies on side; lower half of body becomes pink and upper half is pale	Progressive jaundice, especially in first 24 hours after birth Generalised cyanosis Pallor Mottling Greyness Plethora Haemorrhage, ecchymoses or petechiae that persist Sclerema—hard and stiff skin Poor skin turgor (tenting) Rashes, pustules or blisters Café-au-lait spots—light brown spots Naevus flammeus—port-wine stain Herpetic blister(s) Capillary haemangiomas—bright red, raised, soft, lobulated tumour occurring on the head, neck, trunk or extremities; does not blanch with pressure (see also Birthmarks, Chapter 8)
	Mongolian spots—irregular areas of deep blue pigmentation, usually in sacral and gluteal regions; seen predominantly in newborns of African, Native American, Asian or Hispanic descent (see figure at right)	

TABLE 7.4 Summary of Physical Assessment of the Newborn—cont'd

Usual Findings	Common Variations, Minor Abnormalities	Potential Signs of Distress, Major Abnormalities
	Naevus simplex (stork bite or salmon patch)—flat, deep pink, localised areas usually seen on nape of neck, upper eyelid, glabella or on the upper lip; blanches with pressure and frequently becomes more prominent with crying	
HEAD		
Anterior fontanel—diamond shaped; size varies from barely palpable to 4–5 cm (see Fig 7.4) Posterior fontanel—triangular, 0.5–1 cm Fontanels flat, soft and firm Widest part of fontanel measured from bone to bone, not suture to suture	Moulding after vaginal birth Third sagittal (parietal) fontanel Bulging fontanel because of crying or coughing Caput succedaneum—oedema of soft scalp tissue Cephalhaematoma (uncomplicated)—haematoma between periosteum and skull bone	Fused sutures Bulging or depressed fontanels when quiet Widened sutures and fontanels Craniotabes—snapping sensation along lambdoid suture that resembles indentation of ping-pong ball
EYES		
Lids usually oedematous Colour—slate grey, dark blue, brown Absence of tears Red reflex Corneal reflex in response to touch Pupillary reflex in response to light Blink reflex in response to light or touch Rudimentary fixation on objects and ability to follow to midline	Epicanthal folds in Asian infants Searching nystagmus or strabismus Subconjunctival (scleral) haemorrhages—ruptured capillaries, usually at limbus	Pink colour of iris Purulent discharge Upward slant in non-Asians Hypertelorism (≥ 3 cm) Hypotelorism Congenital cataracts Constricted or dilated fixed pupil Absence of red reflex Absence of pupillary or corneal reflex Inability to follow object or bright light to midline Yellow sclera Leukocoria (white pupil)—possible retinoblastoma
EARS		
Position—top of pinna on horizontal line with outer canthus of eye Startle (Moro) reflex elicited by loud, sudden noise or stimulus Pinna flexible, cartilage present	Inability to visualise tympanic membrane because of filled aural canals Pinna flat against head Irregular shape or size Pits or skin tags	Low placement of ears Absence of startle (Moro) reflex in response to loud noise or stimulus Minor abnormalities possible signs of various syndromes, especially renal
NOSE		
Nasal patency Nasal discharge—thin white mucus Sneezing	Flattened and bruised	Non-patent canals Thick, bloody nasal discharge Flaring of nares (alae nasi) Single nasal canal Copious nasal secretions or stuffiness (may be minor)
MOUTH AND THROAT		
Intact, high-arched palate Uvula in midline Frenulum of tongue Frenulum of upper lip Sucking reflex—strong and coordinated Rooting reflex Gag reflex Extrusion reflex Absent or minimum salivation Vigorous cry	Natal teeth—teeth present at birth; benign but may be associated with congenital defects Epstein pearls—small, white epithelial cysts along midline of hard palate	Cleft lip Cleft palate Large, protruding tongue or posterior displacement of tongue Profuse salivation or drooling Candidiasis (thrush)—white, adherent patches on tongue, palate and buccal surfaces Inability to pass nasogastric tube to stomach Hoarse, high-pitched, weak, absent or other abnormal cry Stridor Micrognathia—small lower jaw seen in Pierre Robin sequence (see Chapter 8)
NECK		
Short, thick, usually surrounded by skinfolds Tonic neck reflex	Torticollis (wryneck)—head held to one side with chin pointing to opposite side	Excessive skinfolds or webbing Resistance to flexion Absence of tonic neck reflex Fractured clavicle; crepitus

Continued

TABLE 7.4 Summary of Physical Assessment of the Newborn—cont'd

Usual Findings	Common Variations, Minor Abnormalities	Potential Signs of Distress, Major Abnormalities
CHEST		
Anteroposterior and lateral diameters equal Slight sternal retractions evident during inspiration Xiphoid process evident Breast enlargement	Funnel chest (pectus excavatum) Pigeon chest (pectus carinatum) Supernumerary nipples Secretion of milky substance from breasts ('witch's milk')	Depressed sternum Marked retractions of chest and intercostal spaces during respiration Asymmetrical chest expansion Redness and firmness around nipples Wide-spaced nipples
LUNGS		
Respirations chiefly abdominal Cough reflex absent at birth, present by 1–2 days Bilateral equal bronchial breath sounds	Rate and depth of respirations may be irregular; periodic breathing Crackles shortly after birth	Inspiratory stridor Expiratory grunting Retractions Persistent irregular breathing Periodic breathing with repeated apnoeic spells Seesaw respirations (paradoxic) Apnoea Unequal breath sounds Persistent fine, medium or coarse crackles Wheezing Diminished breath sounds Peristaltic bowel sounds on one side, with diminished breath sounds on same side
HEART		
Apex—4th–5th intercostal space, lateral to left sternal border S_2 slightly sharper and higher in pitch than S_1	Sinus arrhythmia—heart rate increasing with inspiration and decreasing with expiration Transient cyanosis on crying or straining	Dextrocardia—heart on right side Displacement of apex, muffled heart sound Cardiomegaly Abdominal shunts Murmur Thrill Persistent central cyanosis Hyperactive praecordium
ABDOMEN		
Cylindrical in shape Liver—palpable 2–3 cm below right costal margin Spleen—tip palpable at end of 1st week of age Kidneys—palpable 1–2 cm above umbilicus Umbilical cord—bluish-white at birth with two arteries and one vein Femoral pulses—equal bilaterally	Umbilical hernia Diastasis recti—midline gap between recti muscles 'Wharton's' jelly—unusually thick umbilical cord	Abdominal distension Localised bulging Distended veins Absent bowel sounds Enlarged liver and spleen Ascites Visible peristaltic waves Scaphoid or concave abdomen (possible congenital diaphragmatic hernia) Moist umbilical cord Presence of only one artery in cord Urine, stool or pus leaking from cord or cord insertion site Periumbilical erythema Palpable bladder distension after scant voiding Absent femoral pulses Cord bleeding or haematoma Omphalocele or gastroschisis—protrusion of abdominal contents through umbilical cord or abdominal wall Bladder exstrophy (exteriorised bladder; also associated with epispadias or cloaca)

TABLE 7.4 Summary of Physical Assessment of the Newborn—cont'd

Usual Findings	Common Variations, Minor Abnormalities	Potential Signs of Distress, Major Abnormalities
FEMALE GENITALIA		
Labia and clitoris usually oedematous Urethral meatus behind clitoris Vernix caseosa between labia Urination within 24 hours	Pseudomenstruation—blood-tinged or mucoid discharge Hymenal tag	Enlarged clitoris with urethral meatus at tip Fused labia Absence of vaginal opening Meconium from vaginal opening No urination within 24 hours Masses in labia Ambiguous genitalia Bladder exstrophy
MALE GENITALIA		
Urethral opening at tip of glans penis Testes palpable in each scrotum Scrotum usually large, oedematous, pendulous and covered with rugae; usually deeply pigmented in dark-skinned ethnic groups Smegma Urination within 24 hours	Urethral opening covered by prepuce Inability to retract foreskin Epithelial pearls—small, firm, white lesions at tip of prepuce Erection or priapism Testes palpable in inguinal canal Scrotum small	Hypospadias—urethral opening on ventral surface of penis Epispadias—urethral opening on dorsal surface of penis Chordee—ventral curvature of penis Testes not palpable in scrotum or inguinal canal No urination within 24 hours Inguinal hernia Hypoplastic scrotum Hydrocele—fluid in scrotum Masses in scrotum Meconium from scrotum Discolouration of testes Ambiguous genitalia Bladder exstrophy
BACK AND RECTUM		
Spine intact; no openings, masses or prominent curves Trunk incurvation reflex Anal reflex Patent anal opening Passage of meconium within 48 hours	Green liquid stools in infant under phototherapy Delayed passage of meconium in very-low-birth-weight neonates	Anal fissures or fistulas Imperforate anus Absence of anal reflex No meconium within 36–48 hours Pilonidal cyst or sinus Tuft of hair along spine Spina bifida (any degree)
EXTREMITIES		
10 fingers and toes Full range of motion Nail beds pink, with transient cyanosis immediately after birth Creases on anterior $^{2}/_{3}$ of sole Sole usually flat Symmetry of extremities Equal muscle tone bilaterally, especially resistance to opposing flexion Equal bilateral brachial pulses	Partial syndactyly between 2nd and 3rd toes 2nd toe overlapping 3rd toe Wide gap between 1st (hallux) and 2nd toes Deep crease on plantar surface of foot between 1st and 2nd toes Asymmetrical length of toes Dorsiflexion and shortness of hallux	Polydactyly—extra digits Syndactyly—fused or webbed digits Phocomelia—hands or feet attached close to trunk Hemimelia—absence of distal part of extremity Hyperflexibility of joints Persistent cyanosis of nail beds Yellowing of nail beds Sole covered with creases Transverse palmar (simian) crease Fractures Decreased or absent range of motion Dislocated or subluxated hip Limitation in hip abduction Unequal gluteal or leg folds Unequal knee height (Allis or Galeazzi sign) Audible clunk on abduction (Ortolani's sign) Asymmetry of extremities Unequal muscle tone or range of motion

Continued

TABLE 7.4 Summary of Physical Assessment of the Newborn—cont'd

Usual Findings	Common Variations, Minor Abnormalities	Potential Signs of Distress, Major Abnormalities
NEUROMUSCULAR SYSTEM		
Extremities usually in some degree of flexion Extension of extremity followed by previous position of flexion Head lag while sitting, but momentary ability to hold head erect Ability to turn head from side to side when prone Ability to hold head in horizontal line with back when held prone	Quivering or momentary tremors	Hypotonia—floppy, poor head control, extremities limp Hypertonia—jittery, arms and hands tightly flexed, legs stiffly extended, startles easily Asymmetrical posturing (except tonic neck reflex) Opisthotonic posturing—arched back Signs of paralysis Tremors, twitches and myoclonic jerks Marked head lag in all positions

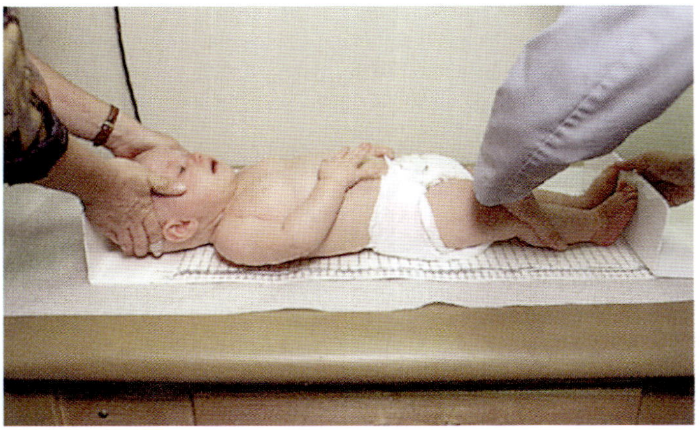

Fig 7.3 Measurement of infant length.

medication treatment regimen. The nurse/midwife should bring neonatal hypertension to the medical practitioner's attention for further evaluation.

Safer Care Victoria recommends routine pulse oximetry screening for critical congenital heart disease (CCHD) for all newborns. Universal screening for CCHD with pulse oximetry has been adopted in many states (see also VAHI & SCV 2020c). Delayed diagnosis of CCHD can result in morbidity or mortality to infants. Research has demonstrated that adding pulse oximetry, a non-invasive, painless technology, to newborn assessment can detect CCHD. Medical practitioners are directed to use motion-tolerant pulse oximeters and to screen infants after 24 hours of age to reduce false-positive results. Because the ductus arteriosus may not be fully closed at 24 hours of age, oxygen saturation must be measured in the right hand (preductal circulation) and in one foot. A reading of 95% or greater in either extremity with a 3% or less difference between the upper and lower extremities (preductal and postduc-

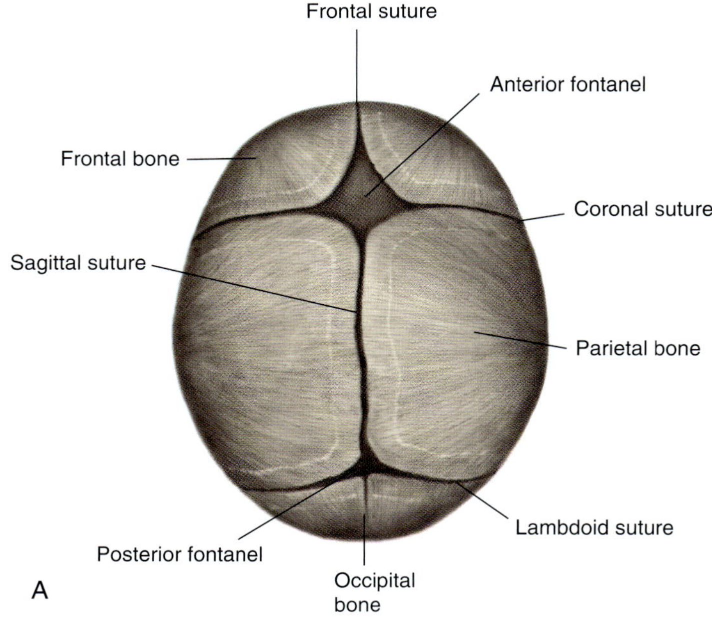

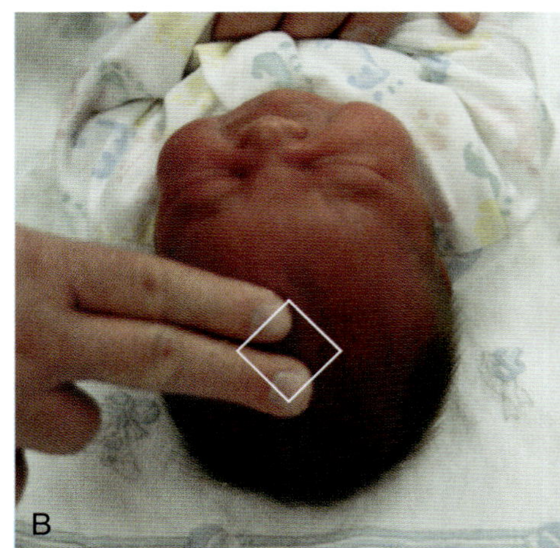

Fig 7.4 (**A**) Location of sutures and fontanels. (**B**) Palpating anterior fontanel.

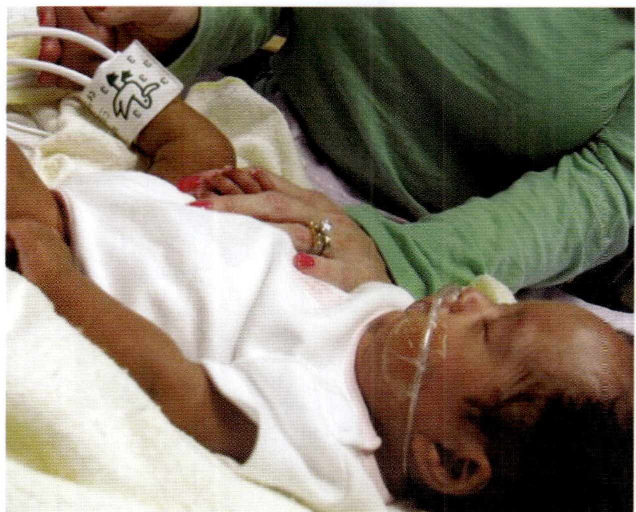

Fig 7.5 Measurement of BP using oscillometry. (Source: Courtesy of E. Jacob, Texas Children's Hospital, Houston.)

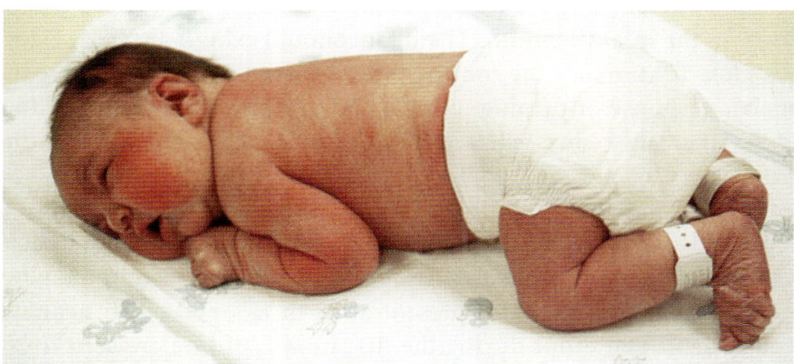

Fig 7.6 Flexion position of neonate. Note: Prone position is avoided for infant sleeping.

tal circulation) is considered to be a 'pass'. Infants with saturation of less than 90% need immediate evaluation.

General Appearance. In the full-term newborn the posture is one of flexion, a result of in utero position (Fig 7.6). Most infants are born in a vertex (head-first) presentation and keep the head flexed, with the chin resting on the upper chest. The arms are flexed at the elbows and rest, folded, on the chest with hands clenched or fisted. The legs are flexed at the knees, the hips are flexed with thighs resting on the abdomen and the feet are dorsiflexed against the anterior aspect of the legs. The vertebral column is also flexed.

Note any deviation from this characteristic fetal position. For example, preterm and hypoxic infants do not assume an attitude of total flexion but rather one of limp or hypotonic extension. Non-vertex presentations also result in variations in posture. In breech presentations the posture depends on the presenting part; a frank breech presentation results in extended legs, abducted and fully rotated thighs, a flattened head on top and a neck that appears elongated.

Observe the infant's behaviour, especially the degree of alertness, drowsiness and irritability, which are common signs of neurological problems. Ask the following questions when assessing behaviour.

- Is the infant easily awakened by a loud noise?
- Is the infant comforted by rocking, sucking or cuddling?
- Does the infant seem to have periods of deep and light sleep?
- When awake, does the infant seem satisfied after a feeding?
- What stimuli elicit responses from the infant?

Skin. The texture of the newborn's skin is velvety smooth and puffy, especially about the eyes, the legs, the dorsal aspect of the hands and feet and the scrotum or labia.

Skin colour depends on racial and familial background and varies greatly among newborns. By the second or third day the skin tone may change, and skin is drier and flakier.

Observe the colour of the skin in relation to activity, position and temperature changes. In general, the infant becomes redder when crying. Table 7.4 describes several other colour changes and minor skin blemishes.

Head. General observation of the head's contour is important because moulding occurs in almost all vaginal births. In a vertex birth the head is usually flattened at the forehead, with the apex rising and forming a point at the end of the parietal bones, and the posterior skull or occiput dropping abruptly. The usual, more oval contour of the head is apparent by 1 or 2 days after birth.

Palpate the skull for any unusual masses or prominences, particularly those resulting from birth trauma, such as caput succedaneum or cephalhaematoma (see Chapter 8). Because of the pliability of the skull, exerting pressure at the margin of the parietal and occipital bones along the lambdoid suture may produce a snapping sensation similar to the indentation of a ping-pong ball. This phenomenon, known as physiological **craniotabes**, may be found normally, especially in newborns of breech birth, but also may be associated with hydrocephalus, congenital syphilis or rickets.

Assess the degree of head control. Although head lag is normal, the full-term newborn has some ability to control the head in certain positions. If the supine infant is pulled by the arms into a semi-Fowler's position, head lag and hyperextension occur (Fig 7.7A). However, as infants are brought forward into a sitting position, they attempt to control their heads in an upright position. As the head falls forwards onto the chest, many infants attempt to right it into the erect position. If they are held in ventral suspension (i.e. held prone above and parallel to the examining surface), the head is held in a straight line with the spinal column (Fig 7.7B). When lying on the abdomen, newborns have the ability to lift the head slightly, turning it from side to side. Marked head lag is seen in neonates with Down syndrome, prematurity, hypoxia and metabolic and neurological disorders.

Eyes. Because newborns tend to keep their eyes tightly closed, begin the examination of the eyes by observing the lids for oedema, which is normally present for 2 days after birth. Observe the eyes for symmetry and for hypertelorism (wide spacing between the eyes), but do not measure the distance between the inner canthi unless there is cause for further investigation. Tears may be present at birth, but purulent discharge from the eyes shortly after birth is abnormal.

To visualise the surface structures of the eye, hold the infant supine and gently lower the head. The eyes will usually open, similar to the mechanism of a doll's eyes. The sclera should be white and clear.

Examine the cornea for any opacities or haziness. The corneal reflex is present at birth but is generally not elicited unless cerebral or eye damage is suspected. The pupil usually responds to light by constricting. Absence of the pupillary reflex, particularly by 3 weeks of age, suggests blindness. A fixed, dilated or constricted pupil may indicate central nervous system damage. A searching nystagmus is common after birth. Strabismus is a normal finding because of the lack of binocularity.

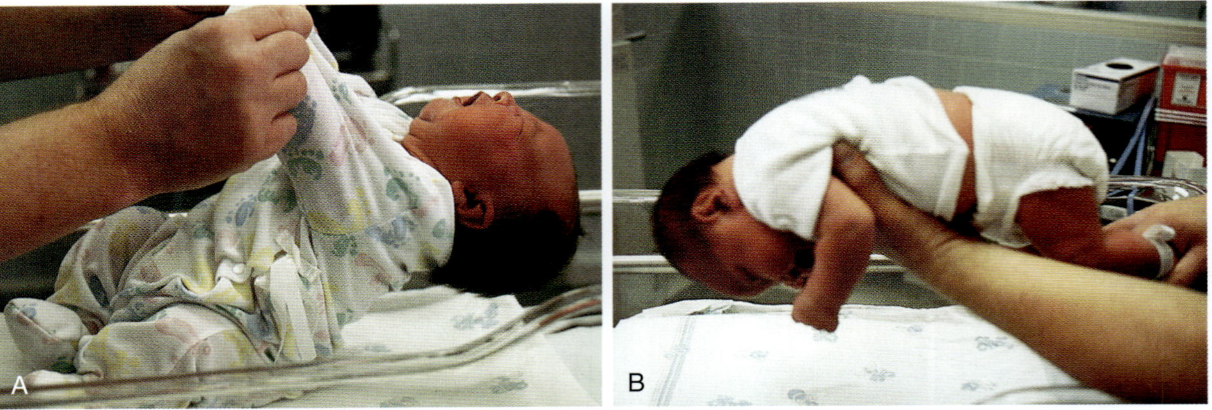

Fig 7.7 Head control in infant. (**A**) Inability to hold head erect when pulled to sitting position. (**B**) Ability to hold head erect when placed in ventral suspension.

Although it is difficult to perform a complete funduscopic examination of the retina, the nurse/midwife should elicit a red reflex.

Ears. Examine the ears for position, structure and auditory function. The pinna is often flattened against the side of the head from pressure in utero. An otoscopic examination may not always be performed because the canals are filled with vernix caseosa and amniotic fluid, making visualisation of the tympanic membrane difficult. Periauricular skin tags, sinuses and misshapen or low-set ears may be familial or associated with other congenital defects such as trisomy 18 and renal defects.

Nose. The newborn's nose is usually quite large for the face. As the face grows, the nose will remain the same size and this discrepancy disappears. The most common congenital abnormality of the nose is choanal atresia, either unilateral or bilateral, which may lead to increased breathing effort or feeding difficulties.

Assess patency of the nasal canals by holding your hand over the infant's mouth and one canal and noting the passage of air through the unobstructed opening. If nasal patency is questionable, report it because most newborns are obligatory nose breathers and are unable to breathe orally in response to nasal occlusion.

Mouth and Throat. Inspect the mouth's existing structures. The palate is normally high arched and somewhat narrow. Inspect the hard and soft palates for any clefts, which warrant further investigation. A common finding is **Epstein pearls**—small, white, epithelial cysts along both sides of the midline of the hard palate. They are insignificant and disappear in several weeks.

The **frenulum** of the upper lip is a band of thick, pink tissue that lies under the inner surface of the upper lip and extends to the maxillary alveolar ridge. It usually disappears as the maxilla grows. It is particularly evident when the infant yawns or smiles.

The **lingual frenulum** attaches the underside of the tongue midway between the ventral surface of the tongue and the tip to the lower palate. It is estimated that 4% to 16% of newborns have a tight lingual frenulum, sometimes referred to as tongue-tie, which may restrict adequate sucking; this is on the increase in Australia (Kapoor et al 2018). Further evaluation may be required to ascertain sucking ability, particularly in breastfed infants. Some medical practitioners recommend frenotomy as a safe and effective surgical procedure that improves comfort, effectiveness and ease of breastfeeding for mother and infant. A recent Cochrane review of five published studies concluded, however, that although a reduction in maternal pain was generally reported, breastfeeding was not consistently improved post procedure (O'Shea et al 2017). Research continues in an effort to determine how best to select which infants may benefit from the procedure and when to perform it (Emond et al 2014, Power & Murphy 2015).

Elicit the **sucking reflex** by placing a nipple or non-latex gloved finger in the infant's mouth. The infant should exhibit a strong, vigorous suck. To stimulate the **rooting reflex**, stroke the cheek and note the infant's response of turning towards the stimulated side and sucking. Assess the **gag reflex** when using a tongue blade to visualise the oropharynx.

Inspect the uvula while the infant is crying and the chin is depressed. However, the uvula may be retracted upwards and backwards during crying. Tonsillar tissue is generally not seen in the newborn. Natal teeth (i.e. teeth present at birth as opposed to neonatal teeth—teeth that erupt during the first month of life) are seen infrequently and erupt chiefly at the position of the lower central incisors. Natal or neonatal teeth can lead to gingivitis, self-mutilation of the tongue and trauma to the mother during breastfeeding; however, they should be extracted only if they are loose enough to involve risk of aspiration or sublingual ulceration or if feeding is severely disturbed. Most will develop normally with normal root structure (Davies & Baddock 2019).

Neck. Because the newborn's neck is short and covered with folds of tissue, for adequate assessment allow the head to fall gently backwards in slight hyperextension while supporting the back in a slightly raised position. Observe for range of motion, shape and any abnormal masses, and palpate each clavicle for possible fractures. (See Fractures, Chapter 8.)

Chest. The shape of the newborn's chest is almost circular, with equal anteroposterior and lateral diameters. The ribs are flexible, and slight **intercostal retractions** are normal on inspiration. The xiphoid process is commonly visible as a small protrusion at the end of the sternum. The sternum is raised and slightly curved.

Inspect the breasts for: size; shape; and nipple formation, location and number. Maternal hormones cause breast enlargement that appears in many newborns of either gender by the second or third day. Occasionally the infant's breasts will secrete a milky substance. Infrequently, more than two nipples are present; if these are found, evaluate the kidneys because of the association of extra nipples with renal anomalies.

Lungs. The newborn's normal respirations are irregular and abdominal, and the rate is between 30 and 60 breaths/min. Periods of **apnoea** lasting more than 20 seconds are abnormal and may be accompanied by **bradycardia**. After the first forceful breaths required to initiate respiration, subsequent breaths should be easy and fairly regular in rhythm. Occasional irregularities occur in relation to crying, sleeping and feeding. **Periodic breathing** is common in full-term newborns and consists of rapid non-laboured respirations followed by pauses of less than 20 seconds; periodic breathing may be more prominent during sleep and is not accompanied by status changes such as cyanosis or bradycardia.

Perform auscultation when the infant is quiet. Bronchial breath sounds should be equal bilaterally. Report any differences in auscultatory findings between symmetrical sites. Crackles soon after birth may indicate areas of atelectasis or the presence of fluid, which represents the normal transition of the lungs to extrauterine life. However, wheezes, persistence of crackles and stridor should be reported.

NURSING CONSIDERATIONS

Signs of respiratory distress include tachypnoea, grunting, nasal flaring, intercostal retractions, stridor, abnormal breath sounds, cyanosis and pallor.

Heart. Heart rate may range from 100 to 180 beats/min shortly after birth and, when the infant's condition has stabilised, from 120 to 140 beats/min. Palpate to find the **point of maximum intensity (PMI)**, which is usually in the fourth to fifth intercostal space, medial to the left midclavicular line. The PMI gives some indication of the location of the heart, which may be displaced in conditions such as congenital diaphragmatic hernia or pneumothorax. **Dextrocardia**, an anomaly wherein the heart is on the right side of the body, should be reported (the abdominal organs may also be reversed), along with associated circulatory abnormalities.

NURSING CONSIDERATIONS

Because auscultation of neonatal breath sounds and heart tones is often difficult for the untrained ear, practise auscultating one parameter at a time. Close your eyes and mentally block out the extraneous sounds heard, such as room noise or neonatal movement; offer the newborn a soother or gloved finger. Auscultation of a murmur and decreased air movement in specific lung fields requires patience and practice; it may require auscultating the heart tones or breath sounds for 1 to 3 minutes each.

Auscultation of the specific components of the heart sounds is difficult because of the rapid rate and effective transmission of respiratory sounds. However, the first (S_1) and second (S_2) sounds should be clear and well defined; the second sound is somewhat higher in pitch and sharper than the first. Murmurs are frequently heard in the newborn as a whooshing, blowing or rasping sound, especially over the base of the heart or at the left sternal border in the third or fourth interspace. Ordinarily they are not associated with specific cardiac defects but frequently represent the incomplete functional closure of fetal shunts. (Chapter 4 discusses grading of heart murmurs.) However, always record and report any murmur or other unusual sounds.

Abdomen. The normal contour of the abdomen is cylindrical and prominent with visible veins. Bowel sounds are audible within the first 15 to 20 minutes after birth. Visible peristaltic waves may be observed in thin newborns but should not be seen in well-nourished infants.

Inspect the umbilical cord to determine the presence of two arteries, which look like papular structures, and one vein, which has a larger lumen than the arteries and a thinner vessel wall. At birth the cord appears bluish-white and moist. After clamping, it begins to dry and appears a dull, yellowish-brown. It progressively shrivels and turns greenish-black. If the umbilical cord appears unusually large in diameter at the base, inspect for the presence of a haematoma or small omphalocele. The cord must not be clamped over an omphalocele because part of the intestine will be clamped, causing tissue necrosis. One practical rule of thumb is to cut the cord distally 10 to 12 cm from a questionable enlargement until further examination is carried out by a medical practitioner. The extra length can be cut once normal anatomy has been identified.

A cord that is draining and erythematous at the base should be investigated by the primary practitioner. The cord undergoes a process of dry gangrene decay, which has an odour; therefore, odour alone may not be a reliable index of suspicion for **omphalitis**.

Palpate after inspecting the abdomen. The liver is normally palpable 1 to 3 cm below the right costal margin. The tip of the spleen can sometimes be felt, but a palpable spleen more than 1 cm below the left costal margin suggests enlargement and warrants further investigation. Although the nurse/midwife should palpate both kidneys, this manoeuvre requires considerable practice. When felt, the lower half of the right kidney and the tip of the left kidney are 1 to 2 cm above the level of the umbilicus. During examination of the lower abdomen, palpate for femoral pulses, which should be strong and equal bilaterally.

Female Genitalia. Normally the labia majora and minora (the minora may be more prominent) and clitoris are oedematous, especially after a breech birth. However, carefully inspect the labia and clitoris to identify any evidence of ambiguous genitalia or other abnormalities. Normally in a girl the urethral opening is located behind the clitoris. Any deviation from this may mistakenly suggest that the clitoris is a small penis, which can occur in conditions such as congenital adrenal hyperplasia.

Vaginal discharge may be noted during the first week of life. This **pseudomenstruation** is a manifestation of the abrupt decrease in maternal hormones and usually disappears by 2 to 4 weeks of age. Faecal discharge from the vaginal opening indicates a rectovaginal fistula and must be reported. Vernix caseosa may be present in large amounts between the labia. Vigorous attempts to remove all the vernix through bathing are avoided to prevent tissue damage. With routine bathing and care, vernix will disappear after several days.

Male Genitalia. Inspect the penis for the urethral opening, which is located at the tip. However, the opening may be totally covered by the prepuce, or foreskin, which covers the glans penis. A tight prepuce is a common finding in newborns and does not indicate phimosis. It should not be forcefully retracted; locating the urinary meatus is usually possible without retracting the foreskin. **Smegma**, a white, cheesy substance, is commonly found around the glans penis, under the foreskin. An erection is common in the newborn. Small, white, firm lesions called **epithelial pearls** may be seen at the tip of the prepuce.

The scrotum may be large, oedematous and pendulous in the full-term neonate, especially in the infant born in breech position. It is more deeply pigmented in dark-skinned infants. A non-communicating **hydrocele** commonly occurs unilaterally and disappears within a few months. Palpate the scrotum for the presence of testes. (See Chapter 4.)

In small newborns, particularly premature infants, the undescended testes may be palpable within the inguinal canal. Absence of the testes may also be a sign of ambiguous genitalia, especially when accompanied by a small scrotum and penis. Inguinal hernias may or may not be manifested immediately after birth. A hernia is easier to detect when the infant is crying. Palpable lymph nodes are most commonly found in the inguinal area. Report a discoloured or dusky scrotum, scrotal oedema or palpation of a small mass to the medical practitioner because these may be a sign of testicular torsion.

Back and Anus. Inspect the spine with the infant prone. The shape of the spine is gently rounded, with none of the characteristic S-shaped curves seen later in life. Any abnormal openings or sinuses, masses, dimples or soft areas are noted. A protruding sac anywhere along the spine, but most commonly in the sacral area, indicates some type of spina bifida. A small sinus, which may or may not be communicating with the spine, is a **pilonidal sinus**; the sinus is usually located on the lower spine at the coccyx. It is frequently covered with a tuft of hair. Although it may have no pathological significance, a pilonidal cyst may indicate the existence of spina bifida occulta or be a portal of entry into the spinal column. With the infant still prone, note the symmetry of the gluteal folds. Report any evidence of asymmetry. Skilled examiners test for developmental dysplasia of the hip. (See Chapter 33.)

The presence of an anal orifice and passage of meconium through the orifice during the first 24 to 48 hours of life indicates anal patency. If the nurse/midwife suspects an imperforate anus, report this to the medical practitioner for further evaluation.

Extremities. Observe range of motion of the extremities throughout the entire examination. The newborn will demonstrate full range of motion in the elbow, hip, shoulder and knee joints. Movements should be symmetrical, smooth and unrestricted. The absence of arm movement signals a potential birth injury paralysis such as Klumpke or Erb-Duchenne paralysis. (See Birth Injuries, Chapter 8.) An asymmetrical or partial Moro reflex should alert the medical practitioner to further evaluate upper extremity mobility. Examine the lower extremities for limb length, symmetry and hip abduction and flexion.

Examine the nails; the nail beds should be pink, although slight blueness is evident in **acrocyanosis.** Persistent cyanosis of the nail beds may indicate hypoxia or vasoconstriction. Yellowing of the nail beds may indicate intrauterine distress (as nails may be stained after intrauterine expulsion of meconium), postterm birth or haemolytic disease. Short or absent nails are seen in preterm infants, whereas long nails, extending over the ends of the fingers, are characteristic of postterm newborns.

The palms of the hands should have the usual creases (see Fig 4.12). A transverse palmar crease (simian crease) suggests Down syndrome but may also be a normal finding. The full-term newborn usually has creases covering the entire sole of the foot. In postterm infants the sole is covered with deep creases, and in preterm infants the creases may partially cover the sole or may be absent. The soles are flat with prominent fat pads. Note any foot abnormalities.

Two reflexes are elicited. The first is the **grasp reflex**. Touching the palms or soles near the base of the digits causes flexion or grasping (Fig 7.8A). The other is **Babinski's' reflex**. Stroking the outer sole of the foot upwards from the heel across the ball of the foot causes the big toe to dorsiflex and the other toes to hyperextend (Fig 7.8B and Table 7.5).

Inspect the extremities for evidence of fractures from birth trauma. The clavicle, humerus and femur are most commonly involved. Limitation of movement, crepitus, visible deformity, asymmetry of reflexes and malposition of the site suggest a fracture.

It is important to assess neonatal muscle tone. By attempting to extend a flexed extremity, determine whether tone is equal bilaterally. Extension of any extremity is usually met with resistance, and when released, the extremity returns to its previous flexed position. **Hypotonia** suggests some degree of hypoxia, neurological or muscular disorder, or condition such as Down syndrome. Asymmetry of muscle tone may indicate a degree of paralysis from damage to the central nervous system. Failure to move the lower limbs suggests a spinal cord lesion or injury. Sustained rhythmic tremors, twitches and myoclonic jerks characterise neonatal seizures or may indicate neonatal abstinence syndrome. (See the sections Neonatal Seizures and Drug-Exposed Infants, Chapter 9.) Sudden asynchronous jerking movements, quivering or momentary tremors are usually normal.

Neurological System. Assessing neurological status is a critical part of the physical examination of the newborn. Much of the neurological testing takes place during evaluation of body systems, such as eliciting localised reflexes and observing posture, muscle tone, head control and

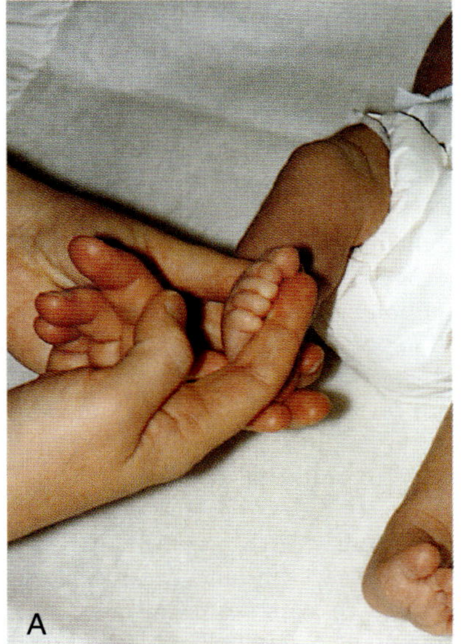

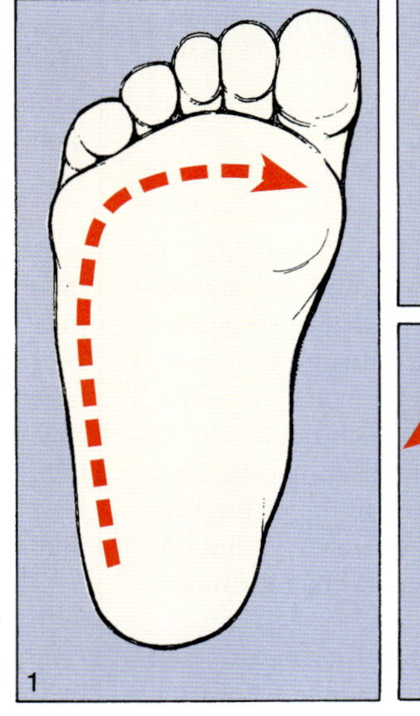

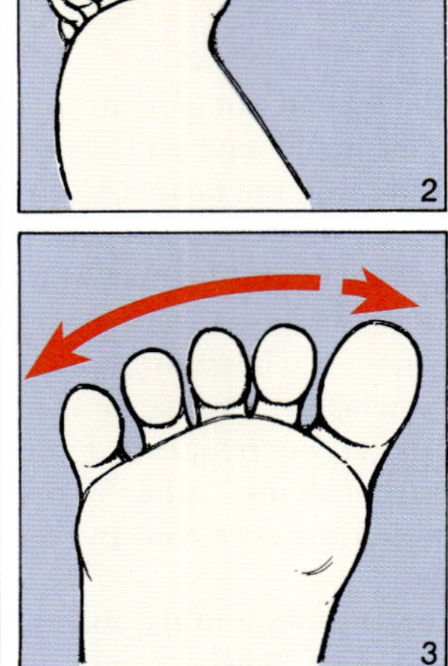

Fig 7.8 (**A**) Plantar or grasp reflex. (**B**) Babinski's reflex. **1** Direction of stroke. **2** Dorsiflexion of big toe. **3** Fanning of toes.

TABLE 7.5 **Assessment of Reflexes in the Newborn**

Reflexes	Expected Behavioural Responses
	LOCALISED
Eyes	
Blinking or corneal reflex	Infant blinks at sudden appearance of bright light or at approach of object towards cornea; persists throughout life.
Pupillary	Pupil constricts when bright light shines towards it; persists throughout life.
Doll's eye	As head is moved slowly to right or left, eyes lag behind and do not immediately adjust to new position of head; disappears as fixation develops; if persists, indicates neurological damage.
Nose	
Sneeze	Nasal passages respond spontaneously to irritation or obstruction; persists throughout life.
Glabellar	Tapping briskly on glabella (bridge of nose) causes eyes to close tightly; usually disappears in infancy.
Mouth and Throat	
Sucking	Infant begins strong sucking movements of circumoral area in response to stimulation; persists throughout infancy, even without stimulation, such as during sleep.
Gag	Stimulation of posterior pharynx by food, suction or passage of tube causes infant to gag; persists throughout life.
Rooting	Touching or stroking cheek along side of mouth causes infant to turn head towards that side and begin to suck; should disappear at about age 3–4 months but may persist for up to 12 months.
Extrusion	When tongue is touched or depressed, infant responds by forcing it outwards; disappears by age 4 months.
Yawn	Infant has spontaneous response to decreased oxygen by increasing amount of inspired air; persists throughout life.
Cough	Irritation of mucous membranes of larynx or tracheobronchial tree causes coughing; persists throughout life; usually present after 1st day of birth.
	EXTREMITIES
Grasp	Touching palms or soles near base of digits causes flexion of hands and toes (see Fig 7.8A); palmar grasp lessens after age 3 months, to be replaced by voluntary movement; plantar grasp lessens by 8 months of age.
Babinski	Stroking outer sole of foot upwards from heel and across ball of foot causes toes to hyperextend and hallux to dorsiflex (see Fig 7.8B); disappears after age 1 year.
Ankle clonus	Briskly dorsiflexing foot while supporting knee in partially flexed position results in 1–2 oscillating movements ('beats'); eventually no beats should be felt.
	MASS
Moro	Sudden jarring or change in equilibrium causes sudden extension and abduction of extremities and fanning of fingers, with index finger and thumb forming a C shape, followed by flexion and adduction of extremities; legs may weakly flex; infant may cry (Fig 7.9A); disappears after age 3–4 months, usually strongest during first 2 months.
Startle	Sudden loud noise causes abduction of arms with flexion of elbows; hands remain clenched; disappears by age 4 months.
Perez	While infant is prone on firm surface, thumb is pressed along spine from sacrum to neck; infant responds by crying, flexing extremities and elevating pelvis and head; lordosis of spine, defecation and urination may occur; disappears by age 4–6 months.
Asymmetrical tonic neck	When infant's head is turned to one side, arm and leg extend on that side and opposite arm and leg flex (Fig 7.9B); disappears by age 3–4 months, to be replaced by symmetrical positioning of both sides of body.
Trunk incurvation (Galant's) reflex	Stroking infant's back alongside spine causes hips to move towards stimulated side; disappears by age 4 weeks.
Dance or step	If infant is held so that sole of foot touches hard surface, there is reciprocal flexion and extension of leg, simulating walking (Fig 7.9C); disappears after age 3–4 weeks, to be replaced by deliberate movement.
Crawl	When placed on abdomen, infant makes crawling movements with arms and legs; disappears at about age 6 weeks (Fig 7.9D).
Placing	When infant is held upright under arms and dorsal side of foot is briskly placed against hard object, such as table, leg lifts as if foot is stepping on table; age of disappearance varies.

movement. However, several important mass (total body) reflexes also need to be elicited. Test these at the end of the examination because they may disturb the infant and interfere with auscultation. Table 7.5 describes these reflexes and several local reflexes. Record and report the absence, asymmetry, persistence or weakness of a reflex.

Maintain a Patent Airway

Establishing a patent airway is the primary objective in the birth room. When the newborn is supine, a neutral neck position (i.e. avoiding neck flexion or hyperextension) is critical to achieving and maintaining a patent airway.

It is recommended to sleep newborns in the supine position at all times. This recommendation is based on the association between sleeping prone and sudden unexpected death in infancy (See Chapter 11.) Since the initial recommendation in 1992 that all infants be placed in the supine position to sleep, there has been no evidence of an increased number of complications, such as choking or vomiting, when infants are placed in a supine sleep position.

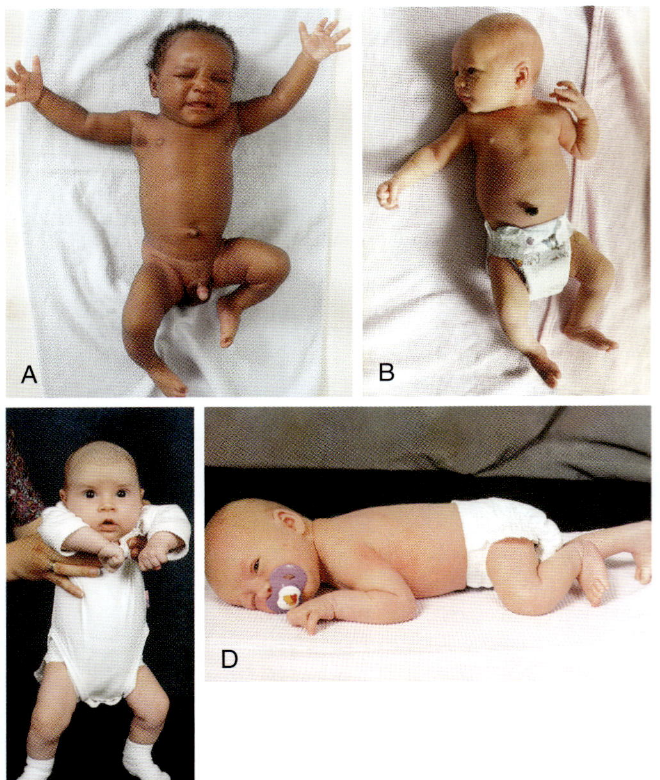

Fig 7.9 (**A**) Moro reflex. (**B**) Tonic neck reflex. (**C**) Dance reflex. (**D**) Crawl reflex. (Source: Courtesy of Paul Vincent Kuntz, Texas Children's Hospital, Houston. Source: *A*, Zitelli, B. J., & Davis, H. W. (2002). *Atlas of pediatric physical diagnosis* (4th ed.). St Louis, MO: Mosby.)

If removal of secretions is required, mechanical suction is used. Use of the proper-sized catheter and correct suctioning technique are essential to prevent mucosal damage and oedema. Gentle suctioning is necessary to prevent laryngospasm, reflex bradycardia and other cardiac arrhythmias from vagal stimulation. Oropharyngeal suctioning is performed for up to 5 seconds with sufficient time between each attempt to allow the infant to reoxygenate. If nasal suctioning is necessary, it must be done *after* oral suctioning to minimise the possibility of aspiration of oropharyngeal contents. Closely monitor vital signs, and report immediately any indication of respiratory distress.

Maintain a Stable Body Temperature

Conserving the newborn's body heat is an essential goal. At birth a major cause of heat loss is **evaporation**, the loss of heat through moisture. The amniotic fluid that bathes the infant's skin favours evaporation. Rapidly drying the skin and hair with a warmed towel and placing the infant in skin-to-skin contact with the mother, covered by a blanket, will minimise heat loss through evaporation.

Another source of heat loss is **radiation**, the loss of heat to cooler solid objects in the environment that are not in direct contact with the infant. Loss of heat through radiation increases as these solid objects become colder and closer to the infant. The temperature of ambient (surrounding) air has no effect on loss of heat through radiation.

Heat loss can also occur through conduction and convection. **Conduction** involves loss of body heat from direct skin contact with a cooler solid object. The nurse/midwife can minimise this by placing the infant on a padded, covered surface rather than directly on a cool hard table and by providing insulation with clothes and blankets.

Convection is similar to conduction, except that heat loss is aided by surrounding air currents. For example, placing the infant in the direct flow of air from a fan or air-conditioner vent causes rapid heat loss through convection. Transporting the neonate in a cot with solid sides reduces airflow around the infant.

Protect from Infection and Injury

Identification

Proper identification of the newborn is essential. The nurse/midwife must verify that identifying bands are securely fastened on the newborn and verify the information (name, sex, mother's admission number and date and time of birth) against the birth records and the child's parent(s).

Eye Care

Newborns have a tearless cry because their lacrimal ducts are not fully mature until approximately 3 months. Most newborns will have grey or blue irises and the sclera may be blue due to its thinness. Infant eyes assume their permanent colour between 3 and 12 months of age.

Studies on maternal attachment suggest that in the first hour of life, a newborn has a greater ability to focus on coordinated movement than at any other time during the next several days.

Vitamin K Administration

Shortly after birth, vitamin K is administered to prevent haemorrhagic disease of the newborn. (See Chapter 8.) The intestinal flora synthesises vitamin K; however, because the infant's intestine is sterile at birth, vitamin K levels are insufficient in newborns. A dose of vitamin K provides protection until the newborn's intestinal flora is established, which usually occurs by 3 to 4 days of age. The major function of vitamin K is to catalyse the synthesis of prothrombin in the liver, which is needed for blood clotting. The vastus lateralis muscle is the traditionally recommended injection site, but the ventrogluteal (not dorsogluteal) muscle may also be used (National Health and Medical Research Council [NHMRC] 2010).

Hepatitis B vaccine Administration

To decrease the incidence of hepatitis B virus (HBV) in children and its serious consequences (cirrhosis and liver cancer) in adulthood, the first of three doses of HBV vaccine is recommended after birth and before hospital discharge for all newborns born to hepatitis B surface antigen (HBsAg)–negative mothers. Refer to the Australian and New Zealand immunisation handbooks and websites for the appropriate schedules relating to gestational age at birth, nationality and additional immunisation requirements and to ensure you are staying informed with updated changes to immunisation policies and procedures (https://immunisationhandbook.health.gov.au/ and https://www.health.govt.nz/our-work/preventative-health-wellness/immunisation/new-zealand-immunisation-schedule).

Newborn Screening

Blood sampling can detect a large number of congenital disorders in the newborn period so that early intervention can take place to decrease the long-term effects and cost of not treating such conditions.

The nurse/midwife's responsibility is to educate parents regarding the importance of screening and to collect appropriate specimens at the recommended time (after 24 hours of age or after the introduction of feedings; hospitalised infants must be screened before 7 days of age). With early newborn discharge before 24 hours, some authorities recommend a repeat screening for phenylketonuria (PKU) within 2 weeks.

NURSING CARE CONSIDERATIONS

Heel Punctures

Heel lancing is necessary to obtain blood for newborn tests, including newborn metabolic screening. Heel lancing is recognised as a painful procedure, and numerous non-pharmacological strategies have demonstrated pain relief potential.

The importance of preventing and minimising pain with this intervention is to initiate non-nutritive sucking, skin-to-skin holding and swaddling/facilitated tucking, and provide breastfeeding or sucrose. These strategies can significantly manage pain behaviours associated with painful procedures in neonates.

Breastfeeding is correlated with pain relief for full-term newborns undergoing painful procedures, as demonstrated by reduction in infants' crying time and reduction in pain scores, but breast milk given by syringe has not shown the same efficacy as breastfeeding itself (Shah et al 2012). Comparison of sucrose with breastfeeding has produced mixed results; thus, it is difficult to determine optimal pain prevention treatment when comparing breastfeeding with sucrose, and more research is needed (Shah et al 2012).

A review of eight randomised controlled studies explored the use of topical anaesthetics such as the eutectic mixture of local anaesthetic (EMLA) cream before venepuncture in term and preterm infants. The authors concluded that analgesic effects were of uncertain clinical significance, and concerns regarding the risk of methaemaglobinaemia need to be further evaluated in future studies (Foster et al 2017).

Having the mother hold the infant in skin-to-skin contact has been shown to significantly reduce the child's distress during painful procedures, as measured by physiological indices such as heart rate and behaviours such as crying. Studies published are diverse with respect to outcomes measured, and it is impossible to have observers be blinded to pain prevention treatments. The authors of a comprehensive review of 25 studies concluded that more research is needed to better understand optimal strategies for, and effects of, skin-to-skin holding for pain prevention and relief (Johnston et al 2017).

There are many effective ways to decrease the pain associated with heel puncture in newborns. It is essential that nurses and midwives use all available resources to advocate for the prevention and management of neonatal pain during such procedures as heel puncture.

The Australian Government Department of Health (2019) provides comprehensive direction for care of mothers affected with HIV and their newborns. Caesarean section performed before the rupture of membranes or the onset of labour may prevent mother-to-child transmission of HIV in optimally treated women, and is associated with a reduction in the risk of mother-to-child transmission among HIV-infected women who are either not receiving antiretroviral therapy or are receiving minimal therapy. For infants whose mother's HIV status is unknown, rapid HIV antibody testing provides information within 12 hours of the infant's birth. Antiretroviral prophylaxis is started as soon as possible, pending completion of confirmatory HIV testing. Breastfeeding is delayed until confirmatory testing is done. If the test is negative, prophylaxis is stopped and breastfeeding may start. If the test is positive, infants should be treated with antiretroviral prophylaxis for 6 weeks, and the mother should not breastfeed.

Universal Newborn Hearing Screening

It is estimated that screening children for hearing loss by risk factors alone fails to identify approximately 50% of all newborns with a congenital hearing loss. Auditory deprivation in early infancy results in structural and functional reorganisation at a cortical level, leading to lifelong deficits (Australian Government Department of Health 2021). Thus without early diagnosis and intervention, hearing loss leads to irreversible deficits in communication and psychosocial skills, cognition and literacy. Where possible screening of hearing is attended to before discharge from the hospital (Sydney Children's Hospital 2021).

Infants may be screened for hearing loss by auditory brainstem response or evoked otoacoustic emissions. For infants born by caesarean birth, it is preferable to delay otoacoustic emission (OAE) testing until after 48 hours of age, as testing earlier than this is associated with significantly higher rates of failure, possibly as a result of retained fluid in the middle ear (Smolkin et al 2012). Newborns who fail the initial screening require referral for outpatient retesting and intervention by 1 month of age; newborns who do not receive initial screening before discharge should also be tested by 1 month of age (Sydney Children's Hospital 2021).

Bathing

Bath time is an opportunity for the nurse/midwife to accomplish much more than general hygiene. It is an excellent time for observing the infant's behaviour, state of arousal, alertness and muscular activity. With the possibility of transmission of organisms such as HBV and HIV via maternal blood and blood-stained amniotic fluid, as part of standard precautions nurses and midwives should wear gloves when handling the newborn until blood and amniotic fluid are removed by bathing.

Early bathing (within the first hour of life) interferes with skin-to-skin holding and breastfeeding, thus compromising basic protection against neonatal infection. In a large study of more than 800 late preterm infants, researchers concluded that early bathing may interfere with transition to extrauterine life and optimal adaptation of body processes, possibly contributing to problems such as hypothermia and hypoglycaemia (Medoff Cooper et al 2012). Time of initial bathing should be based on individualised assessment, and the initial newborn bath is best delayed for at least 24 hours until thermal and cardiorespiratory stabilisation has been achieved and initial skin-to-skin holding and breastfeeding is complete (Chamberlain et al 2019).

The infant's skin surface has a pH of about 5 soon after birth, and the bacteriostatic effects of this pH are significant. In addition, newborn skin is covered with vernix caseosa, a chemical and mechanical skin barrier for newborns. Vernix protects newborns from infection, and assists in the development of the skin's acid mantle. Vernix should not be removed with bathing; allow it to absorb or wear off with normal care and handling (Lund 2016). Consequently, plain warm water is appropriate for routine bathing. If a cleanser is needed, it should be mild and have a neutral pH. Alkaline soaps, oils, powder and lotions are not used because they alter the acid mantle, thus providing a medium for bacterial growth. Talcum or cornstarch powders have the added risk of aspiration if they are applied close to the infant's face.

Care of the Umbilicus

Because the umbilical stump is an excellent medium for bacterial growth, various methods of cord care have been practised to prevent infection. Some methods popular in the past include the use of an antimicrobial agent such as bacitracin or triple dye, or agents such as alcohol or povidone. A Cochrane Review of 21 studies (most of which were conducted in developed countries) found no significant difference between cords treated with antiseptics compared with dry cord care or placebo; there were no reported systemic infections or deaths, and a trend towards reduced colonisation was found in cords treated with antibiotics (Zupan et al 2013). Current recommendations for cord care for infants in the developed world include cleaning the cord initially with sterile water or a neutral pH cleanser, then subsequently cleaning the cord with water (VAHI & SCV 2020d).

Circumcision

Circumcision, the surgical removal of the foreskin on the glans penis, is not a common practice in most countries. The emphasis for circumcision is on parental autonomy to determine what is in the best interest of their newborn, whether the reasons are medical, cultural or personal choice. All policies should encourage the primary care practitioner to ensure that parents have been given accurate and unbiased information about the risks, benefits and alternatives before making an informed choice and that they understand that circumcision is an elective procedure. It is recommended that if parents decide to have their male infant circumcised, procedural analgesia should be provided.

Nurses and midwives are in a unique position to educate parents regarding the care of their newborns, and they must ensure that parents have accurate and unbiased information with which to make an informed decision. Parents should discuss the options for pain control, and the possibility of observing the procedure, with the primary practitioner.

The nurse/midwife should use non-pharmacological interventions as an adjunct to reduce the pain of this operative procedure. Despite adequate scientific evidence that newborns feel and respond to pain, circumcisions may still be performed with either insufficient analgesia or no analgesia at all.

Care of the circumcision depends on the type of procedure. As the area will be tender, the nappy is applied loosely to prevent friction against the penis. The circumcision is evaluated for excessive bleeding in the first few hours after the procedure, and the first void is recorded. A recommended standard is to evaluate the site every 30 minutes for at least 2 hours and then at least every 2 hours thereafter.

Normally, on the second day a yellowish white exudate forms as part of the granulation process. This is not a sign of infection and is not forcibly removed. As healing progresses, the exudate disappears. Parents are educated to report any evidence of bleeding, unusual swelling or absence of voiding to the medical practitioner.

Cultural Influences on Infant Feeding

Cultural beliefs and practices may significantly influence infant feeding methods. Many cultures typically do not give colostrum to newborns and only begin breastfeeding after the milk has 'come in' (i.e. milk is produced in larger volumes than those seen with initial colostrum production). These groups include mothers in Asia, Latin America and sub-Saharan Africa, and often mothers who have emigrated from these areas (Agho et al 2016). Some rationales for this practice include a concern that because colostrum volume is small, the baby may be at risk for dehydration, or that non-milk feeds are needed to 'cleanse' the gastrointestinal tract for digestion. Although perhaps intuitively logical, neither of these rationales is based on evidence. The use of prelacteal feedings significantly increases the risk of infection, particularly in developing countries where sanitation may be poor. In addition, failure to empty the breasts regularly in the early hours and days after delivery contributes to suboptimal milk supply.

A recent study of Chinese immigrant women in Australia reported that Chinese women were more likely to combine breastfeeding with formula and to introduce solids earlier than the general Australian population (Kuswara et al 2016). Chinese mothers shared that although they supported exclusive breastfeeding, grandparents frequently pressured them to use formula, believing that 'a fat baby is a healthy baby'. Wandel and colleagues (2016) reported similar findings after studying a small group of Somali women who immigrated to Norway. Although family support for breastfeeding is generally reported as strong, early formula supplementation is common, as is the belief in the need to introduce water feedings early. Somali culture apparently favours 'chubby' babies, and formula is seen as the best way ensure this weight gain.

 **CULTURAL CONSIDERATIONS**

Acculturation

Acculturation is a process whereby members of one cultural group adopt the beliefs and behaviours of another group. There may be language or literacy issues that interfere with acquisition of up-to-date breastfeeding information. There may be limited family support for immigrant women, and cultural norms may be at odds with information presented by care providers in their new country.

Jones and colleagues (2015) report that although there are potential barriers to breastfeeding common to all women, such as pain, embarrassment, employment or inconvenience, immigrant women often have additional concerns. Strategies to increase the likelihood of breastfeeding success include prenatal breastfeeding education, enhanced breastfeeding support programs in hospitals and linking mothers with non-professional peer supporters (Jones et al 2015).

Human Milk

Human milk is the best option for infant nutrition. Breast milk consists of a number of micronutrients that are bioavailable, meaning these nutrients are available in quantities and qualities that make them easily digestible by the newborn and absorbed for energy and growth. A variety of immunological properties are found exclusively in human milk.

Lysozyme is found in large quantities in human milk with bacteriostatic functions against gram-positive bacteria and *Enterobacteriaceae* organisms. Human milk also contains numerous other host defence factors such as macrophages, granulocytes and T and B lymphocytes. Casein in human milk greatly enhances the absorption of iron, thus preventing iron-dependent bacteria from proliferating in the gastrointestinal tract. Secretory immunoglobulin A (IgA) is found in high levels in colostrum, but levels gradually decrease over the first 14 days of life. Secretory IgA is an immunoglobulin that prevents viruses and bacteria from invading the intestinal mucosa in breastfed newborns, thus protecting them from infection. This whey protein is also believed to play an important role in preventing the development of allergies.

The fat content of human milk is composed of lipids, triglycerides and cholesterol; cholesterol is an essential element for brain growth. The function of these lipids is to allow optimum intestinal absorption of fatty acids and provide essential fatty acids and polyunsaturated fatty acids. Furthermore, lipids contribute approximately 50% of the total calories in human milk. Although the overall fat content in human milk is higher than that of cow's milk–based formula, it is used more efficiently by the infant.

The primary source of carbohydrate in human milk is lactose, which is present in higher concentrations (6.8 g/dL) than in cow's milk–based formula (4.9 g/dL). Other carbohydrates found in human milk include glucose, galactose and glucosamine. The carbohydrates serve not only as a large percentage of the total calories in human milk but also have a protective function; the oligosaccharides (**prebiotic**) in human milk stimulate the growth of *Lactobacillus bifidus* (a **probiotic**) and prevent bacteria from adhering to epithelial surfaces.

Human milk contains the two proteins whey (lactalbumin) and casein (curd) in a whey-dominant ratio of 70 to 80:20 to 30 in early lactation, decreasing to 50:50 in late lactation. Cow's milk is casein-dominant, with a ratio of approximately 20:80 whey to casein ratio. Cow's milk–based formulas vary in their whey:casein ratios, as some have added whey to alter their formulation to more closely resemble human milk (Martin et al 2016). This ratio of whey dominance in human milk makes it more digestible and produces the soft stools seen in breastfed infants. Thus, human milk has a laxative effect, and constipation is uncommon. The whey protein lactoferrin in human milk has iron-binding characteristics with bacteriostatic capabilities, particularly against gram-positive and gram-negative aerobes, anaerobes and yeasts.

Breastfeeding is associated with a decrease in the incidence of type 2 diabetes and obesity, fewer hospital admissions for respiratory tract illnesses in generally healthy infants and higher intelligence scores compared with formula-fed infants (Horta et al 2015, Wang et al 2017). Breastfeeding has an analgesic effect on newborns during painful procedures such as heel puncture and it has also been found to decrease pain scores in full-term and older infants receiving routine childhood immunisations (Modarres et al 2013).

Additional beneficial components of human milk include stem cells, prostaglandins, epidermal growth factor, docosahexaenoic acid (DHA), arachidonic acid (AA), taurine, carnitine, cytokine, interleukins and natural hormones such as thyroid-releasing hormone, gonadotropin-releasing hormone and prolactin.

Breastfeeding

Breastfeeding benefits mothers and babies in many ways and shows a significant change to lifelong health. Australia's infant feeding guidelines suggest to exclusively breastfeed infants up to the age of 6 months, at which time it is recommended that the introduction of solid foods can begin (Australian Breastfeeding Association 2017, New Zealand Breastfeeding Alliance [NZBA] 2021). However, it is recommended to also continue to breastfeed until the age of 12 months and beyond where possible.

Evidence shows that breastfed babies are less likely to suffer from necrotising enterocolitis, diarrhoea, respiratory illness, middle ear infection, type 1 diabetes and childhood leukaemia. Additional evidence has also shown that breastfed babies show improved cognitive development in many stages of development.

Benefits of breastfeeding for the mother are a faster recovery time from childbirth, a reduced risk of breast and ovarian cancer later in life and reduced postnatal depression (NZBA 2021).

The Baby-Friendly Initiative (BFI) is a joint effort of the World Health Organization and UNICEF to encourage, promote and support breastfeeding as the model for optimum infant nutrition. BFI developed 10 research-supported practices as guidelines for caregivers worldwide to promote breastfeeding (World Health Organization, UNICEF & Wellstart International 2009) (Table 7.6). Research indicates that BFI designation is sometimes associated with higher rates of breastfeeding initiation; however, the designation does not appear to affect breastfeeding rates among women with higher educational levels in US populations (Hawkins et al 2014, 2015). Howe-Heyman and Lutenbacher (2016), after reviewing 25 studies published over 23 years, concluded that, although there are more studies that support the BFI as an intervention to increase breastfeeding rates than there are studies that demonstrate no effect, many of the studies are methodologically weak. These authors suggest that peer support, formal prenatal breastfeeding education and needs-based

TABLE 7.6 Ten Steps to Successful Breastfeeding

Every facility providing maternity services and care for newborn infants should:

WHO 10 Steps	BCC Interpretation
1. Have a written breastfeeding policy that is routinely communicated to all healthcare staff.	Have a written breastfeeding policy that is routinely communicated to all healthcare providers and volunteers.
2. Train all healthcare staff in skills necessary to implement this policy.	Ensure all healthcare providers have the knowledge and skills necessary to implement the breastfeeding policy.
3. Inform all pregnant women about the benefits and management of breastfeeding.	Inform all pregnant women and their families about the importance and process of breastfeeding.
4. Help mothers initiate breastfeeding within a half hour of birth (WHO 2009). Place babies in skin-to-skin contact with their mothers immediately following birth for at least an hour. Encourage mothers to recognise when their babies are ready to breastfeed and offer help if needed.	Place babies in uninterrupted skin-to-skin contact with their mothers immediately following birth for at least an hour or until completion of the first feeding or as long as the mother wishes; encourage mothers to recognise when their babies are ready to feed, offering help as needed.
5. Show mothers how to breastfeed and how to maintain lactation even if they are separated from their infants	Assist mothers to breastfeed and maintain lactation should they face challenges including separation from their infants.
6. Give newborn infants no food or drink other than breast milk, unless medically indicated.	Support mothers to exclusively breastfeed for the first 6 months, unless supplements are *medically* indicated.
7. Practise rooming-in—allow mothers and infants to remain together—24 hours a day.	Facilitate 24 hour rooming-in for all mother-infant dyads: mothers and infants remain together.
8. Encourage breastfeeding on demand.	Encourage baby-led or cue-based breastfeeding. Encourage sustained breastfeeding beyond 6 months with appropriate introduction of complementary foods.
9. Give no artificial teats or pacifiers (also called dummies or soothers) to breastfeeding infants.	Support mothers to feed and care for their breastfeeding babies without the use of artificial teats or pacifiers (dummies or soothers).
10. Foster the establishment of breastfeeding support groups and refer mothers to them on discharge from the hospital or clinic.	Provide a seamless transition between the services provided by the hospital, community health services and peer support programs. Apply principles of Primary Healthcare and Population Health to support the continuum of care and implement strategies that affect the broad determinants that will improve breastfeeding outcomes.

Source: The WHO 10 Steps to Successful Breastfeeding (1989) and The Interpretation for Canadian Practice (2011). The Breastfeeding Committee for Canada (BCC). Retrieved from http://www.breastfeedingcanada.ca/documents/2012-05-14_BCC_BFI_Ten_Steps_Integrated_Indicators_Summary.pdf. World Health Organization. (2009). WHO guidelines on hand hygiene in health care, 2009, World Health Organization. http://whqlibdoc.who.int/publications/2009/9789241597906_eng.pdf.

informal postpartum support may be more effective than the BFI for increasing breastfeeding rates (Howe-Heyman & Lutenbacher 2016).

In addition to the physiological qualities of human milk, the most outstanding psychological benefit of breastfeeding is the close mother–child relationship. The infant is nestled close to the mother's skin, can hear the rhythm of her heartbeat, can feel the warmth of her body and has a sense of peaceful security. The mother has a close feeling of union with her child and feels a sense of accomplishment and satisfaction as the infant suckles milk from her owing to oxytocin/prolactin release.

A concern many mothers have is the perceived inconvenience of loss of freedom and independence. Being committed to feeding the infant every 2 to 3 hours can seem overwhelming, especially to women with multiple responsibilities. Many women resume their careers shortly after birth and prefer to bottle-feed. Combining breastfeeding and employment is possible, and many employers provide space for mothers to pump and store their milk. This is an acknowledgment of the demonstrated health benefits of breastfeeding, as a breastfed infant is far less likely to have infection of any sort; thus, the infant's mother is far less likely to need time away from work to care for an ill infant. Although breastfeeding is the preferred form of infant feeding, mothers' decisions regarding their preferences must be respected and supported.

Table 7.7 summarises some common breastfeeding problems and suggested interventions to correct them. Most of these problems are easily prevented or remedied, provided the mother receives education and guidance. Assessment should include a detailed history, examination of the breasts and observation of the breastfeeding (see Nursing Care Guidelines box).

NURSING CARE GUIDELINES

Observing the Breastfeeding Pair

- Position of mother, her body language and any possible tension
- Position of infant—infant's ventral (front) surface is next to mother's ventral surface with the face directly in front of the breast (chest to chest); the infant cannot easily swallow if the head has to turn to the breast
- Position of mother's hand on the breast; using the thumb on top and fingers supporting the breast encircling the areola (the C-hold) facilitates infant's ability to grasp the areola properly
- Stroke the nipple down baby's mouth to get a wide-open mouth
- Flanged position of infant's lips on the areola; the lips should gently grasp most of the areola, with the lower lip covering more of the areola than the upper lip
- Baby's chin, not the nose, touching mother's breast
- Use of alternate breasts and feeding time on each breast
- Technique to break suction; the mother should release suction using fingers between the areola and lips, not pulling infant from the breast abruptly

Encourage frequent feedings and/or expressing to increase milk production; use of supplemental formula, water, glucose water or solid foods will result in decreased breast milk intake and ultimately decreased production.

Many breastfeeding problems respond rapidly to simple interventions, such as correcting the infant's feeding position. However, the mother needs continual reassurance of success and the support that allows her the needed rest and relaxation to breastfeed her infant. Referral to a peer supporter or to supportive agencies, such as local Australian Breastfeeding Association groups or to a lactation consultant, may be beneficial.

Bottle-feeding

Bottle-feeding generally refers to the use of bottles for feeding commercial or evaporated milk formula rather than using the breast, although in some instances human milk may be expressed and fed with a bottle. Bottle-feeding is an acceptable method of feeding. Nurses and midwives should not assume, however, that new parents automatically know how to bottle-feed their infant. Parents who choose bottle-feeding also need support and assistance in meeting their infant's needs.

Feeding Schedules

Ideally, feeding times should be determined by the infant's hunger. Demand feedings are given when the infant signals readiness; scheduled feedings are arranged at predetermined intervals. Although schedules may be satisfactory for bottle-fed infants, they hinder the breastfeeding process. Because of the easy digestibility of human milk, breastfed infants should be fed on demand. At times, breastfed infants will *cluster-feed*; that is, have several short feedings within an hour or two and then sleep for several hours. It is important for mothers to understand that cluster-feeding is a normal, expected pattern for breastfed infants, especially during a growth spurt, to prevent them from worrying that their milk is of insufficient quality or quantity. Cluster-feeding is recognised as a mechanism that facilitates increased milk production to meet the infant's increasing metabolic needs; thus, it is imperative that mothers understand and facilitate cluster-feeding.

Commercially Prepared Formulas

The analysis of human and whole cow's milk indicates that the latter is unsuitable for infant nutrition. Whole cow's milk has a high protein content and low fat content, and may cause intestinal bleeding and lead to iron deficiency anaemia in infants. There has also been some question regarding the unmodified protein content of whole cow's milk, which may trigger an undesired immune response and thus increase the incidence of allergies in children exposed at an early age.

Commercially prepared formulas such as Nan, S26 and Aptami are cow's milk–based formulas that have been modified to more closely resemble the nutritional content of human milk. These formulas are altered from cow's milk by removing butterfat, decreasing the protein content and adding vegetable oil and carbohydrate. Some cow's milk–based formulas have demineralised whey added to yield a whey:casein ratio of 60:40. Standard cow's milk–based formulas, regardless of the commercial brand, have similar compositions of vitamins, minerals, protein, carbohydrates and essential amino acids, with possible variations such as the source of carbohydrate, **nucleotides** to enhance immune function and **long-chain polyunsaturated fatty acids (LCPUFAs)** DHA and AA, which are believed to improve brain function. DHA and AA are both found in large quantities in human milk but until recently were not present in most infant formulas.

A meta-analysis of 15 randomised controlled studies explored outcomes such as physical growth, visual acuity and neurodevelopmental outcomes among term infants fed formula milk fortified with LCPUFAs, compared with infants fed formula that was not enriched with LCPUFAs. The authors concluded that most studies reported no beneficial effects or harms of LCPUFA supplementation on neurodevelopmental outcomes of formula-fed infants, and no consistent beneficial effects on visual acuity (Jasani et al 2017). Thus, routine supplementation of term infant formula with LCPUFAs is not recommended at this time (Jasani et al 2017).

The presence of the probiotics *Lactobacillus rhamnosus* GG and *Bifidobacterium lactis* in breast milk has led to the addition of prebiotic components to some cow's milk–based formula. Prebiotic oligosaccharides are food ingredients that promote the growth and activity of bacteria such as *Lactobacillus* and *Bifidobacterium,* which benefit the host. Although some studies report increasing bifidobacterial counts with prebiotic-supplemented formula, others report that although

TABLE 7.7 Breastfeeding Problems*

Problem	Comments	Interventions
Engorgement	Best intervention is *prevention* with deep areolar latch-on and frequent breastfeeding on both breasts for complete emptying of ducts. If engorgement occurs, infant may be unable to properly grasp distended areola.	Manually express small amount of milk; electric pump may be beneficial for some. Use warm compresses or a warm shower *before feeding;* for severely engorged breasts, cold compresses may be helpful to reduce vascularity *after feeding.* Compress areola with fingers before attempting to latch. This may reduce superficial oedema and facilitate infant's grasp. This is known as *reverse pressure softening.* Use well-fitting nursing bra and wear 24 hours a day. For excessive discomfort, take ibuprofen or paracetamol 30 minutes before feeding. Massage breasts; vary position of infant's mouth on nipple and areola.
Painful nipples	Most common causes are shallow latch, improper care of breasts, bacterial or fungal infection, or infant tongue-tie (tight lingual frenulum). If left untreated, discomfort may cause mother to terminate breastfeeding.	Care of breasts • Avoid soaps, oils or self-prescribed treatments. Gently massage a small amount of expressed breast milk onto sore nipples after feeding. • Expose nipples to air as much as possible. • Change breast pads frequently; avoid plastic-backed pads (may trap moisture). Feeding • Start let-down reflex by manual expression before putting infant to breast. • Begin breastfeeding with less affected breast, then fee on affected side. • Position infant properly at breast to achieve deep areolar grasp. • Vary infant's position during feeding. • Take analgesics 30 min before feeding; apply cool compresses to nipples after feeding.
Delayed let-down reflex	Reflex essential to optimal delivery of milk from alveoli and smaller milk ducts into larger lactiferous ducts; controlled primarily by release of oxytocin. Pain, stress and anxiety can interfere with reflex.	Provide quiet, relaxing atmosphere for breastfeeding (e.g. soothing music, privacy, pillows for positioning, decreased distractions). Stroke breast gently. Apply warmth to breast.
Inadequate milk supply	Production of milk depends primarily on supply and demand. Inadequate supply rarely is related to organic causes, such as decreased glandular tissue, but may occur after breast augmentation or reduction surgery, or as a result of a hormonal imbalance such as polycystic ovarian syndrome.	Continue breastfeeding or expressing every 2–3 hours. Massage breasts before feeding. Apply warm compresses before pumping or feeding. Avoid use of supplemental formula before breastfeeding is well established to prevent nipple preference and satiation (infant will not be hungry enough to breastfeed). Reassure mother that her milk supply is likely to be adequate and it depends on frequent breastfeeding. Encourage more frequent breastfeeding (at least 8–10 times daily, initially at both breasts). Encourage adequate rest, nutrition and fluids. Monitor infant's growth; in some cases formula supplementation may be indicated. An alternative to bottle-feeding is use of a supplemental feeding device consisting of a plastic bag or syringe for formula and a thin feeding tube placed next to mother's nipple during breastfeeding.
Plugged ducts	This may occur at any time, especially during first 6 weeks.	Continue breastfeeding every 2–3 hours. Massage breasts before feeding. Apply warm compresses before pumping or feeding. Alternate feeding positions, positioning infant's chin towards obstructed area.
Mastitis	Inflammation or infection in mammary gland or tissue, most often by *Staphylococcus aureus*; results from inadequate emptying of ducts or from cracks in nipple skin; may be associated with fever and flulike symptoms. Prevention: see Interventions for Plugged ducts, above. If mastitis occurs, current treatment is 10 days of antibiotics (usually amoxicillin or cephalexin, started with onset of symptoms). If symptoms of intense 'burning' in breasts with erythema of nipples, consider *Candida* infection of ducts (oral fluconazole [Diflucan] is treatment).	Continue breastfeeding during this time to keep breast well drained (unless contraindicated for medical reasons such as systemic illness).

Continued

TABLE 7.7 Breastfeeding Problems*—cont'd

Problem	Comments	Interventions
Unsuccessful latch-on	Improper positioning of infant at breast, inability to achieve deep areolar grasp, sleepiness or improper suckling technique may cause this common problem; flat, large or inverted nipples may also be a factor.	Mother and newborn must be positioned so that infant's mouth is in full contact with breast; mother should use C-hold; newborn's mouth is opened wide and most of areola is grasped (see Fig 7.10), especially with lower lip; frequent swallowing should be heard as evidence of spontaneous and successful suckling. Anatomical problems such as flat or inverted nipples may be managed by mother wearing nipple shields to elongate or make nipples more accessible. Additional pumping may be necessary after nursing when shield is used.

*Consult a lactation consultant as needed to resolve problems.

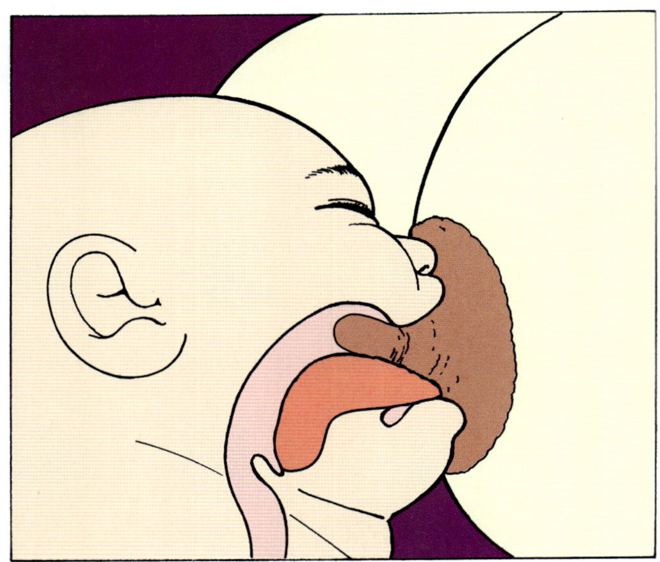

Fig 7.10 The tongue is under the areola, with tip of the nipple at back of the wide-open mouth.

stool frequency is increased, prebiotic infant formula failed to increase bifidobacteria or *Lactobacillus* levels or to decrease the level of pathogens such as *E. coli* (Bertelsen et al 2016). To date, there is insufficient evidence that changes in gastrointestinal microbiota resulting from fortified formula induce a significant clinical benefit for the immune system (Bertelsen et al 2016). Further, long-term health effects of prebiotic formula supplementation are unknown.

Commercially prepared infant formulas fall into four main categories: (1) cow's milk–based formulas (ready to feed), as powder (requires dilution with water) or as a concentrated liquid (requires dilution with water); (2) soy-based formulas, available commercially in ready-to-feed powder and concentrated liquid forms, commonly used for children who are lactose or cow's milk protein intolerant; (3) casein- or whey-hydrolysate formulas, commercially available in ready-to-feed and powder forms and used primarily for children who cannot tolerate or digest cow's milk or soy-based formulas; and (4) amino acid formulas.

The American Academy of Pediatrics Committee on Nutrition (Kleinman & Greer 2014) recommends the use of soy protein–based formulas for infants with galactosaemia and primary (very rare) and secondary lactose intolerance, and in situations where a vegetarian diet is preferred. For infants with documented allergies caused by cow's milk, extensively hydrolysed protein formula should be considered because up to 14% of these infants will also have a soy protein allergy. The casein- or whey-hydrolysate formulas are considered to be less antigenic than either cow's milk or soy-based formulas. The protein hydrolysate formulas (casein and whey) are derived from cow's milk–based formula by a process of heat, filtration and enzyme treatment designed to break the peptide chains into more digestible proteins. There are also amino acid formulas, designed for infants who are extremely sensitive to cow's milk–based, soy-based and partially or extensively hydrolysed casein- and whey-based formulas. A variety of formulas are manufactured for infants and children with special needs.

Follow-up formulas are marketed as a transitional formula for infants older than 6 months who are also eating solid foods. These generally contain a higher percentage of calories from protein and carbohydrate sources, a higher amount of iron and vitamins and a lower amount of fat than standard cow's milk–based formulas. Many nutrition experts and the American Academy of Pediatrics Committee on Nutrition (Kleinman & Greer 2014), however, discount the necessity of follow-up formulas if the infant is receiving an adequate amount of solid food containing sufficient iron, vitamins and minerals.

Goat's milk is a poor source of iron and folic acid. It has an excessively high renal solute load as a result of its high protein content and can cause metabolic acidosis, making it unsuitable for infant nutrition (Kleinman & Greer 2014). Some caretakers believe that goat's milk is less allergenic than other available milk sources and may feed it to their infants to reduce allergic milk reactions. However, infants allergic to cow's milk have experienced anaphylaxis with their first exposure to goat's milk (Pessler & Nejat 2004). Raw, unpasteurised milk from any animal source is not safe for infant nutrition or health.

Promote Parent–Infant Bonding (Attachment)

The process of parenting is based on a relationship between parent and infant. As more is learned of the complexity of neonates and their potential for influencing and shaping their environments, particularly their interaction with significant others, it is apparent that promoting positive parent–child relationships necessitates an understanding of behavioural steps in attachment, including variables that enhance or hinder this process. Nurses and midwives also must be skilled in methods of teaching parents to develop a stronger relationship with their children, especially by recognising potential problems (see Assessment of Attachment Behaviours, p. 144).

Infant Behaviour

Nurses and midwives must appreciate the individuality and uniqueness of each infant. According to the individual temperament, the infant will change and shape the environment, which will undoubtedly influence future development. An infant who sleeps 20 hours a day will be exposed to fewer stimuli than one who sleeps 16 hours a day. In turn, each infant is likely to elicit a different response from parents. The infant who is quiet, undemanding and passive may receive much less

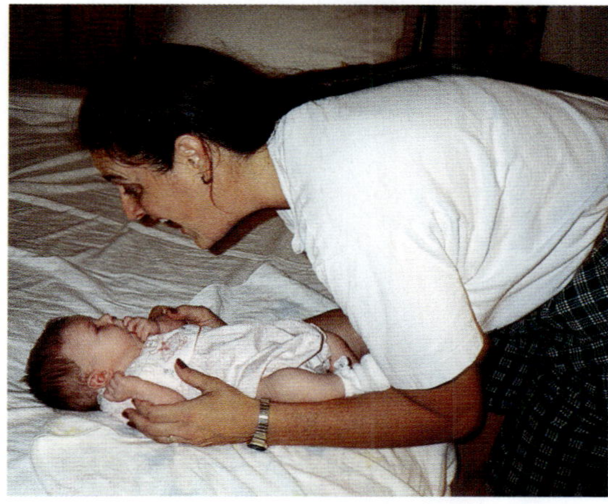

Fig 7.11 En face position between parent and infant can be significant in the attachment process.

attention than the infant who is responsive, alert and active. Behavioural characteristics such as irritability and consolability can influence the ease of transition to parenthood and the parent's perception of the infant.

Nurses and midwives can positively influence the attachment of parent and child. The first step is recognising individual differences and explaining to parents that such characteristics are normal. For example, some people believe that infants sleep throughout the day, except for feedings. For some newborns this may be true, but for many it is not. Understanding that the infant's wakefulness is part of biological rhythm and not a reflection of inadequate parenting can be crucial in promoting healthy parent–child relationships. Another aspect of helping parents involves supplying guidelines on how to enhance the infant's development during awake periods. Placing the child in a cot to stare at the same mobile every day is not exciting, but carrying the infant into each room as one does daily chores can be fascinating.

Maternal Attachment

Mothers often demonstrate a predictable and orderly pattern of behaviour during the attachment process. When mothers are presented with their nude infants, they begin to examine the infant with their fingertips, concentrating on touching the extremities, and then proceed to massage and encompass the trunk with their entire hands. Assuming the **en face** position, in which the mother's and infant's eyes meet in visual contact in the same vertical plane, is significant in the formation of affectional ties (Fig 7.11). Some authors have reported that mothers experiencing depression, as well as adolescent mothers, may have lower rates of secure attachment with their infants (Behrendt et al 2016), necessitating the need for caregivers to monitor such mothers closely and to model attachment behaviours. Nurses and midwives must observe for maternal attachment behaviours and exercise caution in interpreting such behaviours.

The long-term benefits of providing parents with opportunities to bond with their infant during the initial postpartum period are unclear; however, skin-to-skin contact with the mother immediately after birth enhances the likelihood of success in breastfeeding. The nurse/midwife should stress to parents that, although early bonding may be valuable, it does not represent an 'all or none' phenomenon. Throughout the child's life there will be multiple opportunities for the development of parent–child attachment. Bonding is a complex process that develops gradually and is influenced by numerous factors, only one of which is the type of initial contact between the newborn and parent.

One component of successful maternal attachment is **reciprocity** (Brazelton 1974). As the mother responds to the infant, the infant must respond to the mother by some signal, such as sucking, cooing, eye contact, grasping or moulding (conforming to other's body during close physical contact). The first step in this complex process is *initiation,* in which interaction between infant and parent begins. Next is *orientation,* which establishes the partners' expectations of each other during the interaction. Following orientation is *acceleration* of the attention cycle to a peak of excitement. The infant reaches out and coos, both arms jerk forwards, the head moves backwards, the eyes dilate and the face brightens. After a short time, *deceleration* of the excitement and *turning away* occur, in which the infant's eyes shift away from the mother's and the child may grasp his or her own shirt. During this cycle of non-attention, repeated verbal or visual attempts to reinitiate the infant's attention are ineffective. This deceleration and turning away probably prevent the infant from being overwhelmed by excessive stimuli. In a good-quality interaction, both participants have synchronised their attention–non-attention cycles. Parents or other caregivers who do not allow the infant to turn away and who continually attempt to maintain visual contact may encourage the infant to turn off the attention cycle and thus prolong the non-attention phase.

Although this description of reciprocal interacting behaviour is usually observed in the infant by 2 to 3 weeks of age, nurses and midwives can use this information to teach parents how to interact with their newborn infant. Recognising the attention versus non-attention cycles and understanding that the latter is not a rejection of the parent helps parents develop competence in parenting.

Paternal Engrossment

Fathers also show specific attachment behaviours to the newborn. This process of paternal **engrossment**, forming a sense of absorption, preoccupation and interest in the infant, includes: (1) visual awareness of the newborn, especially focusing on the child's beauty; (2) tactile awareness, often expressed in a desire to hold the infant; (3) awareness of distinct characteristics with emphasis on those features of the infant that resemble the father; (4) perception of the infant as perfect; (5) development of a strong feeling of attraction to the child that leads to intense focusing of attention on the infant; (6) extreme elation; and (7) a sense of deep self-esteem and satisfaction. These responses are greatest during the early contacts with the infant and are intensified by the neonate's normal reflex activity, especially the grasp reflex and visual alertness. In addition to behavioural reactions, fathers also demonstrate physiological responses such as increased heart rate and BP during interactions with their newborns.

The process of engrossment has significant implications for nurses and midwives. It is imperative to recognise the importance of early father–infant contact in this process. Fathers need to be encouraged to express their positive feelings, especially if such emotions are contrary to any belief that fathers should remain stoic. If this is not clarified, fathers may feel confused and attempt to suppress the natural sensations of absorption, preoccupation and interest to conform to societal expectations.

Mothers also need to be aware of the responses of the father towards the newborn because one of the consequences of paternal preoccupation with the infant is less overt attention towards the mother. If both parents are able to share their feelings, each can appreciate the process of attachment towards their child and will avoid the unfortunate conflict of being insensitive and unaware of the other's needs. In addition, a father who is encouraged to form a relationship with his newborn is less likely to feel excluded and abandoned once the family returns home and the mother directs her attention towards caring for the infant.

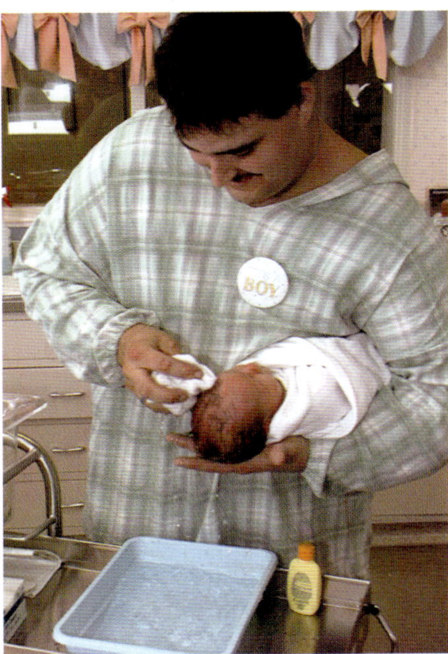

Fig 7.12 A desire to hold the infant and participate in caregiving activities is an important step in the paternal attachment process.

Ideally, the process of engrossment should be discussed with parents before the birth, such as in prenatal classes, to reinforce the father's awareness of his natural feelings towards the expected child. Focusing on the future experience of seeing, touching and holding one's newborn may also help expectant fathers become more comfortable in accepting their paternal feelings. This in turn can assist them in being more supportive towards the mother, especially as labour and birth draw near.

At the infant's birth the nurse/midwife can play a vital role in helping the father express engrossment by assessing the neonate in front of the couple; pointing out normal characteristics; encouraging identification through consistent referral to the child by name; encouraging the father to cuddle, hold and talk to the infant; and demonstrating whenever necessary the soothing powers of caressing, stroking and rocking the child (Fig 7.12).

The father's role in supporting the mother during this period cannot be overemphasised. Once the mother has held the newborn skin-to-skin, the father may also be encouraged to hold the newborn skin-to-skin while the mother rests. Fathers are encouraged to be with the mother during labour and birth, to spend time alone with the mother and newborn after birth and to 'room-in' with the mother and infant. Education programs should be made available to new fathers and include information on holding the newborn, bathing, assisting the mother with breastfeeding, problems associated with breastfeeding and potential solutions and care of the newborn at home (including safety). The integration of the father into the existing dyad of mother–newborn to form a new family—a triad—will help solidify his role as parent and partner in the care and support of his family.

The indications of affection from the father are the same as those expected in the mother, such as visual contact in the en face position and embracing the infant close to the body. When present, such behaviours should be reinforced. If such responses are not obvious, the nurse/midwife needs to assess the father's feelings regarding this birth, cultural beliefs that may prevent his expression of emotions and other factors to facilitate his positive attachment during the newborn period.

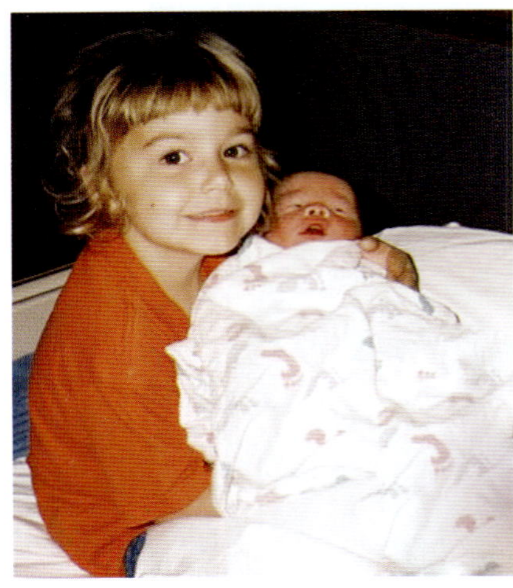

Fig 7.13 Sibling visitation shortly after birth can be significant in the attachment process.

Siblings

Although the attachment process has been discussed almost exclusively in terms of the parents and infants, it is essential that nurses/midwives be aware of other family members, such as siblings, grandparents and members of the extended family, who need preparation for the acceptance of this new child. Young children in particular need sensitive preparation for the birth to minimise sibling jealousy.

In support of **family-centred care**, there is an increasing trend to encourage siblings to visit the mother on the postpartum unit and to hold the newborn (Fig 7.13). Another trend has been the presence of siblings at childbirth. Unlike sibling visitation, this practice has been controversial, yet family-centred care encompasses siblings, grandparents and other significant persons from the extended family unit. Children exhibit different degrees of involvement in the birth process. Some reported benefits include children's increased knowledge of the birth process, less regressive behaviour after the birth and more mothering and caregiving behaviour towards the infant. Some medical practitioners add facilitated family bonding and assimilation of the newborn into the family as positive outcomes. Parents whose children attended the birth have echoed these same benefits and have expressed their desire to repeat the experience should another pregnancy occur. Despite these positive findings, some medical practitioners believe that allowing children to observe a birth could lead to emotional difficulties, although no research supports this contention. Birthing centres that allow siblings at the birth are developing more definitive guidelines, such as an age requirement of at least 4 to 5 years, the presence of a supportive person for the sibling only and an adequate sequence of preparation in which parents explore all options for preparing their other children.

From observations during sibling visitation, there is evidence that sibling attachment occurs. However, the en face position is assumed much less often among the newborn and siblings than between mother and newborn, and when this position is used, it is brief. Siblings focus more on the head or face than on touching or talking to the infant. The siblings' verbalisations are focused less on attracting the infant's attention and more on addressing the mother about the newborn. Children who have established a prenatal relationship with the fetus have demonstrated more attachment behaviours, supporting the suggestion of encouraging prenatal acquaintance. Additional research is needed to establish theories on sibling bonding like those that have been constructed for parental bonding.

Multiple Births and Subsequent Children

A component of attachment that has special meaning for families with multiple births, *monotropy* refers to the principle that a person can become optimally attached to only one individual at a time. If a parent can form only one attachment at a time, how can all the siblings of a multiple birth receive optimum emotional care? In regard to mother–twin bonding, the conclusions of different authors vary. Some report that mothers bond equally to each twin at the time of birth, even if one twin is ill. Others suggest that mothers of twins may take months or even years to form individual attachments and even longer if the twins are identical.

Nurses/midwives can be instrumental in promoting bonding at multiple births. The most important principle is to assist the parents in recognising the individuality of the children, especially monozygotic (identical) twins. The mother should visit with each newborn, including a sick infant, as much as possible after birth. Rooming-in and breastfeeding are encouraged. The nurse/midwife should emphasise any characteristics that are unique to each child and call each infant by name, rather than calling them 'the twins'. Asking the family questions such as 'How do you tell Ashley and Amy apart?' and 'In what ways are Ashley and Amy different and similar?' helps point out their individual characteristics. Behaviours on the Brazelton Neonatal Behavioral Assessment Scale (BNBAS) can be used to illustrate these differences and to stress effective strategies for dealing with multiple personalities at the same time. **Co-bedding** of twins or other multiples in the hospital has at times been suggested to maintain the bond between siblings that was formed in utero. A review of five studies exploring the safety and benefits of the practice of co-bedding stable preterm twins concluded that available evidence is insufficient to recommend this practice (Lai et al 2016). (See also Sudden Infant Death Syndrome, Chapter 11.) The Royal Children's Hospital Melbourne (2020) has also recommended against parents or other family members sleeping in the same bed with infants at home. Because neither the safety nor the benefits of co-bedding for newborns has been documented it is recommended that families be counselled to follow safe sleeping practices, which currently dictate that infants sleep alone for optimal safety.

Another area of attachment that has received minimal attention is maternal bonding of multiparous mothers. Research suggests that 'taking on' a second or third child has several additional tasks:

- promoting acceptance and approval of the second child
- grieving and resolving the loss of an exclusive dyadic relationship with the first child
- planning and coordinating family life to include a second child
- reformulating a relationship with the first child
- identifying with the second child by comparing this child with the first child in terms of physical and psychological characteristics
- assessing one's affective capabilities in providing sufficient emotional support and nurturance simultaneously to two children.

Prepare for Discharge and Home Care

To assess and meet these needs, education must begin early, ideally before the birth. Not only is the postpartum stay sometimes very short (as little as 12 to 24 hours), but mothers are also in the **taking-in phase**, where they may demonstrate passive and dependent behaviours. On the first postpartum day, because of fatigue and excitement about the newborn, mothers may not be able to absorb large amounts of information. This time may need to be spent highlighting essential aspects of care, such as infant safety and feeding. Parents may also be given a list of mother and infant care topics so they can choose issues they wish to review before going home. Education before discharge should focus on newborn feeding patterns, monitoring nappies for stools and voiding, jaundice and infant crying (see Family-Centred Care box).

FAMILY-CENTRED CARE

Healthy Term Newborn Discharge Criteria

- Infant born between 37 and 41 completed weeks of gestation.
- Clinical course and physical examination at discharge have not revealed abnormalities that require continued hospitalisation.
- Vital signs are within normal range and stable for the 6 to 12 hours preceding discharge.
- Infant has urinated regularly and passed at least one stool spontaneously.
- Infant has completed at least two successful feedings. For breastfed infants: A caregiver knowledgeable in breastfeeding must observe a feeding and assess latch, swallow and infant satiety. For bottle-fed infants: Assess ability to coordinate sucking, swallowing and breathing while feeding. These assessments must be documented in the health record.
- Clinical risk of development of hyperbilirubinaemia has been assessed, and follow-up plans per the hospital policy and clinical practice guidelines that are in place.
- Infant has been adequately evaluated and monitored for sepsis based on maternal risk factors, including group B streptococcal disease.
- Maternal blood test and screening results are available and have been reviewed, including syphilis, hepatitis B and HIV as per state regulations.
- Infant blood tests are available and have been reviewed, including cord or infant blood type and direct Coombs test results, as clinically indicated.
- Initial hepatitis B and vitamin K vaccine has been administered.
- If a mother has not previously been vaccinated, she should receive tetanus toxoid, reduced diphtheria toxoid and acellular pertussis vaccine immediately after birth.
- If required the mother will also receive rubella vaccination if low immunity.
- If a mother who births during the flu season has not been previously immunised, she should receive flu vaccine.
- Newborn metabolic, hearing and congenital heart disease screening has been completed per hospital protocol and state regulations if required before discharge.
- Family, environmental and social risk factors have been assessed and proactive management is in place.
- Mother's knowledge, ability and confidence to provide adequate infant care have been assessed for competency.
- An appropriate car seat is available before hospital discharge, and mother has demonstrated competence in its use.
- Continuing medical care is planned; infants discharged sooner than 48 hours should be examined within 48 hours of discharge from the hospital.
- Barriers to adequate follow-up care (e.g. lack of telephone or transportation) have been assessed, and a plan is in place to manage issues.

Follow-up home care within days (or even hours after discharge when minor problems are anticipated) is important to provide adequate mother–newborn care with minimal complications. Despite the changing spectrum of well-newborn healthcare, the nurse/midwife's role continues to be that of providing ongoing assessments of each mother–newborn dyad to ensure a safe transition to home and a successful adaptation into the family unit. The ultimate safety and success of early newborn discharge from the hospital are contingent on using clear discharge criteria and having a high-quality early follow-up program.

REVIEW QUESTIONS

1. Identify the anatomical changes that occur shortly after birth that affect the newborn's adaptation to extrauterine existence. Select all that apply.
   A. Closure of the foramen ovale
   B. Closure of the ductus arteriosus
   C. Increase in pulmonary vascular resistance
   D. Closure of the ductus venosus
   E. Decrease in pulmonary vascular resistance
2. In the newly born infant thermogenesis is achieved by:
   A. shivering
   B. brown fat metabolism
   C. overhead warming unit
   D. skin-to-skin contact with mother.
3. What does the Apgar scoring system assess? Select all that apply.
   A. Respiratory effort
   B. Heart rate
   C. Core temperature
   D. Reflex irritability
   E. Muscle tone
   F. Colour
4. A healthy infant is born to a mother with known high-risk behaviours and whose HIV status is undetermined. The mother states that she wishes to breastfeed her infant. The nurse/midwife's response to the mother's request should be based on which of the following information?
   A. HIV is rarely transmitted to the newborn through maternal milk.
   B. Breastfeeding should be withheld until HIV status (maternal) is determined.
   C. Breastfeeding should be avoided completely in mothers with high-risk behaviours.
   D. In such infants antiretroviral medication should be started within 12 hours of birth.

Correct Answers

1. A, B, D, E; 2. B; 3. A, B, D, E, F; 4. B

REFERENCES

Agho, K. E., Ogeleka, P., Ogbo, F. A., et al. (2016). Trends and predictors of prelacteal feeding practices in Nigeria (2003–2013). Nutrients, 8(8), E462.

Australian Breastfeeding Association. (2017). Is my baby getting enough milk? https://www.breastfeeding.asn.au/bfinfo/my-baby-getting-enough-milk

Australian Breastfeeding Association. (2019). Mastitis. September. https://www.breastfeeding.asn.au/bf-info/common-concerns%E2%80%93mum/mastitis

Australian Government Department of Health. (2019). 33 Human immunodeficiency virus. Pregnancy care guidelines. https://www.health.gov.au/resources/pregnancy-care-guidelines/part-f-routine-maternal-health-tests/human-immunodeficiency-virus

Australian Government Department of Health. (2021). Ear health in Australia. https://www.health.gov.au/health-topics/ear-health

Australian Institute of Health and Welfare. (2020). Australia's mothers and babies data visualisations. Apgar score at 5 minutes. https://www.aihw.gov.au/reports/mothers-babies/australias-mothers-babies-2017-data-visualisations/contents/baby-outcomes/apgar-score-at-5-minutes

Ballard, J. L., Khoury, J. C., Wedig, K., et al. (1991). New Ballard score expanded to include extremely premature infants. The Journal of Pediatrics, 119, 417–423.

Behrendt, H. R., Konrad, K., Goecke, T. W., et al. (2016). Post-natal mother-to-infant attachment in sub-clinically depressed mothers: Dyads at risk? Psychopathology, 49(4), 269–276.

Bergman, N. J. (2013). Neonatal stomach volume and physiology suggest feeding at 1 hour intervals. Acta Paediatrica, 102(8), 773–777.

Bertelsen, R. J., Jensen, E. T., & Ringel-Kulka, T. (2016). Use of probiotics and prebiotics in infant feeding. Best Practice & Research. Clinical Gastroenterology, 30(1), 39–48.

Brazelton, T. B. (1974). Mother-infant reciprocity. In M. H. Klaus, T. Leger, & M. A. Trause (Eds.), Maternal attachment and mothering disorders: A round table. Sausalito, CA: Johnson & Johnson Baby Products.

Canadian Paediatric Society, Community Paediatrics Committee. (updated 2015). Temperature measurement in paediatrics. Retrieved from http://www.cps.ca/en/documents/position.

Casey, M. (2018). Skills for midwifery practice. Elsevier, Melbourne.

Chamberlain, J., McCarty, S., Sorce, J., et al. (2019). Impact on delayed newborn bathing on exclusive breastfeeding rates, glucose and temperature stability, and weight loss. Journal of Neonatal Nursing, 25(2), 74–77.

Davies, L. & Baddock, S. (2019). Supporting the newborn. In Pairman, S., Tracy, S., Dahlen, H., & Dixon, L. Midwifery: Preparation for Practice 4th ed. Sydney: Elsevier Australia.

Dubowitz, L. M. S., & Dubowitz, V. (1977). Gestational age of the newborn. Menlo Park, CA: Addison Wesley.

Emond, A., Ingram, J., Johnson, D., et al. (2014). Randomized controlled trial of early frenotomy in breastfed infants with mild-moderate tongue-tie. Archives of Disease in Childhood. Fetal and Neonatal Edition, 99(3), F189–F195.

Foster, J. P., Taylor, C., & Spence, K. (2017). Topical anaesthesia for needle-related pain in newborn infants. The Cochrane Database of Systematic Reviews, (2), CD010331.

Haddad, L., Smith, S., Phillips, K. D., et al. (2012). Comparison of temporal artery and axillary temperatures in healthy newborns. Journal of Obstetric, Gynecologic, and Neonatal Nursing, 41, 383–388.

Hawkins, S. S., Stern, A. D., Baum, C. F., et al. (2014). Compliance with the Baby-Friendly Hospital Initiative and impact on breastfeeding rates. Archives of Disease in Childhood. Fetal and Neonatal Edition, 99(2), F138–F143.

Hawkins, S. S., Stern, A. D., Baum, C. F., et al. (2015). Evaluating the impact of the Baby-Friendly Hospital Initiative on breast-feeding rates: A multi-state analysis. Public Health Nutrition, 18(2), 179–187.

Horta, B. L., Loret de Mola, C., & Victora, C. G. (2015). Breastfeeding and intelligence: A systematic review and meta-analysis. Acta Paediatrica, 104(467), 14–19.

Howe-Heyman, A., & Lutenbacher, M. (2016). The Baby-Friendly Hospital Initiative as an intervention to improve breastfeeding rates: A review of the literature. Journal of Midwifery & Women's Health, 61(1), 77–102.

Jasani, B., Simmer, K., Patole, S. K., et al. (2017). Long chain polyunsaturated fatty acid supplementation in infants born at term. The Cochrane Database of Systematic Reviews, (3), CD000376.

Johnston, C., Campbell-Yeo, M., Disher, T., et al. (2017). Skin-to-skin care for procedural pain in neonates. The Cochrane Database of Systematic Reviews, (2), CD008435.

Jones, K. M., Power, M. L., Queenan, J. T., et al. (2015). Racial and ethnic disparities in breastfeeding. Breastfeeding Medicine: The Official Journal of the Academy of Breastfeeding Medicine, 10(4), 186–196.

Kapoor, V., Douglas, P., Hill, P., et al. (2018). Frenotomy for tongue-tie in Australian children, 2006–2016: an increasing problem. Medical Journal of Australia, 208(2), 88–89. doi: 10.5694/mja17.00438

Kleinman, R. E., & Greer, F. R. (Eds.) (2014). Pediatric nutrition (7th ed.). Elk Grove Village, IL: American Academy of Pediatrics.

Kuswara, K., Laws, R., Kremer, P., et al. (2016). The infant feeding practices of Chinese immigrant mothers in Australia: A qualitative exploration. Appetite, 105, 375–384.

Lai, N. M., Foong, S. C., Foong, W. C., et al. (2016). Co-bedding in neonatal nursery for promoting growth and neurodevelopment in stable preterm twins. The Cochrane Database of Systematic Reviews, (4), CD008313.

Lund, C. (2016). Bathing and beyond: Current bathing controversies for newborn infants. Advances in Neonatal Care, 16(5S), S13–S20.

Martin, C. R., Ling, P.-R., & Blackburn, G. L. (2016). Review of infant feeding: Key features of breast milk and infant formula. Nutrients, 8(5), 279–290.

Medoff Cooper, B., Holditch-Davis, D., Verklan, M. T., et al. (2012). Newborn clinical outcomes of the AWHONN Late Preterm Infant Research-Based Practice Project. Journal of Obstetric, Gynecologic, and Neonatal Nursing, 41(6), 774–785.

Ministry of Health. (2014). Mastitis and breast abscesses. 7 February. https://www.health.govt.nz/our-work/life-stages/breastfeeding/health-practitioners/mastitis-and-breast-abscesses

Modarres, M., Jazayeri, Q., Rahnama, P., et al. (2013). Breastfeeding and pain relief in full-term neonates during immunization injections: A clinical randomized trial. BMC Anesthesiology, 13(1), 22–28.

National Health and Medical Research Council (NHMRC). (2010). Joint statement and recommendations on vitamin K administration to newborn infants to prevent vitamin K deficiency bleeding in infancy – October 2010 (the Joint Statement). https://ranzcog.edu.au/RANZCOG_SITE/media/RANZCOG-MEDIA/Women%27s%20Health/Vitamin-K.pdf?ext=.pdf

New Zealand Breastfeeding Alliance. (2021). Baby Friendly Aotearoa New Zealand. https://www.babyfriendly.org.nz/

Nugent, J. K. (2013). The competent newborn and the Neonatal Behavioral Assessment State: T. Berry Brazelton's legacy. Journal of Child and Adolescent Psychiatric Nursing, 26, 173–179.

O'Shea, J. E., Foster, J. P., O'Donnell, C. P. F., et al. (2017). Frenotomy for tongue-tie in newborn infants. The Cochrane Database of Systematic Reviews, (3), CD011065.

Pairman, S., Tracy, S., Dahlen, H. & Dixon, L. (2019) Midwifery: Preparation for practice. New Zealand College of Midwives; Australian College of Midwives 4th ed., Australia: Elsevier Health.

Pessler, R. F., & Nejat, M. (2004). Anaphylactic reactions to goat's milk in a cow's milk allergic infant. Pediatric Allergy and Immunology, 15(2), 183–185.

Power, R. F., & Murphy, J. F. (2015). Tongue-tie and frenotomy in infants with breastfeeding difficulties: Achieving a balance. Archives of Disease in Childhood, 100(5), 489–494.

Rabe, H., Gyte, G. M. I., Díaz-Rossello, J. L., et al. (2019). Effect of timing of umbilical cord clamping and other strategies to influence placental transfusion at preterm birth on maternal and infant outcomes. Cochrane Database of Systematic Reviews, CD003248. DOI: 10.1002/14651858.CD003248.pub4

Sasidharan, K., Dutta, S., & Narang, A. (2009). Validity of New Ballard score until 7th day of postnatal life in moderately preterm neonates. Archives of Disease in Childhood. Fetal and Neonatal Edition, 94, F39–F44.

Shah, P. S., Herbozo, C., Aliwalas, L. L., et al. (2012). Breastfeeding or breast milk for procedural pain in neonates. The Cochrane Database of Systematic Reviews, (12), CD004950.

Sim, M. A., Leow, S. Y., Hao, Y., et al. (2016). A practical comparison of temporal artery thermometry and axillary thermometry in neonates under different environments. Journal of Paediatrics and Child Health, 52(4), 391–396.

Smith, J. (2014). Methods and devices of temperature measurement in the neonate: A narrative review of practice recommendations. Newborn and Infant Nursing Reviews, 14(2), 64–71.

Smith, J., Alcock, G., & Usher, K. (2013). Temperature measurement in the preterm and term neonate: A review of the literature. Neonatal Network, 32(1), 16–25.

Smolkin, T., Mick, O., Dabbah, M., et al. (2012). Birth by cesarean delivery and failure of first otoacoustic emissions hearing test. Pediatrics, 130(1), e95–e100.

Sydney Children's Hospital. (2021). Audiology services at Sydney Children's Hospital, Randwick. https://www.schn.health.nsw.gov.au/find-a-service/health-medical-services/audiology-hearing-tests/sch

The Royal Children's Hospital Melbourne. (2020). Safe sleeping. Clinical Guidelines (Nursing). https://www.rch.org.au/rchcpg/hospital_clinical_guideline_index/Safe_sleeping/

The Royal Women's Hospital. (n.d.). NBO: Newborn Behavioural Observations. https://www.thewomens.org.au/health-professionals/clinical-education-training/nbo-australia

Victorian Agency for Health Information (VAHI) and Safer Care Victoria (SCV). (2020a). Resuscitation of neonates. 12 November. https://www.bettersafercare.vic.gov.au/clinical-guidance/neonatal/resuscitation-of-neonates

VAHI & SCV. (2020b). Developmental care for neonates. 12 November. https://www.bettersafercare.vic.gov.au/clinical-guidance/neonatal/developmental-care-for-neonates

VAHI & SCV. (2020c). Oxygen saturation screening for newborns. 12 November. https://www.bettersafercare.vic.gov.au/clinical-guidance/neonatal/oxygen-saturation-screening-for-newborns

VAHI & SCV. (2020d). Umbilical cord care for neonates. 12 November. https://www.bettersafercare.vic.gov.au/clinical-guidance/neonatal/umbilical-cord-care-for-neonates

Wandel, M., Terragni, L., Nguyen, C., et al. (2016). Breastfeeding among Somali mothers living in Norway: Attitudes, practices and challenges. Women and Birth, 29(6), 487–493.

Wang, L., Collins, C., Ratliff, M., et al. (Feb 2017). Breastfeeding reduces childhood obesity risks. Childhood Obesity, 13(3), 197–204.

Widström, A., Brimdyr, K., Svensson, K., et al. (2019). Skin-to-skin contact the first hour after birth, underlying implications and clinical practice. Acta Paediatrica, 108(7), 1192–1204. https://doi.org/10.1111/apa.14754

World Health Organization, UNICEF, Wellstart International. (2009). Baby-friendly hospital initiative: revised, updated and expanded for integrated care, World Health Organization.

Zupan, J., Garner, P., & Omari, A. A. (2004). Topical umbilical cord care at birth. The Cochrane Database of Systematic Reviews, (3), CD001057.

8

Health Problems of the Newborn

Tameeka Mulquiney and Sarah Dechert

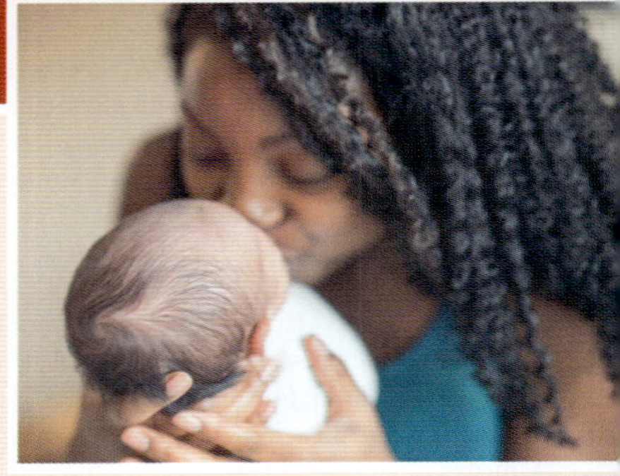

LEARNING OBJECTIVES

- Begin to identify birth injuries and their management
- Begin to identify congenital abnormalities and their management
- Demonstrate the assessment and management skills required for the newborn

BIRTH INJURIES

Several factors predispose an infant to birth injuries. Maternal factors include uterine dysfunction that leads to prolonged or precipitous labour, preterm or postterm labour, and cephalopelvic disproportion. Injury may result from dystocia caused by fetal macrosomia, multifetal gestation, abnormal or difficult presentation (not caused by maternal uterine or pelvic conditions) and congenital anomalies. Intrapartum events that can result in scalp injury include the use of intrapartum monitoring of fetal heart rate and collection of fetal scalp blood for acid–base assessment. Obstetric birth techniques can cause injury. Forceps birth, vacuum extraction and caesarean birth are potential contributory factors. Often more than one factor is present, and multiple predisposing factors may be related to a single maternal condition.

Many injuries are minor and resolve spontaneously in a few days; others, although minor, require some degree of intervention. Still others can be serious or even fatal. Part of the nurse's responsibility is to identify such injuries so that appropriate interventions can be initiated as soon as possible. Birth injuries are classified according to the type of body structure involved (Box 8.1).

Soft Tissue Injury

Infants may sustain various types of soft tissue injury during birth, primarily in the form of bruises and abrasions secondary to dystocia. Soft tissue injury usually occurs when there is some degree of disproportion between the presenting part and the maternal pelvis (**cephalopelvic disproportion**). Box 8.2 lists common types of soft tissue injury. The use of forceps to facilitate a difficult vertex birth may produce discolouration or abrasions with the same configuration as the forceps on the sides of the neonate's face. Petechiae or ecchymoses may be observed on the presenting part after a breech or brow birth. After a difficult or precipitous birth, the sudden release of pressure on the head can produce scleral haemorrhage or petechiae over the face and head. Petechiae and ecchymoses may also appear on the head, neck and face of an infant born with a **nuchal cord**, giving the infant's face a cyanotic appearance. A well-defined circle of petechiae and ecchymoses may also appear on the occipital region of the newborn's head when a vacuum suction cup is applied during birth.

These traumatic lesions generally fade spontaneously and without treatment within a few days. However, petechiae may be a manifestation of an underlying bleeding disorder and require further evaluation.

Nursing Care Management

Nursing care is directed primarily towards assessing the injury, maintaining asepsis of the area to prevent additional skin breakdown and infection and providing an explanation and reassurance to the parents. The nurse should record an accurate description of the injury in writing (e.g. the location, colour, size and shape) and via photographs, when possible, to facilitate subsequent comparative nursing evaluations.

Regardless of how benign the injury, parents may be concerned and mourn the loss of the expected 'perfect' infant. Explanations of the cause and treatment, if any, need to be thorough and repeated frequently. If the injury is temporarily disfiguring, such as extensive facial bruising, nurses can demonstrate acceptance of the child through their example of sensitive, personal care.

Head Injury

Head injury that occurs during the birth process is usually benign but occasionally results in more serious injury. The injuries that produce serious trauma, such as intracranial haemorrhage and subdural haematoma, are discussed in relation to neurological disorders in the newborn (see Chapters 9 and 32). Skull fractures are discussed with other fractures sustained during the birth process. The three most common types of extracranial haemorrhagic injury are caput succedaneum, subgaleal haemorrhage and cephalhaematoma.

Caput Succedaneum

The most commonly observed scalp lesion is **caput succedaneum**, a vaguely outlined area of oedematous tissue situated over the portion of the scalp that presents in a vertex birth (Fig 8.1A). The swelling consists of serum and/or blood that has accumulated in the tissues above the bone. Typically the swelling extends beyond the bone margins (or sutures) and may be associated with overlying petechiae or ecchymosis. It is present at or shortly after birth. No specific treatment is necessary, and the swelling subsides within a few days.

BOX 8.1 Types of Neonatal Physical Injuries at Birth*

Soft tissue injury
- Erythema
- Abrasion
- Petechiae
- Ecchymoses
- Subcutaneous fat necrosis
- Retinal haemorrhage
- Scalp laceration

Head injury
- Caput succedaneum
- Subgaleal haemorrhage
- Cephalhaematoma
- Fracture (depressed or linear)
- Intracranial haemorrhage
- Subdural or epidural haematoma

Nerve injury
- Facial paralysis
- Brachial palsy (Erb-Duchenne paralysis, Klumpke's palsy)
- Phrenic nerve palsy (diaphragmatic paralysis)
- Spinal cord injury
- Vocal cord paralysis

Other
- Fracture-clavicle, femur
- Torticollis
- Scalp abscess
- Subconjunctival (scleral) haemorrhage
- Liver, spleen rupture
- Haemorrhage into abdominal organ(s)

*Partial adaptation from Rozance, P. J., & Rosenberg, A. A. (2012). The neonate. In S. G. Gabbe, J. R. Niebyl, J. L. Simpson, et al (Eds.), *Obstetrics: Normal and problem pregnancies* (6th ed.). Philadelphia, PA: Elsevier/Saunders.

Subgaleal Haemorrhage

Subgaleal haemorrhage is bleeding into the subgaleal compartment (Fig 8.1B). The subgaleal compartment is a potential space that contains loosely arranged connective tissue. It is located beneath the galea aponeurosis, the tendinous sheath that connects the frontal and occipital muscles and forms the inner surface of the scalp. The injury occurs as a result of forces that compress and then drag the head through the pelvic outlet (Parsons et al 2016, Shah & Wusthoff 2016). Instrumented birth, particularly vacuum extraction and forceps delivery, increases the risk of subgaleal haemorrhage. Additional risk factors include prolonged second stage of labour, fetal distress, macrosomia, failed vacuum extraction and maternal primiparity. The bleeding extends beyond bone, often posterior into the neck, and continues after birth, with the potential for serious complications and morbidity.

Early detection of the haemorrhage is vital; serial head circumference measurements and inspection of the back of the neck for increasing oedema and a firm mass are essential. A boggy fluctuant mass over the scalp that crosses the suture line and moves as the baby is repositioned is an early sign of subgaleal haemorrhage (Smith et al 2016). Other signs include pallor, tachycardia, a forward and lateral

BOX 8.2 Common Types of Soft Tissue Injury

Erythema and abrasions—Usually the result of the application of forceps; discolouration the same configuration as the instrument.

Petechiae—Non-raised, pinpoint haemorrhages caused by a sudden increase and then release of pressure during passage through the birth canal; may be seen on the chest, face and head.

Ecchymoses—Small haemorrhagic areas (larger than petechiae) that may occur after traumatic, precipitous or breech delivery.

Subcutaneous fat necrosis—Clearly outlined masses located in the subcutaneous tissues that are firm to the overlying skin but movable over the underlying tissue; most likely caused by traumatic manipulation during delivery.

Subconjunctival (scleral) haemorrhages—The result of rupture of capillaries in the sclera from pressure on the fetal head during delivery; most commonly located in the limbus of the iris.

Retinal haemorrhages—Flame-shaped, irregular or round areas of bleeding in the retina from excessive pressure on the fetal head during delivery; extensive areas possibly indicative of subdural haematoma or brain trauma.

positioning of the newborn's ears as the haematoma extends posteriorly, and increasing head circumference. Computed tomography (CT) or magnetic resonance imaging (MRI) is useful in confirming the diagnosis. Replacement of lost blood and clotting factors is required in acute cases of haemorrhage. Monitoring the infant for changes in level of consciousness and a decrease in the haematocrit is also vital to early recognition and management. An increase in serum bilirubin levels may occur as a result of the degrading red blood cells within the haematoma.

Cephalhaematoma

Cephalhaematoma forms when blood vessels rupture during labour or birth and produce bleeding into the area between the bone and its periosteum. The injury occurs most often with primiparous women and is often associated with forceps birth and vacuum extraction. Unlike caput succedaneum, the boundaries of the cephalhaematoma are distinguishable and do not extend beyond the limits of the bone (Fig 8.1C). The cephalhaematoma may involve one or both parietal bones but rarely affects the occipital and frontal bones. The swelling is usually minimal or absent at birth and increases in size on the second or third day. Blood loss is usually not significant.

No treatment is indicated for uncomplicated cephalhaematoma. Most lesions are absorbed within 2 weeks to 3 months. Lesions that result in severe blood loss to the area or that involve an underlying fracture require further evaluation. Hyperbilirubinaemia may result during resolution of the haematoma. A local infection can develop and is suspected when swelling suddenly increases.

Nursing Care Management

Nursing care is directed towards assessment, observation and accurate documentation of the common scalp injuries. Vigilance in observing for possible associated complications, such as infection or, as in the case of subgaleal haemorrhage, acute blood loss and hypovolaemia, is important. Nursing care of a newborn with a subgaleal haemorrhage includes careful monitoring for signs of haemodynamic instability and shock (Modanlou et al 2016). Because caput succedaneum and cephalhaematoma usually resolve spontaneously, parents need reassurance of their usually benign nature.

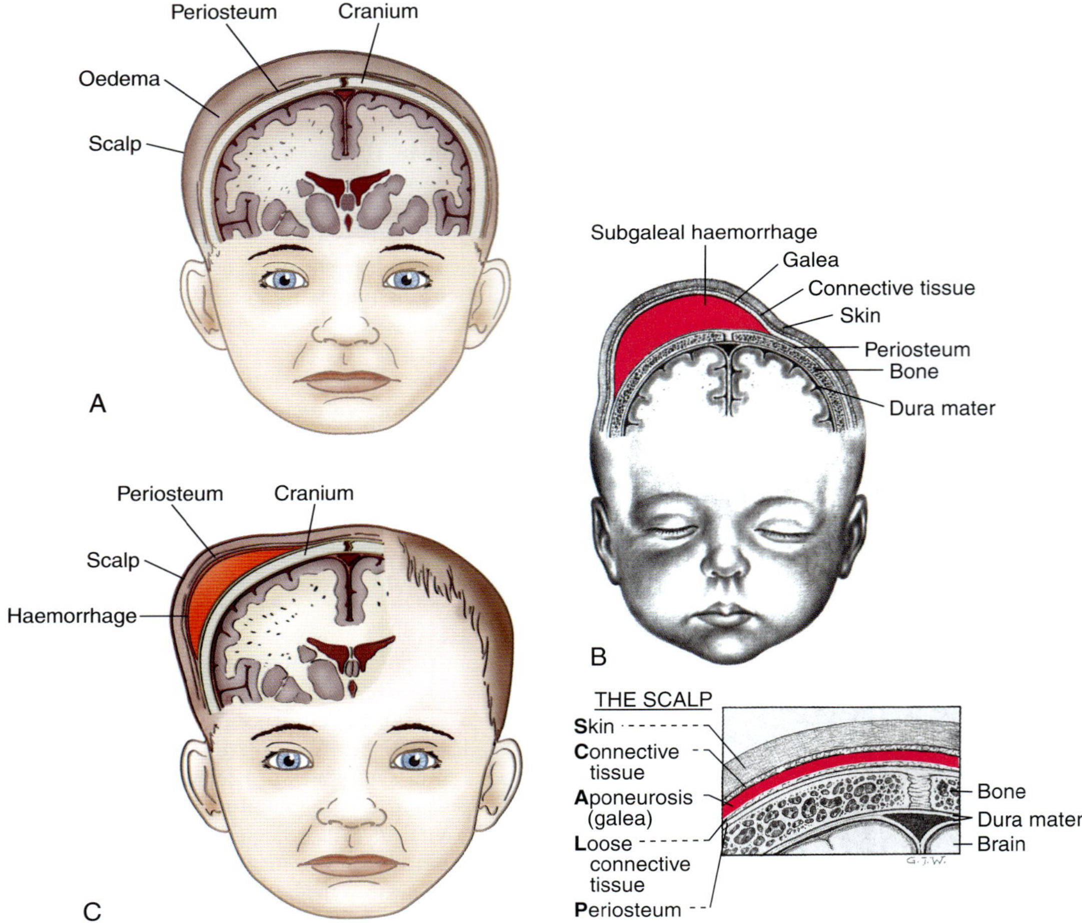

Fig 8.1 (**A**) Caput succedaneum. (**B**) Subgaleal haemorrhage. (**C**) Cephalhaematoma. (Source: *A* and *C*, From Seidel, H. M., Ball, J. W., Dains, J. E., et al (2006). *Mosby's guide to physical examination* (6th ed.). St Louis, MO: Mosby.)

Fractures

Fracture of the clavicle, or collarbone, is the most common birth injury. It is often associated with difficult vertex or breech birth of infants of greater-than-average size. Further examination usually reveals **crepitus** (i.e. the coarse, crackling sensation produced by the rubbing together of fractured bone fragments), and reveals a complete fracture with overriding of the fragments. A palpable spongy mass, representing localised oedema and haematoma, is also a sign of a fractured clavicle.

The newborn with a fractured clavicle may have no symptoms, but the nurse should suspect a fracture if an infant has limited use of the affected arm, malpositioning of the arm, an asymmetrical Moro reflex or focal swelling or tenderness or cries when the arm is moved. Eliciting the scarf sign (i.e. extending arm across chest towards opposite shoulder) for assessment of gestational age is contraindicated if a fractured clavicle is suspected.

In neonates, fractures of long bones, such as the femur or the humerus, are often difficult to detect by radiographic examination. Although osteogenesis imperfecta is a rare finding, assess a newborn infant with a fracture for other evidence of this congenital disorder.

Fractures of the neonatal skull are uncommon. The bones, which are less mineralised and more compressible than bones in older infants and children, are separated by membranous seams that allow the head contour to adjust to the birth canal during birth. Skull fractures usually follow a prolonged, difficult birth or forceps extraction. Most fractures are linear, but some may be visible as depressed indentations that compress or decompress like a Ping-Pong ball. Management of depressed skull fractures is controversial; many resolve without intervention. Surgery may be required in the presence of bone fragments or signs of neurological changes and increased intracranial pressure (ICP). A similar finding in neonates is *craniotabes,* which is usually benign or may be associated with prematurity or hydrocephalus (Johnson 2016). In this condition the cranial bone(s) moves freely on palpation and may be easily compressed.

Nursing Care Management

Often no intervention is prescribed other than proper body alignment, careful dressing and undressing of the infant, and handling and carrying techniques that support the affected bone. If the infant has a fractured clavicle, it is important to support the upper and lower back rather than pull the infant up from under the arms. Occasionally, for immobilisation and relief of pain, the arm on the side of the fractured clavicle may be abducted at more than 60 degrees with the elbow flexed at more than 90 degrees for 7 to 10 days.

Linear skull fractures usually require no treatment. A Ping-Pong–type fracture may require decompression by surgical intervention. The infant is carefully observed for signs of neurological complications. The parents of an infant with a fracture of any bone should be involved in caring for the infant during hospitalisation as part of discharge planning for care at home. Evaluate any newborn large for gestational age and delivered vaginally for a fractured clavicle.

Nerve Injuries

Facial Paralysis

Pressure on the facial nerve (the seventh cranial nerve) during birth may result in injury to the nerve. The primary clinical manifestations are loss of movement on the affected side, such as an inability to completely close the eye, drooping of the corner of the mouth and absence of wrinkling of the forehead and nasolabial fold (Fig 8.2). The paralysis is most noticeable when the infant cries. The mouth is drawn to the unaffected side, the wrinkles are deeper on the normal side and the eye on the involved side remains open.

No medical intervention is necessary. The paralysis usually disappears spontaneously in a few days but may take as long as several months.

Brachial Palsy

Brachial plexus injury results from forces that alter the normal position and relationship of the arm, shoulder and neck. **Erb's palsy** (Erb-Duchenne paralysis) is caused by damage to the upper plexus and usually results from stretching or pulling away of the shoulder from the head, as might occur with shoulder dystocia or with a difficult vertex or breech birth. Other identified clinical situations that are considered to place the baby at risk for brachial palsy include a significantly larger than normal baby with a fetal weight exceeding 5000 g in women without diabetes or 4500 g in women with diabetes, prior recognised shoulder dystocia or a midpelvic operative vaginal birth with a fetal birth weight in excess of 4000 g (The Royal Children's Hospital Melbourne [RCHM] 2018). The less common lower plexus palsy, or Klumpke's palsy, results from severe stretching of the upper extremity while the trunk is relatively less mobile.

The clinical manifestations of Erb's palsy are related to the paralysis of the affected upper extremity and muscles. The arm hangs limp alongside the body. The shoulder and arm are adducted and internally rotated. The elbow is extended and the forearm is pronated, with the wrist and fingers flexed; a grasp reflex may be present because finger and wrist movement remain normal, but the Moro reflex is absent

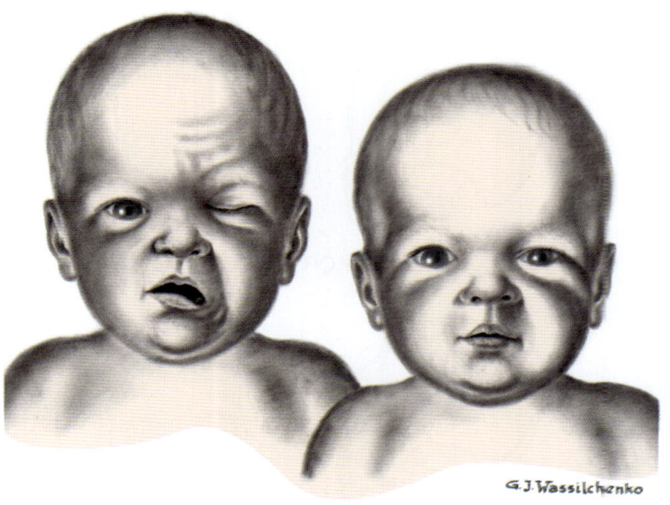

Fig 8.2 **(A)** Paralysis of right side of face 15 minutes after forceps birth. Absence of movement on affected side is especially noticeable when infant cries. **(B)** Same infant 24 hours later.

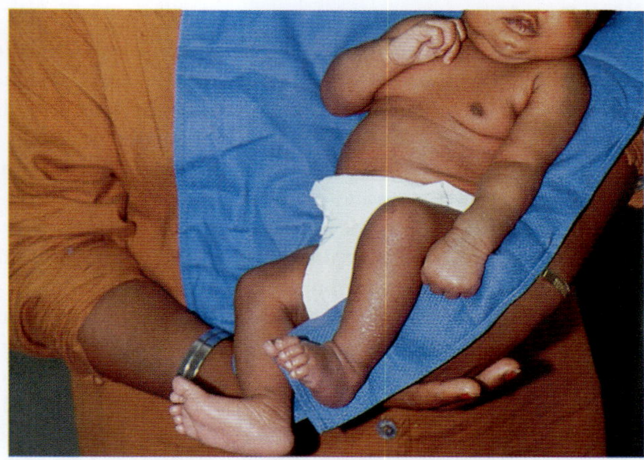

Fig 8.3 Left-sided brachial plexus (Erb-Duchenne) palsy. Note extended, internally rotated arm and pronated wrist on affected side.

(Tappero 2016) (Fig 8.3). In lower plexus palsy the muscles of the hand are paralysed, with consequent wrist drop and relaxed fingers. In a third and more severe form of brachial palsy, total plexus injury, the entire arm and hand are paralysed and hang limp and motionless at the side. The Moro reflex is absent on the affected side for all forms of brachial palsy.

Treatment of the affected arm is aimed at preventing contractures of the paralysed muscles and maintaining correct placement of the humeral head within the glenoid fossa of the scapula. Complete recovery from stretched nerves usually takes 3 to 6 months. Full recovery is expected in the majority of infants (Parsons et al 2016), but there are specific peripartum and neonatal factors associated with persistent neonatal brachial plexus palsy at 1 year (Wilson et al 2016).

A condition that may occur in association with brachial plexus injury is *torticollis.* This symptom, as it is called by many, is observed as a tilting of the head to one side in combination with rotation of the head to the opposite side due to the unilateral contracture of the sternocleidomastoid muscle; it has been reported to occur in as many as 43% of infants with brachial plexus injury (O'Toole & Spiegel 2016). Torticollis may also occur in older infants with positional plagiocephaly (see Chapter 11) and in association with other conditions such as spinal cord tumours, clavicle fracture, congenital scoliosis, Klippel-Feil anomalies and cervical spine subluxation (Hedequist et al 2018). The treatment of torticollis involves massage, stimulation and stretching programs under the supervision of a physiotherapist (Hervey-Jumper et al 2011, O'Toole & Spiegel 2016). Additional pathology associated with torticollis may occur, but it is not within the scope of this section to discuss the range of possibilities.

Phrenic Nerve Paralysis

Phrenic nerve paralysis results in diaphragmatic paralysis as demonstrated by ultrasonography, which shows paradoxical chest movement and an elevated diaphragm. Initially, chest radiography may not demonstrate an elevated diaphragm if the neonate is receiving positive pressure ventilation. The injury sometimes occurs in conjunction with brachial palsy. Respiratory distress is the most common and important sign of injury. Because injury to the phrenic nerve is usually unilateral, the lung on the affected side does not expand, and respiratory efforts are ineffectual. Breathing is primarily thoracic, and cyanosis, tachypnoea or complete respiratory failure may be seen. Pneumonia and atelectasis on the affected side may also occur.

Nursing Care Management

Nursing care of the infant with facial nerve paralysis involves aiding the infant in suckling and helping the mother with feeding techniques. A comprehensive evaluation of the infant's oral motor skills by both a speech pathologist and a lactation consultant are recommended to develop an effective multidisciplinary feeding regimen. The infant may require partial gavage feeding and bottle with a minimum amount of expressed breast milk to prevent aspiration. Breastfeeding is recommended and the mother will need assistance in helping the infant latch to ensure effective milk transfer from the mother to the infant.

Nursing care of the newborn with brachial palsy is concerned primarily with proper positioning of the affected arm. The affected arm should be gently immobilised on the upper abdomen; passive range-of-motion exercises of the shoulder, wrist, elbow and fingers are initiated at 7 to 10 days of age (Carlo & Ambalavanan 2016b, Roland & Hill 2016). Wrist flexion contractures may be prevented with the use of supportive splints or braces. In dressing the infant, give preference to the affected arm. Undressing begins with the unaffected arm, and redressing begins with the affected arm to prevent unnecessary manipulation and stress on the paralysed muscles. Teach parents to use the 'football' position when holding the infant and to avoid picking the child up from under the axillae or by pulling on the arms (The Royal Children's Hospital 2018).

The infant with phrenic nerve paralysis requires the same nursing care as any infant with respiratory distress. The family's emotional needs are also an important part of nursing care; the family needs reassurance regarding the neonate's progress towards an optimal outcome. Follow-up care is also essential because of the extended length of recovery.

CRANIAL DEFORMITIES

In the normal newborn the cranial sutures are separated by membranous seams several millimetres wide. For the first few hours to 1 to 2 days after birth, the cranial bones are highly mobile, which allows the bones to mould and overlap one another, adjusting the circumference of the head to accommodate to the changing shape and character of the birth canal. The principal sutures in the infant's skull are the sagittal, coronal and lambdoid sutures, and the major soft areas at the juncture of these sutures are the anterior and posterior fontanels.

After birth, growth of the skull bones occurs in a direction perpendicular (at right angles) to the line of the suture, and normal closure occurs in a regular and predictable order. Although the age at which closure takes place varies widely in individual children, solid union of all sutures is not completed until late childhood. Normally, sutures and fontanels are ossified by the following ages:

- 8 weeks—posterior fontanel closed
- 6 months—fibrous union of suture lines and interlocking of serrated edges
- 18 months—anterior fontanel closed
- 12 years and older—sutures not separable by ICP.

Closure of a suture before the expected time inhibits the perpendicular growth. Because normal increase in brain volume requires expansion, the skull is forced to grow in a direction parallel to the fused suture. This alteration in skull growth always distorts the head shape when the underlying brain growth is normal. The small head with closed sutures and a normal shape is a result of deficient brain growth; the suture closure is secondary to this brain growth failure. Failure of brain growth is not secondary to suture closure.

Various types of cranial deformities are encountered in early infancy. These include the enlarged head with frontal protrusion, or **bossing** (characteristic of hydrocephalus); the parietal bossing that is seen in chronic subdural haematoma; the small head; and a variety of skull deformities (Fig 8.4). Some occur during prenatal development.

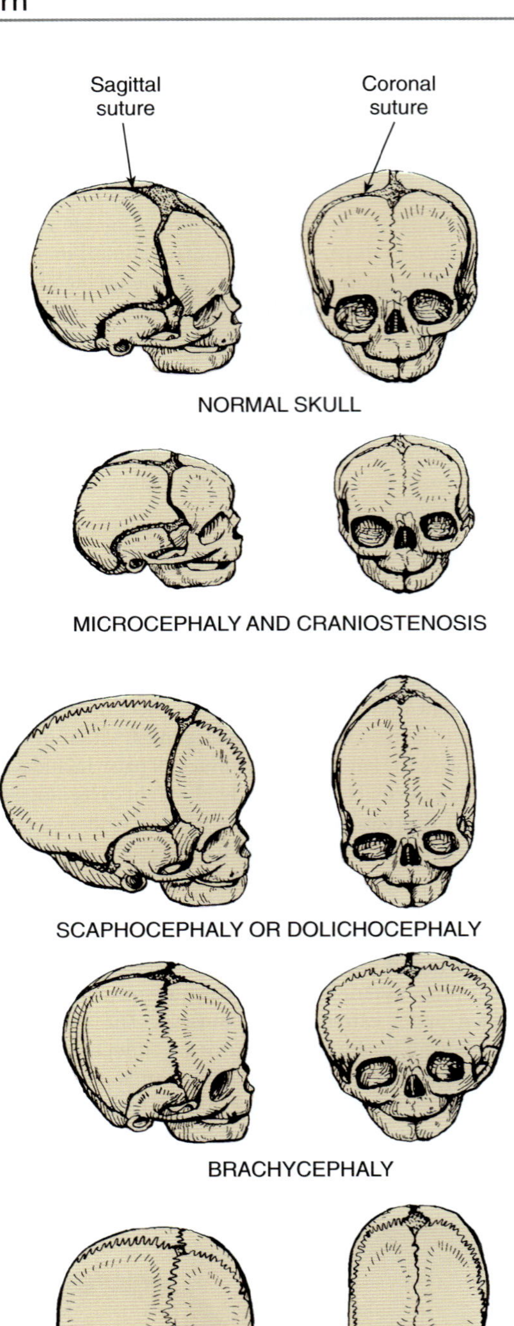

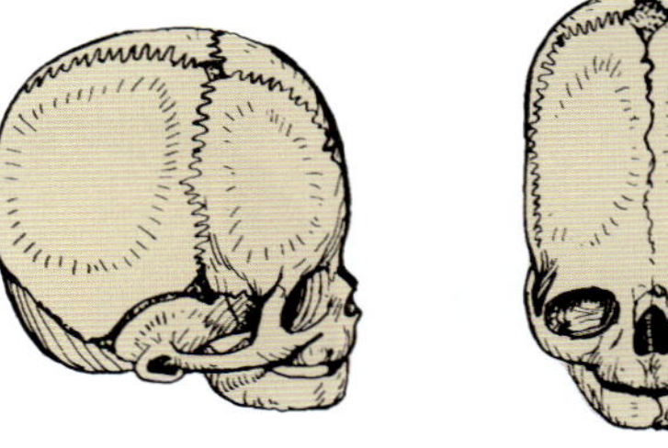

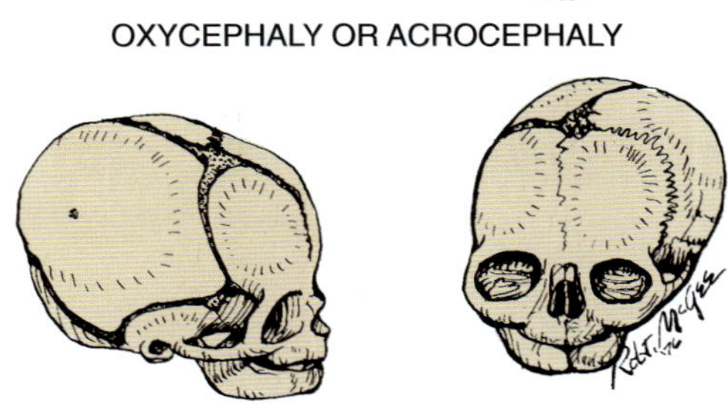

Fig 8.4 Abnormal skull configurations.

In others, head circumference is usually within normal limits at birth, and the deviation from normal development becomes apparent with advancing age.

Microcephaly

Primary (genetic) microcephaly refers to a small head size that may be caused by an autosomal-recessive or autosomal-dominant disorder or a chromosomal abnormality such as Down syndrome or Cornelia de Lange syndrome (Kinsman & Johnston 2016). **Secondary (non-genetic) microcephaly** can result from a variety of insults that occur during the third trimester of pregnancy, the perinatal period or early infancy (Kinsman & Johnston 2016). These stimuli may be irradiation (especially between 4 and 20 weeks' gestation), maternal infection (notably toxoplasmosis, rubella or cytomegalovirus [see Maternal Infections, Chapter 9]), irradiation or chemical agents such as alcohol and tobacco. Other studies have shown a strong association between maternal alcohol ingestion and microcephaly and low birth weight and length (de Araújo et al 2018). Infection, trauma, metabolic disorders and anoxia are all capable of causing decreased brain growth. Microcephaly is defined as an occipitofrontal circumference greater than 3 standard deviations below the mean for age and sex (Thalia et al 2018).

The Zika virus (ZIKV), transmitted by the *Aedes* mosquito, is identified as a causal contributor to microcephaly in infancy (Cauchemez et al 2016, Chibueze et al 2017). In 2016 ZIKV infection was declared a Public Health Emergency of International Concern. Although it causes simple flu-like symptoms in the pregnant mother, ZIKV can lead to serious complications (including microcephaly) in the newborn (Passi et al 2017).

Secondary microcephaly may also occur as a result of maternal diabetes and maternal hyperphenylalaninaemia. Fetal exposure to alcohol and tobacco use was shown to result in a 2.6-fold increase in the risk of isolated secondary microcephaly compared with other causes, including syndromes (Feldman et al 2012).

In both types the neurological manifestations range from decerebration, complete unresponsiveness and autistic behaviour to mild motor impairment, educable neurocognitive impairment and mild hyperkinesis. There appears to be a decided relationship between microcephaly and cognitive delays of varying degrees; however, not all children with microcephaly have cognitive delays.

Nursing Care Management

There is no specific treatment. Nursing care is supportive and may be directed towards helping parents adjust to rearing a child with cognitive impairment when this condition is present. (See Chapter 20.)

Craniosynostosis

Craniosynostosis is defined as the premature closure at birth of one or more cranial sutures (Kinsman & Johnston 2016). The clinical picture depends on which sutures close, the duration of the closure process and the success or failure of the other sutures to compensate by expansion (see Fig 8.4). The condition may be divided according to the number of sutures involved; primary craniosynostosis involves one or more sutures as a result of abnormalities of skull development, whereas secondary craniosynostosis involves the failure of brain growth and expansion (Children's Health Queensland Hospital and Health Service 2018). Focal hydrodynamic mechanisms are involved in the compensatory skull changes seen in craniosynostosis. Brain atrophy and an underlying motor delay account for the position-induced skull changes. Craniosynostosis is also a common feature of children with genetic syndromes such as Crouzon, Apert (Box 8.3), Pfeiffer, Chotzen, Carpenter and Jackson-Weiss syndromes (Kinsman & Johnston 2016). Potential risk factors for craniosynostosis include maternal Caucasian race, advanced maternal age, male infant, use of nitrosatable drugs, fertility treatments and certain paternal occupations (e.g. agriculture, repairmen, mechanics, forestry). Diagnosis is established with CT scan, and MRI is useful in identifying accompanying brain abnormalities. Ultrasound is also shown to be a reliable screening tool to rule out craniosynostosis in newborns with abnormal head shape (Hall et al 2017). Increased ICP is more frequent in children with more than one prematurely fused suture.

The most common form of craniosynostosis is premature closure of the sagittal suture (scaphocephaly) with resulting elongation of the skull in the anteroposterior direction. This occurs more commonly in males and does not result in increased ICP or hydrocephalus. A similar head shape (dolichocephaly) occurs as a result of postnatal position maintenance in some preterm infants (McCarty et al 2016); however, in this case there is no premature closure of sutures. In some types of craniosynostosis an increase in ICP may occur, which may or may not cause cognitive delays but can result in progressive papillo-oedema, optic atrophy and eventual blindness. Other complications include facial asymmetry and malocclusion.

Trigonocephaly, or metopic craniosynostosis, represents a premature closure of the metopic suture in utero, a congenital problem that is familial and often requires surgical treatment to prevent forebrain abnormalities. The metopic suture occurs where the right and left frontal bones meet on the forehead. Craniosynostosis of the metopic suture may be an autosomal dominantly inherited disorder not associated with functional brain or other abnormalities. Other types of craniosynostosis include frontal plagiocephaly (fusion of coronal and sphenofrontal sutures), occipital plagiocephaly (fusion of lambdoid suture or positional), oxycephaly (fusion of coronal and frontoethmoidal sutures) and Kleebattschädel deformity (skull resembles a cloverleaf and hydrocephalus is common) (Kinsman & Johnston 2016).

Therapeutic Management

Treatment involves surgical excision of long bars of bone (strip craniectomy) along or parallel to the fused suture. Various surgical procedures are employed in an effort to release the fused suture and direct growth. Surgery is performed to achieve the best possible cosmetic effect and, in severe cases, to relieve cerebral pressure symptoms and complications. The advised timing of suture release is before 6 months of age for best cosmetic and neurodevelopmental results. For optimal outcomes, it is imperative that a multidisciplinary craniofacial team is involved in the care of the child with craniosynostosis.

BOX 8.3 Cranial Abnormalities Associated with Abnormal Bone Growth

Crouzon syndrome—Craniofacial dysostosis (abnormal ossification of fetal cartilages) with shallow orbits and underdevelopment of the middle third of the face.

Apert syndrome—Craniosynostosis resulting in a prominent forehead; may be extracranial abnormalities, such as syndactyly (webbing) of fingers and toes and cardiac defects.

Treacher Collins syndrome—Asymmetrical facial deformity, including absent cheekbones, underslung jaw and small chin; also downward slant of the eyes and other minor defects.

Pierre Robin sequence—Displacement of the chin as a result of micrognathia (mandibular hypoplasia) or retrognathia (normal-sized mandible positioned posteriorly); also glossoptosis with obstruction of the airway and sometimes a cleft palate.

Nursing Care Management

Nursing care primarily involves the early identification of persistent cranial moulding weeks after regular birth moulding would have resolved and referral for follow-up evaluation. In the postoperative period, nursing care includes observation for changes in neurological status, haemorrhage or infection.

Because of the type of bone surgery involved with craniosynostosis, blood loss can be significant. Therefore, the nurse should carefully monitor haematocrit and haemoglobin after surgery. Nurses should inform and guide parents through this blood bank procedure. With endoscopic surgery, blood loss is minimised, but the child must wear a cranial moulding helmet for 3 to 4 months. The helmet should be worn 23 hours each day and a second helmet may be fitted as a result of rapid head growth; erythematous areas should be examined closely by the orthotist and adjustments made accordingly. Instructions regarding compliance with the helmet and skin care are essential.

Most children have substantial swelling of the eyelids postoperatively; careful handling and talking to the child may help calm fears while the eyelids are swollen shut. Eye care should be limited to gentle cleansing with a moist cloth. Pain management measures should be instituted in infants experiencing postoperative pain as they would be for older children or adults. Fluids and adequate hydration are essential. Oral feedings resume as soon as possible for hydration and for the infant's nutritive sucking needs.

Early surgical management of craniosynostosis allows proper expansion of the brain and the creation of an acceptable appearance. Parents require special support and education during this time, especially from other parents whose infants have undergone similar operations. The nurse can serve as a liaison for this type of parental support.

Craniofacial Abnormalities

Craniofacial abnormalities are those deformities involving the skull and facial bones. They have a low incidence rate in the population, but their effects can be psychologically devastating to affected children and their families. Box 8.3 lists some deformities caused by abnormal growth of cranial bone(s).

Most craniofacial anomalies are compatible with life, and all efforts are made to help the child and family live as normal a life as possible. Advances in microscopic, endoscopic, orthopaedic, neurological and plastic reconstructive surgery techniques have made it possible for children with craniofacial anomalies not only to survive beyond childhood but also to live a fulfilling life without the social stigmas of past decades. These children, however, may continue to face erroneous assumptions of cognitive impairment because of their appearance. Multidisciplinary craniofacial teams are dedicated to helping the child and family achieve optimum potential for intellectual growth, physical competence and social acceptance.

Therapeutic Management

Craniofacial surgical correction involves peeling the patient's face away from the skull and remoulding the understructures. Parts can be brought together, the skull reshaped and remodelled, and bone fragments removed or reshaped. Bone segments from the child's hip or ribs may be used to reshape the skull or facial features. The procedures are performed at various ages, depending on the anomaly, in craniofacial centres specialising in this paediatric problem. The timing of surgery is before school entry and is determined on an individual basis to ensure normal growth and development. Depending on the abnormality, other surgeries are performed, such as mandibular and digit correction.

Nursing Care Management

Direct nursing efforts involve preparation for surgery (often several surgical procedures over time), postoperative care similar to care of any child with cranial surgery and support of the child and family. Frequently this child and family must adjust to the unfamiliar body image, which may be as traumatic as the previous deformity. A helmet may be worn to protect the operative site and bone grafts for 6 months to 2 years. Follow-up care is important.

Pierre Robin Sequence

Pierre Robin sequence (PRS) is a defect characterised by retroposition of the tongue and mandible, which often results in neonatal respiratory and feeding problems. The condition has an incidence of 1 in 8500 to 14,000 live births, and about half of those with PRS have other congenital anomalies (Breugem et al 2016). The tongue may be large (glossoptosis) and frequently falls over the neonate's airway, causing occlusion and respiratory distress. In severe upper airway obstruction a tracheotomy may be required; however, an alternative is to place a modified nasopharyngeal tube and bypass the upper airway obstruction (Alencar et al 2017). From a lateral view the infant's lower jaw can be seen to be positioned posterior (micrognathia) to the upper jaw. PRS may be observed in the newborn nursery when the infant has apnoea and cyanosis in the supine position, due primarily to upper airway obstruction. The neonate is positioned to facilitate an open airway. A tongue-lip adhesion is a common surgical procedure that repositions the tongue anteriorly. Surgical mandibular distraction osteogenesis is another technique used to correct the condition (Cicchetti et al 2012, Scott et al 2011). There are usually no associated neurocognitive defects in isolated (non-syndromic) PRS.

Cleft lip and cleft palate

Cleft lip (CL) with or without cleft palate (CP) is the most common congenital anomaly in Australia and New Zealand and occurs with a frequency of 1 in 800 live births (Health Direct n.d., Health Navigator New Zealand 2020). Isolated CL with or without CP is more common in males, and CP alone is more common in females.

Aetiology

Most cases of CL and/or CP result from a combination of genetic and environmental factors. The gene(s) responsible for clefting in individuals without syndromes is not yet known. However, some genetic syndromes are known to be associated with clefting in approximately 15% of individuals with clefts. Exposure to environmental factors or teratogens may be responsible for clefts at a critical point in embryonic development. Alcohol use, cigarette smoking and prescription drugs, including anticonvulsants, steroids and retinoids, are associated with higher rates of oral clefting. Conversely, folic acid supplements may protect against clefting.

Pathophysiology

Development of the primary and secondary palates takes place at different times and involves different developmental processes, which is why clefts can vary significantly. The primary palate includes the medial portion of the upper lip and the portion of the alveolar ridge that contains the central and lateral incisors. The secondary palate contains the remaining portion of the hard palate and all of the soft palate. A CL can occur unilaterally or bilaterally, and it may present as a simple notch in the upper lip or extend completely to the base of the nose. CL occurs from failure of the maxillary processes to fuse with the nasal elevations on the frontal prominence to form the primary palate, which normally occurs during the sixth week of gestation (Fig 8.5A). A CP is a midline defect and may vary from a bifid uvula (the mildest form of a CP with essentially no functional impact on speech or feeding) to a complete CP that extends from the soft palate into the hard palate.

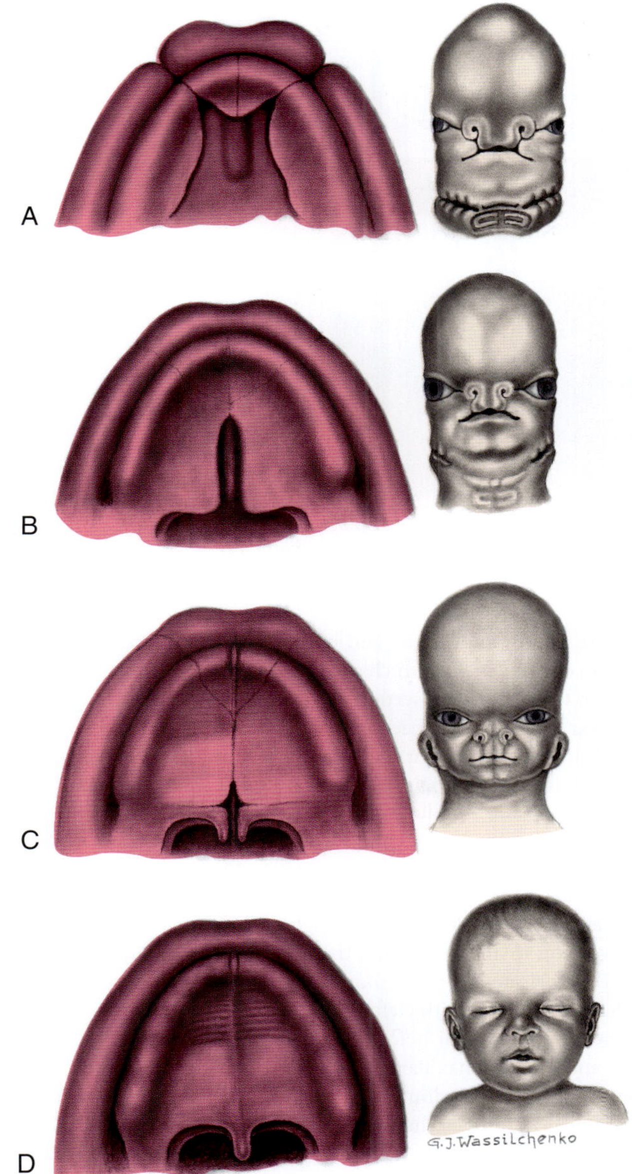

Fig 8.5 (**A–D**) Stages in palatine development. (See text for discussion.)

CP occurs from a failed fusion of the secondary palate (hard and soft palates), which takes place later in development, between the 7th and 12th weeks of gestation (Fig 8.5B–D).

Diagnostic Evaluation

A cleft that involves the lip and/or CP is readily apparent at birth. The CP is detected through visual inspection of the oral cavity or by palpating the hard palate and soft palate with a gloved finger. The degree of malformation of the CL or CP can then be evaluated (Figs 8.6 and 8.7). The presence of a CP is likely to affect feeding even though in most cases the infant's ability to swallow is normal. Poor feeding skills may be an indicator to further evaluate the palate in case a minor palatal defect was not readily detected at birth.

Therapeutic Management

Individuals with clefts should always be treated by a cleft/craniofacial maxillofacial multidisciplinary team, including plastic surgery, otolaryngology, orthodontics, speech-language pathology, paediatrics, nursing, audiology, social work and psychology. Although the initial CL and CP are both repaired within the first year of life, treatment to repair the deformity may continue into early adulthood. Management of both defects is directed towards surgical closure of the cleft, prevention of complications and facilitation of normal growth and development of the child.

Surgical Correction: Cleft Lip. CL repair typically occurs when the baby is between 2 and 3 months of age. Surgical correction is performed when the infant is free of any oral, respiratory or systemic infection and has been reviewed by a paediatric surgeon. Some surgeons work closely with orthodontists and use nasal alveolar moulding (NAM) or taping of the upper lip before surgical repair in order to bring the segments of the lip and alveolus into better alignment before the surgical repair, resulting in less tension on the lip repair following surgery and an improved aesthetic outcome.

Improved surgical techniques have minimised deformity related to scar retraction, but optimum cosmetic results are difficult to obtain in severe defects. Lip, nose and scar revisions may be required at a later age.

Surgical Correction: Cleft Palate. CP repair is typically completed between 6 and 12 months. Although early repair of the CP may restrict skeletal growth of the midface, delaying palate repair after first words emerge may result in significant speech disorders. Children who are younger and less advanced in terms of speech development exhibit better articulation and resonance than those who have their palates

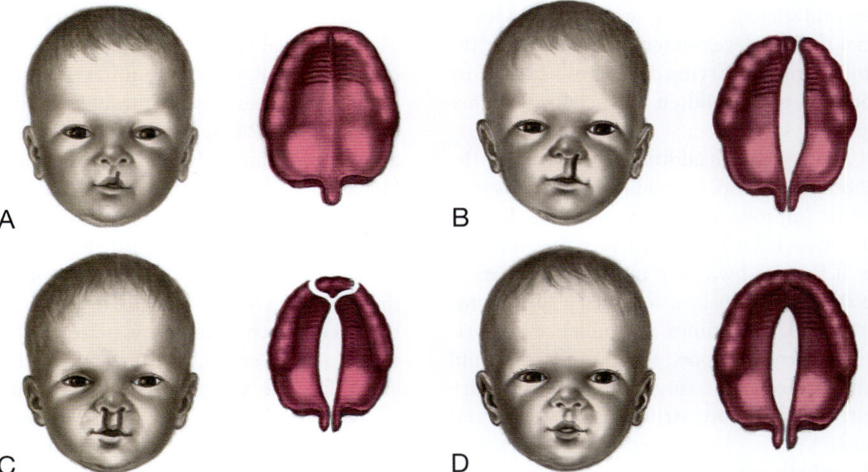

Fig 8.6 Variations in clefts of lip and palate at birth. (**A**) Notch in vermilion border. (**B**) Unilateral cleft lip and cleft palate. (**C**) Bilateral cleft lip and cleft pala-e. (**D**) Cleft palate.

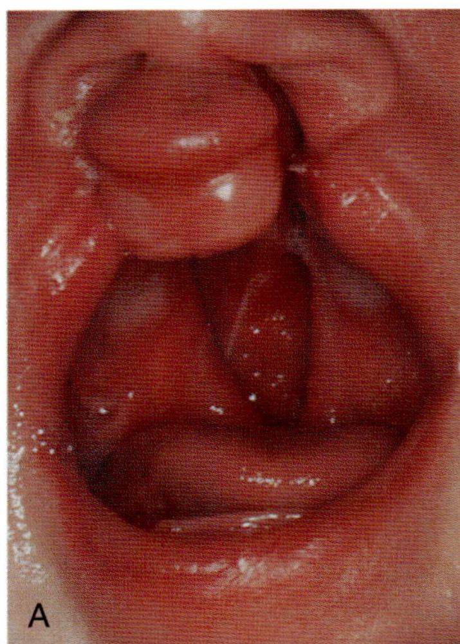

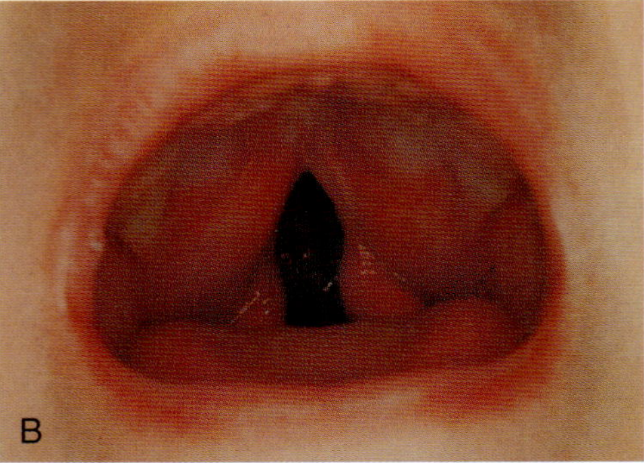

Fig 8.7 (**A**) Bilateral cleft lip with complete cleft palate. Cleft extends from soft to hard palate, exposing nasal cavity. (**B**) Midline cleft of soft palate. (Source: Zitelli, B. J., & Davis, H. W. (2007). *Atlas of pediatric physical diagnosis* (5th ed.). St Louis, MO: Mosby. *B*, Courtesy Barbara Elster, Cleft Palate Center, Pittsburgh.)

repaired when they are older and exhibit more speech and language development. Common techniques used to repair the CP include Veau-Wardill-Kilner V-Y pushback and Furlow double-opposing Z-plasty. Approximately 20% to 30% of patients with repaired CP will exhibit features of velopharyngeal dysfunction such as audible nasal air emission and hypernasality; these features require additional surgery such as levator repositioning, Furlow palatoplasty, pharyngeal flap, sphincter pharyngoplasty or posterior pharyngeal wall augmentation to improve velopharyngeal closure. Nasopharyngoscopy and/or videofluoroscopy should be used to determine which surgery is needed to enhance the function of the velopharynx. Speech pathologists work closely with the team's surgeon to ensure that speech therapy services are provided when the child exhibits speech production errors, and surgery is provided when the child exhibits ongoing velopharyngeal dysfunction that will not respond to therapy.

Long-term Problems. The care of children with CL and CP often involves a team of specialists who meet periodically to examine the child and consult with one another and with the parents. Although the CL and CP are repaired within the first year of life, some children will require additional surgeries to refine the repairs. Many children with CP and/or CL have some degree of speech impairment that requires speech therapy or even further surgery to improve speech if the errors arise from a faulty mechanism. Rotated, missing or malformed teeth, as well as differences in facial skeletal development, may require orthodontic and orthognathic intervention. Varying degrees of hearing loss throughout early childhood also place children with clefts at higher risk for speech and language delays.

Children with CL and CP may require additional surgeries to the lip, nose and palate throughout childhood. CL and nose revisions may be needed to modify scars or improve symmetry. Additionally, the surgeon is likely to perform an alveolar bone graft to repair the cleft defect in the alveolar ridge. If the child with CP exhibits velopharyngeal dysfunction following the initial repair, a secondary surgery for speech will need to be performed. Sometimes an appliance is fabricated to help obturate the velopharyngeal port. Finally, once the child has reached skeletal maturity, orthognathic surgery may be necessary to achieve appropriate alignment of the bony structures of the face and an optimal aesthetic outcome.

Improper drainage of the middle ear, as a result of inefficient function of the eustachian tube secondary to the CP, causes increased pressure in the middle ear and contributes to recurrent middle ear effusion or otitis media, which can lead to hearing impairment in some children with CP. The insertion of grommets/tympanostomy tubes by an otolaryngologist has become standard procedure in the child with CL/CP and is often performed at the same time as other surgical procedures (such as CP repair) to facilitate fluid drainage from the middle ear and prevent middle ear effusion and recurrent otitis media. Audiologists evaluate the child's hearing throughout early childhood and work closely with otolaryngologists to determine whether ear tubes or grommets are needed.

A child with a cleft will go through multiple phases of orthodontic intervention to align teeth and the maxillary arches. At some centres, NAM is fabricated by the orthodontist and used before surgical repair of the CL. Children with clefts may then go through a period of active orthodontic treatment before the alveolar bone graft, at which time they may have maxillary expansion and limited orthodontics. Comprehensive orthodontic treatment of the permanent teeth is then accomplished in much the same manner as for children without clefts, except that children with clefts often have more dental anomalies such as missing teeth, extra teeth, malformed teeth and more teeth out of alignment. Finally, orthognathic surgery to improve alignment of the mandible and maxilla may be completed once the child has reached skeletal maturity (often in the late teen years).

With isolated CL, minimal speech problems are anticipated. The child with CP usually requires the services of a speech-language pathologist at some point throughout childhood. A major problem for a child with CP may be 'cleft palate' speech patterns. Features such as audible nasal air emission and hypernasality are addressed surgically. However, children with repaired CP and/or CL may exhibit active errors relating to velopharyngeal dysfunction or malocclusion. If the child exhibits velopharyngeal dysfunction while developing speech, the child may actively shift the place of articulation to a place lower in the vocal tract that allows him or her to produce a similar sound as the intended speech sound. These errors are often referred to as 'compensatory' speech errors, and the errors will often require speech therapy even after the velopharyngeal mechanism has been surgically corrected. Early intervention that involves the education of parents and the child is critical to ensuring appropriate speech development. In addition to errors relating to velopharyngeal function, children with clefts may exhibit distortions on sounds produced in the front of the mouth if teeth are misaligned or absent, as well as when the mandible and maxilla are not in proper alignment. Finally, hearing loss from middle ear infection or middle ear effusion is an additional impediment because of difficulty in interpreting sounds.

Nursing Care Management

The immediate nursing problems in the care of an infant with CL and CP deformities are related to feeding the infant and dealing with the parental reaction to the defect. Facial deformities are particularly disturbing to parents. CL, especially, is a disfiguring, visible defect that may generate a strong negative response in parents. During the initial phase after birth of an infant with CL or CP, it is important for the nurse to address not only the infant's physical needs but also the parents' emotional needs.

The nurse should encourage expression of parental grief and fears. Such expression may promote attachment in the preoperative period. It is especially important to emphasise the positive aspects of the infant's physical appearance and to express optimism regarding surgical correction while acknowledging the parents' concern and taking into consideration the fact that there may be challenges for rural and remote families.

Feeding. Feeding the newborn with CL/CP can be a challenge, and teaching the parent to successfully feed the child is perhaps one of the most significant and challenging nursing roles. Growth failure in these infants has been attributed to feeding difficulties; however, with appropriate modifications to positioning, infants with non-syndromic CP and/or CL should be able to feed successfully by mouth. Mothers should be encouraged to provide the protective benefits of breastmilk. These infants may require lactation and nutritional counselling and evaluation. Weekly weight checks at the practitioner's office assist in monitoring the infant's weight preoperatively.

Infants with an isolated CL may have difficulty achieving an adequate anterior lip seal (Gailey 2016). The infant with an isolated CL can often breastfeed without difficulty, as the breast tissue is able to conform to the cleft. If bottle-fed, systems that have a wider base such as a NUK (orthodontic) nipple, may allow the baby with a CL to feed more successfully. Finally, cheek support (i.e. squeezing the cheeks together to decrease the width of the cleft) may also help the infant achieve an adequate anterior lip seal during feeding.

Although infants with isolated CL are typically able to breastfeed without difficulty, breastfeeding can be a more difficult process for infants with an unrepaired CP. Infant feeding requires compression and suction. An infant with CP has difficulty creating adequate suction to extract breast milk directly from the breast or a standard bottle. Modified bottles or specialised feeding systems are needed. Accepting that she may not be able to breastfeed can be difficult for a new mother; however, a mother of a child with a cleft should be encouraged to try the following strategies. Have the mother express her milk and provide it with an adaptive bottle made for children with clefts. Skin-to-skin contact should still be encouraged while feeding. Once bottle-feeding has been completed, encourage the infant to still be placed on the mother's breast for non-nutritive sucking to enhance skin-to-skin contact (Australasian Cleft Lip & Palate Association Inc. 2017).

The soft palate must elevate and separate the oral and nasal cavities to achieve negative intraoral pressure and achieve suction. Several specialised bottles are available that do not require suction, including the SpecialNeeds Feeder (formerly Haberman bottle), Pigeon and the Mead Johnson Cleft Palate Nurser (Gailey 2016). The SpecialNeeds Feeder and the Pigeon bottles use a one-way flow valve that allows the infant to feed by compressing the nipple chamber between the tongue and the intact palatal segments. With the one-way flow valve in place, the liquid flows into the baby's mouth rather than back into the bottle chamber when the nipple is compressed. The SpecialNeeds Feeder also has a long nipple chamber that can be compressed by the feeder for additional support. It comes in regular and mini nipple sizes, and also has a slit-cut tip, which the feeder can rotate within the baby's mouth to allow for increased or decreased flow of liquid. The Pigeon bottle has a wide, bulbous nipple and Y-cut tip, which allows for a faster flow of liquid. The SpecialNeeds Feeder and the Pigeon bottle allow the infant to develop relatively independent feeding skills using these bottles. The third modified bottle, the Mead Johnson Cleft Palate Nurser, is a squeezable bottle with a long, thin X-cut nipple; this bottle requires the feeder to compress the bottle in coordination with the infant's suck-swallow-breathe pattern throughout the feeding.

Regardless of the type of nipple used, the person doing the feeding should resist the temptation to remove the nipple because of the noise the infant makes or because of fear that the infant will choke. Infants with clefts do tend to be 'noisy feeders' because they swallow excessive amounts of air throughout the feeding due to their inability to separate the nose and mouth. These infants should be burped frequently or as required. Additionally, they often have some degree of liquid that enters the nasal cavity during the feed, which may alarm the feeder who is not used to feeding babies with clefts. An indication that the infant needs to stop feeding momentarily is the facial signal, which involves elevated eyebrows, a wrinkled forehead or watery eyes; the nipple may be gently removed to allow the infant to swallow milk in the mouth without getting upset.

Mothers will need immediate access to a lactation consultant before discharge from the hospital to assist with positioning and management of milk supply (Australian Breastfeeding Association 2017). Regardless of the feeding method used, the mother and support networks will need ongoing support from the healthcare team before and after discharge from the hospital (Australian Breastfeeding Association 2017).

Preoperative Care. In preparation for the surgical repair, instruct the parents to accustom the infant to some of the needs of the early postoperative period. Some craniofacial surgery teams encourage the transition to cup-feeding before CP surgery, and this feeding method is used postoperatively as well. Alternative methods, such as syringe-feeding, should be introduced several days before surgery. Preoperative preparation, including medication, is determined by the surgical/medical team.

Postoperative Care: Cleft Lip. The major efforts in the postoperative period are directed towards protecting the operative site. Avoid the prone position to prevent suture damage. After CL repair (cheiloplasty), some surgeons allow the infant to return to breastfeeding or bottle-feeding, whereas others require syringe-feeding once the child is awake and alert. CL repair may be performed on an outpatient basis or the child may stay in the hospital overnight for monitoring.

The infant should be positioned to prevent airway obstruction by secretions, blood or the tongue. Gentle aspiration of mouth and nasopharyngeal secretions may be necessary to prevent aspiration and respiratory complications. Because of vascularity of the lip and palate, postoperative care involves monitoring operative sites for bleeding. Excessive swallowing may be a sign of bleeding and swallowing blood.

Postoperative Care: Cleft Palate. Postoperative care varies according to the surgeon's preference. The child should be closely observed postoperatively for signs of airway obstruction, haemorrhage and laryngeal spasm. A face mask is often used to deliver oxygen. A tongue stitch may be used to prevent the tongue from obstructing the airway; it is taped to the cheek and may be removed as per surgeon's preference. Observe the child's vital signs and oxygen saturation for potential airway compromise. Signs of stridor, croup or difficulty breathing and/or swallowing should be carefully evaluated. The child with a CP repair may be placed on clear liquids for 24 hours followed by a liquid diet for 2 weeks. A soft diet may be encouraged for a full 6 weeks following palate repair. Acceptable feeding devices include open cup for liquids, but rigid utensils such as spoons, straws or hard-tipped sippy cups should not be used to avoid accidental injury to the repair.

DERMATOLOGICAL PROBLEMS IN THE NEWBORN

Erythema Toxicum Neonatorum

Erythema toxicum neonatorum, also known as *flea bite dermatitis* or *newborn rash,* is a benign, self-limiting eruption that usually appears within the first 2 days of life. The 1- to 3-mm lesions are firm, pale yellow or white papules or pustules on an erythematous base that resemble flea bites. Erythema toxicum may appear as one or two isolated lesions or as multiple lesions; the rash commonly disappears from one location and reappears elsewhere hours later. The rash appears most commonly on the face, proximal extremities, trunk and buttocks, but it may be located anywhere on the body except the palms and soles. The rash may be more obvious during crying episodes. There are no systemic manifestations, and successive crops of lesions heal without pigmentation changes. The rash usually lasts approximately 5 to 7 days.

The cause is unknown. However, a smear of the pustule shows numerous eosinophils and a relative absence of neutrophils. Obtain bacterial, fungal or viral cultures when the diagnosis is questionable. Although no treatment is necessary, parents are usually concerned about the rash and need to be reassured of the benign and transient nature.

Candidiasis

Candidiasis, also known as moniliasis, is not uncommon in the newborn. *Candida albicans,* the organism usually responsible, may cause disease in any organ system. It is a yeast-like fungus (produces yeast cells and spores) that can be acquired from a maternal vaginal infection during birth; by person-to-person transmission (especially from poor handwashing technique); or from contaminated hands, bottles, nipples or other articles. Mucocutaneous, cutaneous and disseminated candidiasis are observed in this age group. It is usually a benign disorder in the neonate and is often confined to the oral and nappy regions.

Oral Candidiasis

Oral candidiasis (thrush) is characterised by white adherent patches on the tongue, palate and inner aspects of the cheeks (Fig 8.8). Oral candidiasis can be distinguished from coagulated milk when attempts to remove the patches with a tongue blade are unsuccessful. The infant may refuse to suck or may feed poorly because of pain in the mouth. This condition tends to be acute in the newborn and chronic in older infants and young children. Thrush appears when the oral flora is altered as a result of antibiotic therapy or poor handwashing by the infant's caregiver. Although the condition is usually self-limiting, spontaneous resolution may take as long as 2 months, during which time lesions may spread to the larynx, trachea, bronchi and lungs and along the gastrointestinal tract.

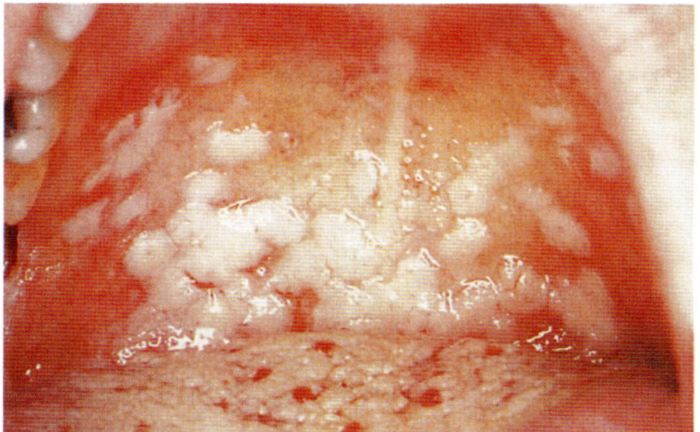

Fig 8.8 Oral candidiasis (thrush). (Source: Courtesy of J.A. Innes. In Goering, R. A., Dockrell, H. A., Zuckerman, M., Chiodini, P. L., Roitt, I. M. (2013). Mims' medical microbiology (5th ed.). Philadelphia: Saunders.)

Oral candidiasis in the newborn is treated with good hygiene and application of a fungicide. The source of infection, usually the mother, should be treated to prevent reinfection. Topical application of 1 mL of nystatin (Mycostatin) over the surfaces of the oral cavity four times a day or every 6 hours is usually sufficient to prevent spread of the disease or prolongation of its course. Oral fluconazole is an alternative for the infant with oesophageal and gastrointestinal candidiasis and for the breastfeeding mother. To prevent relapse, therapy should be continued for at least 2 weeks after the lesions disappear (The Royal Women's Hospital 2018).

Nursing Care Management

Direct nursing care towards preventing spread of the infection and correct application of the prescribed topical medication. For candidiasis in the nappy genital area, teach the caregiver to keep the nappy area clean and dry. Medication should be applied to the affected areas as prescribed. Older infants can introduce *Candida* organisms into their mouths with hands contaminated by contact with nappy dermatitis.

In cases of oral thrush, administer nystatin after feedings. Distribute the medication over the surface of the oral mucosa and tongue with an applicator or syringe; the remainder of the dose is deposited in the mouth to be swallowed by the infant to treat any gastrointestinal lesions. In addition to good hygienic care, other measures to control thrush include rinsing the infant's mouth with plain water after each feeding before applying the medication and boiling reusable teats and bottles for at least 20 minutes after a thorough washing (spores are heat resistant). If using a dummy, boil for at least 20 minutes once daily, and treat the nipples of breastfeeding mothers to prevent reinfection. If the mother is breastfeeding, simultaneous treatment of the infant and mother is recommended if either is infected (Lawrence & Lawrence 2015).

Herpes Simplex Virus

Neonatal herpes is one of the most serious viral infections in the newborn, with a mortality rate of up to 40% in infants with disseminated disease (Victorian Agency for Health Information [VAHI] & Safer Care Victoria [SCV] 2020). The disease may be classified according to the following types: (1) skin, eye and mouth; (2) localised central nervous system (CNS) disease; or (3) disseminated infection involving multiple sites such as the lungs, liver, adrenal glands, CNS, skin, eyes and mouth. Approximately 86% to 90% of herpes simplex virus (HSV) transmission occurs during birth. The rash appears as vesicles or pustules on an erythematous base. Clusters of lesions are common. The lesions ulcerate and crust over rapidly. Fetal scalp monitoring sites are commonly the primary site of infection. The risk of infection during vaginal birth in the presence of genital herpes is estimated to be 25% to 60% with active primary infection at term (VAHI & SCV 2020). Infants born to mothers with a recurrent case of HSV are less likely to contract the virus (VAHI & SCV 2020).

Most infants with neonatal herpes eventually develop this characteristic rash, but many neonates with disseminated disease do not develop a skin rash (Wang et al 2017). Because signs and symptoms resemble those of bacterial sepsis, close assessment is extremely important. Ophthalmological clinical findings include chorioretinitis and micro-ophthalmia; neurological involvement such as microcephaly and encephalomalacia may also develop (Wang et al 2017). Disseminated infections may involve virtually every organ system, but the liver, adrenal glands and lungs are most commonly affected. In HSV meningitis infants develop multiple lesions of cortical haemorrhagic necrosis. It can occur alone or with oral, eye or skin lesions. The presenting symptoms, which may occur in the second to fourth week of life, include lethargy, poor feeding, irritability and local or generalised seizures.

Infants with CNS and disseminated disease have a much higher mortality rate than those initially seen with skin, eye or mouth disease. Neonatal HSV may be difficult to detect in the early newborn period, and non-specific signs such as irritability, fever, poor feeding or lethargy may be seen. When the diagnosis is delayed, mortality rates may be high even with antiviral therapy, and long-term irreversible complications such as seizures, blindness and psychomotor and learning delays are not uncommon.

Nursing Care Management

Neonates with herpes virus or suspected infection (as a result of exposure) should be carefully evaluated for clinical manifestations. The absence of skin lesions in the neonate exposed to maternal herpes virus does not indicate absence of disease. Implement Contact Precautions (in addition to Standard Precautions) according to (VAHI & SCV 2020) guidelines or hospital protocol. It is recommended that swabs of the mouth, nasopharynx, conjunctivae, rectum and any skin vesicles be obtained from the exposed neonate.

Early recognition and treatment with antiviral therapy are essential elements to the prevention of serious and often fatal complications. Closely evaluate infants who are seen in the first 5 or 6 weeks of life with the non-specific signs of poor feeding, lethargy, fever and irritability, with or without the characteristic rash.

Bullous Impetigo

Bullous impetigo is an infectious superficial skin condition most often caused by various strains of *Staphylococcus aureus.* Bullous vesicular lesions erupt on previously untraumatised or intact skin. The lesions may appear on any surface of the body and sometimes become widespread, but the usual distribution involves the buttocks, perineum, trunk, face and extremities. The neonatal form may appear first in the nappy region (Shulman 2016). They vary in size from a few millimetres to several centimetres, contain turbid fluid and are easily ruptured (Shulman 2016). The bullae normally rupture in 1 or 2 days, leaving a superficial red, moist, denuded area with little crusting. In some cases the condition may be mistaken for thermal injury or *staphylococcal scalded skin syndrome* (SSSS).

Nursing Care Management

Once the diagnosis is suspected, the infant is isolated until therapy is instituted to prevent spread of the infection to other infants. Persons who have come in contact with the infant are investigated to determine a possible source of the infecting organism. Scrutinise other infants who have mutual contacts for early detection of any infection. Instruct parents and other visitors regarding precautions for the prevention of infection, especially through handwashing and Standard Precautions. (See Infection Control, Chapter 6.)

Birthmarks

Discolourations of the skin are common findings in the newborn infant. (See Skin, Chapter 4.) Most, such as Mongolian spots or naevus simplex, involve no therapy other than reassuring parents of the benign nature of these discolourations. However, some can be the manifestation of a disease that suggests further examination of the child and other family members (e.g. multiple flat, light-brown café-au-lait spots often characterise the autosomal-dominant hereditary disorder neurofibromatosis and are common findings in Albright syndrome).

Darker or more extensive lesions demand further inspection. Excision of the lesion may be recommended for biopsy. Such lesions include the reddish-brown solitary nodule that appears on the face or upper arm and usually represents a spindle and epithelioid cell naevus (juvenile melanoma); a giant pigmented naevus (bathing trunk naevus), a dark-brown to black irregular plaque that is at risk of transformation to malignant melanoma; and the dark-brown or black macules that become more numerous with age (junctional or compound naevi).

Vascular birthmarks may be divided into vascular malformations and vascular tumours (haemangiomas). Experts now recommend labelling vascular tumours as **haemangiomas of infancy** or **infantile haemangiomas** to differentiate them from other vascular tumours and malformations. A vascular tumour often mislabelled as a haemangioma is a congenital haemangioma; this differs from an infantile haemangioma in that the former is fully formed at birth and may or may not involute over time, whereas the infantile haemangioma typically grows after birth. Haemangiomas may be further classified as localised (sometimes labelled focal), segmental or multifocal (sometimes labelled indeterminate) (Chen et al 2013, Labreze et al 2017). Localised superficial infantile haemangiomas tend to appear early in infancy and spontaneously resolve without therapy within several years, whereas the segmental variety is more likely to cause complications such as ulceration and vital organ compromise and to involve developmental defects. Multifocal haemangiomas are less likely to be associated with the complications seen with the segmental variety (Chen et al 2013).

Vascular stains (malformations) are permanent lesions that are present at birth and are initially flat and erythematous. Any vascular structure—capillary, vein, artery or lymphatic—may be involved. The two most common vascular stains are port-wine stains (naevus flammeus) and transient macular stains (naevus simplex) such as the stork bite or salmon patch, usually located on the glabella or nape of the neck. Port-wine lesions are pink, red or, rarely, purple stains of the skin that thicken, darken and proportionately enlarge as the child grows (Fig 8.9A).

Port-wine stains may also be associated with structural malformations, such as glaucoma or leptomeningeal angiomatosis (i.e. tumour of blood or lymph vessels in the pia arachnoid, or Sturge-Weber syndrome) or bony or muscular overgrowth (Klippel-Trénaunay syndrome). Monitor children with port-wine stains on the eyelids, forehead, cheeks or extremities for these syndromes with periodic ophthalmological examination, neurological imaging and measurement of extremities.

Infantile haemangiomas, also sometimes referred to as strawberry or capillary haemangiomas, are benign cutaneous tumours that involve only capillaries. These are often not apparent at birth but may appear within a few weeks as an erythematous patch, enlarge considerably during the first year of life, and then begin to involute spontaneously. It may take 5 to 9 years for complete resolution. Many patients may be left with residual findings such as telangiectasia, redundant fatty tissue or skin atrophy (Martin 2016). These haemangiomas are bright red, rubbery nodules with a rough surface and a well-defined margin (Fig 8.9B).

Cavernous venous haemangiomas involve deeper vessels in the dermis and have a bluish-red colour and poorly defined margins. These latter forms may be associated with the trapping of platelets (Kasabach-Merritt syndrome) and subsequent thrombocytopenia.

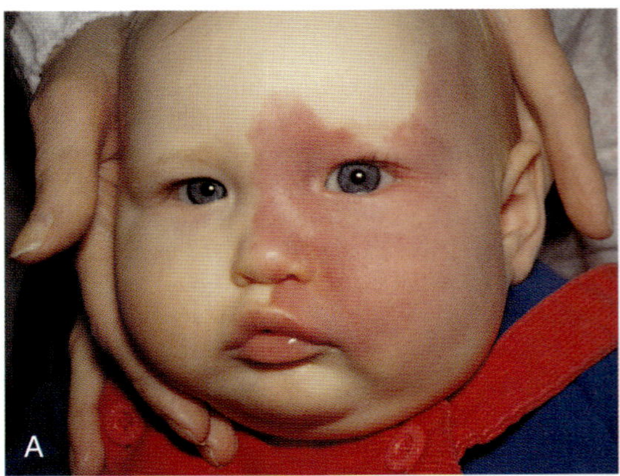
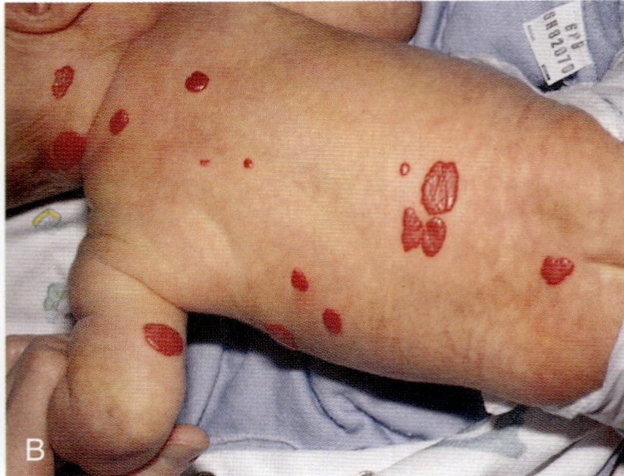

Fig 8.9 (**A**) Port-wine stain. (**B**) Strawberry haemangioma. (Source: Zitelli, B. J., & Davis, H. W. (2002). *Atlas of pediatric physical diagnosis* (4th ed.). St Louis, MO: Mosby.)

Haemangiomas may also occur as part of the PHACE syndrome:

P—Posterior fossa brain malformation
H—Haemangiomas (segmental cervicofacial)
A—Arterial anomalies
C—Cardiac defects, including coarctation of the aorta
E—Eye anomalies.

PHACE syndrome haemangiomas occur predominantly in females, term infants, singleton births and infants of normal birth weight; in addition, PHACE syndrome haemangiomas are primarily large, segmental facial haemangiomas (Labreze et al 2017).

This neurocutaneous syndrome is diagnosed by the presence of a facial haemangioma in addition to either one or several of the other associated conditions; clinical outcomes vary according to the organs involved.

Although many localised superficial haemangiomas require no treatment because of their high rate of spontaneous involution, some vision and airway obstruction may necessitate therapy. Infants with a beard-distribution haemangioma often have airway involvement and must be closely evaluated for airway compromise (Hartzell & Buckmiller 2012). Ulceration is a common complication, especially when the haemangioma is perineal or perioral. This may result in pain, bleeding, infection and scarring. The pulsed-dye laser can effectively reduce some haemangiomas; systemic prednisone administered for 2 to 3 weeks or longer may also deter further growth. Optional treatments may include interferon alfa, imiquimod, propranolol, vincristine, cyclophosphamide and no treatment but simple observation. Propranolol is reported to be the first-line treatment for haemangiomas (Government of South Australia, Department for Health and Wellbeing 2019).

Nursing Care Management

Birthmarks, especially those on the face, are upsetting to parents. Families need an explanation of the type of lesion, its significance and possible treatment (Raising Children Network [Australia] 2021). Parents can benefit from seeing photographs of other infants before and after treatment for port-wine stains or after the passage of time for haemangiomas. Pictures taken to follow the involution process may further help parents gain confidence that progress is taking place.

If laser therapy is performed, the lesion will have a purplish-black appearance for 7 to 10 days, after which the blackness will fade and give way to redness with an eventual lightening of the treated area. During the treatment phase, caution parents to avoid any trauma to the lesion or picking at the scab. Trim the infant's fingernails as an added precaution. Washing the area gently with water and dabbing it dry are adequate, although in some cases a topical antibiotic ointment may be used. Do not give any salicylates during the treatment phase because they decrease the effects of the therapy. Keep the infant out of the sun for several weeks and then protected with a sunscreen of at least sun protection factor 15. Complications associated with laser treatment include possible secondary infection, keloid or pyogenic granuloma formation, localised dermatitis and hyperpigmentation or hypopigmentation.

PROBLEMS RELATED TO PHYSIOLOGICAL FACTORS

Hyperbilirubinaemia

The term **hyperbilirubinaemia** refers to an excessive level of accumulated bilirubin in the blood and is characterised by **jaundice**, or **icterus**, a yellowish discolouration of the skin and other organs. Hyperbilirubinaemia is a common finding in the newborn and in most instances is relatively benign. However, in extreme cases, it can indicate a pathological state.

Hyperbilirubinaemia may result from increased unconjugated or conjugated bilirubin. The unconjugated form (Table 8.1) is the type most commonly seen in newborns. The following discussion of hyperbilirubinaemia is limited to unconjugated hyperbilirubinaemia.

Pathophysiology

Bilirubin is one of the breakdown products of haemoglobin that results from red blood cell (RBC) destruction. When RBCs are destroyed, the breakdown products are released into the circulation, where the haemoglobin splits into two fractions: haem and globin. The globin (protein) portion is used by the body and the haem portion is converted to unconjugated bilirubin, an insoluble substance bound to albumin.

The first two causes, physiological factors and an association with breastfeeding, are discussed in the following sections.

Complications. Unconjugated bilirubin is highly toxic to neurons; therefore, an infant with severe hyperbilirubinaemia is at risk of developing **bilirubin encephalopathy**, a term that describes early varying degrees of acute symptoms of bilirubin toxicity resulting from the deposition of unconjugated bilirubin in brain cells (Blackburn 2013). **Kernicterus**, or **bilirubin-induced neurological dysfunction**, describes the yellow staining of the brain cells and brain cell necrosis that results in chronic, permanent changes to the brain secondary to bilirubin deposition in the brain (Ambalavanan & Carlo 2016, Blackburn 2013). The damage occurs when the serum concentration reaches toxic levels, regardless of cause. There is evidence that a fraction of unconjugated bilirubin crosses the blood–brain barrier in

TABLE 8.1 Comparison of Major Types of Unconjugated Hyperbilirubinaemia*

Physiological Jaundice	Breastfeeding-associated Jaundice (Early Onset)	Breast Milk Jaundice (Late Onset)	Haemolytic Disease
		CAUSE	
Immature hepatic function plus increased bilirubin load from red blood cell (RBC) haemolysis; enterohepatic shunting	Decreased milk intake related to fewer calories consumed by infant before mother's milk is well established; enterohepatic shunting; less frequent stooling	Possible factors in breast milk that prevent bilirubin conjugation Less frequent stooling	Blood antigen incompatibility causing haemolysis of large numbers of RBCs Functional inability of liver to conjugate and excrete excess bilirubin from haemolysis
		ONSET	
After 24 hours (preterm infants, prolonged)	3rd–4th day	4th day	During first 24 hours
		PEAK	
2nd–5th day, depending on ethnic origin, method of feeding	3rd–5th day	10th–15th day	Variable
		DURATION	
Declines on 5th–7th day	Variable	May remain jaundiced for 3–12 weeks or more	Depends on severity and treatment
		THERAPY	
Increase frequency of feedings and avoid supplements. Evaluate stooling pattern. Monitor transcutaneous bilirubin (TcB) or total serum bilirubin (TSB) level. Perform risk assessment (see Fig 8.10). Use phototherapy if bilirubin levels increase significantly or significant haemolysis is present.	Breastfeed frequently (10–12 times/ day); avoid supplements such as water, glucose water or formula. Evaluate stooling pattern; stimulate as needed. Perform risk assessment (see Fig 8.10). Use phototherapy if bilirubin levels increase significantly or significant haemolysis is present. If phototherapy is instituted, evaluate benefits and harm of temporarily discontinuing breastfeeding; additional assessments may be required. Assist mother with maintaining milk supply; feed expressed milk as appropriate. After discharge, follow-up according to age of infant at discharge and hour-specific nomogram bilirubin level at discharge (see p. 186).	Increase frequency of breastfeeding; use no supplementation such as glucose water; cessation of breastfeeding is not recommended. Perform risk assessment (see Fig 8.10). Consider performing additional evaluations: glucose-6-phosphate dehydrogenase, direct and indirect serum bilirubin, family history and others as necessary. May include home phototherapy with a temporary (10–12 hours) discontinuation of breastfeeding; a subsequent TSB may be drawn to evaluate a drop in serum levels (see text). Assist mother with maintenance of milk supply and reassurance regarding her milk supply and therapy. Use formula supplements only at practitioner's discretion.	Monitor TcB or TSB level. Perform risk assessment (see Fig 8.10). Postnatal—Use phototherapy; administer tin mesoporphyrin, administer intravenous immunoglobulin per protocol; if severe, perform exchange transfusion. Prenatal—Perform intrauterine transfusion (fetus). Prevent sensitisation (Rh incompatibility) of Rh-negative mother with Rh immune globulin (RhIg) administration. If mother is breastfeeding, assist with maintenance and storage of milk; may bottle-feed expressed milk as appropriate to therapy. Minimise mother–infant separation, and encourage contact as appropriate.

*Table depicts patterns of jaundice in term infants; patterns in preterm infants will vary according to factors such as gestational age, birth weight and illness.

neonates with physiological hyperbilirubinaemia. When certain pathological conditions exist in addition to elevated bilirubin levels, the infant has an increased permeability of the blood–brain barrier to unconjugated bilirubin and thus potential irreversible damage. The exact level of serum bilirubin required to cause damage is not yet known.

Multiple factors contribute to bilirubin neurotoxicity; therefore serum bilirubin levels alone do not predict the risk of CNS injury. Factors that enhance the development of bilirubin encephalopathy include acidosis, lowered serum albumin levels, intracranial infections such as meningitis and abrupt fluctuations in blood pressure. In addition, any condition that increases the metabolic demands for oxygen or glucose (e.g. fetal distress, hypoxia, hypothermia or hypoglycaemia) also increases the risk of CNS damage despite lower serum levels of bilirubin. The administration of hypertonic solutions such as glucose and sodium bicarbonate in acutely ill infants, which causes a sudden rise in serum osmolality, has also been a contributing factor in the development of bilirubin encephalopathy.

The risk is increased in late-preterm infants, infants born preterm, male infants, inadequately breastfeeding infants and those who are discharged early from the birth hospital without adequate follow-up (Blackburn 2013). Late-preterm infants, especially those who are breastfed, may be at increased risk for hyperbilirubinaemia and should be followed closely. Because of their immaturity, late-preterm infants are less alert, have less stamina and have greater difficulty with latch, suck and swallow than full-term infants (Boies & Vaucher & the

Academy of Breastfeeding Medicine 2016). Proactive lactation management, strategies, support and follow-up for late-preterm infants and some early term infants are important components that affect breastfeeding success (Boies & Vaucher & the Academy of Breastfeeding Medicine 2016).

The signs of bilirubin encephalopathy are those of CNS depression or excitation. Prodromal symptoms consist of decreased activity, increasing lethargy, irritability, poor feeding, hypotonia, high-pitched cry and temperature instability, although some infants, particularly very low-birth-weight infants, may be asymptomatic. Later these subtle findings are followed by development of athetoid cerebral palsy, extrapyramidal symptoms, opisthotonos, dental enamel hyperplasia of the primary teeth, motor delay, seizures and sensorineural hearing deficits (Blackburn 2013). Long-term effects include evidence of neurological damage, such as cognitive impairment, attention-deficit/hyperactivity disorder, delayed or abnormal motor movement (especially ataxia or athetosis), behaviour disorders, perceptual problems or sensorineural hearing loss.

Physiological Jaundice

The most common evidence of hyperbilirubinaemia is the relatively mild and self-limited physiological jaundice, or icterus neonatorum. Unlike haemolytic disease of the newborn (HDN) (see p. 187), physiological jaundice is not associated with any pathological process. Although almost all newborns experience elevated serum bilirubin levels, only about half demonstrate observable signs of jaundice.

Two phases of physiological jaundice have been identified in full-term infants. In the first phase, bilirubin levels of formula-fed Caucasian and Indigenous Australian infants gradually increase to approximately 442 to 530 micromol/L by 2 to 5 days of life, then decrease to a plateau of less than 265 micromol/L by the fifth day. Bilirubin levels maintain a steady plateau state in the second phase without increasing or decreasing until approximately 12 to 14 days, at which time levels decrease to the normal value of 88 micromol/L.

Mechanisms Involved in Physiological Jaundice. On average, newborns produce twice as much bilirubin as do adults because of higher concentrations of circulating erythrocytes and a shorter life span of RBCs (only 70 to 90 days, in contrast to 120 days in older children and adults). In addition, the liver's ability to conjugate bilirubin is reduced because of limited production of glucuronyl transferase. Newborns also have a lower plasma-binding capacity for bilirubin because of lower albumin concentrations than older children. Normal changes in hepatic circulation following birth may contribute to excessive demands on liver function.

Normally, conjugated bilirubin is reduced to urobilinogen by the intestinal flora and excreted in faeces. However, the relatively sterile and less motile newborn bowel is initially less effective in excreting urobilinogen. In the newborn intestine the enzyme beta-glucuronidase is able to convert conjugated bilirubin into the unconjugated form, which is subsequently reabsorbed by the intestinal mucosa and transported to the liver. This process, known as **enterohepatic circulation** or **enterohepatic shunting**, is accentuated in the newborn and is believed to be a significant factor in physiological jaundice (Blackburn 2013). Feeding stimulates peristalsis and produces more rapid passage of meconium, thus diminishing the amount of reabsorption of unconjugated bilirubin, and introduces bacteria to aid in the reduction of bilirubin to urobilinogen. Colostrum, a natural cathartic, facilitates meconium evacuation.

Jaundice in Breastfeeding Infants

The Australian and New Zealand Breastfeeding Associations recommend exclusive breastfeeding for the first 6 months of life. Because breastfeeding can be associated with an increased incidence of jaundice, careful monitoring of the infant while supporting and establishing successful breastfeeding is important (World Health Organization [WHO] 2020). Two types of jaundice have been identified. Breastfeeding-associated jaundice (early-onset jaundice) may begin as early as 2 to 4 days of age. The jaundice is related to the process of breastfeeding and probably results from decreased caloric and fluid intake by breastfed infants before the milk supply is well established, because fasting is associated with decreased hepatic clearance of bilirubin. A decrease in milk (fluid) intake may result in decreased stooling, increased weight loss and increased fatty acid formation, which may interfere indirectly with hepatic uptake of bilirubin and conjugation. Blackburn (2013) asserts, however, that breastfeeding-associated jaundice is most likely to be a result of enterohepatic shunting rather than an increase in new bilirubin formation or abnormal bilirubin conjugation. Supplemental fluids such as glucose water or water do not enhance bilirubin excretion and may delay the excretion process. The current philosophy is to encourage more frequent effective breastfeeding, and thus increase stooling, while monitoring the infant's bilirubin levels with transcutaneous monitoring or serum levels.

Clinical Manifestations

The most obvious sign of hyperbilirubinaemia is jaundice, the yellowish discolouration primarily of the sclera, nails or skin. As a rule, jaundice that appears within the first 24 hours is caused by HDN, sepsis or one of the maternally derived diseases such as diabetes mellitus or infections. Jaundice that appears on the second or third day, peaks on the third to fifth day, and declines on the fifth to seventh day is usually the result of physiological jaundice; as noted earlier, this pattern may vary according to ethnic origin. The intensity of the jaundice is not always related to the degree of hyperbilirubinaemia; therefore, transcutaneous screening or serum bilirubin levels are necessary.

Diagnostic Evaluation

Total serum bilirubin is measured to determine the degree of hyperbilirubinaemia. Normal values of unconjugated bilirubin are 0.2 to 1.4 micromol/L. In the newborn, levels must exceed 5 mg/dL before jaundice (icterus) is observable. However, evaluation of jaundice is not based solely on serum bilirubin levels, but also on the timing of the appearance of clinical jaundice; gestational age at birth; age in days since birth; family history, including maternal Rh factor; evidence of haemolysis; feeding method; infant's physiological status; and progression of serial serum bilirubin levels. The following risk factors are associated with pathological hyperbilirubinaemia in term and late-preterm infants; further investigation is warranted as to the cause, although the exact cause may remain undetermined (Ambalavanan & Carlo 2016, Blackburn 2013):

- appearance of clinical jaundice within 24 hours of birth
- serum bilirubin level or transcutaneous bilirubin in the high-risk zone of the hour-specific nomogram (Fig 8.10)
- blood group incompatibility with a positive direct Coombs test
- hereditary haemolytic disease such as G6PD deficiency
- gestational age 35 to 36 weeks
- East Asian or Asian American race
- cephalhaematoma or significant bruising
- exclusive breastfeeding, especially infants experiencing difficulty breastfeeding or significant weight loss
- history of sibling with hyperbilirubinaemia.

Non-invasive monitoring of bilirubin via cutaneous reflectance measurements (transcutaneous bilirubinometry [TcB]) allows for repetitive estimations of total serum bilirubin and, when used correctly, may decrease the need for invasive monitoring. With shorter maternity stays, the value of transcutaneous bilirubin measurements

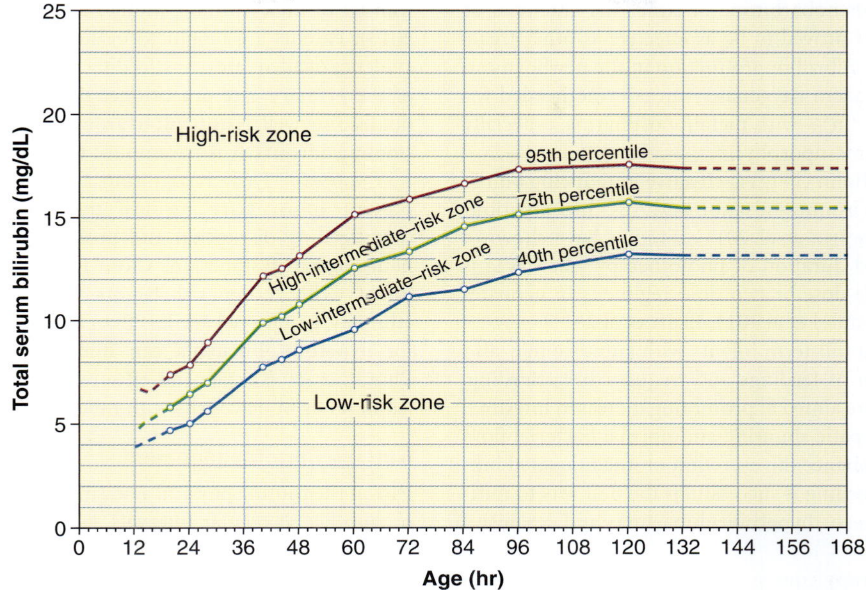

Fig 8.10 Nomogram for designation of risk in 2840 well newborns at 36 or more weeks of gestational age with birth weight of 2000 g or more, or 35 or more weeks of gestational age and birth weight of 2500 g or more, based on the hour-specific serum bilirubin values. (This nomogram should not be used to represent the natural history of neonatal hyperbilirubinaemia.) (Source: From Bhutani, V. K., Johnson, L., & Sivieri, E. M. (1999). Predictive ability of a predischarge hour-specific serum bilirubin for subsequent significant hyperbilirubinaemia in healthy term and near-term newborns. Pediatrics, 103(1), 6–14.)

as a screening tool for evaluating the need for obtaining serum bilirubin levels or closely monitoring the infant has received considerable attention. Regardless of the screening instrument chosen or the decision method used to treat, it is important to note that, to date, no transcutaneous bilirubin meter measures the total serum bilirubin level, and they must be used according to published guidelines as screening tools, not as predictors of need for therapy (Taylor et al 2016). Multiple readings over time at a consistent site (e.g. sternum, forehead) are more valuable than a single reading. Once phototherapy has been initiated, TcB is no longer useful as a screening tool.

The use of hour-specific serum bilirubin levels to predict newborns at risk for rapidly rising levels is now considered the gold standard for monitoring healthy neonates of more than 35 weeks' gestation before discharge from the hospital (American Academy of Pediatrics, Subcommittee on Hyperbilirubinemia 2004). Using a nomogram (see Fig 8.10) with three designated risk levels (high, intermediate or low risk) of hour-specific total serum bilirubin values assists in determining which newborns might need further evaluation before and after discharge. Universal bilirubin screening based on hour-specific total serum bilirubin, performed possibly at the same time as other routine newborn metabolic screening (e.g. phenylketonuria, galactosaemia), has been recommended (American Academy of Pediatrics, Subcommittee on Hyperbilirunbinemia 2004, Bhutani et al 2013). The hour-specific bilirubin risk nomogram is used to determine the infant's risk for developing hyperbilirubinaemia requiring medical treatment or closer screening. Risk factors recognised to place infants in the high-risk category include gestational age of less than 38 weeks, breastfeeding, a sibling who had significant jaundice and jaundice appearing before discharge (American Academy of Pediatrics, Subcommittee on Hyperbilirubinemia 2004). Some experts have recommended universal hour-specific screening in combination with these clinical risk factors, as well as targeted follow-up to prevent further cases of kernicterus (Bhutani et al 2013). A prospective multisite study of ethnically diverse newborns found that the combined use of total serum bilirubin determinations at 24 to 48 hours postnatal age and the hour-specific nomogram, as well as gestational age, were the best predictors for the subsequent use of phototherapy. In this study approximately 90% of the infants were breastfed, but breastfeeding was not found to be an independent risk factor for the development of hyperbilirubinaemia (Bhutani et al 2013).

It is also recommended that healthy late-preterm and term infants ($\geq$ 35 weeks' gestation) receive follow-up care and assessment of bilirubin within 3 days of discharge, if discharged at less than 24 hours, and a risk assessment with the hour-specific nomogram; likewise, newborns discharged at 24 to 47.9 hours should receive follow-up evaluation within 4 days, and those discharged between 48 and 72 hours should receive follow-up within 5 days (American Academy of Pediatrics, Subcommittee on Hyperbilirubinemia 2004). The guidelines for monitoring and treating neonatal hyperbilirubinaemia are published extensively elsewhere, and the reader is referred to the American Academy of Pediatrics, Subcommittee on Hyperbilirubinemia (2004) reference for an in-depth overview of management guidelines. Guidelines have also been published for the management of hyperbilirubinaemia in preterm infants less than 35 weeks' gestation (Maisels et al 2012).

Therapeutic Management

The primary goals in the treatment of hyperbilirubinaemia are to prevent bilirubin encephalopathy and kernicterus, and, as in any blood group incompatibility, to reverse the haemolytic process. The main form of treatment involves the use of phototherapy. Exchange transfusion is generally used for reducing dangerously high bilirubin levels that occur with haemolytic disease.

The pharmacological management of hyperbilirubinaemia with phenobarbital (phenobarbitone) has centred primarily on the infant with haemolytic disease and is most effective when given to the mother several days before delivery. Phenobarbitone promotes hepatic glucuronyl transferase synthesis, which increases bilirubin conjugation and hepatic clearance of the pigment in bile, and protein synthesis, which may increase albumin for more bilirubin binding sites. However, the use of phenobarbitone in either the antenatal or the postnatal period has not proved to be as effective as other treatments in reducing bilirubin. Bilirubin production in the newborn can be decreased by inhibiting haem oxygenase—an enzyme needed for haem breakdown (to biliverdin)—with metalloporphyrins, especially tin protoporphyrin and tin mesoporphyrin.

Intravenous immunoglobulin (IVIg) is effective in reducing bilirubin levels in infants with Rh isoimmunisation and ABO incompatibility (Bratlid et al 2011, Schwartz et al 2011). Studies have shown a decrease in hospital stay and duration of phototherapy when IVIg is administered either as single-dose or two-dose regimens in neonates with haemolytic disease (Demirel et al 2011, Elalfy et al 2011).

Healthy late-preterm and full-term infants with jaundice may also benefit from early initiation of feedings and frequent breastfeeding. These preventive measures are aimed at promoting increased intestinal motility, decreased enterohepatic shunting and normal bacterial flora in the bowel to effectively enhance the excretion of unconjugated bilirubin. Ensuring that breastfeeding is successful is the best way to mitigate the association between hyperbilirubinaemia and exclusive breastfeeding (Maisels 2015).

Phototherapy. **Phototherapy** consists of exposing the infant's skin to an appropriate light source. Light promotes bilirubin excretion by photoisomerisation, which alters the structure of bilirubin to a soluble form (lumirubin). Phototherapy works by enhancing the excretion of bilirubin but does not inhibit its production.

Studies indicate that blue fluorescent light is more effective than white fluorescent in reducing bilirubin levels. However, because blue light alters the infant's colouration, the normal light of fluorescent bulbs in the spectrum of 420 to 460 nm is often preferred so the infant's skin can be better observed for colour (e.g. jaundice, pallor, cyanosis) or other conditions. For phototherapy to be effective, the infant's skin must be fully exposed to an adequate amount of the light source. A nappy and boundary materials for postural support may be left in place; periodically turning the neonate under phototherapy has not been shown to accelerate bilirubin clearance (Stokowski 2011). When serum bilirubin levels are rapidly increasing or approximating critical levels, intensive phototherapy is recommended. Intensive phototherapy with a higher irradiance is considered to be more effective than standard phototherapy for rapid reduction of serum bilirubin levels. The colour of the infant's skin does not influence the efficacy of phototherapy. Best results occur within the first 4 to 6 hours of treatment (Bhutani & American Academy of Pediatrics Committee on Fetus and Newborn 2011, Stokowski 2011). Phototherapy alone is not effective in the management of hyperbilirubinaemia when levels are at a critical level or are rising rapidly; it is designed primarily for the treatment of moderate hyperbilirubinaemia. Available commercial phototherapy delivery systems are numerous and include halogen spotlights, light-emitting diodes, fluorescent tubes or bank lights and fibreoptic mattresses (Stokowski 2011).

The Safer Care Victoria Jaundice in neonates guidelines provide suggestions for initiating phototherapy and for implementing exchange transfusion in infants of 35 weeks' gestation or more. The initiation of phototherapy should always be based on individual clinical judgment rather than serum bilirubin levels alone (VAHI & SCV 2018).

Management of Breastfeeding Jaundice. Recommendations for prevention and management of early-onset jaundice in breastfed infants include: encouraging frequent effective breastfeeding, preferably every 1.5 to 2 hours; avoiding glucose, formula and water supplementation; and monitoring for output. The infant's weight and output should be evaluated along with the breastfeeding pattern and the transfer of milk from the mother to the infant (Lawrence & Lawrence 2015). Parents are taught to evaluate the number of wet nappies as evidence of adequate breastfeeding after the infant is home. Notification of the primary care practitioner if there are indications the infant is not feeding well, is difficult to arouse for feedings or is not voiding and stooling adequately is paramount to breastfeeding success.

Prognosis. Early recognition and treatment of neonatal jaundice prevent unnecessary medical therapies, parent–infant separation, breastfeeding disruption and possibly failure and bilirubin-induced neurological dysfunction. Close follow-up after discharge home in infants with certain risk factors (e.g. exclusive breastfeeding, Asian ethnicity, gestational age less than 38 weeks and increased haemolysis) for hyperbilirubinaemia can minimise risks for a poor outcome. Phototherapy is a safe and effective method of decreasing serum bilirubin levels in newborns with mild to moderate hyperbilirubinaemia.

Nursing Care Management

Part of the routine physical assessment includes observing for evidence of jaundice at regular intervals. Jaundice is most reliably assessed by observing the infant's skin colour from head to toe and the colour of the sclerae and mucous membranes. Applying direct pressure to the skin, especially over bony prominences such as the tip of the nose or the sternum, causes blanching and allows the yellow stain to be more pronounced. Also, bilirubin (especially at high levels) is not uniformly distributed in skin. The nurse should observe the infant in natural daylight for a true assessment of colour.

Prevention of physiological and breastfeeding jaundice may be possible with early introduction of feedings and frequent nursing without water supplementation. Make every effort to provide an optimum thermal environment to reduce metabolic needs.

QUALITY PATIENT OUTCOMES

Neonatal Hyperbilirubinaemia

Total serum bilirubin level will be maintained below the high-risk zone on the hour-specific bilirubin nomogram.

Phototherapy. The infant who receives phototherapy is placed under the light source, exposing as much skin surface as possible, and repositioned frequently to expose all body surface areas to the light. Once phototherapy has been initiated, frequent (every 12 to 24 hours) checks of serum bilirubin levels are necessary because visual and transcutaneous assessments of jaundice are no longer considered valid.

Another reaction to phototherapy is the **bronze-baby syndrome**, in which the serum, urine and skin turn greyish-brown several hours after the infant is placed under the light. This reaction is probably caused by retention of a bilirubin breakdown product of phototherapy, possibly copper porphyrin. The syndrome almost always occurs in infants who have elevated conjugated hyperbilirubinaemia and some degree of cholestasis. The browning generally resolves after discontinuation of phototherapy.

Family Support. Parents need reassurance concerning their infant's progress and comfort due to decreased handling of the newborn and the impact this will have on the parents and family emotionally. The nurse explains all the procedures to familiarise them with the benefits and risks. Reassure parents that the infant under the bilirubin light is warm and comfortable. Remove eye shields and turn off phototherapy when the parents are visiting to facilitate the attachment process. Also reassure parents that the neonate is accustomed to darkness after months of intrauterine existence and benefits a great deal from auditory and tactile stimulation (see Family-Centred Care box).

FAMILY-CENTERED CARE

Phototherapy and Parent–Infant Interaction

The traditional use of phototherapy has evoked concerns regarding a number of psychobehavioural issues, including parent–infant separation, potential social isolation, decreased sensorineural stimulation, altered biological rhythms, altered feeding patterns and activity changes. Parental anxiety is greatly increased, particularly at the sight of the newborn blindfolded and under special lights. The interruption of breastfeeding for phototherapy is a potential deterrent to successful mother–infant attachment and interaction.

Because research has demonstrated that bilirubin catabolism occurs primarily within the first few hours of the initiation of phototherapy, there is increased support for the removal of the infant from treatment for feeding and holding. The benefits of stopping phototherapy for parental feeding and holding outweigh concerns related to the clearance of bilirubin in the healthy full-term newborn with mild to moderate hyperbilirubinaemia.

The initiation of any treatment requires informed consent by the parents; however, in the case of phototherapy, parents may feel considerable anxiety when nurses use such words as 'kernicterus' and 'possible harm to the brain' to describe possible effects of hyperbilirubinaemia. It is imperative that nurses remain sensitive to parents' feelings and information needs during this process. An important nursing intervention is the assessment of the parents' understanding of the treatment involved and clarification of the nature of the therapy.

Discharge Planning and Home Care. With short hospital stays, mothers and infants may be discharged before evidence of jaundice is present. It is imperative that the nurse discuss signs of jaundice with the mother because any clinical symptoms will probably appear at home. Helping parents recognise risk factors and providing suggestions for further surveillance are important aspects of discharge planning. Teach parents to evaluate the number of voids and evidence of adequate breastfeeding once the infant is home, and encourage them to bring the newborn to the hospital, clinic or primary care practitioner if there are problems related to elimination and feeding. Breastfeeding mother–infant dyads must receive appropriate guidance and assistance with breastfeeding to ensure the infant is receiving an adequate amount of breast milk and that stooling is occurring. A follow-up visit to the healthcare practitioner within 2 or 3 days after discharge to evaluate feeding and elimination patterns and jaundice is important in the posthospital care of the full-term newborn (see Diagnostic Evaluation, p. 189, for follow-up recommendations). Some infants may require follow-up for serum bilirubin determination within 24 to 48 hours of discharge.

For every newborn born at 35 or more weeks' gestation, healthcare providers should promote and support successful breastfeeding: nurses should advise mothers to nurse their infants at least 8 to 12 times per day for the first several days; the nurse should recommend against routine supplementation of non-dehydrated breastfed infants with water or glucose (sugar) water (WHO 2020).

Haemolytic Disease of the Newborn

Hyperbilirubinaemia in the first 24 hours of life is most often the result of **haemolytic disease of the newborn (HDN)**, an abnormally rapid rate of RBC destruction. Anaemia caused by this destruction stimulates the production of RBCs, which in turn provides increasing numbers of cells for haemolysis. Major causes of increased erythrocyte destruction are isoimmunisation (primarily RhD) and ABO incompatibility.

Blood Incompatibility

The membranes of human blood cells contain a variety of **antigens**, also known as agglutinogens, substances capable of producing an immune response if recognised by the body as foreign. The reciprocal relationship between antigens on RBCs and antibodies in the plasma causes **agglutination** (clumping). In other words, antibodies in the plasma of one blood group (except the AB group, which contains no antibodies) produce agglutination when mixed with antigens of a different blood group. In the ABO blood group system the antibodies occur naturally. In the Rh system the person must be exposed to the Rh antigen before significant antibody formation takes place and causes a sensitivity response known as **isoimmunisation**.

Rh Incompatibility Isoimmunisation. The Rh blood group consists of several antigens (with D being the most prevalent). For simplicity, only the terms **Rh-positive** (presence of antigen) and **Rh-negative** (absence of antigen) are used in this discussion. (See Autosomal Inheritance Patterns, Chapter 3.) The presence or absence of the naturally occurring Rh factor determines the blood type.

Ordinarily, no problems are anticipated when the Rh blood types are the same in both mother and fetus or when the mother is Rh-positive and the infant is Rh-negative. Difficulty may arise when the mother is Rh-negative and the infant is Rh-positive. Although the maternal and fetal circulations are separate, there is evidence of a bidirectional trafficking of fetal RBCs and cell-free DNA to the maternal circulation (Moise 2012). More commonly, however, fetal RBCs enter into the maternal circulation at the time of birth. The mother's natural defence mechanism responds to these alien cells by producing anti-Rh antibodies.

Under normal circumstances, this process of isoimmunisation has no effect on the fetus during the first pregnancy with an Rh-positive fetus because the initial sensitisation to Rh antigens rarely occurs before the onset of labour. However, with the increased risk of fetal blood being transferred to the maternal circulation during placental separation, maternal antibody production is stimulated. During a subsequent pregnancy with an Rh-positive fetus, these previously formed maternal antibodies to Rh-positive blood cells enter the fetal circulation, where they attach to and destroy fetal erythrocytes (Fig 8.11). Multiple gestations, abruptio placentae, placenta praevia, manual removal of the placenta and caesarean birth increase the incidence of transplacental haemorrhage and subsequent isoimmunisation.

Because the condition begins in utero, the fetus attempts to compensate for the progressive haemolysis by accelerating the rate of erythropoiesis. As a result, immature RBCs (erythroblasts) appear in the fetal circulation—hence the term **erythroblastosis fetalis**.

The development of maternal sensitisation to Rh-positive antigens exhibits wide variability. Sensitisation may occur during the first pregnancy if the woman previously received an Rh-positive blood transfusion. No sensitisation may occur in situations in which a strong placental barrier prevents transfer of fetal blood into the maternal circulation. Approximately 10% to 15% of sensitised mothers have no haemolytic reaction and no adverse effects on the fetus. In addition, some Rh-negative women, even though exposed to Rh-positive fetal blood, are immunologically unable to produce antibodies to the foreign antigen.

In the most severe form of erythroblastosis fetalis (**hydrops fetalis**), the progressive haemolysis causes fetal hypoxia; cardiac failure; generalised oedema (anasarca); and fluid effusions into the pericardial, pleural and peritoneal spaces (hydrops). The fetus may be delivered stillborn or in severe respiratory distress. Maternal Rh immunoglobulin (RhIg) administration, early intrauterine detection of fetal anaemia by ultrasonography (i.e. serial Doppler assessment of the peak velocity

PATHOPHYSIOLOGY REVIEW

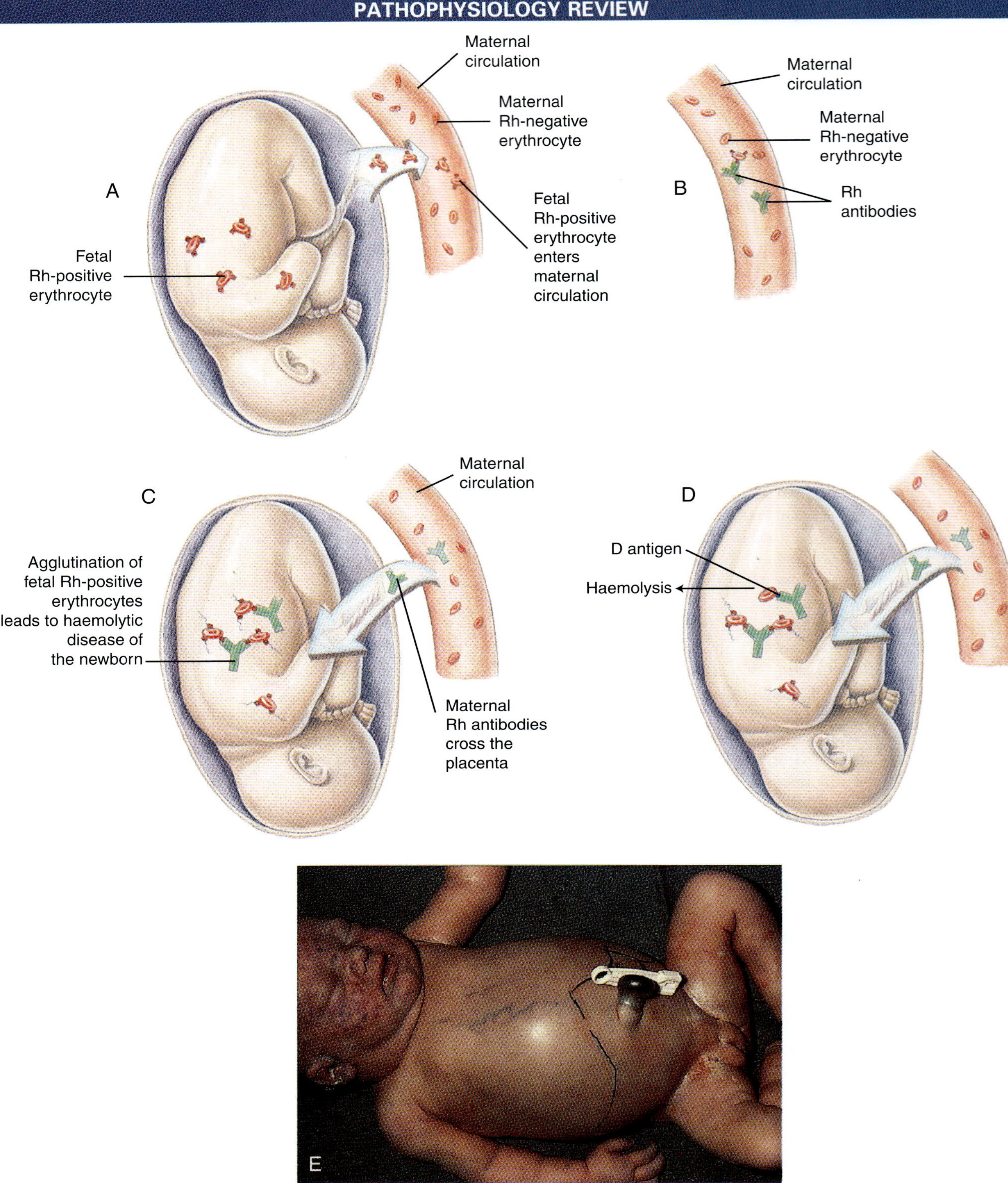

Fig 8.11 Haemolytic disease of the newborn (HDN). (**A**) Before or during birth, Rh-positive erythrocytes from the fetus enter the blood of an Rh-negative woman through a tear in the placenta. (**B**) The mother is sensitised to the Rh antigen and produces Rh antibodies. Because this usually happens after birth, there is no effect on the fetus in the first pregnancy. (**C**) During a subsequent pregnancy with an Rh-positive fetus, Rh-positive erythrocytes cross the placenta, enter the maternal circulation and (**D**) stimulate the mother to produce antibodies against the Rh antigen. (**E**) The Rh antibodies from the mother cross the placenta, causing agglutination and haemolysis of fetal erythrocytes, and HDN develops. (Source: McCance, K., & Huether, S. (2010). *Pathophysiology: The biological basis for disease in adults and children* (6th ed.). St Louis, MO: Mosby.)

in the fetal middle cerebral artery) and subsequent treatment by fetal blood transfusions or high-dose IVIg have dramatically improved the outcome of affected fetuses.

ABO Incompatibility. Haemolytic disease can also occur when the major blood group antigens of the fetus are different from those of the mother. The major blood groups are A, B, AB and O. The incidence of these blood groups varies according to race and geographical location (Better Health Channel 2021).

The presence or absence of antibodies and antigens determines whether agglutination will occur. Antibodies in the plasma of one blood group (except the AB group, which contains no antibodies) will produce agglutination (clumping) when mixed with antigens of a different blood group. Naturally occurring antibodies in the recipient's blood cause agglutination of a donor's RBCs. The agglutinated donor cells become trapped in peripheral blood vessels, where they haemolyse releasing large amounts of bilirubin into the circulation.

The most common blood group incompatibility in the neonate is between a mother with O blood group and an infant with A or B blood group. Haemolysis due to anti-A is more common than for anti-B (see Table 8.2 for possible ABO incompatibilities). Naturally occurring anti-A or anti-B antibodies already present in the maternal circulation cross the placenta and attach to fetal RBCs, causing haemolysis. Unlike the Rh reaction, ABO incompatibility may occur in the first pregnancy. The risk of significant haemolysis in subsequent pregnancies is higher when the first pregnancy is complicated by ABO incompatibility.

Clinical Manifestations

Jaundice usually appears during the first 24 hours after birth, and serum levels of unconjugated bilirubin rise rapidly. Anaemia results from the haemolysis of large numbers of erythrocytes, and hyperbilirubinaemia and jaundice result from the liver's inability to conjugate and excrete the excess bilirubin. Most newborns with HDN are not jaundiced at birth. However, hepatosplenomegaly and varying degrees of hydrops may be evident. If the infant is severely affected, hydrops, anaemia and hypovolaemic shock are apparent. Hypoglycaemia may occur as a result of pancreatic cell hyperplasia.

Diagnostic Evaluation

Early identification and diagnosis of Rh sensitisation is important in the management and prevention of fetal complications. A maternal antibody titre (indirect Coombs test) should be drawn at the first prenatal visit. Genetic testing allows early identification of paternal zygosity at the Rh gene locus, thus allowing earlier detection of the potential for isoimmunisation and avoiding further maternal or fetal testing (Hendrickson & Delaney 2016).

Amniocentesis can be used to test the fetal blood type of a woman whose antibody screen is positive; the use of polymerase chain reaction may determine the fetal blood type, haemoglobin, haematocrit and presence of maternal antibodies. Chorionic villus sampling has drawbacks that preclude its use, including possible spontaneous abortion of the fetus and fetomaternal haemorrhage. With either method the determination of an Rh-negative fetus requires no further treatment. The detection of cell-free fetal DNA in the maternal plasma of Rh-negative women to detect an Rh-positive fetus has been used successfully (Hendrickson & Delaney 2016). Such testing usually negates the necessity for amniocentesis for fetal blood type (Moise & Argoti 2012).

TABLE 8.2 Potential Maternal–Fetal ABO Incompatibilities

Maternal Blood Group	Incompatible Fetal Blood Group
O	A or B
B	A or AB
A	B or AB

Ultrasonography is an important adjunct in the detection of isoimmunisation. Alterations in the placenta, umbilical cord and amniotic fluid volume, as well as the presence of fetal hydrops, can be detected with high-resolution ultrasonography, allowing early, non-invasive treatment before the development of erythroblastosis. Serial Doppler ultrasonography of fetal middle cerebral artery peak velocity is now the gold standard to detect and measure fetal haemoglobin and, subsequently, fetal anaemia (Moise & Argoti 2012). Erythroblastosis fetalis caused by Rh incompatibility can also be assessed by evaluating rising anti-Rh antibody titres in the maternal circulation (indirect Coombs test) or by testing the optical density of amniotic fluid (delta OD 450 test) because bilirubin discolours the fluid. The condition in the newborn is suspected on the basis of the timing and appearance of jaundice (see Table 8.1) and can be confirmed postnatally by detecting antibodies attached to the circulating erythrocytes of affected infants (direct Coombs test or direct antiglobulin test). The Coombs test may be performed on umbilical cord blood samples from infants born to Rh-negative mothers if there is a history of incompatibility or if further investigation is warranted.

Therapeutic Management

The primary aim of therapeutic management of isoimmunisation is prevention. Postnatal therapy usually entails phototherapy for mild cases and exchange transfusion for more severe forms. In severe cases of hydrops, aggressive interventions such as pericardial and pleural fluid aspiration, mechanical ventilatory support and inotropic therapy may be required for stabilisation. Although phototherapy may control bilirubin levels in mild cases, the haemolytic process may continue, causing severe anaemia (if untreated) between 7 and 21 days of life.

Prevention of Rh Isoimmunisation. The administration of RhIg, a human gamma-globulin concentrate of anti-D, to all unsensitised Rh-negative mothers after birth or abortion of an Rh-positive infant or fetus prevents the development of maternal sensitisation to the Rh factor. The injected anti-Rh antibodies destroy (by subsequent phagocytosis and agglutination) fetal RBCs passing into the maternal circulation before the mother's immune system can recognise them. Because the immune response is blocked, anti-D antibodies and memory cells (which produce the primary and secondary immune responses, respectively) are not formed. The inhibition of memory cell formation is especially important because memory cells provide long-term immunity by initiating a rapid immune response once the antigen is reintroduced (McCance & Huether 2014).

To be effective, RhIg must be administered to unsensitised mothers within 72 hours (but possibly as long as 3 to 4 weeks) after the first delivery, miscarriage or abortion and repeated after subsequent pregnancies. The administration of RhIg at 26 to 28 weeks' gestation further reduces the risk of Rh isoimmunisation. RhIg is not effective against existing Rh-positive antibodies in the maternal circulation. RhIg is administered intramuscularly, not intravenously, and only to Rh-negative women with a negative Coombs test—never to the infant.

Studies have demonstrated the effectiveness of neonatal IVIg therapy at decreasing the severity of RBC destruction (haemolysis) in HDN and subsequent development of neonatal jaundice (Elalfy et al 2011). IVIg is believed to attack the maternal cells that destroy neonatal RBCs, slowing the progression of bilirubin production (Hendrickson & Delaney 2016). This therapy, often used in conjunction with phototherapy, may decrease the necessity for exchange transfusion. Maternal administration of high-dose IVIg, alone or in combination with plasmapheresis, decreases the fetal effects of Rh isoimmunisation (Hendrickson & Delaney 2016). The use of a haem-oxygenase inhibitor such as tin mesoporphyrin (administered intramuscularly to the newborn) has proved effective in treating hyperbilirubinaemia in newborns with haemolytic disease (Maisels & Yang 2012).

Intrauterine Transfusion. Infants of mothers already sensitised may be treated by intrauterine transfusion, which consists of infusing blood into the umbilical vein of the fetus. The need for therapy is based on the antenatal diagnosis of fetal anaemia by serial Doppler assessments of middle cerebral artery peak systolic velocity (Moise & Argoti 2012). With the advance of ultrasound technology, fetal transfusion may be accomplished directly via the umbilical vein, infusing type O Rh-negative packed RBCs to raise the fetal haematocrit to 40% to 50%; fetal movement and transfusion risks are minimised by administering a drug such as vecuronium bromide for temporary fetal paralysis. The frequency of intrauterine transfusions may vary according to institution and fetal hydropic status, but one recommendation is in intervals of 10 days, 2 weeks and then 3 weeks for subsequent procedures until the fetus reaches pulmonary maturity at approximately 37 to 38 weeks' gestation (Moise & Argoti 2012). Intraperitoneal blood transfusions are used less commonly for isoimmunisation because of higher associated fetal risks; however, they may be used when intravascular access is impossible.

Exchange Transfusion. Exchange transfusion, in which the infant's blood is removed in small amounts (usually 5 to 10 mL at a time) and replaced with compatible blood (Rh-negative blood), is a standard mode of therapy for treatment of severe hyperbilirubinaemia that is unresponsive to phototherapy or other therapies such as tin mesoporphyrin. However, there are reports that this procedure is less common with closer monitoring of rising bilirubin levels, maternal administration of RhIg, intensive phototherapy and the use of prophylactic phototherapy in preterm infants (Maisels et al 2012). Exchange transfusion removes the sensitised erythrocytes, lowers the serum bilirubin level to prevent bilirubin encephalopathy, corrects the anaemia and prevents cardiac failure. Indications for exchange transfusion include rapidly increasing serum bilirubin levels and haemolysis despite aggressive phototherapy. The criteria for exchange transfusion in preterm infants vary according to associated illness factors. The recommendations are to initiate phototherapy and exchange transfusion in infants of 35 weeks' gestation or more. An infant born with hydrops fetalis or signs of cardiac failure is a candidate for immediate exchange transfusion with fresh whole blood (Better Health Channel 2021).

For exchange transfusion, fresh whole blood is typed and crossmatched to the mother's serum. The amount of donor blood used is usually double the infant's blood volume, which is approximately 85 mL/kg body weight. The double-volume exchange transfusion replaces approximately 85% of the neonate's blood.

An exchange transfusion is a sterile surgical procedure. A catheter is inserted into the umbilical vein and threaded into the inferior vena cava. Depending on the infant's weight, 5 to 10 mL of blood is withdrawn within 15 to 20 seconds, and the same volume of donor blood is infused until the targeted volume (double the estimated blood volume) is reached.

ABO Incompatibility. The treatment for ABO haemolytic disease is early detection and implementation of phototherapy for the reduction of hyperbilirubinaemia. The initial diagnosis is often more difficult because the direct Coombs test may be negative or weakly reactive. The presence of jaundice within the first 24 hours, elevated serum bilirubin levels, RBC spherocytosis and increased erythrocyte production is diagnostic of ABO incompatibility. In some centres IVIg transfusions are used in combination with phototherapy to treat ABO incompatibility. Exchange transfusion is not commonly required for ABO incompatibility except when phototherapy fails to decrease bilirubin concentrations. As stated previously the neonatal administration of tin mesoporphyrin may also serve to decrease the effects of haemolysis associated with ABO incompatibility.

Prognosis. The severe anaemia of isoimmunisation may result in stillbirth, shock, congestive heart failure, poor feeding or poor weight gain. Complications from exchange transfusion are uncommon; however, close monitoring during the procedure is imperative.

Nursing Care Management

The initial nursing responsibility is recognising the early onset of neonatal jaundice. The possibility of haemolytic disease can be anticipated from the prenatal and perinatal history. Prenatal evidence of incompatibility, maternal blood type O and a positive Coombs test are cause for increased vigilance for early signs of jaundice in an infant.

The nursing care of the infant undergoing phototherapy has been described in detail earlier and is no different for infants with hyperbilirubinaemia from haemolytic disease. If an exchange transfusion is required, the nurse prepares the infant and the family and assists the practitioner with the procedure. The infant must remain nil by mouth (NBM) during the procedure; therefore, a peripheral infusion of glucose and electrolytes is established. The nurse documents: blood volumes exchanged, including the amount of blood withdrawn and infused; the time of each procedure; and the cumulative record of the total volume exchanged. The nurse also evaluates vital signs frequently (monitored electronically during the procedure) and correlates them with the removal and infusion of blood. If signs of cardiac or respiratory problems occur, the procedure is stopped temporarily and resumed once the infant's cardiorespiratory function stabilises. The nurse also observes for signs of transfusion reaction (e.g. temperature instability, hypotension, tachycardia, bradycardia, rash) and maintains adequate neonatal thermoregulation, blood glucose levels and fluid balance.

Family Support. Parents often feel guilty because they think they have caused the blood incompatibility. Parents should never be made to feel responsible or negligent. The nurse encourages them to express their thoughts. The nurse should praise parents for actions they took to prevent any problems, such as frequent antepartum examinations and blood tests.

Hypoglycaemia

Neonatal hypoglycaemia has many recognised causes; the following discussion primarily focuses on transient neonatal hypoglycaemia.

Hypoglycaemia is present when the newborn's blood glucose concentration is lower than the body's requirement for cellular energy and metabolism. Other researchers state that the goal of the 'golden hour', the first hour of the preterm newborn after birth, is to maintain a glucose value between 50 and 110 mg/dL (Sharma 2016). The Royal Children's Hospital Melbourne defines neonatal hypoglycaemia as a blood glucose level (BGL) < 2.6 mmol/L. Many neonates with hypoglycaemia present initially asymptomatic and the diagnosis of hypoglycaemia is established via at-risk assessments. Those neonates identified at risk must have a BGL on admission and continue to be monitored as per facility policy and/or in consultation with paediatric management teams (RCHM 2020).

Pathophysiology

After birth the infant must supply nutrients to meet energy requirements for maintaining body temperature, respiration, muscular activity and regulation of blood glucose. Glucose comes primarily from glycogen stores deposited in the liver, heart and skeletal muscles during the last trimester of pregnancy.

The brain is especially dependent on adequate glucose supply for appropriate function. Studies demonstrate that a majority of fetal and neonatal glucose produced is used by neuronal cells; a decreased availability of glucose predisposes both the fetal and the neonatal brain to potential permanent damage (Tam et al 2012). There is evidence of a major shift in energy metabolism from glucose to carbohydrate in newborns during the first several hours of life—hence the importance of providing adequate energy substrate. Although newborns demonstrate the ability to use ketones and amino acids as energy substrate, there are certain limitations. Infants with severe hyperinsulinism are unable to compensate metabolically and require more glucose than normal. Conditions that decrease the availability of substrate or prevent appropriate metabolism of available substrate place the infant at risk for pathological hypoglycaemia. These include: intrauterine growth restriction; preterm birth; gestational diabetes mellitus; maternal use of hypoglycaemic drugs; maternal administration of tocolytics such as terbutaline; intrapartum administration of glucose; perinatal hypoxia; infection; hypothermia; polycythaemia; fetal hydrops; inborn errors of metabolism (IEMs), such as galactosaemia; certain congenital malformations; endocrine disorders; abnormal extrauterine transition; and failure to receive adequate perinatal nutrition.

Both transient neonatal hypoglycaemia and recurrent hypoglycaemia are based on conditions with decreased hepatic glucose production. Transient neonatal hypoglycaemia is associated with intrapartum glucose administration, terbutaline administration, gestational diabetes mellitus, intrauterine growth restriction, perinatal stress or asphyxia, prematurity, cold stress, polycythaemia and large for gestational age. Recurrent hypoglycaemia is observed in neonates with excessive insulin production or hyperinsulinism and includes infants with IEMs, Beckwith-Wiedemann syndrome, nesidioblastosis, Rh isoimmunisation and certain rare endocrine disorders (Sperling 2016).

Clinical Manifestations

The signs of hypoglycaemia are usually vague and often indistinguishable from those observed in other newborn conditions, such as hypocalcaemia, septicaemia, CNS disorders or cardiorespiratory problems. Many newborns with hypoglycaemia, however, are asymptomatic. Because the brain depends on glucose for energy, cerebral signs such as jitteriness, tremors, twitching, weak or high-pitched cry, lethargy, hypotonia, seizures and coma are prominent. Other clinical manifestations are cyanosis, apnoea, rapid and irregular respirations, sweating, eye rolling and refusal to feed. The symptoms often are transient but recurrent.

Diagnostic Evaluation

Diagnosis is confirmed by direct analysis of blood glucose concentration. Two consecutive specimens of blood should be analysed because of the many factors that can affect readings.

Bedside point-of-care blood glucose monitors in neonatal care: must be accurate, rapid and inexpensive; must demonstrate reliability with neonatal haematocrit ranges; must accept small blood volumes; and must provide reliable data for diagnosing neonatal hypoglycaemia and hyperglycaemia (Raizman et al 2016). Strict quality monitoring, regular calibration and adherence to strict protocols are necessary to ensure accuracy.

The most accurate method is the laboratory analysis of serum glucose. Blood specimens may be obtained from heel, arterial or venous punctures.

Proper handling of the specimen is essential because storage at room temperature increases glycolysis. Accurate readings can be facilitated by storing the blood sample on ice to slow cellular metabolism or by removing the RBCs through centrifugation.

Continuous glucose monitoring to measure interstitial glucose levels has been used in preterm and late-preterm infants (McKinlay et al 2015).

Therapeutic Management

Self-limiting or transient hypoglycaemia is common in the first few hours following delivery. In healthy full-term infants who are borderline hypoglycaemic and clinically asymptomatic, the early initiation of feeding (breast or formula) may re-establish normoglycaemia. Most newborns compensate for this low blood glucose with 'counter-regulation' of endogenous fuel production through gluconeogenesis, glycogenolysis and ketogenesis, collectively (Wight et al 2014). Infants at risk for hypoglycaemia should be monitored within the first 2 hours of life and monitoring should continue until acceptable prefeed levels are obtained. Acceptable levels are defined as an infant with at least two consecutive satisfactory glucose measurements (Hawdon 2014).

Oral glucose feedings have been used as a treatment for hypoglycaemia in healthy newborns. However, formula and breast milk are probably more effective because of the carbohydrate content. Hypoglycaemia is preventable in most instances by the initiation of early feeding in healthy, asymptomatic term and late-preterm newborns. Breastfed infants should be put to breast as soon as possible after delivery. (See Infants of Diabetic Mothers, Chapter 9, for management of hypoglycaemia related to transient hyperinsulinaemia.)

The management of neonatal hypoglycaemia can have several outcomes and during this management the initial cause of the hypoglycaemia must be considered before action is taken. Figure 8.12 explains the recommended nursing and medical management taken by the Royal Children's Hospital Melbourne for hypoglycaemia.

Nursing Care Management

Although management strategies for infants with hypoglycaemia remain unclear, the nursing responsibility involves identification of the problem through careful observation of physical status. Another concern is to reduce environmental factors, such as cold stress and respiratory distress, which predispose the infant to the development of a decreased BGL. Infants who are at risk for hypoglycaemia (late-preterm, infants of diabetic mothers/large for gestational age, term small for gestational age) should be carefully screened and observed for symptoms of hypoglycaemia and other comorbidities often observed (e.g. respiratory distress syndrome, feeding intolerance) within the first several hours of life when glucose levels are known to fluctuate. An important nursing intervention is to assist the mother and infant in establishing successful breastfeeding.

An intravenous glucose infusion is required for infants with symptomatic hypoglycaemia who are unable to tolerate oral feedings, infants who are unable to maintain adequate glucose levels with oral feedings and infants with profound hypoglycaemia. Major nursing objectives include preventing, anticipating and recognising potential dangers of concentrated glucose infusion. Too-rapid infusion of the hypertonic solution can cause circulatory overload, hyperglycaemia, glycosuria and intracellular dehydration. Maintaining the ordered flow rate with an intravenous pump and checking and charting hourly intake decrease the chance of such problems.

Because hypoglycaemia may be a symptom of some other underlying pathophysiological process, parents are usually concerned about their infant's progress, particularly because these infants do not feed well or demonstrate behaviours that are typical of healthy infants. Nurses need to be aware of parents' thoughts, allow them to express their feelings and update them on the infant's progress.

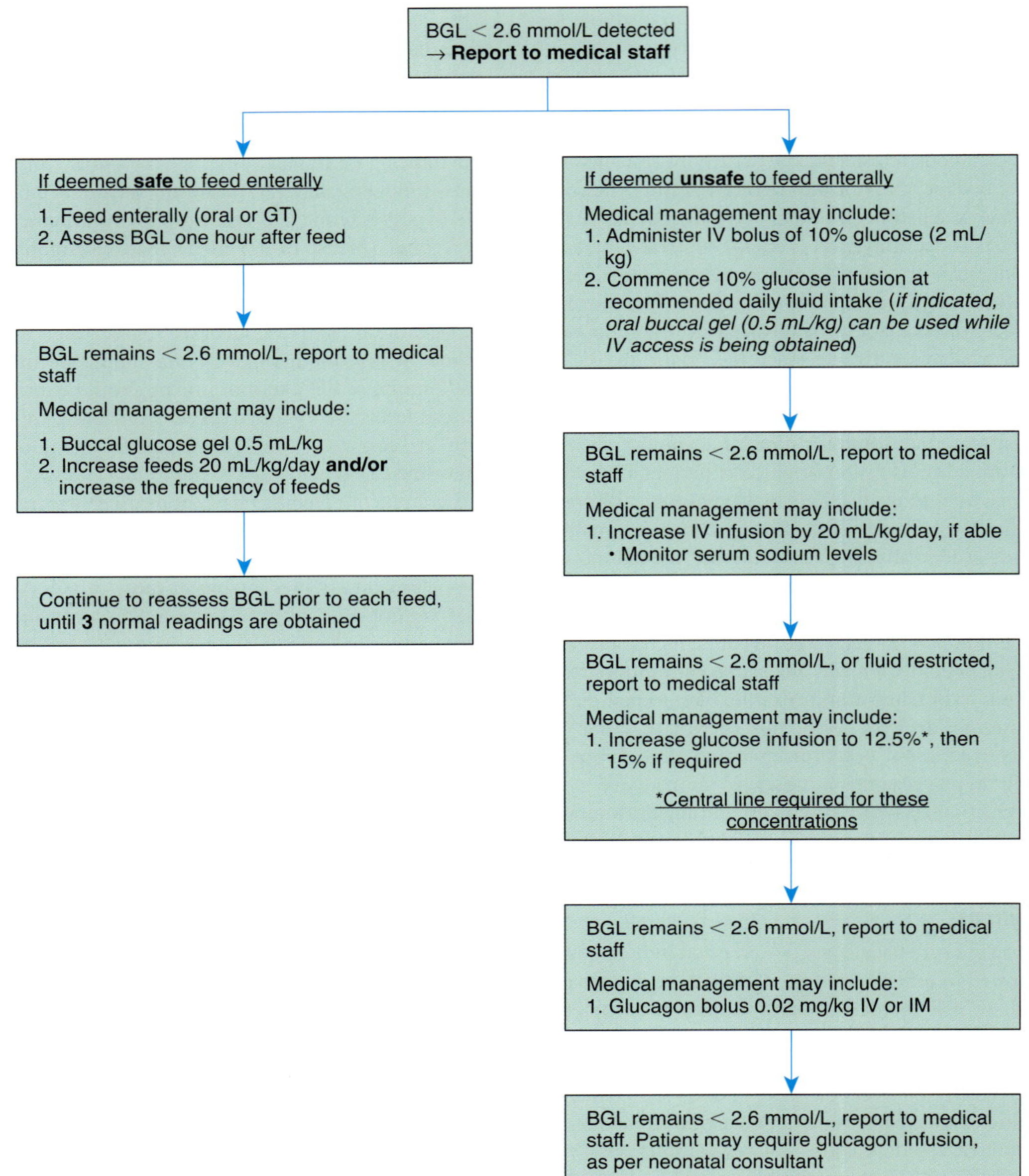

Fig 8.12 Nursing and medical management of neonatal hypoglycaemia (Source: The Royal Children's Hospital Melbourne (RCHM). (2020) Clinical Practice Guidelines (Nursing). Neonatal hypoglycaemia. October. https://www.rch.org.au/rchcpg/hospital_clinical_guideline_index/Neonatal_hypoglycaemia/)

Hyperglycaemia (Transient)

Hyperglycaemia in the newborn is usually defined as a blood glucose concentration greater than > 8.3 mmol/L in the full-term infant or greater than 150 mg/dL in the preterm infant. The condition in preterm infants is associated with increased morbidity and mortality, but the best treatment method to maintain euglycaemia in preterm infants has not been defined (Craig et al 2011). Those affected are usually low-birth-weight infants, particularly those with weights less than 1000 g who are unable to tolerate intravenous glucose infusions at the usual rate. The glucose intolerance is probably related to general immaturity of the usual regulatory mechanisms. Increased blood glucose levels may also occur in infants with sepsis or decreased insulin sensitivity (such as infants with transient diabetes mellitus), infants receiving methylxanthines and infants who are stressed (e.g. infants with respiratory distress syndrome, infants undergoing surgical procedures).

Hyperglycaemia is usually asymptomatic but detected on routine screening. Most often, hyperglycaemia is treated by reducing the infant's glucose intake. Untreated hyperglycaemia may result in an osmotic diuresis with subsequent fluid volume loss and dehydration; if severe, it may result in an intraventricular haemorrhage as a result of fluid shifts in the CNS (Blackburn 2013). Insulin infusion is sometimes administered to very low-birth-weight infants who require but are unable to tolerate intravenous glucose.

Nursing Care Management

Monitor blood glucose frequently, especially in the infant receiving insulin. This requires numerous heel sticks, and sites should be rotated to minimise tissue damage. (See Blood Specimens, Chapter 22, and the Nursing Care Considerations box titled Heel Punctures in Chapter 7.) Closely monitor and measure the infant's urinary output to detect any evidence of glycosuria and possible osmotic diuresis.

Continuous glucose monitoring has the potential to decrease multiple heel puncture or prick to observe glycaemic trends, and to promptly detect episodes of both hypoglycaemia and hyperglycaemia. The utilisation of this technology in very low-birth-weight infants has been described in the literature and found to be safe and reliable (Tiberi et al 2016). However, studies with a larger population of preterm infants are needed to better establish safety, reliability and the therapeutic application of continuous glucose monitoring.

As in the care of all infants, give parents a careful explanation of the therapy, provide frequent progress reports and support them to reduce anxiety. (See Chapter 9.)

Hypocalcaemia

As with many conditions in the neonate, transient hypocalcaemia is difficult to differentiate from other disorders (e.g. sepsis, meningitis, narcotic withdrawal, hypoglycaemia), and the aetiology may not be clear. The incidence is highest at two times during the neonatal period. *Early-onset hypocalcaemia,* which appears within the first 24 to 48 hours, is the more common form and typically affects the preterm or small-for-gestational-age infant and any infant who has experienced perinatal asphyxia. Preterm infants may have hypocalcaemia as a result of inadequate calcium intake, increased calcitonin levels, possible resistance to parathyroid hormone activation preventing calcium removal from bones, acidosis and decreased vitamin D intake and absorption (Blackburn 2013). An infant born to a diabetic mother may also experience early hypocalcaemia, possibly as a result of relative maternal hyperparathyroidism and transient neonatal hypoparathyroidism. Symptoms include jitteriness, prolonged QT interval, apnoea, cyanotic episodes, a high-pitched cry and abdominal distension.

Late-onset hypocalcaemia, which is not apparent until after the first 3 or 4 days of life, is referred to as cow's milk–induced hypocalcaemia or neonatal tetany. Although uncommon in developed countries, it may be observed in well-nourished infants who are fed modified cow's milk, such as evaporated milk formula. Cow's milk, which has a high phosphorus content, produces hyperphosphataemia and a resultant hypocalcaemia by increasing calcium deposition in the bone and soft tissues. Late hypocalcaemia may also be seen in infants with intestinal malabsorption, hyperinsulinaemia, hypoparathyroidism or hypomagnesaemia. Maternal hyperparathyroidism and elevated maternal serum calcium levels may suppress fetal parathyroid gland function, resulting in a transient neonatal hypocalcaemia that may not be apparent (tetany) until 3 or 4 weeks after birth, especially if the newborn is breastfeeding; the mother is usually asymptomatic (Doyle 2016).

The manifestations of neonatal tetany reflect neuromuscular irritation: twitching; tremors; irritability; high-pitched cry; tachycardia; and, rarely, seizures (Blackburn 2013). The preterm neonate with hypocalcaemia may be asymptomatic. Neonatal tetany is rarely seen in industrialised countries because of the prevalent use of commercial formula or human milk as the newborn's primary source of nutrition.

In some preterm neonates, rickets and osteopenia may occur as a result of calcium or phosphorus deficiency in association with vitamin D deficiency, which prevents adequate intestinal absorption of minerals (Blackburn 2013). Very low-birth-weight infants, infants with chronic conditions such as chronic lung disease (bronchopulmonary dysplasia) and infants on prolonged diuretic management are at particular risk for developing rickets and osteopenia (Blackburn 2013). There have been reported cases of vitamin D deficiency in healthy breastfed infants who received minimal ultraviolet light exposure or whose breastfeeding mother had a diet deficient in vitamin D—hence the American Academy of Pediatrics' (2008) recommendation for vitamin D supplementation (400 IU/day, oral) in all newborns exclusively breastfed.

Therapeutic Management

In most instances early-onset hypocalcaemia is transient and resolves in 1 to 3 days. Restoration of a normal calcium level is facilitated by early feedings, physiological correction of hypoparathyroidism and, sometimes, administration of calcium supplements.

Treatment of hypocalcaemia involves intravenous administration (IV bolus) of 10% calcium gluconate (2 mL/kg). Commence 10% glucose infusion at recommended daily fluid intake for BGL to remain < 2.6 mmol/L and report to medical staff. Monitor serum sodium levels and BGL levels to again remain < 2.6 mmol/L, or restrict fluid intake and again report to medical staff. Other treatment may include glucose infusion and further glucagon boluses. Treatment will follow major children's hospital policies (Craig et al 2011). Rapid intravenous calcium administration may cause cardiac arrhythmias and circulatory collapse. The heart rate and blood pressure should be electronically monitored. Take care to ascertain that the infusion device is positioned within the vein because extravasation into surrounding tissue causes local necrosis, calcification and sloughing. Intramuscular administration of calcium gluconate is contraindicated because it precipitates in the tissue, causing necrosis. If the infant can tolerate oral fluids, oral doses of calcium are given with formula. Adequate intake of vitamin D and phosphorus is imperative, especially in low-birth-weight infants. Exercise caution in the use of oral calcium salts because of their hypertonicity and subsequent effects on the bowel of at-risk infants.

Nursing Care Management

Nursing care of the infant with hypocalcaemia is directed towards identifying infants at risk for early hypocalcaemia, observing for clinical manifestations in such infants and administering supplemental calcium, vitamin D and phosphorus. Monitor the infant continuously during intravenous infusions. Calcium gluconate can cause tissue necrosis and scar formation; therefore, it is recommended that superficial veins such as those on the scalp be avoided. To prevent tissue necrosis, carefully observe the infusion site and change it as needed. Calcium gluconate is also incompatible with a number of drugs, most notably sodium bicarbonate.

The nurse also observes for signs of acute hypercalcaemia (e.g. vomiting, bradycardia). If such symptoms occur, discontinue the injection or infusion and notify the practitioner. Seizure precautions must be initiated immediately because seizures are common with acute hypercalcaemia.

To prevent late-onset hypocalcaemia, the nurse provides preventive care and anticipatory guidance regarding the correct use of an infant formula containing the appropriate balance of calcium and phosphorus and assists the parent in planning for meeting the growing infant's nutritional needs through an affordable commercial infant formula. If powder formula is used, ensure that the recommended amount of water is used to avoid inappropriate amounts of calcium and phosphorus ingestion.

If the infant is discharged on formula feedings supplemented with calcium, teach the parents the correct procedure for diluting the mineral in the formula and advise them to use only the prescribed formula. Also teach parents to observe for any signs of hypocalcaemia or hypercalcaemia in the infant receiving supplemental calcium.

Haemorrhagic Disease of the Newborn

Haemorrhagic disease of the newborn, or vitamin K–deficiency bleeding, is a bleeding disorder that occurs as a result of a vitamin K deficiency. Haemorrhagic disease may be classified according to appearance as early, classic or late onset. Newborns' vitamin K stores are virtually absent, and prothrombin activity is moderately deficient, decreases until approximately 72 hours after birth and then begins to increase. Consequently, vitamin K–dependent coagulation factors (e.g. II, VII, IX, X) are significantly reduced. In addition, the newborn's relatively sterile intestinal tract is unable to synthesise the vitamin until feedings have begun.

Signs and symptoms of early haemorrhagic disease typically appear within 1 to 2 days and can include oozing from the umbilicus or circumcision site, bloody or black stools, haematuria ecchymoses on the skin and scalp, epistaxis or bleeding from punctures. Early haemorrhagic disease may occur as late as 14 days after birth. Diagnosis is confirmed by findings of prolonged prothrombin time and partial thromboplastin time accompanied by normal platelet count and fibrinogen level. Factor VII levels may be low in early disease, and levels of undercarboxylated proteins (i.e. proteins induced by vitamin K absence, or PIVKA-II) are elevated with mild disease (Greenbaum 2016).

Another form of haemorrhagic disease occurs in infants born to mothers who are taking the antiepileptic drugs phenytoin and phenobarbitone, or warfarin drugs that cross the placenta and interfere with vitamin K function. The newborn may have a severe form of haemorrhagic disease and should be carefully evaluated and treated accordingly. The bleeding is most severe within the first 24 hours of life and may require treatment with intravenous vitamin K and fresh frozen plasma (Greenbaum 2016).

A late form of haemorrhagic disease (late onset) appears at approximately 2 to 12 weeks of age. This form occurs in totally or predominantly breastfed infants who did not receive adequate vitamin K prophylaxis at birth. Although vitamin K levels in breast milk appear to be lower than in cow's milk–based formulas, previous studies indicate that haemorrhagic disease occurred in infants who were exclusively breastfed and who did not receive the standard prophylaxis at birth or were given a single dose of oral vitamin K (Lawrence & Lawrence 2015). Manifestations of late-onset disease include: evidence of intracranial haemorrhage; jaundice; faltering growth; deep ecchymoses; and bleeding from the gastrointestinal tract, mucous membranes, skin punctures or surgical incisions. The WHO recommend that vitamin K should be given to all newborns as a single, intramuscular dose (Tiberi et al 2016).

Therapeutic Management

The goal of management is prevention of haemorrhagic disease of the newborn with prophylactic administration of vitamin K. The current recommendation to prevent haemorrhagic disease in infants who are breastfed is to provide intramuscular vitamin K at birth. The administration of oral vitamin K is currently not recommended to prevent neonatal haemorrhagic disease (Greenbaum 2016).

In newborns with haemorrhagic disease, treatment is the same as the preventive measures except that the vitamin may be given intravenously to prevent a haematoma at an intramuscular site. Bleeding usually ceases within 2 to 4 hours of vitamin K administration.

Nursing Care Management

Nursing care primarily involves prevention through careful administration of the vitamin into the vastus lateralis or ventrogluteal (not dorsogluteal) muscle. In instances in which this procedure is not routinely carried out (e.g. home births or emergency births), the nurse observes for signs of the bleeding disorder and notifies the practitioner for appropriate diagnosis and treatment. Mothers should be encouraged to consume a healthy, well-balanced diet. However, maternal dietary intake of vitamin K–enriched foods has very little impact on the vitamin K content of breast milk due to varying bioavailability of the food source (Phillippi et al 2016).

PROBLEMS CAUSED BY PERINATAL ENVIRONMENTAL FACTORS

Chemical Agents

Prenatal environmental effects from chemicals such as alcohol, medications or drugs, from infectious disease or from radiation or other environmental factors may be regarded as non-genetic causes of congenital anomalies because these substances can produce congenital structural, functional or growth defects. An agent that produces congenital malformations or increases their incidence is called a **teratogen**.

The relationship of the fetal and maternal circulations allows for the interchange of chemical substances across the placental membrane. Many drugs have been suspected of producing congenital malformations, and some have been definitely implicated. Some of the most recognised teratogenic drugs include alcohol, tobacco, antiepileptic medications (valproic acid, phenytoin), isotretinoin, lithium, methotrexate, cocaine and diethylstilboestrol. (See Chapter 9 for information on drug-exposed infants, fetal alcohol syndrome and alcohol-related birth defects.) The limited metabolic capabilities of the fetal liver and its immature enzyme and transport systems render the unborn child ill equipped for maintaining homeostasis when chemical disturbances are imposed by the mother or the environment. This includes both substances produced by the mother in response to a disease state (such as gestational diabetes mellitus) and exogenous substances ingested or inhaled by the mother. Neural tube defects (e.g. anencephaly, myelomeningocele) may be caused in part by folic acid deficiency, so appropriate supplementation before conception is imperative.

The teratogenic effect of drugs is not believed to affect developing tissue until day 15 of gestation, when tissue differentiation begins to take place. Before that time, drugs usually have little effect because they are believed to have an insignificant affinity for undifferentiated tissue. Also, until implantation takes place, at approximately 7 days after conception, the embryo is not exposed to maternal blood that contains the drug. However, some drugs may affect the uterine lining, making it unsuitable for implantation. Drugs administered between days 15 and 90 may produce an effect if the tissue for which the drug has an affinity is in the process of differentiation at that time. After 90 days, when differentiation is complete, most fetal tissues are relatively resistant to teratogenic effects of drugs. However, the impact on ongoing neurological development is not known.

Nursing Care Management

Caution expectant mothers against ingesting any medication without first consulting a practitioner. To help ensure that fewer women will inadvertently take some chemical that might harm the fetus, medication labels are now required to include information regarding the possible teratogenic effects. Excessive use of some commonplace drugs, such as alcohol, valproic acid and isotretinoin, produces characteristic malformations in the fetus. Nurses should also caution mothers-to-be about appropriate dietary intake and necessary supplements should it be impossible to consume a well-balanced diet. One of the goals of preventing birth defects in diabetic mothers is maintenance of strict glycaemic control and avoidance of excessive weight gain.

Radiation

Ionising radiation in large doses has been shown to be both mutagenic and teratogenic in humans. Pelvic irradiation of pregnant women—from natural background radiation that is present everywhere in varying degrees, from occupational exposure or from diagnostic or therapeutic procedures—is believed to be hazardous to the embryo, although the extent of teratogenicity and the exact dosage required to induce somatic change are not yet known. There is a theoretical risk of carcinogenesis when the fetus is exposed to diagnostic radiation; however, with the radiation levels currently used, there are no known risks for congenital malformations or cognitive impairment. These authors present an extensive review of diagnostic radiation methods used for pregnant and lactating mothers. Carlo and Ambalavanan (2016a) indicate that single diagnostic radiation doses are not adequate to cause harm in the fetus. Diagnostic CT and MRI radiation can be modified to decrease the amount of radiation to the fetus. Radiation may damage the conceptus at any time during its prenatal existence, and it is known that rapidly dividing and differentiating cells, such as those of the embryo, have increased radiosensitivity. As with other teratogens, the type of effect produced is closely correlated with the stage of development at which the radiation exposure occurs.

To help prevent the possibility of radiation damage, it is advisable: (1) to avoid unnecessary radiation exposure, such as elective radiographs to the pelvis and abdomen, in women of childbearing age except during the 2 weeks immediately after menstruation; (2) to ascertain whether pregnancy is a possibility; and (3) to advise both men and women who have lower abdominal or pelvic radiographs to avoid conception for several months. Pregnant women should avoid radioactive iodine exposure because iodine has an affinity for fetal thyroid tissue and can lead to developmental problems such as fetal goitre, microcephaly, intrauterine growth restriction, malignancy and death.

REFERENCES

Alencar, T. R. R., Marques, I. L., Bertucci, A. et al. (2017). The Cleft Palate – Craniofacial Journal; Lawrence 54(3), 256–261. DOI:10.1597/14-228

Ambalavanan, N., & Carlo, W. (2016). Jaundice and hyperbilirubinemia in the newborn. In R. M. Kliegman, B. F. Stanton, J. W. St Geme, et al. (Eds.), Nelson textbook of pediatrics (20th ed.). Philadelphia: Elsevier.

American Academy of Pediatrics. (2008). Prevention of rickets and vitamin D deficiency in infants, children, and adolescents. Pediatrics, 122(5), 1142–1148.

American Academy of Pediatrics, Subcommittee on Hyperbilirubinemia. (2004). Clinical practice guideline: Management of hyperbilirubinemia in the newborn infant 35 or more weeks of gestation. Pediatrics, 114(1), 297–316.

Australian Breastfeeding Association. (2017). Breastfeeding babies with clefts of lip and/or palate. https://www.breastfeeding.asn.au/bf-info/cleft

Australasian Cleft Lip & Palate Association Inc. (2017). General cleft lip & palate information: feeding. https://www.cleft.org.au/members/education/

Better Health Channel. (2021). Blood groups. Summary. State of Victoria. https://www.betterhealth.vic.gov.au/health/ConditionsAndTreatments/blood-groups?viewAsPdf=true

Bhutani, V. K., & American Academy of Pediatrics Committee on Fetus and Newborn. (2011). Phototherapy to prevent severe neonatal hyperbilirubinemia in the newborn infant 35 or more weeks of gestation. Pediatrics, 128(4), e1046–e1052.

Bhutani, V. K., Stark, A. R., Lazzeroni, L. C., et al. (2013). Predischarge screening for severe neonatal hyperbilirubinemia identifies infants who need phototherapy. The Journal of Pediatrics, 162(3), 477–482.

Blackburn, S. (2013). Maternal, fetal, and neonatal physiology: A clinical perspective (4th ed.). St Louis, MO: Saunders.

Boies, E. G., Vaucher, Y. E., & the Academy of Breastfeeding Medicine. (2016). ABM Clinical Protocol #10: Breastfeeding the Late Preterm (34–36 6/7 Weeks of Gestation) and Early Term Infants (37–38 6/7 Weeks of Gestation), Second Revision 2016. Breastfeeding Medicine, 11(10), 494–500.

Bratlid, D., Nakstad, B., & Hansen, T. W. (2011). National guidelines for treatment of jaundice in the newborn. Acta Paediatrica, 100(4), 499–505.

Breugem, C. C., Evans, K. N., Poets, C. F., et al. (2016). Best practices for the diagnosis and evaluation of infants with Robin Sequence. JAMA Pediatrics, 9, 894–902.

Carlo, W. A., & Ambalavanan, N. (2016a). Radiation. In R. M. Kliegman, B. F. Stanton, J. W. St Geme, et al. (Eds.), Nelson textbook of pediatrics (20th ed.). Philadelphia: Elsevier.

Carlo, W. A., & Ambalavanan, N. (2016b). Peripheral nerve injuries. In R. M. Kliegman, B. F. Stanton, J. W. St Geme, et al. (Eds.), Nelson textbook of pediatrics (20th ed.). Philadelphia: Elsevier.

Cauchemez, S., Besnard, M., Bompard, P., et al. (2016). Association between Zika virus and microcephaly in French Polynesia, 2013–15: A retrospective study. Lancet (London, England), 387(10033), 2125–2132.

Chen, T. S., Eichenfield, L. F., & Friedlander, S. F. (2013). Infantile hemangiomas: An update on pathogenesis and therapy. Pediatrics, 131(1), 99–108.

Chibueze, E. C., Tirado, V., Lopes, K., et al. (2017). Zika virus infection in pregnancy: A systematic review of disease course and complications. Reproductive Health, 14(28), 1–14.

Children's Health Queensland Hospital and Health Service. (2018). Craniosynostosis. South Brisbane: Queensland Government. https://www.childrens.health.qld.gov.au/fact-sheet-craniosynostosis/

Cicchetti, R., Cascone, P., Caresta, E., et al. (2012). Mandibular distraction osteogenesis for neonates with Pierre Robin sequence and airway obstruction. The Journal of Maternal-fetal and Neonatal Medicine, 25(Suppl. 4), 141–143.

Craig ME., Twigg SM., Donaghue KC., et al. for the Australian Type 1 Diabetes Guidelines Expert Advisory Group. (2011). National evidence-based clinical care guidelines for type 1 diabetes in children, adolescents and adults, Australian Government Department of Health and Ageing, Canberra. https://www.schn.health.nsw.gov.au/files/attachments/diabetes_in_children.pdf

de Araújo, T.V.B., de Alencar Ximenes R.A., Miranda-Filho, D. de B., et al. (2018). Association between microcephaly, Zika virus infection, and other risk factors in Brazil: final report of a case-control study, The Lancet Infectious Diseases, 18(3). https://doi.org/10.1016/S1473-3099(17)30727-2.

Demirel, G., Akar, M., Celik, I. H., et al. (2011). Single versus multiple dose intravenous immunoglobulin in combination with LED phototherapy in the treatment of ABO hemolytic disease in neonates. International Journal of Hematology, 93(6), 700–703.

Doyle, D. A. (2016). Hypoparathyroidism. In R. M. Kliegman, B. F. Stanton, J. W. St Geme, et al. (Eds.), Nelson textbook of pediatrics (20th ed.). Philadelphia: Elsevier.

Elalfy, M. S., Elbarbary, N. S., & Abaza, H. W. (2011). Early intravenous immunoglobulin (two-dose regimen) in the management of severe Rh hemolytic disease of newborn—a prospective randomized controlled trial. European Journal of Pediatrics, 170(4), 461–467.

Feldman, H. S., Jones, K. L., Lindsay, S., et al. (2012). Prenatal alcohol exposure patterns and alcohol-related birth defects and growth deficiencies: A prospective study. Alcoholism, Clinical and Experimental Research, 36(4), 670–676.

Gailey, D. G. (2016). Feeding infants with cleft and the postoperative cleft management. Oral and Maxillofacial Surgery Clinics of North America, 28, 153–159.

Government of South Australia, Department for Health and Wellbeing. (2019). South Australian Paediatric Clinical Practice Guidelines. Propranolol in infantile haemangioma. Government of South Australia. https://www.sahealth.sa.gov.au/wps/wcm/connect/e1c9ef804233d33986aeeeef0dac2aff/Propranolol+for+Infantile+Haemangioma_Paed_v2_0.pdf?MOD=AJPERES&CACHEID=ROOTWORKSPACE-e1c9ef804233d33986aeeeef0dac2aff-mOX.9Sq

Greenbaum, L. A. (2016). Vitamin K deficiency. In R. M. Kliegman, B. F. Stanton, J. W. St Geme, et al. (Eds.), Nelson textbook of pediatrics (20th ed.). Philadelphia: Elsevier.

Hall, K. M., Besachio, D. A., Moore, M. D., et al. (2017). Effectiveness of screening for craniosynostosis with ultrasound: A retrospective review. Pediatric Radiology, 47(5), 606–612.

Hartzell, L. D., & Buckmiller, L. M. (2012). Current management of infantile hemangiomas and their common associated conditions. Otolaryngologic Clinics of North America, 45(3), 545–556.

Hawdon, J. (2014). Neonatal hypoglycemia: Are evidence-based clinical guidelines available? Neoreviews, 15, 91–98.

Health Direct (n.d.) Cleft lip and cleft palate. https://www.healthdirect.gov.au/cleft-lip-and-cleft-palate

Health Navigator New Zealand. (2020). Birth Defects. Overview. https://www.healthnavigator.org.nz/health-a-z/b/birth-defects/

Hedequist, D., Shah, S. & Yaszay, B. (2018). The Management of Disorders of the Child's Cervical Spine. (1st ed.) New York, NY : Springer US : Imprint: Springer; 2018

Hendrickson, J. E., & Delaney, M. (2016). Hemolytic disease of the fetus and newborn: Modern practice and future investigations. Transfusion Medicine Reviews, 30, 159–164.

Hervey-Jumper, S. L., Justice, D., & Vanaman, M. M. (2011). Torticollis associated with neonatal brachial plexus palsy. Pediatric Neurology, 45(5), 305–310.

Johnson, P. J. (2016). Head, eyes, ears, nose, mouth and neck assessment. In E. P. Tappero & M. E. Honeyfield (Eds.), Physical assessment of the newborn: a comprehensive approach to the art of physical assessment (5th ed.). New York: Springer Publishing Company.

Kinsman, S. L., & Johnston, M. V. (2016). Congenital anomalies of the central nervous system. In R. M. Kleigman, B. F. Stanton, J. W. St Geme, et al. (Eds.), Nelson textbook of pediatrics (20th ed.). Philadelphia: Elsevier.

Labreze, C. L., Harper, H. I., & Hoeger, P. H. (Jan 12, 2017). Infantile haemangioma. Lancet.

Lawrence, R. A., & Lawrence, R. M. (2015). Breastfeeding: a guide for the medical profession (8th ed.). Philadelphia: Elsevier.

Maisels, M. J. (2015). Managing the jaundiced newborn: A persistent challenge. Canadian Medical Association Journal, 187(5), 335–343.

Maisels, M. J., Watchko, J. F., Bhutani, V. K., et al. (2012). An approach to the management of hyperbilirubinemia in the preterm infant less than 35 weeks of gestation. Journal of Perinatology, 32(9), 660–664.

Maisels, M. J., & Yang, H. (2012). Tin-mesoporphyrin in the treatment of refractory hyperbilirubinemia due to Rh incompatibility. Journal of Perinatology, 32(11), 899–900.

Martin, K. L. (2016). Vascular disorders. In R. M. Kliegman, B. F. Stanton, J. W. St Geme, et al. (Eds.), Nelson textbook of pediatrics (20th ed.). Philadelphia: Elsevier.

McCance, K., & Huether, S. (2014). Pathophysiology: The biological basis for disease in adults and children (7th ed.). St Louis, MO: Mosby.

McCarty, D., Peat, J., Malcolm, W., et al. (2016). Dolichocephaly in preterm infants: Prevalence, risk factors, and early motor outcomes. American Journal of Perinatology, 1–7.

McKinlay, C., Alsweiler, J. M., Ansell, J. M., et al, for the Children with Hypoglycemia and their Later Development. (2015). Neonatal glycemia and neurodevelopmental outcomes at 2 years. The New England Journal of Medicine, 373(16), 1507–1518.

Modanlou, H., Hutson, S., & Merritt, A. T. (2016). Early blood transfusion and resolution of disseminated intravascular coagulation associated with massive subgaleal haemorrhage. Neonatal Network, 35(1), 37–41.

Moise, K. J. (2012). Red cell alloimmunization. In S. G. Gabbe, J. R. Niebyl, K. L. Simpson, et al. (Eds.), Obstetrics: Normal and problem pregnancies (6th ed.). London: Churchill Livingstone.

Moise, K. J., & Argoti, P. S. (2012). Management and prevention of red cell alloimmunization in pregnancy: A systematic review. Obstetrics and Gynecology, 120(5), 1132–1139.

O'Toole, P., & Spiegel, D. A. (2016). The neck: Torticollis. In R. M. Kliegman, B. F. Stanton, J. W. St Geme, et al. (Eds.), Nelson textbook of pediatrics (20th ed.). Philadelphia: Elsevier.

Parsons, J. A., Seay, A. R., & Jacobson, M. (2016). Neurologic disorders. In S. L. Gardner, B. S. Carter, M. Enzman-Hines, et al. (Eds.), Merenstein and Gardner's handbook of neonatal intensive care (8th ed.). St Louis, MO: Mosby Elsevier.

Passi, D., Sharma, S., Dutta, S. R., et al. (2017). Zika virus diseases: The new face of an ancient enemy as global public health emergency (2016): Brief review and recent updates. International Journal of Preventive Medicine, 8(6).

Phillippi, J. C., Holley, S. L., Morad, A., et al. (2016). Prevention of vitamin K deficiency bleeding. See comment in PubMed Commons below. Journal of Midwifery and Women's Health, 4, 632–636.

Raising Children Network (Australia). (2021). Birthmarks. A-Z Health Reference. https://raisingchildren.net.au/guides/a-z-health-reference/birthmarks#infantile-strawberry-haemangiomas-nav-title

Raizman, J. E., Shea, J., Daly, C. H., et al. (2016). Clinical impact of improved point-of-care glucose monitoring in neonatal intensive care using Nova StatStrip: Evidence for improved accuracy, better sensitivity, and reduced test utilization. Clinical Biochemistry, 49, 879–884.

Roland, E., & Hill, A. (2016). Neurological problems of the newborn. In R. D. Daruff, J. Jankovic, J. C. Mazziotta, et al. (Eds.), Bradley's neurology in clinical practice (7th ed.). Philadelphia: Elsevier.

Schwartz, H. P., Haberman, B. E., & Ruddy, R. M. (2011). Hyperbilirubinemia: Current guidelines and emerging therapies. Pediatric Emergency Care, 27(9), 884–889.

Scott, A. R., Tibesar, R. J., Lander, T. A., et al. (2011). Mandibular distraction osteogenesis in infants younger than 3 months. Archives of Facial Plastic Surgery, 13(3), 173–179.

Shah, N. A., & Wusthoff, C. J. (2016). Intracranial haemorrhage in the neonate. Neonatal Network, 35(2), 67–72.

Sharma, D. (2016). Golden 60 minutes of newborn's life: Part 1: Preterm neonate. The Journal of Maternal-Fetal & Neonatal Medicine: The Official Journal of the European Association of Perinatal Medicine, the Federation of Asia and Oceania Perinatal Societies, the International Society of Perinatal Obstetricians, 1–12.

Shulman, S. T. (2016). Group A Streptococcus. In R. M. Kliegman, B. F. Stanton, J. W. St Geme, et al. (Eds.), Nelson textbook of pediatrics (20th ed.). Philadelphia: Elsevier.

Smith, A., Kandamany, H., Okafor, I., et al. (2016). Delayed infant subaponeurotic (subgaleal) fluid collections: A case series of 11 infants. The Journal of Emergency Medicine, 50(6), 881–886.

Sperling, M. A. (2016). Hypoglycemia. In R. M. Kliegman, B. F. Stanton, J. W. St Geme, et al. (Eds.), Nelson textbook of pediatrics (20th ed.). Philadelphia: Elsevier.

Stokowski, L. A. (2011). Fundamentals of phototherapy for neonatal jaundice. Advances in Neonatal Care: Official Journal of the National Association of Neonatal Nurses, 11(5S), S10–S21.

Tam, E. W., Haeusslein, L. A., Bonifacio, S. L., et al. (2012). Hypoglycemia associated with increased risk for brain injury and adverse neurodevelopmental outcome in neonates at risk for encephalopathy. The Journal of Pediatrics, 161(1), 88–93.

Tappero, E. (2016). Musculoskeletal system assessment. In E. Tappero & M. A. Honeyfield (Eds.), Physical assessment of the newborn: a comprehensive approach to the art of physical examination (5th ed.). New York: Springer Publishing Company.

Taylor, J. A., Burgos, A. E., Flaherman, V., et al, on behalf of the BORN Investigators. (2016). Utility of decision rules for transcutaneous bilirubin measurements. Pediatrics, 137(5), 1–8.

The Royal Children's Hospital Melbourne (RCHM). (2018). Brachial plexus palsy or Erb's palsy. August. https://www.rch.org.au/kidsinfo/fact_sheets/Brachial_plexus_palsy/

The Royal Children's Hospital Melbourne (RCHM). (2020). Clinical Practice Guidelines (Nursing). Neonatal hypoglycaemia. October. https://www.rch.org.au/rchcpg/hospital_clinical_guideline_index/Neonatal_hypoglycaemia/

The Royal Women's Hospital. (2018). Breast and nipple thrush. June. https://thewomens.r.worldssl.net/images/uploads/fact-sheets/Breast-nipple-thrush-2018.pdf

Tiberi, E., Cota, F., Barone, G., et al. (2016). Continuous glucose monitoring in preterm infants: Evaluation by a modified Clarke error grid. Italian Journal of Pediatrics, 42(29), 1–7.

Victorian Agency for Health Information (VAHI) & Safer Care Victoria (SCV). (2018). Jaundice in neonates. December. https://www.bettersafercare.vic.gov.au/clinical-guidance/neonatal/jaundice-in-neonates

VAHI & SCV. (2020). Herpes simplex virus (HSV) in neonates. 12 November. https://www.bettersafercare.vic.gov.au/clinical-guidance/neonatal/herpes-simplex-virus-hsv-in-neonates

Wang, A., Wohrley, J., & Rosebush, J. (2017). Herpes simplex virus in the neonate. Pediatric Annals, 46(2), e42–e46.

Wight, N., Marinelli, K., & Academy of Breastfeeding Medicine. (2014). Guidelines for blood glucose monitoring and treatment of hypoglycemia in term and late-preterm neonates. Breastfeeding Medicine, 9(4), 173–179.

Wilson, T. J., Chang, K. W. C., Chauhan, S. P., et al. (2016). Peripartum and neonatal factors associated with the persistence of neonatal brachial plexus palsy at 1 year: A review of 382 cases. Journal of Neurosurgery. Pediatrics, 17, 618–624.

World Health Organization (WHO). (2020). e-Library of Evidence for Nutrition Actions (eLENA) Exclusive breastfeeding for optimal growth, development and health of infants. https://www.who.int/elena/titles/exclusive_breastfeeding/en/

9

The High-risk Newborn and Family

Sarah Dechert, Tameeka Mulquiney & Lisa Speedie

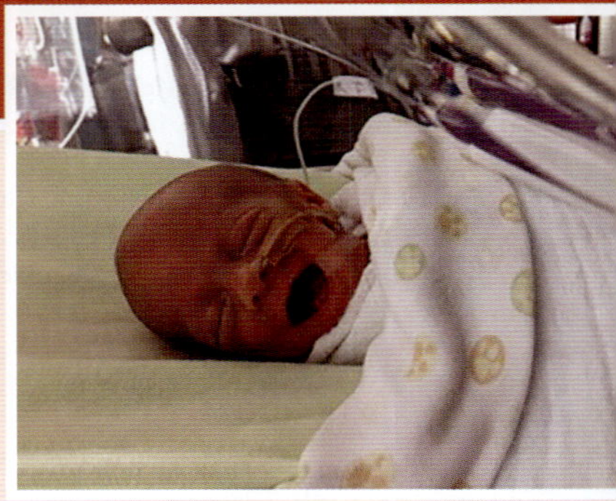

LEARNING OBJECTIVES

- Care of premature and postterm infant
- Describe common illnesses that occur in the high-risk newborn
- Assess the high-risk newborn and plan for the expected outcomes with the family
- Discuss the care of the high-risk newborn and apply family-centred care

GENERAL MANAGEMENT OF HIGH-RISK NEWBORNS

Identification of High-risk Newborns

The **high-risk neonate** is a newborn, regardless of gestational age or birth weight, with a greater-than-average chance of morbidity or mortality, usually because of conditions beyond the normal events related to birth and subsequent adjustment to extrauterine life. The high-risk period begins at the time of viability (i.e. the gestational age at which survival outside the uterus is thought possible, or as early as 24 weeks' gestation) up to 28 days after birth and includes threats to life and health that occur during the prenatal, perinatal and postnatal periods (Queensland Health 2020).

In the past, the late-premature infants of 34 to 36.6 weeks' gestation often received the same treatment as term infants. Late-premature infants actually experience morbidities that are similar to those of premature infants: respiratory distress, hypoglycaemia requiring treatment, jaundice, feeding difficulties and adverse neurodevelopmental outcomes (Gill & Boyle 2017, Natarajan & Shankaran 2016). Assessment and prompt intervention in life-threatening perinatal emergencies often make the difference between a favourable outcome and a lifetime of disability. The nurse/midwife in the neonatal intensive care unit (NICU) knows the characteristics of neonates and recognises the significance of serious deviations from expected observations. The probability of a successful outcome increases when the care team anticipates the need for specialised care and plans for it.

Late-premature Infant

Within the past two decades, several significant changes have occurred in neonatal care. Early postpartum discharge for term and premature infants gained popularity as healthcare institutions attempted to cut healthcare costs. Infants who appeared to be 'near' term began to be treated much like term infants, avoiding the costs of neonatal intensive care for infants who appeared to be healthy. Experts have recommended that infants born between 34 and 36 weeks' gestation be referred to as **late-premature infants** rather than *near-term infants* (Natarajan & Shankaran 2016). Late-premature infants may transition effectively to extrauterine life. However, because of their limited gestation, they remain at risk for problems related to feeding, breathing, neurodevelopment, thermoregulation, hypoglycaemia, hyperbilirubinemia and sepsis (Gill & Boyle 2017, Natarajan & Shankaran 2016). Studies have shown an increased risk for children born at 34 to 36 weeks to be diagnosed with cerebral palsy (CP) (Gill & Boyle 2017, Natarajan & Shankaran 2016). Late- and moderate-premature infants represent an estimated 70% of the total premature infant population. The mortality rate for this group is up to five times higher than that of term infants (Bulut et al 2016, De Carolis et al 2016, Natarajan & Shankaran 2016). Because late-premature infants' birth weights often range from 2000 to 2500 g and they appear relatively mature in comparison to smaller premature infants, they may be cared for in the same way as healthy term infants and their risk factors may be overlooked. Late-premature infants are often discharged early and have a three-fold higher rate of rehospitalisation than term infants (Natarajan & Shankaran 2016). Discussions regarding high-risk infants in this chapter also refer to late-premature infants who are experiencing a delayed transition to extrauterine life.

The *Assessment and Care of the Late Premature Infant* guide (Perry et al 2017) teaches perinatal nurses or midwives about the late-premature infant's risk factors and appropriate care and follow-up (Table 9.1).

Classification of High-risk Newborns

High-risk infants are most often classified according to birth weight, gestational age and main pathophysiological problems. The more common problems related to physiological status involve the infant's maturity and usually chemical disturbances (e.g. hypoglycaemia, hypocalcaemia) and consequences of immature organs and systems (e.g. hyperbilirubinaemia, respiratory distress, hypothermia). Box 9.1 outlines terms describing the developmental status of the newborn.

Weight at birth formerly reflected a reasonably accurate estimation of gestational age; that is, if an infant's birth weight exceeded 2500 g, the infant was considered mature. However, accumulated data have shown that intrauterine growth rates are not the same for all infants and that other factors (e.g. heredity, placental insufficiency and maternal disease) affect intrauterine growth and the infant's birth weight. From these data a more meaningful classification system that encompasses birth weight, gestational age and neonatal outcome has been developed. It has also been found that the lowest perinatal mortality rate occurs in the infant who weighs between 3000 and 4000 g and whose gestational age is between 37 and 42 weeks (Walsh & Fanaroff 2015). (See Fig 7.2 for size comparison of newborn infants.)

TABLE 9.1 Late-premature Infant Assessment and Interventions

Risk Factors	Assessment	Interventions*
Respiratory distress	Assess for cardinal signs of respiratory distress (nasal flaring, grunting, tachypnoea, central cyanosis, retractions) and presence of apnoea, especially during feedings. Assess for hypothermia, hypoglycaemia.	Perform gestational age assessment. Observe for signs of respiratory distress; monitor oxygenation by pulse oximetry; provide supplemental oxygen judiciously.
Thermal instability	Monitor axillary temperature every 30 minutes immediately postpartum until stable; thereafter every 1–4 hours, depending on gestational age and ability to maintain thermal stability.	Provide skin-to-skin care in immediate postpartum period for stable infant. Implement measures to avoid excess heat loss (adjust environmental temperature, avoid draughts). Bathe only after thermal stability has been maintained for 1 hour.
Hypoglycaemia	Monitor for signs and symptoms of hypoglycaemia. Assess feeding ability (latch-on, nipple-feeding). Assess thermal stability and signs and symptoms of respiratory distress. Monitor bedside glucose in infants with additional risk factors (IDM, prolonged labour, respiratory distress, poor feeding).	Initiate early feedings of human milk or formula. Avoid water feedings. Provide IV glucose as necessary for hypoglycaemia.
Jaundice	Observe for appearance of jaundice in first 24 hours. Evaluate maternal–fetal history for additional risk factors that may cause increased haemolysis and circulating levels of unconjugated bilirubin (Rh, ABO, spherocytosis, bruising). Assess feeding method, voiding and stooling patterns.	Monitor transcutaneous or serum bilirubin and note risk zone on hour-specific nomogram (see Fig 8.11).
Feeding problems	Assess suck-swallow and breathing. Assess for respiratory distress, hypoglycaemia, thermal stability. Assess latch-on, maternal comfort with feeding method. Determine weight loss (should be ≤ 10% of birth weight).	Initiate early feedings (human milk or formula). Ensure maternal knowledge of feeding method and signs of inadequate feeding (sleepiness, lethargy, colour changes during feeding, apnoea during feeding, decreased or absent urine output).
Neurodevelopmental problems	Assess for respiratory distress, neonatal jaundice, hypoglycaemia and thermal instability. Assess neurodevelopmental status. Assess for seizure activity.	Perform newborn screening, including hearing test. Implement individualised developmental care. Encourage parents to keep follow-up appointments with primary care provider for evaluation of growth and development (including cognitive function and achievement of appropriate milestones).
Infection	Evaluate maternal–fetal history for risk factors that may contribute to neonatal septicaemia. Assess for signs and symptoms of neonatal infection.	Use standard precautions, especially handwashing between infants and contact with surfaces that may harbour bacteria. Maintain thermal stability. Administer hepatitis B vaccine. Encourage breastfeeding and assist mother–baby pair with breastfeeding. Encourage parents to decrease infant exposure to respiratory viruses post-discharge and obtain vaccines as appropriate to prevent development of respiratory viruses (e.g. influenza).

*This is not an exhaustive list of nursing interventions; additional interventions include those discussed under the care of the high-risk infant in this chapter.

IDM, Infant of diabetic mother; *IV,* intravenous.

Source: Portions adapted from Askin, D. F., Bakewell-Sachs, S., Medoff-Cooper, B., et al (2010). Late premature infant assessment guide. Washington, DC: Association of Women's Health, Obstetric and Neonatal Nurses.

Many perinatal problems can be anticipated before birth. Prenatal testing and labour monitoring have reduced perinatal mortality rate, and specialised care of the distressed newborn is improving the survival rate. If the infant is likely to require special therapy at or soon after birth, plans can be made for the birth to take place at a hospital with the appropriate level of care. This eliminates delay in starting care and avoids some of the dangers associated with transporting the sick newborn. Prenatal evaluation of fetal wellbeing along with advanced surgical and anaesthetic techniques have made intrauterine treatment of certain pathological conditions possible, while enhancing the neonate's chances for survival.

Intensive Care Facilities

Intensive care of the ill and immature newborn requires specialised knowledge and skill in a number of areas. Much of the equipment used in the care of the critically ill adult is unsuited to the needs of the very small infant, so equipment has been modified to meet these needs.

Family-centred care and a quieter environment are often difficult to provide in a busy NICU, so some units have developed step-down and single-room units where staff can observe high-risk infants. Such areas are designed for family-centred care alongside appropriate neurodevelopmental care.

BOX 9.1 Classification of High-Risk Infants

Classification According to Size

Appropriate-for-gestational-age (AGA) infant—An infant whose weight falls between the 10th and 90th percentiles on intrauterine growth curves

Extremely low-birth-weight (ELBW) infant—An infant whose birth weight is less than 1000 g

Intrauterine growth restriction (IUGR)—Found in infants whose intrauterine growth is restricted (sometimes used as a more descriptive term for the SGA infant)

Large-for-gestational-age (LGA) infant—An infant whose birth weight falls above the 90th percentile on intrauterine growth charts

Low-birth-weight (LBW) infant—An infant whose birth weight is less than 2500 g, regardless of gestational age

Small-for-date (SFD) or small-for-gestational-age (SGA) infant—An infant whose rate of intrauterine growth was slowed and whose birth weight falls below the 10th percentile on intrauterine growth curves

Very-low-birth-weight (VLBW) infant—An infant whose birth weight is less than 1500 g

Classification According to Gestational Age

Full-term infant—An infant born between the beginning of 38 weeks and the completion of 42 weeks ofweeks' gestation, regardless of birth weight

Late-premature infant—An infant born between 34 and 36.6 weeks of gestation, regardless of birth weight

Postterm (postmature) infant—An infant born after 42 weeks of gestational age, regardless of birth weight

Premature (premature) infant—An infant born before completion of 37 weeks of gestation, regardless of birth weight

Classification Aaccording to Mortality

Fetal death—Death of the fetus after 20 weeks of gestation and before birth, with absence of any signs of life after birth

Live birth—Birth in which the neonate manifests any heartbeat, breathes or displays voluntary movement, regardless of gestational age

Neonatal death—Death that occurs in the first 27 days of life; early neonatal death occurs in the first week of life; late neonatal death occurs at 7 to 27 days

Perinatal mortality—Describes the total number of fetal and early neonatal deaths per 1000 live births

Postnatal death—Death that occurs at 28 days to 1 year after birth

Organisation of Services

The most efficient organisation of services is a regionalised system. Neonatal intensive care facilities may provide six prescribed levels of care with special equipment, skilled personnel and ancillary services concentrated in a centralised institution (Victoria State Government 2020b).

Current classifications come under six levels: Level 1 and Level 2—primary newborn services; Levels 3, 4 and 5—secondary newborn services; and Levels 6A and 6B—tertiary. Each level increases in care needs for the newborn and length of time of support that the newborn requires. Details of type of care and length of stay may vary within Australia and New Zealand. The following websites are some examples of where further information can be found.

- Newborn care in Victoria: https://www2.health.vic.gov.au/hospitals-and-health-services/patient-care/perinatal-reproductive/maternity-newborn-services/newborn-care-in-victoria
- Maternity care during the birth: https://www.health.govt.nz/your-health/pregnancy-and-kids/services-and-support-during-pregnancy/maternity-care-during-birth

Transporting High-risk Newborns

When an at-risk infant is identified or anticipated, arrangements are made for care in the intensive care facility. The uterus is the ideal transport unit for the infant with anticipated difficulties: whenever possible, transport the mother to where special care is available for giving birth.

The infant must be kept warm, be adequately oxygenated (including intubation if indicated), have vital signs and oxygen saturation monitored and, when indicated, receive an intravenous (IV) infusion. The infant is transported in a specially designed incubator unit that contains a complete life-support system and other emergency equipment that can be carried by ambulance, plane or helicopter.

NURSING CARE OF HIGH-RISK NEWBORNS

Because the majority of infants admitted to intensive care facilities are born before the estimated due date, this chapter focuses primarily on the premature infant. The rate of neonatal complications (e.g. respiratory distress and hypoglycaemia) is highest in this group, and often other high-risk factors (e.g. sepsis and congenital malformations) are associated with prematurity.

Assessment

At birth the newborn is given a thorough assessment to determine any apparent problems and identify those that demand immediate attention. This examination is most concerned with the evaluation of cardiopulmonary and neurological functions. The assessment includes the assignment of an Apgar score (see Chapter 7) and an evaluation for any obvious congenital anomalies or evidence of neonatal distress. The infant is stabilised and evaluated before being transported to the NICU for therapy and more extensive assessment. (See Clinical Assessment of Gestational Age, Chapter 7.)

NURSING CARE CONSIDERATIONS

Physical Assessment

General Assessment

- Using electronic scale, weigh daily or as the baby's condition dictates.
- Measure length and head circumference periodically.
- Describe general body shape and size, posture at rest, ease of breathing, presence and location of oedema.
- Describe any apparent deformities.
- Describe any signs of distress (e.g. poor colour, mottling, hypotonia).

Respiratory Assessment

- Describe shape of chest (e.g. concave, barrel shaped), symmetry, chest tubes or other deviations.
- Describe use of accessory muscles: nasal flaring or substernal, intercostal or suprasternal retractions.
- Determine respiratory rate and regularity.
- Auscultate and describe breath sounds: stridor, crackles, wheezing, areas of absence of sound, grunting, diminished air entry, equality of breath sounds.

NURSING CARE CONSIDERATIONS

Physical Assessment—cont'd

- Determine whether suctioning is needed.
- Describe ambient oxygen and method of delivery; if intubated, describe size of tube, type of ventilator and settings and method of securing tube.
- Determine oxygen saturation by pulse oximetry.

Cardiovascular Assessment

- Determine heart rate and rhythm.
- Describe heart sounds, including any murmurs.
- Determine the point of maximum intensity (PMI), the point at which the heartbeat sounds and palpates loudest (a change in the PMI may indicate a mediastinal shift).
- Describe infant's colour (abnormalities may be of cardiac, respiratory or haematopoietic origin): cyanosis, pallor, plethora, jaundice, mottling.
- Assess colour of mucous membranes and lips.
- Determine blood pressure. Indicate extremity used and cuff size.
- Describe peripheral pulses, capillary refill ($<$ 2 to 3 seconds), peripheral perfusion (mottling).
- Describe monitors, their parameters and whether alarms are in 'on' position.

Gastrointestinal Assessment

- Determine presence of abdominal distension: increase in circumference, shiny skin, evidence of abdominal wall erythema, visible peristalsis, visible loops of bowel, status of umbilicus.
- Determine any signs of regurgitation and time related to feeding; character and amount of residual if gavage fed; if nasogastric tube in place, describe type of suction, drainage (e.g. colour, consistency).
- Describe amount, colour and consistency of any emesis.
- Palpate liver margin.
- Describe amount, colour and consistency of stools.
- Describe bowel sounds: presence or absence.

Genitourinary Assessment

- Describe any abnormalities of genitalia.
- Describe urine amount (as determined by weight), colour, pH and specific gravity (to screen for adequacy of hydration).

Neurological-Musculoskeletal Assessment

- Describe infant's movements (e.g. random, purposeful, jittery, twitching, spontaneous, elicited); level of activity with stimulation; evaluate based on gestational age.
- Describe infant's position or attitude: flexed, extended.
- Describe reflexes observed: Moro, sucking, Babinski's, plantar and other age-appropriate reflexes.
- Determine level of response and consolability.
- Determine changes in head circumference (if indicated); size and tension of fontanels, suture lines.

Temperature

- Determine axillary temperature.
- Determine relationship to environmental temperature.

Skin Assessment

- Describe any discolouration, reddened area, signs of irritation, blisters, abrasions or denuded areas, especially where monitoring equipment, infusions or other apparatus come in contact with skin; also check and note any skin preparation used (e.g. povidone-iodine).
- Determine texture and turgor of skin: dry, smooth, flaky, peeling, etc.
- Describe any rash, skin lesion or birthmarks.
- Determine whether intravenous infusion catheter is in place, and observe for signs of infiltration.
- Describe parenteral infusion lines: location, type (e.g. arterial, venous, peripheral, umbilical, central, peripherally inserted central catheter); type of infusion (e.g. medication, saline, glucose, electrolytes, lipids, total parenteral nutrition); type of infusion pump and rate of flow; type of catheter; and appearance of insertion site.

Monitoring Physiological Data

Most neonates under intensive observation are placed in a controlled thermal environment and monitored for heart rate, respiratory activity and temperature. The monitoring devices are equipped with an alarm system that indicates when the vital signs are above or below preset limits. However, a 'hands-on' assessment, including auscultation of heart tones and breath sounds, is essential.

The placement of electrodes may be challenging because of the lack of flat areas on the neonate's chest, the limited space for alternating sites, the size of the electrodes and irritation from the adhesive.

In the NICU frequent pathology examinations and their interpretation are integral parts of the ongoing assessment of infants' progress. The nurse/midwife keeps accurate intake and output records on all acutely ill infants. An accurate output can be obtained by collecting urine in a plastic urine collection bag specifically made for premature infants (see Urine Specimens, Chapter 22) or by weighing the nappies, which is the simplest and least traumatic means of measuring urinary output. The pre-weighed wet nappy is weighed on a gram scale, and the gram weight of the urine is converted directly to millilitres (e.g. 25 g = 25 mL).

Pathology examinations are a necessary part of the ongoing assessment and monitoring of the sick newborn's progress. The tests most often performed are blood glucose, bilirubin, electrolytes, calcium, haematocrit and blood gases. Samples may be obtained by heel stick, venepuncture, arterial puncture or an indwelling catheter in an umbilical vein, umbilical artery or peripheral artery. When collecting blood samples from the heel, studies have shown that the use of alternative therapies (e.g. non-nutritive sucking, oral sucrose, mechanical vibration, skin-to-skin contact) results in less pain and trauma for infants in the NICU (McGinnis et al 2016, Yin et al 2015). When skilled phlebotomists are available, venepuncture for blood collections may be preferred.

When infants require close monitoring of oxygenation, **pulse oximetry**, a non-invasive measurement of the saturation or per cent of oxygen in haemoglobin, is typically used. The nurse/midwife notes changes in oxygenation (or other aspects being monitored) associated with handling and adjusts the infant's care accordingly. The frequency of taking vital signs depends on the infant's acuity level and response to handling.

Safety Measures

The increased sophistication of supportive technology, including birth systems, monitors, ventilator devices and warmers, creates technology dependence for nurses/midwives providing care to high-risk infants. Although built-in safety systems and better engineering have made these devices more reliable and easier to use, our increasing reliance on them carries with it the additional risks of electrical biohazards and inaccurate function.

Respiratory Support

The primary objective in the care of high-risk infants is to establish and maintain respiration. Many infants require supplemental oxygen and assisted ventilation. All infants require appropriate positioning to ensure an open airway and to maximise oxygenation and ventilation. Oxygen therapy is provided on the basis of the infant's requirements and illness.

Thermoregulation

Along with the establishment of respiration, the most crucial need of the low-birth-weight (LBW) infant is external warmth. Prevention of heat loss in the distressed infant is essential for survival, and maintaining a neutral thermal environment is a challenging aspect of neonatal intensive nursing care. Heat production is a complicated process that involves the cardiovascular, neurological and metabolic systems, and the immature neonate has all the problems related to heat production that are faced by the full-term infant. (See Thermoregulation, Chapter 7.) However, LBW infants are placed at further disadvantage by a number of additional problems. They have an even smaller muscle mass and fewer deposits of brown fat for producing heat, lack insulating subcutaneous fat and have poor reflex control of skin capillaries.

Pathophysiology. The immature neonate, who cannot increase activity and lacks a shivering response, produces heat mainly through increasing metabolic rate. Some heat is generated by liver, heart, brain and skeletal muscles, but the major source of increased heat production during cold stress is **non-shivering thermogenesis**. Noradrenaline, secreted by the sympathetic nerve endings in response to chilling, stimulates fat metabolism in the richly vascularised brown adipose tissue to produce internal heat, which is then conducted through the blood to surface tissues. A significant increase in metabolism requires increased oxygen consumption.

Cold stress poses hazards to the neonate through hypoxia, metabolic acidosis and hypoglycaemia. Increased metabolism in response to chilling creates a compensatory increase in oxygen and calorie consumption.

Noradrenaline released in response to cold stress causes pulmonary vasoconstriction, which further reduces the effectiveness of pulmonary ventilation. Decreased oxygen intake reduces the supply available for glucose metabolism. As a result, glucose is broken down by an alternative, hypoxic pathway (anaerobic glycolysis) that generates increased lactic acid. This, together with acid end-products of brown fat metabolism, contributes to the acidotic state. Anaerobic metabolism consumes glycogen at a faster rate compared with aerobic metabolism, causing hypoglycaemia. This condition is especially marked when glycogen stores are diminished at birth and caloric intake is inadequate after birth.

Maintaining Thermoregulation. To delay or prevent the effects of cold stress, at-risk newborns are placed in a heated environment immediately after birth, where they remain until they are able to independently maintain **thermal stability**—a balance of heat production and conservation and heat dissipation. Because overheating produces an increase in oxygen and calorie consumption, the infant is also compromised in a hyperthermic environment.

An automatically controlled (servocontrolled) incubator is an effective means for maintaining the desired range of temperature in the infant. The mechanism adjusts automatically in response to preset limits and signals from a thermal sensor attached to the abdomen. If the infant's temperature drops, the warming device is triggered to increase heat output. The servocontrol is usually set to a desired skin temperature between 36°C and 36.5°C (Gardner & Hernandez 2016).

Convective heat loss occurs when infants are exposed to increased air flow velocity and turbulence (e.g. draughts from doors, ventilation system, opening and closing incubator portholes and side panels). The infant in a radiant warmer also experiences convective heat losses in response to ventilation draughts and traffic flow around the bed. These losses may be partially countered with plastic wrap placed directly on the infant's body or stretched over the side guards of the warmer unit (Fig 9.1). A plastic bag or bubble wrap that encloses the infant's trunk and lower extremities is also effective in decreasing heat loss in ELBW and VLBW infants. Oxygen or any source of air, such as an oxygen mask or tube, should not blow directly on the infant's face. Oxygen concentrated around the head, such as that supplied to a hood (if used) or nasal cannula, must be warmed and humidified.

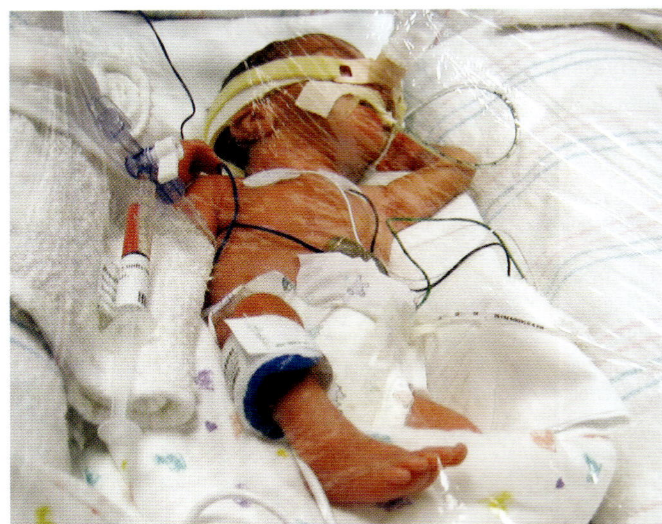

Fig 9.1 Infant under plastic wrap, which produces a draught-free environment. (Source: Courtesy E. Jacobs, Texas Children's Hospital, Houston.)

Radiant heat loss is one of the greatest threats to temperature regulation in the incubator because the temperature of circulating air within has no influence on heat loss to windows, walls or a lower nursery temperature. Such losses can be effectively reduced with the use of double-walled incubators; the infant radiates heat to the inner wall, which is surrounded by the warmed incubator air.

Although the open radiant warmer unit allows easier access to the infant, there is an inherent rise in evaporative water and heat loss from the skin, especially in ELBW and VLBW infants. Transepidermal water losses, a form of insensible weight loss (IWL), may be increased by as much as 50% to 200%, thus predisposing the infant to dehydration; daily fluid requirements are generally increased to compensate for such losses. The use of plastic wrap over the ELBW or VLBW infant in a radiant warmer will help reduce IWL and convective losses.

The infant being cared for in a radiant warmer is kept warm using the servocontrol method. Air temperature manual control should not be used because of the danger of overheating the infant. A reflective aluminium temperature probe cover is used to allow proper function of the servocontrol heating unit. The temperature probe should be placed over a non-bony, well-perfused tissue area such as the abdomen or flank. In general, the probe site is changed when the infant's position is changed to prevent the probe from coming in contact with the bed surface and potentially trapping heat at the probe site, causing an abnormal ambient temperature. Chaseling and colleagues (2016) found that the levels of temperature agreement between the skin (taken at different anatomical sites) and the core body temperature of neonates under a radiant warmer were poorly correlated. The researchers raised two points of concern. First, the feedback provided from a single skin temperature is unlikely to be a reliable representation of true deep core temperature. Second, skin temperature values across the body are non-uniform and the differences between the feet and the forehead/torso have up to a 6°C observed difference (Chaseling et al 2016). Minimising thermal instability is important for infants being cared for in the NICU environment.

Sterile cloth or disposable drapes also block radiant heat waves in a radiant warmer. During such procedures, a warmed blanket or heating pad under the infant is appropriate.

High-risk infants typically have a limited ability to perspire, thus decreasing heat dissipation and increasing risk of hyperthermia. In high-risk neonates hyperthermia is usually a result of overheating rather than increased metabolism. Therefore, knowledge of proper care and use of external heating devices, such as radiant warmers or incubators, is as important as knowing the conditions for which they are being used.

Protection from Infection

Protection from infection is an integral part of all newborn care, but premature and sick neonates are particularly susceptible. Thorough and frequent handwashing is the foundation of a preventive program. This includes all persons who come in contact with infants and their equipment. After handling another infant or equipment, no one should ever touch an infant without first washing hands.

Personnel with infectious disorders are either barred from the unit until they are no longer infectious or are required to wear suitable shields, such as masks or gloves, to reduce the likelihood of contamination. Standard precautions as a method of infection control are instituted in all nursery areas to protect the infants and staff. (See Chapter 6.)

Readmission of infants from home or admission of infants birthed in unsterile conditions or suspected of having communicable illnesses is handled per institutional protocol. Such infants should at least be initially physically isolated from other high-risk infants. For further infection control recommendations, including nursery care of infants with specific communicable diseases, refer to the Australian Guidelines for the Prevention and Control of Infection in Health Care (National Health and Medical Research Council [NHMRC] and Australian Commission on Safety and Quality in Health Care [ACSQHC] 2019) and the New Zealand Healthcare Associated Infections Governance Group website (https://www.health.govt.nz/about-ministry/leadership-ministry/expert-groups/healthcare-associated-infections-governance-group).

Hydration

High-risk infants often receive supplemental parenteral fluids to supply additional calories, electrolytes and/or water. Adequate hydration is particularly important in premature infants because their extracellular water content is higher (70% in full-term infants and up to 90% in premature infants), their body surface area is larger in comparison to their weight and ability to concentrate urine is limited in their underdeveloped kidneys. Therefore, these infants are highly vulnerable to water retention and fluid overload.

Parenteral fluids may be given to the high-risk neonate via several routes depending on the nature of the illness, the duration and type of fluid therapy and unit preference. Common routes of fluid infusion include peripheral, peripherally inserted central venous (or percutaneous central venous), surgically inserted central venous or arterial and, at times, umbilical venous or umbilical arterial catheterisation.

NURSING CARE CONSIDERATIONS

Nurses should be constantly alert for signs of infiltration (e.g. redness, oedema or colour change of tissue; blanching at site) and for signs of overhydration (e.g. weight gain of > 30 g/24 hour, periorbital oedema, tachypnoea, tachycardia and crackles on lung auscultation).

Small, fragile peripheral blood vessels are subject to rupture and subsequent infiltration. This problem is compounded by the use of infusion pumps that may continue to infuse fluid into surrounding tissues. Observations are especially important when using hypertonic solutions (e.g. calcium, sodium bicarbonate, parenteral hyperalimentation) and IV drugs (e.g. antibiotics and vasoactive drugs such as dopamine and dobutamine), which can cause serious tissue damage. With flexible catheters and small IV catheter shields, arm boards and limb restraints are usually unnecessary. If used, restraints should be checked frequently to ensure that no harm to the patient's extremity occurs and that peripheral circulation is adequate.

Infants who are ELBW, tachypnoeic, receiving phototherapy or under a radiant warmer have increased IWL and require appropriate fluid adjustments. Nurses/midwives must monitor fluid status by taking daily (or more frequent) weights; accurately monitoring intake and output of all fluids, including medications and blood products; and evaluating serum electrolyte levels. ELBW infants require more frequent monitoring of these parameters because of their excessive transepidermal fluid loss, immature renal function and tendency to become dehydrated or overhydrated. Intolerance of even glucose 5% is not uncommon in the ELBW infant, with subsequent glycosuria and osmotic diuresis. Alterations in behaviour, alertness or activity level in infants receiving IV fluids may signal an electrolyte imbalance, hypoglycaemia or hyperglycaemia. The nurse/midwife is also alert for tremors or seizures in the VLBW or ELBW infant because these may be a sign of hyponatraemia or hypernatraemia.

A common problem observed in infants who have an umbilical arterial catheter in place is vasoconstriction of peripheral vessels, which can seriously impair circulation. The response is triggered by arterial vasospasm caused by the presence of the catheter, the infusion of fluids or injection of medication. Blanching of the buttocks, genitalia or legs or feet is an indication of vasospasm. The problem must be recognised and reported promptly. The nurse/midwife must also observe for signs of thrombi in infants with umbilical venous or arterial lines. The precipitation of microthrombi in the vascular bed with the use of such catheters is commonly manifested by a sudden bluish discolouration seen in the toes, called 'cath toes'. Failure to alleviate the pathological condition may result in permanent injury to the toes, foot or leg.

Circulatory effects are observed first in the toes but may extend to include the legs and buttocks. The toes first flush and then turn a mulberry colour; if the condition is not corrected, there may be serious complications involving the loss of a limb. The infant with an umbilical venous or arterial catheter should also be observed closely for catheter dislodgment and subsequent bleeding or haemorrhage; urinary output, renal function and gastrointestinal (GI) function are also evaluated in these infants. Although the intent of such catheters is to effectively deliver IV fluids (and sometimes medications) and to obtain arterial blood gas samples, they are not without inherent complications.

Nutrition

Optimum nutrition is critical in the management of premature infants, but difficulties arise in providing for their nutritional needs. The various mechanisms for ingestion and digestion of foods are not fully developed. The problem of providing optimal nutrition to the infant is greatest in the more immature infant.

Physiological Characteristics. The premature infant's need for rapid growth and daily maintenance must be met in the presence of several anatomical and physiological challenges. Although infants demonstrate some sucking and swallowing activities before birth, coordination of these mechanisms does not occur until approximately 32 to 34 weeks' gestation, and they are not fully synchronised until 36 to 37 weeks. Initial sucking is not accompanied by swallowing, and oesophageal contractions are uncoordinated. As infants mature, the suck-swallow pattern develops but is slow and ineffectual, and these reflexes may easily become exhausted.

Nutritional Needs. The demand for nutrients in LBW infants is much higher than that in larger infants. Individual infants vary in activity level, ease of achieving basal energy expenditure, thermoneutrality, physical condition and efficacy of nutrient absorption.

A loss of up to 12% can be expected for the full-term infant in the first week of life. For breastfed babies you would expect to see them regain their birth weight within the two following weeks.

Weight, length and head circumference should all be recorded and charted to give a full picture of the child's overall progress and development. It is not of concern if the child is just on or just below the third percentile, as some children will be proportionately small. The need is for measurements of growth and progress over time. Remember to correct for prematurity (< 37/40) until the child reaches 2 years of age. Fenton growth charts should be used to measure and plot children until 50 weeks gestation (Marks 2015).

Studies regarding the effects of long-chain polyunsaturated fatty acids (LCPUFAs) on cognitive development, visual acuity and physical growth in full-term and premature infants have prompted formula companies to add docosahexaenoic acid (DHA) and arachidonic acid (AA) to their infant formulas. AA and DHA are in human milk, and their presence has been assumed to increase cognitive development in human milk–fed infants compared with infants fed a formula without these fatty acids (Tai et al 2013). A Cochrane review (2016) of 17 trials involving 2260 premature infants concluded that no clear long-term benefit or harm was demonstrated for premature infants receiving LCPUFA-supplemented formula (Moon et al 2016).

Milk from mothers whose infants are born before term contains more protein, sodium, chloride and immunoglobulin A (IgA). Thus mothers are the preferred source of milk for their premature infants. Growth factors, hormones, prolactin, calcitonin, thyroxine, steroids and taurine (an essential amino acid) are also found in human milk. The milk produced by mothers for their infants changes in content over the first 30 days postnatally, at which time it is similar to full-term human milk. Premature infants who received human milk during their hospitalisation demonstrated better intellectual performance scores at 7.5 to 8 years of age compared with children who received formula (Colaizy et al 2012). Improved psychomotor development at 18 months has also been observed in premature infants fed donor human milk compared with formula-fed premature infants. Despite its benefits, LBW infants (< 1500 g) who are exclusively fed unfortified human milk demonstrate decreased growth rates and nutritional deficiencies even beyond the hospitalisation period. These infants often have inadequate calcium, phosphorus, protein, sodium, vitamins and energy intake (Colaizy et al 2012). Specially designed supplements for human milk have been developed to address these deficits. Premature infants fed fortified human milk (FHM) have shorter hospital stays and less infection and necrotising enterocolitis (NEC) than infants given premature formulas. Fortifiers are commercially available, usually as a liquid or powder containing protein, carbohydrate, calcium, phosphorus, magnesium, sodium and varied amounts of zinc, copper and vitamins. Because fortifiers do not contain sufficient iron, an exogenous source must be administered after enteral feeding. Fortifiers should be added to milk as close as possible to feeding time, and FHM should be refrigerated until it is used.

The anti-infection attributes of human milk provide more benefits for premature infants. Secretory IgA concentration is higher in milk from mothers of premature infants than in milk from mothers of full-term infants. IgA is important in the control of bacteria in the intestinal tract, where it inhibits adherence and proliferation of bacteria on epithelial surfaces. Additional protection from infection is provided by leukocytes, lactoferrin and lysozyme, all of which are in human milk. Research suggests that administration of **probiotics**, live microbial supplements, decreases the incidence of NEC by normalising intestinal flora, reducing intestinal permeability and reducing gut inflammation (Dermyshi et al 2017, Sawh et al 2016).

NEC has been shown to occur more often in formula-fed infants than in premature infants fed human milk (Caplan 2015). Research also suggests that NEC is less severe and the prevalence of intestinal perforation lowered when premature infants are fed human milk (Colaizy et al 2012).

Premature infants exclusively fed human milk have demonstrated significantly decreased NEC, fewer positive blood cultures and decreased need for antibiotics (Meier et al 2017). In one study infants fed human milk also received more skin-to-skin contact with their mothers and shorter hospital stays. Neu and Sullivan (2012) suggest that skin-to-skin contact might potentially stimulate the enteromammary immune system to produce specific antibodies against nosocomial (healthcare-associated) pathogens in the nursery. Gastric emptying is improved with human milk feedings for premature infants, primarily because of increased intestinal lactase and possibly decreased intestinal permeability. Finally, the psychological advantages the mother gets from using her own milk cannot be overlooked.

Early feeding (provided that the infant is medically stable) reduces the incidence of complicating factors such as hypoglycaemia and dehydration and reduces the degree of hyperbilirubinaemia. The feeding regimen used varies in different units. One strategy for the prevention of NEC that has been supported by research is the use of standardised feeding protocols. A review of the literature found evidence of a significant reduction in NEC in infants fed by a standard protocol (Gephart & Hanson 2013).

Feeding tolerance and feeding success are not entirely the same concept. **Feeding tolerance** is evaluated by: (1) a soft abdomen; (2) an absence of abdominal distension or visible bowel loops on the skin surface; (3) minimum or no aspirated gastric residual; (4) presence of bowel sounds; (5) usual frequency, colour and consistency of stools; (6) minimum to no spitting up or vomiting; (7) infant's continued interest in feeding; and (8) consistent behaviour pattern. Successful oral feeding should be safe, functional and pleasurable. **Feeding success** can be measured by an infant's ability to: (1) participate in feeding with energy; (2) coordinate sucking and swallowing with adequate pauses for breathing; (3) maintain vital signs and oxygenation within normal limits; (4) maintain normal muscle tone in face and body; (5) complete feeding in about 20 to 25 minutes; (6) manage a liquid bolus with minimum or no loss of liquid from mouth; (7) sustain alertness for feeding; (8) maintain strength and endurance for entire feeding; and (9) measure appropriate-for-age on standard growth curve. A premature infant's success with feeding is first measured in terms of safety and functionality. Nurturing by holding close, but not socialising, during a feeding creates a warm and pleasurable experience. Later, after the infant is a competent feeder, socialisation will enrich both parents' and infant's mealtime enjoyment.

Gavage Feeding. Gavage feeding is a safe means of meeting the nutritional requirements of infants who are not yet ready to feed orally. These infants are usually too weak to suck effectively, are unable to coordinate swallowing or lack a gag reflex. Studies have demonstrated that both bolus and continuous feeding are equally suitable feeding strategies for premature neonates (Bozzetti et al 2016, Rovekamp-Abels et al 2015). Intermittent gavage feeding is used as an energy-conserving technique for infants learning to nipple-feed who become excessively tired, listless or cyanotic.

A correct-sized feeding tube is usually used to instil the feeding, and the usual methods for determining correct placement are used.

(See Chapter 22 for technique.) Although the more relaxed cardiac sphincter makes passage of the tube easier, the heart rate and blood pressure may change in response to vagal stimulation. The procedure is best accomplished when an infant is in a prone or a right side-lying position with the head slightly elevated. Small flexible nasogastric (NG) tubes may be maintained as an indwelling feeding tube and used for prolonged periods without complications of intermittent removal and insertion.

The stomach is aspirated, the contents measured and the aspirate returned as part of the feeding. However, this practice may vary depending on circumstances and individual unit protocol.

Current best practice dictates a radiograph as the only certain way to determine NG tube placement in the stomach. Methods such as auscultation of an air bubble, neck-ear-xiphoid measurements for insertion depth or pH measurements may be the only option for determining placement of feeding tubes in infants in some regional and rural environments when radiography is not an option. Refer to your facility's policy on these occasions to confirm correct protocol on confirming placement.

The infant may be held during gavage feedings by the caregiver or parent. Non-nutritive sucking (NNS) on a pacifier helps infants associate sucking with satiety. A Cochrane review (2016) of NNS demonstrated a significant reduction in length of stay in premature infants receiving an NNS intervention. Other positive outcomes of NNS included enhanced transition from tube- to bottle-feeding and better bottle-feeding performance (Foster et al 2016).

Oral Feeding. Vigorous infants can be fed orally with little difficulty, but compromised premature infants require alternative methods. The amount to be fed is determined largely by the infant's weight gain and tolerance of previous feeding and is increased by small increments until a satisfactory caloric intake is ensured.

The rate of tolerated increase varies from one infant to another, and determining this rate is often a nursing responsibility. Premature infants require more time and patience to feed than full-term infants, and the oropharyngeal mechanism may be stressed by an attempt to feed too rapidly. It is important not to tire the infants or overtax their capacity to retain the feedings. When infants require a prolonged time (25 to > 30 minutes) to complete a feeding, gavage feeding may be considered.

Breastfeeding. It is recommended that human milk is used for all infants, including sick newborns and premature infants (with rare exceptions). The choice of what to feed is the parents' prerogative but it is advised that providers give parents complete and accurate information on the benefits and the risks of not providing breast milk to ensure that an informed decision is made. Barriers to initiation and continuation of breastfeeding include medical practitioner indifference, misinformation, lack of prenatal education about breastfeeding, distracting hospital policies, lack of follow-up, maternal employment, lack of support from family or society, hospital discharge packs with formula or coupons for formula and media portrayal of bottle-feeding (Victoria State Government 2020a).

Premature infants may be able to successfully breastfeed earlier than previously believed (28 to 36 weeks). In addition, premature infants who are breastfed rather than bottle-fed demonstrate fewer oxygen desaturation episodes, an absence of bradycardia, warmer skin temperature and better coordination of breathing, sucking and swallowing (Gardner & Lawrence 2016). The nurse/midwife should carefully evaluate the premature infant for readiness to breastfeed, including assessment of behavioural state, ability to maintain body temperature outside an artificial heat source, respiratory status and readiness to suckle at the mother's breast. The latter may be accomplished with NNS at the breast during skin-to-skin (or kangaroo) contact so the mother and newborn can become accustomed to each other (Gardner & Lawrence 2016, Meier et al 2017). Nasal cannula oxygen may also be provided during breastfeeding if required by the infant.

Time, patience and dedication on the part of the mother and the nursing staff are necessary to ensure breastfeeding success. The process starts slowly, beginning with one oral feeding daily and gradually increasing the feedings as the infant tolerates them. Human milk provides both short-term and long-term advantages in a dose-dependent relationship in that the more breast milk the premature infant receives, the more benefits are gained (Gardner & Lawrence 2016, Meier et al 2017). Supplementary bottle-feeding is inefficient because the infant expends energy and calories to feed twice. Feeding more often and/or supplementing with gavage feeding are more energy and calorie efficient. Breastfeeding the premature infant often requires additional guidance by a lactation consultant and continued support and encouragement by the nursing staff. In addition, post-discharge breastfeeding often requires further guidance, counselling and support.

Nipple-feeding. The infant is positioned in the feeder's arms or placed semi-upright in the lap and is held with the back curved slightly to simulate the position assumed naturally by most full-term newborns. Oral sensitivity can be promoted by the stroking of the infant's lips, cheeks and tongue before feeding.

Brown and colleagues (2016) used the semi-elevated side-lying (ESL) position when introducing bottle-feedings to premature infants between 32 and 36 weeks of age. The ESL position better mimics the breastfeeding position and allows for better coordination of breathing with swallowing.

Feeding Resistance

Any feeding technique that bypasses the mouth prevents the infant from practising sucking and swallowing or experiencing normal hunger and satiation cycles. Infants may demonstrate aversion to oral feedings by averting the head from the nipple, extruding the nipple by tongue thrust, gagging or even vomiting.

Developmental delays have occurred in perceptual-motor performance among infants with feeding refusal as measured by standard tests, although intellectual function remains within normal limits. Other observations include disinterest in or active resistance to oral play, diminished spontaneity and motivation and shallow interpersonal relationships, probably related to the absence of some early incorporative patterns of normal oral experiences.

Infants identified as being at risk for feeding resistance should receive regular oral stimulation based on the child's developmental level. Those who exhibit feeding aversion should begin a stimulation program to overcome resistance and acquire the ability to take nourishment by mouth. Because management requires long-term commitment, successful implementation of a plan for oral stimulation depends on maximum parental involvement and promotion of primary nursing. Key strategies and interventions are in Box 9.2.

Skin Care

Premature infants have immature skin with increased sensitivity and fragility. Alkaline-based soap that might destroy the 'acid mantle' of the skin should be avoided. The increased permeability of the skin facilitates absorption of ingredients. All skin products (e.g. alcohol or povidone-iodine) are used with caution. The skin is rinsed with water afterwards because these substances may cause severe irritation and chemical burns in LBW infants.

Administration of Medications

Administration of therapeutic agents, such as drugs, ointments, IV infusions and oxygen, requires careful attention to detail. The computation, preparation and administration of drugs in minute amounts

BOX 9.2 Strategies to Prevent or Overcome Feeding Resistance

- Minimise noxious stimuli to the mouth
  - Suction only as needed (not routinely)
  - Consider indwelling gastric tube rather than intermittent gavage
  - Use perioral and intraoral stimulation techniques
- Enhance pleasant stimuli to mouth
  - Have infant smell or taste breastmilk
  - Provide non-nutritive suckling while tube feeding
  - Use nipple with proper flow
  - Use perioral and intraoral stimulation
- Use proper position to facilitate swallow and improve suction
  - Hold with feedings
  - Swaddle
  - Facilitate swallowing (e.g. position with chin tucked)
  - Improve formation of suction (e.g. cupping both cheeks for support)
- Timing
  - Do not allow infant to cry before feeding
  - Keep external stimuli to a minimum
  - Feed for short periods at first

Source: Modified from Gardner, S. L., Goldson, E., & Hernandez, J. A. (2016). The neonate and the environment: Impact on development. In S. L. Gardner, B. S. Carter, M. Enzman-Hines, et al (Eds.), *Merenstein and Gardner's handbook of neonatal intensive care* (8th ed.). St Louis, MO: Mosby.

require collaboration among nurses/midwives, medical practitioners and pharmacists to reduce the chance for error. The immaturity of an infant's detoxification mechanisms and inability to demonstrate symptoms of toxicity (e.g. signs of auditory nerve involvement from ototoxic drugs such as gentamicin) complicate drug therapy and require that nurses/midwives be particularly alert for signs of adverse reaction.

Nurses/midwives should be aware of the hazards of administering bacteriostatic and hyperosmolar solutions to infants. Benzyl alcohol, a common preservative in bacteriostatic water, heparin sodium and some saline flushes, is toxic to newborns and should not be used to flush IV catheters or to dilute or reconstitute medications. It is recommended that medications with preservatives such as benzyl alcohol be avoided. Nurses/midwives must read labels carefully to detect the presence of preservatives in any medication administered to an infant.

Hyperosmolar solutions present a potential danger to premature infants. Hyperosmolar solutions given orally to infants can produce clinical, physiological and morphological alterations, the most serious of which is NEC. Oral or parenteral medications should be sufficiently diluted to prevent complications related to hyperosmolality.

Take caution to reduce adverse effects of medication administration in premature infants. Strategies to heighten awareness and decrease unnecessary morbidity in such infants include having two registered nurses/midwives double-check the dosages of potentially lethal medications (high-risk medications) and providing calculators in neonatal units to perform dosage calculations, double-check unit dose medications and have the hospital pharmacy reconstitute medications. Another strategy is to develop computerised guidelines for managing dose ranges based on the neonate's most recent weight so that medications ordered outside the appropriate dose range are re-evaluated by the pharmacist and practitioner. Information technology (e.g. computerised practitioner order entry and clinical participation by a clinical pharmacist) is available to reduce medication errors, yet this technology does not provide the entire solution (Campino et al 2016).

Developmental Outcome

Neonatal intensive care and rapid improvements in technology are associated with improved survival of critically ill newborn and premature infants. Survival rates have increased to 94% for VLBW infants (1001 to 1500 g), 88% for ELBW infants (751 to 1000 g) and 63% for infants weighing 501 g to 750 g (Horbar et al 2012). With decreasing mortality rates, morbidity rates have remained stable. At highest risk for unfavourable outcomes are premature infants compromised during the neonatal period by respiratory distress syndrome (RDS), chronic lung disease (also known as bronchopulmonary dysplasia), NEC, sepsis, anaemia, IVH, hydrocephalus, meningitis or seizures (Rogers & Hintz 2016). These serious sequelae of prematurity correlate with the degree of immaturity, demonstrating the relationship of increasing morbidity associated with decreasing gestational age. A greater incidence of CP, attention-deficit/hyperactivity disorder, visual-motor deficits, mild to severe cognitive disabilities, hearing loss, speech and language impairment and neuromotor problems has been reported in outcome studies of premature infants (Church et al 2012, Rogers & Hintz 2016). Moderate and late-premature infants also exhibit developmental delay compared with their term-born peers, most often noted in the language domain (Cheong et al 2017).

Neurodevelopmental impairment also occurs in premature infants without the complications of IVH, sepsis and hypoxaemia. Conversely, some premature infants do well and function at age level without evidence of neurobehavioural limitations. Improved developmental outcomes are more likely for these infants with the finest medical and nursing care within a developmentally supportive framework. This philosophy requires caregivers to evaluate their own knowledge, skills and attitudes and expand their thinking beyond the traditional medical and nursing models of care.

The rates of survival have increased among infants born at the borderline of viability (22 to 24 weeks' gestation). Younge and colleagues (2017) reported on survival outcomes for periviable infants born at 11 centres across the United States and concluded that the rate of survival without neurodevelopmental impairment increased between 2000 and 2011. Despite these improvements for periviable infants, the incidence of death, neurodevelopmental impairment and other adverse outcomes remains high in this population (Younge et al 2017). The researchers cautioned that despite improvements over time in this periviable population, the incidence of death, neurodevelopmental impairment and other adverse outcomes remains high.

Developmental Assessment. A systematic method for observing NICU infants to collect information concerning each infant's competencies, vulnerabilities and thresholds should be used, such as one based on that similar to Als's (1982) **synactive theory of infant development**. This information forms the basis for planning individualised care appropriate for a particular infant (Table 9.2). The major assumption of this model is that infants, even ELBW infants, can communicate through physical and behavioural responses that provide us with the best information for planning their care. Communication by the infant is seen through three subsystems of function (autonomic, motor and state) that can be readily observed in the clinical setting during rest, care or procedures and during recovery from care or procedures. Responses by an infant's autonomic (physiological), motor and state systems to the environment, physical care or procedures help the nurse/midwife make necessary adjustments to optimise the infant's stability and function.

Individualised developmental care has had positive effects on medical and neurobehavioural outcomes in high-risk newborn infants. A study of developmental care for premature infants found earlier oral feeding; reduced need for mechanical ventilation or supplemental

TABLE 9.2 Synactive Theory of Development: Neurobehavioural Subsystems

Subsystem	Signs of Stress	Signs of Stability
Autonomic	Physiological instability	Physiological stability
Respiratory	Tachypnoea, pauses, gasping, sighing	Smooth, stable respirations; regular rate and pattern
Colour	Mottled, flushed, dusky, pale or grey	Pink, stable colour
Visceral	Hiccups, gagging, choking, vomiting, grunting and straining as if having a bowel movement; coughing, sneezing, yawning	Absence of hiccups, gagging, vomiting, etc.
Autonomic	Tremors, startles, twitches	Absence of tremors, startles, twitches
Motor	Fluctuating tone; lack of control over movement, activity and posture	Consistent tone; controlled or improved movement, activity and posture
Flaccidity	Low tone in trunk; limp, floppy upper and lower extremities; limp, drooping jaw (gape face)	Tone consistent and appropriate for postmenstrual age Well-maintained posture
Hypertonicity	Arm or leg extensions, arm(s) outstretched with fingers splayed in salute gesture, fingers stiffly outstretched, trunk arching, neck hyperextended	Smooth, controlled movements
Hyperflexion activity	Trunk hyperflexion, hyperflexion of extremities, fisting; squirming; frantic diffuse activity or little or no activity or responsiveness	Successful motor strategies for self-regulation (see Self-Regulation below)
State	Disorganised quality to state behaviours, including range of available states, maintenance of state control and transition from one state to another	Easy-to-read state behaviours that are maintained; calm, focused alertness, well-modulated sleep
Sleep	Whimpering sounds, facial twitching, irregular respirations, fussing, grimacing, restless appearance	Clear, well-defined sleep states; periods of quiet, restful sleep
Awake	Glazed unfocused look, staring, worried or pained expression, hyperalert or panicked appearance, eye roving, crying, 'cry-face', actively averting gaze or closing eyes, irritability, prolonged awake periods, inconsolability, frenzy Abrupt or rapid state changes	Alert with bright, shiny eyes; focused attention on object or person; animated expression (e.g. cheek softening, frowning, 'ooh-face', cooing, smiling) Robust crying Good calming, consolability Smooth changes between states, full range of sleep-wake states
Other state-related behaviours and attention-interaction	Efforts to attend to and interact with environmental stimulation eliciting signs of stress and disorganised subsystem functioning	Responsive to auditory, visual and social stimuli
Autonomic	Physiological instability of varying degrees with autonomic, respiratory, colour and visceral responses	Responsiveness to stimuli well maintained and prolonged
Motor	Fluctuating tone, increased motor activity, progressively frantic diffuse activity if stimulation continues	Actively seeking auditory stimulus, minimum motor activity
State	Roving eyes, gaze averted, glazed unfocused look or worried, panicked expression; weak cry; cry-face; irritability Closed eyes and sleeplike withdrawal Abrupt state changes Signs of stress when presented with more than one type of stimulus at a time	Bright, shiny-eyed, alert and attentive expression Sustained awake and alert state Shifting attention smoothly to more than one type of stimulation

Self-regulation—Infant's efforts to achieve, maintain or regain a balanced, stable and relaxed state of subsystem functioning and integration. Success of these efforts will vary among infants depending on maturity, available self-regulatory skills and overall subsystem organisation. Examples of self-regulatory strategies include the following.

- *Motor*—Foot bracing against a boundary or blanket nest, hand holding, clasping hands together, hand to mouth or face, grasping blanket, tubing, tucking trunk, sucking, position changes
- *State*—Lowering state from high arousal to quiet alert or sleep state; releasing energy by rhythmic, robust crying; focused attention and orientation

Facilitation by caregivers—Environmental modifications or developmental care techniques to aid infant's own self-regulatory abilities when environmental challenges exceed infant's capabilities.

Source: Modified from Als, H. (1982). Toward a synactive theory of development: Promise for the assessment and support of infant individuality. Infant Mental Health Journal, 3(4), 229–243; Als, H. (1986). A synactive model of neonatal behaviour organisation: Framework for the assessment of neurobehavioral development in the premature infant and for support of infants and parents in the neonatal intensive care environment. Physical & Occupational Therapy in Pediatrics, 6, 3–55; and Hunter, J. (2010). The neonatal intensive care unit. In J. Case-Smith (Ed.), Occupational therapy for children (6th ed.). St Louis, MO: Mosby.

oxygen; decreased time in the hospital; improved weight gain; enhanced autonomic, motor, state, attention and self-regulatory function; and lowered family stress (Als 2009, Macho 2017). In contrast, a systematic review done by Ohlsson and Jacobs (2013) noted that the evidence did not demonstrate that individualised developmental care improved long-term neurodevelopmental or short-term medical outcomes for premature infants.

Because each infant is unique, supportive developmental care requires ongoing data collection of moment-by-moment responses and flexible care to address the infant's cues. For example, an infant who demonstrates altered vital signs and even apnoea after being weighed might benefit from swaddled weighing to support the infant's competence and organisation during a stressful procedure.

Knowledge of behavioural assessment and infant development assists the nurse/midwife in providing care that supports each infant's ongoing function in a manner consistent with current evidence. Nurses/midwives have the greatest impact on the daily routine experienced by their patients. The CNS is undergoing rapid and significant change during the premature infant's stay in the NICU. This vulnerable period of brain growth, differentiation and organisation is combined with the challenge of developing in environmental conditions that are not typical for the fetus and newborn (Blackburn 2012). Brain organisation peaks from about 20 weeks' gestation to several years after birth. The product of this complex process is establishment of an elaborate circuitry unique to the human brain.

Behavioural State Organisation. Traditional nursing placed emphasis on interpreting physiological data as the basis of caregiving. Developmentally supportive care uses both physiological and behavioural information to better understand the needs of infants in the NICU setting. **Behavioural states** are highly individualised and formed by experience, maturation, circadian rhythms and genetic inheritance. The emerging availability and regulation of arousal states mark a balancing of CNS inhibitory and excitatory processes that affect attention states and also mark executive functions (prefrontal cortex) that influence information processing, learning and socialisation. **State organisation** has been described as a gating mechanism that protects the cortex from overstimulation and promotes coordination among attentional, executive and sensory cortical systems.

Infant responsiveness to environmental stimuli depends on the quality, amount and availability of particular states of arousal. States can be organised into five levels of arousal (Table 9.3). Transitional states such as drowsiness are not considered true states, but are in-between levels of arousal in which the infant either moves towards wakefulness or back into sleep.

Distinct sleep and awake states are observable in infants between 25 and 27 weeks (Buenoa & Menna-Barretob 2016, Guyer et al 2015). Young premature infants spend 70% or more of their time in active sleep. Developmental maturation for the young premature infant is seen by a decrease in the amount of active sleep with an increase in quiet sleep, awake periods and crying. Around 30 to 32 weeks, quiet alert states with some focused attention can occur. Before 32 to 34 weeks, attempts to attend to stimuli may have physiological consequences for the immature infant (Raoof & Ohlsson 2013). Responsiveness to sound and touch is greater during active or light (**rapid eye movement** [REM]) sleep, resulting in longer periods of vulnerability to sleep disturbance (Gardner, Goldson & Hernandez 2016). Maturation continues throughout the first year of life. By 6 months, the amount of quiet sleep is greater than that of active sleep. By 1 year, infants usually sleep 10 to 12 hours at night and take one or two naps during the day. Premature infants generally sleep for shorter periods at night and awaken more frequently than full-term infants. Other maturational changes include organisation of the standard sleep cycle and electroencephalogram sleep patterns comparable to those of adults. Neurological insults, severity of illness, hyperbilirubinaemia and prenatal exposure to drugs can alter behavioural state patterns.

TABLE 9.3 Arousal States

State	Description
Deep sleep	Regular breathing; eyes closed with no movement of eyes under lid; relaxed face; little or no movement or activity except for possible startle response
Active sleep	Sometimes called light sleep; may see rapid eye movements under closed lids, low activity level, breathing regular or irregular, occasional sighing or smiling
Drowsy	Eyes open or closed, unfocused expression; activity level varied
Quiet awake	Different qualities of alerting
• Robust	Bright, shiny appearance to eyes; focused attention; minimum motor activity
• Low level	Dull or unfocused eyes; little energy; appears to look through object or caregiver
• Hyperalert	Wide eyes, panicked expression; may fixate on object or caregiver intensely and have trouble breaking away
Active awake	Active; eyes open or closed; fussy but not crying robustly
Crying	Highest level of arousal; agitated, rhythmic and robust crying

Source: Modified from Als, H. (1995). Manual for the naturalistic observation of newborn behaviour, Newborn Individualized Developmental Care and Assessment Program (NIDCAP). Boston, MA: Harvard Medical School.

Physiological parameters vary depending on level of arousal. Heart rate is higher during waking periods but more variable during active sleep. Blood pressure is higher during wakefulness. Cerebral blood flow is greater during active sleep (greater during quiet sleep in full-term infants). Respiratory rates vary more and are higher in active sleep. Arterial oxygen and carbon dioxide levels are lower in active sleep than in quiet sleep or awake states. Hypoventilation and poorly coordinated chest wall and abdominal movements are reported during active sleep. Apnoeic pauses of less than 20 seconds are more frequent in active than quiet sleep in premature infants.

Nursing care should be timed to the responsiveness of the infant as much as possible to optimise the development of sleep organisation and enhance alerting as it emerges. Sensory stimulation can influence behavioural state as seen by either increased or decreased infant arousal when presented with a stimulus and its removal; the type of stimulus (e.g. loud bell or soft lullaby) also is a factor. The quality of each state, its duration and the movement between states provide information about how well organised the state is and how much state control the infant has. Protection of sleep is an important goal for both the premature and the full-term infant. Environmental modifications and timing of care to provide longer episodes of undisturbed sleep should be planned into care.

Nurses/midwives can also support transitions between states. Gentle arousal to wakefulness by soft speech or gentle touch before caregiving is preferable to the traditional model in which care is begun without warning and with abrupt disruption of sleep. Slow movements and gentle handling support quiet alerting or return to sleep without periods of arousal after care is over. Nurses/midwives should facilitate return to sleep or interact with a quietly alert infant after care events.

An infant's state of arousal allows for communication of responses that are valuable for individualised caregiving. By observing state patterns and individual responses of infants, nurses/midwives can better know their patients and support behavioural state organisation. The nurse/midwife can also share this knowledge with parents to foster intimacy with the child.

Sensory System. Atypical sensory experiences, whether overstimulating or depriving, can modify the developing brain (Gardner, Goldson & Hernandez 2016). In fact, much of the cerebral cortex is associated with the sensory system. Most sensory systems develop prenatally and are capable of functioning before birth. The onset of sensory function proceeds in the same order for each individual (i.e. tactile, vestibular, gustatory-olfactory, auditory and visual). The visual system becomes functional after birth. Sensory input provided before the stimulation would typically occur has been shown to interfere with perceptual and behavioural development (Gardner, Goldson & Hernandez 2016).

The normal experience for the premature infant is within the uterus and for the full-term infant is the home environment with a few primary caregivers. These environments are vastly different from the NICU. The NICU experience for the high-risk infant is made up of external conditions and interactions with caregivers. Often that experience is overstimulating to later-developing sensory systems (i.e. auditory and visual) and understimulating to earlier ones (i.e. tactile, vestibular, gustatory-olfactory). Alterations in the sensory environment may have developmental consequences. The nurse/midwife should consider: (1) timing of stimulation in relation to the infant's current developmental stage; (2) amount of stimulation provided or denied; (3) type of stimulation; and (4) the infant's response to the stimulation (Gardner, Goldson & Hernandez 2016).

By the age of viability, infants in the NICU have sophisticated perioral sensation and perceive pressure, pain and temperature (Gardner, Goldson & Hernandez 2016). Touch in the NICU frequently involves routine, sometimes impersonal, caregiving and procedures that are either intrusive or painful. Even non-painful care has been associated with adverse responses in premature infants.

Premature infants demonstrate cry expression, grimacing and knee and leg flexion during major reposition changes. Hypoxaemia has been reported with non-painful or routine caregiving activities such as suctioning, repositioning, taking vital signs and changing nappies. Other physiological changes involve blood pressure, heart rate and respiratory rhythm (Gardner, Goldson & Hernandez 2016). Nursing activities that are painful or especially intrusive, such as needle puncture, have negative physiological repercussions such as acute decreases in SaO_2 and behavioural state changes in premature infants (Gardner, Enzman-Hines & Nyp 2016). Increased motor activity, agitation, crying and startle reflex have also been described as negative behavioural responses to touch (Gardner, Goldson & Hernandez 2016).

Touch is the first sensory system to develop and forms the basis for early communication between infants and caregivers. In particular, touch is a powerful means of emotional exchange for parents and infants. Positioning and handling techniques promote comfort and minimise stress while creating a balance between nurturing care and necessary interventions.

Therapeutic Handling. Using the developmental model of supportive care, the nurse/midwife closely monitors physiological and behavioural signs to promote organisation and wellbeing of high-risk infants during handling (Box 9.3). The type, timing and amount of handling are carefully considered in terms of the infant's current age, condition, vulnerabilities, thresholds for stress and capabilities. Because touch can be disruptive to maturing sleep-wake states, avoid waking an infant for care or nurturing. Sleep deprivation may affect secretion of growth hormone and interfere with growth and development (Gardner, Goldson & Hernandez 2016).

BOX 9.3 Considerations for Tactile Interventions in the Neonatal Intensive Care Unit

- Modify all handling and touch so that it is supportive and calming.
- Consider sleep-wake states and behavioural cues to determine optimum times for handling and touch.
- Adjust handling and touch based on continual observation of the infant's autonomic and behavioural responses.
- Ensure appropriate touch opportunities for parents aside from routine caregiving.
- Encourage parents to be primary providers of social touch.
- Avoid using massage with vulnerable high-risk infants (e.g. medically unstable, low-birth-weight infants less than 32 weeks' gestation; easily disorganised, low-threshold infants; chronically ill infants with chronic lung disease or cardiac disorders known to display physiological and behavioural disorganisation).
- Assist parents in identifying the most appropriate type of touch and handling for their infant.
- Teach infant cues to parents for monitoring responses to handling and touch.
- Weigh the risks and benefits for any tactile intervention.

Infants who are unable to maintain a gently flexed position during repositioning or care procedures may benefit from containment. Gently holding the infant's arms and legs in a tucked, flexed position close to the body can be accomplished with hands or blanket swaddling. **Facilitated tucking** was shown to decrease physiological and behavioural distress in premature infants during painful procedures (Hartley et al 2015, Lavoie et al 2015). Blanket swaddling and nesting or containment decreased physiological and behavioural stress during routine care procedures such as bathing and heel lance (Hartley et al 2015, Quraishy et al 2013).

Kangaroo care, or skin-to-skin holding, has been advocated for fostering neurobehavioural development and supporting parent–infant intimacy and attachment. Skin-to-skin contact is maintained with the nappy-clad infant resting prone and semi-upright on the bare chest of either parent, who encloses the infant in his or her own clothing to maintain temperature stability. Kangaroo care is reported to reduce the incidence of severe illness and nosocomial infection, support breastfeeding duration until discharge, improve maternal satisfaction and parental interaction and quicken neurological maturation (Gardner, Goldson & Hernandez 2016). Others have reported maintenance of skin temperature, reduction of apnoea and bradycardia, stable $tcPO_2$ level, increased frequency and duration of quiet sleep and less time crying during kangaroo care (Kommers et al 2017). A Cochrane review (2017) examined the effect of kangaroo care on pain from medical and nursing procedures in neonates and determined it to be an effective intervention (Johnston et al 2017).

Therapeutic Positioning. The Red Nose Australia organisation recommends the supine sleeping position for healthy infants in the first year of life as a preventive measure for sudden infant death syndrome (SIDS). (See Sudden Infant Death Syndrome, Chapter 11, for discussion of this and Sudden Unexpected Death in Infancy [SUDI].) Prone sleeping has decreased from more than 73% to about 15% in Australia since the SIDS guidelines were published in 1992 (Red Nose 2018). SIDS is the third highest cause of infant death after the neonatal period (28 days); the rate has decreased by more than 53% with the advent of supine sleeping. (See Sudden Infant Death Syndrome, Chapter 11.) However, after an initial decrease in the 1990s, the overall death rate attributable to sleep-related infant deaths has not declined in more recent years (Huether & McCance 2018, Red Nose 2018).

Infants in the NICU are at increased risk for acquiring position-related deformities for a variety of reasons. Weakness, low tone, immature motor control, the effects of gravity and treatments such as sedation are a few of the factors associated with prolonged immobility or decreased spontaneous movement (Danner-Bowman & Cardin 2015). Common position-related deformities include the following.

- Hyperabduction and flexion of the arms, causing upper extremity external rotation, resulting in a persistent 'W' positioning of the arms, can interfere with later midline skills that form the foundation for feeding, crawling, reaching and midline play with objects (Danner-Bowman & Cardin 2015).
- Lower extremity external rotation deformities occurring when the trunk and pelvis are flat on the mattress, causing extreme hip abduction and outward rotation of the lower limbs or the frog-leg appearance (Gardner, Goldson & Hernandez 2016).
- Neck extension and arching posture often observed in infants pulling away from endotracheal (ET) tubes or nasal prongs during mechanical ventilation or nasal continuous positive airway pressure (CPAP).
- Motor asymmetries reported in premature infants at 32 weeks' gestation or who are small for gestational age, occurring more often than in full-term infants even after 4 months corrected age (Danner-Bowman & Cardin 2015).

Therapeutic positioning reduces the potential for acquired positional deformities that can affect motor development, play skills and social attachment (Danner-Bowman & Cardin 2015). Positioning can affect stability and comfort, and each infant must be observed for the effects of any position or repositioning. A position may also need to be adapted to accommodate necessary medical equipment or particular conditions, such as myelomeningocele, where the supine position is contraindicated before surgical repair of the defect. Deciding on which position and supportive aids to use requires the caregiver to consider the medical and developmental risks and benefits unique to a specific infant and situation (see Nursing Care Considerations box).

NURSING CARE CONSIDERATIONS

General Considerations for Positioning

- Neutral or slightly flexed neck
- Gently rounded shoulders (no flattened posture against bed as in supine or prone positions)
- Elbows flexed
- Hands to face or midline as position allows
- Trunk slightly rounded with pelvic tilt
- Hips partially flexed and adducted to near midline (not medial or neutral alignment) and knee flexion (no frog leg or externally rotated hips flat against bed)
- Lower boundary secured for foot bracing

Source: Danner-Bowman, K. & Cardin, A. (2015). Neuroprotective Core Measure 3: Positioning & Handling — A Look at Preventing Positional Plagiocephaly. Newborn and infant nursing reviews, 15(3), 111–113.

Auditory Environment. The auditory system of the human fetus is mature enough for sound to produce physiological effects as early as 22 to 24 weeks' gestation (Gardner, Goldson & Hernanez 2016). Physical and behavioural responses to sudden, loud NICU noise have been observed in premature and full-term infants (Hassanein et al 2013). Physiological changes include apnoea and bradycardia; fluctuations in heart and respiratory rates, blood pressure and oxygen saturation; and changes in sleep-wake states (Kuhn et al 2013, Pineda et al 2017). These data demonstrate that infants in the NICU are capable of perceiving and responding to sounds around them.

The primary auditory environment in fetal life is made up of the maternal voice, respirations, heartbeat and intestinal sounds. Soon after birth, newborn infants demonstrate preference for their own mother's voice and the language heard in utero (Gardner, Goldson & Hernandez 2016).

Visual Environment. Sight is the least mature of the newborn's senses. The premature infant's eyes undergo significant maturation and differentiation of the retina and its connections to the visual cortex that typically occur in utero during the last trimester of pregnancy (Atkinson & Braddick 2012). Early intense visual stimulation for premature infants could adversely affect visual pathways and alter the developmental course for other sensory systems.

Visual function in premature infants is more limited than that in full-term infants, who, although restricted in ability to focus (accommodation to near and far distances) and discriminate (acuity), will actively explore the environment. Premature infants are less responsive to visual stimulation and have less acuity and accommodation than full-term infants. The ability to visually attend emerges around 30 to 32 weeks, and the infant may become stressed if the visual stimulus is intense and prolonged. Strong visual stimulation such as high-contrast black-and-white patterns can evoke an obligatory staring response by the immature infant who is unable to break away from it. This behaviour is neither appropriate nor desired.

Facilitating Parent–infant Relationships

Because of their physiological instability, premature infants are immediately separated from their mothers and surrounded by a complex barrier of glass windows, mechanical equipment and special caregivers. Increasing evidence indicates that the emotional separation that accompanies the physical separation of mothers and infants interferes with the normal maternal–infant attachment process, discussed in Chapter 7. Maternal attachment is a cumulative process that begins before conception, strengthens by significant events during pregnancy and matures through maternal–infant contact during the neonatal period.

When an infant is sick, the necessary physical separation appears to be accompanied by an emotional estrangement in the parents, which may seriously damage their capacity for parenting their infant. This detachment is further hampered by the tenuous nature of the infant's condition. When survival is in doubt, parents may be reluctant to establish a relationship with their infant, unconsciously preparing themselves for the infant's death. This **anticipatory grief** (see Chapter 19) and hesitancy to embark on a relationship are evidenced by behaviours such as delay in giving the infant a name, reluctance to visit the nursery (or focusing on equipment and treatments rather than on their infant when they do visit) and hesitancy to touch or handle the infant when given the opportunity.

Parents appreciate the support of a nurse/midwife during the initial visit with their infant, but they may also want some time alone with the infant. It is important during the early visits to emphasise the positive aspects of their infant's behaviour and development so that parents can focus on their infant as an individual rather than on the equipment that surrounds the child. For example, the nurse/midwife may describe the infant's spontaneous behaviours during care, such as grasp, sucking and movement, or make comments about the infant's biological functions. Most institutions promote **family-centred care** and have open visiting policies so that parents and siblings can visit as often as they wish. Although paediatric healthcare providers are embracing family-centred care, successful implementation of initiative to support this model is challenging. Christian (2020) demonstrated from parent focus groups evidence of parental stress throughout hospitalisation. Parents reported that uncertainty, fear and lack of control were the predominant factors in this. In the NICU environment, the focus has shifted from parents being participants in performing limited care tasks to being active contributors to the healthcare and management of their infant.

The parents' inability to focus on their infant is a clue for the nurse/midwife to assist the parents in expressing feelings of guilt, anxiety, helplessness, inadequacy, anger and ambivalence. Nurses/midwives can help parents deal with these distressing feelings and recognise that they are normal responses shared by other parents. It is important to point out and reinforce the positive aspects of parents' behaviour and interactions with their infant.

To meet parental needs in the NICU, nurses/midwives must provide accurate information regarding treatment plan and procedures; answer parents' questions honestly; actively listen to parents' fears and expectations; and help parents understand infant responses to hospitalisation (Gardner, Goldson & Hernandez 2016).

Most parents feel shaky and insecure about initiating interaction with their infant. Nurses/midwives can sense parents' level of readiness and offer encouragement in these initial efforts. Parents of premature infants follow the same acquaintance process as do parents of full-term infants. They may quickly proceed through the process or may require several days, or even weeks, to complete it. Parents begin by touching their infant's extremities with their fingertips and poking the infant tenderly, and then proceed to caresses and fondling (Fig 9.2). Touching is the first act of communication between parents and child. Parents need to be prepared for their infant's exaggerated and generalised startle responses to touch so that they will not interpret these as negative reactions to their overtures. It may be necessary to limit tactile stimuli when the infant is critically ill and labile, but the nurse/midwife can offer other options, such as speaking softly or sitting at the bedside.

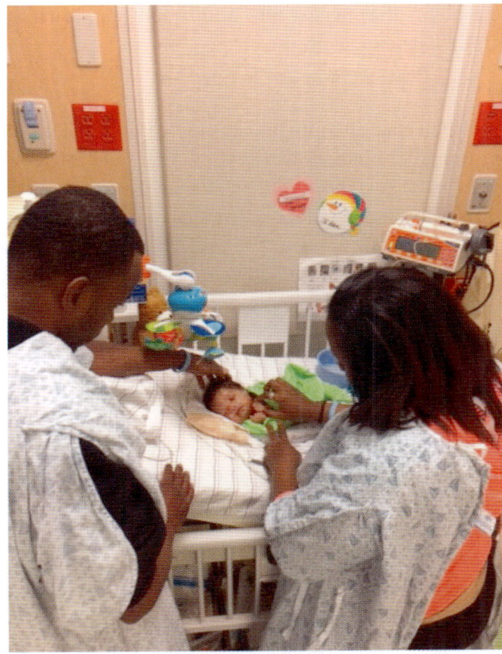

Fig 9.2 Parents interact with their premature infant. (Source: Courtesy K. Fisher, Duke University.)

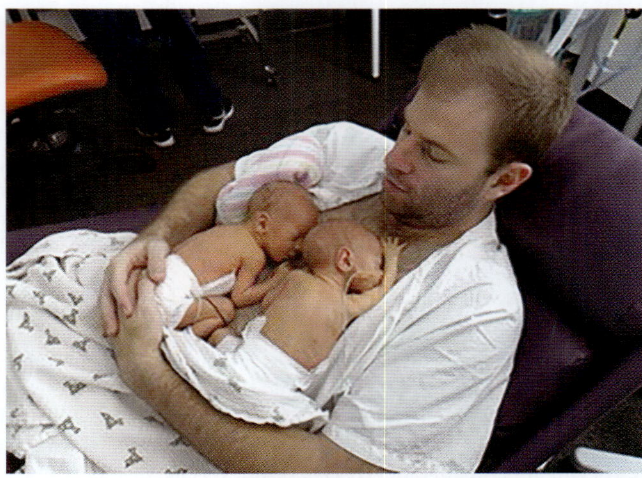

Fig 9.3 Father holding premature twins. (Source: L. Kendrick.)

Above all, nurses/midwives must encourage parents during their caregiving activities and interactions with their infant to promote healthy parent–child relationships (e.g. Fig 9.3); even small amounts of time encourage these relationships. It is also helpful for the parents to have contact and communication with the infant's primary nurse/midwife and associate primary nurse/midwife (according to unit model of nursing care). This decreases the amount of different information given to parents and often instils confidence that, although the parents cannot be at their infant's bedside 24 hours a day, they can call competent and caring nurses/midwives to enquire about the infant's status.

Siblings. In the past, concerns about sibling visitation in the NICU focused on fears of infection and disruption of nursing routines. These fears have not been substantiated, and sibling visits should be a part of the normal operation of NICUs.

The birth of a premature infant is a difficult time for siblings, who rely on the support of understanding parents. When the happy anticipation changes to sadness, worry and altered routines, siblings are bewildered and deprived of their parents' attention. They know something is wrong, but they do not completely understand what it is. Concern about the negative effects on visiting siblings of seeing the ill newborn has not been confirmed. Children have not hesitated to approach or touch the infant, and children less than 5 years of age have been less reluctant than older children. In addition, no measurable differences were found between pre-visit and post-visit behaviours.

The potential benefits of sibling visits must be weighed against the negatives of exposing the child to the NICU environment. Children must be prepared for the unfamiliar NICU atmosphere, but contact with the infant appears to have a positive effect on siblings by helping them deal with the reality rather than the fantasies that are characteristic of young children. Such visits also help bond the family as a unit.

Support Groups. Parents need to feel they are not alone. Parent support groups have been of great value to families of infants in the NICU. Some groups consist of parents who have infants in the hospital and share the same anxieties and concerns. Other groups include parents who have had infants in the NICU and who have dealt with the crisis effectively. The groups are usually under the leadership of a staff person and may involve medical practitioners, nurses/midwives and social workers, but it is the parents who can offer other parents something that no one else can provide.

Discharge Planning and Home Care

Parents become apprehensive and excited as the time for discharge approaches. They have many concerns and insecurities regarding the care of their infant. They fear that the child may still be in danger, that they will be unable to recognise signs of distress or illness and that the infant may not be ready for discharge. Nurses/midwives need to begin early to assist parents in acquiring or increasing their skills in the care of their infant. Appropriate instruction must be provided and sufficient time allowed for the family to take in the information and learn special care requirements. Where rooming-in or other live-in arrangements are available, parents can stay for a few days and nights and assume the care of their infant under the supervision and support of the nursery staff.

Neonatal Loss

The precarious nature of many high-risk infants makes death a real and ever-present possibility. Although infant mortality has been reduced sharply with improved technology, the mortality rate is still greatest during the neonatal period. Nurses/midwives in the NICU must prepare the parents for an inevitable death and facilitate a family's grieving process after an expected or unexpected death.

The loss of an infant has special meaning for the grieving parents. It represents a loss of a part of themselves, a loss of the potential for immortality that offspring represent and a loss of the dream child that they have fantasised about throughout the pregnancy. The parents have a sense of emptiness and failure. In addition, when an infant has lived for such a short time, they may have few, if any, pleasant memories to serve as a basis for the identification and idealisation that are part of the resolution of a loss.

To help parents understand that the death is a reality, it is important that they be given the opportunity to hold their infant before death and, if possible, be present at the time of death so their infant can die in their arms if they choose.

Parents should have the opportunity to actually 'parent' the infant in any manner they wish or are able to before and after the death. This may include seeing, touching, holding, caressing and talking to their infant privately. The parents may also wish to bathe and dress the infant. If parents are hesitant to see their deceased infant, it is advisable to keep the body in the unit for a few hours because many parents change their minds after the initial shock of the death.

Parents may need to see and hold the infant more than once—the first time to say 'hello' and the last time to say 'good-bye'. If parents wish to see the infant after the body has been taken to the morgue, the infant should be retrieved, wrapped in a blanket, rewarmed in a radiant warmer and taken to the mother's room or other private place. The nurse/midwife should plan to stay with the parents but also provide them an opportunity for private time alone with their dead infant if they wish. Individual grief responses of the mother and father should be recognised and handled appropriately. Gender differences and cultural and religious beliefs will affect the parents' grief responses (Koopmans et al 2013).

A photograph of the infant taken before or after death is highly desirable. Parents may wish to have a special family portrait taken with the infant and other family members. This often helps personalise the experience and make it more tangible. The parents may not wish to see the photograph at the time of death, but the chance to refer to it later will help make their infant seem more real, which is a part of the normal grieving process. A photograph of their infant being held by the hand or touched by an adult offers a more positive image than a morgue photograph. The photographs and other personal effects of the deceased infant were perceived as critically important in the grieving process by one group of parents in a survey. Photographs are helpful in remembering the infant's actual appearance during this stressful period (Swaney et al 2016).

A primary nurse/midwife who is familiar to the family should be present during the discussion about the dead or dying infant. A bereavement counsellor is often involved in helping the family through this difficult period. The nurse/midwife should talk with parents openly and honestly about funeral arrangements because few of them have had experience with this aspect of death. Someone from the NICU should take responsibility for acquiring this information. A leader of the appropriate faith may be notified if the parents wish. Issues regarding an autopsy or organ donation (when appropriate) are approached in a multidisciplinary fashion (primary practitioner and primary nurse/midwife) with respect, tact and consideration of the family's wishes. (See also 'Grief and Perinatal Loss' in Gardner, Goldson & Hernandez 2016.)

Before the parents leave the hospital, the nurse/midwife should provide them with the telephone number of the unit (if they do not have it) and invite them to call any time they have any further questions. Many intensive care units make it a point to contact the parents after a neonatal death to assess the parents' coping mechanisms, evaluate the grieving process and provide support as needed.

Nurses/midwives who care for critically ill infants also experience grief. NICU nurses/midwives may feel helpless and sorrowful. It is important that such grief be allowed and that nurses/midwives attend the funeral or memorial service as a part of working through the grieving process. Nurses/midwives may fear that showing emotion is unprofessional and that the expression of grief demonstrates 'loss of control'; these fears are unfounded. Studies have demonstrated that to continue to be effective providers of care, nurses/midwives must be allowed to grieve and support one another through the process (Jonas-Simpson et al 2013).

HIGH-RISK CONDITIONS RELATED TO DYSMATURITY

Premature Infants

Prematurity of infants accounts for the largest number of admissions to the NICU. Immaturity not only places infants at risk for neonatal complications (e.g. hyperbilirubinaemia and RDS, which has the highest incidence in premature infants), but it may also predispose the infant to problems that persist into adulthood (e.g. learning disabilities, growth deficiencies, asthma).

Aetiology

A variety of maternal and pregnancy-related complications increase the risk of premature birth; however, the actual cause of prematurity is not known in most instances. The incidence of prematurity is lowest in the middle to high socioeconomic classes, in which pregnant women are generally in good health, are well nourished and receive prompt and comprehensive prenatal care. The incidence is highest in the lower socioeconomic classes, in which a combination of negative circumstances is present. Other factors, such as multiple pregnancies, gestational hypertension and placental problems that interrupt the normal course of gestation, are responsible for a large number of premature births.

The outlook for premature infants is largely, but not entirely, related to the state of physiological and anatomical immaturity of the various organs and systems at the time of birth. Infants at term have advanced to a state of maturity sufficient to allow a successful transition to the extrauterine environment. Infants born prematurely must make the same adjustments but with functional immaturity proportional to the stage of development reached at the time of birth. The degree to which infants are prepared for extrauterine life can be predicted to some extent by estimated gestational age. (See Clinical Assessment of Gestational Age, Chapter 7.) An understanding of prenatal development provides some concept of the status of the developing systems that must cope with functional changes that occur with birth.

Characteristics

Premature infants have distinct characteristics at various stages of development. Identification of these characteristics provides valuable clues to the gestational age and hence to the infant's physiological capabilities. Physical appearance changes as the fetus progresses to maturity. Skin, posture and tone, distribution of hair and amount of subcutaneous fat provide clues to a newborn's physical development. Observation of spontaneous, active movements and response to stimulation and passive movement contributes to the assessment of neurological status. The appraisal is made as soon as possible after admission to the nursery because much of the observation and management of infants depend on this information.

Therapeutic Management

When birth of a premature infant is anticipated, the intensive care nursery is alerted and a team approach implemented. Ideally, a neonatologist or a neonatal nurse practitioner, a staff nurse and a respiratory therapist are present for the birth. Infants who do not require resuscitation are immediately transferred in a heated incubator to the NICU, where they are weighed and where IV access, oxygen therapy and other therapeutic interventions are initiated as needed. Resuscitation is conducted in the birth area until infants can be safely transported to the NICU. Ongoing care is described elsewhere in the chapter.

Nursing Care Management

As with therapeutic management, individualise nursing care for each infant. See appropriate discussions under Nursing Care of High-Risk Newborns for details of care.

Postterm Infants

Infants born after 42 weeks as calculated from the mother's last menstrual period (or by gestational age assessment) are **postterm**, regardless of birth weight. This constitutes 3.5% to 15% of all pregnancies. The cause of delayed birth is unknown. Postterm infants display the characteristics of infants who are 1 to 3 weeks of age, such as absence of lanugo, little if any vernix caseosa, abundant scalp hair and long fingernails. The skin is often cracked, parchmentlike and peeling. A common finding in postterm infants is a wasted physical appearance that reflects intrauterine nutritional deprivation. Depletion of subcutaneous fat gives them a thin, elongated appearance. The little vernix caseosa that remains in the skin folds may be stained a deep yellow or green, which is usually an indication of meconium in the amniotic fluid.

Fetal and neonatal mortality rates increase significantly in postterm infants compared with those born at term. They are especially prone to fetal distress associated with the decreasing efficiency of the placenta, **macrosomia** and meconium aspiration syndrome. The greatest risk occurs during labour and birth, particularly in infants of primigravidas, or women birthing their first child. Induction of labour is usually recommended when infants are significantly overdue.

HIGH RISK RELATED TO DISTURBED RESPIRATORY FUNCTION

Apnoea of Prematurity

Premature infants are characteristically periodic breathers. They have periods of rapid respiration separated by periods of very slow breathing, and often short periods with no visible or audible respirations.

Apnoea is primarily an extension of this periodic breathing and can be defined as a lapse of spontaneous breathing for 20 or more seconds, or shorter pauses accompanied by bradycardia or oxygen desaturation (Gardner, Enzman-Hines & Nyp 2016).

Apnoea of prematurity (AOP) is a common phenomenon in the premature infant. Rarely observed in full-term infants, apnoeic spells increase in prevalence the younger the gestational age. Most infants less than 32 weeks' gestation and nearly all apparently healthy infants less than 30 weeks' gestation have apnoeic spells (Gardner, Enzman-Hines & Nyp 2016). Apnoea usually resolves as the infant approaches 37 weeks of postmenstrual age, but in those born very prematurely, apnoea can persist up to 43 weeks of postmenstrual age (Alvaro 2012).

AOP may be further classified according to origin. The three recognised types are: (1) central apnoea, an absence of diaphragmatic and other respiratory muscle function that causes a lack of respiratory effort and occurs when the CNS does not transmit signals to the respiratory muscles; (2) obstructive apnoea, when air flow stops because of upper airway obstruction, yet chest or abdominal wall movement is present; and (3) mixed apnoea, a combination of central and obstructive apnoea and the most common form of apnoea seen in premature infants (Gardner, Enzman-Hines & Nyp 2016).

Pathophysiology

AOP reflects the immature and poorly refined neurological and chemical respiratory control mechanisms in premature infants. These infants are not as responsive to hypercarbia and hypoxaemia, and their neurons have fewer dendritic associations than those of more mature infants. The respiratory reflexes of these infants are significantly less mature, which may be a contributing factor in the aetiology. Overall weakness of the muscles of the thorax, diaphragm and upper airway may also contribute to apnoeic episodes in the premature infant. In addition, apnoea is characteristically observed during periods of REM sleep. A variety of factors, including infection, intracranial haemorrhage (ICH) or PDA, can make apnoea worse. Secondary causes of apnoea should be investigated in infants with new-onset apnoea or when there is a significant change in the frequency or severity of apnoeic episodes. Apnoea in full-term infants should always be considered secondary and the cause investigated.

Clinical Manifestations

Factors that contribute to apnoea in premature neonates should be investigated and treated. Apnoea can be anticipated in infants with a variety of conditions (Box 9.4); conversely, one of these disorders may be suspected in infants with persistent apnoeic spells. Although apnoea is an expected event in premature neonates, it should not be designated benign until all other causes have been ruled out. Apnoea is a reason to screen for any of the causes listed in Box 9.4.

Therapeutic Management

Caffeine citrate (methylxanthine) is often effective in reducing the frequency of primary apnoea-bradycardia spells in newborns < 34 weeks. Caffeine acts as a CNS stimulant to breathing. Neonates receiving caffeine must be closely observed for symptoms of toxicity. Caffeine has come to the forefront of pharmacological therapy for AOP because it has fewer side effects than previously used aminophylline or theophylline, requires dosing once daily, has more predictable plasma concentrations, has slower elimination and has a wider therapeutic range (trough, 5 to 20 microgram/mL) (Carlo 2016a).

Nasal CPAP and, more recently, nasal intermittent positive pressure ventilation has been used as an adjunct treatment for AOP. CPAP acts to stabilise the airway and improve lung volumes; hence it is most

BOX 9.4 Possible Causes of Apnoea of Prematurity

- Prematurity
- Airway obstruction with mucus or milk, or poor positioning
- Anaemia, polycythaemia
- Dehydration
- Cooling or overheating
- Hypoxaemia
- Hypercapnia or hypocapnia
- Hypoglycaemia
- Hypocalcaemia
- Hyponatraemia
- Sepsis, meningitis
- Seizures
- Increased vagal tone (in response to suctioning nasopharynx, gavage tube insertion, reflux of gastric contents, endotracheal intubation)
- Central nervous system depression from pharmacological agents
- Intraventricular haemorrhage
- Patent ductus arteriosus, congestive heart failure
- Depression following maternal obstetric sedation
- Respiratory distress as a result of pneumonia, inborn errors of metabolism such as hyperammonaemia, congenital defects of the upper airways

effective for obstructive or mixed apnoea (Royal Children's Hospital Melbourne [RCHM] 2019).

Nursing Care Management

Management of apnoea consists of monitoring respiration and heart rate routinely in all premature infants and preventing contributing conditions. Cardiorespiratory monitors alert the staff to cessation of breathing according to a preset delay time—usually 15 to 20 seconds. Effective monitoring devices do not eliminate the need for alert nursing observation. Nursing observation combined with monitoring is the most effective means of identifying neonatal apnoea.

If begun early, gentle tactile stimulation (e.g. rubbing the back or chest gently, repositioning the infant) will stop most apnoeic spells. If tactile stimulation fails to reinstitute respiration, flow-by oxygen and suctioning of the nose and mouth may be required. If breathing does not begin, the chin is raised gently to open the airway and sufficient positive pressure is applied with a resuscitation mask and bag to lift the rib cage. The infant is never shaken. After breathing is restored, the infant is assessed for possible precipitating factors, such as unstable temperature, abdominal distension (if not observed earlier) or malpositioning of the airway. The use of pulse oximetry has helped detect the onset of an apnoeic episode.

Respiratory Distress Syndrome

Respiratory distress syndrome (RDS) refers to a condition of surfactant deficiency and physiological immaturity of the thorax. The terms *respiratory distress syndrome* and *hyaline membrane disease* are most often applied to this severe lung disorder. It is seen almost exclusively in premature infants but may also be associated with multifetal pregnancies, infants of diabetic mothers, caesarean section birth, cold stress, asphyxia and a family history of RDS (Carlo & Ambalavanan 2016c). The disorder is rarely observed in drug-exposed infants or infants who have been subjected to chronic intrauterine stress (e.g. maternal preeclampsia or hypertension). Respiratory distress of a non-pulmonary origin in neonates may also be caused by sepsis, cardiac defects (structural or functional), exposure to cold, airway obstruction (atresia), IVH, hypoglycaemia, metabolic acidosis, acute blood loss and drugs. Pneumonia in the neonatal period is respiratory distress caused by bacterial or viral agents and may occur alone or as a complication of RDS.

Pathophysiology

Premature infants are born before the lungs are fully prepared to serve as efficient organs for gas exchange. This appears to be a critical factor in the development of RDS. RDS results from a combination of structural and functional immaturity of the lungs.

Because the final unfolding of the alveolar septa, which increases the surface area of the lungs, occurs during the last trimester of pregnancy, premature infants are born with numerous underdeveloped and many uninflatable alveoli. In addition, the fetal chest wall is highly compliant because of the predominance of cartilage rather than bone, and the diaphragm, the dominant respiratory muscle, is prone to fatigue.

Functionally, the fetal lungs are deficient in **surfactant**, a surface-active phospholipid secreted by type II cells in the alveolar epithelium. Surfactant is first produced at about 24 weeks' gestational age, but the type II cells in the lung do not fully mature until about 36 weeks' gestation (Fig 9.4). Acting much like a detergent, this substance reduces the surface tension of fluids that line the alveoli and respiratory passages, resulting in uniform expansion and maintenance of lung expansion at low intra-alveolar pressure. Immature development of these functions seriously compromises respiratory efficiency. Deficient surfactant

PATHOPHYSIOLOGY REVIEW

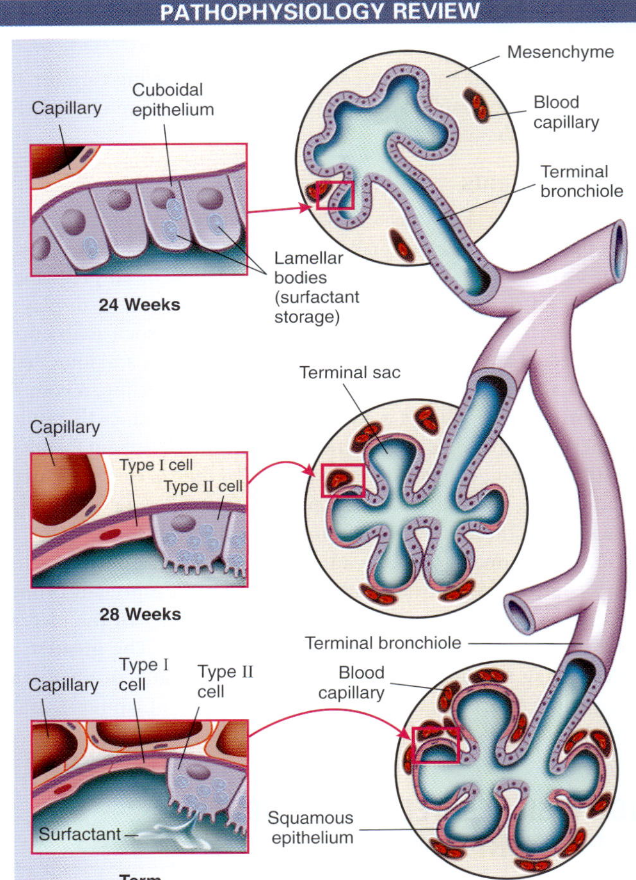

Fig 9.4 Prenatal development of the alveolar unit. (Source: From McCance, K., & Huether, S. [2010]. Pathophysiology: The biological basis for disease in adults and children [6th ed.]. St Louis, MO: Mosby.)

production causes unequal inflation of alveoli on inspiration and the collapse of alveoli on end expiration. Without surfactant, infants are unable to keep their lungs inflated and therefore exert a great deal of effort to re-expand the alveoli with each breath. It has been estimated that each breath requires as much negative pressure (60 to 75 cmH_2O) as the initial lung expansion at birth. With increasing exhaustion they are able to open fewer and fewer alveoli. This inability to maintain lung expansion produces widespread atelectasis.

In the absence of alveolar stability (i.e. normal functional residual capacity) and with progressive atelectasis, pulmonary vascular resistance (PVR) increases, whereas with normal lung expansion it would decrease. Consequently, there is hypoperfusion to the lung tissue with a decrease in effective pulmonary blood flow. The increase in PVR causes partial reversion to the fetal circulation, with a right-to-left shunting of blood through the persisting fetal communications—the ductus arteriosus and foramen ovale.

Inadequate pulmonary perfusion and ventilation produce hypoxaemia and hypercapnia. Pulmonary arterioles, with their thick muscular layer, are markedly reactive to diminished oxygen concentration. Thus a decrease in oxygen tension causes vasospasm in the pulmonary arterioles that is worsened by a decrease in blood pH. This vasoconstriction contributes to a marked increase in PVR. In normal ventilation with increased oxygen concentration, the ductus arteriosus constricts and the pulmonary vessels dilate to decrease PVR (Fig 9.5).

Prolonged hypoxaemia activates anaerobic glycolysis, which produces increased amounts of lactic acid. An increase in lactic acid causes metabolic acidosis. Inability of the atelectatic lungs to blow off excess carbon dioxide produces respiratory acidosis. Lowered pH causes further vasoconstriction. With deficient pulmonary circulation and alveolar perfusion, PaO_2 continues to fall, pH falls and the materials needed for surfactant production are not circulated to the alveoli.

Pulmonary oedema observed in the early stages of RDS also contributes to impaired gas exchange. Factors believed to facilitate this fluid accumulation in the lungs include renal immaturity or insufficiency resulting from hypoxaemia, high fluid intake and PDA, left ventricular dysfunction associated with papillary muscle necrosis, low serum protein concentration and low colloid osmotic pressure, increased alveolar surface tension that enhances the shift of interstitial fluid to alveolar spaces, oxygen toxicity and high plasma vasopressin.

Pulmonary interstitial emphysema (PIE) may develop in premature infants with RDS and immature lungs as a result of overdistension of distal airways. This condition further complicates adequate oxygenation in the immature airways.

Deficiencies in other systems contribute to respiratory distress. For example, a high threshold of the respiratory centre to afferent stimuli and weak or absent gag and cough reflexes reflect the immaturity of the nervous system. In addition, the persistence of fetal haemoglobin may place the infant at a disadvantage during respiratory distress. Although the binding power of fetal haemoglobin for oxygen is much greater than that of adult haemoglobin, this increased affinity also causes less oxygen to be released to the tissues at normal oxygen tension. In the newborn the arterial oxygen concentration must fall to a lower level for bound oxygen to be released from fetal haemoglobin.

A **hyaline membrane** is formed as hypoxaemia and the increased pulmonary vascular pressure cause transudation of fluid into the alveoli. Necrotic cells from damaged alveoli plus the fibrin in the transudate form a membranous layer that lines the alveoli and inhibits gas exchange. The hyaline membrane contributes to respiratory problems by greatly reducing **lung distensibility**, or compliance, the elastic quality of lung tissue that permits expansion in response to a given amount of applied pressure during inspiration. Affected lungs are stiffer and require far more pressure than do normal lungs to achieve an equal

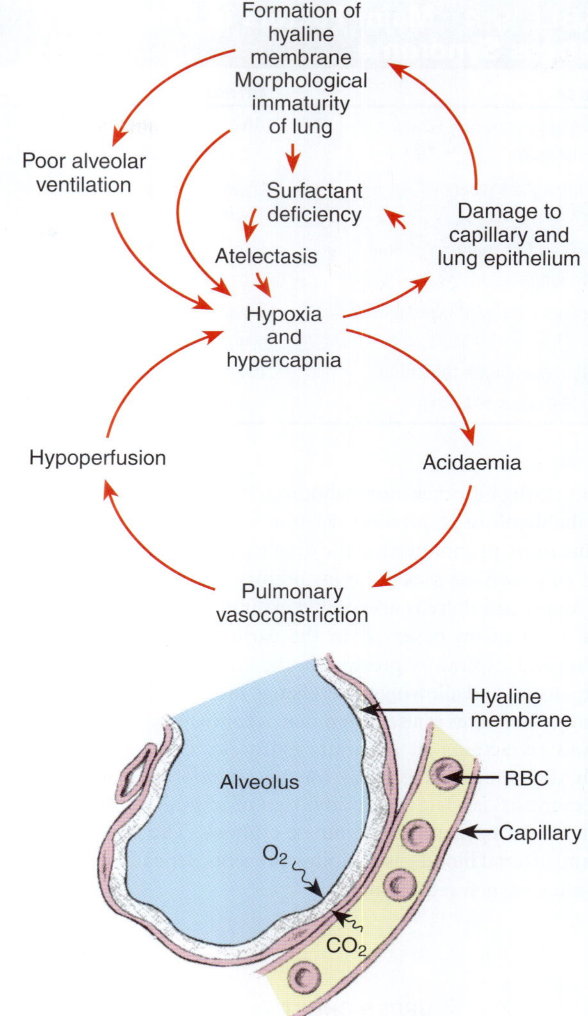

Fig 9.5 Interdependent relationship of factors involved in pathology of respiratory distress syndrome. *CO_2*, carbon dioxide; *O_2*, oxygen; *RBC*, red blood cell. (Source: Pierog, S. H., & Ferrara, A. (1976). Medical care of the sick newborn (2nd ed.). St Louis, MO: Mosby.)

amount of expansion. Table 9.4 summarises the major factors that produce RDS in immature infants.

Clinical Manifestations

Infants with RDS can develop respiratory distress either acutely or over a period of hours, depending on the acuity of pulmonary immaturity, associated illness factors and gestational maturity. The observable signs produced by the pulmonary changes usually begin to appear in infants who apparently achieve normal breathing and colour soon after birth. In a matter of a few hours, breathing gradually becomes more rapid ($>$ 60 breaths/min). Infants may display retractions—suprasternal or substernal, and supracostal, subcostal or intercostal—which result from a compliant chest wall. Weak chest wall muscles and the highly cartilaginous rib structure produce an abnormally elastic rib cage, resulting in indrawing or retraction of the skin between the ribs. During this period the infant's colour may remain good, and auscultation reveals air entry. Some of the criteria for evaluating respiratory distress in infants are illustrated in Fig 9.6.

Within a few hours, respiratory distress becomes more obvious. The respiratory rate continues to increase (to 80 to 120 breaths/min),

TABLE 9.4 Major Factors in Respiratory Distress Syndrome

Cause	Effect
Increased pulmonary vascular resistance	Alveolar collapse; atelectasis; increased difficulty breathing
Impaired gas exchange	Hypoxaemia and hypercapnia with respiratory acidosis
Increased transudation of fluid into lungs	Hypoperfusion of pulmonary circulation
Hypoperfusion (with hypoxaemia)	Tissue hypoxia and metabolic acidosis
Hyaline membrane formation; impaired gas exchange	Increased surface tension of alveoli (surfactant deficiency)

and breathing becomes more laboured. Infants increase the rate rather than the depth of respiration when in distress. Substernal retractions become more pronounced as the diaphragm works hard in an attempt to fill collapsed air sacs. Fine inspiratory crackles can be heard over both lungs, and there is an audible expiratory grunt. This grunting, a useful mechanism observed in the earlier stages of RDS, serves to increase end-expiratory pressure in the lungs, thus maintaining alveolar expansion and allowing gas exchange for an additional brief period. Flaring of the nares is also a sign that accompanies tachypnoea, grunting and retractions in respiratory distress. Central cyanosis (i.e. a bluish discolouration of oral mucous membranes and generalised body cyanosis) is a late and serious sign of respiratory distress. Initially supplemental oxygen may eliminate cyanosis. The use of pulse oximetry and arterial blood gas sampling prevents dependence on colour to determine oxygen requirements.

Severe RDS is often associated with a shocklike state, with diminished cardiac inflow and low arterial blood pressure. As a result of extreme pulmonary immaturity, decreased glycogen stores and lack of accessory muscles, the ELBW and VLBW infant may have severe RDS at birth, bypassing the aforementioned steps in the development of RDS.

Infants with RDS who are treated with exogenous surfactant have a good chance for recovery. Associated complications (of prematurity and RDS) include PDA and congestive heart failure, retinopathy of prematurity, IVH, chronic lung disease, NEC and neurological sequelae.

Diagnostic Evaluation

Laboratory data are non-specific, and the abnormalities observed are identical to those observed in numerous biochemical abnormalities of the newborn (i.e. the findings of hypoxaemia, hypercapnia and acidosis). Specific tests are used to determine complicating factors, such as blood glucose (to test for hypoglycaemia), blood gas measurements for serum pH (to test for acidosis) and PaO_2 (to test for hypoxia). Pulse oximetry is an important component for determining hypoxia. Other special examinations may be used to diagnose or rule out complications.

Radiographic findings characteristic of RDS include: (1) a diffuse granular pattern over both lung fields that resembles ground glass and represents alveolar atelectasis; and (2) dark streaks or air bronchograms, within the ground glass areas that represent dilated, air-filled bronchioles. It is important to distinguish between RDS and pneumonia in infants with respiratory distress.

Prenatal Diagnosis. Fetal lung maturity depends on gestational age and maternal illnesses. Problems such as maternal diabetes delay fetal lung maturation, whereas fetuses exposed to chronic stress (intrauterine growth restriction [IUGR], drug exposure) often have more mature lungs. Antenatal administration of glucocorticoids enhances fetal lung maturity, especially when combined with

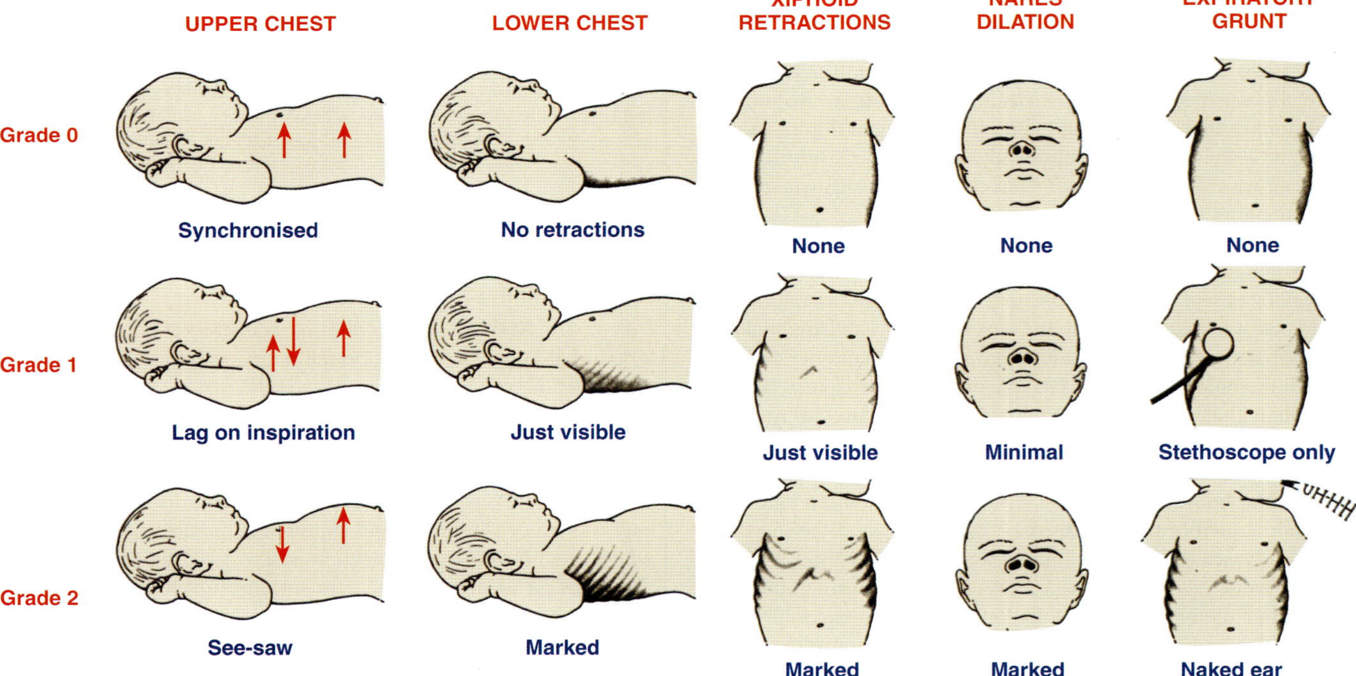

Fig 9.6 Criteria for evaluating respiratory distress. (Source: Modified from Silvermann, W. A., & Anderson, D. H. (1956). A controlled clinical trial of effects of water mist on obstructive respiratory signs, death rate, and necropsy findings among premature infants. Pediatrics, 17, 1.)

postnatal surfactant administration (Gardner, Enzman-Hines & Nyp 2016, Surbek et al 2012).

Functional maturity of the fetal lung is indicated by surfactant phospholipids in amniotic fluid. The most commonly tested is the **lecithin/sphingomyelin** (L/S) ratio, which represents the relationship between these two lipids during gestation. Phospholipids are synthesised by fetal alveolar cells, and the concentrations in amniotic fluid change during gestation. Initially there is more sphingomyelin, but at approximately 32 to 33 weeks the concentrations become equal; sphingomyelin then diminishes and lecithin increases significantly until the fetus has developed sufficient surfactant to maintain alveolar stability at approximately 35 weeks. An **L/S ratio** of 2 : 1 in non-diabetic mothers indicates virtually no risk of RDS.

Other key surfactant compounds (also phospholipids) that are needed to stabilise surfactant are phosphatidylcholine (PC) and phosphatidylglycerol (PG). Without these compounds, lecithin is not functional as a surfactant. Concentrations of PC parallel those of lecithin, peaking at 35 weeks and then gradually decreasing. At 36 weeks PG appears in amniotic fluid and increases until term. By measuring these phospholipids—L/S ratio, PC and PG—the clinician can estimate the maturity of the lungs with a high degree of accuracy. Other, less commonly used methods have been devised to provide rapid, inexpensive and accurate measures of lung maturity. These include the 'shake' or 'bubble' test, in which stable foam or bubbles form when amniotic fluid is shaken in the presence of ethanol, and the tap test, in which abundant bubbles appear in a test tube of amniotic fluid with 6*N*-hydrochloric acid and diethyl ether.

Lamellar bodies, representing the storage form of surfactant, are found in amniotic fluid in increasing quantities with the advancement of gestational age and lung maturity. A quantitative count of lamellar bodies has been reported to be as accurate as the L/S ratio in determining fetal lung maturity. The count can be obtained faster than the L/S ratio, thus making it clinically appealing (Welch et al 2016).

Therapeutic Management

The treatment of RDS includes all the general measures required for any premature infant, as well as those instituted to correct imbalances. The supportive measures most crucial to a favourable outcome are: (1) maintain adequate ventilation and oxygenation with CPAP, high-flow nasal cannula or mechanical ventilation; (2) maintain acid–base balance; (3) maintain a neutral thermal environment; (4) maintain adequate tissue perfusion and oxygenation; (5) prevent hypotension; and (6) maintain adequate hydration and electrolyte status. Nipple and gavage feedings are avoided in any situation that creates a marked increase in respiratory rate because of the greater hazards of aspiration.

Surfactant. The practice of administering exogenous surfactant to premature neonates with RDS is now common therapy in most neonatal ICUs worldwide. Research has demonstrated improvement in blood gas values and ventilator settings, decreased incidence of pulmonary air leaks and a significantly lower infant mortality rate with the use of exogenous surfactant (Saugstad et al 2019). The dependence on ventilation is reduced with the use of surfactant, pneumothorax is reduced, oxygenation is increased and the overall survival rate of premature babies has significantly improved from 30% in the 1970s to 90% today (Saugstad et al 2019).

Studies have compared one surfactant product with another. Bryant and colleagues (2019) found that an investigational synthetic surfactant—lucinactant—mimics the action of human surfactant protein-B (SP-B) and has been shown to be more effective than beractant and colfosceril palmitate at reducing the RDS-related mortality by 14 days of life.

Additional benefits of surfactant replacement therapy include decreased oxygen requirements and mean airway pressure (MAP) within hours of administration and an overall decrease in the incidence of pulmonary air leaks. To date, long-term improvement in the decrease of chronic lung disease and IVH has not been evidenced in all surfactant clinical trials.

Complications seen with surfactant administration include pulmonary haemorrhage and mucus plugging. Use of surfactant in infants with meconium aspiration resulted in a reduction in the severity of respiratory illness and subsequent need for extracorporeal membrane oxygenation (ECMO) support (Gardner, Enzman-Hines & Nyp 2016). Other studies continue to investigate the potential benefits of exogenous surfactant for the treatment of infectious pneumonia and lung hypoplasia associated with congenital diaphragmatic hernia (Zani et al 2016).

Nursing responsibilities with surfactant administration include assistance in the birth of the product, collection and monitoring of arterial blood gases, scrupulous monitoring of oxygenation and assessment of the infant's tolerance of the procedure. Once surfactant is absorbed, there is usually an increase in respiratory compliance that requires adjustment of ventilator settings to decrease MAP and prevent overinflation or hyperoxaemia. Suctioning is usually delayed for an hour or so (depending on the type of surfactant, birth system and unit protocol) to allow maximum effects to occur.

Oxygen Therapy. The goals of oxygen therapy are to provide adequate oxygen to the tissues, prevent lactic acid accumulation resulting from hypoxia and avoid the potentially negative effects of oxygen toxicity. Numerous methods have been devised to improve oxygenation. All require that the gas be warmed and humidified before entering the respiratory tract. If the infant does not require ventilatory assistance, oxygen can be given via nasal prongs to supply variable concentrations of humidified oxygen. If oxygen saturation cannot be maintained at a satisfactory level and the carbon dioxide level ($PaCO_2$) rises, infants will need ventilatory assistance. All nurses and midwives should become familiar with their current policies and procedures in relation to oxygen delivery to neonates. Much attention has been given to high oxygen concentration flow rates for neonates and the effect of free oxygen radicals on the development of conditions such as NED, chronic lung disease and retinopathy of the premature infant (Safe Care Victoria 2021a).

CPAP, the application of 3 to 8 cmH_2O (positive) pressure to the airway, uses the infant's spontaneous respiration to improve oxygenation by helping prevent alveolar collapse and increasing diffusion time. CPAP may be delivered via fitted face mask or nasal prongs (Fig 9.7). Ventilation with CPAP is done entirely by the infant. The use of high-flow nasal cannula (HFNC) at flow rates greater than or equal to 2 L/min is an alternative to nasal cannula for infants with RDS; the infant may be given surfactant shortly after birth then placed on either nasal CPAP or HFNC.

If oxygenation is not improved and the infant requires assisted ventilation, intermittent mandatory ventilation (IMV) is used with positive end-expiratory pressure (PEEP). This allows infants to breathe at their own rate but provides positive pressure breaths with end-expiratory pressure to prevent alveolar collapse and overcome airway resistance. IMV also involves peak inspiratory pressure (PIP) and rate (number of breaths per minute). The PIP is the maximum amount of positive pressure applied to the infant on inspiration. The total amount of pressure transmitted to the airway throughout an entire respiratory cycle is called the *mean airway pressure* (MAP or P_{aw}). Increasing MAP in infants with severe RDS correlates positively with improved oxygenation by maintaining functional residual capacity and overcoming the resistive forces of the atelectatic lung. The MAP is

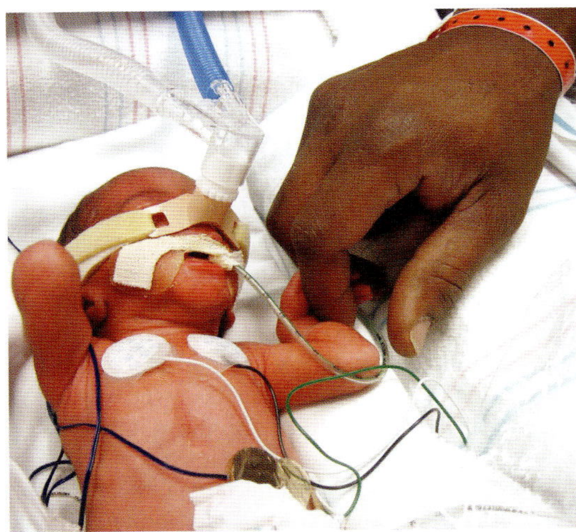

Fig 9.7 Infant on nasal continuous positive airway pressure with father's finger in hand. (Source: Courtesy E. Jacobs, Texas Children's Hospital, Houston.)

affected by changes in the PEEP, PIP and inspiratory/expiratory ratio. Although MAP is now recognised as the major determinant of oxygenation, this does not imply that simply increasing MAP will automatically improve oxygenation (Keszler & Abubakar 2017).

Improved technology has provided to premature or sick neonates a form of mechanical ventilatory assistance previously used in adults: **synchronised intermittent mandatory ventilation** (SIMV). With this method breaths delivered by the ventilator are synchronised to the onset of spontaneous infant breaths. The net effect is to produce full respiratory synchrony rather than asynchronous respiratory efforts (commonly called 'fighting the ventilator') that are believed to significantly impede the ability to adequately oxygenate infants without sedation or muscle paralysis. With SIMV, the operator sets the number of breaths per minute delivered by the ventilator, and the patient may breathe spontaneously between mechanical breaths. In the 'assist-control' mode a mechanical breath is delivered each time a spontaneous respiration is detected; the 'control' mode includes the birth of a mechanical breath at a regular rate if the patient fails to initiate a spontaneous respiration. Additional benefits of SIMV are improved oxygenation, decreased incidence of chronic lung disease and decreased time on mechanical ventilation.

If adequate oxygenation cannot be maintained and hypercarbia persists, infants may benefit from one of the two high-frequency ventilation (HFV) modalities. HFV delivers gas at very rapid rates to provide adequate minute volumes using lower proximal airway pressures by way of high-frequency oscillatory ventilation (HFOV) or high-frequency jet ventilation (HFJV). HFV was initially recommended for intractable respiratory failure, especially for infants with pulmonary air leaks and PIE. Many clinicians have now begun recommending earlier use of HFOV to prevent volutrauma to the lungs of very premature infants (Clark 2017).

Volutrauma is believed to be a key factor in the development of chronic lung disease. Sun and colleagues (2013) reported that HFOV was associated with improved survival and a decreased incidence of neurological disability. HFJV is most often used in the treatment of full-term infants with meconium aspiration, persistent pulmonary hypertension or air leak syndromes.

Complications of Positive Pressure Ventilation. Mechanical ventilation is not without hazards. Positive pressure introduced by mechanical apparatus increases complications such as PIE, pneumothorax and pneumomediastinum. The avoidance of intubation and mechanical ventilation reduces the incidence of chronic lung disease (Gardner, Enzman-Hines & Nyp 2016). Other complications directly related to positive pressure include various problems associated with intubation, such as nasal, tracheal or pharyngeal perforation; stenosis; inflammation; palatal grooves; subglottic stenosis; tube obstruction; and infection.

Medical Therapies. The treatment of the infant with RDS requires one or more IV lines to maintain hydration and nutrition, monitor arterial blood gases and administer medications. Systemic antibiotics may be administered during the acute phase if sepsis is suspected. Caffeine may be used to treat apnoea and to prepare for weaning VLBW and ELBW infants from mechanical ventilation. Inotropes such as dopamine and dobutamine may be required to support the infant's systemic blood pressure and maintain effective cardiac output during the acute phase of illness.

Prevention. The most successful approach to prevention of RDS is prevention of premature birth, especially elective early birth and caesarean section. Improved methods for assessing the maturity of the fetal lung by amniocentesis, although not a routine procedure, allow a reasonable prediction of adequate surfactant formation. Because estimation of a birth date can be miscalculated by as much as 1 month, such tests are particularly valuable when scheduling an elective caesarean section. Studies indicate that the combination of maternal glucocorticoid administration before birth and surfactant administration postnatally has a synergistic effect on neonatal lungs, with the net result being a decrease in infant mortality and incidence of IVH or infection (Gardner, Enzman-Hines & Nyp 2016, Hallman & Saarela 2012).

Nursing Care Management

Care of infants with RDS involves all the observations and interventions previously described for high-risk infants. In addition, the nurse/midwife is concerned with the complex problems related to respiratory therapy and the constant threat of hypoxaemia and acidosis that complicates the care of patients in respiratory difficulty.

The respiratory therapist is often responsible for the maintenance and regulation of respiratory equipment. Nevertheless, nurses/midwives should understand the equipment and be able to recognise when it is not functioning correctly. The most essential nursing function is to observe and assess the infant's response to therapy. Continuous monitoring and close observation are key because an infant's status can change rapidly and because oxygen concentration and ventilation parameters are prescribed according to the infant's blood gas measurements and pulse oximetry readings. Changes in oxygen concentration are based on these observations.

The nurse/midwife determines the amount of oxygen administered, expressed as the fraction of inspired air (FiO_2), on an individual basis according to pulse oximetry and/or arterial oxygen concentration. Capillary samples collected from the heel (see Chapter 22 for procedure) are useful for pH and $PaCO_2$ determinations but not for oxygenation status. Continuous pulse oximetry readings are recorded hourly or more often as required in critically ill infants. Blood sampling is performed after ventilator changes for the acutely ill infant and thereafter when clinically indicated.

In infants with RDS who are acutely ill or extremely premature, an umbilical arterial catheter (UAC) may be used to draw arterial blood for monitoring oxygenation. The catheter is inserted under sterile conditions via one of the umbilical arteries to the premeasured desired position (either at the level of the diaphragm, T6–T10 or between L3 and L4) and rests in the descending aorta. Continuous arterial pressure monitoring may be carried out with an 'in-line' transducer. Practices vary regarding medication administration via a UAC. An umbilical venous catheter (UVC) may be used separately or in conjunction with the UAC, depending on the severity of the infant's illness, the fluid requirements and preferred medical practice.

Mucus may collect in the respiratory tract as a result of the infant's pulmonary condition. Secretions interfere with gas flow and may obstruct the passages, including the ET tube. Suctioning should occur only when necessary and should be based on individual infant assessment, which includes auscultation of the chest, evidence of decreased oxygenation, excess moisture in the ET tube or increased infant irritability. It is recommended that, where possible, an in-line suction device be used on infants who are acutely ill and who do not tolerate any procedure without profound decreases in oxygen saturation, blood pressure and heart rate. The purpose of suctioning an artificial airway is to maintain patency of that airway, not the bronchi. Suction applied beyond the ET tube can cause traumatic lesions of the trachea.

Research indicates that suctioning to a point where the catheter meets resistance and is then withdrawn causes trauma to the tracheobronchial wall. To remove secretions without damage to the tracheobronchial mucosa, the suction catheter is premeasured and inserted to a predetermined depth to avoid extension beyond the ET tube. The practice of suctioning patients on mechanical ventilation has undergone close scrutiny in recent years. Further studies are needed to validate this practice and to determine the best methods for maintaining a patent airway without compromising the patient's wellbeing. All efforts are made to prevent *ventilator-associated pneumonia* in mechanically ventilated high-risk infants.

NURSING CARE CONSIDERATIONS

Suctioning is not an innocuous procedure; it may cause bronchospasm, bradycardia because of vagal nerve stimulation, hypoxia and increased intracranial pressure, predisposing the infant to IVH. It should never be carried out on a routine basis. Improper suctioning technique can also cause infection, airway damage or even pneumothorax.

Nursing care of an infant with RDS is demanding. Pay meticulous attention to subtle changes in the infant's oxygenation status. The importance of attention to detail cannot be overemphasised, particularly in regard to medication administration.

Meconium Aspiration Syndrome

Meconium aspiration syndrome (MAS) occurs when a fetus has been subjected to asphyxia or other intrauterine stress that causes relaxation of the anal sphincter and passage of meconium into the amniotic fluid. Most meconium aspiration occurs with the first breath. However, a severely compromised fetus may aspirate in utero. At birth of the chest and initiation of the first breath, infants inhale fluid and meconium into the nasooropharynx (Fig 9.8).

Pathophysiology

MAS involves the passage of meconium in utero as a result of hypoxic stress. It occurs primarily in full-term and postterm infants but has been reported in infants at less than 37 weeks' gestation. Once the fetus ingests meconium, any gasping activity occurring as a result of intrauterine stress may cause the sticky and tenacious substance to be aspirated into the lower airways. The net results are partial airway obstruction, air trapping, hyperinflation distal to the obstruction and atelectasis caused by surfactant deactivation. A 'ball-valve' situation exists wherein gas flows into the lungs on inspiration but is trapped

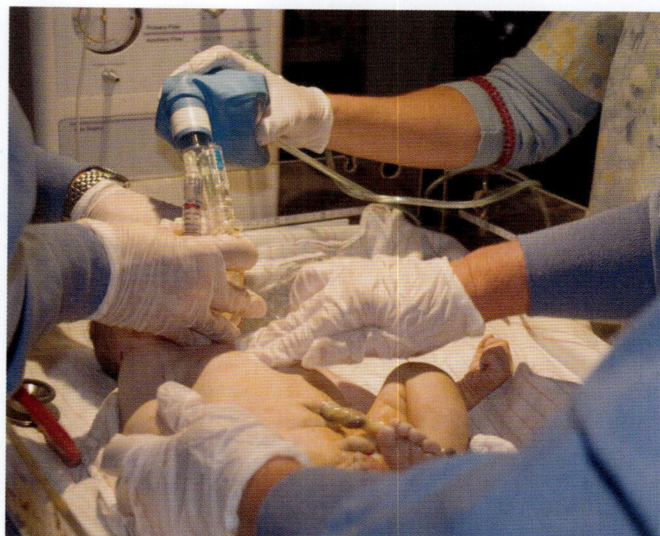

Fig 9.8 Infant being resuscitated at birth. Note presence of meconium on abdomen and umbilical cord. Source: Courtesy Shannon Perry, Phoenix.)

there on exhalation as a result of the small airway diameter. As the infant struggles to take in more air (air hunger), even more meconium may be aspirated. Hyperinflation, hypxaemia and acidaemia result in increased PVR.

In turn, shunting of blood through the ductus arteriosus (right to left) occurs because of increased resistance to blood flow through the pulmonary arteries (and to the lungs), leading to further hypoxaemia and acidosis. Ductal shunting increases with hypoxia; some blood may enter the left atrium (LA) from the right atrium (RA) via the foramen ovale because there is a net decrease in blood returning to the LA via the pulmonary venous system, preventing closure of the foramen ovale. This pathological process is essentially persistence of the fetal circulation, or persistent pulmonary hypertension of the newborn (PPHN), which is discussed later in this chapter. The air trapping of MAS causes overdistension of the alveoli and often air leaks. There is evidence that meconium contributes to the destruction of surfactant, increasing surface tension and further predisposing the alveoli to decreased functional capacity.

Clinical Manifestations

Infants who have released meconium in utero for some time before birth are stained from green meconium stools (those with more recent meconium passage may not be stained), tachypnoeic, hypoxic and often depressed at birth. They develop expiratory grunting, nasal flaring and retractions similar to those of infants with RDS. They may initially be cyanotic or pale, as well as tachypnoeic and they may demonstrate the classic barrel chest from hyperinflation. The infants are often stressed, hypothermic, hypoglycaemic and hypocalcaemic. Severe meconium aspiration progresses rapidly to respiratory failure if untreated. These infants exhibit profound respiratory distress with gasping, ineffective ventilations, marked cyanosis and pallor and hypotonia.

Diagnostic Evaluation

At birth, meconium can often be visualised via laryngoscopy in the respiratory passages and vocal cords. Chest radiographs show uneven distribution of patchy infiltrates, air trapping, hyperexpansion and atelectasis. Air leaks may occur as the illness progresses. Oxygenation will be poor, as evidenced by pulse oximetry and arterial blood gases. These infants may quickly develop metabolic and respiratory acidosis.

Echocardiography assists in the diagnosis of right-to-left shunting of blood away from the pulmonary system.

Therapeutic Management

After birth, the need for tracheal suctioning is based on infant assessment. Infants who are vigorous with strong, stable respiratory effort, good muscle tone and heart rate greater than 100 beats/min should not undergo tracheal suctioning but should be closely monitored (Weiner 2016). On the other hand, infants with poor respiratory effort, low heart rate and poor tone should be rapidly intubated, suctioned and resuscitated according to clinical status after suctioning.

Infants with respiratory distress are admitted to the NICU. Management of MAS consists of ventilatory support, exogenous surfactant administration, IV fluids, systemic antibiotics and in some cases inotropes. Because these infants are prone to development of persistent pulmonary hypertension, they should be supported to maintain normal pH, carbon dioxide and oxygen levels; they may be candidates for ECMO therapy, HFV or nasal oxygen (NO).

Nursing Care Management

Nursing care management is the same as for any high-risk neonate (see nursing care in sections on oxygen therapy, persistent pulmonary hypertension and other complications).

Air Leak Syndromes

Air leaks result from alveolar rupture and subsequent escape of air to tissues in which air is not normally present. Air leaks may occur spontaneously in normal neonates, can result from congenital renal or pulmonary malformations, and often complicate underlying respiratory disease and its therapy (e.g. positive pressure ventilation, especially when high distending pressures are required).

After alveolar rupture, air often vents directly into the pleural space to create a pneumothorax. Air may vent into the perivascular interstitium, a condition termed *pulmonary interstitial emphysema (PIE)*. PIE may be seen on radiographs as early as 2 to 3 hours after birth in ELBW and VLBW infants with severe RDS. Localised PIE may resolve by itself or may lead to pneumothorax. HFV has been reported to improve the outcome in infants with PIE (Ravikumar et al 2019). Air can dissect along the perivascular sheaths to eventually enter the mediastinum and cause pneumomediastinum. More extensive leaks involve the pericardium (manifested as pneumopericardium) or emphysema in the cervical, subcutaneous or retroperitoneal soft tissues.

Clinical Manifestations

Spontaneous **pneumothorax** usually occurs during the first few breaths after birth, primarily in full-term or postterm infants, and is evident by the gradual onset of symptoms of respiratory distress after arrival in the nursey. Use of positive pressure ventilation in resuscitation may cause air leaks. In some cases, such as in extreme prematurity and meconium aspiration, air leaks may not be altogether preventable. The nurse/midwife suspects an air leak on the basis of respiratory manifestations, a decrease in oxygen saturation and a shift in location of maximum intensity of heart sounds and absent or diminished breath sounds (although breath sounds may not be altered because of the small diameter of the chest and auscultation of referred breath sounds).

A **tension pneumothorax** occurs more frequently in infants requiring ventilatory assistance but may also occur in term infants at birth. In premature infants being mechanically ventilated, an air leak may be demonstrated by hypotension, bradycardia, decreased or absent breath sounds unilaterally, decreased oxygenation (by pulse oximetry) and cyanosis, none of which responds to efforts for oxygenation (a resuscitation bag connected to the ET tube and manual ventilations). There may also be chest asymmetry, altered cardiac sounds (diminished, shifted or muffled), a palpable liver and spleen and subcutaneous emphysema. Infants on HFV may demonstrate an air leak by a sudden decrease in systemic blood pressure or an absence of chest movement (because of difficulty in auscultation of the chest with such modalities). The otherwise healthy full-term infant may exhibit only mild to moderate signs of respiratory distress. Air leaks contribute to the risk of an adverse developmental outcome in premature infants (Ravikumar et al 2019).

NURSING CARE CONSIDERATIONS

Early manifestations of pneumothorax include tachypnoea, restlessness and irritability, lethargy, grunting, nasal flaring and retractions. Pneumothorax during ventilatory assistance is evident from abrupt and profound duskiness or cyanosis; significant declines in heart rate, arterial blood pressure and pulse pressure; and poor peripheral perfusion.

Therapeutic Management

Diagnosis is confirmed by transillumination of the chest with a fibreoptic light and/or radiographic examination. In symptomatic infants, treatment is urgent. Trapped air is evacuated by chest tube insertion into the pleural space through a small chest incision. The chest tube is then attached to continuous water-seal or dry suction control drainage. In situations requiring infant transport, a pocket-sized Heimlich valve may be used until an appropriate drainage system can be established. The valve is not effective when fluid drainage is required. Needle aspiration serves as an emergency measure until a chest tube can be inserted. Pneumomediastinum seldom requires treatment, but pneumopericardium is managed by needle aspiration or pericardial tube drainage. The full-term newborn with a small tension pneumothorax may require oxygen therapy and parenteral fluids for a brief period if respiratory distress is not severe.

Nursing Care Management

The most important nursing function is close observation for the possibility of an air leak in susceptible infants. Nurses/midwives have a high level of suspicion in: (1) infants with RDS with or without positive pressure ventilation; (2) infants with meconium-stained amniotic fluid or MAS; (3) infants with radiographic evidence of interstitial or lobar emphysema; (4) infants who required resuscitation at birth; or (5) infants receiving CPAP or positive pressure ventilation.

The general nursing care of the infant with an extraneous air syndrome is the same as that for all high-risk neonates. Respiratory management is similar to that for infants with RDS. Assessing breath sounds frequently, monitoring the efficacy of gas exchange and regulating oxygen therapy according to the infant's needs are vital nursing functions. Pain management is vital in these preverbal and significantly stressed infants (Ravikumar et al 2019).

Persistent Pulmonary Hypertension of the Newborn

Persistent pulmonary hypertension of the newborn (PPHN) results from elevated pulmonary artery pressure with levels equal to or greater than systemic pressure, and large right-to-left shunts through both the foramen ovale and the ductus arteriosus (Mandell et al 2021). Because full development of pulmonary arterial musculature occurs late in gestation, PPHN is primarily a condition of late-premature, full-term or postterm infants, many of whom were products of complicated pregnancies or births. The condition is often associated with meconium aspiration, congenital diaphragmatic hernia with severe respiratory distress, cold stress, respiratory distress (e.g. RDS or pneumonia) and septicaemia (group B streptococci [GBS]). PPHN is believed to be precipitated by perinatal factors, such as perinatal asphyxia, that cause or contribute to constriction of the pulmonary vasculature.

PPHN can be either primary or secondary. Primary PPHN occurs when the pulmonary vessels fail to relax and open with the initial respiration at birth. Secondary PPHN results from hypoxic stress that increases PVR and causes a return to fetal cardiopulmonary circulation. PPHN is most commonly observed in infants at 35 to 44 weeks gestation who have a history of perinatal asphyxia, metabolic acidosis or sepsis and respiratory distress within the first 24 hours. The infants become hypoxic and display marked cyanosis, tachypnoea with grunting and retractions and decreased peripheral perfusion. A loud pulmonary component of the second heart sound and, sometimes, a systolic ejection murmur are present. Diagnosis is established from clinical signs and diagnostic tests, including chest radiography, electrocardiogram and echocardiography (Mandell et al 2021, Steurer et al 2019).

Therapeutic Management

Early recognition and management of conditions that contribute to or cause hypoxia and pulmonary vascular vasoconstriction are the primary goals in the prevention of PPHN. Additional treatment includes careful fluid regulation and evaluation of intravascular fluid volume. Supplemental oxygen reduces hypoxia and decreases pulmonary vasoconstriction. Assisted ventilation, often by HFV, is required if hypoxia is severe. Vasodilators, such as sildenafil (a phosphodiesterase [PDE5] inhibitor) or epoprostenol (prostacyclin), are sometimes prescribed to decrease PVR, thereby avoiding ECMO and NO. Sildenafil administered in intravenous or oral form has been shown to reduce PVR (hypertension) in neonates and improve oxygenation, but further controlled clinical trials are needed (Mandell et al 2021, Buonocore et al 2018).

Nursing Care Management

Nursing care for PPHN is the same as for infants with severe respiratory difficulties and those given mechanical ventilation and cardiovascular support. The infant with PPHN is often the sickest on the unit, depending on the causative factors and reaction to treatment. Because handling for any reason causes a decrease in arterial oxygen concentration, the nurse/midwife must weigh the stresses imposed by routine care against the risk of iatrogenic hypoxia. It is important to decrease noxious stimuli that cause hypoxia and to use clustered nursing interventions that keep non-sedated infants calm. Continuous monitoring of oxygenation, temperature, central venous pressure, vital signs, blood pressure and acid–base balance decreases the need for physical manipulation and disturbance. Infants are further assessed for response to treatments, including IV therapy, fluids, electrolytes and exogenous glucose (Mandell et al 2021, Buonocore et al 2018).

Chronic Lung Disease

Chronic lung disease is a pathological process that develops primarily in ELBW and VLBW infants with RDS. Chronic lung disease may also develop in infants with MAS, persistent pulmonary hypertension, pneumonia and cyanotic heart disease. Infants who develop chronic lung disease are at risk for frequent hospitalisation because of their borderline respiratory reserve, hyperactive airway and increased susceptibility to respiratory infection.

Mild chronic lung disease is operationally defined by the need for supplemental oxygen for 28 days or more but room air by 36 weeks corrected gestational age or at discharge. Moderate chronic lung disease is defined by the need for oxygen for 28 days or more and less than 30% oxygen at 36 weeks corrected gestational age. With severe chronic lung disease infants require more than 30% oxygen at 36 weeks corrected gestational age (Buonocore et al 2018, Botet et al 2012).

The more severe form of chronic lung disease usually begins with severe respiratory failure secondary to RDS or with pneumonia requiring mechanical ventilation with high airway pressure and oxygen supplementation during the first few days of life (Gardner, Enzman-Hines & Nyp 2016, Lowe 2017). Since the advent of antenatal glucocorticoid therapy, surfactant replacement and new ventilator strategies, a 'new' chronic lung disease is emerging. These infants experience a milder initial respiratory course but continue to require ventilatory support or oxygen supplementation and show radiographic pulmonary changes characteristic of chronic lung disease (Lowe 2017).

Pathophysiology

The pathogenesis of chronic lung disease is complex and multifactorial. Chronic lung disease begins when the immature lung undergoes an initial injury, leading to a chronic inflammatory process which results in recurrent injury and abnormal healing (Lowe 2017). A variety of mechanisms have been related to the initial injury, including: (1) prenatal infection (inflammatory process before birth); (2) mechanical ventilation (volutrauma, intubation); (3) supplemental oxygen (oxygen-derived free radicals); (4) increased pulmonary blood flow from PDA; or (5) postnatal infection.

The pulmonary changes are characterised by interstitial oedema and epithelial swelling, followed by thickening and fibrotic proliferation of the alveolar walls and squamous metaplasia of the bronchiolar epithelium. Areas of atelectasis and cystlike foci of hyperaeration are visible on radiographs between 10 and 20 days of life and persist for weeks; however, some infants may not demonstrate cystic foci. Ciliary activity is paralysed by high oxygen concentrations that interfere with the ability to clear the lung of mucus, thus aggravating airway obstruction and atelectasis. As the infant's lungs begin healing, the process is altered, possibly by continuous high oxygenation, inadequate nutrition or vitamin E deficiency, resulting in decreased surface for oxygen and carbon dioxide exchange. The overall results of this process are hypercarbia, hypoxaemia and subsequent inability to wean successfully from oxygen.

As survival of immature premature infants (< 28 weeks' gestation) increases, the occurrence of chronic lung disease also increases.

In addition to chronic lung disease, other diseases associated with similar radiographic findings include congenital heart disease and viral pneumonia caused by cytomegalovirus. There are no laboratory alterations that confirm a diagnosis. Diagnosis is made on the basis of radiographic findings, oxygen therapy or positive pressure ventilation after 28 days, signs of respiratory distress and a history of requiring mechanical ventilation in the first week of life for more than 3 days.

Therapeutic Management

The first approach to management is prevention of the disorder in susceptible infants. A meta-analysis demonstrated that early administration of surfactant (within 2 hours of birth) in ELBW infants with RDS resulted in lower rates of air leak, mortality and chronic lung disease (Polin et al 2014). To reduce the risk of volutrauma with positive pressure ventilation, maintain the lowest PIP necessary to obtain adequate ventilation and use the lowest level of inspired oxygen to maintain adequate oxygenation. Fluid administration is carefully controlled and restricted (Lowe 2017).

No specific treatment exists for chronic lung disease except to maintain adequate arterial blood gases with the administration of oxygen and to avoid progression of the disease. Corticosteroid therapy has been shown to benefit infants with lung disease by decreasing the pulmonary inflammatory response and improving oxygenation and gas exchange, resulting in earlier weaning from mechanical assistance. However, with complications such as sepsis, hypertension and hyperglycaemia and an overall lack of decreased mortality in such infants, this therapy remains controversial. Other adverse effects of this long-acting, potent glucocorticoid have been reported, including growth restriction, GI haemorrhage and cardiomyopathy. In light of studies that show an increased incidence of periventricular leukomalacia, neuromotor abnormalities, CP, decreased cerebral cortical grey matter volume and adverse long-term neurological outcome, the benefits of this treatment may not outweigh the risks (Shah et al 2017). It is possible that inhaling the steroids, so that the drug directly reaches the lung, may reduce the observed adverse events (Shah et al 2017). Research examining whether an alternative dosing regimen of postnatal steroids can reduce the incidence of chronic lung disease without associated neurodevelopmental side effects showed an increased risk of chronic lung disease and adverse neurodevelopmental outcomes for infants receiving a lower cumulative dose (Onland et al 2017).

Weaning infants from oxygen is difficult and must be accomplished gradually. These infants do not tolerate excessive or even normal amounts of fluid well and have a tendency to accumulate interstitial fluid in the lungs, which aggravates the condition. Oral diuretics may be used to control interstitial fluid.

Growth and development are often delayed in infants with chronic lung disease, which is related in part to the difficulties in providing adequate nutrition and in part to the lack of normal sensory stimulation because of prolonged hospitalisation. Infants with chronic lung disease have far greater metabolic needs. This can create a problem for the caregiver, who must ensure adequate nutrition while avoiding overhydration, especially if the infant is ill, eats poorly or has cardiopulmonary instability. The infant may be further compromised by gastro-oesophageal reflux, a frequent complication in premature infants. Adequate intake of protein is particularly important in preventing postnatal growth failure in LBW infants. Protein supplements may be necessary to ensure adequate intake.

Osteopenia may occur in infants with chronic lung disease and in premature infants, with higher incidence among the infants with chronic lung disease, presumably because of low calcium and vitamin D intake secondary to the calciuric effects of diuretic therapy. Dietary supplementation with human milk fortifier, calcium and phosphorus, and vitamin D has reduced the incidence of osteopenia in premature infants.

Prognosis. Reports vary regarding the mortality rate for chronic lung disease. The hospital stay is often long because of the infant's need for supplemental oxygen, although home oxygen therapy provides some infants the opportunity for discharge. A nasal cannula is an acceptable way to administer oxygen for the dependent infant to promote development of motor and social skills. Long-term problems seen in older children who had chronic lung disease as infants include growth failure, airway hyperreactivity, hyperexpansion, increased incidence of respiratory infections and airway obstruction.

Nursing Care Management

Infants with chronic lung disease expend considerable energy in their efforts to breathe, so they must receive plenty of opportunities for rest and additional calories. Growth records provide clues to the need for change in their diets. Some infants require nutritional supplements. Because these infants tire easily and because large quantities of milk might compromise respiration, small, frequent feedings are better tolerated. Reducing environmental stimuli and subsequent hypoxia is an important aspect in the care of these infants. The older infant's behavioural cues may signal carbon dioxide retention.

Adequate hydration is extremely important because a large amount of fluid is lost through respiration, and secretions must be thinned sufficiently to facilitate removal by suctioning. However, because chronic lung disease increases lung permeability, many infants are subject to pulmonary oedema and require fluid restriction. The nurses/midwives must be alert to signs of both overhydration and underhydration, such as changes in weight, electrolytes, output measurements and urine specific gravity and signs of oedema.

Because the growing infant with chronic lung disease has a restricted fluid intake, has higher than average caloric requirements and often requires many oral medications, the nurse/midwife is challenged by the complexity of care involved. Infants with chronic lung disease may become difficult or maladaptive feeders if they are aware of hunger yet compromised by not being able to eat fast enough to satisfy that hunger because of the increased labour of breathing. Individualised nursing efforts to monitor oxygenation requirements during feedings, decrease environmental stimuli, fortify feedings and provide more contact with a primary caregiver may facilitate the infant's care.

Parents are extremely anxious regarding the prognosis when their infant has chronic lung disease. The lengthy hospitalisation interferes with parent–child relationships and deprives the infant of appropriate parental contact and stimulation. The nurse/midwives should encourage the parents to visit the infant and become involved in the routine care. The parents need to be informed regarding medical care, equipment and procedures related to their infant and taught procedures such as suctioning.

Home Care. Because the availability of home cardiac and apnoea monitors and home oxygen therapy has increased, many infants with chronic lung disease can be discharged when they are gaining weight and their oxygen need is low. Home care promotes parent–infant bonding, minimises healthcare costs and prevents nosocomial infections. Preparation for home care requires education and considerable reassurance. Management of home monitoring equipment and home oxygen therapy provokes stress, but most families become comfortable with the machinery while their infant is still in the hospital. Families need reminders about their infant's increased risk of infection and about limiting contact with persons who have respiratory tract infections. Because of their minimum respiratory reserve, even a minor illness can threaten these infants.

Some infants are discharged with a tracheostomy on oxygen supplementation or home ventilators. Discharge teaching and home care nursing (minimum of 2 weeks to several months) is crucial to these infants' safe and successful transition into the community and home setting. Parents need to learn how to advocate for appropriate home care and supplies in anticipation of future needs.

Because of the high mortality rate in the first year, parents should learn cardiopulmonary resuscitation and how to manage any other emergency that might be anticipated for their infant. Helping families cope with their anxieties and reassuring them of their ability to manage the care of their infant are important nursing functions. Parents need follow-up visits in the home and the comfort of knowing that help is only a phone call away.

HIGH RISK RELATED TO INFECTIOUS PROCESSES

Sepsis

Sepsis, or septicaemia, refers to a generalised bacterial infection in the bloodstream. Neonates are highly susceptible to infection because of diminished non-specific (inflammatory) and specific (humoural) immunity, such as impaired phagocytosis, delayed chemotactic response, minimum or absent IgA and immunoglobulin M (IgM), and decreased complement levels. Because of the infant's poor response to pathogenic agents, there is usually no local inflammatory reaction at the portal of entry to signal an infection and the resulting symptoms tend to be vague and non-specific. Consequently, diagnosis and treatment may be delayed.

Although the mortality rate from sepsis has decreased, the incidence has not. Epidemics are not infrequent, and the high-risk infant has a four-times greater chance of developing septicaemia than does the normal neonate. The frequency of infection is almost twice as great in male infants as in females and also carries a higher mortality rate for males. Other risk factors are prematurity, congenital anomalies or acquired injuries that disrupt the skin or mucous membranes, invasive procedures such as placement of IV lines and ET tubes, administration of total parenteral nutrition and nosocomial exposure to pathogens in the NICU. Thorough handwashing is the single most important infection control measure in the NICU. Proper handling of formula and supplies such as syringes and gavage tubes is also vital to prevent infection.

Breastfeeding has a protective effect against infection and should be promoted where possible for all newborns. It is of particular benefit to the high-risk neonate (Lewis et al 2016). Colostrum contains agglutinins that are effective against gram-negative bacteria. Human milk contains large quantities of IgA and iron-binding protein that exert a bacteriostatic effect on *Escherichia coli.* Human milk also contains macrophages and lymphocytes that promote a local inflammatory reaction.

Pathophysiology

The premature withdrawal of the placental barrier leaves infants vulnerable to most common viral, bacterial, fungal and parasitic infections. Immune substances, primarily immunoglobulin G (IgG), are normally acquired from the maternal system and stored in fetal tissues during the final weeks' gestation to provide newborns with passive immunity to a variety of infectious agents. Early birth interrupts this transplacental transmission; thus premature infants have a low level of circulating IgG. The concentrations of immune substances directly relate to the length of gestation. IgA, which plays a role in defence against viral infections, and IgM, with properties that are most efficient in dealing with gram-negative organisms, are not transferred to the fetus, leaving the infant highly vulnerable to invasion by these organisms.

Defence mechanisms of neonates are further hampered by a low level of complement, diminished opsonisation ability, monocyte dysfunction and a reduced number and inefficient function of circulating leukocytes. Furthermore, leukocytes with diminished motility and phagocytic capacity are unable to concentrate their limited numbers selectively at the site of infection. In addition, a hypo-functioning adrenal gland contributes only a meagre anti-inflammatory response. These deficiencies permit rapid invasion, spread and multiplication of organisms. An immature gut mucosal barrier further predisposes the premature infant to bacteria, which may easily cross the mucosa into the bloodstream.

Sources of Infection

Sepsis in the neonatal period can be acquired prenatally across the placenta from the maternal bloodstream or during labour from ingestion or aspiration of infected amniotic fluid. Prolonged rupture of the membranes always presents a risk for maternal–fetal transfer of pathogenic organisms. In utero transplacental transfer can occur with a variety of organisms and viruses such as cytomegalovirus, toxoplasmosis and *Treponema pallidum* (syphilis), which cross the placental barrier during the latter half of pregnancy.

Early-onset sepsis (EOS) ($<$ 3 days after birth) is acquired in the perinatal period. EOS is defined as a positive blood culture in an infant who is less than 72 hours of age. EOS remains an important cause of serious illness and death among neonates of all birth weights and gestational ages.

Infection can occur from direct contact with organisms from the maternal GI and genitourinary tracts. Organisms associated with early-onset infection include GBS, *E. coli* and other gram-negative enteric organisms. Other bacteria noted to cause early-onset infection include *E. coli, Haemophilus influenzae, Enterobacter* organisms and coagulase-negative staphylococci (Pammi et al 2016, Resch et al 2016). Other pathogens that are harboured in the vagina and may infect the infant include gonococci, *Candida albicans,* herpes simplex virus (type II) and chlamydia.

Late-onset sepsis (1 to 3 weeks after birth) is primarily nosocomial and the offending organisms are usually staphylococci, *Klebsiella* organisms, enterococci, *E. coli* and *Candida* species (Pammi et al 2016). Coagulase-negative staphylococci, considered to be primarily a contaminant in older children and adults, is commonly found to be the cause of septicaemia in ELBW and VLBW infants.

Neonatal sepsis is most common in the 'at-risk' infant, particularly the premature infant or the infant born after a difficult or traumatic labour and birth, who is least capable of resisting such bacterial invasion.

Clinical Manifestations

A few neonatal infections (e.g. pyoderma, conjunctivitis, omphalitis and mastitis) are easy to recognise. However, systemic infections are characterised by subtle, vague, non-specific and almost imperceptible physical signs. Often the only complaint concerns an infant's 'failure to do well', not looking 'right' or non-specific respiratory distress. Rarely is there any indication of a local inflammatory response, which would suggest the portal of entry into the bloodstream. The presence of bacteria is indicated by a specific characteristic. For example, group B beta-haemolytic streptococci usually results in severe respiratory distress, periods of apnoea and a chest radiograph similar to that of RDS.

All body systems tend to show some indication of sepsis, although often little correlation exists between the manifestations and the aetiological factors involved. For example, seizures and fever, a universal feature of infection in older children, may be absent in neonates. It is usually the nursing observation of subtle changes in appearance and behaviour that leads to the detection of infection. The non-specific, early signs are hypothermia and changes in colour, tone, activity and feeding behaviour. In addition, sudden episodes of apnoea and unexplained oxygen desaturation (hypoxia) may signal an infection. Significantly, similar signs may be manifestations of a number of clinical conditions unrelated to sepsis, such as hypoglycaemia, hypocalcaemia, opioid withdrawal or a CNS disorder.

Premature infants, particularly ELBW and VLBW infants, are highly susceptible to early sepsis and pneumonia occurring concurrently with RDS. Premature birth has been increasingly shown to be associated with a maternal bacterial pathogen. ELBW and VLBW infants are also highly susceptible to fungal and viral infections. Investigation for such agents should begin when sepsis is suspected in this population. Because meningitis is a common sequela of sepsis, the neonate is evaluated for bacterial growth in cerebrospinal fluid (CSF). Clinical signs of neonatal meningitis, particularly in VLBW infants, may not have typical features of older infants. Clinical signs that may indicate possible neonatal sepsis are listed in Box 9.5.

Diagnostic Evaluation

Because sepsis is easy to confuse with other neonatal disorders, the definitive diagnosis is established by laboratory and radiographic examination. Isolation of the specific organism is always attempted through cultures of blood, urine and CSF. Blood studies may show signs of leukocytosis or leukopenia. Leukopenia is usually an ominous sign because of its frequent association with high mortality rates. An elevated number of immature neutrophils (**left-shift**), decreased or increased total neutrophils and changes in neutrophil morphological characteristics also suggest an infectious process in the neonate. Other diagnostic data that are helpful in the determination of neonatal sepsis include C-reactive protein and interleukins, specifically interleukin-6 (Pammi et al 2016).

Therapeutic Management

In addition to the institution of rigorous preventive measures such as good handwashing, early recognition and diagnosis are essential to increase the infant's chance for survival and reduce the likelihood of permanent neurological damage. Diagnosis of sepsis is often based on suspicion of initial clinical signs and symptoms. Antibiotic therapy is initiated before laboratory results are available for confirmation and identification of the exact organism. Treatment consists of circulatory support, respiratory support and aggressive administration of antibiotics.

Supportive therapy usually involves administration of oxygen (if respiratory distress or hypoxia is evident), careful regulation of fluids, correction of electrolyte or acid–base imbalance and temporary discontinuation of oral feedings. A blood transfusion may be needed to correct anaemia. IV fluids for shock, electronic monitoring of vital signs and regulation of the thermal environment are mandatory.

Antibiotic therapy is continued for 7 to 10 days if cultures are positive, discontinued in 36 to 48 hours if cultures are negative and the infant is asymptomatic and most often administered via IV infusion. Antifungal and antiviral therapies are implemented as appropriate, depending on causative agents.

Prognosis. The prognosis for neonatal sepsis is variable. Severe neurological and respiratory sequelae may occur in ELBW and VLBW infants with early-onset sepsis. Late-onset sepsis and meningitis may also result in poor outcomes for immunocompromised neonates.

The introduction of new markers for neonatal sepsis such as acute phase proteins, cytokines, cell surface antigens and bacterial genomes may prove to be particularly helpful in early differentiation of true sepsis from RDS and in guidance for antibiotic therapy (Camacho-Gonzalez et al 2013, Gilfillan & Bhandari 2017). Future experimental methods being explored to combat infection in neonates include monoclonal antibody therapy, fibronectin infusion and lymphokine enhancement.

BOX 9.5 Manifestations of Neonatal Sepsis

General Signs
- Infant generally 'not doing well'
- Poor temperature control—hypothermia (common), hyperthermia (rare)

Circulatory System
- Pallor, cyanosis or mottling
- Cold, clammy skin
- Hypotension
- Oedema
- Irregular heartbeat—bradycardia, tachycardia

Respiratory System
- Irregular respirations, apnoea or tachypnoea
- Cyanosis
- Grunting
- Dyspnoea
- Retractions

Central Nervous System
- Diminished activity—lethargy, hyporeflexia, coma
- Increased activity—irritability, tremors, seizures
- Full fontanel
- Increased or decreased tone
- Abnormal eye movements

Gastrointestinal System
- Poor feeding
- Vomiting
- Diarrhoea or decreased stooling
- Abdominal distension
- Hepatomegaly
- Haemoccult-positive stools

Haematopoietic System
- Jaundice
- Pallor
- Petechiae, ecchymosis
- Splenomegaly

Nursing Care Management

Nursing care of the infant with sepsis involves observation and assessment as outlined for any high-risk infant. Recognition of the problem is of paramount importance. Awareness of the potential modes of infection transmission also helps the nurse/midwife identify those at risk for developing sepsis. Much of the care of infants with sepsis involves the medical treatment of the illness. Knowledge of the side effects of the specific antibiotic and proper regulation and administration of the drug are vital.

Prolonged antibiotic therapy poses additional hazards for affected infants. Oral antibiotics, if administered, destroy intestinal flora responsible for the synthesis of vitamin K, which can reduce blood coagulability. In addition, antibiotics predispose the infant to growth of resistant organisms and superinfection from fungal or mycotic agents, such as *C. albicans*. Nurses/midwives must be alert for evidence of such complications. Nystatin oral suspension may be administered for prophylaxis against oral candidiasis.

Necrotising Enterocolitis

NEC is an acute inflammatory disease of the bowel with increased incidence in premature and other high-risk infants; it is most common in premature infants. Because the signs are similar to those observed in many other disorders of the newborn, nurses/midwives must constantly be aware of the possibility of this disease.

Pathophysiology

The precise cause of NEC is still uncertain, but it appears to occur in infants whose GI tract has suffered vascular compromise. Contributory factors for NEC include the following: intestinal immaturity, such as gastrointestinal dysmotility; impaired digestive capacity; altered regulation of intestinal blood blow; barrier dysfunction; altered anti-inflammatory control; and impaired host defence (Chang et al 2017).

Frequent use of antibiotic therapy and antacid medications, followed by enteral feeding, are believed to increase the risk of NEC (Chang et al 2017). Prematurity remains the greatest risk factor in this disease (Garg et al 2018).

The damage to mucosal cells lining the bowel wall is great. Diminished blood supply to these cells causes their death in large numbers. They stop secreting protective, lubricating mucus and the thin, unprotected bowel wall is attacked by proteolytic enzymes. It is unable to synthesise protective IgM and the mucosa is permeable to macromolecules (e.g. exotoxins), which further hamper intestinal defences. Gas-forming bacteria invade the damaged areas to produce intestinal **pneumatosis**, air in the submucosal or subserosal surfaces of the bowel.

Clinical Manifestations

The prominent clinical signs of NEC are a distended abdomen, gastric residuals and blood in the stools. Because NEC closely resembles septicaemia, the infant may 'not look well'. Non-specific signs include lethargy, poor feeding, hypotension, apnoea, vomiting (often bile-stained), decreased urinary output and hypothermia. The onset is usually between 4 and 10 days after the initiation of feedings, but signs may be evident as early as 4 hours of age and as late as 30 days. NEC in full-term infants almost always occurs in the first 10 days of life. The early clinical signs of NEC are subtle and non-specific and may often be overlooked for other conditions; the earliest clinical signs include lethargy, abdominal distension and high gastric residuals (Bucher et al 2016, Adams et al 2019). Late-onset NEC is confined primarily to premature infants and coincides with the onset of feedings after they have passed through the acute phase of an illness such as RDS.

Diagnostic Evaluation

Radiographic studies show a sausage-shaped dilation of the intestine that progresses to marked distension and the characteristic intestinal pneumatosis—'soapsuds', or the bubbly appearance of thickened bowel wall and ultralumina. Air may be present in the portal circulation or free air observed in the abdomen, indicating perforation. Laboratory findings may include anaemia, leukopenia, leucocytosis, metabolic acidosis and electrolyte imbalance. In severe cases, coagulopathy (disseminated intravascular coagulation) or thrombocytopenia may be evident. Organisms may be cultured from blood, although bacteraemia or septicaemia may not be prominent early in the course of the disease (Robertson et al 2020).

Therapeutic Management

Prevention is the main line of treatment for NEC. The infant is placed on nil by mouth and a nasal or oral gastric tube is inserted and placed on free drainage. Blood cultures are collected and sent to pathology as soon as possible. Antibiotics are commenced as soon as possible, with current treatment being vancomycin, gentamicin and metronidazole (only if definite NEC confirmed). Gut rest is recommended for 10 to 14 days, along with review for total parenteral nutrition, ongoing fluid management, inotropes, possible ventilation, analgesia, frequent radiology and possible surgery (Safe Care Victoria 2021b).

The administration of maternal antenatal steroids may prevent NEC in some infants by promoting early gut closure and maturation of the gut barrier mucosa (Robertson et al 2020, Wapner et al 2016).

Many meta-analyses of randomised controlled trials have confirmed that oral probiotics effectively prevent NEC when given within the first 7 days and continued for 14 days in premature infants (≤ 34 weeks' gestation) and/or those of a birth weight ≤ 1500 g (Aceti et al 2015, Adams et al 2019, Alfaleh et al 2014, Athalye-Jape et al 2016, Lau & Chamberlain 2015, Uberos et al 2017). Lactoferrin, the major whey protein in human milk, in combination with lysozyme, which is also found in human milk, may have a significant role in the prevention of NEC and neonatal sepsis in high-risk premature infants; both act in the intestine to kill harmful bacteria and enhance intestinal immune properties (Adams et al 2019, Chang et al 2017, Uberos et al 2017).

With early recognition and treatment, medical management is increasingly successful. If there is progressive deterioration under medical management or evidence of perforation, surgical resection and anastomosis are performed. Extensive involvement may necessitate surgical intervention and establishment of an ileostomy, jejunostomy or colostomy. Sequelae in surviving infants include short-bowel syndrome, colonic stricture with obstruction, fat malabsorption and failure to thrive secondary to intestinal dysfunction. Various surgical interventions for NEC are available and depend on the extent of bowel necrosis, associated illness factors and infant stability. Intestinal transplantation has been successful in some former premature infants with NEC-associated short-bowel syndrome who had already developed life-threatening complications related to total parenteral nutrition. More than 50% of these patients survived with improved quality of life. Bowel lengthening procedures and intestinal transplantation may be lifesaving options for infants who previously faced high morbidity and mortality rates (Uberos et al 2017).

Nursing Care Management

Astute nursing care is a key factor in the prompt recognition of the early warning signs of NEC. When the disease is suspected, the nurse/midwife assists with diagnostic procedures and implements the therapeutic regimen. Vital signs, including blood pressure, are monitored for changes that might indicate bowel perforation, septicaemia or cardiovascular shock. Measures are instituted to prevent possible transmission to other infants. It is especially important to avoid rectal temperatures because of the increased danger of perforation. To avoid pressure on the distended abdomen and to facilitate continuous observation, infants are often left without a nappy and positioned supine or on the side.

Because NEC is an infectious disease, one of the most important nursing functions is control of infection. Strict handwashing is the primary barrier to spread, and confirmed multiple cases are isolated. Persons with symptoms of a GI infection should not care for these or any other infants.

The infant undergoing surgery requires the same careful attention and observation as any infant with abdominal surgery, including ostomy care (as applicable). This disorder is one of the most common reasons for performing ileostomies on newborns. Throughout the medical and surgical management of infants with NEC, the nurse/midwife is continually alert for signs of complications, such as septicaemia, disseminated intravascular coagulation, hypoglycaemia and other metabolic derangements.

HIGH RISK RELATED TO CARDIOVASCULAR AND HAEMATOLOGICAL COMPLICATIONS

Patent Ductus Arteriosus

Patent ductus arteriosus (PDA) is a common complication of severe respiratory disease in premature infants. It occurs in the majority of premature infants under 1200 g, and the incidence diminishes in direct relationship to increasing birth weight. During fetal life the ductus remains patent through the vasodilatory action of prostaglandin, which is produced by the placenta and circulated to the fetus. Postnatally the increase in oxygen tension has a constricting effect on the ductus, but it may reopen in premature infants in response to the lowered oxygen tension associated with respiratory impairment.

Lack of ductal smooth muscle in premature infants also prolongs patency of the ductus arteriosus. Functional closure occurs usually within 3 to 4 days, but complete anatomic closure with fibrosis and permanent sealing of the lumen may take up to 2 to 3 weeks.

Clinical Manifestations

Signs of PDA may appear within the first week of life. Early signs are increased $PaCO_2$, decreased PaO_2, increased FiO_2, increased work of breathing and recurrent apnoea. Other signs include: bounding peripheral pulses; wide pulse pressure with decreased diastolic blood pressure; pericardial hyperactivity; cardiomegaly; and a systolic or continuous murmur usually referred to as a 'machinery-type' murmur, heard loudest in systole. If the PDA is wide open, a murmur may not be heard. Spontaneous closure usually occurs within 12 weeks, but in infants with severe lung involvement, the left-to-right shunting of blood leads to pulmonary oedema and may prevent timely weaning from mechanical ventilation. The diagnosis is confirmed by echocardiography.

Therapeutic Management

Therapy consists of careful fluid regulation; respiratory support; and administration of indometacin or ibuprofen, which inhibits prostaglandin synthetase. However, indometacin inhibits platelet function and affects renal function in neonates, so close monitoring for bleeding and renal dysfunction is necessary if this drug is used. If a ductus reopens after cessation of therapy, re-administration of the medication may produce a favourable response. As many as six doses may be used to accomplish ductal closure. Surgical ligation may be necessary if medical therapy is unsuccessful because ductal shunting is perceived as an important contributor to respiratory distress and chronic lung disease.

Nursing Care Management

Nursing observations are important in the recognition and management of PDA. Assisting in early detection, carefully assessing cardiovascular status and monitoring for complications after implementation of therapy are nursing responsibilities. Activities related to therapy include collection of specimens for laboratory examination, continued assessment of renal function (e.g. adequate urinary output, any abnormal laboratory findings such as blood urea nitrogen and creatinine levels) and observation for any bleeding tendencies (e.g. haematest-positive stools or gastric aspirate, oozing from heel sticks or venepuncture sites and laboratory evidence of clotting abnormalities).

Postoperative care includes monitoring for pneumothorax or atelectasis on the affected side, assessment for bleeding and signs or symptoms of infection, supportive respiratory care and pain management. Other nursing observations and management are the same as for the high-risk infant and the infant with congenital heart disease. (See Chapter 27.)

Anaemia

Premature infants tend to develop anaemia that is more severe and appears earlier than in more mature infants. It may be a result of haemorrhage during pregnancy or labour and birth (e.g. loss of placental integrity, anomalies of the umbilical cord, fetomaternal haemorrhage), haemorrhage during the neonatal period (e.g. ICH, visceral trauma) or blood disorders (e.g. haemolytic disease, thrombocytopenia). Anaemia may also be iatrogenic from blood withdrawn in the NICU for laboratory tests. Physiological characteristics of prematurity tend to contribute to the development of anaemia (i.e. a decreased red blood cell mass at birth, a drop in the production of haemoglobin and shortened survival time of red blood cells). This lag in haematopoiesis during continued growth results in physiological anaemia, probably as a consequence of diminished erythropoietin values.

Fortunately, even VLBW infants are able to accommodate the GI absorption of iron required for their high needs. Iron is supplied in iron-fortified formulas or iron supplements as both a preventive and a therapeutic measure. Transfusions with packed red blood cells are often required for severe anaemia, usually for replacement of blood loss from iatrogenic measures. At 4 to 12 weeks of age, 'physiological anaemia' reaches a peak, at which time infants sometimes display signs that suggest true anaemia (e.g. poor feeding, decreased oxygen saturation, pallor).

Nursing Care Management

One of the most common causes of anaemia in acutely ill premature infants is blood loss associated with frequent sampling for blood gas and metabolic analyses. Repeated blood sampling depletes the small total blood volume of premature infants quickly. In light of hepatitis and human immunodeficiency virus (HIV) transmission and the potential for other blood-borne pathogens, measures to reduce iatrogenic blood loss and to minimise the need for transfusions of blood products are important considerations.

The nurse/midwife observes for signs of anaemia in the premature infant: poor feeding, decreased oxygen saturation, systolic murmur, dyspnoea, tachycardia, tachypnoea, diminished activity and pallor. However, some infants may not display all these signs. Poor weight gain may be an indication of a lowered haemoglobin level. (Chapter 28 discusses nursing precautions and observations during blood transfusion.)

Polycythaemia

The current definition of **polycythaemia** is a venous haematocrit of 65% or more (Maheshwari & Carlo 2016). With a haematocrit above 65%, blood flow becomes increasingly sluggish and hyperviscous, resulting in hypoperfusion of organs. Polycythaemia may result from in utero twin-to-twin transfusion and maternal–fetal transfusion, delayed cord clamping or stripping of the umbilical cord, maternal diabetes mellitus or intrapartum asphyxia. The small-for-gestational-age infant is the most at risk for polycythaemia. Increased red blood cell consumption of glucose further predisposes the infant to hypoglycaemia. Infants with polycythaemia have a high incidence of cardiopulmonary distress symptoms (e.g. PPHN, cyanosis and apnoea), seizures, hyperbilirubinaemia and GI abnormalities.

Appropriate therapy for correcting metabolic disturbances (e.g. hypoxia, hypoglycaemia and hyperbilirubinaemia) is implemented. Lowering blood viscosity by partial plasma exchange transfusion may be considered in symptomatic cases.

Nursing Care Management

Nursing care involves watching for signs of polycythaemia (e.g. plethora, peripheral cyanosis, respiratory distress, lethargy, jitteriness or seizure activity, hypoglycaemia, hyperbilirubinaemia) and assisting with diagnostic tests and therapeutic procedures. (Care of the infant with hyperbilirubinaemia is discussed in Chapter 8.)

Retinopathy of Prematurity

Although often discussed in relation to respiratory dysfunction, retinopathy of prematurity (ROP) is a disorder involving immature retinal vasculature. Formerly known as retrolental fibroplasia, ROP is a term used to describe retinal changes observed in premature infants. The incidence and severity of the disease correlate with the degree of the infant's maturity; the younger the gestational age, the greater the likelihood of ROP, with extremely premature infants being most at risk. However, cases have been documented of ROP in full-term infants who received no oxygen therapy (Carter et al 2016).

In addition to immaturity, contributory factors for ROP include oxygenation, respiratory distress, apnoea, bradycardia, heart disease, infections, hypercarbia, acidosis, anaemia and the need for transfusions (Olitsky et al 2016). Previously considered an iatrogenic disease related to hyperoxia, ROP is now believed to be a complex disease of prematurity with multiple causes and therefore difficult to prevent completely. A study done by Owen and colleagues (2017) conducted a comprehensive risk assessment for prediction of ROP and found that severe ROP was best predicted by estimated gestational age (week), the need for any surgery and increased probability of death or moderate/severe chronic lung disease at 7 days. The most predictive model for type 1 ROP included estimated gestational age (week) and the presence of severe chronic lung disease (Owen et al 2017).

Pathophysiology

Severe vascular constriction in the immature retinal vasculature, followed by hypoxia in those areas, is characteristic of ROP. This appears to stimulate vascular proliferation of retinal capillaries into the hypoxic areas, where veins become numerous and dilate. As new vessels multiply towards the lens, the aqueous humour and vitreous humour become turbid. The retina becomes oedematous, and haemorrhages and scarring occur, which separate the retina from its attachment. This process results in irreversible blindness.

Diagnostic Evaluation

Normal vascular growth proceeds in an orderly fashion from the optic disc towards the ora serrata, the irregular anterior margin of the retina. Box 9.6 outlines the stages of ROP. ROP is further classified by location of damage in the retina and by the extent of abnormally developing vascularisation. Infants registered within the Australian and New Zealand Neonatal Network (ANZNN) will continue until the retina is fully vascularised. Ongoing follow-up after discharge of infants who have ROP is important to establish any late sequelae such as refractive errors, strabismus or retinal detachment to name some issues that may occur (Koucheki et al 2020, Safe Care Victoria 2021c).

Therapeutic Management

Studies have shown an association between the development of ROP and high or fluctuating arterial oxygen saturations in ELBW and VLBW infants. Although there is no consensus on the ideal arterial oxygen saturation in premature infants—to prevent either hypoxaemia or hyperoxaemia—evidence is mounting that oxygen saturations of over 94% are undesirable and may have a significant role in the development of ROP (Koucheki et al 2020, Darlow et al 2017, Owen et al 2017). Management and treatment of ROP is primarily aimed at preventing fluctuations in arterial concentrations of oxygen in premature neonates.

The early recognition of ROP, treatment and follow-up care are essential components of disease management. Although prevention is the primary goal of therapeutic management, treatment of retinal pathological conditions is directed towards arresting the proliferation process. Early treatment of high-risk pre-threshold ROP significantly reduced unfavourable outcomes (Koucheki et al 2020, Olitsky et al 2016). Laser photocoagulation therapy is the most common treatment for ROP.

BOX 9.6 Stages of Retinopathy of Prematurity

1. A demarcation line (separates the avascular retina anteriorly from the vascularised retina posteriorly)
2. A ridge (formed from the demarcation line with the height and width, occupies volume and extends beyond the plane of the retina)
3. A ridge with extraretinal fibrovascular proliferation
4. Partial retinal detachment
5. Total retinal detachment

'Plus' disease—increased dilation and tortuosity of peripheral retinal vessels (e.g. stage 2 plus ROP)

Source: Data from International Committee for the Classification of Retinopathy of Prematurity. (2005). The international classification of retinopathy of prematurity revisited. Archives of Ophthalmology, 123(7), 991–999.

Nursing Care Management

The nursing care of extremely premature infants and those at risk for development of ROP should focus on decreasing or avoiding events known to cause fluctuations in systemic blood pressure and oxygenation. The infant's oxygenation status should be carefully monitored and targeted SpO_2 ranges maintained. Individualised care of the premature infant is essential to aid in further decreasing the incidence of ROP. For infants undergoing ophthalmic examination for ROP, concentrated sucrose has proved effective in decreasing pain responses (Gao et al 2016).

Intraoperative nursing care for the infant undergoing laser surgery involves proper infant identification, stabilisation and monitoring of vital signs as required, monitoring of IV therapy and administration of the necessary medications. Postoperative nursing care also includes monitoring the infant for signs of pain and appropriate pain management as needed. After surgery the infant's eyelids will be oedematous and closed; the nurse/midwife informs the parents of this preoperatively. Eye medications are administered as ordered, and the infant's tolerance of these medications is monitored. Most infants are able to feed once awake and alert in the postoperative period. When the infant suffers partial or complete visual impairment, the parents need a considerable amount of support and assistance in meeting his or her special developmental needs. (See Chapter 20.)

HIGH RISK RELATED TO NEUROLOGICAL DISTURBANCE

Neurological complications are observed with increased frequency in premature infants and in infants born after a difficult labour and birth. A disproportionately high incidence of perinatal encephalopathy and psychomotor delay occurs in the high-risk infant population, especially ELBW and VLBW infants. Premature infants are also more vulnerable to cerebral insults (e.g. hypoxia) and chemical alterations (e.g. decreased blood glucose). Fragility and increased permeability of capillaries and prolonged prothrombin time predispose the premature infant's brain to trauma when subjected to increased pressure, such as the forces of labour, high ventilatory pressures, fluid and electrolyte imbalances, sepsis, acidosis and seizure activity. All these factors contribute to intracranial insults, including traumatic bleeding in the newborn, which consists of four major types: intraventricular, subdural, primary subarachnoid and intracerebellar.

Perinatal Hypoxic-ischaemic Brain Injury

Hypoxic-ischaemic brain injury, or hypoxic-ischaemic reperfusion injury, is the most common cause of neurological impairment in term and premature infants. The brain damage usually results from asphyxia before, during or after birth. Ischaemia and hypoxaemia may occur simultaneously, or one may precede the other. The fetal brain is somewhat protected against mild hypoxic events but may be damaged when there is a decrease in cerebral blood flow, systemic blood pressure and oxygen and nutrients such as glucose. Subsequent reperfusion after the event may further result in bleeding of the fragile capillaries and tissue ischaemia.

Hypoxic-ischaemic encephalopathy (HIE) is the resultant cellular damage from hypoxic-ischaemic injury that causes the clinical manifestations observed in each case. Such clinical manifestations are variable and may be mild, moderate or severe. In some infants little or no residual damage may be observed. In general, hypoxia that is severe enough to cause HIE will also damage other organs such as the liver, kidneys, myocardium and GI tract (Carlo & Ambalavanan 2016a, Parsons et al 2016). In the premature infant HIE may occur in conjunction with IVH. Prematurity and general organ and system immaturity may result in hypoxic-ischaemic brain damage in the neonatal period due to altered cerebral blood flow, systemic hypotension and decreased cellular nutrients (blood glucose and oxygen).

The site of the hypoxic-ischaemic injury varies according to the infant's gestational age. In the full-term infant the primary ischaemic damage is parasagittal cerebral injury with cortical necrosis (deeper region of the brain). In the premature infant the primary ischaemic lesion is in the white matter near the ventricles, or periventricular, with resultant periventricular leukomalacia (Miller & Walker 2014).

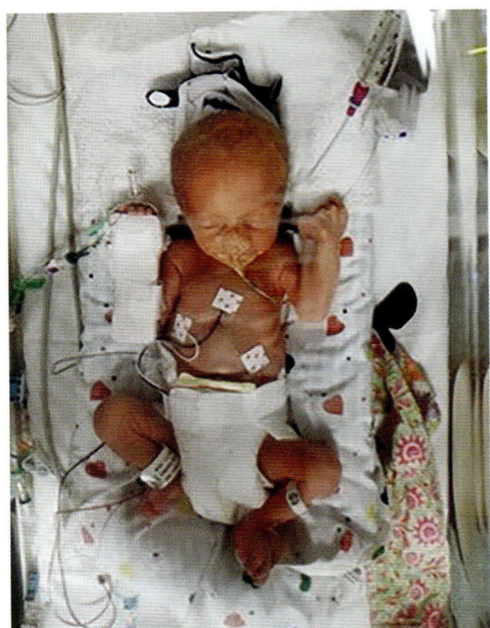

Fig 9.9 Whole body cooling for HIE.

Clinical Manifestations

The neurological signs of encephalopathy appear within the first hours after the hypoxic episode, with manifestations of bilateral cerebral dysfunction. The infant may be stuporous or comatose. Seizures begin after 6 to 12 hours in approximately 50% of the infants, and they become more frequent and severe by 12 to 24 hours. Between 24 and 72 hours the level of consciousness may deteriorate, and after 72 hours persistent stupor, abnormal tone (usually hypotonia) and evidence of disturbances of sucking and swallowing may occur. Muscular weakness of the hips and shoulders occurs in full-term infants and lower limb weakness occurs in premature infants. Apnoeic episodes happen in approximately 50% of the affected infants.

Improvement in neurological deficiencies is highly variable and difficult to predict. Infants who demonstrate the most rapid initial improvement appear to have the best prognosis. Myocardial failure and acute tubular necrosis are frequent complications. The major long-term sequelae of hypoxic-ischaemic injury are cognitive impairment, seizures and CP.

Therapeutic Management

Treatment involves aggressive resuscitation at birth, supportive care to provide adequate ventilation and avoid aggravating the existing hypoxia, and measures to maintain adequate cerebral perfusion and prevent cerebral oedema.

Therapeutic hypothermia provided by either cooling the infant's head or the whole body has been shown to reduce the severity of the neurological damage when it is applied in the early stages of injury (first 6 hours after birth) (Carlo & Ambalavanan 2016b, Parsons et al 2016) (Fig 9.9). Prevention is the most important therapy, and every effort should be made to recognise high-risk pregnancies, monitor the fetus and initiate appropriate therapy early.

Nursing Care Management

Nursing care is primarily the same as for any high-risk infant: careful assessment and observation for signs that might indicate cerebral hypoxia or ischaemia; monitoring of ventilatory and IV therapy; observation and management of seizures; and general supportive care to infants and parents, including guidelines for management in the event of cognitive impairment. During therapeutic hypothermia, the nurse/midwife carefully regulates the infant's body temperature according to the parameters in the cooling protocol being used. The protocol also directs the frequency of blood work, vital signs and other parameters to be monitored. Ensure adequate resuscitation is available including circulation requirements and glucose (Miller 2014).

Intraventricular Haemorrhage

Germinal matrix–intraventricular haemorrhage is known by a variety of terms according to the locus of bleeding: intraventricular haemorrhage, periventricular haemorrhage and subependymal-intraventricular haemorrhage. Most authorities use the term **intraventricular haemorrhage (IVH)** to describe this disorder, which is responsible for a significant percentage of seriously ill infants and neonatal mortality. IVH is said to occur in approximately 30% of premature infants weighing less than 1500 g; the incidence is inversely related to gestational age, with a higher incidence seen in those weighing less than 750 g (Carlo & Ambalavanan 2016a). IVH is extremely common in premature infants, especially ELBW and VLBW infants less than 32 weeks' gestation. The degree of neonatal immaturity correlates with the incidence of haemorrhage, and subsequent neurological handicap is not uncommon.

Pathophysiology

During the early months of prenatal development an extensive but fragile vascular network in the region of the ventricles receives a disproportionately large amount of cerebral blood flow. Blood is directed to the germinal matrix located in the periventricular region near the caudate nuclei of the cerebrum. Premature infants are subject to bleeding in this heavily vascularised region, especially during events that are likely to cause fluctuations in cerebral blood flow, such as hypoxic episodes and the associated increased venous pressure. In IVH the bleeding originates in these capillaries. The blood may rupture through the ependymal lining of the ventricles and fill all or part of the ventricular system. In severe cases the haemorrhage extends into the cerebral parenchyma. Bleeding in the cerebral parenchyma may lead to the development of cystic lesions referred to as periventricular leukomalacia, which is a significant risk factor for CP.

Following bleeding in the ventricle, clots and other debris can obstruct the passages between the ventricles, causing the ventricles to dilate and resulting in the development of hydrocephalus (posthaemorrhagic hydrocephalus).

Several clinical features are associated with IVH: birth asphyxia, early gestational age, LBW, respiratory distress, asynchronous breathing on ventilatory therapy, pneumothorax, low blood glucose, noxious stimuli, hypercarbia, coagulation and platelet disorders, and hypotension. Posthaemorrhagic hydrocephalus and damage to the periventricular white matter of the brain (such as in grade III+) are major determinants of associated chronic problems and prognosis.

Clinical Manifestations

1. **Catastrophic deterioration**—Begins within minutes to hours of the insult with a coma or deep stupor, respiratory abnormalities such as apnoea and hypoventilation, fixed pupils, decerebrate posturing, generalised tonic seizures, flaccid quadriparesis and cardiac arrhythmias.
2. **Saltatory deterioration**—More subtle; signs appear over several hours; may stop altogether, then reappear; signs consist of altered level of consciousness, hypotonia, subtle abnormal eye position and movements, decreased spontaneous or abnormal movements and an abnormally tight popliteal angle; respiratory abnormalities observed in some cases.
3. **Clinically silent deterioration**—Often overlooked clinically; a sudden unexplained decrease in haematocrit may be the only clinical sign of IVH.

Diagnostic Evaluation

In Australia and New Zealand refer to the Royal Prince Alfred Hospital Newborn Care Guidelines to classify intraventricular haemorrhage by grade, ranging from Grade 1 through to Grade IV. It also discusses risk factors and the need for repeated ultrasounds to confirm the grading classification. Check your advising paediatric facility for optimal guidelines; an example of this grading can be found at the following website: https://www.slhd.nsw.gov.au/rpa/neonatal/html/docs/ivh.pdf.

Therapeutic Management

Management of IVH is aimed at prevention, particularly of prematurity and any events that may lead to IVH. The maintenance of adequate oxygenation by decreasing iatrogenic events is the key to keeping ELBW and VLBW infants neurologically intact. Factors associated with prematurity and RDS may predispose the premature infant to IVH: acidosis, electrolyte imbalances and rapid fluid shifts (extracellular to intracellular); administration of hyperosmolar solutions (such as sodium bicarbonate); and hypotension followed by rapid volume expansion. Medical treatments aimed at preventing IVH with vitamin E, maternal vitamin K, pancuronium (to decrease blood pressure fluctuations), ibuprofen, phenobarbitone, magnesium sulfate and surfactant (for RDS) have met with varying degrees of success. Antenatal betamethasone administration has played a significant role in the reduction of IVH in premature infants (Ballabh 2014).

In the event of IVH, treatment is both preventive and supportive. Prompt detection by clinical signs or periodic ultrasonography is a key element in implementing strategies to prevent further damage. Posthaemorrhagic hydrocephalus is a common occurrence within 1 month of the event. Serial lumbar punctures may be used to decrease the amount of CSF and thus decrease ventricular size.

The long-term outcome of IVH is unpredictable and is influenced by the size of the haemorrhage and the extent of parenchymal involvement. Infants with small lesions have an excellent prognosis for neurological outcome (Parsons et al 2016).

Nursing Care Management

In addition to routine observations and management, the nurse/midwife directs care towards prevention of fluctuations in cerebral blood flow. Some nursing procedures increase intracranial pressure. For example, blood pressure increases significantly during ET suctioning in premature infants, and head positioning produces measurable changes in intracranial pressure. Researchers have found that intracranial pressure is highest when infants are in the dependent position and decreases when the head is in a midline position and elevated 30 degrees.

Cerebral pressure is lower when infants are in a midline position as opposed to a side-lying position. When the head is turned to the side without body alignment, the resulting venous congestion creates hydrostatic pressure fluctuations that increase intracranial pressure. Infants encumbered with tubes and monitoring equipment are more difficult to turn while maintaining head–body alignment.

Other interventions that may reduce the risk of increased intracranial pressure include avoiding interventions that cause crying (such as painful procedures). Crying (which essentially creates a Valsalva effect) can impede venous return, increase cerebral blood volume and compromise cerebral oxygenation in LBW infants. Avoid rapid volume expansion following hypotension (primarily in preterms) and administration of hyperosmolar solutions such as sodium bicarbonate. Because air leaks such as pneumothorax produce variable cerebral blood flow, rapid detection and intervention are key components of nursing care of the high-risk infant. Monitoring serum blood glucose levels and preventing hypoglycaemia are also important factors in keeping the infant neurologically intact. Many units practise minimum handling of infants at high risk to avoid fluctuations in cerebral blood flow. In addition, research has suggested that noxious external stimuli (e.g. pain and noise) have a potential role in stimulation that may lead to IVH. Care includes evaluating manipulations and handling and administering analgesics to reduce discomfort.

Intracranial Haemorrhage

ICH in neonates, although manifested in the same ways as in older children, occurs with different frequencies and degrees of severity.

Subdural Haemorrhage

A **subdural haematoma** is a life-threatening collection of blood in the subdural space. The stretching and tearing of the large veins in the tentorium cerebelli, the dural membrane that separates the cerebrum from the cerebellum, is the most common cause. With improved obstetric care this condition has become relatively uncommon; however, it is especially serious because of the inaccessibility of the haematoma to aspiration by subdural tap. Less commonly, haemorrhage occurs when veins in the subdural space over the surface of the brain are torn. (See Head Injury, Chapter 30.)

Subarachnoid Haemorrhage

Subarachnoid haemorrhage, the most common type of ICH, occurs in full-term infants as a result of trauma and in premature infants as a result of the same types of events that cause IVH. Small haemorrhages are the most common. Bleeding is of venous origin, and underlying contusion may also occur.

Intracerebellar Haemorrhage

Intracerebellar haemorrhage is a common finding on postmortem examination of the premature infant and can be a primary haemorrhage in the cerebellum associated with skull compression during abrupt, precipitous birth. It may occur secondary to extravasation of blood into the cerebellum from a ventricular haemorrhage. In the full-term infant the bleeding may follow a difficult birth.

Nursing Care Management

Nursing care is the same as care of the infant with IVH or with perinatal hypoxic-ischaemic brain injury.

Neonatal/perinatal Stroke

Neonatal stroke is reported to occur in 1 in 6000 live term births (Cole et al 2017). Inconsistent terminology and classification of neonatal haemorrhagic stroke (NHS) continues to complicate studies examining NHS (Cole et al 2017).

Neonatal stroke is the second leading cause of seizures in term neonates and may be caused by arterial, thrombotic or ischaemic events that result in altered brain blood flow and infarction. Neonatal stroke is more dominant in males, and there is an increased tendency towards left-sided involvement. Known risk factors for neonatal and perinatal stroke are not clearly defined or described. However, even without clear evidence for risk factors and aetiology, perinatal stroke is a leading cause of cerebral palsy and lifelong neurological morbidity (Cole et al 2017). Diagnosis with MRI is most accurate because head ultrasonography may be negative with an ischaemic event (Cole et al 2017).

Because neonatal stroke can only be diagnosed retrospectively, it is important for the nurse/midwife to be vigilant for apnoea or seizure activity in the first year of life, the time when clinical manifestations will appear.

Neonatal Seizures

Seizures in the neonatal period are usually the clinical manifestation of a serious underlying disease. The most common cause of seizures in the neonatal period (for term and premature infants) is HIE secondary to perinatal asphyxia (Mikati & Hani 2016). Although not life-threatening as an isolated entity, seizures constitute a medical emergency because they signal a disease process that may produce irreversible brain damage. Consequently, it is imperative to recognise a seizure and its significance so that the cause, as well as the seizure, can be treated (Box 9.7).

BOX 9.7 Causes of Neonatal Seizures

Metabolic
- Hypoglycaemia, hyperglycaemia
- Hypernatraemia, hyponatraemia
- Hypocalcaemia
- Hypomagnesaemia
- Pyridoxine deficiency
- Aminoacidurias (e.g. phenylketonuria, maple syrup urine disease)
- Hyperammonaemia

Toxic
- Uraemia
- Bilirubin encephalopathy (kernicterus)

Prenatal Infections
- Toxoplasmosis
- Syphilis
- Cytomegalovirus
- Herpes simplex
- Hepatitis

Postnatal Infections
- Bacterial meningitis
- Viral meningoencephalitis
- Sepsis
- Brain abscess

Trauma at Birth
- Hypoxic brain injury
- Intracranial haemorrhage
- Subarachnoid, subdural haemorrhage
- Intraventricular haemorrhage

Malformations
- Central nervous system agenesis
- Hydranencephaly
- Panencephaly
- Tuberous sclerosis

Miscellaneous
- Degenerative disease
- Benign familial neonatal seizures
- Narcotic withdrawal
- Stroke (fetal, perinatal or neonatal)

Pathophysiology

The features of neonatal seizures are different from those observed in the older infant or child. For example, the well-organised, generalised tonic-clonic seizures seen in older children are rare in infants, especially premature infants. The newborn brain, with its immature anatomical and physiological status and reduced cortical organisation, is developmentally insufficient to allow ready development and maintenance of a generalised seizure. The advanced degree of development of limbic structures with connections to the diencephalon and brainstem probably accounts for the higher frequency of seizure manifestations (such as oral movements, oculomotor deviations and apnoea) that originate in these structures.

Clinical Manifestations

Seizures in newborns may be subtle and barely discernible or grossly apparent. Because most neonatal seizures are subcortical, they do not have the aetiological and prognostic significance of seizures in children. The type of seizure is seldom important because one may produce a variety of manifestations. Neonatal seizures can be divided into four major types: clonic, tonic, myoclonic and subtle seizures. Table 9.5 lists these classifications in order of frequency (Perry et al 2017). Clonic, multifocal clonic and migratory clonic seizures are more common in full-term infants.

Jitteriness or tremulousness in the newborn is a repetitive shaking of an extremity or extremities that may be observed with crying, may occur with changes in sleeping state or may be elicited with stimulation. Jitteriness is relatively common in newborns, and to a mild degree may be considered normal during the first 4 days of life. Jitteriness can be distinguished from seizures by several characteristics: jitteriness is not accompanied by abnormal ocular movement as is a seizure; the dominant movement in jitteriness is tremor, whereas seizure movement is clonic jerking that cannot be stopped by flexion of the affected limb; and jitteriness is highly sensitive to stimulation, whereas a seizure is not. Further evaluation is indicated if jittery

TABLE 9.5 Classifications of Neonatal Seizures

Type	Characteristics
Clonic	Slow, rhythmic jerking movements Approximately 1–3/second
• Focal	Involves face, upper or lower extremities on one side of body May involve neck or trunk Infant is conscious during event
• Multifocal	May migrate randomly from one part of the body to another Movements may start at different times
Tonic	Extension, stiffening movements
• Generalised	Extension of all four limbs (similar to decerebrate rigidity) Upper limbs maintained in a stiffly flexed position (resembles decorticate rigidity)
• Focal	Sustained posturing of a limb Asymmetrical posturing of trunk or neck
Subtle	May develop in either full-term or premature infants but more common in premature Often overlooked by inexperienced observers Signs: • horizontal eye deviation • repetitive blinking or fluttering of the eyelids, staring • sucking or other oral-buccal-lingual movements • arm movements that resemble rowing or swimming • leg movements described as pedalling or bicycling • apnoea (common) Signs may appear alone or in combination
Myoclonic	Rapid jerks that involve flexor muscle groups
• Focal	Involves upper extremity flexor muscle group No electroencephalogram (EEG) discharges observed
• Multifocal	Asynchronous twitching of several parts of the body No associated EEG discharges observed
• Generalised	Bilateral jerks of upper and lower limbs Associated with EEG discharges

Source: Adapted from Volpe, J. (2008). Neonatal seizures. In J. Volpe, Neurology of the newborn (5th ed.). Philadelphia, PA: Saunders.

movements persist beyond the fourth day, if the movements are persistent and prolonged after a stimulus or if they are easily elicited with minimal stimulus.

Spasms are sudden generalised jerks lasting briefly (1 to 2 seconds) that are distinguished from generalised tonic spells by their short duration and by the fact that spasms are most often associated with a single, brief generalised discharge (Mikati & Hani 2016). A **tremor** is repetitive movements of both hands (with or without movement of legs or jaws) at a frequency of 2 to 5 per second and lasting more than 10 minutes. It is common in newborn infants and has a variety of causes, including neurological damage, hypoglycaemia and hypocalcaemia. Tremors are usually of no pathological significance.

Diagnostic Evaluation

Early evaluation and diagnosis of seizures are urgent. In addition to a careful physical examination, the pregnancy and family histories are investigated for familial and prenatal causes. Blood is drawn for glucose and electrolyte examination, and CSF is obtained for examination for gross blood, cell count, protein, glucose and culture. Electroencephalography (EEG) may help identify subtle seizures but is less helpful in establishing a diagnosis; continuous video EEG is the gold standard for monitoring neonatal seizures (Glass 2014, Mikati & Hani 2016). Other diagnostic procedures, such as CT, ultrasonography and echoencephalography, may be indicated. Inborn errors of metabolism should also be evaluated on an individual basis.

Therapeutic Management

Treatment is directed towards the prevention of cerebral damage, correction of metabolic abnormalities, respiratory and cardiovascular support and suppression of the seizure activity. The underlying cause is treated (e.g. glucose infusion for hypoglycaemia, calcium for hypocalcaemia and antibiotics for infection). If needed, respiratory support is provided for hypoxia. Anticonvulsants may be administered, especially when the other measures fail to control the seizures. Buccal or intranasal midazolam can be administered in the emergency management of prolonged seizures when intravenous access cannot be obtained. Buccal or intranasal midazolam may be used in combination with other antiepileptic drugs. Midazolam or diazepam < 1 hour prior to presentation should be regarded as initial doses already given. All states and territories will have protocols and flow charts outlining the desired doses but the standard dose is midazolam 0.15 mg/kg IV/IM (max 10 mg) OR 0.3 mg/kg buccal/IN (max 10 mg), and to also administer diazepam 0.3 mg/kg IV/IO (maximum 10 mg), IV dose preferable OR 0.5 mg/kg PR (maximum 10 mg); do not give IM. Begin second-line treatment with phenytoin (loading dose: 20 mg/kg IV/IO). Infuse undiluted into a large vein over 20 minutes (maximum rate 50 mg/min) in a monitored patient. Do not give in age < 1 month (RCHM 2020).

Nursing Care Management

The major nursing responsibilities in the care of infants with seizures are to recognise when the infant is having a seizure so that therapy can be instituted, to carry out the therapeutic regimen and to observe the response to the therapy and any further evidence of seizures or other symptoms. Assessment and other aspects of care are the same as for all high-risk infants. Parents need to be informed of their infant's status, and the nurse/midwife should reinforce and clarify the practitioner's explanations. The infant's behaviours need to be interpreted for the parents, and the infant's responses to the pharmacological treatment must be anticipated and their significance explained. Encourage parents to visit their infant and perform parenting activities. Parents are also educated regarding the administration of prescribed anticonvulsant drugs and common adverse effects. Seizures generate a great deal of anxiety and fear, and the staff's concern, which is justifiable, can heighten that anxiety. Providing support and guidance is an important nursing function.

HIGH RISK RELATED TO MATERNAL CONDITIONS

Infants of Diabetic Mothers

The morbidity and mortality rates of infants of diabetic mothers (IDMs) have been significantly reduced as a result of effective control of maternal diabetes mellitus and an increased understanding of fetal disorders. However, the offspring of diabetic mothers (type 1, type 2 and gestational) are at risk for a greater number of adverse outcomes. The incidence of congenital anomalies is increased threefold in infants of diabetic mothers (Carlo 2016b, Goldman & Schafer 2020). Cardiac anomalies such as ventriculoseptal defects occur in 30% of IDMs (Goldman & Schafer 2020). Because infants born to women with gestational diabetes mellitus are at risk for many of the same complications as IDMs, the following discussion includes both types of infants.

Hypoglycaemia associated with congenital hyperinsulinism and hypoglycaemia due to inborn metabolic defects is beyond the scope of this discussion.

The severity of the maternal diabetes affects infant survival. Several factors determine the severity: duration of the disease before pregnancy; age of onset; extent of vascular complications; and abnormalities of the current pregnancy such as pyelonephritis, diabetic ketoacidosis, gestational hypertension and non-compliance. *The single most important factor influencing fetal wellbeing is the mother's normoglycaemic status.* Reasonable metabolic control that begins before conception and continues during the first weeks of pregnancy can prevent malformation in an IDM.

Effects of Diabetes on the Fetus

Hypoglycaemia may appear a short time after birth and in IDMs is associated with increased insulin activity in the blood. A standardised definition for neonatal hypoglycaemia remains elusive and controversial. At best, authorities agree that reliance on a single numeric value for every clinical situation is inadequate (see Therapeutic Management section). Hypoglycaemia in the IDM is related to hypertrophy and hyperplasia of the pancreatic islet cells, causing transient hyperinsulinism.

High maternal blood glucose levels during fetal life provide a continuous stimulus to the fetal islet cells for insulin production. This sustained hyperglycaemia promotes fetal insulin secretion that ultimately leads to excessive growth and deposition of fat, which probably accounts for the infants who are large for gestational age, or macrosomic. Maternal hyperlipidaemia and increased lipid transfer to the fetus are responsible for the excessive weight gain and fat deposition seen in such infants. When the neonate's glucose supply is removed abruptly at the time of birth, the continued production of insulin soon depletes the blood of circulating glucose, creating a state of hyperinsulinism and hypoglycaemia within 1.5 to 4 hours, especially in infants of mothers with poorly controlled diabetes. Precipitous drops in blood glucose levels can cause serious neurological damage or death. The birth defects observed in IDMs are thought to occur as a result of multifactorial teratogenic factors rather than hyperglycaemia alone (Goldman & Schafer 2020).

Clinical Manifestations

IDMs have a characteristic appearance (Fig 9.10). They are usually macrosomic for their gestational age, very plump and full faced, liberally coated with vernix caseosa, and plethoric. The placenta and umbilical cord are also larger than average. However, infants of mothers with advanced diabetes may be small for gestational age, have IUGR or be appropriate for gestational age because of maternal vascular (placental) involvement. IDMs have an increased incidence of hypoglycaemia, hypocalcaemia, hyperbilirubinaemia, hypomagnesaemia and RDS. Hyperglycaemia in the diabetic mother and subsequent fetal hyperinsulinism may be a factor in reducing fetal surfactant synthesis, contributing to the development of RDS. Morbidities in IDMs are the result of exposure to elevated glucose and ketone levels, placental insufficiency and prematurity. Although large, these infants may be delivered before term because of maternal complications or increased fetal size.

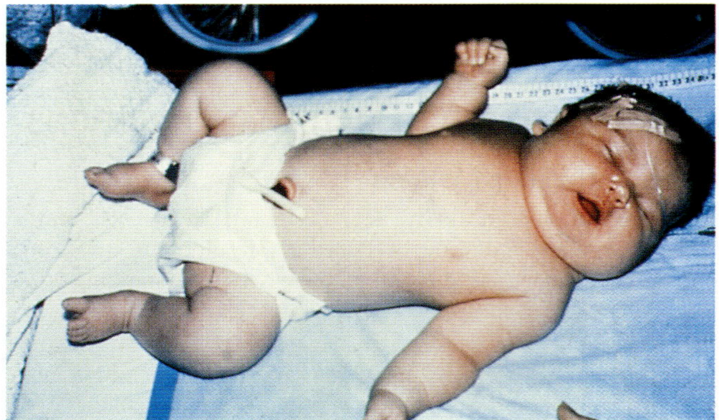

Fig 9.10 Large-for-gestational-age infant. This infant of a diabetic mother weighed 5 kg at birth and exhibits the typical round facies. (Source: Zitelli, B. J. & Davis, H. W. (2007). Atlas of pediatric physical diagnosis [5th ed.]. Philadelphia, PA: Mosby.)

Therapeutic Management

The management of IDMs includes careful monitoring of serum glucose levels and observation for accompanying complications such as RDS. Examine these infants for any anomalies or birth injuries, and regularly obtain blood studies for determinations of glucose, calcium, haematocrit and bilirubin. A common definition of hypoglycaemia has not been established. Several authors have suggested the use of operational thresholds at which hypoglycaemia should be closely monitored and treated. Close observation in infants with known risk factors such as maternal diabetes mellitus or with plasma glucose values below 45 mg/dL (2.5 mmol/L) is recommended (Carlo 2016b). Rozance and colleagues (2016) recommend that therapeutic glucose levels be kept at or above 50 mg/dL in neonates with profound, recurrent or persistent hyperinsulinaemic hypoglycaemia. Studies confirm the importance of maintaining serum glucose levels above 45 mg/dL (2.6 mmol/L) in hyperinsulinaemic infants with hypoglycaemia to prevent serious neurological sequelae (Rozance et al 2016). Recommendations for treatment vary within Australia and New Zealand and all nurses and midwives should consult their own policies and protocols in relation to treatment.

Because the hypertrophied pancreas is so sensitive to blood glucose concentrations, the administration of oral glucose may trigger a massive insulin release, resulting in rebound hypoglycaemia. Therefore, feedings should begin within the first hour after birth provided that the infant's cardiorespiratory condition is stable. Approximately half of IDMs do well and adjust without complications. Infants born to mothers with uncontrolled diabetes may require IV infusion of glucose. Oral and IV intake may be titrated to maintain adequate blood glucose levels. Frequent blood glucose determinations are needed for the first 2 days of life to assess the degree of hypoglycaemia present at any given time.

Nursing Care Management

The nursing care of IDMs involves early examination for congenital anomalies and signs of possible respiratory or cardiac problems, maintenance of adequate thermoregulation, early introduction of carbohydrate feedings as appropriate and monitoring of serum blood glucose levels. The latter is of particular importance because many hypoglycaemic infants may remain asymptomatic. IV glucose infusion requires careful monitoring of the site and the neonate's reaction to therapy. Because macrosomic infants are at risk for problems associated with a difficult birth, they are monitored for birth injuries such as brachial plexus injury and palsy, fractured clavicle and phrenic nerve palsy. Additional monitoring of the infant for associated problems (e.g. RDS, polycythaemia, hypocalcaemia, poor feeding and hyperbilirubinaemia) is also a vital nursing function.

Drug-exposed Infants

Overview

Determining the effects of intrauterine drug and alcohol exposure is difficult for a variety of reasons. Many substance-using women ingest multiple drugs or a combination of drugs and alcohol, and some women who use drugs or alcohol may be undernourished or suffer from chronic medical conditions. Some may not seek prenatal care. For others, the drugs used may be cut with a variety of materials and the strength, dose and duration of exposure are likely to be unknown. Current data from the Australian Institute of Health and Welfare (AIHW) indicate that: 2.2% of pregnant women have used an illicit drug such as marijuana; 0.9% misused prescription analgesics; a further 42% used alcohol; and 15% smoked tobacco (Australian Institute of Health and Welfare [AIHW] 2019).

Substance use by the mother may cause the newborn to have neonatal abstinence syndrome (NAS). Babies affected by NAS will show signs of drug withdrawal due to the women being physically dependent on the drug during pregnancy (The Royal Australian and New Zealand College of Obstetricians and Gynaecologists [RANZCOG] 2021). The syndrome can still be present even if the mother stopped use up to 4 weeks before birth. The newborn is not addicted in a behavioural sense, yet may experience mild to strong physiological signs as a result of the mother's drug use. Therefore, saying that an infant born to a mother who uses substances is addicted is incorrect; drug-exposed newborn is a better term, which implies intrauterine drug exposure.

Clinical Manifestations. Most infants of drug-dependent mothers appear normal at birth but may begin to exhibit signs of drug withdrawal within 12 to 24 hours, depending on the substance and the mother's pattern of use. If mothers have been taking methadone, the signs appear somewhat later—anywhere from 1 or 2 days to 2 to 3 weeks or more after birth. The clinical manifestations of withdrawal may fall into one or all of the following categories: CNS, GI, respiratory and autonomic nervous system signs (RANZCOG 2021, Weiner & Finnegan 2016). The manifestations become most pronounced between 48 and 72 hours of age and may last from 6 days to 8 weeks (Box 9.8).

Signs of withdrawal include increased tone, irritability, increased respiratory rate, disturbed sleep, fever, excessive sucking and loose, watery stools. Other signs observed include projectile vomiting, mottling, crying, nasal stuffiness, hyperactive Moro reflex and tremors (Malcolm 2015). Although these infants suck avidly on fists and display an exaggerated rooting reflex, they are poor feeders with uncoordinated and ineffectual sucking and swallowing reflexes (Kain & Mannix 2018).

One observation in a large percentage of these infants is generalised perspiring, which is unusual in newborn infants. It is significant that although drug-exposed infants may have some tachypnoea, cyanosis or apnoea, they rarely develop RDS when born near term. Narcotics or stress factors in the intrauterine environment apparently accelerate lung maturation even with a high incidence of prematurity.

Not all infants of narcotic-addicted mothers show signs of withdrawal. Because of irregular and varying degrees of drug use, quality of drug and mixed drug usage by the mother, some infants display mild or variable manifestations. Most manifestations are the vague, nonspecific signs characteristic of infants in general; therefore, it is important to differentiate between drug withdrawal and other disorders before instituting specific therapy. Other states (e.g. hypocalcaemia, hypoglycaemia or sepsis) often coexist with the drug withdrawal (Kain & Mannix 2018).

Therapeutic Management. The treatment of the drug-exposed infant initially consists of modulating the environment to decrease external stimuli. Drug therapies to decrease withdrawal side effects are implemented once **neonatal abstinence syndrome (NAS)** is identified. This term is used to describe the behaviours exhibited by the infant exposed to drugs in utero.

Nursing Care Management. When possible, nursery personnel should be alerted to the likelihood of a drug-exposed infant requiring admittance. If the mother has had good prenatal care, the practitioner is aware of the problem and substance abuse treatment may have been instituted before birth. However, a number of mothers deliver their infants without the benefit of adequate care, and the addiction is unknown to healthcare personnel at the time of birth. The degree of narcosis or withdrawal is closely related to the amount of drug the mother has habitually taken, the length of time she has been taking the drug and her drug level at the time of birth. The most severe symptoms occur in the infants of mothers who have taken large amounts of drugs over a long period. In addition, the nearer to the time of birth that the mother takes the drug, the longer it takes the infant to develop withdrawal and the more severe the manifestations. The infant may not exhibit withdrawal symptoms until 7 to 10 days after birth.

Once the presence of NAS is identified in an infant, direct nursing care is provided towards reducing external stimuli that might trigger hyperactivity and irritability (e.g. dimming the lights and decreasing noise levels), providing adequate nutrition and hydration and promoting positive mother–infant relationships. Providing care on demand rather than on a fixed schedule may help reduce irritability for infants. Appropriate individualised developmental care is implemented, such as facilitating self-consoling and self-regulating behaviours (see Table 9.3). Some irritable and hyperactive infants respond to comforting, movement, containment and close contact. Wrapping infants snugly and rocking and holding them tightly limit their ability to self-stimulate. The infant's arms should remain flexed with hands close to the mouth for sucking as appropriate; sucking on fingers or hands is a form of self-control and comfort. Arranging nursing activities to reduce disturbances helps decrease exogenous stimulation.

Each state and territory will have specific guidelines for the management of substance use during pregnancy, birth and the postnatal period. It is advised to follow your state or territory's guidelines or advice from the Ministry of Health in New Zealand to assist with assessment and treatment.

The Neonatal Abstinence Scoring System has been developed to monitor infants in an objective manner and evaluate the infant's response to clinical and pharmacological interventions (Finnegan 1985).

BOX 9.8 Signs of Withdrawal in the Neonate

- Irritability
- Tachypnoea (> 60 beats/min)
- Tremors
- Excoriations (knees, face)
- High-pitched cry
- Mottling (skin)
- Hypertonicity of muscles
- Sneezing
- Frantic sucking of hands
- Yawning
- Poor feeding
- Vomiting, often projectile
- Hyperactivity
- Temperature instability
- Perspiring
- Loose diarrhoeal stools
- Fever
- Seizures
- Nasal stuffiness
- Sleep disturbances

This system also assists nurses, midwives and other healthcare workers in evaluating the severity of the infant's withdrawal symptoms.

Another scoring tool has been developed specifically aimed at measuring neurological behaviour and resultant effects on the neonate when substances are used during pregnancy. The NICU Network Neurobehavioral Scale (NNNS), developed by the National Institutes of Health, provides an assessment of neurological, behavioural and stress-abstinence function in the neonate. The NNNS was designed to provide a comprehensive assessment of both neurological integrity and behavioural function (Kain & Mannix 2018). Most guidelines are lengthy and specific to state/territory. New Zealand currently follows guidelines provided by Australia. The following are some examples of the NSW, Queensland and NZ guidelines.

- New South Wales Government: https://www1.health.nsw.gov.au/pds/ActivePDSDocuments/GL2014_022.pdf
- Department of Health, Queensland: www.health.qld.gov.au/qcg/documents/g-psumat.pdf
- New Zealand: https://practice.orangatamariki.govt.nz/previous-practice-centre/knowledge-base-practice-frameworks/fetal-alcohol-spectrum-disorder/

Breastfeeding. There are very few contraindications to breastfeed: what is recommended is when a woman is using drugs and alcohol during pregnancy, careful and respectful assessment will take place. Where the woman is stable on methadone or buprenorphine and it has been established there is no other drug use, breastfeeding is encouraged. Small amounts of methadone and buprenorphine will be transmitted through the breastmilk to baby, but not in sufficient quantities to affect the baby clinically. However, this is only recommended if the woman is on small doses of methadone or buprenorphine; high doses may precipitate withdrawal in the infant.

Breastfeeding is actively discouraged when the woman is dependent on heroin, methamphetamine, alcohol and most other illicit drugs due to the transfer of substances into breast milk, including possible contaminants. The other concern is the parenting ability, which may be negatively impacted by substance use (Kain & Mannix 2018).

Loose stools and poor intake and regurgitation after feeding predispose the infants to malnutrition, dehydration and electrolyte imbalance. An oral opioid such as morphine may be administered to control loose, watery stools (Weiner & Finnegan 2016). It takes considerable time and patience to ensure that these infants receive sufficient caloric and fluid intake.

Pharmacological treatment is usually based on the severity of withdrawal symptoms, as determined by an assessment tool. Drug therapies to decrease withdrawal side effects include administration of phenobarbitone, morphine, diluted tincture of opium, methadone, buprenorphine or clonidine (Carlo & Ambalavanan 2016b, Weiner & Finnegan 2016). A combination of these drugs may be necessary to treat infants exposed to multiple drugs in utero; careful attention should be given to possible adverse effects (Weiner & Finnegan 2016).

Opiate Exposure

Narcotics have a low molecular weight, allowing them to readily cross the placental membrane and enter the fetal system. When the mother is a habitual user of narcotics, especially heroin or methadone, the unborn child may also become passively physiologically addicted to the drug, which places the infant at risk during the early neonatal period.

Prescription opioids such as oxycodone (OxyContin) have been identified as increasingly popular drugs of abuse, which may cause withdrawal symptoms in neonates. Other chemical substances that may cause neonatal withdrawal include methadone, caffeine and PCP (RANZCOG 2021).

Methadone Exposure

Methadone, a synthetic opiate, has been the therapy of choice for heroin addiction since 1965. Methadone crosses the placenta. An increasing number of infants have been born to methadone-maintained mothers who seem to have better prenatal care and a somewhat better lifestyle than those taking heroin.

Some question exists concerning the benefits of methadone therapy during pregnancy because of its effect on the fetus. Methadone withdrawal resembles heroin withdrawal but tends to be more severe and prolonged. Signs of methadone withdrawal include tremors, irritability, fever, hypertonicity, hyperactive Moro reflex, vomiting and sleep disturbances (Kraft et al 2016). These infants exhibit a disturbed sleep pattern similar to that seen in heroin withdrawal. They have a higher birth weight than those infants in heroin withdrawal, usually appropriate for gestational age. No increased incidence of congenital anomalies is seen.

Late-onset withdrawal occurs at age 2 to 4 weeks and may continue for weeks or months. A higher incidence of SIDS has been reported in these infants (Weiner & Finnegan 2016). This factor is important for perinatal nurses/midwives who coordinate follow-up care for the infant and education for the mother or caregiver. Community health nurses or midwives must know about the potential for withdrawal symptoms.

Therapy for methadone withdrawal is similar to that for heroin withdrawal. The few available follow-up studies of these infants reveal a high incidence of hyperactivity, learning and behaviour disorders and poor social adjustment (RANZCOG 2021).

Methamphetamine Exposure

The fetal and neonatal effects of maternal use of methamphetamines in pregnancy are not well known but appear to be dose related (O'Connor et al 2020). Continuous methamphetamine use during pregnancy is associated with premature birth and low birth weight, both of which contribute to neonatal morbidity and mortality (RANZCOG 2021). Stopping methamphetamine use at any time during pregnancy improves birth outcomes (RANZCOG 2021).

Infants exposed to methamphetamine in utero have significantly smaller head circumferences and birth weights than those not exposed (O'Connor et al 2020). In addition, exposed infants may exhibit agitation, vomiting and tachypnoea. After birth, infants may experience bradycardia or tachycardia that resolves as the drug is cleared from the system. Lethargy may continue for several months, along with frequent infections and poor weight gain. Emotional disturbances and delays in gross and fine motor coordination may occur during early childhood (RANZCOG 2021, O'Connor et al 2020).

Marijuana Exposure

Marijuana is the most common illicit drug used by women ages 18 to 44 years (non-pregnant and pregnant) (RANZCOG 2021). Marijuana crosses the placenta. Some studies have shown that use during pregnancy resulted in decreased birth weight and a need for placement in an NICU (RANZCOG 2021, O'Connor et al 2020). Compounding the issue of the effects of marijuana is multidrug use, which combines the harmful effects of marijuana, tobacco, alcohol, opiates and cocaine (Gunn et al 2016). Long-term follow-up studies on exposed infants are needed.

Fetal Alcohol Spectrum Disorder

Infants and children exposed to alcohol in utero were previously reported to have characteristic facial features, prenatal and postnatal growth failure and neurodevelopmental deficits. This triad of findings, termed **fetal alcohol syndrome (FAS)**, was attributed to excessive ingestion of alcohol by the mother during pregnancy. It has since been shown that infants may not initially display the dysmorphic facial features. These are believed to become more defined with increasing age during childhood. A number of terms (including *alcohol-related neurodevelopmental birth defects* and *fetal alcohol spectrum disorders*) have been proposed to describe the combination of findings. The umbrella term **fetal alcohol spectrum disorder (FASD)** is now recommended to describe the continuum of defects seen in children affected by maternal alcohol intake, including classic FAS at the most severe end of the spectrum.

Categories described by the RANZCOG (2021) for diagnosis of FAS are: growth restriction, both prenatal and postnatal; midfacial dysmorphic facial features; and CNS involvement (i.e. structural, neurological or functional abnormality). Any single one or combination of these may be present in addition to a history of maternal alcohol consumption. The diagnosis of FASD is complicated by the absence of a specific single biological marker and by manifestations that are often seen in other childhood conditions.

The major goal of nursing care is prevention of these disorders through provision of adequate prenatal care for the expectant mother and precautions regarding exposure to potentially harmful infections.

Alcohol (ethanol and ethyl alcohol) interferes with normal fetal development. The effects on the fetal brain are permanent, and even moderate use of alcohol during pregnancy may cause long-term postnatal difficulties, including impaired mother–infant attachment. Because there is no known safe level of alcohol consumption in pregnancy, the current recommendation is that women stop consuming alcohol at least 3 months before they plan to conceive.

Fetal abnormalities are not related to the amount of the mother's alcohol intake, but to the amount consumed in excess of the liver's ability to detoxify it. The liver's capacity to detoxify alcohol is limited and inflexible; when the liver receives more alcohol than it is able to handle, the excess is continually recirculated until the organ is able to reduce it to carbon dioxide and water. This circulating alcohol has a special affinity for brain tissue. There is no specific critical period at which alcohol toxicity may occur, although early gestation is considered the most vulnerable period. Exposure at any period may cause subtle damage to the developing fetus (Tai et al 2017). Other factors that contribute to the teratogenic effects include toxic acetyl aldehyde (a degradation byproduct of ethanol) and other substances that may be added to the alcohol. Poor nutritional state, smoking, polydrug intake and infrequent or lack of prenatal care may compound the problem of alcohol abuse (Reid 2018).

The effects on the fetal brain are reflected in CNS manifestations of FASD (Box 9.9). Cognitive and motor delays, hearing disorders and a variety of defects in craniofacial development are prominent features. MRI studies of children with diagnosed FASD revealed a high incidence of midbrain anomalies, including displacements in the corpus callosum and changes in symmetry in the temporal lobes. Alcohol-exposed infants also demonstrate narrowing in the temporal region and reduced brain growth in portions of the frontal lobe (Lucas et al 2016, Wilhoit et al 2017). Some affected infants display physical features of the syndrome; behaviours, however, are non-specific in newborns and may therefore pass undetected. These include difficulty in establishing respiration, irritability, lethargy, poor suck reflex and abdominal distension.

Nursing Care Management. Nursing care of affected infants involves the same assessment and observations that are employed for any high-risk infant. Poor feeding is characteristic of infants with FASD and is a significant problem throughout infancy. Strategies to provide individualised developmental care are aimed at reducing noxious environmental stimuli and helping the infant achieve self-regulation. Monitoring weight gain, analysing feeding behaviours and devising strategies to promote nutritional intake are especially important.

BOX 9.9 Major Features of Fetal Alcohol Syndrome*

Facial Features

- Short palpebral fissures
- Hypoplastic or smooth philtrum (vertical ridge in upper lip)
- Thinned upper lip (vermilion)
- Short, upturned nose
- Hypoplastic maxilla
- Micrognathia or prognathia in adolescence
- Retrognathia in infancy

Neurological

- Cognitive impairment
- Motor delays
- Microcephaly (head circumference below 10th percentile)
- Poor coordination
- Hypotonia
- Hearing disorders

Behavioural

- Irritability (infancy)
- Hyperactivity (child)

Growth

- Disproportionately low weight to height
- Prenatal growth restriction
- Persistent postnatal growth lag

*For a comprehensive list of fetal alcohol-related birth defects, see Fig. 1 in American Academy of Pediatrics, Committee on Substance Abuse and Committee on Children with Disabilities. (2000). Fetal alcohol syndrome and alcohol-related neurodevelopmental disorders. Pediatrics, 106(2), 358–361.

The effects of FASD have been identified in adolescents and young adults, primarily in relation to growth deficiencies, delayed motor development and cognitive impairment. Children exposed to alcohol prenatally showed more aggressiveness, delinquent behaviour and attention problems (Lucas et al 2016, Wilhoit et al 2017). Facial characteristics in adults tend to be more subtle than in infants and children.

Early diagnosis and intervention are reported to be beneficial for reducing the effects of alcohol exposure on the growing child (Lucas et al 2016, Reid 2018). Nurses should be actively involved in identifying and referring children exposed to alcohol prenatally.

The dangers of heavy drinking are known, and *all* women should be counselled regarding the risks to the fetus. The nurse should emphasise to women of all ages that there is no known 'safe' amount of alcohol intake during pregnancy that will prevent FASD. Furthermore, FASD is a totally preventable congenital anomaly. A change in drinking habits even as late as the third trimester (when brain growth in the fetus is greatest) is associated with improved fetal outcome.

Infants of Mothers Who Smoke

Cigarette smoking during pregnancy is clearly associated with significant birth weight deficits, and there is a definitive dose-response relationship between the number of cigarettes smoked by the mother and these deficits (Abraham et al 2017, AIHW 2018). This dose-related response also affects the Apgar scores. Nearly four times more infants whose mothers smoked three packs per day had low Apgar scores compared with infants whose mothers did not smoke or smoked only one pack per day. Studies indicate that almost 30% of women smoke and the majority of this population are in their childbearing period (AHIW 2018, Sabra et al 2017).

The rate of premature births is increased in mothers who smoke, but the infants are smaller at all stages of gestation. They show fetal growth restriction in length, weight and chest and head circumference; these deficits are not related to maternal appetite or weight gain. The concentration of a pharmacologically active substance found in tobacco—nicotine—has been found to be higher in newborns of mothers who smoke than in the mothers themselves. Nicotine is metabolised to cotinine and secreted in breast milk and has a half-life of 70 to 80 minutes. In addition, it is now recognised that neonates may experience withdrawal symptoms after exposure to nicotine, whether smoked or chewed. It has also been shown that cigarette smoking has detrimental effects beyond the neonatal period, with deficits in growth, intellectual and emotional development and behaviour. Maternal smoking and passive smoking by household members has been correlated with higher rates of SIDS (Cole et al 2020, Tin Tin et al 2016), spontaneous abortion, premature rupture of membranes, premature birth and learning and behaviour deficits (Cole et al 2020, Tin Tin et al 2016).

Nursing Care Management. Nurses/midwives are prime candidates for disseminating information to expectant mothers regarding smoking-related risks. Mothers who stop or substantially reduce smoking during pregnancy improve the quality of life for their unborn infants. In one study, infants of expectant mothers who were given information, support, encouragement, practical guidance and behaviour modification during pregnancy delivered infants with significantly higher birth weights than did controls. If mothers continue to smoke while breastfeeding, encourage them to do so immediately after breastfeeding to reduce the amount of nicotine and cotinine in the breast milk. Smoking decreases milk production in the breastfeeding mother (Mitchell et al 2016). Parents should make all efforts to avoid second-hand smoke around all infants, but especially around those born with respiratory or cardiac problems and those born prematurely.

Maternal Infections

The range of pathological conditions produced by infectious agents is large, and the difference between the maternal and fetal effects caused by any one agent is also great. Some maternal infections, especially during early gestation, can result in fetal loss or malformations because the fetus's ability to handle infectious organisms is limited and the fetal immunological system is unable to prevent the dissemination of infectious organisms to the various tissues.

Not all prenatal infections produce teratogenic effects. Furthermore, disorders caused by transplacental transfer of infectious agents are not always well-defined clinically. Some microbial agents can cause remarkably similar manifestations, and it is not uncommon to test for all when a prenatal infection is suspected. This is the so-called **TORCHS complex**.

T—Toxoplasmosis
O—Other (e.g. hepatitis B, parvovirus, HIV)
R—Rubella
C—Cytomegalovirus infection
H—Herpes simplex
S—Syphilis

To determine the causative agent in a symptomatic infant, perform tests to rule out each of these infections. The *O* category may involve testing for several viral infections (e.g. hepatitis B, varicella-zoster, measles, mumps, HIV, human papillomavirus and human parvovirus). Bacterial infections are not included in the TORCHS workup because they are usually identified by clinical manifestations and readily available laboratory tests. Gonococcal conjunctivitis (ophthalmia neonatorum) and chlamydial conjunctivitis have been significantly reduced by prophylactic measures at birth. HIV infection is discussed in Chapter 28. The major maternal infections, their possible effects and specific nursing considerations are outlined in Table 9.6.

TABLE 9.6 Infections Acquired from Mother Before, During or After Birth*

Fetal or Newborn Effect	Transmission	Nursing Considerations†
Human Immunodeficiency Virus (HIV)		
No significant difference between infected and uninfected infants at birth in some instances Embryopathy reported by some observers: • depressed nasal bridge • mild upward or downward obliquity of eyes • long palpebral fissures with blue sclerae • patulous lips • ocular hypertelorism • prominent upper vermilion border	Transplacental; during vaginal labour and birth; breast milk; feeding infant blood-tinged premasticated food	Administer combination antiretroviral prophylaxis to human immunodeficiency (HIV)–positive mother; prophylaxis to prevent perinatal transmission may begin after first trimester. Choice of regimens is determined by examining a number of factors, including mother's current treatment. Discuss avoidance of premasticated foods given to infant from HIV-infected mother. Caesarean section at 38 weeks' gestation in HIV-positive mothers is recommended to reduce transmission. Avoid breastfeeding in HIV-positive mother. For chemoprophylaxis against *Pneumocystis carinii* pneumonia in HIV-exposed infants, drug of choice is trimethoprim-sulfamethoxazole.
Chickenpox (Varicella-Zoster Virus [VZV])		
Intrauterine exposure—congenital varicella syndrome: limb dysplasia, microcephaly, cortical atrophy, chorioretinitis, cataracts, cutaneous scars, other anomalies, auditory nerve palsy, motor and cognitive delays Severe symptoms (rash, fever) and higher mortality in infant whose mother develops varicella 5 days before to 2 days after birth	First trimester (fetal varicella syndrome); perinatal period (infection)	Use varicella-zoster immune globulin or IVIg to treat infants born to mothers with onset of disease within 5 days before or 2 days after birth. Healthy term infants exposed postnatally to varicella (especially if mother's rash does not appear until after 48 hours of birth) should not receive varicella-zoster immune globulin. (See also Immunisations, Chapter 6, for administration recommendations for premature infants.) Institute isolation precautions in newborn born to mother with varicella up to 21–28 days (latter time if newborn received varicella-zoster immune globulin or IVIg after birth (if hospitalised).† Prevention—Immunise all children with varicella vaccine.

TABLE 9.6 Infections Acquired from Mother Before, During or After Birth—cont'd

Fetal or Newborn Effect	Transmission	Nursing Considerations[†]
Chlamydia Infection (*Chlamydia trachomatis*)		
Conjunctivitis, pneumonia	Last trimester or perinatal period	Standard ophthalmic prophylaxis for gonococcal ophthalmia neonatorum (topical antibiotics, silver nitrate or povidone-iodine) is not effective in treatment or prevention of chlamydial ophthalmia. Treat with oral erythromycin for 14 days.
Coxsackievirus (Group B Enterovirus–non-polio)		
Cytomegalovirus (CMV)		
Variable manifestation from asymptomatic to severe Microcephaly, cerebral calcifications, chorioretinitis Jaundice, hepatosplenomegaly Petechial or purpuric rash Neurological sequelae—seizure disorders, sensorimotor deafness, cognitive impairment	Throughout pregnancy	Infection acquired at birth, shortly thereafter or via human milk is not associated with clinical illness. Affected individuals excrete virus in saliva and other oropharyngeal secretions. Virus is detected in urine or tissue by electron microscopy. Pregnant women should avoid close contact with known cases.
***Erythema Infectiosum* (Parvovirus B19)**		
Fetal hydrops and death from anaemia and heart failure with early exposure Anaemia with later exposure No teratogenic effects established Ordinarily, low risk of ill effect to fetus	Transplacental	First-trimester infection has most serious effects. Pregnant healthcare workers should not care for patients who might be highly contagious (e.g. child with aplastic crisis). Aggressive cardiovascular and respiratory support is required in newborn with hydrops. Routine exclusion of pregnant women from workplace where disease is occurring is not recommended.
Gonococcal Disease (*Neisseria Gonorrhoeae*)		
Ophthalmitis Neonatal gonococcal arthritis, septicaemia, meningitis	Last trimester or perinatal period	Preventive—Apply prophylactic medication to eyes at time of birth. Infant with confirmed ophthalmia, scalp abscess or disseminated infection should be hospitalised and cultures obtained to determine antimicrobial treatment. Consider testing infant for *Chlamydia,* HIV and syphilis. Irrigate infant's eyes with saline until discharge is eliminated. Obtain smears for culture. To treat ophthalmia and non-disseminated infection, administer IV or IM ceftriaxone, once. Disseminated disease requires cefotaxime treatment for 1 week.
Hepatitis B Virus (HBV)		
May be asymptomatic at birth Acute hepatitis, changes in liver function	Transplacental; contaminated maternal fluids or secretions during birth	Administer HBIg to all infants of HBsAG-positive mothers within 12 hours of birth; in addition, administer HepB vaccine at separate site. Prevention—Immunise all infants with HepB vaccine. Infants born to HBsAG-positive mothers and weighing < 2000 g should receive 3-dose vaccine series in addition to birth dose (See Immunisations, Chapter 6.)
Herpes, Neonatal (Herpes Simplex Virus)		
Cutaneous lesions—vesicles at 6–10 days of age; may be no lesions Disseminated disease resembling sepsis—encephalitis in 60%–70% Visceral involvement—granulomas Early non-specific signs—fever, lethargy, poor feeding, irritability, vomiting May include hyperbilirubinaemia, seizures, flaccid or spastic paralysis, apnoeic episodes, respiratory distress, lethargy or coma	History of genital infection in mother or partner in 50% of cases Transmitted intrapartum, either by ascending infection or direct contact, especially primary infection	Absence of skin lesions in neonate exposed to maternal herpesvirus does not indicate absence of disease. Contact precautions (in addition to standard precautions) should be instituted. It is recommended that swabs of mouth, nasopharynx, conjunctivae, rectum and any skin vesicles be obtained from exposed neonate; in addition, urine, stool, blood and CSF specimens should be obtained for culture. Therapy with IV aciclovir is initiated if culture results are positive or if there is strong suspicion of herpesvirus infection; ophthalmic treatment is required for ocular involvement in addition to aciclovir.
Listeriosis (*Listeria Monocytogenes*)		
Maternal infection associated with abortion, premature birth and fetal death Premature birth, sepsis and pneumonia seen in early-onset disease; late-onset disease usually manifests as meningitis	Transplacental, by ascending infection or exposure at birth	Handwashing is essential to prevent nosocomial spread. Treat infected newborn with antibiotics—ampicillin and gentamicin.

Continued

TABLE 9.6 Infections Acquired from Mother Before, During or After Birth—cont'd

Fetal or Newborn Effect	Transmission	Nursing Considerations[†]
Rubella, Congenital (Rubella Virus)		
Eye defects—cataracts (unilateral or bilateral), microphthalmos, retinitis, glaucoma CNS signs—microcephaly, seizures, severe cognitive impairment Congenital heart defects—patent ductus arteriosus Auditory—high incidence of delayed hearing loss Intrauterine growth restriction Hyperbilirubinaemia, meningitis, thrombocytopenia, hepatomegaly	First trimester; early second trimester	Pregnant women should avoid contact with all affected persons, including infants with rubella syndrome. Emphasise vaccination of all unimmunised prepubertal children, susceptible adolescents and women of childbearing age (non-pregnant). Caution women against pregnancy for at least 3 months after vaccination.
Toxoplasmosis (*Toxoplasma Gondii*)		
May be asymptomatic at birth (70%–90% of cases) or have maculopapular rash, lymphadenopathy, hepatosplenomegaly, jaundice, thrombocytopenia Hydrocephaly, cerebral calcifications, chorioretinitis (classic triad) Microcephaly, seizures, cognitive impairment, deafness Encephalitis, myocarditis, hepatosplenomegaly, anaemia, jaundice, diarrhoea, vomiting, purpura	Throughout pregnancy Predominant host for organism is cats May be transmitted through cat faeces or poorly cooked or raw infected meats	Caution pregnant women to avoid contact with cat faeces (e.g. emptying cat litter boxes).

*This table is not an exhaustive representation of all perinatally transmitted infections. For further information regarding specific diseases or treatment not listed here, refer to American Academy of Pediatrics, Committee on Infectious Diseases, Kimberlin, D. W. (Ed.). (2015). 2015 Red Book: Report of the Committee on Infectious Diseases (30th ed.). Elk Grove Village, IL: The Academy.
†Isolation precautions depend on institutional policy.
CNS, Central nervous system; *HBsAg,* hepatitis B surface antigen; *IV,* intravenous.

Nursing Care Management

One of the major goals in care of infants suspected of having an infectious disease is identification of the causative agent. Until the diagnosis is established, implement standard precautions according to institutional policy. In suspected cytomegalovirus and rubella infections, pregnant personnel are cautioned to avoid contact with the infant. Herpes simplex is easily transmitted from one infant to another; therefore, risk of cross-contamination is reduced or eliminated by wearing gloves for patient contact. Careful handwashing is the most important nursing intervention in reducing the spread of any infection.

The major goal of nursing care is prevention of these disorders with provision of adequate prenatal care for the expectant mother and precautions regarding exposure to teratogenic infections.

REFERENCES

Abraham, M., Alramadhan, S., Iniguez, C., et al. (2017). A systematic review of maternal smoking during pregnancy and fetal measurements with meta-analysis. PLoS ONE, 1–13.

Aceti, A., Gori, D., Barone, G., et al. (2015). Probiotics for prevention of necrotizing enterocolitis in premature infants: systematic review and meta-analysis. Italian Journal of Pediatrics, 41, 1–20.

Adams, M., Bassler, D., Darlow, B., et al. (2019). Preventive strategies and factors associated with surgically treated necrotising enterocolitis in extremely preterm infants: an international unit survey linked with retrospective cohort data analysis. BMJ open, 9(10), e031086-e031086

Atkinson, J., & Braddick, O. (2012). Visual and visuocognitive development of children born very prematurely. In V. R. Preedy (Ed.), Handbook of growth and growth monitoring in health and disease (Vol. 1). New York: Springer.

Alfaleh, K., Anabrees, J., Bassler, D., et al. (2014). Probiotics for prevention of necrotizing enterocolitis in premature infants. Cochrane Database of Systematic Review, (4), CD005496.

Als, H. (1982). Toward a synactive theory of development: promise for the assessment and support of infant individuality. Infant Mental Health Journal, 3(4), 229–243.

Alvaro, R. E. (2012). Neonatal Apnea. In D. Fraser (Ed.), Acute respiratory care of the neonate (3rd ed., pp. 51–64). Santa Rosa, CA: NICU Ink Books.

Athalye-Jape, G., Rao, S., & Patole, S. (2016). Lactobacillus reuteri DSM 17938 as a probiotic for premature neonates: A strain-specific systematic review. The Journal of Parenteral and Enteral Nutrition, 40, 783–794.

Australian Institute of Health and Welfare (AIHW). (2019). Alcohol use during pregnancy. Guidelines. https://www.aihw.gov.au/reports-data/population-groups/mothers-babies/resources-for-psychosocial-health-in-pregnancy/alcohol-use-during-pregnancy

Australian Institute of Health and Welfare (AIHW). (2018). Children's Headline Indicators, Smoking during pregnancy. https://www.aihw.gov.au/reports/children-youth/childrens-headline-indicators/contents/indicator-1

Ballabh, P. (2014). Pathogenesis and prevention of intraventricular hemorrhage. Clinics in Perinatology, 41(1), 47–67.

Blackburn, S. T. (2012). Maternal, fetal, and neonatal physiology: a clinical perspective (4th ed.). St. Louis: Elsevier.

Botet, F., Figueras-Aloy, J., Miracle-Echegoyen, X., et al. (2012). Trends in survival among extremely-low-birth-weight infants (less than 1000 g) without significant bronchopulmonary dysplasia. BMC Pediatrics, 63, 63–74.

Bozzetti, V., Paterlini, G., De Lorenzo, P., et al. (2016). Impact of continuous vs bolus feeding on splanchnic perfusion in very low birth weight infants: a randomized trial. Journal of Pediatrics, 176, 86–92.

Brown, L. D., Hendrickson, K., Evans, R., et al. (2016). Enteral nutrition. In S. L. Gardner, B. S. Carter, M. Enzman-Hines, et al. (Eds.), Merenstein & Gardner's handbook of neonatal intensive care (8th ed.). St Louis: Mosby.

Bryant, B., Knights, K., Darroch, S. & Rowland, A. (2019). Pharmacology for health professionals. 5th edition., Chatswood, NSW: Elsevier Australia.

Bucher, B. T., Pacetti, A. S., Lovvorn, H. N., et al. (2016). Neonatal surgery. In S. L. Gardner, B. S. Carter, M. Enzman-Hines, et al. (Eds.), Merenstein & Gardner's handbook of neonatal intensive care (8th ed.). St Louis: Mosby.

Buenoa, C., & Menna-Barretob, L. (2016). Development of sleep/wake, a ctivity and temperature rhythms in newborns maintained in a neonatal intensive care unit and the impact of feeding schedules. Infant Behavior & Development, 44, 21–28.

Bulut, C., Gursoy, T., & Ovali, F. (2016). Short-term outcomes and mortality of late premature infants. Balkan Medical Journal, 33(2), 198–203.

Buonocore, G., Bracci, R. & Weindling, M. (2018). Neonatology A Practical Approach to Neonatal Diseases. 2nd ed. 2018., Champaign, IL: Springer International Publishing.

Camacho-Gonzalez, A., Spearman, P. W., & Stoll, B. J. (2013). Neonatal infectious diseases: evaluation of neonatal sepsis. Pediatric Clinics of North America, 60(2), 367–389.

Campino, A., Santesteban, E., Pascual, P., et al. (2016). Strategies implementation to reduce medicine preparation error rate in neonatal intensive care units. European Journal of Pediatrics, 175, 755–765.

Caplan, M. S. (2015). Neonatal necrotizing enterocolitis: clinical observations, pathophysiology and prevention. In R. J. Martin, A. A. Fanaroff, & M. C. Walsh (Eds.), Fanaroff and Martin's neonatal-perinatal medicine: diseases of the fetus and newborn. St Louis: Elsevier Mosby.

Carlo, W. A. (2016a). Apnea. In R. M. Kliegman, B. F. Stanton, J. W. St Geme, et al. (Eds.), Nelson textbook of pediatrics. Philadelphia: Saunders.

Carlo, W. A. (2016b). Infants of Diabetic Mothers. In R. M. Kliegman, B. F. Stanton, J. W. St Geme, et al. (Eds.), Nelson textbook of pediatrics. Philadelphia: Saunders.

Carlo, W. A., & Ambalavanan, N. (2016a). Intracranial-intraventricular hemorrhage and periventricular leukomalacia. In R. M. Kliegman, B. F. Stanton, J. W. St Geme, et al. (Eds.), Nelson textbook of pediatrics. Philadelphia: Saunders.

Carlo, W. A., & Ambalavanan, N. (2016b). Metabolic disturbances. In R. M. Kliegman, B. F. Stanton, J. W. St. Geme, et al. (Eds.), Nelson textbook of pediatrics. Philadelphia: Saunders.

Carlo, W. A., & Ambalavanan, N. (2016c). Respiratory distress syndrome. In R. M. Kliegman, B. F. Stanton, J. W. St. Geme, et al. (Eds.), Nelson textbook of pediatrics. Philadelphia: Saunders.

Carter, A., Gratny, L., & Carter, B. S. (2016). Discharge planning and follow-up of the neonatal intensive care unit infant. In S. L. Gardner, B. S. Carter, M. Enzman-Hines, et al. (Eds.), Merenstein & Gardner's handbook of neonatal intensive care (8th ed.). St Louis: Mosby.

Chang, H., Chen, J., Chang, J., et al. (2017). Multiple strains probiotics appear to be the most effective probiotics in the prevention of necrotizing enterocolitis and mortality: An updated meta-analysis. PLoS ONE, 12(2), 1–14.

Chaseling, G. K., Molgat-Seon, Y., Daboval, T., et al. (2016). Body temperature mapping in critically ill newborn infants nursed under radiant warmers during intensive care. Journal of Perinatology, 36, 540–543.

Cheong, J. L., Doyle, L. W., Burnett, A. C., et al. (2017). Association between moderate and late premature birth and neurodevelopment and social-emotional development at age 2 years. JAMA Pediatrics, 1–7.

Christian, B. (2020). Translational Research – Parental Stress Associated with Hospitalization of Children with Critical Life-Threatening Conditions and the Long-term Impact. Journal of Pediatric Nursing, 51, 110–113. https://pubmed.ncbi.nlm.nih.gov/32001063/

Church, P. T., Luther, M., & Asztalos, E. (2012). The perfect storm: the high prevalence low severity outcomes of the preterm survivors. Current Pediatric Reviews, 8(2), 142–151.

Clark, R. H. (2017). High-frequency oscillatory ventilation. In S. M. Donn & S. K. Sinha (Eds.), Manual of neonatal respiratory care (4th ed.). New York: Springer.

Colaizy, T., Bell, E., Carlo, W., et al. (2012). Neurodevelopmental effects of donor human milk vs preterm formula in ELBW infants: the MILK trial, 2012, National Institute of Child Health and Human Development. https://www.nichd.nih.gov/sites/default/files/about/Documents/Milk_Protocol.pdf

Cole, L., Dewey, D., Letourneau, N., et al. (2017). Clinical characteristics, risk factors, and outcomes associated with neonatal hemorrhagic stroke: a population-based case-control study. JAMA Pediatrics, 1, 1–9.

Cole, R., Young, J., Kearney, L. & Thompson, J. (2020). Infant care practices and parent uptake of safe sleep messages: a cross-sectional survey in Queensland, Australia. BMC pediatrics, 20(1), 27.

Danner-Bowman, K. & Cardin, A. (2015). Neuroprotective Core Measure 3: Positioning & Handling — A Look at Preventing Positional Plagiocephaly. Newborn and infant nursing reviews, 15(3), 111–113.

Darlow, B. A., Lui, K., Kusuda, S., et al. on behalf of the International Network for Evaluating Outcomes of Neonates. (2017). International variations and trends in the treatment for retinopathy of prematurity. British Journal of Ophthalmology, 0, 1–6.

De Carolis, M. P., Pinna, G., Cocca, C., et al. (2016). The transition from intra to extra-uterine life in late premature infant: a single-center study. Italian Journal of Pediatrics, 42(1), 1–7.

Dermyshi, E., Wang, Y., Yan, C., et al. (2017). The 'golden age' of probiotics: a systematic review and meta-analysis of randomized and observational studies in premature infants. Neonatology, 112(1), 9–23.

Finnegan, L. P. (1985). Neonatal abstinence. In N. Nelson (Ed.), Current therapy in neonatal perinatal medicine (pp. 1985–1986). Toronto: BC Decker.

Foster, J. P., Psaila, K., & Patterson, T. (2016). Non-nutritive sucking for increasing physiologic stability and nutrition in premature infants. Cochrane Database Syst Review, (10), CD001071.

Gao, H., Gao, H., Xu, G., et al. (2016). Efficacy and safety of repeated oral sucrose for repeated procedural pain in neonates: A systematic review. International Journal of Nursing Studies, 62, 118–125.

Gardner, S. L., Enzman-Hines, M., & Nyp, M. (2016). Respiratory diseases. In S. L. Gardner, B. S. Carter, M. Enzman-Hines, et al. (Eds.), Merenstein & Gardner's handbook of neonatal intensive care (8th ed.). St Louis: Mosby.

Gardner, S. L., Goldson, E., & Hernandez, J. A. (2016). The neonate and the environment: impact on development. In S. L. Gardner, B. S. Carter, M. Enzman-Hines, et al. (Eds.), Merenstein & Gardner's handbook of neonatal intensive care (8th ed.). St Louis: Mosby.

Gardner, S. L., & Hernandez, J. A. (2016). Heat balance. In S. L. Gardner, B. S. Carter, M. Enzman-Hines, et al. (Eds.), Merenstein & Gardner's handbook of neonatal intensive care (8th ed.). St Louis: Mosby.

Gardner, S. L., & Lawrence, R. A. (2016). Breast-feeding the neonate with special needs. In S. L. Gardner, B. S. Carter, M. Enzman-Hines, et al. (Eds.), Merenstein & Gardner's handbook of neonatal intensive care (8th ed.). St Louis: Mosby.

Garg, B., Balasubramanian, H., Kabra, N., et al. (2018). Effect of oropharyngeal colostrum therapy in the prevention of necrotising enterocolitis among very low birthweight neonates: A meta-analysis of randomised controlled trials. Journal of human nutrition and dietetics, 31(5), 612–624.

Gephart, S. M., & Hanson, C. K. (2013). Preventing necrotizing enterocolitis with standard feeding protocols: not only possible, but imperative. Advances in Neonatal Care, 13(1), 48–54.

Gilfillan, M., & Bhandari, V. (2017). Biomarkers for the diagnosis of neonatal sepsis and necrotizing enterocolitis: Clinical practice guidelines. Early Human Development, 105, 25–33.

Gill, J. V., & Boyle, E. M. (2017). Outcomes of infants born near term. Archives of Disease in Childhood, 102, 194–198.

Glass, H. C. (2014). Neonatal seizures: advances in mechanisms and management. Clinics in Perinatology, 41(1), 177–190.

Goldman, L. & Schafer, A. (2020). Goldman-Cecil medicine. 26th edition. Philadelphia, PA: Elsevier.

Gunn, J. K., Rosales, C. B., Center, K. E., et al. (2016). Prenatal exposure to cannabis and maternal and child health outcomes: a systematic review and meta-analysis. BMJ (Clinical Research Ed.), 6(4), 1–8.

Guyer, C., Huber, R., Fontijn, J., et al. (2015). Very premature infants show earlier emergence of 24-hour sleep–wake rhythms compared to term infants. Early Human Development, 91, 37–42.

Hallman, M., & Saarela, T. (2012). Respiratory distress syndrome: predisposing factors, pathophysiology, and diagnosis. In G. Buonocore, R. Bracci, & M. Weindling (Eds.), Neonatology: a practical approach to neonatal diseases. New York: Springer.

Hartley, K. A., Miller, C. S., & Gephart, S. M. (2015). Facilitated tucking to reduce pain in neonates: evidence for best practice. Advances in Neonatal Care, 15(3), 201–208.

Hassanein, S., Raggal, N., & Shalaby, A. (2013). Neonatal nursery noise: practice-based learning and improvement. The Journal of Maternal-fetal and Neonatal Medicine, 26(4), 392–395.

Horbar, J. D., Carpenter, J. H., Badger, G. J., et al. (2012). Mortality and neonatal morbidity among infants 501 to 1500 grams from 2000 to 2009. Pediatrics, 129(6), 1019–1026.

Huether, S. & McCance, K. (2018). Pathophysiology: the biologic basis for disease in adults and children. Mosby.

Jonas-Simpson, C., Pilkington, F. B., MacDonald, C., et al. (2013). Nurses' experiences of grieving when there is a perinatal death. SAGE Open, 3(2). http://sgo.sagepub.com/content/3/2/2158244013486116.short.

Johnston, C., Campbell-Yeo, M., Disher, T., et al. (2017). Skin-to-skin care for procedural pain in neonates. Cochrane Database of Systematic Review, (2), CD008435.

Kain, V. & Mannix, T. (2018). Neonatal nursing in Australia and New Zealand: principles for practice. First edition., Chatswood, NSW: Elsevier.

Keszler, M., & Abubakar, K. (2017). Physiologic principles. In J. P. Goldsmith & E. H. Karotkin (Eds.), Assisted ventilation of the neonate (6th ed.). Philadelphia: Elsevier.

Kommers, D. R., Joshi, R., van Pul, C., et al. (2017). Features of heart rate variability capture regulatory changes during kangaroo care in premature infants. Journal of Pediatrics, 182, 92–98.

Koopmans, L., Wilson, T., Cacciatore, J., et al. (2013). Support for mothers, fathers and families after perinatal death. Cochrane Database of Systematic Review, (6), CD000452.

Koucheki, R., Isaac, M., Tehrani, N. et al. (2020). Natural history and outcomes of stage 3 retinopathy of prematurity persisting beyond 40 weeks of postmenstrual age: Dilemma for treatment and follow-up. Melbourne: John Wiley & Sons Australia, Ltd. Clinical & experimental ophthalmology, 48(7), 956–963.

Kraft, W. K., Stover, M. W., & Davis, J. M. (2016). Neonatal abstinence syndrome: Pharmacologic strategies for the mother and infant. Seminars in Perinatology, 40, 203–212.

Kuhn, P., Zores, C., Langlet, C., et al. (2013). Moderate acoustic changes can disrupt the sleep of very preterm infants in their incubators. Acta Paediatrics, 102(10), 949–954.

Lau, C. S., & Chamberlain, R. S. (2015). Probiotic administration can prevent necrotizing enterocolitis in premature infants: A meta-analysis. Journal of Pediatric Surgery, 50, 1405–1412.

Lavoie, P. M., Stritzke, A., Ting, J., et al. (2015). A randomized controlled trial of the use of oral glucose with or without gentle facilitated tucking of infants during neonatal echocardiography. PLoS ONE, 1–11.

Lewis, E. D., Richard, C., Larsen, B. M., et al. (2016). The importance of human milk for immunity in premature infants. Clinics in Perinatology, 3(1), 23–47.

Lowe, T. (2017). Neonatal respiratory outcomes. Combating chronic lung disease in prematurely born infants. The Hive. Summer Edition. Australian College of Nursing. https://www.acn.edu.au/publications/the-hive-2017/neonatal-respiratory-outcomes.

Lucas, B., Doney, R., Latimer, J., et al. (2016). Impairment of motor skills in children with fetal alcohol spectrum disorders in remote Australia: The Lililwan Project: Motor skills impaired in FASD. Drug and alcohol review, 35(6), 719–727.

Macho, P. (2017). Individualized developmental care in the NICU: a concept analysis. Advances in Neonatal Care, 1–13.

Maheshwari, A., & Carlo, W. A. (2016). Plethora in the newborn infant (polycythemia). In R. M. Kliegman, B. F. Stanton, J. W. St Geme, et al. (Eds.), Nelson textbook of pediatrics. Philadelphia: Saunders.

Malcolm, W. (2015). Beyond the NICU: comprehensive care of the high-risk infant. New York: McGraw-Hill.

Mandell, E., Kinsella, J. & Abman, S. (2021). Persistent pulmonary hypertension of the newborn. Wiley Subscription Services, Inc. Pediatric pulmonology, 56(3), 661–669.

Marks, K. (2015). Infant and toddler nutrition. Australian Family Physician. 12(12), 886–889. https://www.racgp.org.au/afp/2015/december/infant-and-toddler-nutrition/

McGinnis, K., Murray, E., Cherven, B., et al. (2016). Effect of vibration on pain response to heel lance: a pilot randomized control trial. Advances in Neonatal Care, 16(6), 439–448.

Meier, P. P., Johnson, T. J., Patel, A. L., et al. (2017). Evidence-based methods that promote human milk feeding of premature infants: an expert review. Clinics in Perinatology, 44(1), 1–22.

Mikati, M. A., & Hani, A. J. (2016). Neonatal seizures. In R. M. Kliegman, B. F. Stanton, J. W. St Geme, et al. (Eds.), Nelson textbook of pediatrics (20th ed.). Philadelphia: Elsevier.

Miller, D. & Walker, K. (2014). The challenge of protecting the perinatal brain against hypoxic ischaemic injury - hasten slowly: Perspectives. The Journal of Physiology, 592(3), 425–426.

Mitchell, E., Cowan, S. & Tipene-Leach, D. (2016). The recent fall in postperinatal mortality in New Zealand and the Safe Sleep programme. Acute Paediatrics, 105(11), 1312–1320.

Moon, K., Rao, S. C., Schulzke, S. M., et al. (2016). Longchain polyunsaturated fatty acid supplementation in premature infants. Cochrane Database of Systematic Review, (12), CD000375.

Natarajan, G., & Shankaran, S. (2016). Short- and long-term outcomes of moderate and late premature infants. American Journal of Perinatology, 33, 305–317.

National Health and Medical Research Council (NHMRC) and Australian Commission on Safety and Quality in Health Care (ACSQHC). (2019). Australian Guidelines for the Prevention and Control of Infection in Health Care. Australian Government. https://www.nhmrc.gov.au/about-us/publications/australian-guidelines-prevention-and-control-infection-healthcare-2019#block-views-block-file-attachments-content-block-1

Neu, J., & Sullivan, S. (2012). Baby and breast: a dynamic interaction. Pediatric Research, 71, 135.

NSW Government. (2018). Guidelines. Infants and Children – Acute Management of Seizures. https://www1.health.nsw.gov.au/pds/ActivePDSDocuments/GL2018_015.pdf

O'Connor, A., Seeber, C., Harris, E., et al. (2020). Developmental outcomes following prenatal exposure to methamphetamine: A Western Australian perspective. Australia: John Wiley & Sons Australia, Ltd. Journal of paediatrics and child health, 56(3), 372–378.

Ohlsson, A. & Jacobs, S. E. (2013). NIDCAP: a systematic review and meta-analyses of randomized controlled trials. Pediatrics, 131(3), 881–893.

Olitsky, S., Hug, D., Plummer, L. S., et al. (2016). Disorders of the retina and vitreous. In R. M. Kliegman, B. F. Stanton, J. W. St Geme, et al. (Eds.), Nelson textbook of pediatrics (20th ed.). Philadelphia: Elsevier.

Onland, W., De Jaegere, A. P. M. C., Offringa, M., et al. (2017). Systemic corticosteroid regimens for prevention of bronchopulmonary dysplasia in premature infants. Cochrane Database of Systematic Reviews, (1), CD010941.

Owen, L. A., Morrison, M. A., Hoffman, R. O., et al. (2017). Retinopathy of prematurity: A comprehensive risk analysis for prevention and prediction of disease. PLoS ONE, 12(2), 1–14.

Pammi, M., Brand, M. C., & Weisman, L. E. (2016). Infection in the neonate. In S. L. Gardner, B. S. Carter, M. Enzman-Hines, et al. (Eds.), Merenstein & Gardner's handbook of neonatal intensive care (8th ed.). St Louis: Mosby.

Parsons, J. A., Seay, A. R., & Jacobson, M. (2016). Neurologic disorders. In S. L. Gardner, B. S. Carter, M. Enzman-Hines, et al. (Eds.), Merenstein & Gardner's handbook of neonatal intensive care (8th ed.). St Louis: Mosby.

Perry, S., Hockenberry, M., Lowdermilk, D., et al. (2017). Maternal child nursing care. 6th edition., St Louis, Missouri: Elsevier Mosby.

Pineda, R., Durant, P., Mathur, A., et al. (2017). Auditory exposure in the neonatal intensive care unit: room type and other predictors. Journal of Pediatrics, 1–11.

Polin, R. A., Carlo, W. A., & Committee on Fetus and Newborn. (2014). Surfactant replacement therapy for premature and term neonates with respiratory distress. Pediatrics, 133(1), 158–163.

Queensland Health. (2020). Queensland Clinical Guidelines. Perinatal care of the extremely preterm baby. Guideline No. MN20.32-V2-R25. http://www.health.qld.gov.au/qcg

Quraishy, K., Bowles, S., & Moore, J. (2013). A protocol for swaddled bathing in the neonatal intensive care unit. Neonatal Therapists, 13(1), 48–50.

Raoof, A., & Ohlsson, A. (2013). Noise reduction management in the neonatal intensive care unit for preterm or very low birthweight infants. Cochrane Database of Systematic Review, (1), CD010333.

Ravikumar, C., McDaniel, D., Quinn, A., et al. (2019). Air Leak Syndrome: Pneumoperitoneum in a Ventilated Neonate. Case reports in pediatrics, 2019, 4238601–4.

Red Nose. (2018). Safe sleeping. What is a safe sleeping environment? https://rednose.org.au/article/what-is-a-safe-sleeping-environment

Reid, N. (2018). Fetal alcohol spectrum disorder in Australia: What is the current state of affairs? FASD in Australia. Drug and alcohol review, 37(7), 827–830.

Resch, B., Renoldner, B., & Hofer, N. (2016). Comparison between pathogen associated laboratory and clinical parameters in early-onset sepsis of the newborn. The Open Microbiology Journal, 10, 133–139.

Robertson, C., Savva, G., Clapuci, R., et al. (2020). Incidence of necrotising enterocolitis before and after introducing routine prophylactic Lactobacillus and Bifidobacterium probiotics. Archives of disease in childhood. Fetal and neonatal edition, 106(4), 380–386.

Rogers, E. E., & Hintz, S. R. (2016). Early neurodevelopmental outcomes of extremely premature infants. Seminars in Perinatology, 40, 497–509.

Rovekamp-Abels, L. W., Hogewind-Schoonenboom, J. E., de Wijs-Meijler, D. P., et al. (2015). Intermittent bolus or semicontinuous feeding for premature infants? Journal of Pediatric Gastroenterol Nutrition, 61(6), 659–664.

Royal Children's Hospital Melbourne (RCHM). (2019). Clinical Guidelines. Apnoea (neonatal). Acute Management. https://www.rch.org.au/rchcpg/hospital_clinical_guideline_index/Apnoea_Neonatal/

Royal Children's Hospital Melbourne (RCHM). (2020). Clinical Practice Guidelines. Afebrile seizures. https://www.rch.org.au/clinicalguide/guideline_index/Afebrile_seizures/

Rozance, P. J., McGowan, J. E., Price-Douglas, W., et al. (2016). Glucose homeostasis. In S. L. Gardner, B. S. Carter, M. Enzman-Hines, et al. (Eds.), Merenstein & Gardner's handbook of neonatal intensive care (8th ed). St Louis: ELSEVIER.

Sabra, S., Gratocos, E., & Gomez Roig, M. D. (2017). Smoking-induced changes in the maternal immune, endocrine, and metabolic pathways and their impact on fetal growth: a topical review. Fetal Diagnosis and Therapy, 1–10.

Safe Care Victoria. (2021a). Better Safer Care. Resuscitation of neonates. https://www.bettersafercare.vic.gov.au/clinical-guidance/neonatal/resuscitation-of-neonates

Safe Care Victoria. (2021b). Better Safer Care. Necrotising enterocolitis (NEC) in neonates. https://www.bettersafercare.vic.gov.au/clinical-guidance/neonatal/necrotising-enterocolitis-nec-in-neonates

Safe Care Victoria. (2021c). Better Safer Care. Retinopathy of prematurity (ROP). https://www.bettersafercare.vic.gov.au/clinical-guidance/neonatal/retinopathy-of-prematurity-rop#goto-screening-criteria

Saugstad, O., Oei, J., Lakshminrusimha, S., et al. (2019). Oxygen therapy of the newborn from molecular understanding to clinical practice. Nature Publishing Group. Pediatric research, 85(1), 20–29.

Sawh, S. C., Deshpande, S., Jansen, S., et al. (2016). Prevention of necrotizing enterocolitis with probiotics: a systematic review and meta-analysis. PeerJ, 10(4), 1–29.

Shah, V. S., Ohlsson, A., Halliday, H. L., et al. (2017). Early administration of inhaled corticosteroids for preventing chronic lung disease in very low birth weight premature neonates. Cochrane Database of Systematic Reviews, (1), CD001969.

Steurer, M., Baer, R., Oltman, S., et al. (2019). Morbidity of persistent pulmonary hypertension of the newborn in the first year of life. The Journal of Pediatrics, 213, 58–65.e4.

Sun, H., Cheng, R., Kang, W., et al. (2013). High-frequency oscillatory ventilation versus synchronized intermittent mandatory ventilation plus pressure support in preterm infants with severe respiratory distress syndrome. Respiratory Care. http://rc.rcjournal.com/content/early/2013/06/13/respcare.02382.abstract.

Surbek, D., Drack, G., Irion, O., et al. (2012). Antenatal corticosteroids for fetal lung maturation in threatened preterm birth: indications and administration. Archives of Gynecology and Obstetrics, 286(2), 277–281.

Swaney, J. R., English, N., & Carter, B. S. (2016). Ethics, values, and palliative care in neonatal intensive care. In S. L. Gardner, B. S. Carter, M. Enzman-Hines, et al. (Eds.), Merenstein & Gardner's handbook of neonatal intensive care (8th ed.). St Louis: Mosby.

Tai, E., Wang, X., & Chen, Z. (2013). An update on adding docosahexaenoic acid (DHA) and arachidonic acid (AA) to baby formula. Food Function, 4, 1767–1775.

Tai, M., Piskorski, A., Kao, J. C., et al. (2017). Placental morphology in fetal alcohol spectrum disorders. Alcohol and alcoholism, 52(2), 138–144.

The Royal Australian and New Zealand College of Obstetricians and Gynaecologists (RANZCOG). (2021). Substance use in pregnancy. https://ranzcog.edu.au/RANZCOG_SITE/media/RANZCOG-MEDIA/Women%27s%20Health/Statement%20and%20guidelines/Clinical-Obstetrics/Substance-use-in-pregnancy-(C-Obs-55)-March-2018.pdf?ext=.pdf

Tin Tin, S., Woodward, A., Saraf, R., et al. (2016). Internal living environment and respiratory disease in children: findings from the Growing Up in New Zealand longitudinal child cohort study. Environmental health, 15(1), 120.

Uberos, J., Aguilera-Rodríguez, E., Jerez-Calero, A., et al. (2017). Probiotics to prevent necrotising enterocolitis and nosocomial infection in very low birth weight preterm infants. Cambridge University Press. British journal of nutrition, 117(7), 994–1000.

Victoria State Government. (2020a). Quality, safety and service improvement. https://www2.health.vic.gov.au/hospitals-and-health-services/quality-safety-service

Victoria State Government. (2020b). Newborn care in Victoria. https://www2.health.vic.gov.au/hospitals-and-health-services/patient-care/perinatal-reproductive/maternity-newborn-services/newborn-care-in-victoria

Walsh, M. C. & Fanaroff, A. A. (2015). Epidemiology for neonatologists. In R. M. Martin, A. A. Fanaroff, & M. C. Walsh (Eds.), Neonatal-perinatal medicine: diseases of the fetus and infant (10th ed.). Philadelphia: Saunders.

Wapner, R. J., Gyamfi-Bannerman, C., & Thom, E., for the Eunice Kennedy Shriver National Institute of Child Health and Human Development Maternal-Fetal Medicine Units Network. (2016). What we have learned about antenatal corticosteroid regimens. Seminars in Perinatology, 40, 291–297.

Weiner, G. M. (Ed.), (2016). Textbook of neonatal resuscitation (7th ed.). Elk Grove Village, IL: American Academy of Pediatrics and American Heart Association.

Weiner, S. M., & Finnegan, L. P. (2016). Drug withdrawal in the neonate. In S. L. Gardner, B. S. Carter, M. Enzman-Hines, et al. (Eds.), Merenstein & Gardner's handbook of neonatal intensive care (8th ed.). St Louis: Mosby.

Welch, R. A., Shaw, M. K., & Welch, K. C. (2016). Amniotic fluid LPCAT1 mRNA correlates with the lamellar body count. Journal of Perinatal Medicine, 44(5), 531–555.

Wilhoit, L. F., Scott, D. A., & Simecka, B. A. (2017). Fetal alcohol spectrum disorders: characteristics, complications, and treatment. Community Mental Health, 1–8.

Yin, T., Yang, L., Lee, T., et al. (2015). Development of atraumatic heel-stick procedures by combined treatment with non-nutritive sucking, oral sucrose, and facilitated tucking: a randomized, controlled trial. International Journal of Nursing Studies, 52(8), 1288–1299.

Younge, N., Goldstein, R., Bann, C. M., et al. for the Eunice Kennedy Shriver National Institute of Child Health and Human Development Neonatal Research Network. (2017). Survival and neurodevelopmental outcomes among periviable infants. The New England Journal of Medicine, 376(7), 617–628.

Zani, A., Eaton, S., Puri, P., EUPSA Network Office, et al. (2016). International Survey on the Management of Congenital Diaphragmatic Hernia. European Journal of Pediatric Surgery, 25(1), 38–46.

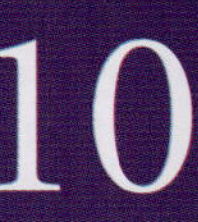

10

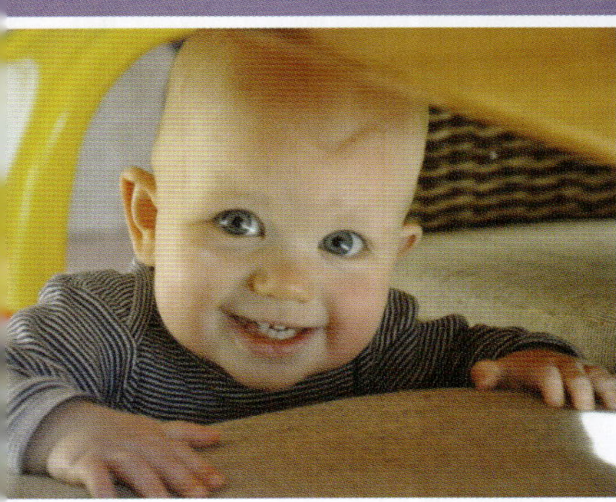

Health Promotion of the Infant and Family

Christine Taylor and Jane Mateer

LEARNING OUTCOMES

- Describe the developmental stages of the infant
- Describe the functional ability of the infant
- Discuss the nutritional needs of the infant with the family
- Demonstrate an understanding of the safety requirements for the infant and educate the family about these

PROMOTING OPTIMUM GROWTH AND DEVELOPMENT

Biological Development

At no other time in life are physical changes and developmental achievements so dramatic as during infancy. All body systems undergo progressive maturation. Concurrent development of skills allows infants to increasingly respond to the environment. Acquisition of these fine and gross motor skills occurs in an orderly head-to-toe and centre-to-periphery (cephalocaudal-proximodistal) sequence.

Proportional Changes

Growth is rapid during the first year, especially during the initial 6 months. Breastfed full-term infants gain an average of 640 g per month until around 5 months of age, when the birth weight has at least doubled (World Health Organization [WHO] 2020). An average weight for a 6-month-old girl is 7.3 kg and 7.9 kg for a boy. Weight gain is slower during the second 6 months. By 1 year of age the infant's birth weight has tripled, to an average of 8.9 kg for girls and 9.6 kg for boys. Infants who are breastfed beyond 4 to 6 months of age typically gain less weight than those who are bottle-fed, yet head circumference is normal.

Height increases by approximately 2.5 cm per month during the first 6 months and by half that amount per month during the second 6 months. Increases in length occur in sudden spurts rather than in a slow, gradual pattern. Average height (length) for girls and boys is around 66 cm at 6 months and 74 cm at 12 months. By 1 year birth length has increased by almost 50%. This increase occurs mainly in the trunk rather than the legs and contributes to the characteristic physique of the older infant (see Fig 10.8A later in this chapter).

Head growth is also rapid and an important determinant of brain growth. Head circumference for girls and boys increases approximately 2 cm per month from birth to 3 months, 1 cm per month from 4 to 6 months and 0.5 cm per month during the second 6 months. The average head size is around 43 cm at 6 months and 46 cm at 12 months. By 1 year of age head size has increased by almost 33%. Closure of the cranial sutures occurs, with the posterior fontanel fusing by 6 to 8 weeks of age and the anterior fontanel closing by 12 to 18 months of age (the average age being 14 months).

It is important to note that genetic, metabolic, environmental and nutritional factors strongly influence infant growth; thus the previous statements are general guidelines only. Use the appropriate growth charts reflecting weight for length and head circumference in each case to determine appropriate growth parameters. It is also important to note the child's growth trajectory: children's growth should follow the growth trajectory for their birth percentile. The WHO growth charts released in 2006 are now recommended as reference growth charts in children 0 to 24 months of age because they represent growth parameters in healthy breastfed full-term infants worldwide and are used as a basis for growth charts in Australia and New Zealand (Turck et al 2013).

Expanding head size reflects the growth and differentiation of the nervous system. By the end of the first year the brain has increased in weight approximately 2.5 times. Maturation of the brain is exhibited in the dramatic developmental achievements of infancy. The primitive reflexes (see Table 7.5) are replaced by voluntary, purposeful movement and new reflexes that influence motor development appear (Box 10.1 and Fig 10.1).

The chest assumes a more adult contour, with the lateral diameter becoming larger than the anteroposterior diameter. The chest circumference approximately equals head circumference by the end of the first year. The heart grows less rapidly than does the rest of the body. Its weight is usually doubled by 1 year of age, whereas body weight triples over the same period. The size of the heart is still large in relation to the chest cavity; its width is approximately 55% of the chest width.

Sensory Changes

During infancy, visual acuity gradually improves and binocular fixation is established. Box 10.2 lists the major developmental characteristics of

BOX 10.1 Neurological Reflexes that Appear During Infancy

Labyrinth righting—Infant in prone or supine position is able to raise head; appears at 2 months, strongest at 10 months.

Neck righting—While infant is supine, head is turned to one side; shoulder, trunk and finally pelvis will turn towards that side; appears at 3 months, until 24 to 36 months.

Body righting—A modification of the neck-righting reflex in which turning hips and shoulders to one side causes all other body parts to follow; appears at 6 months, until 24 to 36 months.

Otolith righting—When body of an erect infant is tilted, head is returned to upright, erect position; appears at 7 to 12 months, persists indefinitely.

Landau—when infant is suspended in a horizontal prone position, the head is raised and legs and spine are extended; appears at 6 to 8 months, lasts until 12 to 24 months.

Parachute—when infant is suspended in a horizontal prone position and suddenly thrust downwards, hands and fingers extend forwards as if to protect against falling (see Fig 10.1); appears at 7 to 9 months, persists indefinitely.

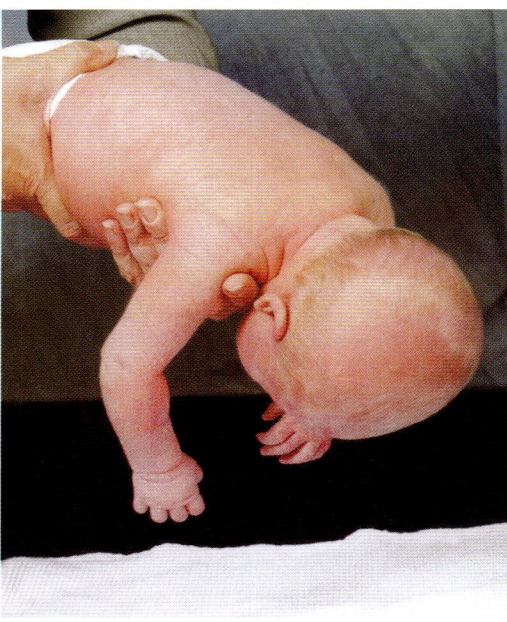

Fig 10.1 Parachute reflex. (Source: Courtesy of Paul Vincent Kuntz, Texas Children's Hospital, Houston.)

vision during infancy. **Binocularity**, or the fixation of two ocular images into one cerebral picture (fusion), begins to develop by 6 weeks of age and should be well established by age 4 months (Fig 10.2). Lack of binocular vision results in strabismus and must be detected early to prevent permanent blindness.

Depth perception (**stereopsis**) begins to develop by age 7 to 9 months but may exist earlier as an innate safety mechanism. At approximately 7 months the parachute reflex appears and may be a protective response during a fall (see Fig 10.1 and Box 10.1).

Infants have a visual preference for looking at the human face; this preference also has a developmental sequence. At age 6 weeks infants show more interest in a picture of a face with eyes than in one without eyes. By 10 weeks of age a picture with both eyes and eyebrows elicits more response, and by 20 weeks of age the mouth is also necessary. By age 6 months infants respond to facial expressions and can distinguish between familiar and strange faces. This is about the time that separation anxiety begins to occur (see information later in this chapter).

BOX 10.2 Major Developmental Characteristics of Vision

Birth

- Visual acuity: 20/100 to 20/400*
- Pupillary and corneal (blink) reflexes present
- Able to fixate on moving object in range of 45 degrees when held 20 to 25 cm away
- Cannot integrate head and eye movements well (doll's eye reflex—eyes lag behind if head is rotated to one side; note that the presence of this reflex at any other time in childhood is abnormal and may indicate a neurological problem)

4 Weeks

- Can follow in range of 90 degrees
- Can watch parent intently as he or she speaks to infant
- Tear glands beginning to function
- Visual acuity hyper-optic because of less spheric eyeball than in adult

6 to 12 Weeks

- Has peripheral vision to 180 degrees
- Has binocular vision beginning at age 6 weeks, well established by age 4 months
- Convergence on near objects beginning by age 6 weeks, developed by age 3 months
- Disappearance of doll's eye reflex

12 to 20 Weeks

- Recognises feeding bottle
- Able to fixate on a 1.25-cm block
- Looks at hand while sitting or lying on back
- Able to accommodate to near objects

20 to 28 Weeks

- Adjusts posture to see an object
- Able to rescue a dropped toy
- Develops colour preference for yellow and red
- Able to discriminate between simple geometrical forms
- Prefers more complex visual stimuli
- Develops hand–eye coordination

28 to 44 Weeks

- Can fixate on very small objects
- Depth perception beginning to develop
- Lack of binocular vision indicative of strabismus

44 to 52 Weeks

- Visual acuity: 20/40 to 20/60
- Visual loss developing if strabismus is present
- Can follow rapidly moving objects

*Measurement of visual acuity differs according to testing procedures. (See Chapter 4.)

With progressive myelination of the auditory pathway, the specific responses of locating sound replace the generalised response of the neonate. Box 10.3 lists the major developmental characteristics of hearing. (See Chapter 7 for further discussion of hearing and the senses of smell, taste and touch.)

Maturation of Systems

Other organ systems also change and grow during infancy. The respiratory rate slows somewhat (see inside back cover) and is relatively stable.

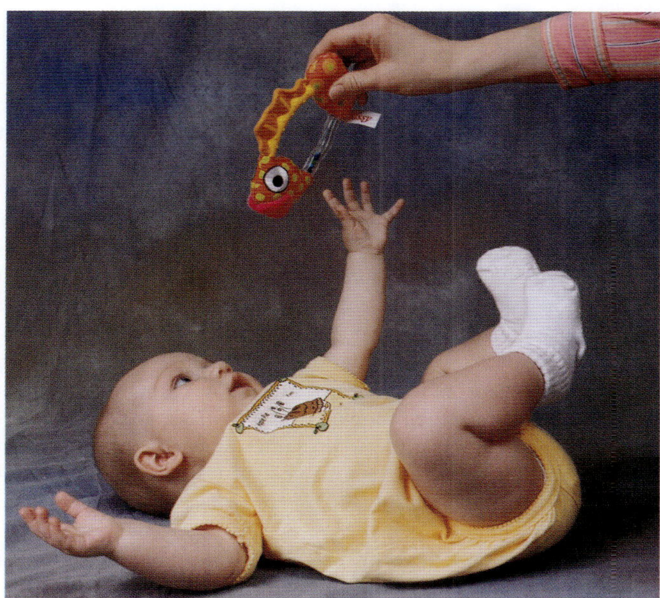

Fig 10.2 Three-month-old infant focuses on visual object and reaches towards it. (Source: Courtesy of Paul Vincent Kuntz, Texas Children's Hospital, Houston.)

BOX 10.3 Major Developmental Characteristics of Hearing

Birth
- Responds to loud noise by startle, or Moro, reflex
- Responds to sound of human voice more readily than to any other sound
- Quieting effect from low-pitched sounds, such as lullaby, metronome or heartbeat

8 to 12 Weeks
- Turns head to side when sound is made at level of ear

12 to 16 Weeks
- Locates sound by turning head to side and looking in same direction

16 to 24 Weeks
- Locates sound by turning head to side and then looking up or down

24 to 32 Weeks
- Locates sounds by turning head in a curving arc
- Responds to own name

32 to 40 Weeks
- Localises sounds by turning head diagonally and directly towards sound

40 to 52 Weeks
- Knows several words and their meaning, such as 'no', and names of family members
- Learns to control and adjust own response to sound, such as listening for the sound to occur again

Respiratory movements continue to be abdominal. Several factors predispose the infant to severe and acute respiratory problems. Given the proximity of the trachea to the bronchi and its branching structures, an infectious agent is rapidly transmitted to the respiratory system and ears. The short, straight eustachian tube closely communicates with the ear, allowing infection to ascend from the pharynx to the middle ear. In addition, the immune system's inability to produce immunoglobulin A (IgA) in the mucosal lining provides less protection against infection in infancy than in later childhood. The entire respiratory tract's ability to produce mucus is diminished, decreasing the humidification of the large volume of inspired air.

Although the lumen of the trachea and bronchi enlarges during infancy, it remains small in comparison with the total size of the lung, maintaining high resistance to the volume of air inspired. The small airways are easily blocked by oedema, mucus or a foreign body. The pliant (flexible) rib cage has less elastic recoil, and during respiratory distress, the work of breathing is increased. In addition, the volume of dead space (i.e. that amount of air needed to fill the respiratory passages with each breath) is large, requiring the infant to breathe approximately twice as fast as the adult to provide the body with the needed amount of oxygen.

As the infant grows, the heart rate slows (see inside back cover), and the rhythm is often **sinus arrhythmia** (rate increases with inspiration and decreases with expiration). Blood pressure also changes during infancy (see inside back cover). Systolic pressure rises during the first 2 months as a result of the left ventricle's increasing ability to pump blood into the systemic circulation. Diastolic pressure decreases during the first 3 months, then gradually rises to values close to those at birth. Fluctuations in blood pressure occur during varying states of activity and emotion.

Significant haematopoietic changes occur during the first year. Fetal haemoglobin (HgbF) is present up to the first 5 months, with adult haemoglobin steadily increasing through the first half of infancy. HgbF results in a shortened survival of red blood cells (RBCs) and thus a decreased number of RBCs. A common result at 3 to 6 months of age is *physiological anaemia*. High levels of HgbF depress the production of **erythropoietin**, a hormone released by the kidney that stimulates RBC production.

Maternally derived iron stores are present for the first 5 to 6 months and gradually diminish, which also accounts for lowered haemoglobin levels towards the end of the first 6 months. The occurrence of physiological anaemia is not affected by an adequate iron supply. However, when erythropoiesis is stimulated, iron stores are necessary for the formation of adequate amounts of haemoglobin.

The digestive processes are relatively immature at birth. Although full-term newborn infants have some limitations in digestive function, human milk has properties that partially compensate for decreased digestive enzymatic activity, thus enabling the infant to receive optimum nutrition during the first several months of life (Lawrence & Lawrence 2016). The enzyme amylase is present in small amounts but usually has little effect on the foodstuffs because of the small amount of time the food stays in the mouth. Gastric digestion in the stomach relies primarily on the action of hydrochloric acid and rennin, an enzyme that acts specifically on the casein in milk to cause the formation of curds (coagulated semisolid particles of milk). The curds cause the milk to be retained in the stomach long enough for digestion to occur.

Digestion also takes place in the duodenum, where pancreatic enzymes and bile begin to break down protein and fat. Secretion of the pancreatic enzyme amylase, which is needed for digestion of complex carbohydrates, is limited until about the fourth to sixth months of life. Lipase is also limited, and infants do not achieve adult levels of fat absorption until 4 to 5 months of age. Trypsin is secreted in sufficient quantities to catabolise protein into polypeptides and some amino acids.

The immaturity of the digestive processes is evident in the appearance of stools. During infancy, solid foods (e.g. peas, carrots, corn, raisins) are passed incompletely broken down in the faeces. An excessive quantity of fibre easily disposes the child to loose, bulky stools. During infancy the stomach enlarges to accommodate a greater volume of food. By the end of the first year the infant is able to tolerate three meals a day and an evening bottle and may have one or two bowel movements daily. However, with any type of gastric irritation, the infant is vulnerable to diarrhoea, vomiting and dehydration.

The liver is the most immature of all the gastrointestinal organs throughout infancy. The ability to conjugate bilirubin and secrete bile is achieved after the first couple of weeks of life. However, the capacities for gluconeogenesis, formation of plasma protein and ketones, storage of vitamins and deaminisation of amino acids remain relatively immature for the first year of life.

Maturation of the sucking, swallowing and breathing reflexes and the later eruption of teeth parallel the changes in the gastrointestinal tract and prepare the infant for the introduction of solid foods.

Sucking activity can occur in utero as early as 15 to 18 weeks of gestation. Weak, mouthing movements may be noted at 27 to 28 weeks' gestation. Complete maturation of sucking, swallowing and breathing patterns are usually synchronised by 34 to 36 weeks, although some sucking and swallowing synchrony skills are seen by 30 to 33 weeks (Lau 2015). Sucking is divided into nutritive and non-nutritive; the latter is observed in infants of all ages and is reported to be primarily for the purpose of satisfying the basic sucking urge. On the other hand, nutritive sucking has as its primary purpose the intake of food. *Suckling* is a term often used for breastfeeding (Lawrence & Lawrence 2016), yet use of the term varies among different sources.

Swallowing (deglutition) is the ability to collect the food (bolus) and propel it into the oesophagus. During the infantile (visceral) swallow reflex food lies in a shallow groove on the top (dorsum) of the tongue. As the tongue is pressed upwards towards the palate, the milk flows by gravity down the sloping tongue and along the sides of the mouth in lateral furrows between the tongue, cheek and gum pads. As the bolus moves downwards, the posterior wall of the pharynx comes forwards to displace the soft palate. This swallowing process is efficient for fluids but not for solids.

As the infant grows, the tongue becomes smaller in proportion to the oral cavity and attains greater motility, the orofacial muscles develop and teeth erupt. Consequently, the mature (somatic) swallow reflex is significantly different. The tongue remains behind the central incisors, and the mandible no longer thrusts forwards. The dorsum of the tongue is less concave and remains higher and parallel, not inclined, against the palate. The lateral furrows are absent because of tooth eruption. Tongue pressure and movement against the hard palate push the bolus back into the pharynx.

Healthy infants also exhibit a special reflex called the *Santmyer swallow.* When a puff of air is directed at the face, the infant will exhibit a reflexive swallow (Khan & Orenstein 2016). This reflex may be useful in the administration of small amounts of fluids or medications, but caution is recommended to prevent aspiration.

The immunological system undergoes numerous changes during the first year. Full-term newborns receive significant amounts of maternal immunoglobulin G (IgG), which for approximately 3 months confers immunity against many antigens to which the mother was exposed. During this time, IgG levels gradually fall as maternal IgG is catabolised, and the newborn produces limited IgG. Infants reach approximately 40% of adult levels by 1 year of age; therefore, during the first 6 to 12 months of life the infant is at higher risk for infections. Significant amounts of immunoglobulin M (IgM) are produced at birth, yet specificity is decreased, thus limiting recognition of certain pathogens. Adult levels of IgM are reached by 9 to 12 months of age. The production of immunoglobulins A, D and E (IgA, IgD and IgE) is much more gradual, and maximum levels are not attained until early childhood.

Prebiotic oligosaccharides found in breast milk produce probiotic bacteria such as bifidobacteria and lactobacilli, which in turn stimulate synthesis and secretion of secretory IgA (sIgA). Secretory IgA is present in large amounts in colostrum; IgA confers protection to the mucous membranes of the gastrointestinal tract (Newburg & He 2015) against many bacteria, such as *Escherichia coli,* and viruses, such as rubella, poliovirus and the enteroviruses. The development of the mucosa-associated lymphoid tissue occurs during infancy; in part, this system is believed to prevent colonisation and passage of bacteria across the infant's mucosal barrier. The function and quantity of T-lymphocytes, lymphokines, interferon-γ, interleukins, tumour necrosis factor–alpha and complement are reduced in early infancy, thus preventing optimal response to certain bacteria and viruses. Probiotics may have a significant role in helping the gastrointestinal tract establish a 'good' bacterial colonisation in the gut to prevent many illnesses, including antibiotic-induced diarrhoea and possibly *Helicobacter pylori* gastritis (Bron et al 2017).

There is evidence that **vernix caseosa**, a white, oily substance that coats the term infant's body and is often found in abundance in the creases of the axillae and groin, has innate immunological properties that serve to protect the newborn from infection (Visscher et al 2015). Vernix also appears to have a role in maintaining the integrity of the stratum corneum and facilitating acid mantle development (Visscher et al 2015). The epidermis of the full-term infant undergoes maturation during the first month of life; the newborn's skin acts as a barrier to infection, assists in thermal regulation and prevents transepidermal water loss in term infants.

During infancy thermoregulation becomes more efficient; the skin's ability to contract and the muscles' ability to shiver in response to cold increases. The peripheral capillaries respond to changes in ambient temperature to regulate heat loss. The capillaries constrict in response to cold, conserving core body temperature and decreasing potential evaporative heat loss from the skin surface. The capillaries dilate in response to heat, decreasing internal body temperature through evaporation, conduction and convection. Shivering (thermogenesis) causes the muscles and muscle fibres to contract, generating metabolic heat, which is distributed throughout the body. Increased adipose tissue during the first 6 months insulates the body against heat loss.

A shift in total body fluid occurs. At birth 75% of the infant's body weight is water and a significant amount of that is extracellular fluid (ECF). As the percentage of body water decreases, so does the amount of ECF—from 40% at term to 20% in adulthood. The high proportion of ECF, which is composed of blood plasma, interstitial fluid and lymph, predisposes the infant to more rapid loss of total body fluid and, consequently, dehydration. The loss of 5% to 10% of the term newborn's initial birth weight in the first 5 days of life is attributed to ECF compartment contraction, enhanced renal tubular function and rapidly increasing glomerular filtration rate (Lindower 2017).

The immaturity of the renal structures also predisposes the infant to dehydration. Complete maturity of the kidney occurs during the latter half of the second year, when the cuboidal epithelium of the glomeruli becomes flattened. Before this time the filtration capacity of the glomeruli is reduced. Infants void urine frequently, and it has a low specific gravity (1.008 to 1.012). At term most infants produce and excrete approximately 45 to 50 mL/kg/24 hr and the volume increases to 60 to 80 mL/kg/24 hr as the infant grows (Lindower 2017). Insensible water loss caused from radiant warmers, increased body temperature and some types of phototherapy may cause the newborn to have little or no urine output in the first 24 hours; however, infants should have at least 1 mL/kg/hr by the second day of life (Lincower 2017).

The endocrine system is adequately developed at birth, but its functions are immature. The interrelatedness of all the endocrine organs has a major effect on the function of any one gland. The lack of homeostatic control because of various functional deficiencies renders the infant especially vulnerable to imbalances in fluid and electrolytes, glucose levels and amino acid metabolism. For example, corticotropin (adrenocorticotropic hormone [ACTH]) is produced in limited quantities during infancy. ACTH acts on the adrenal cortices to produce their hormones, particularly the glucocorticoids and aldosterone. Because the feedback mechanism between ACTH and the adrenal cortex is immature during infancy, there is much less tolerance for stressful conditions, which affect fluid and electrolytes and the metabolism of fats, proteins and carbohydrates. In addition, although the islets of Langerhans produce insulin and glucagon during fetal life and early infancy, blood glucose levels tend to remain labile, particularly under conditions of stress.

Fine Motor Development

Fine motor behaviour includes the use of the hands and fingers in the **prehension** (grasp) of an object. Grasping occurs during the first 2 to 3 months as a reflex and gradually becomes voluntary. At 1 month of age the hands are predominantly closed, and by 3 months they are mostly open. By this time infants demonstrate a desire to grasp an object, but they 'grasp' it more with the eyes than with the hands. If a rattle is placed in the hand, the infant will actively hold onto it. By 4 months of age the infant regards both a small pellet and the hands and then looks from the object to the hands and back again. By 5 months the infant is able to voluntarily grasp an object.

Gradually the palmar grasp (using the whole hand) is replaced with a **pincer grasp** (using the thumb and index finger). By 8 to 9 months of age the infant uses a crude pincer grasp (Fig 10.3), and by 10 months of age the pincer grasp is sufficiently established to enable infants to pick up a raisin and other finger foods. By 11 months the infant has progressed to a neat pincer grasp (Fig 10.4).

By 6 months of age infants have increased manipulative skill. They hold their bottle, grasp their feet and pull them to their mouth. By 7 months they transfer objects from one hand to the other, use one hand for grasping and hold a cube in each hand simultaneously. They enjoy banging objects and will explore the movable parts of a toy. By 10 months of age infants can deliberately let go of an object and will offer it to someone. By 11 months they put objects into a container and like to remove them. By age 1 year infants try to build a tower of two blocks but fail.

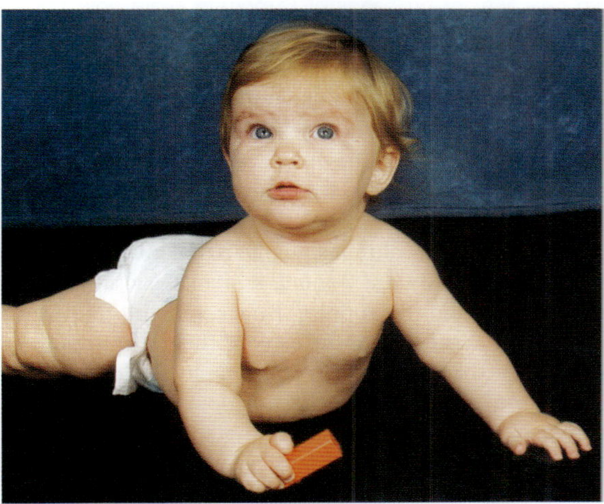

Fig 10.3 Crude pincer grasp at 8 to 10 months of age. (Source: Courtesy Paul Vincent Kuntz, Texas Children's Hospital, Houston.)

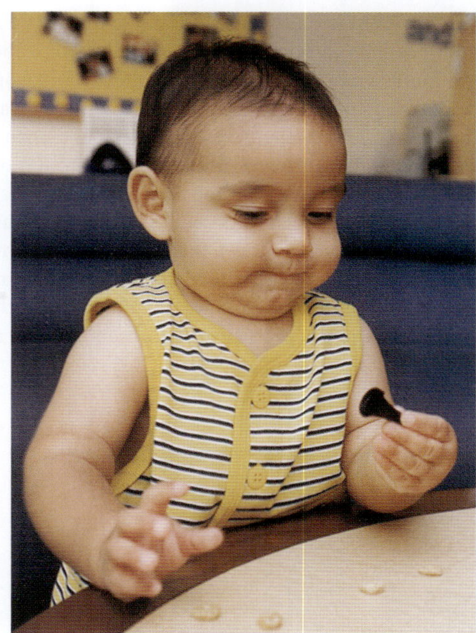

Fig 10.4 Neat pincer grasp at 11 months of age. (Source: Courtesy Paul Vincent Kuntz, Texas Children's Hospital, Houston.)

Gross Motor Development

Gross motor behaviour includes developmental maturation in posture, head balance, sitting, creeping, standing and walking. The full-term neonate is born with some ability to hold the head erect and reflexively assumes the postural tonic neck position when supine. Several of the primitive reflexes have significance in terms of development of later gross motor skills. The righting reflexes elicit certain postural responses, particularly of flexion or extension. They are responsible for certain motor activities, such as rolling over, assuming the crawl position and maintaining normal head-trunk-limb alignment during all activities. The neck-righting reflex, which turns the body to the same side as the head, enables the child to roll over from supine to prone. Other reflexes, such as the otolith-righting and labyrinth-righting reflexes, enable the infant to raise the head (see Box 10.1).

The asymmetrical tonic neck reflex, which persists from birth to 3 months, prevents the infant from rolling over. The symmetrical tonic neck reflex, which is evoked by flexing or extending the neck, helps the infant assume the crawl position. When the head and neck are extended, the extensor tone of the upper extremities and the flexor tone of the lower extremities increase. The child extends the arms and bends the knees. Because of the strong flexor tone of the lower extremities, the infant may initially crawl backwards before crawling forwards. This reflex disappears when neurological maturity allows actual crawling to occur because independent limb movement is required.

Head Control. The full-term newborn can momentarily hold the head in midline and parallel when the body is suspended ventrally and can lift and turn the head from side to side when prone (see Fig 7.8). This is not the case when the infant is lying prone on a pillow or soft surface; infants do not have the head control to lift their head out of the depression of the object and therefore risk possible suffocation. (See Sudden Infant Death Syndrome, Chapter 11.) Marked head lag is evident when the infant is pulled from a lying to a sitting position. By 3 months of age infants can hold their head well beyond the plane of the body. By 4 months of age infants can lift the head and front portion of the chest approximately 90 degrees above the table, bearing their weight on the forearms. Only slight head lag is evident when the infant is pulled from a lying to a sitting position, and by 4 to 6 months head control is well established (Figs 10.5 and 10.6).

Rolling Over. Newborns may roll over accidentally because of their rounded back. The ability to wilfully turn from the abdomen to the back occurs at 5 months, and the ability to turn from the back to the abdomen occurs at 6 months. It is noteworthy that the parachute reflex (see Fig 10.1), which elicits a protective response to falling, appears at 7 months.

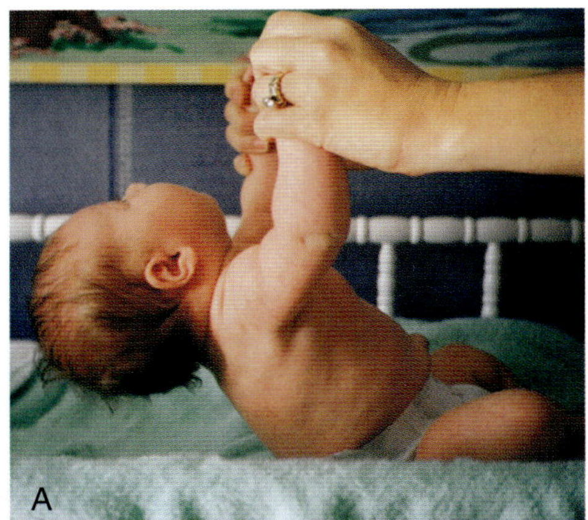

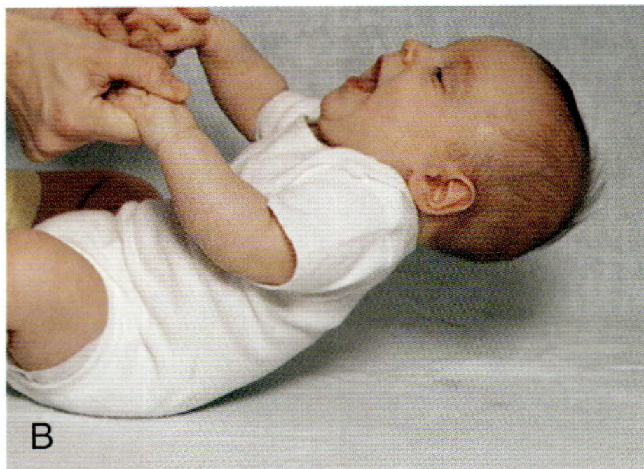

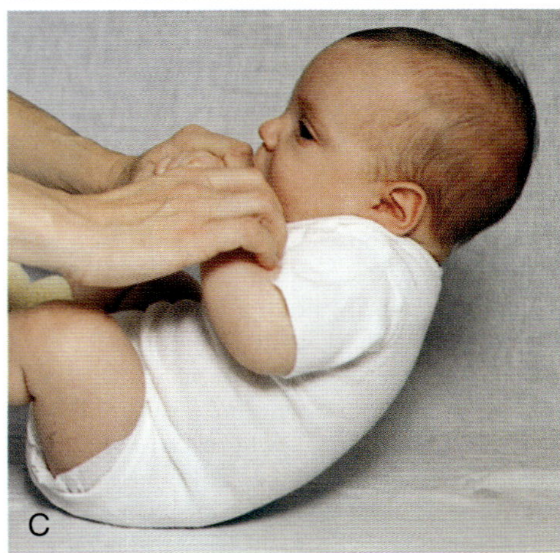

Fig 10.5 Head control while pulled to sitting position. (**A**) Complete head lag at 1 month. (**B**) Partial head lag at 2 months. (**C**) Almost no head lag at 4 months.

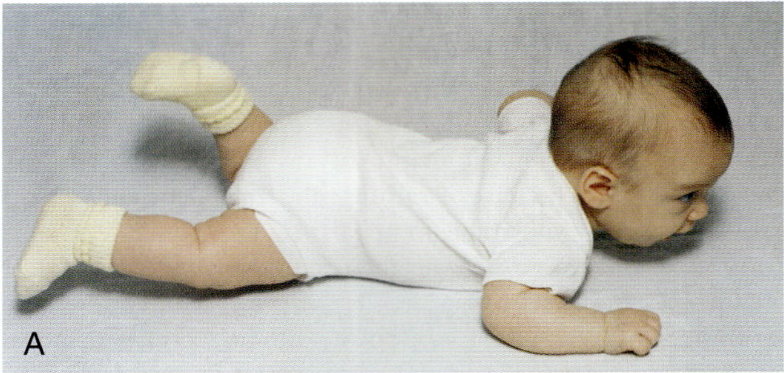

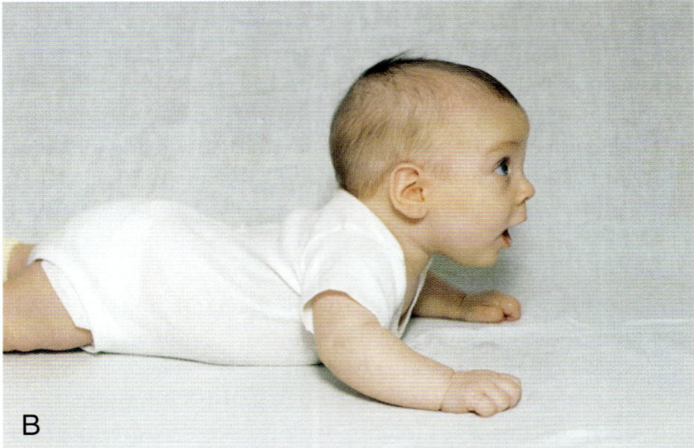

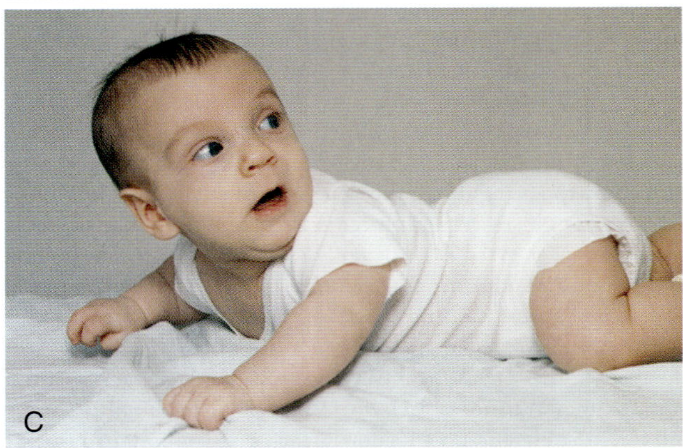

Fig 10.6 Head control while prone. (**A**) Infant momentarily lifts head at 1 month. (**B**) Infant lifts head and chest 90 degrees and bears weight on forearms at 4 months. (**C**) Infant lifts head, chest and upper abdomen and can bear weight on hands at 6 months. Note how this position facilitates turning from abdomen to back.

Sitting. The ability to sit follows progressive head control and straightening of the back (Fig 10.7). For the first 2 to 3 months the back is uniformly rounded. The convex cervical curve forms at approximately 3 to 4 months of age, when head control is established. The convex lumbar curve appears when the child begins to sit, at about age 4 months. As the spinal column straightens, the infant can be propped in a sitting position. By age 7 months infants can sit alone, leaning fowards on their hands for support. By age 8 months they can sit well while unsupported and begin to explore their surroundings in this position rather than in a lying position. By 10 months they can manoeuvre from a prone to a sitting position.

An infant who does not pull to a standing position by 11 to 12 months of age should be further evaluated for possible developmental dysplasia of the hip. (See Chapter 33.) Although infants vary considerably in regard to the achievement of these milestones, they provide guidelines for early intervention. Note that babies born

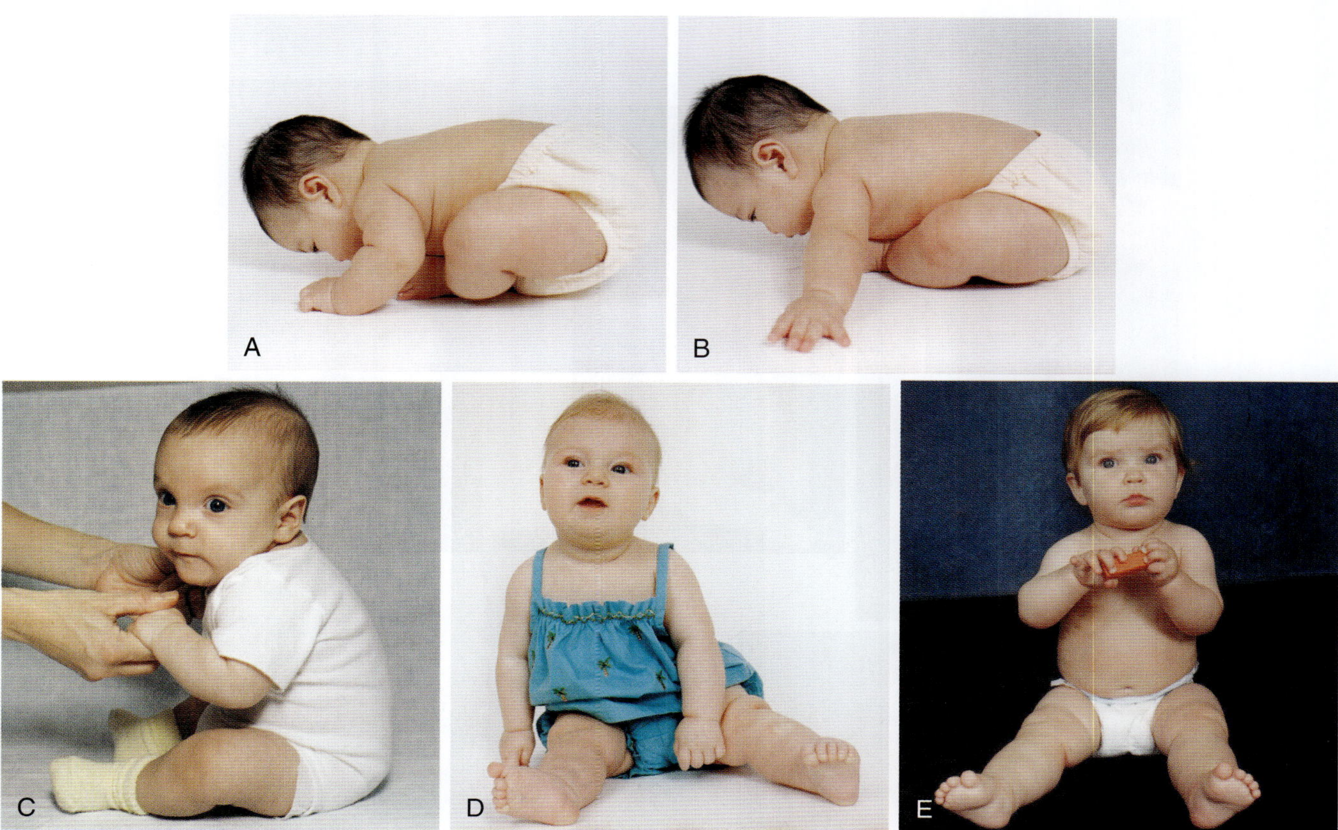

Fig 10.7 Development of sitting. (**A**) Back is completely rounded; infant has no ability to sit upright at 1 month. (**B**) At 2 months, infant exhibits more control; back is still rounded, but infant can try to pull up with some head control. (**C**) Back is rounded only in lumbar area; infant is able to sit erect with good head control at 4 months. (**D**) Infant can sit alone, leaning on hands for support, at 7 months. (**E**) Infant sits without support at 8 months. Note the transferring of objects that occurs at 7 months. (Source: Courtesy Paul Vincent Kuntz, Texas Children's Hospital, Houston.)

prematurely (before 37 weeks of pregnancy) or who have a disability may take longer to reach some milestones.

Locomotion. Locomotion involves acquiring the ability to bear weight, propel forwards on all four extremities, stand upright with support and, finally, walk alone (Fig 10.8). After a cephalocaudal pattern, infants 4 to 6 months old have increasing coordination in their arms. Initial locomotion results in infants propelling themselves backwards by pushing with the arms. By 6 to 7 months of age they are able to bear all their weight on their legs with assistance. **Crawling** (propelling forwards with belly on floor) progresses to **creeping** on hands and knees (with belly off floor) by 9 months. However, not all infants crawl: some achieve locomotion through 'bottom shuffling', and some move directly from sitting to pulling up to standing. At this time they stand while holding onto furniture and can pull themselves to the standing position, but they are unable to manoeuvre back down except by falling. By 11 months they walk while holding onto furniture or with both hands held, and by age 1 year they may be able to walk with one hand held. A number of infants attempt their first independent steps by their first birthday, although all children should be walking by 18 months of age.

Psychosocial Development

Developing a Sense of Trust (Erikson)

Erik Erikson's (1963) phase I (birth to 1 year) is concerned with acquiring a sense of trust while overcoming a sense of mistrust. The trust that develops is a trust of self, of others and of the world. Infants 'trust' that their feeding, comfort, stimulation and caring needs will be met. The crucial element for the achievement of this task is the quality of both the relationship between the parent (or caregiver) and child and the care the infant receives. The provision of food, warmth and shelter by itself is inadequate for the development of a strong sense of self. The infant and parent must jointly learn to satisfactorily meet their needs for mutual regulation of frustration to occur. When this synchrony fails to develop, mistrust is the eventual outcome. Frustration is heightened in situations in which the parent is emotionally immature and does not understand the infant's behavioural cues because of his or her own self-centred phase of development. For example, adolescence is a stage of transition from child to adult where adolescents seek to develop a sense of self and identity. If a teenager focuses on resolving unmet earlier psychological needs then they may not recognise or attend to infant cues.

Failure to learn delayed gratification leads to mistrust. Mistrust can result from either too much or too little frustration. If parents always meet their children's needs before the children signal their readiness, infants will never learn to test their ability to control the environment. If the delay is prolonged, infants will experience constant frustration and eventually mistrust others in their efforts to satisfy them. Therefore, consistency of care is essential.

The trust acquired in infancy provides the foundation for all succeeding phases. Trust allows infants a feeling of physical comfort and security, which assists them in experiencing unfamiliar, unknown

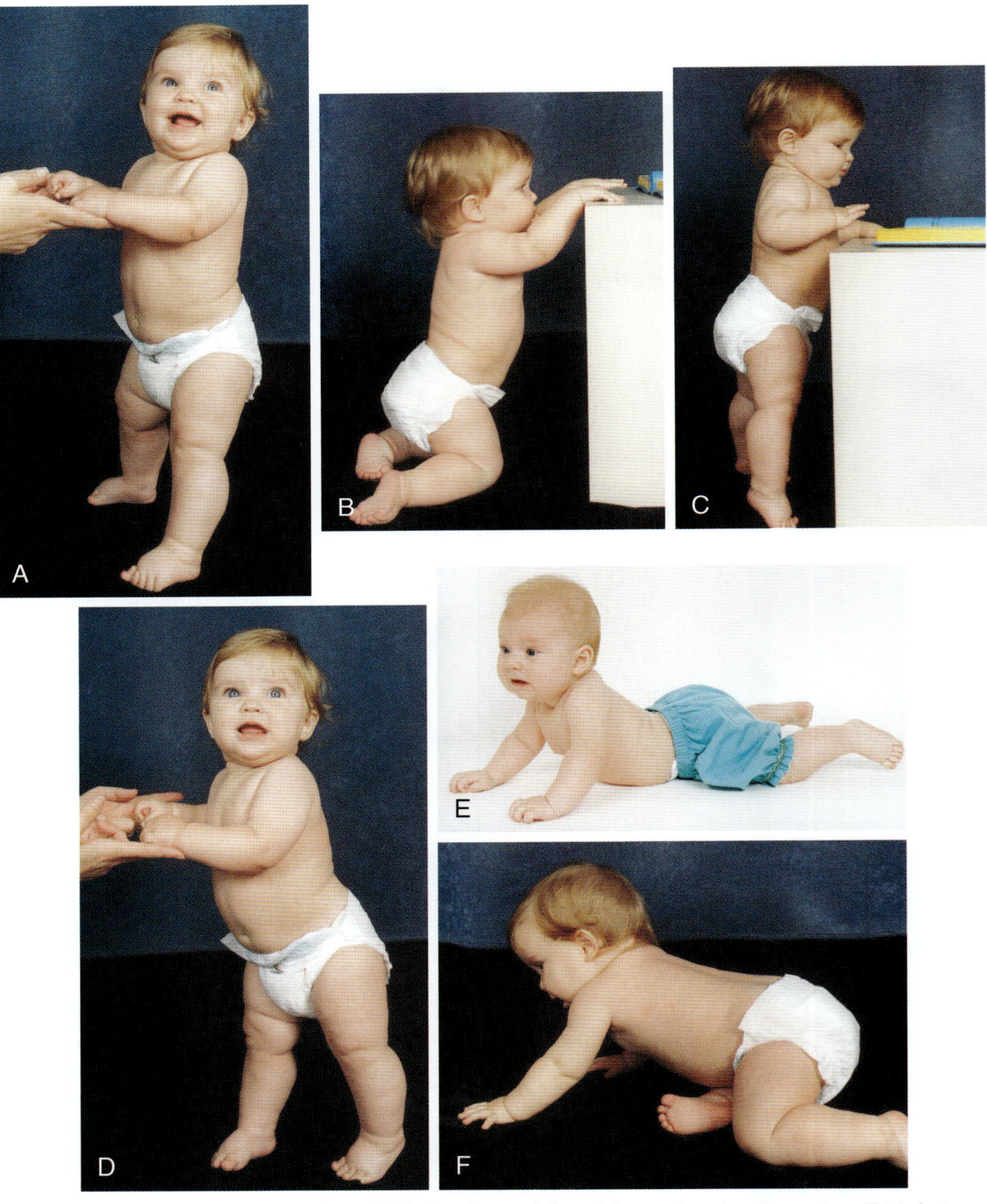

Fig 10.8 Development of locomotion. (**A**) Infant bears full weight on feet by 7 months. (**B**) Infant can manoeuvre from sitting to kneeling position by 8 months. (**C**) Infant can stand holding onto furniture at 8 to 9 months. (**D**) While standing, infant takes deliberate step at 9 to 10 months. (**E**) Infant crawls with abdomen on floor and pulls self forwards and then (**F**) creeps on hands and knees at 9 months. (Source: Courtesy Paul Vincent Kuntz, Texas Children's Hospital, Houston.)

situations with a minimum of fear. Erikson has divided the first year of life into two oral-social stages. During the first 3 to 4 months, food intake is the most important social activity in which the infant engages. The newborn can tolerate little frustration or delay of gratification. **Primary narcissism** (total concern for oneself) is at its height. However, as bodily processes such as vision, motor movements and vocalisation become better controlled, infants use more advanced behaviours to interact with others. For example, rather than cry, infants may put their arms up to signify a desire to be held.

The next social modality involves a mode of reaching out to others through grasping. Grasping is initially reflexive, but even as a reflex it has a powerful social meaning for the parents. The reciprocal response to the infant's grasping is the parents holding on and touching. There is pleasurable tactile stimulation for both the child and the parents.

Tactile stimulation is extremely important in the total process of acquiring trust. The degree of mothering skill, the quantity of food or the length of sucking does not determine the quality of the experience. Rather, it is the total quality of the interpersonal relationship that influences the infant's formulation of trust.

During the second stage, the more active and aggressive modality of biting occurs. Infants learn that they can hold onto what is their own and can more fully control their environment. During this stage infants may be confronted with one of their first conflicts. If they are breastfeeding, they quickly learn that biting causes the mother to become upset and withdraw the breast. Yet biting also brings internal relief from teething discomfort and a sense of power or control.

This conflict has a variety of solutions. The mother may wean the infant from the breast and begin bottle-feeding, or the infant may learn to bite substitute 'nipples' such as a soother, and retain pleasurable breastfeeding. Note that if the mother considers stopping breastfeeding in this case then the nurse can provide support and alternative options that allow infant biting, such as a soother, so breastfeeding can continue. The successful resolution of this conflict strengthens the mother–child relationship because it occurs at a time when infants are recognising the mother as the most significant person in their life.

Cognitive Development

Sensorimotor Phase (Piaget)

The theory most commonly used to explain *cognition,* or the ability to know, is that of Piaget (developed from 1936 to 1952). The period from birth to 24 months is termed the **sensorimotor phase** and is composed of six stages. However, because this discussion centres on ages birth to 12 months, only the first four stages are discussed (Table 10.1; see Table 12.1 for the stages from 13 to 24 months).

During the sensorimotor phase, infants progress from reflexive behaviours to simple repetitive acts to imitative activity. Three crucial events take place during this phase. The first event involves **separation,** in which infants learn to separate themselves from other objects in the

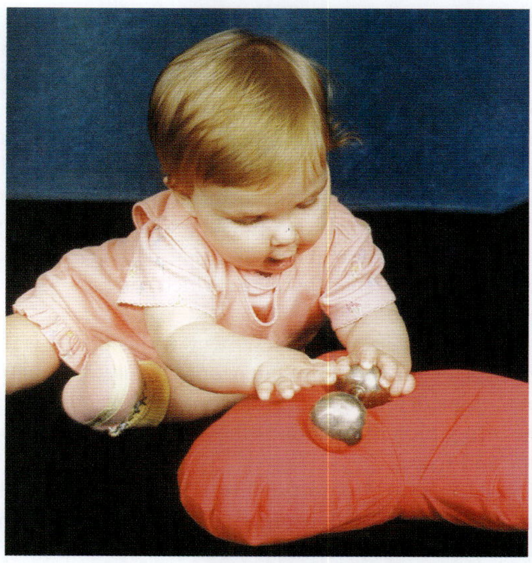

Fig 10.9 Nine-month-old is able to find hidden object under pillow. (Source: Courtesy Paul Vincent Kuntz, Texas Children's Hospital, Houston.)

TABLE 10.1 Sensorimotor Phase During Infancy*

Stage and Age	Cognitive Development	Behaviour
I. Use of reflexes (birth–1 month)	Repetitious use of reflexes establishing pattern of experiences Totally narcissistic (self-centred) being	Mostly reflective (e.g. sucking, swallowing, rooting, grasping, crying) Little or no tolerance for frustration of delayed gratification
II. Primary circular reactions (1–4 months)	Use of reflexes gradually replaced by voluntary activity Recognition of causality occurring when repetition of events causes one stimulus to produce consistent response Beginning notion of temporal space of time as infant realises progression of orderly sequence of events Beginning separation of self from others Learns from type of interaction between objects or individual rather than from object itself Engages in activity for pleasure of the activity more than for its results	Recognises familiar faces and objects (e.g. bottle) Shows anticipation before feeding Shows awareness of strange surroundings, indicating memory Discovers parts of own body—plays with hands, fingers, feet Becomes bored when left alone Shows no separation anxiety unless caregiver's skill differs from usual routine
III. Secondary circular reactions (4–8 months)	Intentional activity replaces repetitious activity that did not produce desired result Beginning of object permanence when object is beyond perceptual range Progressive idea of time; awareness of before and after in sequence of events Able to imitate selective activity from several events Further separation of self from environment Idea of quality and quantity Beginning recognition of symbols as type of communication	Secures objects by pulling on string Searches for objects that have fallen Shows separation anxiety Able to tolerate some frustration and delayed gratification Imitates sounds and simple gestures Shows interest in mirror image (see Fig 10.10) Beginning independence in self-feeding Shows displeasure if activity is inhibited Language development; attracts attention by methods other than crying Realises that parents are present even if not in visual field
IV. Coordination of secondary schemas and their application to new situations (9–12 months)	Concept of object permanence advancing; beginning of intellectual reasoning Associates symbols with events, but classification is based on own experience Distinguishes objects from related activity and perceives them as objects Distinguishes end products from their means; attempts to remove barriers to achieve the end	Actively searches for hidden object (see Fig 10.9) Comprehends meanings of words and simple commands Know that gestures (e.g. bye-bye, kiss) have certain meanings Is able to put objects in container Works to get toy that is out of reach Ventures away from parent to explore surroundings

*For phases during toddlerhood, see Table 12.1.

environment. They realise that others besides themselves control the environment and that certain adjustments must take place for mutual satisfaction to occur. This coincides with Erikson's concept of the formation of trust and mutual regulation of frustration.

The second major accomplishment is achieving the concept of **object permanence**, or the realisation that objects that leave the visual field still exist. A typical example of the development of object permanence is when infants are able to pursue objects they observe being hidden under a pillow or behind a chair (Fig 10.9). This skill develops at approximately 9 to 10 months of age, which corresponds to the time of increased locomotion skills.

The last major intellectual achievement of this period is the ability to use symbols, or **mental representation**. The use of symbols allows the infant to think of an object or situation without actually experiencing it. The recognition of symbols is the beginning of the understanding of time and space.

The first stage, from birth to 1 month, is identified by the infant's use of **reflexes**. At birth the infant expresses individuality and temperament through the physiological reflexes of sucking, rooting, grasping and crying. The repetitious nature of the reflexes is the beginning of associations between an act and a sequential response. When infants cry because they are hungry, a nipple is put in the mouth and they suck, feel satisfaction and sleep. They are assimilating this experience while perceiving auditory, tactile and visual cues. This experience of perceiving certain patterns, or **ordering**, provides a foundation for the subsequent stages.

The second stage, **primary circular reactions**, marks the beginning of the replacement of reflexive behaviour with voluntary acts. During the period from 1 to 4 months, activities such as sucking or grasping become deliberate acts that elicit certain responses. The beginning of accommodation is evident. Infants incorporate and adapt their reactions to the environment and recognise the stimulus that produced a response. Previously they would cry until the nipple was brought to the mouth. Now they associate the nipple with the sound of the parent's voice. They accommodate this new piece of information and adapt by ceasing to cry when they hear the voice—before receiving the nipple. What is taking place is a realisation of causality and recognition of an orderly sequence of events. The infant takes in the environment with all the senses and with whatever motor ability is present.

The **secondary circular reactions** stage is a continuation of primary circular reactions and lasts until 8 months of age. In this stage the primary circular reactions are repeated and prolonged for the response that results. Grasping and holding now become shaking, banging and pulling. Infants shake objects to hear a noise, not solely for the pleasure of shaking. Quality and quantity of an act become evident. 'More' or 'less' shaking produces different responses. Causality, time, deliberate intention and separateness from the environment begin to develop.

Three new processes of human behaviour occur. **Imitation** requires the differentiation of selected acts from several events. By the second half of the first year infants can imitate sounds and simple gestures. Play becomes evident as they take pleasure in performing an act after they have mastered it. Much of infants' waking hours are absorbed in sensorimotor play. **Affect** (outward manifestation of emotion and feeling) is evident as infants begin to develop a sense of permanency. During the first 6 months infants believe that an object exists only for as long as they can visually perceive it; in other words, out of sight, out of mind. A reaction to external objects is evident when the object continues to be remembered even though it is beyond the range of perception. **Object permanence** is a critical component of parent–child attachment and is seen in the development of separation anxiety at 6 to 8 months of age (see discussion later in this chapter).

During the fourth sensorimotor stage, **coordination of secondary schemas and their application to new situations**, infants use previous behavioural achievements primarily as the foundation for adding new intellectual skills to their expanding repertoire. This stage is largely transitional. Increasing motor skills allow for greater exploration of the environment. They begin to discover that hiding an object does not mean that it is gone but that removing an obstacle will reveal the object. This marks the beginning of intellectual reasoning. Furthermore, they can experience an event by observing it, and they begin to associate symbols with events (e.g. 'bye-bye' with 'Mummy goes to work'), but the classification is purely their own. In this stage they learn from the object itself. This is in contrast to the second stage, in which infants learn from the type of interaction between objects or individuals. Intentionality is further developed in that infants now actively attempt to remove a barrier to the desired (or undesired) action (see Fig 10.9). If something is in their way, they attempt to climb over it or push it away, whereas previously they would have given up any attempt to achieve the desired goal.

Another important theorist in cognitive development is Lev Vygotsky (1896–1934), whose work was similar to Piaget's work but proposed that children can be encouraged to progress to a higher stage of development with the assistance of older children or adults. This can be achieved if the child is in a **zone of proximal development** that is close to the next stage (Beloglovsky & Daly 2015).

Development of Body Image

The development of body image parallels sensorimotor development. Infants' kinaesthetic and tactile experiences are the first perceptions of their body, and the mouth is the principal area of pleasurable sensations. Other parts of the body are primarily objects of pleasure—the hands and fingers to suck and the feet to play with. As physical needs are met, they feel comfort and satisfaction with their body. Messages conveyed by the caregivers reinforce these feelings. For example, when infants smile, they receive emotional satisfaction from others who smile back.

Achieving the concept of object permanence is basic to the development of self-image. By the end of the first year infants recognise that they are distinct from their parents. At the same time they have increasing interest in their image, especially in the mirror (Fig 10.10). As motor skills develop, they learn that parts of the body are useful; for example, the hands bring objects to the mouth and the legs help them move to different locations. All these achievements transmit messages

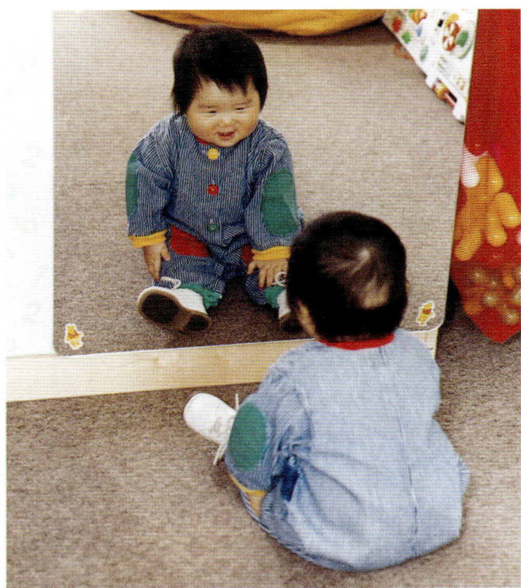

Fig 10.10 Nine-month-old infant enjoying own image in mirror.

to them about themselves. Therefore, it is important to transmit positive messages to infants about their bodies.

Development of Gender Identity

Gender identity is reported to begin in utero because of hormonal influences that are not entirely understood. Such hormones are also thought to influence sexual differentiation of the brain. One's gender identity as being male or female is established by 2 to 3 years of life (Bockting 2016). The final determination of gender identity is influenced by environmental, biological and sociocultural factors. At birth the child is named, and significant others, especially the parents, act certain ways towards the infant because of its gender. Touch is crucial to infant development and plays a primary role in gender development. Infants have great oral sensitivity, which is manifested through sucking and mouthing. They enjoy skin-to-skin contact and explore their own body for pleasure. Infants are capable of genital self-stimulation to orgasm; erections in male infants are common. Parents' responses to these early manifestations of sexuality influence children's evolving attitudes. Therefore, a healthy, accepting response by parents is important.

Social Development

Infants' social development is initially influenced by their reflexive behaviour, such as the grasp, and eventually depends primarily on the interaction between them and the principal caregivers. **Attachment** to the parent is increasingly evident during the second half of the first year. In addition, infants make tremendous strides in communication and personal-social behaviour. Play is a major socialising agent and provides the stimulation needed to learn from interactions with the environment.

Attachment

Human physical contact is extremely important. Parenting is not an instinctual ability but a learned, acquired process. The attachment of parent and child, which begins before birth and assumes even more importance at birth (see Chapter 7), continues during the first year. In the following discussion of attachment, the word *mother* is used in the broad context of the consistent caregiver with whom the child relates more than anyone else. However, in a society with a changing social climate and dissolving sex-role stereotypes, this person may well be the father, grandmother or other family member.

Studies on father–child attachment demonstrate that stages similar to maternal attachment occur and that fathers are more involved in childcare when mothers are employed. Additional research has shown that inexperienced first-time fathers are as capable as experienced fathers of developing a close attachment with their infants. Studies of fathers of high-risk infants demonstrate that fathers experience feelings of love and affection towards their offspring during the newborn period; fathers in one study verbalised more positive feelings of love and affection towards the newborn when they were able to have close physical contact such as holding the child (Logan & Dormire 2018). The father has also been reported to have a significant role in supporting the mother in the perinatal period; fathers of high-risk infants reported concern about their mates' wellbeing in addition to the status of the ill infant (Logan & Dormire 2018). Research demonstrates that fathers develop feelings of attachment with their offspring and that their relationship with the infant is an important factor in the mother's emotional wellbeing.

With many single-parent families in existence, a grandmother (or other significant caretaker) may become the primary caretaker. It is important for nurses to recognise that infant–parent attachments may be present or absent in situations where caretaker roles are less well defined by those involved.

When the infant is not provided a safe haven and consistent and loving care, an insecure attachment develops; such infants do not feel they can trust the world in which they live. This insecure attachment may result in psychosocial difficulties as the child grows and may persist even into adulthood. Perinatal maternal depression has been postulated to alter fetal and neonatal neuroendocrine development, which negatively affects the infant's growth and development (Liu et al 2017).

Attachment progresses during infancy, with the child assuming an increasingly significant role in the family. Two components of cognitive development are required for attachment: (1) the ability to discriminate the mother from other individuals; and (2) the achievement of object permanence. Both these processes prepare the infant for an equally important aspect of attachment: separation from the parent. Separation-individuation should occur as a harmonious, parallel process with emotional attachment.

During the formation of attachment to the parent, the infant progresses through four distinct but overlapping stages. For the first few weeks infants respond indiscriminately to anyone. Beginning at approximately 8 to 12 weeks of age, they cry, smile and vocalise more to the mother than to anyone else but continue to respond to others, whether familiar or not. At approximately 6 months of age, infants show a distinct preference for the mother. They follow her more, cry when she leaves, enjoy playing with her more and feel most secure in her arms. About 1 month after showing attachment to the mother, many infants begin attaching to other members of the family, most often the father.

Infants acquire other developmental behaviours that influence the attachment process. These include: (1) differential crying, smiling and vocalisation (more to mother than to anyone else); (2) visual-motor orientation (looking more at mother, even if she is not close); (3) crying when the mother leaves the room; (4) approaching through locomotion (crawling, creeping or walking); (5) clinging (especially in the presence of a stranger); and (6) exploring away from mother while using her as a secure base.

Effects of Prolonged Separation. Attachment is considered so critical to optimum child development that many researchers have documented the effects of prolonged and early separation on infants in the absence of high-quality parent substitutes. Some of the most famous research on emotional deprivation has been done by John Bowlby, John Robertson and René Spitz. Bowlby (1969) studied the effects of the infant's separation from the mother and noted severe cognitive and physical impairment, particularly if emotional deprivation occurred during the first 3 years of life. He observed that progressive impairment could be arrested or reversed if no further emotional deprivation occurred after the first 2 years, whereas prolonged, severe deprivation beginning early in the first year and lasting for 3 years led to severe, permanent effects. Among these were the inabilities to form trusting, intimate interpersonal relationships; language impairment; and deficiency in abstract thinking. Robertson (1953) and Bowlby (1969) found typical behavioural reactions of infants who were hospitalised and separated from their mothers.

Spitz (1945) studied the effects of emotional deprivation on children raised in foundling homes or institutions. The infants were cared for by one nurse who had responsibility for eight children. Although the caregiver might be a loving, motherly person, she lacked the time to devote individual attention and stimulation to each child. As a result, the children were delayed in physical growth, were more susceptible to disease and demonstrated decreasing developmental quotients over a 2-year period. Spitz found that children developed normally if given one-to-one attention by a mother substitute.

Although these studies represent extreme examples of young children reared in environments essentially devoid of high-quality mothering, rather than temporary separation such as day care, the question remains regarding the long-term effects of separation and other stresses on children.

Severe attachment disorders are psychological and developmental problems that stem from maladaptive or absent attachment between the infant and parent and may persist into childhood and even adulthood (Zeanah & Gleason 2015). Infants at risk for severe attachment disorders include those who have been victims of physical or sexual abuse or neglect; infants exposed to parental alcoholism, mental illness or substance abuse; and infants who have experienced the absence of a consistent primary caregiver as a result of foster care, institutionalisation, parental abandonment or parental incarceration (Zeanah & Gleason 2015). Historically, two different patterns of attachment disorders were described: the emotionally withdrawn–inhibited pattern and an indiscriminate-disinhibited pattern (Zeanah & Gleason 2015). These patterns have been classified into separate disorders: disinhibited social engagement disorder (DSED) and reactive attachment disorder (RAD) of infancy or early childhood. Children with RAD may manifest behaviours such as not being cuddly with parents, failing to seek and respond to comfort when distressed, minimal social and emotional reciprocity and emotional deregulation such as unexplained fearfulness or irritability (Zeanah & Gleason 2015). Children with DSED may exhibit behaviours such as inappropriate approach to unfamiliar adults, lack of suspicion of strangers and poor impulse control (Zeanah & Gleason 2015). Either or both of these complex disorders are diagnosed with maltreated and orphaned children. Without early intervention, some of these children fail to develop a conscience and suffer from an antisocial personality disorder that may lead to criminal acts. Children with autism or other pervasive developmental disorders have behaviours that are categorically different from those with RAD (Zeanah & Gleason 2015).

Based on such findings, nurses need to assess each family with the understanding that stress may or may not be necessarily harmful and that children can adapt even under adverse conditions. The nurse evaluates individual risk factors that influence a child's coping ability, using tools such as the Revised Infant Temperament Questionnaire (see later in this chapter) to assess 'goodness of fit'. When prolonged parental separation occurs, make every effort to help the family provide suitable caregiver substitutes for the child. Individuals who are warm, responsive and interactive with the infant during separation can significantly minimise the physiological and behavioural effects. The nurse should emphasise the child's plasticity and resiliency in coping to minimise the family's feelings of responsibility and guilt.

Separation Anxiety. Between the ages of 4 and 8 months the infant progresses through the first stage of separation-individuation and begins to have some awareness of self and mother as separate beings. At the same time, object permanence is developing and the infant is aware that the parent can be absent. Therefore, **separation anxiety** develops and is manifested through a predictable sequence of behaviours.

During the early second half of the first year, infants protest when placed in their cot, and a short time later they object when the mother leaves the room. Infants may not notice the mother's absence if they are absorbed in an activity. However, when they realise her absence, they protest. From this point on they become very alert to her activities and whereabouts. By 11 to 12 months they are able to anticipate her imminent departure by watching her behaviours, and they begin to protest before she leaves. At this point many parents learn to postpone alerting the child to their departure until just before leaving.

Stranger Fear. As infants demonstrate attachment to one person, they correspondingly exhibit less friendliness to others. Between ages 6 and 8 months fear of strangers and stranger anxiety become prominent and are related to infants' ability to discriminate between familiar and unfamiliar people. Behaviours such as clinging to the parent, crying and turning away from strangers are common (Fig 10.11). Suggestions for coping with stranger fear and separation anxiety are listed later in this chapter.

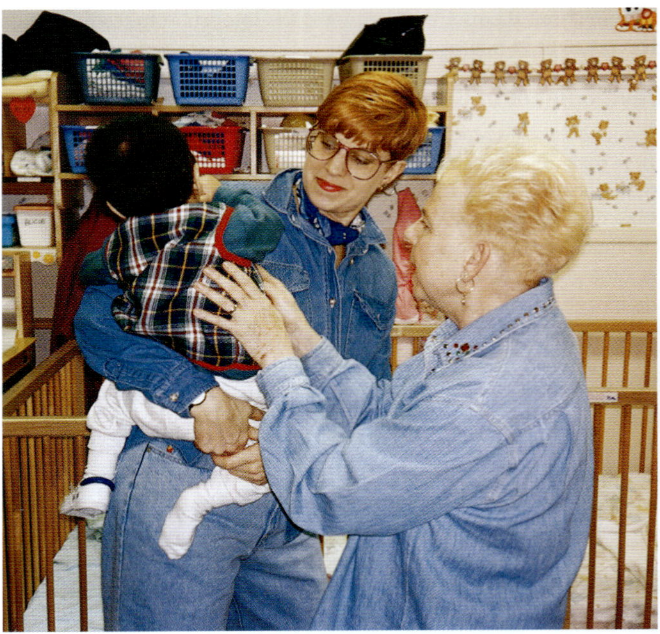

Fig 10.11 Stranger fear behaviours include clinging to the parent and turning away from a stranger.

Language Development

The infant's first means of verbal communication is crying. Crying as a biological sign conveys a message of urgency and signals displeasure, such as hunger. However, crying is also a social event that affects the development of the parent–infant relationship—either by its absence, which usually has a positive effect on parents, or its presence, which may evoke a negative response or persuade parents to minister to the child's physical or emotional needs.

In the first few weeks of life, crying has a reflexive quality and is mostly related to physiological needs. Infants cry for 1 to 1.5 hours per day up to 3 weeks of age and then build up to 2 hours and even 4 hours by 6 weeks. Crying tends to decrease by 12 weeks. It is thought that the increase in crying for no apparent reason during the first few months may be related to the discharge of energy and the maturational changes in the central nervous system. By the end of the first year infants cry for attention; from fear (especially stranger fear); and from frustration, usually in response to their developing but inadequate motor skills.

Personal-social Behaviour

Personal-social behaviour includes the child's personal responses to the environment. It is the area most influenced by external stimuli, but, as in the other fields of behaviour, it follows certain developmental laws. Personal-social behaviour implies communication with one's self and with others. It provides the foundation for the successful mastery of skills such as feeding, control of bodily functions, independence and cooperativeness in play.

Infants have the ability to shape their environment and to elicit certain responses. Newborns show visual preference for the human face and, as early as 1 week of age, begin to watch the parent intently as he or she speaks to them. As they regard the parent's face, activity diminishes, their head bobs up and down and their mouth moves, almost as if they were trying to say something.

By 6 to 8 weeks a social smile in response to pleasurable stimuli is present. This has a profound effect on family members and evokes continued responses from others. By 3 months infants show considerable interest in the environment—excitement when a toy is presented, refusal to be left alone, recognition of parent and demonstration of pleasure by squealing. By 4 months they laugh aloud and enjoy strange, novel stimuli.

By 6 months infants are very personable. They play games such as peek-a-boo when their head is hidden in a towel, signal their desire to be picked up by extending their arms and show displeasure when a toy is removed or their face is washed. They increasingly demonstrate their ability to control the environment. The acquisition of fine and gross motor skills allows much more independence in movement.

By the second half of the first year infants understand simple discipline, such as the meaning of the word 'no' or a scolding remark. They comprehend different facial expressions and are sensitive to emotional changes in others. Imitation is developing during this time. They imitate actions and noises by 7 months, sounds by 8 months and games such as pat-a-cake and peek-a-boo by 10 months.

From 11 months onwards they are increasingly independent. They are learning to feed themselves; are using their fingers, spoon and cup (with much spilling); and can help with dressing by putting the foot out for a shoe or pushing the arm through the sleeve. They not only comprehend the meaning of 'no' but also shake their head to indicate 'no'. They can follow simple directions and gladly perform for others to attract and prolong attention.

Play

Play during infancy represents the various social modalities observed during cognitive development. Infants' activity is primarily narcissistic and revolves around their own body. As discussed under Development of Body Image, body parts are primarily objects of play and pleasure.

During the first year, play becomes more sophisticated and interdependent. From birth to 3 months, infants' responses to the environment are global and largely undifferentiated. Play is dependent; pleasure is demonstrated by a quieting attitude (1 month), a smile (2 months) and a squeal (3 months). From 3 to 6 months infants show more discriminate interest in stimuli and begin to play alone with a rattle or soft stuffed toy or with someone else. They interact much more during play. By 4 months of age they laugh aloud, show preference for certain toys and become excited when food or a favourite object is brought to them. They recognise an image in a mirror, smile at it and vocalise to it.

By 6 months to 1 year, play involves sensorimotor skills. Infants play actual games such as peek-a-boo and pat-a-cake. They demonstrate verbal repetition and imitation of simple gestures. Play is much more selective, not only in terms of specific toys but also in terms of 'playmates'. Although play is **solitary** or one-sided, infants choose with whom they will interact. At 6 to 8 months they usually refuse to play with strangers. Parents are definite favourites, and infants know how to attract their attention. At 6 months they extend the arms to be picked up, at 7 months cough to make their presence known, at 10 months pull the parent's clothing and at 12 months call them by name. This represents a tremendous advance from the newborn who signalled biological needs by crying to express displeasure.

Temperament

The infant's **temperament** or behavioural style influences the type of interaction that occurs between the child and parents and other family members. In assessing a child's temperament, it is the parents' perception of the child and the degree of fit between their expectations and the child's actual temperament that are important. The more dissonance (or lack of harmony) between the child's temperament and the parent's ability to accept and deal with the behaviour, the greater the risk for subsequent parent–child conflicts.

Although many behavioural researchers agree that temperament has a strong biological component, researchers also suggest that the environment, particularly the family, may modify temperament (Gallitto 2015). Family interaction with the infant is perceived as a circular process wherein each family member affects one another and the family as a unit. With these concepts in mind, the nurse has an important role in helping the family understand the infant's temperament as it relates to family dynamics and the eventual wellbeing of the child and family unit (Gallitto 2015).

Several instruments can measure infant temperament. These instruments include the Revised Infant Temperament Questionnaire (Carey & McDevitt 1978), the Infant Behavior Questionnaire (Gartstein & Rothbart 2003) and the Early Infancy Temperament Questionnaire (Medoff-Cooper et al 1993). In discussing test results to parents, it is best to avoid descriptors (e.g. 'difficult'); instead, infants can be described in terms of characteristics (e.g. 'intense' or 'less predictable'). With knowledge of the infant's temperament, nurses are better able to: (1) provide parents with background information that will help them see their child in a better perspective; (2) offer a more organised picture of their child's behaviour and possibly reveal distortions in their perceptions of the behaviour; and (3) guide parents regarding appropriate childrearing techniques.

Appropriate guidance based on awareness of the child's temperament can greatly enhance the quality of interaction between parents and infant. Even just letting parents know that 'difficult' traits are innate can relieve feelings of guilt and incompetence.

Knowledge of the developmental sequence allows the nurse to assess normal growth and minor or abnormal deviations. It also helps parents gain realistic expectations of their child's ability and provides guidelines for suitable play and stimulation. Parents who lack knowledge of child growth and development may set inappropriate behavioural expectations for their child. Emphasising the child's developmental rather than chronological age strengthens the parent–child relationship by fostering trust and lessening frustration. Therefore, thorough understanding and appreciation of children's growth and development are essential.

Because of the complexity of the developmental process during the first 12 months, Table 10.2 is presented to help organise and clarify the data already discussed. Although all milestones are important, some represent essential integrative aspects of development that lay the foundation for achievement of more advanced skills. These essential milestones are designated by an asterisk (*) in the table. The table represents the average monthly age at which various skills are attained. It must be remembered that although the sequence is the same, the rate will vary among children. Because of this variation, it is important for nurses to conduct developmental screening with all children.

Coping with Concerns related to Normal Growth and Development

Separation Anxiety and Stranger Fear

A number of fears can appear during infancy. However, the fear that causes many parents concern is related to strangers and separation. Although some erroneously interpret this as a sign of undesirable, antisocial behaviour, stranger fear and separation anxiety are important components of a strong, healthy parent–child attachment. Nevertheless, this period can present difficulties for the parent and child. Parents may be more confined to the home because the infant violently protests to being left at day care or having a babysitter. To accustom the infant to new people, encourage parents to have close friends or relatives visit often. This provides other persons with whom the child is comfortable and who can give parents time for themselves.

Infants also need opportunities to safely experience strangers. Usually towards the end of the first year infants begin to venture away from the parent and demonstrate curiosity about strangers. If allowed to explore at their own rate, many infants eventually 'warm up'. If

TABLE 10.2 **Growth and Development During Infancy**

Age (Months)	Physical	Gross Motor	Fine Motor	Sensory	Vocalisation	Socialisation/ Cognition
1	Weight gain of 150–210 g weekly for first 6 months Height gain of 2.5 cm monthly for first 6 months Head circumference increases by 1.5 cm monthly for first 6 months Primitive reflexes present and strong Doll's eye reflex and dance reflex fading Obligatory nose breathing (most infants)	Assumes flexed position with pelvis high but knees not under abdomen when prone (at birth, knees flexed under abdomen)* Can turn head from side to side when prone; lifts head momentarily from bed (see Fig 10.6A)* Has marked head lag, especially when pulled from lying to sitting position (see Fig 10.5A) Holds head momentarily parallel and in midline when suspended in prone position Assumes asymmetrical tonic neck reflex position when supine When held in standing position, is limp at knees and hips In sitting position, has uniformly rounded back, absence of head control	Hands predominantly closed Grasp reflex strong Clenches hand on contact with rattle	Able to fixate on moving object in range of 45 degrees when held at distance of 20–25 cm* Visual acuity approaches 20/100† Follows light to midline Quietens when hears a voice	Cries to express displeasure Makes small, throaty sounds Makes comfort sounds during feeding	Is in sensorimotor phase, stage I, use of reflexes (birth–1 month); and stage II, primary circular reactions (14 months) Watches parent's face intently as she or he talks to infant
2	Posterior fontanel closed Crawling reflex disappears	Assumes less flexed position when prone—hips flat, legs extended, arms flexed, head to side* Less head lag when pulled to sitting position (see Fig 10.5B) Can maintain head in same plane as rest of body when held in ventral suspension When prone, can lift head almost 45 degrees off table When held in sitting position, can hold head up, but bends forwards (see Fig 10.7B) Assumes asymmetrical tonic neck reflex position intermittently	Hands often open Grasp reflex fading	Binocular fixation and convergence to near objects beginning When supine, follows dangling toy from side to point beyond midline Visually searches to locate sounds Turns head to side when sound is made at level of ear	Vocalises, distinct from crying* Crying becomes differentiated Coos Vocalises to familiar voice	Demonstrates social smile in response to various stimuli*
3	Primitive reflexes fading	Able to hold head more erect when sitting, but still bobs forwards Has only slight head lag when pulled to sitting position Assumes symmetrical body positioning Able to raise head and shoulders from prone position to 45- to 90-degree angle from table; bears weight on forearms When held in standing position, able to bear slight fraction of weight on legs Regards own hand	Actively holds rattle but will not reach for it* Grasp reflex absent Hands kept loosely open Clutches own hand; pulls at blankets and clothes	Follows objects to periphery (180 degrees)* Locates sound by turning head to side and looking in same direction* Begins to have ability to coordinate stimuli from various sense organs	Squeals aloud to show pleasure* Coos, babbles, chuckles Vocalises when smiling 'Talks' a great deal when spoken to Less crying during periods of wakefulness	Displays considerable interest in surroundings Ceases crying when parent enters room Can recognise familiar faces and objects, such as feeding bottle Shows awareness of strange situations

4	Drooling begins Moro, tonic neck and rooting reflexes disappear*	Has almost no head lag when pulled to sitting position (see Fig 10.5C)* Balances head well in sitting position (see Fig 10.7C)* Back less rounded, curved only in lumbar area Able to sit erect if propped up Able to raise head and chest off surface to angle of 90 degrees (see Fig 10.6B) Assumes predominant symmetrical position Rolls from back to side*	Inspects and plays with hands; pulls clothing or blanket over face in play* Tries to reach objects with hand but overshoots Grasps object with both hands Plays with rattle placed in hand, shakes it, but cannot pick it up if dropped Can carry objects to mouth	Able to accommodate to near objects Binocular vision fairly well established Can focus on a 1.25-cm block Beginning eye-hand coordination	Makes consonant sounds *n, k, g, p, b* Laughs aloud Vocalisation changes according to mood	Is in stage III, secondary circular reactions Demands attention by fussing; becomes bored if left alone Enjoys social interaction Anticipates feeding when sees bottle or mother if breastfeeding Shows excitement with whole body, squeals, breathes heavily Shows interest in strange stimuli Begins to show memory
5	Beginning signs of tooth eruption Birth weight doubles	No head lag when pulled to sitting position When sitting, able to hold head erect and steady Able to sit for longer periods when back is well supported Back straight When prone, assumes symmetrical positioning with arms extended Can turn over from abdomen to back* When supine, puts feet to mouth	Able to grasp objects voluntarily* Uses palmar grasp, bidextrous approach Plays with toes Takes objects directly to mouth Holds one cube while regarding a second one	Visually pursues dropped object Is able to sustain visual inspection of object Can localise sounds made below ear	Squeals Makes cooing vowel sounds interspersed with consonant sounds (e.g. *ah goo*)	Smiles at mirror image Pats bottle or breast with both hands More enthusiastically playful, but may have rapid mood swings Is able to discriminate strangers from family Vocalises displeasure when object is taken away Discovers parts of body
6	Growth rate may begin to decline Weight gain of 90–150 g weekly for next 6 months Height gain of 1.25 cm monthly for next 6 months May begin teething with eruption of two lower central incisors* May chew and bite*	When prone, can lift chest and upper abdomen off surface, bearing weight on hands (see Fig 10.6C) When about to be pulled to sitting position, lifts head Sits in highchair with back straight Rolls from back to abdomen* When held in standing position, bears almost all of weight Hand regard absent	Resecures a dropped object Drops one cube when another is given Grasps and manipulates small objects Holds bottle Grasps feet and pulls to mouth	Adjusts posture to see object Prefers more complex visual stimuli Can localise sounds made above ear Will turn head to side, then look up or down	Begins to imitate sounds* Babbling resembles one-syllable utterances—*ma, mu, da, di, hi** Vocalises to toys, mirror image Takes pleasure in hearing own sounds (self-reinforcement)	Recognises parents; begins to fear strangers Holds arms out to be picked up Has definite likes and dislikes Begins to imitate (cough, protrusion of tongue) Excites on hearing footsteps Laughs when head is hidden in towel Briefly searches for dropped object (object permanence beginning)* Frequent mood swings from crying to laughing with little or no provocation

Continued

TABLE 10.2 **Growth and Development During Infancy—cont'd**

Age (Months)	Physical	Gross Motor	Fine Motor	Sensory	Vocalisation	Socialisation/ Cognition
7	Eruption of upper central incisors Parachute reflex appears (see Fig 10.1)	When supine, spontaneously lifts head off surface Sits, leaning forwards on both hands (see Fig 10.7D)* When prone, bears weight on one hand Sits erect momentarily Bears full weight on feet (see Fig 10.8A) When held in standing position, bounces actively	Transfers objects from one hand to other (see Fig 10.7E)* Has unidextrous approach and grasp Holds two cubes more than momentarily Bangs cubes on table Rakes at small object	Can fixate on very small objects* Responds to own name Localises sound by turning head in curving arch Beginning awareness of depth and space Has taste preferences	Produces vowel sounds and chained syllables—*baba, dada, kaka** Vocalises four distinct vowel sounds 'Talks' when others are talking	Increasing fear of strangers; shows signs of fretfulness when parent disappears* Imitates simple acts and noises Tries to attract attention by coughing or snorting Plays peek-a-boo Demonstrates dislike of food by keeping lips closed Exhibits oral aggressiveness in biting and mouthing Demonstrates expectation in response to repetition of stimuli
8	Begins to show regular patterns in bladder and bowel elimination	Sits steadily unsupported (see Fig 10.7E)* Readily bears weight on legs when supported; may stand holding onto furniture Adjusts posture to reach object	Has beginning pincer grasp using index, fourth and fifth fingers against lower part of thumb Releases objects at will Rings bell purposely Retains two cubes while regarding third cube Secures object by pulling on string Reaches persistently for toys out of reach		Makes consonant sounds *t, d, w* Listens selectively to familiar words Utterances signal emphasis and emotion Combines syllables, such as *dada*, but does not ascribe meaning to them	Exhibits increasing anxiety over loss of parent, particularly mother, and fear of strangers Responds to word 'no' Dislikes dressing, nappy change
9	Eruption of upper lateral incisor may begin	Creeps on hands and knees Sits steadily on floor for prolonged time (10 min) Recovers balance when leaning forwards but cannot do so when leaning sideways Pulls self to standing position and stands holding onto furniture (see Fig 10.8 B and C)*	Uses thumb and index finger in crude pincer grasp (see Fig 10.3)* Grasps third cube Compares two cubes by bringing them together	Localises sounds by turning head diagonally and directly towards sound Depth perception increasing	Responds to simple verbal commands Comprehends 'no-no'	Parent (mother) is increasingly important for own sake Shows increasing interest in pleasing parent Begins to show fears of going to bed and being left alone Puts arms in front of face to avoid having it washed

10	Labyrinth-righting reflex strongest when infant in prone or supine position; is able to raise head	Can change from prone to sitting position Stands while holding onto furniture, sits by falling down Recovers balance easily while sitting While standing, lifts one foot to take step (see Fig 10.8D)	Crude release of an object beginning Grasps bell by handle		Says 'dada' and/or 'mumma' with meaning* Comprehends 'bye-bye' May say one word (e.g. 'hi', 'bye', 'no')	Inhibits behaviour to verbal command of 'no-no' or own name Imitates facial expressions; waves bye-bye Extends toy to another person but will not release it Develops object permanence* Repeats actions that attract attention and cause laughter Pulls clothes of another to attract attention Plays interactive games such as pat-a-cake Reacts to adult anger; cries when scolded Demonstrates independence in dressing, feeding, locomotive skills and testing of parents Looks at and follows picture in book
11	Eruption of lower lateral incisor may begin	When sitting, pivots to reach towards back to pick up an object Cruises or walks holding onto furniture or with both hands held*	Explores objects more thoroughly (e.g. clapper inside bell) Has neat pincer grasp Drops object deliberately for it to be picked up Puts one object after another into container (sequential play) Able to manipulate object to remove it from tight-fitting enclosure		Imitates definite speech sounds	Experiences joy and satisfaction when task is mastered Reacts to restrictions with frustration Rolls ball to another on request Anticipates body gestures when familiar nursery rhyme or story is being told (e.g. holds toes and feet in response to 'This little piggy went to market') Plays games up-down, 'so big', or peek-a-boo Shakes head for 'no'

Continued

TABLE 10.2 **Growth and Development During Infancy—cont'd**

Age (Months)	Physical	Gross Motor	Fine Motor	Sensory	Vocalisation	Socialisation/ Cognition
12	Birth weight tripled* Birth length increased by 50%* Head and chest circumference equal (head circumference 46 cm) Has six to eight deciduous teeth Anterior fontanel almost closed Landau reflex fading Babinski's reflex disappears Lumbar curve develops; lordosis evident during walking	Walks with one hand held* Cruises well May attempt to stand alone momentarily; may attempt first step alone* Can sit down from standing position without help	Releases cube in cup Attempts to build two-block tower but fails Tries to insert pellet into narrow-necked bottle but fails Can turn pages in book, many at a time	Discriminates simple geometrical forms (e.g. circle) Amblyopia may develop with lack of binocularity Can follow rapidly moving object Controls and adjusts response to sound; listens for sound to recur	Says three to five words besides 'dada', 'mumma'* Comprehends meaning of several words (comprehension always precedes verbalisation) Recognises objects by name Imitates animal sounds Understands simple verbal commands (e.g. 'Give it to me', 'Show me your eyes')	Shows emotions such as jealousy, affection (may give hug or kiss on request), anger, fear Enjoys familiar surroundings and explores away from parent Is fearful in strange situation; clings to parent May develop habit of 'security blanket' or favourite toy Has increasing determination to practise locomotor skills Searches for object even if it has not been hidden, but searches only where object was last seen*

*Milestones that represent essential integrative aspects of development that lay the foundation for the achievement of more advanced skills.
†Degree of visual acuity varies according to vision measurement procedure used.

parents hold the child away from their face, the infant can observe while maintaining close physical contact.

A number of factors influence the intensity of a child's stranger fears.

- **Gender, age and size of the stranger**—Female, younger age and smaller size (including kneeling or sitting rather than standing) are less stressful.
- **Approach**—Loud, sudden, intrusive approach causes more distress.
- **Child's proximity to parent**—Being closer to parent (on parent's lap rather than in infant seat) is less stressful.

Consequently, the best approach for the stranger (including the nurse) is to talk softly; meet the child at eye level (to appear smaller); maintain a safe distance from the infant; and avoid sudden, intrusive gestures, such as holding the arms out and smiling broadly.

Parents also may wonder whether they should encourage the child's clinging, dependent behaviour, especially if there is pressure from others who view this as spoiling the child (see following discussion). Parents need reassurance that such behaviour is healthy, desirable and necessary for the child's optimum emotional development. If parents can reassure the infant of their presence, the infant will learn to realise that they are still there even if not physically present. Techniques to reassure infants of the parent's continued presence include talking to infants when leaving the room, allowing them to hear one's voice on the telephone and using transitional objects (e.g. a favourite blanket or toy).

This is no less trying, but a necessary time for infants because parents cannot always be with them. An excellent example of necessary separation is bedtime. Fear of going to bed or being left alone in the dark commonly occurs during the second half of the first year. Fear at bedtime is only one of the many bedtime problems that can occur in young children (see Chapter 11).

Limit Setting and Discipline

As infants' motor skills advance and mobility increases, parents are faced with the need to set safe limits (see Safety Promotion and Injury Prevention later in this chapter). Babies under 12 months of age should not have discipline as they require a warm nurturing environment to promote security. Toddlers do not yet understand consequences or have the skills to change behaviour, so distraction and only introducing one new lesson at a time works best in this age group (Government of South Australia 2015).

Parents must recognise the infant's cognitive and behavioural limitations and implement adequate protection from hazards because infants and toddlers do not understand a cause-and-effect relationship between dangerous objects and physical harm. Additionally, parents may need reassurance that their infant's behaviour is exploratory, not oppositional (at this age) and primarily centred on needs for warmth, love, food, security and comfort. Parents may verbalise that comforting the infant too much or meeting his or her needs will result in a spoiled child; there is no evidence that meeting the infant's basic needs will result in such behaviours later in life. Children will innately test limits and explore during the exploratory phase of growth; instead of discouraging exploration, parents should provide safe alternatives, put away dangerous household items and give children consistent messages and nurturing. Effective teaching for injury prevention optimally begins in infancy by helping parents understand their child's normal development. It must be reiterated continually that infants cry because a need is not being met, not to intentionally irritate an adult. The fussy or irritable infant is a potential victim of traumatic brain injury or **shaken baby syndrome*** (or other bodily harm) because adults and caretakers may not understand the nature of the infant's crying (see also Chapter 11, Colic).

A common concern of parents is that too much attention can spoil a child. Many of the recommendations for promoting attachment, such as attending to the infant's needs to establish trust, accepting fear of strangers and separation from parent, and holding and rocking the crying child, are described by parents as methods of spoiling. However, research on parents' response to crying during early infancy does not support the contention that picking up a crying baby leads to spoiling. Ainsworth (1982) found that the amount an infant cried during the first 3 months had no correlation with the frequency of crying during the rest of the first year. However, the degree of maternal responsiveness to crying did. Parents who were less responsive, such as not picking up the infant immediately on crying, had infants who cried more than those of parents who responded promptly to crying. Parents of colicky infants less than 3 months old who responded to the crying with increased attention successfully decreased the overall crying time.

If too much attention does not cause spoiling in early infancy, parents need to understand what 'spoiling' really is and how it differs from normal behaviour that may mimic aspects of spoiling. The **spoiled child syndrome** has been defined as 'excessive self-centred and immature behaviour, resulting from the failure of parents to enforce consistent, age-appropriate limits' (McIntosh 1989). Spoiled children demand to have their own way; are inconsiderate of others; and have intrusive, obstructive and manipulative behaviour. Indulging children, when combined with clear expectations and limits, does not cause spoiling. However, indulgence with failure to provide guidelines for acceptable behaviour can result in a child who expects to get her or his way all the time. Such expectations are unrealistic and do not help the child in the transition to older childhood, adolescence and adulthood.

Several age-related normal behaviours and child characteristics can be mistaken for evidence of spoiling:

- crying during early infancy that may or may not be associated with colic
- crying associated with unmet basic physical need (e.g. soiled nappy, hunger, physical contact)
- toddler behaviours such as negativism, persistent exploration and temper tantrums
- children experiencing extreme stress from marital discord; physical, emotional or sexual abuse; substance abuse; or mental illness in a parent.

With anticipatory guidance regarding expected but challenging behaviours and situations that may produce extreme stress in children, parents should feel comfortable in loving their infant without fear of spoiling. However, as the infant gets older, parents may need assistance in managing normal, disruptive behaviours, such as temper tantrums, from becoming problems.

Alternative Child Care Arrangements

For many parents, especially working mothers, locating safe and competent childcare facilities for the infant is a challenge—one that is compounded by the number of mothers working outside the home. Over the past 40 years a marked shift has occurred in childcare arrangements, with fewer children cared for at home and more children cared for in group centres or other settings.

Types of Child Care. The basic types of care are in-home care, either in the parents' or caregivers' home (home-based care); and centre-based

*Resource for parents and health care professionals include the Children's Hospital at Westmead's Shaken Baby information (https://kidshealth.schn.health.nsw.gov.au/node/617); KidsHealth New Zealand's Never Ever Shake a Baby (https://www.kidshealth.org.nz/never-ever-shake-baby); and the United States' National Center on Shaken Baby Syndrome and the Period of Purple Crying Program (http://www.dontshake.org).

care, usually in a day care centre. In-home care may consist of a relative or friend who minds the child, or a full-time babysitter who lives in the home, a full-time babysitter who comes to the home or cooperative arrangements such as exchange babysitting. Family day care is where an approved carer provides care in the carer's own home. An approved family day care home typically provides care and protection for up to seven children for part of a day. The seven children include the family day care provider's own children younger than 13 years of age living in the home, but no more than four children are allowed to be preschool age or younger (Department of Social Services [DSS] 2013).

Child centre-based care usually refers to a licensed day care facility that provides care for seven or more children for 6 or more hours a day, although they may also provide occasional and respite care. Work-based group care is another option that is becoming increasingly popular as employers recognise the benefit of providing high-quality and convenient childcare to their employees. Sick-child care may also be available for times when the child is ill. Such programs are often located in community hospitals or in work settings.

Guiding Parents in Selecting Child Care. An important nursing responsibility is guiding parents in locating suitable facilities that have a well-qualified staff. State licensing agencies can help parents identify day care centres that accept children of specific age groups and are convenient to home and work. Their records are available to the public and provide reports from the health, safety and fire departments; periodic evaluations from the licensing agency; complaints filed against the centre; and qualification of the centre's employees. State-licensed programs are supposed to follow established standards, which represent the minimum requirements and safeguards. However, enforcement of the standards is sometimes inadequate. Early childhood programs may also belong to a voluntary accreditation system, the Australian Children's Education and Care Quality Authority (ACECQA); however, all childcare centres must follow the National Quality Standards (ACECQA 2018)* which serves as a model for optimum care. In New Zealand centres follow the licensing criteria and regulations for early childhood education (ECE, https://www.education.govt.nz). References from other parents are also helpful, provided they have investigated the centre carefully and have remained involved with the agency's activities.

Nurses play an important role in infection control and injury prevention. Not only can they advise parents on evaluating a centre's sanitary and safety practices, but they can also take an active part in educating staff in measures to minimise the transmission of infection and injury. Guidelines for nappy changing and toileting recommended by the National Health and Medical Research Council (NHMRC 2013b) include the following:

- personnel washing hands before and after the nappy-changing procedure, after cleaning the change table/mat and after toileting
- wearing disposable gloves on both hands when changing nappies (as well as washing hands as stated above)
- changing nappies as soon as they are soiled
- never rinsing reusable nappies, although faecal contents can be flushed down the toilet
- sending soiled reusable nappies or clothing home in a sealed plastic bag
- cleaning the nappy-changing surface properly with detergent and water after each use and using it only for this purpose
- using child-sized toilets or access to steps and modified toilet seats that provide easier maintenance
- cleaning toilets, seats, potty chairs and nappy-changing areas with detergent and water (if a surface is known to be contaminated then disinfectants can be used, but the area needs to be cleaned before being disinfected; bleach can be used after cleaning if blood spills are present).

Staying healthy preventing infectious diseases in early childhood education and care services (NHMRC 2013b) contains additional infection control guidelines regarding day care: hand hygiene; cleaning sleep equipment and toys; food handling, preparation and disposal; handling, storage and feeding of human milk; care of pets; and conditions or illnesses for which children should be kept out of day care to prevent the spread of illness. In addition, such centres should share information about nationally notifiable infectious diseases that could be communicated to the child or immediate family member (NHMRC 2013b).

Thumb Sucking and Use of Soother

Sucking is the infant's chief pleasure and may not be satisfied by breastfeeding or bottle-feeding. It is such a strong need that infants who are deprived of sucking, such as those with a cleft lip repair, will suck on their tongues. Some newborns are born with sucking blisters on their hands from in utero sucking activity.

Problems arise when parents are overly concerned about the sucking of the fingers, thumb or soother and attempt to restrain this natural tendency. Before giving advice, nurses should investigate the parents' feelings and base guidance on this information.

Soother use (a 'dummy'), particularly in the early days after birth and in the birth hospital, has gained considerable attention in the scientific literature. In the past, experts on breastfeeding recommended that healthcare workers not introduce soothers to breastfed infants unless the parent requested it; however, recent research has shown no effects on soother use and breastfeeding (see Research Focus box). Still, soother use should not replace actual feeding or suckling, and there should be an emphasis on allowing the infant to control the pace, frequency and termination of feeding rather than allowing the soother (or anything else) to become the focus of the interaction.

RESEARCH FOCUS

Soother Use and Breastfeeding

Jaafar and colleagues (2016) performed a meta-analysis on the effects of soother use on healthy full-term newborns whose mothers initiated breastfeeding and concluded that soother use did not adversely affect breastfeeding duration or exclusivity. Others found that restricting soother distribution at the birth hospital did not increase exclusive breastfeeding; instead, they noted a significant increase in the use of supplemental formula feedings in breastfed newborns and a concomitant decrease in the incidence of exclusive breastfeeding (Kair et al 2013).

Soother use has been associated with an increased risk of otitis media in several studies (Ilia & Galanakis 2013, Salah et al 2013). The American Academy of Pediatrics and American Academy of Family Physicians recommend using a soother during the first 6 months because of the benefit with regard to pain management during painful procedures and prevention of sudden infant death syndrome (SIDS), but they recommend that the child be weaned from the soother during the second 6 months of life (American Academy of Pediatrics, Task Force on Sudden Infant Death Syndrome 2016). Australian recommendations by the Red Nose National Scientific Advisory Group (NSAG)

*Information about accreditation criteria and procedures is available from the following: ACECQA (https://www.acecqa.gov.au, the Information for Families section), StartingBlocks.gov.au. Victoria State Government (https://www.education.vic.gov.au, How to choose the best childcare) and New Zealand Government (https://parents.education.govt.nz, Find an early learning service or school).

(2014) also support weaning in the second 6 months; however, they state that Australia and New Zealand have a more conservative approach compared to the United States in urging soother use for SIDS prevention. Non-nutritive sucking such as a soother during painful procedures in neonates has been shown to produce an analgesic effect.

If the child uses a soother, stress safety considerations in purchasing one. Note that soothers must follow the mandatory Australian Standards (AS 2432:1991 Standard for Babies' Dummies Product Safety Australia 2015). Caution parents against altering a soother, thus making it more dangerous (see Aspiration and Suffocation, Chapter 12). Soothers with added decorative gems or 'bling' may be dangerous because the infant or child may remove the decorative object and swallow it or aspirate it into the airway.

During infancy and early childhood there is no need to restrain non-nutritive sucking of the fingers. Malocclusion may occur if thumb sucking persists past approximately 4 years of age, or when the permanent teeth erupt. Some parents may perceive soothers as less damaging because they are discarded by 2 to 3 years of age, whereas thumb sucking may persist well into school-age years. Both soother use and thumb sucking may also have significant cultural variations. Thumb sucking reaches its peak at age 18 to 20 months and is most prevalent when the child is hungry, tired or feeling insecure. Persistent thumb sucking in a listless, apathetic child always warrants investigation. It may be a sign of an emotional problem between parent and child or of boredom, isolation and lack of stimulation.

There is recent evidence that soother use may improve non-nutritive sucking in preterm infants. A randomised control trial with 70 preterm infants found that infants who received a soother had significantly better sucking skills and shorter time to transition to full breastfeeding compared with a control group of preterm infants without soothers (Kaya & Aytekin 2017). Non-nutritive sucking should not be withheld from preterm infants.

Teething

One of the more difficult periods in the infant's (and parents') life is the eruption of the deciduous (primary) teeth, often referred to as teething. The age of tooth eruption shows considerable variation among children, but the order of their appearance is fairly regular and predictable (Fig 10.12). The first primary teeth to erupt are the lower central incisors, which appear at approximately 6 to 10 months of age (average 8 months). These are followed closely by the upper central incisors. The following is a quick guide to assessment of deciduous teeth during the first 2 years: Age of the child in months − 6 = Number of teeth For example, 8 months of age − 6 = 2 teeth at this time.

Teething is a physiological process. Some discomfort is common as the crown of the tooth breaks through the periodontal membrane. Some children show minimum evidence of teething, such as drooling, increased finger sucking or biting on hard objects. Others are irritable and have difficulty sleeping, mild temperature elevation, ear rubbing and decreased appetite for solid foods. Generally, signs of illness such as fever (> 39°C), vomiting or diarrhoea are not symptoms of teething but of illness and may warrant further investigation.

Because teething pain is a result of inflammation, cold is soothing. Giving the child a frozen teething ring or an ice cube wrapped in a washcloth helps relieve the inflammation. An active ingredient in some gels is lidocaine (lignocaine), which has been associated with seizures, death and a rare disorder called methaemoglobinaemia, and prompted a warning from the American Food and Drug Administration. Other commonly used gels may contain salicylates, which have been associated with Reye's Syndrome. Therefore, anaesthetic ointments should only be used under the direct advice and supervision of a healthcare provider (Department of Health Western Australia *n.d.). If persistent irritability affects sleeping and feeding, systemic analgesics such as paracetamol or ibuprofen (if *age appropriate*) can be given for no more than 3 days. However, parents should know that this is a temporary measure and should contact their practitioner if symptoms persist or if the child's condition changes.

PROMOTING OPTIMUM HEALTH DURING INFANCY

Nutrition

Ideally, discussion of optimum nutrition should begin prenatally with the decision to breastfeed or bottle-feed the newborn. The choice for either is highly individual and is discussed in Chapter 7. This section is primarily concerned with infant nutrition during the next 12 months, when growth needs and developmental milestones prepare the child for the introduction of solid foods.

Despite adequate availability of optimum nutrient sources, experts are concerned that infants are not fed appropriately. Infants may be given solid foods when their digestive system is not ready to completely absorb such foods. In addition, drinks that are inappropriate for growing infants may be given in place of enriched infant milk and may only provide 'empty' calories and contribute to childhood and adult cardiovascular disease or obesity and place the infant at risk for iron deficiency anaemia, vitamin D deficiency and rickets. A survey of differences in infant feeding practices between Australian-born and Chinese-born mothers in Australia (Bolton et al 2018) found that about 40% of infants of Chinese-born mothers and 47.5% of infants of Australian-born mothers had consumed food by 4 months of age, despite recommendations that such foods not be introduced until around 6 months of age (Netting et al 2017). There is evidence that early introduction of solid food before 4 months of life is correlated with the development of allergies (Netting et al 2017) and obesity later in life (Barrera et al 2016); however, there is no correlation between length of breastfeeding duration and obesity later in life (Barrera et al 2016, Redsell et al 2016).

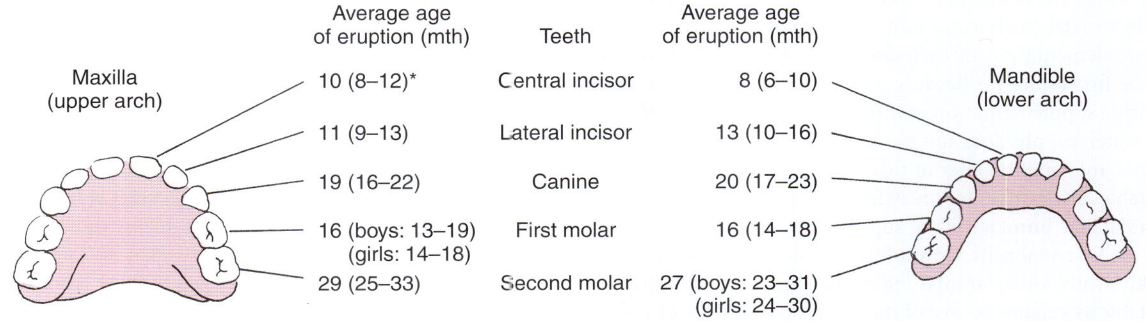

Fig 10.12 Sequence of eruption of primary teeth. *Range represents 1 standard deviation, or 67% of subjects studied. (Source: Data from American Dental Association. http://www.mouthhealthy.org/en/az-topics/e/eruption-charts)

Infant nutrition has a far-reaching, long-term impact on the child's life. Growth and development could be negatively affected, as could the risk of acquiring certain chronic health conditions. Nurses must be proactive in teaching parents what constitutes appropriate infant nutrition and nutritional habits, which provide the child with an optimum opportunity to grow and develop into a healthy child and adult.

The Australian Government produces Australian dietary guidelines (NHMRC 2013a) and infant feeding guidelines (NHMRC 2012) that give recommendations on infant and child feeding, diets and daily nutritional intakes. The New Zealand Ministry of Health has similar recommendations for infants and toddlers and for children and young people, both available on their HealthEd website (https://www.healthed.govt.nz).

The First 6 Months

Human milk is the most desirable complete diet for the infant during the first 6 months. Breastfeeding is rarely contraindicated; the main contraindications to breastfeeding include mothers who are HIV-positive; mothers taking illicit drugs such as heroin, cocaine, methamphetamines or phencyclidine (PCP or 'angel dust'); mothers taking antimetabolites or radioactive medications; and maternal illnesses such as T-cell leukaemia/lymphoma (Lawrence & Lawrence 2016). Although very few routinely prescribed drugs are hazardous to breastfeeding infants, experts recommend consulting with the healthcare provider to determine the benefits and hazards of certain maternal medications (Lawrence & Lawrence 2016).

The healthy term infant receiving breast milk from a well-nourished mother usually requires no specific vitamin and mineral supplements, with a few exceptions. Daily supplements of vitamin D and vitamin B_{12} may be indicated if the mother's intake of these vitamins is inadequate.

A consensus statement by Australian and New Zealand physicians (Munns et al 2006) acknowledged the risks of vitamin D deficiency in infants and children. Infants are at risk from maternal vitamin D deficiency, and older children from a variety of factors including dark skin colour, cultural practices, limited sun exposure and prolonged breastfeeding. Vitamin D supplements are recommended for at-risk children. Note that in Australia 90% of vitamin D comes from sunlight (Sydney Children's Hospital [SCH] 2015); however, care needs to be taken to avoid over-exposure. Babies under 6 months of age should have minimal sun block solution exposure as their skin is very absorbent, and parents should follow the sun safety measure as outlined by Australia's Cancer Council (https://www.cancer.org.au/) or New Zealand's Cancer Society (https://cancernz.org.nz).

Infants, whether breastfed or bottle-fed, do not require additional fluids, especially water or juice, during the first 4 months of life. Excessive intake of water in infants may result in water intoxication and hyponatraemia.

Substituting skim or low-fat milk is unacceptable because the essential fatty acids are inadequate and the solute concentration of protein and electrolytes, such as sodium, is too high.

Fluoride supplementation in exclusively breastfed children is not required for the first 6 months because of the risk of dental fluorosis. However, fluoride supplementation may be necessary if the breastfeeding mother's water supply does not contain the required amount of fluoridation (see information later in this chapter).

An acceptable alternative to breastfeeding is commercial iron-fortified formula. Like human milk, it supplies all nutrients needed by the infant for the first 6 months. Unmodified whole cow's milk, low-fat cow's milk, skim milk, other animal milks and imitation milk drinks are not acceptable as a major source of nutrition for infants because of their limited digestibility, increased risk of contamination and lack of components needed for appropriate growth. Whole milk can cause iron deficiency anaemia in infants, possibly as a result of occult gastrointestinal blood loss (Griebler et al 2015). Pasteurised whole cow's milk is deficient in iron, zinc and vitamin C and has a high renal solute load, which makes it undesirable for infants less than 12 months of age (NHMRC 2012). Dietary fat should not be restricted in infancy unless under medical supervision. Substituting skim or low-fat milk is unacceptable because the essential fatty acids are inadequate and the solute concentration of protein and electrolytes, such as sodium, is too high.

Honey should be avoided in the first 12 months because of the risk of infant botulism (see Chapter 34); soothers should not be coated with honey to encourage the infant to take it. Socialising the infant to food flavours of the family's culture is common in addition to continuing breastfeeding for 2 to 4 years (see Cultural Considerations box). The amount of formula per feeding and the number of feedings per day vary among infants.

CULTURAL CONSIDERATIONS

Multicultural Feeding Practices

Cultural beliefs and values often influence infant feeding practices. Healthcare professionals may benefit from understanding the multicultural feeding practices that parents choose for their infant. Traditional feeding practices include offering a variety of liquids or foods, such as sugared tea, water or honey, during the first few days of life and thereafter.

Employed mothers can continue breastfeeding with guidance and encouragement.* Encourage mothers to set realistic goals for employment and breastfeeding, with accurate information regarding the costs, risks and benefits of available feeding options. Barriers encountered by working breastfeeding mothers include lack of employer or co-worker support, unavailable or inadequate facilities for pumping and storing milk and insufficient time allowed during work time to pump. Many mothers may find that a program of breast-pumping when away from home and bottle-feeding the infant the expressed milk with or without formula supplementation is successful. Expressed breast milk may be stored in the refrigerator (4°C) but should be used within 48 hours (Parks et al 2016). Breast milk should never be thawed or rewarmed in a microwave oven (Parks et al 2016). To thaw the frozen milk, place the container under a lukewarm water bath (40.5°C), use a commercial breast milk warmer or place it in a refrigerator overnight.

The addition of solid foods before 4 to 6 months of age is not recommended. During the early months solid foods are not yet compatible with the ability of the gastrointestinal tract and the infant's nutritional needs. Despite the recommendations not to introduce food into the infant's diet until after 4 to 6 months, studies have found that many parents continue to introduce solid foods sometimes as early as 2 weeks of life (Koletzko et al 2014). Developmentally, infants are not ready for solid food. The extrusion (protrusion) reflex is strong and often causes food to be pushed out of the mouth. Infants instinctively suck when given food. Because of their limited motor abilities, infants are unable to deliberately push food away or avoid feeding.

Early introduction of solid food may also reduce the frequency of breastfeeding or cause eventual cessation of breastfeeding before 6 months of age (NHMRC 2012). Caution parents concerning the excessive use of juices and non-nutritive drinks such as fruit-flavoured drinks or carbonated beverages ('soft drinks') during this period. Many juices

*See also *Breastfeeding & work: your rights at work*, which includes information for breastfeeding in the workplace. This guide can be downloaded at https://www.breastfeeding.asn.au/

and non-nutritive drinks, although readily available to consumers, do not provide sufficient and appropriate caloric intake for infants less than 12 months of age. Such drinks may replace the nutrients in milk (formula) and lead to growth or health problems. Fruit juices are not required in the first 6 months; there are no studies demonstrating benefits of giving fruit juice to infants. Fruit juice drinks also contain sugar, which is not recommended to babies or children as it can lead to obesity and tooth decay in later childhood (Department of Health 2012).

The Second 6 Months

During the second half of the first year, human milk or formula continues to be the primary source of nutrition. Fluoride supplementation begins depending on the infant's intake of fluoridated tap water when mixing commercial formula. Breast milk remains the best source of nutrition well into the second half of the first year; however, if it is discontinued, a commercial iron-fortified formula should be substituted. Formulas specially marketed for older infants, or follow-on formulas, offer no advantages over other infant formulas; however, infant formulas are preferable in infants. The Australian and New Zealand Food Standard 2.9.1 (Australian Government 2016) outlines the composition of infant and follow-on formulas. Both formulas have the same energy, protein and fat minimum content but the maximum content is higher in follow-on formulas. Also, the renal threshold is higher in follow-on formulas, so a formula suited to the infant's age should be used.

Current recommendations from the Australian Infant Feeding Summit in 2015 (Netting et al 2017), based on an international consensus statement, include the early introduction (around 6 months) of allergenic foods (such as peanuts) for preventing food allergies and atopy in later childhood (see also Chapter 11, Food Sensitivity).

Selection and Introduction of Solid Foods

The choice of solid foods to introduce first is variable but should meet the reasons for feeding solids, such as supplying nutrients not found in formula or breast milk. Iron-fortified infant cereal (e.g. rice cereal) is generally introduced first because of its high iron content (7 mg/3 tbsp of prepared dry cereal). Commercially prepared ready-to-serve dry cereals for infants include rice, barley, oatmeal and high-protein cereals. Some of the commercial baby cereals are combined with fruit. These preparations have little nutritional benefit and are more expensive. There is no need to introduce foods slowly, and exposure to a variety of food is recommended to ensure adequate nutrient and energy intake (NHMRC 2012).

The order of introduction of other foods is arbitrary. Iron-rich foods are suggested initially, such as cereal, pureed meat, chicken, fish and cooked plain tofu. The NHMRC guidelines (2012) then suggest foods from each of the five food groups be included, such as vegetables, fruit and dairy products. The rate of introduction depends on the individual infant's tolerance to new foods.

The introduction of solid foods into the infant's diet at this age is essential for adequate growth as breast milk and formula do not provide enough nutrients and energy for the rapidly growing infant, although breast milk or formula feeding continue to be a major source of nutrients (NHMRC 2012). Portion sizes may vary according to the infant's needs. In general, 1 tbsp per year of age (i.e. ½ to ¾ tbsp for most infants under 12 months) is adequate for most infants. In most cases 2 tbsp may be served, but because of the infant's focus on the texture and feel of the food, smaller amounts than those served will be consumed. Another consideration for smaller portions is the concern over feeding habits in early childhood and obesity; early feeding of smaller portions may help prevent the 'clean your plate' or 'eat all your food or you can't get down from the table' concepts, which are known to contribute to overeating in later life. The addition of solids to the diet of exclusively breastfed infants has not been found to significantly increase overall caloric intake or weight gain.

In general, low-calorie milk and foods should not be used in infants and toddlers unless prescribed by a medical officer, such as a general practitioner or paediatrician. The infant's growth during this phase is crucial to future development, and dietary fat is essential for normal growth and development. At the same time it is important to recognise that ingestion of nutrient-poor but high fat, salt or sugar foods are not recommended for infants or children, such as fried potatoes, lollies, ice-cream, cake, soft drink and other sweetened drinks, and other such items do not constitute an appropriate fat intake and may contribute to childhood obesity. Suitable fats include fish, lean meat, nut spreads, oats, legumes, milk and cheese (NHMRC 2013a).

Preferably, home-prepared infant foods should be fresh or frozen because canned foods, except for those prepared for infants, may contain excessive sodium or sugar. Parents are cautioned to avoid reliance on food supplements marketed as iron- or vitamin-fortified as primary sources of minerals. Instead, encourage parents to offer the child a variety of fruits, vegetables and whole grains, including those known to be naturally rich in iron.

Weaning

Defined as the process of giving up one method of feeding for another, **weaning** usually refers to relinquishing the breast or bottle for other liquids and food. In Western societies this is generally regarded as a major task for infants and is often seen as a potentially traumatic experience. It is psychologically significant because the infant is required to give up a major source of oral pleasure and gratification.

Other cultural groups define weaning in relation to significant life events (e.g. teething) or reaching a specific age. No one time for weaning is best for every child, but generally most infants show signs of readiness during the second half of the first year. It is recommended that weaning occur with the infant's needs as a guide (Lawrence & Lawrence 2016). Infants learn that good things come from a spoon. Their increasing desire for freedom of movement may lessen their desire to be held close for feedings. They are acquiring more control over their actions and can easily manipulate a cup to their lips. Imitation becomes a powerful motivator by age 8 or 9 months, and they enjoy using a cup or glass like others do.

Weaning should be gradual by replacing one bottle-feeding or breastfeeding at a time. The night-time feeding is usually the last feeding to be discontinued. If weaning under 6 months of age, parents often feed their babies via a bottle, although some may use a transitional cup.

Sleep and Activity

Sleep patterns vary among infants, with active infants typically sleeping less than milder children. Generally by 3 months of age, most infants' sleep is 15 total hours with a nocturnal pattern of sleep that lasts from 9 to 11 hours and approximately three 1- to 2-hour naps during the day (Feigelman 2016). Consolidation of nocturnal sleep hours occurs during the first 12 months, with decreasing daytime sleep and increasing night-time sleep (approximately 11.7 hours) by 1 year of age. The number of naps per day varies, but infants may take one or two naps by the end of the first year. Daytime naps usually decline during the toddler years to no daytime naps by preschool age. Breastfed infants usually sleep for shorter periods, with more frequent waking, especially during the night, than do bottle-fed infants but fall asleep more quickly (Middlemiss et al 2015). Average total sleep for 4-week-old infants in this study was 14 hours. (For a discussion of sleep position and sleep problems, see Chapter 11.) Others have correlated frequent night-time awakenings in infants to boys, breastfeeding, having a difficult temperament and maternal depression; notably this review found an overall pattern of less frequent wakenings by 6 months of age (Middlemiss et al 2015).

Most infants are naturally active and need no encouragement to be mobile. Problems can arise when devices such as play yards, strollers, commercial swings and walkers are used excessively to limit the infant's naturally curious exploratory nature and activity or to be a 'sitter' while the parent is otherwise occupied. These items restrict movement and prevent infants from exploring and developing necessary gross motor skills. Contrary to popular belief, walkers do not enhance walking and coordination, and they are dangerous if tipped over or placed near the top of stairs, porches, decks, in-ground pools, open fireplaces and other hazardous surfaces.

Dental Health

Good dental hygiene begins with appropriate maternal dental health and counselling during early infancy regarding dietary intake for the promotion of optimal oral hygiene. Counsel parents early regarding feeding practices that increase the risk of poor dental health. Some of these, as previously mentioned, include avoiding propping the milk bottle or giving the milk bottle in the bed, and avoiding fruit juices in a bottle, especially before 6 months of age. These contribute to enamel erosion and **early childhood caries** (previously called *baby bottle tooth decay*).

Once the primary teeth erupt, cleaning should begin. Parents should clean the teeth and gums initially by wiping with a damp cloth; toothbrushing is too harsh for the tender gingiva. The caregiver can stabilise the infant by cradling him or her with one arm and using the free hand to cleanse the teeth. Oral hygiene can be made pleasant by singing or talking to the infant. It is recommended that the infant have a brief oral health examination by 6 months of age from a qualified health practitioner; infants at high risk for caries are identified and oral health counselling is implemented. In Australia parents are encouraged to check their child's mouth for early signs of dental caries. Oral health programs, such as 'Lift the Lip', educate parents about oral health in early childhood, including recognising signs of dental decay, how to examine the child's mouth and actions to promote good oral health (Ministry of Health New South Wales 2014). From 12 months of age a small soft toothbrush without toothpaste can be used on the child's teeth (Oral Health Monitoring Group 2015). Water is advised as a preferred tooth-cleaning solution, as the infant may swallow the toothpaste (and if the toothpaste is fluoridated, the infant may ingest excessive amounts of fluoride). The Australian early childhood oral health guideline (Ministry of Health New South Wales 2014, p. 17) recommends a 'small pea-size' of fluoridated toothpaste for children from 18 months of age to be used and children of any age should spit out after cleaning, not swallow the toothpaste or rinse their mouths after teeth cleaning. The Australian consensus guidelines on fluoride were used to develop the New Zealand guidelines, and they also recommend that low fluoride toothpaste (0.4–0.55 mg/g) be used for children 18 months to 5 years (inclusive), which can be increased to 1 mg/g for children aged 6 years and above (New Zealand Guidelines Group 2009).

Fluoride, an essential mineral for building caries-resistant teeth, is needed beginning at 6 months of age if the infant does not receive water with adequate fluoride content. Tap water should be used rather than bottled water as it contains fluoride, and fluoride supplements are not recommended for children (Ministry of Health New South Wales 2014). If parents believe that their water supply may lack fluoride, then they should seek medical advice about their child's fluoride intake.

Dietary considerations are also important because habits begun during infancy tend to continue into later years. Avoid foods with concentrated sugar (sucrose) in the infant's diet such as soft drinks, chocolates, biscuits, cakes and fruit juice. Parents need to be counselled regarding the detrimental effects of frequent and prolonged bottle-feeding or breastfeeding during sleep, when the milk or other fluid, such as juice, bathes the teeth, producing nursing caries. Babies should be transitioned to a cup for drinks after the age of 6 months to avoid dependency on bottles (Oral Health Monitoring Group 2015). The practice of coating soothers with honey or using commercially available hard-lolly soothers is discouraged. Besides being cariogenic, honey also may cause infant botulism, and parts of the lolly soother can be aspirated. (See Chapter 12 for a more extensive discussion of dental care, including early child caries and fluoride.)

Safety Promotion and Injury Prevention

Injuries are an important cause of death during infancy. In Australia, from 2015 to 2017 unintentional injuries (land transport accidents) were the leading cause of death in children ages 1 to 14 years, and accidental drownings and submersion were the fourth leading cause of death in this age group (Australian Institute for Health and Welfare [AIHW] 2021). The profile is different for New Zealand from 2012 to 2016, where injuries, unintentional and intentional, were the third and fourth leading causes of death (respectively) in infants under 12 months of age, and the second and fourth causes of death in the 1 to 4 years age group (McDonald et al 2018). Under 1 year of age and ages 1 to 4 years most deaths were due to 'transport' causes.

Falls are the leading cause of non-fatal injuries among infants in Australia (Mitchell et al 2018). Furniture, such as cots, highchairs, baby walkers, changing tables and bouncers, are commonly associated with infant falls (Vallmuur & Barker 2016). Constant vigilance, awareness and supervision are essential as children gain increased locomotor and manipulative skills that are coupled with an insatiable curiosity about the environment. Box 10.4 lists the major developmental achievements of each period during infancy and the appropriate injury prevention plan. Table 10.3 lists common types of injuries and associated objects that predispose to such injuries. Suggestions for promoting safety in the home environment are given for specific types of injuries. The acronym SAFE PAD, described in Table 10.3, may be used to identify common types of injuries to infants and older children.

Motor Vehicle Injuries

The use of infant and child safety seats in cars has dramatically reduced motor vehicle–related fatalities, up to 71% in infants younger than 1 year of age (Lee et al 2015). However, a significant number of infants are injured or die from improper restraint within vehicles, either inappropriate restraint or incorrect use of restraint. Australia has national child restraint laws, where it is mandatory for children to be restrained in the car (New South Wales [NSW] Centre for Road Safety 2019). The rules vary for the age of the child: babies (under 6 months) are to be in rear-facing seats; older children from 6 months to 4 years can be in rear or forward-facing child seats; and children 4 to 7 years can use booster seats. Children over the age of 7 years who are too small to be restrained by a seatbelt must use an approved booster seat. Although compliance rates are high (Brown et al 2010), the inappropriate use of the restraints, both in Australia (Brown et al 2010, Koppel et al 2013) and overseas (Bachman et al 2016, Greenwell 2015, Roynard et al 2014), is widespread; for example, incorrect size or insecure attachment of the restraint. There is a car restraint checking system available in Australia and families can take their vehicle with their installed car seat to a checking station for assessment and advice (refer to each state's road transport website for location of the nearest Authorised Restraint Fitting Station).

BOX 10.4 Injury Prevention During Infancy

Birth to 4 Months

Major developmental accomplishments

- Involuntary reflexes, such as the crawling reflex, may propel infant forwards or backwards; the startle reflex may cause the body to jerk.
- May roll over.
- Has increased eye-hand coordination and voluntary grasp reflex.

Injury Prevention

Aspiration

- This is not as great a danger to this age group, but parents should begin practising safeguarding early (see under 4 to 7 months).
- Hold infant for feeding; do not prop bottle.
- Know emergency procedures to relieve choking.
- Use soother with one-piece construction and loop handle.

Suffocation and Drowning

- Keep all plastic bags stored out of infant's reach; discard large plastic garment bags after tying in a knot.
- Do not cover mattress with plastic.
- Use firm mattress and loose blankets; no pillows.
- Make certain cot design follows federal regulations and mattress fits snugly—cot slats 6 cm apart.*
- Do not use drop-side cot. Obtain hardware to permanently secure older drop-side cots to avoid suffocation.
- Position cot away from other furniture and away from radiators.
- Do not tie soother on a string around infant's neck.
- Remove bibs at bedtime.
- Never leave infant alone in bath.
- Do not leave infant under 12 months alone on adult or youth mattress or 'beanbag' type pillows.
- Do not leave infant in a car.

Falls

- Use cot with fixed, raised rails.
- Never leave infant on a raised, unguarded surface.
- When in doubt as to where to place infant, use floor.
- Restrain infant in infant seat and never leave infant unattended while the seat is resting on a raised surface.
- Avoid using a highchair until infant can sit well with support.

Accidental Poisoning

- This is not as great a danger to this age group, but begin practising safeguards early (see under 4 to 7 months).

Burns

- Install smoke detectors in home.
- Avoid warming formula in microwave oven; always check temperature of liquid before feeding.
- Check bath water temperature.
- Do not pour hot liquids when infant is close by, such as sitting on lap.
- Beware of cigarette ashes that may fall on infant.
- Do not leave infant in sun for more than a few minutes; keep exposed areas covered.
- Wash flame-retardant clothes according to label directions.
- Use cool-mist vaporisers.
- Do not leave infant in parked car.
- Check surface heat of car restraint before placing infant in seat.

Motor Vehicles

- Transport infant in federally approved, rear-facing car seat, preferably in back seat.
- Do not place infant on seat of car or in lap.
- Do not place infant in a carriage or stroller behind a parked car.
- Do not place infant or child (in car seat) in front passenger seat with an air bag unless air bag is deactivated.

Bodily Damage

- Keep sharp, jagged objects out of infant's reach.
- Keep nappy pins closed and away from infant.

4 to 7 Months

Major Developmental Accomplishments

- Rolls over
- Sits momentarily
- Grasps and manipulates small objects
- Resecures a dropped object
- Has well-developed eye–hand coordination
- Can focus on and locate small objects
- Can push up on hands and knees
- Crawls backwards
- Places objects in mouth (hand-to-mouth)

Injury prevention

Aspiration

- Keep buttons, beads, syringe caps and other small objects out of infant's reach.
- Keep floor free of any small objects.
- Do not feed infant hard lollies, nuts, food with pits or seeds, or whole or circular pieces of hot dog.
- Exercise caution when giving teething biscuits because large chunks may be broken off and aspirated.
- Do not feed infant while he or she is lying down.
- Inspect toys for removable parts.

Suffocation

- Keep all latex balloons out of reach.
- Remove all cot toys that are strung across cot or play yard when infant begins to push up on hands or knees or is 5 months old.
- Use only cots with well secured cot sides; avoid use of drop-side cots.

Falls

- Restrain in a highchair.

Accidental poisoning

- Make sure that paint for furniture or toys does not contain lead.
- Place toxic substances on a high shelf or in locked cabinet.
- Keep medication vials and bottles locked in a secure place.
- Hang plants or place on high surface rather than on floor.
- Avoid storing large quantities of cleaning fluid, paints, pesticides and other toxic substances.
- Discard used containers of poisonous substances.
- Do not store toxic substances in food containers.
- Keep cosmetic and personal products out of infant's reach.
- Discard used button-size batteries; store new batteries in safe area.
- Know telephone number of local poison control centre.

Burns

- Ensure all taps are out of reach.
- Place hot objects (e.g. cigarettes, candles, incense) on high surface.
- Limit exposure to sun; apply sunscreen.

Motor Vehicles

- See under Birth to 4 Months

Continued

BOX 10.4 Injury Prevention During Infancy—cont'd

Bodily Damage

- Give toys that are smooth and rounded, preferably made of wood or plastic.
- Avoid long, pointed objects as toys.
- Avoid toys that are excessively loud.
- Keep sharp objects out of infant's reach.

8 to 12 Months

Major Developmental Accomplishments

- Crawls, creeps
- Stands holding onto furniture
- Stands alone
- Cruises around furniture
- Walks
- Climbs
- Pulls on objects
- Throws objects
- Picks up small objects; has pincer grasp
- Explores by putting objects in mouth
- Dislikes being restrained
- Explores away from parent
- Has increasing understanding of simple commands and phrases

Injury Prevention

Aspiration

- Keep lint and small objects off floor, off furniture and out of reach of infants.
- When feeding solid table food and only give very small pieces.
- Do not use beanbag toys or allow infant to play with small objects.
- See also under 4 to 7 months.

Suffocation and Drowning

- Keep doors of ovens, dishwashers, refrigerators, coolers and front-loading clothes washers and dryers closed at all times.
- If storing an unused appliance, such as a refrigerator, remove the door.
- Supervise contact with inflated balloons, immediately discard popped balloons and keep uninflated balloons out of reach.
- Fence area around swimming pools.
- Always supervise when near any source of water, such as cleaning buckets, drainage areas, toilets, ponds or other bodies of water within infant's access.
- Keep bathroom doors closed.
- Eliminate unnecessary pools of water.
- Keep one hand on infant at all times when in the bath.
- When swimming keep infant within arm's reach at all times.

Falls

- Avoid walkers, especially near stairs.
- Ensure that furniture is sturdy enough for infant to pull self to standing position and cruise.
- Fence stairways at top and bottom if infant has access to either end.

Accidental Poisoning

- Administer medications as a drug, not as a lolly.
- Avoid use of over-the-counter cough and cold preparations for infants.
- Replace medications and poisons immediately after use; replace caps properly if a child-protector cap is used.
- Keep phone number for poison control centre readily available.

Burns

- Place guards in front of or around any heating appliance, fireplace or furnace.
- Keep electrical wires hidden or out of reach.
- Place plastic guards over electrical outlets; place furniture in front of outlets.
- Keep hanging tablecloths out of reach (infant may pull down hot liquids or heavy or sharp objects).

*Information on many items such as cribs, cots or walkers is available from Product Safety Australia, https://www.productsafety.gov.au

All infants must be secured in approved Australian/New Zealand (AS/NZS) Standards restraint rather than held or placed on the seat of the car. There is no safe alternative. Infant restraints are designed either as an infant-only model or as a convertible infant-toddler model. Either restraint is a semireclined seat that faces the rear of the car. A rear-facing car seat provides the best protection for the disproportionately heavy head and weak neck of an infant (Fig 10.13). This position minimises the stress on the neck by spreading the forces of a frontal crash over the entire back, neck and head; the spine is supported by the back of the car seat. If the seat were faced forwards, the head would whip forwards because of the force of the crash, creating enormous stress on the neck. It is now recommended that all infants and toddlers ride in rear-facing car safety seats until they reach age 2 years or the weight recommended by the car seat manufacturer (NSW Centre for Road Safety 2019). Some infant-only rear-facing infant car safety seats can accommodate children weighing up to a maximum of 16 kg.

The restraint is anchored to the vehicle with the vehicle's seat belt, and the restraint has a harness system for securing the infant. Some harness systems require a clip to keep the shoulder straps correctly positioned. Vehicles manufactured after 1999 have tether straps that attach to anchors in the car seat to better secure the seat and minimise forward movement of the forward-facing convertible seats in the event of an accident. The Australian Standards allow for the ISOFIX anchorage system that has two lower attachment points to minimise movement between the car restraint and the seat belt clip (Australian Competition and Consumer Commission [ACCC] 2015).

Severe injuries and deaths in children have occurred from air bags deploying on impact in the front passenger seat. The back seat is the safest area of the car for children. For restraints to be effective, they must be used properly. Dressing the infant in an outfit with sleeves and legs allows the harness to hold the child securely in the seat. A small blanket or towel rolled tightly can be placed on either side of the head to minimise movement and keep the infant's hips against the back of the seat. Padding between the infant's legs and crotch is added to prevent slouching. Thick, soft padding is not placed under the infant or behind the back because during the impact, the padding will compress, leaving the harness straps loose. Preterm infants being discharged home from the hospital should be placed in appropriate car seat restraints as they would be placed in the car, and their heart rate and oxygen saturation should be monitored to detect any potential problems with airway occlusion.

Although there are child restraint laws, further safety practices are recommended by health experts and authorities. A height of at least 145 cm should be achieved plus a five-step safety test, regardless of the child's age, before using an adult seat belt, and babies and toddlers should be left in rear-facing seats as long as possible (NSW Centre for Road Safety 2019, The Royal Children's Hospital Melbourne 2019). In New Zealand a height of 148 cm is to be achieved before using an adult lap-sash seatbelt (Waka Kotahi NZ Transport Agency 2021).

TABLE 10.3 Common Infant Injuries, Associated Risk Factors and Safety Promotion

Safe Pad	Risk Factors	Suggested Safety Interventions
S—Suffocation, sleep position	Latex balloons	Avoid latex balloons except with close adult supervision.
	Plastic bags	Tie unused plastic bags in a knot and dispose of in a safe container.
	Bed surface (non-infant) such as sofa or adult bed	Avoid placing infants to sleep on sofas, soft bedding or adult bed.
	Pillows	Avoid use of pillows for sleep.
	Soft cushions and blankets	Clear bedding of soft cushions and blankets.
	Prone sleeping	Place infant to sleep on back at all times.
A—Asphyxia, animal bites	Food items: cylindrical items such as hot dogs, hard lollies, peanuts, almonds	Cut hot dogs lengthwise; avoid hard lollies in infants and toddlers. Infants should completely chew up each food item in mouth; do not feed more until item has been swallowed.
	Toys: small toys such as Legos	As a general rule of thumb, if the toy fits into a toilet paper cardboard roll, it can be swallowed by a small child.
	Small objects: batteries, buttons, beads, dried beans, syringe caps, safety pins	Keep out of reach of infants, who are naturally inquisitive.
	Soothers	Soothers should be one piece.
	Baby (talc) powder	Avoid shaking powder over infant; if used, place on adult's hand and then place on infant's skin.
	Domestic dogs, cats	Supervise child around domestic animals; teach not to approach dog that is eating, has puppies or is not feeling well. Animals that are 'tame' can be unpredictable. Small children are the right size for most domesticated animals to come face to face. Closely supervise child around visiting pets. (See Animal Bites, Chapter 32.)
	Window blind cords	Replace cords with rods or keep cords out of reach of children to avoid accidental strangulation.
F—Falls	Stairs	Infants like to climb; place childproof gate at top and bottom of stairs.
	Nappy-changing table	Infants do not have depth perception and cannot perceive a dangerous height from one that is safe. Never leave infants unattended on a flat surface even if not rolling over.
	Cot, bed-cot sides can fall when infant leans on them	In 2011 a mandate was made to stop selling drop-side infant cots because of safety problems with infants being trapped against a wall or mattress and asphyxiation or falling out of bed when the latches do not hold.*
	Infant carriers	Never leave infant unattended in a carrier on top of a surface such as a shopping cart, clothes dryer, washer, kitchen cabinet; place carrier on floor.
	Car seat restraints	Secure infant in car seat restraint securely and never leave unattended.
	Highchair	Restrain infant in highchair; avoid using highchair except for feeding and only if adult supervision is adequate; even restrained infants can squirm out of some restraints and fall.
	Infant walkers	Use only stationary walkers. There is no evidence that walkers help infants 'walk' any sooner. Wheeled walkers can easily be propelled off stairs and other platforms such as balconies or decks, causing significant injury.
	Windows, screens	Avoid placing furniture next to a window. Infants learn to climb and can fall out of open windows, even with screens.
	Television, stereos, sound systems	These must be secured to the stand; infants can pull the stand over, causing the TV or sound system to land on their heads, causing significant injury.
E—Electrical burns or burns	Electrical outlets	Place safety cap over electrical outlets; infants may be burned by placing conductive object into outlet.
	Irons, curlers	Keep out of reach of infant and keep turned off when not in use.
	Water	Infants may turn on tap in bathtub and burn self. Lower the water heater to a safe temperature of 49°C. Before placing infant in bath, check temperature of water and completely turn off tap so child cannot alter temperature of water. NEVER leave infant unattended in bath or sink of water.
	Fireplace	Place a childproof screen in front of fireplace.
	Stove, hot liquids	Keep top front burners off and keep pot handles turned towards back to avoid infant pulling hot pot onto self and causing burn injuries.
	Cigarettes	Avoid smoking and holding infant on lap while smoking cigar or cigarette.

Continued

TABLE 10.3 Common Infant Injuries, Associated Risk Factors and Safety Promotion—cont'd

Safe Pad	Risk Factors	Suggested Safety Interventions
P—Poisoning, ingestions	Medication, ointments, cream, lotions	Medications left in purses or handbags or on a tabletop can often be ingested by the curious infant. **Poisons Information Centre—Australia** Call this number if you think someone has taken an overdose, made an error with medicine or been poisoned. You can call 24 hours a day, 7 days a week from anywhere in Australia. **Telephone:** 131 126 **Website:** https://www.poisonsinfo.nsw.gov.au/ **National Poisons Centre—New Zealand** The National Poisons Centre has a **24-hour freephone 0800 764 766** that you can call to get help and information if you think you or a family member has been exposed to a poison. Don't take risks—call if you have any worries at all. Most things can be poisonous, depending on: • how much is taken • the age and size of the person • whether they're already ill • whether they're taking other medicines that might react.
	Plants: household plants may be a source of accidental poisoning	Keep plants out of child's reach (i.e. at least a metre above ground).
	Cleaning solutions and laundry pods	Store in locked cabinet or in top cabinet where there are no drawers or shelves for infant to climb on. Avoid storing cleaning and caustic solutions in containers such as a soft drink bottle or jar—infants and toddlers cannot differentiate a soft drink from a caustic drain cleaner.
	Inhalation or oral or nasal ingestion of poisonous or harmful chemicals such as methamphetamine, petrol, turpentine	Keep petrol and turpentine stored in a locked cabinet or cupboard out of child's reach. Avoid storing in containers that are also used to keep drinks or food.
A—Motor vehicle safety	Car or truck and hot weather	A motor vehicle–related hazard for infants is overheating (hyperthermia) and subsequent death when left in a vehicle in hot weather (> 26.4°C). Infants dissipate heat poorly, and an increase in body temperature may cause death in a few hours. Caution parents against leaving infants in a vehicle alone for *any reason.*
	Air bags	Avoid placing infant in a car restraint behind an air bag. Deactivate the air bag (available in certain models) or place the infant in the back seat in a proper car seat restraint.
	Car seat restraint	See discussion elsewhere in this chapter.
D—Drowning	Bathtub	NEVER leave infant unattended in bath, sink or pool of water.
	Swimming pools, birdbaths, decorative ponds of water, splash pads	Place fence around pools with gate lock that is out of child's reach. Supervise infants in water at ALL times; an infant may drown in as little as 5 cm of water. Swimming lessons are encouraged but are not foolproof for drowning; use touch supervision—keep child within arm's reach at all times while swimming.
	9 L or larger buckets	Keep buckets empty of water or elevated out of child's reach.

*A number of parent education resources, such as *A parent's guide to Kidsafe homes* and *A parent's guide to Kidsafe roads*, are available from Kidsafe Australia at https://www.kidsafensw.org/.

NURSING CARE CONSIDERATIONS

Rear-facing infant safety seats must NOT be placed in the front seats of cars equipped with an air bag on the passenger side. If an infant safety seat is placed in the passenger seat with an air bag, the child could be seriously injured if the air bag is released because rear-facing infant seats extend closer to the dashboard.

Nurse's Role in Injury Prevention

The task of injury prevention begins to be appreciated only when the potential environmental dangers to which infants are vulnerable are considered. Injury prevention and parent education should be handled on a growth and developmental basis. It is simply impossible to completely protect infants and small children from all potential dangers without placing them in a sterile, impractical environment. However, a large percentage of childhood deaths continue to occur as a result of preventable injuries (Kochanek et al 2016). Nurses must be aware of the possible causes of injury in each age group to provide anticipatory, preventive teaching. For example, the nurse should discuss guidelines for injury prevention during infancy (see Box 10.4) before the child reaches the susceptible age group. Preventive teaching ideally begins during pregnancy.

One-third of all injuries to children occur in the home, and therefore the importance of safety cannot be overemphasised. The Family-Centred Care box summarises a home safety checklist that can be presented to parents to increase their awareness of danger areas in the home and assist them in implementing safety devices and practices *before* their absence can inflict injury on infants. Hands-on displays such as cabinet latches or toilet seat locks can familiarise parents with inexpensive, commercial devices that can be used in the home to prevent injuries. Note that the Australia/New Zealand Standard AS/NZS 3500 requires the outlet of hot water (at the tap) in domestic homes to be less than 50°C, even though the hot water tank is set higher than this to prevent Legionella disease.

FAMILY-CENTRED CARE

Child Safety Home Checklist

Safety: Fire, Electrical, Burns

- ☐ Guards in front of or around any heating appliance, fireplace or gas heater
- ☐ Electrical wires hidden or out of reach
- ☐ No frayed or broken wires; no overloaded sockets
- ☐ Plastic guards or caps over electrical outlets; furniture in front of outlets
- ☐ Hanging tablecloths out of reach and away from open fires
- ☐ Smoke detectors tested and operating properly
- ☐ Kitchen matches stored out of child's reach
- ☐ Large, deep ashtrays throughout house (if used)
- ☐ Small stoves, heaters and other hot objects (e.g. cigarettes, candles, kettles, slow cookers) placed where they cannot be tipped over or reached by children
  - Pot handles turned towards back of stove, centre of table
  - No loose clothing worn near stove
  - No cooking or eating hot foods or liquids with child standing nearby or sitting in lap
- ☐ All small appliances, such as iron, turned off, disconnected and placed out of reach when not in use
- ☐ Cool, not hot, mist vaporiser used
- ☐ Fire extinguisher available on each floor and checked periodically
- ☐ Electrical fuse box and gas shutoff accessible
- ☐ Family escape plan in case of a fire practised periodically and have fire ready plans prepared
- ☐ Emergency telephone number in case of fire and address of home with nearest cross street posted near phone

Safety: Suffocation and Aspiration

- ☐ Small objects stored out of reach
- ☐ Toys inspected for small removable parts or long strings
- ☐ Hanging cot toys and mobiles placed out of reach
- ☐ Plastic bags stored away from young child's reach; large plastic garment bags discarded after tying in knots
- ☐ Mattress or pillow not covered with plastic or in manner accessible to child
- ☐ Household cot design according to Australian Standard AS/NZS 2172:2003 with snug-fitting mattress
- ☐ Cot positioned away from other furniture or windows
- ☐ Portable playpen gates up at all times while in use
- ☐ Accordion-style gates not used
- ☐ Bathroom doors kept closed and toilet seats down
- ☐ Taps turned off firmly
- ☐ Pool fenced with locked gate; fencing complies with local council guidelines and Australian Standard AS 1926.2 – 2012
- ☐ Proper safety equipment at poolside
- ☐ Electric garage door openers stored safely and garage door adjusted to rise when door strikes object
- ☐ Doors of ovens, trunks, dishwashers, refrigerators and front-loading clothes washers and dryers kept closed
- ☐ Unused appliance, such as a refrigerator, securely closed with lock or doors removed
- ☐ Food served in small, non-cylindrical pieces
- ☐ Toy chests without lids or with lids that securely lock in open position
- ☐ Buckets and wading pools kept empty when not in use
- ☐ Clothesline above head level
- ☐ At least one member of household trained in basic life support (cardiopulmonary resuscitation), including first aid for choking

Safety: Accidental Poisoning

- ☐ Toxic substances, including batteries, should be placed on a high shelf, preferably in locked cabinet
- ☐ Toxic plants hung or placed out of reach (i.e. over 1 metre from ground)
- ☐ Excess quantities of cleaning fluid, paints, pesticides, drugs and other toxic substances not stored in home
- ☐ Used containers of poisonous substances discarded where child cannot obtain access
- ☐ Telephone number of local poison control centre and address of home with nearest cross street posted near each phone
- ☐ Medicines clearly labelled in childproof containers and stored out of reach
- ☐ Household cleaners, disinfectants and insecticides kept in their original containers, separate from food and out of reach
- ☐ Cosmetics and personal use items kept out of child's reach.

Safety: Falls

- ☐ Non-skid mats, strips or surfaces in baths and showers
- ☐ Exits, halls and passageways in rooms kept clear of toys, furniture, boxes or other items that could be obstructive
- ☐ Stairs and hallways well lighted, with switches at both top and bottom of stairs
- ☐ Sturdy handrails for all steps and stairways
- ☐ Nothing stored on stairways
- ☐ Treads, risers and carpeting in good repair
- ☐ Glass doors and walls marked with decals
- ☐ Safety glass used in doors, windows and walls
- ☐ Gates on top and bottom of staircases and elevated areas, such as porches and balconies
- ☐ Guardrails on upstairs windows with locks that limit height of window opening and access to areas such as balconies
- ☐ Insect screens on windows higher than the ground floor should be solidly anchored and secured to prevent accidental misplacement and falls from the window
- ☐ Cot side rails raised to full height; mattress lowered as child grows
- ☐ Restraints used in high chairs, walkers or other baby furniture; preferably walkers not used
- ☐ Scatter rugs secured in place or used with non-skid backing
- ☐ Walks, patios and driveways in good repair

Safety: Bodily Injury

- ☐ Knives, power tools and unloaded firearms stored safely or placed in locked cabinet
- ☐ Garden tools returned to storage racks after use
- ☐ Pets properly restrained
- ☐ Swings, slides and other outdoor play equipment kept in safe condition
- ☐ Yard free of broken glass, nail-studded boards, other litter
- ☐ Cement birdbaths placed where young child cannot tip them over
- ☐ Cords of window blinds replaced by rods or placed out of reach of children to prevent accidental strangling

Anticipatory Guidance—Care of Families

Childrearing is no easy task; it presents challenges to both new and seasoned parents. With society's changing roles and mores, combined with a highly mobile population, traditional role models and time-honoured methods of raising children are declining. As a result, parents look to professionals for guidance. Nurses are in an advantageous position to render assistance and offer suggestions. Every phase of a child's life has its particular traumas—toilet training for toddlers, unexplained fears for preschoolers and identity crises for adolescents. For parents of an infant some challenges centre around dependency, discipline, increased mobility and safety. Major areas for parental guidance during the first year are listed in the Family-Centred Care box.

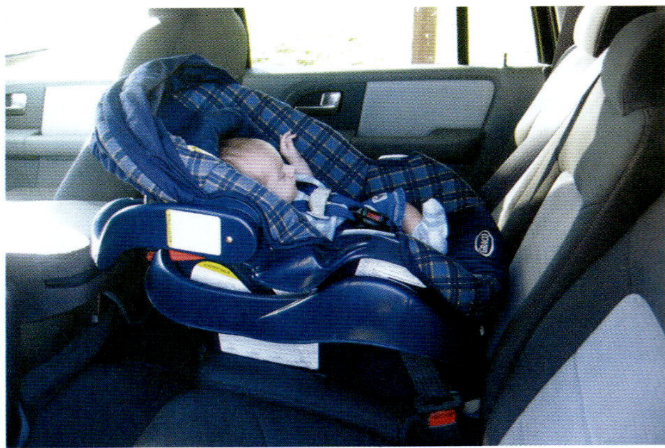

Fig 10.13 Rear-facing infant seat in rear seat of car. (Source: Courtesy Brian and Mayannyn Sallee, Las Vegas.)

FAMILY-CENTRED CARE

Guidance During Infant's First Year

Birth to 6 Months

- Teach parents about car safety with use of approved restraint, facing rearwards, in the middle of the back seat—not in a seat with an air bag.
- Understand each parent's adjustment to newborn, especially mother's postpartum emotional needs.
- Teach care of infant and help parents understand the infant's individual needs and temperament and that the infant expresses wants through crying.
- Reassure parents that infant cannot be spoiled by too much attention during the first 4 to 6 months.
- Encourage parents to establish a schedule that meets needs of infant and themselves.
- Help parents understand infant's need for stimulation in environment.
- Support parents' pleasure in seeing infant's growing friendliness and social response, especially smiling.
- Plan anticipatory guidance for safety.
- Stress need for immunisation.
- Prepare for introduction of solid foods.

6 to 12 Months

- Prepare parents for infant's 'stranger anxiety'.
- Encourage parents to allow infant to cling to them and avoid long separation from either parent.
- Guide parents concerning safety because of infant's increasing mobility.
- Advise parents that babies are too young for discipline and need warm, loving care to feel secure.
- Teach injury prevention because of infant's advancing motor skills and curiosity.
- Encourage parents to leave infant with suitable caregiver to allow some free time.
- Discuss readiness for weaning.
- Explore parents' feelings regarding infant's sleep patterns.

REFERENCES

Ainsworth, M. (1982). Early caregiving and later patterns of attachment. In M. Klaus & M. Robertson (Eds.), Birth, interaction, and attachment. Skillman, NJ: Johnson & Johnson Baby Products.

American Academy of Pediatrics, Task Force on Sudden Infant Death Syndrome. (2016). SIDS and other sleep-related infant deaths: Updated 2016 recommendations for a safe infant sleeping environment. Pediatrics, 138(5), e20162938.

Australian Children's Education and Care Quality Authority (ACECQA). (2018). Child care ratings. Schedule National quality standards. Education and Care Services National Regulations [2011-653]. https://www.startingblocks.gov.au/at-child-care/child-care-ratings/

Australian Competition and Consumer Commission (ACCC). (2015). Keeping Baby Safe. A Guide to Infant and Nursery Products. https://www.accc.gov.au/system/files/639_Keeping%20Baby%20Safe_text_FA4-WEB%20ONLY.pdf

Australian Government. (2016). Australian and New Zealand food Standard 2.9.1 (2016). https://www.legislation.gov.au/Details/F2017C00332

Australian Institute of Health and Welfare (AIHW). (2021). Deaths in Australia. https://www.aihw.gov.au

Bachman, S.L., Salzman G. A., Burke, R. V., et al. (2016). Observed child restraint misuse in a large, urban community: Results from three years of inspection events. Journal of Safety Research, 56, 17–22. Doi: http://dx.doi.org/10.1016/j.jsr.2015.11.005

Barrera, C. M., Perrine, C. G., Li, R., et al. (2016). Age at introduction to solid foods and child obesity at 6 years. Childhood Obesity (Print), 12(3), 188–192.

Beloglovsky, M., & Daly, L. (2015). Early learning theories made visible. St Paul, MN: Redleaf Press.

Bockting, W. (2016). Sexual identity development. In R. M. Kliegman, B. F. Stanton, J. W. St Geme, et al. (Eds.), Nelson textbook of pediatrics (20th ed.). Philadelphia: Elsevier/Saunders.

Bolton, K.A., Kremer, P., Hesketh, K., et al. (2018). Differences in infant feeding practices between Chinese-born and Australian-born mothers living in Australia: A cross-sectional study. BMC Pediatrics, 209. https://doi.org/10.1186/s12887-018-1157-0

Bowlby, J. (1969). Attachment and loss (Vol. 1). New York: Basic Books.

Bron, P.A., Kleerebezem, M., Brummer, R., et al. (2017). Can probiotics modulate human disease by impacting intestinal barrier function? British Journal of Nutrition, 117(1), 93–107. https://doi.org/10.1017/S0007114516004037

Brown, J., Hatfield, J., Du, W., et al. (2010). Population-level estimates of child restraint practices among children aged 0–12 years in NSW, Australia. Accident Analysis and Prevention, 42(6), 2144–2148.

Carey, W. B., & McDevitt, S. C. (1978). Revision of the infant temperament questionnaire. Pediatrics, 61(5), 735–739.

Department of Health. (2012). Health Eating and Physical Activity – Health Eating Guidelines – 6. Good drinks for babies and kids. Australian Government. https://www1.health.gov.au/internet/publications/publishing.nsf/Content/gug-indig-hb~drinks

Department of Health Western Australia (n.d.). Teething and your baby. https://www.healthywa.wa.gov.au/Articles/S_T/Teething-and-your-baby

Department of Social Services (DSS) (2013), Key obligations of a Family Day Care Service. Australian Government. https://www.dss.gov.au/sites/default/files/documents/05_2015/key_obligations_of_a_fdc_service.pdf

Dunford, E., Louie, J., Byrne, C. et al. (2015). The nutritional profile of baby and toddler food products sold in Australian supermarkets. Maternal and Child Health Journal, 19(12), 2598–2604.

Erikson, E. (1963). Childhood and society. New York: WW Norton.

Feigelman, S. (2016). The first year. In R. M. Kliegman, B. F. Stanton, J. W. St Geme, et al. (Eds.), Nelson textbook of pediatrics (20th ed.). Philadelphia: Elsevier/Saunders.

Gallitto, E. (2015). Temperament as a moderator of the effects of parenting on children's behavior. Development and Psychopathology, 27(3), 757–773.

Gartstein, M. A., & Rothbart, M. K. (2003). Studying infant temperament via the Revised Infant Behavior Questionnaire. Infant Behavior and Development, 26(1), 64–86.

Greenwell, N. K. (2015). Results of the national child restraint use special study. (Report No. DOT HS 812 142). May, Washington, DC: National Highway Traffic Safety Administration.

Griebler, U., Bruckmüller, M., Kien, C., et al. (2015). Health effects of cow's milk consumption in infants up to 3 years of age: A systematic review and meta-analysis. Public Health and Nutrition, 19(2), 293-307. https://doi.org/10.1017/S1368980015001354

Ilia, S., & Galanakis, E. (2013). Clinical features and outcomes of acute otitis media in early infancy. International Journal of Infectious Diseases, 17(5), e317–e320.

Jaafar, S. H., Ho, J. J., Jahanafar, S., et al. (2016). Effect of restricted pacifier use in breastfeeding term infants for increasing duration of breastfeeding. Cochrane Database of Systematic Review, (8), CD007202.

Kair, L. R., Kenron, D., Etheredge, K., et al. (2013). Pacifier restriction and exclusive breastfeeding. Pediatrics, 131(4), e1101–e1107.

Kaya, V., & Aytekin, A. (2017). Effects of pacifier use on transition to full breastfeeding and sucking skills in preterm infants: A randomised controlled trial. Journal of Clinical Nursing, 26(13–14), 2055–2063.

Khan, S., & Orenstein, S. R. (2016). The esophagus. In R. M. Kliegman, B. F. Stanton, J. W. St Geme, et al. (Eds.), Nelson textbook of pediatrics (20th ed.). Philadelphia: Elsevier/Saunders.

Kochanek, K. D., Murphy, S. L., Xu, J., et al. (2016). Deaths: Final data for 2014. National Vital Statistics Reports: From the Centers for Disease Control and Prevention, National Center for Health Statistics, National Vital Statistics System, 64(4), 1–122.

Koletzko, B., Poindexter, B., & Uauy, R. (2014). Nutritional Care of Preterm Infants: Scientific Basis and Practical Guidelines. World Review of Nutrition and Dietetics, 4–10. https://doi.org/10.1159/000358453

Koppel, S., Charlton, J. L. & Rudin-Brown, C. M. (2013). The Impact of New Legislation on Child Restraint System (CRS) Misuse and Inappropriate Use in Australia. Traffic Injury Prevention, 14(4), 387–396.

Lau, C. (2015). Development of suck and swallow mechanisms in infants. Annals of Nutrition and Metabolism, 66(suppl5), 7–14.

Lawrence, R. A., & Lawrence, R. M. (2016). Breastfeeding: a guide for the medical profession (8th ed.). Philadelphia: Elsevier.

Lee, L. K., Farrell, C. A., & Mannix, R. (2015). Restraint use in motor vehicle crash fatalities in children 0 year to 9 years old. The Journal of Trauma and Acute Care Surgery, 79, S55–S60.

Lindower, J.B. (2017). Water balance in the fetus and neonate. Seminars in Fetal and Neonatal Medicine, 22(2), 71–75. http://dx.doi.org/10.1016/j.siny.2017.01.002

Liu, Y., Chai, J, Mccoy, D. C., et al. (2017). Maternal depressive symptoms and early childhood cognitive development: A meta-analysis. Psychological Medicine, 47(4), 680–689. https://doi.org/10.1017/S003329171600283X

Logan, R.M. & Dormire, S. (2018). Finding My Way: A phenomenology of fathering in the NICU. Advances in Neonatal Care, 18(2), 154–162. https://doi.org/10.1097/ANC.0000000000000471

McDonald, G. K., Chalmers, S. H., Hii, J., et al. (New Zealand Mortality Review Data Group). 2018. Child and Youth Mortality Review Committee 13th data report 2012–16, p. 20. University of Otago. https://www.hqsc.govt.nz/assets/CYMRC/Publications/CYMRC-13th-data-report-FINAL-Apr-2018.pdf

McIntosh, B. (1989). Spoiled child syndrome. Pediatrics, 83(1), 108–114.

Medoff-Cooper, B., Carey, W. B., & McDevitt, S. C. (1993). The Early Infancy Temperament Questionnaire. Journal of Developmental and Behavioral Pediatrics, 14(4), 230–231.

Middlemiss, S., Yaure, R., & Huey, E. (2015). Translating research-based knowledge about infant sleep into practice. Journal of the American Association of Nurse Practitioners, 27(6), 328–337.

Ministry of Health New South Wales. (2014) Centre for Oral Health Strategy: Early Childhood Oral Health Guidelines for Child Health professionals, 3rd ed, pp. 11–15. SHPN: (COHS) 140370 ISBN: 978-1-74187-066-4 https://www1.health.nsw.gov.au/pds/ActivePDSDocuments/GL2014_020.pdf

Mitchell, R., Curtis, K., & Foster, K. (2018). A 10-year review of child injury hospitalisations, health outcomes and treatment costs in Australia. Injury Prevention, 24(5), 344–350.

Munns, C., Zacharin, M. R., Rodda, C. P., et al. (2006). Prevention and treatment of infant and childhood vitamin D deficiency in Australia and New Zealand: a consensus statement. Medical Journal of Australia, 185(5), 268–272.

National Health and Medical Research Council (NHMRC). (2013a). Australian dietary guidelines. Canberra: NHMRC. https://www.eatforhealth.gov.au

National Health and Medical Research Council (NHMRC). (2013b). Staying healthy preventing infectious diseases in early childhood education and care services [updated 5th edn.], pp. 52–55. Canberra: NHMRC. https://www.nhmrc.gov.au

National Health and Medical Research Council (NHMRC). (2012). Infant Feeding Guidelines: Summary. Canberra: National Health and Medical Research Council. https://www.eatforhealth.gov.au/

Netting, M., Campbell, D., Koplin, J., et al. (2017). An Australian consensus on infant feeding guidelines to prevent food allergy: outcomes from the Australian Infant Feeding Summit. The Journal of Allergy and Clinical Immunology: In Practice, 5(6), 1617–1624. http://dx.doi.org/10.1016/j.jaip.2017.03.013

New Zealand Guidelines Group. (2009). Guidelines for the use of fluorides. Summary. New Zealand Ministry of Health. Wellington. https://www.health.govt.nz/publication/guidelines-use-fluorides

Newburg, D. S., & He Y. (2015). Neonatal Gut Microbiota and Human Milk Glycans Cooperate to Attenuate Infection and Inflammation. Clinical Obstetrics & Gynecology, 58(4), 814–826. https://doi.org/10.1097/GRF.0000000000000156

New South Wales (NSW) Centre for Road Safety. (2019). Child care seats. https://roadsafety.transport.nsw.gov.au/stayingsafe/children/childcarseats/index.html

Oral Health Monitoring Group. (2015). Healthy Mouths, Healthy Lives: Australia's National Oral Health Plan 2015–2024. COAG Health Council. South Australian Dental Service: Adelaide. http://www.coaghealthcouncil.gov.au/

Parks, E. P., Shaikhkhalil, A., Groleau, V., et al. (2016). Feeding healthy infants, children, and adolescents. In R. M. Kliegman, B. F. Stanton, J. W. St Geme, et al. (Eds.), Nelson textbook of pediatrics (20th ed.). Philadelphia: Elsevier/Saunders.

Piaget, J. (1952). The origins of intelligence in children. New York: International University Press.

Product Safety Australia. (2015). Baby dummies. Australian Competition and Consumer Commission. https://www.productsafety.gov.au/standards/baby-dummies-and-dummy-chains

Red Nose. National Scientific Advisory Group (NSAG). (2014). Information Statement: Using a dummy or pacifier. Melbourne, Red Nose. https://rednose.org.au/article/using-a-dummy-or-pacifier

Redsell, S. A., Edmonds, B., Swift, J. A., et al. (2016). Systematic review of randomised controlled trials of interventions that aim to reduce the risk, either directly or indirectly, of overweight and obesity in infancy and early childhood. Maternal and Child Nutrition, 12(1), 24–38.

Robertson, J. (1953). Some responses of young children to loss of maternal care. Nursing Care, 49, 382–386.

Roynard, M., Silverans, P., Casteels, Y., et al. (2014). National roadside survey of child restraint system use in Belgium. Accident Analysis and Prevention, 62(C), 369–376. https://doi.org/10.1016/j.aap.2013.08.021

Salah, M., Abdel-Aziz, M., Al-Farok, A., et al. (2013). Recurrent acute otitis media in infants: Analysis of risk factors. International Journal of Pediatric Otorhinolaryngology, 77(10), 1665–1669.

Spitz, R. A. (1945). Hospitalism: an inquiry into the genesis of psychiatric conditioning in early childhood. In O. Fenichel, P. Greenacre, & H. Hartmann (Eds.), Psychoanalytic studies of the child (Vol. 1). New York: International University Press.

Sydney Children's Hospital (SCH). (2015). Vitamin D therapy – SCH practice guideline. Guideline No: 0/C/15:7004-01:00. http://www.schn.health.nsw.gov.au/_policies/pdf/2015-7004.pdf

Turck, D., Michaelsen, K. F., Shamir, R., et al. (2013). World Health Organization 2006 child growth standards and 2007 growth reference charts: A discussion paper by the committee on nutrition of the European Society for Pediatric Gastroenterology, Hepatology, and Nutrition. Journal of Pediatric Gastroenterology and Nutrition, 57(2), 258–264.

Vallmuur, K., & Barker, R. (2016). Infant product-related injuries: Comparing specialized injury surveillance and routine emergency department data. Australian and New Zealand Journal of Public Health, 40, 37–42.

Visscher, M. O., Adam, R., Brink, S., et al. (2015). Newborn infant skin: Physiology, development, and care. Clinics in Dermatology, 33(3), 271–280. https://doi.org/10.1016/j.clindermatol.2014.12.003

Waka Kotahi NZ Transport Agency. (2021). Requirements for using child restraints in New Zealand. https://www.nzta.govt.nz/safety/what-waka-kotahi-is-doing/education-initiatives/child-restraints/using-child-restraints-in-new-zealand/

World Health Organization (WHO). (2020). The WHO child growth standards. https://www.who.int/childgrowth/standards/en/

Zeanah, C. H., & Gleason, M. M. (2015). Attachment disorders in early childhood—clinical presentation, causes, correlates, and treatment. Journal of Child Psychology and Psychiatry, and Allied Disciplines, 56(3), 207–222.

11

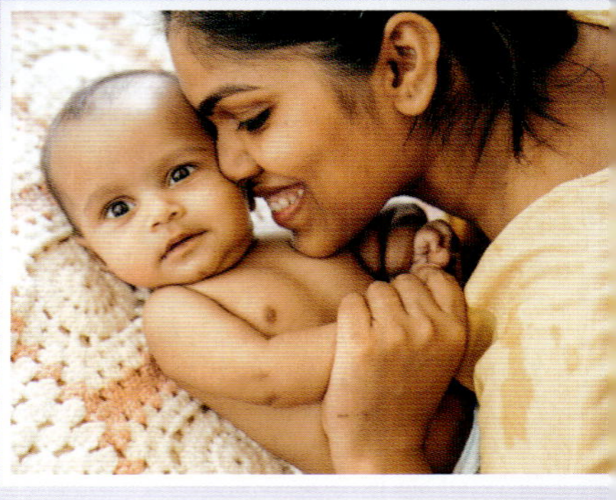

Health Problems of the Infant

Jane Mateer and Christine Taylor

LEARNING OBJECTIVES

- Identify the main risk factors for children in Australia, developing nutritional imbalance and obesity
- Define faltering growth
- Discuss the risk and protective factors for infants and sudden infant death syndrome (SIDS)

NUTRITION IN CHILDREN

Adequate nutrition is essential for optimal growth and development in children, from in-utero and continuing throughout childhood (NSW Health 2021). Health problems arise from over or undernutrition in children. Overnutrition leads to obesity, which is a risk factor for many diseases in later childhood and adulthood. Undernutrition or specific nutritional deficiencies can lead to poor growth and development.

Obesity

Child obesity rates are rising globally. The World Health Organization (WHO) considers childhood obesity as 'one of the most serious public health challenges of the 21st century' (WHO n.d.). The WHO estimate that over 41 million children in the world are obese: this puts them at risk for cardiovascular disease and diabetes at a younger age in adulthood. In Australia during 2017–2018, 25% of children and adolescents aged 2 to 17 years were obese or overweight (Australian Institute of Health and Welfare [AIHW] 2019). From 2012–2013 data, more Aboriginal and Torres Strait Islander children were overweight and obese compared to non-Indigenous children (AIHW 2020). In New Zealand, there is also a marked ethnicity difference between children. In the years 2018–2019, 11.3% of children aged between 2 and 14 years in New Zealand were obese. Child obesity rates in different ethnicities were 28.4% Pacific Island ethnicity, 15.5% Maori, 9.9% Asian ethnicity and 8.2% European/Other (Ministry of Health 2019).

Causes of Obesity

Overweight and obesity is the excess presence of body fat that is usually the result of a greater caloric intake (energy input) than energy expenditure (AIHW 2020). This can be due to excess food intake, a lack of physical activities or a combination of both. However, obesity is a multifactorial disorder that involves a complex interaction between biological and environmental factors that affects the process of gaining weight.

Biological factors include genetics, which generally involves numerous genes and influences aspects such as appetite and metabolism (Singh et al 2017). The field of epigenetics has shown a connection between genetics and the environment, so factors related to a mother during pregnancy are associated with later obesity in the child; for example, famine, smoking, gestational diabetes and maternal obesity (Godfrey et al 2017). These factors can influence the regulation of genes, such as through changes in DNA methylation, which alters the phenotype of genetic expression leading to a susceptibility for developing obesity (Godfrey et al 2017). Another biological factor that has been associated with obesity in children is poor quality or lack of adequate sleep (Kumar & Kelly 2017).

Environmental factors, such as an obesogenic environment, can also influence the development of obesity in children. An obesogenic environment is one which promotes the development of obesity, such as physical, sociocultural, economic and political factors (AIHW 2017). Examples of environments include schools, workplaces, neighbourhoods, media influences and the availability of convenience foods (AIHW 2017). Pressure to eat foods that lead to obesity is seen in social media, television advertising, peer groups or poor parenting choices. Foods that are high in saturated fat and sugar and sugary 'soft' drinks contribute to obesity. Ingestion of soft drinks and fruit juices in excess also contributes to dental decay (AIHW 2020). Factors such as low socioeconomic status and psychological and emotional stress have been also associated with childhood obesity, such as poverty and maternal mental illness (Kumar & Kelly 2017).

Assessment and Management

The WHO considers children overweight if they are one standard deviation above their body mass index (BMI) for their age (WHO n.d.). Waist measurements and other physical measures are recorded while assessing a child for obesity and compared to standard growth charts. Any comorbidities are also identified, such as high blood pressure or sleep apnoea (National Health and Medical Research Council [NHMRC] 2013). A complete history of the child is taken and assessed to rule out genetic, chromosomal or medical conditions, or drug-induced obesity as causes of obesity (Kumar & Kelly 2017). Dietary history and patterns also need to be obtained (NHMRC 2013).

The most recent guidelines in Australia for the management of obesity in children (NHMRC 2013) recommend early weight management as it minimises the effects of obesity into adulthood. Advice recommended to be given includes the benefits of weight management and, importantly, involvement of the family for effective interventions. Communication needs to be respectful and non-judgmental, as this can be a sensitive topic for parents and children. Lifestyle interventions are also recommended, such as changes to the diet and involvement in regular exercise. This may be accompanied by behavioural modification techniques, such as goal setting. Important advice to the parents includes not using food as a reward, separate eating from other activities such as watching television and encouraging children to listen to internal hunger cues. The New Zealand guidelines (Ministry of Health 2016) use the acronym FAB that is useful to remember these interventions: **F**ood and drink, **A**ctivity (reducing the time spent in inactivity and supporting sufficient sleep) and **B**ehavioural changes. If the child has severe obesity, comorbidities or is suspected of having a medical disorder, then recommendations to a specialist health service is needed before intervention (NHMRC 2013).

NUTRITIONAL IMBALANCES

Severe nutritional disorders are uncommon in children who live in developed countries. However, a small number of children remain at risk of a nutritional deficiency of some kind, due to factors such as diet and disease. Areas of concern for nutritional deficiency include iron and vitamin D. Inadequate fat, fibre and general vitamin intake, plus excess sodium intake, are a concern in toddlers (AIHW 2018). Children under 1 year of age who consume breast or formula milk as their main dietary substance are less prone to nutritional deficiency. It is important for nurses who care for infants and children to know what an appropriate diet would be for a child's age and to recognise risk factors for deficiency. Nurses must strive to promote healthy nutritional habits early in childhood through proper education of families and children about healthy lifestyle practices. This includes diet and exercise for health promotion and prevention of morbidities associated with poor micronutrient intake and sedentary lifestyle.

Vitamin Imbalances

Although true vitamin deficiencies are considered rare in Australia and New Zealand, subclinical deficiencies are seen in certain mother–child populations in which dietary intake is imbalanced and contains inadequate amounts of vitamins. **Vitamin D-resistant rickets**, once rarely seen because of the widespread commercial availability of vitamin D–fortified milk, increased before the turn of the century. Populations at risk include the following:

- children who are exclusively breastfed by mothers with an inadequate intake of vitamin D or are exclusively breastfed longer than 6 months without adequate maternal vitamin D intake or supplementation
- children with dark skin pigmentation who: (1) are exposed to minimal sunlight because of socioeconomic, religious or cultural beliefs; (2) live in urban areas with high levels of pollution; or (3) live above or below a latitude of 33 degrees north and south where sunlight does not produce vitamin D (NHMRC, Australian Government Department of Health and Ageing, New Zealand Ministry of Health 2017)
- children whose diets are low in sources of vitamin D and calcium
- children who receive milk products not supplemented with vitamin D (e.g. yoghurt*, raw cow's milk) as their primary dairy source
- children who are overweight or obese (NHMRC, Australian Government Department of Health and Ageing, New Zealand Ministry of Health 2017).

Paediatricians from an Australian paediatric surveillance unit reported that vitamin D-resistant rickets occurred in approximately 4.9/100,000 children 15 years and under per year (The Royal Children's Hospital Melbourne [RCHM] 2018a). Clinical manifestations of vitamin D-deficiency include abdominal pain, seizures, limb pain and weakness. Exclusively breastfed infants may also be at risk for vitamin D-deficiency if maternal levels are inadequate and because human milk has low vitamin D levels (NHMRC, Australian Government Department of Health and Ageing, New Zealand Ministry of Health 2017). Maternal testing during pregnancy can help identify children at risk, in addition to those at risk due to having darker skin, being rarely exposed to sunlight or having an underlying condition which increases the risk of deficiency (RCHM 2018a).

The Australian and New Zealand governments recommend that a child consume 5 microg/day of cholecalciferol for infants and children (NHMRC, Australian Government Department of Health and Ageing, New Zealand Ministry of Health 2017). Food sources that are high in vitamin D are salmon, sardines, tuna and cod liver oil. Vitamin D–fortified foods include orange juice, oatmeal, whole milk, yoghurt and certain breakfast cereals (NHMRC, Australian Government Department of Health and Ageing, New Zealand Ministry of Health 2017).

Children may also be at risk for vitamin deficiencies secondary to special diets, disorders or medical treatments. For example, children on vegetarian diets, especially vegan diets, are at risk of vitamin B_{12} deficiency so it must be ensured that an adequate source of this vitamin is consumed (Pawlak et al 2013, Schürmann et al 2017). Although scurvy (caused by a deficiency of vitamin C) is rare in developed countries, cases have been reported in children who have low intake of vitamin C due to poor oral intake, oral motor dysfunction or feeding problems (Agarwal et al 2014). Vitamin deficiencies of the fat-soluble vitamins A and D may occur in malabsorptive disorders such as cystic fibrosis and short bowel syndrome (NHMRC, Australian Government Department of Health and Ageing, New Zealand Ministry of Health 2017). Preterm infants may develop rickets in the second month of life as a result of inadequate intake of vitamin D, calcium and phosphorus. Children receiving high doses of salicylates may have impaired vitamin C storage. Therefore, children with chronic illnesses resulting in anorexia, decreased food intake or possible nutrient malabsorption as a result of multiple medications should be carefully evaluated for adequate vitamin and mineral intake in some form (parenteral or enteral) (NHMRC, Australian Government Department of Health and Ageing, New Zealand Ministry of Health 2017).

Children with sickle cell disease (SCD) may have suboptimal intakes of calcium, iron and vitamins B_1 and C. This is problematic because low intake of calcium and vitamin B_1 has been correlated with more severe SCD symptoms (Mandese et al 2016). Significant vitamin D deficiencies have also been found in children with intestinal failure who received parenteral nutrition at home; therefore, routine screening and consideration of vitamin D supplementation are recommended (Wozniak et al 2015).

Vitamin A deficiency can occur in children as a result of diarrhoea or infection. Vitamin A deficiency has been associated with an increased risk for blindness in children with measles. However, in a Cochrane review of studies assessing the efficacy of vitamin A in preventing blindness in children with measles, researchers found no evidence specifically related to ocular morbidities (Bello et al 2016).

Excessive doses of vitamins can be concerning as well. In general, an excessive dose is defined as 10 or more times the Recommended Dietary Intake (RDI). Although the water-soluble vitamins, primarily niacin, B_6 and C, can cause toxicity, the fat-soluble vitamins, especially vitamins A and D, tend to cause toxic reactions at lower doses. With the addition of vitamins to commercially prepared foods, the potential for **hypervitaminosis** has increased, especially when combined with excessive use of vitamin supplements. Hypervitaminosis of A and D present the greatest problems because these fat-soluble vitamins are stored in the body and severe anaemia and thrombocytopenia have resulted from mega doses of vitamin A. Hypercalcaemia has been

*Yoghurt does not contain adequate amounts of vitamins A and D, but it is an acceptable source of calcium and phosphorus.

reported in children receiving therapeutic doses of vitamin D for the prevention of rickets (Talarico et al 2016) and in children on high doses of vitamin A for the treatment of autism (Boyd & Moodambail 2016). Vitamin D is the most likely of all vitamins to cause toxic reactions in relatively small overdoses.

Inadequate maternal ingestion of cobalamin (vitamin B_{12}) may contribute to infant neurological impairment when exclusive breastfeeding (past 6 months) is the only source of the infant's nutrition. One vitamin supplementation that is recommended for all women of childbearing age who are planning a pregnancy is that they should take additional folic acid for at least 1 month before and 3 months after conception with a daily dose of 0.4 mg of folic acid, the usual RDI, plus consuming folate-containing food in the diet (NHMRC, Australian Government Department of Health and Ageing, New Zealand Ministry of Health 2017). Folic acid taken before conception and during early pregnancy can reduce the risk of neural tube defects such as spina bifida by as much as 70%. Drugs such as oral contraceptives and antidepressants may decrease folic acid absorption; thus adolescent girls taking these medications should consider supplementation. (See Spina Bifida, Chapter 34.)

Mineral Imbalances

A number of minerals are essential nutrients. **Macrominerals** refer to those with daily requirements greater than 100 mg and include calcium, phosphorus, magnesium, sodium, potassium, chloride and sulfur. **Microminerals**, or **trace elements**, have daily requirements of less than 100 mg and include several essential minerals that have an unclear role in nutrition. The greatest concern with minerals is deficiency, especially iron-deficiency anaemia (see Chapter 28). However, other minerals that may be inadequate in children's diets, even with supplementation, include calcium, phosphorus, magnesium and zinc. Low levels of zinc can cause poor growth in children (NHMRC, Australian Government Department of Health and Ageing, New Zealand Ministry of Health 2017). Some macrominerals may be inadvertently overlooked when a child with intestinal failure or recent surgery is making the transition from total parenteral nutrition to enteral feedings.

An imbalance in the intake of calcium and phosphorus may occur in infants less than 1 year old who are given whole cow's milk instead of infant formula. Whole cow's milk is a poor source of iron, and inadequate intake of iron from other food sources such as iron-fortified cereal may cause iron-deficiency anaemia. Infant formula or breastfeeding is recommended for babies under 12 months of age. However, regardless of whether the baby is breastfed or formula-fed, iron-fortified foods are needed after around 6 months of age due to the rapid growth of babies at this time (NHMRC 2012).

The regulation of mineral balance in the body is a complex process. Dietary extremes of mineral intake can cause a number of interactions that could result in unexpected mineral deficiencies or excesses. Poor outcomes in infants (e.g. fatal hypermagnesaemia) have been associated with mega vitamin therapy with high doses of magnesium oxide. Further, excessive amounts of one mineral, such as zinc, can result in a deficiency of another mineral, such as copper, even if sufficient amounts of copper are ingested. Thus, mega dose intake of one mineral may cause an inadvertent deficiency of another essential mineral, by blocking its absorption in the blood or intestinal wall or by competing with binding sites on protein carriers needed for metabolism (Kang 2018).

Deficiencies can also occur when various substances in the diet interact with minerals. For instance, iron, zinc and calcium can form insoluble complexes with **phytates** or **oxalates** (substances found in plant proteins), which impair the bioavailability of the mineral. This type of interaction is important in vegetarian diets because plant foods such as soy are high in phytates. Also, contrary to popular opinion, spinach is not an ideal source of iron or calcium because of its high oxalate content so only a small proportion of these minerals are absorbed (Kang 2018).

Children with certain illnesses are at greater risk for growth failure, especially in relation to bone mineral deficiency resulting from medical treatments, decreased nutrient intake or decreased absorption of necessary minerals. Those at risk for these deficiencies include children who have: (1) human immunodeficiency virus (HIV); (2) sickle cell disease; (3) cystic fibrosis; (4) gastrointestinal (GI) malabsorption; or (5) nephrosis. Extremely low-birthweight (ELBW) and very-low-birthweight (VLBW) preterm infants and children who are receiving or have received radiation and/or chemotherapy for cancer are also at risk.

Nursing Care Management

A primary goal of paediatric nursing is to ensure adequate nutrition in children. This requires a nutritional assessment based on a thorough dietary history and physical examination for signs of deficiency or excess (see Nutrition, Chapter 12, and Nutritional Assessment, Chapter 4). After assessment data are collected, this information is compared with standardised intakes to identify areas of potential concern. One source of standardised nutrient intakes is the nutrient reference values for Australia and New Zealand (NHMRC, Australian Government Department of Health and Ageing, New Zealand Ministry of Health 2017).

Standardised growth reference charts are used in infants, children and adolescents to compare and assess growth parameters such as height and head circumference with the percentile distribution of other children at the same ages. The WHO growth charts represent standardised growth references now recommended for infants and toddlers up to age 24 months. These growth charts include head circumference, height and weight references that were derived from healthy children in six different countries around the world. These growth standards are based on the growth of healthy infants who were predominantly breastfed for at least 4 months and still breastfeeding to some extent at 12 months (WHO 2009).

Current recommendations for infant feeding include exclusive breastfeeding for the first 6 months with continued breastfeeding for at least 1 year or longer, if desired, with the addition of age-appropriate complementary foods (Australian Breastfeeding Association 2017, NHMRC 2012). The introduction of solid foods is recommended to begin around 6 months and should include introduction of most foods during the first year of life (NHMRC 2012). The exceptions, and foods to avoid, include nuts and hard food to avoid choking, honey as it can cause botulism and cow's milk as it can cause iron deficiency (NHMRC 2012). A variety of foods should be introduced during the early years to ensure a well-balanced nutritional intake. Infants who have a particular nutritional deficiency should be identified. A multidisciplinary approach should be taken to identify the deficiency, determine its aetiology and establish a plan with the caregiver to promote adequate growth and development.

HEALTH PROBLEMS RELATED TO NUTRITION

Severe Acute Malnutrition (Protein–energy Malnutrition)

Malnutrition continues to be a major health problem in the world today, particularly in children younger than 5 years of age. However, lack of food is not always the primary cause of malnutrition. In many developing and underdeveloped nations, diarrhoea (gastroenteritis) is a major factor causing malnutrition (WHO 2017). Additional contributors are:

(1) bottle-feeding (in poor sanitary conditions); (2) inadequate knowledge of proper childcare practices; (3) parental illiteracy; (4) economic and political factors; (5) climate conditions; (6) cultural and religious food preferences; and (7) a lack of adequate food. Poverty and food insecurity, which is the lack of a consistent and reliable food source, play an important role in worldwide malnutrition (US Department of Agriculture 2020). The most extreme forms of malnutrition, or **protein–energy malnutrition**, are **kwashiorkor** and **marasmus**. Some authorities believe that severe malnutrition encompasses more than protein–energy deficits and thus prefer the term *severe childhood undernutrition* (SCU). However, entities such as the WHO (2020) now use the term *severe acute malnutrition* (SAM). SAM may be subdivided into oedematous (kwashiorkor) and non-oedematous with severe wasting (marasmus) types. A third type, marasmic kwashiorkor, has features of both marasmus and kwashiorkor (Médicins Sans Frontières 2020).

In Australia, milder forms of SAM are seen as a result of primary malnutrition, although classic cases of marasmus and kwashiorkor may occur but are rare. Unlike in developing countries, where the main reason for SAM is inadequate food, in Australia SAM may occur despite ample food supplies (see faltering growth, discussed later in this chapter). SAM may also be seen in children with chronic health problems such as: (1) cystic fibrosis; (2) renal disease; (3) cancer; (4) bone marrow transplantation; (5) HIV; (6) inborn errors of metabolism; (7) GI malabsorption; and (8) prolonged, untreated anorexia nervosa. In Australia, infants fed only rice milk, which contains inadequate protein, have been associated with severe malnutrition. Thus it is important for nurses to recognise that SAM can occur in developed countries; therefore, a comprehensive dietary history is essential for any child with clinical features resembling SAM.

Therapeutic Management

The treatment of SAM includes providing a diet with high-quality proteins, carbohydrates, vitamins and minerals. When SAM occurs as a result of persistent diarrhoea, there are three management goals:

1. rehydration with an oral rehydration solution that also replaces electrolytes
2. administration of antibiotics to prevent concurrent infections
3. provision of adequate nutrition by either breastfeeding or a proper weaning diet.

Local protocols are used in developing countries to treat SAM, but experts recommend a three-phase management protocol. The first phase is the **acute or initial phase**, which occurs in the first 2 to 10 days. During this phase, management involves initiation of oral rehydration and treatment of diarrhoea and intestinal parasites. A focus is also placed on prevention of hypoglycaemia and hypothermia and subsequent dietary management. Phase two, **recovery or rehabilitation**, occurs during the next 2 to 6 weeks, and treatment is focused on increasing dietary intake and weight gain. Management in phase 3, the **follow-up phase**, is focused on care after discharge in an outpatient setting to prevent relapse and promote weight gain, provide developmental stimulation and evaluate cognitive and motor development.

In the acute phase of SAM, extreme care must be taken to prevent fluid overload. The child is observed closely for signs of food or fluid intolerance. **Refeeding syndrome** may occur if caloric intake progresses too rapidly. The resulting cardiac failure may cause sudden death in a child who has been malnourished and is fed too rapidly (Ashworth 2016). Because severely malnourished children cannot tolerate a high-protein, high-energy diet, a modest-energy food source is given initially. These children are then slowly progressed to high-protein and high-energy foods as tolerated. A variety of food sources may be used to treat SAM, including oral rehydration solutions, therapeutic milks (e.g. Nutriset) and ready-to-use therapeutic foods (RUTF) that do not require the addition of water, thus preventing exposure to contaminated water sources (see Cultural Considerations box). In addition, parenteral and oral antibiotics are often part of the standard treatment for SAM (MSF 2020).

> **CULTURAL CONSIDERATIONS**
>
> ***World Health Organization Child Growth Standards***
>
> The WHO has published a set of international growth standards, which are based on an expected growth trajectory for children living in an environment which promotes optimal growth. The focus is how infants and children should grow, rather than the effect of a suboptimal environment. The standard, set by the WHO, is based on breastfeeding as the recommended standard for growth and follow a normal growth pattern from birth to the age of 5 years. The growth charts were compiled from a multicentre project conducted in Brazil, Ghana, India, Norway, Oman and the United States, and included 8440 children raised in environments that promoted healthy growth habits, including being breastfed and born to non-smoking mothers. These growth charts and additional information can be accessed at http://www.who.int/childgrowth/standards/en.

Vitamin and mineral supplementations are also required in most cases of SAM with vitamin A, zinc and copper recommended. In contrast, iron supplementation is not recommended until the child can tolerate a steady food source. During recovery, the child is observed for signs of skin breakdown, which should be treated to prevent infection. Breastfeeding is encouraged if the mother and child are able to do so effectively; however, in some cases partial supplementation with a modified cow's milk–based infant formula may be necessary.

The WHO recognises that safe sources of food and water may not be available or adequate for infants after the first 6 months of life and that the risk of malnutrition in these children is greater than their theoretical risk of contracting infections, such as HIV (as a result of breastfeeding). Thus, the organisation recommends breastfeeding continue after 6 months with the introduction of complementary foods, provided there are safe sources of food available (WHO 2020).

Nursing Care Management

SAM appears early in childhood, primarily in children 6 months to 2 years of age, and is associated with early weaning, maternal illiteracy, poverty, large family size and incomplete vaccinations (Mishra et al 2014). It is essential that nursing care focus on the *prevention* of SAM through parent education about feeding practices and infant care during this critical period. Prevention should also focus on the nutritional health of pregnant women as this will directly affect the health and future growth of their unborn children. Breastfeeding is the optimal method of infant feeding for the first 6 months. The immune properties naturally found in breast milk not only nourish infants but also help prevent opportunistic infections that may contribute to SAM. It is essential to ensure the infants' physiological needs are met, including adequate nutrition and hydration, protection from infection and appropriate skin care. Additional nursing care should be focused on educating parents about the importance of: (1) childhood vaccinations to prevent illness; (2) nutrition and wellbeing for lactating mothers; (3) attending well-child visits for infants and toddlers; (4) appropriate food sources for children being weaned from breastfeeding; and (5) sanitation practices to prevent childhood GI illnesses.

Nursing care of young infants should also include appropriate skin care because poor skin integrity contributes to infection, hypothermia, water loss and skin breakdown. If an infant is not well enough to effectively breastfeed or bottle-feed, tube feedings may be required to ensure adequate nutrition. Oral rehydration with an approved oral rehydration solution is commonly used in cases of SAM in which diarrhoea and infection are not immediately life-threatening.

Further, infants may be treated with higher-calorie (100 to 112 kJ per 30 mL) commercial infant formulas when appropriate. One potential drawback of using therapeutic milks (Aptamil Gold, Nan Supreme and S-26 Gold in Australia and Karicare and Aptamil Gold in New Zealand) is that they require water and may become contaminated during mixing if clean water is not used, whereas RUTF, a peanut-based paste containing dried skim milk, vitamins and minerals, has little water content (UNICEF 2013). Therefore, the home-based use of RUTF has gained acceptance for treating childhood malnutrition in developing countries. The packaged RUTF can be stored without refrigeration, has a long shelf-life and improves survival rates in malnourished children (UNICEF 2013). RUTF can also be administered by community health workers and offers the added advantage of home-based treatment of SAM, which can prevent exposure to hospital-acquired infections in already vulnerable children. Finally, by mobilising communities and providing access to RUTF, 80% of children with SAM can be successfully treated at home. Rapid and appropriate care management can lower case-fatality rates to as low as 5% in both the community and the healthcare setting (UNICEF 2013).

It is imperative that nurses be at the forefront of educating and reinforcing healthy nutrition habits with parents of small children to prevent malnutrition. Because children with marasmus may experience emotional as well as nutritional deprivation, care should be consistent with the typical, age-appropriate, developmentally supportive care provided for children with faltering growth.

The WHO has published guidelines for the dietary treatment and management of children with SAM (available at http://www.who.int/elena/titles/full_recommendations/sam_management/en/). These guidelines include 11 recommendations for the management of SAM in infants 6 to 59 months of age, as well as hospital admission and discharge criteria for these infants (WHO 2020).

Food Sensitivity

In Australia, the Australasian Society of Clinical Immunology and Allergy (ASCIA) has published a series of evidence-based dietary guides for food allergy and avoidance of problem foods (ASCIA 2020a). They can be located at: https://www.allergy.org.au/patients/food-allergy. A **food intolerance** exists when a food or food component elicits a reproducible adverse reaction but does not have an established or likely allergic mechanism (ASCIA 2020a). For example, a person with a milk allergy may have an immune-mediated response to cow's milk protein; however, a person who is unable to digest the lactose in cow's milk is intolerant to cow's milk, not allergic to it.

Food allergies are adverse allergic (immunological) reactions to specific components of a food or ingredients in a food, such as a protein, that are recognised by allergen-specific immune cells eliciting an immune reaction that results in the characteristic symptoms of an allergic response. True food allergies may involve anaphylaxis (ASCIA 2020a). Food allergies may also manifest in specific syndromes, such as Heiner syndrome, which is a rare but reversible non–immunoglobulin E (IgE)–mediated hypersensitivity to cow's milk resulting in atypical pulmonary disease in infants and young children (Nowak-Węgrzyn et al 2020). The exact prevalence of food allergies in children is believed to be much lower than what is reported by parents. Food allergy symptoms are most common in infants and young children but can occur at any age. Clinical manifestations of food allergies are as follows:

- **systemic**—anaphylaxis, growth failure
- **GI**—abdominal pain, vomiting, cramping, diarrhoea, colic
- **respiratory**—cough, wheezing, rhinitis, pulmonary infiltrates
- **cutaneous**—urticaria, rash, atopic dermatitis (ASCIA 2020a, WHO 2017).

The most common allergic triggers are egg, cow's milk (dairy), peanut, tree nuts, sesame, soy, wheat, fish and other seafood (ASCIA 2020a). Peanuts are the most prevalent allergen followed by milk and then shellfish. While many children are eventually able to tolerate milk, eggs, soy and wheat by the time they are at school, tree nut, peanut and seafood allergies often persist for life (ASCIA 2020a). There has been a distinct rise in the incidence of food allergies in Australia and New Zealand, with up to 10% of children under 1 year of age and 8% of children up to the age of 5 years having a food allergy (ASCIA 2020a). Since 2010 there has been a five-fold rise in hospital admissions for food allergy-induced anaphylaxis in children under the age of 4 years (ASCIA 2020a). While the evidence is still evolving, research is looking at how the following factors may influence the risk of allergic reaction: the hygiene hypothesis (which suggests that a low exposure to pathogens in early childhood increases the risk of allergy), delayed introduction of foods perceived to produce allergic responses and changes in food preparation (ASCIA 2020a). In addition, there has been a significant increase in Australia, North America and the United Kingdom (World Allergy Organization [WAO] 2017), which suggests the environment and lifestyle choices in the developed world may play a role in allergy development.

Previous recommendations to limit the introduction of solids in the first year of life have now changed, particularly in light of evidence which now demonstrates that a child is less likely to have a significant immune reaction in the first year of life, due to a blunted immune response (NHMRC 2012). The exception has always been honey (due to the risk of botulinum), which should not be introduced until after 12 months of age. Recommendations for the prevention of food allergies in young children include the following (ASCIA 2020b, NHMRC 2012).

- Breastfeeding is recommended for at least the first 6 months of life.
- Exclusion of allergenic foods from the maternal diet during lactation has not been proven to prevent allergies.
- The use of hydrolysed formulas are not recommended for the prevention of allergies. Soy-based infant formulas will not prevent the development of food allergy.
- Introduce complementary solid foods around 6 months of age.
- Introduce allergy-causing foods (including peanut butter, cooked egg, dairy and wheat) in the first year of life, even if the child is at high risk of allergy. Delaying the introduction of these foods will not prevent food allergies and some evidence suggests it may decrease the risk (delaying).

Food allergies usually occur either as IgE-mediated or non–IgE-mediated immune responses. Some toxic reactions may occur because of a toxin found within the food. Food allergy is caused by exposure to **allergens**, usually proteins (but not the smaller amino acids), that are capable of inducing IgE antibody formation (sensitisation) when ingested. **Sensitisation** refers to the initial exposure of an individual to an allergen resulting in an immune response. Subsequent exposure induces a much stronger response that is clinically apparent (Nowak-W grzyn et al 2020). Consequently, food allergy typically occurs after the food has been ingested one or more times. Sensitisation alone is not sufficient to be classified as a food allergy. Rather, an immune-mediated response *and* manifestation of specific signs and symptoms are necessary to categorise an individual as having a food allergy (Nowak-Węgrzyn et al 2020). The most common food allergens are listed in Box 11.1.

BOX 11.1 Hyperallergenic Foods and Sources

Milk*—Ice-cream, butter, margarine (if it contains dairy products), yoghurt, cheese, pudding, baked goods, canned creamed soups, instant breakfast drinks, powdered milk drinks, milk chocolate
Eggs*—Mayonnaise, creamy salad dressing, baked goods, egg noodles, some cake icing, meringue, custard, pancakes, French toast, root beer
Wheat*—Almost all baked goods, pressed or chopped deli meats, gravy, pasta, some canned soups
Legumes—Peanuts*, peanut butter or oil, beans, peas, lentils
Nuts*—Some chocolates, lollies, baked goods, cherry soft drink (may be flavoured with a nut extract), walnut oil
Fish or shellfish*—Cod liver oil, pizza with anchovies, Caesar salad dressing, any food fried in same oil as fish
Soy*—Soy sauce, teriyaki or Worcestershire sauce, tofu, baked goods using soy flour or oil, soy nuts, soy infant formulas or milk, soybean paste, tuna packed in vegetable oil, many margarines
Chocolate—Cola beverages, cocoa, chocolate-flavoured drinks
Buckwheat—Some cereals, pancakes
Pork, chicken—Bacon, frankfurts, sausage, pork fat, chicken broth
Strawberries, melon, pineapple—Gelatine, syrups
Corn—Popcorn, cereal, muffins, cornstarch, cornmeal, corn bread, corn tortilla; many processed foods also contain corn syrup
Citrus fruits—Orange, lemon, lime, grapefruit; any of these in drinks, gelatine, juice or medicines
Tomatoes—Juice, some vegetable soups, spaghetti, pizza sauce
Spices—Chili, pepper, vinegar, cinnamon

*Most common allergens.

Oral allergy syndrome occurs when a food allergen (commonly fruits and vegetables) is ingested and there is subsequent oedema and pruritus involving the lips, tongue, palate and throat. Recovery from these symptoms is usually rapid. **Immediate GI hypersensitivity** is an IgE-mediated reaction to a food allergen that can result in nausea, abdominal pain, cramping, diarrhoea, vomiting, anaphylaxis or all of these (Nowak-Węgrzyn et al 2020). Additional food allergies seen in young children can cause allergic eosinophilic oesophagitis, allergic eosinophilic gastroenteritis, food protein–induced proctocolitis and food protein–induced enterocolitis.

Food allergy or hypersensitivity may also be classified by the interval between ingestion and the manifestation of symptoms: immediate (within minutes to hours) or delayed (2 to 48 hours). Food allergies may occur at any time throughout the life span but are most common during infancy because the immature intestinal tract is more permeable to proteins than the mature intestinal tract thus increasing the likelihood of an immune response. Although food allergies are not inherited, there may be a higher risk of allergies in families (ASCIA 2020a). The hereditary tendency to allergy is referred to as **atopy**. Some infants with atopy can be identified at birth from elevated levels of IgE in the umbilical cord blood.

Deaths have occurred in children who experienced an anaphylactic reaction to food, with onset of a reaction occurring shortly after ingestion (5 to 30 minutes). In Australia and the United States, adolescents and young adults are at the greatest risk of food-induced anaphylaxis deaths (Pouessel et al 2018). In most children affected, the reaction did not begin with skin signs, such as hives, red rash and flushing, but rather mimicked an acute asthma attack (e.g. wheezing, decreased air movement in airways, dyspnoea). This may result in an initial misdiagnosis, leading to delayed treatment. Anaphylaxis responds best with early treatment. Close observation for a sustained response to treatment is essential as a biphasic reaction has been reported in as many as 35% of children, where there is an immediate response to treatment, an apparent recovery and subsequently an acute recurrence of symptoms (O'Loughlin & Hiscock 2020). Children with extremely sensitive food allergies should wear a medical identification bracelet and have an injectable adrenaline cartridge (EpiPen) readily available. (See Emergency Management of Anaphylaxis, Chapter 6.) Any child with a history of food allergy or previous severe reaction to food should have a written emergency treatment plan as well as an EpiPen (O'Loughlin & Hiscock 2020).

Because there is a tendency for children to lose their hypersensitivity, allergenic foods should be reintroduced into the diet after a period of abstinence to evaluate whether the food can be safely added back to the diet. There is evidence that children may tolerate foods to which they were previously allergic when these foods are extensively heated as in muffins or breads. The prolonged or complete avoidance of foods to prevent food allergy is not recommended, as there is some evidence that lack of exposure to antigens may be detrimental (ASCIA 2020b).

NURSING CARE CONSIDERATIONS

The administration of **intramuscular** adrenaline in a child with a life-threatening anaphylactic reaction or one who is experiencing severe symptoms is indicated when the child has any one of the following symptoms (ASCIA 2021):

- difficult noisy breathing, swelling of the tongue, swelling or tightness in throat
- wheeze or persistent cough, difficult talking or hoarse voice
- persistent dizziness or collapse, pale and floppy (young children).

Note that adrenaline is given **before** an asthma reliever in those with known asthma or allergy.

Diagnosis and Therapeutic Management. The diagnosis of food allergy is made based on several factors, including the occurrence of anaphylaxis or any combination of symptoms listed in the ASCIA guidelines within minutes to hours of ingesting food or if such symptoms have occurred after the ingestion of a specific food on one or more occasions. In Australasia, the use of a skin prick test provides a convenient and rapid way to identify the majority of allergies. Where a skin prick test is not available or contraindicated (such as severe eczema), serum allergen-specific IgE measurements may be used in diagnosis (ASCIA 2020a). Intradermal testing is only used for testing allergy where greater sensitivity is needed, such as antibiotic drugs. The atopy patch test may be used for evaluating allergic contact dermatitis and an oral allergen challenge test may be used in certain circumstances (ASCIA 2020a). The oral test is used for specific foods or medications and must be conducted under supervision of an allergy specialist in an environment with resuscitation facilities.

The closest thing to a cure for allergies is a process known as allergen immunotherapy. The process includes regular administration by injection, tablet or sublingual liquid, of increasing doses of an allergen, to a sufferer, over several years (ASCIA 2019a). It works for some allergies, but not all, and it is time consuming. The process aims to switch off the body's response to the allergen, with an end outcome of tolerance.

Where the management of food allergy consists of avoiding a specific food or ingredient, a child may be at risk for inadequate nutrient intake and growth failure. It is therefore recommended that they have an annual nutritional assessment to prevent problems, such as calcium, vitamin D, calorie and protein deficiencies (resulting from dairy omission). Elimination of wheat may result in inadequate intake of the B vitamins, iron and calories.

Nursing Care Management

It is important parents are educated about the importance of breastfeeding and of introducing a broad range of foods from around 6 months of age, including those known to produce allergies (NHMRC 2012). Nursing care of children with a potential food allergy consists of collecting vital health assessment data for the establishment of a diagnosis and assisting with diagnostic testing. It is important for nurses to be informed about food allergy and provide parents and caregivers, as well as older children, with accurate information regarding food allergy. This includes the education of parents, teachers and day care workers regarding signs and symptoms of food allergy and reactions (see Critical Thinking Case Study box). Children with diagnosed food allergy should avoid unfamiliar foods and be wary in restaurants, including those that disclose food ingredients. Labelling guidelines for commercially acquired food requires that food additives such as spices and flavouring be clearly listed. However, hidden ingredients in prepared foods are also potential sources of food allergy. In children with diagnosed allergies to certain foods, a nutritional consultation is imperative for the development of a dietary plan that includes sufficient nutrients for growth and development while avoiding the offending food.

CRITICAL THINKING CASE STUDY

Food Allergy Anaphylaxis

A group of nursing students is holding a health promotion fair at a local primary school for children in Years 1, 2 and 3. The nursing students have several booths set up in the school cafeteria. Three Year 2 boys are playing around in front of one of the booths when Jason, an 8 year old, suddenly starts coughing and clutching his throat. The nursing students observe that he is developing red splotches on his face, neck and throat and that he is scratching. Jason says, 'I'm having trouble breathing!' The school nurse is nearby and comes over to see what the commotion is about. One of the boys with Jason says, 'We didn't mean any harm—we were just goofing around when we put peanuts in his mixed nuts'. One of the student nurses says, 'He's in obvious distress—what should we do?'

1. Evidence—Is there sufficient evidence to draw any conclusions at this time about Jason's condition?
2. Assumptions—Describe some underlying assumptions about the following.
   a. Clinical manifestations of food allergy
   b. The emergency treatment of a food allergy 'reaction', or anaphylaxis
   c. Which one of the following interventions would have highest immediate priority?
      i. Call Jason's parents and ask them to come pick him up from school.
      ii. Call Jason's family practitioner to obtain orders for medication.
      iii. Promptly administer an intramuscular dose of adrenaline.
      iv. Call 000 and wait for the ambulance to arrive.
   d. Based on your answer to item 2c, identify the appropriate medication dosage for this child (his weight is estimated at 24 kg).
3. What implications for nursing care exist in this situation after an intervention in item 2c has been chosen and implemented?
4. Describe the potential results of taking a 'Let's observe Jason for a few minutes before we do anything' stance in this scenario.
5. Is there evidence to support your immediate and secondary nursing interventions?

Provide objective evidence to support your decisions for action.

Answers are available at http://evolve.elsevier.com/AU/Speedie/ncic/

Children with a history of food allergy may spend time in day care; therefore, persons working in day care centres and other children's settings need to be properly educated regarding recognition and management of severe anaphylactic reactions. It is important for schools to ensure that children who have potentially life-threatening food allergies are recognised so plans can be implemented to prevent contact with allergy-producing foods. A written emergency action or food allergy plan should be kept for the child and a self-injectable adrenaline device (EpiPen) should be readily available for these children (ASCIA 2021). Families of children with life-threatening food allergies are at risk for increased psychosocial distress, so healthcare workers should be prepared to meet the families' psychosocial as well as physical needs regarding their child.

Cow's Milk Allergy

Cow's milk allergy (CMA) is a multifaceted disorder representing adverse systemic and local GI reactions to cow's milk protein. Approximately 2% of infants in Australasia develop cow's milk hypersensitivity with the majority growing out of it by age 5 (ASCIA 2019b). This discussion relates to cow's milk protein contained in commercial infant formulas. Whole milk is not recommended for infants younger than 12 months of age. An IgE-mediated allergy to cow's milk may manifest within 15 minutes of consumption or be delayed up to 2 hours, whereas non–IgE-mediated allergies appear more than 2 hours after consumption (ASCIA 2019b). The allergy may manifest within the first 4 months of life through a variety of signs and symptoms (Box 11.2). The diagnosis may initially be made from the history, although the history alone is not diagnostic. The timing and diversity of clinical symptoms vary greatly. For example, CMA may be manifested as colic (see information later in the chapter), diarrhoea, vomiting, GI bleeding, gastro-oesophageal reflux, chronic constipation or sleeplessness in an otherwise healthy infant.

Diagnostic Evaluation. Several diagnostic tests may be performed, including stool analysis for blood (both frank and occult bleeding can

BOX 11.2 Common Clinical Manifestations of Cow's Milk Sensitivity

Gastrointestinal
- Diarrhoea
- Vomiting
- Colic
- Wheezing
- Gastro-oesophageal reflux
- Bloody stools
- Rectal bleeding

Respiratory
- Rhinitis
- Bronchitis
- Asthma
- Sneezing
- Coughing
- Chronic nasal discharge

Other signs and symptoms
- Eczema
- Excessive crying
- Pallor (from anaemia secondary to chronic blood loss in gastrointestinal tract)
- Fussiness, irritability

occur from colitis), eosinophils, leukocytes, serum IgE levels and skin prick testing (Nowak-Węgrzyn et al 2020). Skin testing may help identify the offending food, but the results are not always conclusive. No single diagnostic test is considered definitive for the diagnosis (Kleinman & Greer 2014).

The most definitive diagnostic strategy is elimination of cow's milk in the diet followed by challenge testing after improvement of symptoms. **Challenge testing** involves reintroducing small quantities of milk in the diet to detect resurgence of symptoms. It may also involve the use of a placebo so that the parent is unaware of (or 'blind' to) the timing of allergen ingestion. A double-blind, placebo-controlled food challenge is the gold standard for diagnosing food allergies such as CMA. Careful observation of the child is required during a challenge test because of the possibility of anaphylactic reaction. A clinical diagnosis is made when symptoms improve after removal of milk from the diet and two or more challenge tests produce symptoms (ASCIA 2019b).

Therapeutic Management. Treatment of CMA is elimination of cow's milk–based formula and all other dairy products, as children allergic to cow's milk are often allergic to other dairy milks, such as goat or sheep. For infants who require a milk-based formula, the options are soy, rice, amino acid formula or an extensively hydrolysed formula (EHF). Soy and rice formulas may be useful for children who also react to EHF. Unfortunately, approximately 50% of infants who are sensitive to cow's milk protein will also demonstrate a sensitivity to soy-based formulas. Infants with CMA usually remain on a cow's milk–free diet for 12 months after which time small quantities of milk are reintroduced.

Nursing Care Management. The principal nursing objectives are identification of potential CMA and appropriate counselling of parents regarding substitute infant formulas. Parents often interpret GI symptoms such as spitting up, loose stools or fussiness as CMA and switch the infant to a variety of formulas in an attempt to resolve the problem. Parents need reassurance regarding the needs of non-verbal infants who have an array of symptoms. Endless nights of lost sleep and a crying infant may promote feelings of parenting inadequacy and role conflict, thus aggravating the situation. Nurses can reassure parents that many of these symptoms are common and the reasons are often never discovered, yet the child does achieve appropriate growth and development. Parents should be advised to report acute symptoms to the practitioner for further evaluation. They should be reassured that the infant will receive complete nutrition from the new formula and will have no ill effects from the absence of cow's milk–based formula.

When solid foods are introduced, parents need guidance in avoiding cow's milk products. Carefully reading all food labels helps avoid exposure to prepared foods containing milk products. Although labelled as non-dairy, cream and butter substitutes may contain cow's milk protein.

Lactose Intolerance

The term *lactose intolerance* encompasses at least four different conditions that involve a deficiency of the enzyme lactase, which is needed for the hydrolysis or digestion of lactose in the small intestine. Lactose is hydrolysed into glucose and galactose. **Congenital lactase deficiency** occurs soon after birth when the newborn has consumed lactose-containing milk (human milk or commercial infant formula). This inborn error of metabolism involves the complete absence or severely reduced presence of lactase, is extremely rare and requires a lifelong lactose-free or extremely reduced lactose diet.

Primary lactase deficiency, sometimes referred to as **late-onset lactase deficiency**, is the most common type of lactose intolerance and is manifested usually after 4 or 5 years of age, although the time of onset is variable (Heine et al 2017). Ethnic groups with a high incidence of lactase deficiency include Asians, southern Europeans, Arabs, Israelis and African Americans. Scandinavians tend to have the lowest incidence.

Secondary lactase deficiency may occur secondary to damage that has occurred in the intestinal lumen which decreases or destroys the enzyme lactase (Heine et al 2017). For example, diseases such as cystic fibrosis, sprue, coeliac disease or kwashiorkor and infections such as giardiasis, HIV or rotavirus may cause a temporary or permanent lactose intolerance.

Developmental lactase deficiency refers to the relative lactase deficiency observed in preterm infants of less than 34 weeks of gestation (Albenberg et al 2016). The primary symptoms include abdominal pain, bloating, flatulence and diarrhoea after the ingestion of lactose (Heine et al 2017). The onset of symptoms occurs within 30 minutes to several hours of lactose consumption.

Lactose intolerance can be diagnosed based on the history and improvement of symptoms with a lactose-reduced diet. The breath hydrogen test can be used to diagnose lactase deficiency (Heine et al 2017). However, it is more common to try dietary elimination of lactose and subsequent challenge. The testing of stool pH and glucose content can also be used (Heine et al 2017). Specific to infants, lactose malabsorption may be diagnosed by evaluating faecal pH and reducing substances. Faecal pH in infants is usually lower than in older children, but an acidic pH may indicate malabsorption (Högenauer & Hammer 2016).

Treatment of lactose intolerance is elimination of offending dairy products; however, some advocate decreasing amounts of dairy products rather than total elimination, especially in small children. In infants, lactose-free or low-lactose formula may be used until diarrhoea has resolved (ASCIA 2019b).

One dietary concern is that dairy avoidance in children and adolescents with lactose intolerance will contribute to reduced bone mineral density and osteoporosis later in life (Heine et al 2017). Evidence shows that dietary lactose enhances calcium absorption and that lactose-free diets may negatively affect bone mineralisation (Porto 2016). Therefore, it is recommended that individuals with lactose maldigestion, but no lactose intolerance symptoms, continue to consume small amounts of dairy products with meals to prevent reduced bone mass density and subsequent osteoporosis. Some evidence shows that **probiotics** (i.e. food preparations containing microorganisms such as *Lactobacillus,* which alter the gastrointestinal microflora and thus are beneficial to the host) improve lactose intolerance when live cultures are fermented in dairy products (Canani et al 2016). The positive attributes of probiotics for those with lactose maldigestion include delayed gastrointestinal transit (slower than with milk), positive effects on intestinal and colonic microflora, and a reduction of maldigestion symptoms.

Nursing Care Management. Nursing care is similar to that discussed for CMA and includes: (1) explaining the dietary restrictions to the family; (2) reviewing sources of lactose, including hidden sources; (3) identifying alternative sources of calcium, such as yoghurt; (4) discussing the importance of calcium supplementation; and (5) reviewing strategies for controlling symptoms.

Faltering Growth

Faltering growth is a term which describes a child whose weight or rate of weight gain is slower than what would be expected of a similar child of the same age and gender (Ministry of Health 2021). It has also been called 'failure to thrive', although this term is misleading and can cause some parents distress (RCHM n.d.). Sometimes the term 'poor growth' is also used instead of 'failure to thrive' (RCHM n.d.).

Faltering growth is determined by plotting a child's growth trajectory on a centile chart. A child who is small compared to others, but who is growing and healthy, is not failing to thrive. However, a child whose growth stagnates or declines is failing to grow. This inadequate growth may result from an inability to obtain or use calories required for growth. Faltering growth has no universal definition; however, the objective parameter is usually the deceleration of growth—both height and weight. If faltering growth is severe, poor brain growth may occur as evidenced by a smaller than normal head circumference. The diagnosis is based on growth parameters that: (1) drop more than 2 percentiles from baseline; (2) are persistently below the third to fifth percentiles; or (3) are less than the 80th percentile of median weight-for-height measurement. Weight for length is reported to be a more accurate indicator of undernutrition (Price et al 2020).

Growth measurements alone are not used to diagnose children with faltering growth. Rather, the finding of a pattern of persistent deviation from established growth parameters is cause for concern. Some experts suggest that the previously used classifications of *organic failure to thrive (FTT)* and *non-organic FTT* are too simplistic because in most cases growth failures have mixed causes. Therefore, experts suggest that faltering growth (or FTT) be classified by pathophysiology in the following categories (Homan 2016, McLean & Price 2016, RCHM 2020):

- **inadequate caloric intake**—incorrect formula preparation, neglect, food fads, excessive juice consumption, poverty, breastfeeding problems, behavioural problems affecting eating, parental restriction of caloric intake or central nervous system problems affecting intake
- **inadequate absorption**—cystic fibrosis, coeliac disease, Crohn's disease, vitamin or mineral deficiencies, CMA, biliary atresia or hepatic disease
- **increased metabolism (excessive caloric utilisation)**—hyperthyroidism, congenital heart disease or chronic immunodeficiency
- **defective utilisation**—genetic anomaly such as trisomy 21 or 18, congenital infection or metabolic storage diseases
- **psychosocial factors**—parental depression, substance abuse by parent, attachment issues, behavioural disorders.

Rates of true faltering growth in Australian children is not clearly known. While the primary aetiology of faltering growth is inadequate caloric intake, the cause of faltering growth is often multifactorial and involves a combination of infant organic disease, dysfunctional parenting behaviours, subtle neurological or behavioural problems and disturbed parent–child interactions (Homan 2016, RCHM 2020).

Infants who are born preterm with very low birth weight (VLBW), extremely low birth weight (ELBW) and those with intrauterine growth restriction (IUGR) are often referred for faltering growth within the first 2 years of life. This is because they typically do not grow physically at the same rate as term cohorts even after discharge from the hospital. Catch-up growth is more difficult to achieve in VLBW and ELBW infants. As children, former VLBW and ELBW infants are more likely to have small stature and demonstrate lower cognitive and academic achievement scores than term cohorts (Farajdokht et al 2017). Children with congenital heart disease are also more likely to develop faltering growth in infancy due to inadequate caloric intake, malabsorption, increased energy expenditure that supersedes caloric intake and pulmonary hypertension (McLean & Price 2016).

Other factors that can lead to inadequate caloric intake in infancy include: (1) health or childrearing beliefs such as fad diets; (2) child neglect; (3) child abuse; (4) inadequate nutritional knowledge; (5) financial difficulties; (6) family stress; (7) feeding resistance; and (8) insufficient breast milk intake. In infants younger than 8 weeks of age, breastfeeding problems as a result of inadequate latch or uncoordinated sucking and swallowing may occur (RCHM 2020).

Diagnostic Evaluation

Diagnosis of faltering growth is initially made clinically through identification of signs and symptoms. If faltering growth is acute, the weight, but not the length/height, is below accepted standards (usually the 5th percentile). If faltering growth is chronic, both weight and length/height are low, indicating ongoing malnutrition. The use of weight velocities (according to the WHO growth charts) may be a better indicator of acute growth failure while considering age-dependent changes in growth. Perhaps, as important as anthropometric measurements are, a complete health and dietary history (including perinatal history), physical examination for evidence of organic causes, developmental assessment and family assessment should be undertaken. A dietary intake history, in the form of either a 24-hour dietary recall or a history of food consumed over a 3- to 5-day period, is also essential. In addition, explore the child's activity level, parental stature, perceived food allergies and dietary restrictions.

Therapeutic Management

The primary management of faltering growth is focused on reversing the cause of the growth failure. If malnutrition is severe, the initial treatment is directed at reversing the malnutrition while avoiding refeeding syndrome (see information earlier in this chapter). The goal is to provide sufficient calories to support 'catch-up' growth, which is a rate of growth greater than the expected rate for age. A suggested goal for catch-up growth is 2 to 3 times the average rate of weight gain for the child's corrected age (Kleinman & Greer 2014). In addition to adding caloric density to feedings, the child may require multivitamin supplementation. Any coexisting medical problems must also be addressed.

Prognosis

The prognosis for children with faltering growth is related to the cause. If parents lack knowledge of the infant's needs, teaching may remedy the child's limited caloric intake and permanently reverse the growth failure. Inadequate or infrequent feedings by the infant's primary caretaker, in conjunction with family disorganisation, are often the underlying cause of faltering growth.

There are few long-term studies to provide data on the prognosis of children with faltering growth; however, some researchers have found that children who had faltering growth as infants had shorter statures, lower weights and lower scores on measures of psychomotor development than their peers (Avan et al 2015). Factors that are related to poor prognosis include: (1) severe feeding resistance; (2) lack of awareness in parents; (3) poor parental cooperation; (4) low family income; (5) low maternal educational level; (6) adolescent mothers; (7) preterm birth; (8) IUGR; and (9) early age of onset of faltering growth. Because later cognitive and motor function is affected by malnourishment in infancy, many of these children are below normal in intellectual development resulting in childhood IQ scores that are significantly lower than their peers who have no history of malnourishment (Waber et al 2018). In addition, there is a higher likelihood of eating and behavioural issues among children with a history of malnutrition compared with their peers (Cimino et al 2016). These findings indicate that early identification followed by a long-term plan and regular review of care are needed for the optimum development of these children.

Nursing Care Management

Nurses play a critical role as part of the interprofessional team in the diagnosis of faltering growth through their assessment of the child, parents and family interactions. Knowledge of the characteristics of children with faltering growth and their families is essential in the identification of these children and the rapid confirmation of a diagnosis (Box 11.3). Quality nursing care is underpinned by an ability to accurately and regularly assess weight, head circumference and length/height, keep an accurate record of all intake and document a child's feeding behaviours. In addition, a nurse must document the parent–child interaction during feedings, and assesses other caregiving activities, including play.

Children with faltering growth may have a history of difficult feeding, vomiting, sleep disturbance and excessive irritability. Patterns such as crying during feedings, vomiting, hoarding food in the mouth, ruminating after feeding, refusing to switch from liquids to solids and displaying aversion behaviour, such as turning from food or spitting food, can become attention-seeking behaviours to prolong interaction with caregivers at mealtime. Besides showing signs of malnutrition and delayed social development, children with faltering growth may exhibit altered behavioural interactions with others.

An important primary intervention is to structure the feeding environment to encourage healthful eating, because many children with faltering growth respond to stimuli that have led to negative feeding patterns. Initially, staff members and a dietitian may need to feed these children to thoroughly assess the difficulties encountered during the feeding process and to devise strategies that eliminate or minimise these problems.

There are four primary goals in the nutritional management of children with faltering growth: (1) correct nutritional deficiencies and achieving ideal weight for height; (2) provide adequate calories for catch-up growth; (3) restore optimum body composition; and (4) educate the parents or primary caregivers about the child's nutritional requirements and age-appropriate feeding methods. To determine an individual child's requirements, it is first necessary to work out which centile on the WHO growth charts they should be on. This is done by determining which centile matches their current length/height. This will provide the ideal weight for their current age.

For infants, higher-calorie formulas (e.g. PediaSure) offer a way to increase caloric intake. The nurse should carefully monitor for signs of intolerance to the formula. Calorie intake can also be increased by creating stronger concentrations of standard formula, by adding less water to the mix. Usually only in extreme cases of malnourishment are tube feedings or intravenous therapy required. Finally, carbohydrate additives including fortified cereals and vegetable oil may be indicated. Because vitamin and mineral deficiencies may occur, multivitamin supplementation, including zinc and iron, is recommended.

Maladaptive feeding practices often contribute to growth failure; therefore, parents should be given specific step-by-step directions for formula preparation, as well as a written schedule of feeding times. Fruit juice is restricted in children with faltering growth until adequate weight gain has been achieved using appropriate milk sources. At that time, juice may be reintroduced but limited to no more than 110 g/day.

Behaviour modification techniques may be used with older infants and toddlers to interrupt maladaptive feeding patterns. Feeding times can become a 'war of wills' resulting in food refusal and eventually faltering growth. These behaviours are different from the occasional toddler behaviour of food refusal, which is primarily developmental, not pathological.

In addition to attending to the child's physical needs, the interdisciplinary team must plan care for appropriate developmental stimulation. After an approximate developmental age is established, a planned program of play should be initiated. Ideally, a child life specialist is involved in this plan to implement and supervise the child's play activities. Every effort should be made to educate parents about how to play and interact with their child at a developmentally appropriate level. A paediatric nutrition specialist should also be involved in planning and implementing a diet specifically tailored for the child's growth needs.

Nursing care of children with faltering growth involves a 'family systems' approach. Therefore, if the goal is for the entire family to become healthy, all members should be engaged in the change process. Nursing care of the child's parents is focused on improving their self-esteem and supporting them as they acquire positive, successful parenting skills. Initially, this necessitates providing an environment in which they feel welcomed and accepted.

BOX 11.3 Clinical Manifestations of Failure to Thrive

- Growth failure
- Developmental delays—social, motor, adaptive, language
- Undernutrition
- Apathy
- Withdrawn behaviour
- Feeding or eating disorders, such as vomiting, feeding resistance, anorexia, pica, rumination
- No fear of strangers (at age when stranger anxiety is normal)
- Avoidance of eye contact
- Wide-eyed gaze and continual scan of the environment ('radar gaze')
- Stiff and unyielding or flaccid and unresponsive
- Minimal smiling

SPECIAL HEALTH PROBLEMS

Colic (Paroxysmal Abdominal Pain)

Colic is believed to occur in up to 20% of all infants, yet an organic cause is identified in only a small number of children assessed for excessive crying (Turner & Palamountain 2018). The condition is generally described as abdominal pain or cramping that is manifested by loud crying and drawing the legs up to the abdomen. Parents typically express dissatisfaction with the amount of time the infant spends crying each day. Colic is commonly characterised according to the Wessel criteria, which is crying: (1) greater than 3 hours a day; (2) for more than 3 days per week; and (3) for more than 3 weeks (Sung 2018). Symptoms may increase in the late afternoon or evening (Turner & Palamountain 2018); however, in some infants the onset of symptoms occurs at varying times. Colic is more common in younger infants under the age of 3 months than in older infants. Infants with difficult temperaments are also more likely to exhibit colic.

Aetiology

The potential causes of colic include: (1) feeding too rapidly; (2) overfeeding; (3) swallowing excessive air; (4) improper feeding technique (especially positioning and burping); and (5) emotional stress or tension between parent and infant. Although all of these may occur, there is no evidence that one factor is consistently present. Infants with CMA symptoms have a high rate of colic (44%), and eliminating cow's milk products from these infants' diets can reduce the symptoms.

Therapeutic Management

Management of colic should begin with an investigation of possible organic causes such as CMA, intussusception or GI problems such as sensitivity to lactose. If a milk sensitivity is suspected, a trial of non-cow's milk–based formula is warranted (see section on Cow's Milk Allergy). Oral administration of *Lactobacillus reuteri* to exclusively breastfed infants has been found to be effective in decreasing crying symptoms (Sung 2018). However, the effectiveness of *Lactobacillus reuteri* administration to formula-fed infants is unknown (Ellwood et al 2020, Sung 2018). When no specific cause can be found, the supportive measures discussed in the Nursing Care Management section are used.

The use of hydrolysed formula, a hypoallergenic diet in breastfeeding mothers, increased parental responsiveness and acupuncture may be effective. Simethicone, spinal manipulation, soy, increased carrying of the child and crib vibrators have not been found to be effective (Sung 2018). Behavioural interventions have not proven effective at reducing symptoms of colic either but have helped parents deal with the crying infant in a more positive manner.

NURSING CARE CONSIDERATIONS

To date, there is no evidence to support one remedy that will relieve symptoms in every infant (NHMRC 2012). Dietary changes including the elimination of cow's milk protein in the infant's diet may be effective in reducing the infant's crying, yet these interventions have been found to be only moderately effective (Sung 2018). Probiotics have been found to reduce crying in breastfed infants (Ellwood et al 2020) and may be useful in practice.

If cow's milk sensitivity is suspected, breastfeeding mothers should follow a milk-free diet for a minimum of 3 to 5 days to see if this is effective in reducing the infant's symptoms. If a milk-free diet is helpful, lactating mothers may need calcium supplements to meet requirements (RCHM 2016). Formula-fed infants may improve with the same dietary modifications as for infants with CMA.

Nursing Care Management

The initial step in managing colic is to take a thorough, detailed history of the usual daily events. Areas that should be stressed include the: (1) infant's diet; (2) diet of the breastfeeding mother; (3) timing of the crying; (4) relationship of crying to feedings; (5) presence of a specific family member during crying; (6) habits of family members, such as smoking; (7) activity of the mother or usual caregiver before, during and after crying; (8) characteristics of the cry (e.g. duration, intensity); (9) measures used to relieve crying and their effectiveness; and (10) infant's stooling, voiding and sleeping patterns. Of particular importance is a careful assessment of the feeding process via demonstration by the parent.

Sleep Problems

Sleep problems can be common in young children. The two major categories are the **dyssomnias** and **parasomnias.** With dyssomnias, the child has trouble either falling or staying asleep at night or has difficulty staying awake during the day, and a disorder of amount, quality or timing of sleep. Parasomnias consist of confusional arousals, sleepwalking, sleep terrors, nightmares and rhythmic movement disorders. These typically occur in children 3 to 8 years old (BMJ 2020). This discussion focuses on minor sleep issues in infants such as refusal to go to sleep or frequent waking during the night. Later in this text, other sleep disturbances will be discussed such as obstructive sleep-disordered breathing and sleep terrors.

Concerns regarding sleep are common during infancy. Sometimes these concerns are as basic as parents' questions about whether the infant needs additional sleep. In this case it is best to investigate the reason for their concern, stressing the individual needs of each child. Infants who are active during wakeful periods and growing normally are typically receiving adequate sleep.

However, several more serious concerns require intervention. Sleep disturbances of physiological origin are less common in infants with the exception of colic. The more common sleep disturbances are a learned pattern or developmental characteristic of some infants (Table 11.1). Although many families may report sleep problems typical of these patterns, interventions are offered only when the pattern is disruptive to the family. Sleep problems in early infancy have been positively correlated with higher maternal depression scores, although it may be more related to the mother's perception of her baby's sleep quality rather than the actual sleep the infant achieves (Halal et al 2020); therefore, nurses should discuss infant sleep problems with the mother (and family) in addition to other developmental aspects of newborn care.

Sudden Infant Death Syndrome

Sudden infant death syndrome (SIDS) is defined as the sudden death of an infant younger than 1 year of age that remains unexplained after a complete postmortem examination (autopsy), including an investigation of the death scene and a review of the case history. An autopsy is essential to identify possible natural explanations for sudden unexpected death such as congenital anomalies or infection and to identify a death that was the result of child abuse. The autopsy typically cannot distinguish between SIDS and intentional suffocation, but the scene investigation and medical history may be of help if inconsistencies are discovered.

There has been much debate over the term *SIDS*, yet the definition noted earlier remains for the time being. In Australia, the term *sudden unexpected death in infancy* (SUDI) covers both SIDS and fatal sleeping accidents (Raising Children Network 2020). The risk of SUDI in an infant is particularly high when three key risk factors coincide: (1) vulnerability; (2) age; and (3) environment. This is called the triple risk model. The focus of SIDS prevention is on targeting the risks that can be mitigated; that is, the environment, particularly the one a child sleeps in (Raising Children Network 2020).

In Australia, from 1979 to 2017, the incidence of SIDS decreased by 85% (Red Nose Australia 2020). This is largely due to a safe sleeping campaign promoted through maternal child centres and in paediatric institutions, complemented by improvements in availability of safe bedding options for children. See Table 11.2.

Aetiology

There are numerous theories regarding the aetiology of SIDS, but the cause remains unknown. One hypothesis is that SIDS is related to brainstem abnormalities in the neurological regulation of cardiorespiratory control. This maldevelopment affects arousal and physiological responses to a life-threatening challenge during sleep (Bright et al 2018). Abnormalities include prolonged sleep apnoea, increased frequency of brief inspiratory pauses, excessive periodic breathing and impaired arousal responsiveness to increased carbon dioxide or decreased oxygen. However, *sleep apnoea is not the cause of SIDS.* The majority of infants with apnoea do not die and only a minority of SIDS victims have a documented brief resolved unexplained event (BRUE), which is a term replacing what was previously known as an apparent life-threatening event (ALTE) (see BRUE later in this chapter). Further, the findings of numerous studies indicate that no association exists between SIDS and any childhood vaccine.

A **genetic predisposition** to SIDS has been suspected as a potential cause. In particular, differences in genes pertinent to immune system

TABLE 11.1 Selected Sleep Disturbances during Infancy and Early Childhood

Disorder and Description	Management
NIGHT-TIME FEEDING	
Child has a prolonged need for middle-of-night bottle-feeding or breastfeeding. Child goes to sleep at breast or with bottle. Awakenings are frequent (may be hourly). Child returns to sleep after feeding; other comfort measures (e.g. rocking or holding) are usually ineffective.	Increase daytime feeding intervals to > 4 hr (may need to be done gradually). Offer last feeding as late as possible at night; may need to gradually reduce amount of formula or length of breastfeeding. Offer no bottles in bed. Put to bed awake. When child is crying, check at progressively longer intervals each night; reassure child but do not hold, rock, take to parents' bed or give bottle or soother.
DEVELOPMENTAL NIGHT CRYING	
Child ages 6–12 months with undisturbed night-time sleep now awakens abruptly; may be accompanied by nightmares.	Reassure parents that this phase is temporary. Enter room immediately to check on child but keep reassurances brief. Avoid feeding, rocking, taking to parents' bed or any other routine that may initiate trained night crying.
REFUSAL TO GO TO SLEEP	
Child resists bedtime and comes out of room repeatedly. Night-time sleep may be continuous, but frequent awakenings and refusal to return to sleep may occur and become a problem if parent allows child to deviate from usual sleep pattern.	Evaluate whether hour of sleep is too early (child may resist sleep if not tired). Assist parents in establishing consistent before-bedtime routine and enforcing consistent limits regarding child's bedtime behaviour. If child persists in leaving bedroom, close door for progressively longer periods. Use reward system with child to provide motivation.
TRAINED NIGHT CRYING (INAPPROPRIATE SLEEP ASSOCIATIONS)	
Child typically falls asleep in place other than own bed (e.g. rocking chair or parents' bed) and is brought to own bed while asleep; on awakening, baby cries until usual routine is instituted (e.g. rocking).	Put child in own bed when awake. If possible, arrange sleeping area separate from other family members. When child is crying, check at progressively longer intervals each night; reassure child but do not resume usual routine.
NIGHT-TIME FEARS	
Child resists going to bed or wakes during night because of fears. Child seeks parent's physical presence and falls asleep easily with parent nearby, unless fear is overwhelming.	Evaluate whether hour of sleep is too early (child may fantasise when nothing to do but think in dark room). Calmly reassure frightened child; keeping night-light on may be helpful. Use reward system with child to provide motivation to deal with fears. Avoid patterns that can lead to additional problems (e.g. sleeping with child or taking child to parents' room). If child's fear is overwhelming, consider desensitisation (e.g. progressively spending longer time alone, consult professional help for protracted fears). Distinguish between nightmares and sleep terrors (confused partial arousals).

Source: Modified from Ferber, R. (1987). Behavioural 'insomnia' in the child. Psychiatric Clinics of North America, 10(4), 641–653.

functioning and the development of the autonomic nervous system have been discovered in infants who died of SIDS compared with typical infants (Moon & Hauk 2018). Several 'triple risk factor' hypotheses have been proposed to explain the aetiology of SIDS. The proposed risk factors include an underlying infant vulnerability such as a brain abnormality, a critical incident in the fetal developmental period or in early neonatal life and an environmental stressor such as prone sleep positioning (Raising Children Network 2020).

Risk Factors for Sudden Infant Death Syndrome

Maternal smoking during pregnancy is a major modifiable risk factor for SIDS. The incidence of SIDS is approximately three times greater among infants whose mothers smoked during pregnancy, and risk of death is progressively greater as daily cigarette use increases (Raising Children Network 2020, Moon & Hauk 2018). The effects of smoking by the father and other household members are more difficult to interpret because they correlate highly with maternal smoking. However, an increased risk for SIDS has been found in infants exposed only to postnatal maternal environmental tobacco smoke (Raising Children Network 2020).

Co-sleeping, or an infant sharing a bed with an adult or older child in a non-infant bed, is associated with SIDS. Research has found a significant increase in the risk of SIDS among infants who share a bed, compared with infants who sleep alone (Raising Children Network 2020, Red Nose Australia 2020). There is also an increased risk of accidental suffocation or strangulation when infants were sleeping on a sofa compared with other locations (Red Nose Australia 2020).

Prone sleeping may cause oropharyngeal obstruction or affect thermal balance or arousal state. Rebreathing of carbon dioxide by infants due to sleeping in the prone position is also a possible cause of SIDS. Infants sleeping prone and on soft bedding may be unable to move their heads to the side, thus increasing the risk of suffocation and lethal rebreathing (Moon & Hauk 2018). Therefore, the side-lying position is no longer recommended for infants sleeping at home, day care or hospitals (unless medically indicated). Most preterm infants being discharged from the hospital should be placed in a supine sleeping position unless special factors predispose them to airway obstruction.

Soft bedding (waterbeds, sheepskins, beanbags, pillows and quilts) should be avoided for infant sleeping surfaces. Extra bed linen, stuffed

TABLE 11.2 Epidemiology of Sudden Infant Death Syndrome

Factor	Occurrence
Incidence	In 2017 in Australia there were 87 deaths from SUDI, which equates to 0.3 deaths per 1000 live births (Red Nose Australia 2020); in New Zealand in 2015 there were 2 deaths from SUDI (0.7 per 1000 live births) (Ministry of Health 2015)
Peak age	2–3 months; 95% occur by 6 months; preterm infants die of sudden infant death syndrome (SIDS) at mean age of 6 weeks later than mean age of death from SIDS for term infants
Sex	Higher percentage of boys affected
Time of death	During sleep
Time of year	Increased incidence in winter
Racial	Greater incidence in Aboriginal and Torres Strait and Māori infants
Socioeconomic	Increased occurrence in lower socioeconomic class
Birth	Higher incidence in: • preterm infants, especially infants of extremely and very low birth weight • multiple births* • neonates with low Apgar scores • infants with central nervous system disturbances and respiratory disorders such as bronchopulmonary dysplasia • increasing birth order (subsequent siblings as opposed to firstborn child).
Health status	Infants with a recent history of illness; lower incidence in immunised infants
Sleep habits	Highest risk associated with prone position; use of soft bedding; overheating (thermal stress); co-sleeping with adult, especially on sofa or non-infant bed; higher incidence in co-sleeping with adult smoker Infants co-sleeping with adult at higher risk if younger than 11 weeks
Feeding habits	Lower incidence in breastfed infants
Soother	Lower incidence in infants put to sleep with soother/dummy
Siblings	May have greater incidence in siblings of SIDS victims
Maternal	Young age; cigarette smoking, especially during pregnancy; poor prenatal care; substance abuse (heroin, methadone, cocaine)—a few studies have shown an increased risk in infants exposed to second-hand environmental tobacco smoke

*Although a rare event, simultaneous death of twins from SIDS can occur.
Source: Data from Healthdirect.gov.au https://www.healthdirect.gov.au/sudden-infant-death-syndrome-sids; RedNose.org; AIHW. (2020). Australia's children. https://www.aihw.gov.au/reports/children-youth/australias-children/contents/health/infant-child-deaths; Ministry of Health. (2015). Fetal and infant deaths 2015. New Zealand Government. https://www.health.govt.nz/publication/fetal-and-infant-deaths-2015; Freemantle, J., & Ellis, L. (2018). An Australian perspective. In Duncan, J., & Byard, R. W., (Eds.). SIDS sudden infant and early childhood death: The past, the present and the future (pp. 85–116). University of Adelaide Press.

animals and toys should be removed from the cot while the infant is asleep (Raising Children Network 2020). Also, cot bumper pads should not be used (Red Nose Australia 2020).

Protective Factors for Sudden Infant Death Syndrome

The findings of a meta-analysis indicate that breastfeeding for any duration will significantly reduce SIDS rates; with the effect stronger if exclusive breastfeeding is continued for a long period of time (Moon & Hauk 2018, Red Nose Australia 2020). Soother (dummy) use has also been associated with a lower risk of SIDS, although it is uncertain if this is a direct effect of the soother itself or from associated infant or parental behaviour. To counter concerns over soother use interfering with breastfeeding, parents should be advised to wait until breastfeeding is well established before using a soother. When used, it should be used for each sleep period (Red Nose Australia 2020).

The Raising Children Network (2020) and Red Nose Australia (2020) recommend that *all infants* be placed to sleep in the **supine (on the back) position.** It is also recommended that medically stable preterm infants and infants diagnosed with gastro-oesophageal reflux (GOR) be placed in a supine sleep position unless they have a specific upper airway disorder that places them at greater risk of death than the risk of death from SIDS. Safe sleeping recommendations include encouraging parents to share a bedroom with infants, but not the same sleeping surface, preferably until the infant is a year old, but at least for the first 6 months. Room-sharing decreases the risk of SIDS by as much as 50% (Raising Children Network 2020, Red Nose Australia 2020).

Since the 1990s when advocation of non-prone sleeping for infants began, an increased incidence of positional plagiocephaly has been observed (see later in the chapter). The length of time an infant sleeps for and the total time they sleep each day influences the development of plagiocephaly (Leung et al 2017). Up-to-date childhood immunisation status has also been shown to be protective against SIDS, probably by reducing the incidence of certain diseases.

Although the cause of SIDS is unknown, autopsies reveal consistent pathological findings, such as pulmonary oedema and intrathoracic haemorrhages that confirm the diagnosis. Consequently, autopsies should be performed on all infants suspected of dying of SIDS, and findings should be shared with the parents as soon as possible after the death. Postmortem findings in SIDS and accidental suffocation or intentional suffocation, such as in Munchausen syndrome by proxy (see Child Maltreatment, Chapter 14), are practically the same (Sidebotham et al 2018).

Infant Risk Factors

Certain groups of infants are at increased risk for SIDS:

- low birth weight or preterm birth (< 37 weeks gestation)
- low Apgar scores
- recent viral illness
- siblings of two or more SIDS victims
- male gender.

No diagnostic tests exist to predict which infants, including those in the above-listed groups, will die of SIDS. The next-born sibling of a firstborn infant who died of any non-infectious natural cause are at significantly increased risk for infant death from the same cause, including SIDS. This increased risk for recurrent SIDS in families is consistent with genetic risk factors interacting with environmental risk factors (Red Nose Australia 2020). Home monitoring is not recommended for this group of children, but it is often used by practitioners and may even be requested by parents; even though there is no evidence that home apnoea monitoring prevents SIDS (Hunt & Hauck 2016).

Nursing Care Management

Nurses have a vital role in preventing SIDS by educating families about the risk of prone sleeping in infants from birth to 6 months of age. This starts with being proactive during postpartum discharge planning, newborn discharge teaching, follow-up home visits, well-baby clinic visits and immunisation visits. This education should include the use of appropriate bedding surfaces, the association between SIDS and maternal smoking, the dangers of co-sleeping with adults or other children and where supportive online resources can be found (e.g. Raising Children Network). Further, nurses must continue to take every opportunity to advocate for infants by providing information for parents and caretakers about the modifiable risk factors for SIDS that can be implemented to prevent its occurrence across all sectors of the population. Additionally, nurses have an important role in modelling behaviours for parents that decrease SIDS risk such as placing infants in a supine sleeping position while in the hospital. It is essential nurses maximise opportunities for role-modelling safe sleep practices and providing education to parents before hospital discharge.

Caring for the Family after Sudden Infant Death Syndrome

Loss of a child from SIDS presents several crises for the infant's parents. In addition to grief and mourning the death of their child, the parents must face a tragedy that was sudden, unexpected and unexplained. This discussion focuses primarily on the objectives of care for families experiencing SIDS rather than on the process of grief and mourning, which is explored in Chapter 19.

The first people to arrive at the scene may be the police and emergency medical service personnel. It is expected they should handle the situation by: (1) asking only essential questions (needed at that time); (2) giving no indication of wrongdoing, abuse or neglect; (3) making sensitive judgments concerning any resuscitation efforts for the child; and (4) comforting the family members as much as possible. A compassionate, sensitive approach to the family may help minimise some of the overwhelming guilt and anguish that commonly follow this type of loss (Sidebotham et al 2018).

Until the police have finished processing the scene, the sleep environment should remain as it was when the infant was initially found. If the infant is not pronounced dead at the scene, he or she will be transported to an emergency department to be pronounced dead by a physician. Usually there is no attempt at resuscitation in the emergency department. While in the emergency department the parents should only be asked factual questions such as when they found the infant, how he or she looked and who they called for help. The nurse should avoid any remarks that may suggest responsibility, such as 'Why didn't you go in earlier?' or 'Didn't you hear the infant cry out?' It is the police and coroner's responsibility to document these findings, rather than have parents recount the painful experience in the emergency department. Parents may also express feelings of guilt about administering cardiopulmonary resuscitation (CPR) correctly or the timing of CPR in relation to finding the infant (Sidebotham et al 2018).

The medical practitioner should initiate the discussion of an autopsy, usually with a nurse being present to support the family, ensuring the family understand a diagnosis cannot be confirmed until the postmortem examination is completed. Instructions about the autopsy and funeral arrangements may need to be repeated or put in writing. If the mother was breastfeeding, she will need information about abrupt discontinuation of lactation. The nurse or medical practitioner should contact the primary care practitioner for the infant and the mother to avoid any miscommunications or telephone calls later inquiring about the child's health status.

Parents experiencing perinatal death perceive the response of healthcare workers as having a significant impact on their grieving process. A family-centred approach that involves the sociocultural context and unique needs of the family is essential for perinatal bereavement care, as is adequate training and support for healthcare workers, in how to best deliver care (Perinatal Society of Australia and New Zealand [PSANZ] 2018).

An important aspect of compassionate care for parents is allowing them to say goodbye to their child. These are the parents' last moments with their child, and they should be as quiet, meaningful, peaceful and undisturbed as possible. Encourage parents to hold their infant before leaving the emergency department. Because the parents will be leaving the hospital without their infant, it may be helpful to accompany them to the car or arrange for someone else to take them home. A debriefing session may help healthcare workers who cared for the family cope with troubling emotions.

When the parents return home, a competent, qualified professional should visit them as soon after the death as possible. They should receive printed material that contains accurate information about SIDS (available from the national organisation*). During the initial visit, the nurse should help the parents gain an intellectual understanding of the condition. The nursing objectives are to assess what the parents have been told about SIDS, what they think happened and how they explained the death to the other siblings, family members and friends (Goldstein 2018). One question that the nurse will not be able to answer and therefore should never attempt is, 'Why did this happen to our baby?' or 'Who is responsible for this tragedy?' These and other questions may linger in the parents' minds for months or even years.

When the unexpected death of a child occurs, it is common for one parent to blame the other. Parents may also experience guilt over the child's death. For example, they may feel that if they had checked on their child earlier, he or she might still be alive. It is important that the nurse assist parents in working through these feelings to prevent marital disruption in addition to the loss of the loved child (Goldstein 2018).

Some parents are able to discuss their feelings openly and the nurse should support this coping skill. However, others may be reluctant to express their grief and the nurse can encourage the expression of emotions by asking about crying and feeling sad, angry or guilty. During their interaction, the nurse can help the parents explore their typical coping strategies and, if these are ineffectual, to investigate new approaches. For example, one parent may refrain from discussing the death for fear of upsetting the other parent, but each may need to hear how the other is feeling.

Ideally, the number of visits and plans for subsequent intervention needs to be flexible. Parents facing the question of having a subsequent child will need support. Both the birth of a subsequent child and the survival of that child, especially past the age of death of the previous child, are important transitional stages for parents.

*Red Nose Australia. https://rednose.org.au/section/professionals_hub

Positional Plagiocephaly

Over the last couple of decades, an increase in the incidence of positional plagiocephaly has been reported (Leung et al 2017). The term **plagiocephaly** connotes an oblique or asymmetrical head. Positional plagiocephaly, deformational plagiocephaly or non-synostotic plagiocephaly implies an acquired skull deformity that occurs as a result of cranial moulding during infancy usually as a result of lying in the supine position (RCHM 2018b). Because infants' sutures are not yet fused, the skull is pliable so when infants are placed on their backs to sleep, the posterior occiput flattens over time (Fig 11.1). A typical bald spot develops over the area, which is usually transient. Prolonged pressure on one side of the skull can result in that side becoming misshapen. Mild facial asymmetry may also develop. The sternocleidomastoid muscle may tighten on the preferential side resulting in a condition called *torticollis*. Congenital or acquired torticollis may also cause plagiocephaly. Other causes of deformational plagiocephaly include certain craniofacial syndromes. The following discussion is focused only on positional plagiocephaly (PP) caused by supine sleeping position.

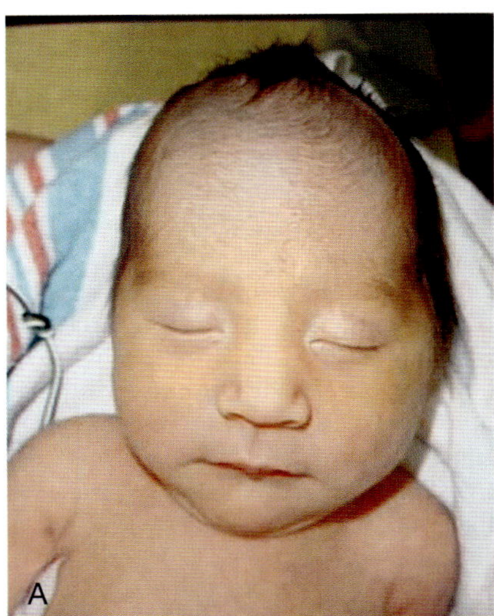

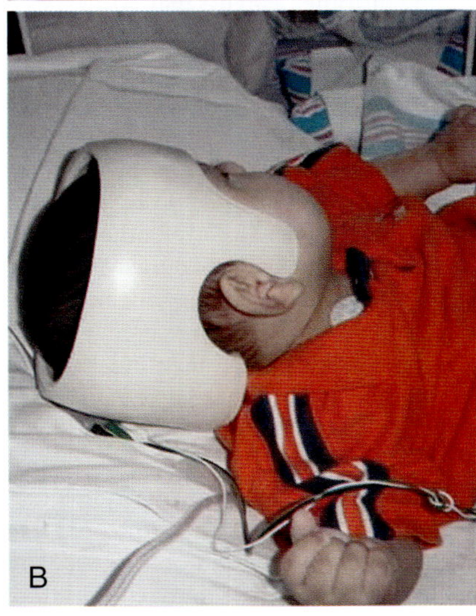

Fig 11.1 (**A**) Plagiocephaly. (**B**) Helmet used to correct plagiocephaly. (Source: Courtesy Dr. Gerardo Cabrera-Meza, Department of Neonatology, Baylor College of Medicine, Houston, TX.)

Diagnostic Evaluation

The diagnosis of PP may be made on physical examination of the infant's head, which is viewed frontally and from above. The typical infant's head shape will resemble a parallelogram with unilateral flattening of the occiput, frontal and parietal bossing, a prominent cheekbone and an anterior ear displacement. An evaluation of neck movement and range of motion is also made to determine the presence of torticollis. In most cases skull films and further radiological studies (CT scan) are used only to rule out craniosynostosis or other cranial deformities that may affect brain growth.

Therapeutic Management

Prevention of PP should begin shortly after birth. The primary recommendation for preventing PP is to ensure an infant is not on their back when awake. This includes avoiding prolonged placement in car safety seats and swings and employing 'tummy time' during awake periods for 10 to 15 minutes three times a day in order to promote prone positioning (Leung et al 2017), a technique originally designed to encourage development of upper shoulder girdle strength.

The watch and wait method of treatment for torticollis and PP is not recommended (Leung et al 2017). Repositioning and physical therapy (RPPT), which includes providing counselling and teaching for parents as to positional changes and tummy time for their child, is recommended. A referral to physical therapy may be needed in the case of congenital torticollis. RPPT is the optimal treatment choice for patients younger than 4 months of age who have mild to moderately severe PP. The earliest types of behavioural modifications can be as simple as increasing tummy time or repositioning the infant's cot in a way that ensures everything interesting in the room is on the side opposite the plagiocephaly (Leung et al 2017).

Moulding therapy (helmet therapy) is the use of an orthotic helmet to promote the resolution of cranial asymmetry while the infant's head is still rapidly growing (Leung et al 2017). Orthotic helmets do not actively mould the skull; instead, they protect the areas that are flattened and allow the child to 'grow into' the flat spots. Studies have shown helmet therapy to achieve correction is three times faster and better than repositioning alone. However, it is also associated with side effects such as irritation, rashes and pressure sores. The findings of recent studies suggest that combined treatment with helmet therapy and physical therapy is the most beneficial for the management of infants older than 4 months who are severely affected or with worsening of mild/moderate plagiocephaly who have been trialled on physical therapy. Infants with severe plagiocephaly should be considered for helmet therapy at any age (Leung et al 2017).

Nursing Care Management

Minor skull deformation is not considered significant, but parents should learn to prevent plagiocephaly by alternating the infant's head position when they sleep (RCHM 2018b). Infants should be placed prone on a firm surface during awake time (tummy time) for at least 10 to 15 minutes three times a day (Leung et al 2017), which prevents plagiocephaly and facilitates development of upper shoulder girdle strength. The latter helps in the progressive development of movements such as rolling over and starting to rise on all fours that are precursors to crawling and eventually walking. Despite the perceived increase in incidence of PP, the supine sleeping position is still recommended because it has led to a significant decrease in loss of infant lives from SIDS. When a nurse or parent notices plagiocephaly, a consultation with the primary practitioner is recommended to evaluate the head shape and ascertain the need for early intervention.

Nurses are in a unique position in well-childcare settings to assess parents' ability to follow guidelines for preventing plagiocephaly by observing them alternating head placement for sleeping, demonstrating sternocleidomastoid muscle exercises (as appropriate to the condition) and implementing tummy time for infants during awake periods. Most importantly, nurses should continue to encourage parents to place the infant in a supine sleep position despite the development of plagiocephaly. Nurses can also assist parents in the proper use of a skull-moulding helmet and reassure them of the high rate of success with the helmet. Allowing parents to verbalise concerns and feelings related to the health status of their child, as well as the provision of current best practice, is an important nursing function.

Brief Resolved Unexplained Event

A **brief resolved unexplained event (BRUE)** is an event in a child under 1 year of age, characterised by marked changes in breathing, tone, colour or consciousness, followed by a return to consciousness in less than a minute. There is no identified cause and it is a diagnosis of exclusion (RCHM 2017). Specifically, one or more of the following must occur: (1) cyanosis or pallor; (2) absent, decreased or irregular breathing; (3) marked change in muscle tone (hypertonia or hypotonia); or (4) altered responsiveness.

A **BRUE** was formerly referred to as *ALTE* or *near-miss SIDS*. However, it is erroneous to characterise ALTE as a near-miss SIDS incident. A history of an unexplained ALTE occurs in 5% to 9% of SIDS victims and the risk of SIDS appears to be higher with two or more unexplained events, but no definitive incidence rates are available. Compared with healthy control infants, the risk for SIDS may be as much as 3 to 5 times greater in infants having experienced an ALTE (RCHM 2017).

Results from the Collaborative Home Infant Monitoring Evaluation (CHIME) study showed that apnoea and bradycardia occurred at both conventional and extreme alarm thresholds in all groups of infants studied: siblings of SIDS infants, infants with ALTEs, symptomatic (of apnoea and bradycardia), asymptomatic preterm infants weighing less than 1750 g at birth and healthy term infants (Hunt & Hauck 2016). Many infants experienced apnoea and bradycardia in each of these groups, yet did not die.

Diagnostic Evaluation

An essential component of the diagnostic process includes a detailed description of the event, including who witnessed the event, where the infant was during the event and what, if any, activities were involved (e.g. during or after a feeding, riding in a car seat restraint, presence of siblings or any minor children, what clothing the infant was wearing). In addition, a prenatal and postnatal history must be obtained. A short period of observation in the emergency department may be appropriate to observe the infant's respiratory pattern and response to feeding. Further, a careful evaluation of late-preterm and preterm infants in their car seat restraint is essential. Upper airway occlusion and subsequent apnoea and cyanosis may occur if the infant is not positioned properly.

If an underlying diagnosis cannot be established, home monitoring may be recommended. The most common monitoring used is continuous recording of cardiorespiratory patterns or inductance plethysmography (Perth Children's Hospital [PCH] 2018). Four-channel pneumocardiograms (or multichannel pneumogram) monitor heart rate, respirations (chest impedance), nasal airflow and oxygen saturation. A more sophisticated test, polysomnography (sleep study), also records brain waves, eye and body movements, oesophageal manometry and end-tidal carbon dioxide measurements. However, none of these tests can predict risk. Some children with normal results may still have subsequent apnoeic episodes.

Therapeutic Management

The treatment of an infant with a BRUE depends on the underlying condition. Several diagnostic tests may be carried out to determine the cause; however, a cause may not be determined in up to 50% of the cases. Testing for seizures, GOR or sepsis is not routine. Clinical suspicion of cause will determine whether pertussis, ECG (electrocardiogram), FBC (full blood count), UEC (urea, electrolytes and creatinine), blood glucose or an NPA (nasopharyngeal aspirate) sample is required (PCH 2018, RCHM 2017).

Nursing Care Management

The diagnosis of a BRUE causes great anxiety and concern in parents, and the initiation of home monitoring presents additional physical and emotional burdens. Parents of infants on home apnoea monitors report experiencing emotional distress, especially depression and hostility, during the first few weeks after hospital discharge. For parents of a SIDS victim who have a new infant on home apnoea monitoring, the anxiety is compounded by the uncertainty of the future of the living child and grief for the lost child. Home apnoea monitoring may offer some predictability and control over the current child's survival through the period of uncertainty.

If home monitoring is required, the nurse can be a major source of support to the family in terms of education about the equipment, education regarding observation of the infant's status and instructions on immediate intervention during apnoeic episodes, including CPR. To help the family cope with the numerous procedures they must learn, adequate preparation before discharge and written instructions are essential. In the first few weeks after discharge, parents may benefit by having a practitioner readily available to answer questions regarding false alarms and for other technical assistance.

Several types of home monitors are available and are set up by either a home monitor equipment company or home health staff. Nurses, especially those involved in the care at home, must become familiar with the equipment, including its advantages and disadvantages. Safety is a major concern because monitors can cause electrical burns and electrocution. The following precautions are recommended.

- Remove leads from infant when not attached to the monitor.
- Unplug the power cord from the electrical outlet when the cord is not plugged into the monitor.
- Use safety covers on electrical outlets to discourage children from inserting objects into sockets.

Additional home use instructions should focus on troubleshooting the monitor alarms. Encourage the parents to look first at the infant if an alarm goes off and ensure that the infant is breathing, and then determine the cause of the alarm. Parents also need information about travelling or running necessary errands with an infant on an apnoea monitor, what to do in case of power failure and who to contact if the monitor alarm goes off continuously but the infant appears well. Siblings should be supervised when near the infant and taught that the monitor is not a toy. Other safety practices include informing local utility services and rescue crews (fire and/or emergency services) of the home monitoring in case of an emergency, especially if the family lives in a remote rural area. Telephone numbers for these services should be posted in the home or set up as speed dial on certain phones if a universal emergency dial system is not available. Post instructions for infant CPR in a central location of the house and encourage parents to tell visitors and other family members about the location of these instructions. If a mobile phone is the main house phone, make sure it stays in a central location for all family members to access in an emergency.

NURSING CARE CONSIDERATIONS

If the infant is apnoeic, gently stimulate the trunk by patting or rubbing it. Call loudly for help even if alone. If the infant is prone, turn to the supine position and flick the heels of the feet. If there is still no response, call for help and immediately begin CPR starting with chest compressions. Never vigorously shake the child. No more than 10 to 15 seconds are spent on stimulation before implementing CPR (Australian Resuscitation Council 2016).

REFERENCES

Agarwal, A., Shaharyar, A., Kumar, A., et al. (2014). Scurvy in pediatric age group—A disease often forgotten. Journal of Orthopaedic Trauma, 6, 101–107.

Albenberg, L., Evans, J., & Piccoli, D. A. (2016). Protracted diarrhea. In R. Wyllie, J. S. Hyams, & M. Kay (Eds.), Pediatric gastrointestinal and liver disease (5th ed.). Pennsylvania: Elsevier.

Ashworth, A. (2016). Nutrition, food security, and health. In R. M. Kliegman, B. F. Stanton, J. W. St Geme, et al. (Eds.), Nelson textbook of pediatrics (20th ed.). Philadelphia: Elsevier/Saunders.

Australasian Society of Clinical Immunology and Allergy (ASCIA). (2019a). Allergen immunotherapy. March. https://www.allergy.org.au/patients/allergy-treatment/immunotherapy

Australasian Society of Clinical Immunology and Allergy (ASCIA). (2019b). Cow's milk (Dairy) allergy. https://www.allergy.org.au/patients/food-allergy/cows-milk-dairy-allergy

Australasian Society of Clinical Immunology and Allergy (ASCIA). (2020a). Allergy testing. July. https://www.allergy.org.au/patients/allergy-testing/allergy-testing

Australasian Society of Clinical Immunology and Allergy (ASCIA). (2020b). ASCIA guidelines – Infant feeding and allergy prevention. November. https://www.allergy.org.au/hp/papers/infant-feeding-and-allergy-prevention

Australasian Society of Clinical Immunology and Allergy (ASCIA). (2021). ASCIA Action Plans and First Aid Plans for Anaphylaxis. https://www.allergy.org.au/hp/anaphylaxis/ascia-action-plan-for-anaphylaxis

Australian Breastfeeding Association. (2017). Health professionals. Information. Is my baby getting enough milk? https://www.breastfeeding.asn.au/bfinfo/my-baby-getting-enough-milk

Australian Institute of Health and Welfare (AIHW). (2017). A picture of overweight and obesity in Australia. https://www.aihw.gov.au/reports/overweight-obesity/a-picture-of-overweight-and-obesity-in-australia/summary

AIHW. (2018). Nutrition across the life stages. Cat. no. PHE 227. Canberra: AIHW. https://www.aihw.gov.au/reports/food-nutrition/nutrition-across-the-life-stages/summary https://www.aihw.gov.au/reports/food-nutrition/nutrition-across-the-life-stages/contents/table-of-contents

AIHW. (2019). Overweight and obesity: overview. https://www.aihw.gov.au/reports-data/behaviours-risk-factors/overweight-obesity/overview

AIHW. (2020). Australia's children: Overweight and obesity. https://www.aihw.gov.au/reports/children-youth/australias-children/contents/health/overweight-and-obesity

Australian Resuscitation Council. (2016). ANZCOR Neonatal Flowchart. Flowcharts. https://resus.org.au/guidelines/flowcharts-3/

Avan, B., Raza, S., & Kirkwood, B. (2015). An epidemiological study of urban and rural children in Pakistan: Examining the relationship between delayed psychomotor development, low birth weight and postnatal growth failure. Transactions of The Royal Society of Tropical Medicine and Hygiene, 109(3), 189–196.

Bello, S., Meremikwu, M. M., Ejemot-Nwadiaro, R. I., et al. (2016). Vitamin A for preventing blindness in children with measles. The Cochrane Database of Systematic Reviews. http://www.cochrane.org/CD007719/ARI_vitamin-preventing-blindness-children-measles.

BMJ. (2020). Dyssomnias in children. BMJ Best Practice. https://bestpractice.bmj.com/topics/en-us/781

Boyd, C., & Moodambail, A. (2016). Severe hypercalcaemia in a child secondary to use of alternative therapies. BMJ Case Reports, 6 October.

Bright, F. M., Vink, R, & Byard, R.W. (2018). Brainstem Neuropathology in Sudden Infant Death Syndrome. In Duncan, J., & Byard, R. W., (Eds.). SIDS sudden infant and early childhood death: The past, the present and the future (pp. 589–614). University of Adelaide Press.

Canani, R. B., Sangwan, N., & Stefka, A. T. (2016). Lactobacillus rhamnosus GG-supplemented formula expands butyrate-producing bacterial strains in food allergic infants. The ISME Journal, 10, 742–750.

Cimino, S., Cerniglia, L., Almenara, C., et al. (2016). Developmental trajectories of body mass index and emotional-behavioral functioning of underweight children: A longitudinal study. Scientific Reports, 6(1), 20211. https:doi.org/10.1038/srep20211

Ellwood, J., Draper-Rodi, J., & Carnes, D. (2020). Comparison of common interventions for the treatment of infantile colic: A systematic review of reviews and guidelines. BMJ Open, 10(2), E035405. http://dx.doi.org/10.1136/bmjopen-2019-035405

Farajdokht, F., Sadigh-Eteghad, S., Dehghani, R., et al. (2017). Very low birth weight is associated with brain structure abnormalities and cognitive function impairments: A systematic review. Brain and Cognition, 118, 80–89. https://doi.org/10.1016/j.bandc.2017.07.006

Godfrey, K. M., Lillycrop, K. A., & Murray, R. (2017). Childhood obesity: epigenetic factors. In M. I. Goran (Ed.), Childhood obesity: Causes, consequences, and intervention approaches (151–158) (ProQuest ebook). Taylor & Francis.

Goldstein, R. D. (2018). Parental grief. In Duncan, J., & Byard, R. W., (Eds.). SIDS sudden infant and early childhood death: The past, the present and the future (pp. 143–154). University of Adelaide Press.

Halal, C., Bassani, D., Santos, I., et al. (2020). Maternal perinatal depression and infant sleep problems at 1 year of age: Subjective and actigraphy data from a population-based birth cohort study. Journal of Sleep Research, E13047.

Heine, R., AlRefaee, F., Bachina, P., et al. (2017). Lactose intolerance and gastrointestinal cow's milk allergy in infants and children – common misconceptions revisited. The World Allergy Organization Journal, 10(1), 41. https://doi.org/10.1186/s40413-017-0173-0

Högenauer, C., & Hammer, H. F. (2016). Maldigestion and malabsorption. In M. Feldman, L. S. Friedman, & L. J. Brandt (Eds.), Sleisenger and Fordtran's gastrointestinal and liver disease (10th ed.). New York: Elsevier.

Homan, G. (2016). Failure to thrive: a practical guide. American Family Physician, 94(4), 295–299.

Hunt, C. E., & Hauck, F. R. (2016). Sudden infant death syndrome. In R. M. Kliegman, B. F. Stanton, J. W. St Geme, et al. (Eds.), Nelson textbook of pediatrics (20th ed.). Pennsylvania: Elsevier.

Kang, J. (2018). Micronutrients and water. In Kang, J., Nutrition and Metabolism in Sports, Exercise and Health (2nd ed., pp. 105–131) (ProQuest ebook). Taylor & Francis.

Kleinman, R. E., & Greer, R. F. (Eds.), (2014). Pediatric nutrition (7th ed.). Elk Grove Village, IL: American Academy of Pediatrics.

Kumar, S. & Kelly, A. (2017). Review of childhood obesity: from epidemiology, etiology, and comorbidities to clinical assessment and treatment. Mayo Clinic Proceedings, 92(2), 251–265. https://doi.org/10.1016/j.mayocp.2016.09.017

Leung, A., Mandrusiak, A., Watter, P., et al. (2017). Impact of Parent Practices of Infant Positioning on Head Orientation Profile and Development of Positional Plagiocephaly in Healthy Term Infants. Physical and Occupational Therapy in Paediatrics. DOI: 10.1080/01942638.2017.1287811

Mandese, V., Marotti, F., Bedetti, L., et al. (2016). Effects of nutritional intake on disease severity in children with sickle cell disease. Nutrition Journal, 15, 46.

McLean, H. S., & Price, D. T. (2016). Failure to thrive. In R. M. Kliegman, J. W. St Geme, et al. (Eds.), Nelson textbook of pediatrics (20th ed.). Pennsylvania: Elsevier.

Médicins Sans Frontières (MSF). (2020). Severe acute malnutrition. https://medicalguidelines.msf.org/viewport/CG/english/severe-acute-malnutrition-16689141.html

Ministry of Health. (2016). Clinical guidelines for weight management in New Zealand children and young people. New Zealand Government. https://www.health.govt.nz/publication/clinical-guidelines-weight-management-new-zealand-children-and-young-people

Ministry of Health. (2019). Obesity statistics. New Zealand Government. https://www.health.govt.nz/nz-health-statistics/health-statistics-and-data-sets/obesity-statistics

Ministry of Health. (2021). Your health. The first year. Vitamin D and your baby. New Zealand Government. https://www.health.govt.nz/your-health/pregnancy-and-kids/first-year/helpful-advice-during-first-year/vitamin-d-and-your-baby

Mishra, K., Kumar, P., Basu, S., et al. (2014). Risk factors for severe acute malnutrition in children below 5 y of age in India: a case-control study. Indian Journal of Pediatrics, 81(8), 762–765.

Moon, R. Y. & Hauck, F. R. (2018). Risk factors and theories. In Duncan, J., & Byard, R. W., (Eds.). SIDS sudden infant and early childhood death: The past, the present and the future (pp. 169–186). University of Adelaide Press.

National Health and Medical Research Council (NHMRC), Australian Government Department of Health and Ageing, New Zealand Ministry of Health. (2017). Nutrient Reference Values. https://www.nhmrc.gov.au/sites/default/files/images/nutrient-refererence-dietary-intakes.pdf

National Health and Medical Research Council (NHMRC). (2012). Eat for health: infant feeding guidelines, information for health workers. Canberra, Australian Government.

National Health and Medical Research Council (NHMRC). (2013). Clinical practice guidelines for the management of overweight and obesity in adults, adolescents and children in Australia. Canberra, Australian Government.

Nowak-Węgrzyn, A., Burks, A. W., & Sampson, H. A. (2020). Reactions to foods. In Burks, A. W., Holgate, S. T., O'Hehir, R. E. et al. Middleton's Allergy: Principles and practices (7th ed., pp. 1294–1325). (Clinical Key ebook). Elsevier.

NSW Health. (2021). Health eating and active living – children. https://www.health.nsw.gov.au/heal/Pages/healthy-eating-and-active-living-children.aspx

O'Loughlin, R. & Hiscock, H. (2020). Presentations to emergency departments by children and young people with food allergy are increasing. Medical Journal of Australia, 213(1), 27–29. https://pubmed.ncbi.nlm.nih.gov/32372419.

Pawlak, R., Parrott, S. J., Raj, S., et al. (2013). How prevalent is vitamin B(12) deficiency among vegetarians? Nutrition Reviews, 71(2), 110–117.

Perinatal Society of Australia and New Zealand (PSNAZ). (2018). Clinical Practice Guideline for Care around Stillbirth and Neonatal Death. 3rd ed. https://www.stillbirthcre.org.au/assets/Uploads/Respectful-and-Supportive-Perinatal-Bereavement-Care.pdf

Perth Children's Hospital (PCH). (2018). Brief Resolved Unexplained Event (BRUE). https://pch.health.wa.gov.au/en/For-health-professionals/Clinical-Practice-Guidelines/Brief-Resolved-Unexplained-event

Porto, A. (2016). Lactose intolerance in infants & children: Parent FAQs. 29 September. https://www.healthychildren.org/English/healthy-living/nutrition/Pages/Lactose-Intolerance-in-Children.aspx

Pouessel, G., Turner, P., Worm, M., et al. (2018). Food-induced fatal anaphylaxis: From epidemiological data to general prevention strategies. Clinical & Experimental Allergy, 48(12), 1584–1593.

Price, A. A., Williams, J. A., Spees, C. K., et al. (2020). Utilization of Current Diagnostic Indicators to Characterize Pediatric Undernutrition among US Children. Nutrients, 12(5), 1409. DOI:10.3390/nu12051409

Raising Children Network. (2020). Sudden unexpected death in infancy (SUDI), SIDS and fatal sleeping accidents. Australia. https://raisingchildren.net.au/guides/a-z-health-reference/sudi

Red Nose Australia. (2020). Facts and Figures. https://rednose.org.au/page/facts-and-figures

Royal Children's Hospital Melbourne (RHCM). (n.d.). Clinical Practice Guidelines. Poor Growth. Background. https://www.rch.org.au/clinicalguide/guideline_index/Poor_growth/

Schürmann, S., Kersting, M., & Alexy, U. (2017). Vegetarian diets in children: A systematic review. European Journal of Nutrition, 56(5), 1797–1817. DOI 10.1007/s00394-017-1416-0

Sidebotham, P., Marshall, D. & Garstang, J. (2018). Responding to unexpected child deaths. In Duncan, J., & Byard, R. W., (Eds.). SIDS sudden infant and early childhood death: The past, the present and the future (pp. 85–116). University of Adelaide Press.

Singh, R., Kumar, P., & Mahalingam, K. (2017). Molecular genetics of human obesity: A comprehensive review. Molecular Biology and Genetics, 340(2), 87–108. http://dx.doi.org/10.1016/j.crvi.2016.11.007

Sung, V. (2018). Infantile Colic, Australian Prescriber, 41(4), 105–110.

Talarico, V., Barreca, M., Galiano, R., et al. (2016). Vitamin D and risk for vitamin A intoxication in an 18-month-old boy. Case Reports in Pediatrics, 2016 (article id 1395718), 1–3.

The Royal Children's Hospital Melbourne (RCHM). (2016). Allergy and immunology: Cows milk allergy. https://www.rch.org.au/uploadedFiles/Main/Content/allergy/Cows%20milk%20allergy.pdf

The Royal Children's Hospital Melbourne (RCHM). (2017). Clinical Practice Guidelines: Brief Resolved Unexplained Event BRUE. https://www.rch.org.au/clinicalguide/guideline_index/Brief_Resolved_Unexplained_Event_BRUE/

The Royal Children's Hospital Melbourne (RCHM). (2018a). Clinical Practice Guidelines: Vitamin D. https://www.rch.org.au/kidsinfo/fact_sheets/Vitamin_D/

The Royal Children's Hospital Melbourne (RCHM). (2018b). Plagiocephaly – misshapen head. https://www.rch.org.au/kidsinfo/fact_sheets/Plagiocephaly_misshapen_head/

Turner, T. & Palamountain, S. (2018). Infantile colic: Clinical features and diagnosis. UpToDate. https://www.uptodate.com/contents/infantile-colic-clinical-features-and-diagnosis

UNICEF. (2013). Position paper, ready-to-use therapeutic food for children with severe acute malnutrition. https://www.unicef.org/media/files/Position_Paper_Ready-to-use_therapeutic_food_for_children_with_severe_acute_malnutrition__June_2013.pdf

US Department of Agriculture. (2020). Economic Research Service: Definitions of food security. https://www.ers.usda.gov/topics/food-nutrition-assistance/food-security-in-the-us/definitions-of-food-security.aspx.

Waber, D., Bryce, C., Girard, J., et al. (2018). Parental history of moderate to severe infantile malnutrition is associated with cognitive deficits in their adult offspring. Nutritional Neuroscience, 21(3), 195–201. https://doi.org/10.1080/1028415X.2016.1258379

World Allergy Organization (WAO). (2017). Food Allergy. https://www.worldallergy.org/education-and-programs/education/allergic-disease-resource-center/professionals/food-allergy

World Health Organisation (WHO). (2009). WHO child growth standards: growth velocity based on weight, length and head circumference: methods and development. https://apps.who.int/iris/handle/10665/44026

World Health Organization (WHO). (2017). Diarrhoeal disease. https://www.who.int/en/news-room/fact-sheets/detail/diarrhoeal-disease

World Health Organization (WHO). (n.d.). Childhood overweight and obesity. https://www.who.int/dietphysicalactivity/childhood/en/

World Health Organization (WHO). (2020). Management of severe acute malnutrition in infants and children. https://www.who.int/features/factfiles/breastfeeding/en/

Wozniak, L. J., Bechtold, H. M., Reyen, L. E., et al. (2015). Vitamin D deficiency in children with intestinal failure receiving home parenteral nutrition. Journal of Parenteral Enteral Nutr, 39(4), 471–475.

12

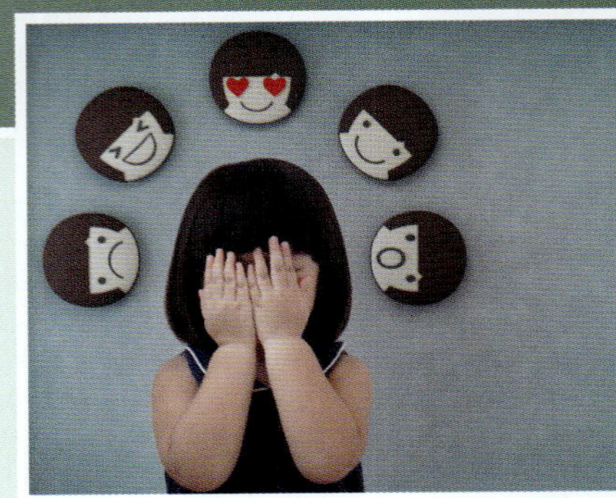

Health Promotion of the Toddler and Family

Julia Laing

LEARNING OBJECTIVES

- Outline usual growth and development of toddlerhood
- Identify challenging areas for the toddler and parent and opportunities for nurses to support healthy growth and development
- Identify key safety concerns for this age group and preventive actions to take.

PROMOTING OPTIMUM GROWTH AND DEVELOPMENT

The term *terrible twos* has often been used to describe the toddler years, the period from 12 to 36 months of age. It is a time of intense exploration of the environment as children attempt to find out how things work; what the word 'no' means; and the effect of frustration and lack of ability to communicate needs can become temper tantrums and negativism, and be seen as obstinacy. 'Getting into things' is their way of learning about their world, especially relationships. Successful mastery of the tasks of this age requires a strong foundation of trust during infancy and frequently necessitates guidance from others when parent and toddler face the struggles of toilet training, limit setting and sibling rivalry. Nurses who understand the dynamics of growth and development of the toddler can help families deal effectively with the tasks of this age.

Biological Development

Proportional Changes

Physical growth slows considerably during toddlerhood. The average weight at 2 years is 12 kg. The average weight gain is 1.8 to 2.7 kg per year. The birth weight is quadrupled by 2½ years of age. The rate of increase in height also slows. The usual increment is an addition of 7.5 cm (3 inches) per year and occurs mainly in elongation of the legs rather than the trunk. The average height of a 2 year old is 86.6 cm. In general, adult height is about twice the child's height at 2 years of age. Accurate measurement of height and weight during the toddler years should reveal a steady growth curve that is *steplike* rather than linear (straight), which is characteristic of the growth spurts during the early childhood years.

The rate of increase in head circumference slows somewhat by the end of infancy, and head circumference is usually equal to chest circumference by 1 to 2 years of age. The usual total increase in head circumference during the second year is 2.5 cm. Then the rate of increase slows until age 5 years, when the increase is less than 1.25 cm per year. The anterior fontanel closes between 12 and 18 months of age.

Chest circumference continues to increase and exceeds head circumference during the toddler years. After the second year the chest circumference exceeds the abdominal measurement which, in addition to the growth of the lower extremities, gives the child a taller, leaner appearance. However, the toddler retains a squat, 'potbellied' appearance because of the less well-developed abdominal musculature and short legs (Fig 12.1). The legs retain a slightly bowed or curved appearance during the second year from the weight of the relatively large trunk.

Sensory Changes

Visual acuity of 20/40 is considered acceptable during the toddler years. Full binocular vision is well developed, and any evidence of persistent strabismus should receive professional attention as early as possible to prevent amblyopia. Depth perception continues to develop, but because of the child's lack of motor coordination, falls from heights remain a persistent danger.

The senses of hearing, smell, taste and touch become increasingly well developed, coordinated with one another and associated with other experiences. All of the senses are used to explore the environment. Toddlers visually inspect an object by turning it over; they may taste it, smell it and touch it several times before they are satisfied with their investigation. They will shake it to see if it makes noise and vigorously test its durability.

Another example of the integrated function of the senses is the toddlers' development of specific taste and texture preferences. Toddlers are much less likely than infants to try a new food because of its appearance or smell, not just its taste. Likewise, a toddler is likely to reject a new food because of its texture. Non-sensory associations with objects also take on significance. For example, if parents refuse to serve a particular food because of their dislike, they will transfer this negative connotation to the child before the child has had an opportunity to taste it. Awareness of these factors is important in several areas of

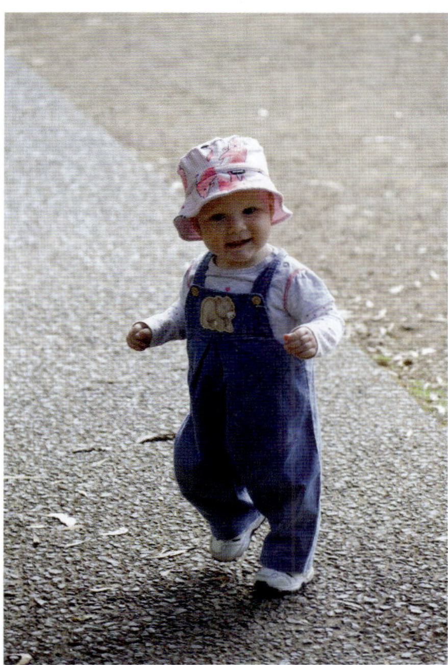

Fig 12.1 Typical toddler gait.

childrearing, such as feeding, teaching socially acceptable habits and reinforcing appropriate behavioural responses to various situations.

Touch continues to be important to the toddler. Descending development of the spinal tract is evidenced by increased sensation in the lower extremities, such as ticklish feet. Pleasant tactile sensations, such as rubbing the back or stroking the hair, soothe and comfort the toddler, especially in times of stress or fatigue.

Maturation of Systems

Most of the physiological systems are relatively mature by the end of toddlerhood. By the end of the first year, all the brain cells are present but continue to increase in size. Myelination of the spinal cord is almost complete by 2 years old, which parallels the completion of most of the gross motor skills associated with locomotion. Brain growth is 75% completed by the end of 2 years.

Development of various areas of the brain seems to correspond with the child's progressive intellectual capacity. As development progresses, specific changes take place in various areas of the cerebral cortex, such as the Broca area for speech and cortical areas for control of the legs, hands, feet and sphincters. Because this neuromotor organisation is so inclusive, complex and intricate, the child is limited in the ability to attend to any one aspect of behaviour for more than a few minutes.

Between 2 and 3 years old, coordination and consolidation of these voluntary functions allow the toddler to listen better, look longer and have an extended attention span. Although postural control is increasingly developed as myelination of the spinal cord advances, the immaturity of this control, combined with the child's limited experiences and lack of visual perception, makes it difficult to do simple acts such as seating oneself in a chair or climbing down stairs.

Volume of the respiratory tract and growth of associated structures continue to increase during early childhood, lessening some of the factors that predisposed the child to frequent and serious infections during infancy. The internal structures of the ear and throat continue to be short and straight, and the lymphoid tissue of the tonsils and adenoids continues to be large. As a result, otitis media, tonsillitis and upper respiratory tract infections are common. The respiratory and heart rates slow, and the blood pressure increases (see inside back cover). Respirations continue to be abdominal.

The digestive processes are fairly complete by the beginning of toddlerhood. The acidity of the gastric contents continues to increase and has a protective function because it destroys many types of bacteria. Stomach capacity increases to allow for the usual schedule of three small meals a day.

One of the more prominent changes of the gastrointestinal system is the voluntary control of elimination. With complete myelination of the spinal cord, control of anal and urethral sphincters is gradually achieved. The physiological ability to control the sphincters occurs somewhere between ages 18 and 24 months old. Bladder capacity also increases considerably. By 14 to 18 months old the child is able to retain urine for up to 2 hours or longer.

The skin functionally matures during early childhood. The epidermis and dermis are more tightly bound together, increasing their resistance to infection and irritation and creating a more effective barrier against fluid loss. Production of sebum is minimal, which contributes to the development of dry skin. The eccrine glands are functional during early childhood and react to changes in temperature, but they produce minimum amounts of sweat. Hair grows thicker and coarser and usually darkens and loses some curliness. Fine hair is evident on the lower arms and legs. Production of adipose tissue declines as hyperplasia of muscle cells increases. With the concurrent growth of the lower extremities, the child assumes more adultlike proportions.

Under conditions of moderate variation in temperature, the toddler rarely has the difficulties of the young infant in maintaining body temperature. The capillaries are able to conserve core body temperature by constricting in response to cold and dilating in response to heat. Shivering, an involuntary act that results in rhythmic muscle contraction, which increases cellular metabolism and produces heat, is much more effective as a source of thermogenesis. The child also learns mechanisms to control body temperature—putting on clothing when cold or removing it when warm.

The defence mechanisms of the tissues and blood, particularly phagocytosis and chemotaxis, are much more efficient in the toddler than in the infant. The production of antibodies is well established. Immunoglobulin G, which neutralises microbial toxins, reaches adult levels by the end of the second year of life. Passive immunity from maternal transfer during fetal life disappears by the beginning of toddlerhood. Immunoglobulin M, which responds to artificial immunising techniques and combats serious infection, attains adult levels during late infancy. Immunoglobulins A, D and E increase gradually, not reaching eventual adult levels until later childhood. However, many young children demonstrate a sudden increase in colds and minor infections when entering day care or preschool because of exposure to new antigens.

Gross and Fine Motor Development

The major gross motor skill during the toddler years is the development of locomotion. By 12 to 13 months old, toddlers walk alone, using a wide stance for extra balance; by age 18 months old, they try to run but fall easily. Between 2 and 3 years of age, refinement of the upright, biped position is evident in improved coordination and equilibrium. At 2 years old toddlers can walk up and down stairs, and by age 2½ years they jump using both feet, stand on one foot for a second or two and manage a few steps on tiptoe. By the end of the second year, they stand on one foot, walk on tiptoe and climb stairs with alternate footing.

Fine motor development is demonstrated in increasingly skilful manual dexterity. Once toddlers achieve pincer grasp, usually at 9 to

10 months old, they combine this skill with other developing sensory and cognitive abilities. For example, by 12 months of age they are able to grasp a very small object. By age 15 months they can drop a pellet into a narrow-necked bottle. Casting or throwing objects and retrieving them become an almost obsessive activity at about 15 months old. By 18 months old, toddlers can throw a ball overhand without losing their balance.

Visual perception of geometrical shapes is also evident at this time. At 12 months old children selectively look at a round hole in a special form board but are unable to insert a round object. By age 15 months they promptly place the round object in the hole, even if the board is revised or turned upside down. Spatial relations also are evident in their ability to build a tower with blocks: by age 18 months, a tower of three or four blocks; by age 24 months, a tower of six or seven blocks; and by age 30 months, a tower of eight blocks or more.

Fine motor skill and visual ability are demonstrated in toddlers' progressive adeptness in manipulating a pencil or crayon. By age 15 months they scribble spontaneously, and by age 24 months they imitate a circular stroke and a vertical line. By the end of the toddler period, the child can copy a circle and imitate a cross.

Mastery of gross and fine motor skills is evident in all phases of the child's activity, such as play, dressing, language comprehension, response to discipline, social interaction and propensity for injuries. Activities occur less in isolation and more in conjunction with other physical and mental abilities to produce a purposeful result. For example, the toddler walks to reach a new location, releases a toy and picks it up again or chooses a new one, and scribbles to look at the image produced. The possibilities of the exploration, investigation and manipulation mastery of the environment—and its hazards—are endless.

Psychosocial Development

Toddlers are faced with the mastery of several important tasks. If the need for basic trust has been satisfied, they are ready to give up dependence for control, independence and autonomy. Some of the specific tasks include the following:

- differentiation of self from others, particularly the mother or primary caregiver
- toleration of separation from parents
- ability to withstand delayed gratification
- control over bodily functions
- acquisition of socially acceptable behaviour
- verbal means of communication
- ability to interact with others in a less egocentric manner.

Mastery of these goals is only begun during late infancy and the toddler years, and such tasks as developing interpersonal relationships with others may not be completed until adolescence. However, crucial foundations for successful completion of such developmental tasks are laid during these early formative years.

Developing a Sense of Autonomy (Erikson)

According to Erikson (1963), the developmental task of toddlerhood is acquiring a sense of **autonomy** while overcoming a sense of doubt and shame. As infants gain trust in the predictability and reliability of their parents, environment and interaction with others, they begin to discover that their behaviour is their own and that it has a predictable, reliable effect on others. Although they are aware of their will and control over others, they are confronted with the conflict of exerting autonomy and relinquishing the much enjoyed dependence on others. Exerting their ideas and independence has definite negative consequences, whereas retaining dependent, submissive behaviour is generally rewarded with affection and approval. On the other hand, continued dependency creates a sense of doubt regarding their potential capacity to control their actions. This doubt is compounded by a sense of *shame* for feeling this urge to revolt against others' will and a fear that they will exceed their own capacity for manipulating the environment. The latter fear is a basis for instituting limit setting and consistent discipline at this age. Without appropriate limits on what is acceptable versus unacceptable behaviour, children have no guidelines for establishing the end points of their ability to control.

Just as the infant has the social modalities of grasping and biting, the toddler has the newly gained modality of holding on and letting go. Holding on and letting go are evident in how the toddler uses the hands, mouth, eyes and, eventually, sphincters when toilet training is begun. Children constantly express these social modalities in play activities such as casting or throwing objects; taking objects out of boxes, drawers or cabinets; holding on tighter when someone says, 'No, don't touch'; and refusing to eat certain foods as taste preferences become strong.

Several characteristics, especially **negativism** and **ritualism**, are typical of toddlers in their quest for autonomy. As toddlers attempt to express their will, they often act with negativism, giving a negative response to requests. The words 'no' or 'me do' can be the sole vocabulary. Emotions become strongly expressed, usually in rapid mood swings. One minute toddlers can be engrossed in an activity, and the next minute they might be violently angry or frustrated because they were unable to manipulate a toy or open a door. If scolded for doing something wrong, they can have a temper tantrum and almost instantaneously pull at the parent's legs to be picked up and comforted. Understanding and coping with these swift changes is often difficult for parents. Many parents find the negativism exasperating and, instead of dealing constructively with it, give in to it, which further threatens the child's search for acceptable methods of interacting with others.

In contrast to negativism, which frequently disrupts the environment, ritualism, the need to maintain sameness and reliability, provides a sense of comfort. Toddlers can venture out with security when they know that familiar people, places and routines still exist. One can easily understand why change, such as hospitalisation, represents such a threat to these children. Without the comfortable rituals, they have little opportunity to exert autonomy. Consequently, dependency and regression occur (see Regression, later in this chapter).

Erikson focuses on the development of the ego, which may be thought of as reason or common sense, during this phase of psychosocial development. The child struggles to deal with the impulses of the id, tolerate frustration and learn socially acceptable ways of interacting with the environment. The ego becomes evident as the child is able to delay gratification.

Toddlers also have a rudimentary beginning of the superego, or conscience, which is the incorporation of the morals of society and the process of acculturation. With the development of the ego, children further differentiate themselves from others and expand their sense of trust in self. But as they begin to develop awareness of their own will and capacity to achieve, they also become aware of their ability to fail. This ever-present awareness of potential failure creates doubt and shame. Successful mastery of the task of autonomy necessitates opportunities for self-mastery while withstanding the frustration of necessary limit setting and delayed gratification. Opportunities for self-mastery are present in appropriate play activities, toilet training, the crisis of sibling rivalry and successful interactions with significant others.

Cognitive Development

Sensorimotor Phase (Piaget)

The period from 12 to 24 months old is a continuation of the final two stages of the sensorimotor phase (Table 12.1). During this time the

TABLE 12.1 Sensorimotor and Preoperational Phases During Toddlerhood*

Stage and Age	Cognitive Development	Behaviour
		SENSORIMOTOR
V. Tertiary circular reactions (13–18 months)	Active experimentation to achieve previously unattainable goals Increased concept of object permanence Differentiation of oneself from objects Early traces of memory Beginning awareness of spatial, causal and temporal relationships Able to enter into an action at any point without reproducing entire sequence	Insatiable curiosity about environment Uses all sensory cues for exploration Ventures away from parent for longer periods Uses physical skills to achieve particular goal Can find hidden objects, but only in first location Able to insert round object into hole Fits smaller objects into each other (nesting) Gestures 'up' and 'down' Puts objects into container and takes them out Realises that 'out of sight' is not out of reach; opens doors and drawers to find objects Gains comfort from parent's voice even if parent is not visible
VI. Invention of new means through mental combinations (19–24 months)	Awareness of object permanence regardless of number of invisible displacements Can infer a cause only while experiencing the effect Imitation increasingly symbolic Beginning sense of time in terms of anticipation, memory and ability to wait Egocentrism in thought and behaviour Global organisation of thought	Searches for object through several hiding places Will infer cause by associating two or more experiences (such as lollies missing, sister smiling) Imitates words and sounds of animals Imitates adult behaviour (domestic mimicry) Follows directions and understands requests Uses words 'up', 'down', 'come' and 'go' with meaning May sit and wait for meals at table for short period Has some sense of time; waits in response to 'just a minute'; may use word 'now' Refers to self by name Engages in parallel play; demonstrates awareness of ownership Concerned with ritualistic, routinised schedule
		PREOPERATIONAL
2–4 years	Increased use of language as mental symbolisation Egocentrism still present in thought, play and behaviour Increased sense of time, space, causality See Box 12.1	Uses two- or three-word phrases Increased vocabulary Refers to self by pronoun Possessive of own toys; uses word 'mine' Begins to use past tense of verbs Uses phrases 'going to', 'in a minute', 'today', 'all done' Uses many future-oriented words, such as 'tomorrow', 'next day', 'afternoon', but has poor concept of passage of time Follows directions using prepositions, such as 'up', 'behind', 'under'

*For the previous four stages during early infancy, see Table 10.1.

cognitive processes develop rapidly and at times seem similar to mature thinking. However, reasoning skills are still primitive and need to be understood to effectively deal with the typical behaviours of this age child. The main cognitive achievement of early childhood is the acquisition of language, which represents mental symbolism.

In the fifth stage, **tertiary circular reactions** (from 13 to 18 months old), the child uses active experimentation to achieve previously unattainable goals. Newly acquired physical skills are increasingly important for the function they serve rather than for the acts themselves. The child incorporates the old learning of secondary circular reactions and applies the combined knowledge to new situations, with emphasis on the results of the experimentation. In this way there is the beginning of rational judgment and intellectual reasoning. During this stage the child further differentiates self from objects. This is evident in the child's increasing ability to venture away from the parent and to tolerate longer periods of separation.

Awareness of a **causal relationship** between two events is apparent. After flipping a light switch, toddlers are aware that a response occurs. However, they are not able to transfer that knowledge to new situations. Therefore, every time they see what appears to be a light switch, they must reinvestigate its function. Such behaviour demonstrates the beginning of categorising data into distinct classes, subclasses and so on. Innumerable examples of this type of behaviour occur as toddlers repeatedly explore the same object each time it appears in a new place. A classic example is their curiosity about electrical outlets. Even if they receive a shock from one of them, they will adamantly poke and inspect every other outlet. This inability to transfer information leaves toddlers particularly vulnerable to injuries. However, traces of memory are evident because they usually avoid the outlet where the shock occurred.

Because classification of objects is still basic, the appearance of an object indicates its function. For example, if the child's toys are stored in a paper bag or large container, the toddler does not perceive a difference between that toy receptacle and the garbage bin or laundry basket. If allowed to turn over the toy receptacle, the child will just as quickly do the same to other similar objects because, in the child's mind, there is no difference. Expecting toddlers to judge which receptacles are permissible to explore and which are not is inappropriate for this age group. Instead, the forbidden object, such as the garbage bin, should be placed out of reach. This has significant implications for prevention of accidents and accidental ingestion of injurious agents.

The discovery of objects as objects leads to an awareness of their **spatial relationships.** Children are able to recognise different shapes and their relationship to one another. For example, they can fit slightly smaller boxes into each other (nesting) and can place a round object into a hole, even if the board is turned around, upside down or reversed. However, they cannot do the same thing with a square until 2 years of age. Children are also aware of space and the relationship of their body to dimensions such as height. They will stretch, stand on a low stair or stool and pull a string to reach an object.

Object permanence has also advanced. Although they still cannot find an object that has been displaced and is no longer visible or has been moved from under one pillow to another without their seeing the change, toddlers are increasingly aware of the existence of objects behind closed doors, in drawers and under tables. Parents are usually acutely aware of this developmental achievement because they find high places and locked cabinets to be the only areas inaccessible to toddlers. Parents also experience toddlers' protest behaviours when the parents leave because toddlers are aware that their parents are absent when they cannot see them.

During ages 19 to 24 months the child is in the final sensorimotor stage, invention of new means through mental combinations. This stage completes the more primitive, autistic thought processes of infancy and prepares the way for more complex mental operations during the phase of preoperational thought. One of the most dramatic achievements of this stage is in the area of object permanence. Toddlers will now actively search for an object in several potential hiding places. In addition, they can infer a cause when only experiencing the effect. They can infer that an object was hidden in any number of places even if they only saw the original hiding place.

Imitation displays deeper meaning and understanding. Earlier, imitation was concrete and action oriented. For example, 'bye-bye' was a behavioural response more than a conceptual gesture of departure. Now it has a broader meaning, such as Mummy is going to work, it is time for a walk or something is no longer present. There is greater symbolisation to imitation.

One type of symbolic imitation is **domestic mimicry**, the imitation of household activity. Toddlers are acutely aware of others' actions and attempt to copy them in gestures and in words. They can imitate the parents' performance of a household task both physically and verbally (Fig 12.2). Parents often remark how accurately they see themselves when the toddler engages in domestic mimicry. Such activity is part of the toddler's learning sex-role behaviour. Identification with the parent

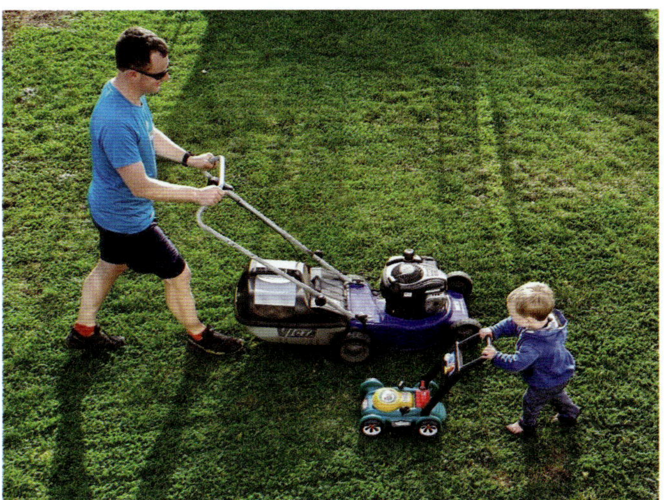

Fig 12.2 Domestic mimicry is common during toddlerhood.

of the same sex becomes apparent by the second year and represents the toddler's intellectual ability to differentiate models of behaviour and to imitate them appropriately.

The concept of time is still embryonic, but toddlers have some sense of timing in terms of anticipation, memory and the limited ability to wait. They may listen to the command 'Just a minute' and behave appropriately. However, their sense of timing is exaggerated—1 minute can last an hour. Toddlers' limited attention spans also indicate their sense of immediacy and concern for the present.

Egocentrism, or the inability to envision situations from perspectives other than one's own, is evident in all aspects of toddlers' behaviour. They see, experience and live every event in reference to themselves. A common example of egocentric behaviour is the toddler who takes a toy away from another child. The toddler is concerned only with playing with the toy and is unable to conceptualise that taking the toy away will make the other child unhappy.

Preoperational Phase (Piaget)

At approximately 2 years of age the child enters the preconceptual phase of cognitive development, which lasts until about age 4 years. The preconceptual phase is a subdivision of the preoperational phase, which spans ages 2 to 7 years. The preconceptual phase is primarily one of transition that bridges the purely self-satisfying behaviour of infancy and the undeveloped socialised behaviour of latency. Preoperational thinking implies that children cannot think in terms of operations—the ability to manipulate objects in relation to each other in a logical fashion. Rather, toddlers think primarily on the basis of their perception of an event. Problem-solving is based on what the toddler sees or hears directly rather than on what the toddler recalls about objects or events. The principal characteristics of this stage are egocentric use of language and dependence on perception in problem-solving.

From ages 2 to 4 years old children learn a variety of words and increasingly use language. In fact, toddlers talk a lot. Speech is primarily of two types: egocentric or socialised. Egocentric speech consists of repeating words and sounds for the pleasure of hearing oneself and is not intended to communicate. This collective monologue reflects the child's lingering self-centredness.

Socialised speech is for communication; however, it is still egocentric in that children communicate about themselves to others. Before age 3 most speech is directed at self-fulfilment or self-reference, such as 'Want drink' or 'I do', and it is directed mostly towards adults. Because children think that everyone else's world is the same as theirs, they expect others to understand their verbal messages even when limited information is conveyed.

Preoperational thinking implies that children cannot think in terms of operations—the ability to manipulate objects in relation to one another in a logical fashion. Rather, toddlers think primarily based on their perception of an event. Problem-solving is based on what they see or hear directly rather than on what they recall about objects and events (Box 12.1).

Within the second year the child increasingly uses language symbolically and is concerned with the 'why' and 'how' of things. For example, a pencil is 'something to write with' and food is 'something to eat'. However, such **mental symbolisation** is closely associated with prelogical reasoning. For instance, a needle is 'something that hurts'. Such painful experiences take on new significance because memory is associated with the specific event, and fears are likely to develop, such as resistance to people who wear hospital uniforms or rooms that look like the medical practitioner's office. Sometimes parents and healthcare practitioners underestimate the child's ability to recall events and give little thought to preparation for visits to a medical practitioner's office or other health facility, resulting in fears that can have a

BOX 12.1 Characteristics of Preoperational Thought

Egocentrism—Inability to envision situations from perspectives other than one's own

Example—If a person is positioned between the toddler and another child, the toddler, who is facing the person, will explain that both children can see the middle person's face. The toddler is unable to realise that the other child views the middle person from a different perspective, the back.

Transductive—Reasoning from the particular to the particular

Example—Child refuses to eat a food because something previously eaten did not taste good.

Global organisation—Belief that a change in any one part of the whole changes the entire whole

Example—Child refuses to sleep in room because location of bed is changed.

Centration—Focusing on one aspect rather than considering all possible alternatives

Example—Child refuses to eat a food because of its colour, even though its taste and smell are acceptable.

Animism—Attributing lifelike qualities to inanimate objects

Example—Child scolds stairs for making child fall down.

Irreversibility—Inability to undo or reverse the actions initiated physically

Example—When told to stop doing something, such as talking, child is unable to think of opposite activity.

Magical—Believing that thoughts are all-powerful and can cause events

Example—Child wishes someone dead; then if the person dies, child feels at fault because of the 'bad' thought that made the death happen.

Example—Calling children 'bad' because they did something wrong makes children feel as though they are bad.

Inability to conserve—Inability to understand the idea that a mass can be changed in size, shape, volume or length without losing or adding to the original mass (instead, children judge what they see by the immediate perceptual clues given to them)

Example—If two lines of equal length are presented in such a way that one appears longer than the other, the child will state that one line is longer even if he or she measures both lines with a ruler and finds that they are the same length.

long-term effect on the child engaging with healthcare. Because of the vulnerability of these early years, it is essential to prepare children for new experiences, whether it is a new babysitter, a general practitioner or a visit to the dentist.

Moral Development: Preconventional or Premoral Level

Toddlers' development of moral judgment is at the most basic level. They have little, if any, concern for why something is wrong. Kohlberg's theory of moral development is influenced by Piaget's theory of moral thought; the first phase of Kohlberg's theory is called the preconventional phase, and it involves punishment and obedience. Young children behave in accordance with the freedom or restriction that is placed on actions. In the punishment and obedience orientation, whether an action is good or bad depends on whether it results in reward or punishment. If children are punished for it, the action is bad. If they are not punished, the action is good, regardless of the meaning of the act. For example, if parents allow hitting, the child will perceive that hitting is good because it is not associated with punishment. By age 36 months, developmental aspects of conscience may be present.

The type of discipline also affects children's moral development. When parents use power to control behaviour, such as physical punishment or withholding privileges, children receive a negative view of morals, especially towards authority figures, such as law enforcement officials. When parents withdraw love or attention, children behave primarily because of guilt, rather than from an internalisation of morals. However, when parents give explanations for the misbehaviour and try to help children change through positive approaches, such as consequences or rewards, children feel less hostility and are more likely to base their actions on an analysis of why an act may be wrong. Of course, the effect of discipline is not limited to the toddler years, and the sole use of explanation is inappropriate during this period. Because parents usually establish disciplinary techniques at this time, the use of constructive approaches should begin early. (See Limit Setting and Discipline, Chapter 2.)

Spiritual Development

Spiritual development in children is often discussed in terms of the child's developmental level because the evolution of spirituality often parallels cognitive development (Lima et al 2013). The child's family and environment strongly influence his or her perception of the world around him or her, and this often includes spirituality. Furthermore, family values, beliefs, customs and expressions of these influence the child's perception of his or her spiritual self (Lima et al 2013). Neuman (2011) proposes that Fowler's stages of faith (Fowler 1981) be used to better understand children and spirituality; she provides an excellent overview of the stages of faith in childhood. The relationship among spirituality, illness in childhood and nursing has been studied in the context of suffering, terminal illness such as cancer and end-of-life care. In the past decade there has been an increased interest in and focus on spiritual care in adults and children as further understanding of the influence of one's spirituality on health, illness and wellbeing has progressed.

Development of Body Image

As in infancy, the development of **body image** closely parallels cognitive development. With increasing motor ability, toddlers recognise the usefulness of body parts and gradually learn their respective names. They also learn that certain body parts have various meanings; for example, during toilet training, the genitalia become significant and cleanliness is emphasised. By 2 years old toddlers recognise gender differences and refer to self by name and then by pronoun. Gender identity is developed by age 3 years old. Also, by this time, children begin to remember events with reference to their personal significance, forming an autobiographical memory that helps establish a continuous identity throughout life's events.

Once they begin preoperational thought, toddlers can use symbols to represent objects, but their thinking may lead to inaccuracies. For example, if someone who is pregnant is called 'fat', they will describe all 'fat' women as having babies. They have a beginning recognition of words used to describe physical appearance, such as 'pretty', 'handsome' or 'big boy'. Such expressions eventually influence how children view their own bodies, and such labelling (negative or positive) becomes part of their body image.

It is evident that body integrity is poorly understood in young children and that intrusive experiences are threatening. For example, toddlers forcefully resist procedures such as examining the ear or mouth and taking an axillary temperature. The procedure itself (e.g. taking vital signs) does not hurt the child, but it represents an intrusion into the child's personal space, which elicits a strong protest. Toddlers also have unclear body boundaries and may associate nonviable parts, such as faeces, with essential body parts. This can be seen in a toddler who is upset by flushing the toilet and watching the stool disappear.

Nurses can help parents foster a positive body image in their child by encouraging them to avoid negative labels, such as 'skinny arms' or 'chubby legs'; such self-perceptions are internalised and can last a lifetime. Body parts, especially those related to elimination and reproduction, should be called by their correct names. Respect for the body should be practised.

Development of Gender Identity

Just as toddlers explore their environment, they also explore their bodies and find that touching certain body parts is pleasurable; this process actually begins in infancy as infants become aware of pleasurable effects of human touch. Genital fondling (masturbation) can occur and involves manual stimulation and posturing movements (especially in young girls) such as tightening the thighs or applying mechanical pressure to the pubic or suprapubic area. Other demonstrations of pleasurable activities include rocking, swinging and hugging people and toys. Parental reactions to toddlers' behaviour influence the children's own attitudes and should be accepting rather than critical. If such acts are performed in public, parents should not condone or bring attention to the behaviour but should teach the child that it is more socially acceptable to perform the behaviour in private.

Children in this age group are learning vocabulary associated with anatomy, elimination and reproduction. Certain associations between words and functions become significant and can influence future attitudes about sexual matters. For example, if parents refer to the genitalia as dirty, especially in the context of elimination, this association between 'genitalia' and 'dirty' may be transferred to sexual functions later in life. Sex-role differences become obvious to children and are evident in much of toddlers' imitative play. Although current research indicates that prenatal exposure to testosterone strongly influences the individual's gender identity, researchers also indicate that there are sensitive periods (e.g. puberty) that may influence the development of gender identity (Hines et al 2015, Stortelder 2014). A sense of maleness or femaleness, or **gender identity**, is formed by age 24 months old when children are able to label their own and other's gender (Steensma et al 2013). Early attitudes are formed about affectionate behaviours between adults from observing parental and other adult intimate activities. (See also Sex Education, Chapter 13.) The quality of relationships with parents is important to the child's capacity for sexual and emotional relationships later in life.

Social Development

Separation and Individuation

A major task of the toddler period is differentiation of self from significant others, usually the mother. The differentiation process consists of two phases: **separation**, the children's emergence from a symbiotic fusion with the mother, and **individuation**, those achievements that mark children's assumption of their individual characteristics in the environment. Although the process begins during the latter half of infancy, the major achievements occur during the toddler years.

Toddlers have an increased understanding and awareness of object permanence and some ability to withstand delayed gratification and tolerate moderate frustration. They begin to lose some of their resistance to separation yet appear even more concerned about the parent's whereabouts. They have learned from experience that parents exist when physically absent. Repetition of events such as going to bed without the parents but waking to find them again reinforces the reliability of such brief separations. Consequently, toddlers are able to venture away from their parents for brief periods because of the security of knowing that the parents will be there when they return. Verbal and visual reassurance from the parent gradually replaces some of the previous need to be physically close for comfort.

Toddlers react differently to strangers than do infants. The appearance of unfamiliar people does not represent such a significant threat to their attachment to their mothers. In addition, toddlers show less fear of strangers, but only when their parents are present. When left alone with a stranger, they are fearful and acutely anxious; manifest depressive behaviour, such as crying and withdrawal; and may become restless, hyperactive or passive, reverting to regressive behaviours. Such reactions may be evident when a child is left with a babysitter; is beginning kindergarten, preschool or day care; or is hospitalised. (See Chapter 22.)

These behaviours are not pathological or harmful if parents realise how desperately their children need them. Indiscriminate friendliness towards strangers and lack of anxiety during separation from parents may be reasons for concern. Sensitive, perceptive parents will be aware of the child's need for increased love, affection and attention when they are together. An attitude such as 'They will get used to the babysitter' will not help young children positively tolerate separation.

The separation-individuation phase encompasses the phenomenon of rapprochement; as the toddler separates from the mother and begins to make sense of experiences in the environment, the child is drawn back to the mother for assistance in verbally articulating the meaning of the experiences (Zimmer-Gembeck et al 2015). Developmentally the term **rapprochement** means the child moves away and returns for reassurance. If the mother's response to the toddler is inappropriate, the toddler may experience insecurity and confusion.

Parents often need help in realising the necessity of preparing children for an inevitable separation. Sometimes with the firstborn, parents tend to overprotect children, shield them from any anxiety-producing experience and insulate them from less than immediate gratification. Although this is not necessarily harmful, especially if opportunities for independence are allowed later, it does not prepare children for unexpected events. A typical example is the birth of a sibling. The child is faced with the crisis of sibling rivalry and separation from the parent. Allowing children to experience brief periods of separation during early infancy prepares them for such experiences later. Indeed, they may still manifest the typical behaviours of protest, but they will also have learned that their mother or father always returns. Therefore, it is important to appreciate the tremendous loss that the death of a parent represents for young children; unlike their other experiences with separation, this time the parent will not return.

Transitional objects, such as a favourite blanket or toy, provide security for young children, especially when they are separated from parents, are dealing with a new stress or are just fatigued (Fig 12.3). Security objects often become so important to toddlers that they refuse to let them be taken away. Such behaviour is normal; there is no need to discourage this tendency. During separations, such as day care or hospitalisation, transitional objects should be provided to minimise any feelings of fear or loneliness.

Learning to tolerate and mastering brief periods of separation are important developmental tasks of children in this age group. In addition, it is a necessary component of parenting because brief periods of separation from their children allow parents to recoup their energy and patience and to avoid directing their irritations and frustrations at the children.

Language Development

The most striking characteristic of language development during early childhood is the increasing level of comprehension. Although the number of words acquired—from about 4 at 1 year of age to approximately 300 at age 2 years—is notable, the ability to understand speech

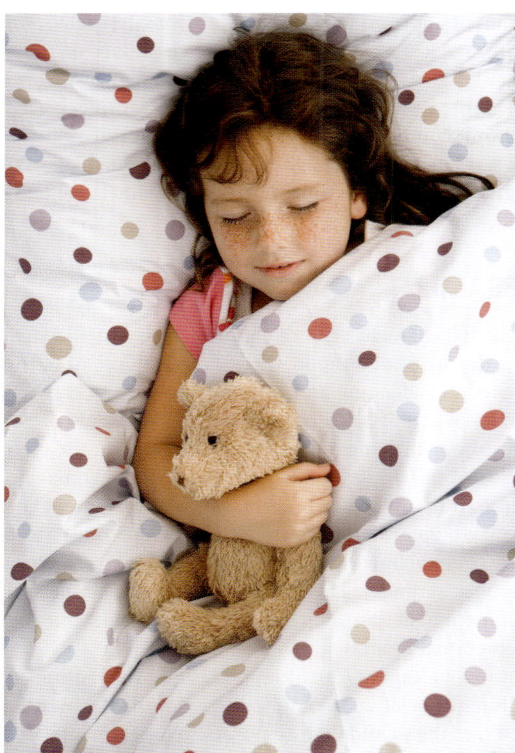

Fig 12.3 Transitional objects, such as a warm and fuzzy stuffed animal, are sources of security to a toddler.

is much greater than the number of words the child can say. Bilingual children can also achieve their early linguistic milestones in each of the languages at the same time and produce a substantial number of semantically corresponding words in each of their two languages from the very first words or signs (Estes & Hay 2015).

At age 1 year the child uses one-word sentences, or holophrases. The word 'up' can mean 'pick me up' or 'look up there'. For the child the one word conveys the meaning of a sentence, but to others it may mean many things or nothing. At this age about 25% of the vocalisations are intelligible. By the age of 2 years the child uses multiword sentences by stringing together two or three words, such as the phrases, 'Mama go bye-bye' or 'all gone', and approximately 65% of the speech is understandable. At 30 months the toddler knows her or his full name. By 3 years the child puts words together into simple sentences, begins to master grammatical rules, acquires five or six new words daily, knows his or her age and gender and can count three objects correctly (Feigelman 2016). Reading books together during this period provides an ideal setting for further language development. Language development among infants and toddlers is positively affected by adult–child conversations including reading, storytelling and interactive adult–child communication. Because of their immature symbolic, memory and attentional skills, infants and toddlers cannot learn from traditional digital media as they do from interactions with caregivers and they have difficulty transferring that knowledge to their three-dimensional experience (Barr 2013). Emerging evidence shows that at 24 months of age, children can learn words from live video-chatting with a responsive adult or from an interactive touchscreen interface that scaffolds the child to choose the relevant answers (Kirkorian et al 2016, Roseberry et al 2014). The Australian Department of Health guidelines discourage the use of any screen media in children under 2 years of age (Tooth et al 2019). However, children 2 to 5 years of age can be introduced to digital media consisting of high-quality programming/apps but should be viewed together with parents and children and should be limited to 1 hour per day Allowing children to use media alone should be avoided.

Gestures (such as putting phone to ear or pointing) precede or accompany each of the language milestones up to 30 months of age. Once language is sufficiently mastered, gestures phase out and the pace of word learning increases.

Personal-Social Behaviour

One of the most dramatic aspects of development in the toddler is personal-social interaction. Parents frequently wonder why their manageable, docile, lovable infant has turned into a determined, strong-willed, volatile-tempered little 'tyrant'. In addition, the tyrant can swiftly and unpredictably revert back to the adorable infant. All this is part of growing up as toddlers acquire an awareness that others' feelings and desires can be different from their own. Through interactions with caregivers, children are able to explore these differences and their consequences which are evident in such areas as dressing, feeding, playing and establishing self-control.

Toddlers are developing skills of independence, which are evident in all areas of behaviour. By 15 months of age children feed themselves, drink well from a covered cup and manage a spoon, with considerable spilling. By 2 years old they use a spoon well and by 3 years old they may be using a fork. Between ages 2 and 3 years old they eat with the family and like to help with chores such as setting the table or removing dishes from the dishwasher, but they lack table manners and may find it difficult to sit through the family's entire meal.

In dressing, toddlers also demonstrate strides in independence. The 15-month-old child helps by putting the arm or foot out for dressing and pulls shoes and socks off. The 18-month-old child removes gloves, helps with pullover shirts and may be able to unzip. By 2 years old toddlers remove most articles of clothing and put on socks, shoes and pants without regard for right or left and back or front. Toddlers still need help to fasten clothes.

Toddlers also begin to develop concern for the feelings of others and develop an understanding of how adult expectations for behaviour apply to specific situations (e.g. causing a sibling to cry while playing rough). As their understanding increases, they develop control. Age-appropriate discipline contributes to healthy social and emotional development. Positive reinforcement, redirection and time-out are appropriate for most toddlers. It is recognised that social and emotional problems can develop in the youngest children. Early screening and intervention promote more positive outcomes as the young child grows and develops.

Play

Play magnifies toddlers' physical and psychosocial development. Interaction with people becomes increasingly important. The solitary play of infancy progresses to **parallel play**: the toddler plays alongside, not with, other children. Although sensorimotor play is still prominent, there is much less emphasis on the exclusive use of one sensory modality. The toddler inspects the toy, talks to the toy, tests its strength and durability and invents several uses for it.

Play assumes many forms and serves several functions. Toddlers benefit from a wide variety of play interactions (e.g. alone, with other children, with adults), environments (e.g. own home, other children's homes, park, playgrounds) and activities (e.g. active, quiet, organised, unstructured).

Imitation is one of the most distinguishing characteristics of play and enriches children's opportunity to engage in fantasy. With less emphasis on sex-stereotyped toys, play objects such as dolls, doll-houses, dishes, cooking utensils, child-sized furniture, trucks and

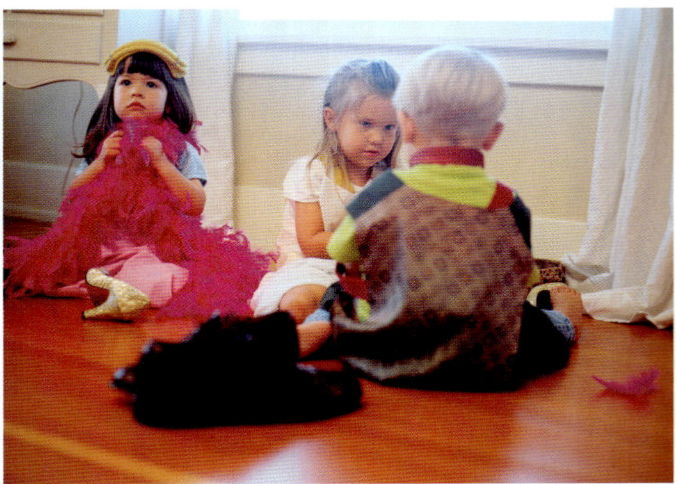

Fig 12.4 Young children enjoy dressing up.

dress-up clothes are used by both sexes; however, boys may be more interested than girls in activities related to trucks, trailers, cars, plastic soldiers or superheroes and building blocks, whereas girls may prefer doll-related activities (Fig 12.4).

Increased locomotive skills make push-pull toys, stick horses, straddle trucks or cycles, a small gym and slide, balls of various sizes and riding toys appropriate for the energetic toddler. Finger paints, thick crayons, chalk, blackboard, paper and puzzles with large, simple pieces use the toddler's developing fine motor skills. Interlocking blocks in varied sizes (but large enough to avoid aspiration) and shapes provide hours of fun and, during later years, are useful objects for creative and imaginative play. The most educational toy is the one that fosters the interaction of an adult with a child in supportive, unconditional play. Parents and other providers are encouraged to allow children to play with a variety of simple toys that foster creative thinking (such as blocks, dolls and clay), rather than passive toys that the child observes (battery-operated or mechanical). Active play time should also be encouraged over the use of computer or video games, which are more passive. Australian Department of Health guidelines encourage toddlers to spend at least 180 minutes a day doing a variety of physical activities including energetic play such as running, jumping and twirling spread throughout the day (Australian Department of Health 2019).

Certain aspects of play are related to emerging linguistic abilities. Talking is a form of play for toddlers, who enjoy musical toys such as 'talking' dolls and animals and toy telephones. Children's television programs are appropriate for some children over 2 years of age who learn to associate words with visual images. However, total media time should be limited to 1 hour or less of quality programming per day. Parents are encouraged to allow the child to engage in unstructured playtime, which is considered much more beneficial than any electronic media exposure (Tooth et al 2019). Toddlers also enjoy 'reading' stories from a picture book and imitating the sounds of animals.

Tactile play is also important for the exploring toddler. Water toys, a sandbox with bucket and shovel, finger paints, soap bubbles and play dough provide excellent opportunities for creative and manipulative recreation. Adults sometimes forget the fascination of feeling slippery textures such as slippery cream, mud or pudding; catching air bubbles; squeezing and reshaping clay; or smearing paints. These types of unstructured activities are as important as educational play to allow children freedom of expression.

Selection of appropriate toys must involve safety factors, especially in relation to size and sturdiness. The oral activity of toddlers puts them at risk for aspirating small objects and ingesting toxic substances. Parents need to be especially vigilant of toys played with in other children's homes and those of older siblings. Toys are a potential source of serious bodily damage to toddlers, who may have the physical strength to manipulate them but not the knowledge to appreciate their danger.

TEMPERAMENT

Temperamental characteristics of children during infancy tend to predominate during toddlerhood. Most challenging or strong-willed infants remain challenging and strong willed during early childhood, but the relaxed infants also become less easy. Parents often perceive toddlers as more challenging, especially considering the typical negativistic traits of this age group. Parents of easy infants may be particularly distressed by the behaviour change, whereas parents of difficult children may be more prepared because of a previously troublesome year, or be overwhelmed by the additional behaviours. For practitioners in a busy setting, asking parents about their impression of the child's temperament can help professionals understand the parent–child interactional process.

Guyer and colleagues (2015) emphasise that parenting style influences children's social and emotional development. Parents are often concerned that their child with an adverse temperament will develop a behavioural dysfunction that persists for a lifetime. The lack of fit between the child's temperament and the parents' expectations is often a source of conflict. The authors point out that behavioural problems in children can be managed appropriately, but the child's temperament cannot be changed (Guyer et al 2015).

Eisenberg and colleagues (2015) found evidence of bidirectional and interactive effects between parenting and children's characteristics of fear, self-regulation, frustration and impulsivity. Children with high frustration levels, impulsivity and low effortful control were more vulnerable to negative parenting behaviours. Such parental behaviours served to predict an increase in children's fearfulness, frustration and effortful control. The authors present information that can be used to evaluate the goodness of fit between the toddler's parents and the toddler's behaviour and make adjustments in parenting style accordingly.

COPING WITH CONCERNS RELATED TO NORMAL GROWTH AND DEVELOPMENT

Table 12.2 summarises the major features of growth and development for the age groups of 15, 18, 24 and 30 months. The key developmental ages are 18 and 24 months, although the chronological ages of 15 and 30 months are also significant. Fifteen months of age is a particularly integrative period of developmental achievement because it represents the completion or fruition of many skills that were unperfected at 1 year of age.

Toilet Training

One of the major tasks of toddlerhood is toilet training. Voluntary control of the anal and urethral sphincters is achieved some time after the child is walking, probably between ages 18 and 24 months. However, complex psychophysiological factors are required for readiness. The child must be able to recognise the urge to let go and hold on and be able to communicate this sensation to the parent. In addition, some motivation is probably involved in the desire to please the parent by holding on rather than pleasing oneself by letting go. Cultural

TABLE 12.2 Growth and Development During the Toddler Years

Physical	Gross Motor	Fine Motor	Sensory	Language	Socialisation/Cognition
AGE 15 MONTHS					
Steady growth in height and weight Head circumference 48 cm Weight 11 kg Height 78.7 cm	Walks without help (usually since age 13 months) Creeps up stairs Kneels without support Cannot walk around corners or stop suddenly without losing balance Assumes standing position without support Cannot throw ball without falling	Constantly casting objects to floor Builds tower of two cubes Holds two cubes in one hand Releases pellet into narrow-necked bottle Scribbles spontaneously Uses cup well but often rotates spoon	Able to identify geometrical forms; places round object into appropriate hole Binocular vision well developed Displays intense and prolonged interest in pictures	Uses expressive jargon Says four to six words, including names Asks for objects by pointing Understands simple commands May shake head to denote 'no' Uses 'no' even while agreeing to the request Uses common gestures such as putting cup to mouth when empty	Tolerates some separation from parent Less likely to fear strangers Beginning to imitate parents, such as cleaning house (sweeping, dusting), folding clothes May discard bottle Manages spoon but rotates it near mouth Kisses and hugs parents; may kiss pictures in book Expresses emotions; has temper tantrums
AGE 18 MONTHS					
Physiological anorexia from decreased growth needs Anterior fontanel closed Physiologically able to control sphincters	Runs clumsily; falls often Walks up stairs with one handheld Pulls and pushes toys Jumps in place with both feet Seats self on chair Throws ball overhand without falling	Builds tower of three or four cubes Release, prehension and reach well developed Turns two or three pages in book at a time In drawing, makes stroke imitatively Manages spoon without rotation		Says 10 or more words Points to common object, such as shoe or ball, and to two or three body parts Forms word combinations Forms gesture-word combinations (points while naming) Forms gesture-gesture combinations	Great imitator (domestic mimicry) Takes off gloves, socks and shoes and unzips zippers Temper tantrums may be more evident Beginning awareness of ownership ('my toy') May develop dependency on transitional objects, such as security blanket

Continued

TABLE 12.2 Growth and Development During the Toddler Years—cont'd

Physical	Gross Motor	Fine Motor	Sensory	Language	Socialisation/Cognition
AGE 24 MONTHS					
Head circumference 49–50 cm Chest circumference exceeds head circumference Lateral diameter of chest exceeds anteroposterior diameter Usual weight gain of 1.8–2.7 kg Usual gain in height of 10–12.5 cm Adult height approximately double height at 2 years May be ready to begin daytime control of bowel and bladder Primary dentition of 16 teeth	Goes up and down stairs alone with two feet on each step Runs fairly well, with wide stance Picks up object without falling Kicks ball forwards without overbalancing	Builds tower of six to seven cubes Aligns two or more cubes like a train Turns pages of book one at a time In drawing, imitates vertical and circular strokes Turns doorknob, unscrews lid	Accommodation well developed in geometrical discrimination; able to insert square block into oblong space	Has vocabulary of approximately 300 words Uses two- or three-word phrases Uses pronouns 'I', 'me', 'you' Understands directional commands Gives first name; refers to self by name Verbalises need for toileting, food or drink Talks incessantly Able to remember and imitate arbitrary sequences of manual actions and gestures	Stage of parallel play Has sustained attention span Temper tantrums decreasing Pulls people to show them something Increased independence from parent Dresses self in simple clothing Develops visual recognition and verbal self-reference ('me big') Develops awareness that feelings and desires of others may be different and begins to explore implications and consequences
AGE 30 MONTHS					
Birth weight quadrupled Primary dentition (20 teeth) completed May have daytime bowel and bladder control	Jumps with both feet Jumps from chair or step Stands on one foot momentarily Takes a few steps on tiptoe	Builds tower of eight cubes Adds chimney to train of cubes Good hand–finger coordination; holds crayon with fingers rather than fist In drawing, imitates vertical and horizontal strokes; makes two or more strokes for cross; draws circles		Gives first and last name Refers to self by appropriate pronoun Uses plurals Names one colour	Separates more easily from parent In play, helps put things away; can carry breakable objects; pushes with good steering Begins to notice gender differences; knows own gender May attend to toilet needs without help except for wiping Emotions expand to include pride, shame, guilt, embarrassment

norms may also affect the age at which children demonstrate readiness (Feigelman 2016).

Three markers signal a child's readiness to toilet train: (1) being aware of the urge to void or stool; (2) interest in and/or motivation to use the toilet and (3) being dry for at least 2 hours during the day (Kimball 2016). According to some experts, physiological and psychological readiness is not complete until ages 24 to 30 months (Rogers 2013); however, parents should begin preparing their children for toilet training earlier than 30 months. By this time the child has mastered the majority of essential gross motor skills, can communicate intelligibly, is in less conflict with parents in terms of self-assertion and negativism and is aware of the ability to control the body and please the parent. One of the nurse's most important responsibilities is to help parents identify the readiness signs in their child (see Nursing Care Guidelines box). On average, girls are developmentally ready to begin toilet training 2 to 3 months before boys (Kimball 2016). Toilet training is a stage which is best led by the child. The child must be ready to achieve this milestone and the process a positive experience for all concerned.

NURSING CARE GUIDELINES

Assessing Toilet Training Readiness

Physical Readiness
- Voluntary control of anal and urethral sphincters, usually by ages 24 to 30 months
- Ability to stay dry for 2 hours; decreased number of wet nappies; waking dry from nap
- Regular bowel movements
- Gross motor skills of sitting, walking and squatting
- Fine motor skills to remove clothing

Mental Readiness
- Recognition of urge to defecate or urinate
- Verbal or non-verbal communication skills to indicate when wet or has urge to defecate or urinate
- Cognitive skills to imitate appropriate behaviour and follow directions

Psychological Readiness
- Expressing willingness to please parent
- Ability to sit on toilet for 5 to 8 minutes without fussing or getting off
- Curiosity about adults' or older sibling's toilet habits
- Impatience with soiled or wet nappies; desire to be changed immediately

Parental Readiness
- Recognition of child's level of readiness
- Willingness to invest the time required for toilet training
- Absence of family stress or change, such as a divorce, moving, new sibling or imminent vacation

Night-time bladder control normally takes several months to years after daytime training begins. This is because the sleep cycle needs to mature so the child can awake in time to urinate. Feigelman (2016) indicates that bedwetting is normal in girls up to age 4 years old and in boys up to age 5 years. Few children have night wetting episodes after daytime dryness is totally achieved; however, children who do not have night-time dryness by the age of 7 years old are likely to require intervention.

Bowel training is usually accomplished before bladder training because of its greater regularity and predictability. The sensation for defecation is stronger than that for urination and easier for children to recognise. A well-balanced diet that includes dietary fibre helps keep stool soft and supports the development and maintenance of regular bowel movements.

A number of techniques are helpful when initiating training, and cultural differences should be considered; however, toilet training must driven by the child, who instigates the process. And as with any developmental task, similar to walking or rolling, the toddler may master it one day and then not be able to master it again for a number of weeks or months.

As the child masters each step of toileting (discussion, undressing, going, wiping, dressing, flushing and hand washing), he or she gains a sense of accomplishment that parents should reinforce. If the parent–child relationship becomes strained, both may need a break to focus on enjoyable activities together. Regression may coincide with a stressful family situation or the child being pushed too hard and too fast. Regression is a normal part of toilet training and does not mean failure but should be viewed as a temporary setback to a more comfortable place for the child.

Temper Tantrums

Toddlers may assert their independence by violently objecting to discipline. They may lie down on the floor, kick their feet and scream as loud as possible. Some have learned the effectiveness of holding their breath until the parent relents. Although holding one's breath may cause fainting from lack of oxygen, the accumulation of carbon dioxide will stimulate the respiratory control centre, resulting in no physical harm. Tantrums are an indication of the child's struggle to control emotions; toddlers are particularly prone to tantrums because their strong drive for mastery and autonomy is frustrated by adult figures or lack of motor, cognitive and communication skills. Temper tantrums commonly occur when the child is ill, hungry, frustrated or tired; some children may use temper tantrums to get parental attention, get something they want or avoid having to do something they do not want to do (El-Radhi 2015). **Temper tantrums** have been linked to two emotional and behavioural processes: anger and distress (Eisbach et al 2014). Anger increases rapidly and peaks near the beginning of the tantrum; components of distress, such as crying and comfort seeking, increase as anger subsides. The majority of temper tantrums (75%) last 5 minutes or less (Eisbach et al 2014).

The best approach towards tapering temper tantrums requires consistency and developmentally appropriate expectations and rewards. Ensuring consistency among all caregivers in expectations, prioritising what rules are important and developing consequences that are reasonable for the child's level of development help manage the behaviour. For example, a popular time for a tantrum is before bedtime. Active toddlers often have trouble slowing down and, when placed in bed, resist staying there. Parents can reinforce consistency and expectations by stating, 'After this story it is bedtime'. Starting at 18 months, time-outs work well for managing temper tantrums.

During tantrums ignore the behaviour, provided the behaviour is not injurious to the child, such as violently banging the head on the floor. Continue to be present to provide a feeling of control and security to the child once the tantrum has subsided. If the tantrum occurs on an outing such as a visit to the shops, the child may need to be removed from the public place until the tantrum has subsided. Provide realistic expectations on such outings; if the child goes into the shop expecting to receive a toy or lollies and does not, a tantrum is likely. Remember that toddlers like routines, so try to adhere to the child's routine for naps, playtime and meals to decrease the child's frustration. During periods of no tantrums, practise developmentally appropriate positive reinforcement.

Other suggestions for handling tantrums include the following (El-Radhi 2015):

- offering the child options instead of an 'all or none' position
- ensuring a consistent response to child's behaviour by all caregivers
- praising the child for positive behaviour when he or she is not having a tantrum or providing a reward system (e.g. sticker chart).

Temper tantrums are common during the toddler years and essentially represent normal developmental behaviours. However, temper tantrums can be signs of serious problems. Temper tantrums that occur past 5 years of age, last longer than 15 minutes or occur more than five times a day are a concern and may indicate a problem (El-Radhi 2015). Nurses should be alert to situations that require further evaluation.

Stress

Adults rarely think of young children as being exposed to stress or suffering its consequences. However, the normal demands of growing up coupled with the usual pressures most families experience mean that few, if any, young children grow up stress-free. Small amounts of stress are beneficial during the early years to help children develop effective coping skills. However, excessive stress is unhelpful, and young children are especially vulnerable because of their limited ability to cope.

To deal with stress in their children's lives, parents must be aware of the signs of stress and be able to identify the source. Any number of other stresses may be imposed on children, such as alternative caregiving arrangements, birth of a sibling, separation and divorce, relocation or illness. Watching children at play can help identify stressors. Other signs of increased stress in a toddler's life may include increased thumb sucking, aggressive behaviour and biting.

The best approach to dealing with stress is prevention—monitoring the amount of stress in children's lives so that levels do not exceed their coping ability. In many instances this is as simple as increasing the child's rest periods to allow for quiet recovery time. Often it involves adequately preparing the child for change, such as day care or a new sibling. It also requires helping the child cope with stress. Unsupervised play is an excellent vehicle for releasing anger or frustration, and toys such as drums, wooden pegs and hammer and play dough provide alternative methods of dissipating anxiety. They also begin to teach socially acceptable ways of dealing with such feelings. Another approach is the use of relaxation and imagery.

Regression

Regression involves a retreat from one's present pattern of functioning to past levels of behaviour. It usually occurs in instances of stress, when one attempts to cope by reverting to patterns of behaviour that were successful in earlier stages of development. Regression is common in toddlers because almost any additional stress-lessens their ability to master present developmental tasks. Any threat to their autonomy, such as illness, hospitalisation, separation or adjustment to a sibling, represents a need to revert to earlier forms of behaviour, such as increased dependency. This can include refusal to use the potty; temper tantrums; demand for the bottle or crib; and loss of newly learned motor, language, social and cognitive skills.

At first, such regression appears acceptable and comfortable for children, but on closer inspection it becomes evident that the loss of newly acquired achievements is frightening and threatening because children are aware of their total helplessness in the recent past. Parents, too, become concerned about regressive behaviour and may force the child to cope with an additional source of stress: the pressure of living up to expected standards. Brazelton (1999) suggests that these predictable times of regression, or **touchpoints**, are an opportunity to prepare parents for the next step in their child's development.

When regression does occur, the best approach is to ignore it while praising existing patterns of appropriate behaviour. The child is saying, 'I can't cope with this present stress and accomplish this new skill as well, but I will eventually if given patience and understanding'. For this reason, it is advisable not to introduce new areas of learning when an additional crisis is present or expected, such as beginning toilet training shortly before a sibling is born or during a brief hospitalisation.

Fears are common during this age and include fear of annihilation, going to sleep, animals and engines, with the greatest fear continuing to be fear of strangers and separation from parents or other caregivers. Because fear of strangers and separation begins in infancy, it is discussed in Chapter 10. The other fears often escalate in the preschool period and consequently are discussed in Chapter 13.

PROMOTING OPTIMUM HEALTH DURING TODDLERHOOD

Nutrition

During the period from 12 to 18 months of age the growth rate slows, decreasing the child's need for calories, protein and fluid. However, the protein (13 g/day) and energy requirements are still relatively high to meet the demands for muscle tissue growth and high activity level. The need for minerals such as iron, calcium and phosphorus may be difficult to meet, considering the characteristic food habits of children in this age group. Parents may be tempted to rely on vitamin supplementation rather than a well-balanced diet to meet these requirements. Toddlers usually require three meals and two snacks per day; however, the portions consumed are generally much smaller compared with those of older children.

At approximately 18 months of age most toddlers manifest this decreased nutritional need with a decreased appetite, a phenomenon known as **physiological anorexia**. They become picky, fussy eaters with strong taste preferences. They may eat large amounts one day and almost nothing the next. They are increasingly aware of the non-nutritive function of food (i.e. the pleasure of eating, the social aspect of mealtime and the control of refusing food). They are influenced by factors other than taste when choosing food. If a family member refuses to eat something, toddlers are likely to imitate that response. If the plate is overfilled, they are likely to push it away, overwhelmed by its size. If food does not appear or smell appetising, they will probably not agree to try it. In essence mealtime is more closely associated with psychological rather than nutritional components. Toddlers like to eat with their fingers and enjoy foods of different colours and shapes (Fig 12.5).

The **ritualism** of this age also dictates certain principles in feeding practices. Toddlers like to have the same dish, cup or spoon every time they eat. They may reject a favourite food simply because it is served in a different dish. If one food touches another, they often refuse to eat it. Mixed foods such as stews or casseroles are rarely favourites. Because toddlers have unpredictable table manners, it is best to use plastic dishes and cups for both economic and safety reasons. For some children a regular mealtime schedule also contributes to their desire and need for predictability and ritualism.

Developmentally by 12 months of age most children eat many of the same foods prepared for the rest of the family. Some may have mastered using a cup with occasional spilling, although most cannot use a spoon adeptly until 18 months of age or later and generally prefer using their fingers (Table 12.3).

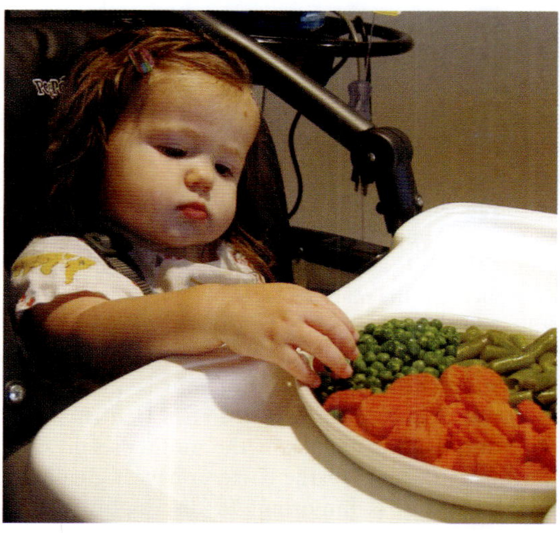

Fig 12.5 Toddlers enjoy finger foods such as green peas. (Source: Courtesy E. Jacobs, Texas Children's Hospital, Houston.)

TABLE 12.3 Developmental Milestones Associated with Feeding

Age (Month)	Development
12–18	Drools less
	Drinks well from cup with lid but may drop it when finished
	Holds cup with both hands
	Begins to use spoon but turns it before reaching mouth
24	Can use straw and cup
	Chews food with mouth closed, and shifts food in mouth
	Distinguishes between finger and spoon foods
	Uses spoon correctly but with some spilling
36	Spills small amount from spoon
	Begins to use fork; holds it in fist
	Uses adult pattern of chewing, which involves rotary action of jaw

Nutritional Counselling

The emphasis on preventing childhood obesity and subsequent cardiovascular disease has prompted a number of changes in dietary recommendations for children and adults alike. It is now recognised that lifetime eating habits are established in early childhood, possibly by the end of the toddler period; healthcare workers are increasingly emphasising the role of food selection choices, exercise, stress reduction and other lifestyle choices (e.g. tobacco and alcohol use) on the quality of adult life and survival. Conditions such as obesity and cardiovascular disease can be prevented by encouraging healthy eating habits in toddlers and their families.

If food is used as a reward or sign of approval, a child may overeat for non-nutritive reasons. If food is forced and mealtime is consistently unpleasant, the usual pleasure associated with eating may not develop. Mealtimes should be enjoyable rather than times for discipline or family arguments. The social aspect of mealtime may be distracting for young children; therefore, an earlier feeding hour may be appropriate. Young children are unable to sit through a long meal and become restless and disruptive. This is particularly common when children are brought to the table just after active play. Calling them in from play 15 minutes before mealtime allows them ample opportunity to get ready for eating while settling down their active minds and bodies.

The method of serving food also takes on more importance during this period. Toddlers need to have a sense of control and achievement in their abilities. Giving them large, adult-size portions can overwhelm them. In general, what is eaten is much more significant than how much is consumed. Toddlers usually restrict their food preference to four or five main foods and rarely try new foods; in some cases, a toddler may insist on one food such as mashed potatoes for lunch and dinner. Small amounts of meat and vegetables supply greater food value than a large consumption of bread or potato. Serving sizes need to be appropriate for age. Young children tend to like less spicy, bland food, although this is a culturally determined preference. Substitutions can be provided for foods that they do not enjoy, although parents need not cater to all of their desires. Frequent, small nutritious snacks can replace a meal.

Mastication (chewing) skills continue to mature, putting children at risk for choking; therefore, large round foods (e.g. hot dogs, grapes, peas, carrots, apple, popcorn) should be avoided until the child is able to chew them effectively. Active play while eating should be discouraged to prevent choking. Appetite and food preferences are sporadic. Often the interest in food parallels a growth spurt; thus, periods of good eating are interspersed with phases of poor eating. If exposed to the same food every day, a young toddler does not learn how to manage the complex sensory information needed to eat new, more difficult foods (e.g. vegetables with a different texture versus pureed, slippery fruits). To help prevent 'food jags' it is recommended that parents present food in various physical forms. The child may need to progress to eating new foods in a stepwise fashion such as visually tolerating the food, interacting with it, smelling it, touching it, tasting it and then eating it.

This period of picky eating can be trying for both parents and child. Many health practitioners consider it to be a developmental phase and stress that most toddlers will consume the necessary amount of food required for growth (Saavedra et al 2013).

Nursing Care Management

Evaluation of adequacy of nutrient intake is the initial nursing goal and requires assessment based on a dietary history and physical examination for signs of deficiency or excess. Once assessment data are collected, this information is evaluated against standard intakes to identify areas of concern. (See Nutritional Assessment, Chapter 4.)

State and federal government dietary guidelines may be used to encourage healthy dietary intakes designed to decrease obesity and cardiovascular risk factors and subsequent cardiovascular disease, which is now known to occur in both young children and adults (Steinberger et al 2016). Such guidelines encourage a variety of fruits, vegetables, wholegrains and low-fat dairy and non-fat dairy products, in addition to fish, beans and lean meat.

The nurse has an important role in evaluating the food intake of infants, children and adolescents and may serve as a resource for parents; the overall nutritional goal should be to provide the best sources of vitamin and mineral intake through food intake rather than rely on supplemental vitamins, which may not always be as well absorbed as food products.

Sleep and Activity

Total sleep time decreases only slightly during the second year and averages about 11 to 12 hours. Most toddlers take one nap a day, and by the end of the second or third year, many relinquish this habit.

Toddlers are more prone to having bedtime resistance (refusal to go to bed) and frequent night waking. Fears can be provoked by a child's daily stressors, such as pressure to toilet train, changes in environment, sibling birth, experiences of loss or separation from parents. Consistent nightly bedtime is associated with better sleep patterns, such as shorter sleep onset latency, decreased waking, longer total sleep and decreased daytime behaviour problems (Mindell et al 2015). In addition, providing transitional objects, such as a favourite stuffed animal or blanket, can ease the child's insecurity at bedtime. Children may need a light snack before bedtime; a heavy meal immediately before bedtime may interfere with sleep. Other suggestions to help small children sleep better include keeping the television out of the child's room, making the hour before bedtime a quiet time of reading stories and avoiding stimulating activities such as computer games and roughhousing (Owens 2016).

A toddler's activity level is high, and rarely is there a problem with too little physical exercise, provided that inappropriate restrictions are not instituted. Recently, however, there has been concern that decreased time spent in actual physical play and more time involved with computers and television watching have increased the tendency towards being overweight. This is especially true in large urban centres during the winter months where there may not be adequate 'safe' play and physical exercise space. With increasing numbers of young children being cared for outside the home, attention to the kinds of activity provided is important. For example, children with high activity levels may benefit from an environment that encourages vigorous play whether outside or in a large indoor play area.

Dental Health

Regular teeth brushing is essential to maintaining good oral health hygiene and reducing the risk of dental decay. It is recommended that children's teeth are wiped or gently brushed as soon as they erupt, and that brushing with fluoridated toothpaste be introduced from 18 months of age (Australian Institute of Health and Welfare [AIHW] 2020). Australia's fluoride guidelines recommend brushing teeth twice a day from 18 months (Armfeld et al 2016).

Diet is critical to developing good teeth because the tooth process depends primarily on fermentable sugars, especially sucrose, and other carbohydrates. Refined table sugar, honey, molasses, corn syrup and dried fruits such as raisins are highly cariogenic. Complex carbohydrates such as breads, potatoes and pasta also contribute to caries because they lower the plaque pH. Sugary beverages that are commonly consumed by children and adolescents and sugar-containing medications are also highly cariogenic (Llena et al 2015).

Ideally, highly cariogenic foods, especially those containing complex sugars, should be eliminated. However, because this is impractical, some suggestions can be helpful. First, *the frequency with which sugar is consumed is more important than the total amount eaten.* Therefore, when sweets are eaten, they are less damaging if consumed immediately after a meal rather than as a snack between meals. When they are served as the dessert, the teeth can be cleaned afterwards, decreasing the amount of time the sugar is in the mouth.

Ideally the teeth should be cleaned after each meal and especially before bedtime, and the child should be given nothing to eat or drink after the night brushing except water. At times when brushing is impractical, the 'swish-and-swallow' method of cleaning the mouth is taught; with a mouthful of water, the child rinses the mouth and swallows, repeating the procedure three or four times. Figure 12.6 from the Australian Dental Association indicates brushing technique for different ages.

A special form of tooth decay in children between 18 months and 3 years of age is **early childhood caries (ECC)** (historically called *nursing caries* or *baby bottle tooth decay*) (Fig 12.7). This often occurs when a child is routinely given a bottle of milk or juice at naptime or bedtime or uses the bottle as a pacifier while awake. The practice of coating a pacifier in honey can also contribute to tooth decay and is not recommended. As the sweet liquid pools in the mouth, the teeth are bathed for several hours in this cariogenic environment. Prolonged bottle-feeding, fruit-juice consumption, lack of periodic dental examination and nocturnal feeding contribute to significant ECC (Ozen et al 2016). The maxillary (upper) incisors and molars are affected most because the mandibular (lower) incisors are protected by the lower lip, tongue and saliva.

ECC is now considered to be an infectious disease of childhood. There is evidence that *Streptococcus mutans* is a highly cariogenic bacterium (American Academy of Pediatric Dentistry 2016). One of the early origins of *S. mutans* is the mother's saliva; infants of mothers with high counts of the bacteria have a greater incidence of ECC. Therefore, it is important to discuss oral hygiene with pregnant women because of its impact on their children's tooth development.

Prevention involves eliminating the bedtime bottle completely, feeding the last bottle before bedtime, not using the bottle as a pacifier and never coating pacifiers in sweet substances. Juice in bottles, especially commercially available ready-to-use bottles, is discouraged; these beverages are especially damaging because the sugar is more readily converted to acid. Juice should always be offered in a cup to avoid prolonging the bottle-feeding habit. Toddlers should be encouraged to drink from a cup at the first birthday and weaned from a bottle by 14 months of age. Nurses are in an excellent position to counsel parents regarding the dangers of this habit and other aspects of dental care.

Tooth decay in children can be prevented by the consumption of fluoridated water which protects teeth against damage, and helps to repair damaged teeth (NHMRC 2017). Fluoridated tap/public water is provided in all Australian states and territories; however, coverage varies across each jurisdiction. The National Child Oral Health Study 2012–14 estimates that 71% of Australian children aged 5 to 14 years had almost all tap/public water as their daily drinking water from age 5 (Do et al 2016). Other families get their water from other sources such as water tanks and private bores.

Infants should visit the dentist when first teeth appear or by the age of 12 months. Some population groups, such as those living in remote areas and those from lower income households, face greater challenges in accessing oral healthcare and experience the greatest burden of poor oral health (AIHW 2019). Children living in remote areas (53%) were more likely to have decay in their primary teeth than children in major cities (39%). Indigenous children were also more likely to have untreated decay in at least one primary tooth (44%) or one permanent tooth (23%) than non-Indigenous children (26% and 10% respectively) (AIHW 2019).

Safety Promotion and Injury Prevention

Injury is the leading cause of death among children ages 1 to 4 years and a major cause of hospitalisation (AIHW 2019). In 2015 to 2017, among children aged 0 to 14 years, the leading causes of injury deaths among children were land transport accidents, which included road traffic fatalities, accidental drowning and assault (AIHW 2019). Other causes of accidental death include suffocation for children less than 1 year of age and drowning for children 1 to 4 years of age (AIHW 2019). Falls are the leading cause of non-fatal injuries among children. These deaths and injuries are preventable, and they highlight the need for public health action and education. There is evidence that one-on-one and face-to-face education in the home, safety interventions and safety

Babies

- Use a damp washcloth and clean your baby's gums by gently rubbing them.
- As teeth appear introduce a soft, child-size toothbrush.
- Do not use toothpaste.
- Visit a dentist when the first teeth appear or by 12 months.

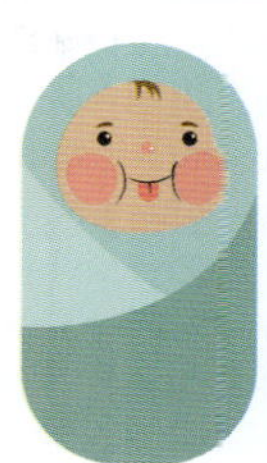

Toddlers

- Brush with a soft child-size toothbrush.
- Use child-strength fluoride toothpaste from 18 months of age.
- Parents should brush and floss their child's teeth.
- Brush twice daily.
- Floss teeth that touch together.

Children (under six years)

- Parents should continue to brush their child's teeth, twice daily.
- Floss teeth that touch together.
- Use child-strength fluoride toothpaste, unless your dentist recommends otherwise.

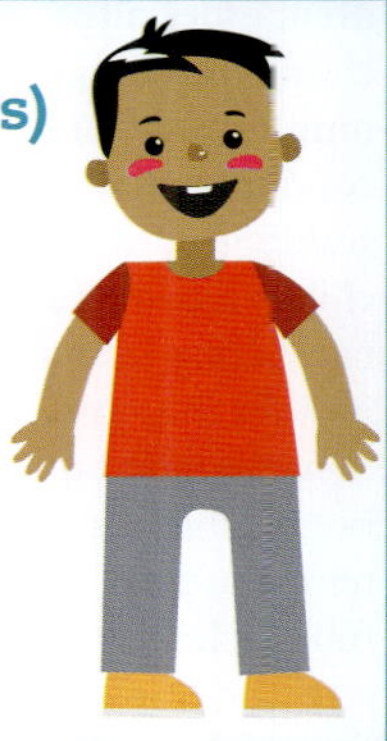

Children (over six years)

- Assist your child with brushing and flossing their teeth twice daily until 8–9 years of age.
- Use adult-strength fluoride toothpaste.

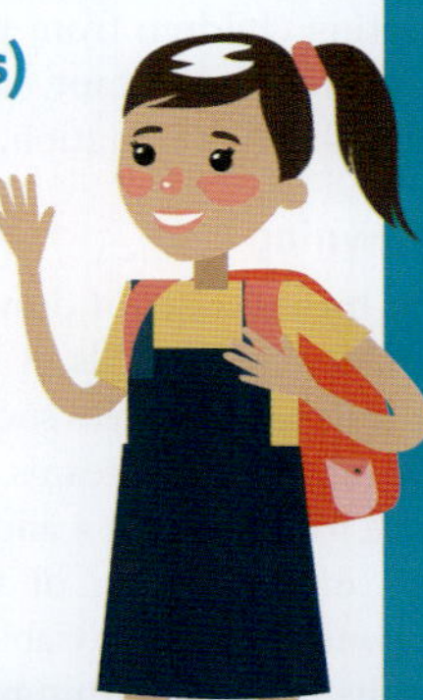

Fig 12.6 Australia Dental Association recommendations for brushing technique at different ages. (Source: Australian Dental Association. (2019). Caring for your child's oral health. https://www.ada.org.au/getattachment/Your-Dental-Health/Resources-for-Professionals/Resources-for-Children-0-11/Children-s-Oral-Health/ADA_OHP_Factsheets_Childrens-Oral-Health-18032019.pdf.aspx)

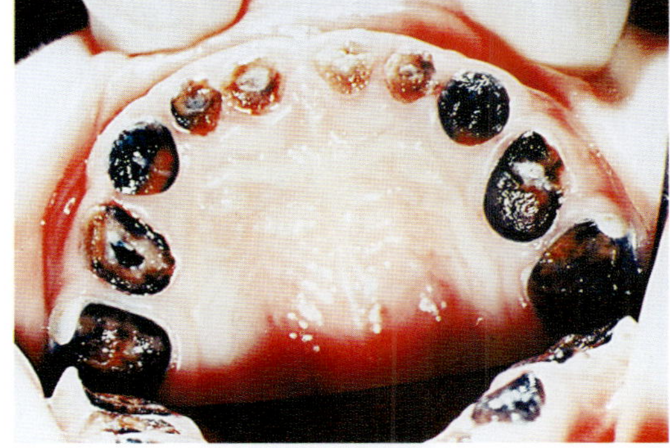

Fig 12.7 Early childhood caries. Note extensive carious involvement of maxillary primary incisors. (Source: Courtesy Bruce Carter, DDS, Texas Children's Hospital, Houston.)

equipment are effective in reducing the number of unintentional childhood injuries (Folger et al 2017).

A major factor in the critical increase of injuries during early childhood compared with the number in preschoolers and school-age children is the unrestricted freedom achieved through locomotion combined with a lack of awareness of danger within the environment. Toddlers are very curious about how things work, and exploration of previously unknown or unseen objects and places is common. Toddlers also have not fully developed or do not understand the cause-and-effect principles and often are unable to gauge danger; poorly developed depth perception may also contribute to falls and tumbles, as does the general bodily structure of toddlers. Specific categories of injuries and appropriate prevention are best understood by associating them with the major developmental achievements of young children. The discussions of injuries in Chapters 2, 10 and 13 are also relevant to safety concerns at this age.

Land Transport Injuries

Land transport injuries cause accidental deaths in children. Many of the deaths are caused by injuries within the car when restraints have not been used or age-related guidelines have not been properly followed. Unrestrained children riding in the vehicle's front seat are at the highest risk for injury. Approved restraints properly installed and applied can reduce the majority of fatalities and injuries.

Toddlers are often involved in pedestrian traffic injuries. Because of their gross motor skills of walking, running and climbing and their fine motor skills of opening doors and fence gates, they are likely to be in hazardous areas unsupervised. Unaware of danger and unable to estimate the speed of a car, children may be hit by moving vehicles. Running after a ball, playing in a pile of leaves or snow or inside a cardboard box, riding a tricycle and playing behind a parked car or near the kerb are common activities that may result in a vehicular tragedy. Being aware of where children are at all times is important especially if the child is naturally curious or courageous.

Another vehicle-related hazard for toddlers is overheating (hyperthermia) and subsequent death when left in a vehicle in hot weather (> 27°C). Small children dissipate heat poorly, and an increase in body temperature can cause death in a few hours. It is estimated that, with the ambient temperature at 22° to 35.5°C, the vehicle interior temperature rises by 10.5° to 11°C for each 10 minutes, even with a window cracked (Duzinski et al 2014). Approximately 50% of adults who left a child in a car either forgot or were unaware that the child was still in the car (Duzinski et al 2014). Parents are cautioned against leaving infants alone in a vehicle for *any reason.*

Preventing vehicular injuries involves protecting and educating children about the danger of moving and parked vehicles. Although toddlers are too young to be trusted to always obey, parents should emphasise looking for moving vehicles before crossing the street and recognising the stop and go colours of traffic lights. Physical barriers limiting children from playing near vehicles help prevent these injuries. Most important, what is preached must be practised. Children learn through imitation, and consistency reinforces learning.

Drowning

The highest rates of drowning occur in children ages 1 to 4 years. With well-developed skills of locomotion, toddlers are able to reach potentially dangerous areas such as bathtubs, toilets, buckets, swimming pools, hot tubs, rivers, streams, beaches and ponds or lakes. Toddlers' intense drive for exploration and investigation, combined with a lack of awareness of the danger of water and their helplessness in water, makes drowning always a viable threat. It is also one category of injury that results in death within minutes, diminishing the chance for rescue and survival. Close adult supervision of children when near any source of water is essential; many drownings in this age group occur when a supervising adult becomes distracted. Kidsafe Australia (2019) recommends remaining within arm's reach of toddlers when around water and in swimming pools to ensure you can get to the child in time if something goes wrong. Teaching swimming and water safety can be helpful but cannot be regarded as sufficient protection. Pool fencing, although critical and mandatory, does not always deter fast-moving children.

Burns

Toddlers' ability to climb, stretch and reach objects above their heads makes any hot surface a potential source of danger. Children pulling pots with hot liquids, especially oil and grease, on top of themselves are a major source of burns. As a precaution, turn pot handles towards the back of the stove and electric pots (e.g. electric kettle, frying pan, slow cooker), including cords, should be placed out of reach. Ideally, the knobs for controlling the stovetop burners should be out of reach, not on the front panel where nimble fingers can turn them on and accidentally touch the hot burner.

Other sources of heat, such as radiators, fireplaces, accessible furnaces, kerosene heaters or wood-burning stoves, should have guards placed in front of them. The tops of some of these heaters are designed to become hot enough to boil water to provide humidity. They are hazardous if touched or if the pan of water is spilled. Portable electric heaters must be placed in a high area, well out of reach of climbing young children.

Hot objects such as candles, incense, hot embers and ashes, cigarettes, cups or pots of tea or coffee, or irons must be placed away from children. Hair curling irons, hair straighteners and hot curlers may also be easily reached and can burn the hands of curious toddlers. Flame burns represent one of the most fatal types of burns and commonly occur when children play with matches or lighters and accidentally set themselves (and the home) on fire. To prevent flame burns, all matches should be stored safely away from children, and parents need to teach children the dangers of playing with matches and lighters. In addition, Australian fire agencies recommend all homes should have smoke detectors installed in all sleeping areas such as bedrooms to alert the occupants of a fire. A safety plan for immediate escape is also essential.

Electrical burns represent an immediate danger to children. With the ability to manipulate small, thin objects, they are able to insert hairpins or other conductive articles into electrical sockets. Young toddlers may explore outlets and wires by mouthing them. Because saliva is an excellent conductor, the chance for a severe circumoral electrical burn is great. Electrical outlets should have protective guards plugged into them when not in use or be made inaccessible by placing furniture in front of them when feasible (Fig 12.8). Children should not be allowed to play with electrical cords, appliances or batteries.

Scald burns are the most common type of thermal injury in children, especially 1 and 2 year olds. Scalding often occurs because the child is reaching towards a stove or other surface and pulling hot water onto himself or herself or because the child has spilled a hot liquid container (such as a parent's coffee or tea) onto himself or herself. A scalding burn is often caused by high-temperature tap water, which children come in contact with as a result of turning on the hot-water tap, falling into a bathtub of hot water or suffering deliberate abuse. Besides the obvious prevention of always supervising children when they are near tap water and checking bathwater temperatures, household water temperatures should be limited to less than 49°C. At this temperature it takes 10 minutes for exposure to the water to cause a full-thickness burn. Conversely, water temperatures of 54°C, the usual setting of most water heaters, expose household members to the risk of full-thickness burns within 30 seconds. Nurses can help prevent such burns by advising parents of this common household danger and recommending that they adjust the water heater to a safe temperature.

Sunburns are a special concern for this age group in Australia and New Zealand. Children spend a large amount of time outdoors, and their increased mobility makes it difficult to prevent sun exposure. Sun safety guidelines should be followed whenever the child is outside: applying a sunscreen with a sun protection factor (SPF) of 15 or greater, dressing in protective clothing (e.g. wide-brimmed hat, protective cotton clothing with a tight weave, sunglasses) and avoiding sun exposure between 10 am and 4 pm.

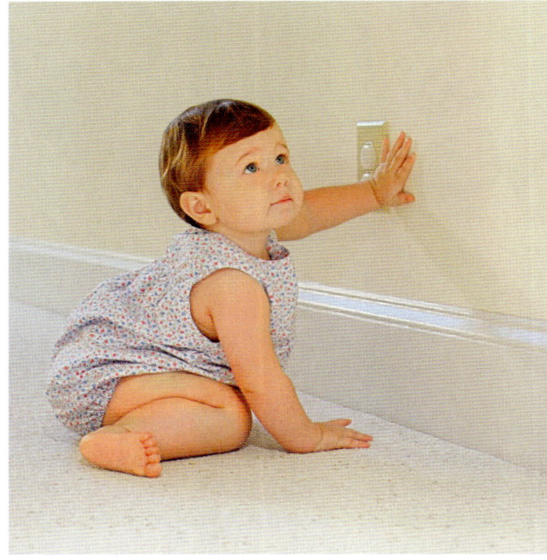

Fig 12.8 Special plastic caps in electrical sockets prevent young fingers from exploring dangerous areas.

Accidental Poisoning

Poison prevention for toddlers is critical. Toddlers are at the highest risk for accidental poisoning because of their innate curiosity and ability to open 'childproof' containers. Because mouthing activity continues to be prevalent after 1 year of age and exploring objects by tasting them is part of children's curious investigation, ingestion is the most common form of exposure (Kostic 2016). Toddlers' curiosity and inability to understand logical consequences further place them at risk for ingesting harmful substances. About 50% of accidental exposures in children involve cosmetics and personal care products, cleaning solutions, plants and foreign bodies, including toys (Kostic 2016). Pharmaceutical agents, such as analgesics, topical preparations, cough and cold products and vitamins, account for most of the other types of ingested agents (Kostic 2016). Although in many instances poisoning does not result in death, it may cause significant morbidity such as oesophageal erosion and stricture from lye ingestion. Toddlers are able to climb most heights, open most drawers or closets and unscrew most lids. By trial and error younger children also manage to undo tops of bottles, plastic containers, aerosol cans and jars, including those with child-resistant lids. Newer forms of drugs such as transdermal patches and cough-suppressant lozenges have created additional dangers because they are not packaged with safety caps and the lozenges look like lollies.

The major reason for poisoning is improper storage (Fig 12.9). The guidelines suggested in Chapter 14 apply to children in this age group as well. However, unlike infants, who are confined to certain heights and unable to unlatch child safety locks, young children manage to find access to many high-level, tight-security places. For this age group only a locked cabinet is safe.

Recent attention has focused on over the counter (OTC) medications used for coughs and colds as a common cause of accidental poisonous ingestion in toddlers. Ingestion of paracetamol is also a common cause of morbidity because it is found in many combination OTC products; caregivers may unknowingly administer a dose of paracetamol in addition to an OTC drug containing the product without knowing the danger.

Nurses and healthcare professionals need to keep up to date with potential toxins readily available to toddlers in society and therefore in the home. Potential poisons such as e-cigarette liquids and other synthetic lifestyle drugs are becoming more prevalent in communities and homes, which in turn make them more accessible to curious and tenacious toddlers.

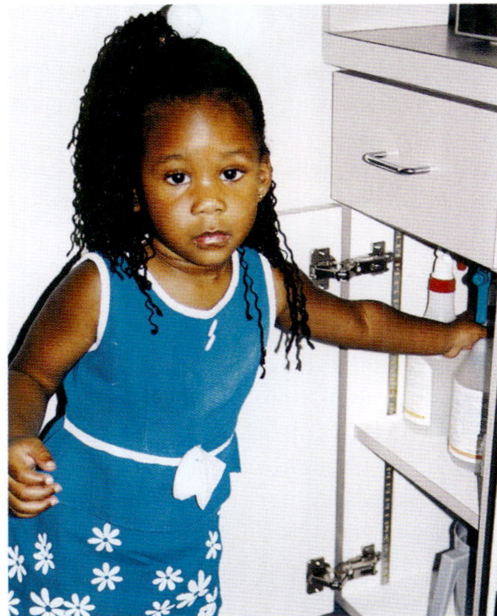

Fig 12.9 Children are most likely to ingest substances that are on their level, such as cleaning agents stored under sinks, rat poison, plants or nappy bin deodoriser.

Emergency and preventive measures for accidental poisoning are further discussed in Chapter 14.

Falls

Falls are still a hazard to children in this age group, although by the later part of early childhood, gross and fine motor skills are well developed, decreasing the incidence of falls down stairs or from chairs. However, playground injuries are common. Children need to learn safety at play areas, such as no horseplay on high slides or jungle gyms, sitting on swings and staying away from moving swings. Prevention includes placement of grass, sand or wood chips under play equipment. Swing seats should be made of plastic, canvas or rubber and have smooth or rounded edges. Slides should have inclines of no more than 30 degrees and have evenly spaced rungs for climbing.

The climbing and running activity of the typical toddler is complicated by total neglect for and lack of appreciation of danger, immature coordination and a high centre of gravity. Falling from furniture is a major cause of injury, with more children in this age group sustaining head injuries than older children. Gates must be placed at both ends of stairs. Accessible windows that are left open during warm weather must be guarded with a rail. Falling from open windows is a major cause of accidental death in urban lower socioeconomic groups; screens are not designed to prevent falls. Doors leading to stairwells or porches must be locked.

Children can fall from highchairs, shopping trolleys, prams, car seats and strollers if not properly restrained or if balance changes when the place where they are sitting is weighed down with heavy objects. Therefore, proper restraint and adequate supervision are essential.

Falls in hospitalised children have received little attention in the scientific literature but are known to occur. In hospital, parents should be shown how to put up and down bedside rails and cot sides and to ensure sides are up if leaving the bedside.

Aspiration and Suffocation

Suffocation deaths usually occur in this age group by choking on food items; other causes include choking on undersized infant pacifiers, small balls and latex balloons (Rivara & Grossman 2016).

Usually by 1 year of age children chew well, but they may have difficulty with large pieces of food, such as meat or whole hot dogs, and with hard foods, such as nuts or dried beans. Small items such as coloured beads, green peas, pellets or beans are often placed into the nose by toddlers and may present a danger if aspirated into the airway. Young children cannot discard pips from fruit or bones from fish as older children can. Lollies that are sealed in plastic wrappers can be difficult to manage, and the plastic wrapper can be aspirated. Therefore, implement the same precautions as discussed for infants regarding food selection. (See Chapter 10.)

Play objects for toddlers must still be chosen with an awareness of the danger of small parts. Large, sturdy toys without sharp edges or removable parts are safest. Coins, paper clips, pull tabs on cans, thumbtacks, nails, screws, jewellery (especially pierced earrings) and all types of pins are common household objects that can cause significant harm if swallowed or aspirated. Because of the danger of aspiration, parents should know emergency procedures for choking.

Suffocation is less frequent from causes seen during infancy but old refrigerators, car trunks, ovens and other large appliances are an ever-present threat. Toddlers can climb inside these appliances and, if they close the door behind them, can become trapped inside. Discarding old appliances and removing all doors during storage can prevent such tragic injuries. Toddlers may also suffocate when toy boxes with heavy, hinged lids accidentally close on their head or neck. Advise parents of this danger and encourage them to buy storage chests with lightweight, removable covers.

Bodily Harm

Toddlers are still clumsy in many of their skills and can seriously harm themselves when walking while holding a sharp or pointed object or having food or objects such as spoons in their mouths. Preventing such occurrences is the best approach with toddlers. Teach the child that when walking with a pointed object, such as a fork, knife or scissors, the pointed end is held away from the face. Dangerous garden or workshop equipment and all firearms should be stored in a locked cabinet. Power lawn mowers are especially dangerous, and young children should not be allowed in an area where a mower is being used, nor should they be taken for a ride on a mower or allowed to operate the device.

Toddlers are often unable to understand that all pets are not as safe as their own; because of toddlers' height, they are often at the eye level of some dogs and may be bitten on the face. It is imperative to teach pet safety to toddlers and keep animals at a safe distance because even the most loving pet may perceive a threat and react accordingly.

Toys can be a source of danger, and safety must be a prime consideration when selecting toys. Most toys have age ranges written on them to designate their safety, but parents should also consider the specific child's readiness.

Strategies for ensuring safety in households with toddlers include the usual precautions recommended for any age group (see Family-Centred Care box). An additional safeguard for young children is the use of safety glass in doors, windows and tabletops and the application of decals on glassed areas to lessen the likelihood of running through glass. Also, children should not be allowed to run, jump, wrestle or play ball in areas where glass litter may be a hazard. (See Injury Prevention, Chapter 13; Animal Bites and Human Bites, Chapter 32.)

Anticipatory Guidance—Care of Families

Understanding toddlers is fundamental to successful childrearing. Nurses, particularly those in ambulatory or child health centres, are in a most favourable position to assist parents in meeting the tasks and needs of children in this age group. Anticipatory guidance in each of the areas presented in the Family-Centred Care box can prevent future problems. Advice is sometimes not the sole answer. Actual assistance, such as being available for telephone consulting, should be a part of the nurse's flexible repertoire of interventions. Whether parents are experiencing the challenges of rearing a first or a subsequent child, they benefit from sharing their feelings, frustrations and satisfactions. They need adult companionship, shared childrearing responsibilities and periodic separation from their children. For single parents such goals can be especially difficult to achieve. Part of a nurse's responsibility is to provide opportunities for parents to express their feelings and to meet their emotional and physical needs.

FAMILY-CENTRED CARE

Guidance During Toddler Years

12 to 18 Months

- Prepare parents for expected behavioural changes of toddler, especially negativism and ritualism.
- Assess present feeding habits and encourage gradual weaning from bottle and increased intake of solid foods.
- Stress expected feeding changes of physiological anorexia, presence of food fads and strong taste preferences, need for scheduled routine at mealtimes, inability to sit through an entire meal and lack of table manners.
- Assess sleep patterns at night, particularly habit of a bedtime bottle, which is a major cause of dental decay, and procrastination behaviours that delay hour of sleep.
- Prepare parents for potential dangers, particularly motor vehicle, poisoning and falling injuries; give appropriate suggestions for childproofing the home.
- Discuss need for firm but gentle discipline and ways to deal with temper tantrums; stress positive benefits of appropriate discipline.
- Emphasise importance for both child and parents of brief, periodic separations.
- Discuss toys that use developing gross and fine motor, language, cognitive and social skills.
- Emphasise need for dental supervision, types of basic dental hygiene at home and food habits that predispose the child to tooth decay; stress importance of supplemental fluoride.

18 to 24 Months

- Stress importance of peer companionship in play.
- Explore need for preparation for additional sibling; stress importance of preparing child for new experiences.
- Discuss present discipline methods, their effectiveness and parents' feelings about child's negativism; stress that negativism is an important aspect of developing self-assertion and independence and is not a sign of spoiling.
- Discuss signs of readiness for toilet training; emphasise importance of waiting for physical and psychological readiness.
- Discuss development of fears, such as fear of darkness or loud noises, and of habits, such as security blanket or thumb sucking; stress normalcy of these transient behaviours.
- Prepare parents for signs of regression in time of stress.
- Assess child's ability to separate easily from parents for brief periods under familiar circumstances.
- Allow parents opportunity to express their feelings of weariness, frustration and exasperation; be aware that it is often difficult to love toddlers at times when they are not asleep!
- Point out some of the expected changes of the next year, such as longer attention span, somewhat less negativism and increased concern for pleasing others.

24 to 36 Months

- Discuss importance of imitation and domestic mimicry and need to include child in activities.
- Discuss approaches towards toilet training, particularly realistic expectations and attitude towards accidents.
- Stress uniqueness of toddlers' thought processes, especially through their use of language, poor understanding of time, causal relationships in terms of proximity of events and inability to see events from another's perspective.
- Stress that discipline still must be structured and concrete and that relying solely on verbal reasoning and explanation leads to confusion, misunderstanding and even injuries.

REFERENCES

Australian Institute of Health and Welfare. (2020). Australia's children. Canberra: AIHW. https://www.aihw.gov.au/reports/children-youth/australias-children/contents/

American Academy of Pediatric Dentistry. (2016). Policy on early childhood caries (ECC): classifications, consequences, and preventive strategies. http://www.aapd.org/assets/1/7/P_ECCClassifications1.PDF

Armfeld, J. M., Chrisopoulos, S., Peres, K. G., et al. (2016). Australian children's oral health behaviours. In: L. G. Do & A. J. Spencer (Eds). Oral health of Australian children: the National Child Oral Health Study 2012–14. Adelaide: University of Adelaide Press.

Australian Department of Health. (2019). Australia's Physical Activity and Sedentary Behaviour Guidelines and the Australian 24-Hour Movement Guidelines. April. http://www.health.gov.au/internet/main/publishing.nsf/content/health-pubhlth-strateg-phys-act-guidelines#npa05.

Barr, R. (2013). Memory constraints on infant learning from picture books, television, and touchscreens. Child Developmental Perspective, 7(4), 205–210.

Brazelton, T. B. (1999). How to help parents of young children: The touchpoints model. Journal of Perinatology, 19(6 Pt. 2), S6–S7.

Do, L. G., Harford, J. E., Ha, D. H., et al. (2016). Australian children's general health behaviours. In: Do, L. G. & Spencer A. J. (Eds). Oral health of Australian children: the National Child Oral Health Study 2012–14. Adelaide, University of Adelaide Press.

Duzinski, S. V., Barczyk, A. N., Wheeler, T. C., et al. (2014). Threat of paediatric hyperthermia in an enclosed vehicle: A year-round study. Injury Prevention: Journal of the International Society for Child and Adolescent Injury Prevention, 20(4), 220–225.

Eisbach, S. S., Cluxton-Keller, F., Harrison, J., et al. (2014). Characteristics of temper tantrums in preschoolers with disruptive behaviour in a clinical setting. Journal of Psychosocial Nursing and Mental Health Services, 52(5), 32–40.

Eisenberg, N., Taylor, Z. E., Widaman, K. F., et al. (2015). Externalizing symptom, effortful control, and intrusive parenting: A test of bidirectional longitudinal relations during early childhood. Development and Psychology, 27(4), 953–968.

El-Radhi, A. S. (2015). Management of common behaviour and mental health problems. British Journal of Nursing, 24(11), 586–590.

Erikson, E. H. (1963). Childhood and society (2nd ed.). New York: Norton.

Estes, K. G., & Hay, J. F. (2015). Flexibility in bilingual infants' word learning. Child Development, 86(5), 1371–1385.

Feigelman, S. (2016). The second year. In R. M. Kliegman, B. F. Stanton, J. W. St Geme, et al. (Eds.), Nelson textbook of pediatrics (20th ed.). Philadelphia: Saunders/Elsevier.

Folger, A., Bowers, K. A., Dexheimer, J. W., et al. (2017). Education of early childhood home visiting to prevent medically attended unintentional injury. Annals of Emergency Medicine, 70(3), 302–310.e1.

Fowler, J. W. (1981). Stages of faith: the psychology of human development and the quest for meaning. San Francisco: Harper & Row.

Guyer, A. E., Jarcho, J. M., Perez-Edgar, K., et al. (2015). Temperament and parenting styles in early childhood differentially influence neural response to peer evaluation in adolescence. Journal of Abnormal Child Psychology, 43(5), 863–875.

Hines, M., Constantinescu, M., & Spencer, D. (2015). Early androgen exposure and human gender development. Biology of Sex Differences, 6, 3.

Kidsafe Australia. (2019). Drowning. https://kidsafe.com.au/wp-content/uploads/2019/03/Drowning-Information-Sheet.pdf

Kimball, V. (2016). The perils and pitfalls of potty training. Pediatric Annals, 45(6), e199–e201.

Kirkorian, H. L., Choi, K., & Pempek, T. A. (2016). Toddlers' word learning from contingent and noncontingent video on touch screens. Child Development, 87(2), 405–413.

Kostic, M. A. (2016). Poisoning. In R. M. Kliegman, B. F. Stanton, J. W. St Geme, et al. (Eds.), Nelson textbook of pediatrics (20th ed.). Philadelphia: Elsevier/Saunders.

Lima, N. N. R., do Nascimento, V. B., de Carvalho, S. M. F., et al. (2013). Spirituality in childhood cancer care. Neuropsychiatic Disease and Treatment, 9, 1539–1544.

Llena, C., Leyda, A., Forner, L., et al. (2015). Association between the number of early carious lesions and diet in children with a high prevalence of caries. European Journal of Paediatric Dentistry, 16(1), 7–12.

Mindell, J. A., Li, A. M., Sadeh, A., et al. (2015). Bedtime routines for young children: A dose-dependent association with sleep outcomes. Sleep, 38(5), 717–722.

Neuman, M. E. (2011). Addressing children's beliefs through Fowler's stages of faith. Journal of Pediatric Nursing, 26(1), 44–50.

NHMRC (National Health and Medical Research Council). (2017). Information paper—water fluoridation: dental and other human health outcomes. Canberra: NHMRC.

Owens, J. A. (2016). Sleep medicine. In R. M. Kliegman, B. F. Stanton, J. W. St Geme, et al. (Eds.), Nelson textbook of pediatrics (20th ed.). Philadelphia: Saunders/Elsevier.

Ozen, B., Van Strijp, A. J., Ozer, L., et al. (2016). Evaluation of possible associated factors for early childhood caries and severe early childhood caries: A multicenter cross-sectional survey. The Journal of Clinical Pediatric Dentistry, 40(2), 118–123.

Rivara, F. P., & Grossman, D. C. (2016). Injury control. In R. M. Kliegman, B. F. Stanton, J. W. St Geme, et al. (Eds.), Nelson textbook of pediatrics (20th ed.). Philadelphia: Elsevier/Saunders.

Rogers, J. (2013). Daytime wetting in children and acquisition of bladder control. Nursing Children and Young People, 25(6), 26–33.

Roseberry, S., Hirsh-Pasek, K., & Golinkoff, R. M. (2014). Skype me: Socially contingent interactions to help toddlers learn. Child Development, 85(3), 956–970.

Saavedra, J. M., Deming, D., Dattilo, A., et al. (2013). Lessons from the feeding infants and toddlers study in North America: What children eat, and implications for obesity prevention. Annals of Nutrition and Metabolism, 62(supp3), 27–36.

Steensma, T. D., Kreukels, B. P., de Vries, A. L., et al. (2013). Gender identity development in adolescence. Hormones and Behaviour, 64(2), 288–297.

Steinberger, J., Daniels, S. R., Hagberg, N., et al. (2016). American Heart Association: Cardiovascular health promotion in children: challenges and opportunities for 2020 and beyond: a scientific statement from the American Heart Association. Circulation, 134, e236–e255.

Stortelder, F. (2014). Varieties of male-sexual identity development in clinical practice: A neuropsychoanalytic model. Frontiers in Psychology, 5, 1512.

Tooth, L., Moss, K., Hockey, R., et al. (2019). Adherence to screen time, recommendations for Australian Children aged 0-12 years. Medical Journal of Australia, 211(4), 181–182.

Zimmer-Gembeck, M. J., Webb, H. J., Thomas, R., et al. (2015). A new measure of toddler-parenting practices and associations with attachment and mothers' sensitivity, competence, and enjoyment of parenting. Early Child Development and Care, 185(9), 1422–1436.

13

Health Promotion of the Preschooler and Family

Emma Collins

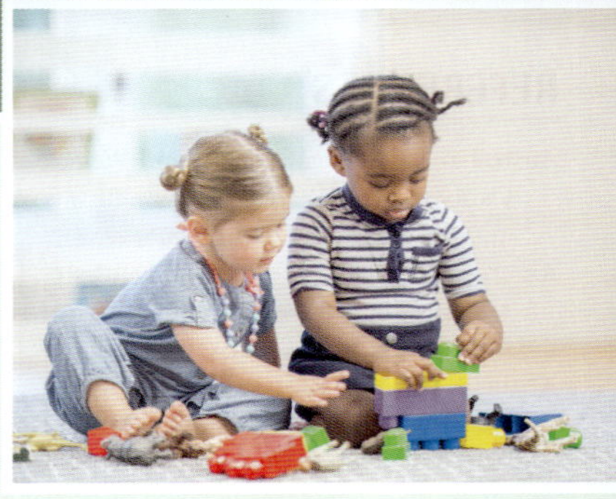

LEARNING OBJECTIVES

- Outline usual growth and development of preschoolers
- Identify challenging areas for the preschooler and parent and opportunities for nurses to support healthy growth and development
- Identify key safety concerns for this age group and preventive actions to take

PROMOTING OPTIMUM GROWTH AND DEVELOPMENT

The combined biological, psychosocial, cognitive, spiritual and social achievements during the preschool period (3 to 5 years of age) prepare preschoolers for their most significant change in lifestyle: entrance into school. Their control of bodily systems, experience of brief and prolonged periods of separation, ability to interact cooperatively with other children and adults, use of language for mental symbolisation and increased attention span and memory prepare them for the next major period: the school years. Successful achievement of previous levels of growth and development is essential for preschoolers to refine many of the tasks that were mastered during the toddler years.

Biological Development

The rate of physical growth slows and stabilises during the preschool years. The average weight is 14.5 kg at 3 years, 16.5 kg at 4 years and 18.5 kg at 5 years. The average weight gain remains approximately 2 to 3 kg per year.

Growth in height also remains steady at a yearly increase of 6.5 to 9 cm. The legs of a preschooler, rather than the trunk, increase in length. The average height is 95 cm at 3 years, 103 cm at 4 years and 110 cm at 5 years.

The preschooler is slender but sturdy, agile and posturally erect. There is little difference in physical characteristics according to sex, except in factors such as dress and hairstyle.

Most organ systems can adjust to moderate stress and change. During this period, most children are toilet trained. For the most part, motor development consists of increases in strength and refinement of previously learned skills, such as walking, running and jumping. However, muscle development and bone growth are still far from mature. Excessive activity and overexertion can injure delicate tissues. Good posture, appropriate exercise and adequate nutrition and rest are essential for optimum development of the musculoskeletal system.

Gross and Fine Motor Behaviour

By 36 months, preschoolers are walking, running, climbing and jumping well. Refinement in eye–hand and muscle coordination is evident in several areas. At age 3 years, the preschooler can ride a balance bike or three-wheeled scooter, walks on tiptoe, balances on one foot for a few seconds and long jumps. By age 4 years, the child skips and hops proficiently on one foot (Fig 13.1) and catches a ball reliably. By age 5 years, the child skips on alternate feet, jumps rope and begins to skate and swim.

Achievement in fine motor development is evident in the child's increasingly skilful manipulation. Drawing shows several advancements in the perception of shape and the development of fine muscle coordination. The 3-year-old child copies a circle and imitates a cross and vertical and horizontal lines. He or she holds the writing instrument with the fingers rather than the fist. The child scribbles or scrawls drawings but can name what has been drawn. The 3 year old is not able to draw a complete stick figure but draws a circle, later adds facial features, and by age 5 or 6 years can draw several parts (head, arms, legs, body and facial features). Between 4 and 5 years of age, the child can trace a cross and copy a square. The triangle and diamond are usually the last geometric figures to be mastered, sometime between ages 5 and 6 years.

As children progress from scribbling to picture making, they advance through four distinguishable stages (Kellogg 1969). In the placement stage, 15-month-old children place their earliest spontaneous scribbling on the paper in a specific placement pattern, such as in the centre, all over, across the lower half or across the page in a diagonal direction (Fig 13.2). Approximately 17 different placement patterns appear by age 2 years and, once developed, are never lost.

By 3 years of age, children are in the shape stage. They draw single-line outline forms such as rectangles, circles, ovals, crosses and other odd shapes. As soon as they draw diagrams, they almost immediately progress to the design stage, in which simple forms are drawn together to make structured designs. When two diagrams are united, the resulting design is called a combine. Three or more united diagrams produce an aggregate. Between ages 4 and 5 years, most children enter the pictorial stage, in which their designs are recognisable as familiar objects. Early pictorial drawings are suggestive of human figures, houses, animals and trees. Later pictorial drawings are more clearly defined and recognisable; they are not representations of the actual object but aesthetically satisfying structures that resemble familiar objects. For example, the initial human figure drawing is a circle with arms attached to the head. It is more an aggregate drawing than any attempt to copy a human figure. Drawings of animals follow the human figure drawing but are only a slight modification, such as attaching ears to the top of the head.

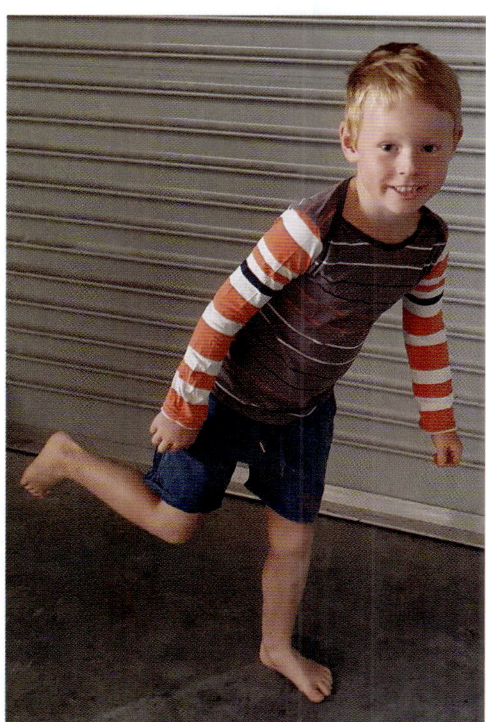

Fig 13.1 A 4-year-old child has sufficient balance to hop on one foot.

Kellogg (1969) suggests that uninhibited scribbling and drawing are necessary for children to learn to read and that children who have been free to experiment and produce abstract forms have developed the mental set required for learning symbolic language. Scribbling and drawing also help develop the fine muscle skills and eye–hand coordination eventually required for making precise letters and numbers.

Drawing is also a tool used for assessing intelligence, personality development and psychosocial adjustment. The precise value of using drawing to measure such concepts is still a nebulous science. However, children (especially school-age children) do reveal thoughts about themselves in their drawings. It is not necessary to have in-depth knowledge of children's drawings to make assumptions about their significance. Being receptive to all the clues, both verbal and non-verbal, is essential to understanding how and what children are communicating to others.

Psychosocial Development

Developing a Sense of Initiative (Erikson)

If preschoolers have mastered the tasks of the toddler period, they are ready to face the developmental challenges of the preschool period. Erikson maintained that the chief psychosocial task of this period is acquiring a sense of initiative. Children are in a stage of energetic learning. They play, work and live to the fullest and feel a real sense of accomplishment and satisfaction in their activities. Conflict arises when children overstep the limits of their ability and inquiry and experience guilt for not having behaved appropriately. Feelings of guilt, anxiety and fear may also result from thoughts that differ from expected behaviour.

A particularly stressful thought is wishing one's parent dead. As a sense of rivalry or competition develops between the child and the same-sex parent, the child may think of ways to get rid of the interfering parent. In most situations, this contest is resolved when the child strongly identifies with the same-sex parent and peers during the school years. However, if that parent dies before the identification process is completed, the preschooler can be overwhelmed with guilt for having wished and therefore 'caused' the death. Clarifying for children that wishes cannot make events occur is essential in helping them overcome their guilt and anxiety.

Development of the **superego**, or conscience, starts towards the end of the toddler years and is a major task for preschoolers. Learning right from wrong and good from bad is the beginning of morality. Children in this age group are generally unable to understand why something is acceptable or unacceptable. They are aware of appropriate behaviour primarily through punishment or reward and rely almost completely on parental principles for developing their own moral judgment. Verbal enforcement of limits is much more effective in this age group than with toddlers. For example, to prevent injuries, parents need to supervise toddlers, keep them contained within protected areas and tell them not to run into the street. The preschooler still needs close supervision but is much more aware of danger and can listen and obey in most instances. If allowed to disagree and question, they will develop socially acceptable behaviour and independence in thought and action.

Oedipal Stage (Freud)

As soon as children comprehend their separateness as persons, they begin to realise that there are categories of objects, such as things, people, males, females, children and adults. One of the principal goals in further differentiation of oneself from others is learning sex differences and sexually appropriate behaviour.

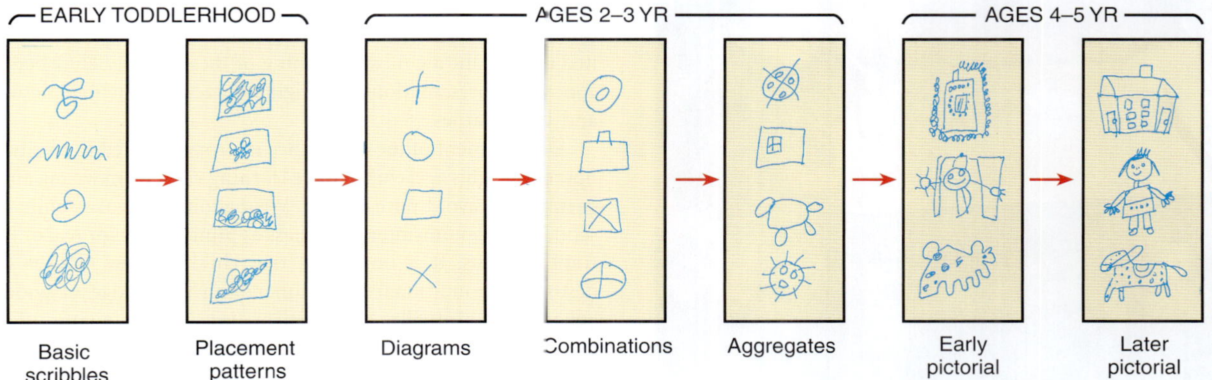

Fig 13.2 Sequential development in self-taught art. (Source: Kellogg, R. (1969). Understanding children's art. In Readings in psychology today. Del Mar, CA: Communications/Research/Machines.)

Cognitive Development

One of the tasks related to the preschool period is readiness for school and scholastic learning. Many of the thought processes of this period are crucial for achieving such readiness, and it is intentional that the child begins school between ages 5 and 6 years, rather than earlier.

Preoperational Phase (Piaget)

Piaget's cognitive theory does not include a period specifically for children 3 to 5 years old. The preoperational phase covers the age span from 2 to 7 years and is divided into two stages: the preconceptual phase, ages 2 to 4 years, and the phase of intuitive thought, ages 4 to 7 years. One of the main transitions during these two phases is the shift from totally egocentric thought to social awareness and the ability to consider other viewpoints (Fig 13.3). Egocentricity, however, is still evident. Children are able to think and verbalise their mental processes without having to act out their thinking. They can think of only one idea at a time and are unable to think of all parts in terms of the whole.

Language continues to develop during the preschool period. Speech remains primarily a vehicle of egocentric communication. Preschoolers assume that everyone thinks as they do and that a brief explanation of their thinking makes them understood by others. Because of this self-referenced, egocentric verbal communication, it is often necessary to explore and understand young children's thinking through other, non-verbal approaches. For children in this age group, the most enlightening and effective method is play, which becomes the child's way of understanding, adjusting to and working out life's experiences. Because of a child's rich imagination and unlimited ability to invent and imitate, all types of play hold therapeutic and communicative value.

Preschoolers increasingly use language without comprehending the meaning of words, particularly concepts of right and left, causality and time. Children may use the concepts correctly but only in the circumstances in which they have learned them. For example, they may know how to put on shoes by remembering that the buckle is always on the outside of the foot. However, if different shoes have no buckles, they cannot reason which shoe fits which foot. They do not understand the concept of right and left.

Superficially, causality resembles logical thought. Preschoolers explain a concept as they have heard it described by others, but their understanding is limited. For example, because preschoolers do not completely understand time, they interpret it according to their own frame of reference, such as 'A long time means until Christmas'.

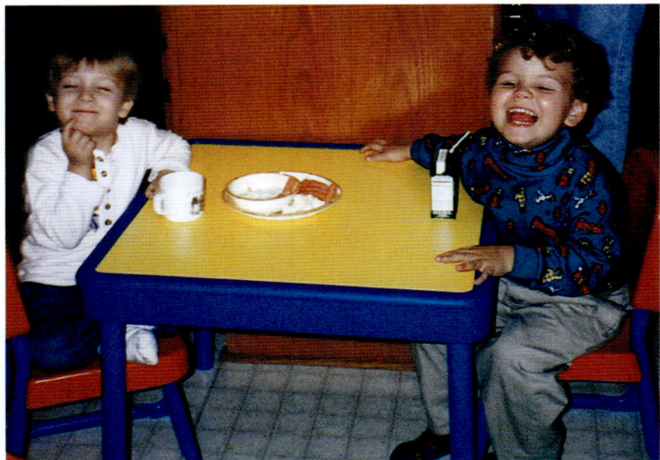

Fig 13.3 Preschool children enjoy friends and often use non-verbal messages to communicate.

Consequently, time is best explained in relation to an event, such as 'Your mother will visit you after you finish your lunch'. Avoiding words such as 'yesterday', 'tomorrow', 'next week' or 'Tuesday' to express when an event is expected to occur and associating time with usual expected daily occurrences help children learn about temporal relationships while increasing their trust in others' predictions.

Preschoolers' thinking is often described as **magical thinking**. Because of their egocentrism and transductive reasoning, they believe that thoughts are all-powerful. Such thinking places them in the vulnerable position of feeling guilty and responsible for bad thoughts that may coincide with the occurrence of a wished event. A typical example is wishing a new sibling dead. If that sibling does die, young children think their wish caused the death. Their inability to reason the cause and effect of illness or injury makes it especially difficult for them to understand such events.

Preschoolers believe in the power of words and accept their meaning literally. A significant example of this type of thinking is calling children 'bad' because they did something wrong. In their minds, telling children that they are bad means that they are bad. For this reason, it is better to relate such words to the act by saying, for example, 'That was a bad thing to do'.

Moral Development (Kohlberg)

Moral development theory is based on cognitive development theory and consists of three major levels: preconventional, conventional and postconventional (Kohlberg 1968). Young children's development of moral judgment is at the most basic level. They have little, if any, concern for why something is wrong. They behave because of the freedoms or restrictions placed on actions. In the punishment and obedience orientation, children (approximately ages 2 to 4 years) judge whether an action is good or bad according to whether it results in reward or punishment. If children are punished for it, the action is bad. If they are not punished, the action is good, regardless of its meaning. For example, if parents allow hitting, the child will perceive that hitting is good because it is not associated with punishment.

From approximately 4 to 7 years of age, children are in the stage of naive **instrumental orientation**, in which actions are directed towards satisfying their needs and, less commonly, the needs of others. They have a concrete sense of justice and fairness during this period of development.

Spiritual Development

Children learn about faith and religion from significant others in their environment, usually from parents and their religious beliefs and practices. However, cognitive level influences young children's understanding of spirituality. Preschoolers have a concrete conception of a god with physical characteristics, often like an imaginary friend. They understand simple stories and memorise short prayers, but have limited understanding of the meaning of these rituals. They benefit from concrete representations of religious practices, such as picture books and small statues.

Development of the conscience is strongly linked to spiritual development. At this age, children are learning right from wrong and behave correctly to avoid punishment. Wrongdoing provokes guilt, and preschoolers often misinterpret illness as punishment for real or imagined transgressions. It is important that children view God as one who bestows unconditional love, rather than as a judge of good or bad behaviour. Spirituality and participation in religious traditions often help children cope during illness and hospitalisation (Drutchas & Anandarajah 2014). Therefore, it is important to address children's spiritual needs to provide the most comprehensive care, especially during times of distress.

Development of Body Image

The preschool years play a significant role in the development of body image. With increasing comprehension of language, preschoolers recognise that individuals have undesirable and desirable appearances. They recognise differences in skin colour and racial identity and are vulnerable to learning prejudices and biases. They are aware of the meaning of words such as 'pretty' or 'ugly', and they reflect the opinions of others regarding their own appearance. By 5 years of age, children compare their size with that of their peers and can become conscious of being large or short, especially if others refer to them as 'so big' or 'so little' for their age. Research indicates that children as young as preschool age experience body dissatisfaction (Tatangelo et al 2016). Because these are formative years, parents should make efforts to instil positive principles regarding body image.

The role families have in developing positive body image is not to be underestimated. Many parents believe that preschoolers are too young to have an awareness of body image, despite research to the contrary, yet agree that body size and shape has an impact on self-esteem of the child (Liechty et al 2016).

Despite the advances in body image development, preschoolers have poorly defined body boundaries and little knowledge of their internal anatomy. Intrusive experiences are frightening, especially those that disrupt the integrity of the skin (e.g. injections and surgery). They fear that all their blood and 'insides' can leak out if the skin is 'broken'. Therefore preschoolers may believe it is critical to use bandages after an injury.

Development of Sexuality

Sexual development during the preschool years is important to a person's overall sexual identity and beliefs. Preschoolers form strong attachments to the opposite-sex parent, while identifying with the same-sex parent. **Sex typing**, or the process by which an individual develops the behaviour, personality, attitudes and beliefs appropriate for his or her culture and sex, occurs through several mechanisms during this period. Probably the most powerful mechanisms are child-rearing practices and imitation. The ways in which parents dress, hold, cuddle, caress, discipline and talk to their child express some aspect of gender-oriented behaviour. Gender identification is a result of complex prenatal and postnatal psychological factors, as well as biological, social and genetic influences. It is believed that most children are aware of their sex and the expected set of related behaviours by 1½ to 2½ years of age. Although toddlers might be aware of their particular sex, they do not possess the language and cognitive skills to investigate sexual identity as fully as preschoolers do.

As sexual identity develops beyond gender recognition, modesty and fears of mutilation may become a concern. Sex-role imitation and 'dressing up' like Mummy or Daddy are important activities. Attitudes and responses of others to role-playing can condition the child to adopt particular views of self or others. For example, comments such as 'Boys shouldn't play with dolls' can influence a boy's masculine self-concept.

Sexual exploration may be more pronounced now, particularly in terms of exploring and manipulating the genitalia. Preschoolers may have questions about sexual reproduction as they search for understanding. (See Sex Education, p. 317, and also Chapters 15 and 17.)

Social Development

During the preschool period, the separation-individuation process is completed. Preschoolers have overcome much of their anxiety associated with strangers and the fear of separation of earlier years. They relate to unfamiliar people easily and tolerate brief separations from parents with little or no protest. However, they still need parental security, reassurance, guidance and approval, especially when entering early childhood education or primary school. Prolonged separation, such as that imposed by illness and hospitalisation, is difficult; however, preschoolers respond well to anticipatory preparation and concrete explanation. They can cope with changes in daily routine much better than toddlers but may develop more imaginary fears. They gain security and comfort from familiar objects such as toys, dolls or photographs of family members. They are able to work through many of their unresolved fears, fantasies and anxieties through play, especially if guided with appropriate play objects (e.g. dolls or puppets) that represent family members, health professionals and other children.

Language

Language becomes more sophisticated and complex during the preschool years. Both cognitive ability and environment, particularly consistent role models, influence vocabulary, speech and comprehension. Language becomes a major mode of communication and social interaction. Vocabulary increases dramatically, from 300 words at age 2 years to more than 2100 words at the end of age 5 years. Sentence structure, grammatical usage and intelligibility also advance to a more adult level. Preschool children may even become bilingual (see Cultural Considerations box).

> **CULTURAL CONSIDERATIONS**
>
> **Bilingual Children**
>
> Some children in Australia and New Zealand are bilingual. Children who learn two languages simultaneously or develop bilingualism in early childhood reach language milestones at similar stages to monolinguals (McCabe et al 2013). The type, quantity and quality of language input determines successful acquisition of each language (McCabe et al 2013). If a child has a language disability, it will manifest in both languages (American Speech-Language-Hearing Association 2017a). Nurses should inquire about each child's language repertoire and identify the child's primary language, especially when assessing a child's development.

Children between ages 3 and 4 years form sentences of approximately three or four words and include only the words most essential to convey meaning. Such speech is often termed *telegraphic* because of its brevity. Three-year-old children ask many questions and use plurals, correct pronouns and the past tenses of verbs. They name familiar objects (such as animals and parts of the body), relatives and friends. They can give and follow simple commands. They talk incessantly, regardless of whether anyone is listening to or answering them. They enjoy musical or talking toys or dolls and imitate new words proficiently.

From ages 4 to 5 years, preschoolers use longer sentences of four or five words and use more words to convey a message, such as prepositions, adjectives and a variety of verbs. They follow simple directional commands, such as 'Put the ball on the chair', but can carry out only one request at a time. They answer questions such as 'What do you do when you are hungry?' by describing the appropriate action. The pattern of asking questions is at its peak, and children usually repeat the question until they receive an answer.

By age 6 years, children can use all parts of speech correctly, except for deviations from the rule. They can define simple objects and actions by describing their use, shape or general category of classification, rather than simply describing their outward appearance. For example, they can define a ball as 'round, something you bounce or a toy', rather than only describing its colour. They can give some examples of opposites, such as 'If Mummy is a woman, Daddy is a man'. They can also describe an object according to its composition, such as 'A spoon is made of metal'.

Personal-social Behaviour

The pervasive ritualism and negativism of toddlerhood gradually diminish during the preschool years. Although self-assertion is still a major theme, preschoolers demonstrate their sense of autonomy differently. They are able to verbalise their request for independence and perform independently because of their much-refined physical and cognitive development. By 4 or 5 years of age, they need little if any assistance with dressing, eating or toileting (Fig 13.4). They can also be trusted to obey warnings of danger, although 3- or 4-year-old children may exceed their boundaries at times.

Preschoolers are much more sociable and willing to please than toddlers. They have internalised many of the standards and values of the family and culture. However, by the end of early childhood, they begin to question parental values and compare them with those of their peer group and other authority figures. As a result, they may be less willing to abide by the family's code of conduct. Preschoolers become increasingly aware of their position and role within the family. Although this is a more secure age for experiencing the addition of another sibling, relinquishing the position of first or youngest is still difficult and requires appropriate preparation.

Play

Various types of play are typical of this period, but preschoolers especially enjoy associative play, group play in similar or identical activities but without rigid organisation or rules. Play should provide for physical, social and mental development (Table 13.1).

Play activities for physical growth and the refinement of motor skills include jumping, running and climbing. Tricycles, wagons, gym and sports equipment, sandpits and wading pools can help develop muscles and coordination. Activities such as swimming, bike riding and obstacle courses teach safety and can also help develop muscles and coordination.

Manipulative, constructive, creative and educational toys provide for quiet activities, fine motor development and self-expression. Easy construction sets, large blocks of various sizes and shapes, a counting frame, alphabet or number flash cards, paints, crayons, simple carpentry tools, musical toys, illustrated books, simple sewing or handicraft sets, large puzzles and clay are suitable toys (Fig 13.5). Electronic games and computer programs can also be valuable in helping children learn basic skills, such as letters and simple words. Although their attention span is still short, preschoolers are beginning to enjoy crafts, especially with the guidance and assistance of adults. A helpful rule in planning creative activities is one simple project per year of age. For example, a 3-year-old child usually has the patience to decorate three eggs but will become bored and restless with more.

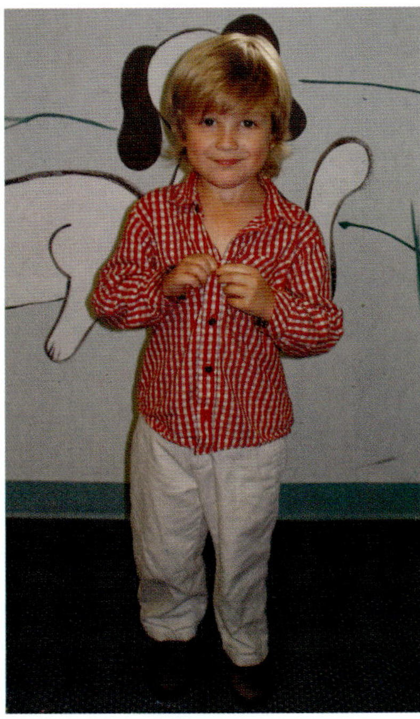

Fig 13.4 Most preschoolers are able to dress themselves but need help with more difficult items of clothing.

Probably the most characteristic and pervasive preschooler activity is imitative, imaginative and dramatic play. Dress-up clothes, dolls, tea sets, dollhouses, telephones, farm animals and equipment, village sets, trains, trucks, cars, planes, hand puppets and medical kits provide hours of self-expression (Fig 13.6). Probably more than any other age group, 4- and 5-year-old children are absorbed in the reproduction of the behaviour of significant adults. Towards the end of the preschool period, children are less satisfied with make-believe or pretend objects and enjoy actually doing the activity, such as cooking and carpentry.

Play is so much a part of the young child's life that reality and fantasy become blurred. The make-believe is reality during play and becomes fantasy only when toys are put away or dress-up clothes are removed. It is no wonder that imaginary playmates are so much a part of this age period. Imaginary companions usually appear between ages 2½ and 3 years and, for the most part, last until the child enters school.

Imaginary companions serve many purposes; they become friends in times of loneliness, they accomplish what the child is still attempting and they experience what the child wants to forget or remember. It is not unusual for the 'friend' to have a myriad of vices and to be blamed for wrongdoing. Sometimes the child hopes to escape punishment by saying, 'My friend Brian broke the glass'. At other times the preschooler may fantasise that the 'companion' misbehaved and play the role of parent. This becomes a way of assuming control and authority in a safe situation.

Parents often worry about their child having imaginary playmates, not realising how normal and useful they are. Parents should be reassured that the child's fantasy is a sign of health that helps differentiate between make-believe and reality. Parents can acknowledge the presence of the imaginary companion by calling him or her by name and even agreeing to simple requests such as setting an extra place at the table, but they should not allow the child to use the playmate to avoid punishment or responsibility. For example, if the child blames the companion for messing up a room, the parents need to clearly state that the child is the only person they see, and therefore the child is responsible for cleaning up.

Children also benefit from play that occurs between them and a parent. Mutual play fosters development from birth through the school years and provides enriched opportunities for learning. Through mutual play, parents can provide tactile and kinaesthetic experiences, can maximise verbal and language abilities and can offer praise and encouragement for exploration of the world. Additionally, mutual play encourages positive interactions between the parent and child, strengthening their relationship. Recommendations for mutual play should reflect the child's developmental level and can incorporate readily available items found in the home or community (e.g. musical CDs, puppets, games and puzzles).

Screen Time

Television programs and other forms of electronic media also have their place in children's play, although each should be only one part of the total repertoire of social and recreational activities. Australian Department of Health (2019) recommend that screen time should be

TABLE 13.1 Growth and Development During Preschool Years

Physical	Gross Motor	Fine Motor	Language	Socialisation	Cognition	Family Relationships
AGE 3 YEARS						
Usual weight gain of 1.8–2.7 kg Average weight of 14.5 kg Usual gain in height of 7.5 cm per year Average height of 95 cm May have achieved night-time control of bowel and bladder	Rides tricycle, balance bike or three-wheeled scooter Jumps off bottom step Stands on one foot for a few seconds Goes up stairs using alternate feet; may still come down using both feet on step Long jumps May try to dance, but balance may not be adequate	Builds tower of 9–10 cubes Builds bridge with three cubes Adeptly places small pellets in narrow-necked bottle In drawing, copies circle, imitates cross, names what has been drawn; cannot draw stick figure but may make circle with facial features	Has vocabulary of about 900 words Uses primarily 'telegraphic' speech Uses complete sentences of three or four words Talks incessantly regardless of whether anyone is paying attention Repeats sentence of six syllables Asks many questions	Dresses self almost completely if helped with back buttons and told which shoe is right or left Pulls on shoes Has increased attention span Feeds self completely Can prepare simple meals, such as cold cereal and milk Can help set table; can dry dishes without breaking any May have fears, especially of dark and going to bed Knows own gender and gender of others Play is parallel and associative; begins to learn simple games, but ofton follows own rules; begins to share	Is in preconceptual phase Is egocentric in thought and behaviour Has beginning understanding of time; uses many time-oriented expressions, talks about past and future as much as about present, pretends to tell time Has improved concept of space, as demonstrated by understanding of prepositions and ability to follow directional command Has beginning ability to view concepts from another perspective	Attempts to please parents and conform to their expectations Is less jealous of younger sibling; may be opportune time for birth of additional sibling Is aware of family relationships and sex-role functions Boys tend to identify more with father or other male figure Has increased ability to separate easily and comfortably from parents for short periods
AGE 4 YEARS						
Pulse and respiration rates decrease slightly Growth rate is similar to that of previous year Average weight of 16.5 kg Average height of 103 cm Length at birth is doubled Maximum potential for development of amblyopia	Skips and hops on one foot Catches ball reliably Throws ball overhead Walks downstairs using alternate footing	Uses scissors successfully to cut out picture following outline Can lace shoes but may not be able to tie bow In drawing, copies square, traces cross and diamond, adds three parts to stick figure	Has vocabulary of 1500 words or more Uses sentences of four or five words Questioning is at peak Tells exaggerated stories Knows simple songs May be mildly profane if associates with older children Obeys prepositional phrases, such as 'under', 'on top of', 'beside', 'behind' or 'in front of' Names one or more colours Comprehends analogies, such as 'If ice is cold, fire is ___'	Very independent Tends to be selfish and impatient Aggressive physically as well as verbally Takes pride in accomplishments Has mood swings Shows off dramatically, enjoys entertaining others Tells family tales to others with no restraint Still has many fears Play is associative Imaginary playmates common Uses dramatic, imaginative and imitative devices Sexual exploration and curiosity demonstrated through play, such as being 'doctor' or 'nurse'	Is in phase of intuitive thought Causality is still related to proximity of events Understands time better, especially in terms of sequence of daily events Unable to conserve matter Judges everything according to one dimension, such as height, width or order Immediate perceptual clues dominate judgment Is beginning to develop less egocentrism and more social awareness May count correctly but has poor mathematic concept of numbers Obeys because parents have set limits, not because of understanding of right or wrong	Rebels if parents expect too much, such as impeccable table manners Takes aggression and frustration out on parents or siblings Do's and don'ts become important May have rivalry with older or younger siblings; may resent older sibling's privileges and younger sibling's invasion of privacy and possessions May 'run away' from home Identifies strongly with parent of opposite sex Is able to run simple errands outside the home

Continued

TABLE 13.1 **Growth and Development During Preschool Years—cont'd**

Physical	Gross Motor	Fine Motor	Language	Socialisation	Cognition	Family Relationships
AGE 5 YEARS						
Pulse and respiration rates decrease slightly Average weight of 18.5 kg Average height of 110 cm Eruption of permanent dentition may begin Handedness is established (about 90% are right-handed)	Skips and hops on alternate feet Throws and catches ball well Jumps rope Skates with good balance Walks backwards with heel to toe Jumps from height of 12 inches and lands on toes Balances on alternate feet with eyes closed	Ties shoelaces Uses scissors, simple tools or pencil well In drawing, copies diamond and triangle; adds seven to nine parts to stick figure; prints a few letters, numbers or words, such as first name	Has vocabulary of about 2100 words Uses sentences of six to eight words, with all parts of speech Names four or more colours Describes drawing or pictures with much comment and enumeration Knows names of days of week, months and other time-associated words Knows composition of articles, such as 'A shoe is made of ____' Can follow three commands in succession	Less rebellious and quarrelsome than at age 4 years More settled and eager to get down to business Not as open and accessible in thoughts and behaviour as in earlier years Independent but trustworthy, not fool-hardy; more responsible Has fewer fears; relies on outer authority to control world Eager to do things right and to please; tries to 'live by the rules' Has better manners Cares for self totally, occasionally needing supervision in dress or hygiene Not ready for concentrated close work or small print because of slight farsightedness and still unrefined eye-hand coordination Play is associative; tries to follow rules but may cheat to avoid losing	Begins to question what parents think by comparing them with age-mates and other adults May notice prejudice and bias in outside world Is more able to view other's perspective, but tolerates differences rather than understanding them May begin to show understanding of conservation of numbers through counting objects regardless of arrangement Uses time-oriented words with increased understanding Cautious about factual information regarding world	Gets along well with parents May seek out parent more often than at age 4 years for reassurance and security, especially when entering school Begins to question parents' thinking and principles Strongly identifies with parent of same sex, especially boys with their fathers Enjoys activities such as sports, cooking and shopping with parent of same sex

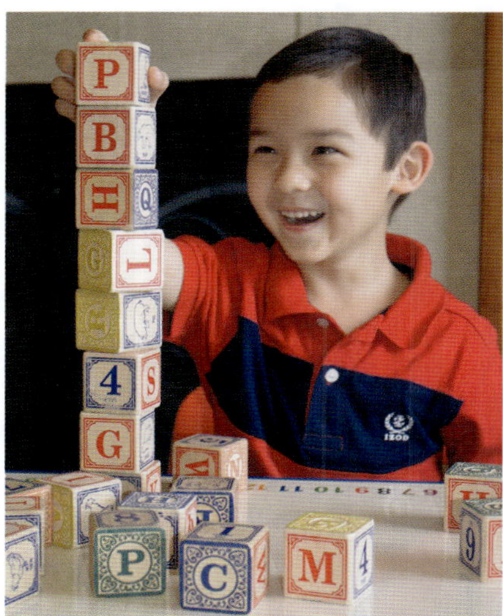

Fig 13.5 Preschoolers enjoy a sense of accomplishment from activities such as stacking blocks.

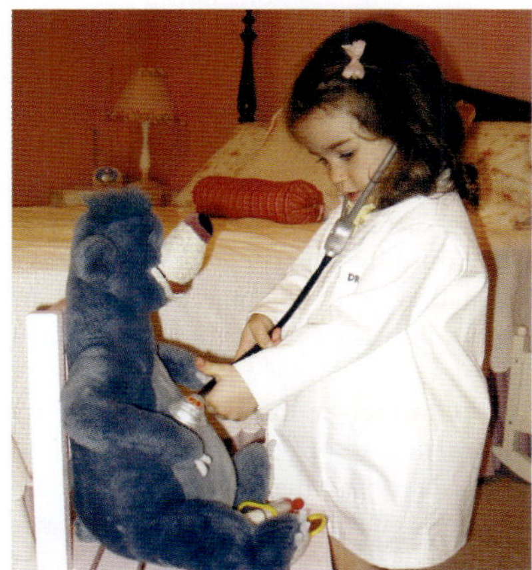

Fig 13.6 Imaginative and imitative play is typical of preschoolers.

limited to one hour per day. Parents and other caregivers should supervise the selection of programs and applications, co-view and discuss programs with their children, co-play games and applications, limit media exposure and set a good example of media use (Tooth et al 2019, Stewart 2019). Children enjoy and learn from educational programs and applications; however, television viewing and other media exposure limit time spent in other meaningful activities such as reading, physical activity and socialisation (Tooth et al 2019). Television viewing and digital play can become an interactive activity when adults participate in these activities with children and discuss the content.

Temperament

Temperament influences children's social development and interactions. Because temperamental characteristics tend to remain stable, the same considerations in terms of childrearing apply during the preschool years. One major concern in the preschool age group is the effect of temperament on adjustment in group situations, especially school, and the long-term consequences of temperamental characteristics. In particular, the degree of adaptability to new situations, intensity of response, distractibility, amount of persistence, mood and activity level influence a child's chances for success in school. Consequently, parents can benefit from suggestions that can promote preschoolers' adjustment. For example, children who are slow to warm up need gradual introduction to new situations and may benefit from the parent's presence until they have settled in. Children with high activity levels tend to adjust better to environments that allow freedom of movement, rather than a structured or regimented classroom. The more aware parents are of their children's unique behaviours, the better they are able to inform teachers or other caregivers of the children's needs and successful approaches to handling the youngsters. In New Zealand, The Strengths and Difficulties Questionnaire is a brief behavioural and emotional screening questionnaire used widely with Well Child providers and other health professionals. It is designed to highlight to the health professional whether or not the parent has any concerns regarding the child's behaviour and emotional status, which could prompt the health professional to investigate concerns further. It is a validated tool that is widely used (Stone et al 2015).

Table 13.1 summarises the major developmental achievements for children 3, 4 and 5 years old.

Coping with Concerns Related to Normal Growth and Development

Preschool and Kindergarten Experience

Many children attend some type of early childhood program, usually kindergarten, home-based care, preschool or a day care centre. Group care has become commonplace with the large number of parents currently employed outside the home. The effects of early education and stimulation on children have increasingly gained recognition. Because social development widens to include age-mates and other significant adults, preschool provides an excellent vehicle for expanding children's experiences with others.

One of the issues that parents face is the child's readiness for early childhood education. School readiness is influenced by a myriad of elements, including: a child's social, emotional and physical development; health status; ability and desire to learn; life experiences; family environment; and parental support. There are no absolute indicators for school readiness. The child's social maturation, especially attention span, is as important as academic readiness.

Nurses can help parents assess a child's readiness in terms of age, physical ability and cognitive and social development (see Table 13.1). For example, a group experience may be difficult for young children with short attention spans. These children may require a different type of experience with more individualised attention.

Sex Education

Preschoolers have assimilated a tremendous amount of information during their short lifetimes. Although their thinking may not be mature, they search constantly for explanations and reasons that are logical and reasonable to them. The word 'why' seems to supplant the word 'no', which was common in toddlerhood. It is only natural that as they learn about 'me', they will also want to know 'why me' and 'how me'. Questions such as 'Where do babies come from?' are as casual as 'Why is the sky blue?', 'What makes it rain?' or 'Who is that?' It is the way in which adults answer questions about procreation that conditions children, even the youngest, to separate these questions from others about their world. If adults answer these questions honestly and as matter-of-factly as any other inquiry, children will feel comfortable asking questions as they explore their bodies and world. If they are answered with a 'tall tale' or an anxious 'You are too young to know about that', children will learn to keep such questions to themselves. Unfortunately, as they harbour these silent mysteries, they formulate their own theories to explain birth. Because magical thinking need not be based on logic or fact, any fantastic and often terrifying explanation can substitute for the truth.

Two rules govern answering sensitive questions about topics such as sex. The first is to find out what children know and think. While investigating the theories children have produced as reasonable explanations, parents can give correct information and also help children understand why their explanations are inaccurate. Another reason for ascertaining what the child thinks before offering any information is to avoid giving an 'unasked for' answer. For example, 4-year-old Lauren asked her father, 'Where did I come from?' Both parents quickly took this inquiry as a clue for offering sex education. After the explanation, Lauren exclaimed, 'I don't know about all that! All I know is Mary came from Auckland, and I want to know where I came from'.

The second rule for giving information is to be honest. True, the preschooler will forget or misunderstand much of the correct information, but the correct information can be restated until the child absorbs and comprehends the facts. Even though the correct anatomical words may be hard to pronounce or difficult to remember, they become important for explaining other concepts later on. Nurses have the opportunity to contribute to early sex education by conveying accurate information regarding genital terms during physical examinations.

When a child does not ask questions, parents and health professionals should take advantage of natural opportunities to discuss reproduction, such as talking about someone who is pregnant or discussing a television program or movie about biological aspects. Many excellent books on sex education are available for preschool children at public libraries and child health centres.

Regardless of whether children are given sex education, they will engage in games of sexual curiosity and exploration. At approximately 3 years of age, children are aware of the anatomical differences between the sexes and are concerned with how the other 'works'. This is not really 'sexual' curiosity because many children are still unaware of the reproductive function of the genitalia. They are curious about the eliminative function of the anatomy. Little boys wonder how girls can urinate without a penis, so they watch girls go to the bathroom. Because they cannot see anything but the stream of urine coming out, they want to observe further. 'Doctor play' is often a game invented for such investigation. Little girls are no less curious about boys' anatomy. They find it intriguing to inspect this 'thing' that girls do not have.

Parents often wonder how to handle such sexual curiosity. A positive approach is to neither condone nor condemn the behaviour, but to tell the children that, if they have questions, they should ask the parents; the parents should then encourage the children to engage in some other activity. In this way, children understand that they can satisfy their sexual curiosity in ways other than playing investigative games. This in no way condemns the act but stresses alternative methods by which to seek solutions and answers. Allowing children unrestricted permissiveness only intensifies their anxiety and concern because exploring and searching usually yield little evidence to satisfy their curiosity.

Another concern for some parents is masturbation, or self-stimulation of the genitalia. This occurs at any age for a variety of reasons and, if not excessive, is normal and healthy. For preschoolers, it is part of sexual curiosity and exploration. If parents are concerned about their child masturbating, it is essential for nurses to investigate the circumstances associated with the activity. Masturbation can be an expression of anxiety, boredom or stress. In the case of excessive masturbation, it may be associated with emotional or behavioural problems and physical or sexual abuse (Strachan & Staples 2012). Management of normal childhood masturbation includes parent education and reassurance, redirection of the child to other activities and discussion with the child regarding appropriate boundaries (Strachan & Staples 2012). In addition, parents should emphasise that masturbation is a private act, thus teaching children socially acceptable behaviour.

Aggression

The term **aggression** refers to behaviour that attempts to hurt a person or destroy property. Aggression differs from anger, which is a temporary emotional state, but anger may be expressed through aggression. Hyperaggressive behaviour in preschoolers is characterised by unprovoked physical attacks on other children and adults, destruction of others' property, frequent intense temper tantrums, extreme impulsivity, disrespect and non-compliance.

A complex set of biological, sociocultural and familial variables influence aggression. Research indicates that types of aggression differ between genders. Boys exhibit more physical aggression than girls during preschool years (Lussier et al 2012). Relational aggression is exhibited at similar rates in boys and girls of this age group; however, differences in the frequency of relational aggression among genders can vary depending on peer interactions in various situations and settings (McEachern & Snyder 2012). Sociocultural factors that are associated with childhood aggression include exposure to community violence (Fleckman et al 2016) and violence in the media (Fitzpatrick et al 2012). Familial variables such as maternal depression, low level of maternal education and low socioeconomic status contribute to childhood aggression (Provençal et al 2015). Family conflict, hostile parenting, low levels of positive interactions and parental warmth, physical and verbal abuse and punitive interactions also contribute to childhood aggression (Jia et al 2016). Other factors that tend to increase aggressive behaviour are frustration, modelling and reinforcement.

Frustration, or the continual thwarting of self-satisfaction by parental disapproval, humiliation, punishment and insults, can lead children to act out against others as a means of release. These children displace their anger on others, particularly peers and other authority figures, especially if they fear their parents. This type of aggression often applies to the child who is well behaved at home but a discipline problem at school or a bully among playmates.

Modelling, or imitating the behaviour of significant others, is a powerful influencing force in preschoolers. Children who are exposed to family violence are observing behaviour that they perceive as acceptable and therefore may exhibit aggressive behaviour with others (Liu 2013). Also, early harsh discipline may lead to aggressive behaviour (Jia et al 2016). Another aspect of modelling is establishing a double-standard for acceptable conduct. For example, in some families aggression is synonymous with masculinity, and boys are encouraged to defend themselves. Although defending one's rights is to be encouraged for both sexes, at times the principle of 'being tough' or 'standing up for yourself' is not tempered with judgment, fairness or equality but becomes an excuse for ruling and dominating others. Such permissive aggression can produce extreme anxiety in children because it makes them feel out of control, even though outwardly they may appear to be the 'boss' or 'bully'.

Another significant source for modelling is media exposure. Numerous studies have found a positive correlation between viewing violent programs and developing aggression; therefore, parents need encouragement to supervise programming, especially for children with aggressive tendencies (Fitzpatrick et al 2012). The Ministry of Health in NZ recommends less than one hour a day of screen time for children aged 2 to 5 years (Stewart et al 2019).

Reinforcement can also shape aggressive behaviour and is closely associated with modelling 'masculine' behaviour. Sometimes the reward for aggressive behaviour is negative (e.g. punishment or disapproval) yet reinforcing because it brings attention. For example, children who are ignored by their parents until they hit a sibling learn that this act attracts attention. Additionally, parents who permit aggressive behaviour by not interfering communicate silent, implicit approval of such acts.

One of the tasks of preschoolers is learning socially acceptable behaviour and the ability to control aggression and redirect their anger. Parents can help children by modelling the appropriate behaviour and encouraging children to express themselves verbally. For example, rather than condoning the hitting of another child for taking a toy, parents can suggest that the child state how he or she feels, such as 'I get angry when you take my ball. Please give it back'.

Children should not be made to feel guilty or ashamed for being angry or frustrated. When children recognise these feelings, they are better able to channel them into constructive, not destructive, outlets. One of the earliest demonstrations of aggression is temper tantrums. (See Chapter 14.) Parents can handle them constructively by not attending to or reinforcing them and by helping children find control through appropriate play situations. In this way, young children learn to acknowledge such feelings and express them in alternative ways, such as pounding on clay or hitting a punching bag. When children are out of control, they may need to be physically restrained or removed from the scene to prevent them from hurting themselves or others.

Sometimes the type of discipline used to extinguish other forms of unacceptable behaviour actually promotes aggressive behaviour. For example, if a child is spanked for an aggressive act, aggression is being used to 'teach' a lesson against aggression. In addition to physically aggressive discipline, inconsistency in disciplinary practices may also foster behaviour problems in children (Duncombe et al 2012). The use of time-out and solitary play are effective disciplinary measures in the preschool years. Additionally, minimising anger and frustration can lead to fewer opportunities for acting out.

When a child exhibits extreme behaviours, such as aggression, parents are often concerned about the need for professional help. Generally, the difference between normal and problematic behaviour is not the behaviour itself but its quantity (number of occurrences), severity (interference with social or cognitive functioning), distribution (different manifestations), onset (when the behaviour started) and duration (at least 4 weeks). When aggressive tendencies are evaluated, these factors are assessed to distinguish between behaviours typically seen at various ages and those that may represent an underlying problem. Extreme aggression requires professional treatment and is often difficult to change.

Speech Problems

The most critical period for speech development occurs between 2 and 4 years of age. During this period, children are using their rapidly growing vocabulary faster than they can produce the words. A failure to master sensorimotor integration results in stuttering or stammering as children try to say the word they are already thinking about. This disfluency in speech pattern is called **developmental stuttering** and is common during language development in children ages 2 to 5 years (Nelson 2013). Stuttering affects boys more frequently than girls, has been shown to have a genetic link and usually resolves during childhood (New Zealand Speech-Language Therapists Association 2020). The New Zealand Speech-Language Therapists Association (2020) encourages parents and caregivers of children who stutter to speak slowly and in a relaxed manner, refrain from interrupting the child's speech, resist completing the child's sentences and take time to listen attentively. When parents or other significant caregivers place undue emphasis on a child's stuttering, they may exacerbate the problem. A speech evaluation is indicated if stuttering persists for 3 to 6 months, there is a family history of stuttering or there is evidence of struggling or distress related to stuttering (National Institute on Deafness and Other Communication Disorders 2016).

The best therapy for speech problems is prevention and early detection. Common causes of speech problems are hearing deficits, developmental delay and physical conditions that impede normal speech production. Referral for evaluation and treatment may be necessary to prevent a problem from interfering with learning. Anticipatory preparation of parents for expected developmental norms may calm caregiver anxiety.

Children pressured into producing sounds ahead of their developmental level may develop dyslalia (articulation problems) or revert to using infantile speech. Prevention involves educating parents regarding the usual achievement of speech production during childhood.

Stress

Although for parents the preschool years generally are less troublesome than toddlerhood, this period presents children with many unique stresses. Some are innate and stem from preschoolers' unique understanding of the world, such as fears. Others are imposed, such as beginning school. Although minimal amounts of stress are beneficial during the early years to help children develop effective coping skills, excessive stress is harmful. Young children are especially vulnerable because of their limited capacity to cope.

To help parents deal with stress in their child's life, they must be aware of signs of stress and be helped to identify the source (Box 13.1). Any number of stresses may be present, such as the birth of a sibling, marital discord, relocation or illness. The best approach to dealing with stress is prevention. It is important to monitor the amount of stress in the child's life so that levels do not exceed ability to cope. In many instances, structuring the child's schedule to allow rest and preparing the child for change, such as entering school, are sufficient measures.

Because stress is a constant aspect of daily living, it is not too early to help preschool children learn to cope with it. They can learn the meaning of the word *stress* and recognise physical signs of a stress reaction, such as a rapid pulse, a pounding heart or fatigue. Teaching children relaxation and imagery is effective. Young children can learn to 'let their bodies go limp like a rag doll'. Parents can use stories to help their child imagine pleasurable events. As language skills improve, parents can encourage preschoolers to talk about their feelings and explore other ways of expressing emotions. Play is an excellent vehicle for venting anger or frustration, and toys such as drums, clay and punching bags provide alternative methods of dissipating anxiety and teaching socially acceptable ways of dealing with such feelings.

Fears

The greatest number and variety of real and imagined fears are present during the preschool years. Preschoolers may fear the dark, being left alone (especially at bedtime), animals (particularly large dogs and snakes), ghosts, sexual matters (castration) and objects or persons associated with pain. The exact cause of children's fears is unknown. Freudians believe that the upsurge of fears during the preschool years results from the anxiety of being injured and mutilated (castration complex). Piaget views fears as a product of the type of thinking in this age group; preschoolers are caught between the egocentric thinking of infants, which protects them from imagined fears, and the more logical thought processes of school-age children, which help explain and dispel potential fears. Children in the preconceptual stage still engage in egocentric thought but are now able to imagine an event without actually experiencing it. For example, seeing someone hurt is sufficient for realising what the hurt must be like and for consequently fearing that hurt. This is commonly observed in medical practice. When watching another child get an injection, the preschooler may become upset, almost as if he or she received the injection.

The concept of animism (i.e. ascribing lifelike qualities to inanimate objects) helps explain why children fear objects. For example, a child may refuse to use the toilet after watching a television commercial in which the toilet bowl is portrayed as turning into a monster.

BOX 13.1 Sources of Stress in Preschoolers

Age 3 Years

- **Stubbornness**—Despite developing interest in social relationships and a concept of 'we', may lapse into uncooperative behaviour
- **Belongings**—Guards possessions
- **Jealousy**—Particularly when it comes to parents' love
- **Separation anxiety**—Difficulty leaving the parent
- **Stranger anxiety**—Expresses fear being around someone unknown
- **Confusion**—Cannot always discriminate between fantasy and reality
- **Fears**—May be precipitated by imagination; may also fear dogs or other animals
- **Speech**—May stutter or stumble over words
- **Activity level**—Seems to be in perpetual motion; may exhaust himself or herself
- **Mealtime**—May forget to eat or lose interest in food
- **Nap or bedtime**—May fear bad dreams, the dark or missing out on some fun while asleep
- **Destructiveness**—May damage or destroy objects
- **Questions**—Continually asks 'Why?' and is upset if trusted adults do not respond or do not know the answer

Age 4 Years

- **Insecurity**—May develop nervous habits such as nail biting, facial tics, thumb sucking, genital manipulation, eye blinking or nose picking; may insist on bringing a familiar item from home to preschool
- **Companionship**—Enjoys interacting with friends, although they may quarrel
- **Belongings**—Protects possessions
- **Sex**—Interested in the human body; may engage in exhibitionism
- **Activity level**—Enjoys running, jumping and slamming doors; may be punished for disruptive behaviour
- **Fears**—Picks up fears from adults; may fear dark room or anything perceived as 'creepy'
- **Attention**—Likes to talk and is frustrated if ignored or put off

Age 5 Years

- **Approval**—Parents' love and acceptance are vital; seeks praise
- **School**—May have difficulty adjusting to kindergarten
- **Separation anxiety**—Particularly fears loss of mother
- **Worrying**—May develop irrational fears; take information out of context; or fret over a misinterpreted, overheard conversation
- **Belongings**—Protects possessions
- **Procrastination**—Delays completing chores or activities
- **Name calling**—Insults others to boost self-image but is upset when he or she is the victim of mockery

Source: Modified from Kuczen, B. (1982). Childhood stress: Don't let your child be a victim. New York: Delacorte.

One fear peculiar to this age is fear of annihilation. Because of poorly defined body boundaries and improved cognitive abilities, young children develop concerns related to loss of body parts, such as their body going down the drain. Because preschool children cannot understand concepts of size, they cannot understand that their body is too large to disappear down the drain.

Preschoolers are also likely to develop parent-induced fears. When parents demonstrate their fears, these concerns are communicated to the children. Such fears tend to be long-lasting and difficult to dispel.

The best way to help children overcome their fears is by actively involving them in finding practical methods to deal with frightening experiences. This may be as simple as keeping a dim night-light in the child's bedroom for reassurance or letting the child bathe a doll so that the child can observe that large objects cannot go down the drain. In this way, the experience that created the fear in the child can be reconstructed without involving the child directly as the victim. The child is allowed alternative methods by which to feel in control while overcoming fear. Medical play is also beneficial, allowing a child to play with a face mask prior to being anaesthetised in theatre or have a puffer or nebuliser can assist with normalising medical equipment.

Usually by 5 or 6 years of age, children relinquish many of their fears. Explaining the developmental sequence of fears and their gradual disappearance may help parents feel more secure in handling preschoolers' fears. However, sometimes fears do not subside with simple measures or developmental maturation. When children experience severe fears that disrupt family life, professional help is required. Successful training programs may include: (1) muscle relaxation; (2) guided imagery; (3) positive self-talk or recitation of brave statements; or (4) thought stopping, or repetition of reassuring statements that block fearful thoughts. Rewards or 'tokens' may be given for 'bravery' and not being afraid. Nurses can apply such interventions in clinical settings to reduce fears (e.g. of being alone or of painful procedures).

PROMOTING OPTIMUM HEALTH DURING THE PRESCHOOL YEARS

Nutrition

Healthy nutrition during childhood should include eating a variety of nutrient-dense foods, ensuring sufficient energy to promote growth and development and balancing energy intake with energy expenditure to maintain a healthy weight. Children should have a range of food from the five core food groups. The Ministry of Health in New Zealand has a number of resources available to families to help them make good food choices for their children and wh nau. The Australian Guide to Healthy Eating is available from most primary healthcare services as well as well child health providers, who can assist with further information on healthy eating. The National Health and Medical Research Council (2013) encourages children to eat a wide variety of nutritious food from the five food groups and drink plenty of water. Figure 13.7 visualises portion sizes and recommendations.

! NURSING ALERT

Obesity in young children has dramatically increased over the past two decades in both Australia and New Zealand, and efforts to provide a healthy diet and to encourage physical activity should begin early to help children achieve optimum health (Ford et al 2013). Healthy food choices should be offered in hospital and schools, and children should be encouraged to make healthy food choices.

The amount and variety of foods young children eat vary greatly from day to day. Consequently, parents sometimes worry about the quantity and quality of food consumed by preschoolers. In general, the quality is much more important than the quantity, which nurses should stress during nutritional counselling. There is some evidence that children self-regulate their caloric intake. If they eat less at one meal, they compensate at another meal or snack.

Sleep and Activity

Sleep patterns vary widely, but the average preschooler sleeps approximately 12 hours a night and infrequently takes daytime naps. Waking during the night is common throughout early childhood. An appropriate and consistent bedtime, nap schedule (as needed) and bedtime

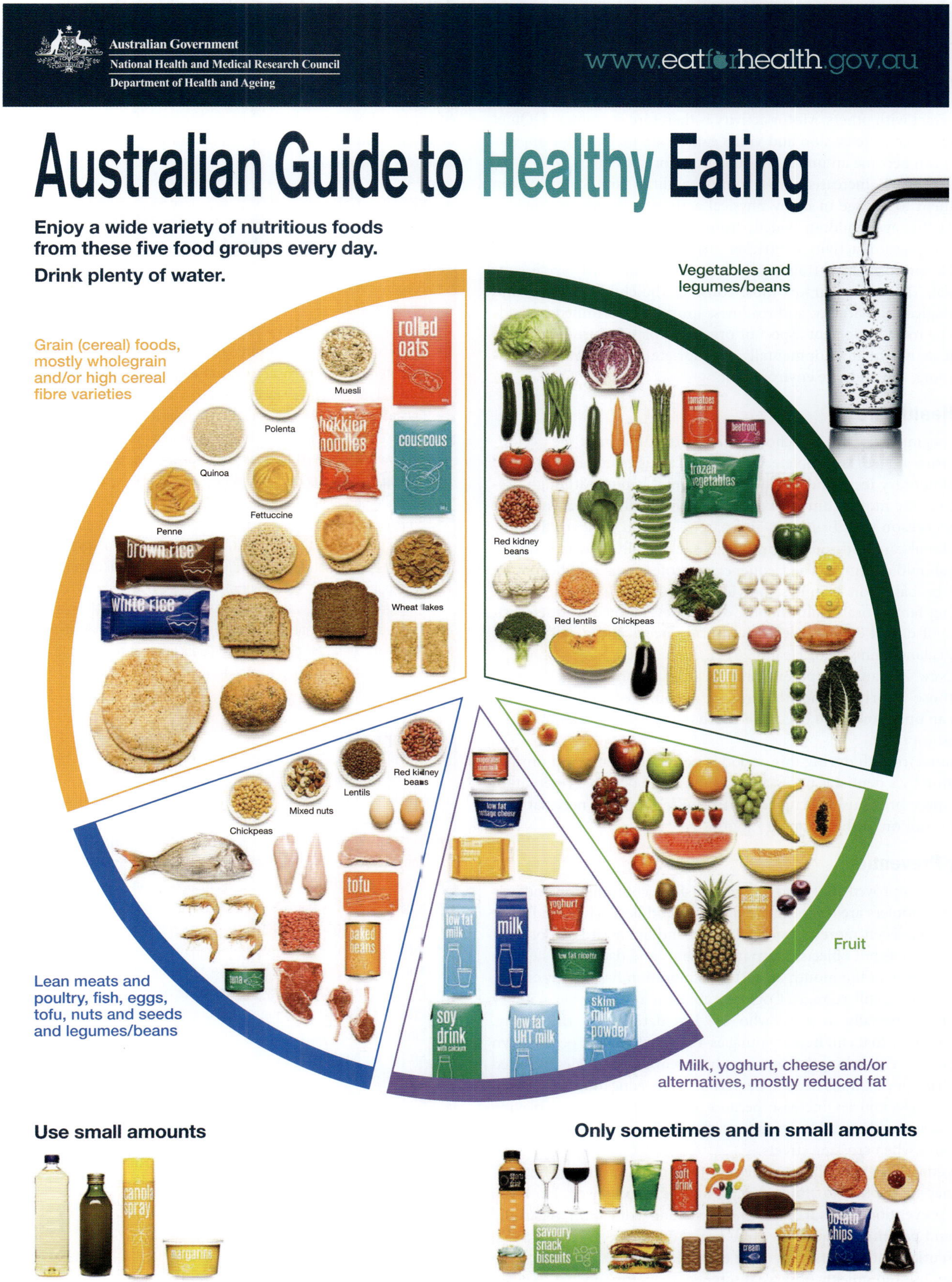

Australian Guide to Healthy Eating

Enjoy a wide variety of nutritious foods from these five food groups every day.

Drink plenty of water.

Grain (cereal) foods, mostly wholegrain and/or high cereal fibre varieties

rolled oats
Muesli
Polenta
hokkien noodles
couscous
Quinoa
Fettuccine
Penne
brown rice
white rice
Wheat flakes

Vegetables and legumes/beans

tomatoes
beetroot
frozen vegetables
Red kidney beans
Red lentils
Chickpeas
corn

Fruit

peaches

Milk, yoghurt, cheese and/or alternatives, mostly reduced fat

evaporated skim milk
low fat cottage cheese
low fat milk
milk
yoghurt
low fat ricotta
soy drink with calcium
low fat UHT milk
skim milk powder

Lean meats and poultry, fish, eggs, tofu, nuts and seeds and legumes/beans

Chickpeas
Mixed nuts
Lentils
Red kidney beans
tofu
baked beans
tuna

Use small amounts

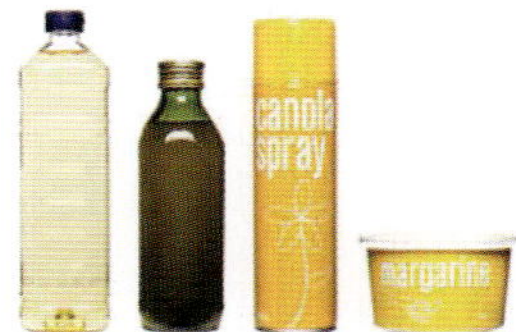

Only sometimes and in small amounts

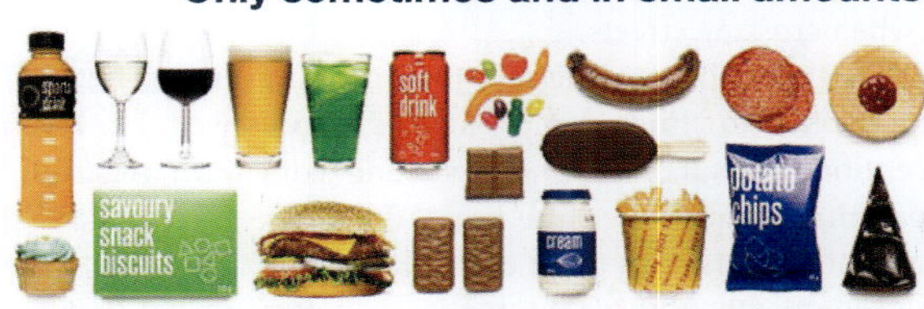

Fig 13.7 Australian Guide to Healthy Eating. (Source: https://healthy-kids.com.au/wp-content/uploads/2013/10/AGTHE.png)

routine can help prevent and treat common sleep problems and night wakings experienced by young children (Honaker & Meltzer 2014). (See Chapter 14 for discussion of sleep problems in preschoolers.)

Motor activity levels continue to be high and allow preschoolers to explore their environment, begin learning physical games and sports and interact with others. Motor activity is therefore encouraged. Quiet activities, such as television and video games, are increasingly appealing and can become an unhealthy substitute for active play.

Preschoolers' increased gross motor abilities and coordination allow them to engage in many physical activities, if only at a novice level. At this age, children benefit from free play and exposure to a variety of physical activities (Stricker 2015). Whether young children should begin formalised training in an activity at this early age is controversial. Training programs must consider the child's physical and psychological immaturity, and readiness must be determined individually. The most important aspect of organised play for preschoolers is that the activity is developmentally appropriate and occurs in a non-threatening, fun and safe environment.

Oral Healthcare

By the beginning of the preschool period, the eruption of the deciduous (primary) teeth is complete. Oral healthcare is essential to preserve these temporary teeth and to teach good dental habits. Although preschoolers' fine motor control is improved, they still require assistance and supervision with brushing, and parents should perform flossing. Professional care and routine prophylaxis, especially fluoride supplements, should continue. The frequency of professional oral healthcare should be based on a child's individual needs and risk assessment, including family oral health habits, dental development, presence or absence of dental disease, special healthcare needs and dietary habits (New Zealand Ministry of Health 2019).

In New Zealand, all parents and healthcare practitioners, especially those in primary health care, are encouraged to 'Lift the Lip'. This is an opportunity to check for tooth decay (New Zealand Dental Association n.d.).

Trauma to teeth during this period is not uncommon, and prompt evaluation by a dentist is necessary if oral trauma occurs. Preservation of the space previously occupied by an avulsed tooth is necessary for proper eruption of the secondary tooth.

Injury Prevention

Because of improved gross and fine motor skills, coordination and balance, preschoolers are less prone to falls than toddlers. They tend to be less reckless; listen more to parental rules; and are aware of potential dangers, such as hot objects, sharp instruments and dangerous heights. Putting objects in the mouth as part of exploration has all but ceased, but poisoning is still a danger. Cognitive ability may play a role in injury avoidance, especially in girls, who are less daring and risk-taking. Inform parents that children as young as 4½ years old have been shown to engage in risk-taking behaviours. Intervention strategies targeted at high-risk populations need to be part of safety education. Pedestrian motor vehicle injuries increase because of activities such as playing in the street, riding bikes, running after balls or forgetting safety regulations when crossing streets.

In general, the guidelines suggested for injury prevention for toddlers may be applied to children in this age group as well. However, injury prevention measures can now include education regarding safety and potential hazards. Because preschoolers are great imitators, it is essential that parents set a good example by 'practising what they preach'. Children quickly observe discrepancies between what they are told to do and what they observe. Establishing habits at this time, such as wearing bicycle helmets, can create long-term safety behaviours.

Anticipatory Guidance—Care of Families

The preschool years present fewer childrearing difficulties than the earlier years, and this stage of development is facilitated by appropriate anticipatory guidance in the areas already discussed (see Family-Centred Care box). Injury prevention also shifts from protection to education. For example, at this age the use of electrical outlet caps may be discontinued, with verbal explanations given of why danger exists and how to avoid it.

FAMILY-CENTRED CARE

Guidance During Preschool Years

Age 3 Years

- Prepare parents for the child's increasing interest in widening personal relationships.
- Encourage enrolment in preschool or other socialisation activities.
- Emphasise importance of setting limits.
- Prepare parents to expect exaggerated tension-reduction behaviours, such as need for 'security blanket'.
- Encourage parents to offer the child choices.
- Prepare parents to expect marked changes at 3½ years, when the child becomes insecure and exhibits emotional extremes.
- Prepare parents for normal dysfluency in speech and advise them to avoid focusing on the pattern.
- Prepare parents to expect extra demands on their attention as a reflection of the child's emotional insecurity and fear of loss of love.
- Warn parents that the equilibrium of a 3 year old will change to the aggressive, out-of-bounds behaviour of a 4 year old.
- Prepare parents to handle anger appropriately and constructively.
- Inform parents to anticipate a more stable appetite with more food selections.
- Stress the need for protection and education of the child to prevent injury. (See Injury Prevention, Chapter 14.)
- Limit screen time.

Age 4 Years

- Prepare parents for more aggressive behaviour, including motor activity and offensive language.
- Prepare parents to expect resistance to parental authority.
- Explore parental feelings regarding the child's behaviour.
- Suggest some type of respite for primary caregivers, such as placing the child in preschool for part of the day.
- Prepare parents for the child's increasing sexual curiosity.
- Emphasise the importance of realistic limit setting on behaviour and appropriate disciplinary techniques.
- Prepare parents for the highly imaginative 4 year old who indulges in 'tall tales' (to be differentiated from lies) and develops imaginary playmates.
- Prepare parents to expect nightmares or an increase in them.
- Provide reassurance that a period of calm begins at 5 years of age.
- Limit screen time.
- Ensure the preschooler gets their 'Before School Check' prior to attending school.

Age 5 Years

- Inform parents to expect a tranquil period at 5 years.
- Help parents prepare the child for entrance into the school environment.
- Make certain immunisations are up to date before entering school.
- Encourage parents to establish safety rules regarding interaction with strangers.
- Suggest that unemployed mothers or fathers consider own activities when child begins school.
- Suggest swimming lessons for child.
- Encourage parents to limit screen time and to screen for inappropriate content.

During this period, an emotional transition between parent and child occurs. Although children are still attached to their parents and accept all their values and beliefs, they are nearing the period of life when they will question previous teachings and prefer the companionship of peers. Entry into school marks a separation for both parents and children. Parents may need help in adjusting to this change, particularly if one parent has focused his or her daily activities on home responsibilities. As a child begins preschool or kindergarten, parents may need to seek activities outside the home, such as community involvement or a career. In this way, all family members are adjusting to change, which is part of the process of growth and development.

REFERENCES

American Speech-Language-Hearing Association. (2017a). The advantages of being bilingual, American Speech-Language-Hearing Association. http://www.asha.org/public/speech/development/The-Advantages-of-Being-Bilingual/.

Australian Department of Health. (2019). Australia's Physical Activity and Sedentary Behaviour Guidelines and the Australian 24-Hour Movement Guidelines. Updated April 2019. http://www.health.gov.au/internet/main/publishing.nsf/content/health-pubhlth-strateg-phys-act-guidelines#npa05 (viewed January 2021).

Drutchas, A., & Anandarajah, G. (2014). Spirituality and coping with chronic disease in pediatrics. Rhode Island Medical Journal, 97(3), 26–30.

Duncombe, M. E., Havighurst, S. S., Holland, K. A., et al. (2012). The contribution of parenting practices and parent emotion factors in children at risk for disruptive behavior disorders. Child Psychiatry and Human Development, 43(5), 715–733.

Fitzpatrick, C., Barnett, T., & Pagani, L. S. (2012). Early exposure to media violence and later child adjustment. Journal of Developmental and Behavioral Pediatrics, 33(4), 291–297.

Fleckman, J. M., Drury, S. S., Taylor, C. A., et al. (2016). Role of direct and indirect violence exposure on externalizing behavior in children. Journal of Urban Health, 93(3), 479–492.

Ford, C. N., Slining, M. M., & Popkin, B. M. (2013). Trends in dietary intake among US 2- to 6-year-old children, 1989-2008. Journal of Nutrition and Dietetics, 113(1), 35–42.

Honaker, S. M., & Meltzer, L. J. (2014). Bedtime problems and night wakings in young children: an update of the evidence. Paediatric Respiratory Reviews, 15(4), 333–339.

Jia, S., Wang, L., Shi, Y., et al. (2016). Family risk factors associated with aggressive behavior in Chinese preschool children. Journal of Pediatric Nursing, 31(6), e367–e374.

Kellogg, R. (1969). Understanding children's art. In Readings in psychology today. Del Mar, CA: Communications/Research/Machines.

Kohlberg, L. (1968). Moral development. In D. L. Sills (Ed.), International encyclopedia of the social sciences. New York: Macmillan.

Kuczen, B. (1982). Childhood stress: Don't let your child be a victim. New York: Delacorte.

Liechty, J. M., Clarke, S., Birky, J. P., et al., & STRONG Kids Team. (2016). Perceptions of early body image socialization in families: Exploring knowledge, beliefs, and strategies among mothers of preschoolers. Body Image, 19, 68–78. https://doi.org/10.1016/j.bodyim.2016.08.010

Liu, J., Lewis, G., & Evans, L. (2013). Understanding aggressive behaviour across the lifespan. Journal of Psychiatric and Mental Health Nursing, 20(2), 156–168.

Lussier, P., Corrado, R., & Tzoumakis, S. (2012). Gender differences in physical aggression and associated developmental correlates in a sample of Canadian preschoolers. Behavioral Sciences and the Law, 30(5), 643–671.

National Health and Medical Research Council. (2013). Australian Guide to Healthy Eating. Canberra: NHMRC; 13 Jan. http://www.nhmrc.gov.au/_files_nhmrc/publications/attachments/n55i_australian_guide_to_healthy_eating.pdf.

New Zealand Dental Association. (n.d.). Common dental problems. https://www.nzda.org.nz/public/your-oral-health/infants-toddlers/common-dental-problems" https://www.nzda.org.nz/public/your-oral-health/infants-toddlers/common-dental-problems

New Zealand Ministry of Health. (2019). Caring for your preschooler's teeth. 4 February. https://www.health.govt.nz/your-health/pregnancy-and-kids/under-fives/3-5-years/caring-your-preschoolers-teeth

New Zealand Speech-Language Therapists' Association. (2020). Stuttering/stammering. https://speechtherapy.org.nz/find-a-therapist/resources-for-families/

McCabe, A., Tamis-LeMonda, C. S., Bornstein, M. H., et al. (2013). Multilingual Children: beyond myths and toward best practices. Social Policy Report, 27(4), 1–36.

McEachern, A. D., & Snyder, J. (2012). Gender differences in predicting antisocial behaviors: developmental consequences of physical and relational aggression. Journal of Abnormal Child Psychology, 40(4), 501–512.

National Institute on Deafness and Other Communication Disorders. (2016). Stuttering. National Institutes of Health. February. https://www.nidcd.nih.gov/health/stuttering.

Nelson, A. (2013). Stuttering, KidsHealth. http://kidshealth.org/en/parents/stutter.html.

Provençal, N., Booij, L., & Tremblay, R. E. (2015). The developmental origins of chronic physical aggression: biological pathways triggered by early life adversity. Journal of Experimental Biology, 218(Pt. 1), 123–133.

Stewart, T., Duncan, S., Walker, C., et al. (2019). Effects of screen time on preschool health and development. Retrieved from https://www.msd.govt.nz/documents/about-msd-and-our-work/publications-resources/research/screen-time-on-preschoolers/children-and-families-research-fund-report-effects-of-screen-time-on-p....pdf

Stone, L., Janssens, J., Vermulst, A., et al. (2015). The Strengths and Difficulties Questionnaire: psychometric properties of the parent and teacher version in children aged 4-7. BMC Psychology, 3(4). https://bmcpsychology.biomedcentral.com/articles/10.1186/s40359-015-0061-8

Strachan, E., & Staples, B. (2012). Masturbation. Pediatrics in Review, 33(4), 190–191.

Stricker, P. R. (2015). Sports goals and applications—preschoolers. American Academy of Pediatrics, https://www.healthychildren.org/English/ages-stages/preschool/nutrition-fitness/Pages/Sports-Goals-and-Applications-Preschoolers.aspx.

Tatangelo, G., McCabe, M., Mellor, D., et al. (2016). A systematic review of body dissatisfaction and sociocultural messages related to the body among preschool children. Body Image, 18, 86–95.

Tooth, L., Moss, K., Hockey, R., et al. (2019). Adherence to screen time, recommendations for Australian Children aged 0-12 years. Medical Journal of Australia, 211(4), 181–182.

14

Health Problems of Early Childhood

Emma Collins

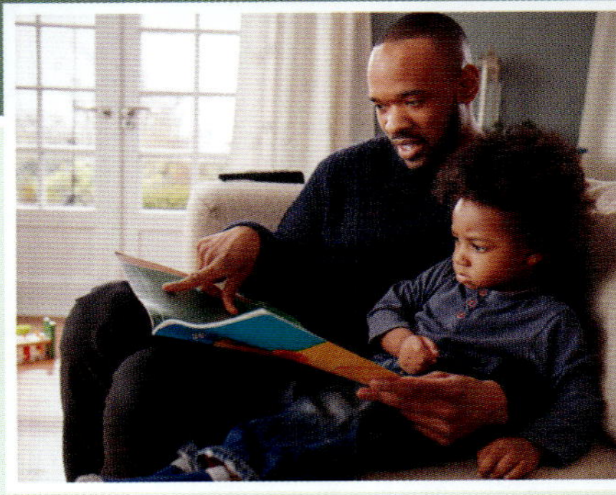

LEARNING OBJECTIVES

- Outline common health problems of early childhood, namely sleep, poisoning and child safety
- Identify areas nurses can support families to enhance the health of infants and children
- Identify key safety concerns for this age group and preventive actions to take

SLEEP PROBLEMS

The preschool years are a prime time for sleep disturbances. Children may have trouble going to sleep, wake during the night, have difficulty resuming sleep after waking during the night, have nightmares or sleep terrors or prolong the inevitable bedtime through elaborate rituals. Such sleep disturbances are typically related to increasing autonomy, negative sleep associations, night-time fears, inconsistent bedtime routines, higher levels of total daily and evening screen time and lack of limit setting (Janssen et al 2020, Babcock 2011).

Media use can also contribute to sleep disturbances. Research has revealed a direct correlation between sleep problems in preschool children, higher levels of total daily and evening media use as well as daytime exposure to violent media content (Janssen et al 2020, Garrison et al 2011). Specific sleep problems associated with media use include delayed sleep onset, nightmares, night waking, daytime tiredness and difficulty waking in the morning (Garrison et al 2011). In addition to limiting the duration of television viewing and other media exposure, parents should ensure that all types of media are age appropriate and are not too frightening or overstimulating.

Consequences of inadequate sleep include daytime tiredness, behaviour changes, hyperactivity, difficulty concentrating, impaired learning ability, poor control of emotions and impulses and strain on family relationships (Bhargava 2011). Nurses should incorporate assessment of sleep patterns and education about the development of healthy sleep behaviours. This includes regular nap, wake and bedtimes. For children admitted to hospital longer term, nurses should maintain consistent sleep behaviours in conjunction with the family or caregiver. Other measures used for sleep, such as a favourite toy or leaving lights on, should be documented in the nursing care plan. Cultural traditions may dictate sleep practices contrary to certain well-accepted professional recommendations. Thus parents may not perceive particular sleep habits as problematic (see Cultural Considerations box).

CULTURAL CONSIDERATIONS

Co-sleeping

Many experts recommend that infants and children be trained to always sleep in their own cot or bed. However, co-sleeping, or the 'family bed' (in which parents allow the children to sleep with them), is an accepted cultural practice among many Māori and Pacific Islander families. Others who have adopted co-sleeping include parents who believe that co-sleeping promotes parent–child bonding, parents who think that co-sleeping diminishes their child's night-time fears or other sleep disturbances and mothers who are breastfeeding. Co-sleeping may be a practical solution to limited numbers of bedrooms or beds in lower socioeconomic families. Controversy exists regarding the medical, developmental and social advantages and disadvantages of co-sleeping. Studies have indicated that co-sleeping is associated with sleep problems, such as frequent night wakings, poor sleep quality and decreased length of sleep (Mindell et al 2010). Parents who are considering co-sleeping should fully investigate the potential risks and benefits. Healthcare providers should be proactive in discussing sleeping arrangements with families at each visit to ensure children's safety and healthy sleep habits. In New Zealand, many midwives and well child practitioners support families to use P pi-Pods or wahakura—these are safe sleeping environments for a baby that can be placed in another bed, to ensure the baby has a safe space to sleep while still co-sleeping.

POISONING

Since the introduction of child-resistant containers, the incidence of poisonings in children has decreased dramatically. However, despite these advances, poisoning remains a significant health concern. In Australia, around 55% of calls to a poisons information centre are child related, with 36% relating to toddlers (Huynh et al 2018). Most calls related to ingestion of non-medicinal and over-the-counter (OTC) medicines, particularly agents containing paracetamol. Calls related to household cleaning agents, namely bleach, were also common (Huynh et al 2018).

Many poisonings reflect the ready accessibility of the products in the home, which is where more than 90% of poisonings occur

(Bronstein et al 2012). There are also many poisons to be aware of outside the house such as snakes, spiders, cane toads and marine animals, particularly bluebottle and Australian tropical jellyfish, blue-ringed octopus and cone shells.

The developmental characteristics of young children predispose them to poisoning by ingestion. Infants and toddlers explore their environment through oral experimentation. Because their sense of taste is not discriminating at this age, they ingest many unpalatable substances. In addition, toddlers and pre-schoolers are developing autonomy and initiative, which increases their curiosity.

This section is primarily concerned with the immediate emergency treatment of ingestion of injurious agents. Box 14.1 summarises specific management of corrosive, hydrocarbon, paracetamol, salicylate, iron and plant poisoning. Appropriate suggestions for poison prevention are discussed in the Nursing Care Considerations, Poison Prevention box. Box 14.2 summaries specific management of bites and stings of Australian animals.

Principles of Emergency Treatment

A poisoning may or may not require emergency intervention, but in every instance medical evaluation is necessary to initiate appropriate action. Advise parents to call the national or state **poisons information centre** *before* initiating any intervention (see Nursing Care Considerations box).

BOX 14.1 Selected Poisonings in Children

Corrosives (strong acids or alkalis)

- Drain, toilet and oven cleaners
- Electric dishwasher detergent (liquid, because of higher pH, is more hazardous than granular)
- Mildew remover
- Batteries
- Denture cleaners
- Bleach

Clinical Manifestations

- Severe burning pain in the mouth, throat and stomach
- White, swollen mucous membranes; oedema of the lips, tongue and pharynx (respiratory obstruction)
- Coughing, haemoptysis
- Drooling and inability to clear secretions
- Signs of shock
- Anxiety and agitation

Comments

- Household bleach is a frequently ingested corrosive but rarely causes serious damage.
- Liquid corrosives are easily ingested and cause more damage than granular/solid preparations. Liquids may also be aspirated, causing upper airway injury.
- Solid products tend to stick to and burn tissues, causing localised damage.

Treatment

- Inducing emesis is contraindicated (vomiting further damages the mucosa).
- Contact the poisons information centre immediately. If the poisons information centre or medical advice and treatment are not immediately available, it may be appropriate to dilute corrosive with water or milk (usually ≤ 120 mL).
- *Do not neutralise.* Neutralisation can cause an exothermic reaction (which produces heat and causes increased symptoms or produces a thermal burn in addition to a chemical burn).
- Maintain patent airway as needed.
- Administer analgesics.
- Give oral fluids when tolerated.
- Oesophageal stricture may require repeated dilations or surgery.

Hydrocarbons

- Petrol
- Kerosene
- Mineral seal oil (found in furniture polish)
- Lighter fluid
- Turpentine
- Paint thinner and remover (some types)

Clinical Manifestations

- Gagging, choking and coughing
- Burning throat and stomach
- Nausea
- Vomiting
- Alterations in sensorium, such as lethargy
- Weakness
- Respiratory symptoms of pulmonary involvement:
  - tachypnoea
  - cyanosis
  - retractions
  - grunting

Comments

- Immediate danger is aspiration (even small amounts can cause bronchitis and chemical pneumonia).
- Petrol, kerosene, lighter fluid, mineral seal oil and turpentine cause severe pneumonia.

Treatment

- Inducing emesis is generally contraindicated.
- Gastric decontamination and emptying are questionable even when the hydrocarbon contains a heavy metal or pesticide; if gastric lavage must be performed, a cuffed endotracheal tube should be in place before lavage because of a high risk of aspiration.
- Symptomatic treatment of chemical pneumonia includes high humidity, oxygen, hydration and paracetamol.

Paracetamol

Clinical Manifestations

Occurs in four stages after ingestion.

1. 0 to 24 hours:
   - nausea
   - vomiting
   - sweating
   - pallor
2. 24 to 72 hours:
   - patient improves
   - may have right upper quadrant abdominal pain
3. 72 to 96 hours:
   - pain in right upper quadrant
   - jaundice
   - vomiting
   - confusion
   - stupor

Continued

BOX 14.1 Selected Poisonings in Children–cont'd

- coagulation abnormalities
- sometimes renal failure, pancreatitis

4. More than 5 days:
   - resolution of hepatoxicity or progress to multiple organ failure
   - may be fatal

Comments

- This is the most common accidental drug poisoning in children.
- Toxicity occurs from acute ingestion. Toxic dose is 150 mg/kg or greater in children.
- Time to commencement of antidote acetylcysteine intravenous infusion is crucial to protect liver from significant toxicity.

Treatment

- Serum paracetamol levels need to be taken 4 hours post ingestion to determine need for acetylcysteine infusion as per nomogram. Serum paracetamol level needs to be below red therapeutic line (Fig 14.1).
  - Acetylcysteine intravenous infusion should be commenced immediately in any child who reports ingestion of > 200 mg/kg or 10 g of sustained-release paracetamol.
  - The decision to cease or continue the acetylcysteine infusion depends on the serum paracetamol level returning to normal, AST and ALT (detecting liver damage) and INR levels declining and urea, electrolytes and creatinine normalising (RCHM 2018b).

Aspirin (acetylsalicylic acid)

Clinical Manifestations

- Acute poisoning (early symptoms):
  - nausea
  - hyperventilation
  - vomiting
  - tinnitus
- Acute poisoning (later symptoms):
  - hyperactivity
  - fever
  - confusion
  - seizures
  - renal failure
  - respiratory failure
- Chronic poisoning:
  - same as listed above but subtle onset and non-specific symptoms (often mistaken for viral illness)
  - bleeding tendencies

Comments

- May be caused by acute ingestion (severe toxicity occurs with 300 to 500 mg/kg).
- May be caused by chronic ingestion (i.e. > 100 mg/kg/day for ≥ 2 days); can be more serious than acute ingestion.
- Time to peak serum salicylate level can vary with enteric aspirin or the presence of concretions (bezoars).

Treatment

- Hospitalisation is necessary for severe toxicity.
- Activated charcoal is given as soon as possible (unless contraindicated by altered mental status). If bowel sounds are present, may be repeated every 4 hours until charcoal appears in the stool.
- Lavage will not remove concretions of aspirin.
- Sodium bicarbonate transfusions are used to correct metabolic acidosis, and urinary alkalinisation may be effective in enhancing elimination; hypokalaemia may interfere with achieving urinary alkalinisation.
- Be aware of the risk of fluid overload and pulmonary oedema.
- Use external cooling for hyperpyrexia.
- Administer anticonvulsants if seizures present.
- Provide oxygen and ventilation for respiratory depression.
- Administer vitamin K for bleeding.
- In severe cases, haemodialysis (not peritoneal dialysis) is used.

Iron

- Mineral supplement or vitamin containing iron

Clinical Manifestations

Occurs in five stages (may have significant variation in symptoms and their progression).

1. Within 6 hours (if child does not develop gastrointestinal symptoms in 6 hours, toxicity is unlikely):
   - vomiting
   - haematemesis
   - diarrhoea
   - haematochezia (bloody stools)
   - abdominal pain
   - severe toxicity may have tachypnoea, tachycardia, hypotension, coma
2. Latency period: up to 24 hours of apparent improvement
3. 12 to 24 hours:
   - metabolic acidosis
   - fever
   - hyperglycaemia
   - bleeding
   - seizures
   - shock
   - death (may occur)
4. 2 to 5 days:
   - jaundice
   - liver failure
   - hypoglycaemia
   - coma
5. 2 to 5 weeks:
   - pyloric stenosis or duodenal obstruction may occur secondary to scarring

Comments

Factors related to frequency of iron poisoning include the following:

- widespread availability
- packaging of large quantities in individual containers
- lack of parental awareness of iron toxicity
- resemblance of iron tablets to lollies (e.g. M&Ms).

Toxic dose is based on the amount of elemental iron ingested. Common preparations include ferrous sulfate (20% elemental iron), ferrous gluconate (12%) and ferrous fumarate (33%). Ingestions of 20 to 60 mg/kg are considered mildly to moderately toxic, and > 60 mg/kg is severely toxic and may be fatal.

Treatment

- Hospitalisation is required when more than mild gastroenteritis is present.
- Use whole bowel irrigation if radio-opaque tablets are visible on abdominal x-ray; may need to be given via nasogastric tube.
- Emesis empties the stomach more effectively than lavage.
- Activated charcoal does not absorb iron.
- Chelation therapy with desferrioxamine should be used in severe intoxication (may turn urine red to orange).
- If IV desferrioxamine is given too rapidly, hypotension, facial flushing, rash, urticaria, tachycardia and shock may occur; stop the infusion, maintain the IV line with normal saline and notify the practitioner immediately.

BOX 14.2 Australian Venomous Bites and Stings

In Australia, there are many spiders, snakes and insects that can bite and sting. Most bites and stings are not life-threatening, but may cause mild pain, redness and/or itching. For most bites and stings, the following first aid treatment will help ease discomfort.

- Wash the area with soap and water and keep it clean and dry.
- Apply ice (wrapped in a thin cotton cloth) or cool running water to reduce the swelling and relieve the pain.
- Seek advice from the poisons information centre.
- If a child is having difficulty breathing, is unconscious or fitting, seek immediate medical assistance (NSW Poisons Information Centre 2017, The Royal Children's Hospital Melbourne [RCHM] 2019).

Snakes

There are many venomous snakes in Australia. Most bites do not result in death; however, all bites should be treated as potentially dangerous.

Treatment

- Apply a firm wide elasticised bandage around the bite and then apply a second bandage over the whole limb. The aim is to prevent lymphatic spread of venom, not to stop blood supply.
- Use a splint to keep the whole limb still.
- Keep the person still and lay them down.
- Ensure child is in a centre with full treatment facilities.
- Consult with clinical toxicologist.
- Child may need to have antivenom (NSW Poisons Information Centre 2017, RCHM 2018b).

Spiders

There are many different types of spiders in Australia. The only venomous species of significance in Australia are the red-back spider and the funnel-web spider.

Clinical Manifestations

- Pain, swelling and/or itching at the bite site
- Sweating
- Nausea and vomiting
- Drooling
- Confusion
- Difficulty breathing

Treatment

For Red-back Spiders

- Wash the area with soap and water and apply an antiseptic if available.
- Administer appropriate analgesia.
- Apply ice or cool running water to relieve pain.
- Consult with clinical toxicologist if required (NSW Poisons Information Centre 2017, RCHM 2019).

For Funnel-web Spiders and Big Black Spiders

- Apply a very firm wide elasticised bandage around the bite and then apply a second bandage over the whole limb. The aim is to prevent lymphatic spread of venom, not to stop blood supply.
- Use a splint to keep the whole limb still to slow the flow of venom around the body.
- Keep the person still.
- Consult with clinical toxicologist to see if antivenom required (NSW Poisons Information Centre 2017, RCHM 2019).

Ticks

Common bush ticks or scrub ticks are often found on people. Ticks bury themselves in the skin and scalp. Some Australian ticks release venom into the blood. Ticks should be killed before removal to reduce the chance of a life-threatening allergic reaction and the development of mammalian meat allergy. Trying to remove the tick before it has been killed may cause the tick to inject more toxin, leading to a serious anaphylactic reaction.

Clinical Manifestations

- Headache
- Blurred vision
- Weak limbs and unsteady walking

Treatment

- Do not pull on the body of the tick or try to remove it with tweezers, as this will inject more toxin.
- To kill the tick safely, the Australasian Society of Clinical Immunology and Allergy (ASCIA 2018) recommends either freezing adult ticks with an ether spray (e.g. Wart-Off spray) or applying permethrin cream (Lyclear cream) to small ticks.
- Wait 10 minutes after treatment for the tick to die, then carefully brush off.
- Wash the area with soap and water and keep the area clean and dry.
- Consult with clinical toxicologist if required (NSW Poisons Information Centre 2017).

Bees, Wasps and Ants

Clinical Manifestations

A bee, wasp or ant sting can cause pain and/or swelling. Some people may have an allergic reaction to the sting, which may cause a rash, vomiting, collapse or difficulty in breathing.

Treatment

- Remove the sting by pulling it out or scraping it away.
- Wash the area with water and keep the area clean and dry.
- Apply ice or cool running water to reduce the swelling and to relieve the pain (do not apply ice to the eye).
- If anaphylaxis occurs administer intra-muscular adrenaline 10 micrograms/kg or 0.01 mL/kg of 1:1000 (maximum 0.5 mL) into the lateral thigh; this should be repeated after 5 minutes if the child is not improving (NSW Poisons Information Centre 2017, RCHM 2017).

Blue-ringed Octopus

The blue-ringed octopus bite is very venomous. A bite may be painless but can cause paralysis, and the person may stop breathing.

Treatment

- Apply a very firm bandage around the bite and then apply a second bandage over the whole limb. Make sure that the bandage is not too tight and cutting off the circulation.
- Seek immediate medical attention.
- Provide resuscitation as required (NSW Poisons Information Centre 2017).

Bluebottle Jellyfish

Clinical Manifestations

Most stings are painful. Blue bottle stings leave a whiplike, red, wavy line on the skin from the tentacle. Allergic reactions are possible.

Treatment

- Clear away the tentacles.
- Immerse or wash the sting area in hot water for 20 minutes, for pain relief.
- If hot water is not available or does not relieve pain, then apply ice or cool running water.
- Avoid using vinegar; it is not useful and may increase pain (NSW Poisons Information Centre 2017).

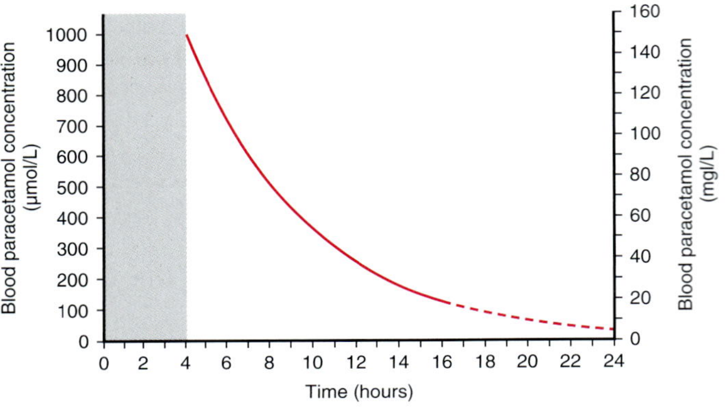

Fig 14.1 Nomogram for acute single-dose paracetamol poisoning

NURSING CARE CONSIDERATIONS

Poisoning

1. Assess the patient.
   - Initiate cardiorespiratory support if needed (airway, breathing, circulation).
   - Assess mental status; re-evaluate routinely.
   - Take vital signs; re-evaluate routinely.
   - Evaluate for possibility of concomitant trauma or illness; treat before initiation of gastric decontamination.
2. Terminate exposure.
   - Empty mouth of pills, plant parts or other material.
   - Flush any body surface (including the eyes) exposed to a toxin with large amounts of moderately warm water or saline.
   - Remove contaminated clothes, including socks and shoes, and jewellery. Ensure protection of rescuers and healthcare workers from exposure.
   - Bring victim of an inhalation poisoning into fresh air.
3. Identify the poison.
   - Question the patient and witnesses.
   - Observe the circumstances surrounding the poisoning (e.g. location, activity before ingestion).
   - Look for environmental clues (empty container, nearby spill, odour on breath) and save all evidence of poison (container, vomitus, urine).
   - Be alert to signs and symptoms of potential poisoning in the absence of other evidence, including symptoms of ocular or dermal exposure.
   - Call the poison information centre or other emergency facility for immediate advice regarding treatment.
4. Prevent poison absorption.
   - Place the child in a side-lying, sitting or kneeling position with the head below the chest to prevent aspiration.

Assessment

The first and most important principle in dealing with a poisoning is to treat the child first, not the poison. This requires an immediate concern for life support. Vital signs are taken, mental status assessed and respiratory or circulatory support is instituted as needed. The child's condition is routinely re-evaluated. Because shock is a complication of several types of household poisons, particularly corrosives, measures to reduce the effects of shock are important, beginning with airway, breathing and circulation support measures. Establishing and maintaining vascular access for rapid intravascular volume expansion is vital in the treatment of paediatric shock.

Gastric Decontamination

Although paediatric poison ingestions are common, they rarely result in significant morbidity or mortality (Bronstein et al 2012). Consider using gastrointestinal decontamination (GID) only after careful evaluation of the potential toxicity of the poison and the risks versus benefits. GID (e.g. activated charcoal, and gastric lavage) is not routinely recommended for most childhood poisonings. Because of continuing controversy regarding the use of these methods, treat each toxic ingestion individually (Albertson et al 2011).

In a minority of poisonings, specific **antidotes** are available to counteract the poison. They are highly effective and should be available in all emergency facilities. Antidotes available to treat toxin ingestion include oxygen for carbon monoxide inhalation, naloxone for opioid overdose, flumazenil for benzodiazepine (diazepam or midazolam) overdose and antivenin for certain poisonous bites.

Prevention of Recurrence

The ultimate objective is to prevent poisonings from occurring or recurring. Home safety education improves poison prevention practices (Kendrick et al 2013). Research supports the effectiveness of parent education on preventing unintentional injuries (Kendrick et al 2013). One effective counselling method is first to discuss the difficulties of constantly watching and safeguarding young children (see Family-Centred Care box). In this way, the challenging task of raising children can lead to a discussion of injury prevention as part of the parental role. This approach also incorporates contributory causes for the incident, such as: inadequate support systems; marital discord; discipline techniques (especially use of physical punishment); and any disruption in the family or family activities, such as holidays, moves, visitors, illnesses or births. A visit to the home, especially after repeat poisonings, is recommended as part of the follow-up care to assess hazards, including family factors, and to evaluate appropriate injury-proofing measures. Another approach is to encourage parents to bend down to the child's eye level and survey the home environment for potential hazards. Have the parents try to open cabinets and reach shelves to access poisons.

FAMILY-CENTRED CARE

Poisoning

A poisoning is more than a physical emergency for the child; it also usually represents an emotional crisis for the parents, particularly in terms of guilt, self-reproach and insecurity in the parenting role. The emergency department is no place to admonish the family for negligence, lack of appropriate supervision or failure to injury-proof the home. Rather, it is a time to calm and support the child and parents while unaccusingly exploring the circumstances of the injury. If the nurse prematurely attempts to discuss ways of preventing such an incident from recurring, the parents' anxiety will block out any suggestions or offered guidance. Therefore, it is preferable for the nurse to delay the discussion until the child's condition is stabilised or, if the child is discharged immediately after emergency treatment, to make a child health nurse or GP referral or send a packet of information.

CHILD MALTREATMENT

The broad term **child maltreatment** includes intentional physical abuse or neglect, emotional abuse or neglect and sexual abuse of children, usually by adults. It is one of the most significant social problems affecting children. In 2019, 11 children and young people died from a non-accidental injury in New Zealand (Child Matters n.d.a). Australia has similar statistics with 22 children dying from assault in 2015 (Child Family Community Australia 2017). Reported statistics only partially represent the actual incidence of child maltreatment because many cases are believed to go unreported.

NURSING CARE CONSIDERATIONS

Poison Prevention

- Assess possible contributing factors in occurrence of injury, such as discipline, parent–child relationship, developmental ability, environmental factors and behaviour problems.
- Institute anticipatory guidance for possible future injuries based on the child's age and developmental level.
- Initiate referral to appropriate agency to evaluate home environment and need for injury-proofing measures.
- Educate parents regarding safe storage of toxic substances.
- Advise parents to take drugs out of sight of children.
- Teach children the hazards of ingesting non-food items.
- Advise parents against using plants for teas or medicine.
- Discuss problems of discipline and children's non-compliance and offer strategies for effective discipline.
- Instruct parents regarding correct administration of drugs for therapeutic purposes and to discontinue drug if there is evidence of mild toxicity.
- Advise parents to contact the poisons information centre or practitioner immediately when a poisoning occurs.

Child Neglect

Child neglect is the most common form of maltreatment. **Neglect** is generally defined as the failure of a parent or other person legally responsible for the child's welfare to provide for the child's basic needs and an adequate level of care.

Important contributing factors for child neglect are lack of knowledge of a child's needs, lack of resources and caregiver substance abuse. For example, neglectful parents often demonstrate poor parenting skills. They may be unaware that an infant needs to be fed every 3 to 4 hours, may not know what to feed the child and may have insufficient funds to buy food. The most serious lack of knowledge is failure to recognise emotional nurturing as an essential need of children. (See also Faltering Growth, Chapter 11.)

Types of Neglect

Neglect takes many forms and can be classified broadly as physical or emotional maltreatment. **Physical neglect** involves the deprivation of necessities, such as food, clothing, shelter, supervision, medical care and education. **Emotional neglect** generally refers to failure to meet the child's needs for affection, attention and emotional nurturance.

Neglect may also include lack of intervention for or fostering of maladaptive behaviour, such as delinquency or substance abuse. **Emotional abuse** or **psychological maltreatment**, an even more difficult aspect of maltreatment to define, refers to the deliberate attempt to destroy or significantly impair a child's self-esteem or competence. Emotional abuse may take the form of rejecting, isolating, terrorising, ignoring, corrupting, verbally assaulting or over-pressuring the child (Hibbard et al 2012).

Physical Abuse

The deliberate infliction of physical injury on a child, usually by the child's caregiver, is termed *physical abuse.* Physical abuse can include anything from bruises and fractures to brain damage. Minor physical injury is responsible for more reported cases of maltreatment than major physical injury, but major physical abuse causes more deaths.

Abusive Head Trauma

Abusive head trauma is a serious form of physical abuse caused by violent shaking of infants and young children. Other commonly used terms include *shaken baby syndrome, inflicted head injury* and *neuro-inflicted brain injury.* This violent shaking would be easily recognised by others as dangerous (American Academy of Pediatrics Committee on Child Abuse and Neglect 2009, Kemp 2011) and is most often a result of the caregiver's frustration with crying, maternal stress or depression (Kemp 2011). In New Zealand, this is the single most preventable cause of serious head injuries in babies under the age of 1 year (Kids Health 2020).

It is important to understand what happens in abusive head trauma. Infants have a large head-to-body ratio, weak neck muscles and a large amount of water in the brain. Violent shaking causes the brain to rotate within the skull, resulting in shearing forces that tear blood vessels and neurons. The characteristic injuries that occur are intracranial bleeding (subdural and subarachnoid haematomas) and, in approximately 80% of cases, bilateral retinal haemorrhages, which are classic results of repetitive acceleration–deceleration head trauma (Maguire et al 2013). Injuries may also include fractures of the ribs and long bones. Most often, there are no signs of external injury, making diagnosis difficult. Clinicians base an abusive diagnosis on patterns of injuries to the infant, but this can be subjective.

Traumatic brain injury is often not an isolated event, with a large number of children showing evidence of a previous injury (Kemp 2011). Victims of traumatic head injury can be seen with a variety of symptoms, from generalised flulike symptoms to unresponsiveness with impending death (Altimier 2008). Many of the presenting symptoms, such as vomiting, irritability, poor feeding and listlessness, are often mistaken for common infant and childhood ailments. In more severe forms, presenting symptoms may include seizures, posturing, alterations in level of consciousness, apnoea, bradycardia or death. The long-term outcomes of traumatic head injury include: seizure disorders; visual impairments, including blindness; developmental delays; hearing loss; cerebral palsy; and mild to profound mental, cognitive or motor impairments (Altimier 2008). Nurses can take an active role in prevention of traumatic head injury by teaching caregivers about care for infants and techniques to cope with inconsolable crying (Kelly et al 2016).

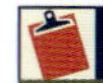

NURSING CARE CONSIDERATIONS

Stress to parents the danger of shaking infants (shaking can cause traumatic head injury). Education must include coping mechanisms on caring for children with inconsolable crying.

Munchausen Syndrome by Proxy

Munchausen syndrome by proxy (MSBP), also known as *medical child abuse* or *factitious disorder by proxy,* is a rare but serious form of child abuse in which caregivers deliberately exaggerate or fabricate histories and symptoms or induce symptoms. It is a form of child maltreatment that may include physical, emotional and psychological abuse for the gratification of the caregiver. In most cases, the perpetrator is the biological mother with some degree of healthcare knowledge and training. Healthcare providers can become easily misled and unknowingly enable the perpetrator (Squires & Squires 2013). Because of the history of symptoms provided by the caregiver, the child endures painful and unnecessary medical testing and procedures. Common symptoms presented are seizures, nausea and vomiting, diarrhoea and altered mental status; they are usually witnessed only by the perpetrator.

Considerations when determining whether a child is a victim of MSBP include the following.

- Is the child's condition consistent with the reported history?
- Does diagnostic evidence support the reported history?
- Has anyone other than the caregiver witnessed the symptoms?
- Is treatment being provided primarily because of the caregiver's demands?

The resolution of symptoms after separation from the perpetrator confirms the diagnosis.

Factors Predisposing to Physical Abuse

The causes of child abuse are multifaceted. Child maltreatment occurs across all socioeconomic, religious, cultural, racial and ethnic groups (AIHW 2020). Three risk factors are commonly identified in child abuse: (1) parental characteristics; (2) characteristics of the child; and (3) environmental characteristics (Child Matters n.d.b). However, no single factor or group of factors is predictive of abuse. Rather, the interaction of these factors is thought to increase the risk of abuse occurring in a particular family.

Parental Characteristics. Some identified characteristics occur more frequently in parents who abuse their children and are therefore considered risk factors. Younger parents more often are abusers of their children. Single-parent families are at higher risk for abuse; and in single-parent families that include an unrelated partner, the partner is sometimes the abuser, although a biological parent is most commonly the perpetrator (Child Matters n.d.b).

Abusive families are often socially isolated and have few supportive relationships. They often have additional stressors, such as low-income circumstances with little education. Parents with substance abuse problems pose a greater risk for abuse and neglect because of a variety of factors. The additional stressors of substance abuse with the demands of normal care of children create situations in which abuse and neglect can occur because these parents have impaired judgment and may react with violence while under the influence of drugs or alcohol (Lyden 2011). With little or no available support system and concurrent stressors imposed by the child or environment, these parents are vulnerable to additional crises of any nature and may strike out at the child as a method of releasing their frustration and anxiety.

Other factors identified in abusive parents include low self-esteem and little knowledge of appropriate parenting skills. Parenting skills are learned behaviours, and parents who grew up with poor parental role models may have difficulty parenting their own children. Often, child abusers were abused themselves or observed some type of abuse in their home (Lyden 2011).

Characteristics of the Child. The onus for child abuse is always on the abuser. However, children who are abused do have some common characteristics. Children from birth to 1 year old are at highest risk for being abused (Child Matters n.d.b). Infants and small children require constant attention and must have all their needs met by others. This can result in parental or caregiver fatigue that results in striking out at the child with physical force, shaking the child or ignoring the child's needs.

The physical and emotional demands placed on the parents or caregiver of an unwanted, brain-damaged, hyperactive or physically disabled child may overwhelm them, resulting in abuse. Children with disabilities may not understand that abusive behaviours are not appropriate, so they may not tell others or defend themselves. Premature infants may be at risk for maltreatment because of failure of parent–child bonding during early infancy, increased physical needs or irritability. One child may be singled out in an abusive family. Removing that child from the home often places the other siblings at risk for abuse. Therefore, no child is safe if left in the abusive environment unless the parents can be helped to learn new parenting skills, to meet the children's needs and to release their frustration through alternatives other than attacking their children. Children who have a physical or developmental disability are also considered to be at greater risk of physical abuse.

Environmental Characteristics. The environment is a significant part of the potentially abusive situation. A typical environment is one of chronic stress, including problems of divorce, family violence, poverty, unemployment, poor housing, frequent relocation, alcoholism and drug addiction. Increased exposure between children and parents, such as that which occurs in crowded living conditions, also increases the likelihood of abuse.

Although most reporting of abuse has been from lower socioeconomic populations, as stated earlier, child abuse is not a problem of any one societal group. Stresses imposed by poverty predispose lower socioeconomic families to abusive situations, and abuse in these groups is more likely to be reported. However, concealed crises may also be present in upper-class families. Families who have substitute caregivers (e.g. day-care providers and babysitters) may also be at risk for child abuse, especially if the family has not fully evaluated the caregiver. Nurses need to be aware of all these factors to identify the less obvious examples of child abuse and neglect.

Sexual Abuse

Sexual abuse is one of the most devastating types of child maltreatment, and estimates indicate that it has increased significantly during the past decade (AIHW 2020). Some of the apparent increase is due to increased awareness and reporting (Evans 2011).

Sexual abuse is defined as acts or behaviours where an adult, older or more powerful person uses a child or young person for a sexual purpose (Child Matters n.d.c). Sexual abuse includes the following types of sexual maltreatment (see also Sexual Assault [Rape], Chapter 18):

- **Incest**—Any physical sexual activity between family members; blood relationship is not required (abusers can include step-parents, unrelated siblings, grandparents, uncles and aunts); it does not include sexual relations between legally sanctioned partners, such as spouses.
- **Molestation**—A vague term that includes 'indecent liberties', such as touching, fondling, kissing, single or mutual masturbation or oral-genital contact.
- **Exhibitionism**—Indecent exposure, usually exposure of the genitalia by an adult man to children or women.
- **Child pornography**—Arranging and photographing, in any media, sexual acts involving children, alone or with adults or animals, regardless of consent by the child's legal guardian; also may denote distribution of such material in any form with or without profit.
- **Child prostitution**—Involving children in sex acts for profit and usually with changing partners.
- **Paedophilia**—Literally means 'love of child' and does not denote a type of sexual activity but rather the preference of an adult for prepubertal children as the means of achieving sexual excitement.

Characteristics of Abusers and Victims

Anyone, including siblings and mothers, can be sexual abusers, but a typical abuser is a man whom the victim knows. Offenders come from all levels of society; however, a higher risk of child abuse has been noted among families with incomes below the poverty level (Breyer & MacPhee 2015). In addition, parents with a high school education are more likely than parents with a university education to be abusers (Breyer & MacPhee 2015). Many offenders hold full-time jobs, are active in community affairs and may not have prior criminal records. Offenders often are employed (or volunteers) in positions such as teaching or coaching that bring them into contact with young girls and boys. Offenders may commit many assaults before being caught.

Incestuous relationships between father or stepfather and daughter are generally prolonged, and the victims are usually reluctant to report the situation because of fear of retaliation and that they will not be believed. Typically, incestuous relationships begin later than other forms of child abuse. The eldest daughter is usually abused, but in her absence another sister may be substituted. Sibling incest may also occur. Sexual abuse by relatives with a strong emotional bond with the victim, such as a parent, is often the most devastating to the child.

Boys are also victims of both intrafamilial and extrafamilial abuse. Compared with female victims, male victims are much less likely to report abuse, and they may suffer much greater emotional harm from incestuous relationships. Boys are likely to be subjected to anal penetration and oral-genital contact. They often have subtle physical findings and are abused by a father, stepfather or mother's boyfriend.

Significant risk factors for child sexual abuse include parental unavailability, lack of emotional closeness and flexibility, social isolation, emotional deprivation and communication difficulties. Most sexual abuse is committed by men and by persons known to the child, such as family members (Forsdike et al 2014).

Initiation and Perpetuation of Sexual Abuse

The cycle of sexual abuse often starts insidiously unless it involves an isolated attack, such as rape. Often offenders spend time with the victims to gain their trust before initiating any sexual contact. Most victims are then pressured into being an accessory to the sexual activity through various means and may be unaware that sexual activity is part of the offer. Children may not reveal the truth for fear that their parents would not believe them if they told, especially if the offender is a trusted member of the family. Some fear that they will be blamed for the situation, and many young children with limited vocabulary have difficulty describing the activity when they do have the courage or opportunity to reveal the abuse. Victims may take years to disclose this abuse.

Nursing care of the Maltreated Child

A critical responsibility of health professionals is identifying abusive situations as early as possible. Nurses who increase their knowledge of the different types of abuse and neglect and underlying causes will enhance their ability to identify, intervene and prevent children from maltreatment and neglect (Lyden 2011). The characteristics that may predispose members of some families to commit abuse can serve as a framework for assessing vulnerability but are never predictive of actual abuse. A careful, detailed history and interview combined with a thorough physical examination are the diagnostic tools needed to identify abuse. Nurses have a special role because they may be the first person to see the child and parent and are the consistent caregivers if the child is hospitalised (see Nursing Care Guidelines box).

NURSING CARE GUIDELINES

Talking with Children Who Reveal Abuse

- Provide a private time and place to talk.
- Do not promise not to tell; tell them that you are required by law to report the abuse.
- Do not express shock or criticise their family.
- Use their vocabulary to discuss body parts.
- Avoid using any leading statements that can distort their report.
- Reassure them that they have done the right thing by telling.
- Tell them that the abuse is not their fault and that they are not bad or to blame.
- Determine their immediate need for safety.
- Let the child know what will happen when you report.

BOX 14.3 Warning Signs of Abuse

- Child has physical evidence of abuse or neglect, including previous injuries.
- History is incompatible with the pattern or degree of injury, such as bilateral skull fractures after being dropped.
- Explanation of how injury occurred is vague or the parent or guardian is reluctant to provide information.
- The patient is brought in with a minor, unrelated complaint and significant trauma is found.
- Histories are contradictory among caregivers.
- The mechanism of injury provided is not possible given age or developmental level of the patient, such as 6 month old turning on hot water.
- Bruising or other injury is present in a non-mobile patient.
- The patient's affect is inappropriate in relation to the extent of injury.
- Evidence of abusive or neglectful parent–child interaction is present.
- The parent, guardian or custodian disappears after bringing in the patient for trauma or a patient with suspicious injury is brought in by an unrelated adult.
- The patient has multiple fractures of differing ages.
- There was a delay in seeking care.
- The parent or caregiver discloses that abuse has or may have occurred.
- The patient makes an outcry of abuse or neglect.

In interviewing the child and family, the nurse must be careful to avoid biasing the child's retelling of the events. Some experts suggest that health professionals limit the interview to the child's physical and mental health concerns and leave topics of the family's social, legal or other problems to the police or Oranga Tamariki (New Zealand's Ministry for Children) (Mollen et al 2012). If this is not possible, make an effort to coordinate the interview process so that all pertinent healthcare professionals can be present for the interview.

Recognition of abuse or neglect necessitates a familiarity with both physical and behavioural signs that suggest maltreatment (Box 14.3). No one indicator can be used to diagnose maltreatment. It is a pattern or combination of indicators that should arouse suspicion and lead to further investigation. It is important to note that some situations (e.g. bleeding disorders, osteogenesis imperfecta or sudden infant death syndrome) may be misinterpreted as abuse. Also, some cultural practices, such as cupping or coin rubbing, may mimic physical abuse. Unintentional injuries, such as burns from metal buckles on car seats, bruising from seat belts or spiral fractures from a twist-and-fall injury, may also be wrongly diagnosed as abuse. Normal variants, such as Mongolian spots and congenital anomalies of genitalia, can be mistaken for abuse.

Caregiver–child Interaction

The nurse can use the initial contact with the family to assess the interaction between the caregiver and the child. Observations of the caregivers should include emotional support for the child, attentiveness to the child's needs and concern for the child's injury. Although caregivers and children may vary in responses to a stressful event, note an unusual caregiver–child relationship and factor this into the overall evaluation of the child.

Certain behavioural responses of the parents to their child and to the interviewer should alert the nurse to the possibility of maltreatment. Abusive parents may have difficulty showing concern towards their child. They may be unable or unwilling to comfort the child. Abusers may blame the child for the injuries or belittle him or her for being clumsy or stupid. When interacting with healthcare workers, the parent may become hostile or uncooperative. During the child's hospitalisation, they may not participate in the child's care and may show little concern for his or her progress, eventual discharge or need for follow-up care.

Abused children's responses to their parents or the injury may also support the suspicion of abuse. Although no one pattern is typical, extremes of behaviour may be observed. Children may be unresponsive to the parent or excessively clinging and intolerant of separation. They may be overly attached to the abusive parent, possibly in the hope of preventing any upset that may precipitate anger and another attack. During care of the injury, children may be passive and accepting of the discomfort or uncooperative and fearful of any physical contact. They may avoid eye contact. Some children maintain a wary watchfulness of all strangers; some shy away from strangers as if frightened; others are unusually affectionate and outgoing.

History and Interview

Child Physical Abuse. It is often difficult to distinguish child maltreatment from accidental injuries. Caregivers whose history of events may be deceptive or incomplete and children who are non-verbal may make the assessment more complex. A purposeful, skilled history and appropriate interview questions help the nurse ensure the right course of action. Knowledge of mechanism of injury and child development is essential. Cases of abuse are often detected when the child or caregiver history of events does not match with physical findings. Children who are verbal can often give a history of the injury. Separating the child from the caregiver may provide a more reliable history. It is important to ask non-leading, open-ended questions. The history should include a narrative of the injury from both caregiver and child (if verbal). Date, time and location where the injury took place, along with who was present at the time of the injury, are essential questions. Family history for bleeding and bone disorders is important. Box 14.4 outlines areas of history that are concerning for abuse.

Neglect and Emotional Abuse. Each child may manifest different responses to neglect, depending on the situation and developmental age of the child. The goal of the interview is to determine whether the child is in a safe environment and whether the caregiver has the skills and resources to care for the child. It is often difficult to determine whether the circumstances constitute poor parenting skills or true neglect. Box 14.4 lists flags for behaviours to look for in neglected and abused children.

Sexual Abuse. An essential component to identifying sexual abuse is the interview. Several dynamics may impede the child's revelation of sexual abuse. Child sexual abuse is often perpetrated by someone known to the child, including family members. In some cases, the child may have been sworn to secrecy. The child may have been told that no one will believe the story or that his or her family would be harmed if he or she told someone about the abuse. Small children may imitate behaviours they have had perpetrated on themselves or have seen others do. The nurse must be able to recognise normal, age-related sexual curiosity and self-stimulating behaviours. Typically, children do not act out specific details of the sexual act or perform intrusive acts on others unless they have sexual knowledge beyond their normal age-related development (Dubowitz & Lane 2016).

Children's reports of sexual abuse may vary from contradictory stories to unwavering versions of the experience. Stories that sound contradictory may reflect the child's experiences in several instances of abuse. Also, children who repeatedly tell identical facts may have been prompted to do so.

Increasing evidence suggests that the types of interrogation children are exposed to after reports of sexual abuse shape their thinking. To avoid biasing the interaction, nurses must be skilful interviewers when questioning children who may be victims of abuse. Medical records should include verbatim statements made by the child and interviewer that reflect appropriate non-leading questions and statements (Lyden 2011). The child may not be emotionally ready to discuss the abuse. Establishing rapport with the child is essential to gaining his or her trust. Interviews should not be rushed. Engaging the child in play activities while encouraging conversation may help the child discuss the abuse. It may take several interviews or psychological counselling for the child to be forthcoming about the abuse. Information regarding the last sexual contact is important because it determines the need for a forensic evaluation. Children who have been sexually abused within the past 72 to 96 hours should be considered for forensic testing.

Unfortunately, there is no typical profile of the victim, and the nurse must have a high index of suspicion to identify these children. Physical signs vary and may include any of those listed for sexual abuse. The victim may exhibit various behavioural manifestations, but none of these behaviours is diagnostic. When abused children exhibit these behaviours, the signs may be incorrectly attributed to the normal stresses of childhood, especially in older school-age children or adolescents. Even signs considered most predictive of sexual abuse (e.g. certain genital findings, sexually inappropriate behaviour for age, enactment of adult sexual activity and intense focus on sexual activity [such as masturbation]) do not always indicate that sexual abuse has occurred. Conversely, abused children may not demonstrate more knowledge of sexual activity than non-abused children. However, one difference in the abused children's explanation of sexual activity may be unusual affective responses. For example, abused children have an increased risk for conduct disorders, aggressive behaviour and poor academic performance (Dubowitz & Lane 2016).

Physical Assessment

Child Physical Abuse. The goal of the physical assessment for child physical abuse is identification of all injuries. A system approach ensures that the whole body is evaluated. In instances of severe abuse and injuries, the assessment should begin with a rapid assessment of airway, breathing, circulation and neurological systems. A systematic head-to-toe examination follows. Attention to areas often overlooked, such as the scalp, behind the ears and the frenulum, is essential. The child's exterior genital area and posterior surface should be completely examined.

Record the location and a detailed description of all injuries. Note the colour, size and location of all bruising. Documentation of any burns found should include the location, pattern, demarcation lines and presence of eschar or blisters. Diagrams of the injuries using a body diagram form are helpful. If possible, obtain photographs of the injuries using a measurement tool.

Not all forms of physical abuse have obvious signs. Intraabdominal organ injury from blunt trauma to the abdomen can occur without signs of external abdominal bruising. Nurses should consider intraabdominal injury in infants and children who have any other signs of abuse.

NURSING CARE CONSIDERATIONS

Incompatibility between the history and the injury is probably the most important criterion on which to base the decision to report suspected abuse.

All evidence collected must adhere to strict guidelines for legal purposes; the chain of custody must be appropriately maintained with local law enforcement personnel. Documentation on the chain of

BOX 14.4 Clinical Manifestations of Potential Child Maltreatment

Physical Neglect

Suggestive Physical Findings

- Growth failure
- Signs of malnutrition, such as thin extremities, abdominal distension, lack of subcutaneous fat
- Poor personal hygiene
- Unclean or inappropriate dress
- Evidence of poor healthcare, such as delayed immunisation, untreated infections, frequent colds
- Frequent injuries from lack of supervision

Suggestive Behaviours

- Dull and inactive affect; excessively passive or sleepy
- Self-stimulatory behaviours, such as finger sucking or rocking
- Begging or stealing food
- Absenteeism from school
- Substance abuse
- Vandalism or shoplifting

Emotional Abuse and Neglect

Suggestive Physical Findings

- Growth failure (faltering growth)
- Eating or feeding disorder
- Enuresis
- Sleep disorder

Suggestive Behaviours

- Self-stimulatory behaviours, such as biting, rocking or sucking
- During infancy, lack of social smile and stranger anxiety
- Withdrawal from environment and people
- Unusual fearfulness
- Antisocial behaviour, such as destructiveness, stealing, cruelty to animals or people
- Extremes of behaviour, such as overcompliant and passive or aggressive and demanding
- Lags in emotional and intellectual development, especially language
- Suicide attempts

Physical Abuse

Suggestive Physical Findings

- Bruises and welts (may be in various stages of healing)
  - On face, lips, mouth, back, buttocks, thighs or areas of torso
  - Regular patterns descriptive of object used, such as belt buckle, hand, wire hanger, chain, wooden spoon, squeeze or pinch marks
  - May be present in various stages of healing
- Burns
  - On soles, palms, back or buttocks
  - Patterns descriptive of object used, such as: round cigar or cigarette burns; sharply demarcated areas from immersion in scalding water; rope burns on wrists or ankles from being bound; burns in the shape of an iron, radiator or electric stove burner
  - Absence of 'splash' marks and presence of symmetrical burns
  - Stun gun injury; that is, lesions circular, fairly uniform (≤ 0.5 cm) and paired about 5 cm apart
- Fractures and dislocations
  - Skull, nose or facial structures
  - Injury denoting type of abuse, such as spiral fracture or dislocation from twisting of an extremity or whiplash from shaking the child
  - Multiple new or old fractures in various stages of healing
- Lacerations and abrasions
  - On backs of arms, legs, torso, face or external genitalia
  - Unusual symptoms, such as abdominal swelling, pain and vomiting from punching
  - Descriptive marks, such as from human bites or pulling out of hair
- Chemical
  - Unexplained repeated poisoning, especially drug overdose
  - Unexplained sudden illness, such as hypoglycaemia from insulin administration

Suggestive Behaviours

- Wary of physical contact with adults
- Apparent fear of parents or going home
- Lying very still while surveying environment
- Inappropriate reaction to injury, such as failure to cry from pain
- Lack of reaction to frightening events
- Apprehensive when hearing other children cry
- Indiscriminate friendliness and displays of affection
- Superficial relationships
- Acting-out behaviour, such as aggression, to seek attention
- Withdrawal behaviour

Sexual Abuse

Suggestive Physical Findings

- Bruises, bleeding, lacerations or irritation of external genitalia, anus, mouth or throat
- Torn, stained or bloody underclothing
- Pain on urination or pain, swelling and itching of genital area
- Penile discharge
- Sexually transmitted disease, non-specific vaginitis
- Difficulty in walking or sitting
- Unusual odour in the genital area
- Recurrent urinary tract infections
- Presence of sperm
- Pregnancy in young adolescent

Suggestive Behaviours

- Sudden emergence of sexually related problems, including excessive or public masturbation, age-inappropriate sexual play, promiscuity or overtly seductive behaviour
- Withdrawn behaviour, excessive daydreaming
- Preoccupation with fantasies, especially in play
- Poor relationships with peers
- Sudden changes, such as anxiety, loss or gain of weight, clinging behaviour
- In incestuous relationships, excessive anger at mother for not protecting son or daughter
- Regressive behaviour, such as bedwetting or thumb sucking
- Sudden onset of phobias or fears, particularly fears of the dark, men, strangers or particular settings or situations (e.g. undue fear of leaving the house or staying at the day-care centre or the babysitter's house)
- Running away from home
- Substance abuse, particularly of alcohol or mood-elevating drugs
- Profound and rapid personality changes, especially extreme depression, hostility and aggression (often accompanied by social withdrawal)
- Rapidly declining school performance

custody form should include the names of persons collecting and receiving evidence (e.g. photographs and DNA samples), types of evidence collected and received and date of receipt (Lyden 2011). It is important that you follow your institution's policies and procedures when completing a physical assessment of this nature.

Neglect and Emotional Abuse. Neglect from deprivation of necessities is easier to identify than emotional neglect or psychological maltreatment because physical signs are usually evident. Assessment of the child's height, weight, nutritional status, hygiene and age-appropriate interactions is important for the overall picture of potential neglect. Emotional maltreatment may be readily suspected, but it is difficult to substantiate. Physical signs are often non-specific, and nurses must rely on behavioural indicators, which range from depression to acting-out behaviour, to help identify a possibly abusive situation. Any persistent and unexplained change in the child's behaviour is an important clue to possible emotional abuse.

Sexual Abuse. Identifying instances of sexual abuse is particularly difficult because, often, few if any obvious physical indications of the activity exist. Physical signs vary and may include any of those listed in Box 14.4 for sexual abuse. The goal of the physical examination is to document genital findings. In most cases, the genital examination findings are normal, which does not mean that sexual abuse did not occur. Fondling or genital-to-genital contact without penetration may leave no physical findings. Forensic evidence obtained directly from a prepubertal victim's body diminishes greatly after 24 hours, with the best chance for evidence collection coming from bed linens or the child's underwear (Girardet et al 2011). The female genital examination should include a description of the vulva, hymen and surrounding tissue. Abnormal findings of concern are injuries to the posterior vulva or the lower half of the hymenal ring or abrasions, bruising or bleeding of the genital or anal tissue. It is often helpful to use a magnifying instrument (colposcope) to detect subtle injuries. There are many variants of normal findings for female genital anatomy, so it is recommended that the examination be done by a practitioner experienced with these types of cases. Contrary to popular myth, the size of the hymenal opening is not predictive of the likelihood of sexual abuse (Adams 2011). For male victims, swelling, abrasions or bruising of the genital tissue raises concerns for abuse. Examine the anal area for symmetry, tone, fissures or scars. Genital tissue heals very quickly and most often without scars. Therefore, unless the child is seen within a few days of injury, the genital tissue may appear normal. In addition, the vaginal and anal mucosa is elastic; therefore, penetration without disruption of tissue is possible. This defies another myth that there is always evidence of female virginity. Consider the collection of specimens for determining the presence of sexually transmitted infections, which may have been contracted during the sexual contact.

Nursing Care Management

Protect the Child From Further Abuse. Initially, identification of instances of suspected abuse or neglect is essential. The nurse may come in contact with abused children in an emergency department, practitioner's office, home, day-care centre or school.

NURSING CARE CONSIDERATIONS

The priority is to remove the child from the abusive situation to prevent further injury.

All states and territories in Australia and New Zealand have laws for mandatory reporting of child maltreatment. Suspected child abuse is reported to the local authorities. Referrals usually come to the state or territory child safety or child protection department and are assigned to a caseworker in an agency, such as Child Safety Services or Child Protection. After a referral has been made, a caseworker is assigned to investigate the report. Based on the findings, the child is left in the home or temporarily removed.

A court proceeding may be necessary before the child can be placed outside the home or when parental rights are to be terminated. When the courts are involved, they usually require firsthand testimony by the referring parties. Nurses may be subpoenaed to appear in court, or their notes may be introduced as evidence in court hearings. Accurate and factual documentation is essential. Behaviours are described, not interpreted, and are recorded daily to establish a progress record (see Nursing Care Guidelines box). Conversations among the nurse, child and parent are recorded verbatim as much as possible.

Australian data suggests that in 2018, 1 in 33 children received child protection care, through investigation, care and protection orders and/or were in out of home care (AIHW 2019). Aboriginal and Torres Strait Islander children were 8 times as likely to receive child protection services than non-Indigenous children (AIHW 2019).

NURSING CARE GUIDELINES

Recording Assessment Data in Suspected Abuse

History of Injury
- Date, time and place of occurrence
- Sequence of events with recorded times
- Presence of witnesses, especially person caring for child at time of incident
- Time lapse between occurrence of injury and initiation of treatment
- Interview with child when appropriate, including verbal quotations and information from drawing or other play activities
- Interview with parent, witnesses and other significant persons, including verbal quotations
- Description of parent–child interactions (verbal interactions, eye contact, touching, parental concern)
- Name, age and condition of other children in home (if possible)

Physical Examination
- Location, size, shape and colour of bruises; approximate location, size and shape on drawing of body outline
- Distinguishing characteristics, such as a bruise in the shape of a hand or a round burn (possibly caused by cigarette)
- Symmetry or asymmetry of injury; presence of other injuries
- Degree of pain; any bone tenderness
- Evidence of past injuries; general state of health and hygiene
- Developmental level of child; screening test

Support the Child. Children suspected of being abused are often hospitalised for medical management of their injuries and to allow further assessment of their safety needs. The needs of these children are the same as those of any hospitalised child. The child should be treated as a child with the usual physical needs, developmental tasks and play interests—not as a victim of abuse. The goal of the nurse–child relationship is to provide a role model for the parents in helping them relate positively and constructively to their child and to foster a therapeutic environment for the child in his or her reprieve from the abusing situation.

Support the Family. The nurse also encourages the child's relationship with non-offending parents. The nurse does not become a substitute parent but rather acts as a role model for parents in helping them relate positively and constructively to their child. When parental ignorance of childrearing practices has played a part in the abuse, the nurse can educate the parent regarding children's physical and emotional needs. Because of the parents' own childrearing, they may not be aware of non-violent methods of discipline, such as time-outs. They may also need help in dealing with their frustration so that they do not vent anger on the child. Because these parents may be sensitive to criticism or resistant to authority figures, teaching is implemented through demonstration and example rather than through lecturing. Praise any competent parenting abilities they demonstrate to promote their sense of parental adequacy.

Advise family members to encourage the child to resume normal activities and observe the child for signs of distress (see Posttraumatic Stress Disorder, Chapter 16). Children express their feelings primarily through behaviour. Parents should be alert for changes in behaviour that indicate distress resulting from the incident, such as remaining in the house, refusal to go to school, changes in sleeping patterns and frequency of dreams and nightmares.

Referral to appropriate child safety agencies is also essential. Many abusive parents live in poverty, and the daily stresses imposed by their circumstances are overwhelming. Seek resources for financial aid, improved housing and child care. Self-help groups also provide important services.

Plan for Discharge. Discharge planning should begin as soon as the legal disposition for placement has been decided, in conjunction with Oranga Tamariki or case worker, which may be temporary foster home placement, return to the parents or permanent termination of parental rights. The latter is the most drastic solution, but it is necessary in situations of life-threatening abuse. Whenever children are sent to a foster home, they must be allowed an opportunity to express their feelings. No matter how severe the abuse, they usually mourn the loss of their parents. They need help to understand why they must not return home and that this new home is in no way a punishment. Whenever possible, foster parents are encouraged to visit in the hospital, and the nurse should take an active role in helping the new parents understand the child, as well as the child's healthcare needs, because studies have shown that the healthcare needs of children in foster care often go unmet (Schneiderman et al 2012).

Prevent Abuse. Prevention of child maltreatment has been an extremely difficult goal. However, nurses have played an important role in such programs. For example, home visits based on identified risk factors (e.g. mothers who are teenagers, unmarried or of low socioeconomic status) were noted to be an effective preventive measure (Selph et al 2013). The nurses provided information on normal child growth and development and routine healthcare needs, served as informal support persons and referred families to appropriate services when a need for assistance was identified.

Nurses in a variety of settings can implement similar activities. For example, nurses in prenatal clinics can prepare expectant families for adjustment to parenthood. Nursery and postpartum nurses can foster the attachment process by encouraging parents to hold and look at their infant, as well as teach coping mechanisms for prolonged crying. Nurses in neonatal intensive care units can minimise the effects of separation by encouraging parents to visit and can help parents become comfortable caring for their child. Nurses in ambulatory settings can teach parents appropriate methods of bathing, feeding, toileting, disciplining and preventing injuries while stressing the normal needs and developmental characteristics of children. Nurses must be sensitive to parental needs for attention, reassurance and reinforcement and should refer parents to community services and self-help groups.

Unlike preventive efforts for neglect and physical abuse, which have been aimed at the potential offender, prevention of child sexual abuse has centred on education of children to protect themselves. Materials are available for parents that describe sexual abuse and its prevention. Helpful games such as 'What if the babysitter wants to wrestle and hug but tells you to keep it a secret?' can be used to explore dangerous situations in advance and help children learn the importance of saying 'no'. They need reassurance that no matter what the other person says or does, the parents want to know about it and will not punish them. Even if children participate in the activity before telling their parents, they must be reassured that it was not their fault. It is equally important to teach children safety in terms of potential risk situations. Several suggestions for parents regarding protecting and educating children against possible molestation are presented in the Family-Centred Care box. The nurse is frequently in a position to discuss the topic of abuse with parents and to provide guidelines. In addition, parents need to be made aware that 'nice' people, including friends and relatives, can be offenders; parents should carefully observe how others act towards the child. Health professionals must alert parents to such dangers and guide them towards an appreciation of the problem, providing concrete guidelines towards child education and protection.

FAMILY-CENTRED CARE

Preventing and Dealing with Sexual Abuse of Children

Sexual assault of children is much more common than most people realise. It may be preventable if children have good preparation. *To provide protection and preparation:*

- Pay careful attention to who is around children. (Unwanted touch may come from someone liked and trusted.)
- Back up a child's right to say no.
- Encourage communication by taking seriously what children say.
- Take a second look at signals of potential danger.
- Refuse to leave children in the company of those who are not trusted.
- Include information about sexual assault when teaching about safety.
- Provide specific definitions and examples of sexual assault.
- Remind children that even 'nice' people sometimes do mean things.
- Urge children to talk about *anybody* who causes them to be uncomfortable.
- Prepare children to deal with bribes, threats and possible physical force.
- Virtually eliminate secrets between children and parents.
- Teach children how to say no, ask for help and control who touches them and how.
- Model self-protective and limit-setting behaviour for children.

If it ever becomes necessary to help a child recover from a sexual assault:

- Listen carefully to understand the child.
- Support the child for telling through praise, belief, sympathy and lack of blame.
- Know local resources and choose help carefully.
- Provide opportunities to talk about the assault.
- Provide opportunities for the entire family to go through a recovery process.

Sexual assault affects everyone. To help deal with this social problem:

- Provide care and support to those who have been victimised.
- Recognise that offenders may not change behaviour even with intervention.
- Organise neighbourhood programs to support each other's efforts to protect children.
- Encourage schools to provide information about sexual assault as a problem of health and safety.
- Organise community groups to support educational treatment and law enforcement programs.

Modified from Adams, C., & Fay, J. (1981). No more secrets: Protecting your child from sexual assault. San Luis Obispo, CA: Impact.

REFERENCES

Adams, J. A. (2011). Medical evaluation of suspected child sexual abuse: 2011 update. Journal of Child Sexual Abuse, 20(5), 588–605.

Albertson, T. E., Owen, K. P., Sutter, M. E., et al. (2011). Gastrointestinal decontamination in the acutely poisoned patient. International Journal of Emergency Medicine, 4, 65.

Altimier, L. (2008). Shaken baby syndrome. Journal of Perinatal and Neonatal Nursing, 22(1), 68–76.

American Academy of Pediatrics Committee on Child Abuse and Neglect. (2009). Abusive head trauma in infants and children. Pediatrics, 123(5), 1409–1411.

Australian Institute of Health and Welfare. (2020). Australia's children. Canberra: AIHW https://www.aihw.gov.au/reports/children-youth/australias-children/contents/

Australian Institute of Health and Welfare. (2019). Child Protection. Canberra: AIHW. https://www.aihw.gov.au/reports-data/health-welfare-services/child-protection/overview

Australasian Society of Clinical Immunology and Allergy (ASCIA). (2018). How to remove ticks to prevent allergic reactions. 8 May. https://allergy.org.au/about-ascia/info-updates/how-to-remove-ticks-to-prevent-allergic-reactions

Babcock, D. A. (2011). Evaluating sleep and sleep disorders in the pediatric primary care setting. Pediatric Clinics of North America, 58(3), 543–554.

Bhargava, S. (2011). Diagnosis and management of common sleep problems in children. Pediatrics in Review, 32(3), 91–98.

Breyer, R. J., & MacPhee, D. (2015). Community characteristics, conservative ideology, and child abuse rates. Child Abuse and Neglect, 41, 126–135.

Bronstein, A. C., Spyker, D. A., Cantilena, L. R., Jr., et al. (2012). 2011 Annual report of the Child Family Community Australia (2017). Child deaths from abuse and neglect. CFCA Resource Sheet. Australian Institute of Family Studies: https://aifs.gov.au/cfca/publications/child-deaths-abuse-and-neglect

Child Matters. (n.d.a). New Zealand child abuse statistics. https://www.childmatters.org.nz/insights/nz-statistics/

Child Matters. (n.d.b). Risk factors of child abuse. https://www.childmatters.org.nz/insights/risk-factors/

Child Matters. (n.d.c). What is child abuse? https://www.childmatters.org.nz/insights/what-is-child-abuse/

Dubowitz, H., & Lane, W. (2016). Abused and neglected children. In R. M. Kliegman, B. F. Stanton, J. W. St Geme, et al. (Eds.), Nelson textbook of pediatrics (20th ed.). Philadelphia: Saunders/Elsevier.

Evans, H. (2011). Pediatrics tackles child sexual abuse. Archives of Pediatrics and Adolescent Medicine, 165(9), 783–784.

Forsdike, K., Tarzia, L., Hindmarsh, E., et al. (2014). Family violence across the life cycle. Australian Family Physician, 43(11), 768–774.

Garrison, M. M., Liekweg, K., & Christakis, D. A. (2011). Media use and child sleep: the impact of content, timing and environment. Pediatrics, 128(1), 29–35.

Girardet, R., Bolton, K., Lohoti, S., et al. (2011). Collection of forensic evidence from pediatric victims of sexual assault. Pediatrics, 128(2), 233–238.

Hibbard, R., Barlow, J., MacMillan, H., et al. (2012). Psychological maltreatment. Pediatrics, 130(2), 372–378.

Huynh, A., Cairns, R., Brown, J., et al. (2018). Patterns of poisoning exposure at different ages: The 2015 annual report of the Australian Poisons Information Centres. Medical Journal of Australia, 209(2), 74–79.

Janssen, X., Martin, A., Hughes, A., et al. (2020). Associations of screen time, sedentary time and physical activity with sleep in under 5s: A systematic review and meta-analysis, Sleep Medicine Reviews, 49, 1–18.

Kelly, P., Wilson, K., Mowjood, A., et al. (2016). Trialling a shaken baby syndrome prevention programme in the Auckland District Health Board. New Zealand Medical Journal, 129(1430), 39–50.

Kemp, A. M. (2011). Abusive head trauma: recognition and the essential investigation. Archives of Disease in Childhood: Education and Practice Edition, 96(6), 202–208.

Kendrick, D., Mulvaney, C. A., Ye, L., et al. (2013). Parenting interventions for the prevention of unintentional injuries in childhood. Cochrane Database of Systematic Review, (3), CD006020.

Kids Health. (2020). Never ever shake a baby. The Paediatric Society of New Zealand and Starship Foundation. https://www.kidshealth.org.nz/never-ever-shake-baby

Lyden, C. (2011). Uncovering child abuse. Nursing Management, 42(Suppl.), 1–5.

Maguire, S. A., Watts, P. O., Shaw, A. D., et al. (2013). Retinal hemorrhages and related findings in abusive and non-abusive head trauma: a systematic review. Eye, 27(1), 28–36.

Mindell, J. A., Sadeh, A., Kohyama, J., et al. (2010). Parental behaviors and sleep outcomes in infants and toddlers: a cross-cultural comparison. Sleep Medicine, 11(4), 393–399.

Mollen, C. J., Goyal, M. K., & Frioux, S. M. (2012). Acute sexual abuse. Pediatric Emergency Care, 28(6), 584–590.

NSW Poisons Information Centre. (2017). Bites and stings. https://www.poisonsinfo.nsw.gov.au/site/files/ul/data_text12/4637545-5600130_Bites_and_Stings_2017.pdf

Schneiderman, J. U., Smith, C., & Palinkas, L. A. (2012). The caregiver as gatekeeper for accessing health care for children in foster care: a qualitative study of kinship and unrelated caregivers. Children and Youth Services Review, 34(10), 2123–2130.

Selph, S. S., Bougatsos, C., Blazina, I., et al. (2013). Behavioral interventions and counseling to prevent child abuse and neglect: a systematic review to update the US Preventative Services Task Force recommendations. Annals of Internal Medicine, 158(3), 179–190.

Squires, J. E., & Squires, R. H. (2013). A review of Munchausen syndrome by proxy. Pediatric Annals, 42(4), 67–71.

The Royal Children's Hospital Melbourne (RCHM). (2019). Spider bite—redback spider. January. https://www.rch.org.au/clinicalguide/guideline_index/Spider_Bite_%E2%80%93_Redback_Spider/

The Royal Children's Hospital Melbourne (RCHM). (2018a). Snakebite. January. https://www.rch.org.au/clinicalguide/guideline_index/Envenomation_and_Bites/

The Royal Children's Hospital Melbourne (RCHM). (2018b). Paracetamol Poisoning. January. https://www.rch.org.au/clinicalguide/guideline_index/Paracetamol_poisoning/

The Royal Children's Hospital Melbourne (RCHM). (2017). Anaphylaxis. August. https://www.rch.org.au/clinicalguide/guideline_index/Anaphylaxis/

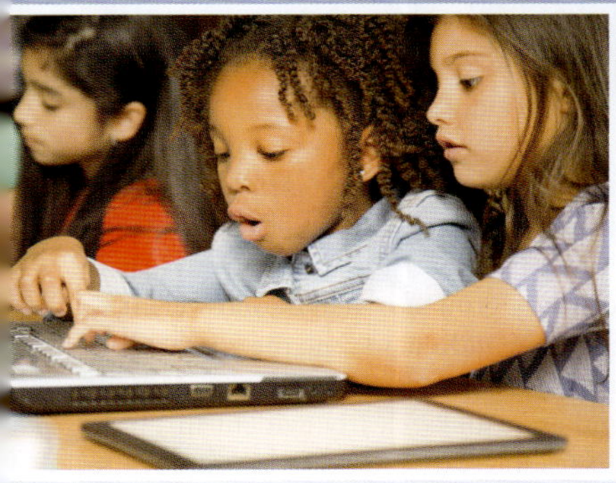

15

Health Promotion of the School-age Child and Family

Andrea Middleton

LEARNING OBJECTIVES

- Outline usual growth and development of school-age children
- Identify challenging areas for the school-age child and family and opportunities for nurses to support healthy growth and development
- Identify key safety concerns for this age group and preventive actions to take

PROMOTING OPTIMUM GROWTH AND DEVELOPMENT

The segment of the life span that extends from age 6 years to approximately age 12 years has a variety of labels, each of which describes an important characteristic of the period. The middle years are most often referred to as school-age or the school years. This period begins with entrance into the wider sphere of influence represented by the school environment, which has a significant impact on development and relationships.

Physiologically the middle years begin with the shedding of the first deciduous tooth and end at puberty with the acquisition of the final permanent teeth (with the exception of the wisdom teeth). In the 5 to 6 years before the school-age period, children progressed from helpless infants to sturdy, complicated individuals with the capacity to communicate, conceptualise in a limited way and become involved in complex social and motor behaviours. Physical growth has been equally rapid. In contrast, the period of middle childhood—between the rapid growth of early childhood and the prepubescent growth spurt—is a time of gradual growth and development, with even more progress in both physical and emotional aspects.

Biological Development

During middle childhood, growth in height and weight assumes a slower but steady pace compared with the earlier years. Between ages 6 and 12 years, children grow an average of 5 cm per year to gain 30 to 60 cm in height and will almost double in weight, increasing 2 to 3 kg per year. The average 6-year-old child is about 116 cm tall and weighs about 21 kg; the average 12-year-old child stands about 150 cm tall and weighs approximately 40 kg. During this age period girls and boys differ little in size, although boys tend to be slightly taller and somewhat heavier than girls. Towards the end of the school-age years both boys and girls begin to increase in size, although most girls begin to surpass boys in both height and weight, to the acute discomfort of both girls and boys.

Physical Changes

School-age children are more graceful than they were as preschoolers, and they are steadier on their feet. Their bodies take on a slimmer look, with longer legs, varying body proportions and a lower centre of gravity. Posture improves over that of the preschool period to facilitate locomotion and efficiency in using the arms and trunk. These proportions make climbing, bicycle riding and other activities much easier. Fat gradually diminishes, and its distribution patterns change, contributing to the thinner appearance of children during the middle years.

Accompanying the skeletal lengthening and fat diminution is an increase in the percentage of body weight represented by muscle tissue. By the end of this age period, both boys and girls double their strength and physical capabilities, and their steady and relatively consistent acquisition of refined coordination increases their poise and skill. However, this increased strength is often misleading. Although strength increases, muscles are still functionally immature compared with those of the adolescent and they are more readily injured by overuse.

The most pronounced changes that seem best to indicate increasing maturity in children are a decrease in head circumference in relation to standing height, a decrease in waist circumference in relation to height and an increase in leg length related to height. These indicators often provide a clue to a child's degree of maturity. Certain physiological and anatomical characteristics are typical of school-age children. Facial proportions change as the face grows faster in relation to the remainder of the cranium. The skull and brain grow very slowly during this period and increase little in size thereafter. Because all of the primary (deciduous) teeth are lost during this age span, middle childhood is sometimes known as the age of the loose tooth (Fig 15.1).

Maturation of Systems

As the gastrointestinal system matures, the child has fewer stomach upsets; better maintenance of blood glucose levels; and an increased stomach capacity, which permits retention of food for longer periods. The school-age child does not need to be fed as carefully, as promptly

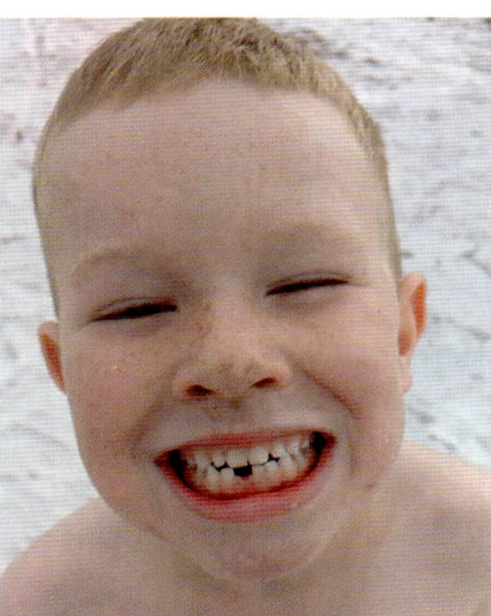

Fig 15.1 Middle childhood is the stage of development when deciduous teeth are shed.

or as frequently as before. Caloric needs are lower than they were in the preschool years and lower than they will be during the coming adolescent growth spurt.

Physical maturation occurs in other body tissues and organs. Bladder capacity, although differing widely among individual children, is generally greater in girls than in boys. There are individual variations in frequency of urination and differences in the same child according to circumstances such as temperature, humidity, time of day, amount of fluids ingested and emotional state.

The heart grows more slowly during the middle years and is smaller in relation to the rest of the body than at any other period of life. Heart and respiratory rates steadily decrease, and blood pressure increases between ages 6 and 12 years.

The immune system becomes more competent in its ability to localise infections and produce an antibody-antigen response. Because of increased exposure to others in school classes, children can have several infections in the first 1 to 2 years of school while immunity develops.

Bones continue to ossify throughout childhood, but because mineralisation is not completed until maturity, children's bones resist pressure and muscles pull less than with mature bones. Consequently, parents must be careful to prevent alterations in bone structure and provide children with well-fitted shoes and with chairs and desks that allow correct sitting posture with the feet able to reach the floor and the hips able to fit well back in the seat. Children should have ample opportunity to move around and be cautious about carrying heavy loads. For example, they should shift books and/or tote bags from one arm to the other. Back packs, when worn correctly, distribute weight more evenly.

Wider differences between children are seen at the end of middle childhood than at the beginning. These differences become increasingly apparent and, if extreme or unique, may create emotional problems. The nurse explains the associated characteristics of height and weight relationships, rapid or slow growth and other important features of development to children and their families. Physical maturity is not necessarily correlated with emotional and social maturity. Seven-year-old children who look like 10-year-old children will think and act like 7 year olds. Expecting behaviour appropriate for 10-year-old children from them is unrealistic and can be detrimental to their development of competence and self-esteem. Conversely, treating 10-year-old children as though they were 7 years old is an equal disservice to them.

Prepubescence

Preadolescence is the period that begins towards the end of middle childhood and ends with the thirteenth birthday. **Puberty** signals the beginning of the development of secondary sex characteristics and **prepubescence**, the 2-year period that precedes puberty, typically occurs during preadolescence.

Towards the end of middle childhood, the discrepancies in growth and maturation between boys and girls become apparent. On average, there is a difference of approximately 2 years between girls and boys in the age of onset of pubescence. For many, especially for girls, preadolescence is a period of rapid growth. For others, mostly boys, it is generally a period of continued steady growth in height and weight.

There is no universal age at which children assume the characteristics of preadolescence. The first physiological signs appear at about 9 years (particularly in girls) and are usually clearly evident in 11- to 12-year-old children. Although preadolescent children do not want to be different, variability in physical growth and physiological changes among children of the same sex, and between the two sexes, is often striking at this time. This variability, especially in relation to the onset of secondary sex characteristics, is of utmost concern to the preadolescent. Either early or late appearance of these characteristics is a source of embarrassment and uneasiness to both sexes. Early appearance of secondary sex characteristics in girls is often associated with dissatisfaction with physical appearance, greater general unhappiness and lower self-esteem. Late-developing boys often have a negative self-concept. Both early appearance of physical characteristics in girls and late appearance in boys have been linked to participation in risk-taking behaviours (e.g. early sexual activity, substance use and reckless vehicle use).

Preadolescence is a time when considerable overlapping of developmental characteristics occurs, with elements of both middle childhood and early adolescence apparent. However, there are sufficient unique characteristics to set this period apart as an age category. Generally, puberty begins at 10 years in girls and 12 years in boys, but its onset in either sex after age 8 years is considered normal. The average age of puberty is 12 years in girls and 14 years in boys. Boys experience little sexual maturation during preadolescence.

Psychosocial Development

Middle childhood is the period of psychosexual development that Freud described as the **latency period**, a time of tranquillity between the oedipal phase of early childhood and the eroticism of adolescence. During this time children experience relationships with same-sex peers following the indifference of earlier years and preceding the heterosexual fascination that occurs for most boys and girls in puberty.

Developing a Sense of Industry (Erikson). Successful mastery of Erikson's first three stages of psychosocial development is probably the most important accomplishment in terms of development of a healthy personality (Erikson 1963). Successful completion of these stages requires a loving environment within a stable family unit that has prepared the child to engage in experiences and relationships beyond this intimate group. During childhood, children affiliate with age-mates, receive the systematic instruction prescribed by their individual cultures and develop the skills needed to become useful, contributing members of their social communities.

A **sense of industry**, or a stage of accomplishment, occurs somewhere between age 6 years and adolescence. The goal of this stage of development is to achieve a sense of personal and interpersonal competence through the acquisition of technological and social skills. School-age children are eager to build skills and participate in meaningful and socially useful work. Interests expand and, with a growing

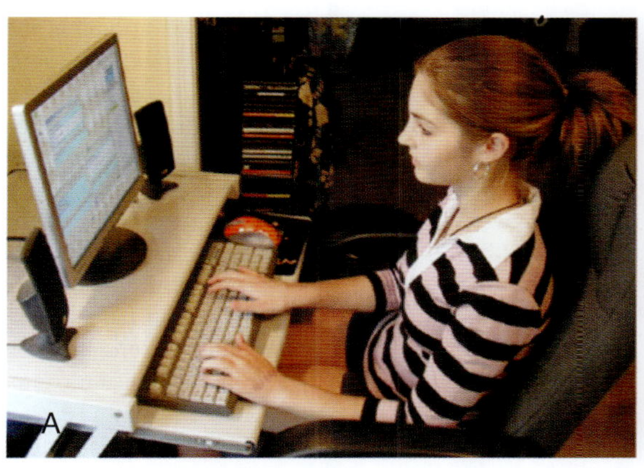
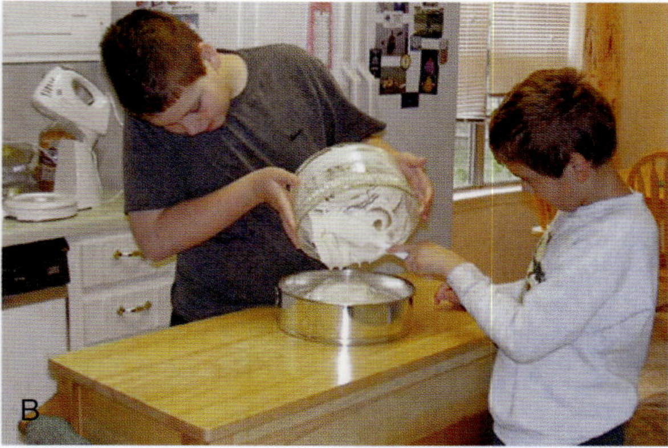

Fig 15.2 School-age children are motivated to complete tasks working alone (**A**) and working with others (**B**).

sense of independence, children want to engage in tasks that they can complete (Fig 15.2). Failure to develop a sense of accomplishment may result in a sense of inferiority.

Many aspects of industry contribute to the child's sense of competence and mastery. Intrinsic motivation is associated with increased competence in mastering new skills and assuming new responsibilities. Children gain a great deal of satisfaction from independent behaviour in exploring and manipulating their environment and from interaction with peers. Extrinsic sources of reinforcement in the form of school marks, material rewards, additional privileges and recognition provide encouragement and stimulation. Often the acquisition of skills is a means for achieving success in special activities such as athletics or social organisations. Peer approval is a strong motivating factor.

The danger inherent in this period of personality development is the occurrence of situations that might result in a sense of inadequacy or **inferiority**. This may happen if the previous stages have not been successfully mastered or if a child is incapable of assuming or unprepared to assume the responsibilities associated with developing a sense of accomplishment. Feelings of inferiority or lack of worth come from children themselves or from the social environment. Children with physical or mental limitations are sometimes at a disadvantage for acquisition of certain skills. When the reward structure is based on evidence of mastery, children who are incapable of developing these skills are at risk for feeling inadequate and inferior.

Even children without chronic disabilities show such a wide range of individual differences in capabilities and preferences that they experience feelings of inadequacy in some areas. No child is able to do well in everything, and children must learn that they will not be able to master each skill that they attempt. All children, even children who usually have positive attitudes towards work and their own capabilities, feel some degree of inferiority in regard to a specific skill that they cannot master.

For some children, success or aptitude in one area may compensate for failure or ineptitude in another. However, the differences in reinforcement provided for success in various areas have significant effects on feelings of adequacy. For example, society places a higher value on success in team sports than on success in repairing a bicycle. Compensating for the inability to excel in more socially valued skills through mastery of other, less valued skills is difficult for children. If the social environment places a negative value on any failure, feelings of inferiority may be increased in the less capable child. Repeated failures can generate such strong feelings that eventually the child is reluctant to attempt any new task or is fearful of not being able to perform as well as his or her peers. Thus intrinsic motivation towards engaging in a task for the pleasure of the challenge conflicts with the external forces that cause feelings of doubt and inferiority. Consequently, the child may no longer try.

A child's concept of success or failure is important. Children who aspire to more than they are capable of usually experience failure. In contrast, children who set their aspirations lower than their level of achievement are likely to experience success. Most accomplishments during the school years are very public. Family, teachers and peers are all aware of success or failure in school. In school and sometimes at home, feelings of inferiority may be produced through comparisons with others that suggest the child is not as good as a peer, sibling or member of another group. This inadequacy becomes a source of embarrassment. The child may even be shamed for the failure. Earlier conflicts of doubt and guilt are closely associated with feelings of inferiority.

A sense of accomplishment also involves the ability to cooperate, to compete with others and to cope effectively with people. Middle childhood is the time when children learn the value of doing things with others and the benefits derived from division of labour in the accomplishment of goals. Children need and want real achievement. When they can accomplish tasks that need to be done and perform well despite individual differences in capacities and emotional development, and when they are suitably rewarded, children develop a sense of industry and accomplishment that prepares them for establishing a stable identity later in life.

Temperament

The reactivity patterns or temperamental traits identified in infancy may continue to influence behaviour in middle childhood. Analysing behavioural patterns observed in past situations can provide clues to the way that a child may react to new situations, although long-range projections are not always successful. Through interaction with the environment, experiences, motives and abilities, many children change. In some children, major temperamental characteristics persist into adolescence; in others they do not.

Many children tend to be identified with one of three broad temperament categories: easy, slow to warm up and difficult. Parents and teachers are in an excellent position to assess a child's behavioural style and to try to make their demands and expectations consonant with the individual child's temperamental characteristics. With easy children this rarely poses a problem. They adapt readily to many childrearing programs and new situations. School entry and other changes usually go smoothly and are accomplished with minimal stress. Difficulties arise with children who are slow to warm up or are difficult or easily distracted.

Slow-to-warm-up children usually exhibit discomfort when introduced to new situations and need time to become accustomed to a new environment, authority figures and expectations. These children may respond with tears, somatic complaints or other manoeuvres to avoid the event. The nurse should encourage them to try new experiences but allow them to adapt to their surroundings at their own speed. Pressure to move quickly into new situations only strengthens the tendency to withdraw. After-school activities can be a cause for reaction, but attending with a friend or contracting for permission to withdraw after a trial of a specified number of times may provide them with sufficient incentive to try.

Difficult or easily distracted children may benefit from 'practice' sessions in which they are prepared for a given event by role playing, visiting the site or reading or listening to stories, or use of other methods to acquaint them with what to expect. Children who are persistent need to know when to stop what they are doing so that the signal to stop will not come as a surprise or trigger a reaction. Nurses need to handle children with difficult temperaments with exceptional patience, firmness and understanding so that they can learn appropriate behaviour in their interactions with others.

Cognitive Development (Piaget)

When children enter the school years, they begin to acquire the ability to relate a series of events and actions to mental representations that they can express both verbally and symbolically. This is the stage that Piaget describes as **concrete operations**, when children are able to use their thought processes to experience events and actions. The term *operation* implies an action that is performed on an object or set of objects; thus a mental operation is an alteration or transformation that an individual carries out in thought rather than in action. Toddlers or preschool children can perform acts that involve ordering, such as correctly arranging a graduated set of circles from largest to smallest on a stick, and can find their way to a friend's house, but they are unable to verbalise the actions involved in the process. School-age children are able to articulate the process and perform the actions mentally without the need to carry out the behaviours.

As children move from the preschool years into the school years, their conceptual abilities become increasingly flexible. During the concrete operational period, they acquire the ability to perform cognitive operations and apply these new skills when thinking about objects, situations and events. Their rigid, egocentric outlook is replaced by thought processes that allow them to see things from another's point of view. They become aware of a variety of perspectives and become more sensitive to the fact that others do not always perceive events exactly as they do. They are able to delay an action until they have evaluated alternative responses to situations. Their steady reduction in egocentricity helps form the basis for logical thought and the development and maturation of morality.

The concrete operational stage occurs between ages 7 and 11 years. During this stage children develop an understanding of relationships between things and ideas. They progress from making judgments based on what they see (perceptual thinking) to making judgments based on what they reason (conceptual thinking). They are increasingly able to master symbols and to use their memories of past experiences to evaluate and interpret the present.

One of the major cognitive tasks of school-age children is mastering the concept of **conservation**—that physical matter does not appear and disappear by magic. They learn that certain properties of the environment are not changed simply by altering their disposition in space. They are able to resist perceptual cues that suggest alterations in the physical state of an object. The nurse can use commonplace items to demonstrate the conservation of liquid, mass, number, length, area and volume (Fig 15.3). To explain the observation that the mass of the clay in the figure has not been altered, children use one of three concepts.

1. Identity—Because nothing has been added and nothing has been taken away, the pancake is still the same clay. Nothing has changed but the shape.
2. Reversibility—The clay can be reshaped into its original form (a ball).
3. Reciprocity—Although the pancake appears larger in circumference, the ball is much thicker. In this instance the child demonstrates the ability to deal with two dimensions at the same time and to comprehend that a change in one dimension compensates for a change in another.

When children are able to use the concepts of identity, reversibility and reciprocity, they can conserve along any physical dimension. They perceive the concept of volume in relation to container size and shape, recognise that size is not necessarily related to weight or volume and are able to manipulate or 'see' in a concrete manner. They recognise that logical operations move in two directions (such as addition and subtraction or multiplication and division) and that certain properties are invariant (e.g. 7 remains 7 whether it is represented by 3 + 4, 2 + 5, seven buttons, seven stars or seven boys).

Children use reversibility in selecting a course of action, which thus provides greater control over themselves and their environment. They have the ability to think through an action sequence, anticipate the consequences and, if needed, return to the beginning and rethink the action in a different direction. They no longer need to experience an action before they can anticipate the results. Reversibility allows mental action and enables children to disassemble and reassemble certain kinds of things in their thoughts.

Classification skills involve the ability to group objects according to the attributes that they have in common. School-age children can place things in a sensible and logical order, group and sort, and hold a concept in their minds while they make decisions based on that concept. In middle childhood children get a great deal of enjoyment from classifying and ordering their environment. They become occupied with numerous and varied collections of objects, such as shells, dolls, cars, stones, cards, stuffed animals and anything that is classifiable. They even begin to order friends and relationships (e.g. first best friend, second best friend).

As children mature, they progress from collecting simply for the sake of collecting and become more selective and discriminating. Their classification systems become more complex and are based on abstract ideas rather than on perception and experience. Much of the pleasure of collections is in the appraising, ordering and reordering of the parts.

During the school-age years children develop combinatorial skills—the ability to manipulate numbers and to learn the skills of addition, subtraction, multiplication and division. They learn to apply the basic operations to any object or quantity. They learn the alphabet and the world of symbols called words that can be arranged in terms of structure and their relationship to the alphabet. They learn to tell time, to see the relationship of events in time (history) and places in space (geography) and to combine time and space relationships (geology and astronomy).

The most significant skill, the ability to read, is acquired during the school years and becomes the most valuable tool for independent enquiry. Children's capacity for exploration, imagination and expansion of knowledge is enhanced by the ability to read as they progress from the repetition and confusion of early efforts to increasing facility and comprehension. Formal academic learning begins at ages 5 to 6 years, when children's intellectual capabilities and cognitive processes allow them to attain intellectual achievements.

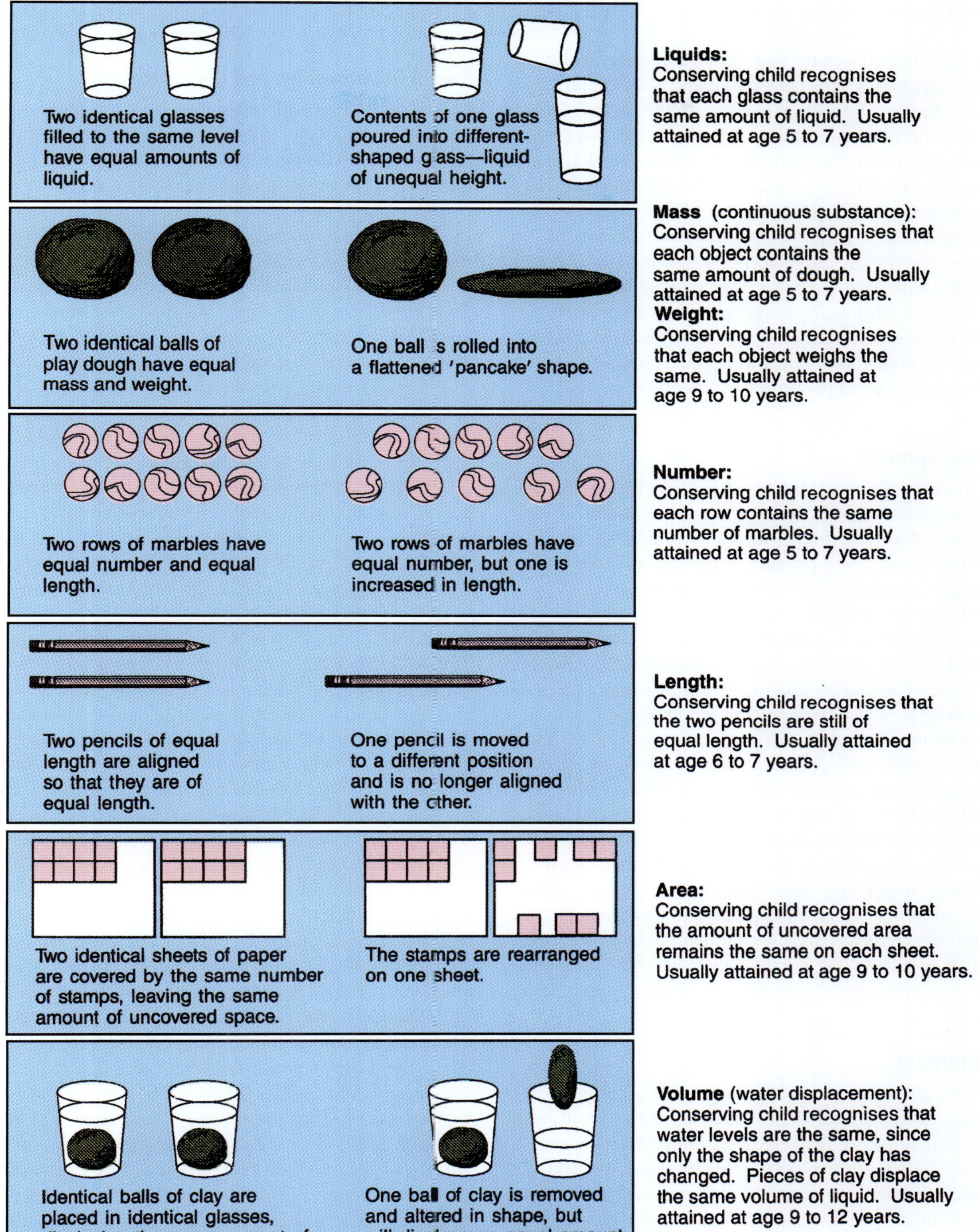

Fig 15.3 Common examples that demonstrate the child's ability to conserve (ages are approximate only).

Moral Development (Kohlberg)

As children move from egocentrism to more logical patterns of thought, they also move through stages in the development of conscience and moral standards. Young children do not believe that standards of behaviour come from within themselves but that others establish and enforce these rules. During preschool years, children perceive rules as definite and require no reason or explanation. Children learn the standards for acceptable behaviour, act according to these standards and feel guilty when they violate the standards. Although children 6 or 7 years old know the rules and behaviours expected of them, they do not understand the reasons behind them. Young children usually judge an act by its consequences. Rewards and punishment guide their judgment; a 'bad' act is one that breaks a rule or causes harm. When a child and an adult differ in judging an act, the adult is right. Children may believe that what other people tell them to do is right and that what they themselves think is wrong. Consequently, children 6 or 7 years old are more likely to interpret accidents and misfortunes as punishment for misdeeds or 'bad' acts.

Older school-age children are able to judge an act by the intentions that prompted it rather than just by the consequences. Rules and judgments become less absolute and authoritarian and begin to be founded more on the needs and desires of others. Rules of conduct are more readily considered in terms of mutual agreement and are based on cooperation and respect for others. Older children are likely to view breaking a rule in relation to the total context in which it appears; reactions are influenced by the situation as well as by the morality of the rule itself. However, it is not until adolescence or beyond that children are able to view morality on an abstract basis with sound reasoning and principled thinking. Although younger children can judge an act only according to whether it is right or wrong, older children take into account a different point of view to make a judgment. They are able to understand and accept the concept of treating others as they would like to be treated.

Language Development

Children enter middle childhood with remarkably efficient language skills, but they make many important linguistic achievements during the school-age years. Word usage and the ability to find and retrieve words quickly when called on to produce what they know in a relatively short time grow considerably during the school years.

Narrative skills improve markedly. School-age children are increasingly able to provide directives that others can correctly interpret without visual data (e.g. explain directions over the telephone). By ages 10 to 12 years the child should be able to use factitive words (such as *know, think* and *believe*), as well as complex pronouns and conjunctions, and be able to form grammatically correct sentences. School-age children gradually become more proficient at making inferences about meanings and learn the subtle exceptions to grammatical rules. This makes them less likely to engage in literal interpretation of messages.

They rapidly develop *metalinguistic awareness*—an ability to think about language and to comment on its properties. This enables them to appreciate jokes, riddles and puns that involve play on words, sounds or double meanings. They are beginning to understand metaphors and figurative statements, such as 'A stitch in time saves nine'. The acquisition of cognitive skills enables them to think about the quality of their own and others' speech and to evaluate and clarify messages.

Social Development

At the beginning of middle childhood, children enter a period of less intense emotions, secure in their dependency on their parents and family and with self-confidence tempered by a more realistic perspective. They have the energy to explore the environment beyond the family, to gradually increase the scope of interpersonal interactions and to invest their curiosity in understanding the world.

Identification with peers is a strong influence in children's gaining independence from parents. The aid and support of peers provides children with enough security to risk the moderate parental rejection brought about by each small victory in their development of independence.

Questions of masculinity and femininity take on importance as sex-role learning assumes more prominence. Boys associate with boys, and girls with girls, each group pursuing its own interests, with communication between the sexes confined to that which is necessary. Much of the child's concept of the appropriate sex role is acquired through relationships with peers. During the early school years there is little difference relative to sex in the play experiences of children. Both girls and boys share games and other activities. However, in the later school years the differences become marked.

Social Relationships and Cooperation

Daily relationships with peers provide the most important social interactions for school-age children. For the first time, children are able to join in group activities with unrestrained enthusiasm and steady participation. Previously, interactions were limited to short periods under considerable adult supervision. With increased skills and wider opportunities, children become involved with one or several peer groups in which they can gain status as respected members.

Valuable lessons are learned from daily interaction with age-mates. First, children learn to appreciate the numerous and varied points of view that are represented in the peer group. As they play together, children discover that there are many occupations for fathers and mothers, more than one version of the same song, different rules for the same game and different customs for celebrating the same holiday. As children interact with peers who see the world in ways that are different to their own, they become aware of the limits of their own point of view. Because age-mates are peers and are not forced to accept one another's ideas as they are expected to accept those of adults, other children have a significant influence on decreasing the egocentric outlook of the individual child. Consequently, children learn to argue, persuade, bargain, cooperate and compromise to maintain friendships.

Second, children become increasingly sensitive to the social norms and pressures of their peer group. The peer group establishes standards for acceptance and rejection, and children may be willing to modify their behaviour to be accepted by the group. They are judged by the physical impression they convey, the skills they possess and other abilities they can demonstrate. The need for peer approval becomes a powerful influence towards conformity. Children learn to dress, talk and otherwise behave in a manner acceptable to the group. A variety of roles, such as class joker or class hero, may be assumed by the individual child to gain approval from the group. However, no child can adapt perfectly to all the requirements of the peer group. If some children find differences between the values of the peer group and the values of their families to be too great, they may relinquish the pleasure of interaction with the group to abide by the regulations established in the home. Thus, in order to diminish conflict within the family, some children may be forced into a position outside the peer group.

Third, the interaction among peers leads to the formation of intimate friendships between same-sex peers (Fig 15.4). School age is the time when children have 'best friends' with whom they share secrets, private jokes and adventures; they come to one another's aid in times of trouble. In the course of these friendships, children also fight, threaten, break up and reunite. These dyadic relationships, in which children experience love for and closeness with a peer, seem to be important as a foundation for relationships in adulthood. The conflicts encountered in the relationship are usually resolved in terms that children are able to control. Because neither child has authority over the other, as in an adult–child relationship, children must work through their differences within the framework of their commitment to each other.

Peer Groups. One of the outstanding characteristics of middle childhood is the formation of formalised peer groups. Initially, children in the early middle years merely hang around the periphery of the formalised group, watching, learning, practising various skills and participating in group activities whenever the members of the group allow them to do so. As they age, children eventually take their places as fully-fledged participating group members.

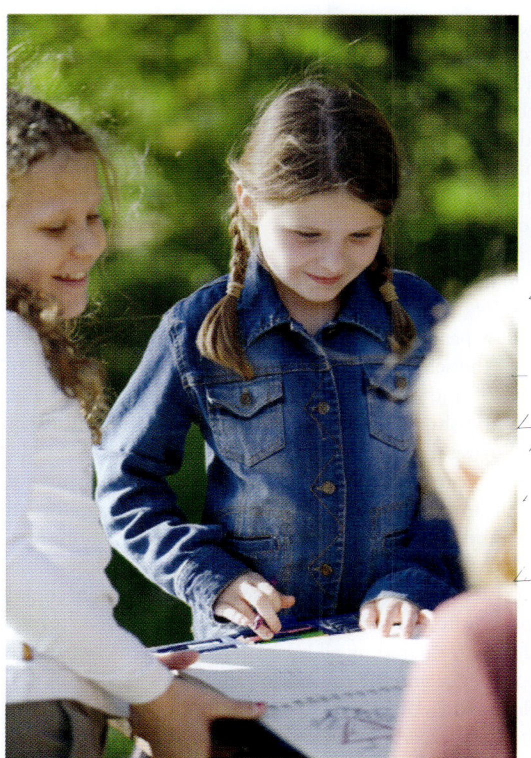

Fig 15.4 School-age children enjoy engaging in activities with a 'best friend'.

A prominent feature of middle childhood groups is the code of rigid rules imposed on the members. Exclusiveness is evident in the selection of persons given the privilege of joining. Acceptance in the group often depends on a pass–fail basis according to social or behavioural criteria. Conformity is the core of the group structure. There are often secret codes, shared interests, special styles of dress and special words that signify membership in the group. Each child must follow a standard of behaviour established by the group. Conforming to the rules provides children with feelings of security and relieves them of the responsibility of making decisions.

Membership in the group provides children with a comfortable place in society. Many of the qualities valued by the group, such as physical strength, daring, ingenuity and comradeship, have not been stressed in the family. However, these are values that contribute to an individual child's total personality. By merging their identity with the identities of their peers, children move from the family group to an outside group as a step towards further independence. They substitute conformity to a peer-group pattern for conformity to a family pattern while they are still too insecure to function independently.

During the early school years, groups are small and loosely organised, with changing membership and no formal structure. They do not demonstrate the elements of cooperation and order that are seen in groups of older children. As a rule, girls' groups are less formalised than boys' groups, and although there may be a mixture of both sexes in groups in the earlier school years, those of later school years are composed predominantly of children of the same sex. Common interests are frequently the central element around which a group is structured.

Children's strong desire not to be different creates problems for those who, for various reasons, are unable to meet the accepted standards of the peer group. Children with disabilities or those who are in some way unable to compete have a difficult time. Children become self-conscious when they are unable to dress like other children, do not have spending money like other children or appear different from other children.

Children who have physical characteristics that are obviously different (such as birthmarks, ears that 'stick out' or physical defects) may be set apart from the peer group and become a target for criticism and ridicule. Peer-group identification and association are essential to socialisation.

Poor relationships with peers and a lack of group identification can also contribute to bullying behaviour. **Bullying** is any recurring activity that intends to cause harm, distress or control towards another individual where there is a perceived imbalance of power between the aggressor(s) and the victim (Rettew & Pawlowski 2016, Australian Education Authorities 2019). Bullying is a complex issue. It can occur in varying degrees of severity in a physical, social or emotional context. Children can be exposed to bullying as victims, perpetrators, bystanders or upstanders. Upstanders attempt to help the victim of bullying in some way such as taking action to stop the bullying or supporting the victim following an incident (Salmivalli 2014, Australian Education Authorities 2019). Although bullying can occur in any setting, it usually takes place in school hallways or on the playground where supervision is minimal but peers are present to witness the attack (Shetgiri 2013).

Cyberbullying involves using an electronic medium to harm or bother another individual and can be more harmful than traditional bullying because the attack can instantly reach a wider audience, while allowing the bully to remain anonymous (Australian Education Authorities 2019, Sticca & Perren 2013). The Longitudinal Study of Australian Children (LSAC) identified 160,000 children aged 12 to 13 experienced at least one bullying-like behaviour within a year and 60% of children experienced two or more bullying behaviours. In the last month, 1 in 5 children experienced online bullying-like behaviours (Australian Institute of Family Studies [AIFS] 2017). The risk for bullying is greater in primary school than high school, but cyberbullying occurs more frequently in high school (Simon & Olson 2014). Children who are targeted for bullying often have internalising characteristics such as anxiety, depression, low self-esteem and reduced assertiveness that may make them an easy target for bullying (Flannery et al 2016). They may also have a disability, be from culturally and linguistically diverse backgrounds or identify as lesbian, gay, bisexual, transgender and/or gender diverse (Australian Education Authorities 2019, Rigby & Johnson 2016).

Bullies are generally defiant towards adults, manipulative and likely to break school rules. They have aggressive attitudes, have a positive view of violence and may experience or witness violence or abuse at home (Simon & Olson 2014). Boys who bully tend to use physical force, referred to as *direct bullying*, but girls usually use bullying methods, such as exclusion, gossip or rumours, which is referred to as *indirect bullying* (Simon & Olson 2014).

The long-term consequences of bullying are significant. Children who bully are more likely to have poor educational and employment outcomes, may engage in antisocial and criminal behaviour or substance abuse and are at higher risk of depression later in life (Australian Education Authorities 2019, Rigby & Johnson 2016). Victims of bullying are at increased risk for low self-esteem, anxiety, depression, feelings of insecurity and loneliness, poor academic performance and self-harm behaviours (Flannery et al 2016). Bullying can be reduced or prevented through supportive relationships with family, intervention of schoolteachers and involvement with positive peer groups. Many schools have developed bullying prevention programs.

Relationships with Families

Although the peer group is highly influential and necessary to normal child development, parents are the primary influence in shaping children's personalities, setting standards for behaviour and establishing value systems. Family values usually predominate when parental and peer value systems come into conflict. Although children may appear to reject parental values while testing the new values of the peer group, ultimately they retain and incorporate many parental values into their own value systems.

As children move into a wider world of peer-group relationships, parents are faced with the task of letting go of control. Parents may find it difficult to face the rejection that children demonstrate as they become more involved with their peer groups. Children may want to spend more time in the company of their peers, may seem eager to leave the house and often prefer activities of the peer group to family activities. During this time, children discover that parents can be wrong, and they begin to question the knowledge and authority of the parents who previously were considered to be all-knowing and all-powerful. Parents can best serve the interests of their children through tolerant understanding and support.

Although increased independence is the goal of middle childhood, children are not yet prepared to abandon parental control. Children need and want restrictions placed on their behaviour; they are not yet prepared to cope with all of the problems of their expanding environment. They feel more secure knowing that there is an authority greater than themselves to implement controls and restrictions. Children may complain loudly about the restrictions and try to break down parental barriers, but they are uneasy if they succeed in doing so. Children feel secure with reasonable, consistent controls. They respect the adults on whom they can rely to prevent them from acting on each and every urge. Children see this behaviour as an expression of love and concern for their welfare.

Children also need their parents as adults, not as 'pals'. Sometimes parents, hurt by their children's rejection, attempt to maintain their children's love and gratitude by assuming the role as a friend. Children need the stable, secure strength provided by mature adults to whom they can turn during troubled relationships with peers or stressful changes in their world. During a disruption in their lives, such as times of failure, periods of illness or a move that separates them from the security of friends, children need the firm, secure anchor of parental interest and concern. With a secure base in a loving family, children are able to develop the self-confidence and maturity needed to stand independently.

Children's relationships with siblings change during the middle years. Children view siblings as equal in power and status. In earlier years, older siblings were influential in the younger siblings' learning. In the middle years, the relationship becomes one of companionship. Positive emotional tone increases, but sibling conflict also increases as the siblings get older. Middle childhood is a period of transition for sibling relationships, a juncture between the open bickering of early childhood and the supportive relationships observed in adult siblings.

Play

As children enter the school years, their play takes on new dimensions that reflect a new stage of development. Not only does play involve increased physical skill, intellectual ability and fantasy, but as children form groups and cliques, they begin to evolve a sense of belonging to a team or club. Belonging to a group is of vital importance. Clubs and organisations are important parts of the culture of childhood.

Rules and Rituals

The need for conformity in middle childhood is strongly manifested in the activities and games of school-age children. Up to this point, they have either played games they have invented themselves or have played in the company of a friend or an adult, and rules more or less evolved with the game. Now they begin to see the need for rules, and the games they play have fixed and unvarying rules that may be bizarre and extraordinarily rigid (especially those made up by the group). But part of the enjoyment of the game is knowing the rules because knowing means belonging. Once the rules are established and agreed on, the demand for conformity is strong.

Conformity and ritual characterise the play of school-age children, not only in games, but also in behaviour and language. Childhood is full of chants and taunts, such as 'Last one is a rotten egg'. Children receive a great deal of pleasure and power from such sayings, which have been handed down with few changes through generations.

Team Play. A more complex form of group play that develops from the need for peer interaction involves the team games and sports that are part of the school years. Such games may require a referee, umpire or person of authority so the rules can be followed more accurately. Team membership has several characteristics that promote child development during the middle years.

Children learn to subordinate personal goals to group goals. Team membership means that each child is accountable to the other team members and that acts may affect the success or failure of the entire group. Each member's behaviour is open to public evaluation, and children risk ostracism, ridicule or scapegoating if they contribute to a team loss. Although individual skills are recognised, team successes and failures are shared by all members. Children learn the concept of interdependence and the reliance of all players on one another.

Children learn that division of labour is an effective strategy for the attainment of a goal. Each person on a team has a specific function, which increases the team's chances of winning. Once children learn that certain goals are best accomplished by dividing tasks among several individuals, they can transfer this knowledge to other social situations. Children also learn that some children are best equipped to perform one part of the task and other children are best suited to another aspect of the task.

Team play helps children learn about the nature of competition. In all team play there is a winning side and a losing side. Because losing is often interpreted as failure, children go to great lengths to avoid the public embarrassment and personal shame that accompany failure. The more a child identifies with the team and values membership in the group, the more distasteful losing becomes. Fear of losing and the failure it implies are strong incentives for group commitment; however, winning is not universally given high value. Some cultures and subcultures emphasise the game and consideration for one's companions rather than the outcome.

Team play also contributes to children's social, intellectual and skill growth (Eime et al 2013). Children work hard to develop the skills needed to become members of a team, to improve their contribution to the group and to anticipate the consequences of their behaviour for the group. Team play helps stimulate cognitive growth because children are called on to learn many complex rules, make judgments about those rules, plan strategies and assess the strengths and weaknesses of members of their own and the opposing teams (Fig 15.5).

Quiet Games and Activities

Although the play of school-age children can be highly active, they also enjoy many quiet and solitary activities. The middle childhood years are the time for collections, and young school-age children's collections are an odd assortment of unrelated objects in messy, disorganised piles. Collections of later years are more orderly and selective and often are organised neatly in scrapbooks, on shelves or in boxes.

School-age children become fascinated with complex board, card, computer and electronic games. Children play these games alone or in groups. As in all games, the adherence to rules is fanatical. Disagreements over the rules can cause much discussion and argument, but are easily resolved by reading the rules of the game.

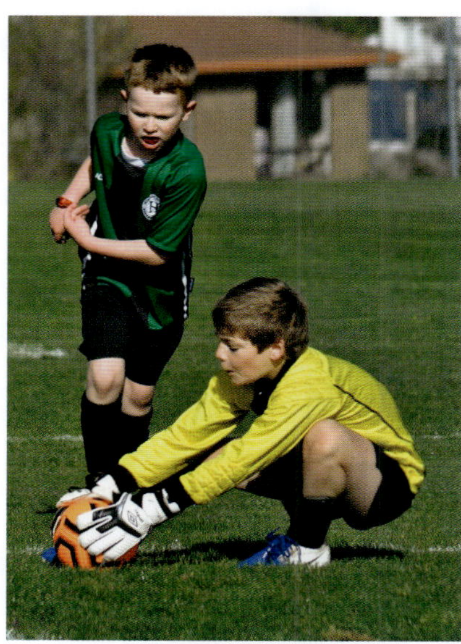

Fig 15.5 Activities engaged in by school-age children, such as junior soccer, vary according to each child's interest and opportunity.

The newly acquired skill of reading becomes increasingly satisfying as school-age children begin to expand their knowledge of the world through books. School-age children never tire of stories and, like preschool children, they love to have stories read aloud. They also enjoy sewing, cooking, carpentry, gardening and creative endeavours, such as painting. Many creative skills, such as those involving music and art, and athletic skills, such as swimming, hiking, dancing and karate, are acquired during childhood and continue to be enjoyed into adolescence and adulthood (Fig 15.6).

Ego Mastery

Play affords children the means to acquire representational mastery over themselves, their environment and others. Through play, children can feel as big, as powerful and as skilful as their imaginations will allow, and they can attain vicarious mastery and power over whomever and whatever they choose. They need to feel in control in their play. School-age children still need the opportunity to use large muscles in exuberant outdoor play and the freedom to exert their newfound autonomy and initiative. They need space in which to exercise and to work off tensions, frustrations and hostility. Physical skills practised and mastered in play help develop a feeling of personal competence, which contributes to a sense of accomplishment and helps provide a place of status in the peer group.

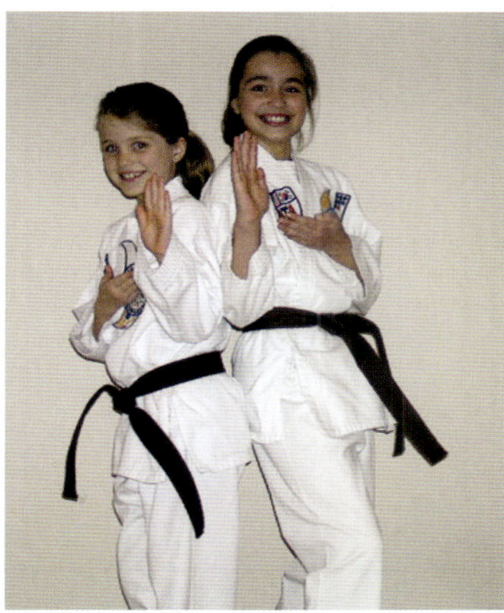

Fig 15.6 School-age children take pride in learning new skills

Table 15.1 presents a summary of growth and development in middle childhood. Because each child has a unique developmental pattern, any descriptions of the typical child of any age group can represent only an average and should not be considered as absolute criteria for any given child.

Development of Self-concept

Closely associated with developing a sense of industry is developing a concept of one's value and worth. With the emphasis on skill building and broadened social relationships, children are continually occupied in the process of self-evaluation. Children's self-concepts are composed of their own critical self-assessments plus their interpretations of the opinions of others. **Self-concept** refers to a conscious awareness of a variety of self-perceptions, such as one's physical characteristics, abilities, values and self-ideals, and one's idea of self in relation to others. It also includes one's body image, sexuality and self-esteem.

Body Image

Body image is what children think about their bodies and is influenced, but not solely determined, by significant others. School-age children are knowledgeable about the human body, and social development during this period focuses to a large extent on the body and its capabilities. School-age children can draw a recognisable human figure, although individually their portrayal of body parts may vary considerably. They are acutely aware of their own body as well as those of their peers and those of adults. It is important that children know body functions and that adults correct any misinformation children have about the body (e.g. what is fat).

During the school years, children focus on peer relationships and conform to group norms. They evaluate how their physical appearance, body configuration and coordination compare with those of their peers. The head is the most noticeable and, to them, important part of the body. They also model themselves after their parents and compare themselves to favoured peers and images observed in the media.

Children are aware of physical disabilities in others, and it is not unusual for them to believe that their own bodies are not the right size or the right shape or are in some way defective. They respond to such concerns in a variety of ways. For example, they will conceal perceived shortcomings of body or performance, as in the obese child who refrains from going swimming, the child who conveniently forgets their sports uniform, the child who conceals an imagined defect or the child with enuresis who declines invitations to sleepover parties. Children seldom express these concerns to families. However, they need reassurance about both the uniqueness and the sameness of their body, while their privacy is respected, and they are allowed appropriate protective strategies. Children who are different become aware of the differences and may find themselves excluded from the group. When children are teased or criticised about being different, the effect can last even into adulthood.

Self-esteem

Self-esteem is children's pictures of their individual worth and consists of both positive and negative qualities. Children actively strive to achieve internalised goals. At the same time, they continually receive feedback on the quality of their performance from individuals they consider to be authorities. By the time they reach school age, children

TABLE 15.1 Growth and Development During School-age Years

Physical and Motor	Mental	Adaptive	Personal–Social
AGE 6 YEARS			
Height and weight gain continues slowly Weight—16–26.3 kg; height—106.7–123.5 cm Central mandibular incisors erupt Loses first tooth Demonstrates gradual increase in dexterity Active age; constant activity Often returns to finger feeding More aware of hand as a tool Likes to draw, print, colour Vision reaches maturity	Develops concept of numbers Can count 13 blocks Knows whether it is morning or afternoon Defines common objects (such as fork and chair) in terms of their use Obeys triple commands in succession Knows right and left hands Says which is pretty and which is ugly of a series of drawings of faces Describes the objects in a picture rather than simply enumerating them Attends Prep or Year 1	At table, uses knife to spread butter or jam on bread At play, cuts, folds, pastes paper; sews crudely if needle is threaded Takes bath without supervision; performs bedtime activities alone Reads from memory; enjoys oral spelling game Likes table games, checkers, simple card games Giggles a lot Sometimes steals money or attractive items Has difficulty owning up to misdeeds Tries out own abilities	Can share and cooperate better Has great need for children of own age Will cheat to win Often engages in rough play Often jealous of younger brother or sister Does what adults are seen doing May have occasional temper tantrums Is a boaster Is more independent, probably influence of school Has own way of doing things Increases socialisation
AGE 7 YEARS			
Begins to grow at least 5 cm in height per year Weight—17.7–30 kg; height—111.8–129.5 cm Maxillary central incisors and lateral mandibular incisors erupt More cautious in approaches to new performances Repeats performances to master them Jaw begins to expand to accommodate permanent teeth	Notices that certain items are missing from pictures Can copy a diamond Repeats three numbers backwards Develops concept of time; reads ordinary clock or watch correctly to nearest quarter-hour; uses clock for practical purposes Attends Year 1 or 2 More mechanical in reading; often does not stop at the end of a sentence, skips words such as *it*, *the* and *he*	Uses table knife for cutting meat; may need help with tough or difficult pieces Brushes and combs hair acceptably without help May steal Likes to help and have a choice Is less resistant and stubborn	Is becoming a real member of the family group Takes part in group play Boys prefer playing with boys; girls prefer playing with girls Spends a lot of time alone; does not require a lot of companionship
AGES 8–9 YEARS			
Continues to gain 5 cm in height per year Weight—19.6–39.6 kg; height—116.8–141.8 cm Lateral incisors (maxillary) and mandibular cuspids erupt Movement fluid; often graceful and poised Always on the go; jumps, chases, skips Increased smoothness and speed in fine motor control; uses cursive writing Dresses self completely Likely to overdo; hard to quiet down after recess More limber; bones grow faster than ligaments	Gives similarities and differences between two things from memory Counts backwards from 20 to 1; understands concept of reversibility Repeats days of the week and months in order; knows the date Describes common objects in detail, not merely their use Attends Year 3 or 4 Reads more; may plan to wake up early just to read Reads classic books, but also enjoys comics More aware of time; can be relied on to get to school on time Can grasp concepts of parts and whole (fractions) Understands concepts of space, cause and effect, nesting (puzzles), conservation (permanence of mass and volume) Classifies objects by more than one quality; has collections Produces simple paintings or drawings	Makes use of common tools such as hammer, saw, screwdriver Uses household utensils and craft materials Helps with routine household tasks such as dusting, sweeping Assumes responsibility for share of household chores Looks after all of own needs at table Buys useful articles; exercises some choice in making purchases Runs useful errands Likes pictorial magazines Likes school; wants to answer all the questions Is afraid of failing a year at school; is ashamed of bad marks Is more critical of self Takes music and sports lessons	Is easy to get along with at home Likes the reward system Dramatises Is more sociable Is better behaved Is interested in boy–girl relationships but will not admit it Goes about home and community freely, alone or with friends Likes to compete and play games Shows preference in friends and groups Plays mostly with groups of own sex but is beginning to mix Develops modesty Compares self with others Enjoys organisations, clubs and group sports

TABLE 15.1 Growth and Development During School-age Years—cont'd

Physical and Motor	Mental	Adaptive	Personal–Social
AGES 10–12 YEARS			
Weight—24.3–58 kg; height—127–162.6 cm Remainder of teeth erupt and tend towards full development (except wisdom teeth) *Boys*—Slow growth in height and rapid weight gain; may become obese in this period *Girls*—Pubescent changes may begin to appear; body lines soften and round out	Writes brief stories Attends Years 5, 6 or 7 Writes occasional short letters to friends or relatives on own initiative Uses telephone for practical purposes Responds to magazine, radio or other advertising Reads for practical information or own enjoyment—stories or library books of adventure, romance, animal stories	Makes useful tools or does easy repair work Cooks or sews in small ways Raises pets Washes and dries own hair, but may need reminding to do so Is sometimes left alone at home for an hour or so Is successful in looking after own needs or those of other children left in his or her care	Loves friends; talks about them constantly Chooses friends more selectively; may have a 'best friend' Enjoys conversation Develops beginning interest in opposite sex Is more diplomatic Likes family; family really has meaning Likes mother and wants to please her in many ways Demonstrates affection Likes father, who is admired and may be idolised Respects parents

have received messages regarding the extent to which they are able to accomplish tasks that have been delegated to them. For example, one child may have been given prestigious responsibilities at home or at school or received special commendation for an achievement. On the other hand, another child may have been sent to a special class for slow learners or may have been the last person selected when children chose sides for a game. These and other signs serve as clues to social worth that children incorporate as part of their self-evaluation.

Children approach the process of self-evaluation from a framework of either self-confidence or self-doubt. Children who have mastered the maturational crises of autonomy and initiative are able to face the world with feelings of pride rather than shame. At first, children's self-concepts are formed exclusively from their perceptions of their parents' evaluation of them. During middle childhood the opinions of peers and teachers are important. Criticisms and peer approval are additional sources of data for evaluation. Parents and other adults are no longer the only persons who respond to their skills, talents and abilities; peers also identify skills and capabilities. Each child soon begins to internalise these outside opinions. If children regard themselves as worthwhile or satisfactory persons, they have high self-esteem, self-confidence and a positive self-concept. If they view themselves as worthless, they have low self-esteem.

Children encounter difficulties assessing their own abilities because they rely on their own expectations or on the expectations expressed by others regarding their performance. They depend almost entirely on external evidence of worth, such as school marks, teachers' comments and parental and peer approval. Children do not yet have the capacity to develop their own independent criteria to evaluate their own accomplishments. It is especially difficult for them to assess their achievement in abstract skills.

Nothing succeeds like success. Significant adults in children's lives can often manage to manipulate the environment so that children meet with success. Each small success can improve a child's self-image. The more positive children feel about themselves, the more confident they feel in trying again for success. All children profit from feeling that they are special to significant adults. A positive self-image makes them feel likeable, worthwhile and capable of valuable contributions. Such feelings lead to self-respect, self-confidence and a general feeling of happiness. Parents can help their school-age children develop self-esteem by being honest, providing opportunities for creativity, helping them succeed in activities and providing positive reinforcement. Nurses can enhance self-esteem by fostering supportive relationships between children and members of their families and by emphasising children's strengths and positive aspects of their behaviour.

Development of Sexuality

Evidence indicates that many children experience some form of sex play during or before preadolescence as a response to normal curiosity, not as a result of love or sexual urge. Children are experimentalists by nature, and this play is incidental and transitory. Any adverse emotional consequences or guilt feelings depend on how the parents manage the behaviour and whether children view their actions as wrong in the eyes of significant persons, particularly their parents.

Children's attitudes towards sex are acquired indirectly at an early age and affect the way they respond to sexual information. Many parents discourage sexual exploration, either through subtle substitution of activities that divert their children's attention from the genitalia or by expressions of anger or disgust at their children's behaviour. These tactics clearly communicate to children that they should not engage in such activities, are being discouraged to ask questions about sex and are being excluded from the sources of information.

Sex Education

Parents may not teach young children the correct terminology for sexual organs or sexual feelings. Often the only vocabulary available to children is one that identifies sexual organs with excretory functions. If children learn that excretory organs and functions are dirty, they may associate 'dirtiness' with the reproductive organs and functions. If children learn the correct terminology for the organs and their functions, this will eliminate or reduce this association. Because parents often either repress or avoid their children's sexual curiosity, sexual information received in childhood is often received almost entirely from peers. One study found that the majority of parents of pre-adolescents and adolescent children believed they were open with sex education discussion; however, only a few parents communicated direct information about safe sex practice (Hyde et al 2013). When peers are the primary source of sexual information, it is often transmitted and exchanged in secret conversation and contains misinformation. These communications can also create anxiety in children and inhibit spontaneous expressions or questioning of their parents.

Sex education programs have been successfully incorporated into a number of primary and high school curriculums. In many of these programs, sexuality is presented in the context of its central role as a biological mechanism for the survival of the culture. Children learn that sexual maturation and reproduction represent each individual's contribution to the natural order of things. This approach provides a natural entry into discussion of sexuality as a basis for family units, marriage and attitudes towards children, as well as an entry into a presentation of the biological facts of sexuality. Many sex education programs also emphasise sexual intimacy as part of close, personal relationship and a means of conveying love.

Nurse's Role in Sex Education

No matter where nurses practise, they can provide information on human sexuality to both parents and children. To discuss the topic adequately, nurses must: understand the physiological aspects of sexuality; know the common myths and misconceptions associated with sex and the reproductive process; understand cultural and societal values; and be aware of their own attitudes, feelings and biases.

When nurses present sexual information to children, they should treat sex as a normal part of growth and development. Nurses should answer questions honestly, matter-of-factly and at the child's level of understanding. School-age children may be more comfortable when boys and girls are segregated for discussions; however, each group needs information about both sexes.

Children need help to differentiate sex and sexuality. Exercises focused on clarifying values, identifying role models, solving problems and practising responsibility are important to prepare school-age children for early adolescence and puberty. In addition, children need explanations of sexual information that is discussed via the media or jokes. A comprehensive sex education program including information about anatomy, pregnancy, contraceptives and sexually transmitted diseases should be presented in simple, accurate terms. Teaching a child to be sexually responsible is an essential component of sex education. Preadolescents need precise and concrete information that will allow them to answer questions such as 'What if I start my period in the middle of class?' or 'How can I keep people from realising I have an erection?' It is important to tell them what they want to know and what they can expect to happen as they mature sexually.

During encounters with parents, nurses can be open and available for questions and discussion. They can set an example by the language they use in discussing body parts and their function and by the way in which they deal with problems that have emotional overtones, such as exploratory sex play and masturbation. Parents need help to understand normal behaviours and to view sexual curiosity in their children as a part of the developmental process. Assessing the parents' level of knowledge and understanding of sexuality provides cues to their need for supplemental information that will prepare them for increasingly complex explanations as their children grow older.

COPING WITH CONCERNS RELATED TO NORMAL GROWTH AND DEVELOPMENT

Discipline

Numerous factors influence the amount and manner of discipline imposed on school-age children: the parents' psychosocial maturity, their own childrearing experiences during childhood, the children's temperament, the context of the children's misconduct and the children's response to rewards and punishments. Discipline serves many purposes: (1) to help the child interrupt or inhibit a forbidden action; (2) to point out a more acceptable form of behaviour so that the child knows what is right in a future situation; (3) to provide some reason, understandable to the child, that explains why one action is inappropriate and another action is more desirable; and (4) to stimulate the child's ability to empathise with the victim of a misdeed.

As children are increasingly able to see a situation from the point of view of another, they are able to understand the effects of their reactions on others and themselves. Disciplinary techniques should help children control their own behaviour.

To be effective, discipline should take place in an environment characterised by positive, supportive parent–child relationships and should involve strategies that educate and guide desired behaviours and eliminate undesired or ineffective behaviours.

Parents should not use punitive actions or corporal punishment because these methods are of limited value and are associated with multiple negative consequences. In particular, physically aggressive parenting practices that involve spanking are linked to children with: poor internalising behaviours such as depression, anxiety and hopelessness; poor externalising behaviours such as aggression and violence; slower cognitive development; and increased risk for physical abuse (Hornor et al 2015). Reasoning, on the other hand, is an effective disciplinary technique for school-age children; however, use of a time-out may be necessary to stop the behaviour acutely.

As their cognitive skills advance, school-age children are able to benefit from more complex disciplinary strategies. For example, withholding privileges, requiring recompense, imposing penalties and contracting can be used with great success. Problem-solving is the best approach to limit setting, and children themselves can be included in the process of determining appropriate disciplinary measures.

Dishonest Behaviour

During middle childhood, children may engage in what is considered to be antisocial behaviour. Lying, stealing and cheating may become manifest in previously well-behaved children. This is especially disturbing to parents, who may have difficulty coping with such behaviour.

Telling lies can occur for a number of reasons. Preschool children often have difficulty distinguishing between fact and fantasy. They do not have the cognitive capacity to deliberately mislead. Sometimes they misperceive or fail to remember an event. By the time they reach school age, they still tell stories but can distinguish between what is real and what is make-believe. If not, they need to learn to distinguish between fantasy and reality. Often children will exaggerate a story or situation as a means to impress their family or friends.

Young children lie to escape punishment or get out of some difficulty, even when the evidence of their misbehaviour is evident. Lying is more common in families in which punishment is severe. When parents model honesty and veracity, the children will often behave in the same way. If parents lie, the children will emulate their behaviour. Older children may lie to meet expectations set by others to which they have been unable to measure up. They may also lie because of low self-esteem or as a means of getting ahead or acquiring something with little effort. However, most children are concerned with the wrongfulness of lying and cheating—especially in their friends. They are quick to tell on others when they detect cheating.

Parents need to be reassured that all children lie sometimes and that they often have difficulty separating fantasy from reality. Healthcare professionals should help parents understand the importance of their own behaviour as role models and of being truthful in their relationships with children. Parents can discuss the issue with the children directly to impress on them how much of their own security and respect is lost when they are not believed.

Cheating is most common in young children ages 5 to 6 years. They find it difficult to lose at a game or contest, and they cheat to win. They have not yet acquired the full realisation of the wrongfulness of this behaviour and do it almost automatically. It usually disappears as they mature. However, when children observe parental behaviours such as boasting about cheating on income taxes, they assume this to be appropriate behaviour. Parents need to be aware of the types of behaviours they model for their children. When they set examples of honesty, children are more likely to conform to these standards.

As with other ethically related behaviour, stealing is not an unexpected event in the younger child. Between ages 5 and 8 years, children's sense of property rights is limited; they tend to take something simply because they are attracted to it, or they take money for what it will buy. They are equally likely to give away something valuable that belongs to them. When young children are caught and punished, they are penitent—they 'didn't mean to' and promise 'never to do it again', but they may well repeat the performance the following day. Often they not only steal but lie about it as well or attempt to justify the act with excuses. It is seldom helpful to trap children into admission by asking directly if they did the offensive thing. Children do not take on such responsibility until nearer the end of middle childhood.

Children steal for several reasons: lack of a sense of property rights, an attempt to acquire the means with which to bribe other children for favours, a strong desire to own the coveted item or a wish for revenge to 'get back at someone' (usually a parent) for what they consider to be unfair treatment. Older children may steal to supplement an inadequate income from other sources. Sometimes stealing is an indication that something is seriously wrong or lacking in the child's life. Children may steal to make up for a perceived lack of love or another satisfaction.

In some settings in which living arrangements are crowded, children have little privacy and much of the family property is communal, children may fail to develop a sense of property rights. Sometimes parents unintentionally confuse children with seemingly conflicting values. In an attempt to teach unselfishness, they may force children to share belongings with others, with the result that the children fail to understand property rights.

If children are told not to take money from their mother's purse or their father's pocket but observe the parents doing the same thing, they receive conflicting messages. Parents may go through a child's pockets or other private areas at night and even discard, without explanation, items of which they do not approve. Children should have a place that is private to them alone that other family members respect. If children's personal rights are respected, they are more likely to respect the rights of others.

It is difficult for many parents to cope with stealing by their children. In most situations it is best not to attempt to find a hidden or deep meaning to the stealing. A reprimand, together with an appropriate and reasonable punishment, such as having the older child pay back the money or return the stolen items, will ordinarily take care of most cases. Most children can learn to respect the property rights of others with little difficulty despite temptations and opportunities. Some children simply need more time to learn the importance of the culture's rules regarding private property.

Coping with Stress

Children today experience significant amounts of stress. This stress comes from a variety of sources. Other sections in this book discuss dealing with specific types of stresses, especially those in which nurses assume a major role, such as hospitalisation, illness, abuse, disabling injuries and death or the threat of death.

In the normal course of growing up, children are pressured by their peers to identify with their friends; to eat, dress and look like their friends; to talk about the same things that their friends talk about; to engage in the same activities as their friends; and yet to compete with them. They are pressured by parents to excel in school, in athletics and in social situations at ever-younger ages. Children in the middle years can be overcommitted with activities such as dance lessons, music lessons, athletics and other activities until the cumulative effect is overwhelming.

Although children receive better treatment than in earlier times, when beatings and child labour were common, their physical and emotional wellbeing is threatened by different stresses. The high divorce rate and the number of single-parent families result in altered relationships and increasing responsibilities for children. Children are stressed by various conflicts within the home.

Children's exposure to household activities such as alcohol or substance abuse, family or domestic violence or criminal activity is a significant problem in Australia and New Zealand. Family violence refers to any violence between family members including extended and kinship relationships (Council of Australian Governments [COAG] 2011). In this form of violence the perpetrator exercises power and control over another person; this can be sexual or non-sexual. Domestic violence is considered a subset of family violence. It refers to violent behaviour between current or previous intimate partners (Australian Institute of Health and Welfare [AIHW] 2018). It is estimated in Australia that 1 in 6 women (16% or 1.5 million) and 1 in 9 men (11% or 992,000) experienced physical and/or sexual abuse before the age of 15 (Australian Bureau of Statistics [ABS] 2016). More than two-fifths of all sexual assaults recorded against children aged 0 to 14 were perpetrated by a family member (ABS 2018). Indigenous women and children, those from culturally and linguistically diverse (CALD) backgrounds and women and children with disabilities are at higher risk of family violence (Frohmader et al 2015) (see Cultural Considerations box).

CULTURAL CONSIDERATIONS

The prevalence of child exposure to family violence is more frequent in Indigenous populations, which is reflected in a higher rate of domestic and family violence within Aboriginal and Torres Strait Islander populations (Human Rights and Equal Opportunity Commission [HREOC] 2006, Steering Committee for the Review of Government Service Provision [SCRGSP] 2011). Indigenous women and girls are 31 times more likely to be hospitalised as a result of domestic and family violence than non-Aboriginal women and girls, and violence is more prevalent in regional and city areas compared to remote areas (SCRGSP 2011). Within Indigenous communities, domestic and family violence needs to be understood in the context of a history of colonisation, dispossession of land, forced child removal, racism and discrimination and the resulting intergenerational trauma that has arisen from this history (Cripps & Davis 2012, Millward 2013). When working with Indigenous children and their families, responses need to be culturally sensitive and community-informed (Cripps & Davis 2012). The nurses should consider:

- breakdown of kinship systems and Aboriginal law
- experiences of racism, discrimination and vilification
- economic exclusion and entrenched poverty
- alcohol and drug abuse
- institutionalisation and child removal policies, and
- the effects of grief and, trauma on parenting (Cripps & Davis 2012).

Being exposed to family violence can have a wide range of detrimental impacts on a child's development, mental and physical health, housing situation and general wellbeing (AIHW 2018). They are at risk of diminished educational attainment, physical and psychological disorders, suicidal ideation, behavioural difficulties and, homelessness and are more likely to display antisocial behaviour and potentially become abusive parents (AIHW 2018, Bland & Shallcross 2015, Campo 2015, Jaffe et al 2012).

However, exposure to family violence alone does not mean a child will necessarily experience negative outcomes. With the right support, children exposed to family violence may have increased resilience later in life (Campo 2015, Jaffe et al 2012).

Exposure to violence in the family, school or community affects children's ability to concentrate and function. Children may be traumatised by witnessing violence and develop fear, insecurity and a sense of helplessness, which can result in social withdrawal and behavioural regression (Levendosky et al 2013). Children exposed to repeated violence can display hyperarousal symptoms leading to posttraumatic stress disorder and symptoms such as nightmares, flashbacks, a fatalistic orientation to the future, depression and anxiety (Levendosky et al 2013).

The school environment may also pose a threat to children's self-image. School-age children have a high fear of failure and criticism (Muris et al 2014). Competing with classmates for marks and teacher recognition, failing an examination, being teased or made fun of in school or being labelled as 'stupid' or 'learning disabled' all result in emotional distress. Teachers or parents may not always recognise or appreciate the worries or sources of stress for school-age children.

Some children are encouraged to feel, think and behave at a level of maturity far beyond what could reasonably be expected of individuals their age. They are expected to take on many adult-type responsibilities, to make decisions they may not be able to make and to achieve more. An emphasis on high test marks can increase stress. Children have little time for being young and enjoying the spontaneous activities of childhood.

When asked to describe sources of worry, school-age children identified concerns such as social threats (e.g. conflicts with friends), medical procedures, danger and death and the unknown (Muris et al 2014). These worries were more prominent in girls versus boys and tend to decrease as children became older (Muris et al 2014). Other potential sources of stress are listed in Box 15.1.

Children respond to stress by using various adaptive and maladaptive coping mechanisms (Skinner et al 2016). Adaptive coping consists of problem-solving, emotional regulation such as mediation or talking with friends and cognitive reappraisal such as reshaping one's thoughts about a situation. Maladaptive coping techniques include internalising symptoms such as withdrawal and helplessness along with externalising symptoms such as aggression and blaming others (Skinner et al 2016). Variables that contribute to children's ability to use adaptive coping include socioeconomic status, family relationships, social support, gender and previous life experiences.

To help children cope with the stresses in their lives, the parent, teacher or healthcare professional must recognise signs that indicate that a child is undergoing stress (see Box 15.1) and identify the source promptly. Children need to learn how to recognise signs of stress in themselves, such as a pounding heart, rapid breathing or 'butterflies' in the stomach. Once they are able to recognise that they are stressed, they can employ techniques for managing their stress. Children can learn relaxation techniques such as deep-breathing exercises, progressive relaxation of muscle groups and positive imagery to reduce stress. Encouraging them to 'blow off steam' through physical activity reduces tension and anxiety. Children need to learn to identify their stress reactions and strategies to reduce stress. Children should list all possibilities to reduce or minimise stress, including those they know will not work. They need to examine what might happen as a consequence of each alternative. The final step is to select what they perceive to be the best option. It is sometimes helpful to have children model their behaviour after that of someone they know who has successfully coped with a similar problem. When children work through this process a few times, they are able to apply problem-solving automatically.

NURSING CARE CONSIDERATIONS

The nurse who observes the following signs of stress in a child should explore the situation further:

- stomach pains or headache
- sleep problems
- bedwetting
- changes in eating habits
- aggressive or stubborn behaviour
- withdrawal or reluctance to participate
- regression to earlier behaviours (e.g. thumb sucking)
- trouble concentrating or changes in academic performance.

Fears

Several anxiety symptoms, including fear of the dark, excessive worry about past behaviour, self-consciousness, social withdrawal and an excessive need for reassurance, are considered normal developmental events for children. School-age children are less fearful of body safety than they were as preschoolers, although they still fear being hurt, kidnapped or having to undergo surgery. They also fear death and are fascinated by all aspects of death and dying. They have less fear of noises, darkness, storms and dogs. Most new fears that trouble school-age children are related to school and family (e.g. fear of failing, fear of teachers and bullies or fear of something bad happening to their parents).

Parents and other persons involved with children should discuss children's fears with them individually or through group activities. Their viewpoints must be respected, and their need to communicate their concerns should be recognised. Sometimes school-age children are inclined to hide their fears to avoid being ridiculed or labelled as a 'baby' or 'chicken'. Hiding fears does not end them, and children who are afraid to communicate their fears may develop displaced fears or phobias. Children need to know that their concerns are heard and understood. Parents who convey this to their children without becoming overprotective help their children feel less lonely and less frightened.

PROMOTING OPTIMUM HEALTH DURING THE SCHOOL YEARS

Health Behaviours

During the middle childhood years, children acquire increased cognitive skills that allow them to make decisions about health behaviours they will select and pursue. In addition to personal traits, children establish health behaviours through social and environmental variables. By the end of middle childhood, children should be able to assume personal responsibility for self-care in the areas of hygiene, nutrition, exercise, recreation, sleep and safety. In general, school-age boys and girls view themselves as healthy and can manage their own care in the areas of seat belt use, exercise, emergency situations and dental health.

Health education is a primary component of comprehensive healthcare, and health education programs should promote desired health behaviour through guided learning and modelling. An optimum program helps children learn about their bodies and about the effect of their behaviour on their health.

BOX 15.1 Potential Sources of Stress in Middle Childhood

Sources of Stress for the 6 Year Old

- **Expectations**—Parents, teachers and other adults beginning to demand more
- **School**—Year 1 introduces the child to the more formal, academic setting; may be the child's first experience away from home all day
- **Activity level**—May find it difficult to sit still for long periods or control impulses
- **Competition**—Wants to be 'first' or best
- **Shyness**—May initially be shy in a new situation but usually recovers quickly
- **Aggression**—May become hostile or aggressive; temper tantrums peak
- **Sensitivity**—Begins to read body language or facial expressions and becomes upset when sensing disapproval
- **Teasing**—Engages in teasing but becomes upset when on the receiving end
- **Decisions**—Has difficulty coping with increasing independence
- **Jealousy**—Sibling rivalry is common
- **Fears**—Usually centre around newly found independence and might include fear of getting lost or fear of making an embarrassing social blunder

Sources of Stress for the 7 Year Old

- **Moodiness**—Is often moody, unhappy or pensive
- **Approval**—Continues to need praise and approval from peer group and parents
- **Modesty**—Demands privacy when in the bathroom or dressing
- **Organisation**—Is comfortable with rules, regulations, routines and order; becomes upset when they are disrupted
- **Interruptions**—Hates to be disturbed when intensely involved in an activity
- **Idols**—Has a desire to be more like an admired idol
- **Friendship**—Becomes more selective about playmates

Sources of Stress for the 8 Year Old

- **Self-criticism**—Is very critical of personal ability and performance
- **Parental authority**—Is beginning to resent parental authority
- **Loneliness**—Likes frequent interaction with friends; may hate to miss school
- **Praise**—Continues to seek approval but can identify when praise is not genuine
- **Independence**—May begin to stay alone for brief periods while parents run errands, with resulting feelings of uneasiness

Sources of Stress for the 9 Year Old

- **Rebelliousness**—Occasionally tests independence by rebelling
- **Opposite sex**—Engages in sex-segregated play; expresses an aversion to the opposite sex
- **Fair play**—Has a keen sense of what is fair and is vehement in demanding personal rights when a situation is perceived as unfair
- **Interruptions**—Continues to dislike interruptions but will usually resume an activity after an interruption
- **Propriety**—Has a sense of propriety and will often be upset if siblings or parents offend the child's notion of decorum or dignity

Sources of Stress for the 10 to 12 Year Old

- **Sexual maturation**—Girls, in particular, may become self-conscious regarding obvious signs of puberty
- **Social issues**—A new level of awareness can generate concern regarding pressing societal problems
- **Stature**—Both boys and girls may be upset by the fact that the girls are taller; the extremely small or extremely large child may be concerned about his or her size
- **Shyness**—If the child already has a problem in this area, it is likely to become more pronounced at this stage
- **Opposite sex**—May become interested, yet shy, around members of the opposite sex
- **Confusion**—Too much freedom can cause the child to flounder or make bad decisions
- **Health**—May become a hypochondriac during this period of development
- **Money**—Is anxious to earn and handle money but often uses poor judgment
- **Competition**—Continues to be highly competitive and looks to peer group for prestige
- **Burnout**—May become vigorously involved in so many activities that he or she finally becomes exhausted
- **Self-concept**—May engage in teasing, scapegoating or vicious attacks to temporarily boost his or her self-image; guilt often ensues; may be self-conscious about attempting a new skill
- **Parents**—Often becomes highly critical or intolerant of parents
- **Idols**—Continues hero worshipping
- **Fair play**—Continues to have a highly developed sense of fair play
- **Drugs and sex**—May be tempted to experiment with drugs or sex because 'everyone' is doing it
- **Peer pressure**—Becomes a powerful motivating force
- **Self-criticism**—May be highly critical of personal performance

*Violence is a universal stress at all ages (see text).
Source: Kuczen, B. (1982). Childhood stress: Don't let your child be a victim. New York: Delacorte Press.

Health promotion projects teach school-age children that social decision-making to promote health is important. Children who engage in healthy behaviours, attain skills in self-control and problem-solving and know others care about them engage in fewer health risk behaviours (Horner et al 2012).

Children can also learn to take a more active role in relationships with healthcare providers. If asked what they would like to ask the health practitioner, most children are able to formulate several questions related to the reason for their visit. Providers can also teach children how to ask these questions so they can learn about their health during well-child visits to the paediatrician, child health nurse and school nurse.

Nutrition

Although caloric needs are diminished in relation to body size during middle childhood, resources are being laid down for the increased growth needs of the adolescent period. It is important to impress on children and their parents the value of a balanced diet to promote growth. When children enter school, they develop an eating style that is increasingly independent from parental influence and scrutiny.

Likes and dislikes established at an early age continue in middle childhood, although the inclination for single-food preferences begins to end and children acquire a taste for an increasing variety of foods. Because children usually eat as the family does, the quality of their diet depends to a large extent on their family's pattern of eating. Other interests and participation in outside activities often compete with mealtime.

Outside Influences

With the influence of the mass media and the temptation of an immense variety of 'junk food', it is all too easy for children to fill up on empty calories—foods that do not promote growth, such as sugars, starches and excess fats. They have more freedom to move without parental supervision and often have small amounts of money to spend on lollies, chocolate, soft drinks and other easily accessible treats. Mid-afternoon snacks are common, and it is wise to encourage consumption of fruit, nuts and other wholesome finger foods to meet this need. Nutrition is a joint responsibility of both the child and the family.

The popularity of fast-food restaurants has aroused the attention of nutritionists and other healthcare professionals concerned with children's nutrition. The restaurants provide fast service, they are relatively inexpensive and appealing to children and their convenience makes them attractive to busy parents as an alternative to eating at home. Because the nutritional content of fast foods is usually available, it is easier for nutrition-conscious parents to help children select appropriate items from the available menu. Nurses can support consumer advocate groups to encourage restaurants to offer items higher in nutritional value (such as skim milk, broiled meats and fresh fruits and vegetables) and to list ingredients and nutritional content on the menu as required for packaged foods.

Childhood obesity is a common health problem in school-age children. In Australia around 1 in 4 (24%) of children aged 5 to 14 years are overweight or obese (AIHW 2020). The availability of inexpensive high-calorie foods, the tendency towards sedentary activities (such as watching television and playing electronic games), insufficient sleep and the trend towards transportation by motor vehicle instead of walking or cycling have reduced caloric expenditure. The consumption of a high-fat diet also contributes to obesity. The problem of childhood obesity is discussed further in Chapter 16. Given the threat of obesity and a diet-conscious society, many school-age children start to diet in an effort to prevent obesity or lose weight or to conform to peer behaviours and pressures. Children need education about food selection and the importance of body-building nutrients as opposed to empty caloric intake.

Sleep and Rest

The amount of sleep and rest required during middle childhood is highly individualised. The specific amount of needed sleep depends on the child's age, activity level and other factors such as health status. The growth rate slows in the school-age years; therefore less energy is expended in growth than during the preceding periods.

Sleep requirements decrease during school-age years; 5 year olds generally require 10 to 13 hours of sleep, whereas 11 year olds require approximately 9 to 11 hours of sleep (Allen et al 2016). School-age children usually do not require a nap. Fewer bedtime problems occur during these years, but occasional difficulties are still associated with the necessary bedtime ritual.

A firm approach to bedtime is usually the most successful. Parents can help children by giving them a little advance warning, but children should realise that when the final bedtime is announced, the parents mean it.

Sleep Problems. During middle childhood, night-time sleep is usually continuous, and the child has developed a repertoire of tactics (such as reading or playing quietly without involving the parents) to deal with occasional difficulties in falling asleep. If a child has a sleep problem, a thorough assessment may be necessary to plan appropriate interventions.

The cause of bedtime resistance is not always clear. For some children it is related to normal fears of their age, such as fear of the dark, strange noises, intruders or other imagined phenomena. Children who are subject to frightening dreams are hesitant to retire, and their sleep is more likely to be disturbed after emotional stimulation before bedtime. Sometimes children are unwilling to give up an exciting or interesting activity, or they are reluctant to leave the protective social circle of the family. Another factor associated with reluctance to go to bed is related to status. For example, older children are given the privilege of a later bedtime than younger children. Promotion to a later bedtime is highly prestigious, and age-mates compare their bedtimes. This may explain why children who believe that playmates enjoy a more privileged position strongly oppose parental decisions. In some situations going to bed is used as a method of control. When going to bed early is imposed as a punishment or when staying up late is a reward, children may view bedtime as punitive or status degrading.

Some children resort to multiple 'curtain calls', such as wanting a drink of water, asking for one more story, needing to go to the bathroom or wanting to watch television. Some children persist in coming out of their rooms repeatedly after being put back to bed. Some voice fears, such as 'there is someone outside the window'. Parents may have difficulty determining whether the fear is legitimate or whether the behaviour is a bid for attention. Consistent reassurance and limit setting usually resolve the problem. Children feel tense and insecure when limits are applied inconsistently, such as when parents grant permission one night and punish the next for the same behaviour.

The night terrors of preschool children may be replaced by sleepwalking and sleep talking. Like night terrors, sleepwalking is associated with the transition from stage 4 to stage 1 of non–rapid eye movement sleep. When children arouse from stage 4 sleep, it is often difficult for them to reach a fully alert, wakeful state rapidly. Sleepwalking occurs in the first 3 to 4 hours of sleep. Children often have no memory of sleepwalking in the morning. The episode begins when the child sits up abruptly and walks, usually with open eyes. During sleepwalking, movements are clumsy and repetitive; parents often observe finger and hand movements. Most commonly, children move about restlessly, then lie down and return to sleep. Children rarely perform purposeful acts during sleepwalking. Any attempts to communicate with the child elicit only mumbled and slurred responses. Sleep talking, like sleepwalking, is not purposeful, and speech is usually incomprehensible and monosyllabic.

The best approach is to leave sleepwalking children alone unless they are in danger or may endanger others. However, clumsiness and stereotyped movements can make sleepwalking very dangerous. If the environment is not safe, children can get hurt. Instruct parents to gently redirect children back to bed without waking them, if possible. If children must be wakened, it is best to call them by name slowly and softly, orient them to where they are, explain that they were walking in their sleep and assure them that it will not happen when they are more relaxed. Preventive measures include avoiding overfatigue in children, making certain they get adequate rest, employing relaxation techniques and relieving any stress the children may be experiencing.

Sleepwalking is usually self-limiting and resolves spontaneously. About 17% of children sleepwalk once during childhood, with a peak onset of 8 to 12 years of age (Carter et al 2014). Persistent sleepwalking occurs in children and adolescents who tend to repress strong emotions, such as anger. They may benefit from learning to express their feelings and from doing self-relaxation before bedtime.

Nightmares are a part of the normal developmental process; up to 50% of children experience nightmares during childhood (Carter et al 2014). Nightmares can begin in children 3 to 6 years of age and peak at 6 to 10 years of age (Carter et al 2014). Repetitive nightmares or increased nightmare frequency may indicate a specific underlying conflict or stressor that is strongly influencing the child's behaviour and thought. Resolving worries or stress will often reduce nightmares. If nightmares become chronic, parents should consider professional counselling (Carter et al 2014).

A traumatic event often produces posttraumatic nightmares, which are anxiety provoking and literal in their depiction of the trauma. As time goes on, the dreams of affected children may consist of 'modified repetitions' that may add more current material to the recurrent dreams (e.g. involving others who were not a part of the traumatic event). Current external stresses, movies or stories may also precipitate a nightmare by reactivating old traumas.

Physical Activity

Exercise is essential for muscle development and tone, refinement of balance and coordination, gaining of strength and endurance, and stimulation of body functions and metabolic processes. Throughout middle childhood, children's increasing capabilities and adaptability permit greater speed and effort in motor activities. Larger, stronger muscles with greater efficiency and skill permit longer and increasingly strenuous play without exhaustion. During this period, children acquire the coordination, timing and concentration that are required to participate in adult-type activities, even though they may lack the strength, stamina and control of the adolescent and adult. Consequently, parents should expect and encourage a larger amount of physical activity during the school years.

Children should have opportunities that provide satisfying experiences to meet individual likes and dislikes. Children need space to run, jump, skip and climb, as well as safe facilities and equipment to use both inside and outside. Appropriate activities that promote coordination and development include running, jumping rope, swimming, dancing and bike riding. Positive reinforcement achieved by experiencing increasingly smooth, rhythmic and efficient use of the body conditions the child towards regular physical activity. However, one must keep in mind that although school-age children are large and appear to be strong, they may not be prepared for strenuous competitive athletics.

Most children need little encouragement to engage in physical activity. They have so much energy that they seldom know when to stop. However, children with disabilities or those who hesitate to become involved in active play, such as obese children, require special assessment and help in determining activities that appeal to them, are compatible with their limitations and meet their developmental needs.

Physical Fitness

The development of physical fitness is a goal for all children. This goal was easy to accomplish in the past when school-age children spent a considerable amount of time each day playing on playgrounds, walking to school and participating in games or sports at school or in their communities. With the advent of technology and the information age, many children are less active physically and spend large portions of their day in front of electronic devices.

Nurses can promote efforts to include physical fitness in school programs and encourage children to engage in aerobic physical activities during their free time. Such activities provide cardiopulmonary benefits, maintain normal weight and have the potential to contribute to lifelong fitness.

Sports. Much controversy has surrounded the trend towards earlier participation in competitive athletics and the amount and type of competitive sports that are appropriate for children in the primary years. The current view is that virtually every child is suited for some type of sport, and authorities do not discourage participation if children are matched to the type of sport appropriate to their abilities and to their physical and emotional constitutions. School-age children enjoy competition, and when teachers, parents and coaches understand children's physical limitations and teach them the proper techniques and safety measures to avoid injury to developing bones and muscles, a safe and appropriate sport can be found for even the most unskilled and uncompetitive child.

BOX 15.2 Goals of Organised Athletics for School-age Children

Organised extracurricular athletic programs for school-age children should focus on helping children develop the following:

- enjoyment of sports and fitness that will be sustained through adulthood
- physical fitness
- fundamental movement skills
- positive self-image and self-regulation
- balanced perspective on sports in relation to the child's school and community life
- commitment to the values of teamwork, fair play and sportsmanship.

Source: Adapted from SPORTAUS, n.d. Nurturing a child's sporting development. Australian Sports Commission. https://www.sportaus.gov.au/athlete_development/top_10_tips_for_parents

During middle childhood, girls have the same basic structure as boys and thus have a similar response to systematic exercise training. At puberty, when boys become larger and have more muscle mass, it is usually recommended that girls compete only against other girls. Before puberty there is no essential difference in strength and size between girls and boys, which makes these precautions unnecessary.

Well-organised extracurricular sports programs based in the community or school encourage enjoyment of sports and fitness in childhood (Box 15.2). Preadolescence is a time to: teach fundamental motor skills; develop fitness in a practical, safe and gradual manner; and promote desired attitudes and values. Activities should include practice sessions and unstructured play. The actual game or event should be managed in a manner that stresses mastery of the sport and enhancement of self-image rather than winning or pleasing others. All children should have an opportunity to participate, and special ceremonies should recognise all participants rather than individuals.

In addition to ensuring the interest, suitability and safety of the sport, parents must make certain that coaches (if involved in the sport) are skilful in managing children and do not engage in abusive behaviour. Coaches, parents and others involved in children's sports play critical roles in shaping children's self-esteem. Any sport for children should emphasise the pleasure of the activity. It is wise to expose children to a variety of individual sports. The overall emphasis of both team and individual sports should be on playing and learning.

Acquisition of Skills

School-age children demonstrate increasing capacity in fine muscle facility and complex artistic skills. Handedness is well established by the beginning of the school years, and children make great strides in writing and drawing during this age period. It is a time of energetic and vibrant creative productivity. With the tools of language and reading, children can create poems, stories and plays. With more advanced fine motor skills, they are able to master an unlimited variety of handicrafts, such as ceramics, needlework, wood carving and beadwork. They avidly pursue these skills in solitude, with a friend or in programs offered through organisations such as boys' or girls' clubs or special interest groups that use crafts as a means to occupy, entertain and educate children.

Music is a favourite form of expression in middle childhood (Fig 15.7). Music stimulates and invigorates school-age children. They can sing in harmony, play instruments in orchestras and bands and manage music at a more complex level. They can compose original songs, learn lyrics almost effortlessly and turn any empty moment into an occasion for singing.

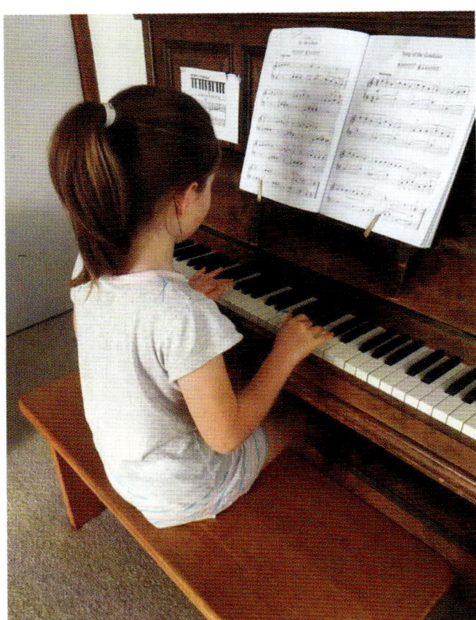

Fig 15.7 Music is a favourite form of expression for school-age children.

School-age children are capable of assuming responsibility for their own needs, although their distaste for soap and water and 'dress' clothes is legendary. School-age children can and want to assume their share of household tasks, which usually are related to the male and female roles that have been defined by their culture. Many also assume responsibility for tasks outside the home, such as babysitting or gardening.

Television, Video Games and the Internet

For some time, child development specialists and parents have been concerned about the effect of media on child development and behaviour. Digital media are integrated into the everyday lives of children and they spend a significant amount of time each day involved in media-related activities, including the use of television, the internet, electronic games and mobile phones. Because of the long periods of exposure, the media have more time to develop children's attitudes than do parents and teachers.

There is no doubt that children learn from various forms of media, but the values and attitudes depicted on these forums are not always realistic and may conflict with values that children were previously taught. School-age children can distinguish fantasy from reality, and some have had sufficient life experience to view information from media with scepticism. However, violence is common in various forms of media, and significant exposure to media violence increases aggressive behaviour, aggressive thoughts and angry feelings in some children (American Academy of Pediatrics, Council on Communications and Media 2016). In addition, repeated exposure to violence can desensitise children to violence, convey a message that violence is acceptable and teach children that initiating violent behaviour is a way to protect themselves (Brockmyer 2015).

Violence in the media can also increase fear and anxiety in children. Events such as terrorist attacks and mass shootings have infiltrated television and the internet, frequently exposing children to real-life violence. Viewing violence in the news can cause immediate effects such as fear, worry and attention difficulty, and can also cause long-term effects such as emotional problems and poor school performance (Leiner et al 2016). Parents should make the ultimate decisions about which programs their child will watch and which sites their child can use on the internet. To reduce exposure to violence and maximise the beneficial effects of television, parents are advised to monitor program selection, view programs with their children and discuss program content when the programs are finished (Leiner et al 2016). (See Chapter 2 for a more in-depth discussion of children and mass media.)

Electronic and internet games have been both criticised and supported in relation to their effect on children and adolescents. Critics maintain that games keep children from schoolwork and can cause tension, sleeplessness and violence. Others support the activity as a means for improving hand–eye coordination and as a substitute for the inactivity of passive television viewing. Benefits may also include development of inductive reasoning (i.e. drawing generalisations from specific observations), improving spatial perception and learning to handle multiple variables that interact simultaneously.

Research suggests that electronic games may affect physical and psychological functioning. Physical effects, including flickering of lights produced by video games, may trigger a reflex seizure (Koepp et al 2016). (See seizure discussion, Chapter 30.) However, research has noted some positive applications of electronic games with dyslexic children (Franceschini et al 2013).

The internet is a popular means for obtaining educational and recreational information. Information technology, particularly the internet, is now used in virtually every home in Australia and is a popular means for obtaining educational and recreational information. Ninety-seven per cent of households with children aged under 15 years have access to the internet, with an average number of seven devices per household (ABS 2016). Although these opportunities provide valuable educational opportunities for children, there are also many risks that parents must acknowledge before children access the internet. Major risks include exposure to inappropriate, dangerous or illegal material; sexual solicitation; exposure to harassment; revelation of financial information that leads to negative consequences; and safety issues relating to sharing personal information or meeting strangers. The best way to eliminate potential risks is discussed in Box 15.3.

Dental Health

The first permanent (secondary) teeth erupt at about 6 years of age. Before their appearance they have been developing in the jaw beneath the deciduous (primary) teeth. The roots of the latter are gradually absorbed, so when a deciduous tooth is shed, only the crown remains. At 6 years of age, all of the primary teeth are present, and those of the secondary dentition are relatively well formed. Eruption of the permanent teeth begins with the 6-year molar, which erupts posterior to the deciduous molars. The others appear in approximately the same order as in eruption of the primary teeth and follow shedding of the deciduous teeth (Fig 15.8).

The pattern of shedding of primary teeth and eruption of secondary teeth is subject to wide variation among children. To allow the larger permanent teeth to occupy the limited space left by shed primary teeth, a series of complicated changes must take place in the jaws. At this time many of the difficulties created by crowding of teeth become apparent. With the appearance of the second permanent (12-year) molars, most of the permanent teeth are present. The third permanent molars, or wisdom teeth, may erupt from 18 to 25 years of age or later. Permanent dentition is somewhat more advanced in girls than in boys.

Because permanent teeth erupt during the school-age years, good dental hygiene and regular attention to dental caries are vital parts of health supervision during this period. Tooth decay is a common problem, and 42% of children ages 2 to 11 years have tooth decay in their primary teeth (AIHW 2020). Children of this age tend to become careless about oral hygiene unless they are carefully supervised. Although children are assuming more responsibility for their own care, they are not as motivated by improved appearance and odour as they will be during adolescence. Nurses should be alert for opportunities to teach correct brushing and flossing techniques; to reinforce avoidance

BOX 15.3 Promoting Healthy Digital Media Use

Healthcare providers can promote healthy digital media use by counselling every family to remember four essential 'Ms'.

- **Manage** screen use. Advise parents to:
  - make and regularly review or revise a family media plan, including individualised time and content limits
  - continue to be present and engaged when screens are used and, whenever possible, co-view and talk about content with children and teens
  - learn about parental controls and privacy settings
  - speak proactively with children and teens about acceptable and unacceptable online behaviours.
- Encourage **meaningful** screen use. Advise parents to:
  - prioritise daily routines, such as interacting face-to-face, sleep and physical activity over screen use
  - prioritise screen activities that are educational, active or social over those that are passive or unsocial
  - help children and teens to choose developmentally appropriate content and to recognise problematic content or behaviours
  - be a part of their children's media lives; for example, join in during video game play and ask about their experiences and encounters online.
- **Model** healthy screen use:
  - encourage parents to review their own media habits, and plan time for alternative hobbies, outdoor play and activities
  - remind parents and adolescents of the dangers of texting or using headphones while driving, walking, jogging or biking
  - encourage daily 'screen-free' times, especially for family meals and socialising
  - remind parents and teens to avoid screens at least 1 hour before bedtime and discourage recreational screen use in bedrooms.
- **Monitor** for signs of problematic screen use at any age, including the following:
  - complaints about being bored or unhappy without access to technology
  - oppositional behaviour in response to screen time limits
  - screen use that interferes with sleep, school or face-to-face interactions
  - screen time that interferes with offline play, physical activity or socialising face-to-face
  - negative emotions following online interactions or video games or while texting.

Source: Adapted from Canadian Paediatric Society. (2019). Digital media: Promoting healthy screen use in school-aged children and adolescents. Paediatric Child Health, 24(6), 402–408.

of fermentable carbohydrates and sticky sweets; and to be alert for problems of malocclusion, toothache and mouth infections.

Comprehensive dental supervision should be an integral part of the health maintenance program. Regular dental prophylaxis (teeth cleaning) by a dentist or dental hygienist and continued fluoride supplementation are essential to decrease the susceptibility of the tooth enamel to acid breakdown. (See Chapter 12 for a discussion of fluoride and other aspects of dental care.)

Brushing

The most effective means of preventing tooth decay is a regimen of proper oral hygiene. Children should learn to carry out their own dental care with the supervision and guidance of parents. Parents should learn proper brushing technique along with their children and should inspect their children's efforts until the children can assume full responsibility for their own care.

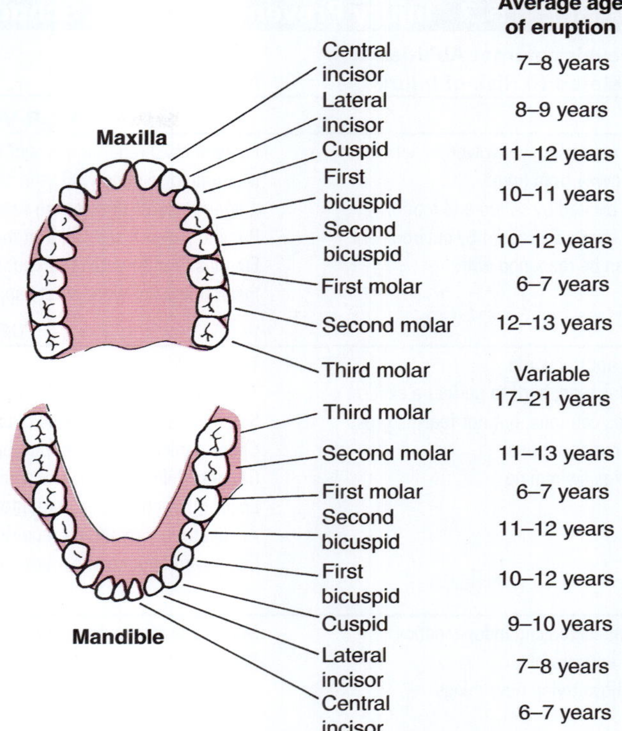

Fig 15.8 Sequence of eruption of secondary teeth.

Most practitioners believe that the majority of children do not possess the fine motor skills needed to brush their teeth properly until approximately 8 years old. Ideally, children should brush teeth after meals, after snacks and at bedtime. The bedtime brushing is especially important because there is more time overnight for interaction between oral bacteria and unremoved substrate on the tooth substance. Children who brush their teeth frequently and become accustomed to the feel of a clean mouth at an early age usually maintain the habit throughout life.

Health Education

Health education of school-age children focuses on providing knowledge of health and influencing habits, attitudes and conduct in relation to health. A viable health education program is based on sound health concepts but should be adjusted to meet specific local needs, objectives and legal requirements. Parents must understand and approve the health education curriculum so that its teaching will be reinforced at home. A comprehensive approach to health education is more successful in developing positive health practices than one in which the subjects are taught in isolation. Many topics presented in health education classes are associated with differing social and cultural attitudes and should be presented accurately and with sensitivity to these attitudes.

Injury Prevention

Because school-age children have developed more refined muscular coordination and control and can apply their cognitive capacities to select a more judicious course of action, the incidence of unintentional injury is diminished in middle childhood compared with the incidence in early childhood. School-age children have exposure to more environments in which they need protection, they acquire skills and interests that expose them to new perils, they have less supervision and they take more responsibility as they begin to participate in the adult world.

Injuries most prevalent in school-age children reflect their developmental stage. Table 15.2 outlines the developmental characteristics and

TABLE 15.2 **Injury Prevention During School-age Years**

Developmental Abilities Related to Risk of Injury	Injury Prevention
	MOTOR VEHICLE CRASHES
Is increasingly involved in activities away from home Is excited by speed and motion Is easily distracted by environment Can be reasoned with	Educate child regarding proper use of seat belts while a passenger in a vehicle. Maintain discipline while the child is a passenger in a vehicle (e.g. ensure that child keeps arms inside, does not lean against doors or interfere with driver). Remind parents and children that no one should ride on the back of a ute. Emphasise safe pedestrian behaviour. Insist that child wear safety apparel (e.g. helmet) when applicable, such as riding a bicycle.
	DROWNING
Is apt to overdo May work hard to perfect a skill Has cautious, but not fearful, gross motor actions Likes swimming	Teach child to swim. Teach basic rules of water safety. Select safe and supervised places to swim. Check sufficient water depth for diving. Caution child to swim with a companion. Ensure that child uses an approved flotation device in water or boat. Advocate for legislation requiring fencing around pools. Learn cardiopulmonary resuscitation.
	BURNS
Has increasing independence Is adventurous Enjoys trying new things	Make sure smoke detectors are in homes. Set water heaters to 48.9°C to avoid scald burns. Instruct child regarding behaviour in areas involving contact with potential burn hazards (e.g. petrol, matches, bonfires or barbecues, lighter fluid, fireworks, cigarette lighters, cooking utensils, chemistry sets). Instruct child to avoid climbing or flying kite around high-tension wires. Instruct child in proper behaviour in the event of fire (e.g. fire drills at home and school). Teach child safe cooking (e.g. use low heat; avoid any frying; be careful of steam burns, scalds or exploding foods, especially from microwaving).
	POISONING
Adheres to group rules May be easily influenced by peers Has strong allegiance to friends	Educate child regarding hazards of taking non-prescription drugs and chemicals, including aspirin and alcohol. Teach child to say 'no' if offered illegal or dangerous drugs or alcohol. Keep potentially dangerous products in properly labelled receptacles, preferably out of reach.
	BODILY DAMAGE
Has increased physical skills Needs strenuous physical activity Is interested in acquiring new skills and perfecting attained skills Is daring and adventurous, especially with peers May play in hazardous places Confidence often exceeds physical capacity Desires group loyalty and has strong need for friends' approval Attempts hazardous feats Accompanies friends to potentially hazardous facilities Delights in physical activity Is likely to overdo Growth in height exceeds muscular growth and coordination	Help provide facilities for supervised activities. Encourage playing in safe places. Keep firearms safely locked up except with adult supervision. Teach proper care of, use of and respect for potentially dangerous devices (e.g. power tools, fireworks). Teach children not to tease or surprise dogs, invade their territory, take dogs' toys or interfere with dogs' feeding. Stress use of eye, ear or mouth protection when using potentially hazardous objects or devices or when engaged in potentially hazardous sports. Teach safety regarding use of trampolines. Teach safety regarding use of corrective devices (glasses); if child wears contact lenses, monitor duration of wear to prevent corneal damage. Stress careful selection, use and maintenance of sports and recreation equipment, such as bicycles. Emphasise proper conditioning, safe practices and use of safety equipment for sports or recreational activities. Caution against engaging in hazardous sports, such as those involving trampolines. Use safety glass and decals on large glassed areas, such as sliding glass doors. Use window guards to prevent falls. Teach name, address and phone number and emphasise that child should ask for help from appropriate people (e.g. cashier, security guard, police) if lost; have identification on child (e.g. sewn in clothes, inside shoe). Teach safety and stranger awareness. • Avoid personalised clothing in public places. • Never go with a stranger. • Have child tell parents if anyone makes child feel uncomfortable in any way. • Teach child to say 'no' when confronted with uncomfortable situations. • Always listen to child's concerns regarding others' behaviour.

accomplishments of middle childhood that predispose children to physical injury and offers guidelines for injury prevention.

The incidence of injury during middle childhood is significantly higher in school-age boys than in school-age girls, and their death rate is twice that of girls (see Chapter 1). Most injuries occur in or near the home or school. The prevalence of injury depends on the dangers present in the environment, the protection offered by adults and the behaviour patterns of the children. Safety helmets, protective eye and mouth shields and protective padding are strongly recommended for children engaging in active sports. Although school-age children are conscious of rules and frequently impose them in relationships with peers, they also tend to challenge established rules. It is often difficult to maintain a balance between the level of supervision and restriction needed by children and their need for freedom and independence.

The incidence of transportation-related injuries is higher in school-age children than in younger children, and the incidence of bicycle injury not involving a motor vehicle is higher than that in teenagers and preschool children. Injuries from burns and poisonings are lowest in school-age children. However, physically active school-age children are susceptible to cuts and abrasions, and the incidence of childhood fractures, strains and sprains is high.

Risk-taking Behaviour

Achieving social acceptance is a primary objective for school-age children. They often attempt dangerous acts (sometimes extreme behaviours) to prove themselves worthy of acceptance and improve their status in the peer group. Peer pressure is a normal part of psychological development, but it is also a major contributor to risk-taking behaviours. Peer challenges often encourage problem behaviours that place children at risk for injury or hazardous habits. School-age children are in the process of moving from preoperational to concrete operational thinking and are only beginning to understand causal relationships. Therefore, they may attempt certain activities without planning or evaluating the consequences.

Children who are risk takers may have inadequate self-regulatory behaviour. These children need to learn the motivation or the incentives for such behaviour and to visualise the possible consequences if the risk-taking behaviour ends in a tragic outcome.

Motor Vehicle Injury

As in all other age groups, the most common cause of severe accidental injury and death in school-age children is involvement in motor vehicle crashes—as either a pedestrian, a passenger or on bicycles. Most of the injuries occur when children misinterpret traffic signs or disobey common traffic safety regulations, cross the street against a red light, cross at places other than designated pedestrian crossings, dart into the street or walk in the same direction as the traffic. Parents consistently overestimate the street-crossing skills of young children ages 5 to 6 years and need education about their children's developmental abilities and competence as pedestrians. Nurses can help parents develop more realistic expectations of their children's behaviour and teach them to model safe street-crossing behaviours through pedestrian skills training programs.

Use of restraint systems, door-lock mechanisms and appropriate passenger seating and behaviour are simple but effective measures for eliminating injuries and reducing the severity of crash injuries. The correct use of seat restraints is essential.

When in the car, school-age children should always be buckled properly in a weight-, height- and age-appropriate seat. Injuries to children ages 5 to 9 years restrained in adult-type seat belts are related to anatomical differences between adults and children. The child's sitting height is less than the adult's, and the child's centre of gravity is located above the level of the lap belt. Consequently, the greater proportion of body mass above the belt may cause more forward motion and jack-knifing over the belt, which increases the risk of head injury from impact with interior vehicle parts. The child's smaller and less developed iliac crests are not suited to serve as an anchor for belts designed to restrain adults, and their intraabdominal organs are less protected by the bony pelvis. The natural behaviour of children, such as readjusting the seating position, moving about and otherwise altering the fit of the restraint, also influences its effectiveness.

All-terrain vehicles (ATVs), designed for off-road use by children and adolescents, are popular with children under 16 years of age but are responsible for a significant number of childhood injuries. These vehicles have a short wheelbase and low profile, which make them relatively unstable and unable to be seen easily. The vehicles can also achieve substantial speed. Most injuries occur when the driver loses control of the vehicle, is thrown from the vehicle or collides with fixed objects or other vehicles. Immature judgment and poorly developed motor skills also contribute to injury. Children under the age of 16 should not use quad bikes, as either a driver or a passenger.

Bicycle Injury

The majority of school-age children have bicycles and love riding them, but this increases their risk of injury on streets and roads. Many injuries are related to the bicyclist breaking traffic laws, including wrong-way riding (facing traffic), failure to give way and turning violations. Others are related to road conditions described as hazardous: bumps, potholes and gravel. Bicycle-related injuries occur in young children playing in their own neighbourhoods and in older children using their bicycles for transportation on streets with heavy traffic.

In addition to major injuries, cuts and bruises from falls and collisions account for a large number of injuries. Other injuries include trauma to internal organs. These injuries initially seem trivial, but injured children can develop serious symptoms (e.g. pain, vomiting or collapse) hours later.

Many of the injuries to school-age children on bicycles occur because of children's developmentally limited range of vision and their inability to process perceptions of road situations sufficiently well and quickly enough to ride safely in traffic. Other important factors are lack of instruction in use of the equipment, lack of safety equipment and unfamiliarity with the bicycle (e.g. having ridden the bicycle for less than a month).

Because head injury is the major cause of bicycle-related fatalities, the single most important aspect of bicycle safety is to encourage the rider to wear a protective helmet. Helmet use has caused a 51% reduction in head injury, 69% reduction in serious head injury, 33% reduction in facial injury and 65% reduction in fatal head injury (Olivier & Creighton 2016).

Other Vehicle-related Injuries

Ride-on mower and other power mower injuries also occur among school-age children. These injuries occur when children are allowed to operate a mower, when they are run over or backed over by another driver or when they fall from a mower or from a trailer pulled by a mower. Although there are no age-specific criteria for the use of lawn mowers, children should not operate lawn mowers until they have appropriate levels of judgment, strength, coordination and maturity, which is usually over age 12 years for walk-behind mowers and over age 16 years for ride-on mowers (American Academy of Orthopaedic Surgeons 2016).

Injuries at School

The risk of injury at school is relatively low, despite the amount of time children spend in that environment. Some injuries occur in gyms, shops and laboratories, as well as on playgrounds and playing fields. Most injuries occur on the way to and from school. Many are related to sports activities (see Chapter 33). Persons concerned with child safety should be alert to hazards in the school environment and should become involved in efforts to make the environment safe in every aspect—physical facilities, equipment, training practices and supervision.

Trampolines and indoor trampoline parks are popular with young children and can cause significant injuries, including fractures, sprains and head injuries. Trampoline injuries result in approximately 1700 visits to the emergency department every year in Australia (Ashby 2015). The most common mechanisms of injury occur during landing (33%), collision with another jumper (8%), performing flips (8%) or coming into contact with the trampoline structure (7%) (Kasmire et al 2016) and mostly resulted in a fracture (81% of fall injuries), predominantly to the upper limb (70% of all fall injuries) (Ashby 2015).

Other Injuries

Falls are still a source of injury in school-age children but less so than in preschool children and toddlers. 'Flipping', a popular activity in which children jump from an elevated surface and perform an aerial flip with the idea of landing upright, has resulted in serious injuries to the face and head and places children at risk for back and spinal cord injury.

Injuries to eyes and teeth are a constant threat to school-age children involved in rough play. (See Chapter 20 [eyes] and Chapter 16 [teeth].) The normally shallow bony orbit of children in this age group makes them particularly vulnerable to eye trauma, especially during contact sports or activities such as basketball, hockey or cricket. Wearing protective eye and mouth gear is essential.

Nurse's Role in Injury Prevention

Nurses are primary advocates for preventive care and guidance. Safety education and anticipatory guidance for both parents and school-age children can be incorporated in all nursing interventions. The most effective means of prevention is education of the child and family regarding the hazards of risk-taking behaviour and improper use of equipment. No piece of equipment is safe unless a child is physically and mentally equipped to use it. A careful history and knowledge of normal growth and development serve as guidelines for both planned and impromptu education.

Parents are often unaware of hazards to their children at various ages, especially those related to normal developmental progress. Susceptibility to injuries and understanding of safety issues are influenced by children's developmental level. Nurses who understand the growth and development of school-age children can provide effective safety education to parents and children and can correct misconceptions before injuries occur. Characteristics of the school-age child and preventive measures are outlined in Table 15.2.

Anticipatory Guidance—Care of Families

The parents of the school-age child find themselves in the position of sharing their child's time and interests with the increasingly important peer group. As a child feels the need to fit into a peer group and gain a sense of industry through individual and cooperative production and performance, he or she moves away from the close, familiar relationships of the family group. It is through these early peer relationships that children prepare for moving from narrow, sheltered family relationships to a broader world of relationships and increased independence. Parents must learn to provide support as unobtrusively as possible without feeling rejected, hurt or angry. The nurse can help parents of the school-age child by providing anticipatory guidance and reassurance throughout this period of child development and maturation (see Family-Centred Care box).

FAMILY-CENTRED CARE

Guidance During School Years

Age 6 Years

- Prepare parents to expect strong food preferences and frequent refusal of specific food items.
- Prepare parents to expect increasingly ravenous appetite.
- Prepare parents for emotional reactions as child experiences erratic mood changes.
- Help parents anticipate continued susceptibility to illness.
- Teach injury prevention and safety, especially bicycle safety and around water.
- Encourage parents to respect child's need for privacy and to provide a separate bedroom for child, if possible.
- Prepare parents for child's increasing interests outside the home.
- Help parents understand the need to encourage child's interactions with peers.

Ages 7 to 10 Years

- Prepare parents to expect improvement in health with fewer illnesses but warn them that allergies may increase or become apparent.
- Prepare parents to expect an increase in minor injuries.
- Emphasise caution in selecting and maintaining sports equipment and re-emphasise safety.
- Prepare parents to expect increased involvement with peers and interest in activities outside the home.
- Emphasise the need to encourage independence while maintaining limit setting and discipline.
- Prepare parents to expect more demands at 8 years.
- Prepare fathers to expect increasing admiration at 10 years; encourage father–child activities.
- Prepare parents for prepubescent changes in girls.

Ages 11 to 12 Years

- Help parents prepare child for body changes of pubescence.
- Prepare parents to expect a growth spurt in girls.
- Make certain child's sex education is adequate with accurate information.
- Prepare parents to expect energetic but stormy behaviour at 11 years, with child becoming more even tempered at 12 years.
- Encourage parents to support child's desire to 'grow up' but to allow regressive behaviour when needed.
- Prepare parents to expect an increase in masturbation.
- Instruct parents that the child may need more rest.
- Help parents educate child regarding experimentation with potentially harmful activities.

Health Guidance

- Help parents understand the importance of regular health and dental care for child.
- Encourage parents to teach and model sound health practices, including diet, rest, activity and exercise.
- Stress the need to encourage children to engage in appropriate physical activities.
- Emphasise providing a safe physical and emotional environment.
- Encourage parents to teach and model safety practices.

REFERENCES

Allen, S. L., Howlett, M. D., Coulombe, J. A., et al. (2016). ABCs of SLEEPING: A review of the evidence behind pediatric sleep practice recommendations. Sleep Medicine Reviews, 29, 1–14.

American Academy of Orthopaedic Surgeons. (2016). Lawn mower injuries in children. http://orthoinfo.aaos.org/topic.cfm?topic = A00611.

American Academy of Pediatrics, Council on Communications and Media. (2016). Virtual violence. Pediatrics, 138, 1–7.

Ashby, K. Pointer, S. Eager, D., Day, L. (2015) Australian trampoline injury patterns and trends Australian and New Zealand Journal of Public Health 39(5), 491494.

Australian Bureau of Statistics (ABS). (2018). Personal Safety Survey, 2016, Canberra: ABS. https://www.abs.gov.au/statistics/people/crime-and-justice/personal-safety-australia/latest-release

Australian Bureau of Statistics (ABS). (2016). Household use of information technology, Australia, 2014–15. Canberra: ABS. www.abs.gov.au/ausstats/abs@.nsf/mf/8146.0

Australian Education Authorities. (2019). Bullying. No Way! https://bullyingnoway.gov.au/

Australian Institute of Family Studies (AIFS). (2017). The Longitudinal Study of Australian Children Annual Statistical Report 2016. Melbourne: AIFS.

Australian Institute of Health and Welfare (AIHW). (2020). Australia's children. Canberra: AIHW. https://www.aihw.gov.au/reports/children-youth/australias-children/contents/

Australian Institute of Health and Welfare (AIHW). (2018). Family, Domestic and Sexual Violence. Canberra: AIHW. https://www.aihw.gov.au/reports/domestic-violence/family-domestic-sexual-violence-in-australia-2018/summary

Bland, D., & Shallcross, L. (2015). Children who are homeless with their family: a literature review for the Queensland Commissioner for Children and Young People. University of Technology, Children and Youth Resource Centre. Brisbane: Queensland. http://eprints.qut.edu.au/84051/4/84051(pub).pdf

Brockmyer, J. F. (2015). Playing violent video games and desensitization to violence. Child Adolescent Psychiatric Clinics of North America, 24, 65–77.

Campo, M. (2015). Children's exposure to domestic and family violence: key issues and responses. Child Family Community Australia (CFCA) paper no. 36. Melbourne: CFCA information exchange, Australian Institute of Family Studies. https://aifs.gov.au/cfca/publications/childrens-exposure-domestic-and-family-violence

Carter, K. A., Hathaway, N. E., & Lettieri, C. F. (2014). Common sleep disorders in children. American Family Physician, 89, 368–377.

Council of Australian Governments (COAG). (2011). The National Plan to Reduce Violence against Women and their Children. Canberra: Department of Social Services.

Cripps, K., & Davis, M. (2012). Communities working to reduce Indigenous family violence. https://apo.org.au/sites/default/files/resource-files/2012-06/apo-nid30379.pdf

Eime, R. M., Young, J. A., Harvey, J. T., et al. (2013). A systematic review of the psychological and social benefits of participation in sport for children and adolescents: Informing development of a conceptual model of health through sport. The International Journal of Behavioral Nutrition and Physical Activity, 10, 98.

Erikson, E. H. (1963). Childhood and society (2nd ed.). New York: Norton.

Flannery, D. J., Todres, J., Bradshaw, C. P., et al. (2016). Bullying prevention: A summary of the report of the National Academies of Sciences, Engineering, and Medicine. Prevention Science, 17, 1044–1053.

Franceschini, S., Gori, S., Ruffino, M., et al. (2013). Action video games make dyslexic children read better. Current Biology, 23, 462–466.

Frohmader, C., Dowse, L., & Didi, A. (2015). Preventing violence against women and girls with disability: Integrating a human rights perspective. Human Rights Defender, 24 (1), 11–15.

Horner, S. D., Rew, L., & Brown, A. (2012). Risk-taking behaviors engaged in by early adolescents while on school property. Issues in Comprehensive Pediatric Nursing, 35, 90–110.

Hornor, G., Bretl, D., Chapman, E., et al. (2015). Corporal punishment: Evaluation of an intervention by PNPs. Journal of Pediatric Health Care, 29, 526–535.

Hyde, A., Drennan, J., Butler, M., et al. (2013). Parents' constructions of communication with their children about safer sex. Journal of Clinical Nursing, 22(23–24), 3438–3446.

Human Rights and Equal Opportunity Commission (HREOC). (2006). Ending family violence and abuse in Aboriginal and Torres Strait Islander communities: Key issues. An overview of the research findings by the Human Rights and Equal Opportunity Commission, 2001–2006. Sydney: HREOC.

Jaffe, P., Wolfe, D., & Campbell, M. (2012). Growing up with domestic violence: assessment, intervention, and prevention strategies for children and adolescents. Cambridge: Hogrefe Publishing.

Kasmire, K. E., Rogers, S. C., & Sturm, J. J. (2016). Trampoline park and home trampoline injuries. Pediatrics, 138, 1–10.

Koepp, M. J., Caciagli, L., Pressler, R. M., et al. (2016). Reflex seizures, traits, and epilepsies: From physiology to pathology. The Lancet. Neurology, 15, 92–105.

Leiner, M., Peinado, J., Villanos, M. T. M., et al. (2016). Mental and emotional health of children exposed to news media of threats and acts of terrorism: The cumulative and pervasive effects. Frontiers in Pediatrics, 4, 1–4.

Levendosky, A. A., Bogat, G. A., & Martinez-Torteya, C. (2013). PTSD symptoms in young children exposed to intimate partner violence. Violence Against Women, 19, 187–201.

Millward, K. (2013). Meeting the needs of our children: Effective community controlled strategies that prevent and respond to family violence (Fact Sheet No. 1). Melbourne: Secretariat of the National Aboriginal and Islander Child Care.

Muris, P., Ollendick, T. H., Roelofs, J., et al. (2014). The short form of the fear survey schedule for children-revised (PSSC-R-SF): An efficient, reliable, and valid scale for measuring fear in children and adolescents. Journal of Anxiety Disorders, 28, 957–965.

Olivier, J., & Creighton, P. (2016). Bicycle injuries and helmet use: A systematic review and meta-analysis. International Journal of Epidemiology, 1–7.

Rettew, D. C., & Pawlowski, S. (2016). Bullying. Child Adolescent Psychiatric Clinics of North America, 25, 235–242.

Rigby, K., & Johnson, K. (2016). The prevalence and effectiveness of anti-bullying strategies employed in Australian Schools. Adelaide, University of South Australia.

Salmivalli, C. (2014). Participant roles in bullying: how can peer bystanders be utilized in interventions? Theory into Practice, 53(4), 286–292.

Shetgiri, R. (2013). Bullying and victimization among children. Advances in Pediatrics, 60(1), 33–51.

Simon, P., & Olson, S. (2014). Building capacity to reduce bullying, workshop summary. Washington, DC: The National Academies Press.

Skinner, E. A., Pitzer, J. R., & Steele, J. S. (2016). Can student engagement serve as a motivational resource for academic coping, persistence, and learning during late elementary and early middle school? Developmental Psychology, 52, 2099–2117.

Steering Committee for the Review of Government Service Provision (SCRGSP). (2011). Overcoming Indigenous disadvantage: Key indicators 2011. Canberra: Productivity Commission.

Sticca, F., & Perren, S. (2013). Is cyberbullying worse than traditional bullying? Examining the differential roles of medium, publicity, and anonymity for the perceived severity of bullying. Journal of Youth and Adolescence, 42, 739–750.

16

Health Problems of the School-age Child

Andrea Middleton

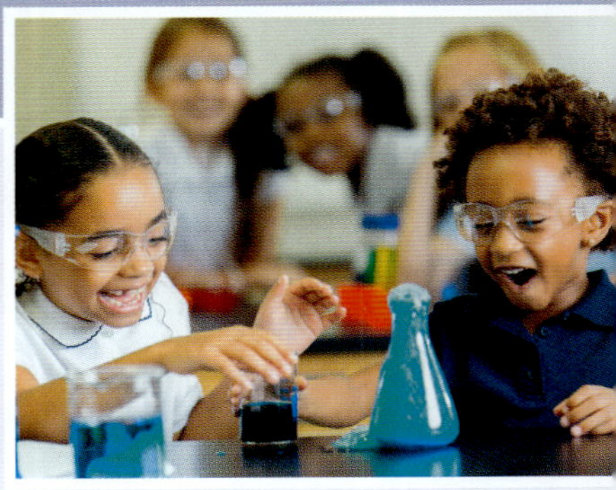

LEARNING OUTCOMES

- Outline common health concerns of school-age children, namely obesity, enuresis and behaviour, emotional and learning disorders.
- Explore the therapeutic management of common health concerns of school-age children.
- Identify opportunities for nurses to advocate for and support children with common health concerns and their family or caregiver.

OBESITY: COMPLICATIONS, TREATMENT AND PREVENTION

Obesity

Few concerns in childhood and adolescence are so obvious to others, are so difficult to treat and have such long-term effects on health as obesity. **Overweight** refers to the state of weighing more than average for height and body build. **Obesity** is defined as an increase in body weight resulting from an excessive accumulation of body fat relative to lean body mass. The **body mass index (BMI)** measurement is recommended as the most accurate method for screening children and adolescents for obesity (Gahagan 2016). Overweight status is described as an age- and gender-specific BMI between the 85th and 94th percentiles based on the Australasian Paediatric Endocrine Group (APEG) Growth Charts for Australia and New Zealand (APEG 2020). Obesity is classified as an age- and gender-specific BMI at or above the 95th percentile for children of the same age and sex. BMI measurements are strongly associated with subcutaneous and total body fat and also with skinfold thickness measurements. However, a subset of adolescents (e.g. athletes) may have a high BMI because of increased muscle mass rather than fat mass. Clinical judgment is needed to understand if the youth is at risk for overweight or obesity.

Aetiology and Pathophysiology

Obesity results from a caloric intake that consistently exceeds caloric requirements and expenditure and may involve a variety of interrelated influences, including metabolic, hypothalamic, hereditary, social, cultural and psychological factors. Because the aetiology of obesity is multifactorial, the treatment requires multilevel interventions. Figure 16.1 illustrates an ecological approach to understanding the multitude of risk factors associated with childhood and adolescent obesity. This framework suggests that the dominant factors, such as the availability of fast-food restaurants, may influence food choices of the children and adolescents who live there. An ecological approach helps promote a better understanding of the roles that institutional, community and societal factors play in the development of children's eating practices and activity levels, thereby taking some of the blame off children for their being overweight.

Energy Balance. A balance between energy intake and energy expenditure is a critical factor in regulating body weight. Factors that raise energy intake or decrease energy expenditure by even small amounts can have a long-term impact on the development of overweight and obesity. For example, eating one small chocolate chip cookie (50 calories) is equivalent to walking briskly for 10 minutes. Factors that raise energy intake or decrease energy expenditure by even small amounts can have a long-term impact on the development of overweight and obesity.

Genetic Factors. Genetic influence is an epidemiological consideration in regard to children's weight. Genetic mutations, such as FTO (fat mass and obesity), are rare but can predispose individuals to becoming overweight or obese (Gahagan 2016). Studies have also suggested a tendency for a combination of genetic and environmental factors. Parental BMI is a more potent predictor of obesity than genetics, suggesting that behaviours and environment play a greater role in obesity (Morandi et al 2012). The increasing rates of obesity within genetically stable populations suggest that environmental and some perinatal factors (e.g. bottle feeding) and possible intrauterine factors (e.g. maternal gestational weight gain and stress) are contributors to the current increases in childhood obesity (Li et al 2012). More research is needed to better understand the influences of family behaviour and adolescent overweight.

Diseases. Fewer than 5% of the cases of childhood obesity can be attributed to an underlying disease. Such diseases include hypothyroidism; adrenal hypercorticoidism; hyperinsulinism; and dysfunction or damage to the central nervous system as a result of tumour, injury, infection or vascular accident. Obesity is a frequent complication of muscular dystrophy, paraplegia, Down syndrome, spina bifida and other chronic illnesses that limit mobility.

Several congenital syndromes have obesity as a feature, including Laurence-Moon-Bardet-Biedl, Prader-Willi and Alström's syndromes and pseudohypoparathyroidism. The most common of these is Prader-Willi syndrome, a disorder characterised by: hypogonadism; slow intellectual development; short stature; and dysmorphic facial features, including a narrowed bifrontal diameter, almond-shaped eyes and triangular mouth. These children are hypotonic and hyperphagic. They lack the internal mechanism that regulates satiety and as a result go to great lengths to obtain food.

Molecular, Metabolic and Endocrine Factors: Regulators of Appetite. A major focus of obesity research has been appetite regulation. The expression of appetite is chemically coded in the hypothalamus

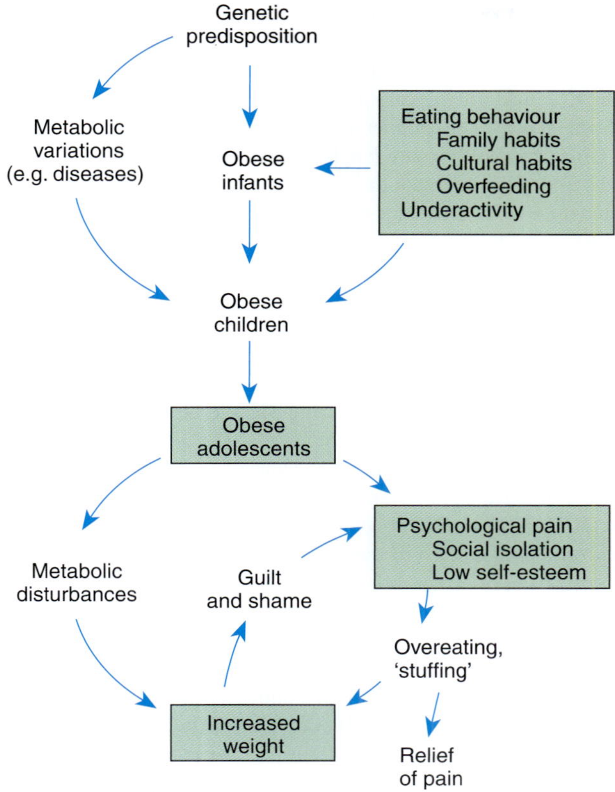

Fig 16.1 Complex relationships in adolescent obesity.

by distinctive circuitry involved in drive and motivation. **Orexigenic** substances produce signals that increase appetite, and **anorexigenic** substances promote the cessation of appetite. Feedback loops between signals have been identified where one signal peptide is able to alter the secretion of another signal peptide. No one signal has been identified as the gatekeeper of appetite. It is apparent that an entire network of signals, including their frequency and amplitude, is responsible for triggering eating behaviours.

This network of appetite signals explains the behavioural observations that appetite and food consumption patterns are dynamic and influenced by biological, environmental and psychological events. Internal cues such as habitual intake, memories of food-related activities and anticipation of consumption easily modify human eating behaviours. External cues that modify the perception of appetite include plate/utensil size, portion sizes served, food aroma, anticipation and the number of food choices (Berthoud 2012, Lee et al 2012).

Researchers have identified a number of hormones and proteins that regulate appetite and weight in animal models. It is likely that these same mechanisms apply to humans. However, the role of hormones and neurotransmitters in determining overweight in humans remains unknown. There is little evidence to support a relationship between obesity and *low metabolism.* There may be small differences in regulation of dietary intake or metabolic rate between obese and non-obese children that could lead to an energy imbalance and inappropriate weight gain, but these small differences are difficult to accurately quantify. Obese children tend to be less active than lean children, but it is uncertain whether inactivity creates the obesity or obesity is responsible for the inactivity. Obesity in adolescents and children can be caused by overeating, low activity levels or both.

Caloric Equilibrium: Sociocultural Factors. The tendency towards obesity occurs whenever environmental conditions are favourable towards excessive caloric intake, such as an abundance of high-calorie/low-nutrient foods, limited access to nutrient-dense foods, reduced or minimum physical activity and snacking combined with excessive screen (e.g. computer, television, video games, mobile phone) time. Family and cultural eating patterns, as well as psychological factors, play an important role. Some families and cultures consider plumpness to be an indication of good health, a status symbol or an indication of affluence. It is not uncommon for obese children to have families that emphasise large portion sizes, admonish children for leaving food on their plates or use food as a reward or punishment. Parents may not have a concept of the amount of food children require and expect them to eat more than they need.

Disparities in obesity rates exist among Indigenous, immigrant and refugee communities, as well as across socioeconomic status. There are higher rates of both overweight and obesity in both Aboriginal and Torres Strait Islander children in Australia and Māori children in New Zealand, particularly boys aged 10 to 14 years (AIHW 2020, Ministry of Health 2012). Lower-socioeconomic groups have a greater prevalence of obesity in both Indigenous and non-Indigenous communities.

Community and Institutional Contributors. Some community factors that influence eating and activity patterns include a lack of a built environment (e.g. food deserts, community gardens, farmers markets, footpaths, parks, bike paths) or affordable and accessible facilities for low-income youth to be active, thus limiting their opportunities to participate in physical activities or eat healthily. Social policies also contribute to obesity. The increased availability of energy-dense foods, pricing strategies that promote unhealthy food choices and overzealous food advertising that targets children and adolescents with high-fat and high-sugar foods are some examples.

The attraction and availability of many sedentary activities, including television, video games, computers, mobile phones and the internet, have greatly influenced the amount of exercise that children get. Studies have shown the association between screen time and obesity among children (Berlin et al 2017, Brown et al 2011, Zhang et al 2016).

Personal and Interpersonal Factors. Psychological factors also affect eating patterns. Infants experience relief from discomfort through feeding and learn to associate eating with a sense of wellbeing, security and the comforting presence of a nurturing person. Eating is soon associated with the feeling of being loved. In addition, the pleasurable oral sensation of sucking provides a connection between emotions and early eating behaviour. Many parents use food as a positive reward for desired behaviours. This practice may become a habit, and the child may continue to use food as a reward, a comfort and a means of dealing with feelings of depression or hostility. Many individuals eat when they are not hungry or in response to stress, boredom, loneliness, sadness, depression or tiredness. Difficulty in determining feelings of satiety can lead to weight problems and may compound the factor of eating in response to emotional rather than physical hunger cues.

Skipping breakfast is associated with a higher BMI. In addition, the frequency of family meals has consistently been shown to be a protective factor for obesity (Gahagan 2016). Family meals tend to provide access to a variety of nutrient-rich foods, particularly fruits and vegetables. Family meals also create a forum for increased family communication and connectedness, both of which promote healthy weight behaviours. This is also a time when parents can model healthy behaviours (Tandon et al 2012).

Diagnostic Evaluation

A careful history is obtained regarding the development of obesity, and a physical examination is performed to differentiate simple obesity from increased fat that results from organic causes. A family history of obesity, diabetes, coronary heart disease and dyslipidaemia should be obtained for all children who are overweight or at risk for overweight. Specific information from the patient and family about the effects of obesity on daily functioning—for example, problems with night-time breathing and sleep, daytime sleepiness, joint pain, ability to keep up with family activities and peers at school—is helpful. The physical examination should focus on identifying comorbid conditions and identifiable causes of obesity. For some, psychological assessment, by interviews and standardised personality tests, may provide insight into the personality and emotional problems that contribute to obesity and that might interfere with therapy.

It is useful to estimate the degree of obesity to determine the component of body weight that can be modified. BMI is currently considered the best method to assess weight in children and adolescents (Gahagan 2016). The calculation is based on the individual's height and weight. In adults, BMI definitions are fixed measures without regard for sex and age. The BMI in children and adolescents varies to accommodate age- and gender-specific changes in growth. The formula for BMI calculation is weight in kilograms divided by height in metres squared (weight (kg)/[height (m)^2]). BMI measures in children and adolescents are plotted on growth charts that enable healthcare professionals to determine BMI-for-age for the patient. The initial assessment of obese children and adolescents should include screening to evaluate for comorbidities. The history is an important guide to determine the workup. A complete physical examination is important. Some areas to focus on include: (1) skin for stretch markings and discolourations (e.g. acanthosis nigricans); (2) joints for swelling and evidence of pain; and (3) airway for evidence of obstruction and enlarged tonsils. Basic laboratory studies include: a fasting lipid panel; fasting insulin level; fasting glucose hepatic enzymes, including gamma-glutamyl transferase (GGT); and, in some institutions, haemoglobin A_{1c}. Other studies, such as a polysomnogram (sleep study), metabolic studies and radiographic evaluations, may be added based on the history and physical examination. These assessments may determine whether the patient needs a referral to specialty services for more focused evaluation and treatment, such as endocrinology (insulin resistance, diabetes), hepatology (elevated liver enzymes, non-alcoholic fatty liver disease), orthopaedics (Blount's disease) or pulmonary medicine (sleep-disordered breathing).

Complications of Obesity

Adults with longstanding obesity are at risk for medical complications that include hypertension, diabetes, coronary heart disease, stroke, fatty liver disease and colorectal cancer. Although obesity-related complications occur frequently in adults, children and adolescents are experiencing significant health consequences as well. Healthcare providers, researchers and government agencies discovered that children and adolescents are developing these complications sooner rather than later in adult life. Childhood obesity has become an increasingly important medical problem, resulting in hypertension, type 2 diabetes, pulmonary complications (e.g. asthma, sleep apnoea), growth acceleration, dyslipidaemia, musculoskeletal problems, fatty liver disease and a potential for psychosocial problems. Diagnostic evaluations of children and adolescents who are overweight or obese have expanded to screen for these complications.

Physical Complications of Obesity

Insulin resistance and type 2 diabetes. Along with obesity, type 2 diabetes mellitus is reaching epidemic proportions in children and adolescents. Up to 45% of all new cases of type 2 diabetes consist of children or adolescents (Temneanu et al 2016). Inactivity and obesity influence insulin resistance. Insulin resistance syndrome, also known as metabolic syndrome, is characterised by hyperinsulinaemia, obesity, hypertension and dyslipidaemia and develops before any of these conditions develops.

Insulin is necessary for the metabolism of fats, proteins and carbohydrates and must be present for glucose to enter the fat and muscle cells. Insulin facilitates the storage of glucose in the form of glycogen in the liver and muscle cells and further prevents the mobilisation of fat from fat cells. The cell membrane has special receptor sites for insulin. Once the receptor site has been established, a chemical reaction results and glucose enters the cell. If the amount of insulin is inadequate, glucose cannot enter the cell. In response to elevated levels of glucose in the body, the pancreas increases the production of insulin, resulting in hyperinsulinaemia. Type 2 diabetes develops when the pancreas is no longer able to lower the blood glucose level by hypersecretion of insulin.

Children and adolescents with type 2 diabetes often have decreased high-density lipoprotein cholesterol levels, increased triglyceride levels and increased blood pressure causing them to be at risk for cardiovascular disease (Berquist 2015).

Fatty liver disease. Recently a growing number of children and adolescents have been diagnosed with **non-alcoholic fatty liver disease (NAFLD)**, which has been recognised as one of the leading causes of chronic liver disease in the general population. Between 10% and 25% of obese children and adolescents are diagnosed with NAFLD, which is the most common liver disease in children (Gahagan 2016). The increased prevalence of NAFLD in the paediatric population appears to coincide with the increasing prevalence of obesity.

NAFLD is generally a benign condition in which a buildup of fat infiltrates the liver. Liver blood tests, including alanine aminotransferase (ALT) and aspartate aminotransferase (AST), are either normal or slightly elevated. Non-alcoholic steatohepatitis (NASH) is a stage within the spectrum of NAFLD where the fatty infiltration causes liver inflammation (steatohepatitis) and may cause scarring. Approximately 25% of paediatric patients with NAFLD will progress to NASH (Temple et al 2016). Although the disease process is not completely understood, some factors contribute to the development of NASH including insulin resistance, diabetes and obesity. People with NASH may feel healthy and show no outward signs of liver disease. NASH and NAFLD are diagnosed by imaging tests such as an ultrasound, CT scan or liver biopsy. NASH can be treated with weight loss for most people; however, for some it will progress leading to cirrhosis and end-stage liver disease, which may require liver transplantation (Temple et al 2016).

Pulmonary complications. Childhood obesity is related to pulmonary complications, including sleep apnoea, exercise intolerance and asthma. Asthma and exercise intolerance can in turn worsen obesity by limiting physical activity and causing further weight gain.

Sleep-disordered breathing is another significant problem with obese adults and children. Obstructive sleep apnoea (OSA) is reported in 20% to 30% of obese children and adolescents (Thompson et al 2016). Evaluating OSA includes assessing for snoring, daytime drowsiness, poor quality of sleep and presence of apnoeic episodes (Thompson et al 2016). Airway obstructions such as enlarged tonsils and adenoids may require assessment and intervention. Continuous positive airway pressure (CPAP) and bilevel positive airway pressure (BiPAP) are used for obese children requiring additional night-time respiratory support.

Musculoskeletal and abnormal growth acceleration. Obesity has been associated with musculoskeletal problems resulting from increased body weight on the supporting structures of the hips, knees and feet. Slipped capital femoral epiphysis is the most common hip disorder among young teenagers and occurs when the cartilage plate (epiphysis) at the top of the femur slips out of place. Blount's disease, another orthopaedic problem, is the overgrowth of the medial aspect of the proximal tibial metaphysis that causes the lower leg to angle inwards (tibia vara). The inner part of the tibia, just below the knee, fails to develop normally, resulting in angulation of the bone. The cause is unknown, but it is thought to be due to the effects of weight on the growth plate (Sabharwal 2015).

Psychological and Social Complications of Obesity. Childhood obesity has been associated not only with metabolic health risk but also with problems in social interactions and relationships. Obese children become targets of early and systematic discrimination. Early studies reported that children at a young age are sensitised to obesity and have begun to incorporate the culture's preference for thinness.

Obesity status is inversely related to several self-perception factors. Many appear to develop a negative self-image and low body satisfaction that persists into adulthood (Rankin et al 2016). Obese children may develop anxiety, depression and a decreased quality of life (Kumar & Kelly 2017). In fact, youth who are obese are more likely to practise unhealthy weight control behaviours (e.g. using diet pills, induced vomiting) that may lead to eating disorders (see Chapter 18) (Rankin et al 2016).

Studies have examined the association between being overweight and obesity and bullying in adolescents. They found that overweight children are more frequently the victims of bullying compared with children of normal weight (Puhl & King 2013, Rankin et al 2016). Bullying behaviours included name calling, teasing, threats, physical harm, rejection, rumours and sexual harassment. Because adolescents are extremely reliant on their peers for social support, identity and self-esteem, they are particularly at risk for the negative consequences of bullying and victimisation. More studies are needed to better understand the effects of overweight and obesity on the psychological and social functioning of children and adolescents.

Therapeutic Management

The best approach to the management of obesity is a preventive one. Early recognition and control measures are essential before the child or adolescent reaches an obese state. Healthcare providers need to educate families about the medical complications of obesity.

Treatments recommended for obese children include diet, exercise, behaviour modification and in some situations pharmacological agents. The treatment of obesity is difficult. Many approaches do not achieve long-term success. The average individual only loses about 5% to 10% of his or her weight with available therapies. Losing weight can have a significant positive effect on many comorbidities, but unfortunately the lost weight is frequently regained in a year or two. A number of multidisciplinary programs offer interventions combining medical, dietary, exercise and psychological support. This therapy is labour intensive and fairly costly.

Diet. Diet modification is an essential part of weight reduction programs. Dietary counselling focuses on improving the nutritional quality of the diet rather than on dietary restriction. Children should avoid fad diets. Most dietitians and nutrition experts recommend a diet with no trans fats, low saturated fat, moderate total fat (≤ 30%), low sodium and at least nine servings of fruits and vegetables, consistent with the Australian Dietary Guidelines (NHMRC 2013) and New Zealand Food and Nutrition Guidelines (Ministry of Health 2020). Many programs recommend using a food diary as a helpful tool to increase awareness of food choices and eating behaviours. The goal is to encourage the individual to make healthier choices in food selection and discourage using food by habit or to appease boredom.

Many dietitians recommend encouraging parents to take charge of family meals and the home food environment to improve their nutritional quality. Getting families to sit down together at the table, away from distractions such as television, makes dinnertime more than just eating. Dinnertime becomes a time to share the events of the day and build relationships. Being able to create an environment in the home where healthy choices are readily available for adolescents is also important. For example, having cut fruit and vegetables in the refrigerator and limiting unhealthy snack foods at home can help adolescents make better choices.

Special Diets. In patients with severe obesity, strict diets have been used, such as the protein-sparing modified fast, hypocaloric diet or **ketogenic diet** (Castaldo et al 2016, Sukkar et al 2013). These diets are designed to provide enough protein to minimise loss of lean body mass during weight loss. Such diets need to be closely monitored and should be used only with multidisciplinary teams that include a physician, nutritionist and behaviour therapist. Generally, the diet consists of 1.5 to 2.5 g of protein per kilogram. The intake of carbohydrates is low enough to induce ketosis. The benefits of the diet are relatively rapid weight loss and anorexia induced by ketosis. Potential complications include protein losses, electrolyte imbalances, hypoglycaemia, inadequate calcium intake, orthostatic hypotension and increased risk for osteoporosis. Low-carbohydrate supplements containing vitamins, minerals and trace minerals, along with therapeutic doses of vitamin D is recommended (Luat et al 2016). It is difficult to sustain these diets over the long term, and the long-term outcomes of using these diets have not been established.

Physical Activity. Regular physical activity is incorporated into all weight reduction programs. Recommendations for physical activity need to consider the patient's current health status and developmental level. Current recommendations encourage children to accumulate 60 minutes or more of moderate to vigorous physical activity per day along with several hours of light physical exercise such as walking (Department of Health 2019, Ministry of Health 2021). The best choice for exercise is any form that is enjoyable and likely to be sustainable. Aerobic and endurance exercises help oxidise body fats. In prepubertal children increasing outdoor play time is likely to be beneficial. Many children find exercise videos and treadmills boring and may not continue these activities. Children and adolescents are more likely to exercise when they have a choice. Individuals can choose from a large variety of physical activities, including team sports and individual sports such as yoga, dance, bike riding and swimming. Limiting sedentary screen time behaviours, such as viewing television, social media sites and video games, is the most effective way to encourage physical activity.

Behaviour Modification. Behaviour modification approaches to weight loss are based on the observation that obese individuals have abnormal eating practices that can be altered. Attention is focused not on food but on the social and behavioural aspects surrounding food consumption. Successful behaviour modification weight programs help children identify and eliminate inappropriate eating habits and include a problem-solving component that enables children to identify problems and determine solutions. Combining behavioural modifications with pharmacological therapy in children 12 years and older has produced mixed results with regard to total weight loss maintained over a significant period of time (Wright & Wales 2016). Programs including family-based behavioural modification, dietary modification and exercise have been shown to be successful in reducing obesity in some children (Altman & Wilfley 2015). Behaviour modification is an important part of multidisciplinary intervention programs.

Surgical Techniques. Surgical techniques (bariatric surgery) that bypass portions of the intestine or occlude a segment of the stomach to produce a marked diet restriction and weight loss are hazardous and cause many metabolic complications. These complications include severe water and electrolyte depletion, persistent diarrhoea, vitamin deficiency, internal herniation and fatty infiltration and degeneration of the liver. In the past, these procedures were considered contraindicated for paediatric patients. Surgical intervention for children and adolescents is being re-evaluated in the context of the significant increase in the prevalence of obesity and concomitant comorbidities within this population. The most common surgical methods used in youth include the Roux-en-Y gastric bypass, adjustable gastric banding and sleeve gastrectomy (Rajjo et al 2017). Minimally invasive surgical techniques are being used with increased frequency.

Bariatric surgery may be the only practical alternative for reducing the increasing numbers of severely overweight adolescents who have failed organised attempts to lose or maintain weight loss through conventional non-operative approaches and who have serious life-threatening conditions. There are few studies in adults and no information for adolescents that suggest surgical weight loss improves the early mortality rates of patients with severe obesity. Therefore, in general, bariatric surgery should be reserved for severely obese adolescents with comorbidities after careful consideration.

Nursing Care Management

Nurses play a key role in the adherence and maintenance phases of many weight reduction programs. Nurse practitioners assess, manage and evaluate the progress of many overweight adolescents. They also play an important role in recognising potential weight problems and assisting parents and adolescents in preventing obesity.

The presence of obesity may not be obvious from appearance alone. Regular assessment of height and weight and computation of the BMI facilitate early recognition of risk. Evaluation includes a height and weight history of the adolescent and family members, eating habits, appetite and hunger patterns and physical activities. A psychosocial history is also helpful in understanding the impact of obesity on the child's life. Steps to approaching behaviour change with youth are described in Box 16.1.

Before initiating a treatment plan, it is important to be certain that the family is ready for change. Lack of readiness may result in failure, frustration and reluctance to address the problem in the future. It may be wiser to defer treatment until the family is ready (Box 16.2). Children need to take a personal responsibility for dietary habits and physical activity. Youth who are forced by their parents to seek help are seldom motivated, become rebellious and are unwilling to control their dietary intake.

Nutritional Counselling. Preventing an increase in body fat during growth is a realistic approach. This is often accomplished by adjusting four aspects of eating: (1) reducing the quantity eaten by purchasing, preparing and serving smaller portions; (2) altering the quality consumed by substituting low-calorie, low-fat foods for high-calorie foods (especially for snacks); (3) eating regular meals and snacks, particularly breakfast; and (4) altering situations by severing associations between eating and other stimuli, such as eating while watching television. Nutrition counselling incorporates health behaviour theories to help motivate and maintain behaviour change. The most successful changes are those that are attainable, reasonable and sustainable.

The nurse teaches children and parents how to incorporate favourite foods into their diet and to select satisfying substitutes. To maintain a healthy diet, it is necessary to encourage the consumption of nutrient-dense foods such as fruits, vegetables, whole grains and low-fat dairy protein products. Keep calories and fat to a healthy level without being significantly restricted. To be successful, a dietary program should be nutritionally sound with sufficient satiety value, produce the desired weight loss and be accompanied by nutrition education and continued support.

Behaviour Therapy. Altering eating behaviour and eliminating inappropriate eating habits are essential to weight reduction, especially in maintaining long-term weight control. Most behaviour modification programs include the following concepts:

- a description of the behaviour to be controlled, such as eating habits
- attempts to modify and control the stimuli that govern eating

BOX 16.1 Paediatric Obesity Prevention Protocol for Primary Care

Step 1: Assess
- Explain and conduct assessments of:
  - weight, height and body mass index percentile
  - dietary intake (fruit, vegetables, sweetened beverages and fast food)
  - activity (screen time, moderate to vigorous activity)
  - eating behaviours (breakfast, portion sizes, family meals).
- Provide and elicit feedback on body mass index and behaviours found to be inside and outside the optimal range.

Step 2: Set Agenda
- Explore interest in changing behaviours not in the optimal range.
- Agree on target behaviours with the patient and caregiver.

Step 3: Assess Motivation and Confidence
- With regard to interest in changing weight status or behaviours, assess:
  - willingness/ability to make change
  - perceived importance
  - confidence in having success.
- Probe the patient regarding ratings of willingness, perceived importance and confidence to explore the advantages and disadvantages of changing.

Step 4: Summarise and Explore Possible Changes
- Summarise the advantages and disadvantages of change.
- Query possible next steps. Allow the adolescent to suggest ideas.
- Provide guidance for getting started in making a change as needed. Encourage achievable goals.
- Summarise the change plan.
- Provide positive feedback.

Step 5: Schedule Follow-up Visit
- If a change plan is made, agree on a follow-up appointment within a specified number of weeks or months.
- If no change plan is made, agree to revisit the topic within a specific number of weeks or months.

Source: Data from Davis, D. M., Gance-Cleveland, B., Hassink, S., et al. (2007). Recommendations for prevention of childhood obesity. Pediatrics, 120, S229–S253.

BOX 16.2 Stages of Change Model

Precontemplation—Not yet acknowledging that there is a problem behaviour that needs to be changed
Contemplation—Acknowledging there is a problem but not yet ready or sure of wanting change
Preparation/determination—Getting ready to change
Action/willpower—Changing behaviour
Maintenance—Maintaining the behaviour change
Relapse—Returning to older behaviours and abandoning the new changes

Source: Data from Prochaska, J. O., & DiClemente, C. C. (1984). The transtheoretical approach: Crossing traditional boundaries of change. Homewood, IL: Dorsey Press.

- development of eating techniques designed to control speed of eating
- positive reinforcement for these modifications through a suitable reward system that does not include food
- create environments where the healthy choice is the easy choice.

Family Involvement. There is a definite connection between family environment, interaction and obesity. The nurse needs to educate parents in the purposes of the therapeutic measures and their role in management. The family needs nutrition education and counselling regarding the reinforcement plan, alterations in the food environment and ways to maintain proper attitudes. They can support their child in efforts to change eating behaviours, food intake and physical activity.

Prognosis. Lifelong eating habits and psychological problems make weight reduction difficult. Compared with normal-weight peers, adolescents with severe obesity are 70% more likely to be obese adults and overweight adolescents are 8% more likely to be obese adults (Kumar & Kelly 2017). Obesity is consistently linked to poorer health outcomes. Obese children have a higher incidence of diabetes and coronary heart disease as adults (Llewellyn et al 2016). Overweight or obese children are almost twice as likely to develop metabolic syndrome as their normal-weight peers (Kim et al 2017). Weight loss in obese children can improve health outcomes. Obese adolescents who had an 8% reduction in weight experienced a reduction in blood glucose and liver fat, resulting in a lower incidence of diabetes and NAFLD (Gow et al 2017). Lifestyle modification approaches to promote energy balance through healthy eating and adequate physical activity have shown modest improvements in risk for obesity; however, interventions that include components about the built environment (e.g. footpaths, fewer fast-food restaurants in the community) have had the greatest impact on obesity (Schmiege et al 2016, Slawson et al 2013).

Prevention. Reducing adolescent obesity has been identified as a national public health priority by the AIHW (2020), the Ministry of Health (2012) in New Zealand and numerous other expert groups. Prevention of obesity should begin in early childhood with the development of healthy eating habits, regular exercise patterns and a positive relationship between parents and children. Prevention of adolescent obesity is best accomplished by early identification of obesity in the preschool, school-age and preadolescent periods. Healthcare professionals should encourage frequent healthcare visits for children who are overweight or obese and incorporate a dietary history and counselling into each well-infant, well-child and well-adolescent visit.

DENTAL DISORDERS

Dental Decay

Dental decay (caries) is one of the most common chronic diseases that affect individuals at all ages, and it is the principal oral problem in children and adolescents. Reducing the incidence and consequences of the disorder remains important. Dental decay, if untreated, results in total destruction of the involved teeth and can lead to significant health risks like endocarditis and sinus and neurological infections.

Pathophysiology

Dental decay is a multifactorial disease. It involves a number of elements: the host, microorganisms, substrate and time.

Host. The prevalence of decay is directly related to the tooth size and morphological characteristics and to the consistency, composition and amount of saliva. The incidence of caries is higher in teeth that are improperly developed, crowded or deeply fissured. The areas most subject to attack by bacteria are grooves and fissures, intradermal areas, gum margins and other smooth surfaces. Newly erupted teeth that have not yet acquired sufficient surface minerals are more susceptible to decay than those that have been erupted for 2 years or longer. Hereditary factors influence resistance and susceptibility, and similar patterns and anatomical characteristics often appear in successive generations. Salivary flow can mechanically clean away bacteria and food debris. It also contains buffering systems, lysozymes, peroxidases and immunoglobulins that influence the development of caries.

Microorganisms. Certain types of microflora contribute to the formation of dental caries. Acidogenic bacteria act on fermentable carbohydrates in dental plaque to produce organic acids that decalcify hard surface tooth enamel. With the inner organic matrix exposed, proteolytic organisms and acids digest and destroy the inner tooth structure. These destructive organisms are harboured and protected in a gelatinous plaque formed on the tooth surface by another group of bacteria that are thought to play no primary role in production of decay.

Substrate. Caries formation is strongly influenced by the two concurrent processes that continually operate on enamel surfaces: acid production and acid neutralisation by saliva. The material on which the acid-forming bacteria act consists essentially of carbohydrates. Among the fermentable carbohydrates, sucrose has been consistently implicated as the most cariogenic. Sucrose-containing substances, especially in acidic forms that cling (such as sour chewy candy) or that promote prolonged contact with the teeth (such as hard candy and lollipops), when ingested between meals, contribute markedly to the development of dental caries. Saliva, some foods and chewing gum after a meal tend to help neutralise much of the acid formed from sucrose.

Time and Other Factors. Bacterial enzymes act on salivary glycoproteins to produce a tenacious protein matrix on the tooth surface. This substance, along with the microorganisms, forms dental plaque. If plaque removal (brushing with a fluoridated toothpaste) is inadequate or non-existent for a significant length of time (a few days), the plaque is metabolised by the bacteria to form acid, which initiates the demineralisation of enamel.

Other factors that contribute to caries formation are heredity, diet, the amount of fluoride in drinking water and acute illnesses. Hereditary factors influence both resistance and susceptibility to dental caries. For example, structural defects, such as deep fissures or crowding of teeth on occlusive surfaces, may be genetically passed from parents to children. The effectiveness of the buffering action of saliva is also highly variable among individuals.

The susceptibility to dental decay is also influenced by the child's general health. Children with special healthcare needs show increased caries activity, likely due to the sugar content of their drug therapy and lower salivary flow (Solanki et al 2016). Children with developmental delays also have an increased incidence of decayed teeth compared with children of similar age without developmental delays (Chi et al 2013). Poor oral hygiene that permits the accumulation of food debris on tooth surfaces allows acid-forming bacteria to thrive and proliferate. Removal of food particles and bacteria-laden plaque inhibits destructive acid formation.

Figure 12.6 from the Australian Dental Association indicates brushing technique for different ages.

Diagnostic Evaluation

Children are more susceptible for the development of dental caries during middle childhood, when permanent teeth erupt. Carious activity is slower and more irregular at later ages but remains a significant health risk to older children and adolescents. Large or extensive caries are usually accompanied by the child's complaint of oral pain and will be apparent on examination to the untrained eye, especially if on visible tooth surfaces. Smaller lesions or cracks in the dentation are best identified by trained dental professionals. Caries between the teeth may not be located without x-ray examination. A common site of decay is the fissures of the molars.

Therapeutic Management

Nurses and other healthcare professionals can provide dental hygiene information and assist families in making periodic dental assessments. However, dentists are the only health professionals qualified to treat caries and most other dental problems. Prevention, including routine daily hygiene and biannual fluoride treatment, is the major thrust of dental therapy. Treatment of dental caries involves removal of all carious portions of the tooth as soon as decay is detected, preparation of a retentive cavity and replacement of the lost portion of the tooth with a material that is durable in the mouth environment. This restoration of involved teeth not only prevents progression of established caries but also reduces the number of harmful bacteria in the oral cavity, reducing the risk of caries to uninvolved teeth.

Nursing Care Management

Oral inspection is an integral part of the nursing assessment of the child. If there is evidence of dental caries or another unhealthy state, the child is referred for dental services. Many families have a family dentist who can provide needed care. However, an alarming number of children do not receive regular preventive dental services; a significant number reach adulthood without being examined or treated by a dentist. Paediatric nurses working in schools and community health centres are instrumental in advocating the importance of oral hygiene and regular dental care.

Restriction of cariogenic foods is important to prevent dental caries, but this should be viewed as an activity in which all family members are involved and not simply a directive for the child to obey. Routinely choosing 'healthy food' rather than sweets should be communicated during health visits so the child interprets caring for his teeth (and smile) as a benefit rather than thinking that limiting sweets is a punishment. Children should be prepared for dental services in such a way that visits to the dentist are a positive experience. Keeping appointments and following through on recommended treatments and practices are habits that extend beyond childhood.

Trauma

Dental injury is common in childhood. Most injuries occur after bicycle accidents, playground mishaps or sports and athletic activities and include fractures of varying degrees of severity, including chipping, dislocation or avulsion. Trauma usually involves the maxillary incisors. Children with protruding teeth, craniofacial abnormalities or neuromuscular disorders are more likely to sustain dental injuries. All tooth injuries require prompt treatment by a dentist to prevent permanent displacement or loss of the tooth or infection.

Nursing Care Management: Tooth Avulsion

A permanent tooth that is avulsed (exarticulated, or 'knocked out') should be reimplanted by the child, adult caregiver or nurse and stabilised as soon as possible so that the blood supply to the tooth can be re-established and the tooth kept alive (see Nursing Care Considerations box). If the avulsed tooth is replaced within 1 hour of the injury, there is a better chance of full recovery (Tinanoff 2016). Avulsed primary teeth are usually not reimplanted.

NURSING CARE CONSIDERATIONS

Avulsed Tooth

1. Recover tooth.
2. Hold tooth by crown; avoid touching root area.
3. If tooth is dirty, rinse it gently under running water or saline; be sure to insert plug in sink or basin (to avoid losing the tooth) and do not scrub the tooth.
4. Insert tooth into gingiva socket.
5. Have child hold tooth in place with tongue or clean finger.
6. Transport child to dentist immediately.
7. Avoid sudden stops or sharp turns to prevent dislodging tooth.

After reimplantation, the tooth usually becomes firmly attached, although endodontic therapy may be required. If permanent reimplantation is not successful, the tooth may be retained anywhere from 6 months to 12 years, which facilitates normal dental growth, development and occlusion.

All mouth trauma, including tooth avulsion, causes a large amount of bleeding due to the vascularity of the tissues. The bleeding can be frightening to children and their families. The nurse should be prepared to effectively manage the emotionality that accompanies tooth avulsion, while also controlling bleeding, pain and reimplantation of a tooth. Using a calm, confident and reassuring approach towards the child and caregivers is often successful in reducing anxiety and ensuring an injury to a tooth or mouth is effectively managed.

DISORDERS OF CONTINENCE

Enuresis

Enuresis (bedwetting) is a common and troublesome disorder that is defined as intentional or involuntary passage of urine in children who are beyond the age when voluntary bladder control should normally have been acquired. Medical evaluation is recommended when inappropriate voiding of urine occurs at least twice a week for a minimum of 3 consecutive months in a child with the chronological or developmental age of at least 5 years (Sinha & Raut 2016). In addition, the urinary incontinence must not be related to the direct physiological effects of a medication (e.g. diuretics) or a general medical condition (e.g. diabetes mellitus or diabetes insipidus, spina bifida or seizure disorder). Enuresis is more common in boys (Sinha & Raut 2016). Enuresis occurs in approximately 20% of children 5 years of age, 10% of children 8 years of age and 3% of children 12 years of age (Caldwell et al 2016, Sinha & Raut 2016). If untreated, enuresis can persist into adulthood.

Enuresis can also be defined as **primary** (bedwetting in children who have never been dry for extended periods) or **secondary** (the onset of wetting after a period of established urinary continence). The passage of urine may occur only during night-time sleep, with the child remaining dry during the day (monosymptomatic), or it may be non-monosymptomatic, where the child has daytime urinary urgency and an occasional daytime incontinence in conjunction with other conditions such as emotional stressors (Elder 2016). Although most children with enuresis do not have coexisting psychopathology, medical evaluation is recommended. Spontaneous recovery occurs in 14% of children (Arda et al 2016).

Enuresis can cause serious psychological problems in affected children. The degree of psychological affect may be related to the impact of enuresis on the child's social life; for example, not being able to attend overnight camps or 'sleep-over' parties with peers. Adolescents with enuresis have described themselves as being anxious or tense, having difficulty sleeping and having bad dreams; many delay or avoid treatment, believing they will eventually 'grow out of it'. Children with enuresis may have significant stress and anxiety in the home environment if parental response to the disorder is harsh or punitive and often demonstrate low self-esteem. In some instances, enuresis may serve as a trigger for child abuse. Although behaviour problems can be associated with these psychological effects, adults who were successfully treated for enuresis as children have normal psychological, social and academic profiles.

Aetiology and Pathophysiology

No clear aetiology for enuresis has been determined. However, several factors and theories are associated with enuresis. There is a high concordance rate of enuresis in monozygotic (identical) twins and an even higher one in dizygotic (non-identical) twins. Additionally, up to 77% of children develop enuresis if both parents were enuretic (Sinha & Raut 2016). Emotional factors may influence enuresis. Some children exhibit temporary regressive behaviour resulting in enuresis after family events such as the birth of a sibling or divorce of parents. Other children, such as those with attention deficit/hyperactivity disorder (ADHD), may have occasional 'accidents' when they become so involved in play that they are unaware of a full bladder or 'forget' to empty the bladder. In other children enuresis may be related to attempts to toilet train before they are developmentally mature enough to maintain bladder control, the emotional atmosphere surrounding the training situation or an excessive amount of emotional dependence on the caregiver.

Several additional theories have been proposed to explain enuresis. The *sleep theory* stems from parental reports that these children sleep more soundly and are difficult to arouse from sleep. The *functional bladder capacity theory* suggests that it is the volume of urine voided after maximum delay of micturition. Another theory suggests that the kidneys of these children fail to concentrate urine during sleep because of insufficient secretion of antidiuretic hormone (ADH). The ADH circadian rhythm may thus be a significant biological marker in enuresis (Arda et al 2016). The *dysfunctional detrusor activity theory* suggests that an unstable bladder detrusor muscle spontaneously contracts to produce bedwetting, either because of abnormal innervation or as a result of other, unknown reasons (Arda et al 2016). Emotional factors may influence the symptom. Some children exhibit temporary regressive behaviour resulting in enuresis after the birth of a sibling or other trauma. Occasionally enuresis can be a behavioural manifestation of a personality disorder.

Clinical Manifestations

The predominant symptom of enuresis is immediate urgency that is accompanied by acute discomfort, restlessness and sometimes urinary frequency. With nocturnal enuresis, the child may or may not feel urgency. If awareness of the urgency is present, the child often reports difficulty awakening to urinate. Spontaneous voiding during sleep occurs, which usually results in multiple nightly incidents. Spontaneous remission of nocturnal enuresis occurs in approximately 15% of cases. However, in some cases nocturnal enuresis continues into adolescence and adulthood.

Diagnostic Evaluation

During the initial phases of evaluation, a routine physical examination is performed to rule out physical causes. These include urinary tract infection, structural disorders of the urinary tract, neurological deficits, disorders that increase the normal output of urine (e.g. diabetes mellitus and diabetes insipidus) and disorders that impair the concentrating ability of the kidneys (e.g. chronic renal failure). If psychological difficulties are evident or a personality disorder is suspected, a routine psychiatric evaluation is warranted.

A detailed history of voiding and bowel habits is obtained, including information about the toilet training process. Assess parental attitudes by listening and asking parents how they have attempted to cope with the bedwetting. An important feature of assessment is a baseline count of enuretic incidents and the time of day when each occurs. This is necessary not only to establish diagnostic reliability but also to confirm outcome success after treatment. It usually consists of a chart or calendar given to the family on which they indicate the date of the incident, the time of the incident and the approximate volume of the urinary output.

The physical examination may be followed by diagnostic evaluation of functional bladder capacity. Functional bladder capacity is determined by having the child hold off voiding until the strongest urgency is felt, at which time the child voids into a measurement container.

Bladder capacity increases with age in children. The normal expected bladder capacity up to the age of 12 is calculated as (age + 1) × 30 mL (with 400 mL being expected for those older than 12 years). Normal daytime voided volumes are usually 65% to 150% of expected bladder capacity (Nankivell & Caldwell 2014).

Therapeutic Management

Enuresis has been treated in several ways. No single method has achieved universal endorsement, and more than one technique is often employed by families coping with enuresis. Therapeutic techniques used to manage nocturnal enuresis include medications, complementary and alternative medicine techniques, such as hypnotherapy, restriction or elimination of fluids after the evening meal, avoidance of caffeinated and sugar-containing beverages after 4 pm, purposeful interruption of sleep to void and motivational therapy. In approximately 14% to 16% of cases, a spontaneous decrease in bedwetting occurs irrespective of the treatments used (Sinha & Raut 2016). Successful treatment is defined as a specified period of dry nights, varying from 7 to 28 consecutive nights.

Initial treatment consists of behavioural therapy such as a reward system, retention control training and a waking schedule treatment. A star chart for every dry night with a reward after a preset number of stars have been earned is an example of a reward system, providing rewards to the child for the desired behaviour. Retention control training was developed after the observation of reduced functional bladder capacity in children who were bedwetters. The child drinks fluids while awake and alert, then delays urination as long as can be tolerated to stretch the bladder to accommodate increasingly larger volumes of urine. The use of Kegel or pelvic muscle exercises may be helpful in children with daytime enuresis. In the waking schedule treatment, the child is awakened during the night at intervals to void. This method has been successful in reducing, but not eliminating, bedwetting incidents.

Conditioning therapy involves training the child to awaken to urinate after a stimulus is given, such as an urine alarm. The device contains a moisture-sensitive wire pad that is placed inside the underpants and is attached to a bell or buzzer. When the system detects moisture, the bell or buzzer sounds, which fully awakens the child. The child is thus conditioned to awaken at the initiation of micturition or to the stimulus of the bell or buzzer and eventually learns to continue voiding in the toilet. The urine alarm can be very effective after a period of at least 6 to 8 weeks, but children may relapse once they stop using it (Arda et al 2016). Relapse is addressed by reinstituting the alarm during sleep. This method is inexpensive compared with drug therapy and has no side effects.

Drug therapy is increasingly being prescribed to treat enuresis; however, drugs are considered second-line management for enuresis. Parents should be cautioned not to think that these agents will cure the condition and should also be advised of the drug's side effects (Elder 2016). Desmopressin and anticholinergic therapy are common medications used in the treatment of enuresis. The selection depends on the interpretation of the cause.

Desmopressin acetate is a synthetic analogue of ADH, which reduces night-time urinary output. Desmopressin acetate is available in tablet form and is the preferred method of delivery. In the past, the medication was delivered in a nasal spray but this formulation caused hyponatraemia and seizures and is no longer recommended (Elder 2016). Response to therapy has been noted to be as high as 70% but the medication must be tapered off because sudden discontinuation has a high relapse rate (Arda et al 2016).

Anticholinergic drugs are indicated for children with an overactive bladder or a poor response to desmopressin. These medications reduce uninhibited bladder contractions and may be helpful for children with daytime urinary frequency. Oxybutynin and imipramine are commonly prescribed anticholinergic medications.

Other therapies and treatment options include stream interruption training, overlearning, fluid restriction and self-monitoring (motivation therapy). Frequently these therapies are coupled with other treatment modalities. Counselling may be beneficial in helping the child, and sometimes the family, adjust to the bedwetting.

It is imperative that punishment not be used to correct enuresis. Supportive therapy such as teaching the child to change soiled pyjamas and bed linens and restriction of fluid intake (especially those containing caffeine) before bedtime should be used instead. Social reinforcement can also be used to enhance the rewards for success. Positive reinforcement in the form of keeping diaries to record dry nights has also been effective in fostering motivation in children.

Nursing Care Management

No matter what therapeutic methods are used, the nurse can support both children and parents who are coping with the problem of enuresis, the treatment plan and the difficulties they may encounter in the process. Both need encouragement and patience. The problem is discussed with both the parent and the child because any treatment involves and requires the child's active participation. In some treatment interventions the child is in charge of the intervention; therefore, parents must learn to support the child rather than intervene themselves. Parents should also be taught to observe for side effects of any medications used. Parents should encourage the child to maintain a regular bowel evacuation regimen; constipation can contribute to nocturnal enuresis (Elder 2016). A calendar with wet and dry nights may be helpful to motivate the child to stay dry and maintain a positive perspective on the problem.

Many parents believe that enuresis is caused by a fear that they have somehow produced the situation by improper childrearing practices. They need reassurance that the bedwetting does not represent wilful misbehaviour. Parents need to understand that punishment such as scolding, shaming and threatening is contraindicated because of their negative emotional impact and limited success in reducing the behaviour. Encourage parents to be patient and understanding and to communicate love and support to the child.

Communication with children is directed towards: eliminating the emotional impact of the problem; relieving feelings of shame, guilt and the burden of parental disapproval; building self-confidence; and motivating them towards independent control. More importantly, the nurse can provide consistent support and encouragement to help children through the inconsistent and unpredictable treatment process. Children need to believe that they are helping themselves and to maintain feelings of confidence and hope.

Encopresis

Encopresis is repeated voluntary or involuntary passage of faeces of normal or near-normal consistency in places not appropriate for that purpose according to the individual's own sociocultural setting. The event must occur at least once a month for a minimum of 3 months, and the child's chronological or developmental age must be at least 4 years (Fiorino & Liacouras 2016). The faecal incontinence must not be caused by physiological effects of a substance (e.g. laxatives) or a general medical condition except through a mechanism involving constipation. The consistency of the stool may vary from normal to liquid, with a more liquid stool seen especially in individuals who have overflow incontinence secondary to faecal retention.

A child 4 years of age or older who has never achieved faecal continence is said to have **primary encopresis**. This type is more frequently observed as a result of neglect, lax training methods, mental subnormalities and familial causes. **Secondary encopresis** is faecal incontinence occurring in a child over 4 years of age after a period of established faecal continence. The disorder is more common in males than in females.

Aetiology

One of the most common causes of encopresis is constipation, which may be precipitated by environmental change, such as having a new sibling, moving to a new house, changing schools or even having to use new or unfamiliar toilet facilities. Chronic, severe constipation has a tendency to impair the usual movement and contractions of the colon, which can lead to faecal obstruction. Abnormalities in the digestive tract (e.g. Hirschsprung's disease, anorectal lesions, malformations, rectal prolapse) and medical conditions (e.g. hypothyroidism, hypokalaemia, hypercalcaemia, lead intoxication, myelomeningocele, cerebral palsy, muscular dystrophy, irritable bowel syndrome) are also associated with constipation, which can lead to encopresis. Voluntary retention of stool may also follow an incident of painful defecation (e.g. in a child with anal fissures). Involuntary retention may be produced by emotional problems caused by the encopresis, which sets up a fear–pain cycle and results in learned abnormal defecation patterns. **Psychogenic encopresis** includes soiling caused by emotional problems.

Normally, children and adolescents have one or two soft-formed stools per day. Children with soiling problems tend to form large-bore stools, which are painful to excrete. Therefore they tend to avoid defecation and withhold stooling. Stool held in the rectum and sigmoid colon loses water and progressively hardens, which causes successively more painful bowel movements and a stretched rectal vault. Over time the child will lose the urge to defecate on his or her own (Colombo et al 2015). A pain–retention–pain cycle is established. Many children have diarrhoea or loose leakage in their clothing and pass small amounts of hard stool, which suggests leakage around an impaction.

Children may experience exacerbations with transitions in the school setting. Some reasons for developing retentive tendencies at this time are fear of using school bathrooms, a busy schedule and the interruption of an established time schedule for bowel evacuation. Children may also react to stress with bowel dysfunction.

Clinical Manifestations

The manifestation of simple constipation is painful expulsion of hard, pellet-like stools. Voluntary retention is usually temporary, with a history of a painful precipitating episode and blood-streaked stools. Involuntary retention is associated with a history of abdominal pain, distension, moodiness, poor appetite and accumulation of stools with periodic passage of voluminous stools. Children display a characteristic posturing during suppression of colonic signals to defecate—stiffening, standing in a corner with straight legs and a bright red face, 'doing a little dance', 'crawling' or hiding behind furniture or behind a tree when playing outdoors. They typically hide soiled underwear. It is not unusual for soiling to take place after bathing because of reflex stimulation.

The child with encopresis often feels ashamed and may wish to avoid social situations (e.g. camp or school) that might lead to embarrassment. School performance and attendance are affected as the child's offensive odour becomes a target for scorn and derision by classmates. The child is not well liked by peers and may be severely rejected by the parents as a result of the symptom. Rejection by peers and parents causes further withdrawal and other behavioural manifestations.

Therapeutic Management

Treatment is aimed towards alleviating the cause of the soiling. To determine the cause, a detailed medical history including risk factors (e.g. negative toilet training, child abuse or neglect, fear of bathrooms), comorbid conditions (e.g. ADHD, cognitive delays, oppositional disorders) and associated symptoms of bowel movements (e.g. retention, overflow soiling, incontinence) are obtained (Mosca & Schatz 2013). Next, a thorough physical examination, including a rectal examination, is completed. An abdominal x-ray film may be obtained to determine the severity of impaction.

Some children may require an extensive and invasive bowel cleansing, to remove the bowel impaction before starting treatment (Colombo 2015). Faecal impaction is relieved by iso-osmotic laxatives such as Movicol, Osmolax or Lactulose. Maintenance dosages are usually insufficient to produce a therapeutic response; a loading dose may be required.

Dietary changes are helpful: elimination of milk and dairy products and consumption of increased amounts of high-fibre foods, such as fruits, vegetables and cereals, as well as increased hydration with water. Behaviour therapy is a vital part of the treatment plan and is indicated to eliminate any fear that has developed as a result of painful defecation. Psychotherapeutic intervention with the child and the family may become necessary.

Nursing Care Management

Education regarding the physiology of normal defecation, toilet training as a developmental process and the treatment outlined for the particular family is a prerequisite to a successful outcome. The regimen prescribed for stimulating elimination is explained to parents. Bowel retraining with a high-fibre diet and a regular toileting routine is essential in treating encopresis.

The child is typically encouraged to sit on the toilet 10 to 15 minutes after meals for intervals of 10 minutes. Placing a footstool below the feet may relax the abdomen and make the child more comfortable. Enemas may be needed for impactions, but long-term use prevents the child from assuming responsibility for defecation. Initially lubricants are given liberally, but stimulant cathartics often cause abdominal cramps that can frighten the child. Positive reinforcement such as giving stickers, praising the child and awarding special activities may encourage the child to participate in the bowel regimen.

Family counselling is directed towards reassurance that most problems resolve successfully, although the child may have relapses during periods of stress, such as vacations or illness. If encopresis persists beyond occasional relapses, the condition needs to be re-evaluated. Behaviour modification techniques are explained, and the family is assisted with a plan suited to the particular situation.

BOX 16.3 Clinical Characteristics of Attention Deficit/Hyperactivity Disorder

- **Inattentive type**—Six or more symptoms (or five for people over 17 years) must be present for at least 6 months:
  - does not pay close attention to details or makes careless mistakes in school or job tasks
  - has problems staying focused on tasks or activities, such as lectures, conversations or long reading
  - does not appear to listen when spoken to (i.e. seems to be elsewhere)
  - does not follow through on instructions and does not complete schoolwork, chores or job duties (may start tasks but quickly loses focus)
  - has problems organising tasks and work (i.e. does not manage time well; has messy, disorganised work; misses deadlines)
  - avoids or dislikes tasks that require sustained mental effort (i.e. preparing reports, completing forms)
  - often loses things needed for tasks or daily life (i.e. school papers, books, keys, wallet, cell phone, eyeglasses)
  - is easily distracted
  - forgets daily tasks, such as doing chores and running errands; older teens and adults may forget to return phone calls, pay bills and keep appointments.
- **Hyperactive/impulsive type**—Six symptoms (or five for people over 17 years) must be present for at least the past 6 months:
  - fidgets with or taps hands or feet, or squirms in seat
  - not able to stay seated (in classroom, workplace)
  - runs about or climbs where it is inappropriate
  - unable to play or do leisure activities quietly
  - always 'on the go', as if driven by a motor
  - talks too much
  - blurts out an answer before a question has been finished (i.e. finishes people's sentences, can't wait to speak in conversations)
  - has difficulty waiting his or her turn while waiting in a line
  - interrupts or intrudes on others (i.e. cuts into conversations, games or activities, starts using other people's things without permission); older teens and adults may take over what others are doing.

DISORDERS WITH BEHAVIOURAL COMPONENTS

Attention Deficit/Hyperactivity Disorder

Attention deficit/hyperactivity disorder (ADHD) refers to developmentally inappropriate degrees of inattention, impulsiveness and hyperactivity (American Psychiatric Association 2013). It is the most prevalent neurodevelopmental disorder in Australia and New Zealand, affecting 1 in every 20 children. ADHD is seen more frequently in boys than in girls. The symptoms of ADHD were first recognised in the early 1900s. Several different names have been applied to the disorder. According to the *Diagnostic and Statistical Manual of Mental Disorders, Fifth Edition* (DSM-5), there are two acknowledged dimensions of ADHD: hyperactivity/impulsivity (HI), represented by symptoms of poor impulse control, difficulty sitting still and fidgeting or squirming; and inattention (IA), represented by symptoms including difficulty sustaining attention, carelessness and disorganisation.

Individuals with ADHD can be very successful in life. However, without identification and proper treatment, ADHD may have serious consequences, including school failure, family stress and disruption, depression, problems with relationships, substance abuse, delinquency, accidental injuries and job failure (ADHD Australia 2019). Difficulties associated with ADHD are most often school related or academic. Children with ADHD are at greater risk for conduct disorders, oppositional defiant disorders, depression, anxiety disorders and developmental disorders such as speech and language delays and learning disabilities than are children without ADHD (ADHD Australia 2019).

Early identification of affected children is important because the characteristics of ADHD significantly interfere with the normal course of emotional and psychological development. Some researchers suggest that poor academic, social and behavioural outcomes are directly related to ADHD; others propose poor outcomes are predicted by co-occurring psychiatric disorders. Therefore, in the evaluation of a child for ADHD, the healthcare provider should assess for coexisting conditions such as emotional or behavioural (e.g. anxiety, depressive, oppositional defiant and conduct disorders), developmental (e.g. learning and language disorders or other neurodevelopmental disorders) and physical (e.g. tics, sleep apnoea) conditions.

Aetiology

The exact cause of ADHD is unknown. A combination of organic, genetic and environmental factors is probably involved. A variety of factors put a child at risk for symptoms of ADHD, including a family history of ADHD. Parents with ADHD have more than 50% chance of having a child with ADHD (ADHD NZ 2021). Other risk factors include exposure to toxins or medications, perinatal complications, infectious diseases such as Lyme disease and paediatric autoimmune neuropsychiatric disorder associated with streptococcus (PANDAS) and head trauma.

Some children may have an absence or insufficiency of noradrenaline, dopamine or serotonin. These neurotransmitters normally occur in high concentrations in the brain and affect activity level, mood and awareness. It is hypothesised that children who lack these neurotransmitters experience learning difficulties in reading, maths and language and are prone to impulsivity. The dopamine system is exquisitely sensitive to hypoxia, particularly in the fetus or infant. Thus any prenatal or postnatal disruption of the flow of blood or oxygen to the brain might set the stage for later ADHD behaviours. Support for a neurochemical aetiology is suggested by the fact that many children with ADHD respond to medications that affect the central nervous system. Many of these children respond to psychostimulants such as methylphenidate hydrochloride, which increases dopamine and noradrenaline levels (ADHD Australia 2019).

Another *neurochemical theory* suggests that symptoms result from an excess of noradrenaline and/or an alteration in the reticular activating system of the midbrain, an area that controls consciousness and attention. This excess or abnormality interferes with the function of filtering out extraneous stimuli. Consequently, children are unable to focus on one stimulus and are compelled to respond to every stimulus in the environment. They demonstrate hyperactive behaviours that result from cognitive 'flooding' and exaggerated arousal that overwhelms the attention filters and overrides inhibitory processes. Other theories maintain that symptoms of ADHD result from dysfunction in the brain circuits of the behavioural inhibition system; structural abnormalities in the prefrontal cortex, caudate and thalamus; and a gene variant known to code for a receptor for dopamine.

The role that environmental factors play in ADHD should not be minimised. Early psychosocial deprivation, such as children who are raised in institutions, can result in ADHD symptoms in later childhood, including increased rates of attention deficit and hyperactivity (Kennedy et al 2016).

Clinical Manifestations

The behaviours exhibited by the child with ADHD are not unusual aspects of child behaviour. The difference lies in the quality of motor activity and the developmentally inappropriate inattention, impulsivity and hyperactivity that the child displays; the degree of severity is highly variable (Parker & Corkum 2016). The manifestations may be numerous or few, mild or severe, and vary with the child's developmental level. Mild manifestations of the symptoms are apparent in at least two settings, usually educational and family environments. Every child with ADHD is different from all other children with ADHD (ADHD NZ 2021).

Children diagnosed with ADHD demonstrate a persistent pattern of inattention and/or hyperactivity-impulsivity that interferes with functioning or development. Box 16.3 lists the clinical characteristics of individuals with inattention and hyperactivity and impulsivity. The symptoms are not solely a manifestation of oppositional behaviour, defiance, hostility or failure to understand tasks or instructions. In addition, symptoms do not occur during the course of schizophrenia or another psychotic disorder and are not better explained by another mental disorder (e.g. mood disorder, anxiety disorder, dissociative disorder, personality disorder, substance intoxication or withdrawal).

Most behavioural manifestations are apparent at an early age, but the learning disabilities may not become evident until the child enters school. A major clinical manifestation is distractibility. The stimuli may come from external sources or internal sources. Children frequently demonstrate immaturity relative to chronological age. Selective attention is often seen, in which the child has difficulty attending to 'non-preferred' tasks, such as completing chores or finishing homework. The child may not consider the consequences of behaviour, may take excessive physical risks (often beginning early in life) and may demonstrate inappropriate social skills.

There is also an increased incidence of comorbid disorders, such as oppositional defiant disorder, mood and anxiety disorders and learning disabilities, in children diagnosed with ADHD (Parker & Corkum 2016). Furthermore, substance abuse and antisocial personality disorders are common in families of children with ADHD.

Course of ADHD. ADHD is relatively stable throughout early adolescence for most children. Some children experience decreased symptoms during adolescence and adulthood, but a significant number of these children carry symptoms into adulthood. The goal for children with ADHD who have any learning disabilities is to help them identify areas of weakness and learn to compensate for them.

Diagnostic Evaluation

There is no single diagnostic test for ADHD. It is important to emphasise the need for a complete and thorough multidisciplinary evaluation of the child, incorporating the efforts of the primary paediatric healthcare provider and the family, as well as possible support from a psychologist, developmental paediatrician, neurologist and classroom teachers. Healthcare providers must first determine whether the child's behaviour is age appropriate or related to a psychiatric disorder.

Before diagnosis, a complete medical and developmental history is obtained. Detailed descriptions of the child's behaviour in the home, in school and in social situations are also obtained from as many observers of the child as possible, particularly from the parents and teachers involved in the child's care.

A physical examination, including vision and hearing screening and a detailed neurological evaluation, is completed. Psychological testing, especially projective tests, is used to identify visual perceptual difficulties, problems with spatial organisation and other phenomena that suggest cortical or diencephalic involvement, and it helps identify the child's intelligence and achievement levels.

Behavioural checklists and adaptive scales should be completed by the child's caregivers and educators and scored by the primary care provider. The assessment tools are also helpful in measuring social adaptive functioning and behavioural concerns in children with ADHD, as well as providing benchmarks for evaluation of improved or worsening behavioural changes once therapy has begun.

Therapeutic Management

Treatment of ADHD depends on the child's age and severity of symptoms. Evidence supports behavioural therapy as the first-line treatment, but other approaches include family education and counselling, medications, environmental manipulation and psychotherapy for the child. The most effective treatment approach is multimodal (Antai-Otong & Zimmerman 2016).

Behaviour Therapy and Psychotherapy. Behaviour therapy focuses on the prevention of undesired behaviours. Families are helped to identify new appropriate contingencies and reward systems to meet the child's developing needs. They may also receive instruction in parenting skills, such as delivering positive reinforcement, rewarding small increments of desired behaviours and providing age-appropriate consequences (e.g. time-out, response cost). Through collaborative teamwork, parents learn techniques to help the child become more successful at home and in school.

Pharmacological Therapy. The most effective and most frequently used medications are stimulants: methylphenidate and dexamfetamine (Weyandt et al 2014). Non-stimulant medications, including noradrenaline reuptake inhibitors and adrenergic agonists, have also shown to be effective with fewer side effects in school-age and adolescent children (Weyandt et al 2014). Children are given a small dosage initially, and the dosage is gradually increased until the desired response is achieved. Children who receive stimulants should be monitored carefully for side effects of medication: appetite loss, abdominal pain, headaches, sleep disturbances and growth velocity. Stimulants are avoided in children who have a history of tic-like behaviours, a family history of Tourette's syndrome (TS) or ADHD combined with TS because these medications may exaggerate tics. Other medications, including tricyclic antidepressants, may be used as adjunct therapy for ADHD, primarily for children with coexisting conditions such as sleep disturbances (American Academy of Pediatrics 2011).

Regularly scheduled re-evaluation of the child is essential with all of these medications to determine medication effectiveness, detect and evaluate any side effects, monitor development and health status (especially growth and blood pressure) and assess family and social status.

Nursing Care Management

It has long been recognised that appropriately educated nurses can assist in the management of ADHD. Nurses, especially school nurses, are active participants in all aspects of management of the child with ADHD. Nurses in the community setting work with families in the home on a long-term basis to help plan and implement therapeutic regimens and to evaluate the effectiveness of therapy. They coordinate services and serve as a liaison between health and education professionals directly involved in the child's therapy program. School nurses understand the child's special needs and work with teachers. Nurses in any setting (e.g. community, school, hospital, practitioner's office) provide support and guidance to children and families during the difficult experience of growing up with a disabling condition and assist in providing education and supportive resources.

To some parents, a diagnosis of ADHD is confirmation of the fear that their child has some irreversible, serious disease; to others it is a relief. All need the opportunity to vent their feelings and suspicions. It is important that they understand that the therapy is not necessarily a panacea and that it will extend over a long period. This has particular significance for changes they need to make in environmental management.

Medication. Two forms of stimulant medications are available: (1) short-acting medications that are immediate release and require administration throughout the day; and (2) intermediate-acting or long-acting medications that are extended release and are administered once a day, usually in the morning. Because the symptoms of ADHD do not disappear on weekends or during vacations, continuous medication may provide therapy that allows them not only to succeed in school but also to function successfully in other social situations and to develop a positive self-image.

Many school-age children take their short-acting medication at home in the morning before going to school and at lunchtime in the school health room. Both parents and school nurses should be sensitive to the issue of peer stigma and children's feelings about taking these medications at school.

Parents need to be informed of the possible side effects of medications. The use of caffeine decreases the efficacy of these drugs, and insulin requirements for children with diabetes may also be altered. If decreased appetite is a concern, giving the psychostimulants with or after meals rather than before, encouraging consumption of nutritious snacks in the evening when the effects of the medication are decreasing and serving frequent small meals with healthy 'on-the-go' snacks are helpful interventions. Sleeplessness is reduced by administering medication early in the day and using the minimal effective dosages.

The issue of stimulants and their relationship to growth suppression is another area of concern for parents. Long-term use of dexamfetamine may result in suppression of growth. Nurses monitor growth closely and provide information on the child's growth, as well as discuss options for diet and nutrition to the child and caregivers.

Parents often express concern that their child will become addicted to the psychostimulants or the antidepressant drugs. Both types of drugs have the potential for abuse, and all children taking these drugs should be monitored closely for psychological dependence, tolerance, depression and other adverse behaviour changes or idiosyncratic effects. A potential exists for misuse and dependence with stimulant medications due to the pharmacological action on neurotransmission. The level of misuse of prescribed stimulants is increasing. Adolescents with ADHD may misuse their medication to augment cognitive function for academic purposes. Nurses must explore this potential with their patients and caution parents to keep these drugs safely stored.

Environmental Manipulation. Encourage families to learn how to modify the environment to allow the child to be more successful. Consistency is especially important for children with ADHD. Consistency between families and teachers in terms of reinforcing the same goals is essential. Fostering improved organisational skills requires a more highly structured environment than most children need. The child should be encouraged to make more appropriate choices and to take responsibility for his or her actions.

Other helpful interventions include teaching parents how to make organisational charts (e.g. listing all activities that must be performed before leaving for school), suggesting how to decrease distractions in the environment while the child is completing homework (e.g. turning off the TV, having a consistent study area equipped with needed supplies) and helping parents understand ways to model positive behaviours and problem-solving. The focus is on strategies to help the child succeed and cope with deficits while emphasising strengths.

Psychiatric, Psychological and Social Therapies. Counselling or therapy can be helpful for children who demonstrate signs of anxiety or depression. Therapy can help the child develop a healthier self-esteem and practise problem-solving strategies. The adolescent may benefit from group work focusing on social skill development. Parents of children with ADHD can face a lot of stress, and therapy may be indicated for parents and other family members.

Learning Disability

Learning disabilities consist of three characteristics: (1) lower intellectual ability; (2) childhood onset; and (3) significant impairment of social functioning or adaptation (Blows et al 2016). The disabilities are related to communication, reading, writing and/or learning new things requiring individualised support and resources (Blows et al 2016). The types of disabilities include dyslexia (difficulty with reading, letter reversal), dysgraphia (difficulty with writing), dyscalculia (difficulty with calculation), right–left confusion and short attention span. Not included are learning problems that result primarily from visual, hearing or motor disabilities; cognitive impairment; emotional disturbances; or environmental disadvantage.

A comprehensive battery of tests is needed to confirm a learning disability. These include intelligence tests (these children tend to have normal or above-average intelligence); hand–eye coordination tests; and measurements of auditory and visual perception, comprehension and memory. Often a wide gap exists between verbal and performance scores on intelligence tests.

Therapeutic Management

Nurses must understand which type of learning disability a child has to best provide direction for the child, parents and teachers. Children with an auditory perceptual deficit appear unable to follow directions or to comprehend large amounts of verbal teaching. These children need to learn with diagrams, pictures, demonstrations and written lists. Children with a visual perceptual deficit may have difficulty reading, lining up numbers for mathematical operations or judging distance. These children may have dyslexia and may do better with demonstration and a verbal approach. Children with an integrative deficit may have difficulty sequencing data or storing and retrieving sensory data. Multisensory techniques should be used, and comprehension should be checked frequently throughout instruction. Children with motor deficits may need to use computers in the classroom because their handwriting will not improve. They may need to find alternatives to physical competition that requires coordination of movement. Children with learning disorders grow up to be adults with learning disorders. The goal is to help them identify their area of weakness and to compensate for it.

Tic Disorders

A **tic** is an involuntary, recurrent, random, rapid, highly stereotyped movement or vocalisation. The condition affects 1 in 100 Australian children (Tourette Syndrome Association of Australia [TSAA] 2014) and 6 in 1000 New Zealander children (Tourette Association of New Zealand [TANZ] 2020).

Tics can be simple or complex and can involve eye movements, other motor movements or vocalisations (Box 16.4). Tics decrease during concentration, are markedly diminished during sleep and become more exaggerated when the affected children are experiencing stress or excitement. Obsessive-compulsive behaviours in the form of ritualistic activities may also be present and can occur in individuals free of tics. A number of medications can precipitate or exacerbate tics.

Almost all mild, transient tic disorders of childhood are self-limiting and disappear within a few months, usually less than a year. The most common tics involve the eyes, head and face, and treatment does not affect recovery. Tic disorders can begin at any time during childhood.

BOX 16.4 Types of Tics

Simple motor—Eye blinking, grimacing, neck jerking, shoulder jerking

Complex motor—Jumping, squatting, stamping the foot, thrusting out the arm, hitting or biting self, ritualistic movements (smelling an object, touching own or another's body, obsessive or compulsive patterns of behaviour), grooming behaviours

Simple vocal—Throat clearing, sniffing, grunting, coughing, snorting, lip noises

Complex vocal—Echolalia (repeating last-heard sound, word or phrase of another), palilalia (repeating own sounds or words), coprolalia (use of socially unacceptable words, often obscene), shouting of words out of con-

PANDAS is the abbreviation for *paediatric autoimmune neuropsychiatric disorders associated with streptococcal infections* (National Institute of Mental Health 2016). The term is used to describe a subset of children and adolescents who have obsessive-compulsive disorder and/or tic disorders and in whom symptoms worsen after strep. The disorder results from postinfectious autoimmunity after a streptococcal infection. Diagnostic criteria for PANDAS are as follows (National Institute of Mental Health 2016):

- presence of obsessive-compulsive disorder and/or a tic disorder
- paediatric onset of symptoms (age 3 years to puberty)
- episodic course of symptom severity
- association with group A beta-haemolytic streptococcal infection (a positive throat culture for strep or history of scarlet fever)
- association with neurological abnormalities (motoric hyperactivity or adventitious movements, such as choreiform movements).

Motor or vocal tics are considered chronic if they persist for longer than 1 year. The most severe of the chronic tic disorders is Gilles de la Tourette's syndrome, more commonly referred to as Tourette's syndrome (American Psychiatric Association 2013). Diagnosis of a tic disorder is based on clinical observations.

Therapeutic Management

Most tic disorders resolve by late childhood or adolescence without treatment and cause no physical harm to the child. Therapeutic management consists primarily of support to the child and family, reassurance about the prognosis and education regarding expectations (of the child) for control. Although the child is able to suppress the manifestations to some degree, persistent pressure for control constitutes an additional stress to an affected child. Medications may provide some relief of symptoms of chronic tics. Therapeutic plasma apheresis to remove the offending autoantibodies is under investigation for children with PANDAS. Genetic counselling is advisable for families of children with chronic tics.

Gilles de la Tourette's Syndrome

Tics are the defining feature of Gilles de la Tourette's syndrome (GTS). GTS is the most complex and severe of the tic disorders (American Psychiatric Association 2013). According to DSM-5 criteria, the presence of motor and vocal (or phonic) tics manifesting before 18 years of age for more than 12 months in the absence of secondary causes warrants diagnosis of GTS (American Psychiatric Association 2013). It begins between ages 2 and 16 years, is more common in boys than girls, persists throughout life and is characterised by rapidly repetitive multiple motor and vocal movements. The prevalence of GTS is approximately 0.8% between the ages of 6 and 18 years. GTS is complicated by psychiatric comorbidities (ADHD, obsessive-compulsive disorder, anxiety/depressive disorders and autism spectrum disorders) in about 90% of cases.

Secondary tic disorders are less frequent than primary tic disorders and should be suspected in older onset (> 20 years) and associated neurological abnormalities. Various conditions may present with secondary tics, including neurodevelopmental disorders, acute brain lesions, neurodegenerative illnesses, immune-mediated conditions and drugs or toxins. A later age at onset (e.g. late adolescence or adulthood), abrupt onset and association with other neurological manifestations represent red flags that should prompt the exclusion of secondary causes of tics (Ganos 2016).

The cause of GTS is uncertain; most theories implicate abnormalities of various neurotransmitters or a dysregulation in brain circuits that connect the basal ganglia to the motor cortex. Family research illustrates a genetic influence for GTS (Ong et al 2016).

The manifestations of GTS wax and wane in intensity and exhibit a continuing pattern of change in which old tics disappear and new tics develop. The onset is usually mild, and the initial tic is of brief duration. The minor tics then come and go, becoming more intense and lasting longer. Some tics may be severe from the onset, often with no symptom-free periods. A high percentage of children with GTS have associated obsessive-compulsive symptoms (e.g. recurring thoughts or the need to arrange and rearrange objects, repeatedly turn the light switch off and on, tie and retie their shoes, and so on). Other problems associated with GTS include ADHD, disruptive behaviour and learning disabilities. For some children, these associated symptoms may be more disturbing than the tics. Diagnosis is based on clinical observations, especially if other family members are affected. The tics do not lead to physical deterioration or affect the child's life expectancy.

Therapeutic Management

Treatment of GTS is primarily symptomatic and consists of child and family education and support. Children with more severe tics sometimes obtain symptomatic relief from medications. Various α_2-agonists (guanfacine) are first-line medications for the treatment of tics. Antipsychotic medications (mostly risperidone, haloperidol) are also effective, but with a less favourable side-effect profile. The goal is to use the lowest dose of medication that reduces symptoms to an acceptable level while enhancing the child's development. Genetic counselling is also advised for families of children affected by GTS (Ganos 2016).

Nursing Care Management

Education of children, families, teachers and others involved in the affected child's everyday life is a major aspect of therapy. Affected children are often quick to become angry or easily frustrated. They may also have temper tantrums. These children need to be guided towards acceptable substitute behaviours to develop normally, both socially and emotionally. Punishment for the behaviours is inappropriate because these actions are involuntary.

Children with GTS are in a constant, ongoing battle to control their impulses and need positive relationships with their parents, peers, healthcare providers and educators to become well adjusted. A child's self-concept can be damaged if parents react to the disability with controlling behaviours, guilt, anger or hostility.

School nurses can help children with GTS cope with their condition by advocating positive support from peers, ensuring the child has access to extracurricular activities and academic support or classroom accommodations, and educating teachers and classmates about GTS.

Nurses can assist families in long-term monitoring of symptoms and determining whether symptoms interfere with the child's development or require more intensive therapy. Families of children taking medication need to be alert to possible side effects, including lethargy, personality change, increased appetite and weight gain, depression or parkinsonian symptoms (e.g. tremor; muscle rigidity; shuffling gait; hypokinesia; and difficulty chewing, swallowing and speaking) and anticholinergic symptoms (e.g. confusion, excitement, dilated pupils, blurred vision, dry mouth and dysphagia).

The nurse may advocate for additional family support by referral to health agencies such as the local health departments, social services and parent groups.

Posttraumatic Stress Disorder

Posttraumatic stress disorder (PTSD) refers to the development of characteristic symptoms after exposure to an extremely traumatic experience or catastrophic event. The traumatic experience or catastrophic event is typically life-threatening to self or a significant other and may involve witnessing mutilation or death, experiencing or witnessing a serious injury, or physical coercion. The disturbance causes clinically significant distress or impairment in social, occupational or other important areas of functioning and is not attributable to the physiological effects of a medication or illicit substance or another medical condition (Connor et al 2014). It is important to note that PTSD is not limited to children who have lived in war-torn countries. Events such as motor vehicle, school and recreational accidents and bullying have been identified as causes of PTSD.

After a horrific event, the child's response involves intense fear, helplessness or horror, resulting in behaviour that is disorganised, depressed or agitated. The characteristic symptoms include persistent reexperiencing of the traumatic event, persistent avoidance of stimuli associated with the trauma, numbing of general responsiveness and persistent symptoms of increased arousal. The response to the event occurs in three stages. The initial response to the stressor is intense arousal, which usually lasts from a few minutes to 1 or 2 hours, depending on the stressor and the individual. The stress hormones are at the maximum as the individual prepares for 'fight or flight'. A prolonged arousal phase may indicate psychosis.

The second phase, which lasts approximately 2 weeks, is one in which defence mechanisms are mobilised. It is a period of calm in which the event appears to have produced no impression. The victim feels numb, and stress hormone secretion is absent. The reaction is outside the individual's awareness, is not well controlled and involves some type of behaviour pattern. Defence mechanisms are less adaptive to specific situations and may not be what the situation demands. Denial that anything is wrong is a frequently observed defence mechanism. Without professional support, the child may develop severe depression, aggression or psychosis (Gerson & Rappaport 2013).

The third phase is one of coping, which normally extends over 2 to 3 months. This is a phase of consciously directed inquiry. The victim wants to know what happened and appears to be getting worse, when actually he or she is getting better. Numerous psychological symptoms such as depression, repetitive phenomena, phobic symptoms, anxiety symptoms and conversion reactions may be apparent. Children frequently display repetitive actions. They play out the situation over and over again in an attempt to come to terms with their fear. Flashbacks are common. This phase can be self-perpetuating, and a prolonged reaction can develop into an obsession with the traumatic event. Some traumatic effects remain indefinitely.

Nursing Care Management

Healthcare providers are often the first to identify and treat traumatised children. Appropriate interventions early can decrease the sequelae of the traumatic event such as PTSD. There are various brief systematic tools that providers can use to screen children after a traumatic event for symptoms of PTSD (Connor et al 2014). Children need to deal with any traumatic event; much hinges on the intensity of the event and their reactions to it. Children's reactions depend heavily on their social environment and the way in which their caretaking adults react to the event. Children usually react in the same manner as their caregivers (contagious pathology); therefore, it is important to be aware of these reactions. In the second, or defence, phase of PTSD, the appropriateness of the defence mechanism must be assessed, and children must be assisted in coping with their emotions.

Coping is a learned response, and children in the third phase can be helped to use their coping strategies to deal with their fears. Children usually are willing to accept reasoning. Those who are assisted in their catharsis and allowed expression will survive without serious lasting effects. Encourage them to play out the stress and/or discuss their feelings about the event.

Children need professional help if any of the phases of PTSD are prolonged. Boys are more likely to have a prolonged defence phase than girls. Occasionally the precipitating event will go unrecognised (bullying and psychological abuse are most common in school-age children), and the affected child will engage in what is considered to be unusual behaviour. Children exhibiting any sudden change in behaviour need to be assessed for exposure to a traumatic event. When the change in behaviour is determined to be caused by a traumatic event, treatment should be implemented immediately to prevent or reduce the long-term emotional and psychological effects of PTSD (Gerson & Rappaport 2013).

School Phobia

Children other than beginning students who resist going to school or who demonstrate extreme reluctance to attend school for a sustained period as a result of severe anxiety or a fear of school-related experiences are said to have school phobia. The terms *school refusal* and *school avoidance* are also used to describe this behaviour. School phobia occurs in children of all ages, but it is more common in children 10 years of age and older. School avoidance behaviours occur in both boys and girls and in children from all socioeconomic levels.

Anxiety that verges on panic is a constant manifestation, and children can develop symptoms as a protective mechanism to keep them from facing the situation that distresses them. Physical symptoms are prominent and may affect any part of the body; headache, nausea, vomiting, diarrhoea, dizziness, anorexia, leg pains or abdominal pains are most common. The children may even develop a low-grade fever. A striking feature of school phobia is the prompt subsiding of symptoms when it is evident that the child can remain at home. Another significant observation is absence of symptoms on weekends and holidays, unless they are related to other places such as parties. Occasional mild reluctance to attend school is not uncommon among schoolchildren, but if the fear continues for longer than a few days, it must be considered a serious problem.

The onset is usually sudden and precipitated by a school-related incident. By taking a careful history, nurses find out whether a poor attendance record is due to trivial reasons.

Aetiology

A number of factors can cause school phobia. Sometimes the complaints are related to: a transient, specific cause, such as fear of a mismatched or overcritical teacher; fear of failing an examination or giving an oral presentation for a painfully shy child; or discrimination based on race, dress or physical appearance. School avoidance may also be related to a safety concern, such as a bully, cyberbullying or a threatening gang. An insecure home situation in which children fear that they may be deserted by a parent may be the basis of anxiety, especially if the parent has previously threatened to leave.

A frequent source of fear is separation anxiety growing out of a strong, dependent relationship between the mother and child in which the child is reluctant to leave the mother and she is equally reluctant to have the child leave her (although this feeling may be unconscious on the mother's part). The intense need for closeness between mother and child is normal in infancy, but the persistence of this type of relationship into childhood is inappropriate.

Characteristically, these children are not afraid to go to school; rather, they are afraid to leave home. They fear that something dreadful might happen while they are separated from their families. These symptoms may be precipitated by a situation that intensifies the mutual dependency between the mother and the child, such as illness, arrival of a new baby, a move to a new neighbourhood or school, or parental discord.

In some instances children have an unrealistic, exaggerated view of their abilities and achievements. When they feel threatened by incidents that challenge their estimates of themselves, such as a minor episode that leads to embarrassment, return to school after an absence, transfer to another class or even imagined social or academic failure, they become anxious and withdraw, frequently seeking proximity to the mother. Sometimes the step-up in expectations at school or a change in important personnel at school (e.g. teacher or principal) is a contributing factor. Occasionally the child may be suffering from an undiagnosed learning disability.

Therapeutic Management

The treatment for school phobia depends on the cause. If the reason for the problem is an examination, a relationship with a bully or a mismatch between teacher and child, it can be dealt with accordingly. When the child is helped to understand and cope with the fear, the symptoms usually disappear. In severe cases when returning to school is unsuccessful, professional psychiatric consultation is usually desirable to help identify possible distorted family relationships or a personality disturbance in the child and to help both the child and the family understand the sources of the problem.

Some children with a moderately severe separation anxiety disorder and school refusal may be treated with an antidepressant. However, medical and psychiatric evaluation is always required before anxiolytic agents are prescribed.

Nursing Care Management

School nurses play a vital role in the identification and management of school phobia as many of these students will visit the school nurse. Treatment of school phobia depends on the cause but all students should be treated with support and reassurance. Parents must be convinced gently but firmly that immediate return to school is essential and that it is their responsibility to insist on school attendance.

Prevention. School phobia and other dependency problems can be avoided by encouraging independence at appropriate times during infancy and early childhood. For example, by 6 months of age children can be left with a babysitter for a few hours. Two year olds can be left at home (while awake) with a sitter. By 3 years of age children should experience being left somewhere other than their home (e.g. grandparents' home or child care). As soon as they are able, they should be able to feed, dress and wash themselves. By 3 to 4 years of age children can be allowed to play in the garden by themselves, and later they should be allowed to play in the neighbourhood by themselves.

For most first-time school fears, simple reassurances and a little advance preparation are all that is necessary. Direct contact with the school and teachers is an excellent way to allay anticipatory anxiety. Parents can take the child to visit the school about a month before school starts, introduce the child to the teacher and let the child experience the classroom firsthand.

Bedtime is also an excellent time to help children resolve first-day jitters. Bedtime stories and books suited to the occasion are available from bookshops and libraries. Several videotapes and tape recordings are also available to help children cope with a variety of common fears (e.g. dark, nightmares, babysitters, doctors, dentists, monsters).

Parents who suspect that their child may be especially frightened may want to accompany the child to school and wait outside the classroom on the first day. A gradual breakaway over succeeding days should relieve their child's and their own anxiety. If the distress extends over a long period, professional help may be necessary.

Functional Abdominal Pain

Functional abdominal pain (FAP) is a complaint of childhood that is often attributed to psychogenic causes, although it can be a symptom of either psychosomatic or organic disease. The disorder commonly affects school-age children and is more common in children over 8 years of age and in girls more often than in boys (Sood & Matta 2016). FAP is traditionally defined as three or more separate episodes of abdominal pain at least 3 months before diagnosis that interferes with functioning. FAP can be diagnosed by a primary care provider in children 4 to 18 years of age with chronic abdominal pain when there are no warning symptoms or signs, the physical examination is normal and the stool sample tests are negative for occult blood. Warning symptoms and signs include involuntary weight loss, deceleration of linear growth, gastrointestinal blood loss, persistent vomiting, chronic severe diarrhoea, persistent right upper or right lower quadrant pain, unexplained fever, family history of inflammatory bowel disease or abnormal or unexplained physical findings (Korterink et al 2015). Any of these symptoms or signs is indication to pursue diagnostic testing for specific anatomical, infectious, inflammatory or metabolic aetiologies on the basis of specific symptoms in an individual case. Significant vomiting includes bilious emesis, protracted vomiting, cyclic vomiting or a pattern worrisome to the healthcare provider. Alarm signs on abdominal examination include localised tenderness in the right upper or right lower quadrants, a localised fullness or mass effect, hepatomegaly, splenomegaly, abdominal distension and perianal abnormalities (e.g. tags, fissures or fistulas) (Almadhoun 2012).

Aetiology and Pathophysiology

Only a minority of youngsters with FAP have an organic basis for their pain. Organic causes include inflammatory bowel disease, peptic ulcer disease, lactose intolerance, pelvic inflammatory disease, urinary bladder infection and pancreatitis. Psychogenic causes of abdominal pain, such as school phobia, depression, acute reactive anxiety and conversion reaction, account for a small number of cases.

In cases in which no organic disorder is identifiable, the abdominal pain of FAP has been attributed to dysfunction. Dysfunctional conditions causing FAP include constipation, chronic stool retention, overeating, irritable colon and intestinal gas, with heightened awareness of intestinal motility or dysmotility. Normally, intestinal contents arrive at the distal portion of the intestine with a relatively high fluid content, and fluid is extracted in the distal colon and rectum. If the normally relaxed distal intestine fails to relax and prevents the flow of its contents towards the rectum, the resulting excessive distension and spasms of the distal intestinal musculature produce pressure on nerve endings, causing pain.

The symptoms of FAP may result from multiple causes, and it is important to assess a number of factors that could place a child at risk for this condition, including: somatic predisposition, dysfunction or disorder; lifestyle and habit, including routines, diet and life tempo; temperament and learned response patterns, such as the child's behaviour style, personality and learned coping skills; and milieu and critical events (i.e. the child's intimate surroundings [familial, social and cultural norms] and unexpected sources of stress or gratification).

Children at risk for FAP tend to be high achievers who have extensive personal goals or whose parents have unusually high expectations. They are described as being more mature and sensitive than others or as worriers. At risk are children who are overly concerned about what others think about them but have difficulty meeting the expectations of parents, teachers and others. They are uncomfortable with expressions of anger or argument, especially directed at those persons who are significant in their lives. School attendance is adversely affected, and these children generally exhibit poor learning performance. It is not uncommon for symptoms to be aggravated during school days.

Clinical Manifestations

Children with FAP have real pain that is usually located in the periumbilical and/or epigastric area. On palpation the pain is more likely to be experienced in the epigastric area or in the lower right or left quadrant and is accompanied by vague tenderness without muscle guarding. The pain is irregular in time, duration and intensity and is associated with either loose or pellet-formed stools. Other symptoms that may accompany the abdominal pain are headache, flushing, pallor, dizziness and fatigue. Nausea, vomiting, diarrhoea and dysuria are sometimes part of the syndrome. The symptoms reflect the heightened intensity of response to stimulation of the autonomic bowel sites. Loose stools are a result of the exaggerated propulsive motility, and the pain is caused by the sharply increased mechanical tension in the gut.

Pain on morning wakening, which improves in the afternoon and becomes severe again before bedtime, suggests FAP. A hallmark of FAP is school absenteeism whereas children with organic diseases attend school regularly. Children with FAP rarely remain in bed, instead lying on the couch watching television. At night, pain may delay the onset of sleep but seldom wakes the child (Brett et al 2012).

Diagnostic Evaluation

Diagnosis is based on a complete family history, the child's health history, physical examination and laboratory tests. The family history may provide evidence of a hereditary disorder or mimicry of adult symptoms. The child is evaluated for evidence of an organic basis for symptoms, such as pain that radiates to the back, pain that awakens the child from sleep, persistent right upper or right lower quadrant pain, unexplained or recurrent fever, weight loss, gastrointestinal blood loss, significant vomiting, chronic severe diarrhoea or family history of inflammatory bowel disease (Korterink et al 2015). Pain is assessed for location, quality, frequency, duration, any associated symptoms, alleviating factors and exacerbating factors. Pain diaries can assist in clarifying details of abdominal pain and triggering factors. An organic cause is found in less than 10% of children diagnosed with FAP.

Therapeutic Management

Treatment involves providing reassurance and reducing or eliminating symptoms. Initial efforts are directed towards ruling out organic causes of the pain, relieving discomfort and attempting to determine the situations that precipitate attacks.

Emphasise a high-fibre diet, and bowel training for pain associated with bowel patterns. Treatment may also include acid-reduction therapy for pain associated with dyspepsia, antispasmodic agents, smooth muscle relaxants or low doses of psychotropic agents for pain. Dietary modifications may include removal of dairy products, fructose and gluten for 2 to 3 weeks to rule out lactose intolerance, sensitivity to high sugar content, and coeliac disease. Other treatments include cognitive-behavioural therapy and biofeedback.

Nursing Care Management

The nurse is instrumental in assessment and management of FAP in children. Many techniques used in a routine assessment elicit information that might help identify factors that contribute to the child's symptoms. Evaluate the child's social and psychological adjustment, and obtain the details of the pain directly from the child. Questions that provide clues to parent–child relationships and the way the family deals with angry feelings provide information for diagnosis and management. Relationships with peers, school problems and other concerns of the child need to be explored. Note any evidence of depression.

Once the diagnosis has been established, the parents and the child need an explanation of the pain, which can be compared with a skeletal muscle cramp or a headache for easier comprehension. Reassurance that the symptoms are not unique to their child and that the pain is rarely associated with a severe disease can help relieve parental fears and anxieties.

Discuss a high-fibre diet with the child and family, and emphasise bowel training. The child is encouraged to establish a pattern of sitting on the toilet for 10 to 15 minutes immediately after breakfast to take advantage of the increased colonic activity after meals. If necessary, have the child use stimulatory suppositories to induce early-morning defecation.

Once parents are reassured that there is no organic cause for the pain, they need guidance on what to do during a pain episode. Often they feel helpless and anxious, which tends to compound the child's distress. The simple measure of having the child rest in a peaceful, quiet environment and providing comfort will often relieve the symptoms in a short time. Application of a heat pack may also ease the discomfort. If pain is not relieved by these simple measures, teach parents how to administer antispasmodics, if prescribed. For example, if pain is precipitated by meals, having the child take the medication 20 to 30 minutes before mealtime may prevent an episode.

The most valuable assistance that the nurse can provide is support and reassurance to the family. When open communication is established and families are able to see a relationship between stress-provoking situations and the child's symptoms, the chance for remedial action is enhanced.

Childhood Depression

Depression in childhood is often difficult to detect because many children may be unable to adequately express their feelings and tend to act out their problems and concerns rather than identify them verbally. Adult caregivers, healthcare professionals and educators may not recognise early warning signs of depression in children or may delay referral and treatment, believing symptoms of depression in children are 'just a stage of development' and will resolve with maturation. Childhood depression does exist, but the manifestations often differ from those in depressed adults. The characteristics of depression are largely determined by parallel developments in symbolism, language and cognitive development. Younger children demonstrate a more cause-and-effect relationship between the stressors and the depressive manifestations. In older children the relationships between stressful events and depression are less clear. Their reactions are less physiological and more cognitively complex, and the observed behaviours tend to be age-specific. Depressed children often exhibit a distinctive style of thinking characterised by low self-esteem, hopelessness, poor social engagement with peers and a tendency to explain negative events in terms of personal shortcomings.

Some states of depression are temporary (e.g. acute depression precipitated by a traumatic event). The causative event might be a period of hospitalisation, loss of a parent through death or divorce, or loss of a significant relationship with something (a pet), someone (a friend or family member) or a place (move from a familiar home, neighbourhood or city). The easily identified manifestations include a sad, downcast face; tearfulness; irritability; and withdrawal from previously enjoyed activities and relationships. The child tends to spend more time in solitary activities, especially television viewing. Schoolwork is impaired. Some children become more dependent and clinging, whereas others become more aggressive and disruptive. Sleeplessness or hypersomnia, changes in appetite or weight (either increased or decreased), constipation, tiredness and non-specific complaints of not feeling well are common reactions. Responses are not sustained and can be modified with social and family support.

More serious and less common are depressive responses to more chronic stress and loss. These are frequently observed in children with chronic illness or disability. There is no apparent precipitating event, but a history of frequent disruptions in important relationships often occurs. A history of depressive illness in one or both parents during the child's lifetime is also common. The manifestations are similar to those seen in acute reactions. Major depressive disorders in childhood have a number of similarities with several other psychological disorders. Some forms of depression develop under unique circumstances, such as the following.

1. **Persistent depressive disorder** (also called *dysthymia*) is a depressed mood that lasts for at least 2 years. A person diagnosed with persistent depressive disorder may have episodes of major depression along with periods of less severe symptoms, but symptoms must last for 2 years (National Institute of Mental Health 2016).
2. **Psychotic depression** occurs when a person has severe depression plus some form of psychosis, such as having disturbing false fixed beliefs (delusions) or hearing or seeing upsetting things that others cannot hear or see (hallucinations). The psychotic symptoms typically have a depressive 'theme', such as delusions of guilt, poverty or illness (National Institute of Mental Health 2016).
3. **Seasonal affective disorder** is characterised by the onset of depression during the winter months, when there is less natural sunlight. This depression generally lifts during spring and summer; however, the depression predictably returns every winter. Winter depression is typically accompanied by social withdrawal, increased sleep and weight gain (National Institute of Mental Health 2016).
4. **Bipolar disorder** is different from depression, but it is included here because individuals experience episodes of extremely low moods that meet the criteria for major depression (called *bipolar depression*). A person with bipolar disorder also experiences extreme high—euphoric or irritable—moods called *mania* or a less severe form called *hypomania* (National Institute of Mental Health 2016).

Examples of other types of depressive disorders added to the diagnostic classification of DSM-5 include disruptive mood dysregulation disorder (diagnosed in children and adolescents) and premenstrual dysphoric disorder (American Psychiatric Association 2013).

Therapeutic Management

Depressed children are managed by a health team specially trained in the care of children with mental disorders. Treatment is highly individualised and should be undertaken in the least constrictive environment, usually an outpatient setting. Suicidal children are admitted to the hospital for protection if the family is unable to provide constant monitoring (see Suicide, Chapter 18). Hospitalisation may also be advised for children with associated disruptive behaviour, such as

BOX 16.5 Characteristics of Children With Depression

Behaviour
- Predominantly sad facial expression with absent or diminished range of affective response
- Solitary play or work; tendency to be alone; disinterest in play
- Withdrawal from previously enjoyed activities and relationships
- Lowered grades in school; lack of interest in doing homework or achieving in school
- Diminished motor activity; tiredness
- Tearfulness or crying
- Dependent and clinging or aggressive and disruptive behaviour

Internal States
- Utterance of statements reflecting lowered self-esteem, sense of hopelessness or guilt
- Suicidal ideations

Physiological Manifestations
- Constipation
- Non-specific complaints of not feeling well
- Change in appetite resulting in weight loss or gain
- Alterations in sleeping pattern, sleeplessness or hypersomnia

fighting with peers or family. Most therapeutic regimens focus on various combinations of counselling, psychotherapy, family therapy, cognitive therapy, education (teaching social and life skills that facilitate coping), environmental improvement and pharmacotherapy.

Nursing Care Management

Nurses should be aware that depression is a problem that can easily be overlooked in the school-age child and one that can interrupt normal growth and development. Recognising depression (Box 16.5) and making appropriate referrals are important nursing functions. Identification of the depressed child requires: a careful history taking (e.g. health, growth and development, social family health); interviews with the child; and observations by the nurse, parents and teachers. If antidepressants are prescribed, the child and family need to know that antidepressants must be at a therapeutic level for 2 to 4 weeks to achieve a beneficial effect. The child and family also need to monitor the child for side effects of the specific drug prescribed and any interactions with other drugs.

Childhood Schizophrenia

Childhood schizophrenia refers to severe deviations in ego functioning and is generally reserved for psychotic disorders that appear in children younger than 15 years of age. Childhood schizophrenia is a very rare illness among children in the general population; only about 2 in every 1000 children with mental illness have childhood schizophrenia.

The cause of schizophrenia is unknown, but three risk factors have been identified: genetic characteristics, gestational and birth complications and winter birth. Biological relatives of affected individuals have an increased chance of developing the disorder. For example, the risk for the children if both parents have schizophrenia is 40%. The rate of concordance is 10% for dizygotic (non-identical) twins and 40% to 50% for monozygotic (identical) twins.

Altered development of the central nervous system is an aetiological factor. Psychosocial theories, especially those focusing on the parent–child relationship, have not been supported, but certain social and environmental factors may play a role in a child's vulnerability to developing schizophrenia.

BOX 16.6 Characteristics of Childhood Schizophrenia

- Bizarre behaviour patterns and stereotyped movements such as robotlike walking, whirling or graceful gyrations
- Periods of hypoactivity alternating with periods of hyperactivity
- Inappropriate affect that ranges from flatness to explosiveness
- Common occurrence of temper tantrums
- Language disturbances such as speaking in fragmented sentences, parrot-like repetition of words, development of a private language and altered tone of voice; for some schizophrenic children, muteness or uttering only a single word on rare occasions
- Distorted time orientation with a blending of past, present and future
- Distorted sense of and use of the body
- Apparent denial of the human quality in people, such as attempting to use a person as a step stool to reach an object
- Conveying of a non-human identity by action, sounds or posture, such as barking or calling self a vacuum cleaner
- Frequent occurrence of compulsive behaviour and phobias

Childhood schizophrenia is characterised by symptoms that last at least 6 months and that seriously interfere with the child's functioning at school, at home or in other social situations. However, the basic core disturbance is the child's lack of contact with reality and the subsequent development of a world of his or her own.

The most common manifestations are language disturbances, impaired interpersonal relationships and inappropriate affect (outward expression of emotion) (Box 16.6). Treatment involves management of symptoms, prevention of relapse and social and occupational rehabilitation of the young person. In some individuals drug therapy produces dramatic improvement in symptoms and social adjustment. Antipsychotic drugs that may be used include haloperidol, clozapine, chlorpromazine and risperidone. Family interventions and family therapy often result in improvements in psychotic symptoms, thought disorders and social functioning among children with schizophrenia.

Nursing Care Management

Nursing of psychotic children is a highly specialised area, but because such problems are occurring with increasing frequency, nurses should recognise children who consistently demonstrate abnormal behaviour and refer them for evaluation.

Nurses should also instruct family members of children taking antipsychotic drugs to observe for possible side effects. Common side effects of these drugs include dizziness, drowsiness, tachycardia, hypotension and extrapyramidal effects such as abnormal movements and seizures. Agranulocytosis occurs in 1% of patients who take clozapine in the first few months of treatment (Clozapine is not recommended for children under 16 years of age). Therefore a mandatory monitoring program requires that patients taking clozapine have a white blood cell (WBC) count performed every week during the first 6 months of therapy and every other week for the second 6 months of therapy. Pharmacies and clinicians report the weekly WBC count and cannot dispense clozapine to the patient without evidence of a safe WBC count.

Anxiety Disorders

Anxiety disorders include a range of conditions characterised by excessive fear and anxiety (Ege & Reinholdt-Dunne 2016). They are the most common type of mental health disorder in childhood, affecting up to 31% of all children and adolescents (Ege & Reinholdt-Dunne

2016). There are many types of anxiety disorders that affect youth, the most common being generalised anxiety disorder, panic disorder, separation anxiety disorder, social anxiety disorder and phobic disorders. Comorbid disorders, in particular ADHD and depression, commonly occur with anxiety disorders.

Symptoms of anxiety disorders include recurring fears and worries about routine parts of everyday life including social situation, leaving home or separation from a loved one. They could have trouble sleeping or concentrating and refuse to go to school. Evaluation for an anxiety disorder often begins with a discussion with the primary care provider. Some physical health conditions (i.e. thyroid dysfunction or hypoglycaemia) and some medications can imitate or worsen an anxiety disorder. A thorough mental health evaluation is also helpful because anxiety disorders often coexist with other related conditions, such as depression or obsessive-compulsive disorder (National Institute of Mental Health 2016).

Therapeutic Management

Anxiety disorders are treated with psychotherapy, medication or both (Dillon-Naftolin 2016). Cognitive-behavioural therapy (CBT) is an effective psychotherapy for people with anxiety disorders by teaching individuals different ways of thinking, behaving and reacting to anxiety-producing and fearful situations. CBT also teaches social skills, which is vital for treating social anxiety disorder (National Institute of Mental Health 2016). Two specific components of CBT used to treat social anxiety disorder are **cognitive therapy** and **exposure therapy**. Cognitive therapy focuses on identifying, challenging and then neutralising unhelpful thoughts underlying anxiety disorders. Exposure therapy focuses on confronting the fears underlying an anxiety disorder to help people engage in activities they have been avoiding. Exposure therapy is used along with relaxation exercises and/or imagery (National Institute of Mental Health 2016).

Medications are sometimes used as the initial treatment of an anxiety disorder, or for an insufficient response to psychotherapy. The most common classes of medications are antidepressants, antianxiety drugs and beta-blockers. Antidepressants may be risky for children, adolescents and young adults. Therefore a black box warning for suicide and suicide ideation is added to the labels of antidepressants. Any child, adolescent or young adult taking an antidepressant should be monitored closely, especially during the initial phase of the medication (National Institute of Mental Health 2016).

Conduct Disorders

Conduct disorder is categorised under the broad heading of disruptive behaviour disorders and is defined as repetitive behaviours through which the rights of others are violated and societal rules are broken (American Psychiatric Association 2013). The disruptive behaviour causes clinically significant impairment in social, academic or occupational functioning. A pattern of three or more specific criteria must be present for at least 12 months and one criterion for 6 months to make the diagnosis. Table 16.1 lists the criteria and examples.

Children who exhibit these behaviours should receive a comprehensive evaluation by an experienced mental health professional. Children with a conduct disorder may have coexisting conditions such as mood disorders, anxiety, PTSD, substance abuse, ADHD, learning problems or thought disorders. Without treatment, many children with conduct disorder are unable to adapt to the demands of adulthood and continue to have problems with relationships and holding a job. They often break laws or behave in an antisocial manner (American Academy of Adolescent and Child Psychiatry 2013).

Therapeutic Management

Children with conduct disorder are likely to have ongoing problems if they and their families do not receive early and comprehensive

TABLE 16.1 Criteria for Conduct Disorder Diagnosis

Diagnostic Criteria	Examples
A. A repetitive and persistent pattern of behaviour in which the basic rights of others or other age-appropriate societal norms or rules are violated, as manifested by the presence of at least three of the following 15 criteria in the past 12 months from any of the categories below, with at least one criterion present in the past 6 months.	
Aggression to people and animals	1. Often bullies, threatens or intimidates others. 2. Often initiates physical fights. 3. Has used a weapon that can cause serious physical harm to others (e.g. a bat, brick, broken bottle, knife and gun). 4. Has been physically cruel to people. 5. Has been physically cruel to animals. 6. Has stolen while confronting a victim (e.g. mugging, purse snatching, extortion, armed robbery). 7. Has forced someone into sexual activity.
Destruction of property	8. Has deliberately engaged in fire setting with the intention of causing serious damage. 9. Has deliberately destroyed others' property (other than by fire setting).
Deceitfulness or theft	10. Has broken into someone else's house, building or car. 11. Often lies to obtain goods or favours or to avoid obligations (i.e. 'cons' others). 12. Has stolen items of non-trivial value without confronting a victim (e.g. shoplifting without breaking and entering; forgery).
Serious violations of rules	13. Often stays out at night despite parental prohibitions, beginning before age 13 years. 14. Has run away from home overnight at least twice while living in the parental or parental surrogate home, or once without returning for a lengthy period. 15. Is often truant from school, beginning before age 13 years.
B. The disturbance in behaviour causes clinically significant impairment in social, academic or occupational funding.	
C. If the individual is age 18 years or older, criteria are not met for antisocial personality disorder.	

Source: From American Psychiatric Association. (2013). Diagnostic and statistical manual of mental disorders: DSM (5th ed.). Washington, DC: American Psychiatric Publishing.

treatment. Treatment of children with conduct disorder can be complex and challenging depending on the severity of the behaviours. Adding to the challenge of treatment may include the child's uncooperative attitude, fear and distrust of adults. The paediatric psychiatrist uses information from the child, family, teachers, community (including the legal system) and other healthcare providers to identify the causes of the disorder (American Academy of Adolescent and Child Psychiatry 2013).

Treatment options include psychotherapy, behavioural therapy, family therapy and pharmacotherapy. Although there is no medication approved for the treatment of conduct disorder, medications may relieve specific symptoms. Stimulant medications including methylphenidate and risperidone have a large effect on childhood aggression, whereas antipsychotics have clinical efficacy on conduct disorders (Balia et al 2017).

REFERENCES

ADHD Australia. (2019). ADHD in Children. https://www.adhdaustralia.org.au/about-adhd/adhd-in-children/

ADHD New Zealand (ADHD NZ). (2021). Children and Teens with ADHD. https://www.adhd.org.nz/children-and-teens-with-adhd.html

Almadhoun, O. (2012). Managing chronic abdominal pain in children. Contemporary Pediatrics, 29(3), 18–20.

Altman, M., & Wilfley, D. E. (2015). Evidence update on the treatment of overweight and obesity in children and adolescents. Journal of Clinical Child and Adolescent Psychology, 44(4), 521–537.

American Academy of Adolescent and Child Psychiatry. (2013). Conduct Disorder. https://www.aacap.org/AACAP/Families_and_Youth/Facts_for_Families/FFF-Guide/Conduct-Disorder-033.aspx

American Academy of Pediatrics. (2011). ADHD: Clinical practice guideline for the diagnosis, evaluation and treatment of the school-aged child with attention-deficit/hyperactivity disorder in children and adolescents. Pediatrics, 128(5), 1007–1022.

American Psychiatric Association. (2013). Diagnostic and statistical manual of mental disorders (5th ed.). Arlington, VA: American Psychiatric Association.

Antai-Otong, D., & Zimmerman, M. L. (2016). Treatment approaches to attention deficit hyperactivity disorder. The Nursing Clinics of North America, 51, 199–211.

Arda, E., Cakiroglu, B., & Thomas, D. T. (2016). Primary nocturnal enuresis: A review. Nephro-Urology Monthly, 8(4), e35809.

Australasian Paediatric Endocrine Group (APEG). (2020). Growth and Growth Charts. https://apeg.org.au/clinical-resources-links/growth-growth-charts/

Australian Institute of Health and Welfare (AIHW). (2020). Overweight and Obesity. https://www.aihw.gov.au/reports/children-youth/australias-children/contents/health/overweight-obesity

Balia, C., Carucci, S., Coghill, D., et al. (2017). The pharmacological treatment of aggression in children and adolescents with conduct disorder; do callous-unemotional traits modulate the efficacy of medication? Neuroscience and Biobehavioral Reviews, 91, 218–238.

Berlin, K. D., Kamody, R. C., Thurston, I. B., et al. (2017). Physical activity, sedentary behaviors, and nutritional risk profiles and relations to body mass index, obesity, and overweight in eighth grade. Behavioral Medicine (Washington, D.C.), 43(1), 31–39.

Berquist, M. J. (2015). Understanding type 2 diabetes in students with obesity and the role of the school nurse. NASN School Nurse, 30(2), 81–84.

Berthoud, H.-R. (2012). The neurobiology of food intake in an obesogenic environment. The Proceedings of the Nutrition Society, 1(1), 1–10.

Blows, E. S., Teoh, L., & Paul, S. P. (2016). Recognition and management of learning disabilities in early childhood by community practitioners. Community Practitioner, 89(5), 32–35.

Brett, T., Rowland, M., & Drumm, B. (2012). An approach to functional abdominal pain in children and adolescents. The British Journal of General Practice, 62(600), 386–387.

Brown, J., Nicholson, J. M., Broom, D. H., et al. (2011). Television viewing by school-age children: associations with physical activity, snack food consumption and unhealthy weight. Social Indicators Research, 101, 221–225.

Caldwell, P. H. Y., Sureshkumar, P., & Wong, W. C. F. (2016). Tricyclic and related drugs for nocturnal enuresis in children. Cochrane Database of Systematic Reviews, CD02117.

Castaldo, G., Palmieri, V., Galdo, G., et al. (2016). Aggressive nutritional strategy in morbid obesity in clinical practice: Safety, feasibility, and effects on metabolic and haemodynamic risk factors. Obesity Research & Clinical Practice, 10(2), 169–177.

Chi, D. L., Rossitch, K. C., & Beeles, E. M. (2013). Developmental delays and dental caries in low-income preschoolers in the USA: A pilot cross-sectional study and preliminary explanatory model. BMC Oral Health, 13, 53.

Colombo, J. M., Wassom, M. C., & Rosen, J. M. (2015). Constipation and encopresis in childhood. Pediatrics in Review, 36(9), 393–402.

Connor, D. F., Ford, J. D., Arnsten, A. F. T., et al. (2014). An update on posttraumatic stress disorder in children and adolescents. Clinical Pediatrics, 54(6), 517–528.

Department of Health. (2019). National Physical Activity, Sedentary Behaviour and Sleep Recommendations for Children and Young People (5-17 years). https://www1.health.gov.au/internet/main/publishing.nsf/Content/health-pubhlth-strateg-phys-act-guidelines

Dillon-Naftolin, E. (2016). Identification and treatment of generalized anxiety disorder in children in primary care. Pediatric Annals, 45(10), e349–e355.

Ege, S., & Reinholdt-Dunne, M. L. (2016). Improving treatment response for paediatric anxiety disorders: An information-processing perspective. Clinical Child and Family Psychology Review, 19, 392–402.

Elder, J. S. (2016). Enuresis and voiding dysfunction. In R. M. Kliegman, B. F. Stanton, J. W. St Geme, et al. (Eds.), Nelson textbook of pediatrics (20th ed.). Philadelphia: Saunders/Elsevier.

Fiorino, K. N., & Liacouras, C. A. (2016). Encopresis and functional constipation. In R. M. Kliegman, B. F. Stanton, J. W. St Geme, et al. (Eds.), Nelson textbook of pediatrics (20th ed.). Philadelphia: Saunders/Elsevier.

Gahagan, S. (2016). Overweight and obesity. In R. M. Kliegman, B. F. Stanton, J. W. St Geme, et al. (Eds.), Nelson textbook of pediatrics (20th ed.). Philadelphia: Saunders/Elsevier.

Ganos, C. (2016). Tics and Tourette's: Update on pathophysiology and tic control. Current Opinion in Neurology, 29(4), 513–518.

Gerson, R., & Rappaport, N. (2013). Traumatic stress and posttraumatic stress disorder in youth: Recent research findings on clinical impact, assessment and treatment. The Journal of Adolescent Health, 52(2), 137–143.

Gow, M. L., Baur, L. A., Johnson, N. A., et al. (2017). Reversal of type 2 diabetes in youth who adhere to a very-low-energy diet: A pilot study. Diabetologia, 60(3), 406–415.

Kennedy, M., Kreppner, J., Knights, N., et al. (2016). Early severe institutional deprivation is associated with a persistent variant of adult attention-deficit/hyperactivity disorder: Clinical presentation, developmental continuities and life circumstances in the English and Romanian adoptees study. Journal of Child Psychology and Psychiatry, and Allied Disciplines, 57(10), 1113–1125.

Kim, J., Lee, I., & Lim, S. (2017). Overweight or obesity in children aged 0 to 6 and the risk of adult metabolic syndrome: A systematic review and meta-analysis. Journal of Clinical Nursing, 26, 23–24.

Korterink, J., Devanarayana, N. M., Rajindrajith, S., et al. (2015). Childhood functional abdominal pain: Mechanisms and management. Nature Reviews. Gastroenterology & Hepatology, 12, 159–171.

Kumar, S., & Kelly, A. S. (2017). Review of childhood obesity: From epidemiology, etiology, and comorbidities to clinical assessment and treatment. Mayo Clinic Proceedings. Mayo Clinic, 92(2), 251–265.

Lee, N. M., Carter, A., Owen, N., et al. (2012). The neurobiology of overeating. European Molecular Biology Organization Reports, 13(9), 785–790.

Li, R., Magadia, J., Fein, S. B., et al. (2012). Risk of bottle-feeding for rapid weight gain during the first year of life. Archives of Pediatrics and Adolescent Medicine, 166(5), 431–436.

Llewellyn, A., Simmonds, M., Owen, C. G., et al. (2016). Childhood obesity as a predictor of morbidity in adulthood: A systematic review and meta-analysis. Obesity Reviews: An Official Journal of the International Association for the Study of Obesity, 17(1), 56–67.

Luat, A. F., Coyle, L., & Kamat, D. (2016). The ketogenic diet: A practice guide for pediatricians. Pediatric Annals, 45(12), e446–e450.

Ministry of Health. (2012). The Health of New Zealand Children 2011/12: Key findings of the New Zealand Health Survey. https://www.moh.govt.nz/NoteBook/nbbooks.nsf/0/35624B64BEC88496CC257AFA0069BF2A/$file/health-of-new-zealand-child-2011-12-v2.pdf

Ministry of Health. (2020). Current Food and Nutrition Guidelines. https://www.health.govt.nz/our-work/eating-and-activity-guidelines/current-food-and-nutrition-guidelines

Ministry of Health. (2021). Physical Activity. https://www.health.govt.nz/our-work/preventative-health-wellness/physical-activity

Morandi, A., Meyre, D., Lobbens, S., et al. (2012). Estimation of newborn risk for child or adolescent obesity: Lessons from longitudinal birth cohorts. PLoS ONE, 7(11), e49919.

Mosca, N. W., & Schatz, M. L. (2013). Encopresis, not just an accident. NASN School Nurse, 28(5), 218–221.

Nankivell, G., & Caldwell, P. (2014). Paediatric urinary incontinence. Australian Prescriber, 37, 192–195.

National Health and Medical Research Council (NHMRC). (2013). Eat for Health: Australian Dietary Guidelines. https://www.health.gov.au/sites/default/files/australian-dietary-guidelines.pdf

National Institute of Mental Health. (2016). PANDAS – question and answers. https://www.nimh.nih.gov/health/publications/pandas/index.shtml

Ong, M. T., Mordekar, S. R., & Seal, A. (2016). Fifteen minute consultation: Tics and Tourette syndrome. Archives of Disease in Childhood. Education and Practice Edition, 101, 87–94.

Parker, A., & Corkum, P. (2016). ADHD diagnosis: As simple as administering a questionnaire or a complex diagnostic process? Journal of Attention Disorders, 20(6), 478–486.

Puhl, R. M., & King, K. M. (2013). Weight discrimination and bullying. Best Practice & Research. Clinical Endocrinology & Metabolism, 27(2), 117–127.

Rajjo, T., Mohammed, K., Alsawas, M., et al. (2017). Treatment of pediatric obesity: An umbrella systematic review. Journal of Clinical Endocrinology and Metabolism, 102(3), 763–775.

Rankin, J., Matthews, L., Cobley, S., et al. (2016). Psychological consequences of childhood obesity: Psychiatric comorbidity and prevention. Adolescent Health, Medicine and Therapeutics, 7, 125–146.

Sabharwal, S. (2015). Blount disease: An update. The Orthopedic Clinics of North America, 46(1), 37–47.

Schmiege, S. J., Gance-Cleveland, B., Gilbert, L., et al. (2016). Identifying patterns of obesity risk behavior to improve pediatric primary care. Journal for Specialists in Pediatric Nursing, 21, 18–28.

Sinha, R., & Raut, S. (2016). Management of nocturnal enuresis – myths and facts. World Journal of Nephrology, 5(4), 328–338.

Slawson, D. L., Fitzgerald, N., & Morgan, K. T. (2013). Position of the Academy of Nutrition and Dietetics: The role of nutrition in health promotion and chronic disease prevention. Journal of the Academy of Nutrition & Dietetics, 113(7), 972–979.

Solanki, N., Kumar, A., Awasthi, N., et al. (2016). Assessment of oral status in pediatric patients with special health care needs receiving dental rehabilitation procedures under general anesthesia: A retrospective analysis. The Journal of Contemporary Dental Practice, 17(6), 476–479.

Sood, M. R., & Matta, S. R. (2016). Approach to a child with functional abdominal pain. Indian Journal of Pediatrics, 83(12), 1452–1458.

Sukkar, S. G., Signori, A., Borrini, C., et al. (2013). Feasibility of protein-sparing modified fast by tube (ProMoFasT) in obesity treatment: A phase II pilot trial on clinical safety and efficacy (appetite control, body composition, muscular strength, metabolic pattern, pulmonary function test). Mediterranean Journal of Nutrition and Metabolism, 6, 165–176.

Tandon, P. S., Zhou, C., Sallis, J. F., et al. (2012). Home environment relationships with children's physical activity, sedentary time, and screen time by socioeconomic status. The International Journal of Behavioral Nutrition and Physical Activity, 9, 88.

Temneanu, O. R., Trandafir, L. M., & Purcarea, M. R. (2016). Type 2 diabetes mellitus in children and adolescents: A relatively new clinical problem within pediatric practice. Journal of Medicine and Life, 9(3), 235–239.

Temple, J. L., Cordero, P., Li, J., et al. (2016). A guide to non-alcoholic fatty liver disease in childhood and adolescence. International Journal of Molecular Sciences, 17(6), 947.

Thompson, N., Mansfield, B., Stringer, M., et al. (2016). An evidence-based resource for the management of comorbidities associated with childhood overweight and obesity. Journal of the American Association of Nurse Practitioners, 28(10), 559–570.

Tinanoff, N. (2016). Dental caries. In R. M. Kliegman, B. F. Stanton, J. W. St Geme, et al. (Eds.), Nelson textbook of pediatrics (20th ed.). Philadelphia: Saunders/Elsevier.

Tourette Syndrome Association of Australia (TSAA). (2014). Tourette Syndrome. https://tourette.org.au/

Tourette Association of New Zealand (TANZ). (2020). About Tourette Syndrome. https://tourettes.org.nz/about-ts/" https://tourettes.org.nz/about-ts/

Weyandt, L. L., Marraccini, M. E., Gudmundsdottir, B. G., et al. (2014). Pharmacological interventions for adolescents and adults with ADHD: Stimulant and nonstimulant medications and misuse of prescription stimulants. Psychology Research and Behavior Management, 9(7), 223–249.

Wright, N., & Wales, J. (2016). Assessment and management of severely obese children and adolescents. Archives of Disease in Childhood, 101(12), 1161–1167.

Zhang, G., Wu, L., Zhou, L., et al. (2016). Television watching and risk of childhood obesity: A meta-analysis. European Journal of Public Health, 26(1), 13–18.

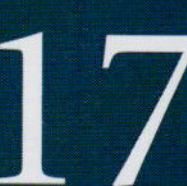

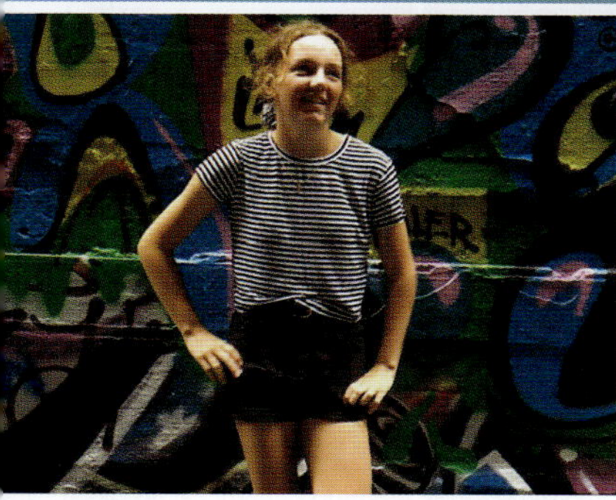

Health Promotion of the Adolescent and Family

Lisa Speedie

LEARNING OBJECTIVES

- Be able to describe normal growth and development for the adolescent.
- Demonstrate an understanding of family-centred care for the family and the adolescent.
- Demonstrate an understanding of adolescent reproduction and educate the adolescent and their family in relation to sexuality.
- Assist the adolescent and family with mental health assessment and conditions that may arise during adolescence.
- Educate the adolescent and family on areas of safety during adolescence.
- Develop an understanding of what is health promotion for the adolescent and their family.

PROMOTING OPTIMUM GROWTH AND DEVELOPMENT

Adolescence is a dynamic period of transition from childhood to adult maturity; a time of profound biological, intellectual, psychosocial and economic change—this phase of rapid growth and development is second only to the first of life. During this period individuals progress through phases of physical and sexual maturity, gradually develop more sophisticated intellectual and reasoning capabilities and make critical social, emotional, educational and occupational decisions that will ultimately shape their adult careers and health outcomes. The changes that occur during adolescence have important health risk implications. Young people are exposed to a wide variety of opportunities and behaviours that could have long-term health consequences, underlining the key role nurses have in promoting safety and health practices among this population.

When examining widely accepted theories of adolescent development, researchers have challenged many popular notions. For example, a common belief is that teenagers' behaviours are overwhelmingly negative, controlled by 'raging hormones', and that adolescence is a period when rebellious and risky behaviour is the norm causing struggles with adult caregivers. Although these notions are mistaken, the foundational ideal is not benign; choices and behaviours that some adolescents make during this period have detrimental effects on their long-term health outcomes, so healthcare provider attitudes, interactions with adolescents and the application of consistent, safety-first policies and program development are vital. Current research supports a positive view of this developmental period, confirming that adolescence involves a complex interplay of biological, cognitive, psychological and social change. These changes occur at predicable but highly variable individual timeframes that are interdependent on multiple variables, including the social determinates of health. On the individual level, changes include biological maturation, cognitive development and psychological development. Change also occurs in the social contexts of adolescents' families, peer groups, schools, faith communities and workplaces.

Adolescence progresses for each child in three distinct phases: (1) early adolescence, also termed *pubescent,* typically ages 11 to 14 years; (2) middle adolescence, typically ages 15 to 17 years; and (3) late adolescence, also termed *young adulthood,* typically ages 18 to 22 years. Many researchers feel that neurodevelopment is not complete until 25 years old, so consideration has been given to young adulthood extending later into the third decade of life (McCormick & Scherer 2018). The physical, emotional and psychological changes, opportunities, challenges, social pressures and resources available to young people differ during these three unique phases. Early adolescence is characterised primarily by the physical changes of puberty and the emotional responses to those changes. Middle adolescence is characterised by transition from adult-caregiver to peer-dominant orientation, often with intense self-focus preoccupations and experimentation with music, technology, dress and physical appearance. Wide variations of cognitive development, gender, peer and future-career exploration, as well as experimental social behaviours, including sexuality and recreational drug use, typically occur at this time. Late adolescence features full physical maturation and the transition towards adult behaviours, sustainable emotional and intimate relationships and critical thinking skills to independently manage healthcare, career and responsibilities (Table 17.1).

TABLE 17.1 Growth and Development During Adolescence

Early Adolescence (11–14 Years)	Middle Adolescence (15–17 Years)	Late Adolescence (18–20 Years)
	GROWTH	
Rapidly accelerating growth Reaches peak velocity Secondary sexual characteristics appear	Growth decelerating in girls Stature reaches 95% of adult height Secondary sexual characteristics well advanced	Physically mature Structure and reproductive growth almost complete
	COGNITION	
Explores newfound ability for limited abstract thought Clumsy groping for new values and energies Comparison of 'normality' with peers of same sex	Developing capacity for abstract thinking Enjoys intellectual powers, often in idealistic terms Concern with philosophic, political and social problems	Established abstract thought Can perceive and act on long-range options Able to view problems comprehensively Intellectual and functional identity established
	IDENTITY	
Preoccupied with rapid body changes Trying out of various roles Measurement of attractiveness by acceptance or rejection by peers Conformity to group norms Decline in self-esteem	Modified body image Self-centred; increased narcissism Tendency towards inner experience and self-discovery Rich fantasy life Idealistic Able to perceive future implications of current behaviour and decisions; variable application	Body image and gender-role definition nearly secured Mature sexual identity Phase of consolidation of identity Increase in self-esteem Comfortable with physical growth Social roles defined and articulated
	RELATIONSHIPS WITH PARENTS	
Defining independence–dependence boundaries Strong desire to remain dependent on parents while trying to detach No major conflicts over parental control	Major conflicts over independence and control Low point in parent–child relationship Greatest push for emancipation; disengagement Final and irreversible emotional detachment from parents	Emotional and physical separation from parents completed Independence from family with less conflict Emancipation nearly secured
	RELATIONSHIPS WITH PEERS	
Seeks peer affiliations to counter instability generated by rapid change Upsurge of close, idealised friendships with members of same sex Struggle for mastery within peer group	Strong need for identity to affirm self-image Behavioural standards set by peer group Acceptance by peers extremely important—fear of rejection Exploration of ability to attract opposite sex	Peer group recedes in importance in favour of individual friendship Testing of romantic relationships against possibility of permanent alliance Relationships characterised by giving and sharing
	SEXUALITY	
Self-exploration and evaluation Limited dating, usually group Limited intimacy	Multiple plural relationships Internal identification of heterosexual, homosexual or bisexual, pansexual and other attractions Exploration of 'self-appeal' Feeling of 'being in love' Tentative establishment of relationships	Forms stable relationships and attachment to another Growing capacity for mutuality and reciprocity Dating as a romantic pair May publicly identify as gay, lesbian or bisexual, transgender, intersex, queer or other (not limited to LGBTIQ+) Intimacy involves commitment rather than exploration and romanticism
	PSYCHOLOGICAL HEALTH	
Wide mood swings Intense daydreaming Anger outwardly expressed with moodiness, temper outbursts and verbal insults, and name calling	Tendency towards inner experiences; more introspective Tendency to withdraw when upset or feelings are hurt Vacillation of emotions in time and range Feelings of inadequacy common; difficulty asking for help	More constancy of emotion Anger more likely to be concealed

Biological Development

Neuroendocrine Events of Puberty

The fundamental biological changes of adolescence are collectively referred to as puberty. **Puberty** involves a predictable sequence of physical changes that occur sequentially during adolescence that results in sexual and physical maturation. The events of puberty are triggered by hormonal influences and are controlled by the anterior pituitary gland in response to stimulus from the hypothalamus.

Puberty begins as the hypothalamus produces increased levels of gonadotropin-releasing hormone (GnRH). GnRH travels through a network of capillaries to the anterior pituitary gland, where it stimulates the production and secretion of follicle-stimulating hormone (FSH) and luteinising hormone (LH) (Fig 17.1). Increasing levels of FSH and LH in the blood stimulate gonadal response. The sequential response varies for the two genders: for females, FSH stimulates growth of ovarian follicles and production of oestrogen.

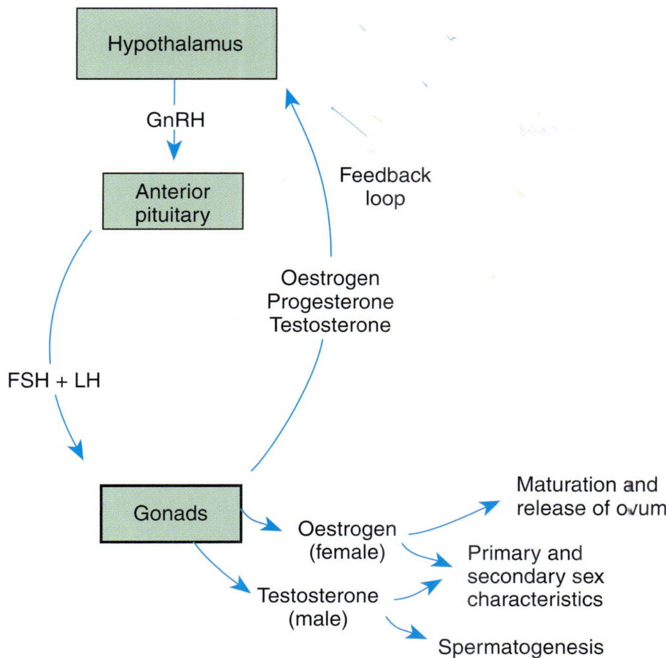

Fig 17.1 Hormonal interaction among hypothalamus, pituitary and gonads. (*GnRH,* Gonadotropin-releasing hormone; *FSH,* follicle-stimulating hormone; *LH,* luteinising hormone.)

LH initiates ovulation, the formation of the corpus luteum and progesterone production. For males, LH acts on testicular Leydig cells, prompting maturation of the testicles and testosterone production. FSH, acting with LH, stimulates sperm production. Sex steroids—oestrogen, progesterone and testosterone and other androgens—are released from the gonads and effect biological changes in various organs, including muscles, bones, skin and hair follicles. Increasing serum levels of sex steroids also provide feedback to the hypothalamus, causing decreases in GnRH secretion. When serum sex hormone levels decrease, the hypothalamus is stimulated to increase GnRH secretion, again initiating the sequence that produces the appropriate gonadal responses.

Initiation of Puberty. The precise mechanism that institutes the changes at puberty is not completely understood. Although the pituitary gland and gonads are capable of mature function and can respond to stimuli at any age, the hypothalamic–pituitary–gonadal system is kept in a dormant state throughout childhood by some central nervous system inhibitory mechanism in the region of the hypothalamus. It is believed that the receptor sites in the hypothalamus are so sensitive that minute quantities of circulating sex hormones are sufficient to inhibit the secretion of GnRH during childhood. The hypothalamus loses this negative sensitivity at puberty, which allows the hypothalamic–pituitary–gonadal mechanism to attain full secretory function. As puberty progresses, the pituitary and gonads become increasingly sensitive to positive hormonal stimulation.

Changes in Reproductive Hormones

Females. The primary sexual characteristic in girls is the development and release of an egg, or ovum, from the ovaries approximately every 28 days. Beginning in early puberty, FSH stimulates oestrogen production by the ovaries. However, concentrations of oestrogen do not reach levels high enough to cause ovulation. By the time girls reach midpuberty, the body produces oestrogen in larger amounts. This quantity of oestrogen production results in the building of an endometrial lining of the uterus and first menstruation, or menarche. At menarche, ova still do not generally mature enough to be released. However, as puberty progresses, usually one ovarian follicle becomes dominant during each menstrual cycle and produces increasing amounts of oestrogen during the early-cycle, follicular phase. This follicle then releases an ovum, a process termed *ovulation,* around day 14 of the menstrual cycle. After ovulation the follicle involutes and its oestrogen production decreases. This leads to a drop in serum oestrogen and progesterone. The pituitary gland responds to the drop in these hormone levels with increased production of FSH, initiating the start of a new menstrual cycle.

By direct action, oestrogens cause growth and development of the vagina, uterus and fallopian tubes. The skin of the labia majora, as well as that of the breast areola and nipples, grows and darkens under the influence of oestrogen. Oestrogen is responsible for breast enlargement. Oestrogen also promotes the growth of pubic and axillary hair, and widening of the hips. At low levels oestrogen tends to stimulate skeletal growth in both boys and girls, but at higher levels it inhibits growth.

Males. The primary male sexual characteristic is the development of viable sperm. During puberty, FSH acts on testicular cells, stimulating the production of viable sperm. FSH and LH also act on a different group of testicular cells, resulting in increased production and secretion of testosterone. In this process of sexual development, boys do not experience a discrete event analogous to menstruation or ovulation in girls. However, just as the production of a mature ovum tends to occur 1 year or more after menarche in girls, the production of viable sperm tends to follow boys' first ejaculations. The capacity to ejaculate appears relatively early in boys' sexual development, approximately 1 year after initial testicular enlargement and the appearance of pubic hair. From a clinical perspective, however, an adolescent should be considered potentially fertile with a first menstrual period or a first ejaculation.

Testosterone and other androgens have a direct impact on growth of the penis, scrotum, prostate and seminal vesicles of the testicles. The tremendous growth-promoting properties of these hormones also result in rapid increases in muscle mass, skeletal growth, bone age and bone density. In both sexes androgens are responsible for the development of pubic, axillary, facial and body hair. Clinically, increased activity of androgens is associated with pubertal conditions such as acne, body odour, deepening of the voice, a spurt in height and an increase in red blood cell levels.

Pubertal Sexual Maturation

Increases in reproductive hormones are responsible for dramatic changes in secondary sexual characteristics that occur during puberty. As with general growth, development of secondary sexual characteristics occurs in a predictable sequence. This sequence has been divided into a series of five phases termed the **Tanner stages** (Box 17.1 and Figs 17.2 to 17.5). Although the sequence of sexual

BOX 17.1 Tanner Stages

The Tanner stages were developed by Dr. J. M. Tanner and colleagues. Tanner stages describe the stages of pubertal growth and are numbered from stage 1 (immature) to stage 5 (mature) for both males and females. In females the Tanner stages describe pubertal development based on breast size and the shape and distribution of pubic hair. In males the Tanner stages describe pubertal development based on the size and shape of the penis and scrotum and the shape and distribution of pubic hair.

Source: Data from Tanner, J. M. (1962). Growth of adolescents. Oxford: Blackwell Scientific Publications.

Height spurt
9.5–14.5
Menarche
10.5–15.5
Breast
2 3 4 5
7–13
12–18
Pubic hair
2 3 4 5
7 8 9 10 11 12 13 14 15 16 17 18
Age (yr)

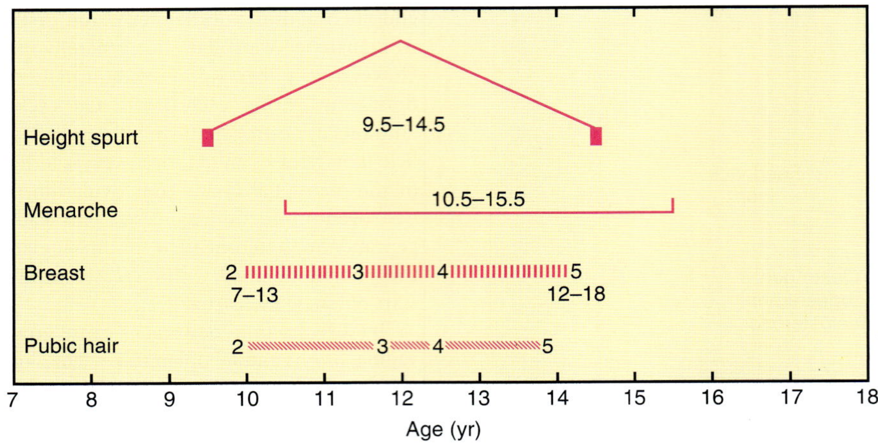

Fig 17.2 Approximate timing of developmental changes in girls. Numbers indicate stages of development. Range of ages during which some of the changes occur is indicated by inclusive numbers below them. See Figs 17.3 and 17.4 for explanation. (Source: Based on revised data from Herman-Giddens, M., Slora, E. J., Wasserman, R. C., et al. (1997). Secondary sexual characteristics and menses in young girls seen in office practice: A study from the Pediatric Research in Office Settings Network. Pediatrics, 99(4), 505–512.)

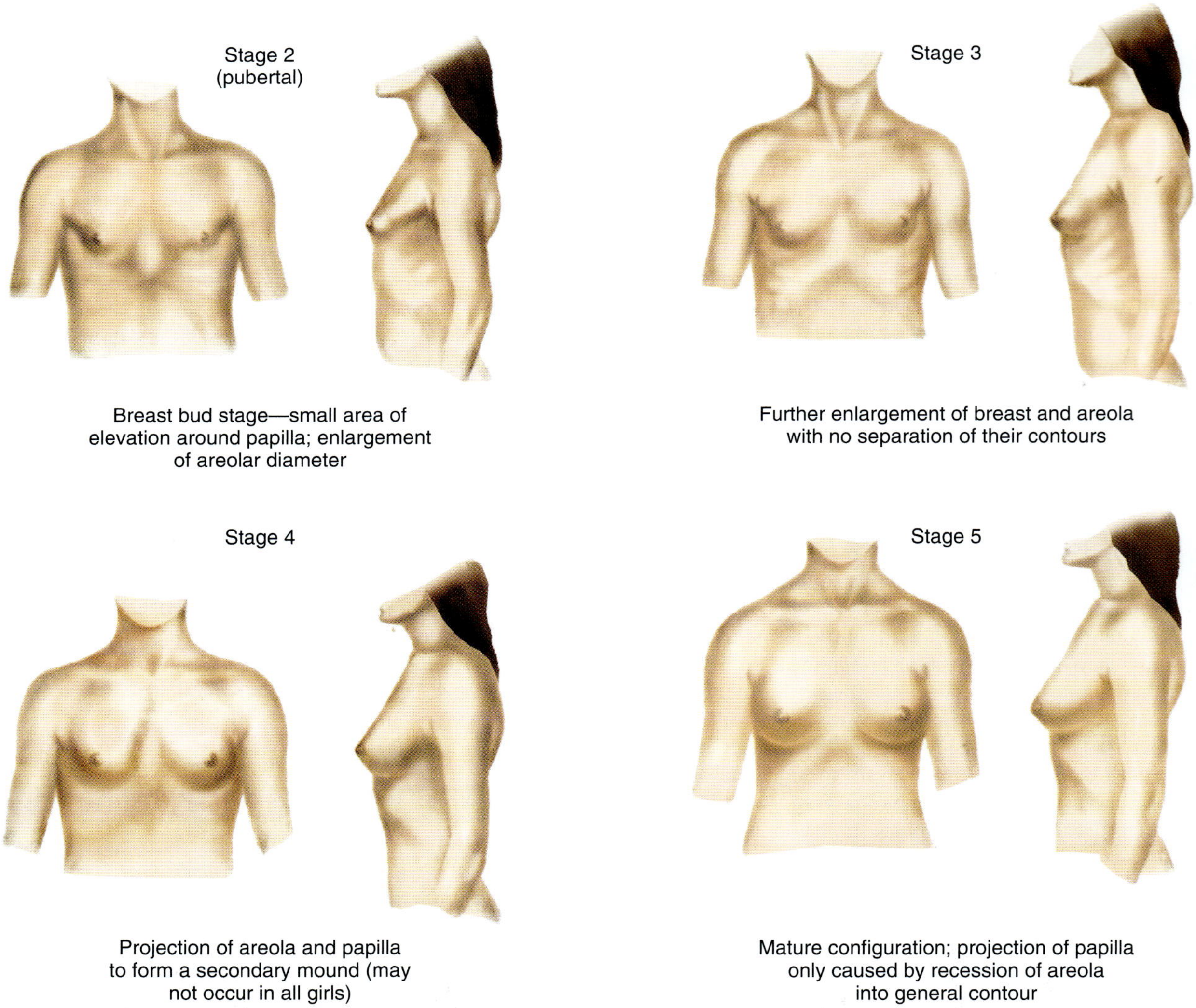

Stage 2
(pubertal)
Breast bud stage—small area of elevation around papilla; enlargement of areolar diameter
Stage 3
Further enlargement of breast and areola with no separation of their contours
Stage 4
Projection of areola and papilla to form a secondary mound (may not occur in all girls)
Stage 5
Mature configuration; projection of papilla only caused by recession of areola into general contour

Fig 17.3 Development of breasts in girls. Average age span is 8 to 12¾ years. Stage 1 (prepubertal—elevation of papilla only) is not shown. (Source: Modified from Marshall, W. A., & Tanner, J. M. (1969). Variations in pattern of pubertal changes in girls. Archives of Disease in Childhood, 44(235), 291–303; and Daniel, W. A., & Paulshock, B. Z. (1979). A physician's guide to sexual maturity. Patient Care, 13, 122–124.)

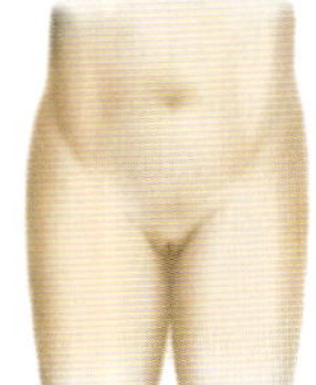
Stage 1 (prepubertal)

No pubic hair; essentially the same as during childhood; no distinction between hair on pubis and over the abdomen

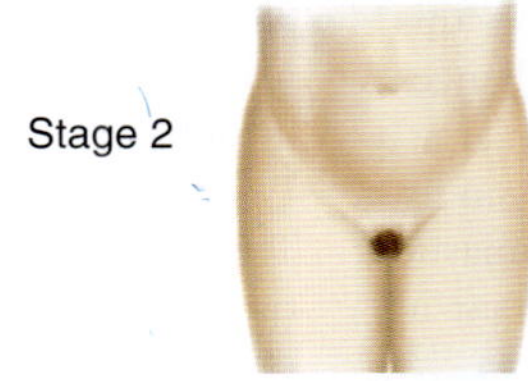
Stage 2

Sparse growth of long, straight, downy and slightly pigmented hair extending along labia; between stages 2 and 3 begins to appear on pubis

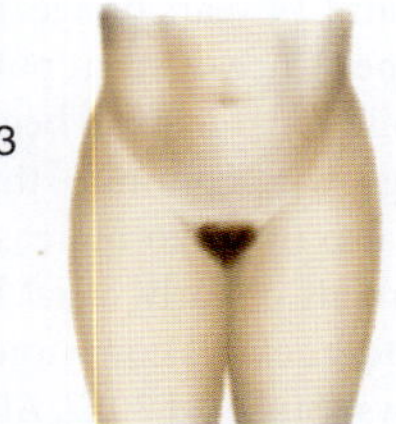
Stage 3

Hair darker, coarser and curly and spread sparsely over entire pubis in the typical female triangle

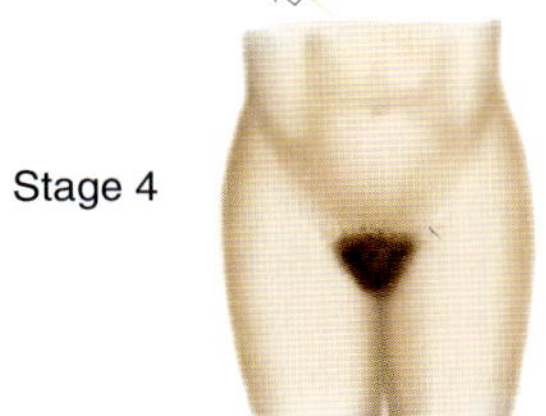
Stage 4

Pubic hair denser, curled and adult in distribution but less abundant and restricted to the pubic area

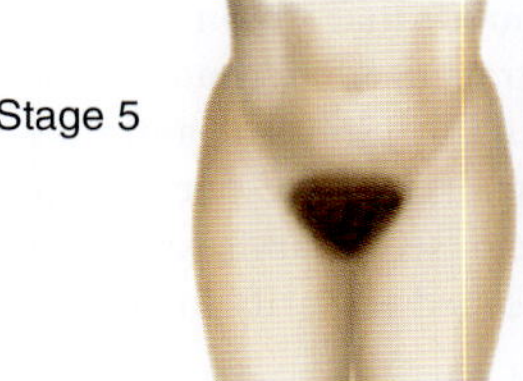
Stage 5

Hair adult in quantity, type and pattern with spread to inner aspect of thighs

Fig 17.4 Growth in pubic hair in girls. Average age span for stages 2 through 5 is 11 to 14 years. (Source: Modified from Marshall, W. A., & Tanner, J. M. (1969). Variations in pattern of pubertal changes in girls. Archives of Disease in Childhood, 44(235), 291–303; and Daniel, W. A., & Paulshock, B. Z. (1979). A physician's guide to sexual maturity. Patient Care, 13, 122–124.)

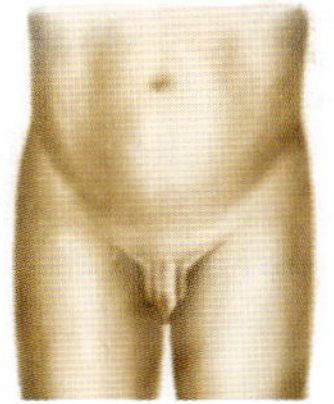
Stage 1 (prepubertal)

No pubic hair; essentially the same as during childhood; no distinction between hair on pubis and over the abdomen

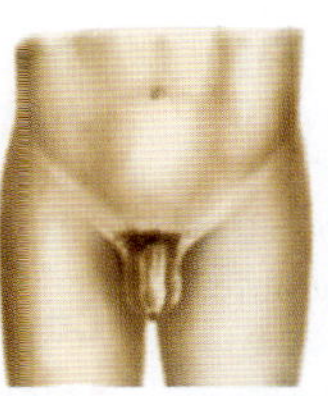
Stage 2 (pubertal)

Initial enlargement of scrotum and testes; reddening and textural changes of scrotal skin; sparse growth of long, straight, downy and slightly pigmented hair at base of penis

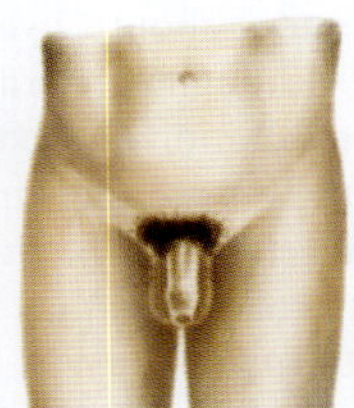
Stage 3

Initial enlargement of penis, mainly in length; testes and scrotum further enlarged; hair darker, coarser and curly and spread sparsely over entire pubis

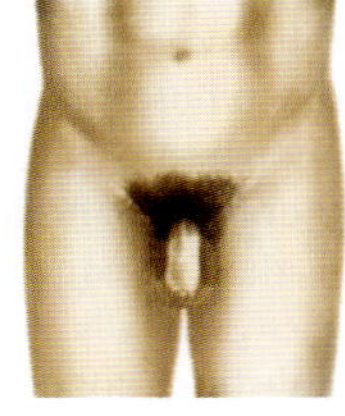
Stage 4

Increased size of penis with growth in diameter and development of glans; glans larger and broader; scrotum darker; pubic hair more abundant with curling but restricted to pubic area

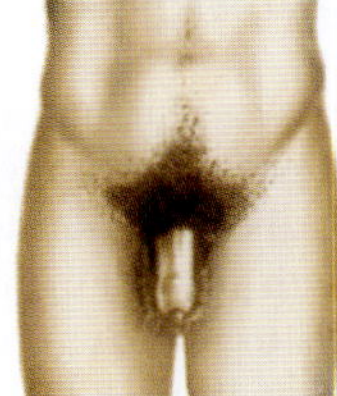
Stage 5

Testes, scrotum, and penis adult in size and shape; hair adult in quantity and type with spread to inner surface of thighs

Fig 17.5 Developmental stages of secondary sexual characteristics and genital development in boys. Average age span is 12½ to 16 years. (Source: Modified from Marshall, W. A., & Tanner, J. M. (1970). Variations in the pattern of pubertal changes in boys. Archives of Disease in Childhood, 45(239), 13–23; and Daniel, W. A., & Paulshock, B. Z. (1979). A physician's guide to sexual maturity. Patient Care, 13, 122–124.)

development is predictable, the age at which these changes occur and the rate of developmental progression vary considerably among individuals.

Sexual Maturation in Girls. The earliest, most easily visible changes of puberty in girls are changes in the nipple and areola and development of a small bud of breast tissue (thelarche). The average age of thelarche varies among ethnic groups.

Sexual Maturation in Boys. The first pubescent changes in boys are testicular enlargement accompanied by thinning, reddening and increasing looseness of the scrotum. These events usually occur between 9½ and 14 years of age. Early puberty is also characterised by the initial appearance of scant pubic hair, which continues throughout puberty. Penile enlargement begins, and testicular enlargement and pubic hair growth continue throughout midpuberty. During this period boys also undergo increasing muscularity, early voice changes and development of early facial hair. Gynaecomastia (breast enlargement and tenderness) is common during midpuberty, occurring in up to 70% of boys (Sun et al 2017, Ali & Donohoue 2016). Gynaecomastia disappears within 2 years of development; however, it may persist in obese individuals. By midpuberty there is a definite increase in the length and width of the penis, testicular enlargement continues and first ejaculation occurs. Axillary hair develops, and facial hair extends to cover the anterior neck. Final voice changes occur secondary to the growth of the larynx.

Sun et al (2017) found that secondary sexual characteristics occurred earlier in Australian adolescents than those described in Tanner's studies in England in 1969. The authors suggest that genetic factors, environmental factors and lifestyle changes may be the cause for the earlier appearance of secondary sexual characteristics but note that further studies are needed to clarify these findings.

Physical Growth During Puberty

Along with increases in reproductive hormones and sexual maturation, major changes in skeletal and lean body mass occur during puberty. The final 20% to 25% of linear growth is achieved during puberty, and up to 50% of ideal adult body weight is gained during this time as well. The **pubertal growth spurt** refers to the general increase in growth of the skeleton, muscles and internal organs, which reaches a peak rate at about 12 years of age in girls and about 14 years of age in boys. Although accelerated growth occurs in all adolescents, the age of onset, duration and extent vary among individuals. Genetic endowment is the most important determinant of the onset, rate and duration of pubertal growth, although adequate nutrition, environment and health status also play important roles.

Normal Patterns of Growth. Once the process of growth begins, the sequence of changes is progressive and usually predictable. Awareness of this sequence is not only important for reassuring concerned adolescents and parents but also useful in diagnosing conditions associated with abnormal growth. In general, girls begin puberty and reach maturity about 2 years earlier than boys. The pubertal growth spurt begins as early as 9½ years or as late as 14½ years in girls, and as early as 10½ years and as late as 16 years in boys.

General growth includes accumulation of body mass, along with increases in height and weight. Lean body mass, primarily muscle mass, increases in both girls and boys during early puberty. For girls, the rate of muscle mass growth peaks at menarche and then slows. For boys, muscle mass continues to increase throughout puberty, resulting in the attainment of significantly higher lean body mass in boys than in girls. In girls, gain in fat mass increases markedly early in puberty and continues to increase after menarche. In boys there is a peak deceleration in the rate of fat mass accumulation at the time of their growth spurt, and thereafter a slower and much less dramatic increase than in girls.

Other Physiological Changes

In addition to the sexual development changes of puberty, numerous body systems mature as well. The size and strength of the heart, blood volume and systolic blood pressure increase, and the heart rate decreases. Consistent with the general developmental timetable, these changes appear earlier in girls, who establish a slightly higher pulse rate and a slightly lower systolic blood pressure than boys. Blood volume and values in blood components steadily increase during childhood to reach adult levels in adolescence. There is an increase in serum iron, the number of red blood cells, haemoglobin and haematocrit levels more so in boys compared with girls, which is likely to be related to the increased muscle mass in pubertal boys.

The lungs increase in both diameter and length during puberty. The respiratory rate, decreasing steadily throughout childhood, reaches the adult rate in adolescence. Respiratory volume, vital capacity and other physiological properties related to respiratory function are increased, and to a greater extent in boys than in girls. The differences between the sexes are a result of the greater lung growth associated with boys' increased shoulder and chest size.

The rate of steady decline in basal metabolic rate from birth to adulthood slows during puberty, coinciding with the growth spurt in both sexes, reflecting the increase in physiological activities. A slightly higher metabolic rate in boys than in girls is probably a function of differences in androgenic hormones. Basal body temperature gradually decreases with age in both sexes, reaching adult values by 12 years of age in girls and somewhat later in boys.

Adolescence is also a time of continued brain growth. Although the number of neurons does not increase, there is a proliferation of the support cells that brace and nourish the neurons and an increase in the number of neural connections. Development of these connections within the cortex of the brain continues during adolescence and may not reach adult levels until 26 years old. In addition, the growth of the myelin sheath around the nerve cells continues through and beyond puberty, enabling faster neural processing. This 'fine-tuning' of the neurosystem, also called neuroplasticity, coincides with development of the more advanced cognitive capacities of youth and continues into early adulthood. Recent studies have shown that the frontal cortex areas of the brain, associated with executive functions, continue myelinisation throughout adolescence and may not be complete until as late as age 26 years (McCormick & Scherer 2018).

Cognitive Development

Emergence of Formal Operational Thought (Piaget)

Jean Piaget (1972) described the shift from childhood to adolescence as a movement from concrete to formal operational thought. Children's thinking is oriented to things and events that they can observe directly. Unable to think in terms of abstract possibilities, they process information based on what is directly observable. For most young people, emergence of formal operational thinking occurs between the ages of 11 and 14 years. **Formal operational thought** includes being able to think in abstract terms, consider consequences to actions and hypothesise possibilities. Adolescents gradually become able to symbolically associate behaviours with abstract concepts such as attractiveness, adult status, responsibilities or happiness. They also become capable of conceptualising a future time perspective rather than being tied to the concrete thinking of 'here-and-now' that is common during the latency period. They are able to imagine a sequence of future events that might occur including college or occupational opportunities, or how current situations, such as relationships with parents or friends, could change to meet an imagined ideal.

Even with the best framework for health promotion, persons who are capable of formal operational thought and reasoned decision-making do not always choose safe, healthy options of behaviour. This is especially true for developing adolescents; when faced with time constraints, personal stress from home, community and school settings, sleep deprivation, social media influences or overwhelming peer pressure, young people are more likely to abandon their rational thought processes.

Unfortunately, many of the health-related decisions adolescents confront, such as those related to illicit substance use, safety practices or sexual behaviour, involve issues that are personally stressful, emotionally overwhelming or new and novel/interesting to adolescents. Under such conditions, young people tend to diminish their capacities for abstract formal reasoning even if they typically use advanced decision-making skills.

Adolescent Conceptions of Self

With development of formal operational thought, adolescents begin thinking in more abstract capacities and are able to verbalise personal and interpersonal characteristics, beliefs and emotional states. Compared with children, they develop a more differentiated self-concept, recognising that their behaviour and performance vary from setting to setting and that they are separate with varied thoughts and ideals from their parents. Over time, adolescents integrate these disparate observations of their selves into abstract personal characterisations (e.g. 'I am a sensitive person').

Psychological theories help explain how adolescents use these powerful new cognitive tools to make the transition to adult roles and relationships (Elkind 1978, Lapsley 1993). Being able to think about one's own thoughts and emotions can lead to periods of extreme self-absorption, what Elkind called *adolescent egocentrism*. This self-absorption has also been described by Lapsley as a way of imagining and 'trying on' various personas and practising hypothetical interactions in an attempt to develop a separate sense of self.

There is growing evidence that the inward-focused or narcissistic egocentrism of early adolescence may be an important developmental mechanism that leads to positive mental health among mature adults, but adolescents with a strong sense of invulnerability to danger in their personal fable are more likely to engage in risky behaviours that can lead to significant morbidity and mortality. Teens who feel invincible to danger have more delinquent behaviours and drug use, whereas teens with psychological invulnerability have better mastery and coping skills (Baams et al 2015).

Changes in Social Cognition

Gains in cognitive abilities also have an impact on perspective-taking capacities of young people. As adolescents mature, they are increasingly able to 'step into the shoes' of others. Preadolescents develop limited perspective-taking skills, first learning to step into the shoes of their closest friends and then, during adolescence, the skills develop towards considering the experiences of other peers and family members, and finally people outside their social circle. Perspective-taking capacities develop further as adolescents engage in mutual role-taking. As they mature, teens are able to discuss various issues highlighting points of importance to people in various social roles (e.g. 'From a parent's perspective, having a curfew is important because it means I'm safely home'). Older adolescents also realise that the perspectives people hold are influenced by a range of intrapersonal, interpersonal and sociocultural factors and can be acceptable but varied from their own. They are typically able to consider the choices, behaviours and outcomes experienced by other people while making their own health-related choices. The ability to consider alternative choices that may or may not apply to the teen significantly expands the opportunities to develop health-promoting behaviours or adapt new strategies of self-care.

Development of Value Autonomy

With advances in cognitive development, adolescents' beliefs become more abstract and increasingly rooted in general ideological principles with gradual independence from their parents' beliefs and values. Adolescents progress towards greater behavioural independence as they encounter new social situations and make independent decisions. They face a variety of cognitive conflicts as they compare past experiences and the advice of their parents to the views and influence of peers and deal with competing pressures to behave in given ways. Earlier in life most teens accept the decisions or points of view of their parents while maturing adolescents begin to 'test', substitute or adopt a set of values distinct from those significant adults in their lives. This struggle to clarify values, created in part by an expanded behavioural independence, is a large part of the process of developing what has been termed **value autonomy** (Steinberg 1990). The development of a personal value system is a gradual process, with evidence that value autonomy occurs relatively late in adolescence, between the ages of 18 and 20 years (Steinberg 1990).

Moral Development

Moral development parallels advances in reasoning and social cognition. With the attainment of abstract thought and the realisation that people's perspectives and opinions may differ, the ways adolescents approach moral issues change. According to one theory of moral development (Kohlberg & Gilligan 1972), older children and young adolescents function at a conventional level of moral reasoning in which absolute moral guidelines are seen to emanate from authorities such as parents or teachers. Thus judgments of right and wrong are made according to a set of concrete rules. A major concern is to act or behave in ways that will gain or maintain the approval of others.

Elements of **principled moral reasoning** emerge during adolescence. With this level of reasoning, adolescents question absolutes and rules and view moral standards as subjective and based on points of view that are subject to disagreement. One may have a moral duty to abide by social standards for behaviour, but only insofar as those standards support and serve human ends. Thus occasions arise in which social conventions should be questioned and when principles such as justice, caring or quality of life take precedence over established social norms. Empirical research on Kohlberg's theory has demonstrated that aspects of both conventional and principled reasoning are present during adolescence, and different levels of reasoning are used at different times and in different situations.

Kohlberg's scheme of moral development focuses on an orientation to justice. This orientation holds as its ideal a morality based on reciprocity and equal respect. From this orientation the most important consideration in making moral decisions would be whether the individuals involved were treated 'fairly' by the ultimate decision. Gilligan (1982) proposes that an equally valid alternative to the justice orientation is one that emphasises caring. From this perspective, the ideal is a morality of attention to others and responses to human need. As opposed to the justice orientation, which assumes that moral decisions are best made from a detached position of objectivity, the caring orientation is rooted in the belief that moral decisions should be shaped by attachments and responsiveness to others. Studies have found that although both men and women are capable of approaching moral problems from the perspectives of justice and caring, women may be more likely to give caring-oriented responses before justice-oriented ones, whereas men are more likely to follow the opposite pattern (Gilligan 1986, Walker et al 1987).

Spiritual Development

Religious beliefs also become more abstract and principled during the adolescent years. Specifically, adolescents' beliefs become more oriented towards spiritual and ideological matters and less oriented towards rituals, practice and the strict observance of religious customs. Compared with children, adolescents place more emphasis on the internal aspects of religious commitment, such as what a person believes, and less on the external manifestations, such as whether an individual attends religious worship (Elkind 1978).

Consistent with developmental changes in value autonomy, the religious beliefs of young people are likely to become more personalised and less bound to the traditional religious practices they may have been exposed to when they were younger. As adolescents mature and form an identity, they may either reject or conform to their family's traditional beliefs (Chester et al 2019).

Psychosocial Development

Identity Development

The task of **identity** formation is to develop a stable, coherent picture of oneself that includes integrating one's past and present experiences with a sense of where one is headed in the future. Erik Erikson (1968) describes identity achievement as one of the main psychosocial tasks of the adolescent years; 'From among all possible and imaginable relations [the adolescent] must make a series of ever-narrowing selections of personal, occupational, gender-related and ideological commitments'.

The cognitive development and social environment that occur during adolescence push individuals to reflect on their place in society, the way others view them, their own sense of self-worth and their options regarding career, service and contributions in the future. For most individuals, the formation of a coherent self-identity occurs at some time during late adolescence and early adulthood.

Erikson (1968) suggests that the key to identity achievement lies in adolescents' interactions with others—role model adults, caregivers and, most significantly, peers. Cultural influences, the environmental surroundings and the society norms in which an adolescent lives play important roles in determining the range of available alternatives for identity formation. Optimally, adolescents have the opportunity to explore a range of possible options related to ideological, occupational and interpersonal roles before making an identity commitment.

It is critical for the nurse to be sensitive to variations in family systems and cultural variations among their adolescent patients, as well as in general within the community where they serve. Asking the adolescent about the home and school environment as well as cultural beliefs helps establish therapeutic communication.

Development of Autonomy

Becoming an autonomous, self-governing person is another fundamental psychosocial task of adolescence. Autonomy includes emotional, cognitive and behavioural components. Emotional autonomy is that aspect of independence related to changes in an individual's close relationships, and behavioural autonomy is the capacity to make independent decisions and follow through with them. Individuals generally begin the process of emotional autonomy during early adolescence by becoming more emotionally independent from their parents but remain cohesive with their friends. In the process of separating from their parents, younger adolescents often shift a portion of their emotional ties to other adults, often developing 'crushes' on teachers, coaches, celebrities or the parent/caregiver of a trusted friend while gradually becoming less emotionally dependent.

Sexuality

Adolescence represents a critical time in the development of sexuality. Hormonal, physical, cognitive and social changes that occur during adolescence all have an impact on sexual development and ultimately sexual orientation and gender identity. Of all the developmental changes that affect adolescent sexuality, none is more obvious than the impact of puberty. Adolescents must come to terms with hormonal influences, physiological manifestations such as menstruation and ejaculation and physical changes such as breast and genital development. All these changes have a profound impact on the way teenagers perceive their bodies (i.e. body image). In addition to transitions in body image, increasing levels of pubertal hormones contribute to emotional liability and increased levels of sexual motivation among both boys and girls. The degree to which adolescents feel comfortable with their bodies may affect sexual behaviours and varies widely among teens.

Changes in sexual motivations and feelings, happening at the same time as shifts in cognitive skills, contribute to painful conjectures ('Is what I'm feeling normal?'), self-conscious concerns ('Am I good looking enough?') and hypothetical thinking ('What if he/she wants to have sex?'). The emergence of formal operational thinking also increases adolescents' decision-making capabilities concerning sexual issues. The important task of successfully incorporating sexuality into developing or establishing an intimate relationship is made possible by the advanced cognitive abilities that emerge over the course of adolescence.

Part of adolescent identity formation involves the development of sexual identity. For young adolescents, the process of sexual identity development usually involves forming close friendships with same-gender peers with whom they may discuss various sexual topics or experiment sexually, often to satisfy curiosity. Sexual activity among young teenagers varies by gender. Masturbation provides an opportunity for sexual self-exploration; participation in this behaviour is influenced by learned cultural attitudes and sex-role expectations. Boys typically begin masturbating during early adolescence; the age of first masturbation varies greatly for girls. Although some girls begin masturbating during early adolescence, many do not masturbate until after they have had intercourse. Once sexual exploration begins, approximately 33% of teens engage in oral sex and sexual intercourse in the same year (Doornwaard et al 2015).

The sixth National Survey of Australian Secondary Students and Sexual Health released in 2018 reported that many students aged 15 to 18 years at some point had all engaged in some form of sexual activity. The students reported this was from deep kissing (74%) to sexual intercourse (47%). Within the report, the students that were sexually active reported that they were discussing intercourse (81%) and how they planned to protect their sexual health (77%) prior to having sexual intercourse. The survey found that 57% reported using condoms and 41% reported the use of oral contraception; 33% reported 'sexting' within the last 2 months but mostly with a partner or friend (Australian Institute of Health and Welfare [AIHW] 2020a).

An integrated sexual identity often emerges during late adolescence as individuals incorporate sexual experiences, feelings and knowledge. For most, this identity is consistent with their own physical and mental capacities and with societal limits and expectations. Whatever their orientation, most older teenagers possess the capacity to have intimate relationships that satisfy the emotional and sexual needs of both partners (Fig 17.6).

Sexual Orientation. Sexual orientation is an important aspect of sexual identity. **Sexual orientation** is defined as a pattern of sexual arousal or romantic attraction:

- towards persons of the opposite gender (heterosexual)
- towards persons of the same gender (homosexual, often called gay, lesbian or queer)
- towards both their own gender and the opposite genders (bisexual)
- based on personality and not limited to a specific gender (pansexual).

This list is not exhaustive as there are many other types of attraction; for example, asexual people are not sexually aroused by any

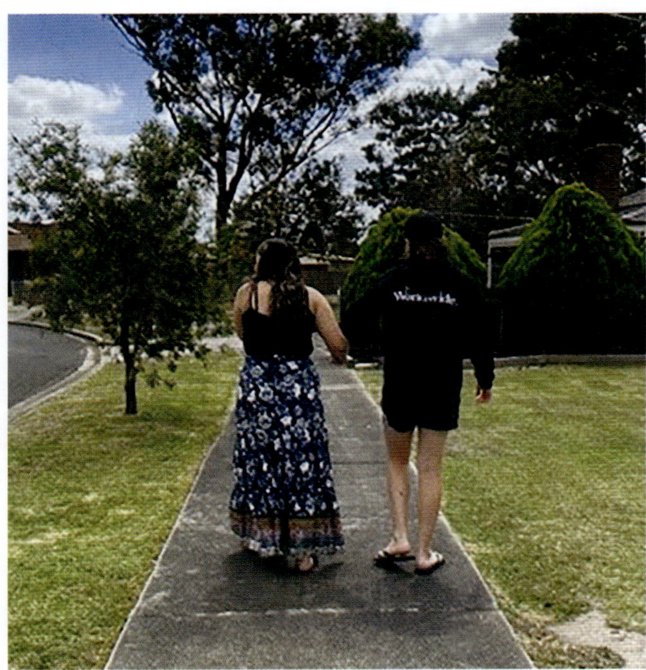

Fig 17.6 Romantic relationships are an important part of adolescence.

gender. The way a person describes their sexual orientation can also be influenced by their gender identity, such as people in the process of gender transition (transgender). Being transgender is related to your gender identity, referring to your internal sense of belonging, whether that is male, female, man, women, boy or girl. It is not an indication of your sexual orientation which is someone's sexual attraction to others who may be of the same sex, opposite sex or either sex.

Sexual orientation encompasses several dimensions: (1) sexual orientation identity that consists of how an individual defines their sexual orientation; (2) sexual attraction that includes the gender to which the individual is romantically and physically attracted; and (3) sexual behaviour that consists of whom an individual has sexual relationships with (O'Neill & Wakefield 2017). In individuals, the direction and intensity of each dimension are not necessarily consistent with any of the others.

The development of sexual orientation as part of sexual identity includes several developmental milestones during late childhood and throughout adolescence. These milestones do not necessarily occur in the same order for everyone, nor are they completed in the same amount of time. They include: (1) the realisation of romantic or erotic attraction to people of one (or both) genders; (2) erotic daydreaming about one or both genders; (3) romantic partners or dates without sexual activity; (4) sexual activity with people of the preferred gender or genders (also, for some teens, sexual activity with a non-preferred gender, due to curiosity or social pressure); (5) self-identification of the orientation that best fits one's current circumstances and understanding; (6) publicly self-identifying that orientation, usually to intimate friends and family first, then the wider social group; and (7) an intimate, committed sexual relationship with a person of the gender appropriate to one's orientation. The order of these milestones varies greatly among adolescents.

Gender. Nurses who ask teens what gender term (pronoun) they prefer as identification in healthcare settings demonstrate support and understanding of emerging gender issues. The information is also important as the provider considers clinical management and screening for risks. Transgender expression and sexual orientation are separate and distinct concepts, and it is the role of the nurse to support the growth of the child, adolescent and family through this continuum to ensure more positive outcomes. The nurse needs to become educated in the correct terminology and be aware that there is a range of gender identities on the gender spectrum.

For many young people their gender identity—their internal sense of being male or female—matches their assigned gender. These young people are called 'cisgender', with 'cis' being Latin prefix meaning 'on the same side', pertaining to their gender is on the same side as their biological sex. For other young people their gender identity is not 'on the same side' and their gender identity does not correspond with the assigned gender and biological sex, so these young people are referred to as transgender ('trans' being the Latin prefix for 'across or over'). In saying this, other young people may not identity or define themselves specifically as male or female; they may identity as both or neither. Young people communicate their gender identity in a way that is comfortable for them. This may be through clothing, hair styles, outward presentation or behaviour. The important message is that gender identity neither relates to, nor determines their sexual orientation; therefore, the healthcare professional must be aware of communication gender stereotype gestures, language and communication. Cisgender young people and young people who are transgender can identify as straight, LGBTIQ+ (lesbian, gay, bisexual, transgender, queer, intersex or other) or asexual. As healthcare professionals, to meet their needs we need to focus not on their sexual orientation but also on their gender identity.

Sharing Self-identity. Adolescents who identify as LGBTIQ+ tend to publicly self-identify ('come out') later than their heterosexual/binary peers. Without positive LGBTIQ+ role models or a supportive family member or peer group, sexual and gender minority teens can feel isolated, confused and depressed, and they may delay or avoid sharing their sexual orientation and/or gender identity with anyone for fear of rejection or violence. For example, when adolescents who would otherwise identify as bisexual can only find a peer group of gay and lesbian teens, they may focus on their same-gender dimensions of orientation and adopt the label of lesbian or gay; later, they may self-label as bisexual. Likewise, some gay and lesbian adolescents may first identify as heterosexual, then bisexual, before identifying as gay or lesbian. Gender identity may also develop over time through increased access to information and support, allowing an adolescent to find the language to express their sense of self.

It is vital to remember the usual rules of confidentiality, and that it is up to the individual to decide when, how and to whom they will come out regardless of age. No-one (including healthcare professionals and family) should reveal this information without the adolescent's consent or assume that their family/carers, peers or other health professionals are aware of their sexual orientation and/or gender identity. Transgender young people are among the most marginalised in the community and due to this face higher rates of homelessness, unemployment, social isolation, prejudices and discrimination, family rejection and mental health issues (The Gender Centre 2021). Many services offered are metropolitan based and not-for-profit-funded in Australia and New Zealand and there is little available for regional and rural transgender young people. Therefore, the nurse's role in offering support is one of great importance.

A person's gender may be anywhere on the masculine to feminine continuum and may not meet society's 'norm' which is often based on biological sex characteristics. Gender variants for young people exist and they may identify as many terms, of which only some have been discussed in this chapter. The promotion and use of positive and correct language is critical when discussing this topic with the young person and others. Lead by example and communicate with feelings of honesty and empathy to the best of your ability to support the young person and their family. As a nurse you play an important role in the mental health of LGBTIQ+ young people and are an avenue and advocate for resources and support.*

Intimacy

Intimate relationships are emotional attachments between two people characterised by concern for each other's wellbeing; a willingness to disclose private, possibly sensitive topics; and a sharing of common interests and activities. Intimate relationships are distinct from sexual relationships; it is possible for individuals to have close intimate relationships without becoming sexually involved. At the same time, people can be involved in sexual relationships that are not particularly intimate.

Social Environments

Although all adolescents experience similar biological and cognitive changes and face similar psychosocial tasks, the health-related effects of these changes are not the same for all people. Why are individuals not affected in the same ways by puberty, by changes in thinking patterns and by changes in social and legal status? The answer lies in the fact that biological, cognitive and social changes of adolescence are shaped by the social environment in which the changes take place. The social environment provides the opportunities, barriers, role models and support for individuals' development and health. Systems within the social environment, including family, peers, schools, community, social determinates of health, social media community and the larger society, all contribute uniquely to an adolescent's development and health.

Families

Over the past several decades, changes have taken place within the family microsystem that have important implications for adolescent health. Higher rates of divorce and remarriage, increasing numbers of single parents, same-gender parents, older parents (including grandparents) and blended families have affected youth. There is also an increasing percentage of dual-parents or working mothers among contemporary society. Higher rates of divorce and the decisions of single women to have children have increased the number of children spending at least part of their childhood in a single-parent family. Correspondingly, many young people find themselves in blended families, thus developing relationships with step-parents during their adolescent years. A growing number of same-gender couples are raising their own or adopted children as well (McCormick & Scherer 2018). Changes in family structure have been accompanied by changes in parent employment patterns and a dramatic increase in the percentage of mothers who work outside the home.

Peer Groups

One hallmark of adolescence is the increasing value young people place on friendships and relationships with peers (Fig 17.7). Adolescents spend more time with their peers than do children. Compared with younger children, adolescent peer groups are more autonomous and more likely to include members of the opposite gender. Because of the changes that have taken place within family systems in contemporary society, peer groups play a significant role in the socialisation of adolescents.

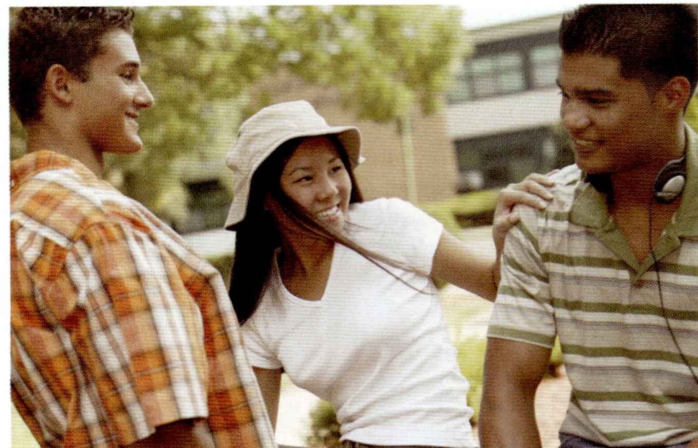

Fig 17.7 The peer group is a major influence in adolescent development.

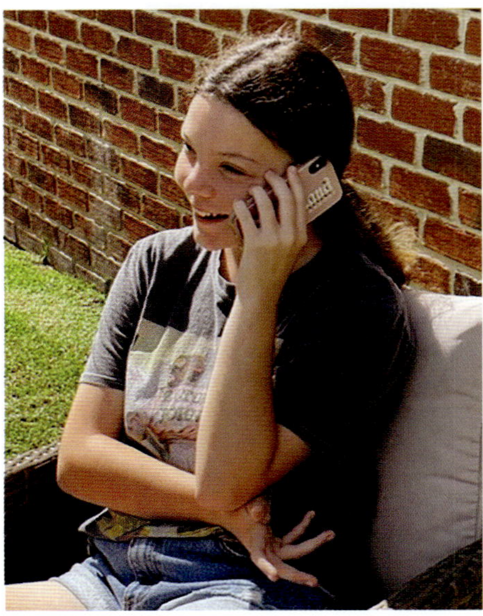

Fig 17.8 The smartphone allows adolescents to talk or message with peers for hours.

Peers serve as credible sources of information, serve as role models of social behaviours and provide sources of social reinforcement or a bridge to alternative lifestyles. Close and supportive peer friendships have beneficial effects for young people (Fig 17.8); however, adolescents with greater peer identification than parental identification, especially when the peers model or promote risky behaviours, are more prone to negative and health-compromising behaviours.

Schools

In contemporary society, schools play an increasingly important role in preparing young people for adulthood. Schooling is essential for a successful future for both boys and girls. Failure to complete high school reduces employment opportunities and the probability of earning an adequate income. Yet many schools do not meet the developmental

---

*Online resources for support include:

- ReachOut.com—https://au.reachout.com/identity/gender
- Trans Youth Equality Foundation—http://www.transyouthequality.org/
- The Gender Centre Inc.—http://www.gendercentre.org.au
- Minus18—https://www.minus18.org.au/about
- InsideOUT—http://insideout.org.nz/
- Rainbow Youth—https://ry.org.nz/
- OK2BME (Canada)—http://ok2bme.ca/resources/kids-teens/
- GLAAD (United States)—http://www.glaad.org/transgender/resources

needs of all young people. Because of a variety of reasons, including safety, academic performance and access issues, some families choose alternatives to mainstream schools, such as community school programs and homeschooling.

Technology as a Social Environment

Social media and advanced technology are prominent in the lives of most adolescents. The widespread availability of the internet and access to social networking sites such as Instagram, Twitter, Facebook, email, blogs and countless others that are rapidly evolving have created virtual communities and multiple opportunities for young people to interact with one another. Smartphones offer mobile opportunities to talk on the phone or send text messages, photos or videos. Other forms of social media such as TikTok have become the norm as a means of communicating. Even though many of the 'forms' of communication are physical on these platforms, physical activity overall has declined, especially in organised sport, particularly in the younger adolescent age group 10 to 13 (Kemp et al 2020).

Social networking sites have created a more public arena for trying out identities, having multiple identities and developing interpersonal skills with a wider network of people, occasionally with anonymity. These virtual opportunities provide a source for socialisation for young people who have limited access to friends (because of rural location, shyness or chronic conditions) to interact with people like themselves. However, many adolescents use the online social environment to interact with the same peers they spend their day with at school.

Text messaging via smartphones is also a common activity and can be disruptive during school. Both the online and the text environment can create opportunities for **cyberbullying**, in which teens engage in insults, harassment and publicly humiliating statements online or on smartphones. There is a recognised danger of adolescents coming in contact and sharing personal information with sexual predators who pose as adolescents in an attempt to make personal contact with underage victims or engage them in 'sexting' (i.e. sending sexually explicit or suggestive pictures or messages online). Adolescent sexting, rather than being an innocent anonymous activity, has been linked to risky sexual behaviours (Morelli et al 2016).

There is increased concern focusing on adolescent vehicle driving and distractions such as texting or concurrent handheld smartphone usage. More than 76% of teens in Australia own smartphones and more than 43% reported having texted or emailed while driving (Kemp et al 2020). Studies have shown that drivers using handheld devices are considerably more distracted and spend less time looking at the road or paying attention to driving conditions (Bagot et al 2018, George & Odgers 2015).

PROMOTING OPTIMUM HEALTH DURING ADOLESCENCE

Health promotion involves empowering individuals, families and communities to take developmentally and contextually appropriate actions towards realising their potential. It includes physical, cognitive, emotional and social dimensions. Health promotion involves helping youth acquire the power (including knowledge, attitudes and skills), authority (permission to use their power) and opportunities to make choices that increase the likelihood of creating positive expressions of health for themselves in their contexts.

A comprehensive approach to health promotion combines activities aimed at individuals with interventions focused on changing norms, attitudes and behaviours of peer groups, families, communities and society at large. Major causes of adolescent morbidity include the use of motor and recreational vehicles, sexual and physical abuse, sexual activity such as unwanted pregnancy and sexually transmitted infection (STIs) and substance use. Mental disorders, chronic illness, eating disorders and oral health problems are other important sources of morbidity (Kannet 2016). Chapter 18 provides further information about threats to adolescent health and wellbeing.

Contexts for Adolescent Health Promotion

A consensus is growing that the most effective adolescent health promotion efforts involve multiple systems and address multiple issues. Interventions integrating programs and expertise from healthcare, school and community-based settings can effectively increase adolescents' prevention skills, improve their access to healthcare services, build adult motivation and support for adolescent prevention practices, and change physical environments and social norms to support healthy behaviour. Such a comprehensive approach to health promotion requires a great deal of cooperation and coordination on the part of complex institutions. On the other hand, by not limiting the responsibility for adolescent health to one person or one setting, multiple opportunities for health promotion arise. Individual efforts reinforce important themes and become an integral part of an overall health promotion strategy.

Schools. Schools are a primary site for adolescent health promotion and disease prevention. Large numbers of young people can be affected by school-based health promotion efforts because virtually all teenagers attend school, at least through the early adolescent years. Group interventions offer adolescents a sense of anonymity, which they prefer when obtaining information about sensitive topics. School personnel often have special expertise and experience with health education. Through daily contact, school staff can develop supportive relationships with a limited number of students. Parent–teacher associations and school boards also link schools with the larger community in ways that can be used to expand the scope of adolescent health promotion efforts.

School-based health promotion interventions include classroom health education, school-level policies and environmental changes. School systems often offer classroom programs which include components that focus on building students' knowledge and skills and establish peer support for health-enhancing behaviours.

Healthcare Settings. Consistent, supportive, one-on-one interactions over time between adolescents and members of the healthcare team provide significant opportunities for health promotion. These relationships can create 'safe environments' in which adolescents can disclose sensitive information related to health risk. In turn, this information should be incorporated into preventive interventions specific to individual adolescent needs.

Healthcare settings offer the advantage of being able to provide confidential services, which are especially important in sensitive situations such as those involving substance use and sexual behaviour. Interventions provided through healthcare settings can include parents and help create social environments that support adolescents' health-enhancing behaviours. Another advantage is that healthcare settings have resources available to address various components of health, including physical, emotional and social needs.

To be effective, healthcare services for adolescents must be accessible and appropriate. To be accessible, services must be available, affordable and approachable. Services must include outreach to adolescents and their parents, informing them of the availability of services. Mechanisms for low- or no-cost services must be developed because cost is a major barrier to adolescents receiving appropriate care. Locating healthcare services in places such as schools, youth services centres, shopping centres and detention facilities and offering convenient clinical hours are two strategies that increase accessibility for teenagers who may not use traditional services.

The Internet and Other Technologies. A growing number of health promotion activities use the communication technologies that adolescents surround themselves with. Health-related websites designed to appeal to youth (often designed with youth) offer extensive information on nearly every topic that can affect adolescent health, although the accuracy and quality of such websites varies greatly. Social networking sites have been created to help youth with specific health issues. Some youth clinics offer text message reminders of appointments and smartphone calls to return for STI testing results. Other programs even offer text messages or emails with: encouragements for youth who are trying to quit smoking; reminders about safer sex practices; or tips to improve nutrition, exercise and weight management. Although clinicians need to consider carefully the levels of privacy and confidentiality in the use of different forms of technology, there is growing evidence of effectiveness in engaging youth through the technology they use to communicate.

Adolescent Health Screening

One strategy for health promotion by nurses and other professionals in healthcare settings is one-on-one health screening. Through information gained during a health screening interview, the health professional can identify both assets and threats to an adolescent's health and wellbeing. The health screening interview also offers an opportunity for health professionals to build trusting relationships with adolescents. This sense of trust may be critical for adolescents to act on information, attitudes and skills that are shared to help them successfully negotiate particular stressors.

Health Concerns of Adolescence

Effective health education for adolescents should incorporate a developmentally appropriate, multifaceted approach. Motivational interviewing improves adherence to healthcare advice by using a collaborative approach. In this process, the adolescent is encouraged to introspectively explore ambivalence and develop solutions for effecting change. Education alone is not enough to change behaviour. Effective programs for adolescents must include opportunities to improve communication and empowerment skills (Hoying et al 2016).

Several professional organisations have published guidelines aimed at improving and maintaining healthcare for adolescents and young adults. Australia has released the *Young Australians: their health and wellbeing 2011* as the last full longitudinal study and report. The report is the fourth in a series of national statistical reports on young people aged 12 to 24 years, produced by the Australian Institute of Health and Welfare (AIHW 2011). It provides the latest available information on how Australia's young people are faring according to a set of national indicators of health and wellbeing. Death rates have fallen considerably among young people, mainly due to declines in injury deaths. Most young people are achieving national minimum standards for reading, writing and numeracy, are fully engaged in study or work and have strong support networks. There are some favourable trends in risk and protective factors, such as declines in smoking and illicit substance use. But it is not all good news. There is a high rate of mental disorders among young people, and road transport crashes, although continuing to decline, are still a major cause of death among young males. Too many young people are overweight or obese, are not doing sufficient physical activity or eating enough fruit and vegetables, and are drinking alcohol at risky levels. Aboriginal and Torres Strait Islander young people are far more likely to be disadvantaged across a broad range of indicators.

In 2016, New Zealand released a full report on adolescent health and key findings, Pathways to child health, development and wellbeing: Optimal environments for orchids and dandelions. An overview of the evidence (Kvalsvig et al 2016). The report outlined areas of concern in relation to child and adolescent health due to the increase in childhood poverty, infectious diseases, family violence, inequities in health experience particularly by Māori and Pacific Islander children and adolescents and increased pressure on low-income families to meet the needs of their children's growth and development (Kvalsvig et al 2016). This report review used a 'biodevelopmental framework', an evidence-based approach to assist policy makers to begin to develop equitable and effective early childhood policies and programs to address these concerns.

Psychosocial Adjustment

As adolescents experience the many changes of adolescence, they redefine who they are and what they want out of life. Most individuals progress through the changes of their adolescent years with minimum emotional upheaval, countering the belief that this period in life is one of 'storm and stress'. Some adolescents, however, do have difficulty coping and exhibit emotional distress, especially when multiple normative events happen simultaneously and are combined with non-normative life events.

Adolescence is characterised by change within multiple domains. Changes associated with pubertal development typically take place during the early adolescent years. Early- and late-maturing adolescents who feel they are 'out of sync' with their age-mates' growth patterns may have a more difficult time emotionally than those who develop 'on time' with their peers.

Intentional and Unintentional Injury

Injuries. In Australia in 2016–17 falls accounted for approximately half of the hospitalised injury cases for young adolescents, with motor vehicle crashes the second leading cause of intentional and unintentional injury for older adolescents (AIHW 2020b). Assault cases account for almost the remainder, with 48% being from bodily force where the perpetrator was a parent, carer or other family member (AIHW 2020b). The rate of hospitalisation of injury cases is almost twice as high for children residing in very remote regions compared to those in major cities. It is higher again among Indigenous compared to non-Indigenous children and adolescents across all age groups from 0 to 18 years (AIHW 2020b). The incidence of intentional harm was also higher in regional and outer regional areas compared to major cities and, again higher among Indigenous adolescents than non-Indigenous adolescents. Intentional harm was cited as higher in females than males in all areas (AIHW 2020b).

Unfortunately, Māori adolescents also had a higher rate of both unintentional and intentional injury than non-Māori children and respectively higher rates of hospitalisation (Ministry of Health 2018). Motor vehicle crashes were again a leading cause, followed by accidental poisoning and falls. Intentional injury rates were again almost twice as high as those of non-Māori adolescents, with number of females almost double that of males (Ministry of Health 2020).

Deaths. In 2018, the death rate among young people aged 15 to 24 was 35 deaths per 100,000. Overall, the death rate among young people has fallen over time from 42 deaths per 100,000 in 2009 to 35 deaths per 100,000 in 2018. Death rates were higher among young males (49 per 100,000) than females (20 per 100,000) (AIHW 2020a). The leading cause of death among young people was injuries (74%). In 2018, injuries contributed 845 deaths of young people aged 15 to 24—a rate of 26 per 100,000 people. The leading causes of injury deaths were intentional self-harm (51%), land transport accidents (26%) and accidental poisoning (8.0%). Also in 2018, the age-specific rate of suicide among young people was 13.5 per 100,000. Young people accounted for

14% of suicide deaths. The rate of suicide was higher among young males (20 per 100,000) than females (6.4 per 100,000). Between 2009 and 2018, the rate of suicide among young people increased from 9.1 per 100,000 in 2009 to 14 per 100,000 in 2018 (AIHW 2020a).

Māori adolescents have a higher overall death rate due to suicide and to self-harm than non-Māori adolescents. What was also noticeable was the increase in the death rate due to unintentional injury through incidents of suffocation/accidental threats to breathing, and this was present in both males and females in the young adolescent age group 10 to 14 years (Ministry of Health 2018). The second leading cause of death was motor vehicle crashes.

Dietary Habits and Eating Disorders

Overweight and Obesity. According to estimates from the Australian Bureau of Statistics (ABS) National Health Survey 2017–18, 41% (1.3 million) of young people aged 15 to 24 were overweight or obese. This proportion was higher among males than females—47% (737,000) of males aged 15 to 24 were overweight or obese compared with 36% (543,000) of females (AIHW 2020c).

In 2019–20 in New Zealand, 1 in every 10 children were classed as obese (9.4%). This can be broken down into ethnicity, with 29% being Pacific Islander, 13.2% Māori, 3.4% Asian and 7.2% of European/Other children. Children within lower socioeconomic areas were almost one-third more likely to be obese. This is a decrease from the previous year but is too early to accredit to any health promotion interventions introduced into schools as yet (Ministry of Health 2020).

Puberty marks the beginning of accelerated physical growth, which can as much as double adolescents' nutritional requirements for iron, calcium, zinc and protein. At the same time, growing independence, the need for peer acceptance, concern with physical appearance and an active lifestyle may affect eating habits, food choices, nutrient intake and thus nutritional status. Iron-deficiency anaemia and obesity are increasingly common among adolescents; they are found in all income and racial/ethnic groups and both genders (Fig 17.9). Inadequate intake of certain vitamins (e.g. folic acid, vitamin B_6, vitamin A) and minerals (e.g. iron, calcium, zinc) is also evident, particularly among girls and teenagers of low socioeconomic status. In combination with other factors, these dietary patterns could result in increased risk for chronic diseases such as heart disease, osteoporosis and some types of cancer later in life. Girls, in particular, are susceptible to iron deficiency at menarche. Maximum bone mass is also acquired during adolescence; therefore, the calcium deposited during these years determines the risk of osteoporosis.

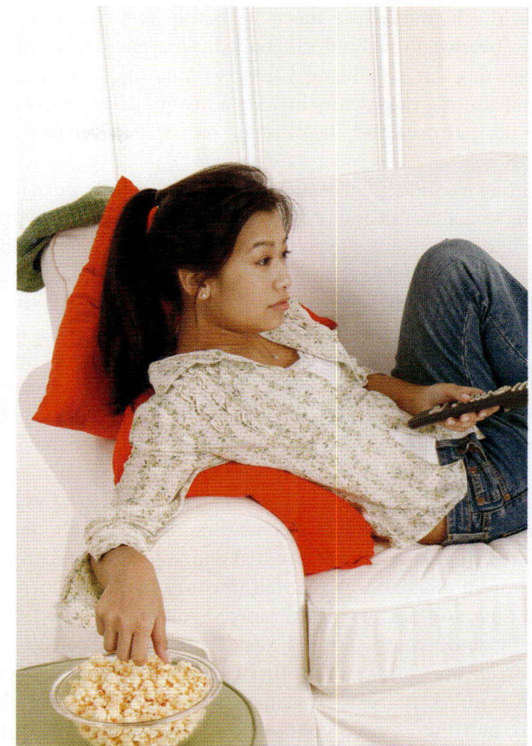

Fig 17.9 Snacking on empty calories is common among adolescents, especially during inactivity.

Physical Activity

Physical activity is important for an adolescent's health, development and psychosocial wellbeing. Limiting screen time and sedentary behaviour is also essential to encourage wellbeing. Regular activity assists with brain development, bone strength, muscle tone and control, coordination and maintaining healthy weight. The other benefits of being active, particularly for an adolescent, are that it assists with concentration, mental health, self-esteem and sleep (AIHW 2020c) (Fig 17.10).

As noted above, when obesity is rising, being physical also assists with long-term cardiovascular, metabolic and musculoskeletal health. The adolescent who is active is more likely to continue to be active to some level into adulthood and decrease risk factors for illnesses such as type 2 diabetes and some cancers (AIHW 2020c).

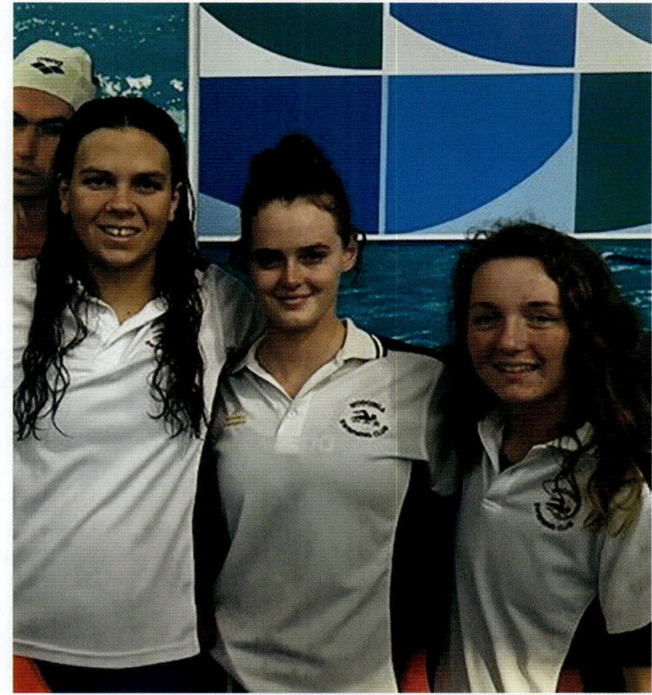

Fig 17.10 Adolescents should be encouraged to participate in activities that contribute to lifelong physical activity.

Sexual Behaviour, Sexually Transmitted Infections and Unintended Pregnancy

The success of lowering unwanted pregnancies and the prevalence of STIs among young people rely heavily on the knowledge about reproductive matters and access to and use of effective contraception. Use of condoms is the most effective method of protection against STIs among sexually active people, and is effective in preventing unintended pregnancies. Rates of STIs have been increasing over the past decade, with chlamydia the most frequently reported STI in 2018. Chlamydia overwhelmingly affects young heterosexual men and women, with those most at risk being young women aged 15 to 29 years. Other contributing risk factors include a history of prior STIs, new or multiple sex partners and inconsistent use of barrier contraceptives (Fisher 2019).

Obtaining a confidential sexual history can be an important step in promoting sexual health and preventing STIs and unintended pregnancies among young people. Given their sensitive nature, questions about sexuality should be prefaced by an explanation of their purpose and the limits of confidentiality. Initial questions can cover less sensitive topics, such as milestones in pubertal development and, for girls, the menstrual history (including the age at menarche, timing of menstrual cycles, duration of menstrual flow and symptoms of dysmenorrhoea). Questions should also address dating behaviour, same- and other gender attractions and same- and other gender sexual behaviour (e.g. 'There are many ways people can be sexual with others, such as kissing; touching; and having oral, vaginal and anal sex. In what ways have you been sexual with others?'). Adolescents should be asked about a history of uninvited or non-consensual sexual contact (e.g. 'Has anyone ever touched you in a sexual way that felt uncomfortable or when you did not want them to? Has anyone ever forced you to have sex?').

Sexually active youth should be asked about their consistency and motivation to use condoms or other barrier methods for preventing STIs; the number of sexual partners they have had over the past 6 months; and the use of alcohol or other substances in connection with sexual activity. The use of birth control pills or other forms of hormonal contraception is not protective against STIs. Sexually active adolescents should also be asked about any history of pregnancies or STIs. Adolescents who reveal a history of physical or sexual abuse, who admit to heavy use of alcohol or other drugs, or who have unstable social or economic support systems should also be asked whether they have ever exchanged sex for money, shelter or drugs.

Use of Tobacco, Alcohol and Other Substances

Young adolescents choosing to drink under the age of 15 years are at the greatest risk of harm from drinking and tend to engage in risk-taking behaviour, putting them at a higher risk of injury (Azzopardi et al 2018). Choosing to drink at an early age tends to lead to more likelihood of drinking heavily in adulthood and increasing risk factors of certain disease processes and health disorders (AIHW 2020d).

Approximately 7% of 12- to 14-year-old adolescents in 2017 had had at least one drink on a single occasion in the last week and rates were similar for males and females (AIHW 2020d). Of this group, 1% had engaged in risk-taking drinking, where they had drunk five or more standard drinks on one occasion in the last week, which significantly increases their risk of harm to themselves and others (Azzopardi et al 2018). Males were more likely to be the ones take this risk and almost twice as more likely to engage in risk-taking drinking; this was more evident in Indigenous and Māori young people than non-Indigenous and non-Māori young people (Azzopardi et al 2018).

Young people in lower and disadvantaged socioeconomic areas were more likely to drink and smoke than those living in less-disadvantaged areas, but this was not statistically significantly high. What is significantly noticeable is there is higher rates of Indigenous and Māori young people smoking than non-Indigenous and non-Māori (Azzopardi et al 2018, Azzopardi et al 2019).

In 2016–17, around 14% of young adolescents had used some type of illicit substance by the age of 12 to 15 years, and males (15%) were slightly more likely to have done so than females (13%). There has been little shift in this figure over the last 10 years; what has shifted is the type of illicit drug used (AIHW 2020d, Azzopardi 2019).

Data from the 2019 National Drug Strategy Household Survey (NDSHS) are available in a report on substance use among young people aged 14 to 24. Self-reported data from the 2019 NDSHS found that 97% of young people aged 14 to 17 and 80% of people aged 18 to 24 had never smoked tobacco (AIHW 2020e).

Fewer Young People are Taking Up Smoking. The proportion of people aged 14 to 17 who had never smoked increased from 82% in 2001 to 97% in 2019. The proportion of 14 to 17 year olds who were daily smokers decreased from 11% in 2001 to 1.9% in 2019. However, the estimate for 2019 should be interpreted with caution as the relative standard error (RSE) is between 25% and 50%. In 2019, two-thirds (66%) of young people aged 14 to 17 had never had a full serve of alcohol, compared with only 15% of those aged 18 to 24. The proportion of 14 to 17 year olds consuming five or more drinks at least monthly remained stable between 2016 and 2019 (8.0% and 8.9%, respectively) but has declined since 2001 (30%) (AIHW 2020d).

There were no significant declines among 14 to 17 year olds in recent illicit drug use (at least once in the past 12 months) between 2016 and 2019. However, recent use was considerably lower in 2019 (9.7%) than in 2001 (23%); use of cannabis fell from 21% to 8.2% (AIHW 2020d).

Depression and Suicide

Based on information from the second Australian Child and Adolescent Survey of Mental Health and Wellbeing (also known as the Young Minds Matter survey) undertaken in 2013–14, around 14% of children aged 12 to 17 met the clinical criteria for one or more mental disorders in the previous 12 months (Lawrence et al 2015). Anxiety disorders (7.0%) were the most common. Young males were more likely than young females to have attention deficit hyperactivity disorder (ADHD) or conduct disorder, while young females were more likely than young males to have anxiety or a major depressive disorder.

It is crucial to explore thoughts about and possible plans for suicidal acts with all troubled adolescents. Once an assessment of the immediate risk of suicide is completed, the nurse can construct a management scheme that ensures safety. If the adolescent has a specific plan, immediate referral for acute intervention with a psychiatrist or other mental health professional is indicated. (See Suicide, Chapter 18.)

Physical, Sexual and Emotional Abuse

Adolescents who have been physically, sexually or emotionally abused during childhood or adolescence face challenges to healthy development. Around 1 in 4 adolescents reports having been physically abused, primarily by family members and less commonly by someone outside the family. Certain groups of adolescents, such as LGBTIQ+ youth or those who are developmentally delayed, may be especially vulnerable to abuse (Lawrence et al 2015).

A common constellation of symptoms among adolescents who have been victims of sexual abuse includes substance abuse, depression, withdrawn mood, violence and somatic complaints. Adolescents who have been abused are more likely than non-abused adolescents to engage in health-compromising behaviours such as self-mutilation, suicide attempts, injection drug use and early sexual activity (Ferrara et al 2016, Maquire et al 2015) and are at higher risk of being sexually exploited.

School and Learning Problems

In 2019, most Year 7 and Year 9 students met the minimum standards for reading (ranging from 90% to 96%), writing (83% to 96%) and numeracy (95% each), similar results to 2018. A higher proportion of female than male students achieved at or above the national minimum standards for reading and writing, while for numeracy the proportions were similar for males and females. The proportion of students who met the standards for literacy declined with increasing years of schooling, particularly for writing among males (89% in Year 7 falling to 83% in Year 9). For numeracy, the rates remained relatively stable across the years (AIHW 2020f).

Data from the national literacy and numeracy tests are not directly comparable with data from previous state- and territory-based tests. For the period 2001 to 2007, the proportion of students meeting the literacy and numeracy benchmarks remained much the same from year to year (ACARA 2018).

Completion of secondary school is the first step along the pathway to either further education or entry into the labour market and is considered important preparation for participation in many aspects of adult life. Students who fail to complete Year 12 may have fewer employment opportunities and are more likely to experience extended periods of unemployment than Year 12 graduates. According to the ABS 2019 Survey of Education and Work, nearly one-third of school leavers aged 15 to 24 years did not complete Year 12, and those who left school without completing Year 10 were twice as likely to be unemployed than those who completed Year 12 (25% compared with 12% respectively). To address this issue, the Council of Australian Governments (COAG) has introduced a youth participation requirement from 1 January 2010, which requires young people to be in school until they complete Year 10 and then to participate in full-time education, training or employment until they reach age 17 (COAG 2019).

Aboriginal and Torres Strait Islander and Māori Young People. Young Aboriginal and Torres Strait Islander people were less likely to have achieved the Year 7 and Year 9 reading, writing and numeracy minimum standards—73%, 70% and 76% for Year 7 students and 67%, 59% and 75% for Year 9 students, respectively, in 2019—30 percentage points lower than for non-Indigenous students. They were also far less likely to remain in school to Year 12, with an apparent retention rate of 45% compared with 77% for non-Indigenous students in 2019. However, the gap in apparent retention rates has narrowed over the last decade, from 39 percentage points in 2010 to 32 percentage points in 2019 (COAG 2019).

New Zealand Education has developed a very different approach to education to build on engagement in education at all year levels, but particularly at the early to late adolescent age group. To assist with engaging Māori adolescents and ensuring cultural needs are meet, the New Zealand Education Department have put into place several education systems, one being Māori-medium education (Kura Kaupapa Māori). Students are taught all or some of the curriculum in the Māori language for at least 51% of the time. This has seen an improvement in retention of students aged 13 to 15 years double in the last 7 years (Ministry of Education 2021). These schools are based on Māori philosophies but also cover the National Curriculum for the remaining 19% of the curriculum. Students also have the options of Te Aho o Te Kura Pounmau (Te Kura) which is home or distance learning, to accommodate for those that may not have the means to travel to school or if Māori medium education is not an option for them. Data has shown the reintroduction of Youth Guarantee, which allows 16- to 19-year-old students to study level 1 to 3 trade certificates free of charge, has also increased school attendance for Māori young people (Ministry of Education 2021). The other major education provider to young Māori people is Wānanga. New Zealand has three wānanga, and these teach according to āhuatanga Māori (Māori tradition) and tikanga Māori (Māori custom). They offer certificates, diplomas and degrees. Some teach in specialised areas up to doctorate level.

Remoteness. Students in Years 7 and 9 in remote and very remote areas were less likely to meet the minimum standards for reading, writing and numeracy than those in metropolitan areas in 2009. These patterns may be influenced by the high proportion of Indigenous students in remote and very remote areas, and the poorer performance of these students. Remoteness is classified according to the Ministerial Council on Education, Employment, Training and Youth Affairs (MCEETYA) Schools Geographic Location scale. Young people aged 18 to 24 years living in major cities were twice as likely to be studying for a qualification as those living in outer regional and remote areas combined: 43% and 22% respectively, according to the ABS General Social Survey (2016).

Hypertension

As adolescents experience sexual maturation, along with increases in height and weight, blood pressure increases from the onset of adolescence and continues to rise until the end of pubertal growth. Approximately 1% of adolescents have sustained hypertension, defined as a blood pressure greater than the 95th percentile of standards. The detection of hypertension during adolescence is important because hypertension is one of the major preventable risk factors for adult cardiovascular disease. With increasing levels of obesity, there have been reports of increasing incidence of hypertension among adolescents (Cheung et al 2017).

Infectious Diseases and Immunisation

An immunisation update is an important part of adolescent preventive care. Obtaining a record of the teenager's prior immunisation is important.

Vaccination initiates the body's natural defence mechanism—the immune response—to build resistance to specific infections (immunise). It is a safe and effective way to protect against harmful communicable diseases.

Vaccines are a powerful and cost-effective public health intervention, significantly reducing the risk of disease, disability and death, particularly in childhood (McGovern & Canning 2015, Orenstein & Ahmed 2017, WHO 2021). Successful immunisation interventions include the worldwide eradication of smallpox and the widespread elimination of poliomyelitis (polio).

The Australian Government Department of Health Australian Immunisation Handbook digital and hard copy is available to assist with all immunisation requirements for adolescents at https://immunisationhandbook.health.gov.au/. The New Zealand immunisation information for adolescents is available via the Immunisation Handbook 2020 at https://www.health.govt.nz/publication/immunisation-handbook-2020.

Body Art. Body art (piercing and tattooing) is an aspect of adolescent identity formation. The skin has become the latest source of parent–adolescent conflict. Adolescents often seek body art as an expression of their personal identity and style. Tattoos may mark significant life events such as new relationships, births and deaths. Piercing the ear, nose, lip, nipple, eyebrow, labia, navel, penis or tongue may sometimes create a health problem. It is a nursing responsibility to caution adolescents against having piercing performed by friends, parents or themselves. Although in most cases piercings have few, if any, serious side effects, there is always a risk for complications such as infection, cyst or keloid formation, bleeding, dermatitis or metal allergy. Using the same unsterilised needle to pierce body parts of multiple teenagers presents the same risk for HIV, hepatitis C virus and hepatitis B virus transmission as occurs with other needle-sharing activities. Furthermore, there is a danger of contaminated tattoo ink that occurred in association with skin infections, such as non-tuberculous *Mycobacterium chelonae* (Mudedla et al 2015).

Sleep Deprivation and Insomnia

The changing social environment of adolescents can often change their sleep patterns at a time when their growth and development require additional sleep for health. Although adolescents should generally get around 9 hours of sleep each night, early-morning school scheduling, extracurricular activities, homework, employment and desired social time with peers or on the internet can make it difficult for them to get sufficient sleep. Recent studies into sleep among adolescents have shown that nearly half may not get the recommended amounts of sleep, and as many as 1 in 4 are regularly sleep deprived—that is, report 7 hours or less of sleep per night (Kann et al 2016, Tarokh et al 2016). Sleep deprivation can affect physical and mental health and has been associated with higher rates of overweight and obesity, depression, somatic complaints such as headaches and stomach-aches, fatigue and difficulties with concentration. These physical and psychological effects of inadequate sleep can also affect school performance and thus contribute to school problems. Health teaching and health promotion should include information to promote sufficient sleep.

Homeless youth, youth who go to bed hungry because of insufficient access to food and those with anxiety disorders are all more likely to experience sleep disturbances. However, the high rate of young people who do not get enough sleep and the health consequences of inadequate sleep suggest that nurses should regularly assess all adolescents for the amount and quality of sleep they are getting. Health teaching and health promotion should include information to promote sufficient sleep.

Health Promotion among Special Groups of Adolescents

Certain groups of adolescents experience health problems at disproportionate rates and face barriers to healthcare because of a lack of financial resources, limited availability of appropriate resources or other factors.

Aboriginal and Torres Strait Islander Adolescents

Aboriginal and Torres Strait Islander children vary in their ability to meet growth and development milestones and the challenges of adolescence and young adulthood. To be most effective, future health promotion interventions must include strategies that increase health promotion factors in the lives of other children and adolescents growing up in high-risk environments.

However, too many Indigenous adolescents experience predictable outcomes associated with living in environments where risk factors outweigh protective factors. Non-Indigenous adolescents have higher learning, emotional and physical challenges. They are more likely to drop out of school and have limited opportunities for higher education, become parents at an early age, are incarcerated in youth detention facilities or die as a result of homicide or unintentional injuries before reaching adulthood. The increase in health risk behaviours during adolescence, in combination with limited access to healthcare and effective preventive services, places these adolescents at significantly higher risk for adolescent pregnancy, STIs, HIV/AIDS, chronic or other infectious diseases (hypertension, tuberculosis [TB] and hepatitis), substance abuse, emotional problems and violence. All these health problems, which often lead to premature death or chronic disorders, are preventable.

Effective health promotion programs can make important contributions to the prevention of health problems among Indigenous adolescents. A consensus is growing that health promotion programs will be most effective if they are culturally competent. A culturally competent approach is one that recognises the importance of culture and incorporates—at all levels—the assessment of relations across cultures, with attention to dynamics that result from cultural differences, the expansion of cultural knowledge and the adaptation of programs to meet culture-specific needs. Nurses, working with other healthcare professionals and community leaders, can develop or adapt culture-specific health promotion interventions.

Health and Wellbeing of Indigenous Young People

Aboriginal and Torres Strait Islander peoples generally have poorer health, are more likely to experience disability and reduced quality of life and typically die at much younger ages due to ill health. This health disadvantage begins at an early age and often continues to adversely affect their wellbeing throughout life. The burden of disease and injury among Indigenous Australians is higher than for other Australians for all ages. For Indigenous young people, this burden is largely attributable to the high rates of mental disorders, such as anxiety and depression, substance use and injuries (AIHW 2018).

A strong sense of identity as an Aboriginal or Torres Strait Islander person is also vital to the wellbeing of Indigenous young people. A study in Western Australia found that having a strong sense of self, connection to family, kin, Aboriginal language and Aboriginal culture and inheritance were recognised as important contributors to an Aboriginal person's racial identity (Kickett-Tucker & Shaouli Shahid 2019). Indigenous adolescents' identification with local cultures is a protective factor in their social and emotional wellbeing; however, peer influences (e.g. encouraging alcohol consumption) may override the protective influence of cultural identity (AIHW 2018).

There are various measures of health status that can provide information on both Indigenous health and the health inequality that exists between Indigenous and non-Indigenous Australians. These are self-assessed health status, life expectancy, mortality, hospitalisations, injuries and poisoning and health conditions. These measures all show that young Indigenous Australians tend to have poorer health outcomes than non-Indigenous young people.

Self-assessed Health Status

Young people's self-assessed health status can be affected by a number of factors such as levels of education, remoteness, Indigenous status and socioeconomic status. The proportion of Indigenous young people rating their health as 'excellent', 'very good' or 'good' is similar to that for all young people (90% for Indigenous and 93% for all young people). Indigenous young people aged 15 to 24 years were almost equally likely as all young people to rate their health as 'excellent' (25% and 27% respectively) but less likely to rate their health as 'very good' (33% and 40% respectively). Furthermore, higher proportions of Indigenous young people rated their health as 'good' (32% and 26% respectively) and fair or poor (10% and 7% respectively) than all young people.

Injury and poisoning is the leading cause of death and disease burden among Indigenous young people and is among the top three causes of hospitalisation. Information from prevalence surveys and disease registers indicate the burden of particular health conditions among Indigenous young people, as well as identifying conditions that are particularly prevalent such as trachoma, skin infections, diabetes, rheumatic heart disease and hearing problems or infections, which are relatively uncommon in the general population. Among Indigenous young people aged 15 to 24 years in 2013, the leading causes of disease burden among males were mental health disorders (27%), intentional injury (20%) and unintentional injury (17%), and among females mental health disorders (29%), intentional injury (10%) and communicable disease (10%) (AIHW 2018).

Indigenous young people also experience higher rates of hospitalisation for mental and behavioural disorders. In 2018–19, there were 2643 hospital separations for mental and behavioural disorders among Indigenous young people aged 12 to 24 years—a rate almost three times as high as for other young people (1858 and 678 respectively per 100,000, excluding the Australian Capital Territory, Tasmania and private hospitals in the Northern Territory). The leading causes of these hospital separations for Indigenous young people were schizophrenia (306 per 100,000), mental and behavioural disorders due to use of alcohol (348 per 100,000) and reactions to severe stress (266 per 100,000). These rates were two to three times as high as for other young people, with corresponding rates of 83, 125 and 119 per 100,000 respectively.

Indigenous young people aged 18 to 24 years were more likely to experience physical or threatened violence than all young people (33% compared with 24% respectively), according to the 2016 General Social Survey (ABS 2016). The disparity is even greater for young Indigenous females, where the rate of physical or threatened violence was twice that of all young females (34% and 17% respectively) (AIHW 2016b).

LGBTIQ+ Adolescents

Although adolescents may participate in same-gender sexual activity or have same-gender attractions, they will not necessarily be lesbian, gay, bisexual or transgender adults. In 2015 approximately 273,000 high school students had sexual contact only with the same sex and 739,000 students had sexual contact with both sexes (Zaza et al 2016). Assigning sexual orientation labels to adolescents is complex and should be approached cautiously. Nurses should confidently and consistently ask teens their gender identity when interviewing them and acknowledge their choice of gender terms and, if applicable, preferred name. Screening questions regarding sexual attractions and experiences should be phrased in ways that allow adolescents to discuss same-gender, opposite-gender and cis and non-binary attractions, such as using the term *partner* rather than *boyfriend* or *girlfriend*.

The population of lesbian, gay, bisexual, transgender, queer, intersex or other (LGBTQI+) adolescents has unique developmental issues and health challenges. Most of the health challenges of sexual minority teens are responses to negative societal attitudes and messages about homosexual or bisexual orientation. Compared with their heterosexual peers, there is a higher prevalence of being bullied at school or cyberbullied, and experiencing physical or sexual dating violence (Zaza et al 2016). They may use alcohol, marijuana and other substances to escape their anxieties. They are less likely to participate in sports and belong to exercise facilities, and there is an increased prevalence of eating disorders, especially among lesbians and transgender teens (O'Neill & Wakefield 2017). Furthermore, they are at much greater risk for suicidal behaviours than their heterosexual peers. Although nurses should screen all youth about suicidal thoughts and history of suicide attempts, it is especially critical for an adolescent who identifies as gay, lesbian, bisexual or transgender or one who is questioning their sexual orientation or gender. Also, LGBTQI+ adolescents need the same sexuality education and information on pregnancy prevention and STI transmission and prevention that is appropriate for all other adolescents, as much education is only oriented towards heterosexual and binary gender individuals.

As mentioned earlier, publicly disclosing an LGBTQI+ orientation (sexual and/or gender) during adolescence ('coming out') brings additional challenges. Many adolescents disclose their orientation to a close peer, then a sibling and finally a parent (Steever et al 2014). Adolescents face hostility, violence and even rejection from their peers and families. For many young people who are also raised with religion, there is added guilt and shame in coming out and often the young person is isolated from family and friends even further when coming out if they need to leave the religion (Prior & Cusack 2016, Witoslawski 2020). For many young people living in regional and rural Australia, the prevailing culture, perceptions and stigmas still associated with the LGBTQI+ community, along with a lack of support services, there are considerable barriers for them to feel safe and supported to come out (Lewis 2020). Nurses should not encourage teens to disclose their sexual orientation and/or gender to their families without first forming a safety plan in case the reaction is not supportive.

Adolescents who acknowledge same-gender sexual attractions/relationships or non-binary gender are also at risk for violence and harassment from schoolmates, neighbours and even strangers. Others show rejection in more subtle ways, but even these non-supportive responses can have an effect on adolescents' healthy development. Sexual/gender minority adolescents fear similar uncaring attitudes among healthcare providers and avoid disclosing their sexual orientation, gender identity and emotional health during primary care visits (Snyder et al 2017). To provide sensitive, professional care for LGBTQI+ adolescents, nurses should be sensitive in their choice of language and use of preferred name (if applicable), and be non-judgmental and caring in their communication.

Rural Adolescents

Except for higher rates of accidental injuries (related in part to farm accidents) and lower rates of delinquency among rural adolescents compared with urban ones, few known differences in health problems exist. Research on the health status of rural adolescents is limited, but rural adolescents experience many of the same health problems as adolescents in metropolitan areas. However, rural adolescents face barriers to health promotion because they have more limited access to appropriate healthcare services.

Rural adolescents' access to healthcare is limited by shortages of professionally staffed mental and physical health services, inadequately trained providers and transportation problems. Rural communities often lack adequately trained nurses, medical practitioners, dentists, psychologists, social workers and allied health professionals, in addition to modern equipment. Rural health professionals often feel inadequately prepared to address adolescents' physical and psychosocial health issues. In metropolitan areas, providers who are unwilling or unable to address adolescents' concerns can refer to colleagues with expertise in adolescent health issues. The absence of adolescent health specialists, combined with a limited network of agencies focused on adolescent health promotion, exacerbates rural youths' problems in obtaining appropriate services.

Nursing Care Management

With continued increases in the numbers of adolescents and rising rates of health-related problems of youth, there is an unprecedented need for adolescent health promotion. Nursing professionals can make significant contributions to health promotion among adolescents and their families. Because nurses understand the biological, cognitive, psychosocial and social transitions of adolescence and their impact on health behaviour, they can address adolescents' developmental and health needs. Working with colleagues from other disciplines, community members, parents and adolescents themselves, nurses must become part of a comprehensive approach that delivers consistent messages across clinical, school and community-based settings. Nurses should be at the forefront of developing and disseminating culturally appropriate health promotion interventions among special populations, including minority adolescents; gay, lesbian and bisexual youth; and rural teenagers.

REFERENCES

Ali, O., & Donohoue, P. A. (2016). Gynecomastia. In R. M. Kliegman, B. F. Stanton, J. W. St Geme, et al. (Eds.), Nelson textbook of pediatrics (20th ed.). Philadelphia: Saunders/Elsevier.

Australian Bureau of Statistics (ABS). (2016). General Social Survey: Summary Results, Australia. Summary of findings. https://www.abs.gov.au/statistics/people/people-and-communities/general-social-survey-summary-results-australia/2016

Australian Curriculum, Assessment and Reporting Authority (ACARA). (2018). National Report on Schooling in Australia. 13th Edition. https://www.acara.edu.au/reporting/national-report-on-schooling-in-australia/national-report-on-schooling-in-australia-2018

Australian Institute of Health and Welfare (AIHW). (2011). Young Australians: their health and wellbeing 2011. Cat. no. PHE 140 Canberra: AIHW. https://www.aihw.gov.au/reports/children-youth/young-australians-their-health-and-wellbeing-2011/summary

Australian Institute of Health and Welfare (AIHW). (2018). Aboriginal and Torres Strait Islander adolescent and youth health and wellbeing 2018: in brief. Cat. no. IHW 198. Canberra: AIHW. https://www.aihw.gov.au/getmedia/e9434481-c52b-4a79-9cb5-94f72f04d23e/aihw-ihw-198.pdf.aspx

Australian Institute of Health and Welfare (AIHW). (2020a). Health of young people. Profile of young people. Sexual and reproductive health. https://www.aihw.gov.au/reports/australias-health/health-of-young-people

Australian Institute of Health and Welfare (AIHW). (2020b). Australia's children. Injuries. https://www.aihw.gov.au/reports/children-youth/australias-children/contents/health/injuries

Australian Institute of Health and Welfare (AIHW). (2020c). Australia's children. Physical activity. https://www.aihw.gov.au/reports/children-youth/australias-children/contents/health/physical-activity

Australian Institute of Health and Welfare (AIHW). (2020d). Australia's children. Smoking and drinking behaviour. https://www.aihw.gov.au/reports/children-youth/australias-children/contents/health/physical-activity

Australian Institute of Health and Welfare (AIHW). (2020e). National Drug Strategy Household Survey 2019. Drug Statistics series no. 32. PHE 270. https://www.aihw.gov.au/reports/illicit-use-of-drugs/national-drug-strategy-household-survey-2019/contents/summary

Australian Institute of Health and Welfare (AIHW). (2020f). Australia's children. Child Learning and Development. https://www.aihw.gov.au/reports/children-youth/australias-children/contents/education/child-learning-development

Australian Institute of Health and Welfare (AIHW): Kreifeld, R. & Harrison, J. E. (2020). Indigenous injury deaths: 2011–12 to 2015–16. Injury research and statistics series no. 130. Cat. no. INJCAT 210.

Azzopardi, P., Hearps, S., Francis, K., et al. (2019). Progress in adolescent health and wellbeing: tracking 12 headline indicators for 195 countries and territories, 1990–2016. The Lancet, 393(10176), 1101–1118.

Azzopardi, P., Sawyer, S., Carlin, J., et al. (2018). Health and wellbeing of Indigenous adolescents in Australia: a systematic synthesis of population data. The Lancet, 391(10122), 766–782.

Baams, L., Dubas, J., Overbeek, G., et al. (2015). Transitions in body and behavior: a meta-analytic study on the relationship between pubertal development and adolescent sexual behavior. Journal of Adolescent Health, 56(6), 586–598.

Bagot, K., Matthews, S., Mason, et al. (2018). Current, future and potential use of mobile and wearable technologies and social media data in the ABCD study to increase understanding of contributors to child health. Developmental Cognitive Neuroscience, 2018, 32, 121–129.

Chester, K., Klemera, E., Magnusson, J., et al.(2019). The role of school-based health education in adolescent spiritual moral, social and cultural development. SAGE Publications. Health Education Journal, 78(5), 582–594.

Cheung, E. L., Bell, C. S., Samuel, J. P., et al. (2017). Race and obesity in adolescent hypertension. Pediatrics, 139(5), e20161433.

Council of Australian Governments (COAG). (2019). Education Council. Developing a new national children's education and care workforce strategy. http://www.educationcouncil.edu.au/EC-Reports-and-Publications.aspx

Doornwaard, S., ter Bogt, T., Reitz, E., et al. (2015). Sex-Related Online Behaviors, Perceived Peer Norms and Adolescents' Experience with Sexual Behavior: Testing an Integrative Model. PloS one, 10(6), e0127787.

Drummond, M. B., & Upson, D. (2014). Electronic cigarettes: Potential harms and benefits. Annals of the American Thoracic Society, 11(2), 236–242.

Elkind, D. (1978). Understanding the young adolescent. Adolescence, 13(49), 128–134.

Erikson, E. (1968). Identity: Youth in crisis. New York: Norton.

Ferrara, P., Guadagno, C., Sbordone, A., et al. (2016). Child abuse and neglect: A review of the literature. Current Pediatric Reviews, 12(4), 301–310.

Finkelhor, D., & Jones, L. (2012). Have sexual abuse and physical abuse declined since the 1990s? Lebanon: University of New Hampshire Press.

Gao, Z., Chen, S., Pasco, D., et al. (2015). A meta-analysis of active video games on health outcomes among children and adolescents. Obesity Reviews: An Official Journal of the International Association for the Study of Obesity, 16(9), 783–794.

George, M. & Odgers, C. (2015). Seven Fears and the Science of How Mobile Technologies May Be Influencing Adolescents in the Digital Age. Perspectives on Psychological Science, 10(6), 832–851.

Gilligan, C. (1982). In a different voice. Cambridge, Mass: Harvard University Press.

Gilligan, C. (1986). Adolescent development reconsidered. Paper presented at Invitational Conference on Health Futures of Adolescents, Daytona Beach, FL.

Hare, D. (2019). LGBTQI experiences of seeking help and justice in the wake of sexual harm. Wellington: The New Zealand Women's Studies Association. Women's Studies Journal, 33(1), 25–32.

Hoying, J., Melnyk, B. M., & Arcoleo, K. (2016). Effects of the COPE cognitive behavioral skills building TEEN program on the healthy lifestyle behaviors and mental health of Appalachian early adolescents. Journal of Pediatric Health Care, 30(1), 65–72.

Kann, L., McManus, T., Harris, W. A., et al. (2016). Youth risk behavior surveillance – United States, 2015. Morbidity and Mortality Weekly Report. Surveillance Summaries (Washington, D.C.: 2002), 65, 1–177.

Kemp, B., Parrish, A. & Cliff, D. (2020). 'Social screens' and 'the mainstream': longitudinal competitors of non-organized physical activity in the transition from childhood to adolescence. The International Journal of Behavioral Nutrition and Physical Activity, 17(1), 5.

Kickett-Tucker, C. & Shaouli Shahid, S. (2019). In the Nyitting Time: The Journey of Identity Development for Western Australian Aboriginal Children and Youth and the Interplay of Racism: Handbook of Children and Prejudice. Champaign, IL: Springer.

Kohlberg, L., & Gilligan, C. (1972). The adolescent as philosopher: the discovery of the self in a post-conventional world. In J. Kagan & R. Coles (Eds.), Twelve to sixteen: Early adolescence. New York: Norton.

Kvalsvig, A., D'Souza, A., Duncanson, M., et al. (2016). Pathways to child health, development and wellbeing: Optimal environments for orchids and dandelions. An overview of the evidence. Wellington: Ministry of Health. https://www.health.govt.nz/publication/pathways-child-health-development-and-wellbeing-optimal-environments-orchids-and-dandelions-overview

Lapsley, D. K. (1993). Toward an integrated theory of adolescent ego development: The 'new look' at adolescent egocentrism. The American Journal of Orthopsychiatry, 63(4), 562–571.

Lawrence, D., Johnson, S., Hafekost, J., et al. (2015). The Mental Health of Children and Adolescents. Report on the second Australian Child and Adolescent Survey of Mental Health and Wellbeing. Department of Health. https://www1.health.gov.au/internet/main/publishing.nsf/Content/mental-pubs-m-child2.

Ledbetter, D. & Johnson, P. (2018). Endocrine Surgery in Children. Berlin Heidelberg: Springer. https://link-springer-com.ezproxy.csu.edu.au/book/10.1007%2F978-3-662-54256-9

Lewis, C. (2020). Rethinking access for minority segments in rural health: An LGBTQI+ perspective. The Australian Journal of Rural Health, 28(5), 509–513.

Maquire, S. A., Williams, B., Naughton, A. M., et al. (2015). A systematic review of the emotional, behavioural and cognitive features exhibited by school-aged children experiencing neglect or emotional abuse. Child Care, Health and Development, 41(5), 641–653.

McCormick, C. & Scherer, D. (2018). Child and adolescent development for educators. Second edition. New York: Guilford Press.

McGovern, M. & Canning, D. (2015). Vaccination and all-cause child mortality from 1985 to 2011: global evidence from the demographic and health surveys. American Journal of Epidemiology, 182(9), 791–798. https://doi.org/10.1093/aje/kwv125

Ministry of Education. (2021). Education in New Zealand. About our Education System. https://www.education.govt.nz/our-work/our-role-and-our-people/education-in-nz/#:~:text=New%20Zealand's%20education%20system%20has,education%220%E2%80%93%20higher%20and%20vocational%20education.

Ministry of Health. (2018). Suicide and intentional self-harm. Our Work. New Zealand Government. https://www.health.govt.nz/our-work/populations/maori-health/tatau-kahukura-maori-health-statistics/nga-mana-hauora-tutohu-health-status-indicators/suicide-and-intentional-self-harm

Ministry of Health. (2020). Indicator of potentially avoidable hospitalisations for the Child and Youth Wellbeing Strategy: A brief report on methodology. July. New Zealand Government.

Morelli, M., Bianchi, D., Baiocco, R., et al. (2016). Sexting, psychological distress and dating violence among adolescents and young adults. Psicothema, 28(2), 137–142.

Mudedla, S., Avendano, E. E., & Raman, G. (2015). Non-tuberculous mycobacterium skin infections after tattooing in healthy individuals: A systematic review of case reports. Dermatology Online Journal, 21(6).

O'Neill, T., & Wakefield, J. (2017). Fifteen-minute consultation in the normal child: Challenges relating to sexuality and gender identity in children and young people. Archives of Disease in Childhood. Education and Practice Edition, 102(6), 298–303.

Orenstein, W. & Ahmed, R. (2017). Simply put: vaccination saves lives. Proceedings of the National Academy of Sciences, 114(16), 4031–4033. https://doi.org/10.1073/pnas.1704507114

Prior, J. H. & Cusack, C. M. (2016). Public theologies of love in the Civitas Dei and Civitas Terrena: Sexuality and the transformation of Sydney, Australia 1960–2010. Theology & Sexuality, 21(2), 85–104. https://doi.org/10.1080/13558358.2016.1206681

Snyder, B. K., Burack, G. D., & Petrova, A. (2017). LGBTQ youth's perceptions of primary care. Clinical Pediatrics, 56(5), 443–450.

Steever, J., Francis, J., Gordon, L. P., et al. (2014). Sexual minority youth. Primary Care, 41(3), 651–669.

Steinberg, L. (1990). Autonomy, conflict and harmony in the family relationship. In S. Feldman & G. Elliot (Eds.), At the threshold: The developing adolescent. Cambridge, MA: Harvard University Press.

Sun, Y., Mensah, F., Azzopardi, P., et al. (2017). Childhood social disadvantage and pubertal timing: a national birth cohort from Australia. Pediatrics (Evanston), 139(6), e20164099.

Tarokh, L., Saletin, J. M., & Carskadon, M. A. (2016). Sleep in adolescence: Physiology, cognition and mental health. Neuroscience and Biobehavioral Reviews, 70, 182–188.

The Gender Centre. (2021). Explore Gender. https://gendercentre.org.au/resources/support-resources/youth-support

Walker, L., de Vries, B., & Trevethan, S. (1987). Moral stages and moral orientations in real-life and hypothetical dilemmas. Child Development, 58, 842–858.

World Health Organization (WHO). (2021).Vaccines and immunisation. Overview. https://www.who.int/health-topics/vaccines-and-immunization#tab=tab_1

Zaza, S., Kann, L., & Barrios, L. C. (2016). Lesbian, gay, and bisexual adolescents: Population estimate and prevalence of health behaviors. The Journal of the American Medical Association, 316(22), 2355–2356.

18

Health Problems of the Adolescent

Lisa Speedie

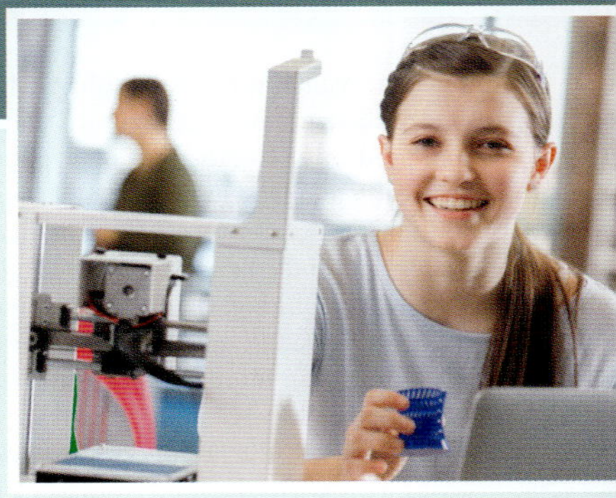

LEARNING OUTCOMES

- Describe the main conditions that cause concern with the reproductive system and process of adolescence
- Identify and manage the appropriate care of interpersonal violence occurring for adolescence
- Identify and plan care management that is family centred for the adolescent and their family relating to stress and safety

HEALTH CONDITIONS OF THE MALE REPRODUCTIVE SYSTEM

Penile Conditions

Common congenital anomalies of the penis are almost always detected and corrected in infancy or early childhood. In some cases boys who need an operative procedure to repair hypospadias (the most common congenital deformity of the penis) may reach adolescence with a penis that looks different from those of their friends. A few who have received no medical care have uncorrected deformities that can cause serious psychological problems during this sensitive period of development. These young boys need to be identified for surgical repair of the defect.

Uncircumcised males may encounter some problems during adolescence related to a tight foreskin that cannot be retracted over the enlarging glans *(paraphimosis).* Necrosis and tissue necrosis of the glans may occur if the condition is not treated properly; in most cases the glans oedema can be reduced by gentle manual compression, but other non-invasive techniques include the use of ice or compression wraps (Pohlman et al 2013). Eventually the foreskin is returned to its original position. Uncircumcised males are at higher risk for infections such as balanitis and prosthitis. Penile carcinoma (penile intraepithelial neoplasia) is associated with numerous human papillomavirus (HPV) types, but only one HPV type, HPV-16, is associated with 76% of penile neoplasias (Diorio & Giuliano 2016). HPV types 6 and 11 are commonly associated with genital warts, which may be benign or malignant (Diorio & Giuliano 2016).

Trauma to the penis, including burns and accidental injuries, can occur in various ways. The frenulum (the fold on the lower surface of the glans that connects it with the prepuce) can be torn after retraction of the foreskin, unusually rough masturbation or coitus. It can be frightening to the young boy but usually heals spontaneously with minimum care. However, any extensive bleeding may require suturing of the tissues. Penile fracture is a rupture of the corpus cavernosum as a result of blunt trauma to the erect penis, usually during vigorous sexual intercourse or masturbation. The condition is considered a urological emergency, and surgical repair is recommended to prevent further complications (Chahal et al 2016).

Drugs such as trazodone (Desyrel), taken alone or in combination with cocaine or Ecstasy (MDMA [3-4 methylenedioxymethamphetamine]), may cause a prolonged erection (priapism), which can be extremely uncomfortable and in some cases may require surgical intervention to release blood trapped in the corpus cavernosum. Drugs available to adults for erectile dysfunction or other drugs not intended for recreational uses may have unintentional and undesirable side effects requiring immediate medical attention. Antidepressant and antipsychotic drugs may also cause an ischaemic priapism requiring emergent treatment (Armstrong et al 2015). Other conditions that may be seen include zipper injury or entrapment, entrapment by metal or glass objects, balanitis, prosthitis and STIs.

Varicocele

A varicocele is a congenital condition characterised by elongation, dilation and tortuosity of the veins of the spermatic cord superior to the testicle. The finding is rare in prepubertal children, but the incidence increases to 5% to 15% in adolescent boys (Elder 2016). Idiopathic varicocele is the most common treatable cause of male-related impaired fertility, especially if caught and treated early (Elder 2016). Varicoceles occur most often on the left side because of the greater length of the left spermatic vein and its entry into the left renal artery; the right spermatic vein enters the vena cava directly and at a lesser angle, which may be a source of future difficulty. A varicocele can be palpated as a wormlike mass situated above the testicle that decreases in size when the male is recumbent and becomes distended and tense when he is upright. Some males may experience discomfort during sexual stimulation.

Varicocele repair has shown improvement in semen parameters among adult patients but there is no established set of semen parameters for adolescents, making semen analysis difficult to interpret (Garcia-Roig & Kirsch 2015). Varicocelectomy is currently indicated for adolescents based on testicular volume differences and not abnormal semen parameters (Garcia-Roig & Kirsch 2015).

Epididymitis

Epididymitis is an inflammatory reaction of the epididymis of the testicle primarily as a result of an infection (bacterial or viral), a chemical irritant (urine) or a non-specific cause (local trauma). The clinical presentation is slow and insidious with unilateral scrotal pain, redness and swelling. Associated symptoms include urethral discharge, dysuria, fever and pyuria. Epididymitis is not associated with gastrointestinal symptoms as found in testicular torsion. The causative factor in sexually active males 14 to 35 years of age is predominantly *Chlamydia trachomatis* and *Neisseria gonorrhoeae* (McConaghy & Panchal 2016). Some experts recommend reserving antibiotic therapy only for infants and children under the age of 14 years with pyuria or positive urine cultures due to the small amount of those with epididymitis who actually have positive urine cultures (McConaghy & Panchal 2016). In children 14 years and older, empiric antibiotics are recommended based on the most likely causative organism (McConaghy & Panchal 2016). Mild presentation of symptoms may mimic testicular torsion, which requires immediate surgical intervention. Therefore, immediate evaluation by a practitioner is indicated. Treatment consists of supportive therapy with analgesics, anti-inflammatories and scrotal elevation. If anatomical abnormalities are suspected, refer to a urologist. For adolescent males who test positive for chlamydia or gonorrhoea, conduct an assessment for other STIs and inform the adolescent that his partner will also require treatment.

Testicular Torsion

Torsion of the testicle is a condition in which the tunica vaginalis, which normally encases the testicle, fails to do so and the testis hangs free from its vascular structures. This condition can result in partial or complete venous occlusion with rotation around this vascular axis. In severe torsion the organ can become swollen and painful; the scrotum becomes red, warm and oedematous and appears to be immobile or fixed as a result of spasm of the cremasteric fibres.

Rapid growth and increasing vascularity of the testicle are thought to be precursors to torsion, accounting for the occurrence at puberty. Typically, the adolescent complains of pain that is severe and acute; nausea, vomiting and abdominal pain may accompany the pain. On examination, the scrotum is swollen and red, and the cremasteric reflex is often absent. Fever and urinary symptoms are generally not present. If the pain duration is less than 6 hours, manual detorsion may be attempted; however, prompt surgical treatment is necessarily for unsuccessful manual attempts or if pain duration is longer than 6 hours (Elder 2016).

Nursing Care Management

Nurses should be alert to the possibility of testicular torsion in adolescents who complain of scrotal pain. Because torsion may result from trauma to the scrotum, nurses should refer the child or adolescent for medical evaluation immediately.

Gynaecomastia

Some degree of bilateral or unilateral breast enlargement occurs frequently in boys during puberty. Approximately half of adolescent boys have transient gynaecomastia, which usually lasts less than 1 year and subsides spontaneously. When gynaecomastia has a prepubertal onset, the adolescent should be evaluated for rare adrenal or gonadal tumours or Klinefelter's syndrome. Gynaecomastia may also be drug induced; spironolactone, cimetidine, ketoconazole, oestrogens and antiandrogens have all been shown to cause the disorder.

If gynaecomastia persists or is extensive enough to cause embarrassment, plastic surgery is indicated for cosmetic and psychological reasons. Administration of testosterone has no effect on breast development or regression and may even aggravate the condition.

Nursing Care Management

Management usually consists of assuring the adolescent and his parents that this situation is benign and temporary. However, all adolescents with gynaecomastia should receive a careful medical evaluation to rule out pathological causes. The adolescent may benefit from the knowledge that it occurs in up to 70% of his peers.

HEALTH CONDITIONS OF THE FEMALE REPRODUCTIVE SYSTEM

Gynaecological Examination

Whether it is her first experience or one of many, adolescent girls are often apprehensive before a pelvic examination. Adolescents are self-conscious about their bodies and the changes taking place. The adolescent needs anticipatory guidance regarding what to expect and what she can do to help herself relax during the procedure. Many fears and apprehensions are a result of information she has obtained from family members and friends. The discussion should begin by addressing these anxieties.

The initial reproductive preventive healthcare visit should consist of a general examination, a visual breast examination, an external pelvic examination as indicated and education regarding healthy behaviours such as normal pubertal development and menstruation. A confidential portion of the visit should include discussion of sexual activity, contraception and sexually transmitted diseases. Indications for an internal examination are started in asymptomatic women at 21 years of age but should be performed earlier if the adolescent is experiencing any female genital tract, pelvic, urological or rectal problems. The initial visit provides an excellent opportunity for teaching about hygiene and body functions. Encourage the girl to ask questions about changes in her body and the implications. The pelvic examination should be as non-stressful as possible. Nurses should attempt to make the initial pelvic examination a positive experience for the adolescent because this can increase the likelihood of compliance with annual visits. The adolescent should have the option of choosing a supportive person to be present during the examination. Suggested individuals might include a parent, best friend, partner or other health professional.

Menstrual Disorders

Amenorrhoea

Menarche, or the first menstrual period, occurs relatively late in female pubertal development. Although girls vary in the onset and rate of progression of pubertal development, the sequence and tempo should be the same. When an adolescent is seen with a complaint of absence of menses, a careful history of the timing of her pubertal development will help determine whether there is a need for further evaluation or if reassurance is all that is necessary.

Primary amenorrhoea is an absence of any secondary sex characteristics by 13 years old or absence of uterine bleeding with secondary sex characteristics by 15 years old (Sucato & Burstein 2016). Primary amenorrhoea is also characterised when menarche has not occurred 4 years after thelarche (Sucato & Burstein 2016). The cause of primary amenorrhoea may be anatomical, hormonal, genetic or idiopathic. A thorough patient and family history and physical examination provide clues to the aetiology.

Secondary amenorrhoea is defined as the absence of menses after menstruation was previously established for more than three menstrual cycles or irregular menses for 6 months after the establishment of normal menses (Berz & McCambridge 2016). Irregular menstrual cycles are common within the first year after menarche because these early cycles may be anovulatory, resulting in regular, irregular or absent bleeding. Girls with a later onset of menarche take longer to establish regular ovulatory cycles. Pregnancy is the most common cause of secondary amenorrhoea and should be ruled out in both types of amenorrhoea even if the adolescent denies sexual activity.

Hypogonadotropic Amenorrhoea

Functional hypogonadotropic amenorrhoea reflects a problem in the central hypothalamic–pituitary axis and often results from hypothalamic suppression as a result of stress (in the home, school or workplace) or a sudden and severe weight loss, eating disorders or strenuous exercise (Berz & McCambridge 2016). Women who are more than 20% underweight for height or who have had rapid weight loss and women with eating disorders such as anorexia nervosa may report amenorrhoea.

Exercise-associated amenorrhoea can occur in women undergoing vigorous physical and athletic training and is thought to be associated with many factors, including: body composition (height, weight and percentage of body fat); type, intensity and frequency of exercise; nutritional status; and presence of emotional or physical stressors.

Assessment of amenorrhoea begins with a thorough history and physical examination. Specific components of the assessment process depend on a patient's age—adolescent, young adult or perimenopausal—and whether she has menstruated previously.

An important initial step, often overlooked, is to be sure that the female is not pregnant. Once pregnancy has been ruled out by a beta human chorionic gonadotropin (hCG) pregnancy test, diagnostic tests may include follicle-stimulating hormone level, thyroid-stimulating hormone and prolactin levels, and screening for an eating disorder (Berz & McCambridge 2016).

Nursing Care Management

When amenorrhoea is caused by hypothalamic disturbances, the nurse is an ideal health professional to assist women because many of the causes are potentially reversible (e.g. stress, weight loss for non-organic reasons). Counselling and education are primary interventions and appropriate nursing roles. When a stressor known to predispose a woman to hypothalamic amenorrhoea is identified, initial management involves addressing the stressor.

If an adolescent's exercise program is thought to contribute to her amenorrhoea, several options exist for management. Treatment options include a decrease in the intensity or duration of training or modifications in her diet to include the appropriate nutrition for her age. Accepting the former alternative may be difficult for one who is committed to a strenuous exercise regimen. Many young female athletes may not understand the consequences of low bone density or osteoporosis; nurses can point out the connection between low bone density and stress fractures. The nurse and adolescent should also investigate other factors that may be contributing to the amenorrhoea and develop plans for altering lifestyle and decreasing stress.

Dysmenorrhoea

Dysmenorrhoea, pain during or shortly before menstruation, is one of the most common gynaecological problems in women of all ages. Dysmenorrhoea begins for most women in adolescence, within the first 3 to 5 years after menarche once ovulation is established (Rani et al 2016). Menstrual problems, including dysmenorrhoea, are relatively more common in women who smoke and are obese. Dysmenorrhoea is also associated with menarche before 12 years old, nulliparity and menstrual flow more than 7 days (Yu 2014).

Primary Dysmenorrhoea

Primary dysmenorrhoea is a condition associated with ovulatory cycles. Primary dysmenorrhoea has a biochemical basis and arises from the release of prostaglandins with menses. During the luteal phase and subsequent menstrual flow, prostaglandin F_2-alpha ($PGF_{2\alpha}$) is secreted. Excessive release of $PGF_{2\alpha}$ increases the amplitude and frequency of uterine contractions and causes vasospasm of the uterine arterioles, resulting in ischaemia and cyclic lower abdominal cramps. Systemic responses to $PGF_{2\alpha}$ include backache, weakness, sweats, gastrointestinal symptoms and central nervous system symptoms (dizziness, syncope, headache and poor concentration). Pain usually begins at the onset of menstruation and lasts 8 to 48 hours.

Nursing Care Management

Management of primary dysmenorrhoea depends on the severity of the problem and the individual woman's response to various treatments. Important components of nursing care are information and support. Because menstruation is so closely linked to reproduction and sexuality, menstrual problems such as dysmenorrhoea can have a negative influence on sexuality and self-worth.

Exercise helps relieve menstrual discomfort through increased vasodilation and subsequent decreased ischaemia. It also releases endogenous opiates (specifically beta-endorphins), suppresses prostaglandins and shunts blood flow away from the viscera, resulting in reduced pelvic congestion. Specific dietary changes, such as decreasing salt and refined sugar, and maintaining good nutrition are helpful in decreasing some of the systemic symptoms associated with dysmenorrhoea. Medications used to treat primary dysmenorrhoea include prostaglandin synthesis inhibitors, primarily non-steroidal anti-inflammatory drugs (NSAIDs) such as ibuprofen or naproxen (Yu 2014). NSAIDs are most effective if started several days before menses or at least by the onset of bleeding but are associated with many adverse effects, such as drowsiness, dizziness, nausea and indigestion. NSAIDs should only be used short term.

Secondary Dysmenorrhoea

Secondary dysmenorrhoea is defined as painful menses associated with a pathological condition, such as adenomyosis, endometriosis, pelvic inflammatory disease, endometrial polyps or fibroids. Women with secondary dysmenorrhoea often have other symptoms that may suggest the underlying cause. In contrast to primary dysmenorrhoea, the pain of secondary dysmenorrhoea is often characterised by dull, lower abdominal aching that radiates to the back or thighs and feelings of bloating or pelvic fullness. In addition to a physical examination with a careful pelvic examination, diagnosis may be assisted by ultrasound examination, dilation and curettage, endometrial biopsy or laparoscopy. Treatment is directed towards removal of the underlying pathology. Many of the measures described for pain relief of primary dysmenorrhoea are also helpful for women with secondary dysmenorrhoea.

Endometriosis

Endometriosis is characterised by the presence and growth of endometrial tissue outside of the uterus. The tissue may be implanted on: the ovaries; anterior and posterior cul-de-sac; broad, uterosacral and round ligaments; rectovaginal septum; sigmoid colon; appendix; pelvic peritoneum; cervix; and inguinal area (Fig 18.1). A cystic lesion of endometriosis found in the ovary is sometimes described as a chocolate cyst because of the dark colouring of the contents of the cyst caused by the presence of old blood.

Endometrial tissue contains glands and stoma and responds to cyclic hormone stimulation in the same way that the uterine

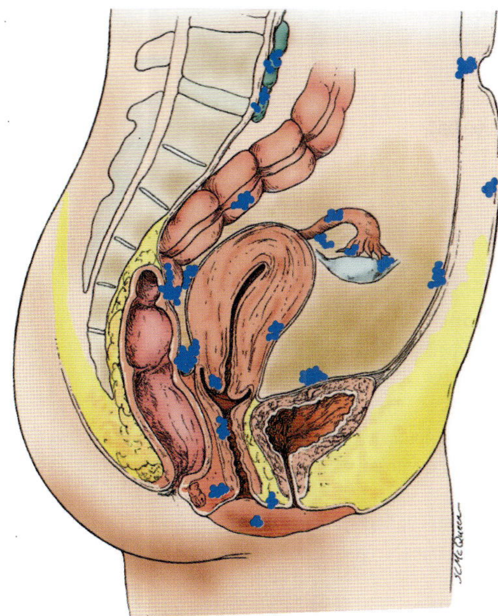

Fig 18.1 Common sites of endometriosis. (Source: Lentz, G. M., Lobo, R. A., Gershenson, D. M., et al. (Eds.). (2012). Comprehensive gynecology (6th ed.). Philadelphia, PA: Mosby.)

endometrium does but often out of phase with it. The tissue grows during the proliferative and secretory phases of the cycle. During or immediately after menstruation the tissue bleeds, resulting in an inflammatory response with subsequent fibrosis and adhesions to adjacent organs.

Symptoms vary among women and range from non-existent to incapacitating. Severity of symptoms can change over time and may not reflect the extent of the disease. The major symptoms of endometriosis are pelvic pain, dysmenorrhoea and dyspareunia (painful intercourse). Women may also have chronic non-cyclic pelvic pain, pelvic heaviness or pain radiating into the thighs. Many women report bowel symptoms such as diarrhoea, pain with defecation and constipation caused by avoiding defecation because of the pain.

Nursing Care Management

Treatment is based on the severity of symptoms and the goals of the woman or couple. Women without pain who do not want to become pregnant need no treatment. In women with mild pain who may desire a future pregnancy, treatment may be limited to use of NSAIDs during menstruation.

Women who have early symptomatic disease and who can postpone pregnancy may be treated with oral contraceptive pills (OCPs) that have a low oestrogen-to-progestin ratio to shrink endometrial tissue. Any low-dose OCPs can be used if taken for 15 weeks, followed by 1 week of withdrawal. Continuous combined hormone therapy (e.g. OCPs, oestrogen/progestin patch, oestrogen/progestin vaginal ring) for menstrual suppression and administration of NSAIDs are the usual treatment for adolescents under the age of 16 years who have endometriosis.

Surgical intervention is often needed for severe, acute or incapacitating symptoms. Decisions regarding the extent and type of surgery are influenced by a woman's age, the desire for children and the location of the disease. For women who do not want to preserve their ability to have children, the only definite cure is total abdominal hysterectomy with bilateral salpingo-oophorectomy (TAH with BSO). In women in their childbearing years who want children and in whom the disease does not prevent bearing children, reproductive capacity should be retained through careful removal by laparoscopic surgery or laser therapy (e.g. coagulation, vaporisation or resection) of all endometrial tissue possible, with retention of ovarian function.

Endometriosis recurs in approximately 40% of women. Thus for many women endometriosis is a chronic disease with conditions such as chronic pain or infertility. Counselling and education are critical components of nursing care for women with endometriosis. Women need an honest discussion of treatment options, with review of the potential risks and benefits of each option. Because pelvic pain is a subjective, personal experience that can be frightening, support is important. Sexual dysfunction resulting from dyspareunia is common and may necessitate referral for counselling. Support groups for women with endometriosis may be found in some locations.

Premenstrual Syndrome

Premenstrual dysphoric disorder (PMDD) is a more severe variant of premenstrual syndrome (PMS) in which 2% to 6% of women have significant physical and behavioural symptoms that interfere with daily living (Sucato & Burstein 2016). Based on a large body of evidence, PMDD is included in the *Diagnostic and Statistical Manual of Mental Disorders, Fifth Edition* (DSM-5) as a distinct diagnosis. There are several validated screening tools, such as the Premenstrual Symptoms Screening Tool (PSST), that can help identify PMS and PMDD. To obtain an accurate history, encourage the woman to keep a daily log of her symptoms.

The causes of PMS and PMDD continue to be investigated. A number of biological and neuroendocrine aetiologies have been suggested; however, none has been conclusively substantiated as the causative factor. It is likely that biological and psychosocial factors contribute to PMS and PMDD (Craner et al 2014).

Therapeutic and Nursing Care Management

There is little agreement on management. Any changes that help a woman with PMS exert control over her life have a positive effect. For this reason, lifestyle changes are often effective in its treatment.

Nurses can advise women that self-help modalities often result in significant symptom improvement. Regular exercise and regular sleep can provide symptom relief for some women.

Medications often used in the treatment of PMS include diuretics, prostaglandin inhibitors (NSAIDs) and OCPs. However, research with diuretics has only been performed with adults (Akgul & Kanbur 2015). Studies of progesterone have not shown that it is an effective treatment (Ford et al 2012). Serotonergic-activating agents, including the selective serotonin reuptake inhibitors (SSRIs), are approved by the Food and Drug Administration (FDA) as first-line pharmacological therapy for PMS and PMDD (Sucato & Burstein 2016). The drugs have a rapid onset, so either intermittent or continuous use is effective for symptom relief (Sucato & Burstein 2016).

Abnormal Uterine Bleeding

Abnormal uterine bleeding (AUB) is any form of uterine bleeding that is irregular in amount, duration or timing and is not related to regular menstrual bleeding. Box 18.1 lists possible causes of AUB. Although often used interchangeably, the terms *AUB* and *dysfunctional uterine bleeding (DUB)* are not synonymous. DUB is any AUB that does not have a pathogenic cause (Deligeoroglou et al 2013).

AUB can be anovulatory or ovulatory but is most commonly caused by anovulation. When no surge of luteinising hormone (LH) occurs or if insufficient progesterone is produced by the corpus luteum to support the endometrium, it will begin to involute and shed. This process most often occurs at the extremes of a woman's reproductive years, when the menstrual cycle is just becoming established at menarche or when it

BOX 18.1 Possible Causes of Abnormal Uterine Bleeding

Pregnancy-related Conditions
- Threatened or spontaneous miscarriage
- Retained products of conception after elective abortion
- Ectopic pregnancy
- Placenta praevia/placenta abruptio
- Trophoblastic disease

Lower Reproductive Tract Infections
- Cervicitis
- Endometritis
- Mesometritis
- Salpingitis

Benign Anatomical Abnormalities
- Adenomyosis
- Leiomyomata
- Polyps of the cervix or endometrium

Neoplasms
- Endometrial hyperplasia
- Cancer of cervix and endometrium
- Hormonally active tumours (rare)
- Vaginal tumours (rare)

Malignant Lesions
- Cervical squamous cell carcinoma
- Endometrial adenocarcinoma
- Oestrogen-producing ovarian tumours
- Testosterone-producing ovarian tumours
- Leiomyosarcoma

Trauma
- Genital injury (accidental, coital trauma, sexual abuse)
- Foreign body
- Lacerations

Systemic Conditions
- Adrenal hyperplasia and Cushing's disease
- Blood dyscrasias
- Coagulopathies
- Hypothalamic suppression (from stress, weight loss, excessive exercise)
- Polycystic ovary disease
- Thyroid disease
- Pituitary adenoma or hyperprolactinaemia
- Severe organ disease (renal or liver failure)

Iatrogenic Causes
- Medications with oestrogenic activity
- Anticoagulants
- Exogenous hormone use (oral contraceptives, menopausal hormone therapy)
- Selective serotonin reuptake inhibitors
- Tamoxifen
- Intrauterine devices
- Herbal preparation (ginseng)

Source: Data from De Silva, N. K. (2016). Abnormal uterine bleeding in adolescents: Evaluation and approach to diagnosis. *UpToDate.* https://www.uptodate.com/contents/abnormal-uterine-bleeding-in-adolescents-evaluation-and-approach-to-diagnosis; American College of Obstetricians and Gynecologists. (2015). Committee Opinion No. 651: Menstruation in girls and adolescents: Using the menstrual cycle as a vital sign. Obstetrics and Gynecology, 126(6), e143–e146.

draws to a close at menopause. AUB also occurs with any condition that gives rise to chronic anovulation associated with continuous oestrogen production. Such conditions include obesity, hyperthyroidism and hypothyroidism, polycystic ovarian syndrome and any of the endocrine conditions discussed in the sections on amenorrhoea. A diagnosis of AUB is made only after ruling out all other causes of abnormal menstrual bleeding.

Therapeutic Management

For mild cases, give iron supplements and ask the adolescent to keep a diary to monitor menstrual patterns (Sucato & Burstein 2016). The most effective medical treatment of acute bleeding episodes is administration of combined oral contraceptives (oestrogen and progestin) (Sucato & Burstein 2016). Adolescents with severe bleeding may require intravenous oestrogen along with a combined oral contraceptive. The oral contraceptive is given for at least 3 to 6 months after the acute phase has passed. Such long-term treatment will help prevent recurrence of the pattern of AUB and haemorrhage. If the woman wants contraception, she should continue to take OCPs. If she has no need for contraception, the treatment may be stopped to assess the woman's bleeding pattern.

Nursing Care Management

Nursing assessments for adolescents or young women who have a menstrual disorder include the following:
- taking a thorough menstrual, obstetric, sexual and contraceptive history
- exploring the adolescent's perceptions of her condition, cultural or ethnic influences, lifestyle and patterns of coping
- evaluating the amount of pain or bleeding experienced and its effect on daily activities
- noting any home remedies and prescriptions to relieve discomfort; a symptom diary, in which the adolescent records emotions, behaviours, physical symptoms, diet, and exercise and rest patterns, is a useful diagnostic tool.

Expected outcomes for the adolescent are that she will do the following:
- verbalise her understanding of reproductive anatomy, cause of her disorder, medication regimen and diary use
- verbalise her understanding and accept her emotional and physical responses to her menstrual cycle
- develop personal goals that benefit her emotionally and physically
- choose appropriate therapeutic measures for her menstrual problems
- adapt successfully to the condition if cure is not possible.

In addition to the medical, surgical and nursing interventions discussed with each problem, additional nursing interventions may include the following:
- accepting the woman's symptoms as valid
- correlating data from the daily diary of emotional status, subjective feelings and physical state with physiological changes
- encouraging the woman to express her feelings about her symptoms

- providing information about therapeutic options (pharmacological and non-pharmacological) so the woman or she and her partner can make choices considered best for them
- providing information about local support groups.

Care has been effective when the woman reports improvement in the quality of her life, skill in self-management and a positive self-concept and body image.

Vulvar Pain

There are two new classifications in relation to vulval pain, divided into: (1) vulval pain with an identified cause; and (2) vulvodynia, consisting of vulval pain present for at least 3 months with nil identifiable cause but possible associated features.

Symptoms described as distressing vaginal pain in the pre-pubertal population are now being treated separately to adult-presenting symptoms. This genital pain is not present in either adolescent or adult women and differs from vulval pain in its aetiology and treatment. Often pre-pubertal pain presents nocturnally as a shooting or stabbing pain, lasting for several hours, and can wake the child from sleep. Post menarche the pain changes again, and associated issues such as difficulty inserting tampons and pain while tampons are inserted (Dunford et al 2019).

This shows there are differences in associations, pathophysiology and management of vulval pain between paediatric, adolescent and adult women, so nurses must take this into consideration when caring and educating.

Vaginal Infections

Vaginal discharge and itching of the vulva and vagina are among the most common reasons a woman seeks help from a healthcare provider. More women complain of vaginal discharge than any other gynaecological symptom; however, vaginal discharge resulting from infection must be distinguished from normal secretions. Normal vaginal secretions (or physiological leukorrhoea) are clear to cloudy in appearance, non-irritating and have a mild, inoffensive odour. The discharge may turn yellow after drying. Normal vaginal secretions are acidic, with a pH range of 4.0 to 5.0. The amount of leukorrhoea differs with phases of the menstrual cycle, with greater amounts occurring at ovulation and just before menses. Leukorrhoea is also increased during pregnancy. Normal vaginal secretions contain lactobacilli and epithelial cells.

Vaginitis, or abnormal vaginal discharge, is an infection caused by a microorganism. The most common vaginal infections are bacterial vaginosis (BV), candidiasis and trichomoniasis. Although group B *Streptococcus* is considered normal vaginal flora, it may also cause infection. Vulvovaginitis (i.e. inflammation of the vulva and vagina) may be caused by: vaginal infection; copious leukorrhoea, which can cause maceration of tissues; and chemical irritants, allergens and foreign bodies, which may produce inflammatory reactions.

Bacterial Vaginosis

BV is the most common gynaecological infection in Australia and New Zealand (Ratten et al 2021). It is associated with preterm labour in pregnant women and postoperative infections after a hysterectomy (Ratten et al 2021). The exact cause of BV is unknown. It is a syndrome in which normal, hydrogen peroxide–producing lactobacilli are replaced with high concentrations of anaerobic and gram-negative bacteria. With the increase of anaerobes, the level of vaginal amines is raised and the normal acidic pH of the vagina is altered. Epithelial cells slough off, and numerous bacteria attach to their surfaces (clue cells). When the amines are volatilised, the characteristic odour of BV occurs. BV discharge is usually profuse, thin and white, grey or milky in appearance. Some women also may experience mild irritation or pruritus, although some women with BV remain asymptomatic.

Screening and Diagnosis. A focused history may help distinguish BV from other vaginal infections if the young woman is symptomatic. Reports of fishy odour and increased thin vaginal discharge are most significant, and a report of increased odour after intercourse is also suggestive of BV. You should question women with previous occurrence of similar symptoms, diagnosis and treatment because women with BV often have been treated incorrectly because of misdiagnosis.

Therapeutic Management. First-line treatment of BV includes oral metronidazole (Flagyl), although vaginal preparations (e.g. metronidazole gel, clindamycin cream) are also used (Bradshaw & Sobel 2016). When the woman is taking oral metronidazole, advise her to avoid drinking alcoholic beverages or she will experience severe side effects of abdominal distress, nausea, vomiting and headache.

Candidiasis

Vulvovaginal candidiasis, or yeast infection, is the second most common type of vaginal infection. The most common organism is *Candida albicans.* It is estimated that 80% to 90% of yeast infections in women are caused by this organism (Mendling et al 2016). The most common non-*albicans Candida* species is *Candida glabrata* (Sobel 2016).

Screening and Diagnosis. In addition to noting the woman's symptoms, their onset and their course, the history is a valuable screening tool for identifying predisposing risk factors. Physical examination should include a thorough inspection of the vulva and vagina.

Therapeutic Management. A number of antifungal preparations are available for the treatment of *C. albicans.* Oral medications include a variety of azole medications. The first time a woman suspects that she may have a yeast infection, she should see a healthcare provider for confirmation of the diagnosis and treatment recommendation. If she has another infection, she may wish to purchase an over-the-counter preparation and self-treat. Women should always be counselled to seek care for numerous recurrent or chronic yeast infections.

Adolescents who have extensive irritation, swelling and discomfort of the labia and vulva may find sitz baths helpful in decreasing inflammation and increasing comfort. Completing the full course of treatment prescribed, even during menstruation, is essential to removing the pathogen.

Sexually Transmitted Infections

Sexually transmitted infections (STIs) are infections or infectious disease syndromes transmitted primarily by sexual contact. The term *sexually transmitted infection* includes more than 25 infectious organisms that are transmitted through sexual activity and the dozens of clinical syndromes that they cause (Box 18.2). STIs are among the most common health problems today, with an estimated 1 million people in Australia being infected with a new STI every year (Australian Institute of Health and Welfare [AIHW] 2011). Adolescents and young adults between the ages of 15 and 24 years acquire half of all new STIs each year (AIHW 2011). The following discussion focuses on the most common STIs in adolescents and young women.

Prevention

Preventing infection (primary prevention) is the most effective way of reducing the adverse consequences of STIs for adolescents and young women. Risk-free options include complete abstinence from sexual activities that transmit semen, blood or other body fluids. Involvement in a mutually monogamous relationship with an uninfected partner also eliminates the risk of contracting STIs. Prompt diagnosis and

BOX 18.2 Sexually Transmitted Infections

Bacteria
- Chlamydia
- Gonorrhoea
- Syphilis
- Chancroid
- Lymphogranuloma venereum
- Genital mycoplasmas
- Group B streptococci

Protozoa
- Trichomoniasis

Viruses
- HIV
- Herpes simplex virus, types 1 and 2
- Cytomegalovirus
- Viral hepatitis A and B
- Human papillomavirus

Parasites
- Pediculosis (may or may not be sexually transmitted)
- Scabies (may or may not be sexually transmitted)

treatment of current infections (secondary prevention) can also prevent personal complications and transmission to others.

STIs may disproportionately affect young people who are socio-economically and geographically disadvantaged and those from different cultural backgrounds. Aboriginal and Torres Strait Islander young women are over-represented among adolescent mothers as well as for chlamydia and gonorrhoea notifications (Kang et al 2017). Research suggests that limited access to family planning information and services may contribute to relatively high numbers of teenage births in rural communities (Amjad et al 2019). Homeless and incarcerated youths may also have higher rates of chlamydia. Young people who undertake same-sex activity may be more vulnerable to STIs (Kang et al 2017).

Sexually Transmitted Infections/Human Immunodeficiency Virus Prevention Strategies

An essential component of primary prevention is counselling the woman regarding sexual practices so she can avoid acquiring or transmitting STIs, including attaining knowledge of her partner, reducing her number of partners, practising low-risk sex, avoiding the exchange of body fluids and obtaining vaccinations.

Adolescents and young women should be taught low-risk sexual practices and which sexual practices to avoid. Sexual fantasising is safe, as are caressing, hugging, body rubbing and massage. Mutual masturbation is low risk as long as there is no contact with a partner's semen or vaginal secretions. All sexual activities are safe when both partners are monogamous, trustworthy and known (by testing) to be free of disease. Anal-genital intercourse, anal-oral contact and anal-digital activity are high-risk sexual behaviours and should be avoided.

The physical barrier promoted for the prevention of STIs, including human immunodeficiency virus (HIV), is the latex male condom. The nurse should remind women to: use a condom with every sexual encounter; use latex or polyurethane male condoms; use a condom with a current expiration date; use each one only once; and handle it carefully to avoid damaging it with fingernails, teeth or other sharp objects.

The female condom (i.e. a lubricated polyurethane sheath with a ring on each end that is inserted into the vagina) is an effective mechanical barrier for STIs, including HIV. The consistent use of condoms (male or female) for every act of sexual intimacy when there is the possibility of transmission of disease is stressed by nurses.

The National HPV Vaccination Program was established in Australia in 2007, and offers a course of three injections to be given over a 6-monthly period, with individuals considered fully immunised after the third injection. Until 31 December 2009 the program included both a school-based program to cover girls aged 12 to 18 years and a community-based catch-up program for those aged 18 to 26 years and younger females not in the education system. From 1 January 2010, the catch-up program was completed, with the school-based program for 12 to 13 year old girls continuing as part of the National Immunisation Program Schedule. Infection with HPV is not restricted to women and there is growing evidence that the virus is a cause of some cancers among men (principally throat, anal and penile cancers) (Cristaudo & Giuliani 2020). Therefore, the HPV vaccination program was extended to include young men as well as young women.

Since 1 January 2017, HPV immunisation in New Zealand has been funded for everyone aged 9 to 26 years (inclusive) including boys and young men. Gardasil 9 has replaced the existing Gardasil vaccine. The vaccine is given as two doses to those aged 14 years and under, and three doses to those aged 15 years and older. The vaccine is offered to boys and girls through participating schools at Year 8, around age 12. HPV immunisation is also available free through general practices from 9 years of age (Ministry of Health 2017).

Sexually Transmitted Protozoa Infections

Trichomoniasis

Trichomonas vaginalis is an STI and is the third most common cause of vaginal infection after BV and candida (Gibson et al 2014). Trichomoniasis is caused by *T. vaginalis,* an anaerobic, one-celled protozoan with characteristic flagella. Although trichomoniasis may be asymptomatic, men present with urethritis whereas women commonly experience characteristically yellowish to greenish, frothy, malodorous discharge. Inflammation of the vulva, vagina or both may be present, and the woman may complain of irritation. The cervix and vaginal walls may demonstrate characteristic 'strawberry spots' or tiny petechiae, and the cervix may bleed on contact. In severe infections the vaginal walls, the cervix and occasionally the vulva are acutely inflamed.

Screening and Diagnosis. In addition to obtaining a history of current symptoms, obtain a thorough sexual history. Note any history of similar symptoms in the past and the treatment used. Determine whether partners were treated.

Therapeutic Management. The recommended treatment is metronidazole or tinidazole orally in a single dose (Gibson et al 2014). Although the male partner is usually asymptomatic, he should receive treatment also because trichomonads often harbour in the urethra or prostate. If partners are not treated, the infection is likely to recur.

Sexually Transmitted Bacterial Infections

Chlamydia

Chlamydia trachomatis is the most frequently reported bacterial STI in Australia and New Zealand, yet most cases are still undiagnosed (AIHW 2020a). These infections are often silent and highly destructive; their sequelae and complications are very serious. Chlamydial infections are difficult to diagnose; the symptoms, if present, are non-specific, and the organism is expensive to culture.

The most serious complication of chlamydial infections is pelvic inflammatory disease leading to infertility, ectopic pregnancy and chronic pelvic pain (AIHW 2020a). Chlamydial infection of the cervix causes inflammation, resulting in microscopic cervical ulcerations that may increase the risk of acquiring HIV. Infants born to mothers with chlamydia may develop ophthalmia neonatorum (conjunctivitis) or pneumonia after perinatal exposure (AIHW 2020a).

Screening and Diagnosis. In addition to obtaining information regarding the presence of risk factors (e.g. younger than 25 years old, no use of barrier contraceptives, new or multiple partners), enquire about the presence of any symptoms. Although infection is usually asymptomatic, some women may experience vaginal bleeding, mucoid or purulent cervical discharge, abdominal pain or dysuria; men may report testicular pain, penile discharge or dysuria.

Chlamydia PCR testing is recommended for all sexually active young people about once a year. First-pass urine chlamydia PCR is adequate, as is a self-collected lower vaginal swab for chlamydia PCR. Alternatively, an endocervical swab in a female or urethral swab in a male can be done for chlamydia PCR. Chlamydia screening can be done quickly and incorporated into routine preventive health practice. If the young person is Aboriginal or Torres Strait Islander, additional screening for gonorrhoea (first-pass urine PCR is adequate for screening) and syphilis is recommended, because these infections are more prevalent among sexually active Aboriginal people. If a urethral or cervical swab is collected, gonorrhoea culture rather than PCR is recommended.

Therapeutic Management. The treatment of chlamydial infections includes doxycycline or azithromycin (Gibson et al 2014). Because chlamydia is often asymptomatic, caution the woman to take all medication prescribed. Individuals should abstain from sexual intercourse for 7 days after treatment and all exposed sexual partners should be treated. Adolescents should be screened again in 3 to 6 months after treatment to evaluate for reinfection (Gibson 2014).

Gonorrhoea

The majority of individuals with gonorrhoea are young people ages 15 to 24 years old (AIHW 2020a). Gonorrhoea is caused by the aerobic, gram-negative diplococci *Neisseria gonorrhoeae.* It is almost exclusively transmitted by sexual contact. The bacteria infects mucosal membranes, including the cervix, uterus, fallopian tubes, urethra, rectum, mouth, throat and eyes.

Women are often asymptomatic, but when they are symptomatic, they may have a greenish-yellow purulent endocervical discharge or vaginal bleeding. Women may complain of pain (i.e. chronic or acute severe pelvic or lower abdominal pain). Infected men usually have symptoms and report purulent discharge and dysuria (Gibson et al 2014). Individuals with rectal gonorrhoea may be completely asymptomatic or conversely may experience severe symptoms with profuse purulent anal discharge, rectal pain and blood in the stool. Rectal itching, fullness, pressure and pain with bowel movements are also common symptoms. Pharyngeal infection is usually asymptomatic but may cause a sore throat. A diffuse vaginitis with vulvitis is the most common form of gonococcal infection in prepubertal girls. There may be few signs of infection, but vaginal discharge, dysuria or swollen, reddened labia are sometimes present.

Screening and Diagnosis. First-pass urine PCR is adequate when screening for gonorrhoea. Gonococcal infection cannot be diagnosed reliably by clinical signs and symptoms alone. Individuals may have 'classic' symptoms, vague symptoms that may be attributed to a number of conditions or no symptoms at all. Nucleic acid amplification tests (NAATs) are used to diagnose gonorrhoea. Vaginal specimens are the preferred testing in women, but urine, oral swabs or anal swabs can also be used (Gibson et al 2014).

Therapeutic Management. Management of gonorrhoea is becoming more challenging as drug-resistant strains are increasing. The treatment of choice for uncomplicated urethral, endocervical and rectal infections in pregnant and non-pregnant women is ceftriaxone given intramuscularly once. Gonorrhoea is highly communicable. Recent (past 60 days) sexual partners should be examined, cultured and treated with appropriate regimens.

Syphilis

Syphilis, one of the earliest described STIs, is caused by *Treponema pallidum,* a motile spirochaete. Transmission is thought to be by entry through microscopic abrasions in the subcutaneous tissue, which can occur during sexual intercourse. The disease can also be transmitted through kissing, biting or oral-genital sex. Transplacental transmission may occur at any time during pregnancy; the degree of risk is related to the quantity of spirochaete in the maternal bloodstream. Syphilis is a complex disease that can lead to serious systemic disease and even death when untreated.

Infection manifests itself in distinct stages with different symptoms and clinical manifestations. Primary syphilis is characterised by a primary lesion, the chancre, which appears 14 to 21 days after infection. This lesion often begins as a painless papule at the site of inoculation and erodes to form a non-tender, shallow, ulcer that is accompanied by lymphadenopathy. Secondary syphilis occurs 6 weeks to a few months after the appearance of the chancre. It is characterised by a widespread, symmetrical, maculopapular rash on the abdomen and extremities including the palms and soles and generalised lymphadenopathy. The infected individual also may experience fever, headache and malaise. Condylomata lata (i.e. broad, painless, pink-grey, wartlike infectious lesions) may develop on the vulva, perineum or anus. If untreated, the individual enters a latent phase that is primarily asymptomatic. Neurological, cardiovascular, musculoskeletal or multiorgan system complications can develop in the latent stage (AIHW 2021).

Screening and Diagnosis. All women who are diagnosed with another STI or with HIV should be screened for syphilis. A test for antibodies may not be reactive in the presence of active infection because it takes time for the immune system of the body to develop antibodies to any antigens. Up to one-third of people in early primary syphilis may have non-reactive serological tests.

If the young person is Aboriginal or Torres Strait Islander, a sex worker of either gender, a young man who has had sex with men or an injecting drug user, additional screening for syphilis is recommended, because this infection is prevalent among these sexually active groups.

Therapeutic Management. Penicillin G is the preferred drug for treating patients with all stages of syphilis, including pregnant women (Gibson et al 2014). Individuals with a penicillin allergy should be desensitised rather than offered treatment with an alternative medication (Gibson et al 2014).

Pelvic Inflammatory Disease

Pelvic inflammatory disease (PID) is an infectious process that most commonly involves: the uterine tubes, causing salpingitis; the uterus, causing endometritis; and, more rarely, the ovaries and peritoneal surfaces. Multiple organisms have been found to cause PID and common agents include *Neisseria gonorrhoeae, C. trachomatis* and a variety of other aerobic and anaerobic bacteria. It is estimated that each year approximately 1 million women experience an episode of PID, with the highest rates occurring in women ages 15 to 19 years old (AIHW 2021, Spain & Rheinboldt 2017). It encompasses a wide variety of pathological processes; the infection can be acute, subacute or chronic and can have a wide range of symptoms.

Most PID results from the ascending spread of microorganisms from the vagina and endocervix to the upper genital tract. This spread most commonly happens at the end of or just after menses after reception of an infectious agent. During the menstrual period several factors facilitate the development of an infection: the cervical os is slightly open, the cervical mucus barrier is absent and menstrual blood is an excellent medium for growth. PID also may develop after a miscarriage or an induced abortion, pelvic surgery or childbirth.

Risk factors for acquiring PID are those associated with the risk of contracting an STI, including under the age of 25 years, multiple partners, high rate of new partners and low socioeconomic status (Spain & Rheinboldt 2017). Women who have a long-term indwelling intrauterine device (IUD) are at increased risk for PID (AIHW 2021, Spain & Rheinboldt 2017). PID tends to recur.

Women who have had PID are at increased risk for ectopic pregnancy, infertility and chronic pelvic pain. Other problems associated with PID include dyspareunia, pyosalpinx (pus in the uterine tubes), tubo-ovarian abscess and pelvic adhesions.

The symptoms of PID vary, depending on whether the infection is acute, subacute or chronic; however, pain is common to all types of infection. It may be dull, cramping, intermittent (subacute) or severe, persistent and incapacitating (acute). Women may also report fever, chills, abdominal pain, nausea and vomiting, increased vaginal discharge, urinary tract infection symptoms and irregular bleeding.

Screening and Diagnosis. PID is difficult to diagnose because of the accompanying wide variety of symptoms. Treatment is recommended for PID in all sexually active young women and others at risk for STIs if the following criteria are present and no other cause or causes of the illness are found: lower abdominal tenderness, in combination with adnexal tenderness, uterine tenderness or cervical motion tenderness. Other criteria to support the diagnosis of PID include an oral temperature of 38.3°C or above, abnormal cervical mucopurulent discharge, microscopic presence of abundant white blood cells in vaginal fluid, elevated erythrocyte sedimentation rate, elevated C-reactive protein or laboratory documentation of cervical infection with *N. gonorrhoeae* or *C. trachomatis* (The Royal Women's Hospital *n.d.).

Therapeutic and Nursing Care Management. Perhaps the most important nursing intervention is prevention counselling. Primary prevention includes education in avoiding contracting STIs; secondary prevention involves preventing a lower genital tract infection from ascending to the upper genital tract. Instructing women in self-protective behaviours such as practices to avoid contracting STIs and using barrier methods is critical.

Although treatment regimens vary with the infecting organism, generally a broad-spectrum antibiotic is used (Spain & Rheinboldt 2017). Treatment for mild to moderately severe PID may be oral (e.g. ceftriaxone plus doxycycline and metronidazole) or parenteral (e.g. cefotetan or cefoxitin plus doxycycline [oral]), and regimens can be administered in inpatient or outpatient settings. Hospitalisation and parenteral antibiotics are recommended for women unresponsive to or unable to tolerate an oral regimen, severe illness, pregnancy, tubo-ovarian abscess or inability to exclude a surgical emergency (Das et al 2016).

Sexually Transmitted Viral Infections

Human Papillomavirus

Human papillomaviruses (HPV) can cause cancers such as cervical cancer, anal cancer and head and neck cancers, affecting both women and men. They can also cause genital warts and skin warts. The HPV types that infect the genitals can be spread by direct contact during sexual activity with a person who has the virus. HPV infection is very common, with 4 in 5 persons infected in their lifetime before the vaccine was introduced (The Royal Women's Hospital *n.d.).

Screening and Diagnosis. A woman with HPV lesions may complain of symptoms such as a profuse, irritating vaginal discharge; itching; dyspareunia; or postcoital bleeding. She also may report 'bumps' on her vulva or labia. History of a known exposure is important; however, because of the potentially long latency period and the possibility of subclinical infections in men, the lack of a history of known exposure cannot be used to exclude a diagnosis of HPV infection.

Physical inspection of the vulva, the perineum, the anus, the vagina and the cervix is essential whenever HPV lesions are suspected or seen in one area. Because speculum examination of the vagina may block some lesions, it is important to rotate the speculum blades until all areas are visualised. When lesions are visible, the characteristic appearance previously described is considered diagnostic. However, in many instances cervical lesions are not visible, and some vaginal or vulvar lesions also may be unobservable to the naked eye. Because of the potential spread of vulvar or vaginal lesions to the anus, gloves should be changed between vaginal and rectal examinations.

The only definitive diagnostic test for the presence of HPV is histological evaluation of a biopsy specimen. The HPV-DNA test can be used to screen for the high-risk types of HPV that are likely to cause cancer.

Therapeutic Management. Many warts may resolve on their own so treatment may not be necessary. Treatment does not eradicate HPV but may reduce the signs and symptoms of warts. No one of the treatments is superior to all other treatments, and no one treatment is ideal for all warts (Smith & Angarone 2015).

Patient counselling is essential. Women must understand the virus, how it is transmitted, that no immunity is conferred with infection, and that reinfection is likely with repeated contact. Encourage all sexually active women with multiple partners or a history of HPV to use latex condoms for intercourse to decrease acquisition or transmission of the infection. Semi-annual or annual health examinations are recommended to assess disease recurrence and screening for cervical cancer.

Herpes Simplex Virus

Women are more likely than men to become infected with herpes simplex virus (HSV), especially if they have multiple partners. Most persons infected with HSV-2 have not been diagnosed, and many infections are transmitted by persons unaware that they are infected.

HSV infection is caused by two different antigen subtypes of HSV: HSV type 1 (HSV-1) and HSV type 2 (HSV-2). HSV-2 is usually transmitted sexually, and HSV-1 non-sexually. Although HSV-1 is more commonly associated with gingivostomatitis and oral labial ulcers (fever blisters) and HSV-2 with genital lesions, neither type is exclusively associated with the respective sites.

Many HSV infections are asymptomatic or have very mild symptoms; however, some may experience one or more painful lesions, fever, chills, malaise, lymphadenopathy and headaches lasting 2 to 3 weeks. Typically the lesions initially appear as macules and papules that progress to form vesicles, pustules and ulcers. Women may have a more severe clinical course than do men and may have itching, inguinal tenderness and vulvar oedema. HSV cervicitis is common with initial HSV-2 infections. The cervix may appear normal or be friable, reddened, ulcerated or necrotic. A heavy, watery-to-purulent vaginal discharge is common. Extragenital lesions may be present because of autoinoculation. Urinary retention and dysuria may occur secondary to autonomic involvement of the sacral nerve root.

Individuals with recurrent episodes of HSV infections commonly have only local symptoms that are usually less severe than those associated with the initial infection. Systemic symptoms are usually absent, although the characteristic prodromal genital tingling is common. Recurrent lesions involve a small number of lesions that are less severe and last 8 to 10 days (Sauerbrei 2016). Few women with recurrent disease have cervicitis.

The HSV-2 can be passed from the mother to the infant during pregnancy, childbirth or the newborn period with a higher risk of transmission if the mother is having the first outbreak versus a recurrent outbreak. Exposure to HSV-2 may lead to a potentially fatal neonatal herpes infection (The Department of Health *n.d.).

Screening and Diagnosis. Although a diagnosis of herpes infection may be suspected from the history and physical examination, it is confirmed by laboratory studies. A viral culture is obtained by swabbing exudate during the vesicular stage of the disease.

Therapeutic Management. Genital herpes is a chronic and recurring disease for which there is no known cure. Management is directed towards specific treatment during primary and recurrent infections, prevention, self-help measures and psychological support.

Oral medications used for treating the first clinical HSV infection include aciclovir, famciclovir and valaciclovir. These medications are considered for episodic or suppressive therapy for recurrent HSV. Intravenous aciclovir may be used for individuals with a compromised immune system or severe disease (Sauerbrei 2016).

Because neonatal HSV infection is such a devastating disease, prevention is critical. Current recommendations include carefully examining and questioning all women about symptoms at onset of labour (The Department of Health *n.d.). If visible lesions are not present at onset of labour, vaginal birth is acceptable. Caesarean birth after labour begins or membranes rupture is recommended if visible lesions are present. Infants who are born through an infected vagina should be observed carefully and cultured.

The emotional effect of contracting an incurable STI such as herpes is considerable. At diagnosis many emotions may surface—helplessness, anger, denial, guilt, anxiety, shame or inadequacy. Women need the opportunity to discuss their feelings and help in learning to live with the disease. Herpes can affect a woman's sexuality, her sexual practices and her current and future relationships. She may need help in raising the issue with her partner or future partners.

Hepatitis

Five different viruses (hepatitis viruses A, B, C, D and E) account for almost all cases of viral hepatitis in humans. These are discussed in Chapter 25.

Human Immunodeficiency Virus

Human immunodeficiency virus (HIV) is a bloodborne pathogen and transmission of the virus can occur in the perinatal period, through sexual intercourse with an infected person or by sharing needles with an infected person. HIV is discussed in Chapter 28.

HEALTH CONDITIONS RELATED TO REPRODUCTION

The biological maturation that forms the foundation of adolescent development and the transition to adulthood is accompanied by conflicting feelings, attitudes and social practices related to developing sexuality. During adolescence the sexual drive emerges, and adolescents begin to explore their ability to attract a partner.

Adolescent Pregnancy

In 2017, births to teenage mothers made up 2.2% of all live births. Births to teenage mothers decreased by more than 40% between 2006 and 2017 from 17.6 to 9.2 live births per 1000 females aged 15 to 19 years. Motherhood for women under the age of 20 can be a positive and maturing experience. For many young people, becoming a parent can have a transformative impact, particularly with changing unhealthy behaviours and relationships (Australian Human Rights Commission [AHRC] 2019).

Recent findings also show some positive birth outcomes for teenage mothers compared with mothers aged 20 to 24 years with teenage mothers:

- more likely to have a spontaneous labour (and less likely to have a caesarean section)
- less likely to have diabetes
- less likely to have gestational diabetes (AHRC 2019).

However, mothers who give birth under the age of 20 are also a vulnerable population group, who may experience lower education and reduced employment. This may increase the risk of socioeconomic disadvantage for both child and mother (AHRC 2019). Children of vulnerable young parents are also at risk of becoming teenage parents themselves (AHRC 2019, AIHW 2020a).

Teenage motherhood is associated with a number of poorer health and wellbeing outcomes for both mother and baby. In the short term, babies born to teenage mothers are at greater risk of being born preterm, with a low birthweight, stillbirth and neonatal death (AIHW 2020a, Marino et al 2016). Children of teenage mothers may go on to have behavioural, emotional and cognitive disadvantages (Marino et al 2016). Depression is more prevalent among pregnant adolescents than adult pregnant women or adolescents in general, and teenage motherhood can have a long-lasting effect on mental health (AIHW 2020a, Amjad et al 2019).

Teenage motherhood, particularly at younger ages, can pose significant long-term risks to both mother and child. Teenage mothers often delay having their pregnancy confirmed and/or seeking antenatal care, and are more likely to engage in risky behaviour, including smoking and drinking alcohol during pregnancy. Consequently, teenage mothers face increased risk of miscarriage, preterm birth, low birthweight and other complications of pregnancy and birth and perinatal mortality (AIHW 2020a). A number of factors are associated with teenage birth including family history of teenage pregnancy, sexual abuse in childhood, unstable housing arrangements, poor school attendance and performance, socioeconomic disadvantage, living in rural and remote areas and being Aboriginal and Torres Strait Islander (AIHW 2020a).

Medical Aspects

Adolescents often receive delayed or inadequate prenatal care. Prenatal care may be delayed because the adolescent does not realise she is pregnant or denies the pregnancy until the second or third trimester. Medical concerns of adolescent pregnancies include gestational diabetes, anaemia, preeclampsia and low platelet syndrome (Kawakita et al 2016).

The obstetric risk and risk to the infant during a second pregnancy for the adolescent is much higher. An adolescent with a poor outcome in the first pregnancy has a three-fold risk of repeating the poor outcome in the second pregnancy. In adolescents the risk for a preterm delivery recurring is double the rate found in older women.

Complications of Pregnancy

Bleeding can occur early in pregnancy with an incidence ranging from 7% to 21% (Sapra et al 2017). The risk of a spontaneous abortion is higher in women with bleeding than without bleeding (Sapra et al 2017).

When a young woman is seen with bleeding and abdominal pain, an **ectopic pregnancy** must be ruled out.

Structural Factors. Labour may be prolonged in younger adolescents, particularly those 12 to 16 years of age; this is directly related to fetopelvic incompatibility and is a reflection of the adolescent's smaller stature and incomplete growth process. The incidence of prolonged labour is highest in girls younger than age 14 years. Girls who are 12 to 13 years old have the highest rate of caesarean births, primarily because of cephalopelvic disproportion. However, older adolescents 15 to 21 years of age, especially those who have previously delivered a baby, often have labours that are shorter than average. The transition between pelvic disproportion and pelvic adequacy appears to occur around 15 years of age in the average adolescent.

Nutritional Needs. Caloric requirements during adolescence closely parallel the growth curve, and the need for protein, calcium and iron is increased. Young adolescents tolerate caloric restriction poorly, and the anabolic need for calories during pregnancy places an added burden on their bodies.

Mother–Infant Relationship

Adolescents often have unrealistic expectations for the child. The young mother may view the infant as a plaything or a love object for herself. Children of adolescent mothers experience more developmental problems than children of adult mothers. The amount of cognitive stimulation in the child's early home environment is associated with the child's level of cognitive attainment. Nurses need to stress the importance of the adolescent caring for the child even when other adults (e.g. mother or grandmother) are involved. The other adults present need education and support to allow optimum development of the infant and adolescent mother.

Adolescent Fathers

Little information is available about adolescent fathers. Most studies have small sample sizes and rely on reporting from the mother rather than the young man himself. Most teen fathers have a strong emotional commitment to and interest in their child (Lau 2016). This involvement has positive effects on the mother's self-esteem and decreases her level of distress and depression.

Nursing Care Management

It is evident from the preceding discussion that nurses play a central role in meeting the needs of pregnant adolescents. The nurse may be the one to whom the young girl turns for help and guidance in her dilemma and on whom she relies for support and reassurance.

The first goal in nursing care of the pregnant adolescent is to help her obtain healthcare whether she elects to continue or terminate the pregnancy. Typically, adolescents are reluctant to seek medical help, in part because of anxiety but more often because of a tendency to deny the pregnancy. Early prenatal care is essential for the welfare of both mother and infant. For guidelines, teaching and general support measures during pregnancy, the reader is directed to the textbooks available on nursing care throughout the maternity cycle.

Adolescent Abortion

Abortion legislation is different in every Australian state and territory and differs again in New Zealand. Surgical abortion is a low-risk procedure most commonly used for first-trimester abortion (7 to 12 weeks) in Australia. Known as suction aspiration or suction curette, it involves removing the lining and contents of the uterus (womb). A range of other surgical techniques are used for abortion later in pregnancy.

Medication abortion offers an alternative to surgical abortion for women in the early weeks of pregnancy. Medication abortion uses a combination of two medications, mifepristone and misoprostol, to end a pregnancy up to 9 weeks. Mifepristone was previously known as RU 486 and is sometimes called the 'abortion pill'.

Medication abortion is a low-risk, non-invasive way to terminate (end) a pregnancy. It is around 99% effective at ending a pregnancy. Around 2% to 5% of women who have a medication abortion will need some follow-up treatment to complete the abortion.

Information about abortion services in Australia and New Zealand are listed in Box 18.3.

BOX 18.3 Abortion Services in Australia and New Zealand

Australia

Victoria

My Options: 1800 696 784, 1800 555 660 (National Relay Service), 13 14 50 (interpreter); Monday to Friday, 10 am to 4 pm; info@1800myoptions.org.au
Marie Stopes Australia: 1300 867 104

NSW

Family Planning and Marie Stopes Australia: Contact the Family Planning NSW Talkline on 1300 658 886; Monday to Friday, 8.30 am to 5 pm
Marie Stopes Australia: 1300 867 104

Tasmania

Family Planning Tasmania
South: 421 Main Rd, Glenorchy: 6273 9117
North: 269 Wellington St, Launceston: 6343 4566
North-West: 199 Mount St, Upper Burnie: 6431 7692

Queensland

Women's Health: 1800 017 676
Children by Choice: 1800 177 725
Pregnancy, Birth and Baby: 1800 882 436
Marie Stopes Australia: 1300 867 104

Northern Territory

Family Planning Welfare Association of NT: (08) 8948 0144
Marie Stopes Australia:1300 867 104

Western Australia

Marie Stopes Australia: 1300 866 130

South Australia

Pregnancy Advisory Centre: (08) 7117 8999

Australia Capital Territory

Marie Stopes Australia, Sexual Health and Family Planning ACT Incorporated: 1300 867 104

New Zealand

Whangarei Family Planning Clinic: (09) 438 1986 or 0800 372 546
Auckland Medical Aid Centre: (09) 638 6040
Tauranga Family Planning: 07 578 8539
The Women's Clinic, Palmerston North: 0800 226 784
Wellington Hospital, Te Mahoe Unit: Phone 04 806 0761
Nelson Hospital: 03 546 1800
Wairau Hospital: 03 520 9999
Ashburton Hospital: 03 308 4149
Christchurch Women's Hospital: 03 346 4699
Dunedin Hospital: 03 470 9400 (Day Surgery Unit) or 0800 TOPSDHB
The Women's Clinic, Invercargill: 0800 226 784

Nursing Care Management

The adolescent considering an abortion will need help to explore the meaning of the various alternatives for elective abortion and consequences to herself and her significant others. It is often difficult for a woman to express her true feelings (e.g. what abortion means to her now and in the future and what support or regret her friends and peers may demonstrate). A calm, matter-of-fact approach on the part of the nurse can be helpful. Clarifying, restating and reflecting statements; open-ended questions; and feedback are communication techniques that can be used to maintain a realistic focus on the situation and bring the woman's problems into the open. If family or friends cannot be involved, scheduling time for nursing personnel to give the necessary support is an essential component of the care plan.

Contraception

Family planning services have developed and expanded during recent years, but the need for contraceptive services as part of the healthcare of adolescents remains great. The birth control pill and condom remain the most popular methods for adolescents; 3-month injectable contraception is more popular among lower-income adolescents. Adolescents commonly delay seeking contraceptive information. The adolescent should be given accurate information about the risks and benefits of each method before making a choice.

The choice of a safe and effective contraceptive method must be suited to the individual (Table 18.1). The choice is based on preference after the adolescent is informed of the benefits and disadvantages.

Nursing Care Management

Nurses are often involved in providing education about contraception. Such education is ideally combined with ongoing sex education. Although sexual abstinence is a highly desirable form of contraception for adolescents, nurses working with adolescents must recognise that teens feel multiple pressures to engage in sexual intercourse.

Sexual Assault (rape)

Typically, stranger rape is what comes to mind when one thinks of sexual assault; however, more than half of assaults are committed by someone known to the survivor. Although both males and females can be sexually assaulted, females are at greatest risk. Adolescents are at high risk for sexual assault; other high-risk groups include: survivors of childhood sexual or physical abuse; persons who are disabled; persons with substance abuse problems; sex workers; persons who are poor or homeless; and persons living in prisons, institutions or areas of military conflict. Sexual assault remains underreported for multifactorial reasons.

Nurses can obtain information about their state statutory rape reporting responsibilities from state or local child protective services agencies, legal counsel, rape crisis organisations or state or territory health services.

Diagnostic Evaluation

Rape victims may exhibit a variety of reactions, and the circumstances of the initial medical evaluation may be frightening and stressful. The initial contact with the rape victim must be supportive because the interrogation and associated activities have the potential to add to the trauma of the sexual assault. First of all, the victim needs to know that they are: (1) all right and (2) not being blamed for the situation. A physical examination is carried out as soon as possible because physical evidence deteriorates rapidly. This examination will be attended to by a health professional who is trained appropriately in this area where possible. The victim should not bathe or shower before the examination.

The young person is always told in advance in understandable terms exactly what to expect in the way of tests and procedures, and the explanation is accompanied by strong emotional support. The victim is examined thoroughly, including non-genital areas, for evidence of injury that might substantiate the use of force.

The forensic examination of a sexual assault victim must follow strict legal requirements. The medical record may provide key evidence for the legal case. Practitioners specially trained for rape examination should be used when possible. Nurses are often members of this group. Evaluation for STIs is an important part of the evaluation.

Therapeutic Management

Adolescents who have been raped arrive under a variety of circumstances. They are usually brought by parents, friends or police officers, but some may seek medical help on their own. It is advisable to obtain parental consent for examination, but the examination may be performed without parental consent if the adolescent is mature and the parents are unavailable. A female observer or chaperone should be present during the history and examination of female victims who are examined by a male practitioner. Whether a parent should be present during the examination is determined on an individual basis. The parent's presence is usually encouraged if the parent is supportive and the young person agrees.

Nursing Care Management

Many of the approaches that have been described for sexually abused children (see Chapter 14) also apply to adolescents. Sexual assault is a devastating experience with long-lasting effects. The primary goal of nursing care is to avoid inflicting further stress on the adolescent, who is often angry, confused, frightened, embarrassed and filled with self-blame. The nurse must do everything possible to reduce the stress of the interrogation and examination. Although most health professionals and police officers are sensitive to the needs of adolescents and attempt to make the process as non-stressful as possible, the nurse should be alert to cues that indicate the victim is being overstressed.

Follow-up care of the rape victim is essential and extends over a long period. The health-compromising responses to sexual assault include posttraumatic stress disorder (PTSD), anxiety and depression. PTSD is the most common mental health sequela of sexual violence, with rates of 16% to 60% among women (Ullman & Peter-Hagene 2016). Aside from the universal need for emotional support, the needs of rape victims vary widely and depend on the nature of the incident, the victim's age when the rape occurred, the physical and emotional injuries sustained by the victim, the legal actions being considered as a result, the resources available for informal support and the anticipated reactions of persons in the informal support network.*

In addition to the needs of the adolescent rape victim, the nurse should also be sensitive to the needs and reactions of the adolescent's parents. Some parents will be angry and blame the adolescent; others will feel guilty and embarrassed.

*NSW Rape Crisis Centre: 1800 424 017
Sexual Assault Counselling Australia: 1800 211 028
LGBTIQ+ Violence Service: 1800 497 212
Sexual Assault Crisis Line: 1800 806 292
Victorian Sexual Assault Crisis Line (SACL): 1800 806 292 or 8345 3495
NZ National free helpline: 0800 88 33 00
Wellington Rape Crisis: 04 801 8973, https://wellingtonrapecrisis.org.nz/

TABLE 18.1 Advantages and Disadvantages of Contraceptive Methods in Adolescents

Method	Advantages	Disadvantages
	BEHAVIOURAL METHODS	
Abstinence	100% effective in preventing STIs and pregnancy	Peer pressure to conform Relatively high failure rate from non-compliance
Withdrawal (coitus interruptus) Withdrawal of penis before ejaculation	No medical visit necessary	High failure rate Some seminal fluid often released before ejaculation Ejaculate at vaginal orifice may enter vagina No STI protection
Calendar method Refrain from intercourse during fertile period (time of ovulation)	Teaches adolescent girls about their menstrual cycle Encourages couple participation	High failure rate Requires a regular, predictable menstrual cycle (irregular menses are common for first 2 years after menarche) No STI protection
	BARRIER METHODS	
Condom	Minimal side effects Easy to use Available without prescription Portable Provides protection against STIs	Requires consistent use Requires premeditated intent for sexual union May decrease sensation Misuse results in failure Decreased spontaneity
Male—Penile covering to trap sperm	Spermicidal condoms increase effectiveness for pregnancy and STI prevention Inexpensive compared with female condom	Latex sensitivity or allergies in a small percentage of people Improper use may lead to pregnancy or development of STI
Female—Inserted into vagina with base covering part of perineum; may be inserted 8 hours before intercourse	Female participation Made of polyurethane; no latex sensitivities and can be used with oil-based lubricants Provides protection from STIs	May be difficult to insert Noisy
Diaphragm Cervical covering to prevent sperm from reaching egg Must be used in conjunction with spermicidal jelly May be inserted 4–6 hours before intercourse If inserted early, should be checked for placement before intercourse	Can be fitted in virgins Low failure rate when used correctly Few contraindications May be reused	High failure rate in adolescents because of inconvenience of use Requires consistent use Requires fitting and instruction by medical personnel Requires premeditated intent for sexual union Requires body awareness and comfort with touching oneself for insertion Minimal STI protection May increase incidence of urinary tract infection
Cervical cap Soft rubber dome with a firm but pliable rim; fits over base of the cervix close to the junction of the cervix and vaginal fornixes	May be inserted hours before intercourse Insertion and removal similar to diaphragm	Available in only four sizes Must remain in place at least 6 hours after intercourse but no longer than 48 hours Not recommended for women with abnormal Papanicolaou test result, history of toxic shock syndrome or difficulty with proper fitting No STI protection
	CHEMICALS	
Spermicidal foam, jelly, cream and suppositories Substance inserted into vagina to kill sperm	Available without prescription Inexpensive Easy to use No major health concerns	High failure rate unless combined with condom Possible for sperm to be ejaculated directly into uterine os, bypassing spermicide in vagina Must be used shortly before coitus; therefore, requires interruption of sexual experience Repeated sexual union requires repeated application Requires premeditated intent for sexual union Messy Nonoxynol-9 associated with increased transmission of HIV to women; should not be used with anal sex in male partner sex for same reason No STI protection

TABLE 18.1 Advantages and Disadvantages of Contraceptive Methods in Adolescents—cont'd

Method	Advantages	Disadvantages
HORMONAL METHODS		
Oral contraceptives Oestrogen and progesterone-like compounds Inhibit ovulation by blocking release of gonadotropins from anterior pituitary gland	99% effective if used correctly Safe for adolescents Method of choice for most adolescents Administered by mouth Becomes a ritual not associated with sexual activity Regulates menses, decreases dysmenorrhoea and acne, decreases menstrual flow Prevents ovarian and endometrial cancers Prevents functional ovarian cysts	Higher failure rate in adolescents than in older women Need to follow precise instructions; requires continued motivation, consistent use Requires prescription Price substantial for adolescent No STI protection Possible side effects include headaches, missed or scanty periods, breakthrough bleeding, blood clot
Medroxyprogesterone acetate (Depo-Provera) Progestin that suppresses hormonal cycle and prevents ovulation Injection given every 3 months	No interruption of intercourse Invisible method	No STI protection Possible side effects include significant weight gain, decreased bone density, decreased HDLs, irregular menses or amenorrhoea, decreased libido, depression Fertility perhaps delayed after discontinuation Must return to care provider every 3 months for injection US Food and Drug Administration recommends discontinuation after 2 years because of decreased bone density
Levonorgestrel intrauterine system (Mirena) T-shaped intrauterine device that releases 20 microg/dL of levonorgestrel Inserted within 7 days of menses and remains in place for 5 years Thickens cervical mucus and inhibits sperm mobility and function	> 99% effective Effectively prevents fertilisation, resulting in low rates of ectopic pregnancy Reduced length and quantity of menstrual bleeding Reduced dysmenorrhoea No weight gain	Risk of perforation at time of insertion 2–12% expulsion rate Not recommended in nulliparous women or women not in monogamous relationships Possible side effects include abdominal pain, headache, vaginal discharge and breast pain No STI protection
Etonogestrel implant (Implanon) 40 × 2 mm implanted rod Progestin-only method Suppresses ovulation	> 99% effective Efficacy not user dependent Provides 3 years of protection Single rod insertion and removal Palpable but not visible after insertion	Irregular menstrual bleeding Other less common side effects include headache, vaginitis, weight gain No STI protection
EMERGENCY OR POSTCOITAL CONTRACEPTION		
Emergency contraception works in one of three ways: by suppressing or delaying ovulation, by preventing the meeting of sperm and egg or by preventing implantation Progestin-only pill given within 72 hours of intercourse *or* Insertion of a copper-releasing intrauterine device up to 7 days after unprotected intercourse	Useful in unplanned sexual intercourse or contraceptive failure May be given in advance for emergency use Available without prescription for adults	No STI protection May cause nausea if combination method used May change timing of next menstrual cycle

HDL, High-density lipoprotein; *HIV,* human immunodeficiency virus; *STI,* sexually transmitted infection.

HEALTH CONDITIONS WITH A BEHAVIOURAL COMPONENT

Anorexia Nervosa and Bulimia Nervosa

Anorexia nervosa (AN) is an eating disorder characterised by a refusal to maintain a minimally normal body weight, intense fear of gaining weight along with behaviour that interferes with weight gain and a body image disturbance (Herpertz-Dahlmann 2015). It is a disorder with social, psychological, behavioural, cultural and physiological components resulting in significant morbidity and mortality. AN is characterised by a distorted body image with adolescents' self-confidence relying on their weight and body shape. The disorder is a clinical diagnosis listed in the *Diagnostic and Statistical Manual of Mental Disorders, Fifth Edition* (DSM-5) with two distinct subtypes: restricting type and binge-eating/purging type (Herpertz-Dahlmann 2015). Individuals with AN are described as perfectionists, academically high achievers, conforming and conscientious.

Bulimia nervosa (BN; from the Greek meaning 'ox hunger') refers to an eating disorder similar to AN. BN is characterised by repeated episodes of binge eating followed by inappropriate compensatory behaviours, such as: self-induced vomiting; misuse of laxatives, diuretics or other medications; fasting; or excessive exercise (Herpertz-Dahlmann 2015). The binge behaviour consists of secretive, frenzied consumption of large amounts of high-calorie (or 'forbidden') foods during a brief time (usually about 2 hours). The binge is counteracted by a variety of weight-control methods (purging), including self-induced vomiting, diuretic and laxative abuse and rigorous exercise. These binge–purge cycles are followed by self-deprecating thoughts, a depressed mood and an awareness that the eating pattern is abnormal.

Other Specified Feeding or Eating Disorder (OSFED) was formerly recognised as Eating Disorder Not Otherwise Specified (EDNOS) in the Diagnostic and Statistical Manual of Mental Disorders (DSM-IV).

According to the DSM-5, a person with OSFED may present with many of the symptoms of other eating disorders such as AN, BN or binge eating disorder (BED) but will not meet the full criteria for diagnosis of these disorders. Around 30% of people who seek treatment for an eating disorder have OSFED. People with OSFED commonly present with extremely disturbed eating habits and/or a distorted body image and/or overvaluation of shape and weight and/or an intense fear of gaining weight (if underweight). OSFED is the most common eating disorder diagnosed for adults as well as adolescents, and affects both males and females (The Butterfly Foundation 2020a).

Epidemiology

Eating disorders and disordered eating together are estimated to affect over 16% of the Australian population. BED and OSFED are the most common eating disorders, affecting approximately 6% and 5%, respectively, while AN and BN each occur in below 1% of the general population. Many people with eating disorders also present with at least one other lifetime psychiatric disorder.

Among adolescents, individuals with BN, BED and individuals with AN have one or more comorbid psychiatric conditions at some point in their lives. The most common and significant psychiatric comorbidities for adolescents and adults with BN and BED, as well as adults with AN, are mood, anxiety and substance-use disorders. In contrast, the only psychiatric disorder that commonly co-occurs with AN is oppositional defiant disorder (The Butterfly Foundation 2020b).

Pathophysiology

No consensus exists on the pathophysiology of AN and BN. A combination of genetic, neurochemical, psychodevelopmental, sociocultural and environmental factors appear to cause the disorder (Campbell & Peebles 2014). Dieting and body dissatisfaction appear to be common to the initiation of both AN and BN.

The prominent physiological changes that occur as a result of weight loss have raised suspicions of a prominent physiological disturbance as a causative factor. Because most of these physiological disturbances resolve with the normalisation of body weight and healthy eating, this argues against their role as a primary cause. The neurotransmitter serotonin affects appetite control, sexual and social behaviour, stress responses and mood and possibly accounts for some of the changes seen in patients with AN. BED is also associated with dopamine in the nucleus accumbens portion of the brain that is programmed for reward and motivation. The significance of these changes and their connection to eating disorders are not well understood (Kreipe 2016).

Individuals with eating disorders commonly have psychiatric problems, including affective disorder, anxiety disorder, obsessive-compulsive disorder and personality disorder. Adult women with eating disorders were found to have higher rates of obsessive-compulsive behaviour traits in their childhood. Persons with eating disorders have also been found to have higher reported rates of substance abuse, with alcohol problems being more common in those with BN than AN (Kreipe 2016, The Butterfly Foundation 2020b). It is important to note that many of the clinical findings are directly related to the state of starvation and improve with weight gain. Research continues in an effort to better understand the aetiology and pathogenesis of eating disorders.

Clinical Manifestations

The most obvious manifestation of AN is the severe and profound weight loss induced by self-imposed starvation. The adolescents identify with this skeleton-like appearance and do not regard this body type as abnormal or ugly. Adolescents with AN often eat small amounts of food or play with food on their plates to give the impression that they are eating adequately and not experiencing disturbances in their eating habits. This can lead friends and family to disregard the possibility of AN. The adolescents can display a marked preoccupation with food—preparing meals for others, talking about food, hoarding food. Many become obsessed with fasting and engage in frequent strenuous exercise. The binge–purge subtype of AN is characterised with chewing then spitting out the food rather than swallowing, or laxative usage to speed up the weight-loss process (Kreipe 2016) (see Critical Thinking Case Study box).

CRITICAL THINKING CASE STUDY

Anorexia Nervosa

Jaspreet is a 13-year-old girl whose grades have been excellent and whom the teachers describe as a 'model student'. Recently, Jaspreet's teacher told the school nurse that Jaspreet's parents were in the middle of a moving and obtaining new employment, both of which were very stressful for them. In addition, several of Jaspreet's friends told the teacher and nurse that they are concerned about Jaspreet because she runs every day at lunchtime and seldom eats lunch with them. Jaspreet told her friends that she gained weight over the winter months and that she is running because she wants to qualify for the athletic team this spring. The school nurse asks to see Jaspreet and takes a health history and set of vitals including her weight and notes that Jaspreet's oral temperature is 36°C and that she weighs 34 kg. Jaspreet states she has lost 9 kg over winter and that she is very happy as this is almost halfway to her weight loss.

1. Evidence—Is there sufficient evidence to draw any conclusions about Jaspreet's behaviour?
2. Assumptions—Describe some underlying assumptions about the following:
   a. personality characteristics of individuals with anorexia nervosa (AN)
   b. factors influencing the development of AN
   c. clinical manifestations of AN
   d. treatment of AN.
3. What priorities for nursing care should be established for Jaspreet at this time?
4. Does the evidence objectively support your argument (conclusion)?

Young people with AN tend to withdraw from peer relationships and engage in self-imposed social isolation. They continually strive for perfection, which may be demonstrated in other compulsive behaviours. They are usually overachievers, and their schoolwork is very important to them.

In the wake of the severe weight loss, these young females exhibit physical signs of altered metabolic activity. They develop secondary amenorrhoea, bradycardia, lowered body temperature, decreased blood pressure and cold intolerance. They have dry skin and brittle nails and develop lanugo. The changes are usually reversible with adequate weight gain and improved nutritional status.

Bulimia is more common in older adolescent girls and young women; males with bulimia are less common. BN patients may be of average or slightly above-average weight. The diagnosis is confirmed, according to the DSM-5, by at least one binge-eating episode per week for the preceding 3 months.

The frequency of bingeing can be anywhere from once per week to seven or eight times per day. Because persons with bulimia usually binge on high-calorie foods, especially sweets, ice-cream and pastries, insulin production is stimulated to cope with the added carbohydrates. When the food is vomited, the unused insulin stimulates hunger and the desire to eat.

Diagnostic Evaluation

There are four eating disorders that are recognised by the Diagnostic and Statistical Manual of Mental Disorders (DSM), which are:

- other specified feeding and eating disorders
- bulimia nervosa
- binge eating disorder
- anorexia nervosa.

History and Physical Examination. A complete history and physical examination are important to rule out other causes for weight loss. The medical assessment of an eating disorder focuses on the complications of altered nutritional status and purging. A careful history assesses weight changes, dietary patterns and the frequency and severity of purging and excessive exercise. Purging behaviours include vomiting or other methods such as abuse of laxatives, enemas, diuretics, anorexic drugs, caffeine or other stimulants. Measure the patient's weight and height and evaluate it for appropriateness according to standard weight for height, age and sex determined according to the percentile of his or her expected body weight or body mass index (BMI).

Particularly important parts of the physical examination are vital sign measurement (heart rate and blood pressure, both supine and standing, and body temperature). Hypotension, bradycardia and hypothermia are often seen in association with extremely low weight. Dry skin, lanugo, acrocyanosis and breast atrophy are findings that have been associated with AN. Distinctive hand lesions (Russell's sign) have also been observed; the backs of the hands are often scarred and cut from repeated abrasion of the skin against the maxillary incisors during self-induced vomiting. Other findings include swelling of the parotid and submandibular glands and erosion of the enamel of the anterior teeth because of chronic acid exposure from vomiting.

Prolongation of the QT interval may be detected in some patients. Mitral valve prolapse (MVP) may also develop. An abdominal examination is important to detect intestinal dilation from chronic severe constipation as a result of decreased intestinal motility. Finally, a neurological examination assesses for other causes of weight loss or vomiting such as evidence of brain tumour.

Complications of Eating Disorders

Many potential complications can occur as a result of starvation and persistent purging. Some of these are osteoporosis, cardiac impairments, cognitive changes, difficulties in psychological functioning, gastrointestinal dysfunction (e.g. slowed motility, symptoms of nausea and bloating), endocrinological changes, electrolyte abnormalities (especially hypokalaemia and metabolic alkalosis), dental erosions, enlarged salivary glands and infertility.

AN has been associated with MVP, QT-interval prolongation and heart failure. MVP is a common finding in patients with AN, affecting 32% to 60% of patients compared with 6% to 22% in the general population. This may be because of an increased ability to detect the disorder in patients with intravascular volume depletion consistent with the state of starvation.

The risk of heart failure is greatest in the first 2 weeks of refeeding in patients with an eating disorder. Patients with moderate to severe AN (e.g. approximately 10% below ideal body weight) are at risk for the refeeding syndrome during the first 2 to 3 weeks of treatment. **Refeeding syndrome** consists of cardiovascular, neurological and haematological complications that occur because of shifts in phosphate from extracellular to intracellular spaces in individuals who have total body phosphorus depletion as a result of malnutrition. Refeeding syndrome can cause cardiac arrest and delirium. The risk is reduced by slower refeeding, replacing phosphorus and carefully avoiding a high sodium intake. Carefully monitoring serum electrolytes and observing for signs of oedema or congestive heart failure are important during refeeding.

Amenorrhoea used to be a diagnostic criterion for AN in the DSM-IV; however, many women do not experience amenorrhoea and were at risk for being underdiagnosed. In addition, men were excluded from the AN diagnoses with the DSM-IV amenorrhoea criteria. Amenorrhoea may occur with AN patients as a result of low levels of follicle-stimulating hormone and luteinising hormone. Menses is usually restored within 6 months of achieving 90% of the ideal body weight.

Therapeutic Management

The treatment and management of AN involve three major thrusts: (1) reinstitution of normal nutrition or reversal of the severe state of malnutrition; (2) resolution of disturbed patterns of family interaction; and (3) individual psychotherapy to correct deficits and distortions in psychological functioning. Treatment of eating disorders requires interventions of an interdisciplinary team composed of a primary practitioner, nurse, dietitian and mental health provider with paediatric and adolescent healthcare experience. Because of the psychogenic nature of the disorder, the treatment may be long.

Nutrition Interventions. The initial goal is to treat the life-threatening malnutrition and to restore dietary stability and weight gain. This may necessitate intravenous or tube feeding if the malnutrition is severe. The patient should avoid rapid weight gain because it has been associated with severe metabolic abnormalities in some patients, such as refeeding syndrome, which consists of cardiovascular, neurological and haematological complications that occur when nutritional replacement is given too rapidly.

Dietary interventions are combined with behavioural therapy to improve the underlying psychological misconception about the weight loss. Another aspect of treatment is to relieve the anxiety related to eating and the depression that accompanies the disorder. Weight gain alone cannot be considered a cure for the disease and is an unreliable sign of progress. Relapses are frequent as the person reverts to previous eating patterns when removed from the therapeutic environment.

Psychotherapy. Individual psychotherapy is aimed at helping the young person resolve the adolescent identity crisis, particularly as it relates to a distorted body image. It is essential that adolescents rely on their own thinking, become more realistic in self-appraisal and become capable of living as self-directed, competent individuals who enjoy life without manipulating the body and its functions. Psychotherapy focuses on helping the young person resolve the adolescent identity crisis, particularly when it results in a distorted body image.

Behavioural Therapy. Behavioural modification, usually through cognitive behavioural therapy or motivational interviewing, has met varying degrees of success. The goal is to increase the patient's feelings of control and responsibility towards achieving recovery. Providing privileges or activities for weight gain or positive eating behaviours may be successful, but treatment should also address the conflict precipitating the disorder (The Butterfly Foundation 2002b).

Pharmacotherapy. Pharmacotherapy in the treatment of eating disorders lacks evidence of efficacy. The few studies that have been done have primarily evaluated medications' efficacy in the treatment of comorbid disorders such as obsessive-compulsive disorders and depression. Anxiolytic medications may be helpful before meals to relieve some AN patients' anxiety.

Prognosis. Predictors of more favourable outcomes are: having BN rather than AN; having a purging type of AN rather than a restricting type; having a short duration of illness; and having a higher discharge weight after hospitalisation. Current research reports that BMI at the start or end of treatment and severity of the eating disorder have no effect on the outcome of individuals with an eating disorder; however, individuals 19 years and older and individuals who participate in an inpatient treatment program have significantly lower rates of relapse (Berends et al 2016).

AN has the highest mortality rate of any mental health disorder (Harrington et al 2015, The Butterfly Foundation 2020a). The most common cause of non-natural mortality was suicide, with higher rates among adolescents with BN compared with AN (Fichter & Quadflieq 2016, The Butterfly Foundation 2020a). Although the changes associated with AN are often reversible, the physical complications can involve every organ system in the body and the effects of severe malnutrition are often obvious for many years. For example, adolescents with eating disorders are at risk of developing osteopenia or osteoporosis associated with a two-fold to seven-fold higher fracture risk in later life because most of the bone mass is built up during adolescence.

Nursing Care Management

Nurses need to adopt and maintain a kind and supportive, yet firm, manner in managing the care of the adolescent with eating disorders without creating a passive-dependent attitude. The individual requires sustained support and reassurance to cope with ambivalent feelings related to body concept and the desire to be seen as cooperative, reliable and worthy of receiving kindness. Encouraging the adolescent with education and activities that strengthen self-esteem facilitates the resocialisation process and promotes social acceptance among peers.

It is important that nurses be aware of the physical side effects of AN. Patients with AN frequently limit their fluid intake. Urinary tract problems are frequent, and ketones and proteins are commonly detected in the urine as a result of fat and protein breakdown. Vital sign instability can be severe and can include orthostatic hypotension; the pulse becomes irregular and may decrease markedly. Bradycardia and hypothermia can result in cardiac arrest.

Eating disorders are complex and multifaceted. Because patients often deny their illness, they may refuse the treatment efforts of health providers. The treatment plan needs to be developed carefully and with patience and empathy. Power struggles with patients may escalate the eating disorder symptomatology in that control issues are often central to the development of eating disorders. Implementing less intrusive interventions first and allowing them time to develop is important before applying more restrictive interventions. If possible, treatment should match patients' readiness to change. The care team needs to agree about the treatment philosophy and protocol to avoid sending mixed messages to the patient. It is important to motivate and treat eating disorder patients with respect and support while being direct with expectations on their eating behaviours (Beukers et al 2015).

Nurses, patients and families can find assistance and information the National Eating Disorders Collaboration (NEDC).

Prevention. There are no easy ways to prevent an eating disorder. However, public and professional awareness of signs and symptoms can facilitate early identification and treatment to prevent or reduce the long-term adverse consequences. Providing parents with the tools to support positive self-image and tools to create health home environments may help contradict personal or medial influences that lead to eating disorders. Additionally, media literacy on the societal drive for thinness and overall nutrition education may help. Box 18.4 outlines the early signs of AN.

SUBSTANCE ABUSE

Although experimentation with drugs during childhood and adolescence is widespread, most children and teens do not become high-risk users. There has been a reduction in the use of illicit drugs by young people in Australia and New Zealand in the last 2 years, but unfortunately both countries have seen a rise in the risk-taking behaviour of consuming on average more than four standard drinks on one occasion (AIHW 2020b, Ministry of Health 2016).

Motivation

Most drug use begins with experimentation. The drug may be used only once, may be used occasionally or may become part of a drug-centred lifestyle. Children and adolescents initiate drug use out of curiosity. Adolescents who use drugs may fall into one of two broad categories—experimenters and compulsive users—or they may fall into a third category somewhere on the continuum between these extremes, referred to as *recreational users*, principally of drugs such as marijuana, cocaine, alcohol and prescription drugs.

Types of Drugs Abused

Any drug can be abused, and most are potentially harmful to adolescents still going through formative life experiences. Drugs with mind-altering abilities that are available on the 'street' and are of medical and

BOX 18.4 Early Signs of Anorexia Nervosa

The adolescent:

- consumes an inappropriate diet (excessively strict) or may refuse to eat altogether
- develops peculiar eating habits such as toying with food, performing food 'rituals', preparing and forcing food on family members without eating any themself
- denies hunger even after eating very little/almost nothing for days or even weeks
- engages in excessive exercise, such as compulsive jogging, running up and down stairs, rigorous calisthenics to burn off calories—often to the point of exhaustion
- takes laxatives, diuretics or enemas to speed intestinal transit time, to lose added weight and to empty intestines
- vomits deliberately; may go to bathroom after a meal and turn on taps to avoid being heard
- develops a distorted body image; states that they 'feels fat' as they become increasingly thin
- loses weight; fails to achieve the 25th percentile on normal growth curves or jumps across several growth channels on the curve
- withdraws from social interaction; starts to spend time in room studying, exercising or otherwise occupied
- displays personality traits such as perfectionism or obsessive-compulsive disorder tendencies.

legal concern are the hallucinogenic, narcotic, hypnotic and stimulant drugs. In addition, healthcare professionals are concerned about the use of alcohol and volatile substances that are inhaled to achieve altered sensation (e.g. petrol, antifreeze, plastic model aeroplane cement, organic solvents). Cough and cold preparations are common substances abused by adolescents and young adults. Many of the medications are often found in the medicine or kitchen cabinet at home and are available at a decreased cost compared with the more exotic drugs of abuse. The abuse of prescription and synthetic drugs such as opioids, benzodiazepines such as Xanax, and stimulants is increasing among adolescents and young people (Stager 2016). Websites also promote the 'safe use' of some psychoactive drugs and supply information on new 'designer' drugs that are not detectable on a standard urine drug screening test.

Tobacco

According to data from ASSAD, in 2017, 2.2% of secondary school students aged 12 to 14 years were current smokers, and rates were similar for boys (2.6%) and girls (1.8%). Smoking was more common among 14 year olds (3.6%) than 12 year olds (1.5%) (Guerin & White 2020). The proportion of students aged 12 to 14 years who were current smokers and lived in areas of greater socioeconomic disadvantage (lowest socioeconomic areas) was higher than the proportion who lived in areas of least disadvantage (highest areas) (2.9% and 1.4%, respectively). However, the difference was not statistically significant (AIWH 2020b, Ministry of Health 2016).

Cigarette smoking is still considered a chief avoidable cause of death. The hazards of smoking at any age are undisputed; however, a preventive approach to teenage smoking is especially important. Because of its addictive nature, smoking begun in childhood and adolescence can result in a lifetime habit, with increased morbidity and early mortality.

The increased popularity of electronic cigarettes has reached into Years 7 to 10 (13 to 16 years of age); high school students and e-cigarettes are the most commonly used tobacco product among 13- to 16-year-old secondary school students (AIHW 2020b, Singh et al 2016). There is concern that these products are used to promote smoking cessation, yet there is no evidence to support this claim. In fact, a recent study found that 98.7% of flavoured e-cigarette products and 99.4% of non-flavoured e-cigarette products contained nicotine (Marynak et al 2017).

Children living in areas of greatest socioeconomic disadvantage (4.4%) were more likely exposed to second-hand smoke than those in areas of least disadvantage (0.8%). There was no statistically significant difference across remoteness areas for exposure to second-hand smoke in the home (AIHW 2020b, Ministry of Health 2016).

Aetiology

Adolescents begin smoking for a variety of reasons, including: imitation of adult behaviour; peer pressure; a desire to imitate behaviours and lifestyles; and a desire to control weight, especially among young women. Adolescents who do not smoke usually have family members and friends who do not smoke or who oppose smoking. Most teens who refrain from smoking have a desire to succeed in academics or athletics.

Nursing Care Management

Prevention of regular smoking in adolescents is the most effective way to reduce the overall incidence of smoking. A variety of methods have been used. Posters, charts, displays, statistics and the use of examples of actual damaged lungs to communicate the hazards of smoking all have their supporters and doubters.

For the most part, smoking prevention programs that focus on the negative, long-term effects of smoking on health have been ineffective.

Alcohol

In 2017, 6.8% of secondary school students aged 12 to 14 had at least one drink on a single occasion in the last week and rates were similar for boys and girls (Guerin & White 2020). Drinking was more common among 14 year olds (10.4%) compared with 12 year olds (4.2%) (AIHW 2020b, Ministry of Health 2016).

In 2017, around 1% of secondary school students aged 12 to 14 years engaged in single occasion risky drinking (i.e. drank five or more standard drinks on one occasion in the past week), putting them at risk of injury. There was no statistically significant difference between rates of risky drinking in boys (1.2%) and girls (0.8%). Drinking at this level was again more common among 14 year olds (1.9%) compared with 12 year olds (0.2%) (AIHW 2020b, Ministry of Health 2016).

Severe physical and psychological symptoms accompany abrupt withdrawal, and long-term use leads to slow tissue destruction, especially of the brain and liver cells. The most noticeable effects of alcohol occur within the central nervous system and include changes in cognitive and autonomic functions such as judgment, memory, learning ability and other intellectual capacities. Young people with alcoholism often drink alone and cannot control their use of alcohol. They often rely on the substance as a defence against depression, anxiety, fear or anger.

Cocaine

Although cocaine is not pharmacologically considered a narcotic, it is legally categorised as such. Cocaine is available in two forms: water-soluble cocaine hydrochloride, which is administered by 'snorting' or intravenous injection, and non-soluble alkaloid (freebase) cocaine, which is used primarily for smoking. Crack, or 'rock', is a purer, more menacing form of the drug. It can be produced cheaply and smoked in either water pipes or mentholated cigarettes.

Narcotics

Narcotic drugs include opiates, such as heroin and morphine, and opioids (opiate-like drugs), such as hydromorphone, hydrocodone, fentanyl and codeine. These drugs produce a state of euphoria by removing painful feelings and creating a pleasurable experience and a sense of success accompanied by clouding of the consciousness and a dreamlike state. Physical signs of narcotic abuse include constricted pupils, respiratory depression and, often, cyanosis. Needle marks may be visible on the arms or legs in chronic users. Physical withdrawal from opiates is extremely unpleasant unless controlled with supervised tapering doses of the opioid or substitution of methadone.

Central Nervous System Depressants

Central nervous system depressants include a variety of hypnotic drugs that produce physical dependence and withdrawal symptoms on abrupt discontinuation. They create a feeling of relaxation and sleepiness but impair general functioning. Drugs in this category include barbiturates, non-barbiturates and alcohol. Barbiturates combined with alcohol produce a profound depressant effect. Flunitrazepam (Rohypnol), known as the 'date rape drug', is a hypnotic drug abused by adolescents. Many women and men report being raped after unknowingly being given Rohypnol in a drink. Rohypnol is 10 times more powerful than diazepam (Valium). It produces prolonged sedation, a feeling of wellbeing and short-term memory loss.

Central Nervous System Stimulants

Amphetamines and cocaine do not produce strong physical dependence and can be withdrawn without much danger. However, psychological dependence is strong, and acute intoxication can lead to violent aggressive behaviour or psychotic episodes characterised by paranoia, uncontrollable agitation and restlessness. When combined with barbiturates, the euphoric effects are particularly addictive.

Methamphetamine can be snorted, injected, swallowed or smoked and produces a burst of energy in its users, along with intense, alternating attacks of boldness and paranoia. It provokes excitement far more intense than that caused by cocaine. The drug, with the street names *crank, meth* and *crystal,* is inexpensive and has a longer period of action than cocaine. Instead of a short (few minutes) high, as achieved with cocaine, a user can remain 'up' for hours on a similar dose of crank.

Mind-altering Drugs

Hallucinogens (psychedelics, psychotomimetics, psychotropics or illusionogenics) are drugs that produce vivid hallucinations and euphoria. These drugs do not produce physical dependence, and they can be abruptly withdrawn without ill effect. However, the acute and long-term effects are variable, and in some individuals the dissociative behaviour may be prolonged. Cannabis (marijuana, hashish) and lysergic acid diethylamide (LSD) are also included in this category of drugs.

Nursing Care Management

Nurses who have contact with children and adolescents are in an excellent position to provide information about substance abuse and to serve as patient advocates. Nurses most often encounter young substance abusers when they are: (1) experiencing overdose or withdrawal symptoms; (2) manifesting bizarre behaviour or confusion secondary to drug ingestion; (3) worried that they are or will become addicted; or (4) worried about a friend or family member who is addicted.

SELF-HARM

Self-harm is defined as a direct and intentional damage to one's body without the intent to die (Doyle et al 2017, Stanford et al 2016, Zubrick et al 2016). It is also referred to as *self-injury* and *self-mutilation.* This definition excludes indirect self-injury behaviours such as eating disorders or drug abuse and excludes socially accepted behaviours such as tattooing and piercing (Brown & Plener 2017). The most common methods of self-harm are listed in Box 18.5.

The prevalence of self-harm among adolescents ranges from 1.5% to 65.9%; the wide range of frequencies is due to inconsistencies among researchers on how self-harm is defined, how self-harm is measured and how age is defined among adolescents (Chan et al 2018, Thabrew et al 2018, Zubrick et al 2016). Self-harm peaks at 15 to 16 years of age and starts to decline by 18 years of age. Self-harm is more prominent in females, among individuals with sexual orientation confusion and among individuals with a history of physical or sexual abuse. Factors associated with self-harm include a suicide attempt or self-harm among a friend or family member, fighting with parents or friends, and being bullied at school (Chan et al 2018, Thabrew et al 2018, Zubrick et al 2016).

BOX 18.5 Types of Self-harm Behaviours

- Cutting
- Poisoning
- Strangulation
- Branding
- Scratching or scraping
- Hitting or banging
- Pulling hair or skin
- Biting
- Burning

Aetiology

Adolescents engage in self-harm to get relief from life stressors or abate emotions such as anger, frustration or depression. Inflicting physical pain in the form of self-harm provides distraction from stress and feelings. Adolescents also experience euphoria when self-harming. Endorphins are released when the body is injured, resulting in a pleasurable sensation. Self-harming behaviours can become addictive.

Because the hypothalamic–pituitary–adrenocortical (HPA) axis is involved in stressful situations, it has been suggested that individuals who self-harm have an altered HPA axis (Brown & Plener 2017, Thabrew et al 2018). More research is needed with this association.

Diagnostic Evaluation

Most adolescents who self-harm do not seek treatment because they feel the incident is not serious enough to require help, they do not want any help or they do not want others to know about their behaviour (Thabrew et al 2018). Adolescents who do seek help primarily go to a friend or family member; thus, most self-harm actions are not discussed with healthcare professionals. Nurses must be aware of the potential for self-harm among adolescents and educate family and friends about warning signs. These signs include the following:

- multiple cuts/burns on arms, legs, hips or stomach
- wearing baggy clothes or long sleeves/pants to conceal wounds
- finding razors, scissors, lighters or knives hidden in the adolescent's room
- spending long periods of time in a locked bedroom or bathroom, especially after conflicts with friends or family

Therapeutic Management

No specific treatment effectively eliminates self-harm behaviours. Adolescents are referred to mental health professionals to confront negative thinking, assist with mood management and encourage healthy activities to manage stress. The most effective treatment includes family therapy with goals to improve communication, teach conflict-resolution and problem-solving skills, and foster positive relationships.

SUICIDE

Suicide is defined as the deliberate act of self-injury with the intent that the injury results in death. Most experts distinguish among suicidal ideation, suicide attempt (or parasuicide) and suicide.

Suicidal ideation involves a preoccupation with thoughts about committing suicide and may be a precursor to suicide. Although it is common for adolescents to experience occasional suicidal thoughts, expressions of preoccupation with suicide should be taken seriously and an assessment should be conducted for appropriate referral. A **suicide attempt** is intended to cause injury or death. The term *parasuicide* is used to refer to behaviours ranging from gestures to serious attempts to kill oneself. *Parasuicide* is a preferred term because it makes no reference to intent and because a person's motive may be too difficult or complex to determine. However, all parasuicidal activity should be taken seriously.

All nurses should follow through with a referral to the most appropriate service for the child or adolescent in their community or via telehealth as soon as possible. The referral will need to take into consideration cultural needs and the means the child/adolescent's family has to attend the appointment. Many services have waiting lists; therefore, information in relation to phone support services should be provided, contact made with the family doctor if possible for support and any other relevant support services available to the child/adolescent and family within their community for support.

NURSING CARE CONSIDERATIONS

A history of a previous suicide attempt is a serious indicator for possible suicide completion in the future. Studies of adolescent suicides have found that as many as half of the adolescents had made previous attempts.

Aetiology

Individual, family and social or environmental factors have all been implicated in suicide. The single most important individual factor is the presence of an active psychiatric disorder (e.g. depression, bipolar disorder, psychosis, substance abuse or conduct disorder). Alcohol use in particular has been associated with more than 50% of suicides (Thompson & Swartout 2018, Thabrew et al 2018, Chan et al 2018).

Family factors influencing suicide include: parental loss; family disruption; a family history of suicide, depression, substance abuse or emotional disturbance; child abuse or neglect; unavailable parents; poor communication and isolation within the family; family conflict; and unrealistically high parental expectations or parental indifference with low expectations.

Methods

Firearms are by far the most commonly used instruments in completed suicides among adolescent males, whereas cutting or piercing is the most common method among females (Chan et al 2018, Clapperton 2019, Heerde et al 2015, Matthews et al 2016). For adolescent males, the other common means of suicide are cutting/piercing, jumping and hanging/suffocating; for females, the other common means are jumping, hanging/suffocating and firearms.

The most common method of suicide *attempt* is overdose or ingestion of a potentially toxic substance, such as drugs. The second most common method of suicide attempt is self-inflicted laceration.

NURSING CARE CONSIDERATIONS

Given what is known about youth suicide, nurses should ask parents, especially those with at-risk adolescents, if firearms are available in the house and, if so, recommend their removal. Parents must ensure that their children—especially those who are depressed, have poor problem-solving skills or use drugs or alcohol—do not have access to firearms. Parents must also be educated on the warning signs of suicide (Box 18.6).

Motivation

Suicidal ideation is common in adolescents. It represents numerous fantasies, such as relief from suffering, a means of gaining comfort and sympathy, or a means of revenge against those who have hurt them. Adolescents have the erroneous perception that the act of suicide will evoke remorse and pity and that they will be able to return and witness the grief. Angry children or adolescents who are unable to directly punish those who have injured or insulted them may take revenge on those who love them through self-destruction ('They'll be sorry when they find me dead'; 'They'll be sorry they were mean to me').

For adolescents who are severely depressed, suicide seems to be the only release from their despair. These adolescents rarely provide evidence of their intent and frequently conceal their suicidal thoughts. Many adolescents, however, tell their peers of their suicidal thoughts or plans but avoid telling adults. Social isolation is a significant factor in distinguishing adolescents who will kill themselves from those who will not. It is also more characteristic of those who complete suicide than of those who make attempts or threats (Clapperton 2019).

BOX 18.6 Warning Signs of Suicide

- Preoccupation with themes of death—focuses on morbid thoughts
- Wants to give away cherished possessions
- Talks of own death, desire to die
- Loss of energy, loss of interest, listlessness
- Exhaustion without obvious cause
- Changes in sleep patterns—too much or too little
- Increased irritability, argumentativeness or stubbornness
- Physical complaints—recurrent stomach-aches, headaches
- Repeated visits to medical practitioner, nurse practitioner or emergency department for treatment of injuries
- Reckless behaviour
- Antisocial behaviour—engages in drinking, uses drugs, fights, commits acts of vandalism, runs away from home, becomes sexually promiscuous
- Sudden change in school performance—lowered marks, cutting classes, dropping out of activities
- Resists or refuses to go to school
- Remains distant, sad, remote—flat affect, frozen facial expression
- Describes self as worthless
- Sudden cheerfulness after deep depression
- Social withdrawal from friends, activities, interests that were previously enjoyed
- Impaired concentration
- Dramatic change in appetite

Therapeutic Management

Threats of suicide should always be taken seriously. There has been a tendency to dismiss suicide attempts as impulsive acts resulting from temporary crises or depression. If a suicide attempt fails to draw attention to their problems or makes them worse, the child or adolescent may conclude that suicide is the only answer. Children and adolescents need to know that someone cares and must be provided with swift and efficient crisis intervention. Although ordinary practitioners can manage an acute depressive reaction without difficulty, the adolescent who has made a serious attempt or has a specific plan for suicide should receive immediate attention and competent psychiatric care.

Nursing Care Management

Nurses play a pivotal role in reducing adolescent suicide. Nurses have the opportunity to provide anticipatory guidance to parents and adolescents. They can teach parents to be supportive and to develop positive communication patterns that help teens feel connected with and loved by their families. To foster healthy development, parents can be encouraged to provide teens with creative outlets and to assist young people in accepting strong emotions—pain, anger and frustration—as a normal part of the human experience.

Care of suicidal adolescents includes early recognition, management and prevention. The most important aspect of management is the recognition of warning signs that indicate that an adolescent is troubled and might attempt suicide. The nurse must take any suicidal remarks seriously and not leave the young person alone until the degree of suicidality is assessed.

Healthcare professionals must be alert to the signs of depression, and anyone who exhibits such behaviour should be referred for thorough psychological assessment. Depression is manifested differently in children and adolescents than in adults. In teens, it may be masked by impulsive aggressive behaviours. Defiance, disobedience, behaviour problems and psychosomatic disturbances can indicate underlying depression, suicidal ideation and impending suicide attempts.

Peers and other confidants are valuable observers and excellent sources of information about potential suicide attempts. They may not be able to diagnose depression, but they are able to sense when a friend has undergone a marked personality change. It is important to emphasise that the peer who detects any changes in a friend is a potential rescuer and should not remain silent about the observations. Friendship does not imply collusion. A peer who believes that a friend may be suicidal should alert someone who can help (e.g. a parent, teacher, guidance counsellor).

Routine health assessments of adolescents should include questions that assess the presence of suicidal ideation or intent. The following questions can be asked (Clapperton 2019).

1. Do you consider yourself a happy person, an unhappy person or somewhere in the middle?
2. Have you ever been so unhappy or upset that you felt like being dead?
3. Have you ever thought about hurting yourself?
4. Have you ever developed a plan to hurt yourself or kill yourself?
5. Have you ever attempted to kill yourself?

If adolescents answer 'yes' to questions 2, 3 or 4, they should be asked if they feel that way now to assess for current suicidality. If teens say they have attempted suicide in the past, assess the number of times and ask them to describe what they were feeling, which method they used, what happened, if they would make a similar attempt and how they would handle their despair now. Any previous suicide attempt indicates an increased risk for a future attempt. The risk for a suicide attempt in the near future increases as the frequency of suicidal ideation increases. For any expression of suicidal intent, the child or adolescent should receive immediate attention and competent psychiatric care.

Relevant mental health contacts for Australia and New Zealand are listed in Box 18.7.

BOX 18.7 Mental Health Services in Australia and New Zealand

Australia

Lifeline: 13 11 14
Kids Helpline Phone Counselling Service: 1800 55 1800
Beyond Blue: 1300 22 4636

New Zealand

Safe Talk NZ: 0800 044334 (24/7 helpline); webchat at www.safetotalk.nz
Youth Helpline: 0800 787 984
Māori Helpline: 0800 787 798
Pacific Helpline: 0800 787 799; 0800 What's Up: online counsellors available 3.00 pm to 10.00 pm, 7 days a week; www.whatsup.co.nz
Youth Line: 0800 376 633; free text 234; talk@youthline.co.nz
Lifeline (including Suicide Crisis Helpline Tautoko and Kidsline): 0800 LIFELINE (0800 54 33 54); free text HELP (4357)
0508 Tautoko (0508 82 88 65); Kidsline: 0800 54 37 54

REFERENCES

Akgul, S., & Kanbur, N. (2015). Premenstrual disorder and the adolescent: Clinical case report, literature review, and diagnostic and therapeutic challenges. International Journal of Adolescent Medicine and Health, 27(4), 363–368.

Amjad, S., MacDonald, I., Chambers, T., et al. (2019). Social determinants of health and adverse maternal and birth outcomes in adolescent pregnancies: A systematic review and meta-analysis. Paediatric and Perinatal Epidemiology, 33(1), 88–99.

Armstrong, W. R., Grimsby, G. M., & Jacobs, M. A. (2015). Pediatric priapism secondary to psychotherapeutic medications. Urology, 86(2), 376–378.

Australian Human Rights Commission (AHRC). (2019). Annual Report 2018-2019. The year in review. https://humanrights.gov.au/our-work/commission-general/publications/annual-report-2018-2019

Australian Institute of Health and Welfare (AIHW). (2011). Young Australians: their health and wellbeing 2011. Cat. no. PHE 140 Canberra: AIHW. https://www.aihw.gov.au/getmedia/14eed34e-2e0f-441d-88cb-ef376196f587/12750.pdf.aspx?inline=true

Australian Institute of Health and Welfare (AIHW). (2020a). Health of young people. Sexual and reproductive health. 23 July. https://www.aihw.gov.au/reports/australias-health/health-of-young-people

Australian Institute of Health and Welfare (AIHW). (2020b). Alcohol, tobacco & other drugs in Australia. Younger people. Key findings. 15 December. https://www.aihw.gov.au/reports/alcohol/alcohol-tobacco-other-drugs-australia/contents/priority-populations/younger-people

Australian Institute of Health and Welfare (AIHW). (2021). Health status: Health conditions. Incidence of sexually transmissible infections and blood-borne viruses. https://www.aihw.gov.au/reports-data/australias-health-performance/australias-health-performance-framework/national/all-australia/conditions/health-conditions/3_1_3

Berends, T., van Meijel, B., Nugteren, W., et al. (2016). Rate, timing and predictors of relapse in patients with anorexia nervosa following a relapse prevention program: A cohort study. BMC Psychiatry, 16(1), 316.

Berz, K., & McCambridge, T. (2016). Amenorrhea in the female athlete: What to do and when to worry. Pediatric Annals, 45(3), e97–e102.

Beukers, L., Berends, T., de Man–van Ginkel, J. M., et al. (2015). Restoring normal eating behaviour in adolescents with anorexia nervosa: A video analysis of nursing interventions. International Journal of Mental Health Nursing, 24(6), 519–526.

Bradshaw, C. S., & Sobel, J. D. (2016). Current treatment of bacterial vaginosis–limitations and need for innovation. The Journal of Infectious Diseases, 214(Suppl. 1), S14–S20.

Brown, R. C., & Plener, P. L. (2017). Non-suicidal self-injury in adolescence. Current Psychiatry Reports, 19(3), 20.

Campbell, K., & Peebles, R. (2014). Eating disorders in children and adolescents: State of the art review. Pediatrics, 134(3), 582–592.

Chahal, A., Gupta, S., & Das, C. (2016). Penile fracture. BMJ Case Reports, 2016.

Chan, S., Denny, S., Fleming, T., et al. (2018). Exposure to suicide behaviour and individual risk of self-harm: Findings from a nationally representative New Zealand High School Survey. SAGE Publications. Australian and New Zealand Journal of Psychiatry, 52(4), 349–356.

Clapperton, A. (2019). Identifying typologies among persons admitted to hospital for non-fatal intentional self-harm in Victoria, Australia. Springer Berlin Heidelberg. Social Psychiatry and Psychiatric Epidemiology, 54(12), 1497–1504.

Craner, J. R., Sigmon, S. T., Martinson, A. A., et al. (2014). Premenstrual disorders and rumination. Journal of Clinical Psychology, 70(1), 32–47.

Cristaudo, A. & Giuliani, M. (2020). Sexually Transmitted Infections Advances in Understanding and Management. Champaign, IL: Springer International Publishing.

Das, B. B., Ronda, J., & Trent, M. (2016). Pelvic inflammatory disease: Improving awareness, prevention and treatment. Infection and Drug Resistance, 9, 191–197.

Deligeoroglou, E., Karountzos, V., & Creatsas, G. (2013). Abnormal uterine bleeding and dysfunctional uterine bleeding in pediatric and adolescent gynecology. Gynecological Endocrinology, 29(1), 74–78.

Diorio, G. J., & Giuliano, A. R. (2016). The role of human papilloma virus in penile carcinogenesis and preneoplastic lesions: A potential target for vaccinations and treatment strategies. The Urologic Clinics of North America, 43(4), 419–425.

Doyle, L., Sheridan, A., & Treacy, M. P. (2017). Motivations for adolescent self-harm and the implications for mental health nurses. Journal of Psychiatric and Mental Health Nursing, 24(2–3), 124–142.

Dunford, A., Rampal, D., Kielly, M., et al. (2019). Vulval Pain in Pediatric and Adolescent Patients. Journal of Pediatric and Adolescent Gynecology, 32(4), 359–362. https://doi.org/10.1016/j.jpag.2019.03.005

Elder, J. S. (2016). Disorders and anomalies of the scrotal contents. In R. M. Kliegman, B. F. Stanton, J. W. St Geme, et al. (Eds.), Nelson textbook of pediatrics (20th ed.). Philadelphia: Saunders/Elsevier.

Fichter, M. M., & Quadflieq, N. (2016). Mortality in eating disorders – results of a large prospective clinical longitudinal study. The International Journal of Eating Disorders, 49(4), 391–401.

Ford, O., Lethaby, A., Roberts, H., et al. (2012). Progesterone for premenstrual syndrome. Cochrane Database of Systematic Review, (3), CD003415.

Garcia-Roig, M. L., & Kirsch, A. J. (2015). The dilemma of adolescent varicocele. Pediatric Surgery International, 31(7), 617–625.

Gibson, E. J., Bell, D. L., & Powerful, S. A. (2014). Common sexually transmitted infections in adolescents. Primary Care, 41(3), 631–650.

Guerin, N. & White, V. (2020). ASSAD 2017 Statistics & Trends: Australian Secondary Students' Use of Tobacco, Alcohol, Over-the-counter Drugs, and Illicit Substances. 2nd ed. Cancer Council Victoria. https://www.health.gov.au/sites/default/files/documents/2020/07/secondary-school-students-use-of-tobacco-alcohol-and-other-drugs-in-2017.pdf

Harrington, B. C., Jimerson, M., Haxton, C., et al. (2015). Initial evaluation, diagnosis, and treatment of anorexia nervosa and bulimia nervosa. American Family Physician, 91(1), 46–52.

Heerde, J., Toumbourou, J., Hemphill, S.A., et al. (2015). Incidence and Course of Adolescent Deliberate Self-Harm in Victoria, Australia, and Washington State. Elsevier Inc. Journal of Adolescent Health, 57(5), 537–544.

Herpertz-Dahlmann, B. (2015). Adolescent eating disorders: Update on definitions, symptomatology, epidemiology, and comorbidity. Child & Adolescent Psychiatric Clinics of North America, 24(1), 177–196.

Ratten, L., Plummer, E., Murray, G., et al. (2021). Sex is associated with the persistence of non-optimal vaginal microbiota following treatment for bacterial vaginosis: a prospective cohort study. BJOG: An International Journal of Obstetrics and Gynaecology, 128(4), 756–767.

Hilbert, D. W., Smith, W. L., Chadwick, S. G., et al. (2016). Development and validation of a highly accurate quantitative real-time assay for diagnosis of bacterial vaginosis. Journal Clinical Microbiology, 54(4), 1017–1024.

Kang, M., Rochford, A., Skinner, S., et al. (2014). Sexual behaviour, sexually transmitted infections and attitudes to chlamydia testing among a unique national sample of young Australians: baseline data from a randomised controlled trial. BMC Public Health, 14(1), 12.

Kawakita, T., Wilson, K., Grantz, K. L., et al. (2016). Adverse maternal and neonatal outcomes in adolescent pregnancy. Journal of Pediatric and Adolescent Gynecology, 29(2), 130–136.

Kreipe, R. E. (2016). Eating disorders. In R. M. Kliegman, B. F. Stanton, J. W. St Geme, et al. (Eds.), Nelson textbook of pediatrics (20th ed.). Philadelphia: Saunders/Elsevier.

Lau, C. C. (2016). The lives of young fathers: A review of selected evidence. Social Policy and Society: A Journal of the Social Policy Association, 15(1), 129–140.

Marynak, K. L., Gammon, D. G., Rogers, T., et al. (2017). Sales of nicotine-containing electronic cigarette products: United States, 2015. American Journal of Public Health, 107(5), 702–705.

Matthews, E. M., Woodward, C. J., Musso, M. W., et al. (2016). Suicide attempts presenting to trauma centers: Trends across groups using the national trauma data bank. The American Journal of Emergency Medicine, 34(8), 1620–1624.

McConaghy, J. R., & Panchal, B. (2016). Epididymitis: An overview. American Family Physician, 94(9), 723–726.

Mendling, W., Weissenbacher, E.R., Gerber, S., et al. (2016). Use of locally delivered dequalinium chloride in the treatment of vaginal infections: A review. Archives of Gynecology and Obstetrics, 293(3), 469–484.

Ministry of Health. (2016). Research Report: The New Zealand Drug Harm Index 2016 (2nd ed.). 7 April. https://www.health.govt.nz/publication/research-report-new-zealand-drug-harm-index-2016

Ministry of Health. (2017). Your health. Questions and answers about HPV immunisation. New Zealand Government. https://www.health.govt.nz/your-health/healthy-living/immunisation/immunisation-older-children/human-papillomavirus-hpv/questions-and-answers-about-hpv-immunisation

Pohlman, G. D., Phillips, J. M., & Wilcox, D. T. (2013). Simple method of paraphimosis reduction revisited: Point of technique and review of the literature. Journal of Pediatric Urology, 9(1), 104–107.

Rani, A., Sharma, M. K., & Singh, A. (2016). Practices and perceptions of adolescent girls regarding the impact of dysmenorrhea on their routine life. International Journal of Adolescent Medicine and Health, 28(1), 3–9.

Sauerbrei, A. (2016). Optimal management of genital herpes: Current perspectives. Infection and Drug Resistance, 9, 129–141.

Sapra, K. J., Joseph, K. S., Galea, S., et al. (2017). Signs and symptoms of early pregnancy loss. Reproductive Sciences, 24(4), 502–513.

Singh, T., Arrazola, R. A., & Corey, C. G. (2016). Tobacco use among middle and high school students—United States, 2011–2015. Morbidity and Mortality Weekly Report, 65(14), 361–367.

Smith, L., & Angarone, M. P. (2015). Sexually transmitted infections. The Urologic Clinics of North America, 42(4), 507–518.

Sobel, J. D. (2016). Recurrent vulvovaginal candidiasis. American Journal of Obstetrics and Gynecology, 214(1), 15–21.

Spain, J., & Rheinboldt, M. (2017). MDCT of pelvic inflammatory disease: A review of the pathophysiology, gamut of imaging findings, and treatment. Emergency Radiology, 24(1), 87–93.

Stager, M. M. (2016). Substance abuse. In R. M. Kliegman, B. F. Stanton, J. W. St Geme, et al. (Eds.), Nelson textbook of pediatrics (20th ed.). Philadelphia: Saunders/Elsevier.

Stanford, S., Jones, M. P. & Hudson, J. (2016). Rethinking pathology in adolescent self-harm: Towards a more complex understanding of risk factors. Journal of Adolescence (London, England.), 54, 32–41.

Sucato, G. S., & Burstein, G. R. (2016). Menstrual problems. In R. M. Kliegman, B. F. Stanton, J. W. St Geme, et al. (Eds.), Nelson textbook of pediatrics (20th ed.). Philadelphia: Saunders/Elsevier.

Thabrew, H., Gandeza, E., Bahr, G., et al. (2018). The management of young people who self-harm by New Zealand Infant, Child and Adolescent Mental Health Services: cutting-edge or cutting corners? SAGE Publications. Australasian psychiatry: bulletin of the Royal Australian and New Zealand College of Psychiatrists, 26(2), 152–159.

The Butterfly Foundation. (2020a). Eating Disorders: Mental health first aid guidelines. April. https://mhfa.com.au/sites/default/files/MHFA_eatdis_guidelines_A4_2013.pdf

The Butterfly Foundation. (2020b). Butterfly. Let's talk eating disorders: The reality of eating disorders in Australia. https://butterfly.org.au/wp-content/uploads/2020/12/The-reality-of-eating-disorders-in-Australia-2020.pdf

The Department of Health. (n.d.). Programs and Campaigns. Sexual and reproductive health. Sexually transmitted infections. https://www1.health.gov.au/internet/publications/publishing.nsf/Content/womens-health-policy-toc~womens-health-policy-four~womens-health-policy-four-sexual

The Royal Women's Hospital. (n.d.). Health information. Sexually Transmitted Infections. About STI's. https://www.thewomens.org.au/health-information/sex-sexuality/sexually-transmitted-infections/about-stis/

Thompson, M. P., & Swartout, K. (2018). Epidemiology of suicide attempts among youth transitioning to adulthood. Journal of Youth and Adolescence, 47(4), 807–817.

Ullman, S. E., & Peter-Hagene, L. C. (2016). Longitudinal relationships of social reactions, PTSD symptoms, and revictimization in sexual assault survivors. Journal of Interpersonal Violence, 31(6), 1074–1094.

Yu, A. (2014). Complementary and alternative treatments for primary dysmenorrhea in adolescents. The Nurse Practitioner, 39(11), 1–12.

Zubrick, S., Hafekost, J., Johnson, S., et al. (2016). Self-harm: Prevalence estimates from the second Australian Child and Adolescent Survey of Mental Health and Wellbeing. London, England: SAGE Publications. Australian and New Zealand Journal of Psychiatry, 50(9), 911–921.

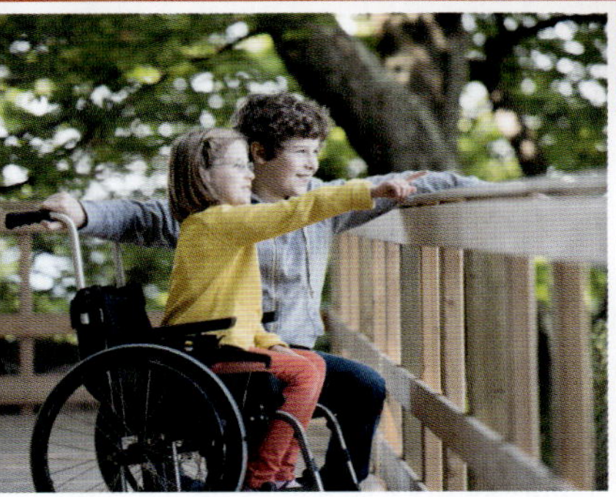

Impact of Chronic Illness, Disability or End-of-life Care for the Child and Family

Lisa Speedie

LEARNING OUTCOMES

- Discuss the concepts of care of a child with special needs
- Discuss the concepts of death and dying
- Describe how patient-centred care is provided to the child and family in death and dying
- Discuss child and parental needs in relation to disabilities, chronic illness and death and dying

PERSPECTIVES ON THE CARE OF CHILDREN AND FAMILIES LIVING WITH OR DYING FROM CHRONIC OR COMPLEX DISEASES

Scope of the Problem

Advances in medical and nursing care, such as the increasing viability of extremely preterm infants, the portability of life-sustaining technology (e.g. total parental nutrition, ventilator support) and life-extending treatments for children with conditions that previously would have led to an early death (e.g. malignancies, genetic conditions), have led to an exponential rise in the prevalence of children with complex and chronic diseases (Downing 2020). These children have complex conditions involving several organ systems and requiring multiple specialists, technological supports and community services to assist them to function to their healthiest potential. The complex and high level of skills required to meet their daily healthcare needs and the continuous nature and potential volatility of the condition sets this group apart from the broader population of children with special healthcare needs (Downing 2020, Yu et al 2019).

The nature and severity of childhood chronic and complex conditions is widely heterogeneous. Table 19.1 is a non-exhaustive sampling of conditions organised by specialty. However, these children and families are similar in the vulnerability that they experience due to the health and developmental consequences of these diagnoses on the child, such as ongoing functional impairment, neurodevelopmental disability, dependence on medical technology and the need for ongoing skilled, supportive care from healthcare providers and family members. Although many authors have described the rise in prevalence that has come about because of advances in medical care (Downing 2020, Yu et al 2019, Sercu et al 2018), accurate estimates of the numbers of affected families are not known. However, the impact of chronic and complex illness in children is wide ranging. The family experiences significant challenges necessitated by the child's care requirements (Downing 2020, Yu et al 2019, Sercu et al 2018). A child's activity level and developmental opportunities can be affected. Days can be lost from school. Children with complex chronic conditions may be at increased risk for behaviour or emotional problems. Parents may lose days from work, experience financial strain and be challenged both emotionally and physically as they cope with care of the child.

Siblings are also affected by having a 'different' brother or sister, and they may simultaneously feel guilt, anger or jealousy towards their ill sibling. Clinicians need to know that siblings of children with chronic illnesses are at risk for negative psychological effects (Hartling et al 2014). Parents need encouragement and assistance with understanding the reactions of siblings to having a chronically ill family member (e.g. behavioural regression, anxiety, withdrawal, apathy). Additionally, secondary losses (such as the ability to participate in extracurricular activities or social events) occur because of routines imposed by the affected child's chronic condition. Chronic conditions can often be complex and expensive and take a psychological, social and economic toll on children affected and their families. The management of chronic conditions can interrupt a child's normal development and the risk of long-term vulnerabilities increase as the complexities increase (Hiscock et al 2020, Australian Institute of Health and Welfare [AIHW] 2020). Health professionals play a key role in the management of these chronic conditions and management of how they impact on growth and development.

In 2017–2018 around 43% of children in Australia had at least one long-term condition. Up to 20% had two or more long-term complex conditions. Of these children boys were more likely to have one long-term condition than girls in Australia (46% compared to 39%) (AIHW 2020). The overall picture for Māori children and young people with chronic conditions and disabilities was much more mixed. For complex conditions such as intellectual disabilities, epilepsy, non-insulin–dependent diabetes, rates for Māori children and young people were significantly higher than for non-Māori non-Pacific children and young people. Whereas conditions such as rheumatic fever and bronchiectasis for Māori children and young people far exceed those for non-Māori and non-Pacific children and young people (acute

TABLE 19.1 Chronic Conditions of Childhood

Specialty	Examples of Chronic Conditions
Cardiology	Complex congenital heart disease, congestive heart failure, cardiac dysrhythmias, Kawasaki disease, rheumatic fever, hyperlipidaemia
Endocrinology	Diabetes, congenital adrenal hyperplasia, Cushing's syndrome
Gastroenterology	Short bowel syndrome, biliary atresia, inflammatory bowel disease, hepatitis, cirrhosis, peptic ulcer disease, coeliac disease
Haematology	Sickle cell anaemia, thalassaemia, aplastic anaemia, hereditary anaemias, haemophilia
Immunology	Immune deficiency, human immunodeficiency virus, Wiskott-Aldrich syndrome, severe combined immunodeficiency disease
Nephrology	Prune belly syndrome, renal disease
Neurology	Cerebral palsy, ataxia-telangiectasia, muscular dystrophy, seizure disorder, spina bifida, traumatic brain injury
Oncology	Brain tumour, leukaemia, lymphoma, solid tumours, bone tumours, rare tumours
Pulmonology	Asthma, chronic lung disease, cystic fibrosis, tuberculosis
Rheumatology	Systemic lupus erythematosus, juvenile rheumatoid arthritis, dermatomyositis

rheumatic fever 23.0 times higher; bronchiectasis 5.4 times higher) (Craig et al 2012).

In 2006, 14% of children living in households had a disability (condition) and nearly one-third of these children were Māori. At the same time, 14% (28,000) of Māori children aged 0–14 years were reported to have a disability; 49% were reported to have more than one type of disability (condition). In this age group, 17% of Māori boys and 12% of Māori girls were disabled, compared to 11% and 8% of non-Māori, respectively (Craig et al 2012).

Trends in Care

Family-centred Care

Children's physical and emotional health, as well as their cognitive and social functioning, is strongly influenced by how well their families function (Xafis et al 2015, Leemann et al 2020). The importance of family-centred care—a philosophy that considers the family as the constant in the child's life—is especially evident in the care of children with special needs (see also Family-Centred Care, Chapter 1). As parents learn about the child's healthcare needs, they often become experts in delivering care. Healthcare providers, including nurses, are adjuncts to the child's care and need to form partnerships with parents. Effective communication and negotiation between parents and nurses are essential to forming trusting and effective partnerships and finding the best ways to meet the needs of the child and family. Collaborative relationships are characterised by communication, dialogue, active listening, awareness and acceptance of others' differences (Leemann et al 2020).

Family Healthcare Provider Communication

The disclosure of a serious chronic or complex condition of a child is one of the most stressful aspects of communication between families and healthcare professionals. Often, parents have suspected for some time that something is wrong with their child and believe that their concerns were minimised or ignored by healthcare professionals (Leemann et al 2020). After a diagnosis is made, factors that influence parent dissatisfaction with the way in which information is communicated include disrespectful attitudes, breaking bad news in an insensitive manner, withholding information and changing a treatment course without preparing the child and family (Barnes et al 2012, Leemann et al 2020). Conversely, parents report satisfaction when they perceived healthcare providers to be available, demonstrate competence and engage the child and parent in care decision-making (Barnes et al 2012, Xafis et al 2015). Similar factors are important in communication of changes in the child's condition throughout the course of the illness.

Establishing Therapeutic Relationships

Another important aspect of family-centred care of children with chronic and complex conditions is establishing a therapeutic relationship with the child and family, which has been shown to predict improved health-related outcomes (Leemann et al 2020). Families, most often the mother, take on enormous responsibility in providing technical care and symptom management of their child's condition outside of the healthcare institution (Goudie et al 2014). To build successful therapeutic relationships with families, it is necessary for nurses to recognise parents' expertise with regards to their child's condition and needs.

The Role of Culture in Family-centred Care

Issues of culture, ethnicity and race affect access to services, utilisation and follow-through with referrals and recommendations (Leemann et al 2020, Toomey et al 2013). For some ethnic and minority populations, cultural understandings of illness, the structure of family life, social roles for individuals with disabilities and other factors related to the perception of children may differ from those of mainstream Australian and New Zealand culture.

Shared Decision-making

Shared decision-making among the child, family and healthcare team can result from open, honest, culturally sensitive communication and the establishment of a therapeutic relationship among the family and healthcare providers. In a shared decision-making model, the healthcare professionals provide honest, clear information regarding diagnosis, prognosis, treatment options and risk–benefit assessment. The patient and family then share information with the healthcare team regarding important family values, acceptable levels of discomfort or inconvenience and the ability to comply with treatments being recommended (Wiener et al 2013, Wyatt et al 2015). This process allows them to discuss all options in terms of the risks and benefits to the child and family, the prognosis or expected course of the illness and the impact on the family's resources (Box 19.1). Together, the parents and healthcare team can make decisions that are best for the family and child at the time the decision is made.

Normalisation

Normalisation refers to the efforts family members make to create a normal family life, their perceptions of the consequences of these efforts and the meanings they attribute to their management efforts (Leemann et al 2020). For chronically ill children, such efforts may include attending school, pursuing hobbies and recreational interests and achieving employment and a level of independence. For their families, it may entail adapting the family routine to accommodate the ill or disabled child's health and physical needs (Leemann et al 2020, Downing 2020).

BOX 19.1 Facilitating Shared Decision-Making

- Continually assess the impact of the child's illness and treatment on the family.
- Provide honest, accurate information regarding the trajectory of the disease, anticipated complications and prognostic information.
- Discuss what the family desires for the child's quality of life.
- Avoid personal opinion or judgment of the family's questions and decisions.
- Be aware of nurses' personal and cultural assumptions and the ways these assumptions impact communication, decision-making and judgment.

Home care represents the return to a system and set of priorities in which family values are as important in the care of a child with a chronic health problem as they are in the care of other children. Home care seeks to achieve goals that are consistent with the developmental model (Stein 1985).

THE FAMILY OF THE CHILD WITH A CHRONIC OR COMPLEX CONDITION

A major goal in working with the family of a child with chronic or complex illness is to support the family's coping and promote their optimal functioning throughout the child's life. Long-term, comprehensive care involves forming parent–professional partnerships that can support a family's adaptation across the trajectory of the illness to the many changes that may be necessary in day-to-day life, determine expectations of and for the child and provide a long-term perspective (Box 19.2).

Often the impact of a child's medical or developmental condition is first experienced as a crisis at the time of diagnosis, which may occur at birth, after a long period of diagnostic testing or immediately after a tragic injury. But the impact may also be felt before the diagnosis is made, when parents are aware that something is wrong with their child but before medical confirmation (Downing 2020, Yu et al 2019).

The diagnosis and initial discharge home are critical times for parents. Several factors can make this particularly difficult, including a long duration of uncertainty in the diagnostic process, negative perceptions of chronic illness, insufficient information and lack of mutual trust between parents and their child's healthcare team (Downing 2020, Yu et al 2019). Parental feelings of shock, helplessness, isolation, fear and depression are common. Throughout the first year, parents struggle to accept the child's diagnosis, care and uncertainty of the future (Barnes & Rowe 2013). Optimal support at the time of diagnosis and initial discharge home can be encouraged by providing explicit and uncomplicated information to parents in an empathic way (Barnes & Rowe 2013); assessing the family's daily routine, living conditions, background knowledge, skills and abilities and coping behaviours; and evaluating the family's understanding of the information. It is also necessary to reassess parents' needs for information and support on a routine basis (Barnes & Rowe 2013, Yu et al 2019).

BOX 19.2 Adaptive Tasks of Parents Having Children with Chronic Conditions

1. Accept the child's condition.
2. Manage the child's condition on a day-to-day basis.
3. Meet the child's normal developmental needs.
4. Meet the developmental needs of other family members.
5. Cope with ongoing stress and periodic crises.
6. Assist family members to manage their feelings.
7. Educate others about the child's condition.
8. Establish a support system.

Source: Canam C. (1993). Common adaptive tasks facing parents of children with chronic conditions. Journal of Advanced Nursing, 18, 46–53.

Impact of the Child's Chronic Illness

Each member in the family of a child with a chronic or complex illness is affected by the experience (Goudie et al 2014). The effects on the parents and their responses may be so intense that they directly influence the other members' reactions and the child's own coping.

Parents

In addition to the stress of grieving for the loss of hope for a perfect child, parents are affected by whether or not they receive positive feedback from interactions with their child. Many parents feel satisfaction and fulfilment from the parenting role. For others, parenting may be a series of unrewarding experiences that contribute to feelings of inadequacy and failure (Box 19.3). These responses may be most evident in parents who are responsible for the child's care.

Parental Roles. Parenting a child with a complex chronic condition requires attending to the routine aspects of parenting with the added responsibility of performing complex technical care, symptom management, advocating for their child and seeking and coordinating health and social services for their ill or disabled child. These added responsibilities must then be balanced with the needs of other family members, extended family and friends, and personal health and obligations to minimise consequences to the overall functioning of the family.

Often one parent or partner remains at home to manage existing family responsibilities while the other remains with the ill child. The partner who is not included in the caregiving activities may feel neglected because all of the attention is directed towards the child and be resentful that he or she is not sufficiently informed to be competent in the care. Without active participation in the child's care, the parent has little appreciation of the time and energy involved in performing these activities. When this partner does attempt to participate, the other parent may criticise the less skilful efforts. As a result, communication and support for each other may be adversely affected.

Parental Differences. Parents of a child with a complex condition often adjust and cope differently. One parent will often take on a

BOX 19.3 Anticipated Parental Stress Points

Diagnosis of the condition—Parents require considerable education while dealing with an emotional response.

Developmental milestones—Times that children normally achieve walking, talking and self-care are delayed or impossible for the child.

Start of schooling—Particularly stressful are situations in which appropriate schooling will not be in a regular class placement.

Reaching the ultimate attainment—Parents must handle situations such as realising that ambulation will be impossible or that the child will not learn to read.

Adolescence—Issues such as sexuality and independence become prominent.

Future placement—Decisions about placement must be made when the child becomes an adult or when the parents can no longer care for the child.

Death of the child—Parents need to make decisions about end-of-life choices for the child. They will need to anticipate the child may die before them. Parents will need to plan for the child's death and begin preparations.

primary caregiver role and are more likely to give up their employment to care for their children, often resulting in social isolation (Barnes & Rowe 2013). This parent often has the greatest need for social support and positive appraisal of the situation than the working parent.

Some working parents of children with disabilities struggle with issues that may be distinct from those of the caring parent. Leemann and colleagues (2020) gives the example that fathers may think that their role as protector is challenged because they do not know how to help and cannot protect their family from seemingly overwhelming problems. Within same-sex families, the same concerns may also be present and must be acknowledged and supported.

Single-parent Families. Single-parent families are of special concern. As the only parent of a child who may require extensive, sophisticated and lifelong care, the single parent may feel an enormous burden. Available financial and emotional resources may already be stretched to the limit. A special effort should be made to assist the single parent in finding financial and support services that can ease the burden of care. Nurses can also assist the single parent in identifying helping roles that may be acceptable to relatives and friends.

Siblings

Results of studies are less clear regarding the ways that siblings are affected by having a brother or sister with a complex condition (Downing 2020, Hartling et al 2014). Most evidence shows a negative effect on siblings of children with chronic illnesses compared with siblings of healthy children (Downing 2020, Hartling et al 2014). Siblings of children with chronic illnesses report psychosocial problems more often than their peers (Downing 2020). A number of factors increase the risk of negative effects for siblings of ill children. Responsibility for caregiving, differential treatment by parents and limitations in family resources and recreational time are often the experiences of siblings of ill or disabled children (Box 19.4).

Coping with Ongoing Stress and Periodic Crises

Professionals can help families cope with stress by providing anticipatory guidance, providing emotional support, assisting the family in assessing and identifying specific stressors, aiding the family in developing coping mechanisms and problem-solving strategies and working collaboratively with parents so that they become empowered in the process (Downing 2020, Yu et al 2019).

Concurrent Stresses within the Family

The ability to deal with the overwhelming stress of a chronic illness is challenged further when additional stresses are present. Stressors may be situational or developmental. They may be related to marital difficulties, sibling needs, homelessness or social isolation. Some families may simultaneously be struggling with a family member's alcohol or other drug problem. Even relatively minor stressors, such as arranging care for siblings, managing the home and travelling to distant treatment centres, can challenge a family's ability to cope successfully.

BOX 19.4 Supporting Siblings of Children with Special Needs

Promote Healthy Sibling Relationships

- Value each child individually and avoid comparisons. Remind each child of his or her positive qualities and contribution to other family members.
- Help siblings see the differences and similarities between themselves and the child with special needs. Create a climate in which children can achieve successes without feeling guilty.
- Teach siblings ways to interact with the child.
- Seek to be fair in terms of discipline, attention and resources; require the affected child to do as much for himself or herself as possible.
- Let siblings settle their own differences; intervene only to prevent siblings from hurting one another.
- Legitimise reasonable anger. Even children with special needs behave badly sometimes.
- Respect a sibling's reluctance to be with or to include the child with special needs in activities.

Help Siblings Cope

- Listen to siblings to let them know that their thoughts and suggestions are valued.
- Praise siblings when they have been patient, have sacrificed or have been particularly helpful. Do not expect siblings to always act in this manner.
- Acknowledge the personal strengths siblings have and their ability to cope with stress successfully.
- Provide age-appropriate information about the child's condition and update it when appropriate.
- Let teachers know what is happening so that they can be understanding and helpful.
- Recognise special stress times for siblings and plan to minimise negative effects.
- Schedule special time with siblings; have a friend or family member substitute when parent is unavailable.
- Encourage siblings to join or help establish a sibling support group.
- Use the services of professionals when needed. If parent feels that such a service is necessary, it should be provided in as vigorous a manner as a service for the child with special needs.

Involve Siblings

- Seek out ways to realistically include siblings in the care and treatment of the child with special needs.
- Limit caregiving responsibilities and give recognition when siblings perform them.
- Develop a library of children's books on special needs.
- Invite siblings to attend meetings to develop plans for the child with special needs (e.g. individualised educational program [IEP], individualised family service plan [IFSP]).
- Discuss future plans with them.
- Solicit their ideas on treatment and service needs.
- Have them visit professionals who work with the child.
- Help them develop competencies to teach the child new skills.
- Provide opportunities for siblings to advocate for the child.
- Allow siblings to set their own pace for learning and involvement.

Sources: World Health Organization (WHO). (2018). Integrating palliative care and symptom relief into paediatrics: a WHO guide for health care planners, implementers and managers. Annex 3, Child-friendly health care: a manual for health workers (excerpts). https://www.who.int/publications/i/item/integrating-palliative-care-and-symptom-relief-into-paediatrics; Southall DP, Burr S, Smith RD, et al. (2000). The Child-Friendly Healthcare Initiative (CFHI): Healthcare provision in accordance with the UN Convention on the Rights of the Child. Child Advocacy International. Department of Child and Adolescent Health and Development of the World Health Organization (WHO); Royal College of Nursing (UK); Royal College of Paediatrics and Child Health (UK). United Nations Children's Fund (UNICEF). Pediatrics, 106(5), 1054–1064. https://pubmed.ncbi.nlm.nih.gov/11061775/

Most families, regardless of their income or insurance coverage, have financial concerns. The costs of caring for a child with a complex illness can be overwhelming.

Coping Mechanisms

Coping mechanisms are behaviours aimed at reducing the tension caused by a crisis. **Approach behaviours** are coping mechanisms that result in movement towards adjustment and resolution of the crisis. **Avoidance behaviours** result in movement away from adjustment and represent maladaptation to the crisis.

Parental Empowerment

Empowerment can be seen as a process of recognising, promoting and enhancing competence. For parents of children with chronic conditions, empowerment may occur gradually as strength and capabilities are drawn on to master the child's care, manage family life and plan for the future. Advocating for the child and developing parent–professional partnerships are part of taking charge (Sercu et al 2018).

Assisting Family Members in Managing their Feelings

Although some previous research has postulated stages of adaptation to a chronic illness, there is a great deal of individual variation in responses to the diagnosis, adjustments made and timeframes for coming to terms with a diagnosis. It is important that professionals recognise and respect a wide range of reactions and coping mechanisms. In fact, members of the family of a child with a complex chronic condition may experience a number of difficult emotions, including fear, guilt, anger, resentment and anxiety. Learning to manage these emotions promotes adaptive coping. Support from professionals, other family members and friends can assist family members in managing their feelings. The following discussion examines some common phases of adjustment and emotional reactions.

Shock and Denial

The initial diagnosis of a chronic illness or complex condition is often met with intense emotion and is characterised by shock, disbelief and sometimes denial. Denial as a defence mechanism is a necessary cushion to prevent disintegration and is a normal response to grieving for any type of loss. Probably all family members experience various degrees of adaptive denial as they learn of the impact that the diagnosis has on their lives.

In children, the importance of denial has repeatedly been demonstrated as a factor in their positive coping with the diagnosis. Denial allows the child to maintain hope in the face of overwhelming odds and to function adaptively and productively. Similar to hope, denial may be an adaptive mechanism for dealing with loss that persists until a family or patient is ready or needs other responses.

Denial is probably the least understood and most poorly dealt-with reaction. If denial is labelled as maladaptive, it can lead to inappropriate attempts to strip away the reaction by repeated and sometimes blunt explanations of the prognosis. However, denial becomes maladaptive only when it prevents recognition of treatment or rehabilitative goals necessary for the child's optimal survival or development.

Adjustment

For most families, adjustment gradually follows shock and is usually characterised by an open admission that the condition exists. This stage may be accompanied by several responses, which are normal parts of the adaptation process. Probably the most universal of these feelings are **guilt** and **self-accusation**. Guilt is often greatest when the cause of the disorder is directly traceable to the parent, as in genetic diseases or accidental injury. However, it can occur even without any scientific or realistic basis for parental responsibility. Frequently, the guilt stems from a false assumption that the child's condition is a result of personal failure or wrongdoing, such as not doing something correctly during pregnancy or the birth. Guilt may also be associated with cultural or religious beliefs. Some parents are convinced that they are being punished for some previous misdeed. Others may see the illness as a trial sent by God to test their religious strength and faith. With correct information, support and time, most parents master guilt and self-accusation.

Children, too, may interpret their serious illness as retribution for past misbehaviour. The nurse should be particularly sensitive to the child who passively accepts all painful procedures. This child may believe that such acts are inflicted as deserved punishment. It is vital that parents and healthcare professionals reassure children that their illnesses are not their fault.

Other common and normal reactions to a diagnosis are bitterness and anger. Anger directed inwards may be evident as self-reproaching or punitive behaviour, such as neglecting one's health and verbally degrading oneself. Anger directed outwards may be manifested in either open arguments or withdrawal from communication and may be evident in the person's relationship with any number of individuals, such as the spouse, the child and siblings. Passive anger towards the ill child may be evident in decreased visiting, refusal to believe how sick the child is or an inability to provide comfort. Healthcare providers are among the most common targets for parental anger. Parents may complain about the nursing care, the insufficient time paediatricians spend with them or the lack of skill of those who draw blood or start intravenous infusions.

Children are apt to respond with anger as well, and this includes the affected child and the well siblings. Children are aware of the loss engendered by their illness or complex condition and may react angrily to the restrictions imposed or the feelings of being different. Siblings may also feel anger and resentment towards the ill child and parents for the loss of routine and parental attention. It is difficult for older children and almost impossible for younger children to comprehend the plight of the affected child. Their perception is of a brother or sister who has the undivided attention of their parents, is showered with cards and gifts and is the focus of everyone's concern.

Reintegration and Acknowledgment

For many families, the adjustment process culminates in the development of realistic expectations for the child and reintegration of family life with the illness or complex condition in a manageable perspective. Because a large portion of this phase is one of grief for a loss, total resolution is not possible until the child dies or leaves home as an independent adult. Therefore, one can regard adjustment as 'increased comfort' with everyday living rather than a complete resolution.

This adjustment phase also involves social reintegration in which the family broadens its activities to include relationships outside of the home with the child as an acceptable and participating member of the group. This last criterion often differentiates the reaction of gradual acceptance during the adjustment period from total acceptance or perhaps is more descriptive of the acknowledgment process.

Establishing a Support System

The diagnosis of a child with a complex chronic condition is a major situational crisis that affects the entire family system. However, families can experience positive outcomes as they successfully deal with the many challenges that accompany a child with chronic illness (Sercu et al 2018, Leemann et al 2020).

THE CHILD WITH A CHRONIC OR COMPLEX CONDITION

The child's reaction to chronic illness depends to a great extent on his or her developmental level, temperament and available coping mechanisms; on the reactions of family members or significant others; and, to a lesser extent, on the condition itself. A child's conceptual understanding of his or her own illness is based not only on age and developmental level but also on the duration and type of experience accumulated with the disease. Knowledge of these variables is essential in providing the kind of information and support needed by these children to cope with an often overwhelming situation.

Developmental Aspects

The impact of a complex chronic illness is influenced by the age at onset. Chronic illness affects children of all ages, but the developmental aspects of each age group dictate particular stresses and risks for the child. The nurse must also recognise that children need to redefine their condition and its implications as they develop and grow. For example, appearance, skills and abilities are highly valued by peers (Fig 19.1). A teenager who is limited in any of these qualities is subject to rejection. This is especially marked when an illness interferes with sexual attractiveness.

Children's developmental concepts of illness are discussed in Chapter 21. An understanding of these developmental factors facilitates planning care to support the child and minimise the risks. Developmental aspects of chronic illness on children are described in Table 19.2.

Coping Mechanisms

Children with chronic conditions tend to use five distinct patterns of coping (Box 19.5). Children with more positive and accepting attitudes about their chronic illness use a more adaptive coping style characterised by optimism, competence and compliance. They show fewer behaviour problems at home and at school. The two maladaptive coping patterns—'Feels different and withdraws' and 'Is irritable, is moody and acts out'—are associated with poorer adaptation; children using these strategies have poorer self-concepts, more negative attitudes about their conditions and more behaviour problems at home and at school.

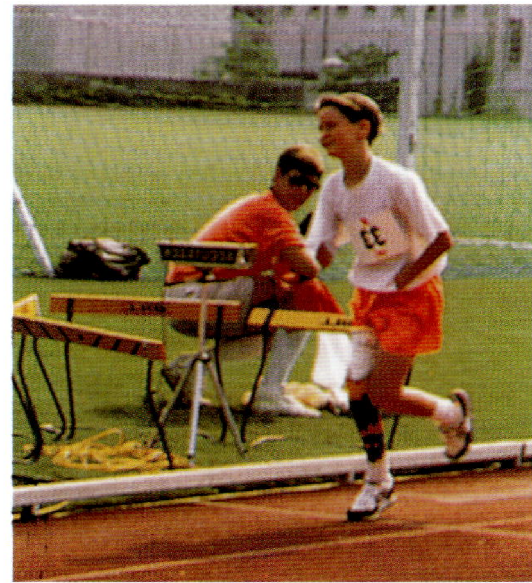

Fig 19.1 Children with any type of impairment should have the opportunity to develop their skills. (Source: Courtesy of Poyo/Hinton Photography.)

Hopefulness

Children, particularly adolescents, are sensitive to the presence or absence of hope. Hopefulness is an internal quality that mobilises humans into goal-directed action that may be satisfying and life sustaining. A sense of hopefulness can produce increased participation in health-seeking behaviours and an improved sense of wellbeing.

NURSING CARE OF THE FAMILY AND CHILD WITH A CHRONIC OR COMPLEX CONDITION

Assessment

Because the nurse may meet a family during any phase of the adjustment process, several assessment areas are important. The family's ability to cope with previous stresses influences the current situation and answers to questions about their usual coping skills are enlightening. Knowledge of concurrent stresses, such as financial, marital or non-marital and career or unemployment, helps identify families who may have fewer resources to cope with the child's needs.

Provide Support at the Time of Diagnosis

The diagnosis is a critical time for parents and can influence how they perceive their healthcare providers across the trajectory of care. Although they may not hear or remember all that is said to them, they frequently sense a certain attitude of acceptance, rejection, hope or despair that may influence their ability to absorb the shock and begin adapting to the family's altered future.

Parents may be encouraged to be together when they are informed of their child's condition, thus avoiding the problem of one parent having to interpret complex information and deal with the initial emotional reaction of the other. The informing session should take place in a private, comfortable setting free of distractions and interruptions in an atmosphere in which the parents feel free to express their emotions. Their emotional needs are acknowledged by showing acceptance of expressions, such as crying, sadness, anger and disappointment.

The informing session does not end with the presentation of devastating news. Instead, the child's strengths, appealing behaviours and potential for development are stressed, as are available rehabilitation efforts or treatments. Parents can be encouraged to view their experiences as a series of challenges that they are capable of handling, particularly with available professional feedback. The parents are assured that the nurse will be available to answer questions and to provide further assistance as needed.

The preceding discussion relates primarily to the initial informing interview. However, because of the need for long-term follow-up, it is only one in a series of continuing discussions. In all interactions, the family's input is solicited and incorporated into the care plan. Some situations require consideration of special problems.

Support the Family's Coping Methods

For the family to meet the stresses of optimally adjusting to the child's condition, each member must be individually supported so that the family system is strong. Although the family can indefinitely support a member who is in need of assistance, its greatest strength lies in every member supporting each other. The nurse should bear in mind that the family member in greatest need is not necessarily the affected child but may be a parent or sibling who is dealing with stresses that require intervention.

Parents

The nurse can provide support by being attentive to families' responses to their children. Mothers and fathers need to experience success, joy

TABLE 19.2 **Developmental Effects of Chronic Illness or Disability on Children**

Developmental Tasks	Potential Effects of Chronic Illness or Disability	Supportive Interventions
	INFANCY	
Develop a sense of trust	Multiple caregivers and frequent separations, especially if hospitalised	Encourage consistent caregivers in hospital or other care settings.
	Deprived of consistent nurturing	Encourage parental presence, 'rooming in' during hospitalisation and participation in care.
Bond, or attach, to parent	Delayed because of separation; parental grief for loss of 'dream' child; parental inability to accept the condition, especially a visible defect	Emphasise healthy, perfect qualities of infant. Help parents learn special care needs of infant for them to feel competent.
Learn through sensorimotor experiences	More exposure to painful experiences than pleasurable ones	Expose infant to pleasurable experiences through all senses (touch, hearing, sight, taste, movement).
	Limited contact with environment from restricted movement or confinement	Encourage age-appropriate developmental skills (e.g. holding bottle, finger feeding, crawling).
Begin to develop a sense of separateness from parent	Increased dependency on parent for care	Encourage all family members to participate in care to prevent overinvolvement of one member.
	Overinvolvement of parent in care	Encourage periodic respite from demands of care responsibilities.
	TODDLERHOOD	
Develop autonomy	Increased dependency on parent	Encourage independence in as many areas as possible (e.g. toileting, dressing, feeding).
Master locomotor and language skills	Limited opportunity to test own abilities and limits	Provide gross motor skill activity and modification of toys or equipment, such as modified swing.
Learn through sensorimotor experience; beginning preoperational thought	Increased exposure to painful experiences	Give choices to allow simple feeling of control (e.g. choice of what book to look at, what kind of sandwich to eat). Institute age-appropriate discipline and limit setting. Recognise that negative and ritualistic behaviours are normal. Provide sensory experiences (e.g. water play, sandpit play, finger painting).
	PRESCHOOL AGE	
Develop initiative and purpose Master self-care skills	Limited opportunities for success in accomplishing simple tasks or mastering self-care skills	Encourage mastery of self-help skills. Provide devices that make tasks easier (e.g. self-dressing).
Begin to develop peer relationships	Limited opportunities for socialisation with peers; may appear 'like a baby' to age mates Protection within tolerant and secure family, causing child to fear criticism and withdraw	Encourage socialisation (e.g. inviting friends to play, day care experience, trips to park). Provide age-appropriate play, especially associative play opportunities. Emphasise child's abilities; dress appropriately to enhance desirable appearance.
Develop sense of body image and sexual identification	Awareness of body centring on pain anxiety and failure	Encourage healthy relationships
Learn through preoperational thought (magical thinking)	Guilt (thinking he or she caused the illness or disability or is being punished for wrongdoing)	Help child deal with criticisms; realise that too much protection prevents child from realities of world. Clarify that cause of child's illness or disability is not his or her fault or a punishment.
	SCHOOL AGE	
Develop a sense of accomplishment	Limited opportunities to achieve and compete (e.g. many school absences, inability to join regular athletic activities)	Encourage school attendance; schedule medical visits at times other than school; encourage child to make up missed work.
Form peer relationships	Limited opportunities for socialisation	Educate teachers and classmates about child's condition, abilities and special needs. Encourage sports activities (e.g. Special Olympics). Encourage socialisation
Learn through concrete operations	Incomplete comprehension of the imposed physical limitations or treatment of the disorder	Provide child with information about his or her condition. Encourage creative activities
	ADOLESCENCE	
Develop personal and sexual identity	Increased sense of feeling different from peers and reduced ability to compete with peers in appearance, abilities, special skills	Help child realise that many of the difficulties the teenager is experiencing are part of normal adolescence (rebelliousness, risk taking, lack of cooperation, hostility towards authority).

Continued

TABLE 19.2 Developmental Effects of Chronic Illness or Disability on Children—cont'd

Developmental Tasks	Potential Effects of Chronic Illness or Disability	Supportive Interventions
Achieve independence from family	Increased dependency on family; limited job or career opportunities	Provide instruction on interpersonal and coping skills. Encourage increased responsibility for care and management of the disease or condition (e.g. assuming responsibility for making and keeping appointment [ideally alone], sharing assessment and planning stages of healthcare delivery, contacting resources). Discuss planning for future and how condition can affect choices.
Form healthy relationships	Limited opportunities for friendships; less opportunity to discuss sexual concerns with peers Increased concern with issues such as why did they get the disorder and whether they will marry and have a family	Encourage socialisation with peers, including peers with special needs and those without special needs. Encourage activities appropriate for age. Be alert to cues that signal readiness for information regarding implications of condition on sexuality and reproduction. Understand that adolescent has same sexual needs and concerns as any other teenager.
Learn through abstract thinking	Decreased opportunity for earlier stages of cognition impeding achievement of level of abstract thinking	Provide instruction on decision-making, assertiveness and other skills necessary to manage personal plans.

BOX 19.5 Coping Patterns Used by Children with Special Needs

Develops competence and optimism—Accentuates the positive aspects of the situation and concentrates more on what he or she has or can do than on what is missing or on what he or she cannot do; is as independent as possible

Feels different and withdraws—Sees self as being different from other children because of the chronic health condition; views being different as negative; sees self as less worthy than others; focuses on things he or she cannot do and sometimes over-restricts activities needlessly

Is irritable, is moody and acts out—Uses proactive and self-initiated coping behaviours, although usually counterproductive in that the behaviours are not ego enhancing or socially responsible and do not result in desired outcomes; acts out irritability, which may or may not be associated with the condition's symptoms

Complies with treatment—Takes necessary medications, treatments; adheres to activity restrictions; also uses behaviours that indicate developing independence (e.g. assumes responsibility for taking medication)

Seeks support—Talks with adults, children, paediatricians and nurses; develops plans to handle problems as they occur; uses downward comparison (i.e. realises that others have it worse)

Source: Modified from Austin, J., Patterson, J., Huberty, T. (1991). Development of the coping health inventory for children. Journal of Pediatric Nursing, 6(3), 166–174.

and pride in their children to give the support they need. It is important for nurses to examine their attitudes to determine their ability to engage in parent–professional partnerships.

Parents can be encouraged to discuss their feelings towards the child, the impact of this event on their marriage and associated stresses such as financial burdens. For most families, regardless of their income or insurance coverage, financial concerns exist. The costs of caring for a child with special needs can be overwhelming.

Parent-to-parent Support

Just being with another parent who has shared similar experiences is helpful. It may not need to be a parent of a child with the same diagnosis because parents in the process of adjusting to a child with special needs—or finding respite services, educational or rehabilitative services, special equipment vendors and financial counselling—tread a common path.

Advocate for Empowerment

Nurses can advocate for methods that foster opportunities for parent empowerment. For example, nurses can suggest reimbursement for travel and child care plus stipends to enable parents' voices to be heard at meetings and conferences. They can encourage parent membership on committees and advisory boards.

The Child

Through ongoing contacts with the child, the nurse: (1) observes the child's responses to the disorder, ability to function and adaptive behaviours within the environment and with significant others; (2) explores the child's own understanding of his or her illness or condition; and (3) provides support while the child learns to cope with his or her feelings. Children are encouraged to express their concerns rather than allowing others to express them for them because open discussions may reduce anxiety.

Siblings

The presence of a child with special needs in a family may result in parents paying less attention to the other children. Siblings may respond by developing negative attitudes towards the child or by expressing anger in different forms. The nurse can help by using anticipatory guidance, questioning the parents about what they believe is the best way to have siblings respond to the child and guiding them through ways to meet their other children's needs for attention. This questioning should take place before serious negative effects occur.

Siblings may also experience embarrassment associated with having a brother or sister with a chronic or complex condition. Parents are then faced with the difficulty of responding to this embarrassment in an understanding and appropriate manner without punishing the siblings for how they feel. Parents are encouraged to talk with the siblings about how they view their affected sibling.

Educate about the Disorder and General Healthcare

Educating the family about the disorder is actually an extension of revealing the diagnosis. Education involves not only supplying technical information but also discussing how the condition will affect the child. Parents may only be able to process limited information at any one time. It may be helpful to provide essential information and then follow by asking, 'What else would you like to know about your child's condition?' Responding to parents' questions and concerns ensures that their information needs are met.

Activities of Daily Living

Parents also need guidance in how the condition may interfere with or alter activities of daily living, such as eating, dressing, sleeping and toileting. One area frequently affected is nutrition. Common problems are undernutrition resulting from food being inappropriately restricted or loss of appetite, vomiting or motor deficits that interfere with feeding; overnutrition may also occur, usually because of a caloric intake in excess of energy expenditure because of boredom and lack of stimulation in other areas. Although the child requires the same basic nutrients as other children, the daily requirements may differ. Special nutritional considerations are discussed as appropriate throughout the text.

Safe Transportation

Modifications may also be needed regarding car safety. Children with conditions such as low birth weight (see Discharge Planning and Home Care, Chapter 8) or orthopaedic, neuromuscular or respiratory impairments often cannot safely use conventional car restraints. For example, children with hip spica casts cannot sit properly in child safety seats (see Developmental Dysplasia of the Hip, Chapter 33). Modifications can be made to some commercial models, and for older children a special vest is available that secures the child to the back seat in a lying-down position.

Primary Healthcare

Children with special needs require all the usual healthcare recommended for any child. Attention to injury prevention, immunisations, dental health and regular physical examinations is essential. Nurses can play an important role in reminding parents of these aspects of care that are so often neglected when the concern is focused on the child's chronic condition. Specific discussions of nutrition, sleep and activity, dental health and injury prevention are presented in the chapters on health promotion for specific age groups. Immunisations are discussed in Chapter 25.

Promote Normal Development

Aside from knowledge of the condition and its effect on the child's abilities, the family must be guided towards fostering appropriate development in their child. Although each stage may take longer to achieve, parents are guided towards helping the child fully realise his or her potential in preparation for the next developmental stage. Table 19.2 outlines developmental aspects of complex conditions and supportive interventions. With appropriate planning and knowledge of strategies to improve the child's functional abilities, most children can live fulfilling and productive lives.

One important aspect of promoting normal development is to encourage the child's self-care abilities in both activities of daily living and the medical regimen. An assessment of the child's age and physical, emotional and mental capacities, as well as the support and structure provided by the family, should be considered in determining the appropriate level of self-care in the medical regimen. Even toddlers can be involved in their own care by holding supplies for the parent during a procedure. Over time, children should be encouraged towards greater autonomy in the self-care arena.

Early Childhood

During infancy, the child is achieving basic trust through a satisfying, intimate, consistent relationship with his or her parents. However, affected children's early existence may be stressful, chaotic and unsatisfying. Consequently, they may need more parental support and expressions of affection to achieve trust. Likewise, the parents require assistance in finding ways to meet the infant's needs, such as how to hold a rigid or flaccid infant, how to feed a child with tongue thrust or episodes of dyspnoea and how to stimulate a child who seems incapable of achieving any skills. If hospitalisations are frequent or prolonged, every effort is made to preserve the parent–child relationship (see also Chapter 21).

School Age

For school-age children, the major tasks are entry into school and achieving a sense of industry. Although the importance of school in the life of all children is well known, school absences are significantly higher among children with chronic illnesses than among their healthy peers. The more school absences the child experiences, the more difficult it is to resume attendance and school phobia may result. The child should return to school as soon as possible after diagnosis or treatments.

Adolescence

Adolescence can be a particularly difficult period for the teenager and family. All of the needs discussed previously apply to this age group as well. Developing **independence** or **autonomy**, however, is a major task for the adolescent as planning for the future becomes a prominent concern. Although the emphasis in the past has been on achieving independence from physical assistance, recent developments in the fields of special education, adolescent development and family systems suggest redefining autonomy in terms of individuals' capacities to take responsibility for their own behaviour, to make decisions regarding their own lives and to maintain supportive social relationships. Given this understanding, even individuals with severe impairments can be viewed as autonomous if they perceive their own needs and take responsibility for meeting them, either directly or by engaging the assistance of others. As adolescents become more autonomous, the nurse can help them articulate their needs, participate in developing their own care plans and discover and express how others can be of greatest assistance.

Establish Realistic Future Goals

One of the most difficult adjustments is setting realistic future goals for the child that are based on the child's own goals and values.

Planning for the future should be a gradual process. All along, the parents should cultivate realistic vocations for the child. For example, if children have physical disabilities, they can be directed towards intellectual, artistic or musical pursuits. Children with developmental disabilities can be taught manual skills. In this way, the child's development proceeds in the direction of self-support through gainful employment.

With prolonged survival, young people with chronic illnesses must deal with new decisions and problems, such as marriage, employment and insurance coverage. With appropriate guidance, individuals with disabilities can attain gainful employment, marriage and a family. For those whose conditions are genetic, counselling is needed regarding future offspring.

PALLIATIVE CARE IN CHILDHOOD TERMINAL ILLNESS

Scope of the Problem

The number of children living with chronic, life-limiting illnesses has increased exponentially as advances in technology and pharmacology have led to improved treatments (AIHW 2020). These chronic conditions often result in substantial suffering, symptom distress and healthcare needs that increase the possibility of death (Box 19.6) (AIHW 2020, Downing 2020). The majority of the children who die do so while undergoing intensive treatments in a hospital setting (Keele et al 2013), having been mechanically ventilated and often experiencing acute and chronic pain and other distressing symptoms (Barnes & Rowe 2013).

Palliative care is now widely recognised as a critical part of excellent care for children with complex, chronic or life-limiting diseases, but patients continue to receive this care very late in their illness trajectory. Many healthcare professionals lack clinical education in the principles of making the transition with children from curative to palliative care or methods of adequately managing the pain and suffering experienced by children and their families during the dying process (Downing 2020). As our ability to treat disease, disability and trauma advances, we must also improve our care of those children who live with the spectre of chronic life-threatening illness and premature death.

BOX 19.6 Conditions Contributing to Childhood Death

- Cancer
- Complications of prematurity
- Congenital anomalies
  - Trisomy 13, 18
  - Anencephaly
  - Holoprosencephaly
  - Lissencephaly
  - Inborn errors of metabolism
- Cystic fibrosis
- Human immunodeficiency virus infection/acquired immunodeficiency syndrome
- Major organ dysfunction or failure
  - Congenital or acquired heart disease or defects
  - Liver defects
  - Renal failure
- Neurodegenerative diseases
  - Muscular dystrophy
  - Spinal muscular atrophy
  - Adrenoleukodystrophy
  - Ataxia-telangiectasia
- Severe neurological and/or physical disability
- Severe gastrointestinal disorder or malformation
- Epidermolysis bullosa
- Severe immunodeficiencies
- Severe forms of osteogenesis imperfecta
- Trauma
  - Accidents

Principles of Palliative Care

Palliative care involves an interdisciplinary approach to the management of a child's life-threatening or life-limiting illness from diagnosis through death and focuses on preventing or relieving the child's symptoms and support of the child. The World Health Organization (WHO 2014) defines paediatric palliative care as the 'active total care of the child's body, mind and spirit, and also involv[ing] giving support to the family. It begins when illness is diagnosed, and continues regardless of whether or not a child receives treatment directed at the disease'. Palliative care interventions do not serve to hasten death; rather, they provide pain and symptom management, attention to issues faced by the child and family with regard to death and dying and promotion of optimal functioning and quality of life. The implementation of neonatal and paediatric palliative care consulting services within hospitals has led to enhanced quality of life and end-of-life care for children and their families and support for their care providers (Enguidanos et al 2014, Younge et al 2015).

Several principles are hallmarks of palliative care (Levine et al 2013). The child and family are the unit of care in which services are coordinated across all sites of care. An interdisciplinary team of healthcare professionals consisting of social workers, chaplains, nurses, nurse consultants and paediatricians skilled in caring for children with life-threatening or life-limiting conditions assists the family by focusing care on the complex interactions between physical, emotional, social and spiritual needs.

Goals of Care

Palliative care seeks to relieve the physical, emotional, social and spiritual distress produced by life-limiting conditions, to assist in complex decision-making and to enhance the quality of life (Downing 2020). To do so most effectively, providers must guide realistic goal setting for the patient. Frequent, periodic and timely discussions between the healthcare provider team and parents (and child when developmentally appropriate) regarding the goals of care are critical (Hill et al 2014). The possibility that a child's illness or condition is not curable and that death may be an inevitable outcome causes everyone involved a great deal of stress (Brandon et al 2014). Paediatricians, other members of the healthcare team and families consider all information regarding the child's situation and make difficult choices regarding treatment options. These decisions can have a profound impact on the child and family. Whenever possible, the goals of the child should be solicited and respected. Establishing goals of care has become an essential component of quality palliative medicine (Hill et al 2014, Downing 2020) and should address the physical, emotional, social and spiritual distress experienced by patients and their families. Nurses are often best situated to evaluate suffering and the impact of the goals of care because of the amount of time they spend with patients and their families compared with other medical team members (Mastro et al 2015).

Uncertainty about the child's prognosis among healthcare providers is often a barrier to the provision of optimal palliative care (Friedrichsdorf 2017, Coad et al 2014). As a result, many families have not always received the option of shifting the focus of treatment to the child's comfort and quality of life when cure is unlikely (see Research Focus box). Although current American Academy of Pediatrics (2014) guidelines recommend collaborative integrated care that includes clear and honest discussions with patients and families about the goals of treatment and any concerns they may have, specific discussions about the burden of treatment and the benefits of end-of-life care planning is often absent.

RESEARCH FOCUS

Palliative Care

Results of landmark studies of medical practitioner decision-making regarding when to change the focus of care to palliation and comfort show high variability across paediatricians and settings (Randolph et al 1999, Thompson et al 2009). In one survey of over 300 paediatricians, only 15% of participating paediatricians would recommend early referral for palliative care for children with cancer. In contrast, 44% would make such a recommendation at the end of life (Thompson et al 2009). This reluctance to change to a focus on palliative care by paediatricians occurs for a number of reasons, including the belief that not being able to 'save' a child is a 'failure'. Also, the paediatrician and other members of the healthcare team may lack knowledge of and experience with the principles of palliative care (Davies et al 2008). Paediatric nurses, empowered with the skills and understanding of quality palliative care, can help the care team focus on palliative care goals and ensure that these principles are integrated into the care model throughout the entire clinical course, even when formal palliative care consultation is not solicited.

Effective communication is critical for quality palliative care. Barriers to effective communication are among the most important factors perceived to interfere with optimal end-of-life paediatric care (Coad et al 2014). Parents almost always want clinicians to discuss advance care options and to assist them in such complex decision-making. Although the nurse may not be the one spearheading such discussions, the nurse can be instrumental in advocating for discussions to occur and that patient preferences are verbalised. First, the nurse provides information about the child and family to the healthcare team, provides information to the child and family about treatment plans and goals and coordinates discussions between the family and healthcare team. Second, the nurses provides an important source of emotional support to the child and family as they attempt to comprehend and assess the impact of the information they are given. Third, the nurses actively engage as advocates in palliative care planning by challenging the status quo and by assisting all invested parties to understand the overall patient care mission. This level of advocacy in which the child and family are given assistance with interpreting and understanding goals will lead to valid and shared decision-making. The foundation for good decision-making depends on establishing clear goals of care based on individual preferences and beliefs that are attainable given a child's clinical condition (Downing 2020, Broden et al 2020).

Earlier acknowledgment by both paediatricians and parents that children have no realistic chance for cure is often associated with implementation of do-not-resuscitate (DNR) orders, and greater provision of palliative care measures, but even when paediatricians recommend limiting or withdrawing life-sustaining interventions many parents disagree. Current factors influencing paediatricians' and nurses' resuscitation decisions include: (1) patient characteristics (96%); (2) personal experience/biases (85%); (3) family's wishes and desires (81%); (4) disease characteristics (74%); and (5) societal perspectives (36%) (Dupont-Thibodeau et al 2017). Factors found to influence parents' decisions to limit or withdraw life-sustaining measures include: parents' prior end-of-life decision-making for loved ones; observations of pain and suffering of their child and other hospitalised children; various emotions, including guilt and sorrow; and awareness of their child's desire to forgo life-sustaining measures (Downing 2020). The use of a paediatric advance directive for older minors may raise awareness of children's wishes as part of the family decision-making process (Broden 2020), but parents find engagement in advance care planning to be difficult (Lotz et al 2017), especially when they do not agree with their child. Three strategies have been posited for providers to manage differences between parent and child preferences: deference, advocative and arbitrative. Parental decision-making preferences are deferred to in the deference strategy, whereas child preferences are advocated in the advocative strategy. The arbitrative strategy is used to work to resolve the differences between parents and the child (Sisk et al 2017) (see Research Focus box, Box 19.7 and Table 19.3).

BOX 19.7 Communicating with Families

Listen for an 'invitation' to talk about the situation.

- 'Sometimes I wonder if I am doing the right thing.'
- 'What have other parents done in this situation?'
- 'Do you know of other children who have survived this?'
- 'I think the doctor is not telling me everything.'

Use open-ended, non-judgmental questions to explore families' wishes.

- 'Can you tell me more about how you are feeling?'
- 'What questions do you (or your child) have that I can answer for you?'
- 'What are your concerns (or worries, fears) right now?'
- 'What is important to you (or your child, family) at this time?'

RESEARCH FOCUS

Importance of Honest Communication

Numerous studies have found that families facing the impending death of a child depend on information provided to them by the healthcare team, particularly an honest appraisal of the child's prognosis, to make difficult decisions regarding care options for their child and care measures after life-sustaining measures were eliminated (Cole & Foito 2019).

As the group of health professionals who are most involved with families, nurses are in an excellent position to ensure that families know the options available to them. The nurse's first responsibility is to explore the patient's and family's wishes. This is best done with the medical practitioner, but at times nurses need to initiate the process. When discussing difficult issues, nurses are open to the child's or family's indirect comments that communicate uncertainty or concerns about the course of care. Nurses answer questions honestly, and if they do not know the answer, reassure the family that they will arrange for a discussion with the medical practitioner. It is important to address any fantasies or misunderstandings by seeking to clarify what the family has heard. Finally, it is important for the nurse to remain neutral and avoid giving personal opinions or experiences. The goal of communication is to facilitate the identification of the family's wishes, based on their unique values and beliefs (see Table 19.3).

Awareness of Dying in Children with Life-threatening Illness

One of the initial reactions of parents (and some healthcare professionals) to the discovery of a life-threatening illness is to protect the child from the impact of the diagnosis (Ferrell et al 2016, Larcher et al 2015, Lotz et al 2017). However, it is now widely understood that terminally ill children develop an awareness of the seriousness of their diagnosis, even when protected from the truth (Jalmsell et al 2015, Lotz et al 2017). The avoidance of talking openly and honestly with children with life-threatening illnesses and their siblings can lead to fear, guilt, misconceptions and the pain of grieving alone. Surviving siblings may experience psychiatric sequelae as children and into adulthood.

TABLE 19.3 **Communicating Bad News to Families**

Approach	Effective Techniques
Provide a setting conducive to communication.	Ensure privacy; use appropriate body language; make eye contact.
	Have parents choose who will attend.
Determine what the parent knows.	Ask questions ('What have you made of all this?' or 'What were you told?').
	Listen to the vocabulary and comprehension of the parents.
	Recognise denial but do not acknowledge it at this stage.
Determine what the parent wants to know.	Obtain a clear invitation to share information (if this is what the parent wants). Use questions such as 'Are you the sort of person who likes to know every detail or just the basic facts?'
Give information (aligning and educating).	Start at level of parents' comprehension and use the same vocabulary. Give information slowly, concisely and in simple language. Avoid medical jargon. Check regularly to be certain that content is understood.
Respond to parents' reactions.	Acknowledge all reactions and feelings, particularly using the emphatic response technique (identifying emotion, identifying cause of emotion and responding appropriately).
	Expect tears, anger and other strong emotions.
Close.	Briefly summarise major areas discussed.
	Ask parents if they have other important issues to discuss at this time.
	Make an appointment for the next meeting.

Discussing Death with Children

Children need honest and accurate information about their illness, treatments and prognosis. There is broad consensus across research and practice that it is important to involve children, regardless of age, in discussions about their illness and care plans (Cohen et al 2016, Jacobs et al 2015, Broden et al 2020). The appropriate timing and approach for these discussions are less clear (Broden et al 2020, Cohen 2016). This information needs to be given in clear, simple language. In most situations this best occurs as a gradual process, characterised by increasingly open dialogue among parents, professionals and the child. Providing an atmosphere of open communication early in the course of an illness facilitates answering difficult questions as the child's condition worsens. Providing appropriate literature about the disease, as well as about the experience of illness and possible death, is also helpful. How and when to involve children in decisions regarding care during their dying process and death are individual matters. In general, the nurse should ask parents how they would like their child to be told of the prognosis and how they want to be included in their child's care. Some parents may request that their child not be told that he or she is dying, even if the child asks. This often places healthcare providers in a difficult situation. Children, even at a young age, are perceptive. Despite not being told outright that they are dying, they realise that something is seriously wrong and that it involves them. Children deserve to be provided with the truth.

Children and families often have an unspoken anxiety related to the fear of dying and/or the dying process. Children and their families will share some similar fears and worries, but others will be unique (Cohen et al 2016). Identifying the specific fears and fostering candid discussion of them will allow the nurse to minimise the suffering associated with this anxiety as much as possible.

Anxiety and fear may also lead to a range of emotional expressions on the part of the child that may be disturbing to families, particularly if they are not prepared. This may include emotional liability, aggression and expressions of anger, depression and withdrawal. Helping families to understand that such expressions are not unexpected or abnormal may ease anxiety for the family and facilitate better coping. The nurse may provide further reassurance by both practising and introducing families to the concepts of active listening, simple relaxation and therapeutic touch. The bedside nurse can also structure the hospital or home environment to allow for maximum control and independence within the limitations imposed by the developmental level and physical condition of the child. Nurses can mitigate the suffering of anxiety by explaining all procedures and therapies, detailing the physical effects the child is likely to experience and answering all questions in a frank, honest manner.

Children's Understanding of and Reactions to Dying

The use of chronological age and/or the child's stage of development as a marker for timing and content of discussions about death can be problematic due to the variability in cognitive development within particular ages and stages. Ages and stages may be helpful as a general guide, but communication should be based on the cognitive developmental capabilities of the individual child and his or her readiness for such discussion. This individualised approach not only takes into consideration the cognitive abilities of the child but also includes assessment of potential vulnerabilities, experiences with the illness, readiness for information and relationships with parents and/or caregivers (Broden et al 2020, Downing 2020). Influences also include nationality, religion, life-limiting illness, personal experiences with death and family members' explanations and attitudes surrounding death (Weaver et al 2016). By approximately 7 years of age most children understand the key bioscientific components of death (Box 19.8). Studies have found that children ranging in age from 4 to 12 years have an adultlike understanding of death (Wolfelt 2013). However, anyone working with children must be aware of significant developmental variations related to their understanding and fears of death. Cultural, national and religious differences in beliefs about an afterlife have also been found to influence a child's understanding of death. Sensitive assessment of the child's developmental understanding of death and the family's cultural and spiritual beliefs related to dying and death is an important but often overlooked aspect of care.

Children ask very difficult questions at unexpected times and often to nurses. This can be very confronting and nurses can be unsure how to respond. Listen to the child and find out exactly what the child is asking of you, such as 'Am I dying?', 'What have my mum and dad been told?' or 'What is wrong with me?' Children will have many questions. Normalise these questions and feelings and reassure the child/adolescent that they are safe to ask these questions. Children are very aware of discrepancies between verbal and non-verbal expression and

BOX 19.8 Children's Development of the Subconcepts of Death

Universality

- All living things eventually die.
- Death is all inclusive; everyone dies.
- Death is inevitable, unavoidable.
- Death is unpredictable; exact timing is unknown.

Before Universality

- They themselves, children in general and/or their family or friends may be viewed as excluded.
- Understanding that *they* will die precedes understanding that *everyone* will die.
- Death is avoidable if you are clever.
- Death occurs in the remote future only.

Irreversibility

- Once the physical body dies, it cannot be made alive again.

Before Irreversibility

- Death is temporary (e.g. falling asleep and waking up, leaving for and returning from a trip) and reversible.

Non-functionality

- Once a living thing dies, all life-defining capabilities (e.g. eating, sleeping, seeing, hearing) of the body cease.

Before Non-functionality

- The dead continue external functions (e.g. eating, speaking).

Causality

- External and internal events can cause one's death.

Before Causality

- Death results from unrealistic causes (e.g. misbehaving), concrete causes (e.g. poison, guns) or external causes (e.g. accidents, murder).

Non-corporeal Continuation

- Some form of personal continuation exists after death of the physical body (e.g. reincarnation, ascension of the soul to heaven).

Before Non-corporeal Continuation

- Unknown.

communication and may be asking for clarification due to mixed messages from non-verbal communication. Open and honest communication is required and parents need to be educated and supported to provide this also.

Infants and Toddlers

Exactly how preverbal children view death is a mystery because there is no way of reliably assessing their views of death. On the basis of their cognitive abilities, it is likely that they have no concept of death. The egocentricity of toddlers and their vague separation of fact and fantasy make it impossible for them to comprehend absence of life. Although they may repeat what initially sounds like a correct definition of death, such as 'Grandpa is dead; he went to heaven', they may expect Grandpa's return for several months before accommodating themselves to the absence. They can perceive events only in terms of their own frame of reference: living.

Reactions to Dying. Separation from parents and alterations in their routine represent threats to the toddler who is seriously ill and to the well-toddler sibling. Behavioural responses may include regression to less independent levels of behaviour related to speech, toileting, eating, drinking, crying, clinging, biting, hitting, withdrawal and physical illness. Toddlers may perceive the seriousness of their condition from the parents' reactions of anxiety, sadness, depression or anger. Although young children are unaware of the reason for such emotions, they often find their parents' behaviour disturbing and upsetting. Helping parents deal with their feelings allows them more emotional reserve to meet the needs of their children. Encouraging parents to stay in the hospital as much as possible and to participate in the child's care promotes the parents' and child's adjustment to a serious, potentially fatal illness or injury.

Preschool Children

Several characteristics of preschoolers' cognitive and psychological development affect their concept of death. Because they are egocentric at this age, they often have a tremendous sense of self-power and omnipotence. Therefore, they believe that their thoughts are sufficient to cause events. The consequence of such magical thinking is feelings of guilt, shame and punishment.

Concept of Death. Children between 3 and 5 years of age have usually heard the word *death* and have some sense of its meaning. They see death as a departure, possibly as a type of sleep. They may recognise the fact of physical death but do not separate it from living abilities. The dead person in the coffin still breathes, eats and sleeps. Death is temporary and reversible; life and death can change places with one another. Because of the immature concept of time, they have no real understanding of the universality and inevitability of death. Words such as *forever* and *everyone* have meaning only in the child's egocentric thinking. Waiting until Christmas may be 'forever', and anybody the child denotes is 'everyone'. Children of this age take the literal meaning of words, and euphemisms are avoided. Preschoolers who are told that Grandma has 'gone to sleep' may fear going to sleep themselves.

Reactions to Dying. If preschoolers become seriously ill, they may conceive of the illness as punishment for their thoughts or actions. The usual diagnostic and treatment procedures, in combination with enforced hospitalisation, can confirm their belief that they are being punished. If their parents do not stay with them during hospitalisation or prevent the traumatic procedures, they may believe that the parents are retaliating for previous misdeeds or bad thoughts.

The same principles of magical thinking and omnipotence affect preschoolers when a sibling becomes critically ill or dies. One of the most significant types of death is sudden unexpected death in infancy (SUDI) of which sudden infant death syndrome (SIDS) is considered a subtype (see the section Sudden Infant Death Syndrome, Chapter 11). Because it occurs unexpectedly to a healthy infant (who may have been rejected and unwanted by a jealous sibling), preschoolers find no evidence to support a physical cause of death. Indeed, the parents often are unaware of the reason for the fatality and may question any possible cause. If preschoolers are in any way accused or suspected of having harmed the infant, they may feel extremely guilty and responsible for the tragedy. On observing their parents' acute grief, they may interpret the anger or depression as a rejection of them.

School-age Children

Although school-age children have a better understanding of causality, less egocentricity and an advanced perception of time, they may still associate misdeeds or bad thoughts with causing death and feel intense guilt and responsibility for the event. However, because of their higher cognitive abilities, they respond well to logical explanations and comprehend the figurative meaning of words better than children in younger age groups. Although they are less likely to interpret explanations in a purely literal sense, they are still prone to self-referenced definitions. For this reason, it is important for adults to clarify the meanings of statements and to repeatedly ask the children what they think.

Concept of Death. Much of the discussion on the preschool child's understanding of death also relates to the younger school-age child. However, these children have a deeper understanding of death in the concrete sense. Children of this age attempt to ascribe a more comprehensible meaning to the event by personifying death as a devil, God, ghost or bogeyman. Naturalistic-physiological explanations of why death occurs and what happens to the dead body may also be a preoccupation in this age group. Factual explanations, such as 'When you die, your body decays in the ground' are consistent with their concrete thinking.

By age 7 years, most children have an increasingly adult concept of death. They realise that it is universal, irreversible and non-functional; children with cancer gain a more mature, biological understanding of death at an earlier age than their well peers. Their attitudes towards death are greatly influenced by the reactions and attitudes of others, particularly their parents.

Reactions to Dying. The increased ability of school-age children to comprehend and reason poses additional risks for them. They may fear the reason for the illness, communicability of the disease to themselves or others, consequences of the disease on their functioning and relationships with others and the process of dying and death itself. They tend to fear the expectation of the event more than its realisation. Their fear of the unknown is greater than that of the known. Like preschoolers, their fantasy explanations for the unexpected or the unknown are usually much more frightening and extreme than the actual situation. For this reason, anticipatory preparation is both necessary and effective. These children respond well to explanations of the disease, names of drugs and so on. The developmental task of this age is industry; thus, helping children who may be facing their own death to maintain control over their body—by understanding what is happening to them and participating in what is done to them—allows them to achieve independence, self-worth and self-esteem and to avoid a sense of inferiority.

The realisation of impending death or failure to recover is a tremendous threat to school-age children's sense of security and ego strength. These children are likely to exhibit their fear more through verbal uncooperativeness. Additional behavioural responses for the well sibling may include worrying about the health and safety of other family members and having problems in school. Encouraging children to talk about their feelings, allowing control where possible and appropriate and providing outlets for aggression through play are means of dealing with this expression of anger and fear.

Adolescents

By the time most children reach adolescence, they have a mature understanding of death. As abstract thinking develops, there is more questioning of death and related topics, such as the religious meaning of afterlife. However, other developmental needs, especially formation of the child's own identity, make this an exceptionally difficult time for young people to cope with the loss of a loved one or with their own impending death.

Concept of Death. Although adolescents have a mature understanding of death, they tend to think they will not die as a young person. The search for the spiritual meaning of what follows death is typical at this age.

Reactions to Dying. Adolescents may have a great deal of difficulty in coping with death. Although they have reached the level of adult comprehension of the concept of death, they are least likely of all age groups to accept cessation of life, particularly their own. Developmentally, the rejection of death is understandable because adolescents' tasks are to establish an identity by finding out who they are, what their purpose is and where they belong.

Adolescents strive for group acceptance and independence from parental constraints. As a result, they rely on peer rules and beliefs for personal direction and reject opposing parental demands. However, when faced with the crisis of serious illness, they may consider themselves alienated from peer associations and unable to communicate with their parents for emotional support. Therefore, they may feel virtually alone in their struggle. Support groups or other means of networking with adolescents facing death may be useful.

Healthy adolescents must deal with several maturational crises, such as the acceptance of bodily changes and socialisation of intensifying sexual impulses. Any threat to either task increases their vulnerability to the stress of coping with such crises. The devastation of a terminal illness and the effects of chemotherapy may be greater concerns than the prospect of dying. Adolescents' orientation to the present compels them to worry about physical changes even more than the prognosis for future recovery.

Nurses can help parents communicate with adolescents by: providing information on typical adolescent responses and coping patterns; acting as role models; avoiding alliances with either parent or child; and allowing parents the opportunity to vent their feelings of frustration, incompetence or failure in an atmosphere of acceptance and without judgment.

Delivery of Palliative Care Services

Once the healthcare team and family have discussed the likelihood of death as the outcome of a child's medical condition or illness, it is necessary to determine the child's and family's preference for the location of palliative care. The circumstances of the child's illness may influence the location in which palliative care is provided. Regardless of the circumstances of the illness or the location of care, it is important to focus on interventions that address all aspects of the child's and family's comfort. This requires attention to the child's physical comfort and the social, emotional and spiritual needs of the child and family. Based on the decision by the child and family regarding their wishes for care, the family has several options from which to choose.

Hospital

Families may choose to remain in the hospital to receive care if the child's illness or condition is unstable and home care is not an option, or the family is uncomfortable with providing care at home. If a family chooses to remain at the hospital for terminal care, make the setting as homelike as possible. Families can bring familiar items from the child's room at home. In addition, develop a consistent and coordinated care plan for the child's and family's comfort.

Community Care

Many children who require palliative care will be looked after in, and by, families, and their choice is often within their local community. There is often a sense of community care and support early in the child's illness which is then well established and in a position to respond as the child's care needs increase. There can be challenges in providing a community care approach due to distance and access to services. There needs to be a collaborative approach to care and good communication in both directions to ensure family-centred care is meet.

Religious and Cultural Considerations

Cultural and religious beliefs influence how a family reacts to illness and death, and often lead to rituals that will be performed at the time of death and in bereavement. Nurses caring for children and their families at these times need to have understanding of and respect for these cultural and religious needs. In saying that, it is important that assumptions are not made on the grounds of ethnicity or religion due to anything that may be encountered within any given group. The most effective way of understanding is to communicate with the family and be aware of their cultural and religious needs. Seek out the assistance of written material in different languages or interpreter services where needed to assist with this information gathering. Palliative Care Australia has produced Multicultural Palliative Care Guidelines which serve as a useful guide to some of the issues that may be encountered (Taylor & Box 1999). Ministry of Health—Manatū Hauora revised and updated the National Framework for Palliative Care Nursing in Aotearoa New Zealand which assists with specific strategies for children and families (Palliative Care Nurses New Zealand 2014).

NURSING CARE OF THE CHILD AND FAMILY AT THE END OF LIFE

Management of Pain and Suffering

Unfortunately, terminally ill children commonly report the presence of unrelieved pain and other distressing symptoms (Downing 2020, Broden et al 2020). One of the great fears for children and families dealing with terminal illness is that of unrelieved pain. However, in the majority of circumstances it is possible to effectively control pain with analgesic/pain relieving medications.

Distressing symptoms can have detrimental effects on the child's quality of life and long-lasting negative effects on the family after the child's death. Parents report that having their child in pain was unendurable and resulted in feelings of helplessness and a sense that they must be present and vigilant to get the necessary pain medications. Persistent pain also has an impact on the family as a whole. Nurses can alleviate the fear of pain and suffering by providing interventions aimed at treating the pain and symptoms associated with the terminal process in children. It is important to adopt an individualised approach to pain relief, taking into account the unique circumstances of each child and family. Each symptom should be addressed, with consideration given to aetiology and the most effective therapy.

Pain and Symptom Management

When the pain and symptoms experienced by dying children are being managed, it is important to clearly communicate the intent of any interventions proposed. For example, many children with progressive cancer may be given 'palliative chemotherapy' or 'palliative radiotherapy'. The healthcare team and family must understand that the goal of these treatments is either to increase comfort by slowing the progression of an incurable tumour (palliative chemotherapy) or to reduce swelling or pressure from a tumour that is causing pain (palliative radiation).

Occasionally children require very high doses of opioids to control pain. This may occur for several reasons. The child on long-term opioid pain management can become tolerant of the drug, so more drug must be given to maintain the same level of pain relief. This is not to be confused with addiction, which is a psychological dependence on the side effects of opioids. Addiction is not a factor in managing terminal pain in a child, and the nurse plays an important role in educating parents that their child will not become addicted. Other reasons for increasing dosages of opioids include progression of disease and other physiological causes of pain. It is important to understand that there is no maximum dosage that can be given to control pain. However, nurses often express concern that administering dosages of opioids that exceed those with which they are familiar will hasten the child's death. The **principle of double effect** addresses such concerns. It provides an ethical standard that supports the use of interventions that have the intention of relieving pain and suffering even though there is a foreseeable possibility that death may be hastened. In cases in which the child is terminally ill and in severe pain, using large doses of opioids and sedatives to manage pain is justified when no other treatment options are available that would relieve the pain but make the possibility of death less likely. (See Chapter 5 for an extensive discussion of pain assessment and management.)

In addition to medications, non-pharmacological interventions may also reduce the perception of pain and can sometimes decrease the amount of pain medication that is needed, thereby reducing unwanted side effects. These interventions include providing soothing surroundings, avoiding excessive lighting, ensuring a pleasant room temperature and having pleasant smells in the room. Other techniques such as music therapy, distraction and guided imagery should be combined with medications to provide the child and family strategies to control pain. Often families will have insight into the things that comfort their child, and this input should be encouraged because it not only helps the child but may also provide the family with comfort (Downing 2020, Kain & Mannix 2018). Children may be empowered and find added relief with the use of complementary techniques such as acupuncture, guided imagery, relaxation training, meditation and distraction (stories, videos, music, bubble blowing and singing). Children can also be taught techniques to use during painful procedures. A range of physical therapies could also be considered for the child in pain. Touch, massage, warmth, cold and electrical therapies are all used in the management of various types of pain (Kain & Mannix 2018).

Children may experience a variety of symptoms besides pain during their terminal course, either as a result of their disease process or as a side effect of medicines used to maintain their comfort (Box 19.9). The underlying disease and previous treatment history will contribute to the types and severity of symptoms the individual child experiences during the dying process. Nurses caring for children who are receiving palliative care for a terminal condition or illness assess frequently for any symptoms that are causing the child physical distress. Assessment includes information regarding the symptom's onset, severity, duration and effect on the child's quality of life.

Parents' and Siblings' Need for Education and Support through the Caregiving Process

Often, as the child's illness worsens, parents and other family members are the primary caregivers while the child is at home. This role can create physical, emotional and financial strain on the larger family system. Therefore, parents and other family members caring for dying children have a number of educational and support needs.

Educational Needs

Family caregivers need comprehensive education about various aspects of the care that they are providing to their child. This preparation can ease feelings of helplessness and anxiety and provide a sense of competence as they move from caring for an ill child to caring for a dying child. This education begins early in the transition from curative to palliative care. Table 19.4 provides some common areas of educational needs of family caregivers and suggestions on how nurses can assist families in meeting these needs. Education about physical care is best provided as the need arises. Instructing parents too early in the signs and symptoms of respiratory distress or the method of stopping a nosebleed can increase the parents' anxiety.

BOX 19.9 Common Symptoms Experienced by Dying Children

Pain
- Visceral pain
- Bone pain
- Neuropathic pain

Gastrointestinal
- Anorexia
- Nausea and vomiting
- Constipation
- Diarrhoea

Genitourinary
- Urinary tract infections
- Urinary retention

Haematological
- Anaemia
- Bleeding

Respiratory
- Cough
- Congestion
- Secretions
- Shortness of breath
- Wheezing

Central nervous system
- Fatigue
- Fevers, chills
- Sleep disturbance
- Restlessness, agitation
- Seizures

Integumentary
- Dry skin
- Rash, itching
- Pressure sores
- Oedema

Emotional
- Fear
- Anxiety
- Depression

Emotional Support

Members of the family can be overwhelmed by powerful emotions that can threaten their ability to cope. Anger, guilt, anxiety and helplessness are normal feelings that many parents experience and often project onto other members of the family or healthcare team. Nurses assisting these families cannot prevent parents from feeling this way; however, they can assist the family in recognising the normalcy of these emotions and in identifying ways in which to cope. A wide network of emotional support is important to parents, such as family members, nurses, paediatricians and other healthcare providers, but parents also find comfort in support from non-familiar individuals through social media (Tan et al 2012, Broden et al 2020).

Spiritual and Religious Support

Meeting the spiritual or religious needs of the child and family is as important as teaching caregiving techniques. Because many families rely on religion or spirituality for emotional support, the degree to which these needs are met successfully may determine how well the child and family cope with the dying process (Broden et al 2020). Parents say religion and spirituality both sustain hope for a positive outcome and provide a way to cope with less desirable circumstances and outcomes. Additionally, many families use religion and spirituality as a source of guidance during complex medical decision-making.

Sibling Support

It is important to consider the needs of siblings experiencing the death of a brother or sister (Fig 19.2). As mentioned earlier, the developmental stage and level of maturity of the siblings will have a strong influence on the feelings and behaviours exhibited as their brother's or sister's illness progresses and their care intensifies. Siblings may feel isolated and displaced during the time that a brother or sister is dying. Parents devote the majority of their time to the care and comfort of the dying child, which causes siblings to feel left out. Siblings may become resentful of their sick brother or sister and begin to feel guilty or ashamed about such feelings. Simultaneously, siblings may appreciate having responsibilities in the care of their brother or sister and desire to be included to a greater degree (Russell et al 2018). Regular visits by siblings to see their sick sibling in hospital allows them to see what is happening for themselves and to process that their brother or sister is very sick and that they need special care. It is important, however, that they are adequately prepared for what they might see. In the situation where siblings cannot visit, regular updates, video calls and use of digital media can be helpful. It is important to ensure siblings feel included in their sick sibling's lives.

Siblings may benefit from the opportunity to be included in the care of the sick child and be part of the family's care process. Children can help in many ways such as assist with schoolwork, update on TV shows or social media or just assist siblings with drawings or reading. Staff involved in caring for the family may also find opportunities to include siblings, whether this is in the hospital or in the community setting.

Caregiver Support

As the care of the dying child becomes the primary focus of the parent, personal and household needs often take on secondary significance. These tasks, however, can become burdensome and increase the family's stress if not attended to. Nurses can help the family identify ways for friends, community service organisations and extended family members to assist with tasks such as household chores, shopping, meal preparation and laundry.

Care at the Time of Death

Few parents have cared for a dying child, and thus parents are not prepared to lead their child through the dying process (Fig 19.3). Awareness that the child's death is near allows the parents and family to determine the location and circumstance of the child's death. This allows the family to create a meaningful death for their child, which improves their ability to cope in the difficult days, weeks and years after the child has died. Nurses have an important role in helping parents recognise the changes in their child that signal that death may be near (see Applying Evidence to Practice box). Further resources to support families can be found in most Australian states and territories and in New Zealand. The main contacts are Palliative Care Australia (02 6232 0700) and National Paediatric Palliative Care Network: Starship (New Zealand; General Enquiries 09 367 0000, ssfis@adhb.govt.nz).

Physical Changes

Physical changes can vary widely among children and are often more pronounced in children dying of prolonged illness or disability. Generally, as the child progresses through the dying process, there is an overall decline in the child's physical condition.

TABLE 19.4 Preparation and Education of Family Caregivers

Needs of Family Caregivers	Professional Interventions
PRACTICAL NEEDS	
Is home care or care in the hospital appropriate for my child?	Explore the family's preferences for home care or hospital care as appropriate.
How will we pay for end-of-life care at home, in the hospital or in a hospice?	Evaluate the family's funding source and provide resources and assistance as necessary.
Where do I get equipment and supplies? How does the equipment work? Whom do I call if equipment malfunctions?	Provide the family with appropriate telephone numbers and contact people for questions about equipment and medical care.
How should we arrange our house to best meet the needs of our child? Will there be help available to us at home?	Plan for availability of caregivers (i.e. parents, family, friends, professionals) and help coordinate a schedule for provision of care.
Whom do I call for medical questions?	Provide a contact person for the family to call with concerns or questions.
PERSONAL CARE	
How do I give my child a bed bath? How do I wash my child's hair in bed? How do I change linen with my child in bed? How do I perform skin care? How do I perform mouth care? How do I administer medications?	Instruct all caregivers about providing daily care to the child. Provide written instruction and reference material for caregivers to review.
What do I do if my child does not want to eat? Is there something I can do to get my child to eat? Does my child need supplements or a special diet?	Assess the child's nutritional status and parents' view on supplemental nutrition. Educate the family on decreased nutritional needs and potential complications from overfeeding or overhydration.
PHYSICAL CARE	
How do I assess my child's pain? When should I give pain medications? What do I do when pain management is ineffective?	Assess the child's current comfort status and educate the family on current interventions. Educate the family about assessing the child's comfort level. Instruct the family that the child may be uncomfortable for a variety of reasons (e.g. constipation, anxiety, fever, headache, muscle cramp, disease) and educate the family about the appropriate interventions for particular circumstances.
What should I do when our child is constipated or has diarrhoea? How do I control nausea and vomiting? What do I do if my child has a fever? What do I do if my child has seizures? What do I do if my child has trouble breathing?	Provide an accessible supply of medications that can help alleviate discomfort (e.g. laxatives, sedatives, antipyretics). Encourage the caregiver to telephone a contact person about questions or ineffective interventions.
ACTIVITY AND SOCIAL INTERACTIONS	
Can we safely travel and enjoy family gatherings with our child? In which activities can we engage our child?	Encourage the family to engage in fun and memorable activities with the child.
Should friends and family be encouraged to visit?	Encourage visitors when appropriate.
What interventions can I do to help my child relax and rest comfortably?	Encourage the family to use relaxation techniques that have previously been beneficial to the child.

Emotional Changes

As children approach death, they may begin to recall events that were important with their families. They may want to draw pictures or leave messages for important friends and family. Often children begin to reassure their parents and other significant people that they are not afraid and are ready to die.

During the final few days to hours of death, children may experience visions of 'angels' or people and talk with them (Barnes & Rowe 2013). They may mention that they are not afraid and that someone is waiting for them. Often these visions are of family members or friends who have preceded them in death. In most instances these visions provide a comforting presence and reassurance for the child and family. Not all children will express these types of experiences.

Care of the Family Experiencing Unexpected Childhood Death

In cases of long-term, potentially fatal illnesses, families may experience anticipatory grief. Parents mourn the loss of their child long before the death. They are reminded of their child's uncertain future each time they see the pain the child must endure or experience the sudden loss of hope during a relapse. This prolonged period of anticipatory grief provides families with the opportunity to complete 'unfinished business', such as helping the child and siblings understand and cope with a fatal prognosis. Many families reflect on their changed perspective of time after learning of the diagnosis, particularly their heightened awareness of the value of each day.

Death resulting from accident or trauma, or from acute illness in settings such as the emergency department or intensive care unit, often

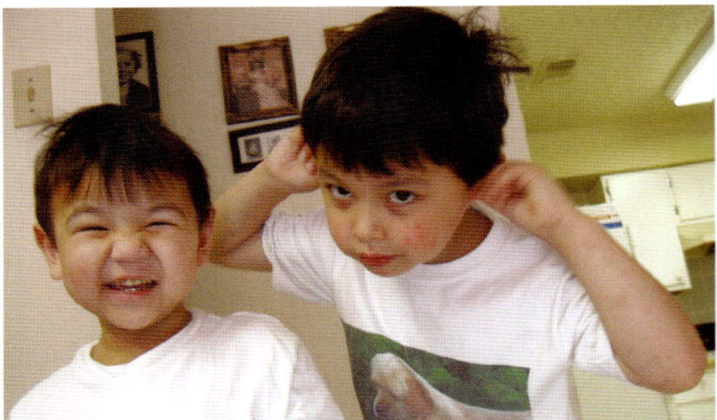

Fig 19.2 It is important to consider the needs of siblings experiencing the death of a brother or sister.

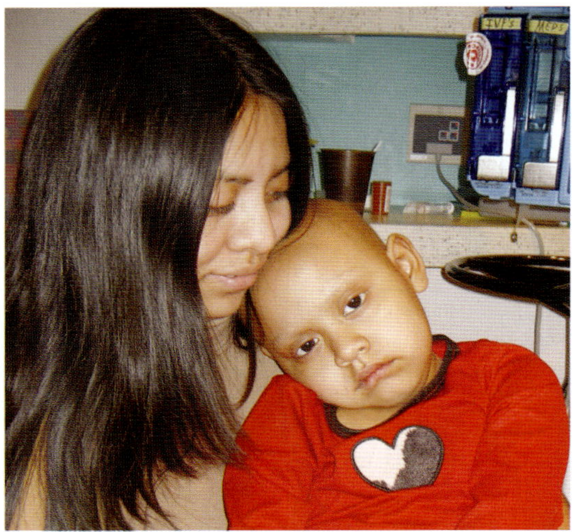

Fig 19.3 For the dying child there is no greater comfort than the security and closeness of a parent.

requires the active withdrawal of some form of life-supporting intervention, such as a ventilator or bypass machine. These situations frequently raise difficult ethical issues, and parents are often less prepared for the actual moment of death (Box 19.10). Nurses can assist parents by providing detailed information about what will happen as supportive equipment is withdrawn, ensuring that appropriate pain medications are administered to prevent pain during the dying process and allowing the parents time to be with and speak to their child before the start of the withdrawal.

SPECIAL DECISIONS AT THE TIME OF DYING AND DEATH

People are often unprepared to cope with the numerous decisions that must be made when a loved one is dying or dies. When the death is expected, there is the opportunity to make plans in advance, such as where the child should spend the last days or what types of funeral arrangements are desired. When death is unexpected, the shock is sufficient to render the survivors incapable of making even simple decisions. Those in attendance at the death and those caring for the dying child can be instrumental in initiating decisions that may facilitate the grief process. The following is a brief review of selected instances in which nurses can guide parents in making decisions related to the expected or unexpected death.

BOX 19.10 Strategies for Intervention with Survivors After Sudden Childhood Death

Arrival of the Family

- Meet the family immediately and escort to a private area.
- A healthcare worker with bereavement training should remain with the family.
- Provide information about the extent of illness or injury and treatment efforts.
- If the healthcare worker must leave the family or if the family requests privacy, return in 15 minutes so the family does not feel forgotten.
- Provide tissues, telephone and tea/coffee.

Pronouncement of Death

- When available, the family's own medical practitioner should inform them of the child's death.
- Alternatively, the medical practitioner or nurse should introduce himself or herself and establish calm, reassuring eye contact with the parents.
- Honest, clear communication that avoids misinterpretation is essential.
- Non-verbal communication such as remaining with the family in silence may be most empathetic.
- Acknowledge the family's guilt, attempt to alleviate it and deal openly and non-judgmentally with anger.
- Provide information, answer questions and offer reassurance that everything possible was done for the child.

Viewing of the Body

- Offer the parents the opportunity to see the body; repeat the offer later if they decline.
- Before viewing, inform the parents of bodily changes they should expect (tubes, injuries, cold skin).
- A single staff member should accompany the family but remain inconspicuous.
- Offer the opportunity to hold the child.
- Allow the family as much time as they need.
- Offer parents the opportunity for siblings to view the body.

Formal Concluding Process

- Discuss and answer questions concerning autopsy and funeral arrangements; obtain signatures on the body release and autopsy forms.
- Provide anticipatory guidance regarding symptoms of grief response and their normalcy.
- Provide written materials about grief symptoms.
- Escort the family to the exit or to their car if necessary.
- Provide a follow-up phone call in 24 to 48 hours to answer questions and provide support.
- Provide referral for community health nursing visit.
- Provide referrals to local support and resource groups (e.g. bereavement groups, bereavement counsellors, sudden infant death syndrome groups).

Advance Care Planning

Discussing advance care planning with children and families is one of the most difficult—but unfortunately the most important—things a paediatrician must do for the dying child and the family. It can bring feelings of sadness, guilt and fear to the forefront and make the situation very raw and death of a child close. It is a conversation that must occur and the nurse often needs to be the one to begin this conversation. Avoiding this discussion denies children and families the opportunity to voice an opinion, and to have a choice about the care they really want to receive and where and how they want that care provided. Advance care planning is 'a process of discussions between families and healthcare providers about preferences for care. It enables treatments and goals in the context of the patient's current and anticipated future health' (Xafis et al 2015). The objective is to determine the overall goal of not just medical care, and also the interventions that the child and family wish to have provided, but also, just as importantly, what they do not wish to have provided and implemented. This then guides treatment, particularly when the child begins to show signs of deterioration in condition. These decisions and discussions may evolve and progress over time and possibly change but the process must begin as soon as possible. This process of thinking ahead is becoming increasingly important as technological advances see more children survive with chronic and complex medical conditions (Broden et al 2020).

Viewing of the Body

Although most institutions recognise the need for parents to hold and spend time with the dead child, a dilemma may arise when the body is mutilated. Although the memory of the child's disfigurement can be extremely upsetting and can generate concern regarding how much the child suffered, not seeing the body can leave the parents with imagined ideas of how their child looked. This can be worse than the reality, and it can delay the acceptance of the death. When family members choose to view the body, they need preparation for this upsetting experience. The nurse should inform them about what to expect and why certain parts of the body are covered or bandaged.

Organ or Tissue Donation and Autopsy

For some families this may be a meaningful act—one that benefits another human being despite the loss of their child. Unfortunately, initiating a discussion about tissue donation is often stressful for staff, and there may be confusion regarding whose responsibility this is. In centres in which transplants are performed, a full-time transplant coordinator is usually available to inform the family about organ donation and to take care of details. When possible, the topic is raised before death occurs.

Discussion of the option to donate organs is always separate from communication of impending or actual death.

Nurses need to be aware of common questions about organ donation so they can help families make an informed decision. Healthy children who die unexpectedly are excellent candidates for organ donation. Children who have cancer, chronic disease or infection or who have suffered prolonged cardiac arrest may not be suitable candidates, although this is individually determined.

In cases of unexplained death, violent death or suspected suicide, autopsy is required by law.

Siblings' Attendance at Funeral Services

One of the most frequent concerns of parents is whether young or school-age children should attend funeral or burial services. Sharing moments of deep significance with parents helps children understand

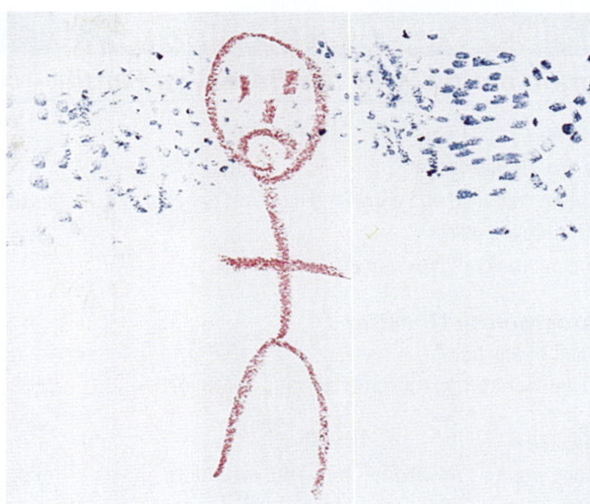

Fig 19.4 Drawing made by a 7-year-old child whose sister died in a car crash. The drawing shows the boy sad and crying (dots are tears) because he was not allowed to see his dead sibling.

the experience and deal with their own feelings, and depriving them of this opportunity may leave children with lifelong regrets (Fig 19.4). However, a child should never be forced to attend a post-death service. Children need preparation for post-death services (Downing 2020). They should be told what to expect, particularly how the deceased person will look if the coffin is open. Ideally, a parent explains the details to the child. If the parent's grief prevents this communication, a significant family member or friend should substitute.

CARE OF THE GRIEVING FAMILY

No event is more devastating for families than the threatened or actual loss of a child. Families, especially parents, are deprived of the joy and fulfilment of watching a child grow. All family members are affected by the loss, and their needs must be recognised to facilitate their grief process.

In expected death, the child and family are generally involved in the plan for interventions both before and after the death. In unexpected death, the survivors face the tremendous task of integrating the loss into their lives, with no opportunity for anticipatory grief. In either situation nurses can facilitate the grief process by having a basic understanding of the process. Helpful strategies include being aware of expected reactions, talking with family members, ascertaining their needs and supporting their efforts to cope, adapt and grieve (see Applying Evidence to Practice box). Applying the principles of family-centred care is as important at this time as at any other.

APPLYING EVIDENCE TO PRACTICE

Communicating with the Bereaved Family

Examples of Non-therapeutic Statements

Advice

- You should get out more.
- Stop feeling sorry for yourself.
- You need to be strong for your family.

Cheerfulness

- Now, now, don't cry; cheer up.
- Cheer up, you can always have another baby.

Interpretation

- It was God's will.
- It's better now because she is at peace.

Reassurance

- I know how you feel.
- Don't worry, everything will work out.
- At least you still have the rest of your family.

Argument

- How can you say that?
- It's wrong to blame anyone.
- You should be glad his suffering is over.

Ignoring the Loss

- Remember, you're young and can still have another baby.
- It could be worse; he could have lived with severe brain damage.

Continued

APPLYING EVIDENCE TO PRACTICE

Communicating with the Bereaved Family—cont'd

Examples of Therapeutic Statements

Focus on Feelings
- You seem confused and angry; tell me what is happening for you.
- You are feeling pain.
- Tell me more about how you are feeling.

Non-judgmental Questions
- Can I be of any help?
- Can I contact anyone for you or assist if possible?

Clarification
- Correct me if I'm wrong, but you intend to make all the arrangements.
- I'm not sure I understand. Tell me more about __________.

Explanations
- You can touch her and hold her if you wish.

Concern, Support, Empathy
- Your daughter's birthday is near. That must be painful to deal with.
- It's okay to cry.
- It sounds like you have been doing some painful thinking.

Support, Silence
- I'm here if you want to talk. (Silence)
- Hello. (Touch, silence)

Assessment of Coping and Support
- Do you have friends and family who can help you now?
- You have been through a lot. How are you doing now?
- Is there someone who can drive you home?

Validation of Loss
- You have been through a very tough time.
- He was a special boy to all the staff. I will miss him.

Grief

Grief is not a single event, but is rather the process of experiencing physiological, psychological, behavioural, social and spiritual reactions to the loss of a child. Grief is highly individualised, encompassing a broad range of manifestations from person to person. It is a natural and expected reaction to loss. It is neither orderly nor predictable. Grieving is often necessary for healing to occur. When death is the expected or a possible outcome of a disorder, the child and family members may experience anticipatory grief. Anticipatory grief may be manifested in varying behaviours and intensities. It may be characterised by denial, anger, depression and other psychological and physical symptoms. Anticipatory guidance may assist grieving family members. Healthcare professionals emphasise that grief reactions such as hearing the dead person's voice, feeling distant from others or seeking reassurance that they did everything possible for the lost person are normal, necessary and expected. These reactions in no way signify poor coping or an approaching mental breakdown. On the contrary, such behaviours signify that the survivor is working through the acute grief. They are a necessary part of grief work. Anticipatory guidance regarding the mourning process may be helpful to families so that they can recognise the normalcy of their experiences.

It is important to recognise that some family members may experience 'complicated' grief. **Complicated grief reactions** (those that continue more than a year after the loss) include such symptoms as intense intrusive thoughts, pangs of severe emotion, distressing yearnings, feelings of being excessively alone and empty, unusual sleep disturbance and maladaptive levels of loss of interest in personal activities. An unexpected, sudden death is a risk factor for complicated grief (Haley 2016). Bereaved persons experiencing such prolonged and complicated grief are referred to an expert in grief and bereavement counselling.

Parental Grief

The grief of parents after the death of a child has been found to be a more intense, complex, long-lasting and fluctuating grief experience than that of other bereaved individuals. Although parents experience the primary loss of their child, many secondary losses are felt, such as the loss of part of one's self, hopes and dreams for the child's future, the family unit, prior social and emotional community supports and often spousal support. It is common for parents of the same child to experience different grief reactions.

Studies involving bereaved parents have shown that grieving does not end by the severing of the bond with the deceased child but rather involves a continuing bond between the parent and the dead child (Scholtes & Browne 2015). Parental resolution of grief is a process of integrating the deceased child into daily life in which the pain of losing a child is never completely gone but lessens. There are occasions of brief relapse but not to the degree experienced when the loss initially occurred. Thus parental grief work is never completed and is a timeless process of accepting the new reality of being without a child, as it changes over time. Although parents are expected to grieve the loss of their child, parental grief is often minimised, which leaves parents to work through their grief in isolation and silence.

Sibling Grief

Each child grieves in his or her own way and on his or her own timeline. Children, even adolescents, grieve differently from adults. Adults and children differ more widely in their reactions to death than in their reactions to any other phenomenon. Children of all ages grieve the loss of a loved one, and their understanding and reactions to death depend on their age and developmental level (Table 19.5). Children often grieve for a longer duration than adults, revisiting their grief as they grow and develop new understandings of death. However, rather than grieving continually, they tend to grieve in spurts and can be emotional and sad one moment and then, just as quickly, off and playing.

Children express their grief through play and other behaviours. They can be exquisitely attuned to their parents' grief and try to protect them by not asking questions and avoiding upsetting them. This can set the stage for the sibling to try to become the 'perfect child'. Children exhibit many of the grief reactions of adults, including physical sensations and illnesses, anger, guilt, sadness, loneliness, withdrawal, acting out, regression, sleep disturbances, isolation and search for meaning. Again, nurses are attentive for signs that siblings are struggling with their grief and provide guidance to parents when possible.

TABLE 19.5 Children's Understanding of and Reactions to Death

Concepts of Death	Reactions to Death	Interventions
	INFANTS AND TODDLERS	
Death has least significance to children younger than 6 months of age. After parent–child attachment and the development of trust is established, the loss, even if temporary, of the significant person is profound. Prolonged separation during the first several years is thought to be more significant in terms of future physical, social and emotional growth than at any subsequent age. Toddlers are egocentric and can only think about events in terms of their own frame of reference: living. Their egocentricity and vague separation of fact and fantasy make it impossible for them to comprehend absence of life. Instead of understanding death, this age group is affected more by any change in lifestyle.	With the death of someone else, they may continue to act as though the person is alive. As children grow older, they will be increasingly able and willing to let go of the dead person. Ritualism is important; a change in lifestyle could be anxiety producing. This age group reacts more to the pain and discomfort of a serious illness than to the probable fatal prognosis. This age group also reacts to parental anxiety and sadness.	Help parents deal with their feelings, allowing them more emotional reserve to meet the needs of their children. Encourage parents to remain as near to the child as possible, yet be sensitive to the parents' needs. Maintain as normal an environment as possible to retain ritualism. If a parent has died, encourage the establishment of a consistent caregiver for the child. Promote primary nursing.
	PRESCHOOL CHILDREN	
Children of this age believe their thoughts are sufficient to cause death; the consequence is a feeling of guilt, shame and punishment. Their egocentricity implies a tremendous sense of self-power and omnipotence. They usually have some sense of the meaning of death. Death is seen as a departure, a kind of sleep. They may recognise the fact of physical death but do not separate it from living abilities. Death is seen as temporary and gradual; life and death can change places with one another. There is no understanding of the universality and inevitability of death.	If they become seriously ill, they conceive of the illness as a punishment for their thoughts or actions. They may feel guilty and responsible for the death of a sibling. Their greatest fear concerning death is separation from their parents. They may engage in activities that seem strange or abnormal to adults. With fewer defence mechanisms to deal with loss, young children may react to a less significant loss with more outward grief than to the loss of a significant person. The loss is so deep, painful and threatening that the child must deny it for the time being to survive its overwhelming impact. Behavioural reactions such as giggling, joking, attracting attention or regressing to earlier developmental skills indicate children's need to distance themselves from tremendous loss.	Help parents deal with their feelings, allowing them more emotional reserve to meet the needs of their children. Help parents to understand behavioural reactions of their children. Encourage parents to remain near the child as much as possible, to minimise the child's great fear of separation from parents. If a parent has died, encourage establishment of a consistent caregiver for the child. Promote primary nursing.
	SCHOOL-AGE CHILDREN	
These children still associate misdeeds or bad thoughts with causing death and feel intense guilt and responsibility for the event. Because of their higher cognitive abilities, they respond well to logical explanations and comprehend the figurative meaning of words. They have a deeper understanding of death in a concrete sense. They particularly fear the mutilation and punishment they associate with death. They personify death as the devil, a monster or the bogeyman. They may have naturalistic-physiological explanations of death. By age 9 or 10, children have an adult concept of death, realising that it is inevitable, universal and irreversible.	Because of their increased ability to comprehend, they may have more fears; for example: • the reason for the illness • communicability of the disease to themselves or others • consequences of the disease • the process of dying and death itself • fear of the unknown, which is greater than their fear of the known. The realisation of impending death is a tremendous threat to their sense of security and ego strength. They are likely to exhibit fear through verbal uncooperativeness rather than actual physical aggression. They are interested in post-death services. They may be inquisitive about what happens to the body.	Help parents deal with their feelings, allowing them more emotional reserve to meet the needs of their children. Encourage parents to remain near the child as much as possible, yet be sensitive to the parents' needs. Because of children's fear of the unknown, anticipatory preparation is very important. Because the developmental task of this age is industry, interventions of helping children maintain control over their bodies and increasing their understanding allow them to achieve independence, self-worth and self-esteem and avoid a sense of inferiority. Encourage children to talk about their feelings and provide aggressive outlets. Encourage parents to honestly answer questions about dying rather than avoiding questions or fabricating euphemisms. Encourage parents to share their moments of sorrow with their children. Provide preparation for post-death services.

Continued

TABLE 19.5 Children's Understanding of and Reactions to Death—cont'd

Concepts of Death	Reactions to Death	Interventions
	ADOLESCENTS	
Adolescents have a mature understanding of death. They are still very much influenced by remnants of magical thinking and are subject to feelings of guilt and shame. They are likely to see deviations from accepted behaviour as the reason for their illness.	Adolescents straddle transition from childhood to adulthood. They have the most difficulty in coping with death. They are least likely to accept the cessation of life, particularly if it is their own. Concern for the present is much greater than for the past or the future. They may consider themselves alienated from their peers and unable to communicate with their parents for emotional support, feeling alone in their struggle. Adolescents' orientation to the present compels them to worry about physical changes even more than the prognosis. Because of their idealistic view of the world, they may criticise funeral rites as barbaric, money making and unnecessary.	Help parents deal with their feelings, allowing them more emotional reserve to meet the needs of their children. Avoid alliances with either parent or child. Structure hospital admission to allow for maximum self-control and independence. Answer adolescents' questions honestly, treating them as mature individuals and respecting their needs for privacy, solitude and personal expressions of emotions. Help the parents understand their child's reactions to death and dying, especially that concern for present crises, such as loss of hair, may be much greater than concern for future ones, including possible death.

Mourning

Shock and Disbelief

Shock, numbness and disbelief are seen during the immediate phase of grief. As one parent described, 'We were as prepared for our son's death as anyone could be, but it was a shock when in a moment his life was finished. I just can't get over the rapidity with which life ends'. This temporary numbness protects the survivors from the overwhelming pain associated with grief. Decisions are often made automatically, and only certain details are remembered.

Expression of Grief

When the numbness fades, a period of intense grief begins, characterised by loneliness and yearning for the deceased. During this stage many of the signs of acute grief are evident, and physical complaints such as appetite changes and an inability to sleep are common. There is a tendency to review the events of the deceased's life and to evaluate the relationship with the loved one. Feelings of guilt and anger are common at this time.

Disorganisation and Despair

During the stage of disorganisation and despair, the pain of the loss is replaced primarily by emptiness, apathy and deep depression. There is a feeling that life has no meaning and that the pain will never end. This is particularly relevant for parents. For example, mothers often comment that they feel they have suffered a double loss—loss of their child and loss of the mothering role. Feelings of estrangement from other loved ones are common, and social isolation may foster the depression.

Reorganisation

Reorganisation refers to recovery from the loss. During this gradual process the survivors again find meaning in living, readjust to life without the deceased, develop new or renewed relationships and learn to live with the memory of the deceased with much less pain. This never means that the loved one is forgotten and the pain is gone. There always remains a deep ache that is never totally replaced with happiness and one that returns more intensely; for example, on holidays or anniversaries.

A Grandparent's Grief

Grandparents experience a unique 'double grief' when a child dies. Not only do they lose a grandchild, they witness the pain and suffering that their own child is experiencing. They generally experience feelings of helplessness and hopelessness as they cannot console their own child who is feeling great pain and grief, while dealing with their own grief.

When a grandchild dies, grandparents may feel a range of emotions such as hurt, pain and suffering but often the attention is on grieving parents and siblings and grandparents often are forgotten or seen as the 'rocks' of the family and depended on to keep the family together. It is important to acknowledge the intensity and the range of feeling that they too are experiencing. They too need understanding, support and information. Grandparents often share a special bond with their grandchild and experience a very unique loss of their dreams and hopes for their grandchild's future.

Grandparents may also feel great sadness and guilt due to regret that they did not spend a lot of time with their grandchild. This may compound the grief experienced when a grandchild dies in this situation and bring some tension to the family. Inclusion of all family members must be acknowledged.

THE NURSE AND THE CHILD WITH LIFE-THREATENING ILLNESS

Nurses' Reactions to Caring for Children with Life-threatening Illnesses

Nurses experience grief and moral distress as they become aware that a child's death is inevitable. Furthermore, nurses experience compassion fatigue as a result of cumulative losses over time as children they care for die and inflict unnecessary pain (Green et al 2016). Reflection on these experiences and feelings, knowledge of the grief process and care of oneself are essential for the nurse to provide effective care to dying children and their families (Brandon et al 2014, Bloomer et al 2016).

Denial

When children are admitted to a paediatric unit with a suspected diagnosis of a serious illness, the initial response from some nurses is shock and denial. However, their behavioural reaction may be withdrawal from the child and family. They choose the 'cure' philosophy over the 'care' philosophy as a method of distancing themselves from the implications of emotional involvement. Because of their own dependency on denial, some nurses may inappropriately support denial in parents. There are several methods of conveying this message, such as emphasising only optimistic 'survival statistics', negating the seriousness of the illness, focusing on 'cheering up' the family and engaging in casual conversation to avoid meaningful dialogue. Although this increases nurses' comfort in caring for the dying child, it does little to help family members progress beyond denial and begin anticipatory grieving.

Anger and Depression

Some nurses may be angry for having been assigned to the 'leukaemia case', for example, because the very exposure to potential failure in a fatal illness is extremely threatening. Others may feel angry for having to subject the child to painful procedures or for being unable to relieve the child's physical and emotional suffering. Instead of anger, some nurses may feel depression for any of these reasons.

Without understanding the reason for the emotion, however, nurses may project the anger onto others, particularly family members. They may be unable to tolerate the child's uncooperative behaviour or the parents' continual requests for information. Anger fuels more anger, and parents react with hostility and think the members of the nursing staff are rejecting them. A vicious circle of resentment, mistrust and frustration may result.

Depression also has adverse effects on the therapeutic relationship because nurses may withdraw from the child and parents as a method of controlling their sadness. Unaware of the reason for the avoidance, family members interpret it as evidence of inadequate care. This reaction also fosters a non-supportive cycle of avoidance, withdrawal, resentment and frustration. However, the messages are usually more covert than when the nurses' reaction is anger and may prevent a climax that could result in a solution to the problem.

Guilt

Nurses who feel unable to deal with fatal illness in a child often experience guilt. Nurses who become angry or depressed when caring for a dying child often reveal that they are uncomfortable with this response, but they feel unable to choose a more direct and constructive approach. They express guilt for having been intolerant of the child's or parents' behaviours, and they realise the missed opportunity to provide these individuals with professional support and guidance.

The one important difference between a dying child and an ill child is that there may be no second chance to meet the needs of the dying child. This finality is difficult to comprehend but can lead to a better understanding of one's own responses to dying. For example, when guilt makes an individual uncomfortable enough to seek alternative behaviour patterns, there is an opportunity for change, provided the individual is given some assistance and support.

Ambivalence

One of the most universal reactions of nurses is ambivalence in their feelings towards a dying child. There is the fluctuating adherence to hope for a cure and fear of a relapse. Sometimes the motivations for both are more for personal needs. For example, the nurse may hope that the child recovers to avoid readmissions. Such thoughts are certainly understandable in light of the emotional toll of nursing a dying child.

Coping with Stress

Paediatric critical care and oncology nurses surveyed about work stresses ranked patient death as the most stressful, yet one of the most rewarding, experiences. The less experienced the nurse, the more likely that death is rated as a stressor. Furthermore, nurses overestimated the percentage of deaths on their units, which suggests that the experience overwhelms them.

One stress-related outcome of caring for dying children is **burnout**—a state of physical, emotional and mental exhaustion. It occurs as a result of prolonged involvement with individuals in situations that are emotionally demanding. Nurses working in intensive care units are particularly prone to this occupational hazard, but staff nurses also can experience it when dealing with certain groups of children, such as those who may die. Avoiding burnout and coping constructively, effectively and therapeutically with children who are dying and their families require a deliberate and concerted effort on the part of the nurse.

Self-awareness

The initial step in effectively caring for a dying child is making a deliberate choice to become involved. Many nurses react negatively to the word *involvement* because they believe that professionals must remain uninvolved to maintain objectivity. Involvement does not displace objectivity. On the contrary, allowing oneself to feel with the other person expands one's ability to comprehend the meaning and depth of their emotion (see Family-Centred Care box). Ideally the nurse achieves detached concern, which allows sensitive, understanding care because the nurse is sufficiently detached to make objective, rational decisions.

Knowledge and Practice

Intervening therapeutically with terminally ill children and their families demands more than self-awareness. It also requires that nursing practice be based on sound theoretical formulations and empirical observations that provide a general, concise analysis of the typical reactions of families.

Involvement does carry the potential risk of clouding objectivity, but awareness of one's reactions and investments in the care of a dying child minimise this hazard. Developing awareness requires the willingness to investigate one's motivations for choosing to work in such an area, to understand the stresses inherent in the role, to review one's resolution of past losses and to contemplate one's own fears of death. Often nurses who have a cold, impersonal reaction to dying patients come to realise that their reaction stems from previous unresolved conflicts or losses. Once they are able to talk about such experiences, they are usually able to gain insight into their behaviour and begin to develop alternative methods of reacting.

Nurses also must explore ethical issues surrounding the definition of death, the use of extraordinary and lifesaving measures versus allowing the child to die and patients' rights to know and choose their own destinies. Once nurses have soundly formulated the principles by which to practise, they need opportunities for decision-making. When a team approach is used, nurses can be valuable members of the group if their own values have been clarified and they have critically assessed the family's responses.

Support Systems

Support systems are essential to continued functioning in a high-stress environment. They allow nurses to regenerate energies by sharing feelings and concerns with others. Dealing with feelings about death in isolation can lead to repressed feelings such as denial, anger and depression. These feelings may be manifested in poor interactions among staff, inappropriate or non-supportive interactions with families, an inability to evaluate care plans or advocate for families and a need to control. Support is an important catalyst for processing feelings about death.

Social supports may be personal family members such as parents or spouses, extended relatives and friends. Professional supports include colleagues, consultants, teachers and supervisors. Peers may be sources of technical and practical advice. Because the death of a patient is more stressful for a less experienced nurse, a mentoring relationship between a senior nurse and the less experienced nurse may provide support and role modelling and assist in the development of effective coping strategies. Forums for staff support and opportunities for debriefing after deaths have been shown to facilitate adaptive coping responses and enhance provider–patient relationships.

Other Strategies

Any number of other strategies may be used to reduce stress. These include maintaining good general health practices, especially regular exercise, and participating in diversionary activities that are of personal interest beyond the workplace. Distancing techniques are also effective, such as leaving work at work, informing other staff not to contact one on one's days off, periodically assuming less demanding assignments and taking time off when needed (Koy et al 2017). Mindfulness-based meditation may be another effective strategy to decrease stress and regain a sense of control among nurses experiencing compassion fatigue and burnout.

A final technique is to focus on the positive aspects of the caregiving role. Despite the difficult times in caring for these children and families, many rewarding experiences must be remembered. Dedicated efforts reap numerous rewards, and these must not be forgotten or minimised. Reflection on positive feedback from appreciative families can revitalise self-esteem and job satisfaction.

Some nurses find shared remembrance rituals useful in resolving grief. Similarly, attending the funeral services can be a supportive act for both the family and the nurse and in no way detracts from the professionalism of care. For the family it conveys a sense of worth and caring by the nurse. For the nurse it can provide a sense of closure with the family and facilitate the grief process (Box 19.11).

BOX 19.11 Nurses Experiencing the Stress of Caregiving: Strategies that Help

Recognise the inevitability of the child's death—One's own unrealistic expectations can cause the greatest grief due to the belief that something more should or could have been done to prevent the child's death. Shift the focus of care to providing guidance and comfort for the child and family to increase a sense of accomplishment. Avoid self-blame for situations over which you have no control.

Develop knowledge and apply it—Increase personal knowledge about caring for dying children and their families. Apply this knowledge to provide the best possible care to the patient and family.

Identify ways the work setting can provide support—Ask for relief from highly emotional or conflicted situations, take time off and have a holiday, seek mentorship and make use of institutional support services such as multidisciplinary team meetings or employee assistance personnel.

Provide briefings—Inform others involved in the child's care about the child's condition and changes as they occur. After the death, notify caregivers who were closely involved to allow them the opportunity to grieve for the child.

Provide debriefings—Organise staff remembrance services to share experiences and feelings, 'bereavement' rounds and multidisciplinary team review of care.

Find meaning—Accept that even the death of a child is a part of life and find meaning in the caregiving experience with the child and family. Reflect on the experience, what it meant and how it influenced your view on nursing care.

Separate work and personal life—Develop strategies to leave work behind when at home with family. Avoid trips to the hospital on days off.

Take care of yourself—Recognise the stress of caring for dying children and find healthy activities to help manage that stress. Exercise, good nutrition and rest are important when work stress is high.

Say goodbye—Identify comfortable ways to say goodbye to the dead child. Attending memorial or funeral services, keeping a memento, journalling, making plantings and so on are all individual ways to acknowledge the importance of the child to the caregiver.

REFERENCES

Australian Institute of Health and Welfare (AIHW). (2020). Australia's Children. Chronic conditions and burden of disease. Australian Government. https://www.aihw.gov.au/reports/children-youth/australias-children/contents/health/chronic-conditions

Barnes, S., Gardiner, C., Gott, M., et al. (2012). Enhancing patient-professional communication about end-of-life issues in life-limiting conditions: a critical review of the literature. Journal of Pain and Symptom Management, 44(6), 866–879.

Barnes, M. & Rowe, J. (2013). Child, Youth and Family Health: Strengthening Communities. (2nd Ed). Churchill Livingstone, Elsevier.

Bloomer, M., Endacott, R., Copnell, B. et al. (2016). 'Something normal in a very, very abnormal environment' – Nursing work to honour the life of dying infants and children in neonatal and paediatric intensive care in Australia. Intensive & Critical Care Nursing, 33, 5–11.

Brandon, D. H., Ryan, D., Sloane, R. et al. (2014). Impact of a Pediatric Quality of Life Program on providers' patterns of moral distress. The American Journal of Maternal Child Nursing, 39, 189–197. PMID:24759312.

Broden, E., Deatrick, J., Ulrich, C., et al. (2020). Defining a 'Good Death' in the Pediatric Intensive Care Unit. American Journal of Critical Care, 29(2), 111–121.

Coad, J., Patel, R., & Murray, S. (2014). Disclosing terminal diagnosis to children and their families: palliative professionals' communication barriers. Death Studies, 38(1–5), 302–307.

Cohen, J. A., Mannarino, A. P., & Deblinger, E. (2016). Treating trauma and traumatic grief in children and adolescents. Guilford Publications.

Cole, M. & Foito, K. (2019). Pediatric end-of-life simulation: preparing the future nurse to care for the needs of the child and family. Journal of Pediatric Nursing, 44, e9–e12.

Craig, E., McDonald, G., Adams, J., et al. (2012). Te Ohonga Ake. The Health of Māori Children and Young People with Chronic Conditions and Disabilities in New Zealand. Dunedin: New Zealand Child and Youth Epidemiology Service, University of Otago.

Davies, B., Sehring, S. A., Partridge, J. C., et al. (2008). Barriers to palliative care for children: perceptions of pediatric health care providers. Pediatrics, 121(2), 282–288.

Downing, J. (2020). Children's Palliative Care: An International Case-Based Manual. Champaign, IL: Springer International Publishing: Imprint: Springer.

Dupont-Thibodeau, A., Hindié, J., Bourque, C. J., et al. (2017). Provider perspectives regarding resuscitation decisions for neonates and other vulnerable patients. The Journal of Pediatrics, 188, 142–147.e3.

Enguidanos, S., Housen, P., Penido, M. et al. (2014). Family members' perceptions of inpatient palliative care consult services: a qualitative study. Palliative Medicine, 28(1), 42–48.

Ferrell, B. R., Wittenberg, E., Battista, V., et al. (2016). Exploring the spiritual needs of families with seriously ill children. International Journal of Palliative Nursing, 22(8), 388–394.

Friedrichsdorf, S. J. (2017). Contemporary Pediatric Palliative Care: Myths and Barriers to Integration into Clinical Care. Current Pediatric Reviews 13(1), 8–12.

Goudie, A., Narcisse, M. R., Hall, D. E., et al. (2014). Financial and psychological stressors associated with caring for children with disability. Families, Systems and Health: The Journal of Collaborative Family Healthcare, 32(3), 280–290.

Green, J., Darbyshire, P., Adams, A., et al. (2016). It's agony for us as well: Neonatal nurses reflect on iatrogenic pain. Nursing Ethics, 23(2), 176–190.

Haley, C. (2016). Pillitteri's Child and Family Health Nursing in Australia and New Zealand. (2nd Ed). Wolters Kluwer.

Hartling, L., Milne, A., Tjosvold, L., et al. (2014). A systematic review of interventions to support siblings of children with chronic illness or disability. J Paediatric Child Health, 50(10), E26–E38.

Hill, D. L., Miller, V., Walter, J. K., et al. (2014). Regoaling: a conceptual model of how parents of children with serious illness change medical care goals. BMC Palliative Care, 13(1), 9.

Hiscock, H., O'Loughlin, R., Pelly, R., et al. (2020). Strengthening care for children: pilot of an integrated general practitioner–paediatrician model of primary care in Victoria, Australia. Collingwood: CSIRO. Australian Health Review, 44(4), 569–575.

Jacobs, S., Perez, J., Cheng, Y. I., et al. (2015). Adolescent end-of-life preferences and congruence with their parents' preferences: Results of a survey of adolescents with cancer. Pediatric Blood Cancer, 62(4), 710–714.

Jalmsell, L., Kontio, T., Stein, M., et al. (2015). On the child's own initiative: Parents communicate with their dying child. Death Studies, 39(2), 111–117.

Kain, V. & Mannix, T. (2018). Neonatal nursing in Australia and New Zealand: principles for practice. Chatswood, NSW: Elsevier.

Keele, L., Keenan, H. T., Sheetz, J., et al. (2013). Differences in characteristics of dying children who receive and do not receive palliative care. Pediatrics, 132(1), 72–78.

Koy, V., Yunibhand, J., Angsuroch, Y., et al. (2017). Relationship between nursing care quality, nurse staffing, nurse job satisfaction, nurse practice environment, and burnout: literature review. International Journal of Research in Medical Sciences, 3(8), 1825–1831.

Larcher, V., Craig, F., Bhogal, K., et al. (2015). Making decisions to limit treatment in life-limiting and life-threatening conditions in children: a framework for practice. Archives of Disease in Childhood, 100, s1–s23.

Leemann, T., Bergstraesser, E., Cignacco, E., et al. (2020). Differing needs of mothers and fathers during their child's end-of-life care: secondary analysis of the 'Paediatric end-of-life care needs' (PELICAN) study. London: BioMed Central. BMC Palliative Care, 19(1), 1–118.

Levine, D., Lam, C. G., Cunningham, M. J., et al. (2013). Best practices for pediatric palliative cancer care: a primer for clinical providers. The Journal of Supportive Oncology, 11(3), 114–125.

Lotz, J. D., Daxer, M., Jox, R. J., et al. (2017). 'Hope for the best, prepare for the worst': A qualitative interview study on parents' needs and fears in pediatric advance care planning. Palliative Medicine, 31(8), 764–771.

Mastro, K. A., Johnson, J. E., McElvery, N., et al. (2015). The benefits of a nurse-driven, patient- and family-centred pediatric palliative care program. The Journal of Nursing Administration, 45(9), 423–428.

Palliative Care Nurses New Zealand. (2014). A National Professional Development Framework for Palliative Care Nursing Practice in Aotearoa New Zealand. Wellington: Ministry of Health. https://www.health.govt.nz/publication/national-professional-development-framework-palliative-care-nursing-aotearoa-new-zealand

Randolph, A. G., Zollo, M. B., Egger, M. J., et al. (1999). Variability in physician opinion on limited pediatric life support. Pediatrics, 103, e46.

Russell, C. E., Widger, K., Beaune, L. et al. (2018). Siblings' voices: a prospective investigation of experiences with a dying child. Death Studies, 42(3), 184–194.

Scholtes, D., & Browne, M. (2015). Internalized and externalized continuing bonds in bereaved parents: their relationship with grief intensity and personal growth. Death Studies, 39(2), 75–83.

Sercu, M., Beyens, I., Cosyns, M., et al. (2018). Rethinking end-of-life care and palliative care: learning from the illness trajectories and lived experiences of terminally ill patients and their family carers. Qualitative Health Research, 28(14), 2220–2238.

Sisk, B. A., DuBois, J., Kodish, E., et al. (2017). Navigating Decisional Discord: The Pediatrician's Role When Child and Parents Disagree. Pediatrics, 139(6), e20170234.

Stein, R. E. K. (1985). Home care: a challenging opportunity. Children's Health Care: Journal of the Association for the Care of Children's Health, 14(2), 90–95.

Tan, J., Docherty, S. L., Barfield, R. et al. (2012). Addressing parental bereavement support needs at the end of life for infants with complex chronic conditions. Journal of Palliative Medicine, 15(5), 579–584.

Taylor, A. & Box, M. (1999). Multicultural Palliative Care Guidelines. Palliative Care Australia. https://palliativecare.org.au/wp-content/uploads/2015/05/Multicultural-palliative-care-guidelines.pdf

Thompson, L. A., Knapp, C., Madden, V., et al. (2009). Pediatricians' perceptions of and preferred timing for pediatric palliative care. Pediatrics, 123(5), e777–e782.

Toomey, S. L., Chien, A. T., Elliott, M. N., et al. (2013). Disparities in unmet need for care coordination: the national survey of children's health. Pediatrics, 131(2), 217–224.

Weaver, M. S., Heinze, K. E., Bell, C. J., et al. (2016). Establishing psychosocial palliative care standards for children and adolescents with cancer and their families: An integrative review. Palliative Medicine, 30(3), 212–223.

Wiener, L., McConnell, D. G., Latella, L., et al. (2013). Cultural and religious considerations in pediatric palliative care. Palliative and Supportive Care, 11(1), 47–67.

Wolfelt, A. (2013). Helping children cope with grief. Routledge.

World Health Organization (WHO). (2018). Integrating palliative care and symptom relief into paediatrics: a WHO guide for health care planners, implementers and managers. https://www.who.int/publications/i/item/integrating-palliative-care-and-symptom-relief-into-paediatrics

Wyatt, K. D., List, B., Brinkman, W. B., et al. (2015). Shared decision making in pediatrics: a systematic review and meta-analysis. Academic Pediatrics, 15(6), 573–583.

Xafis, V., Wilkinson, D., & Sullivan, J. (2015). What information do parents need when facing end-of-life decisions for their child? A meta-synthesis of parental feedback. BMC Palliative Care, 14(1), 19.

Younge, N., Smith, P. B., Godlberg, R. N., et al. (2015). Impact of a palliative care program on end-of-life care in a neonatal intensive care unit. Journal of Perinatology, 35(3), 218–222.

Yu, J., Schenker, Y., Maurer, S., et al. (2019). Pediatric palliative care in the medical neighborhood for children with medical complexity. Families Systems & Health, 37(2), 107–119.

20

Impact of Cognitive or Sensory Loss on the Child and Family

Andrea Middleton

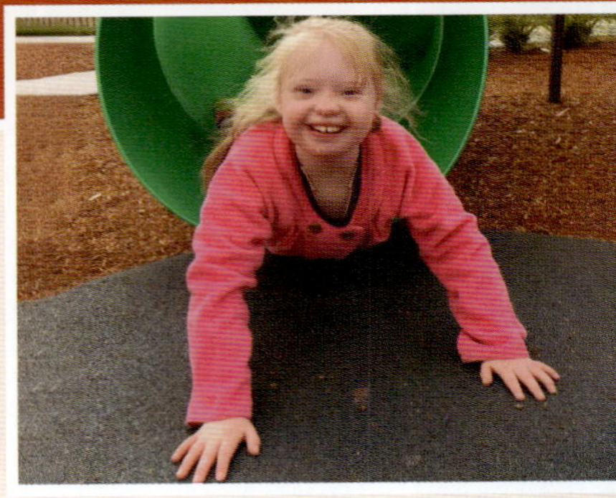

LEARNING OUTCOMES

- Outline common conditions that affect cognition and sensory perception of infants, children and adolescents.
- Understand the challenges faced by infants, children and adolescents with cognitive or sensory losses and their families.
- Explore the therapeutic management of common conditions that impact on cognition and sensory perception of infants, children and adolescents.
- Identify opportunities for nurses to advocate for and support infants, children or adolescents with common conditions that impact cognition and sensory perception.

COGNITIVE DISABILITY

General Concepts

Cognitive disability (CD) is a general term that encompasses any type of intellectual disability and affects from 2.5% to 3% of the population (Ageranioti-Belanger et al 2012, Bellman et al 2013, Shapiro & Batshaw 2016). The term *intellectual disability* (formerly *mental retardation*) has become the most common internationally used term (American Psychiatric Association 2013, Tasse et al 2013). In this chapter, the term CD is used synonymously with *intellectual disability.*

Intellectual disability is a disability that is present from birth or occurs in the developmental period and is characterised by significant subaverage intellectual functioning and limitations in adaptive functioning. Intellectual functioning is measured by the intelligence quotient (IQ) test score. The American Psychiatric Association's *Diagnostic and Statistical Manual of Mental Disorders, Fifth Edition* (DSM-5) criteria recommend moving away from exclusively relying on IQ testing towards using additional measures of adaptive functioning (American Psychiatric Association 2013, Moran 2013). The DSM-5 is the diagnostic standard used in Australia and New Zealand and states that the child with CD must demonstrate deficits in adaptive functioning that result in failure to meet developmental and sociocultural standards for personal independence and social responsibility (Moran 2013).

Diagnosis and Classification

The diagnosis of CD is usually made after professionals or the family suspects that the child's developmental progress is delayed. In some cases, it is confirmed at birth because of recognition of distinct syndromes. At the other extreme, the diagnosis is made when problems such as speech delays or school problems arouse concern. In all cases a high index of suspicion for developmental delay and behavioural signs is necessary for early diagnosis, and routine developmental screening can assist in early identification. Delays are typically seen in gross and fine motor and speech development, although the latter is most predictive. Developmental disability can be described as any significant lag or delay in a child's physical, cognitive, behavioural, emotional or social development when compared against developmental norms. CD is an impairment encompassing intellectual ability and adaptive behaviour that are functioning significantly below average. In the absence of clear-cut evidence of CD, it is more appropriate to use a diagnosis of developmental disability.

Results of standardised tests are helpful in contributing to the diagnosis of CD. Tests for assessing adaptive behaviours include the Vineland Adaptive Behaviour Scale (Vineland-3) and the Adaptive Behaviour Assessment System (ABS–third edition). Informal appraisal of adaptive behaviour may be made by those fully acquainted with the child (e.g. teachers, parents, other care providers). Frequently, these observations lead parents to seek evaluation of the child's development.

Aetiology

The causes of severe CD are primarily genetic, biochemical and infectious. Although the aetiology is unknown in the majority of cases, familial, social, environmental and organic causes may predominate. Among individuals with CD, a sizeable proportion of the cases are linked to Down syndrome, fragile X syndrome (FXS) or fetal alcohol syndrome. General categories of events that may lead to CD include the following (Gilissen et al 2014, Hoyme et al 2016, Katz & Lazcano-Ponce 2008, Mefford et al 2012):

- infection and intoxication, such as congenital rubella, syphilis, maternal drug consumption (e.g. fetal alcohol syndrome), chronic lead ingestion or kernicterus
- trauma or physical agent (e.g. injury to the brain experienced during the prenatal, perinatal or postnatal period)
- inadequate nutrition and metabolic disorders, such as phenylketonuria or congenital hypothyroidism
- gross postnatal brain disease, such as neurofibromatosis and tuberous sclerosis
- unknown prenatal influence, including cerebral and cranial malformations, such as microcephaly and hydrocephalus

- chromosomal abnormalities resulting from radiation; viruses; chemicals; parental age; and genetic mutations that occur in disorders such as Down syndrome and FXS
- gestational disorders, including prematurity, low birth weight and postmaturity
- psychiatric disorders that have their onset during the child's developmental period up to age 18 years, such as autism spectrum disorders (ASDs)
- environmental influences, including evidence of a deprived environment associated with a history of intellectual disability among parents and siblings.

NURSING CARE OF CHILDREN WITH IMPAIRED COGNITIVE FUNCTION

Nurses play a major role in identifying children with CD. In the newborn and early infancy periods, few signs are present, except in such disorders as Down syndrome (discussed later in this chapter). However, delayed developmental milestones are the major clues to CD. In addition, nurses must have a high index of suspicion for early behaviour patterns that may suggest CD. Parental concerns, such as delayed development compared with siblings, need to be taken seriously. All children should receive regular developmental assessment, and the nurse is often the person responsible for performing such assessments. When delays are found, the nurse must use sensitivity and discretion in revealing this finding to parents.

Educate Child and Family

To teach children with CD, one must investigate their learning abilities and deficits. This is important for the nurse who may be involved in a home care program or who may be caring for the child in a school or healthcare setting. The nurse who understands how these children learn can effectively teach them basic skills or prepare them for various health-related procedures.

Children with CD have a marked deficit in their ability to discriminate between two or more stimuli because of difficulty in recognising the relevance of specific cues. However, these children can learn to discriminate if the cues are presented in an exaggerated, concrete form and if all extraneous stimuli are eliminated. For example, the use of colours to emphasise visual cues or the use of singing or rhymes to stress auditory cues can help them learn. Their deficit in discrimination also implies that concrete ideas are learned much more effectively than abstract ideas. Therefore demonstration is preferable to verbal explanation, and learning should be directed towards mastering a skill rather than understanding the scientific principles underlying a procedure.

Another cognitive deficit is in short-term memory. Whereas children of average intelligence can remember several words, numbers or directions at one time, children with CD are less able to do so. Therefore they need simple, one-step directions. Learning through a step-by-step process requires a task analysis in which each task is separated into its necessary components and each step is taught completely before proceeding to the next activity.

One critical area of learning that has had a tremendous impact on education for cognitively impaired individuals is motivation or the use of positive reinforcement to encourage the accomplishment of specific tasks or behaviours. Advances in technology have greatly aided in providing reinforcement, especially in children with severe disabilities and who may have physical disabilities that limit their range of capabilities.

Early intervention program is a systematic program of therapy, exercises and activities designed to address developmental delays in children with disabilities to help achieve their full potentials (Bull 2011, Crnic et al 2017, Guralnick 2017). Considerable evidence indicates that these programs are valuable for cognitively impaired children. Nurses working with these families need to be aware of the types of programs in their community.

Parents should enquire about these programs by contacting the appropriate agencies. Early intervention exposure includes structured educational programs, parent training and family-intervention training with available family resources that tend to be associated with more positive developmental and behavioural outcomes in children with CD (Crnic et al 2017, Guralnick 2017, Wallander et al 2014). As children grow older, their education should be directed towards vocational training that prepares them for as independent a lifestyle as possible within their scope of abilities.

Teach Child Self-care Skills

When a child with CD is born, parents often need assistance in promoting normal developmental skills that other children learn easily. There is no way to predict when a child should be able to master self-care skills, such as feeding, toileting, dressing and grooming because a wide age variability exists in the cognitively impaired child who is able to accomplish such functions.

Teaching self-care skills also necessitates a working knowledge of the individual steps needed to master a skill. For example, before beginning a self-feeding program, the nurse performs a task analysis. After a task analysis, the child is observed in a particular situation, such as eating, to determine what skills are possessed and the child's developmental readiness to learn the task. Family members are included in this process because their 'readiness' is as important as the child's. Numerous self-help aids are available to facilitate independence and can help eliminate some of the difficulties of learning, such as using a plate with suction cups to prevent accidental spills.

Promote Child's Optimal Development

Optimal development involves more than achieving independence. It requires appropriate guidance for establishing acceptable social behaviour and personal feelings of self-esteem, worth and security. These attributes are not simply learned through a stimulation program. Rather, they must arise from the genuine love and caring that exist among family members. However, families need guidance in providing an environment that fosters optimal development. Often the nurse can provide assistance in these areas of childrearing.

Another important area for promoting optimal development and self-esteem is ensuring the child's physical wellbeing. Any congenital defects, such as cardiac, gastrointestinal or orthopaedic anomalies, should be repaired. Plastic surgery may be considered when the child's appearance can be substantially improved. Dental health is significant, and orthodontic and restorative procedures can improve facial appearance immensely.

Encourage Play and Exercise. Children who are cognitively impaired have the same need for play and exercise as any other child. However, because of the children's slower development, parents may be less aware of the need to provide such activities. Therefore the nurse will need to guide parents towards selection of suitable play and exercise activities. Because play has been discussed for children in each age group in earlier chapters, only the exceptions are presented here.

The type of play is based on the child's developmental age, although the need for sensorimotor play may be prolonged. Parents should use every opportunity to expose the child to as many different sounds, sights and sensations as possible. Appropriate toys include musical mobiles, stuffed toys, floating toys, a rocking chair or horse, a swing, bells and rattles. The child should be taken on outings, such as trips to

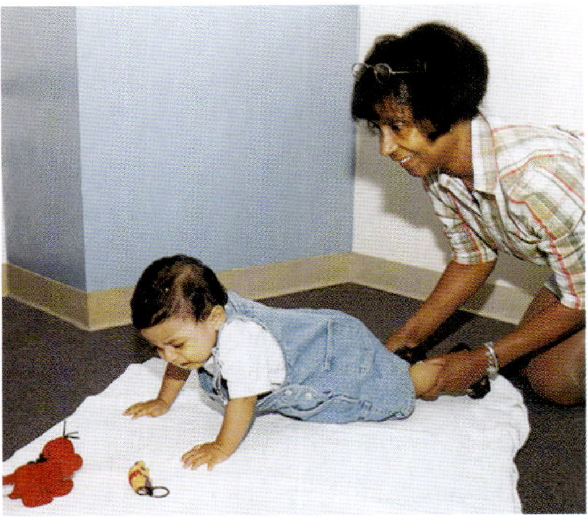

Fig 20.1 Placing an attractive object outside the child's reach encourages crawling movements. (Source: Courtesy of James DeLeon, Texas Children's Hospital, Houston, TX.)

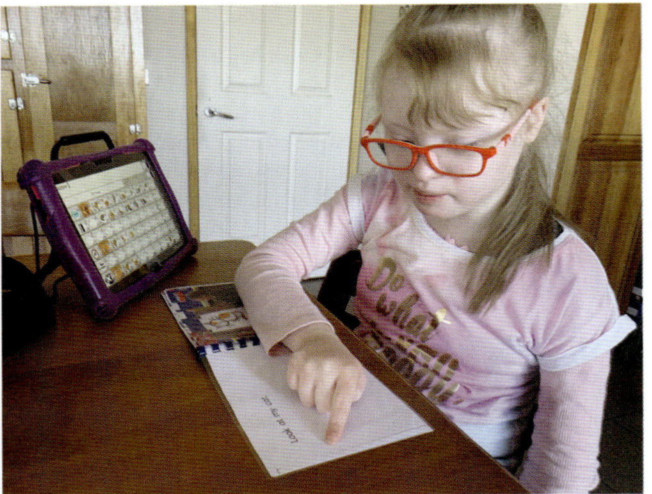

Fig 20.2 A young child can use technology for educational needs.

the grocery store or shopping centre. Other people should be encouraged to visit in the home, and individuals should relate directly to the child through means such as cuddling, holding, rocking and talking to the child in the face-to-face fashion.

Toys are selected for their recreational and educational value. For example, a large inflatable beach ball is a good water toy; it encourages interactive play and can be used to learn motor skills, such as balance, rocking, kicking and throwing. Attractive toys encourage a child to reach, therefore assisting in the development of motor skills (see Fig 20.1). Musical toys that mimic animal sounds or respond with social phrases are excellent ways of encouraging speech. A doll with removable clothes and different types of fasteners can help the child learn dressing skills. Toys should be simple in design so that the child can learn to manipulate them without help. For children with severe cognitive and physical impairment, electronic switches can be used to allow them to operate toys (Figs. 20.2 and 20.3).

Suitable activities for physical activity are based on the child's size, coordination, physical fitness and maturity, motivation and health (see Fig 20.3). Some children may have physical problems that prevent participation in certain sports, such as atlantoaxial instability in children with Down syndrome (discussed later in this chapter). These

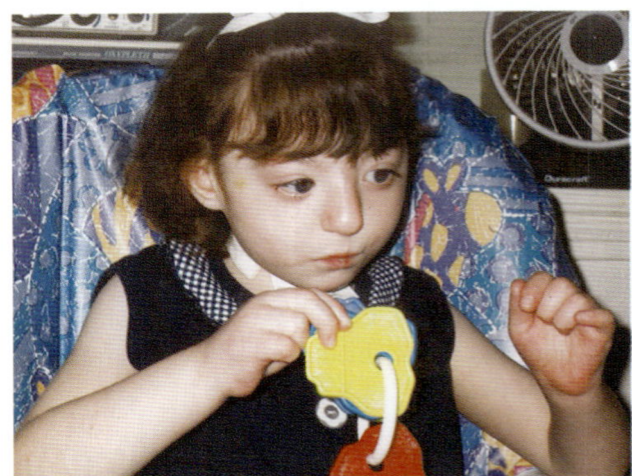

Fig 20.3 A favourite toy provides stimulation for a young child.

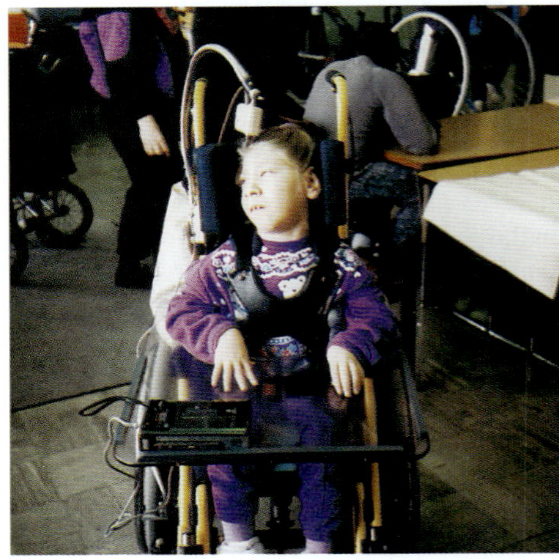

Fig 20.4 A child with cognitive and physical difficulties can activate electronic and communication equipment by moving a device near her head.

children often have greater success in individual and dual sports than in team sports and enjoy themselves most with children of the same developmental level.

Safety is a major consideration in selecting recreational and exercise activities. For example, toys that may be appropriate developmentally may present dangers to a child who is strong enough to break them or use them incorrectly.

Provide Means of Communication. Verbal skills are typically delayed more than other physical skills. Speech requires adequate hearing and interpretation (receptive skills) and facial muscle coordination (expressive skills). Because both receptive and expressive skills may be impaired, these children need frequent audiometric testing and should be fitted with hearing aids if indicated. In addition, they may need help in learning to control their facial muscles. For example, some children may need tongue exercises to correct the tongue thrust or gentle reminders to keep the lips closed.

Non-verbal communication may be appropriate for some of these children, and various devices are available. For children with physical limitations, several adaptations or types of communication devices are available to facilitate selection of the appropriate picture or word (Fig 20.4). Some children may be taught sign language or Blissymbols—a highly stylised system of graphic symbols representing words, ideas and concepts. Although the symbols require education to learn their meaning, no reading skill is required. The symbols are typically arranged on a board, and the person points or uses some type of selector to convey a message.

Establish Discipline. Discipline must begin early. Limit-setting measures need to be simple, consistently applied and appropriate for the child's mental age. Control measures are based primarily on teaching a specific behaviour rather than on understanding the reasons behind it. Stressing moral lessons is of little value to a child who lacks the cognitive skills to learn from self-criticism or evaluation of previous mistakes. Behaviour modification, especially reinforcement of desired actions, and use of time-out procedures are appropriate forms of behaviour control.

Encourage Socialisation. Acquiring social skills is a complex task, as is learning self-care procedures. Active rehearsals with role-playing and practice sessions and positive reinforcement for desired behaviour have been the most successful approaches. Parents should be encouraged early to teach their child socially acceptable behaviour: waving goodbye, saying 'hello' and 'thank you', responding to their name, greeting visitors and sitting modestly. The teaching of socially acceptable sexual behaviour is especially important to minimise sexual exploitation. Parents also need to expose the child to strangers so that he or she can practise manners because there is no automatic transfer of learning from one situation to another.

Dressing and grooming are also important aspects of self-esteem and social acceptance. Clothes should be clean, age appropriate and well fitted with self-adhering fasteners and elastic openings to facilitate self-dressing.

Opportunities for social interaction and infant stimulation programs should began at an early age. As soon as possible, parents should enrol their child in early intervention or other appropriate preschool programs. Not only do these programs provide education and training, but they also offer an opportunity for social interaction with other children and adults. As children grow older, they should have peer experiences similar to those of other children, including group outings, sports and organised activities (Bull 2011, Sanchack & Thomas 2016, Shapiro & Batshaw 2016).

Provide Information on Sexuality. Adolescence may be a particularly difficult time for parents, especially in terms of the child's sexual behaviour, possibility of pregnancy, future plans to marry and ability to be independent. Frequently, minimal anticipatory guidance has been offered to parents to prepare the child for physical and sexual maturation. The nurse should help in this area by providing parents with information about sexuality education that is geared to the child's developmental level. For example, adolescent girls need a *simple* explanation of menstruation and instructions on personal hygiene during the menstrual cycle.

These adolescents also need practical sexual information regarding anatomy, physical development and conception. Because they are easy to persuade and lack judgment, they need a well-defined, concrete code of conduct with specific instructions for handling certain situations. The subtleties of social sexual behaviour are less beneficial than specific instructions for handling certain situations. For example, an adolescent should be firmly told never to go alone anywhere with any person that he or she does not know well. To protect the child or adolescent from sexual abuse, parents must closely observe their child's or adolescent's activities and associates. The question of contraceptive protection for these adolescents is often a parental concern (Quint & O'Brien 2016).

Help Family Adjust to Future Care

Not all families are able to cope with home care of children who have a cognitive disability, especially those who have severe or profound CD or multiple disabilities. Older parents may not be able to continue care responsibilities after they reach retirement or older age. The decision regarding residential placement is a difficult one for families, and the availability of such facilities varies widely. The nurse's role includes assisting parents in investigating and evaluating programs and helping parents adjust to the decision for placement.

Care for the Child During Hospitalisation

Caring for the child during hospitalisation can be a special challenge. Frequently, nurses are unfamiliar with children who are cognitively impaired, and they may cope with their feelings of insecurity and fear by ignoring or isolating the child. Not only is this approach non-supportive; it may also be destructive to the child's sense of self-esteem and optimum development, and it may impair the parents' ability to cope with the stress of the experience. To prevent engaging in this non-therapeutic approach, nurses are encouraged to use the mutual participation model in planning the child's care.

When the child is admitted, a detailed history is taken, with special focus on all self-care abilities. Questions about the child's abilities are approached positively. For example, rather than asking, 'Is your child toilet trained yet?' the nurse may state, 'Tell me about your child's toileting habits'. The assessment should also focus on any special devices that the child uses, effective measures of limit setting, unusual or favourite routines and any behaviours that may require intervention. If the parent states that the child engages in self-stimulatory or self-enjurious activities (e.g. head banging, self-biting), the nurse should enquire about events that precipitate them and techniques (e.g. distraction, medication) that the parents use to manage them (Morano et al 2017, Oliver & Richards 2010).

The nurse also assesses the child's functional level of eating and playing; ability to express needs verbally; progress in toilet training; and relationship with objects, toys and other children. The child is encouraged to be as independent as possible in the hospital.

Explain procedures to the child using methods of communication that are at the appropriate cognitive level. Generally, explanations should be simple, short and concrete, emphasising what the child will physically experience. Demonstration either through actual practice or with visual aids is always preferable to verbal explanation. Include parents in preprocedural teaching to aid in the child's learning and to help the nurse learn effective methods of communicating with the child.

During hospitalisation, the nurse should also focus on growth-promoting experiences for the child. For example, hospitalisation may be an excellent opportunity to emphasise to parents abilities that the child does have but has not had the opportunity to practise, such as self-dressing. It may also be an opportunity for social experiences with peers, group play or new educational and recreational activities. For example, one child who had the habit of screaming and kicking demonstrated a definite decrease in those behaviours after he learned to pound pegs and use a punching bag. Hospitalisation may also offer parents a respite from everyday care responsibilities and an opportunity to discuss their feelings with a concerned professional.

Assist in Measures to Prevent Cognitive Disability

Besides having a responsibility to families with a child with CD, nurses also need to be involved in programs aimed at preventing CD. Many of the familial, social and environmental factors known to cause mild impairment are preventable. Counselling and education can reduce or eliminate such factors (e.g. poor nutrition, cigarette smoking, chemical abuse) which increase the risk of prematurity and intra-uterine growth restriction. Interventions are directed towards improving maternal health by educating women regarding the dangers of chemicals, including prenatal alcohol exposure, which affects organogenesis, craniofacial development and cognitive ability. Other preventive strategies that play an important role include adequate prenatal care; optimal medical care of high-risk newborns; rubella immunisation; genetic counselling; and prenatal screening, especially in terms of Down syndrome or FXS. The use of folic acid supplements prevents neural tube defects during pregnancy and during the child-bearing years; the use of newborn screening for treatable inborn errors of metabolism (e.g. congenital hypothyroidism, phenylketonuria and galactosaemia) is appropriate to prevent developmental disabilities in children.

Down Syndrome

Down syndrome is the most commonly occurring chromosomal abnormality. It is estimated that 1 in every 1100 babies born in Australia will have Down syndrome, and 1 in every 1000 births in New Zealand (Down Syndrome Australia [DSA] 2021, New Zealand Down Syndrome Association [NZDSA] n.d.). It occurs in people of all cultures and backgrounds.

Aetiology

The cause of Down syndrome is not known, but evidence from cytogenetical and epidemiological studies supports the concept of multiple causality. Although the cause is unclear, the cytogenetics of the disorder is well established. In most cases, Down syndrome is attributable to an extra chromosome 21 (group G), hence the name non-familial trisomy 21. Although children with trisomy 21 are born to parents of all ages, there is a statistically greater risk in older women, particularly those older than 35 years of age. For example, in women 35 years old, the chance of conceiving a child with Down syndrome is about 1 in 350 live births; but in women 40 years old, it is about 1 in 100. However, the majority (approximately 80%) of infants with Down syndrome are born to women younger than 35 years old because younger women have higher fertility rates (Arumugam et al 2016, DSA 2021, Lee 2016, NZDSA n.d.). About 4% of the cases may be caused by translocation of chromosomes 15 and 21 or 22. This type of genetic aberration is usually hereditary and is not associated with advanced parental age. About 2% to 4% of affected persons demonstrate mosaicism, which refers to a mixture of normal and abnormal chromosomes in the cells. The degree of cognitive and physical impairment has been related to the percentage of cells with the abnormal chromosome makeup. However, numerous other interacting factors are likely to contribute to individual differences and cognitive-level outcomes in Down syndrome, such as early neural development, dietary factors, lifestyle and the environment (Coppede 2016, Karmiloff-Smith et al 2016).

Diagnostic Evaluation

Down syndrome can usually be diagnosed by the clinical manifestations alone (Box 20.1 and Fig 20.5), but a chromosome analysis should be done to confirm the genetic abnormality.

Several physical problems are associated with Down syndrome. Many of these children have congenital heart malformations, the most common being septal defects. Respiratory tract infections are prevalent and, when combined with cardiac anomalies, are the chief causes of death, particularly during the first year of life. Hypotonicity of chest and abdominal muscles and dysfunction of the immune system probably predispose the child to the development of respiratory tract infection. Other physical problems include thyroid dysfunction, especially congenital hypothyroidism and an increased incidence of leukaemia.

Therapeutic Management

Although no cure exists for Down syndrome, a number of therapies are advocated, such as surgery to correct serious congenital anomalies (e.g. heart defects, strabismus). These children also benefit from evaluative echocardiography soon after birth and regular medical care. Evaluation of sight and hearing is essential, and treatment of otitis media is required to prevent auditory loss, which can influence cognitive function. Periodic testing of thyroid function is recommended, especially if growth is severely delayed.

Prognosis

Life expectancy for those with Down syndrome has improved in recent years but remains lower than for the general population. The majority of individuals with Down syndrome survive to approximately 60 years old and beyond (Englund et al 2013, Weijerman & de Winter 2010). As the prognosis continues to improve for these individuals, it will be important to provide for their long-term healthcare and social and leisure needs.

Nursing Care Management

Support the Family at the Time of Diagnosis

Because of the unique physical characteristics, infants with Down syndrome are usually diagnosed at birth, and parents should be informed of the diagnosis at this time. Most parents usually prefer that both of them be present during the informing interview so that they can support one another emotionally. Parents appreciate receiving reading material about the syndrome and being referred to parent groups and/or professional counselling.

Parental responses to the child may greatly influence decisions regarding future care. Whereas some families willingly take the child home, others consider foster care or adoption. The nurse must answer questions regarding developmental potential carefully because the responses may influence the parents' decision. The nurse should share the available informative sources (e.g. parent groups, professional counselling and literature) to help the family learn about Down syndrome (see Critical Thinking Case Study box).

> **CRITICAL THINKING CASE STUDY**
>
> ***Diagnosis of Down Syndrome***
>
> The parents of Melissa, a newborn diagnosed as having Down syndrome, ask the nurse, 'What are we supposed to do with her?' They further state that they already have three other children at home.
>
> 1. What evidence should you consider regarding this condition?
> 2. What additional information is required at this time?
> 3. List the nursing intervention(s) that have the highest priority.
> 4. Identify important patient-centred outcomes with reference to your nursing interventions.
>
> Answers are available at http://evolve.elsevier.com/AU/Speedie/ncic/.

Assist the Family in Preventing Physical Problems. Many of the physical characteristics of infants with Down syndrome present challenges and nursing problems. The hypotonicity of muscles and hyperextensibility of joints complicate positioning. The limp, flaccid extremities resemble the posture of a rag doll; as a result, holding the infant is difficult and cumbersome. Sometimes parents perceive this lack of the infant's moulding to their bodies as evidence of inadequate parenting. The extended body position promotes heat loss because more surface area is exposed to the environment. Encourage the parents to swaddle or wrap the infant snugly in a blanket before picking up the child to provide security and warmth. The nurse also discusses with parents their feelings concerning attachment to the child, emphasising that the child's

BOX 20.1 Clinical Manifestations of Down Syndrome

Head and Eyes
- Separated sagittal suture
- Brachycephaly
- Rounded and small skull
- Flat occiput
- Enlarged anterior fontanel
- Oblique palpebral fissures (upward, outward slant)*
- Inner epicanthal folds
- Speckling of iris (Brushfield's spots)

Nose and Ears
- Small nose*
- Depressed nasal bridge (saddle nose)*
- Small ears and narrow canals
- Short pinna (vertical ear length)
- Overlapping upper helices
- Conductive hearing loss

Mouth and Neck
- High, arched, narrow palate*
- Protruding tongue
- Hypoplastic mandible
- Delayed teeth eruption and microdontia
- Alignment teeth abnormalities (common)
- Periodontal disease
- Neck skin excess and laxity*
- Short and broad neck

Chest and Heart
- Shortened rib cage
- Twelfth rib anomalies
- Pectus excavatum or carinatum
- Congenital heart defects (common; e.g. atrial septal defect, ventricular septal defect)

Abdomen and Genitalia
- Protruding, lax and flabby abdominal muscles
- Diastasis recti abdominis
- Umbilical hernia
- Small penis
- Cryptorchidism
- Bulbous vulva

Hands and Feet
- Broad, short hands and stubby fingers
- Incurved little finger (clinodactyly)
- Transverse palmar crease
- Wide space between big and second toes*
- Plantar crease between big and second toes*
- Broad, short feet and stubby toes

Musculoskeletal and Skin
- Short stature
- Hyperflexibility and muscle weakness*
- Hypotonia
- Atlantoaxial instability
- Dry, cracked and frequent fissuring
- Cutis marmorata (mottling)

Other
- Reduced birth weight
- Learning difficulty (average IQ of 50)
- Hypothyroidism (common)
- Impaired immune function
- Increased risk of leukaemia
- Early-onset dementia (in one-third)

*Most common findings in modified chart (Arumugam et al 2016, Pueschel 1999).

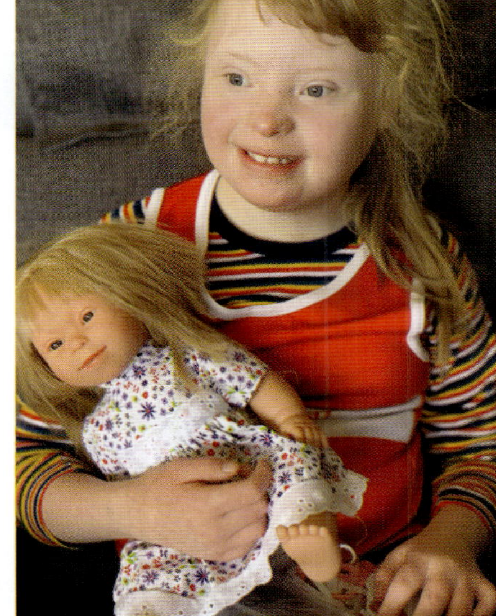

Fig 20.5 A young child with Down syndrome holding a doll with Down syndrome.

lack of clinging or moulding is a physical characteristic and not a sign of detachment or rejection.

Decreased muscle tone compromises respiratory expansion. In addition, the underdeveloped nasal bone causes a chronic problem of inadequate drainage of mucus. The constant stuffy nose forces the child to breathe by mouth, which dries the oropharyngeal membranes, increasing the susceptibility to upper respiratory tract infections. Measures to lessen these problems include clearing the nose with a bulb-type syringe, rinsing the mouth with water after feedings, increasing fluid intake and using a cool-mist vaporiser to keep the mucous membranes moist and the secretions liquefied. Other helpful measures include changing the child's position frequently, practising good hand washing and properly disposing of soiled articles, such as tissues. Inadequate drainage resulting in pooling of mucus in the nose also interferes with feeding. Because the child breathes by mouth, sucking for any length of time is difficult. When eating solids, the child may gag on the food because of mucus in the oropharynx. Parents are advised to clear the nose before each feeding; give small, frequent feedings; and allow opportunities for rest during mealtime.

The protruding tongue also interferes with feeding, especially of solid foods. Parents need to know that the tongue thrust is not an indication of refusal to feed but a physiological response. Parents are advised to use a small but long, straight-handled spoon to push the food towards the back and side of the mouth. If food is thrust out, it should be refed.

Dietary intake needs supervision. Decreased muscle tone affects gastric motility, predisposing the child to constipation. Dietary measures, such as increased fibre and fluid, promote evacuation. The child's eating habits may need careful scrutiny to prevent obesity. Height and weight measurements should be obtained on a serial basis.

During infancy, the child's skin is pliable and soft. However, it gradually becomes rough and dry and is prone to cracking and infection. Skin care involves the use of minimum soap and application of lubricants. Lip balm is applied to the lips, especially when the child is outdoors, to prevent excessive chapping.

Assist in Prenatal Diagnosis and Genetic Counselling. Prenatal diagnosis of Down syndrome is possible through chorionic villus sampling and amniocentesis because chromosome analysis of fetal cells can detect the presence of trisomy or translocation. However, advances in development of non-invasive prenatal testing have resulted in a measurement of cell-free deoxyribonucleic acid (DNA) from the plasma of pregnant women, detecting nearly all cases of Down syndrome (Huang et al 2014, Lee 2016, Lewis et al 2014, Liao et al 2012).

Prenatal testing with genetic counselling should be offered to all women, including those of advanced maternal age (greater than 35 years) and those of younger age (less than 35 years) because most children with Down syndrome are born to younger mothers due to their higher overall birth rate (Lee 2016). If prenatal testing indicates that the fetus is affected, the nurse must allow the parents to express their feelings concerning elective abortion and support their decision to terminate or proceed with the pregnancy. It is important for nurses to be aware of their own attitudes regarding testing and related decisions.

Fragile X Syndrome

Fragile X syndrome (FXS) is the most common inherited cause of CI and the second most common genetic cause of CI or intellectual disability after Down syndrome. It has been described in all cultures, affecting around 1 in 3600 to 4000 males and about 1 in 5000 to 6000 females in Australia and New Zealand (Fragile X Association of Australia [FXAA] 2021, Fragile X New Zealand [FXNZ] 2021). The incidence of carrier girls is 1 in 151, and the incidence of carrier boys is 1 in 468 worldwide (FXNZ 2021, Mink 2016).

The syndrome is caused by an abnormal gene on the lower end of the long arm of the X chromosome. Chromosome analysis may demonstrate a fragile site (a region that fails to condense during mitosis and is characterised by a non-staining gap or narrowing) in the cells of affected males and females and in carrier females. This fragile site has been determined to be caused by a gene mutation that results in excessive repeats of nucleotide in a specific DNA segment of the X chromosome. The number of repeats in a normal individual is between 6 and 50. An individual with 50 to 200 base-pair repeats is said to have a permutation and is therefore a carrier. When passed from a parent to a child, these base-pair repeats can expand to more than 2000, which is termed a *full mutation.* This expansion occurs only when a carrier mother passes the mutation to her offspring; it does not occur when a carrier father passes the mutation to his daughters.

The inheritance pattern has been termed X-linked dominant with reduced penetrance. This is in distinct contrast to the classic X-linked recessive pattern in which all carrier females are normal, all affected males have symptoms of the disorder and no males are carriers. Consequently, genetic counselling of affected families is more complex than that for families with a classic X-linked disorder, such as haemophilia. Both affected sexes are capable of transmitting the fragile X disorder. Prenatal diagnosis of the fragile X gene mutation is possible with direct DNA testing in a family with an established history using amniocentesis or chorionic villus sampling (Finucane et al 2017). The FMR1 mutation testing is highly accurate and is being researched regarding the incorporation into the newborn universal screening program (Abrams et al 2012, Bagni et al 2012, Finucane et al 2012, Sorensen et al 2013).

Clinical Manifestations

The classic trend of physical findings in adult men with FXS consists of a long face with a prominent jaw (prognathism); large, protruding ears; and large testes (macro-orchidism). In prepubertal children, however, these features may be less obvious, and behavioural manifestations may initially suggest the diagnosis (Box 20.2). In carrier females, the clinical manifestations are extremely varied.

Therapeutic Management

FXS has no cure. Medical treatment may include the use of serotonin agents, such as carbamazepine (Tegretol) or fluoxetine (Prozac), to control violent temper outbursts and the use of central nervous system stimulants or clonidine (Catapres) to improve attention span and decrease hyperactivity. Two possible treatments of FXS being investigated are reactivation of the affected gene and protein replacement (Bagni et al 2012, Kuehn 2011).

All affected children require referral to early intervention programs that include speech and language therapy, occupational therapy and special education assistance. A multidisciplinary assessment of common medical problems associated with FXS such as cardiac, neurological and orthopaedic anomalies and gastrointestinal problems is imperative to improve comprehensive care that may lead to better quality of life for these patients and their families (Kidd et al 2014).

Prognosis

Individuals with FXS are expected to live a normal life span. Their CI may be improved by behavioural and educational interventions that usually begin in preschool-age children.

Nursing Care Management

Because CI is a fairly consistent finding in individuals with FXS, the care given to these families is the same as for any child with intellectual disability. Because the disorder is hereditary, genetic counselling is

BOX 20.2 Clinical Manifestations of Fragile X Syndrome

Physical Features

- Increased head circumference
- Long, wide or protruding ears
- Long, narrow face with prominent jaw
- Strabismus
- Mitral valve prolapse, aortic root dilation
- Hypotonia
- In postpubertal males, enlarged testicles

Behavioural Features

- Mild to severe cognitive impairment
- Speech delay; may be rapid speech with stuttering and word repetition
- Short attention span, hyperactivity
- Hypersensitivity to taste, sounds, touch
- Intolerance to change in routine
- Autistic-like behaviours, such as social anxiety and gaze aversion
- Possible aggressive behaviour

important to inform parents and siblings of the risks of transmission. In addition, any male or female with unexplained or non-specific mental impairment should be referred for genetic testing and, if needed, counselling.

SENSORY LOSS

Deafness and Hard of Hearing

Hearing loss is one of the more common disabilities in Australia and New Zealand. Hearing Australia (n.d.) cares for around 14,000 children up to the age of 12 who use a hearing aid or cochlear implant. For infants admitted to neonatal intensive care units, the incidence rises sharply to approximately 2 to 4 per 100 neonates (Almadhoob & Ohlsson 2015, Colella-Santos et al 2014). Incidence is also higher for Aboriginal and Torres Strait Islander children in Australia. Among children aged 0 to 14 years, Indigenous Australians are twice as likely to have a long-term ear/hearing problem and three times as like to have otitis media (Australian Institute of Health and Welfare [AIHW] 2020) (see Otitis Media, Chapter 26). Māori and Pacific Islander children in New Zealand have a higher prevalence of mild-moderate hearing loss (Digby 2014).

Definition and Classification

People who are *deaf* or *hard of hearing* may range in severity from slight to profound hearing loss. *Slight to moderately severe hearing loss* describes a person who has residual hearing sufficient to enable successful processing of linguistic information through audition, generally with the use of a hearing aid. *Severe to profound hearing loss* describes the situation where hearing precludes successful processing of linguistic information through audition with or without a hearing aid. People who are deaf or hard of hearing and have a difficulty with speech tend not to have a physical speech defect other than that caused by the inability to hear.

Hearing defects may be classified according to aetiology, pathology or symptom severity. Each is important in terms of treatment, possible prevention and rehabilitation.

Aetiology. Hearing loss may be caused by a number of prenatal and postnatal conditions. These may include a family history of childhood hearing loss, anatomical malformations of the head or neck, low birth weight, severe perinatal asphyxia, perinatal infection (cytomegalovirus, rubella, herpes, syphilis, toxoplasmosis, bacterial meningitis), maternal prenatal substance abuse, chronic ear infection, cerebral palsy, Down syndrome, prolonged neonatal oxygen supplementation or administration of ototoxic drugs (Colella-Santos et al 2014, Gan et al 2016, Haddad & Keesecker 2016, Singh 2015).

In addition, high-risk neonates who survive the once fatal prenatal or perinatal conditions may be susceptible to hearing loss from the disorder or its treatment. For example, sensorineural hearing loss may be a result of continuous humming noises or high noise levels associated with incubators, oxygen hoods or intensive care units, especially when combined with the use of potentially ototoxic antibiotics.

Environmental noise is a special concern. Sounds loud enough to damage sensitive hair cells of the inner ear can produce irreversible hearing loss. Very loud, brief noise (e.g. gunfire) can cause immediate, severe and permanent loss of hearing. Longer exposure to less intense but still hazardous sounds (e.g. loud persistent music via headphones, sound systems, concerts or industrial noises) may also produce hearing loss (Biassoni et al 2014, Guest et al 2017, Liberman & Kujawa 2017, Pawlaczyk-Luszczynska et al 2017). Hearing loss caused by toxic substances (e.g. smoking or second-hand smoke) or when combined with loud noises, tends to produce a synergistic effect on hearing that causes hearing dysfunction (Fabry et al 2011, Talaat et al 2014).

Pathology. Disorders of hearing are divided according to the location of the defect. Conductive or middle-ear hearing loss results from interference of transmission of sound to the middle ear. It is the most common of all types of hearing loss and most frequently a result of recurrent serous otitis media. Conductive hearing loss involves mainly interference with loudness of sound.

Sensorineural hearing loss involves damage to the inner ear structures or the auditory nerve. The most common causes are congenital defects of inner ear structures or consequences of acquired conditions, such as kernicterus, infection, administration of ototoxic drugs or exposure to excessive noise. Sensorineural hearing loss results in distortion of sound and problems in discrimination. Although the child hears some of everything going on around them, the sounds are distorted, severely affecting discrimination and comprehension.

Mixed conductive-sensorineural hearing loss results from interference with transmission of sound in the middle ear and along neural pathways. It frequently results from recurrent otitis media and its complications.

Central auditory imperception includes all hearing losses that are not linked to defects in the conductive or sensorineural structures. They are usually divided into organic or functional losses. In the organic type of central auditory imperception, the defect involves the reception of auditory stimuli along the central pathways and the expression of the message into meaningful communication. Examples are aphasia, the inability to express ideas in any form, either written or verbal; agnosia, the inability to interpret sound correctly; and dysacusis, difficulty in processing details or discriminating among sounds. In the functional type of hearing loss, no organic lesion exists to explain a central auditory loss. Examples of functional hearing loss are conversion hysteria (an unconscious withdrawal from hearing to block remembrance of a traumatic event), infantile autism and childhood schizophrenia.

Symptom Severity. Hearing is expressed in terms of a decibel (dB), a unit of loudness, and is measured at various frequencies, such as 500, 1000 and 2000 cycles/second, the critical listening speech range. Hearing loss can be classified according to hearing threshold level (the measurement of an individual's hearing threshold by means of an audiometer) and the degree of symptom severity as it affects speech (Table 20.1). These classifications offer only general guidelines regarding the effect of the loss on any individual child because children differ greatly in their ability to use residual hearing.

Therapeutic Management

Conductive Hearing Loss. Treatment of hearing loss depends on the cause and type of hearing defect. Many conductive hearing defects respond to medical or surgical treatment, such as antibiotic therapy for acute otitis media or insertion of tympanostomy tubes for chronic otitis media. When the conductive loss is permanent, hearing can be improved with the use of a hearing aid to amplify sound.

The nurse should be familiar with the types, basic care and handling of hearing aids, especially when the child is hospitalised. Types of aids include those worn in or behind the ear, models incorporated into an eyeglass frame and types worn on the body with a wire connection to the ear (Fig 20.6). One of the most common problems with a hearing aid is acoustic feedback, an annoying whistling sound usually caused by improper fit of the ear mould. Sometimes the whistling may be at a frequency that the child cannot hear but that is annoying to others. In this case, if children are old enough, they are told of the noise and asked to readjust the aid.

TABLE 20.1 Classification of Hearing Loss Based on Symptom Severity

Hearing Level (dB)	Effect
Slight: 16–25	Has difficulty hearing faint or distant speech Usually is unaware of hearing difficulty Likely to achieve in school but may have problems No speech defects
Mild to moderate: 26–55	May have speech difficulties Understands face-to-face conversational speech at 0.9–1.5 m
Moderately severe: 56–70	Unable to understand conversational speech unless loud Considerable difficulty with group or classroom discussion Requires special speech training
Severe: 71–90	May hear a loud voice if nearby May be able to identify loud environmental noises Can distinguish vowels but not most consonants Requires speech training
Profound: 91	May hear only loud sounds Requires extensive speech training

dB, Decibels.

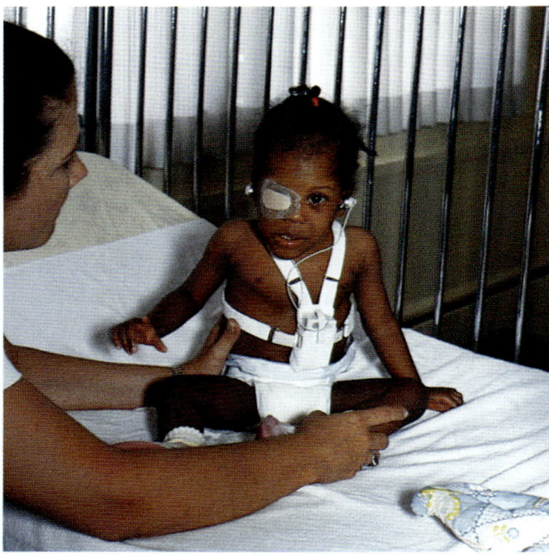

Fig 20.6 On-the-body hearing aids are convenient for young children, such as this child with severe bilateral hearing loss. Note eye patching for strabismus.

As children grow older, they may be self-conscious about the device. Efforts may be made to make the aid inconspicuous, such as styling the hair to cover behind-the-ear aids or the use of in-the-ear or miniature digital models, or encourage the use of attractive frames for glasses with connected hearing aids. Give children responsibility for the care of the device as soon as they are able because fostering independence is a primary goal of rehabilitation.

NURSING CARE CONSIDERATIONS

Stress to parents the importance of storing batteries for hearing aids in a safe location out of reach of children and teaching children not to remove the battery from the hearing aid (or supervising young children when they do so). Battery ingestion requires immediate emergency management.

Sensorineural Hearing Loss. The treatment aim for sensorineural hearing loss is to improve hearing and communication with hearing aids or cochlear implants. Sensorineural hearing loss has been associated with damaged auditory hair cells or nerve fibres or abnormal development of the inner ear structures. Because conventional hearing aids only amplify sound that may not be processed by a damaged inner ear, some children may not benefit from hearing aids and require a referral for a cochlear implant. A cochlear implant bypasses the hair cells to directly stimulate surviving auditory nerve fibres so that they can send signals to the brain. These signals can be interpreted by the brain to produce sound and sensations (Easwar et al 2017, Gan et al 2016, Grindle 2014). The cochlear implant consists of an internal surgically implanted prosthetic device (receiver and electrode array) and external device (microphone, speech processor and transmitter coil) (Gan et al 2016). The cochlear implant provides a sensation of hearing for individuals who have severe or profound hearing loss (Farinetti et al 2014, Lantos 2012, Pettinato et al 2017).

Multichannelled implants are sophisticated devices that stimulate the auditory nerve at a number of locations with differently processed signals. This type of stimulation allows a person to use the pitch information present in speech signals, leading to better understanding of speech. The trend is towards early use of cochlear implants, usually by 12 months old, to give the child maximum opportunity to develop listening, language and speaking skills.

The cochlear implantation is a safe hearing surgical technique associated with a low complication rate. A reported global complication rate comprised minor complications that were mainly infectious in children (acute otitis media) and cochleovestibular in adults (tinnitus and vertigo) and major complications, including mostly reimplantation after revision surgery or device failure (Farinetti et al 2014). However, cases of meningitis, particularly pneumococcal meningitis, have been reported. Therefore, it has been recommended that all children receiving a cochlear implant must be vaccinated with the pneumococcal polyvalent vaccine (Haddad & Keesecker 2016).

Nursing Care Management

Assess for Hearing Concerns. Assessment of children for hearing loss is a critical nursing responsibility. Identification of hearing loss before the first 3 months of age with intervention no later than 6 months old is essential to improve the language and educational development for children who are deaf or hard of hearing (Lammers et al 2015, Rohlfs et al 2017). Auditory testing is discussed in Chapter 4.

At birth, the nurse can observe the neonate's response to auditory stimuli, as evidenced by the startle reflex, head turning, eye blinking and cessation of body movement. The infant may vary in the intensity of the response, depending on the state of alertness. However, a consistent absence of a reaction should lead to suspicion of hearing loss. Box 20.3 summarises other clinical manifestations of hearing loss in infants.

Children who are profoundly deaf or hard of hearing are much more likely to be diagnosed during infancy than the child who is less severely affected. If the defect is not detected during early childhood, it is likely to become evident during entry into school, when the child has difficulty learning. Unfortunately, some of these children are erroneously placed in special classes for students with learning disabilities or CI. Therefore, it is essential that the nurse suspect a hearing loss in any child who demonstrates the behaviours listed in Box 20.3.

BOX 20.3 Clinical Manifestations of Deafness or Being Hard of Hearing

Infants

- Lack of startle or blink reflex to a loud sound
- Failure to be awakened by loud environmental noises
- Failure to localise a source of sound by 6 months old
- Absence of babble or voice inflections by 7 months old
- General indifference to sound
- Lack of response to the spoken word; failure to follow verbal directions
- Response to loud noises as opposed to the voice

Children

- Use of gestures rather than verbalisation to express desires, especially after 15 months old
- Failure to develop intelligible speech by 24 months old
- Monotone and unintelligible speech; lessened laughter
- Vocal play, head banging or foot stamping for vibratory sensation
- Yelling or screeching to express pleasure, needs or annoyance
- Asking to have statements repeated or answering them incorrectly
- Greater response to facial expression and gestures than to verbal explanation
- Avoidance of social interaction; prefer to play alone
- Enquiring, sometimes confused facial expression
- Suspicious alertness alternating with cooperation
- Frequent stubbornness because of lack of comprehension
- Irritability at not making themselves understood
- Shy, timid and withdrawn behaviour
- Frequent appearance of being 'in a world of their own' or markedly inattentive

NURSING CARE CONSIDERATIONS

When parents express concern about their child's hearing and speech development, refer the child for a hearing evaluation. Absence of well-formed syllables *(da, na, yaya)* by 11 months old should result in immediate referral.

During early childhood, the primary importance of hearing loss is the effect on speech development. A child with a mild conductive hearing loss may speak fairly clearly but in a loud, monotone voice. A child with a sensorineural defect usually has difficulty in articulation. Communication may be difficult, leading to frustration when words are not understood. For example, an inability to hear higher frequencies may result in the word *spoon* being pronounced 'poon'. Children with articulation problems need to have their hearing tested.

Lip-reading. Although the child may become an expert at lip-reading, only about 40% of the spoken word is understood, less if the speaker has an accent, moustache or beard. Exaggerating pronunciation or speaking in an altered rhythm further lessens comprehension. Parents can help the child understand the spoken word by using the suggestions in the Nursing Care Guidelines box. The child learns to supplement the spoken word with sensitivity to visual cues, primarily body language and facial expression (e.g. tightening the lips, muscle tension, eye contact).

Sign language. Sign language, such as Auslan or New Zealand Sign Language (NZSL), is a visual-gestural language that uses hand signals that roughly correspond to specific words and concepts in the English language. Encourage family members to learn signing because using or watching hands requires much less concentration than lip-reading or talking. Also, a symbol method enables some children who are deaf or hard of hearing to learn more and to learn faster.

Speech-language therapy. The most formidable task in the education of a child who is profoundly deaf or hard of hearing is learning to speak. Speech is learned through a multisensory approach using visual, tactile, kinaesthetic and auditory stimulation. Encourage parents to participate fully in the learning process.

Additional aids. Everyday activities present problems for older children who are deaf or hard of hearing. For example, they may not be able to hear the telephone, doorbell or alarm clock. Several commercial devices are available to help them adjust to these dilemmas. Flashing lights can be attached to a telephone or doorbell to signal its ringing. Trained hearing ear dogs can provide great assistance because they alert the person to sounds, such as someone approaching, a moving car, a signal to wake up or a child's cry. Special teletypewriters or telecommunications devices for the Deaf (TDD or TTY) help people who are deaf or hard of hearing communicate with each other over the telephone; the typed message is conveyed via the telephone lines and displayed on a small screen.

Any audiovisual medium presents dilemmas for these children, who can see the picture but cannot hear the message. However, with closed captioning a special decoding device is attached to the television, and the audio portion of a program is translated into subtitles that appear on the screen.

Socialisation. Socialisation is extremely important to children's development. If children attend a special school for people who are deaf or hard of hearing, they are able to socialise with peers in that setting. Classmates become a potential source of close friendships because they communicate more easily among themselves. Encourage parents to promote these relationships whenever possible.

Children who are deaf or hard of hearing may need special help with school or social activities. For children wearing hearing aids, keep background noise to a minimum. Because many of these children are able to attend regular classes, the teacher may need assistance in adapting methods of teaching for the child's benefit. The school nurse is often in an optimal position to emphasise methods of facilitated communication, such as lip-reading (see Nursing Care Guidelines box). Because group projects and audiovisual teaching aids may hinder the learning of a child who is deaf or hard on hearing, carefully evaluate the use of these educational methods.

In a group setting, it is helpful for the other members to sit in a semicircle in front of the child who is deaf or hard of hearing. Because one of the difficulties in following a group discussion is that the child is unaware of who will speak next, someone should point out each speaker. Speakers can also be given numbers, or their names can be written down as each person talks. If one person writes down the main topic of the discussion, the child is able to follow lip-reading more closely. Such practices can increase the child's ability to participate in sports, organisations such as Scouts and group projects.

Support Child and Family. Once the diagnosis of hearing loss is made, parents need extensive support to adjust to the shock of learning about their child's disability and an opportunity to realise the extent of the hearing loss. If the hearing loss occurs during childhood, the child also requires sensitive, supportive care during the long and often difficult adjustment to this sensory loss. Early rehabilitation is one of the best strategies for fostering adjustment. Progress in learning communication, however, may not always coincide with emotional adjustment. Depression or anger is common, and such feelings are a normal part of the grieving process.

Care for the Child During Hospitalisation. The needs of the hospitalised child who is deaf or hard of hearing are the same as those of any other child, but the disability presents special challenges to the nurse. For example, verbal explanations must be supplemented by tactile and visual aids, such as books or actual demonstration and practice.

Children's understanding of the explanation needs to be constantly reassessed. If their verbal skills are poorly developed, they can answer questions through drawing, writing or gesturing. When communicating with the child, the nurse should use the same principles as those outlined for facilitating lip-reading. Ideally, nurses without foreign accents should be assigned to the child. The child's hearing aid is checked to ensure that it is working properly. If it is necessary to awaken the child at night, the nurse should gently shake the child or turn on the hearing aid before arousing the child. The nurse should always make certain that the child can see him or her before any procedures, even routine ones such as changing a nappy or regulating an infusion. It is important to remember that the child may not be aware of the nurse's presence until alerted through visual or tactile cues.

Ideally, parents are encouraged to room with the child. However, the nurse must convey to them that this is not to serve as a convenience to the nurse but as a benefit to the child. Although the parents' aid can be enlisted in familiarising the child with the hospital and explaining procedures, the nurse should also talk directly to the youngster, encouraging expression of feelings about the experience. If the child's speech is difficult to understand, try to become familiar with their pronunciation of words. Parents often can be helpful by explaining the child's usual speech habits. Non-verbal communication devices that use pictures or words that the child can point to are also available. The nurse can make boards by using pictures or writing the words on cardboard representing common needs, such as *parent, food, water* or *toilet.*

The nurse has a special role as child advocate and is in a strategic position to alert other health team members and other patients to the child's special needs regarding communication. For example, the nurse should accompany other practitioners on visits to the child's room to ensure that they speak to the child and that the child understands what is said. Caregivers may forget that the child has the abilities to perceive and learn despite a hearing loss, and consequently they communicate only with the parents. As a result, the child's needs and feelings remain unrecognised and unaddressed.

Because children who are deaf or hard of hearing may have difficulty forming social relationships with other children, introduce the child to roommates and encourage them to engage in play activities. The hospital setting can provide growth-promoting opportunities for social relationships. With the assistance of a play specialist, the child can learn new recreational activities, experiment with group games and engage in therapeutic play. Playing with puppets or dollhouses, role-playing with dress-up clothes, building with blocks or Legos, finger painting and water play can help the child express feelings that previously were suppressed.

Assist in Measures to Prevent Hearing Loss. A primary nursing role is prevention of hearing loss. Because the most common cause of hearing loss is chronic otitis media, it is essential that appropriate measures be instituted to treat existing infections and prevent recurrences. Children with a history of ear or respiratory infections or any other condition known to increase the risk of hearing loss should receive periodic auditory testing. Aboriginal and Torres Strait Islander children and Māori or Pacific Islander children have an increased prevalence of conductive hearing loss attributed to chronic ear disease such as otitis media (AIHW 2020, Digby 2014).

To prevent the causes of hearing loss that begin prenatally and perinatally, pregnant women need counselling regarding the necessity of early prenatal care, including genetic counselling for known familial disorders; avoidance of all ototoxic drugs, especially during the first trimester; tests to rule out syphilis, rubella or blood incompatibility; medical management of maternal diabetes; strict control of alcohol intake; adequate dietary intake; and avoidance of smoke exposure. Stress the necessity of routine immunisation during childhood to eliminate the possibility of acquired sensorineural hearing loss from rubella, mumps or measles (encephalitis).

Exposure to excessive noise pollution is a well-established cause of sensorineural hearing loss. The nurse should routinely assess the possibility of environmental noise pollution and advise children and parents of the potential danger. A recent randomised single-blind clinical trial supported the use of earplugs in preventing temporary hearing loss associated with loud music exposure (Ramakers et al 2016).

Blindness and Low Vision

Low vision is a common problem during childhood. Causes of low vision such as refractive error, strabismus and amblyopia occur in 5% to 10% of all preschoolers, who are usually identified through vision screening programs (Alley 2013, Rahi et al 2010). The nurse's role is one of assessment, detection, prevention, referral and (in some instances) rehabilitation.

Definition and Classification

Low Vision is a general term that encompasses partial sight or partial visual loss. *Partial sight* or *partial visual loss* is defined as a visual acuity between 20/70 and 20/200. The child can generally use normal-sized print because near vision is almost always better than distance vision. *Legal blindness* or *severe permanent visual loss* is defined as a visual acuity of 20/200 or lower or a visual field of 20 degrees or less in the better eye.

Aetiology

Low vision can be caused by a number of genetic and prenatal or postnatal conditions. These include perinatal infections (herpes, chlamydia, gonococci, rubella, syphilis, toxoplasmosis); retinopathy of prematurity; trauma; postnatal infections (meningitis); and disorders such as sickle cell disease, juvenile rheumatoid arthritis, Tay-Sachs disease, albinism and retinoblastoma. In many instances, such as with refractive errors, the cause of the defect is unknown.

Refractive errors are the most common types of visual disorders in children. The term *refraction* means bending and refers to the bending of light rays as they pass through the lens of the eye. Normally, light rays enter the lens and fall directly on the retina. However, in refractive disorders, the light rays either fall in front of the retina (myopia) or beyond it (hyperopia). Other eye problems, such as strabismus, may or may not include refractive errors, but they are important because, if untreated, they result in severe permanent low vision from amblyopia. These, along with other less frequent visual disorders, are summarised in Box 20.4. In addition to these disorders, other visual problems can be a result of infection or trauma.

Trauma. Trauma is a common cause of low vision in children. Injuries to the eyeball and adnexa (supporting or accessory structures, such as eyelids, conjunctiva or lacrimal glands) can be classified as penetrating or non-penetrating. Penetrating wounds are most often a result of sharp instruments (e.g. sticks, knives or scissors) or propulsive objects (e.g. firecrackers, guns, arrows or slingshots). Non-penetrating injuries may be a result of foreign objects in the eyes, lacerations, a blow from a blunt object such as a ball (cricket ball, basketball, tennis ball) or fist or thermal or chemical burns.

Treatment is aimed at preventing further ocular damage and is primarily the responsibility of the ophthalmologist. It involves adequate examination of the injured eye (with the child sedated or anaesthetised in severe injuries); appropriate immediate intervention, such as removal of the foreign body or suturing of the laceration; and prevention of complications, such as administration of antibiotics or steroids and complete bed rest to allow the eye to heal and blood to reabsorb (see Nursing Care Considerations box). The prognosis varies according to the type of injury. It is usually guarded in all cases of penetrating wounds because of the high risk of serious complications.

BOX 20.4 Types of Low Vision

Refractive Errors

Myopia

Nearsightedness: Ability to see objects clearly at close range but not at a distance

Pathophysiology

Results from eyeball that is too long, causing images to fall in front of the retina

Clinical Manifestations

- Headaches
- Dizziness
- Excessive eye rubbing
- Head tilt or forward head thrusts
- Difficulty in reading or doing other close work
- Clumsiness; walking into objects
- Blinking more than usual or irritability when doing close work
- Inability to see objects clearly
- Poor school performance, especially in subjects that require demonstration, such as arithmetic

Treatment

- Corrected with biconcave lenses that focus rays on retina
- May be corrected with laser surgery

Hyperopia

Farsightedness: Ability to see objects at a distance but not at close range

Pathophysiology

- Results from eyeball that is too short, causing image to focus beyond retina

Clinical manifestations

- Because of accommodative ability, child can usually see objects at all ranges
- Most children are normally hyperopic until about 7 years old

Treatment

- When required, corrected with convex lenses that focus rays on retina
- May be corrected with laser surgery

Astigmatism

- Unequal curvatures in refractive apparatus

Pathophysiology

- Results from unequal curvatures in cornea or lens that cause light rays to bend in different directions

Clinical Manifestations

- Depend on severity of refractive error in each eye
- Possible clinical manifestations of myopia

Treatment

- Corrected with special lenses that compensate for refractive errors
- May be corrected with laser surgery

Anisometropia

- Different refractive strength in each eye

Pathophysiology

- May develop amblyopia because weaker eye is used less

Clinical Manifestations

- Depend on severity of refractive error in each eye
- Possible clinical manifestations of myopia

Treatment

- Treated with corrective lenses, preferably contact lenses, to improve vision in each eye so that they work as a unit
- May be corrected with laser surgery

Amblyopia

Lazy eye: Reduced visual acuity in one eye

Pathophysiology

- Results when one eye does not receive sufficient stimulation
- Each retina receives different images, resulting in diplopia (double vision)
- Brain accommodates by suppressing less intense image
- Visual cortex eventually does not respond to visual stimulation, with resultant loss of vision in that eye

Clinical Manifestations

- Poor vision in affected eye

Treatment

- Preventable if treatment of primary visual defect, such as anisometropia or strabismus, begins before 6 years old

Strabismus

'Squint' or malalignment of eyes
Esotropia: Inward deviation of eye
Exotropia: Outward deviation of eye

Pathophysiology

- May result from muscle imbalance or paralysis, poor vision or congenital defect
- Because visual axes are not parallel, brain receives two images and amblyopia can result

Clinical Manifestations

- Squints eyelids together or frowns
- Difficulty in focusing from one distance to another
- Inaccurate judgment in picking up objects
- Inability to see print or moving objects clearly
- Closing one eye to see
- Tilting head to one side
- If combined with refractive errors, may see any of the manifestations listed for refractive errors
- Diplopia
- Photophobia
- Dizziness
- Headaches

Treatment

- Depends on cause of strabismus
- May involve occlusion therapy (patching stronger eye) or surgery to increase visual stimulation to weaker eye
- Early diagnosis essential to prevent vision loss

Cataracts

- Opacity of crystalline lens

Pathophysiology

- Prevents light rays from entering eye and refracting on retina

Clinical Manifestations

- Gradual decrease in ability to see objects clearly
- Possible loss of peripheral vision

Continued

BOX 20.4 Types of Low Vision—cont'd

- Nystagmus (with permanent vision loss)
- Grey opacities of lens
- Strabismus
- Absence of red reflex

Treatment
- Requires surgery to remove cloudy lens and replace lens (with intraocular lens implant, removable contact lens, prescription glasses)
- Must be treated early to prevent permanent visions loss from amblyopia

Glaucoma

Increased intraocular pressure

Pathophysiology
- Congenital type results from defective development of some component related to flow of aqueous humour
- Increased pressure on optic nerve causes eventual atrophy and severe permanent vision loss

Clinical Manifestations
- Loss of peripheral vision—mostly seen in acquired types
- Possible bumping into objects
- Perception of haloes around objects
- Possible complaint of pain or discomfort (severe pain, nausea or vomiting if sudden rise in pressure)
- Eye redness
- Excessive tearing (epiphora)
- Photophobia
- Spasmodic winking (blepharospasm)
- Corneal haziness
- Enlargement of eyeball (buphthalmos)

Treatment
- Requires surgical treatment (goniotomy) to open outflow tracts
- May require more than one procedure

NURSING CARE CONSIDERATIONS

Eye Injuries

Foreign Object
- Examine the eye for presence of a foreign body (evert upper eyelid to examine upper eye).
- Remove a freely movable object with the pointed corner of gauze pad lightly moistened with water.
- Do not irrigate the eye or attempt to remove a penetrating object (see Penetrating Injuries).
- Caution the child against rubbing the eye.

Chemical Burns
- Irrigate the eye copiously with tap water for 20 minutes.
- Evert upper eyelid to flush thoroughly.
- Hold the child's head with eye under a tap of running lukewarm water.
- Take the child to the emergency department.
- Have the child rest with eyes closed.
- Keep the room darkened.

Ultraviolet Burns
- If skin is burned, patch both eyes (make certain eyelids are completely closed); secure dressing with crepe bandages wrapped around head rather than with tape.
- Have the child rest with eyes closed.
- Refer to an ophthalmologist.

Haematoma ('Black Eye')
- Use a torch to check for gross hyphema (haemorrhage into anterior chamber; visible fluid meniscus across iris; more easily seen in light-coloured than in brown eyes).
- Apply ice for first 24 hours to reduce swelling if no hyphema is present.
- Refer to an ophthalmologist immediately if hyphema is present.
- Have the child rest with eyes closed.

Penetrating Injuries
- Take the child to the emergency department.
- Never remove an object that has penetrated the eye.
- Follow strict aseptic technique in examining the eye.
- Observe for the following:
  - aqueous or vitreous leaks (fluid leaking from point of penetration)
  - hyphema
  - shape and equality of pupils, reaction to light, prolapsed iris (not perfectly circular).
- Apply a Fox shield if available (not a regular eye patch) and apply patch over unaffected eye to prevent bilateral movement.
- Maintain bed rest with the child in a 30-degree Fowler's position.
- Caution child against rubbing eye.
- Refer to an ophthalmologist.

Infections. Infections of the adnexa and structures of the eyeball or globe may occur in children. The most common eye infection is conjunctivitis. Treatment is usually with ophthalmic antibiotics. Severe infections may require systemic antibiotic therapy. Steroids are used cautiously because they exacerbate viral infections such as herpes simplex, increasing the risk of damage to the involved structures.

Nursing Care Management

Nursing care of the child who is blind or has low vision is a critical nursing responsibility. Discovery of low vision as early as possible is essential to prevent social, physical and psychological damage to the child. Assessment involves: (1) identifying those children who by virtue of their history are at risk; (2) observing for behaviours that indicate a vision loss; and (3) screening all children for visual acuity and signs of other ocular disorders such as strabismus. This discussion focuses on clinical manifestations of various types of visual problems (see Box 20.4). Vision testing is discussed in Chapter 4.

Infancy. At birth, the nurse should observe the neonate's response to visual stimuli, such as following a light or object and cessation of body movement. The infant may vary in the intensity of the response, depending on the state of alertness.

Of special importance in detecting low vision during infancy are the parents' concerns regarding visual responsiveness in their child.

Their concerns, such as lack of eye contact from the infant, must be taken seriously. During infancy, the child should be tested for strabismus. Children with lack of binocularity after 2 to 4 months of age or not fixating and following an object by 6 months should be referred to a paediatric ophthalmologist or an eye care specialist (Rogers & Jordan 2013).

Childhood. Because the most common cause of low vision during childhood is refractive error, testing for visual acuity is essential. In addition to assessing for refractive errors, the nurse should be aware of signs and symptoms that indicate other ocular problems. Learning that their child is blind or has low vision precipitates an immense crisis for families. Encourage the family to investigate appropriate early intervention and educational programs for their child as soon as possible.

Promote Parent–Child Attachment. A crucial time in the life of infants who or blind or have low vision is when the infant and the parents are getting acquainted with each other. Pleasurable patterns of interaction between the infant and parents may be lacking if there is not enough reciprocity. For example, if the parent gazes fondly at the infant's face and seeks eye contact but the infant fails to respond because he or she cannot see the parent, a troubled cycle of responses may occur. The nurse can help parents learn to look for other cues that indicate the infant is responding to them, such as whether the eyelids blink; whether the activity level accelerates or slows; whether respiratory patterns change, such as faster or slower breathing, when the parents come near; and whether the infant makes throaty sounds when the parents speak to the infant. In time, parents learn that the infant has unique ways of relating to them. Encourage the parents to show affection using non-visual methods, such as talking or reading, cuddling and walking the child.

Promote the Child's Optimal Development. Promoting the child's optimum development requires rehabilitation in a number of important areas. These include learning self-help skills and appropriate communication techniques to become independent. Although nurses may not be directly involved in such programs, they can provide direction and guidance to families regarding the availability of programs and the need to promote these activities in their child.

Development and independence. Motor development depends on sight almost as much as verbal communication depends on hearing. From earliest infancy, parents are encouraged to expose the infant to as many visual-motor experiences as possible, such as sitting supported in an infant seat or swing and being given opportunities for holding up the head, sitting unsupported, reaching for objects and crawling.

Despite blindness or low vision, the child can become independent in all aspects of self-care. The same principles used for promoting independence in sighted children apply, with additional emphasis on non-visual cues. For example, the child may need help in dressing, such as special arrangement of clothing for style coordination and braille tags to distinguish colours and prints.

The child with permanent blindness or low vision also must learn to become independent in navigational skills. The two main techniques are the tapping method (use of a cane to survey the environment for direction and to avoid obstacles) and guides, such as a sighted human guide or a guide dog. Children who are partially sighted may benefit from ocular aids, such as a monocular telescope.

Play and socialisation. Children who are blind or have severe low vision do not learn to play automatically. Because they cannot imitate others or actively explore the environment as children with full vision can do, they depend much more on others to stimulate and teach them how to play. Parents need help in selecting appropriate play materials, especially those that encourage fine and gross motor development and stimulate the senses of hearing, touch and smell. Toys with educational value are especially useful, such as dolls with various clothing fasteners.

Children who are blind or have severe low vision have the same needs for socialisation as children who have full vision do. Because they have little difficulty in learning verbal skills, they are able to communicate with age mates and participate in suitable activities. The nurse should discuss with parents the opportunities for socialisation outside the home, especially regular preschools. The trend is to include these children with children with full vision to help them adjust to the outside world for eventual independence.

To compensate for inadequate stimulation, these children may develop self-stimulatory activities, such as body rocking, finger flicking or arm twirling. Discourage such habits because they delay the child's social acceptance. Behaviour modification is often successful in reducing or eliminating self-stimulatory activities.

Education. The main obstacle to learning is the child's total dependence on non-visual cues. Although the child can learn via verbal lecturing, he or she is unable to read the written word or to write without special education. Therefore the child must rely on braille, a system that uses raised dots to represent letters and numbers. The child can then read braille with the fingers and can write messages using a braille writer. However, this system is not useful for communicating with others unless others read braille. A more portable system for written communication is the use of a braille slate and stylus or a microcassette tape recorder. A recorder is especially helpful for leaving messages for others and taking notes during classroom lectures.

Books on CDs and tapes are significant sources of reading material in addition to braille books, which are large and cumbersome.

Children with partial sight benefit from specialised visual aids that produce a magnified retinal image. The basic methods are accommodative techniques, such as bringing the object closer; and devices such as special plus lenses, handheld and stand magnifiers, telescopes, video projection systems and large-print materials. Children with diminished vision often prefer to do close work without their glasses and compensate by bringing the object very near to their eyes.

Care for the Child During Hospitalisation. Because nurses are more likely to care for children who are hospitalised for procedures that involve temporary loss of vision than for children who have severe permanent low vision, the following discussion concentrates primarily on the needs of such children. The nursing care objectives in either situation are to: (1) reassure the child and family throughout every phase of treatment; (2) orient the child to the surroundings; (3) provide a safe environment; and (4) encourage independence. Whenever possible, the same nurse should care for the child to ensure consistency in the approach.

When children with full vision temporarily lose their vision, almost every aspect of the environment becomes bewildering and frightening. They are forced to rely on non-visual senses for help in adjusting to the reduced vision without the benefit of any special training. Nurses have a major role in minimising the effects of temporary loss of vision. They need to talk to the child about everything that is occurring, emphasising aspects of procedures that are felt or heard. They should always identify themselves as soon as they enter the room and before they approach the child. Because unfamiliar sounds are especially frightening, these are explained. Encourage the parents to room with their child and participate in the care. Familiar objects, such as a teddy bear or doll, should be brought from home to help lessen the strangeness of the hospital. As soon as the child is able to be out of bed, orient the child to the immediate surroundings. If the child is able to see on admission, this opportunity is taken to point out significant aspects of the room. Encourage the child to practise ambulating with the eyes closed to become accustomed to this experience.

The room is arranged with safety in mind. For example, place a stool next to the bed to help the child climb in and out of bed. The furniture is always placed in the same position to prevent collisions. If the child has difficulty navigating by feeling the walls, a rope can be attached from the bed to the point of destination, such as the bathroom. Attention to details (e.g. well-fitting slippers and robes that do not drag on the floor) is important in preventing tripping. Unlike the child who has low vision, these children are not familiar with navigating with a cane.

The child is encouraged to be independent in self-care activities, especially if the visual loss may be prolonged or potentially permanent. For example, during bathing, the nurse sets up all of the equipment and encourages the child to participate. At mealtimes, the nurse explains where each food item is on the tray, opens any special containers, prepares cereal or toast and encourages the child in self-feeding. Favourite finger foods (e.g. sandwiches, hamburgers, hot dogs or pizza) may be good selections. Praise the child for efforts at being cooperative and independent. Any improvements made in self-care, no matter how small, are stressed.

Appropriate recreational activities are provided, and if a child play specialist is available, such planning is done jointly. Because children with temporary low vision have a wide variety of play experiences to draw on, they are encouraged to select activities. For example, if they like to read, they may enjoy listening to audiobooks or having someone read to them. If they prefer manual activity, they may appreciate playing with clay or building blocks or feeling different textures and naming them. If they need an outlet for aggression, activities such as pounding or banging on a drum can be helpful.

Occasionally, children who are blind or have low vision come to the hospital for procedures to restore their vision. Although this is an extremely happy time, it also requires intervention to help them adjust to sight. They need an opportunity to take in all that they see. They should not be bombarded with visual stimuli. They may need to concentrate on people's faces or their own to become accustomed to this experience. They often need to talk about what they see and to compare the visual images with their mental ones. The children may also go through a period of depression, which must be respected and supported. Encourage the children to discuss how it feels to see, especially in terms of seeing themselves.

Children who increase their vision also need time to adjust and engage in activities that were impossible before. For example, they may prefer to use braille to read rather than learning a new 'visual approach' because of familiarity with the touch system. Eventually, as they learn to recognise letters and numbers, they will integrate these new skills into reading and writing. However, parents and teachers must be careful not to push them before they are ready. This applies to social relationships and physical activities as well as learning situations.

Assist in Measures to Prevent Low Vision. An essential nursing goal is to prevent low vision. This involves many of the same interventions discussed for hearing loss:

- prenatal screening for pregnant women at risk, such as those with rubella or syphilis infection and family histories of genetic disorders associated with visual loss
- adequate prenatal and perinatal care to prevent prematurity
- periodic screening of all children, especially newborns through preschoolers, for congenital and acquired low vision caused by refractive errors, strabismus and other disorders
- rubella immunisation of all children
- safety counselling regarding the common causes of ocular trauma, including safe practices when working with, playing with and carrying objects such as scissors, knives and balls.

After detection of eye problems, the nurse should encourage the family to prevent further ocular damage by undertaking corrective treatment. For the child with strabismus, this often necessitates occlusion patching of the stronger eye. Compliance with the procedure is greatest during the early preschool years. It is more difficult to encourage school-age children to wear the occlusive patch because the poor visual acuity of the uncovered weaker eye interferes with school work and the patch sets them apart from their peers. In school, they benefit from being positioned favourably (closer to the whiteboard or other visual media) and allowed extra time to read or complete an assignment. If treatment of the eye disorder requires instillation of ophthalmic medication, the family is taught the correct procedure.

Children who need glasses to correct refractive errors need time to adjust to wearing glasses. Young children who often pull off glasses benefit from temporal pieces that wrap around the ears or an elastic strap attached to the frames and around the back of the head to hold the glasses on securely. Once children appreciate the value of clear vision, they are more likely to wear the corrective lenses.

Glasses should not interfere with any activity. Special protective guards are available during contact sports to prevent accidental injury, and all corrective lenses should be made from safety glass, which is shatterproof. Often, corrective lenses improve visual acuity so dramatically that children are able to compete more effectively in sports. This in itself is a tremendous inducement to continue wearing glasses.

Contact lenses are a popular alternative to conventional glasses, especially for adolescents. Contact lenses offer several advantages over glasses, such as greater visual acuity, total corrected field of vision, convenience (especially with the extended-wear type) and optimal cosmetic benefit.

Hearing Loss and Low Vision

The most traumatic sensory loss is loss of both vision and hearing, which may have profound effects on the child's development. These losses interfere with the normal sequence of physical, intellectual and psychosocial growth. Although such children often achieve the usual motor milestones, their rate of development is slower. These children learn communication only with specialised training. Finger spelling is one desirable method often taught to these children. Words are spelled letter by letter into the child's hand, and the child spells into the other person's hand. Some children with residual hearing or low vision can learn to speak. Whenever possible, encourage speech because it allows communication with other individuals.

The future prospects for children who are deaf or hard of hearing and blind or has low vision are, at best, unpredictable. Congenital hearing loss and low vision are accompanied by other physical or neurological problems, which further diminish the child's learning potential. The most favourable prognosis is for children who have acquired hearing and visual loss with few, if any, associated disabilities. Their learning capacity is greatly potentiated by their developmental progress before the sensory losses. Although total independence, including gainful vocational training, is the goal, some children who are deaf or hard of hearing and blind of have low vison are unable to develop to this level. They may require lifelong parental or residential care. The nurse working with such families helps them deal with future goals for the child, including possible alternatives to home care during the parents' advancing years.

COMMUNICATION DIFFICULTIES

Autism Spectrum Disorders

Autism spectrum disorders (ASDs) are complex neurodevelopmental disorders of unknown aetiology. The American Psychiatric Association's

Diagnostic and Statistical Manual of Mental Disorders, Fifth Edition (DSM-5) revised the definition for ASD based on two behaviour domains that include difficulties in social communication and social interaction, and unusually restricted, repetitive behaviour, interest or activities (American Psychiatric Association 2013, Brentani et al 2013, Lai et al 2014).

ASD is now frequently diagnosed in toddlers because their atypical development is being recognised early (Lai et al 2014, Zwaigenbaum et al 2015). It occurs in 1 in 150 children in Australia (AIHW 2017) and 1 in 100 children in New Zealand (Ministry of Health 2021); it is about four times more common in boys than in girls and is not related to socioeconomic level, culture or parenting style (AIHW 2017).

Aetiology

The cause of ASD is unknown. Researchers are investigating a number of theories, including a link between hereditary, genetic, medical, immune dysregulation/neuroinflammation, oxidative stress (damage to cellular tissue) and environmental factors (De Rubeis et al 2014, Lai et al 2014, Ng et al 2017, Posar & Visconti 2017, Wong et al 2016). Individuals with ASD may have abnormal electroencephalograms, epileptic seizures, delayed development of hand dominance, persistence of primitive reflexes, metabolic abnormalities (elevated blood serotonin), cerebellar vermis hypoplasia (part of the brain involved in regulating motion and some aspects of memory) and infantile abnormal head enlargement (Raviola et al 2016, Rutter 2011).

There is a relatively high risk of recurrence of ASD in families with one affected child (Chawarska et al 2014, Rutter 2011, Yoder et al 2009, Zwaigenbaum et al 2015). Several genes have been suggested as possible causative factors in ASD (Talkowski et al 2014, Willsey & State 2015, Wong et al 2016).

The scientific evidence to date shows no link between measles, mumps and rubella (MMR) and thimerosal-containing vaccines and ASDs (Barile et al 2012, Goin-Kochel et al 2016, Price et al 2010, Taylor et al 2014, Uno et al 2015). Recent reports have retrospectively tied ASD to prenatal and perinatal events, such as maternal and paternal ages over 40 years old (for fathers, 1 in 116 births; for mothers, 1 in 123 births), uterine bleeding during pregnancy, low Apgar score fetal distress and neonatal hyperbilirubinaemia (Amin et al 2011, Kolevzon et al 2007, Rutter 2011). These same researchers, however, urge caution in interpreting these findings.

Clinical Manifestations and Diagnostic Evaluation

Children with ASD demonstrate core deficits primarily in social interactions, communication and behaviour. Failure of social interaction and communication development is one of the hallmarks of ASD. Parents of autistic children have reported that their child showed less interest in social interaction (e.g. abnormal eye contact, decreased response to own name, decreased imitation, usual repetitive behaviour) and had verbal and motor delays (Bolton et al 2012, Sanchack & Thomas 2016). Children with ASD may have significant gastrointestinal symptoms. Constipation is a common symptom and can be associated with acquired megarectum in children with ASD (Buie et al 2010).

Children with ASD do not always have the same manifestations, from mild forms requiring minimal supervision to severe forms in which self-abusive behaviour is common. The majority of children with ASD have some degree of CI, with scores typically in the moderate to severe range. Despite their relatively moderate to severe disability, some children with autism (known as savants) excel in particular areas, such as art, music, memory, mathematics or perceptual skills, such as puzzle building.

Communication difficulties are a common sign in children with ASD that may range from absent to delayed speech. Any child who does not display language skills such as babbling or gesturing by 12 months old, single words by 16 months old and two-word phrases by 24 months old is recommended for immediate hearing and language evaluation. Autism regression is when the child seems to develop normally but then regresses suddenly; this is a red-flag event that has been frequently displayed in expressive language (Fernell et al 2013, Raviola et al 2016, Sanchack & Thomas 2016).

Early recognition, referral, diagnosis and intensive early intervention tend to improve outcomes for children with ASD (Adelman & Kubiszyn 2016, Reichow et al 2012, Peterson & Barbel 2013, Zwaigenbaum et al 2015). Unfortunately, diagnosis is often not made until 2 to 3 years after symptoms are first recognised. However, in a retrospective study, the majority of parents observed atypical development in their ASD children before 24 months old (Lemcke et al 2013).

The Modified Checklist for Autism in Toddlers (M-CHAT) is a widely used screening tool for autism in Australia and New Zealand that is completed during child nurse appointments. Children whose screening results are concerning should receive a comprehensive developmental evaluation from a developmental paediatrician, child neurologist, child psychiatrist or child psychologist.

Prognosis

Although ASD is usually a lifelong condition with often devastating comorbid conditions, with early and intensive interventions the symptoms associated with autism can be greatly improved, and in some cases reported symptoms were completely overcome (Sanchack & Thomas 2016, Wodka et al 2013). Some ultimately achieve independence, but most require lifelong adult supervision. Aggravation of psychiatric symptoms occurs in about half of the children during adolescence, with girls having a tendency for continued deterioration.

Early recognition of behaviours associated with ASD is critical to implement appropriate interventions and family involvement. There is a growing body of evidence that parent-delivered interventions are associated with some improved outcomes, yet further research is needed in this area incorporating consistent measures (Bearss et al 2015, Brentani et al 2013, Oono et al 2013). The prognosis is most favourable for children with higher intelligence, functional speech and fewer behavioural issues (Orinstein et al 2014, Raviola et al 2016, Solomon et al 2011).

Nursing Care Management

Therapeutic intervention for ASD and associated comorbidities is a specialised area involving professionals with advanced training. Although there is no cure for ASD, numerous therapies have been used. The most promising results have been through highly structured and intensive behaviour modification programs. In general, the objective in treatment is to promote positive reinforcement, increase social awareness of others, teach verbal communication skills and decrease unacceptable behaviour. Providing a structured routine for the child to follow is a key in the management of ASD.

ASD is associated with comorbidities (e.g. aggression, explosive outburst, self-injury, asthma, epilepsy, gastrointestinal/digestive disorders, immune disorders, feeding disorders, anxiety disorder, bipolar disorder, sleeping disorders) that have been treated not only with early behavioural modification programs but also with medical and complementary and alternative medicine (Sanchack & Thomas 2016). Complementary and alternative medicine has emerged as a treatment of ASD ranging from parent-massage and therapeutic horseback riding to the implementation of elimination diets (e.g. gluten-free diet and casein-free diet); vitamin and omega-3 supplementation; and high-fat, low-carbohydrate ketogenic diet; however, there is a need for further research to validate these therapeutic approaches (Cheng et al 2017, Gabriels et al 2015, Lee et al 2014, Lofthouse et al 2012, Ly et al 2017).

When these children are hospitalised, the parents are essential to planning care and ideally should stay with the child as much as possible. Nurses should recognise that not all children with ASD are the same and that they require individual assessment and treatment. Decreasing stimulation by using a private room, avoiding extraneous auditory and visual distractions, and encouraging the parents to bring in possessions the child is attached to may lessen the disruptiveness of hospitalisation. Because physical contact often upsets these children, minimal holding and eye contact may be necessary to avoid behavioural outbursts. Take care when performing procedures on, administering medicine to and feeding these children because they may be either fussy eaters who wilfully starve themselves or gag to prevent eating, or indiscriminate hoarders who swallow any available edible or inedible items, such as a thermometer. Eating habits of ASD children may be particularly problematic for families and may involve food refusal accompanied by mineral deficiencies, mouthing objects, eating non-edibles and smelling and throwing food (Herndon et al 2009).

Children with ASD need to be introduced slowly to new situations, with visits with staff caregivers kept short whenever possible. Because these children have difficulty organising their behaviour and redirecting their energy, they need to be told directly what to do. Communication should be at the child's developmental level, brief and concrete.

Family Support. ASD, as with so many other chronic conditions, involves the entire family and often becomes 'a family disease'. Nurses can help alleviate the guilt and shame often associated with this disorder by stressing what is known from a biological standpoint and by providing family support. It is imperative to help parents understand that they are not the cause of the child's condition.

Parents need expert counselling early in the course. As much as possible, the family is encouraged to care for the child in the home. Families are often able to provide home care and assist with the educational services the child needs. As the child approaches adulthood and the parents become older, the family may require assistance in locating a long-term placement facility.

REFERENCES

Abrams, L., Cronister, A., Brown, W. T., et al. (2012). Newborn, carrier, and early childhood screening recommendations for fragile X. Pediatrics, 130(6), 1126–1135.

Adelman, C. R., & Kubiszyn, T. (2016). Factors that affect age of identification of children with autism spectrum disorder. Journal of Early Intervention. https://doi.org/10.1177/1053815116675461.

Ageranioti-Belanger, S., Brunet, S., D'Anjou, G., et al. (2012). Behavior disorders in children with an intellectual disability. Paediatrics & Child Health, 17(2), 84–88.

Alley, C. L. (2013). Preschool vision screening: Update on guidelines and techniques. Current Opinion in Ophthalmology, 24(5), 415–420.

Almadhoob, A., & Ohlsson, A. (2015). Sound reduction management in the neonatal intensive care unit for preterm or very low birth weight infants. Cochrane Database of Systematic Review, (1), CD010333.

American Psychiatric Association. (2013). Diagnostic and statistical manual of mental disorders (5th ed.). (DSM-V). Arlington, VA: American Psychiatric Association.

Amin, S. B., Smith, T., & Wang, H. (2011). Is neonatal jaundice associated with autism spectrum disorders: A systematic review. Journal of Autism and Developmental Disorders, 41(11), 1455–1463.

Arumugam, A., Raja, K., Venugopalan, M., et al. (2016). Down-syndrome-A narrative review with a focus on anatomical features. Clinical Anatomy, 29, 568–577.

Australian Institute of Health and Welfare (AIHW). (2017). Autism. https://www.aihw.gov.au/reports/disability/autism-in-australia/contents/autism

Australian Institute of Health and Welfare (AIHW). (2020). Indigenous hearing health. https://www.aihw.gov.au/reports/australias-health/indigenous-hearing-health

Bagni, C., Tassone, F., Neri, G., et al. (2012). Fragile X syndrome: Causes, diagnosis, mechanisms, and therapeutics. The Journal of Clinical Investigation, 122(12), 4314–4322.

Barile, J. P., Kuperminc, G. P., Weintraub, E. S., et al. (2012). Thimerosal exposure in early life and neuropsychological outcomes 7-10 years later. Journal of Pediatric Psychology, 37(1), 106–118.

Bearss, K., Burrell, T. L., Stewart, L., et al. (2015). Parent training in autism spectrum disorder: What's in a name? Clinical Child and Family Psychology Review, 18(2), 170–182.

Bellman, M., Byrne, O., & Sege, R. (2013). Developmental assessment of children. British Medical Journal (Clinical Research Ed.), 346, e8687.

Biassoni, E. C., Serra, M. R., Hinalaf, M., et al. (2014). Hearing and loud music exposure in a group of adolescents at the ages of 14-15 and retested at 17-18. Noise and Health, 16(72), 331–341.

Bolton, P. F., Golding, J., Emond, A., et al. (2012). Autism spectrum disorder and autistic traits in the Avon Longitudinal Study of Parents and Children: Precursors and early signs. Journal of the American Academy of Child and Adolescent Psychiatry, 51(3), 249–260.

Brentani, H., Paula, C. S., Bordini, D., et al. (2013). Autism spectrum disorders: An overview on diagnosis and treatment. Revista Brasileira de Psiquiatria (Sao Paulo, Brazil: 1999), 35(Suppl. 1), S62–S72.

Buie, T., Campbell, D. B., Fuchs, G. J., 3rd, et al. (2010). Evaluation, diagnosis, and treatment of gastrointestinal disorders in individuals with ASDs: A consensus report. Pediatrics, 125(Suppl. 1), S1–S18.

Bull, M. J. (2011). Committee on Genetics: Health supervision for children with Down syndrome. Pediatrics, 128(2), 393–406.

Cheng, N., Rho, J. M., & Masino, S. A. (2017). Metabolic dysfunction underlying autism spectrum disorder and potential treatment approaches. Frontiers in Molecular Neuroscience, 10.

Chawarska, K., Shic, F., Macari, S., et al. (2014). 18-month predictors of later outcomes in younger siblings of children with autism spectrum disorder: A baby siblings research consortium study. Journal of the American Academy of Child and Adolescent Psychiatry, 53(12), 1317–1327.

Colella-Santos, M. F., Hein, T. A., de Souza, G. L., et al. (2014). Newborn hearing screening and early diagnostic in the NICU. BioMed Research International, 845308.

Coppede, F. (2016). Risk factors for Down syndrome. Archives of Toxicology, 90, 2917–2929.

Crnic, K. A., Neece, C. L., McIntyre, L. L., et al. (2017). Intellectual disability and developmental risk: Promoting intervention to improve child and family wellbeing. Child Development, 88(2), 436–445.

De Rubeis, S., He, X., Goldberg, A. P., et al. (2014). Synaptic, transcriptional and chromatin genes disrupted in autism. Nature, 515, 209–215.

Digby, J., Purdy, S. C., Kelly, A. S., et al. (2014). Are hearing losses among young Māori different to those found in the young NZ European population? The New Zealand Medical Journal, 127(1398), 98–110.

Down Syndrome Australia (DSA). (2021). Statistics. https://www.downsyndrome.org.au/about-down-syndrome/statistics/

Easwar, V., Yamazaki, H., Deighton, M., et al. (2017). Cortical representation of interaural time difference is impaired by deafness in development: Evidence from children with early long-term access to sound through bilateral cochlear implants provided simultaneously. The Journal of Neuroscience, 37(9), 2349–2361.

Englund, C. K., Jonsson, B., Zander, C. S., et al. (2013). Changes in mortality and causes of death in the Swedish Down syndrome population. American Journal of Medical Genetics. Part A, 161, 642–649.

Fabry, D. A., Davila, E. P., Arheart, K. L., et al. (2011). Secondhand smoke exposure and the risk of hearing loss. Tobacco Control, 20(1), 82–85.

Farinetti, A., Gharbia, D. B., Mancini, J., et al. (2014). Cochlear implant complications in 403 patients: Comparative study of adults and children and

review of the literature. European Annals of Otorhinolaryngology, Head and Neck Diseases, 131, 177–182.
Fernell, E., Eriksson, M. A., & Gillberg, C. (2013). Early diagnosis of autism and impact on prognosis: A narrative review. Clinical Epidemiology, 5, 33–43.
Finucane, B., Abrams, L., Cronister, A., et al. (2012). Genetic counseling and testing for FMRI gene mutations: Practice guidelines of the National Society of Genetic Counselors. Journal of Genetic Counseling, 21(6) 752–760.
Finucane, B., Lincoln, S., Bailey, L., et al. (2017). Prognostic dilemmas and genetic counseling for prenatally detected fragile X gene expansions. Prenatal Diagnosis, 37, 37–42.
Fragile X Association of Australia (FXAA). (2021). Fragile X Syndrome. https://www.fragilex.org.au/fragile-x-disorders/fragile-x-syndrome/
Fragile X New Zealand (FXNZ). (2021). About Fragile X Syndrome. https://fragilex.org.nz/about-fragile-x-syndrome/
Gabriels, R. L., Pan, Z., Dechant, B., et al. (2015). Randomized controlled trial of therapeutic horseback riding in children and adolescents with autism spectrum disorder. Journal of the American Academy of Child and Adolescent Psychiatry, 54(7), 541–549.
Gan, R., Rowe, A., Benton, C., et al. (2016). Management of hearing loss in children. Paediatrics & Child Health, 26(1), 15–20.
Gilissen, C., Hehir-Kwa, J., Thung, D. T., et al. (2014). Genome sequencing identifies major causes of severe intellectual disability. Nature, 11, 344–347.
Goin-Kochel, R. P., Mire, S. S., Dempsey, A. G., et al. (2016). Parental report of vaccine receipt in children with autism spectrum disorder: Do rates differ by pattern of ASD onset? Vaccine, 34, 1335–1342.
Grindle, C. R. (2014). Pediatric hearing loss. Pediatrics in Review, 35(11) 456–463.
Guest, H., Munro, K. L., Prendergast, G., et al. (2017). Tinnitus with a normal audiogram: Relation to noise exposure but no evidence for cochlear synaptopathy. Hearing Research, 344, 265–274.
Guralnick, M. J. (2017). Early intervention for children with intellectual disabilities: An update. Journal of Applied Research in Intellectual Disabilities, 30, 211–229.
Haddad, J., & Keesecker, S. (2016). Hearing loss. In R. M. Kliegman, R. F. Stanton, I. I. I. St Geme, et al. (Eds.), Nelson textbook of pediatrics (20th ed.). Philadelphia: Elsevier Inc.
Hearing Australia. (n.d.). Children and Young Adults. https://www.hearing.com.au/Hearing-loss/Children-young-adults
Herndon, A. C., DiGuiseppi, C., Johnson, S. L., et al. (2009). Does nutritional intake differ between children and autism spectrum disorders and children with typical development? Journal of Autism and Developmental Disorders, 39(2), 212–222.
Hoyme, H. E., Kalberg, W. O., Elliot, A. J., et al. (2016). Updated clinical guidelines for diagnosing fetal alcohol spectrum disorders. Pediatrics, 138.
Huang, X., Zheng, J., Chen, M., et al. (2014). Noninvasive prenatal testing of trisomies 21 and 18 by massively parallel sequencing of maternal plasma DNA in twin pregnancies. Prenatal Diagnosis, 34(4), 335–340.
Karmiloff-Smith, A., Al-Janabi, T., D'Souza, H., et al. (2016). The importance of understanding individual differences in Down syndrome[version 1; referees: 2 approved]. F1000Research, 5(F1000 Faculty Rev), 389.
Katz, G., & Lazcano-Ponce, E. (2008). Intellectual disability: Definition, etiological factors, classification, diagnosis, treatment and prognosis. Salud Publica de Mexico, 50(Suppl. 2), S132–S141.
Kidd, S. A., Lachiewicz, A., Barbouth, D., et al. (2014). Fragile X syndrome: A review of associated medical problems. Pediatrics, 134(5), 995–1005.
Kolevzon, A., Gross, R., & Reichenberg, A. (2007). Prenatal and perinatal risk factors for autism: A review and integration of findings. Archives of Pediatrics and Adolescent Medicine, 161(4), 326–333.
Kuehn, B. M. (2011). Scientists find promising therapies for fragile X and Down syndromes. The Journal of the American Medical Association, 305(4), 344–346.
Lai, M. C., Lombardo, M. V., & Baron-Cohen, S. (2014). Autism. Lancet, 383(9920), 896–910.
Lammers, M. J., Jansen, T. T., Grolman, W., et al. (2015). The influence of newborn hearing screening on the age at cochlear implantation in children. The Laryngoscope, 125(4), 985–990.
Lantos, J. D. (2012). Ethics for the pediatrician: The evolving risk of cochlear implants in children. Pediatrics in Review, 33(7), 323–326.
Lee, B. (2016). Cytogenetics: Down syndrome and other abnormalities of chromosome number. In R. M. Kliegman, R. F. Stanton, I. I. I. St Geme, et al. (Eds.), Nelson textbook of pediatrics (20th ed.). Philadelphia: Elsevier Inc.
Lee, Y. J., Oh, S. H., Park, C., et al. (2014). Advanced pharmacology evidenced by pathogenesis of autism spectrum disorder. Clinical Psychopharmacology and Neuroscience, 12(1), 19–30.
Lemcke, S., Juul, S., Parner, E. T., et al. (2013). Early signs of autism in toddlers: A follow-up study in the Danish National Birth Cohort. Journal of Autism and Developmental Disorders, 43(10), 2366–2375.
Lewis, C., Hill, M., Silcock, C., et al. (2014). Non-invasive prenatal testing for trisomy 21: A cross-sectional survey of service users' views and likely uptake. An International Journal of Obstetrics and Gynaecology, 121(5), 582–594.
Liao, G. J., Chan, K. C., Jiang, P., et al. (2012). Noninvasive prenatal diagnosis of fetal trisomy 21 by allelic ratio analysis using targeted massively parallel sequencing of maternal plasma DNA. PLoS ONE, 7(5), e38154.
Liberman, M. C., & Kujawa, S. G. (2017). Cochlear synaptopathy in acquired sensorineural hearing loss: Manifestations and mechanisms. Hearing Research, 349, 138–147.
Lofthouse, N., Hendren, R., Hurt, E., et al. (2012). A review of complementary and alternative treatments for autism spectrum disorders. Autism Research and Treatment, 870391.
Ly, V., Bottelier, M., Hoekstra, P. J., et al. (2017). Elimination diet's efficacy and mechanisms in attention deficit hyperactivity disorder and autism spectrum disorder. European Child and Adolescent Psychiatry, 26(9), 1067–1079.
Mefford, H. C., Batshaw, M. L., & Hoffman, E. P. (2012). Genomics, intellectual disability, and autism. The New England Journal of Medicine, 366, 733–743.
Ministry of Health. (2021). Autism Spectrum Disorder. https://www.health.govt.nz/your-health/conditions-and-treatments/disabilities/autism-spectrum-disorder
Mink, J. W. (2016). Congenital, developmental, and neurocutaneous disorders: Fragile X syndrome. In M. K. Crow, J. H. Doroshow, J. M. Drazen, et al. (Eds.), Goldman-Cecil Medicine (25th ed.). Philadelphia: Elsevier-Saunders.
Moran, M. (2013). DSM-5 provides new take on neurodevelopment disorders. Psychiatric News, 48(2), 6–23.
Morano, S., Ruiz, S., Hwang, J., et al. (2017). Meta-analysis of single-case treatment effects on self-injurious behavior for individuals with autism and intellectual disabilities. Autism & Developmental Language Impairments, 2, 1–26.
New Zealand Down Syndrome Association (NZDSA). (n.d.). What is Down Syndrome. https://nzdsa.org.nz/what-is-ds/
Ng, M., de Montigny, J. G., Ofner, M., et al. (2017). Environmental factors associated with autism spectrum disorder: A scoping review for the years 2003-2013. Health Promotion and Chronic Disease Prevention in Canada: Research, Policy and Practice, 37(1), 1–23.
Oliver, C., & Richards, C. (2010). Self-injurious behavior in people with intellectual disability. Current Opinion in Psychiatry, 23(5), 412–416.
Oono, I. P., Honey, E. J., & McConachie, H. (2013). Parent-mediated early intervention for young children with autism spectrum disorders (ASD). Cochrane Database of Systematic Review, (4), CD009774.
Orinstein, A. J., Helt, M., Troyb, E., et al. (2014). Intervention for optimal outcome in children and adolescents with a history of autism. Journal of Developmental and Behavioral Pediatrics, 35(4), 247–256.
Pawlaczyk-Luszczynska, M., Zamojska-Daniszewska, M., Dudarewicz, A., et al. (2017). Exposure to excessive sounds and hearing status in academic classical music students. International Journal of Occupational Medicine and Environmental Health, 30(1), 55–75.
Pettinato, M., De Clerck, I., Verhoeven, J., et al. (2017). Expansion of prosodic abilities at the transition from babble to words: A comparison between children with cochlear implants and normally hearing children. Ear and Hearing, 38(4), 475–486.
Peterson, K., & Barbel, P. (2013). On alert for autism spectrum disorders. Nursing, 43(4), 28–34.

Posar, A., & Visconti, P. (2017). Autism in 2016: The need for answers. Jornal de Pediatria, 93(2), 111–119.

Quint, E. H., & O'Brien, R. F. (2016). Committee on Adolescence and The North American Society for Pediatric and Adolescent Gynecology. Pediatrics, 138. doi:10.1542/peds.2016-0295.

Price, C. S., Thompson, W. W., Goodson, B., et al. (2010). Prenatal and infant exposure to thimerosal from vaccines and immunoglobulins and risk of autism. Pediatrics, 126(4), 656–664.

Rahi, J. S., Cumberland, P. M., Peckham, C. S., et al. (2010). Improving detection of blindness in childhood: The British Childhood Vision Impairment study. Pediatrics, 126(4), e895–e903.

Ramakers, G. G. J., Kraaijenga, V. J. C., van Zanten, G. A., et al. (2016). Effectiveness of earplugs in preventing recreational noise-induced hearing loss – A randomized clinical trial. JAMA Otolaryngology– Head and Neck Surgery, 142(6), 551–558.

Raviola, G., Trieu, M. L., DeMaso, D. R., et al. (2016). Autism spectrum disorder. In R. M. Kliegman, B. F. Stanton, I. I. I. St Geme, et al. (Eds.), Nelson textbook of pediatrics (20th ed.). Philadelphia: Elsevier/Saunders.

Reichow, B., Barton, E. E., Boyd, B. A., et al. (2012). Early intensive behavioral intervention (EIBI) for young children with autism spectrum disorders (ASD). Cochrane Database of Systematic Review, (10), CD009260.

Rogers, G. L., & Jordan, C. O. (2013). Pediatric vision screening. Pediatrics in Review, 34(3), 126–133.

Rohlfs, A., Friedhoff, J., Bohnert, A., et al. (2017). Unilateral hearing loss in children: A retrospective study and review of the current literature. European Journal of Pediatrics, published on line: 28 January.

Rutter, M. L. (2011). Progress in understanding autism: 2007-2010. Journal of Autism and Developmental Disorders, 41(4), 395–404.

Sanchack, K. E., & Thomas, C. A. (2016). Autism spectrum disorder: Primary care principles. American Family Physician, 94(12), 972–979.

Shapiro, B. K., & Batshaw, M. L. (2016). Intellectual disability. In R. M. Kliegman, B. F. Stanton, I. I. I. St Geme, et al. (Eds.), Nelson textbook of pediatrics (20th ed.). Philadelphia: Elsevier/Saunders.

Singh, V. (2015). Newborn hearing screening: Present scenario. Indian Journal of Community Medicine, 40(1), 62–65.

Solomon, M., Buaminger, N., & Rogers, S. J. (2011). Abstract reasoning and friendship in high functioning preadolescents with autism spectrum disorders. Journal of Autism and Developmental Disorders, 41(1), 32–43.

Sorensen, P. L., Gane, L. W., Yarborough, M., et al. (2013). Newborn screening and cascade testing for FMR1 mutations. American Journal of Medical Genetics. Part A, 161A(1), 59–69.

Talaat, H. S., Metwaly, M. A., Khafagy, A. H., et al. (2014). Does passive smoking induce sensorineural hearing loss in children? International Journal of Pediatric Otorhinolaryngology, 78(1), 46–49.

Talkowski, M. E., Minikel, E. V., & Gusella, J. F. (2014). Autism spectrum disorder genetics: Diverse genes with diverse clinical outcomes. Harvard Review of Psychiatry, 22(2), 65–75.

Tasse, M. J., Luckasson, R., & Nygren, M. (2013). AAIDD proposed recommendations for ICD-11 and the condition previously known as mental retardation. Intellectual and Developmental Disabilities, 51(2), 127–131.

Taylor, L.E., Swerdfeger, A.L., & Eslick, G.D. (2014). Vaccines are not associated with autism: An evidence-based meta-analysis of case-control and cohort studies. Vaccine, 32(29), 3623–3629.

Uno, Y., Uchiyama, T., Kurosawa, M., et al. (2015). Early exposure to the combined measles-mumps-rubella vaccine and thimerosal-containing vaccines and risk of autism spectrum disorder. Vaccine, 33(21), 2511–2516.

Wallander, J. L., Biasini, F. J., Thorsten, V., et al. (2014). Dose of early intervention treatment during children's first 36 months of life is associated with developmental outcomes: An observational cohort study in three low/low-middle income countries. BMC Pediatrics, 14, 281.

Weijerman, M. E., & de Winter, J. P. (2010). Clinical practice: The care of children with Down syndrome. European Journal of Pediatrics, 169(12), 1445–1452.

Willsey, A. J., & State, M. W. (2015). Autism spectrum disorders: From genes to neurobiology. Current Opinion in Neurobiology, 30, 92–99.

Wodka, E. L., Mathy, P., & Kalb, L. (2013). Predictors of phrase and fluent speech in children with autism and severe language delay. Pediatrics, 131(4), e1128–e1134.

Wong, S., Napoli, E., Krakowiak, P., et al. (2016). Role of p53, mitochondrial DNA deletions, and paternal age in autism: A case-control study. Pediatrics, 137(4), e20151888.

Yoder, P., Stone, W. L., Walden, T., et al. (2009). Predicting social impairment and ASD diagnostic in younger siblings of children with autism spectrum disorder. Journal of Autism and Developmental Disorders, 39(10), 1381–1391.

Zwaigenbaum, L., Bauman, M. L., Stone, W. L., et al. (2015). Early identification of autism spectrum disorder: Recommendations for practice and research. Pediatrics, 136, S10–S40.

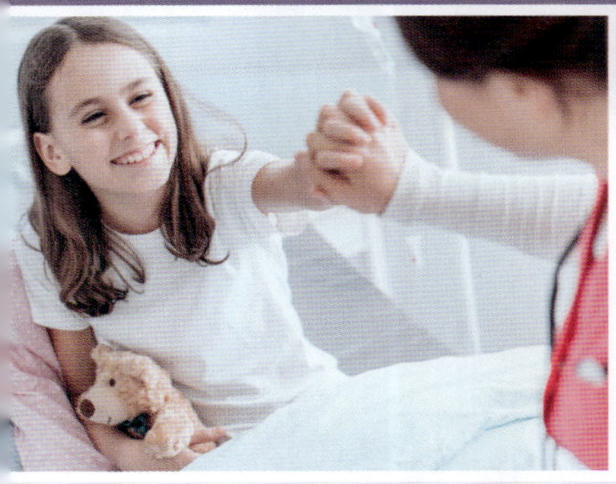

21 Family-centred Care of the Child During Illness and Hospitalisation

Deb Surman and Julia Laing

LEARNING OBJECTIVES

- Identify stressors experienced by the infant, child and young person undergoing treatment/care in hospital
- Identify coping behaviours experienced by infants, children and young people while hospitalised
- Discuss effective communication techniques to cater for the various stages of child development
- Recognise and acknowledge the importance of maintaining cultural safety when caring for infants, children and young people
- Understand the strategies to encourage and facilitate family-centred care

STRESSORS OF HOSPITALISATION AND CHILDREN'S REACTIONS

Often, illness and hospitalisation are the first crises children must face. Children are particularly vulnerable to these stressors because stress represents a change from the usual state of health and environmental routine and children have a limited number of coping mechanisms to resolve stressors. Major stressors of hospitalisation include separation, loss of control, bodily injury and pain. Children's reactions to these crises are influenced by their developmental age. Previous experience with illness, separation or hospitalisation and innate and acquired coping skills, as well as the seriousness of the diagnosis and current support systems, also affect their reactions. Children express fears caused by the unfamiliar environment or lack of information and control; child-staff relations; and the physical, social and symbolic environment (Lerwick 2016, Fraser & Rosina 2017).

Separation Anxiety

The major stress from middle infancy throughout the preschool years, especially for children ages 6 to 30 months, is separation anxiety, also called anaclitic depression. The principal behavioural responses to this stressor during early childhood are summarised in Box 21.1. During the initial stage of protest, children react aggressively to the separation from the parent. They cry and scream for their parents, refuse the attention of anyone else and are inconsolable in their grief (Fig 21.1). In contrast, the second stage is the stage of despair. In despair, the crying stops and depression is evident. The child is much less active, is uninterested in play or food and withdraws from others.

The third stage of detachment is where the child superficially appears to adjust to the loss. The child becomes more interested in the surroundings, plays with others and seems to form new relationships. However, this behaviour is the result of resignation and is not a sign of contentment. The child detaches from the parent to escape the emotional pain of desiring the parent's presence and copes by forming shallow relationships with others, becoming increasingly self-centred and attaching primary importance to material objects. This is the most serious stage in that reversal of the potential adverse effects is less likely to occur after detachment is established. The temporary separations imposed by hospitalisation do not cause such prolonged parental absences that the child enters detachment. Although progression to the stage of detachment is uncommon, the initial stages are frequently observed even with brief separations from either parent. Unless health team members understand the meaning of each stage of behaviour, they may erroneously label the behaviours as positive or negative. For example, they may see the loud crying of the protest phase as 'bad' behaviour. Because the protests increase when a stranger approaches the child, they may interpret that reaction as meaning they should stay away. During the quiet, withdrawn phase of despair, health team members may think that the child is finally 'settling in' to the new surroundings, and they may see the detachment behaviours as proof of a 'good adjustment'. The faster this stage is reached, the more likely it is that the child will be regarded as the 'ideal patient'.

Such reactions are distressing to parents, who are unaware of their meaning (Fig 21.2). If parents are regarded as intruders, they will see their absence as 'beneficial' to the child's adjustment and recovery. They may respond to the child's behaviour by staying for only short periods, visiting less frequently or deceiving the child when it is time to leave. The result is a destructive cycle of misunderstanding and unmet needs. Considerable evidence suggests that even with stressors, children are remarkably adaptable and permanent ill effects are rare.

Early Childhood

Separation anxiety is the greatest stress imposed by hospitalisation during early childhood. If separation is avoided, young children have a

BOX 21.1 Manifestations of Separation Anxiety in Young Children

Stage of Protest

- Behaviours observed during later infancy include the following:
  - cries
  - screams
  - searches for parent with eyes
  - clings to parent
  - avoids and rejects contact with strangers.
- Additional behaviours observed during toddlerhood include the following:
  - verbally attacks strangers (e.g. 'Go away')
  - physically attacks strangers (e.g. kicks, bites, hits, pinches)
  - attempts to escape to find parent
  - attempts to physically force parent to stay.
- Behaviours may last from hours to days.
- Protest, such as crying, may be continuous, ceasing only with physical exhaustion.
- Approach of stranger may precipitate increased protest.

Stage of Despair

- Observed behaviours include the following:
  - is inactive
  - withdraws from others
  - is depressed, sad
  - lacks interest in environment
  - is uncommunicative
  - regresses to earlier behaviour (e.g. thumb sucking, bedwetting, use of soother (dummy), use of bottle).
- Behaviours may last for a variable length of time.
- Child's physical condition may deteriorate from refusal to eat, drink or move.

Stage of Detachment

- Observed behaviours include the following:
  - shows increased interest in surroundings
  - interacts with strangers or familiar caregivers
  - forms new but superficial relationships
  - appears happy.
- Detachment usually occurs after prolonged separation from parent; it is rarely seen in hospitalised children.
- Behaviours represent a superficial adjustment to loss.

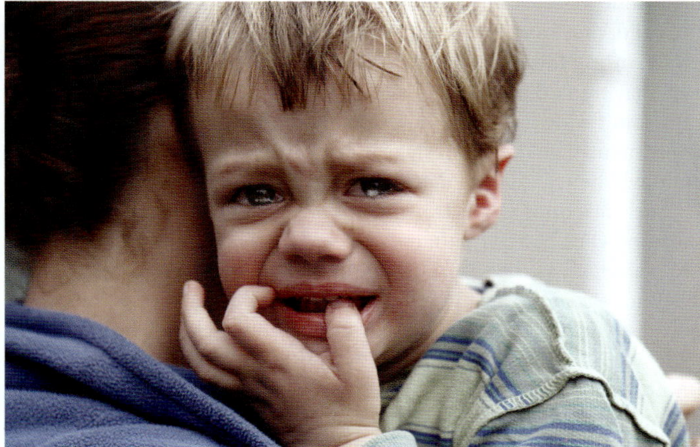

Fig 21.1 In the protest phase of separation anxiety, children cry loudly and are inconsolable in their grief for the parent.

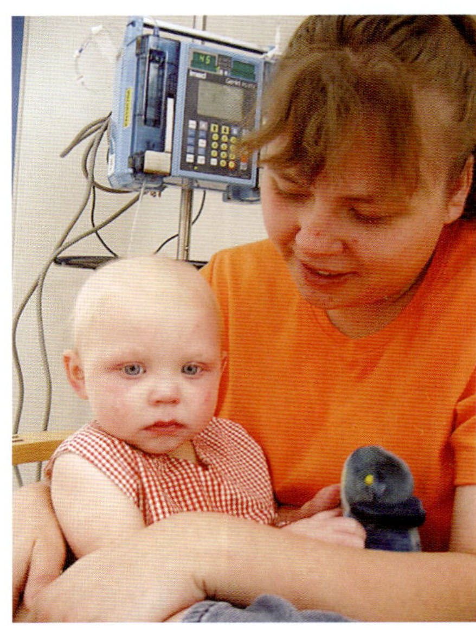

Fig 21.2 Young children may appear withdrawn and sad even in the presence of a parent. (Source: Courtesy of E. Jacob, Texas Children's Hospital, Houston, Texas.)

tremendous capacity to withstand any other stress. During this age period, these typical reactions are seen. Children in the toddler stage demonstrate more goal-directed behaviours. For example, they may plead with the parents to stay and physically try to keep the parents with them or try to find parents who have left. They may demonstrate displeasure on the parents' return or departure by: having temper tantrums; refusing to comply with the usual routines of mealtime, bedtime or toileting; or regressing to more primitive levels of development. Temper tantrums, bedwetting or other behaviours may also be expressions of anger, a physiological response to stress or symptoms of illness.

Later Childhood and Adolescence

In a study that asked children about their fears when hospitalised, children listed their greatest fears regarding hospitalisation as being separated from family and friends, being in an unfamiliar environment, receiving treatments and losing self-determination or choices (Coyne 2006, Öztürk Şahin & Topan 2019). In a qualitative study of children 5 to 9 years old, children described hospitalisation in stories that focused on being alone and feeling scared, angry or sad. These children also described the need for protection and companionship while hospitalised (Lambert et al 2014, Livesley & Long 2013, Wilson et al 2010).

Although school-age children are better able to cope with separation in general, the stress and regression imposed by illness or hospitalisation may increase their need for parental security and guidance. This is particularly true for younger school-age children who have only recently left the safety of the home and are struggling with the crisis of school adjustment. Older children may react more to the separation from their usual activities and peers than to the absence of their parents. These children may not like school but admit to missing its routine and worry that they will not be able to compete or 'fit in' with their classmates when they return. Feelings of loneliness, boredom, isolation and depression are common. Such reactions may occur more as a result of separation than of concern over the illness, treatment or hospital setting.

Loss of Control

One of the factors influencing the amount of stress imposed by hospitalisation is the lack of control. Lack of control increases the perception of threat and can affect children's coping skills. Additional hospital stimuli of sight, sound and smell may be overwhelming. Without an insight into the type of environment conducive to children's optimal growth, the hospital experience can at best temporarily slow development and at worst permanently restrict it.

Effects of Hospitalisation on the Child

Children may react to the stresses of hospitalisation before admission, during hospitalisation and after discharge. A recent qualitative study found that children 5 to 6 years of age were able to understand the association between stress and illness; this understanding is related to the child's developmental age and illness experience (Cheetham et al 2016). This may or may not be affected by the duration of the condition or prior hospitalisations. Nurses should avoid assuming the child has learned how to cope from prior medical experiences (Box 21.2).

Individual Risk Factors

Several risk factors make certain children more vulnerable to the stresses of hospitalisation, including the environment they live in and their personality traits (Box 21.3). Some children may exhibit significantly greater degrees of psychological upset than other children. Because separation is such an important issue surrounding hospitalisation for young children, children who are active and strong willed tend to fare better when hospitalised than those who are passive. Consequently, nurses should be alert to children who passively accept all changes and requests; these children may need more support than 'oppositional' children.

BOX 21.2 Post-hospital Behaviours in Children

Young Children

- They show initial aloofness towards parents; this may last from a few minutes (most common) to a few days.
- This is frequently followed by dependency behaviours:
  - tendency to cling to parents
  - demands for parents' attention
  - vigorous opposition to any separation (e.g. staying at preschool or with a babysitter).
- Other negative behaviours include the following:
  - new fears (e.g. nightmares)
  - resistance to going to bed, night waking
  - withdrawal and shyness
  - hyperactivity
  - temper tantrums
  - food peculiarities
  - attachment to blanket or toy
  - regression in newly learned skills (e.g. self-toileting).

Older Children

- Negative behaviours include the following:
  - emotional coldness followed by intense, demanding dependence on parents
  - anger towards parents
  - jealousy towards others (e.g. siblings).

BOX 21.3 Risk Factors that Increase Children's Vulnerability to the Stresses of Hospitalisation

- 'Difficult' temperament
- Lack of fit between child and parent
- Age (especially between 6 months old and 5 years old)
- Male gender
- Below-average intelligence
- Multiple and continuing stresses (e.g. frequent hospitalisations)

The stressors of hospitalisation may cause young children to experience short- and long-term negative outcomes. Adverse outcomes may be related to the length and number of admissions, multiple invasive procedures and the parents' anxiety. Common responses include regression, separation anxiety, apathy, fears and sleeping disturbances, especially for younger children. Supportive practices, such as family-centred care and frequent family visiting, may lessen the detrimental effects of such admissions.

Changes in the Paediatric Population. The paediatric population in hospitals has changed dramatically over the past two decades. With a growing trend towards shortened hospital stays and outpatient surgery, a greater percentage of the children hospitalised today have more serious and complex problems than those hospitalised in the past. Many of these children are fragile newborns and children with severe injuries or disabilities who have survived because of major technological advances, yet they have been left with chronic or disabling conditions that require frequent and lengthy hospital stays. The nature of their conditions increases the likelihood that they will experience more invasive and traumatic procedures while they are hospitalised. These factors make them more vulnerable to the emotional consequences of hospitalisation and result in their needs being significantly different from those of the short-term patients of the past. The majority of these children are infants and toddlers, which is the age group most vulnerable to the effects of hospitalisation. (Refer to Chapter 19 for further discussion on children with special needs.)

Beneficial Effects of Hospitalisation

Although hospitalisation is stressful for children, it can also be beneficial. The most obvious benefit is the recovery from illness, but hospitalisation also can present an opportunity for children to master stress and feel competent in their coping abilities. The hospital environment can provide children and families with new socialisation experiences that can broaden their interpersonal relationships. In addition, hospitalisation can provide access to supportive resources that they may never have had access to otherwise. Appropriate nursing strategies to recognise psychological benefits are presented later in the chapter.

STRESSORS AND REACTIONS OF THE FAMILY OF THE CHILD WHO IS HOSPITALISED

Parental Reactions

The crisis of childhood illness and hospitalisation affects every member of the family. Parents' reactions to illness in their child depend on a variety of factors. An association was found between coping abilities and the variables of income range, information provided to the family on admission to the facility and preparation for hospitalisation (Galeano & Carvajal 2016). A number of factors affecting parent's reactions to variables are identified in Box 21.4.

BOX 21.4 Factors Affecting Parents' Reactions to Their Child's Illness

- Seriousness of the threat to the child
- Previous experience with illness or hospitalisation
- Medical procedures involved in diagnosis and treatment
- Available support systems
- Personal ego strengths
- Previous coping abilities
- Additional stresses on the family system
- Cultural and religious beliefs
- Communication patterns among family members
- Information and education provided to family throughout hospitalisation
- Socioeconomic status

Research has identified common themes among parents whose children were hospitalised, including feeling an overall sense of helplessness, questioning the skills of staff, accepting the reality of hospitalisation, needing to have information explained in simple language, dealing with fear, coping with uncertainty and seeking reassurance from caregivers. A qualitative study of parents experiencing care for their child in a paediatric intensive care unit found that they desired continuity of nursing care, needed assurance that the bedside nurse valued their child as an individual and needed preparation for the complexities of the child's care regimen (Baird et al 2016). Reassurance from the healthcare team can be in the form of collaboration, information sharing, preparation for procedures, ensuring formal and informal support for the family and providing information in an unbiased and culturally sensitive manner (Eichner & Johnson 2012, COAG 2015).

Sibling Reactions

Various factors have been identified that influence the effects of the child's hospitalisation on siblings. Siblings' reactions to a sister's or brother's illness or hospitalisation differ little when a child becomes temporarily ill. Siblings experience loneliness, fear and worry, as well as anger, resentment, jealousy and guilt. Illness may also result in children's loss of status within either their family or their social group. It has been found that parents of siblings of children with chronic illness tended to rate sibling health and quality of life better than the siblings' self-reports. The greater disease severity of affected child and older sibling age may be risk factors for impaired well sibling quality of life (Jessup et al 2018, Limbers & Skipper 2014).

Parents are often unaware of the number of effects that siblings experience during the sick child's hospitalisation and the benefit of simple interventions to minimise such effects, such as explicit explanations about the illness and provisions for the siblings to remain at home. Sibling visitation is usually beneficial to the patient, sibling and parent but should be evaluated on an individual basis. Siblings should be prepared for the visit with developmentally appropriate information and be given the opportunity to ask questions.

NURSING CARE OF THE CHILD WHO IS HOSPITALISED

Preparation for Hospitalisation

Children and families require individualised care to minimise the potential negative effects of hospitalisation. One method that can decrease negative feelings and fear in children is preparation for hospitalisation. The rationale for preparing children for the hospital experience and related procedures is based on the principle that a fear of the unknown exceeds fear of the known. When children do not have paralysing fear to cope with, they are able to direct their energies towards dealing with the other, unavoidable stresses of hospitalisation.

Admission Assessment

The nursing admission history refers to a systematic collection of data about the child and family that allows the nurse to plan individualised care. The nursing admission history presented in Box 21.5 is organised according to the functional health patterns outlined by Gordon (2002). This assessment framework is a guideline for formulating nursing diagnoses. One of the main purposes of the history is to assess the child's usual health habits at home to promote a more normal environment in the hospital. Therefore, questions related to activities of daily living in the nutritional/metabolic, elimination, sleep/rest and activity/exercise patterns are a major part of the assessment. The questions found under the health perception/health management pattern are directed towards evaluation of the child's preparation for hospitalisation and are key factors in determining whether additional preparation is needed. The questions included in the self-perception/self-concept and role/relationship patterns offer insight into the child's potential reaction to hospitalisation, especially in terms of separation.

The nurse should also enquire about the use of any medications at home, including complementary medicine practices (Box 21.6). Many families use alternative or complementary therapies simultaneously with or after conventional treatments. It is important that the use of any herbal or complementary therapy be noted in a preoperative assessment because of possible anaesthesia or surgical complications related to herbal products.

In addition to completing the nursing admission history, nurses should also perform a physical assessment (see Chapter 4) before planning care. At the very least, the nurse's physical assessment of the child should include observation of the body for any bruises, rashes, signs of neglect, deformities or physical limitations. The nurse should also listen to the heart and lungs to assess overall physical status. For example, it is impossible to evaluate improvement in respiratory function in a child admitted with pulmonary disease unless there are baseline data with which to compare subsequent findings.

Preparing the Child for Admission

The preparation that children require on the day of admission depends on the kind of prehospital counselling they have received. If they have been prepared in a formalised program, they usually know what to expect in terms of initial medical procedures, inpatient facilities and nursing staff. However, prehospital counselling does not preclude the need for support during procedures, such as obtaining blood specimens, x-ray tests or physical examination. For example, undressing young children before they feel comfortable in their new surroundings can be upsetting. Causing needless anxiety and fear during admission may adversely affect the nurse's establishment of trust with these children. Therefore, nursing assistance during the admission procedure is vital regardless of how well prepared any child is for the experience of hospitalisation. In addition, spending this time with the child gives the nurse an opportunity to evaluate the child's understanding of subsequent procedures (Fig 21.3). Ideally, a primary nurse is assigned whenever possible to allow for individualised care and to provide an additional support person for the child.

BOX 21.5 Nursing Admission History According to Functional Health Patterns*

Health Perception/Health Management Pattern

- Why has your child been admitted?
- How has your child's general health been?
- What does your child know about this hospitalisation?
  - Ask the child why he or she came to the hospital.
  - If the answer is 'For an operation or for tests', ask the child to tell you about what will happen before, during and after the operation or tests.
- Has your child ever been in the hospital before?
  - How was that hospital experience?
  - What things were important to you and your child during that hospitalisation? How can we be most helpful now?
- What medications does your child take at home?
  - Why are they given?
  - When are they given?
  - How are they given (if a liquid, with a syringe or medicine cup; if a tablet, swallowed with water; or other)?
  - Does your child have any trouble taking medication? If so, what helps?
  - Is your child allergic to any medications?
- What, if any, forms of complementary medicine practices are being used?

Nutrition/Metabolic Pattern

- What is the family's usual mealtime?
- Do family members eat together or at separate times?
- What are your child's favourite foods, beverages and snacks?
  - Average amounts consumed or usual size of portions
  - Special cultural practices, such as family eats only ethnic food
- What foods and beverages does your child dislike?
- What are your child's feeding habits (bottle, cup, spoon, eats by self, needs assistance, any special devices)?
- How does your child like the food served (warmed, cold, one item at a time)?
- How would you describe your child's usual appetite (hearty eater, picky eater)?
  - Has being sick affected your child's appetite? In what ways?
- Are there any known or suspected food allergies?
- Is your child on a special diet?
- Are there any feeding problems (excessive fussiness, spitting up, colic); any dental or gum problems that affect feeding?
  - What do you do for these problems?

Elimination Pattern

- What are your child's toileting habits (nappy, toilet trained—day only or day and night, use of word to communicate urination or defecation, potty chair, regular toilet, other routines)?
- What is your child's usual pattern of elimination (bowel movements)?
- Do you have any concerns about elimination (bedwetting, constipation, diarrhoea)?
  - What do you do for these problems?
- Have you ever noticed that your child sweats a lot?

Sleep/Rest Pattern

- What is your child's usual hour of sleep and awakening?
- What is your child's schedule for naps; length of naps?
- Is there a special routine before sleeping (bottle, drink of water, bedtime story, night light, favourite blanket or toy, prayers)?
- Is there a special routine during sleep time, such as waking to go to the bathroom?
- What type of bed does your child sleep in?
- Does your child have a separate room or share a room; if shared, with whom?
- Does your child sleep with someone or alone (e.g. sibling, parent, other person)?
- What is your child's favourite sleeping position?
- Are there any sleeping problems (falling asleep, waking during night, nightmares, sleep walking)?
- Are there any problems in awakening and getting ready in the morning?
  - What do you do for these problems?

Activity/Exercise Pattern

- What is your child's schedule during the day (preschool, day-care centre, regular school, extracurricular activities)?
- What are your child's favourite activities or toys (both active and quiet interests)?
- What is your child's usual television-viewing schedule at home?
- What are your child's favourite programs?
- Are there any television restrictions?
- Does your child have any illness or disabilities that limit activity? If so, how?
- What are your child's usual habits and schedule for bathing (bath in tub or shower, sponge bath, shampoo)?
- What are your child's dental habits (brushing, flossing, fluoride supplements or rinses, favourite toothpaste); schedule of daily dental care?
- Does your child need help with dressing or grooming, such as hair combing?
- Are there any problems with these patterns (dislike of or refusal to bathe, shampoo hair or brush teeth)?
  - What do you do for these problems?
- Are there special devices that your child requires help in managing (eyeglasses, contact lenses, hearing aid, orthodontic appliances, artificial elimination appliances, orthopaedic devices)?
- Note: Use the following code to assess functional self-care level for feeding, bathing and hygiene, dressing and grooming and toileting.
  - **0**—Full self-care
  - **I**—Requires use of equipment or device
  - **II**—Requires assistance or supervision from another person
  - **III**—Requires assistance or supervision from another person and equipment or device
  - **IV**—Is totally dependent and does not participate

Cognitive/Perceptual Pattern

- Does your child have any hearing difficulty?
  - Does the child use a hearing aid?
  - Have 'tubes' been placed in your child's ears?
- Does your child have any vision problems?
  - Does the child wear glasses or contact lenses?
- Does your child have any learning difficulties?
- What is the child's grade in school?
- For information on pain, see Chapter 5

Self-perception/Self-concept Pattern

- How would you describe your child (e.g. takes time to adjust, settles in easily, shy, friendly, quiet, talkative, serious, playful, stubborn, easy-going)?
- What makes your child angry, annoyed, anxious or sad? What helps?
- How does your child act when annoyed or upset?
- What have your child's experiences been with and reactions to temporary separation from you (parent)?
- Does your child have any fears (places, objects, animals, people and situations)?
  - How do you handle them?
- Do you think your child's illness has changed the way he or she thinks about himself or herself (e.g. shyer than normal, embarrassed about appearance, less competitive with friends, stays at home more)?

Continued

BOX 21.5 Nursing Admission History According to Functional Health Patterns—cont'd

Role/Relationship Pattern

- Does your child have a favourite nickname?
- What are the names of other family members or others who live in the home (relatives, friends, pets)?
- Who usually takes care of your child during the day and night (especially if other than parent, such as babysitter, relative)?
- What are the parents' occupations and work schedules?
- Are there any special family considerations (adoption, foster child, step-parent, divorce, single parent)?
- Have any major changes in the family occurred lately (death, divorce, separation, birth of a sibling, loss of a job, financial strain, mother beginning a career, other)? Describe child's reaction.
- Who are your child's play companions or social groups (peers, younger or older children, adults or prefers to be alone)?
- Do things generally go well for your child in school or with friends?
- Does your child have 'security' objects at home (soother, bottle, blanket, stuffed animal or doll)? Did you bring any of these to the hospital?
- How do you handle discipline problems at home? Are these methods always effective?
- Does your child have any condition that interferes with communication? If so, what are your suggestions for communicating with your child?
- Will your child's hospitalisation affect the family's financial support or care of other family members (e.g. other children)?
- What concerns do you have about your child's illness and hospitalisation?
- Who will be staying with your child while hospitalised?
- How can we contact you or another close family member outside of the hospital?

Sexuality/Reproductive Pattern

(Answer questions that apply to your child's age group.)

- Has your child begun puberty (developing physical sexual characteristics, menstruation)? Have you or your child had any concerns?
- Does your daughter know how to do a breast self-examination?
- Does your son know how to do a testicular self-examination?
- How have you approached topics of sexuality with your child?
- Do you think you might need some help with some topics?
- Has your child's illness affected the way he or she feels about being a boy or a girl? If so, how?
- Do you have any concerns with behaviours in your child, such as masturbation, asking many questions or talking about sex, not respecting others' privacy or wanting too much privacy?
- Initiate a conversation about an adolescent's sexual concerns with open-ended to more direct questions and using the terms 'friends' or 'partners' rather than 'girlfriend' or 'boyfriend'.
  - Tell me about your social life.
  - Who are your closest friends? (If one friend is identified, could ask more about that relationship, such as how much time they spend together, how serious they are about each other, if the relationship is going the way the teenager hoped.)
  - Might ask about dating and sexual issues, such as the teenager's views on sexuality education, 'going out', 'living together' or premarital sex.
  - Which friends would you like to have visit you in the hospital?

Coping/Stress Tolerance Pattern

(Answer questions that apply to your child's age group.)

- What does your child do when tired or upset?
  - If upset, does your child want a special person or object?
  - If so, explain.
- If your child has temper tantrums, what causes them and how do you handle them?
- Whom does your child talk to when worried about something?
- How does your child usually handle problems or disappointments?
- Have there been any big changes or problems in your family recently? If so, how have you handled them?
- Has your child ever had a problem with drugs or alcohol or tried to commit suicide?
- Do you think your child is 'accident-prone'? If so, explain.

Value/Belief Pattern

- What is your religion?
- How is religion or faith important in your child's life?
- What religious practices would you like continued in the hospital?

* The focus of the admission history is the child's psychosocial environment. Most of the questions are worded in terms of parental responses. Depending on the child's age, they should be addressed directly to the child when appropriate.

BOX 21.6 Complementary Medicine Practices and Examples

Nutrition, diet and lifestyle of behavioural health changes—Macrobiotics, megavitamins, diets, lifestyle modification, health risk reduction and health education, wellness

Mind-body control therapies—Biofeedback, relaxation, prayer therapy, guided imagery, hypnotherapy, music or sound therapy, massage, aromatherapy, education therapy

Traditional and ethnomedicine therapies—Acupuncture, ayurvedic medicine, herbal medicine, homeopathic medicine, natural products, traditional Asian medicine,

Structural manipulation and energetic therapies—Acupressure, chiropractic medicine, massage, reflexology, rolfing, therapeutic touch, Qi Gong

Pharmacological and biological therapies—Antioxidants, cell treatment, chelation therapy, metabolic therapy, oxidising agents

Bioelectromagnetic therapies—Diagnostic and therapeutic application of electromagnetic fields (e.g. transcranial electrostimulation, neuromagnetic stimulation, electroacupuncture)

Nursing Interventions

Preventing or Minimising Separation

A primary nursing goal is to prevent separation, particularly in children younger than 5 years old. Many hospitals have developed a system of family-centred care. Efforts to collaborate with families and encourage their involvement in the patient's care include optimising family visitation, family-centred rounding, family presence during procedures or interventions and opportunities for formal and informal family conferences (Meert et al 2013). Family-centred care started in paediatrics with the increased recognition of child and family separation trauma in the inpatient setting. Policies were adapted first in paediatrics to allow for rooming-in, longer visiting hours, sibling visits and systems to allow families to accompany patients off the unit for procedures (ACSQHC 2018, HUSH Foundation n.d.).

Parental Absence During Infant Hospitalisation

Familiar surroundings also increase the child's adjustment to separation. If the parents cannot stay with the child, they should leave favourite articles from home with the child, such as a blanket or a toy. Children gain comfort and reassurance from holding onto these

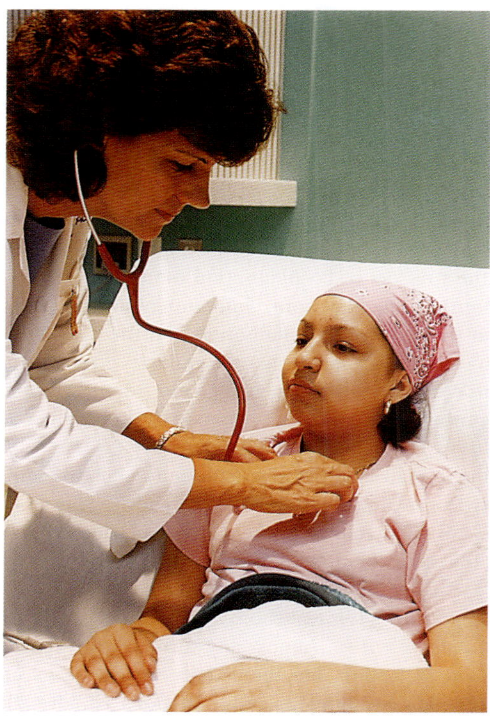

Fig 21.3 The initial admission procedures give the nurse an opportunity to get to know the child and to assess the child's understanding of the hospital experience.

possessions. They make the association that if the parents left this, the parents would surely return. Placing an identification band on the toy lessens the chances of its being misplaced and provides a symbol that the toy is experiencing the same needs as the child. Other reminders of home include photographs and video recordings of family members reading a story or singing a song. These reminders can be brought out at lonely times, such as on awakening or before sleeping. Some units allow pets to visit, which can have therapeutic benefits for a child. Often the importance of treasured objects to school-age children or adolescents can be overlooked or criticised. However, these older children have a special object to which they formed an attachment in early childhood. Therefore, treasured or transitional objects can help even older children feel more comfortable in a strange environment.

Minimising Loss of Control

Children feel a loss of control due to physical restrictions, changed routines and enforced dependency. Some of these stressors cannot be prevented, although most can be minimised through individualised nursing care to help minimise their impact.

Promoting Freedom of Movement. Younger children react most strenuously to any type of physical restriction or immobilisation. Although temporary immobilisation may be necessary for some interventions such as maintaining an intravenous line, most physical restrictions can be prevented if the nurse gains the child's cooperation.

For young children, particularly infants and toddlers, preserving parent–child contact is the best means of decreasing the need for restraint. Nearly the entire physical examination can be done in a parent's lap with the parent hugging the child for procedures, such as an otoscopic examination. For painful procedures, the nurse should assess the parents' preferences for assisting, observing or waiting outside the room.

Maintaining the Child's Routine. Altered daily schedules and loss of rituals are particularly stressful for toddlers and early preschoolers and may increase the stress of separation. The nursing admission history provides a baseline for planning care around the child's usual home activities. A frequently neglected aspect of altered routines is the change in the child's daily activities. A typical child's day, especially during the school years, is structured with specific times for eating, dressing, going to school, playing and sleeping. However, this time structure vanishes when the child is hospitalised. Although nurses have a set schedule, the child is frequently unaware of it and the new schedules that are imposed may be rigid.

Encouraging Independence. The dependent role of the hospitalised patient imposes tremendous feelings of loss for older children. Principal interventions should focus on respect for individuality and the opportunity for decision-making. Although these sound simple, their efficacy lies with nurses who are flexible and tolerant. It is also important for the nurse to empower the patient while not feeling threatened by a sense of lessened control.

Enabling children's control involves helping them maintain independence and promoting the concept of self-care. Self-care refers to the practice of activities that individuals personally initiate and perform on their own behalf in maintaining life, health and wellbeing (Orem 2001).

Promoting Understanding. Loss of control can occur from feelings of having too little influence on one's destiny or from sensing overwhelming control or power over fate. Although preschoolers' cognitive abilities predispose them to magical thinking and delusions of power, all children are vulnerable to misinterpreting causes for stress, such as illness and hospitalisation.

Most children feel more in control when they know what to expect because the element of fear of the unknown is reduced. Anticipatory preparation and provision of information help lessen stress and increase understanding (see Chapter 19).

Informing children of their rights while hospitalised fosters greater understanding and may relieve some of the feelings of powerlessness they typically experience. An increasing number of hospitals and organisations have developed a patient charter that is prominently displayed throughout the hospital or is presented to children and their families on admission (Box 21.7).

Preventing or Minimising Fear of Bodily Injury

Beyond early infancy, all children fear bodily injury from mutilation, bodily intrusion, body image change, disability or death. In general, preparation of children for painful procedures decreases their fears and increases cooperation. Modifying procedural techniques for children in each age group also minimises fear of bodily injury. Whenever procedures are performed on young children, the most supportive intervention is to do the procedure as quickly as possible while maintaining parent–child contact.

Because of toddlers' and preschool children's poorly defined body boundaries, the use of bandages may be particularly helpful. For example, telling children that the bleeding will stop after the needle is removed does little to relieve their fears, but applying a small Band-Aid usually reassures them. The size of bandages is also significant to children in this age group; the larger the bandage, the more importance is attached to the wound. Watching their surgical dressings become successively smaller is one way young children can measure healing and improvement. Prematurely removing a dressing may cause these children considerable concern for their wellbeing. Specific pain management strategies are discussed in Chapter 5.

BOX 21.7 Charter on the Rights of Children and Young People in Healthcare Services in Australia

Every child and young person has a right:

- to consideration of their best interests as the primary concern of all involved in his/her care
- to express their views and to be heard and taken seriously
- to the highest attainable standard of healthcare
- to respect for themselves as a whole person, as well as respect for their family and the family's individual characteristics, beliefs, culture and contexts
- to be nurtured by their parents and family and to have family relationships supported by the service in which the child or young person is receiving healthcare
- to information in a form that is understandable to them
- to participate in decision-making and as appropriate to their capabilities to make decisions about their care
- to be kept safe from all forms of harm
- to have their privacy respected
- to participate in education, play creative activities and recreation if this is difficult due to their illness or disability
- to continuity of healthcare including well planned care that takes them beyond the paediatric context.

Source: Australia Children's Healthcare Australasia (CHA) and Association for the wellbeing of Children in Healthcare (AWCH). (2017). Charter on the rights of children and young people in healthcare services in Australia. https://children.wcha.asn.au/publications/charter-rights-children-and-young-people-healthcare-services-australia

Providing Developmentally Appropriate Activities

A primary goal of nursing care for the child who is hospitalised is to minimise threats to the child's development. Many strategies (e.g. minimising separation) have been discussed and may be all that the short-term patient requires. However, children who experience prolonged or repeated hospitalisation are at greater risk for developmental delays or regression. The nurse who provides opportunities for the child to participate in developmentally appropriate activities further normalises the child's environment and helps reduce interference with the child's ongoing development.

Interference with normal development may have long-term implications for developing infants and toddlers. The nurse plays a primary role in identifying children at risk and helping plan, implement and evaluate developmental intervention. (See Chapters 9 and 11.)

School is an integral part of development for the school-age child and adolescent. Accreditation standards for hospitals serving children consider access to appropriate educational services a key factor in the accreditation decision process when a child's treatment requires a significant absence from school (ACSQHC 2018). The nurse can encourage children to resume schoolwork as quickly as their condition permits, help them schedule and protect a selected time for studies and help the family coordinate hospital educational services with their children's schools. Children should have the opportunity to continue art and music classes, as well as their academic subjects.

To meet the unique developmental needs of adolescents, special units may be developed that provide privacy, increased socialisation and appropriate activities for these young people. Typically, these units can be set apart from the general paediatric facility so that the teenagers do not share space with younger children, who are often perceived as a threat to their maturity.

Providing Opportunities for Play and Expressive Activities

Play is one of the most important aspects of a child's life and one of the most effective tools for managing stress. Because illness and hospitalisation constitute crises in a child's life and often involve overwhelming stresses, children need to act out their fears and anxieties as a means of coping with these stresses. Play is essential to children's mental, emotional and social wellbeing; however, play does not stop when children are ill or in the hospital. On the contrary, play in the hospital serves many functions (Box 21.8). Of all hospital facilities, no room probably alleviates the stressors of hospitalisation more than the playroom (or activity room). In the playroom, children temporarily distance themselves from their illness, hospitalisation and the associated stressors. This room should be a safe haven for children, free from medical or nursing procedures (including medication administration), strange faces and probing questions. The playroom then becomes a sanctuary in an otherwise frightening environment.

Engaging in play activities gives children a sense of control. In the hospital environment, most decisions are made for the child; play and other expressive activities offer the child much-needed opportunities to make choices for themselves. Even if a child chooses not to participate in a particular activity, the nurse has offered the child a choice, perhaps one of only a few real choices the child has had that day.

Diversional Activities. Almost any form of play can be used for diversion and recreation, but the activity should be selected on the basis of the child's age, interests and limitations. Children do not necessarily need special direction for using play materials. All they require is the raw materials with which to work and adult approval and supervision to help keep their natural enthusiasm and expression of feelings. Small children enjoy a variety of small, colourful toys that they can play with in bed or in their room or more elaborate play equipment, such as playhouses, sandboxes, rhythm instruments or large boxes and blocks that may be a part of the hospital playroom.

When supervising play for ill or convalescent children, it is best to select activities that are simpler than would normally be chosen for the child's specific developmental level. These children usually do not have the energy to cope with more challenging activities. Other limitations also influence the type of activities. Special consideration must be given to children who are confined in terms of movement, have a restricted extremity or are isolated. Toys for isolated children must be disposable or need to be disinfected after every use.

Toys. Parents of hospitalised children often ask nurses about the types of toys that would be best to bring for their child. Although parents often want to buy new toys for the hospitalised child to offer cheer and comfort, it is often better to wait. Small children need the comfort and reassurance of familiar things, such as the stuffed animal the child hugs for comfort and takes to bed at night. These familiar items are a

BOX 21.8 Functions of Play in the Hospital

- Provides diversion and brings about relaxation
- Helps the child feel more secure in a strange environment
- Lessens the stress of separation and the feeling of homesickness
- Provides a means for release of tension and expression of feelings
- Encourages interaction and development of positive attitudes towards others
- Provides an expressive outlet for creative ideas and interests
- Provides a means for accomplishing therapeutic goals
- Places child in active role and provides opportunity to make choices and be in control

link with home and the world outside the hospital. All toys brought into the hospital should be assessed for safety.

Expressive Activities. Play and other expressive activities provide one of the best opportunities for encouraging emotional expression, including the safe release of anger and hostility. Non-directive play that allows children freedom for expression can be tremendously therapeutic. Therapeutic play, however, should not be confused with play therapy, a psychological technique reserved for use by trained and qualified therapists as an interpretative method with emotionally disturbed children. Therapeutic play, on the other hand, is an effective, non-directive modality for helping children deal with their concerns and fears, and at the same time, it often helps the nurse gain insights into children's needs and feelings.

Creative Expression. Although all children derive physical, social, emotional and cognitive benefits from engaging in art and other creative activities, children's need for such activities is intensified when they are hospitalised. Drawing and painting are excellent media for expression. Children are more at ease expressing their thoughts and feelings through art because humans think first in images and later learn to translate these images into words. Children need only to be supplied with the raw materials, such as crayons and paper, large brushes and an ample supply of art and craft materials while in hospital.

Although interpretation of children's drawings requires special training, observing changes in a series of the child's drawings over time can be helpful in assessing psychosocial adjustment and coping. The nurse can use children's drawings, stories, poetry and other products of creative expression as a springboard for discussion of thoughts, fears and understanding of concepts or events (see Chapter 4). A child's drawing before surgery, for example, may reveal unvoiced concerns about mutilation, body changes and loss of self-control.

Nurses can incorporate opportunities for musical expression into routine nursing care. For example, simple musical instruments, such as bracelets with bells, can be placed on infants' legs for them to shake to accompany mealtime music or dressing changes. Dance and movement suggestions may encourage a child to ambulate.

Dramatic Play. Dramatic play is a well-recognised technique for emotional release, allowing children to re-enact frightening or puzzling hospital experiences. Through use of puppets, replicas of hospital equipment or some actual hospital equipment, children can act out the situations that are a part of their hospital experience. Dramatic play enables children to learn about procedures and events that concern them and to assume the roles of the adults in the hospital environment.

Play must consider any limitations imposed by the child's condition. For example, small children are prone to explore their environment by placing things in their mouth. Therefore, a child who is allergic to wheat should not be given modelling dough made with flour. A child on a restricted salt intake should not play with modelling dough because salt is one of its major constituents. At home the play program can be planned around the therapy regimen. Play can be satisfactorily incorporated into the child's care if the nurse and others involved allow some flexibility and use creativity in planning for play.

Maximising Potential Benefits of Hospitalisation

Although hospitalisation generally represents a stressful time for children and families, it also represents an opportunity for facilitating positive change within the child and among family members. For some families, the stress of a child's illness, hospitalisation or both can lead to strengthening of family coping behaviours and the emergence of new coping strategies.

Fostering Parent–Child Relationships. The crisis of illness or hospitalisation can mobilise parents into more acute awareness of their child's needs. For example, hospitalisation provides opportunities for parents to learn more about their children's growth and development. When parents are helped to understand children's usual reactions to stress, such as regression or aggression, they are not only better able to support the child through the hospital experience but also may extend their insights into childrearing practices once home.

Difficulties in parent–child relationships that existed before hospitalisation that are characterised by feeding problems, negative behaviour and sleep disturbances may decrease during hospitalisation. The temporary cessation of such problems sometimes alerts parents to the role they may be playing in propagating the negative behaviour. With assistance from health professionals, parents can restructure ways of relating to their children to foster more positive behaviour.

Hospitalisation may also represent a temporary reprieve or refuge from a disturbed home. Typically, abused or neglected children's dramatic physical and social improvement during hospitalisation is proof of the benefits and potential growth that can occur during hospitalisation. These children can temporarily seek support, reassurance and security from new relationships, particularly with nurses and hospitalised peers.

Providing Educational Opportunities. Illness and hospitalisation represent excellent opportunities for children and other family members to learn more about their bodies, each other and the health professions. For example, during a hospital admission for a diabetic crisis, the child may learn about the disease; the parents may learn about the child's needs for independence, normalcy and appropriate limits; and each of them may find a new support system in the hospital staff.

Promoting Self-mastery. The experience of facing a crisis such as illness or hospitalisation can provide an opportunity for self-mastery of coping skills. Younger children have the chance to test fantasy versus reality fears. They realise that they were not abandoned, mutilated or punished. In fact, they were loved, cared for and treated with respect for their individual concerns. It is not unusual for children who have undergone hospitalisation or surgery to tell others that 'it was nothing' or to display proudly their scars or bandages. For older children, hospitalisation may represent an opportunity for decision-making, independence and self-reliance. They are proud of having survived the experience and may feel a genuine self-respect for their achievements. Nurses can facilitate such feelings of self-mastery by emphasising aspects of personal competence in the child and not focusing on uncooperative or negative behaviour.

Providing Socialisation. Hospitalisation may offer children a special opportunity for social acceptance. Lonely, asocial and even delinquent children find a sympathetic environment in the hospital. Children who have a physical disability or are in some other way 'different' from their age mates may find an accepting social peer group. Although this does not always spontaneously occur, nurses can structure the environment to foster a supportive child group. For example, selection of a compatible roommate can help children gain a new friend and learn more about themselves. Forming relationships with significant members of the healthcare team, such as the medical practitioner, nurse, child life specialist or social worker, can greatly enhance children's adjustment in many areas of life.

Supporting Family Members

Support involves the willingness to stay and listen to parents' verbal and non-verbal messages. Sometimes the nurse does not give this support directly. For example, the nurse may offer to stay with the child to allow the parents time alone or may discuss with other family members the parents' need for extra relief. Often relatives and friends want to help but do not know how. Suggesting ways, such as babysitting, preparing meals, doing laundry or transporting the siblings to school, can prompt others to help reduce the responsibilities that burden parents.

Support may also be provided through the clergy. Parents with deep religious beliefs may appreciate the counsel of a clergy member, but because of their stress, they may not have enough energy to initiate the contact. Nurses can be supportive by arranging for clergy to visit, upholding parents' religious beliefs and respecting the individual meaning and significance of those beliefs.

Providing Information

Important nursing interventions to provide to the family should include information regarding the disease process, its treatment, prognosis and home care. In addition, anticipatory guidance regarding the child's emotional and physical reactions to illness and hospitalisation should be discussed.

For many families, the child's illness is the first contact they have with the hospital experience. Often parents are not prepared for the child's behavioural reactions to hospitalisation. Reactions can include separation behaviours, regression, aggression and hostility. Providing the parents with information about these normal and expected behavioural responses can lessen the parents' anxiety during the hospital admission. The family is equally unfamiliar with hospital rules, which often compounds their confusion and anxiety. Therefore, the family needs clear explanations about what to expect and what is expected of them.

Parents also need to be aware of the effects of illness on the family and strategies that prevent negative changes. If appropriate, parents should keep their families well informed and communicate with everyone as much as possible. They should treat all the children equally and as normally as before the illness occurred. Discipline, which initially may not have been a priority for an ill child, should be continued to provide a measure of security and predictability. When ill children know that their parents expect certain standards of conduct from them, they feel certain that they will recover. Conversely, when all limits are removed, they fear that something catastrophic will happen.

Helping parents understand the meaning of post hospitalisation behaviours in the sick child is necessary for them to tolerate and support such behaviours. In addition, parents should be forewarned of the common reactions after discharge (see Box 21.2). Parents who do not expect such reactions may misinterpret them as evidence of the child's 'being spoiled' and demand perfect behaviour at a time when the child is still reacting to the stress of illness and hospitalisation. If the behaviours, especially the demand for attention, are dealt with in a supportive manner, most children can relinquish them and assume prior levels of functioning.

Encouraging Parent Participation

Preventing or minimising separation is a key nursing goal with the child who is hospitalised but maintaining parent–child contact is also beneficial for the family. One of the best approaches is encouraging parents to stay with their child and to participate in the care whenever possible. Although some health facilities provide special accommodations for parents, the concept of rooming-in can be instituted anywhere. The first requirement is the staff's positive attitude towards parents. In a qualitative study of 24 mothers of hospitalised children, mothers expected nurses to provide physical support and emotional support in terms of having a friendly rather than critical attitude, and being approachable and receptive of mothers' questions and anxieties (Konuk Şener & Karaca 2017).

When hospital staff members genuinely appreciate the importance of continued parent–child attachment, they foster an environment that encourages parents to stay. When parents are included in the care planning and understand that they are a contributing factor to the child's recovery, they are more inclined to remain with their child and have more emotional reserves to support themselves and the child through the crisis. An empowerment model allows the nurse to focus on parents' strengths and seek ways to promote growth and family functioning so that the parents become empowered in caring for their child. Strategies such as bedside reporting have allowed parents to be involved as active members of the team moving closer to family-centred care. Allowing parents of sick children to participate during rounds can reduce parents' anxiety and improve communication (Blankenship et al 2015).

Because the mother may tend to be the primary family caregiver, she may spend more time in the hospital than the father. Not all parents feel equally comfortable assuming responsibility for their child's care. Some may be under such great emotional stress that they need a temporary reprieve from total participation in caregiving activities. Others may feel insecure in participating in specialised areas of care, such as bathing the child after surgery. On the other hand, some mothers may feel a great need to be in control of their child's care. This seems particularly true of young mothers, mothers of young children and ethnic or minority mothers. Individual assessment of each parent's preferred involvement is necessary to prevent the effects of separation while supporting parents in their needs as well.

With lifestyles and gender roles changing, fathers may assume all or some of the usual parenting roles in the household. In these cases, it may be the father–child relationship that requires preservation. Fathers need to be included in the care plan and respected for their parental role. For some fathers, the child's hospitalisation may represent an opportunity to alter their usual caregiving role and increase their involvement. In single-parent families, the caregiver may not be a parent but an extended family member, such as a grandparent or aunt.

One of the potential problems with continuous parent involvement is neglect of the parent's need for sleep, nutrition and relaxation. Often the sleeping accommodations are limited to a chair, and sleep is disrupted by nursing procedures. Encouraging the parents to leave for brief periods, arranging for sleeping quarters on the unit but outside the child's room and planning a schedule of alternating visits with another family member can minimise the stresses for the parent.

CULTURAL CONSIDERATIONS

Nurses need to consider the cultural requirements and obligations of their patient and family and refer to the resources available to assist with the family's needs (ACSQHC 2018). For example, Aboriginal liaison officers are available in many hospitals and provide emotional, social, spiritual and cultural support to Aboriginal and Torres Strait Islander families with any concerns during their stay and discharge planning. In Aotearoa/New Zealand Kai Tiaki are available in every hospital to support Māori in their health.

Preparing for Discharge and Home Care

Discharge preparation often involves education of the family for continued care and follow-up in the home. Depending on the diagnosis, this may be relatively simple or highly complex. Preparing the family for home care demands a high degree of competence in planning and implementing discharge instructions.

Nurses are key individuals in the discharge process as they collaborate with others in the planning and implementation phases to ensure appropriate care after hospitalisation. Throughout the hospitalisation, the nurse should be aware of the need for discharge planning and those factors that affect the family's ability to provide home care. A thorough assessment of the family and home environment should be performed to ensure that the family's emotional and physical resources are enough to manage the tasks of home care. (For a discussion of family and home assessment strategies, see Chapter 4.) Consultation with social workers regarding available community services, including respite care, is needed to ensure that appropriate support agencies are available, such as emergency facilities, home health agencies and equipment vendors. Financial resources are also a consideration. To coordinate the immense task of assessment and to plan implementation, a care coordinator or manager should be included early in the discharge process.

The preparation for hospital discharge and home care begins during the admission assessment. Short- and long-term goals are established to meet the child's physical and psychosocial needs. For children with complex care needs, discharge planning focuses on obtaining appropriate equipment and healthcare personnel for the home. Discharge planning is also concerned with treatments that parents or children are expected to continue at home. In planning appropriate teaching, nurses need to assess the actual and perceived complexity of the skill, the parents' or child's ability to learn the skill and the parents' or child's previous or present experience with such procedures.

The discharge teaching plan incorporates levels of learning, such as observing, participating with assistance and finally acting without help or guidance. The skill is divided into discrete steps, and each step is taught to the family member until it is learned. Return demonstration of the skill is requested before new skills are introduced. A record of teaching and performance provides an efficient checklist for evaluation. All families should receive detailed *written* instructions about home care, with telephone numbers for assistance, before they leave the hospital. Communication between the nurse and home healthcare, if applicable, is essential for ensuring a smooth transition for the child and family on discharge.

After the family is competent in performing the skill, they are given responsibility for the care. When possible, the family should have a transition or trial period to assume care with minimal healthcare supervision. This may be arranged on the unit or in a location near the hospital. Such transitions provide a safe practice period for the family, with assistance readily available when needed, and are especially valuable when the family lives far from the hospital.

In many instances, parents need only simple instructions and understanding of follow-up care. However, the overwhelming care assumed by some families, coupled with other stressors that they may be experiencing, necessitates continued professional support after discharge. A follow-up home visit or telephone call gives the nurse an opportunity to individualise care and provide information in perhaps a less stressful learning environment than the hospital. Appropriate referrals and resources may include visiting nurse or home health agencies, private nurse services, school system, physical therapist, mental health counsellor, social worker and any number of community agencies. Sharing the important issues surrounding the child's and family's needs is essential. Referral summaries should be concise, specific and factual. When numerous support services are required, periodic collaboration among the professionals involved and the family is an excellent strategy to ensure efficient usage and comprehensive delivery of services.

CARE OF THE CHILD AND FAMILY IN SPECIAL HOSPITAL SITUATIONS

In addition to a general paediatric unit, children may also receive care in special facilities, such as an intensive care unit, an isolation room or in the ambulatory setting.

Ambulatory or Outpatient Setting

The ambulatory or outpatient setting provides needed medical services for the child while eliminating the necessity of overnight admission. The benefits of ambulatory care are: to minimise stressors of hospitalisation, especially separation from the family; reduced chances of infection; and increased cost savings. Admission to the ambulatory or outpatient hospital setting is usually for surgical, therapeutic or diagnostic procedures, such as insertion of tympanostomy tubes, hernia repair, tonsillectomy or bronchoscopy.

In the ambulatory or outpatient setting, adequate preparation is particularly challenging. Ideally, the child and parents should receive preadmission preparation, including a tour of the facility and a review of the day's events. Parents need information in advance to help prepare the child and themselves for surgery and enable them to care for the child at home after the procedure. Parents also appreciate suggestions for items to bring to the hospital, such as blankets or stuffed animals. When preadmission preparation is not possible, time should be allowed on the day of the procedure for children to become acquainted with their surroundings and for nurses to assess, plan and implement appropriate teaching.

Explicit discharge instructions are important after outpatient surgery (refer to the previous section Preparing for Discharge and Home Care). Parents need guidelines on when to call their healthcare provider regarding a change in the child's condition. A follow-up telephone call system allows for nurses to check on the child's progress within 48 to 72 hours after discharge. It also provides an opportunity for the nurse to review discharge information and answer additional questions.

Isolation

Admission to an isolation room increases all of the stressors typically associated with hospitalisation. There is further separation from familiar persons, additional loss of control and added environmental changes, such as sensory deprivation and the strange appearance of visitors. Orientation to time and place is affected. These stressors are compounded by children's limited understanding of isolation. Preschool children have difficulty understanding the rationale for isolation because they cannot comprehend the cause-and-effect relationship between germs and illness. They are likely to view isolation as punishment. Older children understand the causality better but still require information to decrease fantasising or misinterpretation.

When a child is placed in isolation, preparation is essential for the child to feel in control. With young children, the best approach is a simple explanation, such as: 'You need to be in this room to help you get better. The germs made you sick, and you could not help that. This is a special place to make all the germs go away'.

All children, but especially younger ones, need preparation in terms of what they will see, hear and feel in isolation. Therefore, they are shown the mask, gloves and gown and are encouraged to 'dress up' in them. Playing with the strange apparel lessens the fear of seeing 'ghost-like' people walk into the room. Before entering the room, nurses and other health personnel should introduce themselves and let the child see their faces before donning masks. In this way, the child gains a sense of familiarity in an otherwise strange and lonely environment.

Emergency Admission

One of the most traumatic hospital experiences for the child and parents is an emergency admission. The sudden onset of an illness or the occurrence of an injury leaves little time for preparation and explanation. Sometimes the emergency admission is compounded by admission to an intensive care unit (ICU) or the need for immediate surgery. However, even in instances requiring only outpatient treatment, the child is exposed to a strange, frightening environment and to experiences that may elicit fear or cause pain.

There is a wide discrepancy between what constitutes a medically defined emergency and a patient-defined emergency. A growing concern is the use of major emergency departments for routine primary care health visits. To offset overcrowding in emergency departments, many facilities have opened urgent care centres for after-hours healthcare. Telephone triage for minor illnesses for patients is also emerging as a healthcare delivery mode to differentiate illnesses such as a common cold from true life-threatening conditions that require immediate provider attention and intervention. Other factors contributing to the overuse of emergency departments (as opposed to the primary care provider's office) include the increasing number of households where both parents work full-time and cannot afford to take time off during the day to take the sick child to a healthcare provider.

In paediatric populations, most visits to an emergency department are for respiratory infections; skin conditions, gastrointestinal disorders and trauma (e.g. poisoning) account for the remainder of cases. The most common reason parents give for bringing the child to the emergency department is concern about the illness worsening. However, healthcare providers may not think that the progressive symptoms necessitate immediate or emergency care. One of the nurse's primary goals is to assess the parents' perception of the event and their reasons for considering it serious or life-threatening.

Lengthy preparatory admission procedures are often inappropriate for emergency situations. In such instances, nurses must focus their nursing interventions on the essential components of admission counselling (Box 21.9) and complete the process as soon as the child's condition has stabilised.

Unless an emergency is life-threatening, children need to participate in their care to maintain a sense of control. Because emergency departments are frequently hectic, there is a tendency to rush through

BOX 21.9 Guidelines for Special Hospital Admission

Emergency Admission

- Lengthy preparatory admission procedures are often impossible and inappropriate for emergency situations.
- Focus assessment on airway, breathing and circulation; weigh child whenever possible for calculation of drug dosages.
- Unless an emergency is life-threatening, children need to participate in their care to maintain a sense of control.
- Focus on essential components of admission counselling, including the following:
  - appropriate introduction to the family
  - use of child's name, not terms such as 'honey' or 'dear'
  - determination of child's age and some judgment about developmental age (if the child is of school age, asking about the grade level will offer some evidence of intellectual ability)
  - information about child's general state of health, any problems that may interfere with medical treatment (e.g. allergies) and previous experience with hospital facilities
  - information about the chief complaint from both the parents and the child.

Admission to Intensive Care Unit

- Prepare child and parents for elective intensive care unit (ICU) admission, such as for postoperative care after cardiac surgery.
- Prepare child and parents for unanticipated ICU admission by focusing primarily on the sensory aspects of the experience and on usual family concerns (e.g. persons in charge of child's care, schedule for visiting, area where family can stay).
- Prepare parents regarding child's appearance and behaviour when they first visit child in ICU.
- Accompany family to bedside to provide emotional support and answer questions.
- Prepare siblings for their visit; plan length of time for sibling visitation; monitor siblings' reactions during visit to prevent them from becoming overwhelmed.
- Encourage parents to stay with their child.
  - If visiting hours are limited, allow flexibility in schedule to accommodate parental needs.
  - Give family members a written schedule of visiting times.
  - If visiting hours are liberal, be aware of family members' needs and suggest periodic respites.
  - Assure family they can call the unit at any time.
- Prepare parents for expected role changes and identify ways for parents to participate in child's care without overwhelming them with responsibilities:
  - help with bath or feeding
  - touch and talk to child.
  - help with procedures
- Provide information about child's condition in understandable language.
  - Repeat information often.
  - Seek clarification of understanding.
  - During bedside conferences, interpret information for family members and child or, if appropriate, conduct report outside room.
- Prepare child for procedures even if it involves explanation while procedure is performed.
- Assess and manage pain; recognise that a child who cannot talk, such as an infant or child in a coma or on mechanical ventilation, can be in pain.
- Establish a routine that maintains some similarity to daily events in child's life whenever possible.
  - Organise care during normal waking hours.
  - Keep regular bedtime schedules, including quiet times when television or radio is lowered or turned off.
  - Provide uninterrupted sleep cycles (60 minutes for infants; 90 minutes for older children).
  - Close and open curtains and dim lights to allow for day and night.
  - Place curtain around bed for privacy.
  - Orient child to day and time; have clocks or calendars in easy view for older children.
- Schedule a time when child is left undisturbed (e.g. during naps, visit with family, playtime or favourite program).
- Provide opportunities for play.
- Reduce stimulation in environment.
  - Refrain from loud talking or laughing.
  - Keep equipment noise to a minimum.
  - Turn alarms as low as safely possible.
  - Perform treatments requiring equipment at one time.
  - Turn off bedside equipment that is not in use, such as suction and oxygen.
  - Avoid loud, abrupt noises.

procedures to save time. However, the extra few minutes needed to allow children to participate may save many more minutes of useless resistance and uncooperativeness during subsequent procedures. Other supportive measures include ensuring privacy, accepting various emotional responses to fear or pain, preserving parent–child contact, explaining all events before or as they occur and personally remaining calm. Pain management strategies are discussed in Chapter 5.

At times, because of the child's physical condition, little or no preparatory counselling for emergency treatment can be done. In such situations, counselling subsequent to the event has therapeutic value. The counselling should focus on evaluating children's thoughts regarding admission and related procedures. It is similar to pre-counselling techniques; however, instead of supplying information, the nurse listens to the explanations offered by the child. Projective techniques such as drawing, doll play or storytelling are especially effective. The nurse then bases additional information on what has already been understood.

Intensive Care Unit

Admission to an ICU can be traumatic for both the child and the parents (Fig 21.4). The nature and severity of the illness and the circumstances surrounding the admission are major factors. Parents experience significantly more stress when the admission is unexpected rather than expected. Stressors for the child and parent are described in Box 21.10. An effective strategy to help enhance parents' ability to cope is to simply ask them what is stressful and implement interventions specific to their stress.

The family's emotional needs are paramount when a child is admitted to an ICU. A major stressor for parents of a child in the ICU is the child's appearance (Latour et al 2008). Although the same interventions discussed earlier for the stressors of separation and loss of control apply here, additional interventions may also benefit the family and child. Nurse behaviours that exemplified caring and affection were perceived as helpful in decreasing stress (Baird et al 2016). Behaviours perceived as not helpful included separating the child from the parents and communicating poorly with parents. Therefore, even critical care must be centred on the family. It is important that visiting hours be liberal and flexible enough to accommodate parental needs and involvement.

Critically ill children become the focus of the parents' lives, and parents' most pressing need is for information. They want to know if their child will live and, if so, whether the child will be the same as before. They need to know why various interventions are being done for the child, that the child is being treated for pain or is comfortable and that the child may be able to hear them even though not awake. When parents first visit the child in the ICU, they need preparation regarding the child's appearance. Ideally, the nurse should accompany the parents to the bedside to provide emotional support and answer any questions.

Despite the stresses normally associated with ICU admission, a sense of security develops from being carefully monitored and receiving individualised care. Therefore, planning for transition to the non-ICU is essential and should include the following:

- assignment of a primary nurse
- explanation of the differences between the two units and the rationale for the change to less intense monitoring of the child's physical condition
- selection of an appropriate room, such as one that is close to the nursing station, and a compatible roommate.

BOX 21.10 Neonatal or Paediatric Intensive Care Unit Stressors for the Child and Family

Physical Stressors

- Pain and discomfort (e.g. injections, intubation, suctioning, dressing changes, other invasive procedures)
- Immobility (e.g. use of restraints, bed rest)
- Sleep deprivation
- Inability to eat or drink
- Changes in elimination habits

Environmental Stressors

- Unfamiliar surroundings (e.g. crowding)
- Unfamiliar sounds
  - Equipment noise (e.g. monitors, telephone, suctioning, computer printout)
  - Human sounds (e.g. talking, laughing, crying, coughing, moaning, retching, walking)
- Unfamiliar people (e.g. healthcare professionals, patients, visitors)
- Unfamiliar and unpleasant smells (e.g. alcohol, adhesive remover, body odours)
- Constant lights (disturb day/night rhythms)
- Activity related to other patients
- Sense of urgency among staff
- Unkind or thoughtless comments from staff

Psychological Stressors

- Lack of privacy
- Inability to communicate (if intubated)
- Inadequate knowledge and understanding of situation
- Severity of illness
- Parental behaviour (expression of concern)

Social Stressors

- Disrupted relationships (especially with family and friends)
- Concern with missing school or work
- Play deprivation

Source: Data primarily from Tichy, A. M., Braam, C. M., Meyer, T. A., et al. (1988). Stressors in paediatric intensive care units. Pediatric Nursing, 14(1), 40–42; Abela, K. M., Wardell, D., Rozmus, C., et al. (2020). Impact of paediatric critical illness and injury on families: An updated systematic review. Journal of Pediatric Nursing, 51, 21–31.

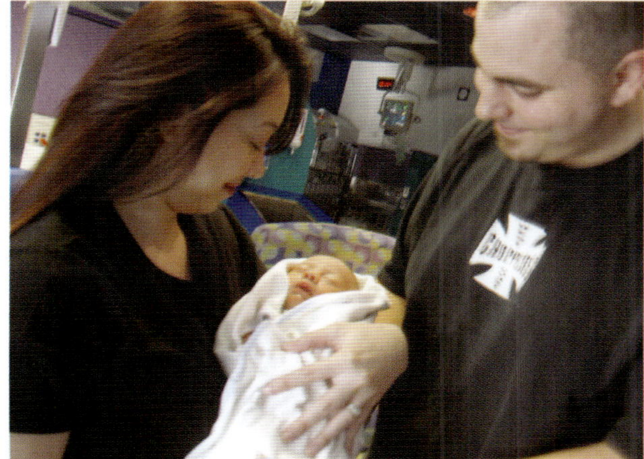

Fig 21.4 Parental presence during hospitalisation provides emotional support for the child and increases the parent's sense of empowerment in the caregiver role. (Source: Courtesy of E. Jacob, Texas Children's Hospital, Houston, TX.)

REFERENCES

Australian Commission on Safety and Quality in Health Care (ACSQHC). (2018). National Safety and Quality Health Service Standards. User guide for acute and community health service organisations that provide care for children. https://www.safetyandquality.gov.au/sites/default/files/migrated/National-Safety-and-Quality-Health-Service-Standards-User-Guide-for-Acute-and-Community-Health-Service-Organisations-the-Provide-Care-for-Children.pdf

Baird, J., Rehm, R. S., Hinds, P. S., et al. (2016). Do you know my child? Continuity of nursing care in the paediatric intensive care unit. Nursing Research, 65(2), 142–150.

Blankenship, A., Harrison, S., Brandt, S., et al. (2015). Increasing parental participation during rounds in a paediatric cardiac intensive care unit. American Journal of Critical Care, 24(6), 532–538.

Cheetham, T. J., Turner-Cobb, J. M., & Gamble, T. (2016). Children's implicit understanding of the stress-illness link: Testing development of health cognitions. British Journal of Health Psychology, 4, 781–795.

Council of Australian Governments (COAG). (2015). National Framework for child and family health services—secondary and tertiary services. Canberra.

Coyne, I. (2006). Children's experiences of hospitalization. Journal of Child Health Care: For Professionals Working with Children in the Hospital and Community, 10(4), 326–336.

Eichner, J. M., & Johnson, B. H. (2012). Patient- and family-centered care and the pediatrician's role. Pediatrics, 129(2), 394–404.

Fraser, J. & Rosina, R. (2017). Chapter 4: Psychosocial development and response to illness. In: Fraser, J., Waters, D., Forster, E., et al. Paediatric Nursing in Australia: Principles for Practice. (2nd edn.). Melbourne: Cambridge.

Galeano, M. D., & Carvajal, B. V. (2016). Coping in mothers of premature newborns after hospital discharge. Newborn and Infant Nursing Reviews, 16(3), 105–109.

Gordon, M. (2002). Manual of nursing diagnosis (10th ed.). St Louis, MO: Mosby.

Jessup, M., Smyth, W., Abernethy, G., et al. (2018). Family-centred care for families living with cystic fibrosis in a rural setting: A qualitative study. Journal of Clinical Nursing, 27(3–4), e590–e599. https://onlinelibrary.wiley.com/doi/abs/10.1111/jocn.14105

Konuk Şener, D., & Karaca, A. (2017). Mutual Expectations of Mothers of Hospitalized Children and Pediatric Nurses Who Provided Care: Qualitative Study. Journal of Pediatric Nursing, S0882-5963(16), 30159-2.

Lambert, V., Coad, J., Hicks, P., et al. (2014). Young children's perspectives of ideal physical design features for hospital-built environments. Journal of Child Health Care, 18(1), 57–71.

Latour, J. M., van Goudoever, J. B., & Hazelzet, J. A. (2008). Parent satisfaction in the pediatric ICU. Pediatric Clinics of North America, 55(3), 779–790.

Lerwick, J. L. (2016). Minimizing pediatric healthcare-induced anxiety and trauma. World Journal of Clinical Pediatrics, 5(2), 143–150.

Limbers, C., & Skipper, S. (2014). Health-related quality of life measurement in siblings of children with physical chronic illness: A systematic review. Families, Systems and Health: The Journal of Collaborative Family Healthcare, 32(4), 408–415.

Livesley, J. & Long, T. (2013). Children experiences as hospital in-patients: Voice, competence and work. Messages for nursing from a critical ethnographic study.

International Journal of Nursing Studies, 50(10), 1292–1303.

Meert, K. L., Clark, J., & Eggly, S. (2013). Family-centered care in the pediatric intensive care unit. Pediatric Clinics of North America, 60(3), 761–772.

Orem, D. (2001). Nursing: Concepts of practice (5th ed.). New York: Mosby.

Öztürk Şahin, Ö., & Topan, A. (2019). Investigation of the fear of 7–18-year-old hospitalized children for illness and hospital. Journal of Religion and Health, 58(3), 1011–1023.

Wilson, M. E., Megel, M. E., Enenbach, L., et al. (2010). The voices of children: Stories about hospitalization. Journal of Pediatric Health Care, 24(2), 95–102.

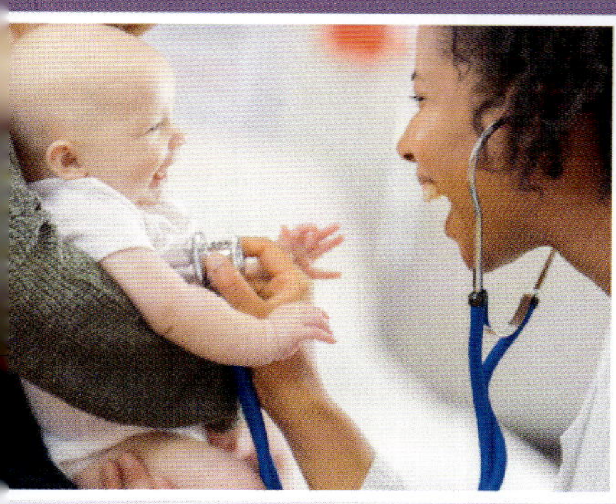

22

Paediatric Nursing Interventions and Skills

Deb Surman

LEARNING OBJECTIVES

- Consider the legal and ethical responsibilities when planning and implementing nursing interventions
- Understand the developmental requirements for children of specific ages when planning procedures/nursing care
- Demonstrate an understanding of cultural requirements of children and their families when planning care
- Develop a sound understanding of the common procedures undertaken in paediatric nursing
- Demonstrate knowledge and skills regarding safe administration of medication to paediatric patients

GENERAL CONCEPTS RELATED TO PAEDIATRIC PROCEDURES

Informed Consent

Before undergoing any invasive procedure, the patient or the patient's legal surrogate must receive sufficient information on which to make an informed healthcare decision. **Informed consent** should include: the nature of the illness or condition, proposed care or treatment; potential risks, benefits and alternatives; and what might happen if the patient chooses not to consent. Additionally, discussions should include the procedure team roles, including trainees involved in care (Firdouse et al 2017). To obtain valid informed consent, healthcare providers must meet the following three conditions.

1. The person must be capable of giving consent; he or she must be over the age of majority (usually age 18 years) and must be considered competent (i.e. possessing the mental capacity to make choices and understand their consequences).
2. The person must receive the information needed to make an intelligent decision.
3. The person must act voluntarily when exercising freedom of choice without force, fraud, deceit, duress or other forms of constraint or coercion.

The patient has the right to accept or refuse any healthcare. If a patient is treated without consent, the hospital or healthcare provider may be charged with assault and held liable for damages. Additionally, consent is a two-way process that requires both the healthcare provider to share all required information and the patient to hear and understand the information. Healthcare providers must deliver information in the appropriate language and health literacy level for the patient and family. There must also be adequate time for questions and opportunity to clarify concerns. Informed consent and medical decision-making is not a one-time event but an ongoing process that requires continual communication among the healthcare team, patient and caregivers (CFCA 2017).

Requirements for Obtaining Informed Consent

Written informed consent of the parent or legal guardian is usually required for medical or surgical treatment of a minor, including many diagnostic procedures. One universal consent is not sufficient. Separate informed permissions must be obtained for each surgical or diagnostic procedure, including the following:

- major surgery
- minor surgery (e.g. cutdown, biopsy, dental extraction, suturing a laceration [especially one that may have a cosmetic effect], removal of a cyst, closed reduction of a fracture)
- diagnostic tests with an element of risk (e.g. bronchoscopy, angiography, lumbar puncture, cardiac catheterisation, bone marrow aspiration)
- medical treatments with an element of risk (e.g. blood transfusion, thoracentesis or paracentesis, radiotherapy).

Other situations that require patient or parental consent include the following:

- photographs for medical, educational or public use
- removal of the child from the healthcare institution against medical advice
- postmortem examination, except in unexplained deaths, such as sudden infant death, violent death or suspected suicide
- release of medical information.

Decision-making involving the care of older children and adolescents (greater than 7 years with appropriate age, maturity and psychological state) should include the patient's **assent** (if feasible), as well as the parent's consent (Poston 2016). Assent means the child or adolescent has been informed about the proposed treatment, procedure or research and is willing to permit a healthcare provider to perform it. If the child or adolescent merely fails to object, this does not equate assent. Assent should include the following:

- helping the patient achieve a developmentally appropriate awareness of the nature of his or her condition
- telling the patient what he or she can expect
- making a clinical assessment of the patient's understanding
- soliciting an expression of the patient's willingness to accept the proposed procedure.

Healthcare providers should use multiple methods to provide information, including age-appropriate methods (e.g. videos, peer discussion, diagrams and written materials). The nurse should provide an assent form for the child to sign, and the child should keep a copy.

By including the child in the decision-making process and gaining his or her acceptance, staff members demonstrate respect for the child. Assent is not a legal requirement but an ethical one to protect the rights of children. Chapter 19 provides further discussion on the dying child's right to refuse treatment.

Eligibility for Giving Informed Consent

Informed Consent of Parents or Legal Guardians. Parents have full responsibility for the care and rearing of their minor children, including legal control over them. As long as children are minors, their parents or legal guardians are required to give informed consent before medical treatment is rendered or any procedure is performed. If the parents are married to each other, consent from only one parent is required for non-urgent paediatric care. If the parents are divorced, consent usually rests with the parent who has legal custody (CFCA 2017). Emergency care of a paediatric patient should never be withheld due to the absence of a parent or legal guardian. Parents also have a right to withdraw consent later. If the legal caregivers disagree on the treatment course, it is within the healthcare providers' scope to request consultation of a hospital ethics board to determine what care is in the best interest of the patient (Dahl et al 2015).

Evidence of Consent. Regulations on obtaining informed consent vary from state to state, and policies differ at each healthcare facility. It is the medical practitioner's legal responsibility to explain the procedure, risks, benefits and alternatives. The nurse witnesses the patient's, parent's or legal guardian's signature on the consent form and may reinforce what the patient has been told. A signed consent form is the legal document that signifies that the process of informed consent has occurred. If parents are unavailable to sign consent forms, verbal consent may be obtained via the telephone in the presence of two witnesses. Both witnesses record that informed consent was given and by whom. Their signatures indicate that they witnessed the verbal consent.

Informed Consent of Mature and Emancipated Minors. State laws differ regarding the age of majority; that is, the age at which a person is considered to have all the legal rights and responsibilities of an adult. The age of consent is 16 years of age in the Australian Capital Territory, New South Wales, Northern Territory, Queensland, Victoria and Western Australia. In Tasmania and South Australia the age of consent is 17 years of age. In New Zealand a young person aged 16 years and over can consent to their treatment as if they were an adult. Competent adults can give informed consent on their own behalf. An **emancipated minor** is one who is legally under the age of majority but is recognised as having the legal capacity or social status of an adult under circumstances prescribed by state law, such as pregnancy, marriage, high school graduation or independent living. A **mature minor** exception to consent laws is recognised for children 14 years and older who possess the maturity and cognitive abilities to understand all elements of informed consent and make a choice based on the information. Legal action may be required for designation as a mature minor (CFCA 2017, RACP 2019).

Treatment without Parental Consent. Exceptions to requiring parental consent before treating minor children occur in situations in which children need urgent medical or surgical treatment and a parent is not readily available to give consent or refuses to give consent. For example, a child may be brought to an emergency department accompanied by a grandparent. In the absence of parents or legal guardians, persons in charge of the child may be given permission by the parents to give informed consent by proxy. In emergencies, including danger to life or the possibility of permanent injury, appropriate care should not be withheld or delayed because of problems obtaining consent (CFCA 2017, RACP 2019). The nurse should document any efforts made to obtain consent.

Parental refusal to give consent for lifesaving treatment or to prevent serious harm can occur and requires notification to child protective services to render emergency treatment. For example, Jehovah's Witnesses commonly choose to avoid receiving blood products due to religious beliefs. In cases where a blood product is crucial for the child's survival, it is important to work together with the family, medical team and child protective services to determine the course of action that is in the best interest of the child. Where possible, family's rights and decisions will be upheld and the focus of care. Parents are primarily responsible for all decisions about their own children; however, when the child's life is at risk, the focus will shift onto the child's life and wellbeing and this may conflict with the parents' choices and decisions (CFCA 2017).

Adolescents, Consent and Confidentiality. The *Privacy Act 1988* (Cwlth) was passed to help protect and safeguard the security and confidentiality of health information. Because adolescents are not yet adults, parents have the right to make most decisions on their behalf and receive information. Adolescents, however, are more likely to seek care in a setting in which they believe their privacy will be maintained.

Preparation for Diagnostic and Therapeutic Procedures

Technological advances and changes in healthcare have resulted in more paediatric procedures being performed in a variety of settings. Many procedures are both stressful and painful experiences. For many procedures, the focus of care is psychological preparation of the child and family. However, some procedures require the administration of sedatives and analgesics.

Therapeutic play, procedural preparation and support, developmentally appropriate education and promoting normalcy are all significant ways the child life specialist can have a positive impact on the healthcare experience for the child and family. Child life specialists and nursing staff can work together to implement evidence-based interventions to decrease fear, anxiety and discomfort experienced by children in the healthcare environment (Association of Child Life Professionals 2017).

Psychological Preparation

Preparing children for procedures decreases their anxiety, promotes their cooperation, supports their coping skills and may teach them new ones, and facilitates a feeling of mastery in experiencing a potentially stressful event.

Children differ in their 'information-seeking dimension'. Some actively ask for information about the intended procedure, but others characteristically avoid information. Parents can often guide nurses in deciding how much information is enough for the child because parents know whether the child is typically inquisitive or satisfied with short answers. Asking older children their preferences about the amount of explanation is also important.

The exact timing of the preparation for a procedure varies with the child's age, developmental level and the type of procedure. No exact guidelines govern timing, but in general, the younger the child, the closer the explanation should be to the actual procedure to prevent undue fantasising and worrying. Concurrent preparation is a strategy that can be used during a procedure to explain what a child can expect to occur and sense immediately before it happens (Blaney et al 2016). This can be helpful for emergency procedures, for a highly anxious child or for younger age groups where extensive prior preparation is not possible or beneficial. With complex procedures, more time may be needed for assimilation of information, especially with older children. For example, the explanation for an injection can immediately precede the procedure for all ages, but preparation for surgery may begin the day before for young children and a few days before for older children, although the nurse should elicit older children's preferences.

Establish Trust and Provide Support. The nurse who has spent time with and established a positive relationship with a child usually finds it easier to gain cooperation. If the relationship is based on trust, the child will associate the nurse with caregiving activities that give comfort and pleasure most of the time rather than discomfort and stress. If the nurse does not know the child, it is best for the nurse to be introduced by another staff member whom the child trusts. The first visit with the child should not include any painful procedure and ideally should focus on the child first and then on an explanation of the procedure. A simple way to begin the process of creating trust is by engaging in play with the patient through favourite activities or toys. Body language is another key element of promoting trust. Positive body language, such as sitting instead of standing, and avoiding the use of technical medical terminology in conversation can enhance the therapeutic caregiver relationship with the child and family (Lidgett 2016).

Parental Presence and Support. Children need support during procedures, and for young children, the greatest source of support is the parents. They represent security, protection, safety and comfort. Parental presence has a positive impact on the level of pain, stress and negative behaviour experienced by the child, as well as parental distress and satisfaction (Bice & Wyatt 2017). Additionally, there is no difference in technical complications when parents remain with children. However, controversy exists regarding the role parents should assume during the procedure, especially if discomfort is involved. The nurse should assess the parents' preferences for assisting, observing or waiting outside the room, as well as the child's preference for parental presence. Respect the child's and parents' choices. Give parents who wish to stay appropriate explanation about the procedure, and coach them about where to sit or stand and what to say or do to help the child through the procedure. Support parents who do not want to be present in their decision, and encourage them to remain close by so they can be available to support the child immediately after the procedure. It can be helpful for parents to assist the healthcare team in identifying an alternative support person for their child, such as a child life therapist nurse, if they are unable to be present during the procedure. Parents should know that someone will be with their child to provide support. Ideally, this person should inform the parents after the procedure about how the child did.

Provide an Explanation. Age-appropriate explanations are one of the most widely used interventions for reducing anxiety in children undergoing procedures. Before performing a procedure, explain what is to be done, what sensations the child may feel, what is expected of the child and why the procedure is being done. It is important that the child understand the procedure is not punishment. The explanation should be short, simple and appropriate to the child's level of comprehension. Long explanations may increase anxiety in a young child. When explaining the procedure to parents with the child present, the nurse uses language appropriate to the child because unfamiliar words can be misunderstood (Table 22.1). If the parents need additional preparation, it is done in an area away from the child. Teaching sessions are planned at times most conducive to the child's learning (e.g. after a rest period) and for the usual span of attention.

Special equipment is not necessary for preparing a child, but for young children who cannot yet think conceptually, using objects to supplement verbal explanation is important. Children often learn through behaviour modelling such as seeing a doll experience the procedure, watching a video or seeing a picture. Additionally, allowing children to handle actual items that will be used in their care, such as a stethoscope, sphygmomanometer or oxygen mask, helps them develop familiarity with these items and reduces the fear often associated with their use. Miniature versions of hospital items such as gurneys and x-ray and intravenous (IV) equipment can be used to explain what the children can expect and permit them to safely experience situations that are unfamiliar and potentially frightening. Written and illustrated materials are also valuable aids to preparation.

TABLE 22.1 Selecting Non-threatening Words or Phrases

Words and Phrases to Avoid	Suggested Substitutions
Shot, bee sting, stick	Medicine under the skin, poke that will feel like a pinch
Organ	Place in body
Test	To see how (specify body part) is working
Incision, cut	Make an opening
Oedema	Puffiness
Stretcher, gurney	Rolling bed, bed on wheels
Stool/urine	Child's usual term
Dye	Medicine to help place in your body (show on a picture)
Pain	Hurt, discomfort, 'owie', 'boo-boo', sore, achy, scratchy, pinch
Deaden, numb	Not feel body part as much
Fix	Make better
Take (as in 'take your temperature')	See how warm you are
Take (as in 'take your blood pressure')	Check your pressure; hug your arm
Put to sleep, anaesthesia	Different kind of sleep so you won't feel anything
Catheter	Soft tube, small straw
Monitor	Television screen
Electrodes	Stickers, ticklers
Specimen	Take some blood

Physical Preparation

One area of special concern is the administration of appropriate sedation and analgesia before stressful procedures.

Performance of the Procedure

Supportive care continues during the procedure and can be a major factor in a child's ability to cooperate. Ideally, the same nurse who explains the procedure should perform or assist with the procedure. The child may also benefit from a parent or trusted caregiver who can offer coaching techniques and support during the procedure. Before beginning, all equipment is assembled and the room is readied to prevent unnecessary delays and interruptions that increase the child's anxiety. Minimising the number of people present and allowing one person to speak during the procedure also can decrease the child's anxiety.

To promote long-term coping and adjustment, give special consideration to the patient's age, coping skills and procedure to be performed in determining where a procedure will occur. Treatment rooms should be used for procedures requiring sedation, such as bone marrow aspirates and lumbar punctures in younger children. Traumatic procedures should never be performed in 'safe' areas, such as the playroom. If the procedure is lengthy, avoid conversation that could be misinterpreted by the child. As the procedure is nearing completion, the nurse may inform the child 'this is the last piece of tape' or simply inform the child when the procedure is completed.

Expect Success. Nurses who approach children with confidence and who convey the impression that they expect to be successful are less likely to encounter difficulty. It is best to approach a child as though cooperation is expected. Children sense anxiety and uncertainty in an adult and respond by striking out or actively resisting. Although it is not possible to eliminate such behaviour in every child, a firm approach with a positive attitude tends to convey a feeling of security to most children.

Involve the Child. Involving children helps gain their cooperation. Permitting choices gives them some measure of control. However, a choice is given only in situations in which one is available. Asking children, 'Do you want to take your medicine now?' leads them to believe they have an option and provides them the opportunity to legitimately refuse or delay the medication. This places the nurse in an awkward, if not impossible, position. It is much better to state firmly, 'It's time to drink your medicine now'. Children usually like to make choices, but the choice must be one that they do indeed have (e.g. 'It's time for your medicine. Do you want to drink it plain or with a little water?').

Many children respond to tactics that appeal to their maturity or courage. This also gives them a sense of participation and achievement. For example, preschool children will be proud that they can hold the dressing during the procedure or remove the tape. The same is true for school-age children, who often cooperate with minimal resistance.

Provide Distraction. Distraction is a powerful coping strategy during painful procedures (Bice & Wyatt 2017). It is accomplished by focusing the child's attention on something other than the procedure. Singing favourite songs, listening to music with a headset, counting aloud or blowing bubbles to 'blow the hurt away' are effective techniques. (For other non-pharmacological interventions, see Chapter 20.)

Allow Expression of Feelings. The child should be allowed to express feelings of anger, anxiety, fear, frustration or any other emotion. It is natural for children to strike out in frustration or to try to avoid stress-provoking situations. The child needs to know that it is all right to cry. Behaviour is children's primary means of communication and coping and should be permitted unless it inflicts harm on them or those caring for them. Harmful behaviour should be acknowledged, and appropriate limitations should be set to promote patient and caregiver safety.

Postprocedural Support

After the procedure, the child continues to need reassurance that he or she performed well and is accepted and loved. If the parents did not participate, the child is united with them as soon as possible so they can provide comfort.

Preparing the Family

The process of patient education involves giving the family information about the child's condition, the regimen that must be followed and why, and other health teaching as indicated. The goal of this education is to enable the family to modify behaviours and adhere to the regimen that has been mutually established (see Applying Evidence to Practice box).

APPLYING EVIDENCE TO PRACTICE

General Principles of Family Education

- Establish a rapport with the family.
- Avoid using confusing specialised terms or jargon. Clarify all terms with the family and use the term that is clear to the child.
- When possible, allow family members to decide how they want to be taught (e.g. all at once or over a day or two). This gives the family a chance to incorporate the information at a rate that is comfortable.
- Provide accurate information to the family about the illness.
- Assist family members in identifying obstacles to their ability to comply with the regimen and in identifying the means to overcome those obstacles. Then help family members find ways to incorporate the plan into their daily lives.

If equipment will be needed at home (e.g. suction machines, syringes), begin making the necessary arrangements in advance so that discharge can proceed smoothly. Whenever possible, make arrangements for the family to use the same equipment in the home that they are using in the hospital. This allows them to become familiar with the items. In addition, the staff can help troubleshoot the equipment in a controlled environment. Plan the teaching sessions well in advance of the time the family will be responsible for performing the care. The more complex the procedure, the more time is needed for training.

Review the instructions with family members (see Applying Evidence to Practice box). Encourage note taking if they desire. Allow ample practice time under supervision. At least one family member, but preferably two members, should demonstrate the procedure before they are expected to care for the child at home. Provide the family with the telephone numbers of resource individuals who are available to assist them in the event of a problem.

APPLYING EVIDENCE TO PRACTICE

Family Preparation for Procedures

Family education for specific procedures is included throughout this unit. General concepts applicable to most family education sessions include the following:

- name of the procedure
- purpose of the procedure
- length of time anticipated to complete the procedure
- anticipated effects
- signs of adverse effects
- assess the family's level of understanding
- demonstrate and have family return demonstration (if appropriate).

Surgical Procedures

Preoperative Care

Children experiencing surgical procedures require both psychological and physical preparation. An important concern is restriction of food and fluids before surgery to avoid pulmonary aspiration during anaesthesia. Additionally, fasting too long can cause discomfort, headache, dehydration or hypoglycaemia and can delay recovery and hospital discharge (Dolgun et al 2017). Infants require special attention to fluid needs. They should not be without oral fluids for an extended period preoperatively to avoid glycogen depletion and dehydration. If surgical procedures are delayed, it is the nurse's responsibility to communicate with the surgical

TABLE 22.2 Fasting Recommendations to Reduce the Risk of Pulmonary Aspiration*

Ingested Material	Minimum Fasting Period (hr)†
Clear liquids‡	> 2
Breast milk	4
Infant formula	6
Non-human milk§	6
Light meal¶	6

*These recommendations apply to healthy patients who are undergoing elective procedures. They are not intended for women in labour. Following the guidelines does not guarantee that complete gastric emptying has occurred.
†Fasting periods noted in chart apply to all ages.
‡Examples of clear liquids include water, fruit juices without pulp, carbonated beverages, clear tea and black coffee.
§Because non-human milk is similar to solids in gastric emptying time, the amount ingested must be considered when determining appropriate fasting period.
¶A light meal typically consists of toast and clear liquids. Meals that include fried or fatty foods or meat may prolong gastric emptying time. Both the amount and the type of foods ingested must be considered when determining an appropriate fasting period.
Source: American Society of Anesthesiologists, Committee on Standards and Practice Parameters. (2011). Practice guidelines for preoperative fasting and the use of pharmacological agents to reduce the risk of pulmonary aspiration: Application to healthy patients undergoing elective procedures. Anesthesiology, 114(3), 495–511.

team to adjust fasting guidelines appropriately (Williams et al 2014). Table 22.2 contains current preoperative fasting guidelines.

In general, psychological preparation is similar to that discussed earlier for any procedure and uses many of the same techniques used in preparing a child for hospitalisation, such as films, books, brochures, play and tours (see Chapter 21). Stress points before and after surgery include the admission process, blood tests, administration of preoperative medication (if prescribed), transport to the operating room, the mask on the face during induction and the stay in the post-anaesthesia care unit. Wearing a hospital gown without the security of underpants or pyjama bottoms can also be traumatic. Therefore, these articles of clothing should be allowed to be worn into the operating room and removed after induction of anaesthesia. Children are at higher risk of ineffective response to anaesthesia and complications in the recovery period because of higher anxiety in the preoperative period associated with stranger anxiety (infants), separation anxiety (toddlers and preschoolers) and fear of injury or death (adolescents) (Al-Yateem et al 2016).

Individualised psychological intervention consisting of systematic preparation, rehearsal of the forthcoming events and supportive care at each of these points has shown to be more effective than a single-session preparation or consistent supportive care without systematic preparation and rehearsal (Fortier et al 2015). A family-centred preoperative preparation program may consist of a tour of the perioperative areas with short explanations of the events 5 to 7 days before surgery, a link to a webpage may be provided or written material to review a couple of times with additional explanations and demonstrations of perioperative processes, a mask to take home and practise with, pamphlets to guide parents on supporting children during induction, phone calls to coach parents on preparing children 1 or 2 days before surgery, toys and supplies in the holding area, and smartphone applications with interactive tours and videos.

Parental Presence. Some institutions support parental presence during induction of anaesthesia. Benefits of well-prepared children and parents along with parental presence during induction of anaesthesia include reduced anxiety for children and parents, lower doses of postoperative analgesia, lower incidence of severe emergence delirium symptoms, decreased postoperative maladaptive behaviours and shorter discharge time for short procedures (Fortier et al 2015). Other studies have not supported a reduction in children's anxiety (Pomicino et al 2018).

Concern exists regarding the appropriateness of parental presence during induction for all parents. Some parents may become upset by the rapid succession of induction events, by observing their child becoming limp and by leaving the child in the care of strangers. Although parents who are anxious before surgery tend to become even more anxious after the induction, the reverse is true of parents with little anxiety. There is little evidence to suggest that parental presence during induction provides decreased anxiety for parents and caregivers (Al-Yateem et al 2016). Appropriate education is essential to help parents understand the stages of anaesthesia, what to expect and how to support their child.

Preoperative Sedation. The goals for using preoperative medications include anxiety reduction, amnesia, sedation, antiemetic effect and reduction of secretions (Manworren & Fledderman 2000). (Chapter 5 includes a discussion of pain management strategies for children undergoing surgery.) When drugs are administered, they should be delivered traumatically via oral, intranasal or IV routes. Numerous pre-anaesthetic drug regimens are used with children, and no consensus exists on the optimal method. Some institutions promote distraction or parental support instead of medications due to the incidence of postoperative medication delirium (Batawi 2015).

Intraoperative Care

The role of the paediatric operating room nurse is to advocate for care of the patient in surgery through the verification of procedure and laterality, implants, skin preparation, necessary instrumentation and supplies. The operating room nurse assesses, recognises and intervenes for the paediatric surgical patient at high risk for pressure injury due to patient diagnosis, patient anatomy, general anaesthesia, intraoperative positioning, immobility, moisture and nil-by-mouth (NBM) status. Clear communication is used through collaboration with the interdisciplinary team (anaesthesia, surgeon, scrub technician, nurses, radiology, etc.) to coordinate the intraoperative and postoperative disposition of the surgical patient. Family-centred care is provided through engaging the family in the preoperative procedure verification and updating them throughout the procedure (Herd & Rieben 2014).

Postoperative Care

Various psychological and physical interventions and observations help prevent or minimise possible unpleasant effects from anaesthesia and the surgical procedure. Although serious postoperative complications in healthy children undergoing surgery are rare, continuous monitoring of the child's cardiopulmonary status is essential during the immediate postoperative period to reduce this risk (Pawar 2012). Postanesthetic complications such as airway obstruction, postextubation croup, laryngospasm and bronchospasm make maintaining a patent airway and maximum ventilation critical.

Monitoring the patient's oxygen saturation and providing supplemental oxygen as needed, maintaining body temperature and promoting

TABLE 22.3 Potential Causes of Postoperative Vital Sign Alterations in Children

Alteration	Potential Cause	Comments
	HEART RATE	
Increase	Decreased perfusion (shock) Elevated temperature Pain Respiratory distress (early) Medications (atropine, morphine, adrenaline [epinephrine]) Hypoxia	Heart rate may increase to maintain cardiac output.
Decrease	Vagal stimulation Increased intracranial pressure Respiratory distress (late) Medications (neostigmine)	Bradycardia is of more concern in young child than tachycardia.
	RESPIRATORY RATE	
Increase	Respiratory distress Fluid volume excess Hypothermia Elevated temperature Pain	Body responds to respiratory distress primarily by increasing rate.
Decrease	Anaesthetics, opioids Pain	Decreased respiratory rate from opioids may be compensated for by increased depth of respiration.
	BLOOD PRESSURE	
Increase	Excess intravascular volume Increased intracranial pressure Carbon dioxide retention Pain Medication (ketamine, adrenaline [epinephrine])	This is serious in premature infants because it increases risk of intraventricular haemorrhage.
Decrease	Vasodilating anaesthetic agents (halothane, isoflurane) Opioids (e.g. morphine)	Decreased blood pressure is late sign of shock because of elasticity and constriction of vessels to maintain card ac output.
	TEMPERATURE	
Increase	Shock (late sign) Infection Environmental causes (warm room, excess coverings) Malignant hyperthermia	Fever associated with infection usually occurs later than fever of non-infectious origin. Absence of fever does not rule out infection, especially in infants. Malignant hyperthermia requires immediate treatment.
Decrease	Vasodilating anaesthetic agents (halothane, isoflurane) Muscle relaxants Environmental causes (cool room) Infusion of cool fluids or blood	Neonates are especially susceptible to hypothermia, with serious or fatal consequences.

fluid and electrolyte balance are important aspects of immediate postoperative care. Vital signs are continuously monitored, and each vital sign is evaluated in terms of side effects from anaesthesia, shock or respiratory compromise (Table 22.3).

A change in vital signs that demands immediate attention in the perioperative period is caused by **malignant hyperthermia (MH)**, a potentially fatal pharmacogenetic disorder of muscle metabolism. In susceptible children, inhaled anaesthetics and the muscle relaxant suxamethonium trigger the disorder, producing hypermetabolism. Symptoms of MH include hypercarbia (increasing end-tidal carbon dioxide), elevated temperature, tachycardia, tachypnoea, acidosis, muscle rigidity, hyperkalaemia and rhabdomyolysis. A family or previous history of sudden high fever associated with a surgical procedure and myotonia increase the risk for MH. Children who have successfully undergone prior surgery without adverse effects may still be considered susceptible (Salazar et al 2014).

Treatment of MH includes immediate discontinuation of the triggering agent, hyperventilation with 100% oxygen and IV dantrolene sodium. If the child is hyperthermic, initiate cooling measures such as ice packs to the groin, axillae and neck and iced nasogastric (NG) lavage. The surgery may be discontinued, or if it is emergent, it may be continued with a different anaesthetic agent. The patient should be transferred to an intensive care unit for at least 36 hours and closely monitored for stabilisation of vital signs, metabolic state and possible recurrence of symptoms.

Managing pain is a major nursing responsibility after surgery. The nurse should assess pain frequently and administer analgesics to provide comfort and facilitate cooperation with postoperative care such as ambulation and deep breathing. Opioids are the most used analgesics. Routinely scheduled IV analgesics, patient-controlled analgesia, regional blocks and epidural infusions, rather than as-needed orders, provide excellent analgesia in postoperative paediatric patients.

Non-pharmacological postoperative recovery interventions include the use of distraction, videos, interactive game applications and therapy dogs. Therapy dogs can facilitate decreased pain perception, increase in activity and emotional stabilisation in the postoperative period (Calcaterra et al 2015).

NURSING CARE CONSIDERATIONS

Because deep breathing is usually painful after surgery, be certain that the child has received analgesics. Have the child splint the operative site (depending on its location) by hugging a small pillow or a favourite stuffed animal.

Because respiratory tract infections are a potential complication of anaesthesia, make every effort to aerate the lungs and remove secretions. The lungs are auscultated regularly to identify abnormal sounds or any areas of diminished or absent breath sounds. To prevent pneumonia, encourage respiratory movement with incentive spirometers or other motivating activities. If these measures are presented as games, the child is more likely to comply. The child's position is changed every 2 hours, and deep breathing is encouraged. Patients with preexisting pulmonary disease may be advised to begin incentive spirometry before the day of surgery (Azhar 2015). Early respiratory movement can decrease the patient's need for supplemental oxygen and promote discharge home sooner (Shaughnessy et al 2015).

Many paediatric patients are discharged shortly after surgery. Preparation for discharge begins with the preadmission preparation visit. Thorough discharge processes and education can greatly assist in the prevention of unplanned readmissions (Payne & Flood 2015). The nurse should discuss instructions for postoperative care and review them throughout the perioperative visit. After discharge, the nursing staff often makes phone calls to check the patient's status. Patient education and compliance with discharge instructions can also be assessed during these phone calls (Flippo et al 2015) (see Applying Evidence to Practice box)

Compliance

Compliance, also termed **adherence**, refers to the extent to which the patient's behaviour coincides with the prescribed regimen in terms of taking medication, following diets or executing other lifestyle changes. In developing strategies to improve compliance, the nurse must first assess level of compliance. Because many children are too young to assume partial or total responsibility for their care, parents are usually primarily responsible for home management.

When enquiring about a patient's compliance, it can be helpful to ask details about how medication administration or other interventions are carried out instead of asking yes-or-no questions. For example, a healthcare provider could ask about what time of day patients performs their prescribed interventions, what beverage they prefer to take their medications with or how many doses were missed this week (Brown & Sinsky 2013). Several methods exist, each with advantages and disadvantages. The most successful approach includes a combination of at least two of the following methods.

- **Clinical judgment**—This is subject to bias and inaccuracy unless the nurse carefully evaluates the criteria used in assessment.
- **Self-reporting**—Most people overestimate their compliance even when they admit to lapses.
- **Direct observation**—This is difficult to use outside the healthcare setting, and awareness of being observed frequently affects performance.
- **Monitoring appointments**—Keeping appointments indirectly indicates compliance with the prescribed care.
- **Monitoring therapeutic response**—Few treatments yield directly measurable results (e.g. decreased blood pressure, weight loss); record on a graph or chart.
- **Pill counts**—The nurse counts the number of pills remaining in the original container and compares the number missing with the number of times the medication should have been taken. Although this is a simple method, families may forget to bring the container or deliberately alter the number of pills to avoid detection. This method is also poorly suited to liquid medication. Another technique is the use of pill container caps that record every opening as a presumptive dose.

APPLYING EVIDENCE TO PRACTICE

Postoperative Care

- Ensure that preparations are made to receive the child.
  - Bed or cot is ready.
  - IV pumps and poles, suction apparatus and oxygen flow meter are at bedside.
- Obtain baseline information.
  - Take vital signs, including blood pressure; keep blood pressure cuff in place and deflated to lessen disturbance to child.
  - Take and record vital signs more frequently if any value fluctuates.
- Inspect operative area.
- Check dressing if present.
- Outline any bleeding area on dressing or cast with pen.
- Reinforce, but do not remove, loose dressing.
- Observe areas below surgical site for blood that may have drained towards bed.
- Assess for bleeding and other symptoms in areas not covered with a dressing, such as throat after tonsillectomy.
- Assess skin colour and characteristics.
- Assess level of sedation and activity.
- Notify medical practitioner of any irregularities in child's condition.
- Assess for evidence of pain.
- Review surgeon's orders after completing initial assessment and check that any preoperative orders, such as seizure or cardiac medications, have been reordered and can be given by available routes (oral preparations may be contraindicated).
- Monitor vital signs as ordered and more often if indicated.
- Check dressings for bleeding or other abnormalities.
- Check bowel sounds.
- Observe for signs of shock, abdominal distension and bleeding.
- Assess for bladder distension.
- Observe for signs of dehydration.
- Detect presence of infection.
  - Take vital signs every 2 to 4 hours as ordered.
  - Collect or request needed specimens.
  - Inspect wound for signs of infection—redness, swelling, heat, pain and purulent drainage.

- **Chemical assay**—For certain drugs, such as digoxin, measurement of plasma drug levels provides information on the amount of drug recently ingested. However, this method is expensive, indicates only short-term compliance and requires precise timing of the assay for accurate results.

Compliance Strategies

Strategies to improve compliance involve interventions that encourage families to follow the prescribed treatment regimen. Some evidence suggests that higher levels of self-esteem and increased autonomy favourably affect adolescent compliance (Letitre et al 2014). Additionally, anxiety, depression and self-esteem can be negatively affected when treatment regimens are inadequately followed. However, family factors are important, and characteristics associated with good compliance include family support, family reminders, good communication and expectations for successful completion of the therapeutic regimen. No one approach is always successful, and the best results occur when at least two strategies are used.

Organisational strategies involve the care setting and the therapeutic plan. This may involve increasing the frequency of appointments, designating a primary provider, reducing the cost of medication by prescribing generic brands, reducing the treatment's disruption of the family's lifestyle and using 'cues' to minimise forgetting.

The nurse instructs the family about the treatment plan. Although education is an important factor in enhancing compliance, and patients who are more knowledgeable about their condition are more likely to comply, education alone does not ensure compliant behaviour. The nurse should incorporate teaching principles known to enhance understanding and retention of material. Individualised teaching strategies appropriate for developmental and cognitive levels of the individual, as well as involvement of the immediate and extended family (e.g. grandparents) in education sessions, may enhance compliance.

Treatment strategies relate to the child's refusal or inability to take the prescribed medication. The family may also have difficulty following a prescribed treatment regimen. They may remember and understand the instructions but may not be able to give the medicine as prescribed. Assess the reason for refusal. For example, the child may not be able to swallow pills. In this case perhaps pills could be a liquid medication substituted (always review medication to ensure that crushing is acceptable before giving this instruction).

Assess the treatment and medication schedule to determine whether it is reasonable for a home situation. Although an every-6-hour or every-8-hour schedule is reasonable for hospitals, a parent would have difficulty getting up once or twice nightly. Instead, the patient could take a medication during the day at times that would be easy to remember.

Behavioural strategies are designed to modify behaviour directly. Nurses can use several effective strategies with children to encourage the desired behaviour. Positive reinforcement is one strategy that strengthens the behaviour.

SKIN CARE AND GENERAL HYGIENE

Maintaining Healthy Skin

Maintaining an IV line, removing a dressing, positioning a child in bed, changing a nappy, using electrodes and using restraints all have the potential to contribute to skin injury. General guidelines for skin care are listed in the Applying Evidence to Practice box.

Assessment of the skin is easiest to accomplish during the bath. Examine for early signs of injury. Risk factors include impaired mobility, protein malnutrition, oedema, incontinence, sensory loss, anaemia, infection, failure to turn the patient and intubation. Identification of risk factors helps determine children who need a more thorough skin assessment. Several risk assessment scales are available for use in paediatrics, such as the Braden Q Scale, the Neonatal Skin Risk Assessment Scale, the Waterlow Scale and the Glamorgan Scale (Razmus & Bergquist-Beringer 2017). Initial assessment should occur on admission to identify pressure ulcers and wounds that occurred before admission.

Pressure ulcers, a form of pressure injuries, are localised damage to the skin and/or underlying soft tissue due to decreased perfusion as a result of increased pressure. Pressure ulcers most often occur over bony prominences or related to medical or other devices. Pressure injuries are staged to classify the amount of tissue damage that has occurred.* Necrotic tissue must be removed so the tissue depth can be assessed accurately. Accurate documentation of redness or obvious

APPLYING EVIDENCE TO PRACTICE

Skin Care

- Keep skin free of excess moisture (e.g. urine or faecal incontinence, wound drainage, excessive perspiration).
- Cleanse skin with mild non-alkaline soap or soap-free cleaning agents for routine bathing.
- Provide daily cleansing of eyes, oral and nappy or perineal areas, and any areas of skin breakdown.
- Apply non–alcohol-based moisturising agents after cleansing to retain moisture and rehydrate skin.
- Use minimum amount of tape and adhesives. On very sensitive skin, use a protective, pectin-based or hydrocolloid skin barrier between skin and tape or adhesives.
- Place pectin-based or hydrocolloid skin barriers directly over excoriated skin. Leave barrier undisturbed until it begins to peel off or for 5 to 7 days. With wet, oozing excoriations, place a small amount of stoma powder on site, remove excess powder and apply skin barrier. Hold barrier in place for several minutes to allow barrier to soften and mould to skin surface.
- Alternate electrode and probe placement sites and thoroughly assess underlying skin typically every 8 to 24 hours.
- Eliminate pressure secondary to medical devices such as tracheostomy tubes, wheelchairs, braces and gastrostomy tubes.
- Be certain fingers or toes are visible whenever extremity is used for IV or arterial line.
- Use a draw sheet to move child in bed or onto a stretcher; do not drag child from under the arms.
- Position in neutral alignment; pillows, cushions or wedges may be needed to prevent hip abduction and pressure to bony prominences, such as heels, elbows and sacral and occipital areas. When child is positioned laterally, pillows or cushions between the knees, under the head and under the upper arm will help promote neutral body alignment. Avoid donut cushions because they can cause tissue ischaemia. Elevate the head of bed 30 degrees or less to reduce pressure unless contraindicated.
- Do not massage reddened bony prominences because this can cause deep tissue damage; provide pressure relief to bony prominences.
- Routinely assess the child's nutritional status. A child who is nil by mouth (NBM) for several days and is receiving only IV fluid is nutritionally at risk, which can also affect the skin's ability to maintain its integrity. Consider parenteral nutrition.

*Staging of pressure ulcers and guidelines for prevention and management of pressure ulcers are available online from the Australian Commission on Safety and Quality in Health Care: Comprehensive Care Standard & Hospital Acquired Complications at https://www.safetyandquality.gov.au/our-work/comprehensive-care/related-topics/pressure-injuries

skin breakdown is essential. Colour, size (diameter and depth), location, presence of sinus tracts, odour, exudate and response to treatment are observed and recorded at least daily.

Friction and shear contribute to pressure ulcers. **Friction** occurs when the surface of the skin rubs against another surface, such as bed sheets. The skin may have the appearance of an abrasion. The skin damage is usually limited to the epidermal and upper layers. It most often occurs over the elbows, heels or occiput. Prevention of friction injury includes the use of: customised splinting or foam-padded boots over the heels; gel pillows under the heads of infants and toddlers; moisturising agents; protective, transparent barrier dressings over susceptible areas; and soft, smooth bed linens and clothing (August et al 2020). By itself, friction does not cause tissue necrosis, but when it acts with gravity, it results in shear injury.

Shear is the result of the force of gravity pushing down on the body and friction of the body against a surface, such as the bed or chair. For example, when a patient is in the semi-Fowler's position and begins to slide to the foot of the bed, the skin over the sacral area remains in the same place because of the resistance of the bed surface. The blood vessels, bone and muscle in the area are stretched and slide parallel to the stationary skin, which may cause small-vessel thrombosis and tissue death (Singh et al 2017). Prevention of shear injury includes using lift sheets when repositioning a patient, elevating the bed no more than 30 degrees for short periods and elevating the knees to interrupt the pull of gravity on the body towards the foot of the bed.

Epidermal stripping results when the epidermis is unintentionally removed when tape is pulled off the skin. These lesions are usually shallow and irregularly shaped. Babies are at increased risk for epidermal injury. Prevention includes using no tape when possible or securing dressings with self-adherent cohesive bandage or stretchy netting (stockinette). Using porous or low-tack tapes (e.g. Micropore, paper, hydrogel), using alcohol-free skin sealants (No Sting Barrier Film) or picture framing wounds with hydrocolloid or wafer barriers (e.g. DuoDERM, Coloplast, Stomahesive) and then taping on top of the barrier will also reduce epidermal stripping.

Chemical factors can also lead to skin damage. Faecal incontinence (especially when mixed with urine), wound drainage or gastric drainage around gastrostomy/percutaneous endoscopic gastrostomy (PEG) tubes can erode the epidermis. The skin can quickly progress from redness to denudement if exposure continues. Moisture barriers, gentle cleansing with alcohol-free cleansers or wipes as soon after exposure as possible, and skin barriers can be used to prevent damage caused by chemical factors. For non-intact skin, a barrier cream with zinc oxide should be applied (Singh et al 2017). It is important to only cleanse the stool and urine during nappy changes, not the paste. In addition, foam dressings that wick moisture away from the skin are helpful around gastrostomy tubes and tracheostomy sites.

Bathing

Most infants and children can be bathed at the bedside or in a standard bathtub or shower. Assess the child and family's preferences for bath time frequency and family involvement. For infants and young children confined to bed, use commercially available bath cloths or the towel method. Immerse two towels in a dilute soap solution and wring them damp. With the child lying supine on a dry towel, place one damp towel on top of the child and use it to gently clean the body. Discard the towel and dry the child and turn him or her prone. Repeat the procedure using the second damp towel. If bar soap is used, discard the basin and bar soap after a single bath (Marchaim et al 2012) because they can serve as a reservoir for pathogens in the hospital setting.

Oral Hygiene

Mouth care is an integral part of daily hygiene and should be continued in the hospital. Oral hygiene can prevent infection and promote comfort, adequate nutrition and verbal communication. For some young children, this is their first introduction to the use of a toothbrush. Infants and debilitated children require the nurse or a family member to perform mouth care. For infants who do not yet have teeth, a soft moistened cloth or swab can be used to gently clean the gums. Children should begin brushing their teeth after the first teeth emerge around 6 months of age. For children less than 3 years of age, a grain-sized amount of fluoride toothpaste should be used. For children 3 to 6 years of age, a pea-sized amount of fluoride toothpaste should be used (Australian Dental Association 2020). Although young children can manage a toothbrush and are encouraged to use it, most need assistance to perform satisfactorily. Older children, although capable of brushing and flossing without assistance, sometimes need to be reminded.

Hair Care

Children should have their hair brushed and combed at least once daily. The hair is styled for comfort and in a manner pleasing to the child and parents. The hair should not be cut without parental permission, although clipping hair to provide access to a scalp vein for IV insertion may be necessary.

FEEDING THE SICK CHILD

Loss of appetite is a symptom common to most childhood illnesses. Decreased appetite can be a result of pain or discomfort, nausea and vomiting, emotional concerns or loss of control. Because an acute illness is usually short, the nutritional state is seldom compromised. Urging food on the sick child may precipitate nausea and vomiting. In most cases, children can usually determine their own need for food.

Refusing to eat may also be one way children can exert power and control in an otherwise helpless situation. For young children, loss of appetite may be related to depression caused by separation from their parents. Parents' concern with eating can intensify the problem. Forcing a child to eat meets with rebellion and reinforces the behaviour as a control mechanism. Encourage parents to relax any pressure during an acute illness. Although it is best to provide high-quality, nutritious foods, the child may desire foods and liquids that contain mostly empty or non-nutritional calories. Some well-tolerated foods include jelly, diluted clear soups, carbonated drinks, flavoured ice blocks, dry toast and crackers. Even though these substances are not nutritious, they can provide necessary fluid and calories.

Dehydration is always a hazard when children have a fever or anorexia, especially when accompanied by vomiting or diarrhoea. Fluids should not be forced, and the child should not be awakened to take fluids. Forcing fluids may create the same difficulties as urging the child to eat unwanted food. Gentle persuasion with preferred beverages will usually meet with success. Using play techniques can also be effective (see Applying Evidence to Practice box).

Regardless of the type of diet, charting the amount consumed is an important nursing responsibility. Descriptions need to be detailed and accurate, such as '125 mL of orange juice, one pancake and 250 mL of milk'. Comments such as 'ate well' or 'ate poorly' are inadequate. Charting the percentage of the meal eaten is also inadequate unless food is measured before serving. For infants, assess the duration, amount and frequency of breastfeeding or bottle-feeding and the possible addition of solid foods to determine whether nutrition is adequate.

Although sick children's appetites may be poor and not characteristic of their home eating habits, the hospital stay provides numerous opportunities for nurses to assess the family's knowledge of good

APPLYING EVIDENCE TO PRACTICE

Feeding a Sick Child

- Take a dietary history (see Chapter 4) and use information to make eating time as similar to eating at home as possible.
- Encourage parents or other family members to feed child or to be present at mealtimes.
- Make mealtimes pleasant; avoid any procedures immediately before or after eating; make certain child is rested and pain free.
- Serve small, frequent meals rather than three large meals or serve three meals and nutritious between-meal snacks.
- Provide finger foods for young children.
- Involve children in food selection and preparation whenever possible.
- Serve small portions and serve each course separately, such as soup first, followed by meat, potatoes and vegetables and ending with dessert. With young children, camouflage size of food by cutting meat thicker so less appears on plate or by folding a cheese slice in half. Offer second helpings.
- Ensure a variety of foods, textures and colours.
- Provide food selections that are favourites of most children, ham and cheese sandwiches, hot dogs, hamburgers, chicken nuggets, pasta, pizza and fruit yoghurt.
- Avoid foods that are highly seasoned, have strong odours or are all mixed unless typical of cultural practices.
- Provide fluid selections that are favourites of most children, such as fruit juice, soft drinks, flavoured ice blocks, ice-cream, milk, milkshakes, pudding, jelly, clear broth or yoghurt.
- Offer nutritious snacks, such as frozen yoghurt or pudding, ice-cream, cereal or sweet or dry biscuits and cheese slices, pieces of raw vegetable or fruit and dried fruit or cereal.
- Make food attractive and different—for example:
  - serve a 'picnic lunch' in a paper bag
  - pack food in a Chinese takeaway container; decorate container
  - put a 'face' or a 'flower' on a hamburger or sandwich with pieces of vegetable
  - use a cookie cutter to shape a sandwich
  - serve pudding, yoghurt or juice frozen as an ice block
  - make slushies or snow cones by pouring flavoured syrup on crushed ice
  - serve fluids through brightly coloured or unusually shaped straws
  - make 'bowtie' sandwiches by cutting them in triangles and placing two points together
  - slice sandwiches into 'fingers'
  - grate mounds of cheese
  - cut apples horizontally to make circles
  - break uncooked spaghetti into toothpick lengths and skewer cheese, cold meat, vegetables or fruit chunks.
- Praise children for what they do eat.
- Do not punish children for not eating by removing their dessert or putting them to bed.

nutrition and to implement teaching as needed to improve nutritional intake.

CONTROLLING ELEVATED TEMPERATURES

An elevated temperature, most frequently from fever but occasionally caused by hyperthermia, is one of the most common symptoms of illness in children. This manifestation is a great concern to parents. To facilitate an understanding of fever versus hyperthermia, the following terms are defined.

- **Set point**—The temperature around which body temperature is regulated by a thermostat-like mechanism in the hypothalamus.
- **Fever (hyperpyrexia)**—An elevation in set point such that body temperature is regulated at a higher level; may be arbitrarily defined as rectal temperature above 38°C.
- **Hyperthermia**—Body temperature exceeding the set point, which usually results from the body or external conditions creating more heat than the body can eliminate, such as in heat exhaustion, heat-stroke, aspirin toxicity, seizures or hyperthyroidism.

Body temperature is regulated by a thermostat-like mechanism in the hypothalamus. This mechanism receives input from centrally and peripherally located receptors. When temperature changes occur, these receptors relay the information to the thermostat, which either increases or decreases heat production to maintain a constant set point temperature. However, during an infection, pyrogenic substances cause an increase in the body's normal set point, a process that is mediated by prostaglandins. Consequently, the hypothalamus increases heat production until the core temperature reaches the new set point.

During the fever (febrile) state, shivering and vasoconstriction generate and conserve heat during the chill phase of fever, raising central temperatures to the level of the new set point. The temperature reaches a plateau when it stabilises in the higher range. When the temperature is greater than the set point or when the pyrogen is no longer present, a crisis, or defervescence, of the temperature occurs.

Most fevers in children are of brief duration with limited consequences and are viral in origin. Children may experience warm, flushed skin, chills, aches, malaise or irritability during a fever. However, children who appear very ill, immunocompromised children and neonates are at high risk for serious bacterial illness, such as urinary tract infections or bacteraemia, and are likely to receive a sepsis workup, antibiotics and hospitalisation (Häusler et al 2018).

Fever has physiological benefits, including increased white blood cell activity, interferon production and effectiveness and antibody production and enhancement of some antibiotic effects such as penicillin (Patricia 2014). Contrary to popular belief, neither the rise in temperature nor its response to antipyretics indicates the severity or aetiology of the infection, which casts doubt on the value of using fever as a diagnostic or prognostic indicator.

Therapeutic Management

Treatment of elevated temperature depends on whether it is attributable to a fever or hyperthermia. Because the set point is normal in hyperthermia but increased in fever, different approaches must be used to lower body temperature successfully.

Fever

The principal reason for treating fever is the relief of discomfort. However, children with cardiopulmonary disease or immunocompromised children may not tolerate the increase in metabolic demand from a fever and should receive antipyretic therapy. Relief measures include pharmacological and environmental intervention. The most effective intervention is the use of antipyretics to lower the set point.

Antipyretics include paracetamol, aspirin and non-steroidal anti-inflammatory drugs (NSAIDs). Paracetamol is the preferred drug. Aspirin should not be given to children because of its association in children with influenza virus or chickenpox and Reye's syndrome. One non-prescription NSAID, ibuprofen, is approved for fever reduction in children as young as 6 months of age.

Another antipyretic, paracetamol, can be given every 4 hours but no more than four times in 24 hours due to the risk of hepatotoxicity.

Because body temperature normally decreases at night, three or four doses in 24 hours will control most fevers. The temperature is usually retaken 30 to 60 minutes after the antipyretic is given to assess its effect but should not be repeatedly measured. The child's level of discomfort is the best indication for continued treatment.

The nurse can use environmental measures to reduce fever if they are tolerated by the child and if they do not induce shivering. Shivering is the body's way of maintaining the elevated set point by producing heat. Compensatory shivering greatly increases metabolic requirements above those already caused by the fever.

Traditional cooling measures—such as wearing minimum clothing; exposing the skin to air; reducing room temperature; increasing air circulation; and applying cool, moist compresses to the skin (e.g. the forehead)—are effective if used approximately 1 hour after an antipyretic is given so the set point is lowered. Cooling procedures such as sponging or tepid baths are ineffective in treating febrile children (these measures are effective for hyperthermia) either when used alone or in combination with antipyretics, and they cause considerable discomfort (Lim et al 2018).

Seizures associated with a fever occur in 2% to 5% of all children, usually in those between 6 months and 5 years of age. About 30% to 50% of children have subsequent febrile seizures; a younger age at onset and a family history of febrile seizures are associated with increased incidence of recurring episodes. Evidence does not support the use of antipyretic drugs or anticonvulsants to prevent a second febrile seizure. Nursing interventions should focus on ways to provide care and comfort during a febrile illness (Rosenbloom et al 2013). Simple febrile seizures lasting less than 10 minutes do not cause brain damage or other debilitating effects (Kubota et al 2020). (See Febrile Seizures, Chapter 30.)

Hyperthermia

Unlike in fever, antipyretics are of no value in hyperthermia because the set point is already normal. Consequently, cooling measures are used. If a child is severely hyperthermic with a core temperature above 40°C, it may be necessary to perform continuous monitoring of vital signs including core temperature and urinary output and administer IV fluids in a critical care environment (Chan & Mamat 2015). Cool applications to the skin help reduce the core temperature. Cooled blood from the skin surface is conducted to inner organs and tissues, and warm blood is circulated to the surface, where it is cooled and recirculated. The surface blood vessels dilate as the body attempts to dissipate heat to the environment and facilitate this cooling process.

Traditionally, cool compresses decrease high temperature. For tepid baths in a bath tub, it is usually best to start with warm water and gradually add cool water until the desired water temperature of 37°C is reached to acclimatise the child to the lower water temperature. Generally, the temperature of the water must only be 1°C less than the child's temperature to be effective. The child is placed directly in the tub of tepid water for 15 to 20 minutes, while water is gently squeezed from a washcloth over the back and chest or gently sprayed over the body from a sprayer. In the bed or cot, cool washcloths or towels are used, exposing only one area of the body at a time. Continue sponging for approximately 20 minutes.

After the tub or sponge bath, the child is dried and dressed in lightweight pyjamas, a nightgown or a nappy and placed in a dry bed. The child is dried by gently rubbing the skin surface with a towel to stimulate circulation. The temperature is retaken 30 minutes after the tub or sponge bath. The tub or sponge bath should not be continued or restarted until the skin surface is warm or if the child feels chilled. Chilling causes vasoconstriction, which defeats the purpose of the cool applications. In this condition, little blood is carried to the skin surface; the blood remains primarily in the viscera to become heated.

Whether a temperature elevation in the critically ill child is caused by fever or hyperthermia, it should be treated aggressively. The metabolic rate increases 10% for every 1°C increase in temperature and three to five times during shivering, thus increasing oxygen, fluid and caloric requirements. If the child's cardiovascular or neurological system is already compromised, these increased needs are especially hazardous. In all children with an elevated temperature, attention to adequate hydration is essential. Most children's needs can be met through additional oral fluids.

Family Teaching and Home Care

Fever is one of the most common problems for which parents seek healthcare. High levels of parental anxiety (fever phobia) surrounding potential complications of fever such as seizures and dehydration are prevalent and can result in overusing antipyretics. Parents need to know that sponging is indicated for elevated temperatures from hyperthermia rather than fever and that ice water and alcohol are inappropriate, potentially dangerous solutions (Lim et al 2018). Parents should know how to take the child's temperature, how to read the thermometer accurately and when to seek professional care (see Family-Centred Care box). Oral temperatures should not be taken within 15 minutes of the child eating or drinking hot or cold food. Some of the newer temperature-measuring devices, such as plastic strip or digital thermometers, may be better suited for home use. (See Temperature, Chapter 4.) If the use of paracetamol or ibuprofen is indicated, the parents need instructions in administering the drug. Emphasise accuracy in both the amount of drug given and the time intervals at which the drug is administered. Along with reduced activity, encourage small, frequent sips of clear liquids. Dress the child in light clothing; use a light blanket for children who are cold or shivering (Monsma et al 2015, Ward 2019).

FAMILY-CENTRED CARE

The Child with Fever

Call the Doctor Immediately if

- Your child is younger than 3 months old and has a temperature of 38°C or higher.
- The fever is over 40°C.
- Your child looks or acts very sick or sleepy, or has a stiff neck, severe headache, severe ear pain, severe sore throat, repeated vomiting or diarrhoea, unexplained rash on the skin, confusion, trouble breathing or inability to be comforted.
- Your child has had a recent seizure.
- Your child has a history of immune system problems such as cancer or sickle cell disease.
- Your child has been in a very hot place such as a car.
- Your child has taken steroid medication.
- The fever continues for more than 24 hours in a child younger than 2 years or more than 3 days in a child older than 2 years.

Source: The Royal Children's Hospital Melbourne (RCHM). (2020). Fever in children. July. https://www.rch.org.au/kidsinfo/fact_sheets/Fever_in_children/

SAFETY

Safety is an essential component of any patient's care, but children have special characteristics that require an even greater concern for safety. Because small children in the hospital are separated from their usual environment and do not possess the capacity for abstract thinking and reasoning, it is the responsibility of everyone who meets them to maintain protective measures throughout their hospital stay. Nurses need to understand the age level at which each child is operating and plan for safety accordingly.

Identification bands and the use of three patient identifiers are particularly important for children. Infants and unconscious patients are unable to tell or respond to their names. Toddlers may answer to any name or to a nickname only. Older children may exchange places, give an erroneous name or choose not to respond to their own names as a joke, unaware of the hazards of such practices. Additionally, allergy bands for medications and food should be worn by all patients.

Environmental Factors

All the environmental safety measures for the protection of adults apply to children, including good illumination, floors that are clear of fluid and objects that might contribute to falls and non-skid surfaces in showers and tubs. All staff members should be familiar with the area-specific fire plan. Lifts and stairways should be made safe.

All windows should be secured. Window blind and curtain cords should be out of reach, with split cords to prevent strangulation. Soothers (dummies) should not be tied around the neck or attached to an infant by a string.

Electrical equipment should be in good working order and used only by personnel familiar with its use. It should not be in contact with moisture or situated near tubs. Electrical outlets should have covers to prevent burns in small children, whose exploratory activities may extend to inserting objects into the small openings.

Staff members should practise proper care and disposal of small objects such as syringe caps, needle covers and temperature probes. Staff also must carefully check bathwater before placing the child in it and never leave children alone in a bathtub. Infants are helpless in water, and small children (and some older ones) may turn on the hot water tap and be severely burned.

Furniture is safest when it is scaled to the child's proportions, is sturdy and is well balanced to prevent its being easily tipped over. A special hazard for children is the danger of entrapment under an electronically controlled bed when it is activated to descend. Infants and small children must be securely strapped into infant seats, feeding chairs and strollers. Baby walkers should not be used because they provide access to hazards, resulting in burns, falls and poisonings. Infants, young children and children who are weak, paralysed, agitated, confused, sedated or cognitively impaired should never be left unattended on treatment tables, on scales or in treatment areas. Even premature infants are capable of surprising mobility; therefore, portholes in incubators must be securely fastened when not in use.

Cot sides should always be raised and fastened securely. Use cots that meet federal safety standards (Australian Competition and Consumer Commission 2007). Anyone attending an infant or small child on a stretcher or table should never turn away without maintaining hand contact with the child; that is, keeping one hand on the child's back or abdomen to prevent rolling, crawling or jumping from the open cot (Fig 22.1). A child who is likely to climb over the sides of the cot is safest when placed in a specially constructed cot with a cover over the top. Never tie nets to the movable cot sides or use knots that do not permit quick release.

The safest sleeping position to prevent sudden infant death syndrome is wholly supine until at least 1 year of age (Cole et al 2021). No pillows should be placed in a young infant's cot while the infant is sleeping. A firm sleep surface with no other bedding or any soft items in the cot in a shared room (not a shared bed) and the avoidance of overheating, exposure to tobacco smoke, alcohol and illicit drugs further increase the safety of an infant's sleeping environment. Car seats, strollers, swings or other sitting devices should not be used for routine sleep. Additionally, swaddling is not recommended for infants over 2 months of age due to the risk of death if the infant rolls into the prone position. In accordance with the Red Nose Australia guidelines to avoid extra bedding in the cot, many institutions recommend an infant sleep sack for adequate warmth and safety.

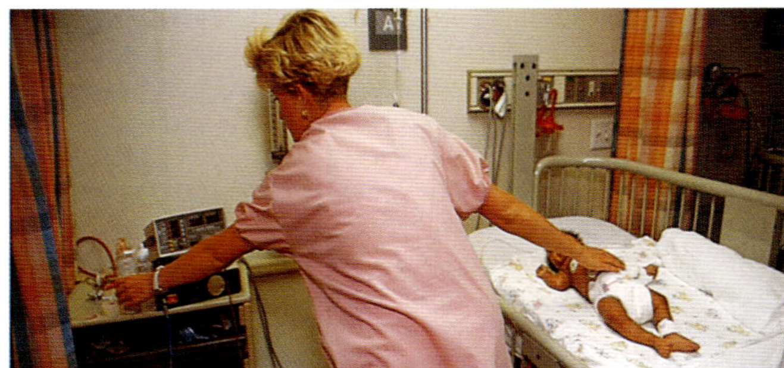

Fig 22.1 The nurse maintains hand contact when her back is turned.

Toys

Toys play a vital role in the everyday lives of children, and they are no less important in the hospital setting. Nurses are responsible for assessing the safety of toys brought to the hospital by well-meaning parents and friends. Toys should be appropriate to the child's age, condition and treatment. For example, if the child is receiving oxygen, electrical or friction toys or equipment are not safe because sparks can cause oxygen to ignite. Inspect toys to ensure they are non-allergenic, washable and unbreakable and that they have no small, removable parts that can be aspirated or swallowed or can otherwise inflict injury on a child. All objects within reach of children younger than 3 years of age should pass the choke tube test. A toilet paper roll is a handy guide. If a toy or object fits into the cylinder (items less than 3 cm across or balls less than 4.5 cm in diameter), it is a potential choking danger to the child. Latex balloons pose a serious threat to children of all ages. If the balloon breaks, a child may put a piece of the latex in his or her mouth. If it is aspirated or swallowed, the latex piece is difficult to remove, resulting in choking. Latex balloons should never be permitted in the hospital setting.

Preventing Falls

Although children have a known predisposition to falls based on normal growth and development, falls risk identification and prevention for children with medical conditions is especially important due to greater risk for injury from a fall (Murray et al 2016). Falls prevention begins with identification of children most at risk for falls. Paediatric hospitals use various methods to identify a child's risk of falls. After a risk assessment is performed, multiple interventions are needed to minimise paediatric patients' risk of falling, including education of patient, family and staff (Australian Commission on Safety and Quality in Health Care [ACSQHC] 2019a).

To identify children at risk of falling, perform a fall risk assessment on patients on admission and throughout hospitalisation. Risk factors for hospitalised children include the following.

- **Medication effects**—Post-anaesthesia or sedation; analgesics or narcotics, especially in those who have never had narcotics in the past and in whom effects are unknown
- **Altered mental status**—Secondary to seizures, brain tumours or medications
- **Altered or limited mobility**—Reduced skill at ambulation secondary to developmental age, disease process, tubes, drains, casts, splints or other appliances; new to ambulation with assistive devices such as walkers or crutches

- **Postoperative children**—Risk of hypotension or syncope secondary to large blood loss, a heart condition or extended bed rest
- History of falls
- Infants or toddlers in cots with side rails down or on the bed with family members
- Changes to the patient's environment

Once children at risk of falls have been identified, alert other staff members by posting signs on the door and at the bedside, applying a special-coloured armband labelled 'Fall Precautions', labelling the chart with a sticker or documenting information on the chart.

Preventing falls also relies on age-appropriate education of patients. Assist the child with ambulation even though he or she may have ambulated well before hospitalisation. Patients who have been lying in bed need to get up slowly, sitting on the side of the bed before standing.

The nurse also needs to educate family members in the following

- Call the nursing staff for assistance, and do not allow patients to get up independently.
- Keep the side rails of the cot or bed up whenever the patient is in the cot or bed.
- Do not leave infants on the bed; put them in the cot with the side rails up.
- When all family members need to leave the bedside, notify the staff and ensure that the patient is in the bed or cot with the side rails up and call bell within reach (if appropriate).

In the event of a fall, it is important to immediately respond to the needs of the patient, notify appropriate personnel (including caregivers) and document the event.

Infection Control

According to the ACSQHC and the Centres for Disease Control and Prevention, nosocomial (healthcare-associated) infections pose a significant threat to patient safety. These infections occur when there is interaction among patients, healthcare personnel, equipment and bacteria. Healthcare-associated infections include infections such as *Clostridium difficile* or hospital-onset methicillin-resistant *Staphylococcus aureus*, as well as central line-associated bloodstream infections (CLABSIs), catheter-associated urinary tract infections (CAUTIs) and some surgical site infections. Healthcare-associated infections can be preventable if caregivers practise meticulous cleaning and disposal techniques.

Standard precautions synthesise the major features of universal (blood and body fluid) precautions (designed to reduce the risk of transmission of blood-borne pathogens) and body substance isolation (designed to reduce the risk of transmission of pathogens from moist body substances). Standard precautions involve vigilant hand hygiene and the use of barrier protection, such as gloves, goggles, gown or mask, to prevent contamination from: (1) blood; (2) all body fluids, secretions and excretions except sweat, regardless of whether they contain visible blood; (3) non-intact skin; and (4) mucous membranes. Standard precautions are designed for the care of all patients to reduce the risk of transmission of microorganisms from both recognised and unrecognised sources of infection.

Transmission-based precautions are designed for patients with documented or suspected infection or colonisation (i.e. presence of microorganisms in or on patient but without clinical signs and symptoms of infection) with highly transmissible or epidemiologically important pathogens for which additional precautions beyond standard precautions are needed to interrupt transmission in hospitals. There are three types of transmission-based precautions: airborne precautions, droplet precautions and contact precautions. They may be combined for diseases that have multiple routes of transmission. They are to be used in addition to standard precautions.

Airborne precautions reduce the risk of airborne transmission of infectious agents. Airborne transmission occurs by dissemination of either airborne droplet nuclei (small-particle residue [$<$ 5 mm] of evaporated droplets that may remain suspended in the air for long periods) or dust particles containing the infectious agent. Microorganisms carried in this manner can be dispersed widely by air currents and may become inhaled by or deposited on a susceptible host within the same room or over a longer distance from the source patient, depending on environmental factors. Individuals may become infected who have not had direct face-to-face contact with the source individual. Special air handling and ventilation are required to prevent airborne transmission. Airborne precautions apply to patients with known or suspected infection with pathogens transmitted by the airborne route such as measles, varicella and tuberculosis.

Droplet precautions reduce the risk of droplet transmission of infectious agents. Droplet transmission involves contact of the conjunctivae or the mucous membranes of the nose or mouth of a susceptible person with large-particle droplets ($>$ 5 mm) containing microorganisms generated from a person who has a clinical disease or who is a carrier of the microorganism. Droplets are generated from the source person primarily during coughing, sneezing or talking and during procedures such as suctioning and bronchoscopy. Transmission requires close contact between source and recipient persons because droplets do not remain suspended in the air and generally travel only short distances, usually within 1 m up to 3 m, through the air. Due to changes relating to COVID-19, the need for 1.5 m social distancing is required where possible in all healthcare settings. Wearing of masks is at present still required in all healthcare settings and, where required, full personal protective equipment is to be worn. Because droplets do not remain suspended in the air, special air handling and ventilation are not required to prevent droplet transmission. Droplet precautions apply to any patient with known or suspected infection with pathogens that can be transmitted by infectious droplets.

Contact precautions reduce the risk of transmission of microorganisms by direct or indirect contact. Direct-contact transmission involves skin-to-skin contact and physical transfer of microorganisms to a susceptible host from an infected or colonised person, such as occurs when turning or bathing patients. Direct-contact transmission also can occur between two patients (e.g. by hand contact). Indirect contact transmission involves contact of a susceptible host with a contaminated intermediate object, usually inanimate, in the patient's environment. Contact precautions apply to specified patients known or suspected to be infected or colonised with microorganisms that can be transmitted by direct or indirect contact. All healthcare settings require all healthcare staff to follow strict COVID-19 precautions for infection control and will be guided appropriately by their state/territory health departments on specific requirements as needed due to the nature of COVID-19 and ongoing outbreaks still being experienced and changes to the situation.

Transporting Infants and Children

Infants and children need to be transported within the unit and to areas outside the paediatric unit. Infants and small children can be carried for short distances within the unit, but for more extended trips, the child should be securely transported in a suitable conveyance.

Special care is needed in transporting critically ill patients in the hospital. Critically ill children should always be transported on a stretcher or bed (rather than carried) by at least two appropriately trained staff members with monitoring continued during transport. A blood pressure monitor (or standard blood pressure cuff), pulse oximeter and cardiac monitor/defibrillator should accompany every patient (Alamanou & Brokalaki 2014). Airway equipment, oxygen and emergency medications should accompany the patient. The monitoring and staff members required for transport will vary depending on the acuity and clinical status of the patient. Additionally, it is important for the nurse to be familiar with emergency transport of patients in the event of severe weather, fire or security threats when power or lifts may be unavailable.

Restraining Methods

The ACSQHC has established regulations to minimise the use and ensure safety of patients in restraints. It defines *restraint* as 'any manual method, physical or mechanical device, material or equipment that immobilises or reduces the ability of a patient to move his or her arms, legs, body or head freely ... or a drug or medication when it is used as a restriction to manage the patient's behaviour or restrict the patient's freedom of movement and is not a standard treatment or dosage for the patient's condition' (ACSQHC 2019b). A restraint should only be applied by a healthcare team member with demonstrated competency in restraint management. The physical force may be human, mechanical devices or a combination of the two. Examples of restraints include limb restraints, elbow restraints, vest restraints and tight tucking of sheets to prevent movement in bed.

Mechanical supports such as immobilisers for fractures, orthopaedic devices to maintain proper body alignment, leg braces, protective helmets and surgical dressings are not considered restraints. An arm board to secure a peripheral IV line is not considered a restraint unless it is tied down to the bed or immobilises the entire limb such that the patient cannot access his or her body. Hand mitts are not considered a restraint unless tied down to the bed or used in conjunction with a wrist restraint. Developmentally age-appropriate safety interventions for infants, toddlers and preschoolers, such as net enclosures on beds, cot domes, cot side rails and highchair lap safety belts, are generally not considered restraints. Picking up, redirecting or holding an infant, toddler or preschooler is not considered restraint. Interventions that would typically be employed by a childcare provider outside of a healthcare environment to ensure safety in young children are not considered restraints.

Before initiating restraints, the nurse completes a comprehensive assessment of the patient to determine whether the need for a restraint outweighs the risk of not using one. Restraints can result in loss of dignity, violation of patient rights, psychological harm, physical harm and even death. Consider alternative methods first and document them in the patient's record.

Restraints for violent, self-destructive behaviour are limited to situations with a significant risk of patients physically harming themselves or others because of behavioural reasons and when non-physical interventions are not effective. Before initiating a behavioural restraint, the nurse should assess the patient's mental, behavioural and physical status to determine the cause for the child's potentially harmful behaviour. If behavioural restraints are indicated, a collaborative approach involving the patient (if appropriate), the family and the healthcare team should be used. Behavioural restraints can include personal restraints, such as a physical hold, or mechanical restraints, such as secured anklets and wristlets or bilateral arm immobilisers.

Children in behavioural restraints must be observed and assessed according to facility policy—typically continuously, every 15 minutes or every 2 hours. Assessment components include signs of injury associated with applying restraint, nutrition and hydration, circulation and range-of-motion of extremities, vital signs, hygiene and elimination, physical and psychological status and comfort and readiness for discontinuation of restraint. The nurse must use clinical judgment in setting a schedule within the facility's policy for when each of these parameters needs to be evaluated.

Non-violent/non–self-destructive patients may also require restraints to support medical healing. Examples of situations where a non-behavioural restraint may be necessary for the patient's safety include removal of an artificial airway or airway adjunct for delivery of oxygen, indwelling catheters, tubes, drains, lines, pacemaker wires or disruption of suture sites. The medical-surgical restraint is used to ensure that safe care is given to the patient. Patient confusion, agitation, unconsciousness and developmental inability to understand direct requests or instructions may warrant the use of non-behavioural restraints to maintain patient safety. The potential risks of the restraint are offset by the potential benefit of providing safer care.

Mummy Restraint or Swaddle

When an infant or small child requires short-term restraint for examination or treatment that involves the head and neck (e.g. venepuncture, throat examination, gavage feeding), a mummy wrap effectively controls the child's movements. When used only for the duration of the test or procedure, this is not considered a restraint. The mummy restraint or swaddle should not be used for behaviour or long-term restraint. A blanket or sheet is opened on the bed or cot with one corner folded to the centre. The infant is placed on the blanket with the shoulders at the fold and feet towards the opposite corner. With the infant's right arm straight down against the body, the right-shoulder side of the blanket is pulled firmly across the infant's right shoulder and chest and secured beneath the left side of the body. The left arm is placed straight against the infant's side, and the left-shoulder side of the blanket is brought across the shoulder and chest and locked beneath the body on the right side. The lower corner is folded and brought over the body and tucked. To modify the mummy restraint for chest examination, bring the folded edge of the blanket over each arm and under the back and then fold the loose edge over and secure it at a point below the chest to allow visualisation and access to the chest (Fig 22.2).

POSITIONING FOR PROCEDURES

Infants and small children are unable to cooperate for many procedures. Therefore, the nurse is responsible for minimising their movement and discomfort with proper positioning. It can also be helpful to involve the caregivers or child life therapists during procedures to minimise distress in the child. Older children usually need only minimal, if any, positioning hold or movement restrictions. Careful explanation and preparation beforehand and support and simple guidance during the procedure are usually enough. For painful procedures, the child should receive adequate analgesia and sedation to minimise pain and the need for excessive restraint. For local anaesthesia, use buffered lidocaine (lignocaine) to reduce the stinging sensation or a topical anaesthetic.

Femoral Venepuncture

The nurse places the child supine with the legs in a frog position to provide extensive exposure of the groin area. A towel can also be placed under the hips. The infant's legs can be effectively controlled by the nurse's forearms and hands (Fig 22.3). Only the side used for the venepuncture is uncovered, so the practitioner is protected if the child urinates during the procedure. Apply pressure to the site to prevent oozing from the site.

Extremity Venepuncture or Injection

The most common sites of venepuncture are the veins of the extremities, especially the arm and hand. A convenient position is to place the child in the parent's (or assistant's) lap with the child facing the parent and in the straddle position. Next, place the child's arm for venepuncture on a firm surface, such as a treatment table. The nurse can

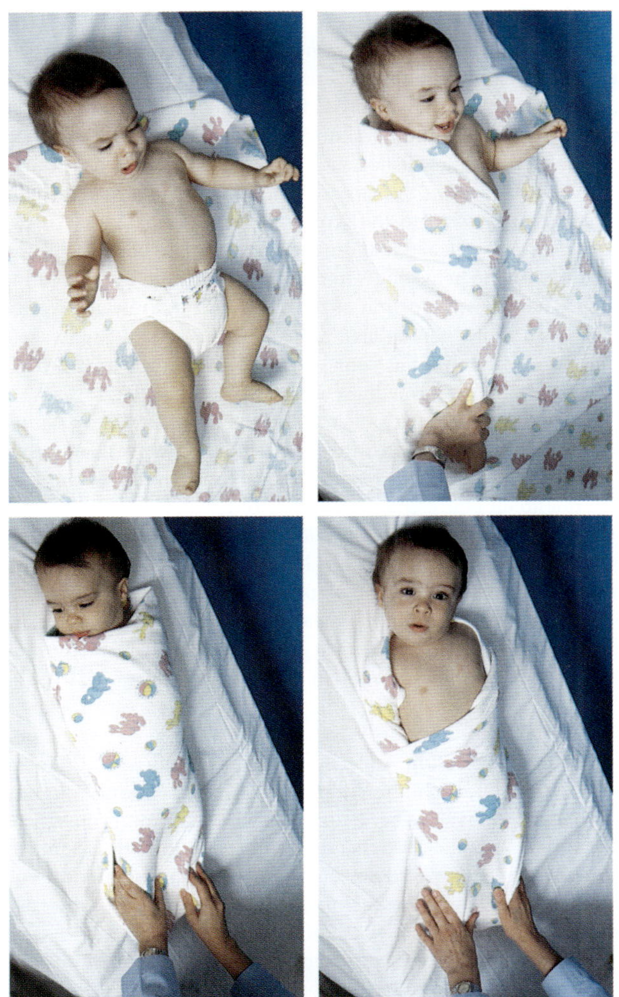

Fig 22.2 Mummy restraint.

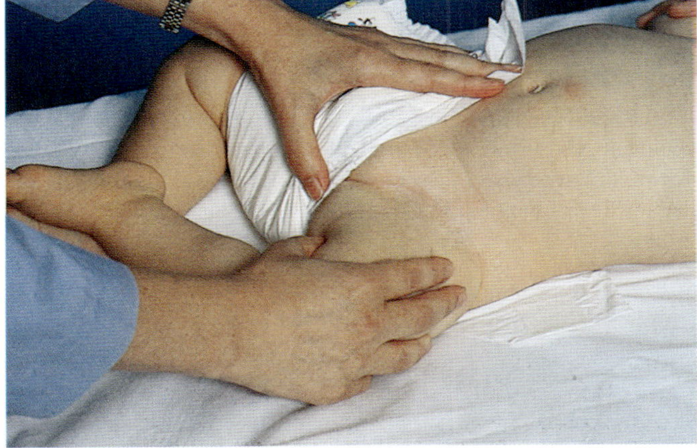

Fig 22.3 Positioning infant for femoral venepuncture.

partially stabilise the child's outstretched arm and have the parent hug the child's upper body, preventing movement; the nurse can then use the parent's arm to immobilise the venepuncture site. This type of comfort hold also comforts the child because of the close body contact, allows for distraction techniques for the child and allows each person to maintain eye contact (Fig 22.4).

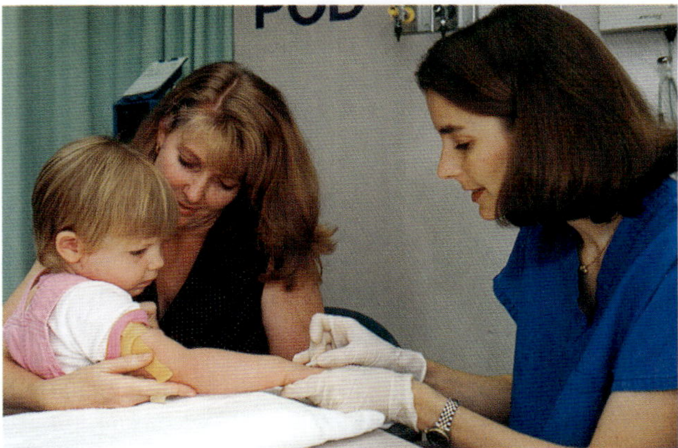

Fig 22.4 Therapeutic comfort hold of child for extremity venepuncture with parental assistance.

Lumbar Puncture

Paediatric lumbar puncture (LP) sets contain smaller spinal needles, but sometimes the provider will specify a different size or type of needle depending on the child's size or obesity. The technique for the LP procedure in infants and children is like that in adults, although modifications are suggested in neonates, who have less distress in a side-lying position with modified neck extension than in flexion or a sitting position.

Children can be positioned in a side-lying or sitting position. Children are usually easiest to control in the side-lying position, with the head flexed and the knees drawn up towards the chest. Even cooperative children need to be held gently under the knees and around the shoulders to prevent possible trauma from unexpected, involuntary movement. They can be reassured that, although they are trusted, holding will serve as a reminder to maintain the desired position. It also provides a measure of support and reassurance to them (Fig 22.5).

A flexed sitting position may be used, depending on the child's ability to cooperate and whether sedation will be used. In the sitting position with the hips flexed and spine curved forwards, the interspinous space is maximised between L3 and L5 (Ford 2016). The child is placed with the buttocks at the edge of the table. For an infant, the nurse's hands immobilise the arms and legs. Neck flexion has not been shown to enhance the interspinous space opening in children.

Specimens and spinal fluid pressure are obtained, measured and sent for analysis in the same manner as for adult patients. Take vital signs as ordered throughout and after the procedure and observe the child for any changes in level of consciousness, motor activity and other

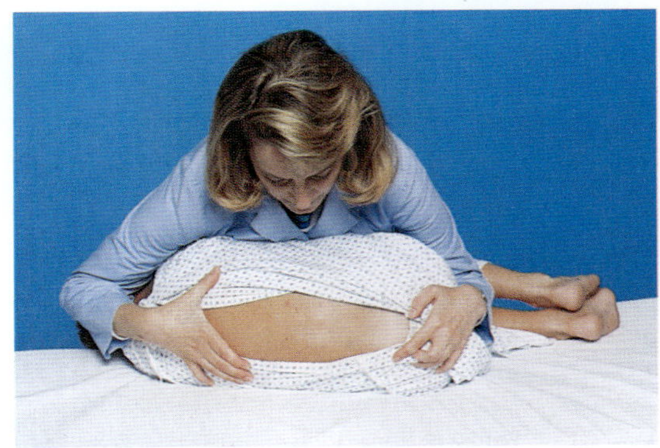

Fig 22.5 Side-lying position for lumbar puncture.

neurological signs. Post-LP headache may occur and can be related to larger needle size, prior history of headaches and postural changes. There is insufficient evidence to support the use of bed rest after LP to reduce post-LP headaches (Rusch et al 2014). Treatment generally includes rest and oral analgesics that do not inhibit platelet function.

Bone Marrow Aspiration or Biopsy

The position for a bone marrow aspiration or biopsy depends on the chosen site. In children, the posterior or anterior iliac crest is most frequently used, but in infants less than 18 months old, the tibia may be selected because the iliac crest has not yet ossified.

If the posterior iliac crest is used, the child is positioned prone and if the anterior iliac crest is used, the child is typically positioned side-lying or supine. Sometimes a small pillow or folded blanket is placed under the hips to facilitate obtaining the bone marrow specimen. Children should receive adequate analgesia or anaesthesia to relieve pain and should be monitored appropriately throughout the procedure. If the child might awaken, he or she may need to be held, preferably by two people—one person to immobilise the upper body and a second person to immobilise the lower extremities. A pressure dressing is applied to the puncture site on completion of the procedure and maintained for 24 hours.

COLLECTION OF SPECIMENS

Many of the specimens needed for diagnostic examination of children are collected in much the same way as they are for adults. Older children can cooperate if given proper instructions on what is expected of them. Infants and small children, however, are typically unable to follow directions or control body functions sufficiently to help in collecting some specimens.

Urine Specimens

There are many diagnostic situations that warrant urine specimens. The age of the child will affect the collection technique, as well as developmental considerations. Children will better understand what is expected if the nurse uses familiar terms, such as 'wee-wee'. Preschoolers and toddlers are usually unable to void on request. It is often best to offer them water or other liquids that they enjoy and wait about 30 minutes until they are ready to void voluntarily. Some have difficulty voiding in an unfamiliar receptacle. Placing a potty chair on the toilet is usually satisfactory. Toddlers who have recently acquired bladder control may be especially reluctant because they undoubtedly have been admonished for 'going' in places other than those approved by parents. Enlisting the parents' help usually leads to success.

Urine Collection Bags

For infants and toddlers who are not toilet trained, special urine collection bags with self-adhering material around the opening at the point of attachment may be used. To prepare the infant, the genitalia, perineum and surrounding skin are washed and dried thoroughly because the adhesive will not stick to a moist, powdered or oily skin surface. The collection bag is easiest to apply if attached first to the perineum, progressing to the symphysis pubis (Fig 22.6). With girls, the perineum is stretched taut during application to ensure a leakproof fit. With boys, the penis and sometimes the scrotum are placed inside the bag. The adhesive portion of the bag must be firmly applied to the skin all around the genital area to avoid leakage. The bag is checked frequently and removed as soon as the specimen is available because the moist bag may become loosened on an active child.

Management of urinary tract infections in infants 2 to 24 months old recommend that any positive screen obtained from a bag specimen be confirmed by culture via bladder catheterisation or suprapubic aspiration due to an unacceptably high rate of false-positive results (Royal Children's Hospital Melbourne [RCHM] 2020). Although the bag specimen collection method is less invasive and traumatic to an infant, some families and clinicians may prefer to collect only one definitive specimen and avoid additional delay in obtaining a second specimen. Urine bag specimens may be most appropriate for a urine dipstick or urinalysis, not urine cultures (Stein et al 2015, Kaufman 2020).

Twenty-four-hour Collection

For a 24-hour collection, collection bags are required in infants and small children. Older children require special instruction about notifying someone when they need to void or have a bowel movement so that urine can be collected separately and is not discarded. Some older school-age children and adolescents can take responsibility for collection of their own 24-hour specimens and can keep output records and transfer each voiding to the 24-hour collection container.

The collection period always starts and ends with an empty bladder. At the time the collection begins, instruct the child to void and discard the specimen. All urine voided in the subsequent 24 hours is saved in a container with a preservative or is placed on ice. Twenty-four hours from the time the pre-collection specimen was discarded, the child is again instructed to void, the specimen is added to the container and the entire collection is taken to the laboratory.

Bladder Catheterisation and Other Techniques

Bladder catheterisation or suprapubic aspiration is used when a specimen is urgently needed or a child is unable to void or otherwise provide an adequate specimen. The Royal Children's Hospital Melbourne recommends that a urine specimen be obtained by bladder

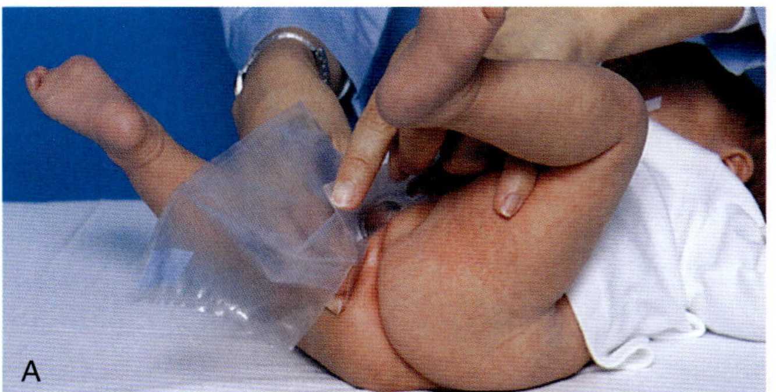

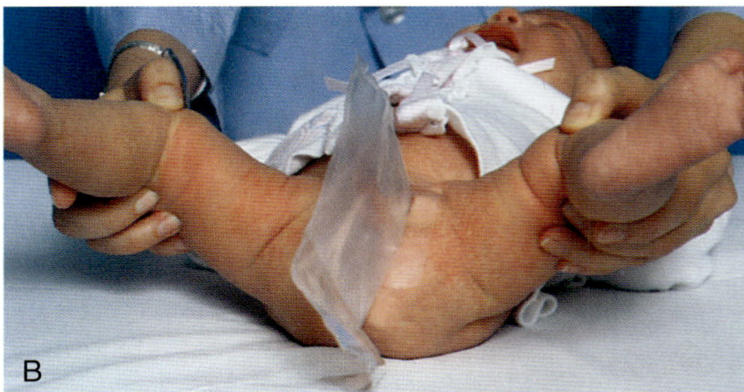

Fig 22.6 Application of urine collection bag. (**A**) On female infants, the adhesive portion is applied to the exposed and dried perineum first. (**B**) The bag adheres firmly around the perineal area to prevent urine leakage.

catheterisation or suprapubic aspiration in ill-appearing febrile infants with no apparent source of infection before antimicrobial administration and to confirm a positive screen for infection (RCHM 2019).

Catheterisation is a sterile procedure, and standard precautions for body substance protection should be followed. If the catheter is to remain in place, a Foley catheter is used. Table 22.4 gives guidelines for choosing the appropriate-size catheter and length of insertion.

Adolescent boys and children with a history of urethral surgery may be catheterised with a curved, Coudé-tipped catheter to assist with guiding the catheter past tight or partially blocked urethral openings. Children with myelodysplasia and those who have been identified as being sensitive or allergic to latex are catheterised with catheters manufactured from an alternative material. When an indwelling catheter is indicated for urinary drainage, a lubricious-coated or silicone catheter is selected because these materials produce less irritation of the urethral mucosa compared with Silastic or latex catheters when left in place for more than 72 hours.

Sterile anaesthetic gel lubricant with applicator is assembled according to the manufacturer's instructions, and several drops of the lubricant are placed at the meatus. The child is advised that the lubricant is used to reduce any discomfort associated with inserting the catheter and that introduction of the catheter into the urethra will produce a sensation of pressure and a desire to urinate (Australia and New Zealand Urological Nurses Society Catheterisation Guideline Working Party 2013).

TABLE 22.4 Straight Catheter or Foley Catheter*

	Size (Length of Insertion [cm]) for Girls	Size (Length of Insertion [cm]) for Boys
Term neonate	5–6 (5)	5–6 (6)
Infant to 3 years	5–8 (5)	5–8 (6)
4–8 years	8 (5–6)	8 (6–9)
8 years to prepubertal	10–12 (6–8)	8–10 (10–15)
Pubertal	12–14 (6–8)	12–14 (13–18)

*Foley catheters are approximately 1 Fr size larger because of the circumference of the balloon. Example: 10-Fr Foley catheter = approximately 12-Fr calibration.

TRANSLATING EVIDENCE INTO PRACTICE

The Use of Lidocaine (Lignocaine) Lubricant for Urethral Catheterisation

Ask the Question

PICOT Question

In children, does a lidocaine (lignocaine) lubricant decrease the pain associated with urethral catheterisation?

Search for the Evidence

Search Strategies

Search selection criteria included English-language publications, research-based studies and review articles on the use of the lidocaine (lignocaine) lubricant before urethral catheterisation.

Databases Used

Cochrane Collaboration, PubMed, MD Consult, BestBETs, American Academy of Pediatrics

Critically Analyse the Evidence

- Gray (1996) published a review of strategies to minimise distress associated with urethral catheterisation in children and supported intraurethral instillation of a local anaesthetic that contains 2% lidocaine (lignocaine) before catheter insertion.
- One prospective, double-blind, placebo-controlled trial evaluated the use of lidocaine (lignocaine) lubricant for discomfort in 20 children before urethral catheterisation. Two doses of lidocaine (lignocaine) lubricant instilled into the urethra 5 minutes apart significantly reduced pain and distress during urethral catheterisation (Gerard et al 2003).
- Boots and Edmundson (2010) conducted a randomised controlled trial in 200 children in a follow-up to the study by Gerard and colleagues. Conclusions were that a topical application of 2% lidocaine (lignocaine) gel followed by urethral instillation of lidocaine (lignocaine) gel is effective in reducing discomfort before urinary catheterisation, and two urethral instillations offered no significant difference over a single instillation.
- Mularoni and colleagues (2009) found in a three-armed placebo-controlled, double-blind, randomised controlled trial of 43 children younger than 2 years of age that topical and intraurethral lidocaine (lignocaine) lubricant was superior to the placebos of topical aqueous lubricant alone and topical and intraurethral aqueous lubricant in lowering distress, but it did not fully alleviate pain.
- A placebo-controlled, double-blind, randomised controlled trial of 115 children younger than 2 years of age found no significant difference when 2% lidocaine (lignocaine) gel was compared with a non-anaesthetic lubricant. The lubricant was applied to the genital mucosa for 2 to 3 minutes and liberally applied to the catheter but not instilled into the urethra (Vaughn et al 2005).
- A randomised controlled trial of 126 children ages 4 days to 23 months found a significant decrease in pain response in children who received topical and intraurethral 2% lidocaine (lignocaine) gel compared with children who received a non-anaesthetic lubricant (Castelo et al 2014).
- A randomised controlled trial of 133 children ages 0 to 24 months found no difference in pain response in children who received intraurethral 2% lidocaine (lignocaine) gel lubricant compared with children who received a non-anaesthetic lubricant during urethral catheterisation. However, there was significantly increased pain response in children during instillation of the lidocaine (lignocaine) lubricant compared with the non-anaesthetic lubricant. Additionally, there was no difference in parent satisfaction scores between the non-anaesthetic lubricant and lidocaine (lignocaine) lubricant (Poonai et al 2015).

Apply the Evidence: Nursing Implications

There is moderate-quality evidence with strong recommendations (Guyatt et al 2008) for using a lidocaine (lignocaine) lubricant to decrease pain associated with urethral catheterisation.

Four published research studies were found to support the use of anaesthetic before urethral catheterisation, one found topical application alone insufficient to reduce pain and one found no difference in pain response between anaesthetic and non-anaesthetic application. Several publications support the effectiveness of lidocaine (lignocaine) gel lubricant in clinical practice. Topical application followed by one or two transurethral instillations of 2% lidocaine (lignocaine) gel before urethral catheterisation minimises distress and reduces pain before urinary catheterisation.

Quality and Safety Competencies: Evidence-based Practice*

Knowledge

- Differentiate clinical opinion from research and evidence-based summaries.
- Describe use of lidocaine (lignocaine) gel for pain reduction during urethral catheterisation.

Continued

TRANSLATING EVIDENCE INTO PRACTICE

The Use of Lidocaine (Lignocaine) Lubricant for Urethral Catheterisation—cont'd

Skills

- Base individualised care plan on patient values, clinical expertise and evidence.
- Integrate evidence into practice by using lidocaine (lignocaine) gel for pain reduction during urethral catheterisation in children.

Attitudes

- Value the concept of evidence-based practice (EBP) as integral to determining best clinical practice.
- Appreciate the strengths and weakness of evidence for using lidocaine (lignocaine) gel for pain reduction during urethral catheterisation in children.

*Adapted from Quality and Safety Education for Nurses (QSEN) at http://www.qsen.org.

Suprapubic aspiration is mainly used when the bladder cannot be accessed through the urethra (e.g. with some congenital urological birth defects, severe phimosis or labial adhesions) or to reduce the risk of contamination that may be present when passing a catheter. With the advent of small catheters (5- and 6-French straight catheters), the need for suprapubic aspiration has decreased. Access to the bladder via the urethra has a much higher success rate than suprapubic aspiration, in which success depends on the practitioner's skill at assessing the location of the bladder and the amount of urine in the bladder. However, suprapubic aspiration remains a more accurate specimen collection method for urine cultures and should be considered for infants who have unsatisfactory urine collection or inconclusive results (Eliacik et al 2016).

Suprapubic aspiration involves aspirating bladder contents by inserting a 20- or 21-gauge needle in the midline approximately 1 cm above the symphysis pubis and directed vertically downward. The nurse prepares the skin as for any needle insertion, and the bladder should contain an adequate volume of urine. This can be assumed if the infant has not voided for at least 1 hour or the bladder can be palpated above the symphysis pubis or verified via ultrasound. This technique is useful for obtaining sterile specimens from young infants because the bladder is an abdominal organ and is easily accessed. Suprapubic aspiration is painful; therefore, pain management during the procedure is important (see Nursing Care Considerations box).

Stool Specimens

Stool specimens are frequently collected from children to identify parasites and other organisms that cause diarrhoea, assess gastrointestinal function and check for occult (hidden) blood. Ideally, stool should be collected without contamination with urine, but in children wearing nappies, this is difficult unless a urine bag is applied. Children who are toilet trained should urinate first, flush the toilet and then defecate into a bedpan (preferably one that is placed on the toilet to avoid embarrassment) over the toilet. Stool specimens should never be contaminated with toilet water to avoid inaccurate results.

Stool specimens should be large enough to obtain an ample sampling, not merely a faecal fragment. Specimens are placed in an appropriate container, which is covered and labelled. If several specimens are needed, mark the containers with the date and time and keep them in a specimen refrigerator. Exercise care in handling the specimen because of the risk of contamination. If a stool specimen cannot be obtained, some laboratory tests may allow for internal rectal swab.

Blood Specimens

Whether the blood specimen is collected by the nurse or by others, the nurse is responsible for making certain that specimens such as serial examinations and fasting specimens are collected on time and that the proper equipment is available. Collecting, transporting and storing specimens can have a major impact on laboratory results. For accurate results, blood must be collected in the proper tube for the test. When preparing for blood specimen collection, the nurse should consult the institution's laboratory reference guide to determine appropriate tubes for specimen collection, as well as the volume of blood required for the test. Inadequate sample size will result in rejected specimens and may require repeat venepuncture in order to obtain accurate samples, causing additional discomfort for the patient. When multiple blood tests are ordered for a patient and there is concern about the total volume of blood that may be needed, the nurse should be aware that the World Health Organization advises that the maximum volume of blood collected over any 24-hour period should not exceed 3 mL/kg (Clinical Laboratory Standards Institute 2017, Howie 2011). When collecting multiple samples via vacutainer system, the order of sample collection also has an impact on test results because the additive from one tube may inadvertently be transferred to subsequent tubes, affecting sample integrity (Clinical Laboratory Standards Institute 2017). The order of collection is different if collecting blood in capillary tubes or microtainers.

Venous blood samples can be obtained by direct venepuncture or by aspiration from a peripheral venous catheter or central venous access device. Evidence for best practice supports use of direct venepuncture as the preferred method for venous blood collection because it minimises risk for haemolysis of specimen (Braniff et al 2014). However, when venous access is difficult or repeated specimens are necessary, sampling blood from an indwelling catheter may be warranted. Benefits of using an existing catheter include decreased anxiety, decreased discomfort and improved patient/caregiver satisfaction (Infusion Nurses Society 2016). Withdrawing blood specimens through peripheral lock devices in small peripheral veins has varying degrees of success. Although it avoids an additional venepuncture for the child, attempting to aspirate blood from the peripheral lock may shorten the life of the device and may cause haemolysis of the blood specimen, leading to ambiguous results. Factors to consider when deciding to use an IV catheter for blood collection include difficulty of venous access, vein size, location of existing IV catheter, catheter size, type of IV fluid infusing, ease of aspiration and frequency of blood sampling. Any of these factors may increase the risk of haemolysis of the specimen. Before obtaining laboratory specimens, 1 to 2 mL of blood must be withdrawn from the catheter to clear any saline, heparin or IV fluids from the tubing. When using an IV infusion site for specimen collection, pause the infusion before collecting the blood sample because the type of fluid being infused may affect test results. For example, a specimen collected for glucose determination would be inaccurate if removed from a catheter through which glucose-containing solution was infusing.

Blood Collection from Central Venous Catheters

Central lines can be used to withdraw blood specimens; however, risks include catheter occlusion and catheter-associated bloodstream infection. When collecting blood specimens from a central line, a small volume of blood must first be withdrawn and discarded to clear the line of any IV fluids, heparin or other fluids that might erroneously affect test results. The Infusion Nurses Society (2011) recommends withdrawing and discarding 1.5 to 2 times the fill volume of the central venous access device (CVAD) before obtaining laboratory specimens. Limited research supports using the initial discard volume as a blood culture specimen (see Research Focus box). Some facilities allow reinfusion of the blood initially withdrawn from the CVAD, especially when blood conservation is essential. Another technique that conserves blood is the push-pull method in which blood is withdrawn into a syringe and reinfused into the CVAD three times. A new sterile syringe is then attached and the laboratory specimen is withdrawn; no blood is discarded. If drawing blood from a multi-lumen central line, ensure that all lumens are clamped, except for the lumen being used to draw blood.

RESEARCH FOCUS

Central Venous Access Device

In 62 paediatric oncology emergency patients, the initial 5 mL of blood drawn from a CVAD was used to inoculate blood culture bottles instead of the usual practice of discarding this first 5 mL of blood. A second specimen was obtained (as per standard of care) and used to inoculate separate blood culture bottles. In the 186 paired blood cultures, 4.8% were positive. In all positive cultures, both specimens contained the same organism. In 4 pairs, the first specimen (the one that is usually discarded) grew organisms earlier than the standard of care specimen, allowing for earlier administration of definitive antibiotics. The results of this study could lead to a change in practice, allowing the first 5 to 10 mL of blood obtained from CVADs to be used for blood cultures, rather than discarding this initial sample (Winokur et al 2014).

Blood Collection from Peripheral Veins

When venepuncture is performed, the needed specimens are collected as quickly as possible and after the needle is withdrawn, pressure is applied to the puncture site with dry gauze until bleeding stops (see Nursing Care Considerations box). When the venepuncture site is in the antecubital fossa, pressure should be applied with the arm extended, not flexed, to reduce bruising. The nurse then covers the site with an adhesive bandage. In young children, adhesive bandages pose an aspiration hazard, so avoid using them or remove the adhesive bandage as soon as the bleeding stops. If bruising or haematoma develops after venepuncture, applying warm compresses to the ecchymosis area increases circulation, helps remove extravasated blood and decreases pain.

Blood Collection from Arterial Vessels

Arterial blood samples are sometimes needed for blood gas measurement, although non-invasive techniques, such as transcutaneous oxygen monitoring and pulse oximetry, are used frequently. Arterial samples may be obtained by arterial puncture using the radial, brachial or femoral arteries or from indwelling arterial catheters. Assess adequate circulation before arterial puncture by observing capillary refill or performing the **Allen test**, a procedure that assesses the circulation of the radial, ulnar or brachial arteries. When collecting a blood

NURSING CARE CONSIDERATIONS

Guidelines for Skin and Vessel Punctures

To Reduce Pain from Heel, Finger, Venous or Arterial Punctures

- Apply EMLA cream (a eutectic mix of lidocaine [lignocaine] and prilocaine) topically over the site if time permits (> 60 minutes). LMX cream (lidocaine [lignocaine]) also may be used and requires a shorter application time (30 minutes). The cream should be covered with a small transparent dressing or a piece of plastic wrap (e.g. cling wrap) for the specified time interval. To remove the transparent dressing atraumatically, grasp opposite sides of the film and pull the sides away from each other to stretch and loosen the film. After the film begins to loosen, grasp the other two sides of the film and pull. If unable to wait 30 to 60 minutes for topical creams to be effective, use a vapocoolant spray or buffered lidocaine (lignocaine) (injected intradermally near the vein with a 30-gauge needle) to numb the skin more quickly.
- Use non-pharmacological methods of pain and anxiety control (e.g. ask the child to take a deep breath when the needle is inserted and again when the needle is withdrawn, to exhale a large breath or blow bubbles to 'blow hurt away' or to count slowly and then faster and louder if pain is felt).
- Keep all equipment out of sight until used.
- Encourage parental presence or assistance, if they wish.
- Restrain the child *only as needed* to perform the procedure safely; use comfort positioning (see p. 494).
- Allow the skin preparation agent to dry completely before penetrating the skin.
- Use the smallest-gauge needle (e.g. 25 gauge) that permits free flow of blood; for neonates and infants, a 27-gauge needle may be sufficient for obtaining 1 to 1.5 mL of blood and for prominent veins (needle length is only 1.25 cm).
- If possible, avoid putting an IV line in the dominant hand or the hand the child uses to suck the thumb.
- Use an automatic lancet device for precise puncture depth of the finger or heel; press the device lightly against the skin; avoid steadying the finger against a hard surface.
- Have a 'two-try-only' policy to reduce excessive insertion attempts—two operators each have two insertion attempts. If insertion is not successful after four punctures, consider alternative venous access, such as a peripherally inserted central catheter (PICC).
- Have a policy for proactively identifying children with difficult access and appropriate interventions (e.g. most experienced operator for the first attempt, use transilluminator or ultrasonography for insertion guidance).

For Multiple Blood Samples

- Use an intermittent infusion device (e.g. saline lock) to collect additional samples from an existing IV line.
- Consider PICC lines early, not as a last resort.
- Coordinate care to allow several tests to be performed on one blood sample; use micro methods of collection whenever possible.
- Cluster orders for bloodwork to minimise painful venepunctures and/or line entries.
- Anticipate tests (e.g. drug levels, chemistry, immunoglobulin levels) and ask the laboratory to save blood for additional testing.
- Maximum blood collection volumes for any 24-hour period should not exceed 3 mL/kg; limits should be lower for children who are acutely or chronically ill (Clinical Laboratory Standards Institute 2017, Howie 2011).

For Heel Punctures in Newborns

- Heel punctures have been shown to be more painful than venepuncture (Shah & Ohlsson 2011).
- Kangaroo care (placing the nappy-clad newborn against the parent's bare chest in skin-to-skin contact) 10 to 15 minutes before and during heel puncture reduces pain (Johnston et al 2017).
- Breastfeeding during a neonatal heel puncture is effective in reducing pain and has been found to be more effective than sucrose in some studies (Benoit et al 2017).
- If breast milk is unavailable, administer sucrose and encourage the newborn to suck a soother (Stevens et al 2016). When commercially manufactured 24% sucrose solution is unavailable, add 1 teaspoon of sugar to 4 teaspoons of sterile water. Use this solution to coat the soother or administer 2 mL to the tongue 2 minutes before the procedure.
- Although safe for use in preterm infants when applied correctly, EMLA has been found to be no more effective than placebo in preventing pain during heel puncture (Anand & Hall 2006).

sample from an established arterial line, use the in-line sampling port and follow institutional policy. Because unclotted blood is required, use only heparinised collection tubes or syringes for arterial blood samples. In addition, no air bubbles should enter the collection tube or syringe because they can alter blood gas concentration. Crying, fear and agitation can also affect blood gas values; therefore, make every effort to comfort the child. Pack arterial blood samples in ice to reduce blood cell metabolism and transport to the laboratory immediately.

Blood Collection by Capillary Methods

Take capillary blood samples from children by finger-prick or heel puncture. When using a finger for capillary blood collection, use the second or third finger. Cleanse the area with alcohol or chlorhexidine and allow to dry. After performing the finger-prick, wipe once with dry gauze before beginning collection. Gently massage the entire finger to maintain blood flow. Avoid squeezing just the tip of the finger. Hold the finger-prick site facing downwards to facilitate blood collection. A common method for taking peripheral blood samples from infants younger than 6 months of age is by heel puncture. Before the blood sample is taken, cleanse the area with alcohol or chlorhexidine. Holding the infant's foot firmly with the free hand, the nurse then punctures the heel with an automatic lancet device. An automatic device delivers a more precise puncture depth and is less painful than using a manual lancet (Sorrentino et al 2017). Several studies demonstrate that the automatic lancet is safer and has been shown to require fewer heel punctures, less collection time and lower recollection rates (Sorrentino et al 2017). A surgical blade of any kind is contraindicated. Although obtaining capillary blood gases is a common practice, this method may not accurately reflect arterial values.

The most serious complications of infant heel puncture are necrotising osteochondritis from lancet penetration of the underlying calcaneus bone, resulting in infection and abscess of the heel. To avoid osteochondritis, the puncture should be no deeper than 2 mm and should be made at the outer aspect of the heel. The boundaries of the calcaneus can be marked by an imaginary line extending posteriorly from a point between the fourth and fifth toes and running parallel with the lateral aspect of the heel and another line extending posteriorly from the middle of the great toe and running parallel with the medial aspect of the heel (Fig 22.7). Repeated trauma to the walking surface of the heel can cause fibrosis and scarring that may interfere with locomotion.

Children do not like the discomfort associated with venous, arterial and capillary punctures. These procedures have been identified by children as the most frequent causes of pain during hospitalisation. Arterial puncture was identified as being one of the most painful of all procedures experienced. Toddlers are most distressed by venepuncture, followed by school-age children and then adolescents. Consequently, nurses should use developmentally appropriate language when preparing a child for venepuncture (see Table 22.1) and use developmentally appropriate pain reduction techniques to lessen the discomfort of these procedures.

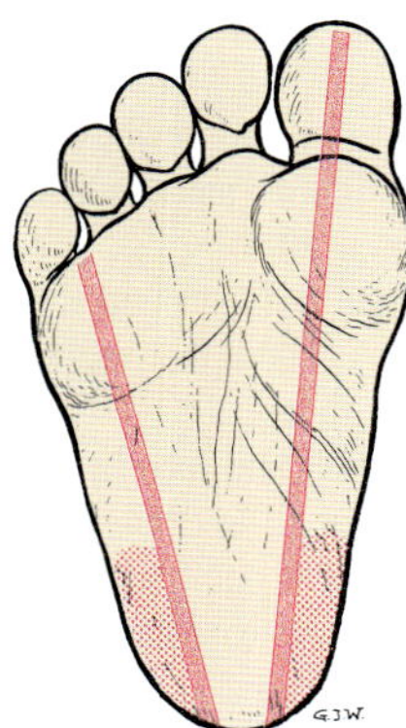

Fig 22.7 Puncture site (coloured stippled area) on the sole of an infant's foot.

Respiratory Secretion Specimens

Collection of sputum is sometimes required for the diagnosis of respiratory infections, especially tuberculosis. Because the infectious organisms are in the lungs and lower airways, the sputum specimen must be produced by deep cough, not just spitting oral secretions into a container. Older children and adolescents can cough forcefully and supply sputum specimens when given proper directions. The nurse must make it clear to the child that a coughed specimen is needed, not merely mucus cleared from the throat. It is helpful to demonstrate a deep cough. Infants and small children are unable to follow directions to cough on demand.

Sometimes a satisfactory sputum specimen can be obtained using a suction device such as a mucus trap, if the catheter is inserted into the trachea and the cough reflex elicited. This procedure can be uncomfortable for the child, so the nurse should be sure to provide developmentally appropriate comfort measures. A catheter inserted into the back of the throat is not sufficient. For children with a tracheostomy, a specimen is easily aspirated from the trachea or major bronchi by attaching a collecting device to the suction apparatus.

Viral pathogens, such as influenza or respiratory syncytial virus, may be detected by nasal washings or by nasopharyngeal swab. However, these two collection methods are not always interchangeable, and the nurse must clarify the proper collection method for the test ordered. A specimen collected by an improper method will be rejected by the laboratory and the patient will have to endure the discomfort of repeat collection.

Other respiratory secretion collection methods include nasopharyngeal and oropharyngeal swabs used to test for strep pharyngitis, *Bordetella* and other pathogens. Swab sticks should have plastic, not wooden, shafts. The nurse swabs both tonsils and the posterior pharynx when obtaining an oropharyngeal specimen. Touching the teeth, gums and tongue with the swab stick should be avoided. The swab stick is immediately inserted into the culture tube, taking care that the swab does not come in contact with the outside of the container or the hands of the nurse collecting the sample. Some culture kits require squeezing an ampoule within the culture tube to release the culture medium. Viral testing usually requires that the specimen be placed in a special container and be transported on ice, so the nurse should ensure that the correct container is on hand before obtaining the specimen.

ADMINISTRATION OF MEDICATION

Determination of Drug Dosage

Nurses must have an understanding of the safe dosages of the medications they administer to children, as well as the expected actions, possible side effects and signs of toxicity. Unlike the standardised doses for adult medications, dosing for paediatric medications is usually presented as a recommended dose range, based on age, weight or body surface area. Differences between adult and paediatric dosing of medications are related to physiological differences. Factors related to growth and maturation affect an individual's capacity to metabolise and excrete drugs. Immaturity or defects in any of the important processes of absorption, distribution, biotransformation or excretion can significantly alter the pharmacodynamics of a drug, resulting in increased toxicity or inadequate effect. Newborn and premature infants are particularly vulnerable to the harmful effects of drugs due to immature enzyme systems in the liver (where most drugs are broken down and detoxified), lower concentrations of plasma proteins (necessary for binding and transporting drugs) and immature functioning of kidneys (where most drugs are excreted). Children metabolise many drugs more rapidly than adults. Consequently, children may require larger doses (per weight) than adults and/or more frequent administration to achieve a therapeutic effect. This is particularly important in pain control, when the dosage of analgesics may need to be increased or the interval between doses decreased in order to meet the needs of the child.

Nurses are accountable for the medications that they administer. An important part of that responsibility is having a working knowledge of drug actions and potential side effects. In addition, nurses should know the safe dose ranges for the drugs with which they work. Before giving any medication, the paediatric nurse must be vigilant to verify that the drug has been dispensed in a dose that is within the recommended range for the child. Paediatric dosages are most often expressed in units of measure per body weight (mg/kg). Some medications, such as chemotherapy, are more precisely dosed using **body surface area (BSA)**, which historically is believed to be a more accurate reflection of metabolic rate and less affected by adipose tissue than weight-based calculations. The ratio of BSA to weight varies inversely with length; therefore, an infant who is shorter and weighs less than an older child or adult has relatively more BSA than would be expected from the weight. BSA can be determined by using the **West nomogram** or the commonly used Mosteller formula: square root of (height [cm] × weight [kg]) ÷ 3600. Conversion programs are also widely available on the internet.

Checking Dosage

Administering the correct dosage of a drug is a shared responsibility between the provider who orders the drug and the nurse who carries out that order. Children react with unexpected severity to some drugs, and ill children may be especially sensitive to drugs. When a dose is ordered that is outside the usual range, or when there is some question regarding the preparation or the route of administration, the nurse should check with the prescribing provider before proceeding with the administration because the nurse is legally liable for any drug administered.

Even when given at the correct dosage, many drugs are potentially hazardous or lethal. For this reason, the Institute for Safe Medical Practices (2020) and the ACSQHC (n.d.a) have identified a list of 'high-alert' medications. Most facilities have regulations requiring that these high-alert medications be double-checked by another nurse before giving them to the child. Among drugs that require such safeguards are antiarrhythmics, anticoagulants, chemotherapeutic agents and insulin. Other high-alert medications include adrenaline, opioids and sedatives. A misplaced decimal point placement could result in a 10-fold or greater dosing error. So even if this precaution is not mandatory, nurses are wise to incorporate this safe practice and take the additional time to independently check and recheck drug dose calculations.

Another category of high-alert medications are the 'look-alike, sound-alike' drugs that have similar names but significantly different doses and side effects. To emphasise these differences, Tall Man lettering is recommended by the Australian Commission on Safety and quality in healthcare and ACSQHC. Examples of Tall Man lettering include DOBUTamine and DOPamine, and predniSONE and predniSOLONE (ACSQHC 2017).

Identification

Before the administration of any medication, the child must be correctly identified using three identifiers (e.g. name and medical record number and birth date). With an infant, young child or non-verbal child, the parent or guardian (if present) can verify the child's identity. After verbal verification of the child's identity (by the parent, guardian or child), the identification band should be verified using three identifiers. Bedside computers and handheld barcode scanners can be used to verify the identification (ID) bracelet directly with the patient's electronic record.

Preparing the Parents

Nearly all parents have given some type of medication to their child and can describe the approaches they have found successful. In some cases, it is less traumatic for the hospitalised child if a parent gives the medication, provided that the nurse prepares the medication and supervises its administration. Children that take daily medications at home are accustomed to the parent functioning in this capacity and may be less likely to fuss than if a stranger administers the medication. Individual decisions need to be made regarding parental presence and participation for other procedures, such as holding the child during injections.

Preparing the Child

Every child requires developmentally appropriate preparation for parenteral administration of medication and supportive care during the procedure. Even if the child has received several injections, rarely does a child become accustomed to the discomfort. With every dose of medication, the nurse should be cognisant of the developmental needs of the child, whether it is the first dose or the 200th dose for that child.

Oral Administration

The oral route is preferred for giving medications to children because of the ease of administration. Oral medications are available in a variety of dosing formulations, including tablets, capsules, chewable tablets, orally dissolving tablets, sprinkles and oral liquids. Although some children can swallow or chew solid medications at an early age, solid preparations are not recommended for younger children because of the danger of aspiration. Determining when a child is old enough to swallow pills depends on the developmental age of the child, the size of the pill and the child's past experiences with medications. The nurse should ensure that the formulation of any prescribed medication will be appropriate for the child, based on developmental level, swallowing ability and available formulations of the medication.

Many paediatric medications come in liquid preparations for added ease of administration. Some liquids may have an unpleasant aftertaste. The taste can be camouflaged whenever necessary, by mixing the medication with a small amount of juice or apple sauce.

Preparation

The most accurate means for measuring small amounts of medication is the plastic disposable calibrated oral/enteral syringe. Oral/enteral syringes are single-use only, distinguished by colour (either orange or purple depending on the brand) and are available in sizes from 1 mL to 60 mL. Not only does the syringe provide a reliable measure, but it also serves as a convenient means for transporting and administering the medication. The medication can be placed directly into the child's mouth from the syringe.

Paper cups are totally unsuitable for liquid medications because they collapse easily, are likely to have irregularly shaped or crumpled bottoms and retain considerable amounts of thick medication. Moulded plastic cups with measuring lines are often supplied with over-the-counter medications for cough and fever, but the vast majority of families in one study could not measure a 5-mL dose within 0.5 mL (Ryu & Lee 2012, Yin et al 2016). Measures less than 1 teaspoon are impossible to determine accurately with a medicine cup. The teaspoon is also an inaccurate measuring device and is subject to error. Teaspoons vary greatly in capacity, and different persons using the same spoon will pour different amounts, resulting in potentially dangerous dosing errors (Beckett et al 2012, Torres et al 2018).

Because of the risk of inaccurate dosing when using medicine cups and teaspoons, all liquid oral medications, over-the-counter and prescription, should be dosed only in millilitres and never in teaspoons or other non-metric units. Syringes are the preferred device for dosing accuracy. Measuring cups with metric markings may be used as an alternative.

Another unreliable device for measuring liquids is the dropper, which varies to a greater extent than the teaspoon or measuring cup. The volume of a drop varies according to the viscosity (thickness) of the liquid measured (Peacock et al 2010). Viscous fluids produce much larger drops than thin liquids. Many medications are supplied with caps or droppers designed for measuring each specific preparation. These are accurate when used to measure that specific medication but are not reliable for measuring other liquids. Emptying dropper contents into a medicine cup invites additional error. Because some of the liquid clings to the sides of the cup, a significant amount of the drug can be lost.

Young children and some older children have difficulty swallowing tablets or pills. For these children, tablets may need to be crushed. Commercial devices are available or simple methods can be used for crushing tablets. Some pills can be crushed and mixed with apple sauce or a small amount of juice. Some drugs, such as medication with an enteric or protective coating or formulated for slow release, should not be crushed because crushing will alter the amount of drug that is absorbed. In some cases this might result in an overdose of medication. Before crushing any paediatric medication, where consultation with pharmacy is available, do so. Where possible you need to consult with the prescriber to discuss all other prescribed medication and possible interactions by crushing the medication and alteration to absorption rates. If this is not possible, and pharmacy is not available for consultation, consult with either your state/territory's children's hospital medication guidelines or use telehealth for further guidance.

When children need to take solid oral medication for an extended period, the nurse can help teach the child how to swallow tablets or capsules. Training sessions include using verbal instruction, demonstration, reinforcement for swallowing progressively larger lollies or capsules, paying no attention for inappropriate behaviour and gradual withdrawal of guidance after children can swallow their medication. Helpful tips for patients of all ages can be found at http://www.pillswallowing.com.

In some situations, paediatric doses may require splitting pills or tablets. The nurse should be vigilant to ensure that the divided dose is accurate. With tablets, only those that are scored can be halved or quartered accurately. If the medication is soluble, the tablet or contents of a capsule can be mixed in a small, pre-measured amount of liquid and the appropriate portion given (Valizadeh et al 2015). For example, if half a dose is required, the tablet is dissolved in 5 mL of water and 2.5 mL is given.

Administration

Although administering liquids to infants is relatively easy, the nurse must take care to prevent aspiration. While holding the infant in a semireclining position, place the medication in the mouth using an oral syringe (without a needle). It is best to place the syringe along the side of the infant's tongue and administer the liquid slowly in small amounts, waiting for the child to swallow between increments.

Medicine cups can be used effectively for children, toddlers and older infants who are able to drink from a cup. Because of the natural outward tongue thrust in infancy, medications may need to be retrieved from the lips or chin and refed. Allowing the infant to suck the medication that has been placed in an empty nipple or inserting the syringe or dropper into the side of the mouth, parallel to the nipple, while the infant nurses is another convenient method for giving liquid medications to infants. Medication is not added to the infant's formula feeding because the child may subsequently refuse the formula. Dispose of any plastic covers that may be on the ends of syringes because these covers are choking hazards.

Intramuscular Administration

Selecting the Syringe and Needle

The volume of medication prescribed for intramuscular injections in small children necessitates selection of a syringe that can measure small amounts of solution. For volumes less than 1 mL, the tuberculin syringe, calibrated in 0.01 mL increments, is appropriate. Doses smaller than 0.5 mL may be facilitated using a 0.5 mL low-dose syringe. These syringes, along with specially constructed needles, minimise the possibility of inadvertently administering incorrect amounts of a drug because of **dead space**, which allows fluid to remain in the syringe and needle after the plunger is pushed completely forward. A minimum of 0.2 mL of solution remains as dead space in a standard needle hub; therefore, when very small amounts of two drugs are combined in the syringe, such as mixtures of insulin, the ratio of the two drugs can be altered significantly, due to dead space. Measures that minimise the effect of dead space are: (1) when two drugs are combined in the syringe, always draw them up in the same order to maintain a consistent ratio between the drugs; (2) use the same brand of syringe (dead space may vary between brands); and (3) use one-piece syringe units (needle permanently attached to the syringe).

Dead space is also an important factor to consider when injecting medication because flushing the syringe with an air bubble adds an additional amount of medication to the prescribed dose. This can be hazardous when very small amounts of a drug are given. Consequently, flushing is not recommended, especially when less than 1 mL of medication is given. Syringes are calibrated to deliver a prescribed drug dose, and the amount of medication left in the hub and needle is not part of the syringe barrel calibrations.

Certain drugs such as iron polymaltose, diphtheria and tetanus toxoid may cause irritation when tracked into the subcutaneous tissue. The Z-track method is recommended for use in infants and children rather than an air bubble. In the Z-track method, slight traction is applied to the skin over the injection site, so that it shifts slightly; while maintaining the skin taut, the injection is administered, skin traction is released and the needle is removed.

The **needle length** must be enough to penetrate the subcutaneous tissue and deposit the medication into the body of the muscle. The needle gauge should be as small as possible to deliver the fluid safely. Smaller-diameter (25 to 30 gauge) needles cause the least discomfort, but larger gauges are needed for viscous medication and prevention of accidental bending of longer needles.

Determining the Site

Factors to consider when selecting a site for an intramuscular (IM) injection on an infant or child include the following:

- the amount and viscosity of the medication to be injected
- the amount and general condition of the muscle mass
- the frequency or number of injections to be given during the course of treatment
- the type of medication being given
- factors that may impede access to or cause contamination of the site
- the child's ability to assume the required position safely.

Older children and adolescents usually pose few problems in selecting a suitable site for IM injections, but infants, with their small and underdeveloped muscles, have fewer available options. It is sometimes difficult to assess the amount of fluid that can be safely injected into a single site. Usually 1 mL is the maximum volume that should be administered in a single IM site to small children and older infants. The muscles of small infants may not tolerate more than 0.5 mL. As the child approaches adult size, the nurse can use volumes approaching those given to adults. However, the larger the amount of solution, the larger the muscle at the injection site must be.

Injections must be administered in muscles large enough to accommodate the quantity of medication, while avoiding major nerves and blood vessels. The IM immunisation site recommended by the Centers for Disease Control and Prevention, World Health Organization, for infants is the anterolateral thigh or vastus lateralis. However, immunisations at the ventrogluteal site have been found to have fewer local reactions and fever (Yapucu Güneş et al 2016). Studies have also found fewer systemic reactions (e.g. irritability and persistent crying or screaming) and greater parental acceptance for the ventrogluteal site. The ventrogluteal site is relatively free of major nerves and blood vessels, is a relatively large muscle with less subcutaneous tissue than the dorsal site, has well-defined landmarks for safe site location and is easily accessible in several positions. Distraction and prevention of unexpected movement may be more easily achieved by placing the child supine on a parent's lap for ventrogluteal site use (Atay et al 2017).

The deltoid muscle, a small muscle near the axillary and radial nerves, can be used for small volumes of fluid in children as young as 18 months of age. Its advantages are less pain and fewer side effects from the injectate (as observed with immunisations), compared with the vastus lateralis. Table 22.5 summarises the three major injection sites, and Figure 22.8 illustrates the location of the preferred IM injection sites for children.

Administration

Although injections that are executed with care seldom cause trauma to children, there have been reports of serious disability related to IM injections in children. Repeated use of a single site has been associated with fibrosis of the muscle with subsequent muscle contracture. Injections close to large nerves, such as the sciatic nerve, have been responsible for permanent disability, especially when potentially neurotoxic drugs are administered. For this reason, the dorsogluteal site (buttocks) is no longer recommended as a site for IM injections for children under the age of 10 years (Brown et al

TABLE 22.5 Intramuscular Injection Sites in Children

	Vastus Lateralis (Fig. 22.8, A)	Ventrogluteal (Fig. 22.8, B)	Deltoid (Fig. 22.8, C)
Location*	Palpate to find greater trochanter and knee joints; divide vertical distance between these two landmarks into thirds; inject into middle third	Palpate to locate greater trochanter, anterior superior iliac tubercle (found by flexing thigh at hip and measuring up to 1–2 cm above crease formed in groin), and posterior iliac crest; place palm of hand over greater trochanter, index finger over anterior superior iliac tubercle and middle finger along crest of ileum posteriorly as far as possible; inject into centre of V formed by fingers	Locate acromion process; inject only into upper third of muscle that begins about two finger breadths below acromion
Needle Insertion and Size	Insert needle perpendicular to knee in infants and young children or perpendicular to thigh or slightly angled towards anterior thigh. 22–25 gauge (15–25 mm)	Insert needle perpendicular to site but angled slightly towards iliac crest. 22–25 gauge (13–25 mm)	Insert needle perpendicular to site but angled slightly towards shoulder. 22–25 gauge (13–25 mm)
Advantages	Large, well-developed muscle that can tolerate larger quantities of fluid (0.5 mL [infant] to 2.0 mL [child]) Easily accessible if child is supine, side lying or sitting	Free of important nerves and vascular structures Easily identified by prominent bony landmarks Thinner layer of subcutaneous tissue than in dorsogluteal site, thus less chance of depositing drug subcutaneously rather than intramuscularly Can accommodate larger quantities of fluid (0.5 mL [infant] to 2.0 mL [child]) Easily accessible if child is supine, prone or side lying Less painful than vastus lateralis	Faster absorption rates than gluteal sites Easily accessible with minimal removal of clothing Less pain and fewer local side effects from vaccines compared with vastus lateralis
Disadvantages	Thrombosis of femoral artery from injection in midthigh area Sciatic nerve damage from long needle injected posteriorly and medially into small extremity More painful than deltoid or gluteal sites	Health professionals' unfamiliarity with site	Small muscle mass; only limited amounts of drug can be injected (0.5–1.0 mL) Small margins of safety with possible damage to radial nerve and axillary nerve (not shown; lies under deltoid at head of humerus)

*Locations are indicated by asterisks in Fig. 22.13.

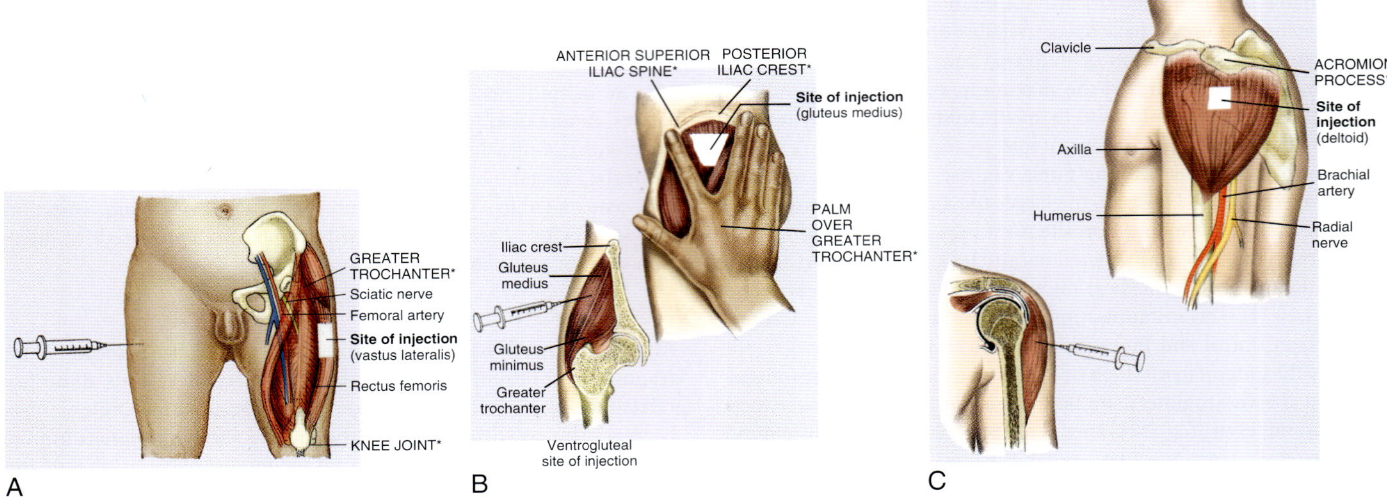

Fig 22.8 Injection sites in children. (**A**) Vastus lateralis. (**B**) Ventrogluteal. (**C**) Deltoid.

2015). When such drugs are injected, use great care in locating the correct site.

Aspiration during intramuscular vaccine administration is no longer recommended by the World Health Organization (Kroger et al n.d., Sisson 2015). Aspiration for routine injections into deltoid or vastus lateralis is not indicated because there are no large blood vessels in these locations. Aspiration may still be indicated before injection of medications such as penicillin into larger muscle groups such as the ventrogluteal site (Crawford & Johnson 2012). One study of IM injection techniques revealed that the straighter the path of needle insertion (e.g. 90-degree angle), the less displacement and shear to tissue, causing less discomfort.

APPLYING EVIDENCE TO PRACTICE

Intramuscular Administration of Medication

- Apply EMLA (a eutectic mix of lidocaine [lignocaine] and prilocaine) or LMX cream (lidocaine [lignocaine]) topically over site if time permits.
  - Prepare medication.
  - Select appropriately sized needle and syringe.
  - If withdrawing medication from an ampoule, use a needle equipped with a filter that removes glass particles; then use a new, non-filter needle for injection.
  - Maximum volume to be administered in a single site is 1 mL for older infants and small children.
  - Have medication at room temperature before injection.
  - Determine site of injection; make certain that muscle is large enough to accommodate volume and type of medication.
  - For infants and small or debilitated children, use the vastus lateralis or ventrogluteal muscles; the dorsogluteal muscle is insufficiently developed to be a safe site for infants and small children.
  - Obtain sufficient help in restraining child.
  - Explain briefly what is to be done and, if appropriate, what child can do to help.
  - Expose injection area for unobstructed view of landmarks.
  - Select a site where skin is free of irritation and danger of infection; palpate for and avoid sensitive or hardened areas.
  - With multiple injections, rotate sites. When giving multiple injections at the same time (immunisations, for example), the Centers for Disease Control and Prevention recommends that injection sites in the same muscle group must be at least 2.5 cm apart.
  - Place child in a lying or sitting position; child is not allowed to stand because landmarks are more difficult to assess, restraint is more difficult and the child may faint and fall.
  - **Ventrogluteal**—on side with upper leg flexed and placed in front of lower leg.
  - **Vastus lateralis**—supine, lying on side or sitting.
- Use a new, sharp needle (not one that has pierced rubber stopper on vial) with smallest diameter that permits free flow of the medication.
- Grasp muscle firmly between thumb and fingers to isolate and stabilise muscle for deposition of drug in its deepest part; in obese children, spread skin with thumb and index finger to displace subcutaneous tissue and grasp muscle deeply on each side.
- Allow skin preparation to dry completely before penetrating skin.
- Decrease perception of pain.
  - Distract child with conversation.
  - Give child something on which to concentrate (e.g. squeezing a hand or side rail, pinching own nose, humming, counting, yelling 'Ouch!').
  - Spray vapocoolant on site before injection, place a cold compress or wrapped ice cube on site about 1 minute before injection or apply cold to contralateral site.
  - Studies have shown that applying manual pressure to the injection site for 10 seconds before injection can reduce post-injection pain (Derya et al 2015, Öztürk et al 2017).
  - Have child hold a small adhesive bandage and place it on puncture site after intramuscular injection is given.
  - Insert needle quickly using a dartlike motion at a 90-degree angle unless contraindicated.
- Avoid tracking any medication through superficial tissues:
  - Replace needle after withdrawing medication.
  - Use the Z-track or air-bubble technique as indicated.
  - Avoid any depression of the plunger during insertion of the needle.
  - The Centers for Disease Control and Prevention no longer recommends aspiration before intramuscular injections.
  - Remove needle quickly; hold gauze firmly against skin near needle when removing it to avoid pulling on tissue.

APPLYING EVIDENCE TO PRACTICE

Intramuscular Administration of Medication—cont'd

- Apply firm pressure to site after injection; massage site to hasten absorption unless contraindicated, as with irritating drugs.
- Place a small adhesive bandage on puncture site; with young children, decorate it by drawing a smiling face or other symbol of acceptance.
- Hold and cuddle young child and encourage parents to comfort child; praise older child.
- Allow expression of feelings.
- Discard syringe and uncapped, uncut needle in sharps container located near site of use.
- Record time of injection, drug, dose and injection site.

Subcutaneous and Intradermal Administration

Subcutaneous and intradermal injections are frequently administered to children, but the technique differs little from the method used with adults. Examples of **subcutaneous injections** include insulin, hormone replacement, allergy desensitisation and some vaccines. Tuberculin testing, local anaesthesia and allergy testing are examples of frequently administered **intradermal injections**.

Techniques to minimise the pain associated with these injections include changing the needle if it pierced a rubber stopper on a vial, using 26- to 30-gauge needles (only to inject the solution) and injecting small volumes ($\leq$ 0.5 mL). The angle of the needle for the subcutaneous injection is typically 90 degrees. In children with little subcutaneous tissue, some practitioners insert the needle at a 45-degree angle. However, the benefit of using the 45-degree angle rather than the 90-degree angle remains controversial.

Although subcutaneous injections can be given anywhere there is subcutaneous tissue, common sites include the centre third of the lateral aspect of the upper arm, the abdomen and the centre third of the anterior thigh. Some providers believe it is not necessary to aspirate before injecting subcutaneously; for example, this is an accepted practice in the administration of insulin. Automatic injector devices do not aspirate before injecting.

When giving an intradermal injection into the volar surface of the forearm, the nurse should avoid the medial side of the arm, where the skin is more sensitive.

Intravenous Administration

The IV route for administering medications is frequently used in paediatric therapy. For some drugs, it is the only effective route. This method is used for giving drugs to children who:

- have poor absorption as a result of diarrhoea, vomiting or dehydration
- need a high serum concentration of a drug
- have resistant infections that require parenteral medication over an extended time
- need continuous pain relief
- require emergency treatment.

The nurse needs to consider several factors in relation to IV medication. When a drug is administered intravenously, the effect is almost instantaneous and further control of side effects is limited. Most drugs for IV administration require a specified minimum dilution, rate of flow or both, and many drugs are highly irritating or toxic to tissues outside the vascular system. In addition to the precautions and nursing observations commonly related to IV therapy, factors to consider when preparing and administering drugs to infants and children by the IV route include the following:

- amount of drug to be administered
- minimum dilution of drug and whether child is fluid restricted
- type of solution in which drug can be diluted
- length of time over which drug can be safely administered
- rate limitations of child, vascular system and infusion equipment
- time that this or another drug is to be administered
- compatibility of all drugs that child is receiving intravenously
- compatibility with infusion fluids.

Before any IV infusion, check the site of insertion for patency, which includes flushing easily without resistance and brisk blood return. Never flush against resistance and if encountered, the integrity of the access should be further evaluated (Gorski et al 2016, Gorski et al 2021). Never administer medications in the same IV tubing with blood products. Only one antibiotic should be administered at a time. Extra fluids needed to administer IV medications can be problematic for infants and fluid-restricted children. Syringe pumps are often used to deliver IV medication because they minimise fluid requirements and more precisely deliver small volumes of medication compared with large-volume infusion pumps. Regardless of the technique, the nurse must know the minimum dilutions for safe administration of IV medications to infants and children.

Peripheral Intermittent Infusion Device

When extended access to a vein is required without the need for continuous fluid, a **peripheral lock**, also known as an **intermittent infusion device** or **saline** or **heparin lock**, is an alternative. The peripheral lock allows a child more freedom than being connected to a continuous IV infusion. It is most frequently used for intermittent infusion of medication, such as antibiotics, via peripheral venous route. A short, flexible catheter is used as the lock device, and a site is selected where there will be minimal movement, such as the forearm. The catheter is inserted and secured in the same manner as for any peripheral IV infusion device, but the hub is capped with a stopper or injection cap. When it is time for medication administration, the injection cap is disinfected, the lock is flushed to ensure patency and then IV tubing, primed with either normal saline or medication, is connected.

The type of device used may vary, and the care and use of the peripheral lock are carried out according to the protocol of the institution or unit. However, the general concept is the same. The catheter remains in place and is flushed with saline before and after infusion of the medication, to maintain patency.

Central Venous Catheters

Children with acute or chronic illnesses who require repeated blood sampling or medications, long-term chemotherapy, intensive care or frequent hyperalimentation or antibiotic therapy are best managed with a central venous catheter. Because the large central veins (such as the subclavian, femoral or superior vena cava) allow more rapid diffusion of fluids and medications, they offer a more durable venous access than peripheral IV catheters. However, central venous catheters also have a greater risk of bloodstream infection.

Short-term or **non-tunnelled central venous catheters** are used in acute care, emergency and intensive care units. These catheters are made of polyurethane and are placed in large veins such as the subclavian, femoral or jugular. Insertion is by surgical incision or percutaneous threading. A chest radiograph should be taken to verify that the catheter tip is properly located in a large central vein before administration of fluids or medications.

Peripherally inserted central catheters (PICCs) can be used for short-term and moderate-length therapy. These catheters consist of silicone or polymer material and are placed by specially trained nurses, medical practitioners or interventional radiologists. The most common insertion site is above the antecubital area using the median, cephalic or basilic vein. The catheter is threaded either with or without a guidewire into the superior vena cava.

Children with chronic illnesses who require long-term venous access, for months or years, are best managed with a CVAD. CVADs have several different characteristics. They can be tunnelled or non-tunnelled, external or internal and inserted peripherally or centrally. Factors that influence selection of the type of CVAD for a child include the reason for placement of the catheter (diagnosis), length of therapy, risk to the patient in placement of the catheter and availability of resources to assist the family in maintaining the catheter.

Long-term CVADs include tunnelled catheters and implanted infusion ports (Fig 22.9). They may have single, double or triple lumens. Several lumen (multi-lumen) catheters allow more than one therapy to be administered at the same time. Reasons to use multi-lumen catheters include repeated blood sampling, total parenteral nutrition (TPN), administration of blood products or infusion of large quantities or concentrations of fluids, administration of incompatible drugs or fluids at the same time (through different lumens) and central venous pressure monitoring.

With any of the central venous catheters, medication is easily instilled through the injection cap. Maintenance of the catheter includes dressing changes, flushing to maintain patency and prevention of occlusion or dislodgement.

To access the implanted CVAD, the port must be palpated and stabilised. The overlying skin should be cleansed. The port should only be accessed with a special non-coring Huber needle. The needle is inserted through the diaphragm of the port, which is usually located on the top or side, depending on the style. If the port needs to be accessed for several days, a special infusion set with a Huber needle and extension tubing with a Luer connection can be inserted and an occlusive dressing applied to keep the needle in place (see Fig 22.9). When the infusion set is used, the procedure for administration of fluids and medications is the same as for an intermittent infusion device or a central venous catheter. To prevent infection, meticulous aseptic technique must be used any time the CVAD is entered, including instillation of heparin or saline to prevent clotting. Huber needles need to be changed at established intervals, usually 5 to 7 days.

The children and parents are taught the procedure for care of the CVAD before discharge from the hospital, including preparation and injection of the prescribed medication, the flush and dressing changes. A protective device may be recommended for some active children to prevent them from accidentally dislodging the needle. Many children take responsibility for preparing and administering medications. Both verbal and written step-by-step instructions are provided for the learners.

Infection and catheter occlusion are two of the most common complications of central venous catheters. They require treatment with antibiotics for infection and a fibrinolytic agent, such as alteplase, for thrombus formation (Scott et al 2017). When the line is not in use, the catheter should be clamped. The parents are cautioned to keep scissors away from the child to prevent accidental cutting of the catheter. If the catheter leaks, the parents are instructed to tape it above the leak and then clamp the

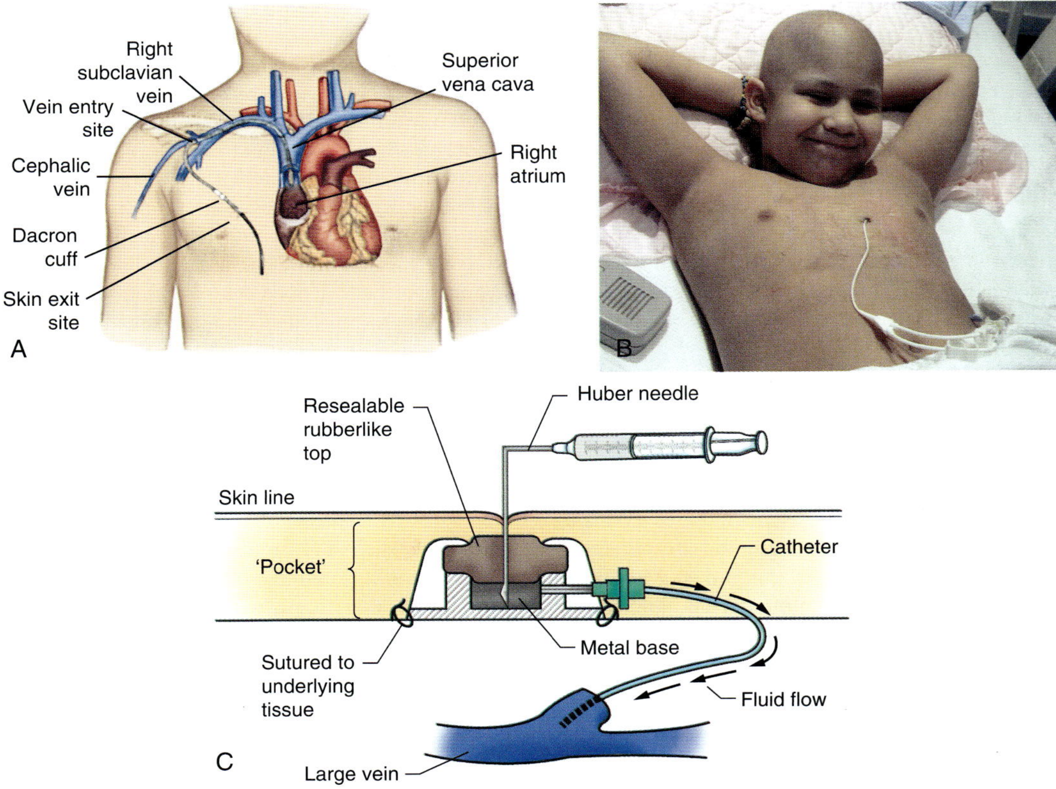

Fig 22.9 Venous access devices. (**A**) External central venous catheter insertion and exit site. (**B**) Child with an external central venous catheter (dressing removed for photo). (**C**) Side view of an implanted port.

catheter at the taped site. The child should be taken to the provider as soon as possible to prevent infection or clotting after a catheter leak.

Intraosseous Infusion

Situations may occur in which rapid establishment of systemic access is vital and venous access is complicated by peripheral circulatory collapse, hypovolaemic shock (secondary to vomiting or diarrhoea, burns or trauma), cardiopulmonary arrest or other conditions. It is recommended that intraosseous access be obtained if venous access cannot be readily achieved after three unsuccessful attempts or 90 seconds in a paediatric resuscitation (Chameides et al 2012). Intraosseous infusion provides a rapid, safe and lifesaving alternative route for administration of fluids and medications until intravascular access is possible. This procedure is usually reserved for children who are unconscious or for those receiving analgesia because the procedure is painful. Local anaesthesia should be used for a semiconscious patient. Contraindications for placement of an intraosseous catheter include concurrent problems involving that extremity, such as skin rash, bone fracture, osteogenesis imperfecta or osteosarcoma.

A large-bore rigid needle such as an intraosseous needle (e.g. Cook) or a bone marrow aspiration needle (e.g. Jamshidi) is inserted into the medullary cavity of a long bone. The anteromedial aspect of the tibia—1 to 3 cm below the tibial tuberosity—is the preferred site for children of all ages because it is flat and has a large marrow cavity. In newborns, the distal third of the femur may be used. The distal tibia is an alternative site. A battery-powered intraosseous needle driver (EZ-IO) is also available for use in prehospital and hospital settings and has a high rate of success in paediatric resuscitation and stabilisation (RCHM 2020).

Once established, the intraosseous route can be used during resuscitation to administer the same medications that could be given through the IV route. During infusion through an intraosseous needle, monitor the extremity closely for swelling or oozing of fluid at the insertion site. Give attention to the dependent tissue of the leg. Extravasation of fluid from the bone marrow may be hidden under the leg. Check for swelling of the entire lower leg when the intraosseous bone marrow needle is in the tibia or ankle, and check the entire upper leg when the intraosseous needle is in the femur. Compartment syndrome has resulted from an infiltrated intraosseous line. Other complications, although rare, include fractures, skin necrosis, osteomyelitis and cellulitis (Molacek et al 2018).

Once the intraosseous needle is in place, it should stand alone and feel secure. The needle should be secured using tape and gauze. If a bone marrow aspirate needle is used, gauze should be built up around the needle to provide support and prevent trauma or dislodgement. Drugs may be pushed and fluids delivered via an infusion pump. The intraosseous line may be discontinued after IV access has been achieved.

MAINTAINING FLUID BALANCE

Measurement of Intake and Output

Accurate measurements of fluid intake and output (I&O) are essential to the assessment of fluid balance. Measurements from all sources—including gastrointestinal, parenteral, urine, stools, vomitus, fistulas, NG suction, sweat and drainage from wounds—must be included in assessment of fluid balance. Although the provider usually indicates when I&O measurements are to be recorded, it is a nursing responsibility to keep an accurate I&O record on children in certain situations, including the following:

- receiving IV therapy
- recently underwent major surgery
- receiving diuretic or corticosteroid therapy
- with severe thermal burns or injuries
- with renal disease or damage
- with congestive heart failure
- with dehydration
- with diabetes mellitus
- with oliguria
- in respiratory distress
- with chronic lung disease.

Infants and small children who are unable to use a bedpan and those who have bowel movements with every voiding require the application of a collecting device. If collecting bags are not used, wet nappies or pads are carefully weighed to ascertain the amount of fluid lost. This includes liquid stool, vomitus and other losses. The volume of fluid in millilitres is equivalent to the weight of the fluid measured in grams. The specific gravity as a measure of osmolality assists in assessing the degree of hydration.

Special Needs when the Child is Not Permitted to Take Fluids by Mouth

Infants or children who are unable or are to be nil by mouth (NBM) have special needs. To ensure that they are not inadvertently given oral fluids, a sign can be placed in some obvious place, such as over their beds or on their shirts, to alert caregivers and other hospital personnel to the NBM status. To prevent the temptation to drink, fluids should not be left at the bedside. Older children may try to sneak a drink when out of sight of caregivers, so nurses would be wise to keep an eye on NBM children if they go into bathrooms or other locations where they are not easily observed.

Parenteral Fluid Therapy

Site and Equipment

The site selected for peripheral IV infusion depends on accessibility and convenience. Although it is possible to use any accessible site in older children, the child's developmental, cognitive and mobility needs must be considered when selecting a site. Ideally, in older children, the superficial veins of the forearm should be used, leaving the hands free. An older child can help select the site and thereby maintain some measure of control. For veins in the extremities, it is best to start with the most distal site and avoid the child's favoured hand to reduce the disability related to the procedure. Restrict the child's movements as little as possible, and avoid a site over a joint in an extremity, such as the antecubital space. In small infants, a superficial vein of the hand, wrist, forearm, foot or ankle is usually most convenient and most easily stabilised (Fig 22.10). Foot veins should be avoided in children learning to walk and in children already walking. Superficial veins of the scalp have no valves, insertion is easy and they can be used in infants up to about 9 months of age, but they should be used only when other site attempts have failed.

A transilluminator (Fig 22.11), also known as near-infrared imaging, aids in finding and evaluating veins for access. Although not as powerful as ultrasound, a transilluminator requires minimal training and experience to use (Bahl et al 2016). Small veins that may not be visible or palpable (especially in infants and toddlers) are often more readily visualised using a transilluminator. The cephalic vein in the proximal forearm may be the optimal vein for ultrasound-guided placement (Takeshita et al 2015). Because veins stand out so clearly with transillumination, they appear more superficial than they are. Although visualisation of veins is improved with transillumination, an increase in successful venepuncture is not guaranteed (Rothbart et al 2015). Some devices require assistance to hold them in place. Commercial devices have not caused burns in infants or children. Practice in this technique is necessary for optimal outcomes (Stolz et al 2016).

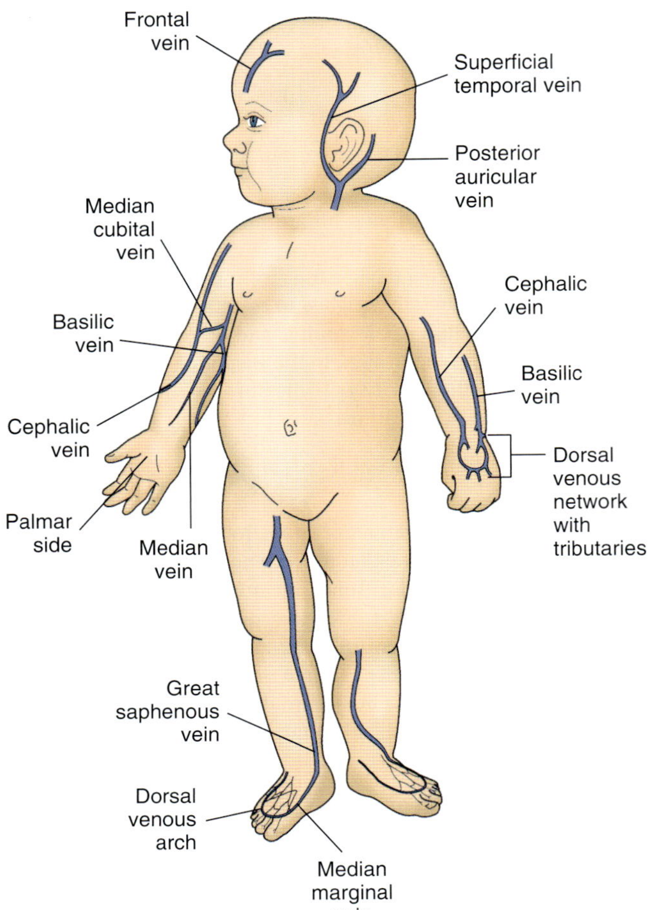

Fig 22.10 Preferred sites for venous access in infants.

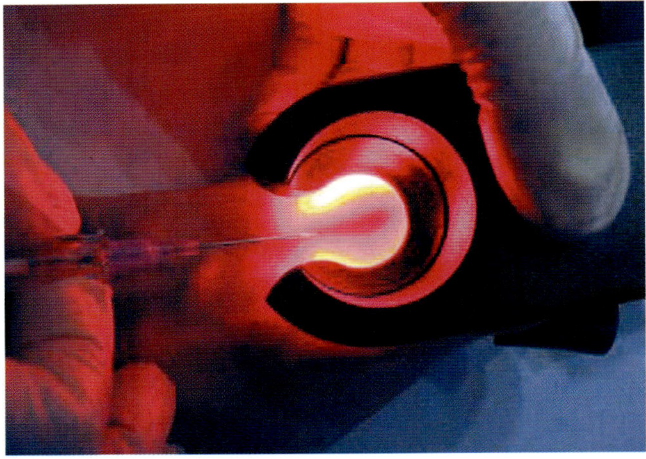

Fig 22.11 Transilluminator: low-heat light-emitting diode (LED) light placed on the skin to illuminate veins; an opening allows cannulation of vein. (Source: Professor Mark Waltzman, Children's Hospital, Boston.)

Selection of a scalp vein may require clipping the hair in the area around the site to better visualise the vein and provide a smoother surface on which to tape the catheter hub and tubing. Clipping a portion of the infant's hair may be upsetting to parents; therefore, they should be told what to expect and be reassured that the hair will grow back. Remove as little hair as possible directly over the insertion site and taping surface. Save the clipped hair because parents often wish to keep it. A rubber band slipped onto the head from brow to occiput will usually suffice as a tourniquet, although if the vessel is visible, a tourniquet may not be necessary.

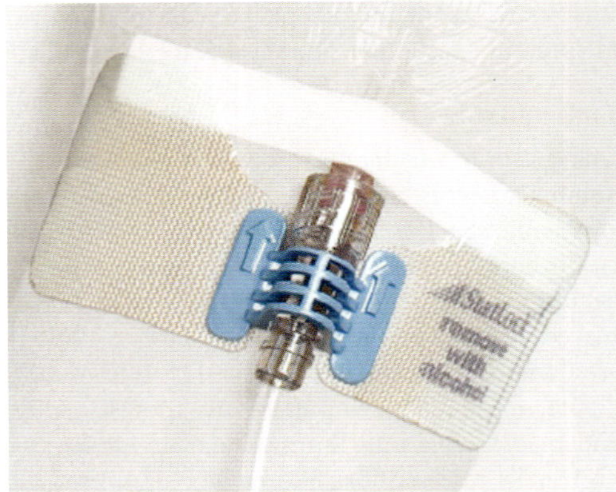

Fig 22.12 StatLock securement devices enhance peripheral intravenous line dwell time and decrease phlebitis.

For most IV infusions in children, a 22- to 24-gauge catheter may be used if therapy is expected to last 6 days or less. The smallest-gauge and shortest-length catheter that will accommodate the prescribed therapy should be chosen. The length of the catheter may be directly related to infection or embolus formation; the shorter the catheter, the fewer the complications. The gauge of the catheter should be enough to maintain adequate flow of the IV fluids into the cannulated vein, while allowing adequate blood flow around the catheter walls to promote proper haemodilution of the infusate.

Determining the best catheter for the patient early in the therapy provides the best chance of avoiding catheter-related complications. As the duration of therapy increases, decisions regarding the type of infusion device (short peripheral, midline, PICC or central venous catheter) should be explored. Guidelines such as flow charts and algorithms are available to help in these decisions.

Securement of a Peripheral Intravenous Line

Catheters must be stabilised for easy monitoring and evaluation of the access site, to promote delivery of therapy and to prevent damage, dislodgement or migration of the catheter (Marsh et al 2018).

To maintain the integrity of the IV line, adequate protection of the site is required. The catheter hub is firmly secured at the puncture site with a transparent dressing and commercial securement device (e.g. StatLock) (Fig 22.12) or clear non-allergenic tape. Transparent dressings are ideal because the insertion site is easily observed. Minimal tape should be used at the puncture site and on 2 to 5 cm of skin beyond the site to avoid obscuring the insertion site for early detection of infiltration. The catheter insertion site and 2 to 5 cm along the vein proximal to the site should be readily visible so the area can be monitored for signs of infiltration, irritation or leakage.

A protective clear dressing is applied to the insertion site to protect the catheter from dislodgement and to allow for easy visual site checks which will be requireed no less than hourly for paediatric IV cannulation site checks (Fig 22.13). Easy access to the IV site for frequent (hourly) assessments must be considered (Kleidon et al 2020). It is important to safely secure the IV tubing to prevent infants and children from becoming entangled in the tubing and accidentally pulling out the catheter or needle. Securing the tubing in this manner also eliminates movement of the catheter hub at the insertion site (mechanical manipulation). A colourful and interesting sticker can be applied to the protecting device to add a positive note to the procedure.

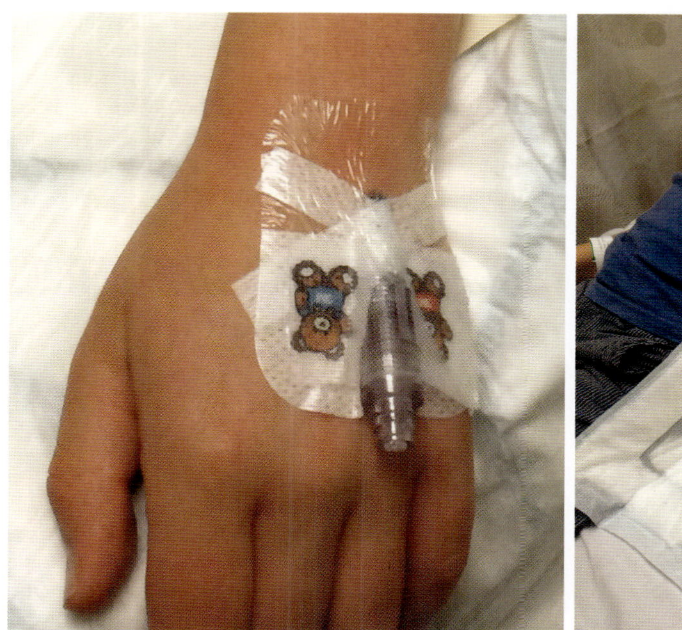
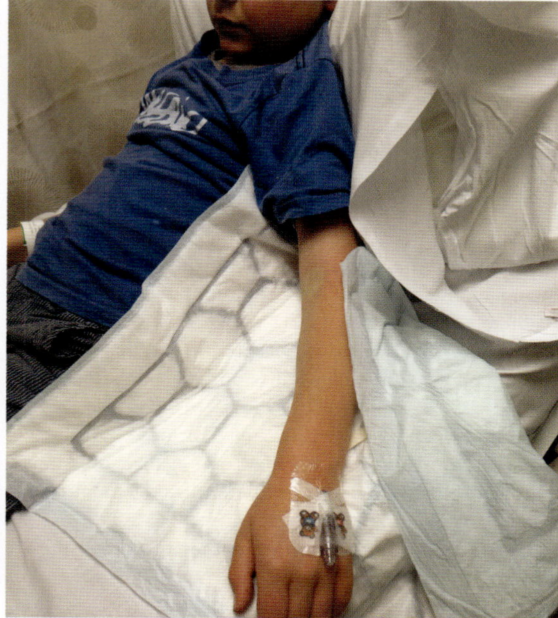

Fig 22.13 Young child with intravenous cannula with clear dressing to ensure visual access to site. If required, splint underneath hand and arm to secure (Source: Courtesy Emma Collins.)

Finger and toe areas are left uncovered by dressings or tape to allow for assessment of circulation. The thumb is never immobilised because of the risk of developing contractures with prolonged limitation of movement. An extremity should never be encircled with tape. The use of roll gauze, self-adhering stretch bandages (Coban) and crepe bandages should also be avoided because these products can cause constriction and hide signs of infiltration.

> **NURSING CARE CONSIDERATIONS**
>
> Opaque covering should be avoided; however, if any type of opaque covering is used to secure the IV line, the insertion site and extremity distal to the site should be visible to detect an infiltration. If these sites are not visible, they must be checked frequently to detect problems early.

Safety Catheters and Needleless Systems

Needlestick injuries are a serious risk for nurses and other healthcare professionals who provide IV therapy to their patients. Current technologies, including safety catheters and needleless systems, have minimised the risk of exposure to blood-borne pathogens by needlestick injury. Safety catheters employ retractable needle mechanisms to prevent accidental needlesticks when using over-the-needle peripheral IV catheters.

Needleless IV systems are designed to prevent needlestick injuries during administration of IV push medications and IV piggyback medications. There are three general types of needleless systems, based on how the connector displaces fluid:

- negative displacement systems, including blunt-tip cannulas for use with pre-slit injection caps; these cause a backflow of blood into the catheter when a syringe is disconnected
- positive displacement systems, a valve system that pushes a small amount of IV fluid back into the cap when disconnecting; this action prevents inadvertent catheter occlusion
- neutral displacement systems.

Flushing and disconnection procedures are different for each type of system. There is no way to know which type of mechanism is used by simply looking at the connectors. Therefore, the nurse must have an understanding of the mechanics of the system in use at the institution. Some needleless devices can be used with any tubing, but other devices can only be used with compatible IV delivery systems. There is some evidence that positive-pressure systems (blunt cannula systems) are associated with lower CLABSI rates and decrease the risk of catheter-related clots.

> **NURSING CARE CONSIDERATIONS**
>
> Misconnections of tubing have occurred, resulting in patient deaths. Many needleless IV systems allow other types of tubing such as blood pressure and oxygen tubing to connect and instil air directly into the IV line. Before tubing is connected or reconnected to a patient, trace it completely from the patient to the point of origin for verification.

Infusion Pumps

A variety of infusion pumps are available and used in nearly all paediatric infusions to accurately administer medication and minimise the possibility of overloading the circulation. It is important to calculate the amount to be infused in a given length of time, set the infusion rate and monitor the apparatus frequently (at least every 1 to 2 hours) to make certain that the desired rate is maintained, the integrity of the system remains intact, the site remains intact (free of redness, oedema, infiltration or irritation) and the infusion does not stop. Smart infusion pump technology provides built-in safety features that can alert nurses when pump settings are outside of programmed parameters, thereby reducing infusion errors and improving patient safety. Smart pump software within the infusion pump is programmed with dose and infusion rate information for commonly used drugs. The smart pump can recognise drug information in its database, check dosing, calculate infusions, monitor line pressure and report errors back to nursing.

Continuous infusion pumps, although convenient and efficient, are not without risks. Overreliance on the accuracy of the machine can cause either too much or too little fluid to be infused; therefore, its use does not eliminate careful periodic assessment by the nurse. Excess pressure can build up if the machine is set at a rate faster than the vein is able to accommodate (or if the machine continues to pump when the catheter is no longer in the vein).

Maintenance

In a consensus guideline of 16 organisations and professional associations, the following maintenance recommendations were made for central venous catheters (O'Grady et al 2011).

- Use transparent dressings to allow site visualisation. If diaphoresis, bleeding or oozing prevents adequate adhesion, gauze dressings can be used.
- Replace any dressing when damp, visibly soiled or loose. Routinely replace transparent dressings every 7 days and gauze dressings every 2 days unless the risk of central catheter dislodgement outweighs the benefits of the dressing change.
- Do not apply ointments to the insertion site; they promote fungal growth and antimicrobial resistance.
- Replace IV administration sets at the following frequencies:
  - continuous infusions of crystalloids at no less than 96-hour intervals, but at least every 7 days
  - blood product or lipid emulsion sets within 24 hours of starting the infusion
  - propofol sets every 6 to 12 hours and when the vial is changed.
- No recommendation was made on the frequency of intermittent set changes.
- In paediatric patients, peripheral IV catheters may remain in place until a complication occurs or the therapy is complete.
- Promptly remove temporary central catheters or peripheral IV catheters as soon as they are no longer needed.

Complications

The same precautions regarding maintenance of asepsis, prevention of infection and observation for infiltration are carried out with patients of any age. However, infiltration is more difficult to detect in infants and small children than in adults. The increased amount of subcutaneous fat and the amount of tape used to secure the catheter often obscure the early signs of infiltration. When the fluid appears to be infusing too slowly or ceases, the usual assessment for obstruction within the apparatus—kinks, screw clamps, shutoff valve and positioning interference (e.g. a bent elbow)—often locates the difficulty. When these actions fail to detect the problem, it may be necessary to carefully remove some of the dressing to obtain a clear view of the venepuncture site. Dependent areas, such as the palm and undersides of the extremity or the occiput and behind the ears, should be examined because infiltrations in these areas may not be readily visible.

IV therapy in paediatrics can be difficult to maintain because of mechanical factors such as vascular trauma resulting from the catheter, the insertion site, vessel size, vessel fragility, pump pressure, the patient's activity level, operator skill and insertion technique, forceful administration of boluses of fluid and infusion of irritants or vesicants through a small vessel. These factors cause infiltration and extravasation injuries. **Infiltration** is defined as inadvertent administration of a non-vesicant solution or medication into surrounding tissue. **Extravasation** is defined as inadvertent administration of vesicant solution or medication into surrounding tissue (Murphy et al 2019). A **vesicant** or **sclerosing agent** causes varying degrees of cellular damage when even minute amounts escape into surrounding tissue. Guidelines are available for determining the severity of tissue injury by staging characteristics, such as the amount of redness, blanching, the amount of swelling, pain and the quality of pulses below infiltration, capillary refill and warmth or coolness of the area (Murphy et al 2019).

Treatment of infiltration or extravasation varies according to the type of drug involved. Guidelines are available outlining the sequence of interventions and specific treatment of infiltration or extravasation with antidotes.

NURSING CARE CONSIDERATIONS

When infiltration or extravasation is observed (signs include erythema, pain, oedema, blanching, streaking on the skin along the vein and darkened area at the insertion site), immediately stop the infusion, elevate the extremity, notify the provider and initiate the ordered treatment as soon as possible. Remove the IV line when it is no longer needed (e.g. after infusing an antidote).

Phlebitis, or inflammation of the vessel wall, may also develop in children who require IV therapy. There are three types of phlebitis: (1) mechanical (caused by rapid infusion rate, manipulation of the IV); (2) chemical (caused by medications); and (3) bacterial (caused by staphylococcal organisms). The initial sign of phlebitis is erythema (redness) at the insertion site. Pain may or may not be present.

Peripheral IV catheters are the most used intravascular device. Heavy cutaneous colonisation of the insertion site is the single most important predictor of catheter-related infection with all types of short-term, percutaneously inserted catheters. Phlebitis, largely a mechanical rather than infectious process, remains the most important complication associated with the use of peripheral venous catheters.

Removal of a Peripheral Intravenous Line

When the time comes to discontinue an IV infusion, many children are distressed by the thought of catheter removal. Therefore, they need a careful explanation of the process and suggestions for helping. Encouraging children to remove or help remove the tape from the site provides them with a measure of control and often fosters their cooperation. The procedure consists of turning off any pump apparatus, occluding the IV tubing, removing the tape, pulling the catheter out of the vessel in the opposite direction of insertion and exerting firm pressure at the site. A dry dressing (adhesive bandage strip) is placed over the puncture site.

When removing the needle from an implanted port, the line should be flushed with 5 mL of heparin, 100 units/mL, before removal of the needle, to ensure patency during the interim between accesses.

Non-tunnelled central lines can be removed by specially trained nurses with orders by provider. Tunnelled lines and implanted ports should be removed by the surgical team.

Rectal Administration

The rectal route for administration of medications is useful when a child is unable to take oral medications due to vomiting, altered gastrointestinal motility or altered mental status. Advantages to medication administration via the rectal route include absence of need to coax a child to swallow unpleasant-tasting medications and relative ease of accessibility for giving medications during an emergency if the patient is unconscious or vomiting and there is no venous access. Some of the drugs available in suppository form are paracetamol, aspirin, sedatives, analgesics (morphine), antiemetics and laxatives. Absorption by rectal mucosa is dependent on several factors, including gut motility, amount of time that the drug remains in the rectum and amount of stool present at time of drug administration. The difficulty in using the rectal route is that unless the rectum is empty at the time of insertion, the absorption of the drug may be delayed, diminished or prevented by the presence of faeces. Sometimes the drug is later evacuated, securely surrounded by stool. If the patient is neutropenic, immunosuppressed or thrombocytopenic, the rectal route may be contraindicated due to risk of introducing bacteria into the bloodstream.

Optic, Otic and Nasal Administration

There are few differences in administering eye, ear and nose medication to children and to adults. The major difficulty is in gaining children's cooperation. Older children need only an explanation and direction. Although the administration of optic, otic and nasal medication is not painful, these drugs can cause unpleasant sensations, which can be eliminated with various techniques.

Instilling eye drops in infants can be difficult because they often clench the eyelids tightly closed. One approach is to place the drops in the nasal corner where the eyelids meet. The medication pools in this area, and when the child opens the eyelids, the medication flows onto the conjunctiva. For young children, playing a game can be helpful, such as instructing the child to keep the eyes closed to the count of three and then open them, at which time the drops are quickly instilled. Ointment can be applied by gently pulling down the lower eyelid and placing the ointment in the lower conjunctival sac.

Ear drops are instilled with the child in the prone or supine position and the head turned to the appropriate side. To avoid uncomfortable stimulation of vertigo, ensure that ear medications are at room temperature before instilling. For children younger than 3 years of age, the external auditory canal is straightened by gently pulling the pinna downwards and straight back. The pinna is pulled upwards and back in children older than 3 years of age.

Nose drops are instilled in the same manner as in the adult patient. Remove mucus from the nose with a clean tissue or a washcloth. Unpleasant sensations associated with medicated nose drops are minimised when care is taken to position the child with the head extended well over the edge of the bed or pillow (Fig 22.14).

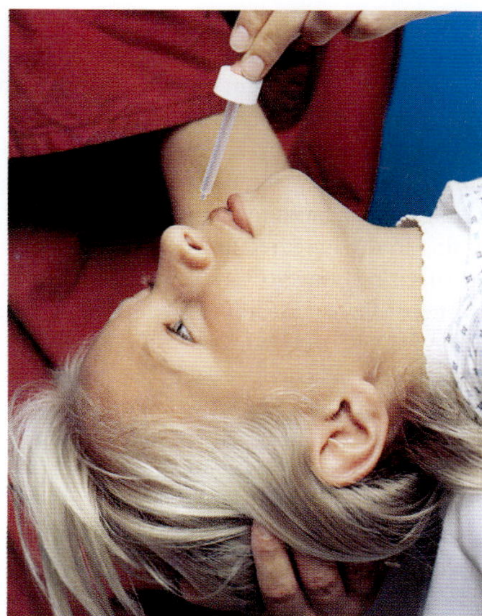

Fig 22.14 Proper position for instilling nose drops.

Aerosol Therapy

Aerosol therapy can be an effective method for administering medication directly into the airway. Bronchodilators, steroids, mucolytics and antibiotics, suspended in particulate form, can be inhaled so that the medication reaches the small airways. This route of administration can be useful in avoiding the systemic side effects of certain drugs and in reducing the amount of drug necessary to achieve the desired effect. Aerosol therapy is particularly challenging in children who are too young to cooperate with controlling the rate and depth of breathing. Administration of aerosolised medications to children requires skill, patience and creativity. Because many children with airway diseases, such as asthma, use aerosol therapies on a regular basis, it is important for families to have an understanding of the home plan of care, including drugs to use for maintenance and drugs to use for rescue.

Breath sounds and work of breathing should be assessed before and after treatments. Young children who become upset by having a mask held close to the face may become fatigued with fighting the procedure and may appear worse during and immediately after the therapy It may be necessary to spend a few minutes calming the child after the procedure and allowing the vital signs to return to baseline to accurately assess changes in breath sounds and work of breathing.

Family Teaching and Home Care

The nurse usually assumes responsibility for preparing families to administer medications at home. The family should understand why the child is receiving the medication and the effects that might be expected, as well as the amount, frequency and length of time the drug is to be administered.

> **NURSING CARE CONSIDERATIONS**
>
> If parents have difficulty reading or if there is a language barrier, use colours and/or pictures to convey instructions. For example, mark each drug with a colour and place the appropriate colour on a calendar chart or on a drawing of a clock to identify when the drug needs to be given. If a liquid medication and syringe are used, also mark the syringe at the place the plunger needs to be with colour-coded tape. Several websites and smartphone applications are available to help create patient-specific medication calendars.

Nasogastric, Orogastric and Gastrostomy Administration

When a child has an indwelling feeding tube or a gastrostomy, oral medications are usually given via that route. An advantage of this method is the ability to administer oral medications around the clock without disturbing the child. A disadvantage is the risk of occluding, or clogging, the tube, especially when giving viscous solutions through small-bore feeding tubes. The most important preventive measure is adequate flushing after the medication is instilled.

ALTERNATIVE FEEDING TECHNIQUES

Some children are unable to take nourishment by mouth because of: anomalies of the throat, oesophagus or bowel; impaired swallowing capacity; severe debilitation; respiratory distress; or unconsciousness. These children are frequently fed by way of a tube inserted orally or nasally into the stomach (**orogastric** [OG] or **NG gavage**) or duodenum-jejunum (**enteral gavage**) or by a tube inserted directly into the stomach (**gastrostomy**) or jejunum (**jejunostomy**). Such feedings may be intermittent or by continuous drip. During gavage or gastrostomy feedings, infants are given a soother. Non-nutritive sucking has several advantages, such as increased weight gain and decreased crying. However, only soothers with a safe design can be used to prevent the possibility of aspiration. Using improvised soothers made from bottle nipples is not a safe practice.

When a child is concurrently receiving continuous-drip gastric or enteral feedings and parenteral (IV) therapy, the potential exists for inadvertent administration of the enteral formula through the circulatory system. The possibility for error increases when the parenteral solution is a fat emulsion, a milky-appearing substance. Safeguards to prevent this potentially serious error include the following.

- Be sure that the feeding bag and all tubings are cleaned on a regular basis, according to the manufacturer's recommendations.
- Use enteral-specific connectors (ENFit) that are not compatible with Luer or needleless connections used for IV tubing (Guenter & Lyman 2016, ACSQHC n.d.b).
- Use a separate, specifically designed enteral feeding pump mounted on a separate pole for continuous-feeding solutions.
- Label all tubing of continuous enteral feeding with brightly coloured tape or labels.
- Use specifically designed continuous-feeding bags to contain the solutions instead of parenteral equipment, such as a burette.
- Whenever access or connections are made, trace the tubing all the way from the patient to the bag to ensure that the correct tubing source is selected.

Gavage Feeding

Infants and children can be fed simply and safely by a tube passed into the stomach through either the nares or the mouth. The tube can be left in place or inserted and removed with each feeding. In older children, it is usually less traumatic to tape the tube securely in place between feedings. For long-term enteral tube feedings, the tube should be removed and replaced with a new tube according to hospital policy, manufacturer recommendations, specific orders and the type of tube used. Meticulous hand washing is practised during the procedure to prevent bacterial contamination of the feeding, especially during continuous-drip feedings.

Not all feeding tubes are the same. Polyethylene and polyvinylchloride types lose their flexibility and need to be replaced frequently, usually every 3 or 4 days. Polyurethane and silicone tubes remain flexible, so they can remain in place up to 30 days. Advantages of small-bore tubes include a reduced incidence of pharyngitis, otitis media, aspiration and discomfort. Disadvantages include difficulty during insertion (may require a stylet or metal guide wire), collapse of the tube during aspiration of gastric contents to test for correct placement, dislodgement during forceful coughing, migration out of position, knotting, occlusion and unsuitability for thick feedings.

Procedure

Infants are easier to control if they are first wrapped in a mummy restraint (see Fig 22.2). Even tiny infants with random movements can grasp and dislodge the tube. Preterm infants do not ordinarily require restraint, but if they do, a small blanket folded across the chest and secured beneath the shoulders is usually enough. Take care that breathing is not compromised.

TRANSLATING EVIDENCE INTO PRACTICE

Confirming Nasogastric Tube Placement in Paediatric Patients

Ask the Question

PICOT Question

In children, how should correct placement of NG tubes be assessed during hospitalisation?

Search for Evidence

Search Strategies

Search selection criteria included English, research-based articles and children and adolescents requiring NG tube placement. Search areas included aspirate, auscultation and radiology methods, NG tube length prediction methods, age-related height-based methods and accurate NG tube placement. Searches excluded newborns and preterm infants.

Databases Used

PubMed, Cochrane Collaboration, MDConsult, Joanna Briggs Institute, AHRQ–National Guideline Clearinghouse, TRIP database Plus, PedsCCM, BestBETS

Critical Appraisal of the Evidence

- Studies compared various methods used to evaluate correct placement of the NG tube.
- Accurate NG tube length measurement:
  - children 8 years, 4 months of age or younger—use age-related height-based (AHRB) equation for NG length predictions
  - children older than 8 years, 4 months of age; of short stature; or when you cannot obtain accurate height—use nose-ear-midxiphoid-umbilicus (NEMU) (Beckstrand et al 2007)
  - no significant difference between AHRB and NEMU methods of tube placement; using nose-ear-xiphoid only resulted in increased risk of misplaced tube (Cirgin Ellett et al 2012).

Radiographs

- Although abdominal x-ray provides confirmation of enteral tube location, the results can sometimes be equivocal. In addition, this method cannot be used for ongoing, frequent placement verification basis due to the risk of radiation exposure to the child (Irving et al 2014). Alternative methods of verification have evidence-based support in the literature (Cincinnati Children's Hospital Medical Center 2011).

Non-radiological Verification Methods

- A pH of 5 or less supports that the tip of the tube is in the gastric location (Cirgin Ellett et al 2005, Huffman et al 2004, Nyqvist et al 2005, Phang et al 2004, Society of Pediatric Nurses Clinical Practice Committee et al 2011, Westhus 2004).
- A pH greater than 5 does not reliably predict correct distal tip location. This may indicate respiratory or oesophageal placement or the presence of medications to suppress acid secretion. Gastric aspirate pH means are statistically significantly lower compared with means from intestinal and respiratory pH aspirates (Cirgin Ellett et al 2005, Gilbertson et al 2011, Phang et al 2004, Society of Pediatric Nurses Clinical Practice Committee et al 2011, Westhus 2004).

Visual Inspection of Aspirate

- Visual inspection is less accurate than pH to confirm placement. Aspirate colours are specific to the intended placement location. Gastric contents are clear, off-white or tan or may be brown-tinged if blood is present. Respiratory secretions may look the same. Intestinal contents are often bile stained, light to dark yellow or greenish-brown (Phang et al 2004, Society of Pediatric Nurses Clinical Practice Committee et al 2011, Westhus 2004).

Enzyme Testing

- Aspirate testing of enzyme levels for bilirubin, pepsin and trypsin is highly accurate but limited to laboratory assessment (Cirgin Ellett et al 2005, Westhus 2004).

CO_2 Monitoring

- CO_2 monitoring is a reliable method to determine incorrect tube placement in the respiratory tract; it requires a capnograph monitor (Cirgin Ellett et al 2005).

Continued

TRANSLATING EVIDENCE INTO PRACTICE

Confirming Nasogastric Tube Placement in Paediatric Patients—cont'd

- CO_2 monitoring is useful to determine whether or not the enteral tube is in the respiratory tract; however, CO_2 monitoring does not provide information for determining whether the tube is in the intestines, stomach or oesophagus (Cirgin Ellett et al 2012).

Gastric Auscultation

- Auscultation as a verification tool is reliable only 60% to 80% of the time and should not be used without additional methods (Neumann et al 1995).
- Although evidence shows auscultation alone is not a reliable confirmatory test, it is still widely used by nurses for evaluation of enteral tube placement (Lyman et al 2016, Northington et al 2017).
- Using aspirate and non-aspirate NG tube placement verification methods in combination increases the likelihood for accurate NG tube placement to 97% to 99%, similar to the radiological chest radiography gold standard of 99% (Cirgin Ellett et al 2005, Phang et al 2004, Society of Pediatric Nurses Clinical Practice Committee et al 2011, Westhus 2004).

Electromagnetic Device

- An electromagnetic tracing device demonstrated 100% accuracy in enteral feeding tubes in a study of both adults and children; however, the device requires special training for use and cannot detect enteral tubes smaller than 8 French (Bourgault et al 2015, Powers et al 2011).

Apply the Evidence: Nursing Implications

There is good evidence with strong recommendations (Guyatt et al 2008) that a combination of verification methods to confirm NG tube placement will reduce the required number of x-rays in children (Society of Pediatric Nurses Clinical Practice Committee et al 2011). These methods include pH testing and visual inspection of the pH aspirate. There is also good evidence that improving the accuracy of predicting NG tube length before insertion will enhance the precision of successful NG tube placement. Auscultation is used in combination with other NG tube verification methods. Further investigation of additional non-invasive, user-friendly, portable verification methods is warranted, including ultrasound and electromagnetic tracer (Powers et al 2011).

Quality and Safety Competencies: Evidence-Based Practice*

Knowledge

- Differentiate clinical opinion from research and evidence-based summaries.
- Describe the various verification methods to confirm NG tube placement.

Skills

- Base individualised care plan on patient values, clinical expertise and evidence.
- Integrate evidence into practice by using the techniques for NG and OG tube placement verification in clinical care.

Attitudes

- Value the concept of evidence-based practice as integral to determining best clinical practice.
- Appreciate the strengths and weakness of evidence for confirming NG tube placement.

NG, nasogastric; OG, orogastric.
*Adapted from the QSEN at http://www.qsen.org.

APPLYING EVIDENCE TO PRACTICE

Nasogastric Tube Feedings in Children

- Place child supine with head slightly hyper-flexed or in a sniffing position (nose pointed towards ceiling).
- Measure the tube for approximate length of insertion and mark the point with a small piece of tape (Fig 22.15A).
- Consider using lidocaine (lignocaine) nasal spray to numb the nostril before tube insertion.
- Insert a tube that has been lubricated with sterile water or water-soluble lubricant through either the mouth or one of the nares to the predetermined mark. Because most young infants are obligatory nose breathers, insertion through the mouth causes less distress and helps stimulate sucking. In older infants and children, the tube is passed through the nose and alternated between nostrils. An indwelling tube is almost always placed through the nose (Fig 22.15B).
    - When using the nose, slip the tube along the base of the nose and direct it straight back towards the occiput.
    - When entering through the mouth, direct the tube towards the back of the throat.
    - If the child can swallow on command, synchronise passing the tube with swallowing.
- Confirm placement (see Translating Evidence into Practice: Confirming Nasogastric Tube Placement in Paediatric Patients box).
- Stabilise the tube by holding or taping it to the cheek, not to the nose or forehead because of possible damage to the nostril. To maintain correct placement, measure and record the amount of tubing extending from the nose or mouth to the distal port when the tube is first positioned. Recheck this measurement before each feeding (Fig 22.15C).
- Warm the formula to room temperature. Do *not* microwave! Pour formula into the barrel of the syringe attached to the feeding tube. To start the flow, give a gentle push with the plunger but then remove the plunger and allow the fluid to flow into the stomach by gravity. The rate of flow should not exceed 5 mL every 5 to 10 minutes in premature and very small infants and 10 mL/min in older infants and children to prevent nausea and regurgitation. The rate is determined by the diameter of the tubing and the height of the reservoir containing the feeding and is regulated by adjusting the height of the syringe. A usual feeding may take 15 to 30 minutes to complete.
- Flush the tube with sterile water (1 or 2 mL for small tubes to 5 to 15 mL or more for large ones).
- Cap or clamp indwelling tubes to prevent loss of feeding.
    - If the tube is to be removed, first pinch it firmly to prevent escape of fluid as the tube is withdrawn. Withdraw the tube quickly.
- Position the child with the head elevated 30 to 45 degrees or on the right side for 30 to 60 minutes in the same manner as after any infant feeding to minimise the possibility of regurgitation and aspiration. If the child's condition permits, bundle the youngster after the feeding.
- Record the feeding, including the type and amount of residual, the type and amount of formula and how it was tolerated.
    - For most infant feedings, any amount of residual fluid aspirated from the stomach is refed to prevent electrolyte imbalance and the amount is

Continued

APPLYING EVIDENCE TO PRACTICE

Nasogastric Tube Feedings in Children—cont'd

subtracted from the prescribed amount of feeding. For example, if the infant is to receive 30 mL and 10 mL is aspirated from the stomach before the feeding, the 10 mL of aspirated stomach contents is refed along with 20 mL of feeding. Another method can be used in children. If residual fluid is more than a quarter of the last feeding, return the aspirate and recheck in 30 to 60 minutes. When residual fluid is less than a quarter of the last feeding, give the scheduled feeding. If large amounts of aspirated fluid persist and the child is due for another feeding, notify the provider.

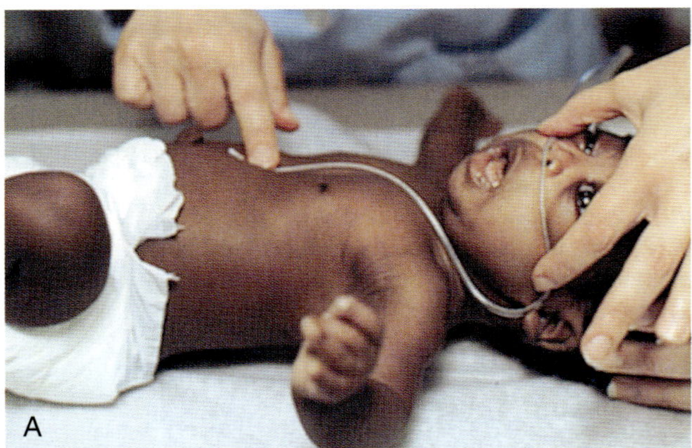

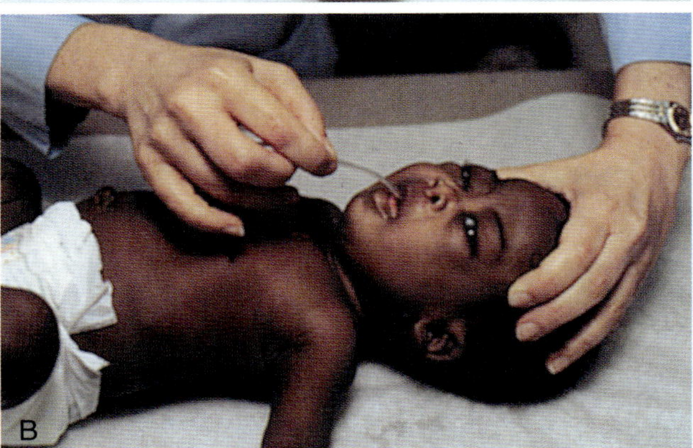

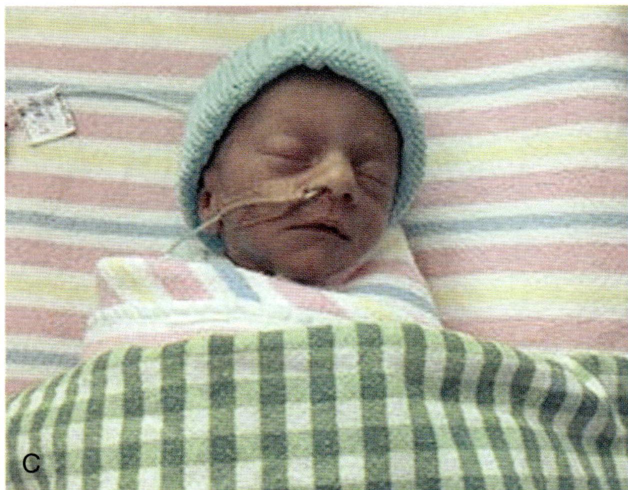

Fig 22.15 Gavage feeding. (**A**) Measuring the tube for orogastric feeding from the tip of the nose to the earlobe and to the midpoint between the end of the xiphoid process and the umbilicus. (**B**) Inserting the tube. (**C**) Completed insertion of nasal gastric tube.

Gastrostomy Feeding

Feeding by way of gastrostomy, or PEG tube, is often used for children in whom passage of a tube through the mouth, pharynx, oesophagus and cardiac sphincter of the stomach is contraindicated or impossible. It is also used to avoid the constant irritation of an NG tube in children who require tube feeding over an extended period. A gastrostomy tube may be placed with the child under general anaesthesia or percutaneously using an endoscope with the patient sedated and under local anaesthesia (percutaneous endoscopic gastrostomy). The tube is inserted through the abdominal wall into the stomach about midway along the greater curvature and secured by a purse-string suture. The stomach is anchored to the peritoneum at the operative site. The tube used can be a Foley, wingtip or mushroom catheter. Immediately after surgery, the catheter may be left open and attached to gravity drainage for 24 hours or more.

Direct postoperative care of the wound site towards prevention of infection and irritation. Cleanse the area with soap and water at least daily or as often as needed to keep the area free of drainage. After healing, meticulous care is needed to keep the area surrounding the tube clean and dry to prevent excoriation and infection. Exercise care to prevent excessive pull on the catheter that might cause widening of the opening and subsequent leakage of highly irritating gastric juices. Use barrier ointments such as zinc oxide, petrolatum-based ointment and non-alcohol skin barrier film to control leakage; add absorptive powders and pectin-based skin barrier wafers if skin irritation is present (RCHM n.d.). Secure the tube to the abdomen using a commercial stabiliser, polyurethane foam or the H tape method, and leave a small loop of tubing at the exit site to prevent tension on the site.

Granulation tissue may grow around a gastrostomy site (Fig 22.16). This moist, beefy-red tissue is not a sign of infection. However, if it continues to grow, the excess moisture can irritate the surrounding skin. The use of hydrogen peroxide for routine site cleansing has been identified as one of the possible causes of hypergranulation tissue,

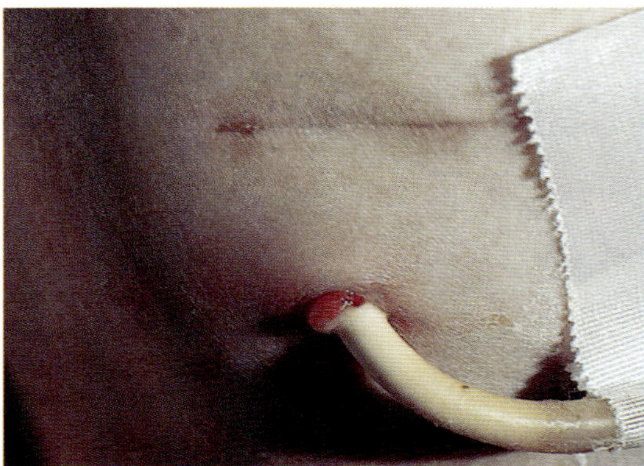

Fig 22.16 Appearance of healthy granulation tissue around a stoma.

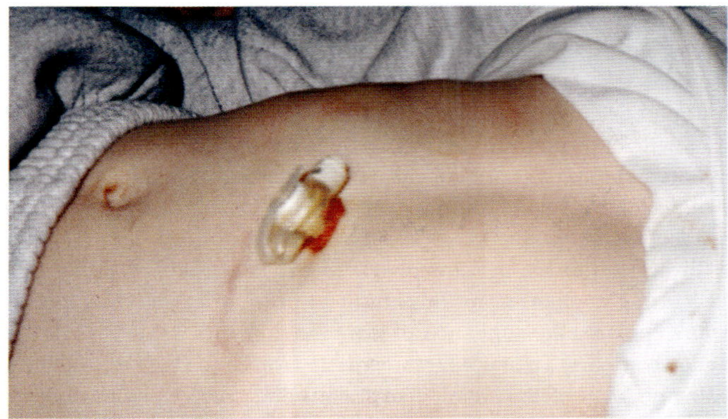

Fig 22.17 Child with a skin-level gastrostomy device (MIC-KEY), which provides for secure attachment of extension tubing to the gastrostomy opening.

corrosion and excessive drying of the tissue and disruption of wound healing. Clinical guidelines issued by the Royal Children's Hospital Melbourne (RCHM n.d.) recommend managing hypergranulation by stabilising the tube, keeping the peristomal area dry by applying polyurethane foam and using triamcinolone (0.5%) three times a day. Silver nitrate may also be used for hypergranulation.

For children receiving long-term gastrostomy feeding, a **skin-level device** (e.g. MIC-KEY, Bard Button) offers several advantages. The small, flexible silicone device protrudes slightly from the abdomen, is cosmetically pleasing, affords increased comfort and mobility to the child, is easy to care for and is fully immersible in water. The one-way valve at the proximal end minimises reflux and eliminates the need for clamping. However, the skin-level device requires a well-established gastrostomy site and is more expensive than the conventional tube. In addition, the valve may become clogged. When functioning, the valve prevents air from escaping; therefore, the child may require frequent bubbling. With some devices, during feedings, the child must remain still because the tubing easily disconnects from the opening if the child moves. With other devices, extension tubing can be securely attached to the opening (Fig 22.17). The feeding is instilled at the other end of the tubing in a manner like that for a regular gastrostomy. The extension tubing may also have a separate medication port. Both the feeding and the medication ports have plugs attached. Some skin-level devices require a special tube to be able to decompress the stomach (to check residual or decompress air).

Feeding of water, formula or pureed foods is carried out in the same manner and rate as for gavage feeding. A mechanical pump may be used to regulate the volume and rate of feeding. After feedings, the infant or child is positioned on the right side or in the Fowler's position and the tube may be clamped or left open and suspended between feedings, depending on the child's condition. A clamped tube allows more mobility but is only appropriate if the child can tolerate intermittent feedings without vomiting or prolonged backup of feeding into the tube. Sometimes a Y tube is used to allow for simultaneous decompression during feeding. If a Foley catheter is used as the gastrostomy tube, apply very slight tension. The tube is securely taped to maintain the balloon at the gastrostomy opening and prevent leakage of gastric contents and the tube's progression towards the pyloric sphincter, where it may occlude the stomach outlet. As a precaution, the length of the tube is measured postoperatively and then remeasured each shift to be certain it has not slipped. The nurse can make a mark above the skin level to further ensure its placement. When the gastrostomy tube is no longer needed, it is removed; the skin opening usually closes spontaneously by contracture.

NURSING CARE CONSIDERATIONS

If a gastrostomy button or tube is accidentally pulled out, a Foley catheter can be gently inserted in the tract to maintain patency until a new tube can be inserted.

Nasoduodenal and Nasojejunal Tubes

Children at high risk for regurgitation or aspiration, such as those with gastroparesis, mechanical ventilation or brain injuries, may require placement of a postpyloric feeding tube. A trained provider inserts the nasoduodenal or nasojejunal tube because of the risk of misplacement and potential for perforation in tubes requiring a stylet. Accurate placement is verified by radiography. Small-bore tubes may easily clog. Flush the tube when feeding is interrupted, before and after medication administration and routinely every 4 hours or as directed by institutional policy. Tube replacement should be considered monthly to ensure optimal tube patency. Continuous feedings are delivered by a mechanical pump to regulate their volume and rate. Bolus feeds are contraindicated. Tube displacement is suspected in children showing signs of feeding intolerance such as vomiting. In these cases, stop the feedings and notify the provider.

Total Parenteral Nutrition

Total parenteral nutrition (TPN) provides for the total nutritional needs of infants and children whose lives are threatened because feeding by way of the gastrointestinal tract is impossible, inadequate or hazardous.

Total parenteral nutrition therapy involves IV infusion of highly concentrated solutions of protein, glucose and other nutrients. The solution is infused through conventional tubing with a special filter attached to remove particulate matter or microorganisms that may have contaminated the solution. The highly concentrated solutions require infusion into a vessel with enough volume and turbulence to allow for rapid dilution. The wide-diameter vessels selected are the superior vena cava and innominate or intrathoracic subclavian veins approached by way of the external or internal jugular veins. The highly irritating nature of concentrated glucose precludes the use of the small peripheral veins in most instances. However, dilute glucose-protein hydrolysates that are appropriate for infusing into peripheral veins are being used with increasing frequency. When peripheral veins are used, intralipid becomes the major calorie source. For long-term alimentation, central venous catheters are usually used.

The major nursing responsibilities are the same as for any IV therapy and include control of sepsis, monitoring of the infusion rate and assessment of the patient. The TPN solution must be prepared under rigid aseptic conditions, which is best accomplished by specially trained technicians. Nurses should change the TPN, lipids and tubing on a frequent basis. More frequent tubing changes are required for TPN and lipids because these solutions can increase risk of microbial growth. Meticulous aseptic precautions should be used whenever the line is entered or changed. In some institutions, this may be a nursing responsibility. If so, the procedure is carried out according to hospital protocol.

The infusion is maintained at a constant rate by means of an infusion pump to ensure the proper concentrations of glucose and amino acids. Accurate calculation of the rate is required to deliver a measured amount in each length of time. Because alterations in flow rate are relatively common, the drip should be checked frequently to ensure an even, continuous infusion. The TPN infusion rate should not be increased or decreased without the provider being informed because alterations can cause hyperglycaemia or hypoglycaemia.

General assessments, such as vital signs, I&O measurements and checking results of laboratory tests, facilitate early detection of infection or fluid and electrolyte imbalance. Additional amounts of potassium and sodium chloride are often required in hyperalimentation; therefore, observation for signs of potassium or sodium deficit or excess is part of nursing care. This is rarely a problem except in children with reduced renal function or metabolic defects. Hyperglycaemia may occur during the first day or two as the child adapts to the high-glucose load of the hyperalimentation solution. Although hyperglycaemia occurs infrequently, insulin may be required to help the body adjust. When this occurs, nursing responsibilities include blood glucose testing. To prevent hypoglycaemia when the hyperalimentation is disconnected, the rate of the infusion and the amount of insulin are decreased gradually.

Family Teaching and Home Care

When alternative feedings are needed for an extended period, the family needs to learn how to feed the child with an NG, gastrostomy or TPN feeding regimen. The same principles apply as discussed earlier in this chapter for compliance, especially in terms of education, and in Chapter 21 for discharge planning and home care. Plan ample time for the family to learn and perform the procedures under supervision before they assume full responsibility for the child's care. Refer the family to community agencies that provide support and practical assistance. To further support the family there are some organisations that are able to provide ongoing support for the child and family such as The Oley Foundation in Australia (http://www.oley.org) and The Paediatric Society of New Zealand and Starship Foundation (https://www.kidshealth.org.nz/tube-feeding).

PROCEDURES RELATED TO ELIMINATION

Enema

The procedure for giving an enema to an infant or child does not differ essentially from that for an adult except for the type and amount of fluid administered and the distance for inserting the tube into the rectum. Depending on the volume, use a syringe with rubber tubing, an enema bottle or an enema bag.

An isotonic solution is used in children. Plain water is not used because, being hypotonic, it can cause rapid fluid shift and fluid overload. The Fleet enema (paediatric or adult sized) is not advised for children because of the harsh action of its ingredients (sodium biphosphate and sodium phosphate). Commercial enemas can be dangerous to patients with megacolon and to dehydrated or azotaemic children. The osmotic effect of the Fleet enema may produce diarrhoea, which can lead to metabolic acidosis. Several case studies have reported additional complications such as extreme hyperphosphataemia, hypernatraemia and hypocalcaemia, which may lead to neuromuscular irritability and coma.

Ostomies

Children may require stomas for various health problems. The most frequent causes in infants are necrotising enterocolitis and imperforate anus and, less often, Hirschsprung's disease. In older children, the most frequent causes are inflammatory bowel disease, especially Crohn's disease (regional enteritis) and ureterostomies for distal ureter or bladder defects.

Care and management of ostomies in older children differ little from the care of ostomies in adult patients. The major emphasis in paediatric care is preparing the child for the procedure and teaching care of the ostomy to the child and family.

Children with ileostomies are fitted immediately after surgery with an appliance to protect the skin from the proteolytic enzymes in the liquid stool. Infants may not be fitted with a pouch in the immediate postoperative period. When stomal drainage is minimal, as is often the case in small or preterm infants, a gauze dressing will suffice. Give the parents a choice of caring for the colostomy with or without an appliance. Paediatric appliances are available in a variety of sizes to ensure an adequate fit.

Protection of the peristomal skin is a major aspect of stoma care. Well-fitting appliances are important to prevent leakage of contents. Before applying the appliance, prepare the skin with a skin sealant that is allowed to dry. Then apply stoma paste around the base of the stoma or to the back of the wafer. The sealant and paste work together to prevent peristomal skin breakdown.

In infants with a colostomy left unpouched, skin care is similar to that of any child wearing a nappy. However, protect the peristomal skin with a barrier substance (e.g. zinc oxide ointment [Sensi-Care] or a mixture of zinc oxide ointment and stoma powder [Stomahesive]). A nappy larger than the one usually worn may be needed to extend upwards over the stoma and absorb drainage. If the skin becomes inflamed, denuded or infected, the care is similar to the interventions used for nappy dermatitis. A zinc-based product helps protect healthy skin, heal excoriated skin and minimise pain associated with skin breakdown. The skin protectant adheres to denuded, weeping skin. The nurse can apply zinc-based products over topical antifungal and antibacterial agents if infection is present. No-sting barrier film is a skin sealant that has no alcohol base and can be used on open skin without stinging.

Children with familial adenomatous polyposis may require a colectomy with ileoanal reservoir to prevent or treat carcinoma of the colon. Peristomal skin care for these children is particularly challenging because of increased liquid stools, increased digestive enzymes that may cause skin breakdown and the stoma being at skin level rather than raised. Additional care with this condition includes close monitoring of fluid and electrolyte status and increased incidence of bowel obstruction.

An enterostomal therapy nurse specialist is an important member of the healthcare team and will have additional suggestions and assistance with skin care information and ostomy pouching options. The nurse can obtain further information by contacting the Australian Association of Stomal Therapy Nurses Site (https://www.stomaltherapy.com/) and The Paediatric Society of New Zealand's Gastroenterology, Hepatology and Nutrition Special Interest Group (https://www.paediatrics.org.nz/our-work/special-interest-groups/gastroenterology).

Family Teaching and Home Care

Because these children are almost always discharged with a functioning colostomy, preparation of the family should begin as early as possible in the hospital. The nurse instructs the family in the application of the device (if used), care of the skin and appropriate action in case skin problems develop. Early evidence of skin breakdown or stomal complications, such as ribbonlike stools, excessive diarrhoea, bleeding, prolapse or failure to pass flatus or stool, is brought to the attention of the medical practitioner, nurse or stoma specialist. The same principles are applied as discussed earlier in this chapter for compliance, especially in terms of education, and in Chapter 21 for discharge planning and home care.

REFERENCES

Alamanou, D. G., & Brokalaki, H. (2014). Intrahospital transport policies: The contribution of the nurse. Health Science Journal, 8(2), 166–178.

Al-Yateem, N., Brenner, M., Shorrab, A. A., et al. (2016). Play distraction versus pharmacological treatment to reduce anxiety levels in children undergoing day surgery: A randomized controlled non-inferiority trial. Child: Care, Health and Development, 42(4), 572–581.

Anand, K. J., & Hall, R. W. (2006). Pharmacological therapy for analgesia and sedation in the newborn. Archives of Diseases in Childhood Fetal and Neonatal Edition, 91(6), 448–453.

Association of Child Life Professionals. (2017). Mission, values, vision. Association of Child Life Professionals. http://www.childlife.org/child-life-profession/mission-values-vision.

Atay, S., Yilmaz Kurt, F., Akkaya, G., et al. (2017). Investigation of suitability of ventrogluteal site for intramuscular injections in children aged 36 months and under. Journal for Specialists in Pediatric Nursing, 22(4), e12187.

August, D., Ray, R., Kandasamy, Y., et al. (2020). Neonatal skin assessments and injuries: Nomenclature, workplace culture and clinical opinions—Method triangulation a qualitative study. Journal of Clinical Nursing, 29(21–22), 3986–4006.

Australia and New Zealand Urological Nurses Society Catheterisation Guideline Working Party. (2013). Catheterisation Clinical Guidelines. ANZUS, Victoria. https://www.rch.org.au/clinicalguide/guideline_index/Urinary_tract_infection/

Australian Commission on Safety and Quality in Health Care (ACSQHC). (2017). National Tall Man Lettering List. ACSQHC: Sydney. https://www.safetyandquality.gov.au/sites/default/files/2019-04/National-Tall-Man-Lettering-List-Nov-2017.pdf

Australian Commission on Safety and Quality in Health Care (ACSQHC). (2019a). Action 5.24: Preventing falls and harm from falls. NSQHS Standards. ACSQHC: Sydney. https://www.safetyandquality.gov.au/standards/nsqhs-standards/comprehensive-care-standard/minimising-patient-harm/action-524

Australian Commission on Safety and Quality in Health Care. (2019b). Standards. Strategies for improvement. Para 3. https://www.safetyandquality.gov.au/standards/nsqhs-standards/comprehensive-care-standard/minimising-patient-harm/action-53

Australian Commission on Safety and Quality in Health Care (ACSQHC). (n.d.a). High risk medicines resources. ACSQHC: Sydney. https://www.safetyandquality.gov.au/our-work/medication-safety/high-risk-medicines/high-risk-medicines-resources

Australian Commission on Safety and Quality in Health Care (ACSQHC). (n.d.b). National standard for user-applied labelling of injectable medicines fluids and lines. ACSQHC: Sydney. https://www.safetyandquality.gov.au/our-work/medication-safety/safer-naming-labelling-and-packaging-medicines/national-standard-user-applied-labelling-injectable-medicines-fluids-and-lines

Australian Competition and Consumer Commission. (2007). Safety alert: Cots. ACCC Publishing Unit: Canberra. January. https://www.accc.gov.au/system/files/Cot%20safety%20-%20safety%20alert.pdf

Australian Dental Association. (2020). New Australian Fluoride Guidelines released. https://www.ada.org.au/News-Media/News-and-Release/Latest-News/New-Australian-Fluoride-Guidelines-released

Azhar, N. (2015). Pre-operative optimisation of lung function. Indian Journal of Anaesthesia, 59(9), 550–556.

Bahl, A., Pandurangadu, A. V., Tucker, J., et al. (2016). A randomized controlled trial assessing the use of ultrasound for nurse-performed IV placement in difficult access ED patients. The American Journal of Emergency Medicine, 34(10), 1950–1954.

Batawi, H. E. (2015). Effect of preoperative oral midazolam sedation on separation anxiety and emergence delirium among children undergoing dental treatment under general anesthesia. Journal of International Society of Preventive & Community Dentistry, 5(2), 88–94.

Beckett, V. L., Tyson, L. D., Carroll, D., et al. (2012). Accurately administering oral medication to children isn't child's play. Archives of Disease in Childhood, 97(9), 838–841.

Beckstrand, J., Cirgin Ellett, M., & McDaniel, A. (2007). Predicting internal distance to the stomach for positioning nasogastric and orogastric feeding tubes in children. Journal of Advanced Nursing, 59, 274–289.

Benoit, B., Martin-Misener, R., Latimer, M., et al. (2017). Breast-feeding analgesia in infants: An update on the current state of evidence. The Journal of Perinatal & Neonatal Nursing, 31(2), 145–159.

Bice, A. & Wyatt, T. (2017). Holistic comfort interventions for pediatric nursing procedures: a systematic review. Journal of Holistic Nursing, 35(3), 280–295. DOI:10.1177/0898010116660397

Boles, J. (2016). Preparing Children and Families For Procedures or Surgery. Pediatric Nursing, 42(3), 147–149.

Boots, B. K., & Edmundson, E. E. (2010). A controlled, randomised trial comparing single to multiple application lidocaine analgesia in paediatric patients undergoing urethral catheterisation procedures. Journal of Clinical Nursing, 19(5–6), 744–748.

Bourgault, A. M., Heath, J., Hooper, V., et al. (2015). Methods used by critical care nurses to verify feeding tube placement in clinical practice. Critical Care Nurse, 35(1), e1–e7.

Braniff, H., DeCarlo, A., Haskamp, A., et al. (2014). Pediatric blood sample collection from a pre-existing peripheral intravenous (PIV) catheter. Journal of Pediatric Nursing, 29(5), 451–456.

Brown, J., Gillespie, M., & Chard, S. (2015). The dorso-ventro debate: In search of empirical evidence. The British Journal of Nursing, 24(22), 1132–1139.

Brown, M., & Sinsky, C. A. (2013). Medication adherence: We didn't ask and they didn't tell. Family Practice Management, 20(2), 25–30.

Calcaterra, V., Veggiotti, P., Palestrini, C., et al. (2015). Post-operative benefits of animal-assisted therapy in pediatric surgery: A randomised study. PLoS ONE, 10(6), 1–13.

Castelo, M., Li, J., Taddio, A., et al. (2014). A randomized controlled trial of 2% lidocaine gel compared to current standard of care in infants undergoing urinary catheterization. Annals of Emergency Medicine, 64(Suppl. 4), S105.

Chameides, L., Samson, R. A., Schexnayder, S. M., et al. (Eds.) (2012). Pediatric advanced life support provider manual. American Heart Association.

Chan, Y. K., & Mamat, M. (2015). Management of heat stroke. Trends in Anaesthesia and Critical Care, 5(2–3), 65–69.

Child Family Community Australia (CFCA). (2017). Age of consent laws. CFCA Resource Sheet, July – 2017. https://aifs.gov.au/cfca/publications/age-consent-laws

Cincinnati Children's Hospital Medical Center. (2011). Confirmation of nasogastric/orogastric tube (NGT/OGT) placement—BeST Evidence Statement. https://www.childrensmn.org/departments/webrn/pdf/ng-og-verification-clinical-standard-preview-2015.pdf.

Cirgin Ellett, M. L., Cohen, M. D., Perkins, S. M., et al. (2012). Comparing methods of determining insertion length for placing gastric tubes in children 1 month to 17 years of age. Journal for Specialists in Pediatric Nursing, 17(1), 19–32.

Cirgin Ellett, M. L., Croffie, J. M., Cohen, M. D., et al. (2005). Gastric tube placement in young children. Clinical Nursing Research, 14, 238–252.

Clinical Laboratory Standards Institute. (2017). Collection of diagnostic venous blood specimens. In CLSI standard GP41 (7th ed.). Wayne, PA: Clinical and Laboratory Standards Institute.

Cole, R., Young, J., Kearney, L., et al. (2021). Priority setting: Consensus for Australia's infant safe sleeping public health promotion programme. Journal of Paediatrics and Child Health, 57(2), 219–226. doi:10.1111/jpc.15178

Crawford, C. L., & Johnson, J. A. (2012). To aspirate or not: An integrative review of the evidence. Nursing, 42(3), 20–25.

Dahl, A., Sinha, M., Rosenberg, D. I., et al. (2015). Assessing physician-parent communication during emergency medical procedures in children: An observational study in a low-literacy Latino patient population. Pediatric Emergency Care, 31(5), 339–342.

Derya, E. Y., Ukke, K., Taner, Y., et al. (2015). Applying manual pressure before benzathine penicillin injection for rheumatic fever prophylaxis reduces pain in children. Pain Management Nursing, 16(3), 328–335.

Dolgun, E., Yavuz, M., Eroğlu, B., et al. (2017). Investigation of preoperative fasting times in children. Journal of Perianesthesia Nursing, 32(2), 121–124.

Eliacik, K., Kanik, A., Yavascan, O., et al. (2016). A comparison of bladder catheterization and suprapubic aspiration methods for urine sample collection from infants with a suspected urinary tract infection. Clinical Pediatrics, 55(9), 819–824.

Firdouse, M., Wajchendler, A., Koyle, M., et al. (2017). Checklist to improve informed consent process in pediatric surgery: A pilot study. Journal of Pediatric Surgery, 52(5), 859–863.

Flippo, R., NeSmith, E., Stark, N., et al. (2015). Reduction of 30-day preventable pediatric readmission rates with postdischarge phone calls utilizing a patient- and family-centered care approach. Journal of Pediatric Health Care, 29(6), 492–500.

Ford, J. M. (2016). Lumbar puncture (Pediatric). Elsevier. https://lms.elsevier-performancemanager.com/ContentArea/NursingSkills/GetNursingSkillsDetails?skillid=CCP_081&skillkeyid=809&searchTerm=lumbar%20puncture&searchContext=nursingskills.

Fortier, M. A., Kain, Z. N., & Morton, N. (2015). Treating perioperative anxiety and pain in children: A tailored and innovative approach. Pediatric Anesthesia, 25(1), 27–35.

Gerard, L. L., Cooper, C. S., Duethman, K. S., et al. (2003). Effectiveness of lidocaine lubricant for discomfort during pediatric urethral catheterization. Journal of Urology, 170, 564–567.

Gilbertson, H. R., Rogers, E. J., & Ukoumunne, O. C. (2011). Determination of a practical pH cutoff level for reliable confirmation of nasogastric tube placement. Journal of Parenteral and Enteral Nutrition, 35(4), 540–544.

Gorski, L. A., Hadaway, L., Hagle, M., et al. (2016). 2016 infusion therapy standards of practice. Journal of Infusion Nursing, 39(Suppl. 1), S1–S159.

Gorski, L., Hadaway, L., Hagle, M., et al. (2021). Infusion Therapy Standards of Practice, 8th Edition. Journal of infusion nursing, 44(1S), S1–S224.

Gray, M. (1996). Atraumatic urethral catheterization of children. Pediatric Nursing, 22(4), 306–310.

Guenter, P., & Lyman, B. (2016). ENFit enteral nutrition connectors. Nutrition in Clinical Practice, 31(6), 769–772.

Guyatt, G. H., Oxman, A. D., Vist, G. E., et al. (2008). GRADE: An emerging consensus on rating quality of evidence and strength of recommendations. British Medical Journal, 336, 924–926.

Häusler, D., Häusser-Kinzel, S., Feldmann, L., et al. (2018). Functional characterization of reappearing B cells after anti-CD20 treatment of CNS autoimmune disease. Proceedings of the National Academy of Sciences, 115(39), 9773–9778. DOI: 10.1073/pnas.1810470115

Herd, H. A., & Rieben, M. A. (2014). Establishing the surgical nurse liaison role to improve patient and family member communication. Association of Perioperative Registered Nurses Journal, 99(5), 594–599.

Howie, S. R. C. (2011). Blood sample volumes in child health research: Review of safe limits. Bulletin of the World Health Organization, 89, 46–53.

Huffman, S., Pieper, P., Jarczyk, K. S., et al. (2004). Methods to confirm feeding tube placement: Application of research in practice. Pediatric Nursing, 30, 10–13.

Infusion Nurses Society. (2011). Infusion nursing standards of practice. Journal of Infusion Nursing, 34(Suppl. 1), S63–S64.

Infusion Nurses Society. (2016). Policies and procedures for infusion therapy (5th ed.). Infusion Nurses Society. author.

Institute for Safe Medication Practices. (2020). Oral dosage forms that should not be crushed. 21 February. https://www.ismp.org/recommendations/do-not-crush

Institute for Safe Medication Practices. (2016). FDA and ISMP lists of look-alike drug names with recommended Tall Man letters. https://www.ismp.org/Tools/tallmanletters.pdf.

Irving, S. Y., Lyman, B., Northington, L., et al. (2014). Nasogastric tube placement and verification in children: Review of the current literature. Critical Care Nurse, 34(3), 67–78.

Johnston, C., Campbell-Yeo, M., Disher, T., et al. (2017). Skin-to-skin care for procedural pain in neonates. Cochrane Database of Systematic Reviews, (2), CD008435.

Kaufman, J. (2020) How to... collect urine samples from young children. Archives of disease in childhood. Education and practice edition, 105(3), 164–171.

Kleidon, T., Rickard, C., Gibson, V., et al. (2020). Smile - Secure my intravenous line effectively: A pilot randomised controlled trial of peripheral intravenous catheter securement in paediatrics. Journal of Tissue Viability, 29(2), 82–90. doi: 10.1016/j.jtv.2020.03.006.

Kroger, A. T., Duchin, J., & Vazquez, M. (n.d.). General best practice guidelines for immunization: best practice guidance of the Advisory Committee on Immunization Practices (ACIP). https://www.cdc.gov/vaccines/hcp/acip-recs/general-recs/downloads/general-recs.pdf.

Kubota, J., Higurashi, N., Hirano, D., et al. (2020). Predictors of recurrent febrile seizures during the same febrile illness in children with febrile seizures. Journal of the Neurological Sciences, 411, 116682. https://doi.org/10.1016/j.jns.2020.116682

Letitre, S. L., DeGroot, E. P., Draaisma, E., et al. (2014). Anxiety, depression and self-esteem in children with well-controlled asthma: Case-control study. Archives of Disease in Childhood, 99(8), 744–748.

Lidgett, C. D. (2016). Improving the patient experience through a commit to sit service excellence initiative. Journal of Patient Experience, 3(2), 67–72.

Lim, J., Kim, J., Moon, B., et al. (2018). Tepid massage for febrile children: A systematic review and meta-analysis Australia. International Journal of Nursing Practice, 24(5), e12649. DOI: 10.1111/ijn.12649

Lyman, B., Kemper, C., Northington, L., et al. (2016). Use of temporary enteral access devices in hospitalized neonatal and pediatric patients in the United States. Journal of Parenteral and Enteral Nutrition, 40(4), 574–580.

Manworren, R., & Fledderman, M. (2000). Preparation of the child and family for surgery. In B. V. Wise, C. McKenna, G. Garvin, et al. (Eds.), Nursing care of the general pediatric surgical patient. Gaithersburg, MD: Aspen.

Marchaim, D., Taylor, A. R., Hayakawa, K., et al. (2012). Hospital bath basins are frequently contaminated with multidrug-resistant human pathogens. American Journal of Infection Control, 40(6), 562–564.

Marsh, N., Larsen, E., Genzel, J., et al. (2018). A novel integrated dressing to secure peripheral intravenous catheters in an adult acute hospital: a pilot randomised controlled trial. Trials, 19(1), 596. https://trialsjournal.biomedcentral.com/track/pdf/10.1186%2Fs13063-018-2985-9.pdf

Molacek, J., Houdek, K., Opatrný, V., et al. (2018). Serious complications of intraosseous access during infant resuscitation. European Journal of Pediatric Surgery Reports, 6(1), e59–e62.

Monsma, J., Richerson, J., & Sloand, E. (2015). Empowering parents for evidence-based fever management: An integrative review. Journal of the American Association of Nurse Practitioners, 27(4), 222–229.

Mularoni, P. P., Cohen, L. L., DeGuzman, M., et al. (2009). A randomized clinical trial of lidocaine gel for reducing infant distress during urethral catheterization. Pediatric Emergency Care, 25(7), 439–443.

Murphy, A., Gilmour, R., & Coombs, C. (2019). Extravasation injury in a paediatric population. ANZ Journal of Surgery, 89(4), E122–E126.

Murray, E., Edlund, B. J., & Vess, J. (2016). Implementing a pediatric fall prevention policy and program. Pediatric Nursing, 42(5), 256–259.

Neumann, M. J., Meyer, C. T., Dutton, J. L., et al. (1995). Hold that x-ray: Aspirate pH and auscultation prove tube placement. Journal of Clinical Gastroenterology, 20, 293–295.

Northington, L., Lyman, B., Guenter, P., et al. (2017). Current practices in home management of nasogastric tube placement in pediatric patients: A survey of parents and homecare providers. Journal of Pediatric Nursing, 33, 46–53.

Nyqvist, K. H., Sorell, A., & Ewald, U. (2005). Litmus tests for verification of feeding tube location in infants: Evaluation of their clinical use. Journal of Clinical Nursing, 14, 486–495.

O'Grady, N. P., Alexander, M., Burns, L. A., et al. (2011). Guidelines for the prevention of intravascular catheter-related infections. Clinical Infectious Diseases, 52(9), e162–e193.

Öztürk, D., Baykara, Z. G., Karadag, A., et al. (2017). The effect of the application of manual pressure before the administration of intramuscular injections on students' perceptions of postinjection pain: A semi-experimental study. Journal of Clinical Nursing, 26(11–12), 1632–1638.

Patricia, C. (2014). Evidence-based management of childhood fever: What pediatric nurses need to know. Journal of Pediatric Nursing, 29(4), 372–375.

Pawar, D. (2012). Common post-operative complications in children. Indian Journal of Anaesthesia, 56(5), 496–501.

Payne, N. R., & Flood, A. (2015). Preventing pediatric readmissions: Which ones and how? The Journal of Pediatrics, 166(3), 519–520.

Peacock, G., Parnapy, S., Raynor, S., et al. (2010). Accuracy and precision of manufacturer-supplied liquid medication administration devices before and after patient education. Journal of the American Pharmacists Association, 50(1), 84–86.

Phang, J. S., Marsh, W. A., Barlows, T. G., et al. (2004). Determining feeding tube location by gastric and intestinal pH values. Nutrition in Clinical Practice, 19, 640–644.

Pomicino, L., Maccacari, E. & Buchini, S. (2018). Levels of anxiety in parents in the 24 hr before and after their child's surgery: A descriptive study. Journal of Clinical Nursing, 27(1–2), 278–287. DOI: 10.1111/jocn.13895

Poonai, N., Li, J., Langford, C., et al. (2015). Intraurethral lidocaine for urethral catheterization in children: A randomized controlled trial. Pediatrics, 136(4), 880–886.

Poston, R. D. (2016). Assent described: Exploring perspectives from the inside. Journal of Pediatric Nursing, 31(6), 353–365.

Powers, J., Luebbehusen, M., Spitzer, T., et al. (2011). Verification of an electromagnetic device compared with abdominal radiograph to predict accuracy of feeding tube placement. Journal of Parenteral and Enteral Nutrition, 35(4), 535–539.

Powers, J., Peed, J., Burns, L., et al. (2012). Chlorhexidine bathing and microbial contamination in patients' bath basins. American Journal of Critical Care, 21(5), 338–342.

Razmus, I., & Bergquist-Beringer, S. (2017). Pressure ulcer risk and prevention practices in pediatric patients: A secondary analysis of data from the national database of nursing quality indicators. Ostomy/Wound Management, 63(2), 26–36.

Rosenbloom, E., Finkelstein, Y., Adams-Webber, T., et al. (2013). Do antipyretics prevent the recurrence of febrile seizures in children? A systematic review of randomized controlled trials and meta-analysis. European Journal of Paediatric Neurology, 17(6), 585–588.

Rothbart, A., Yu, P., Müller-Lobeck, L., et al. (2015). Peripheral intravenous cannulation with support of infrared laser vein viewing system in a pre-operation setting in pediatric patients. BMC Research Notes, 8, 463.

Royal Australasian College of Physicians (RACP). (2019). Royal Australasian College of Physician's submission to the Medical Council of New Zealand. Draft statement of Information, choice of treatment and informed consent. June 2019. https://www.racp.edu.au//docs/default-source/advocacy-library/racp-submission-to-the-medical-council-of-new-zealand-statement-on-information-choice-of-treatment-and-informed-consent.pdf?sfvrsn=afa81a1a_6

Rusch, R., Schulta, C., Hughes, L., et al. (2014). Evidence-based practice recommendations to Prevent/Manage post-lumbar puncture headaches in pediatric patients receiving intrathecal chemotherapy. Journal of Pediatric Oncology Nursing, 31(4), 230–238.

Ryu, G. S., & Lee, Y. J. (2012). Analysis of liquid medication dose errors made by patients and caregivers using alternative measuring devices. Journal of Managed Care Pharmacy, 18(6), 439–445.

Salazar, J. H., Yang, J., Shen, L., et al. (2014). Pediatric malignant hyperthermia: Risk factors, morbidity, and mortality identified from the nationwide inpatient sample and kids' inpatient database. Pediatric Anesthesia, 24(12), 1212–1216.

Scott, D., Ling, C., MacQueen, B., et al. (2017). Recombinant tissue plasminogen activator to restore catheter patency: efficacy and safety analysis from a multihospital NICU system. Journal of Perinatology, 37(3), 291–295.

Shah, V., & Ohlsson, A. (2011). Venepuncture versus heel lance for blood sampling in term neonates. Cochrane Database of Systematic Reviews, (5), CD001452.

Shaughnessy, E. E., White, C., Shah, S. S., et al. (2015). Implementation of postoperative respiratory care for pediatric orthopedic patients. Pediatrics, 136(2), 505–512.

Sisson, H. (2015). Aspirating during the intramuscular injection procedure: A systematic literature review. Journal of Clinical Nursing, 24(17–18), 2368–2375.

Society of Pediatric Nurses Clinical Practice Committee, SPN Research Committee, & Longo, M. A. (2011). Best evidence: Nasogastric tube placement verification. Journal of Pediatric Nursing, 26(4), 373–376.

Sorrentino, G., Fumagalli, M., Milani, S., et al. (2017). The impact of automatic devices for capillary blood collection on efficiency and pain response in newborns: A randomized controlled trial. International Journal of Nursing Studies, 72, 24–29.

Stein, R., Dogan, H. S., Hoebeke, P., et al. (2015). Urinary tract infections in children: EAU/ESPU guidelines. European Urology, 67(3), 546–558.

Stevens, B., Yamada, J., Ohlsson, A., et al. (2016). Sucrose for analgesia in newborn infants undergoing painful procedures. Cochrane Database of Systematic Reviews, (7), CD001069.

Stolz, L. A., Cappa, A. R., Minckler, M. R., et al. (2016). Prospective evaluation of the learning curve for ultrasound-guided peripheral intravenous placement. The Journal of Vascular Access, 17(4), 366–370.

Takeshita, J., Nakayama, Y., Nakajima, Y., et al. (2015). Optimal site for ultrasound-guided venous catheterisation in paediatric patients. Critical Care, 19(1), 15.

The Royal Children's Hospital Melbourne (RCHM). (2019). Urinary tract infection. July. https://www.rch.org.au/clinicalguide/guideline_index/Urinary_tract_infection/

The Royal Children's Hospital Melbourne (RCHM). (2020). Clinical Guidelines (Nursing) Adrenaline and fluid bolus administration in resuscitation. https://www.rch.org.au/rchcpg/hospital_clinical_guideline_index/Adrenaline_and_fluid_bolus_administration_in_resuscitation/#Definition%20of%20terms

The Royal Children's Hospital Melbourne (RCHM). (n.d.). Gastronomy—common problems. https://www.rch.org.au/clinicalguide/guideline_index/Gastrostomy_Common_problems/

Torres, A., Parker, R. M., Sanders, L. M., et al. (2018). Parent preferences and perceptions of milliliters and teaspoons: Role of health literacy and experience. Academic Pediatrics, 18(1), 26–34.

Valizadeh, S., Rasekhi, M., Hamishehkar, H., et al. (2015). Medication errors in oral dosage form preparation for neonates: The importance of preparation technique. Journal of Research in Pharmacy Practice, 4(3), 147–152.

Vaughn, H., Paton, E. A., Bush, A., et al. (2005). Does lidocaine gel alleviate the pain of bladder catheterization in young children? A randomized, controlled trial. Pediatrics, 116(4), 917–920.

Westhus, N. (2004). Methods to test feeding tube placement in children. MCN The American Journal of Maternal Child Nursing, 29, 282–291.

Williams, C., Johnson, P. A., Guzzetta, C. E., et al. (2014). Pediatric fasting times before surgical and radiologic procedures: Benchmarking institutional practices against national standards. Journal of Pediatric Nursing, 29(3), 258–267.

Winokur, E. J., Pai, D., Rutledge, D. N., et al. (2014). Blood culture accuracy: Discards from central venous catheters in pediatric oncology patients in the emergency department. Journal of Emergency Nursing, 40(4), 323–329.

Yapucu Güneş, Ü., Ceylan, B. & Bayındır, P. (2016). Is the ventrogluteal site suitable for intramuscular injections in children under the age of three? Journal of Advanced Nursing, 72(1), 127–134.

Yin, H. S., Parker, R. M., Sanders, L. M., et al. (2016). Liquid medication errors and dosing tools: A randomized controlled experiment. Pediatrics, 138(4), e20160357.

23

The Child with Fluid and Electrolyte Imbalance

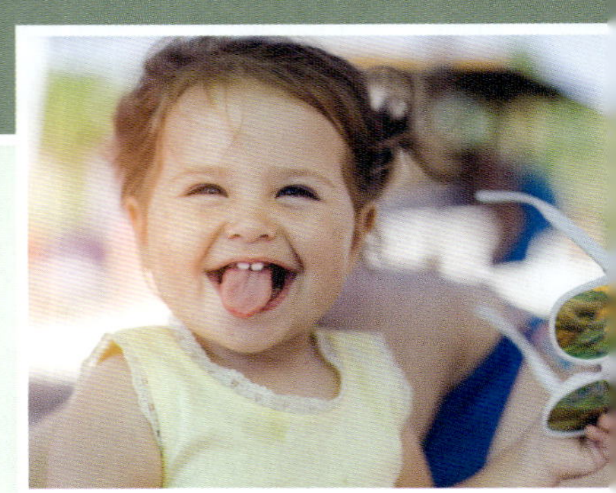

Patience Mayo

LEARNING OBJECTIVES

- Describe the normal distribution, mechanisms of movement and regulation of fluids and electrolytes in the body
- Describe the role of lungs, kidneys and chemical buffers in regulating the acid–base balance in the body
- Describe the aetiology, clinical manifestations, nursing diagnoses, outcomes and interventions for a paediatric patient with altered fluid, electrolyte and acid–base balances
- Discuss the various types of shock, describe the pathophysiology, clinical manifestations and subsequent management of shock in paediatric patients
- Describe the pathophysiology of burns, assessment, immediate resuscitation, subsequent management of burn injuries in paediatric patients

INTRODUCTION

This chapter will focus on fluid and electrolyte imbalances, shock and burn injuries in children. Fluid and electrolyte balance is achieved through numerous physiological processes which are crucial for achieving homeostasis. Disturbances in fluid and electrolyte balance result from most illnesses, extreme temperatures, vigorous activities and therapeutic interventions such as use of diuretics. Therefore, it is important that nurses develop an understanding of the physiology of fluid, electrolyte and acid–base balance to appropriately anticipate, recognise and respond to any disturbances to each of these elements. Shock or circulatory failure is time critical as the progression of shock can lead to cell death due to inadequate tissue perfusion and the cells cannot be regenerated, so an understanding of the mechanisms of shock is essential. This chapter will discuss the various types of shock and describe the pathophysiology, clinical manifestations and subsequent management of shock. Burn injuries occur among children in Australia/New Zealand, remaining potentially life-threatening and as such, healthcare staff need to be better prepared to manage patients with burn injuries. Therefore, this chapter will also discuss the occurrence of burn injuries, pathophysiology, immediate resuscitation, postresuscitation care, rehabilitation and burn preventive measures.

DISTRIBUTION OF BODY FLUIDS

The distribution of body fluids, or **total body water** (TBW), involves the presence of **intracellular fluid** (ICF) and **extracellular fluid** (ECF). Water is the major constituent of body tissues, and the TBW in an individual ranges from 45% (in late adolescence) to 75% (in term newborn) of total body weight.

The ICF refers to the fluid contained within the cells, whereas the ECF is the fluid outside the cells. The ECF is further broken down into several components: intravascular (contained within the blood vessels), interstitial (surrounding the cell; the location of most ECF) and transcellular (contained within specialised body cavities such as cerebrospinal, synovial and pleural fluid). In the newborn about 50% of the body fluid is contained within the ECF, whereas 30% of the toddler's body fluid is contained within the ECF.

Body water is important in body function not only because of its abundance but also because it is the medium in which body solutes are dissolved and all metabolic reactions take place. Because even small alterations in fluid composition affect these metabolic processes, precise regulation of the volume and composition of the fluid is essential. In healthy individuals, body water remains singularly constant, but marked alterations in either its volume or its distribution, which occur in many disease states, can produce severely damaging physiological consequences.

Water Balance

Under normal conditions the amount of water ingested closely approximates the amount of urine excreted in a 24-hour period, and the water in food and from oxidation approximates the amount lost in faeces and through evaporation. In this way, the body maintains equilibrium.

Mechanisms of Fluid Movement

Water is retained in the body in a relatively constant amount and, with few exceptions, is freely exchangeable among all body fluid compartments. The proximity of the extravascular compartment to the cells allows for continuous change in volume and distribution of fluids, largely determined by solutes (especially sodium) and physical forces

PATHOPHYSIOLOGY REVIEW

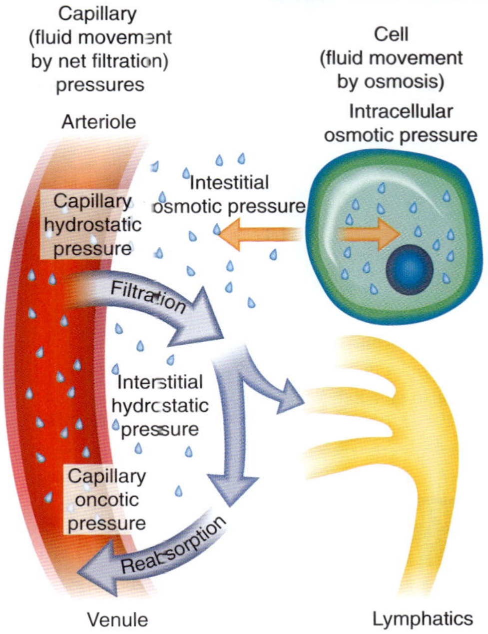

Arterial Capillary Pressures	
Capillary hydrostatic pressure	35 mm Hg
Interstitial fluid hydrostatic pressure	2 mm Hg
Net hydrostatic pressure	**33 mm Hg**
Capillary oncotic pressure	24 mm Hg
Interstitial fluid oncotic pressure	0 mm Hg
Net oncotic pressure	**24 mm Hg**
Net filtration pressure	**+9 mm Hg**

Venous Capillary Pressures	
Capillary hydrostatic pressure	18 mm Hg
Interstitial fluid hydrostatic pressure	1 mm Hg
Net hydrostatic pressure	**17 mm Hg**
Capillary oncotic pressure	25 mm Hg
Interstitial fluid oncotic pressure	0 mm Hg
Net oncotic pressure	**25 mm Hg**
Net filtration pressure	**–8 mm Hg**

Fig 23.1 Pathophysiology review. Capillary filtration forces. Water, electrolytes and small molecules exchange freely between the vascular compartment and the interstitial space at the site of capillaries and small venules. The rate and amount of exchange are driven by the physical forces of hydrostatic and oncotic pressures and the permeability and surface area of the capillary membranes. The two opposing hydrostatic pressures are capillary hydrostatic pressure and interstitial hydrostatic pressure. The two opposing oncotic pressures are capillary oncotic pressure and interstitial oncotic pressure. The *forces that favour filtration* from the capillary are capillary hydrostatic pressure and interstitial oncotic pressure, and the *forces that oppose filtration* are capillary oncotic pressure and interstitial hydrostatic pressure. The sum of their effects is known as *net filtration pressure.* In the example of normal exchange above, a small amount of fluid moves to the lymph vessels, which accounts for the net filtration difference between the arterial and venous ends of the capillary. (Source: McCance, K., & Huether, S. (2014). Pathophysiology: The biological basis for disease in adults and children (7th ed.). St Louis, MO: Mosby.)

(Fig 23.1). Transport mechanisms are the basis for all activity within the cells, and because the cells have limited ability to store materials, movement in and out of cells must be rapid. Internal control mechanisms are responsible for distribution and maintenance of fluid balance (Box 23.1).

Maintaining Water Balance. Maintenance water requirement is the volume of water needed to replace obligatory fluid loss such as that from insensible water loss (through the skin and respiratory tract), evaporative water loss and losses through urine and stool formation. The amount and type of these losses may be altered by disease states such as fever (with increased sweating), diarrhoea, gastric suction and pooling of body fluids in a body space (often referred to as **third spacing**).

Nurses should be alert for altered fluid requirements in various conditions.

- Increased requirements
  - Fever (add 12% per rise of 1°C)
  - Vomiting, diarrhoea
  - High-output kidney failure
  - Diabetes insipidus
  - Diabetic ketoacidosis
  - Burns
  - Shock
  - Tachypnoea
  - Radiant warmer (preterm infant)
  - Phototherapy (infants)
  - Postoperative bowel surgery (e.g. gastroschisis)
- Decreased requirements
  - Heart failure

BOX 23.1 Internal Control Mechanisms Influencing Fluid Balance

Thirst—The impetus to ingest water is stimulated by increased solute concentration (osmolality) of extracellular fluid and/or diminished intravascular volume.

Antidiuretic hormone (ADH)—ADH is released from the posterior pituitary gland in response to increased osmolality and decreased volume of intravascular fluid; it promotes water retention in the renal system by increasing the permeability of renal tubules to water.

Aldosterone—Aldosterone is secreted by the adrenal cortex; it enhances sodium reabsorption in renal tubules, thus promoting osmotic reabsorption of water.

Renin–angiotensin system—Diminished blood flow to the kidneys stimulates renin secretion, which reacts with plasma globulin to generate angiotensin, a powerful vasoconstrictor. Angiotensin also stimulates the release of aldosterone.

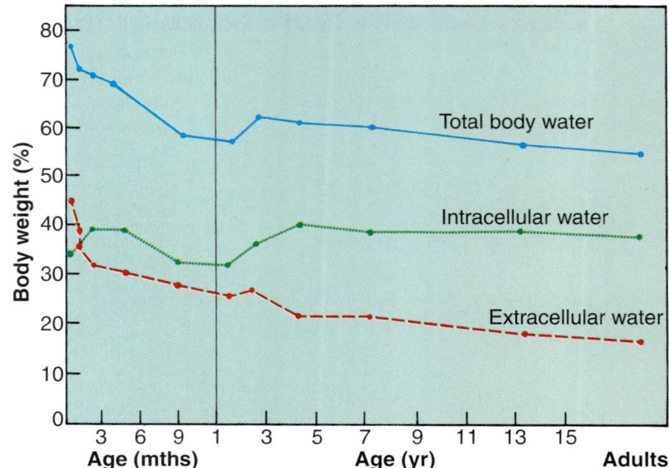

Fig 23.2 Changes in total body water, intracellular water and extracellular water in percentages of body weight. (Source: Based on data from Friis-Hansen, B. (1961). Body water compartments in children: Changes during growth and related changes in body composition. Pediatrics, 28, 169–181.)

TABLE 23.1 Daily Maintenance Fluid Requirements*

Body Weight	Amount of Fluid Per Day
3–10 kg	100 mL/kg
11–20 kg	1000 mL plus 50 mL/kg for each kg > 10 kg
> 20 kg	1500 mL plus 20 mL/kg for each kg > 20 kg

*Not appropriate for neonatal use.

- Syndrome of inappropriate antidiuretic hormone
- Mechanical ventilation
- After surgery
- Oliguric renal failure
- Increased intracranial pressure

Basal maintenance calculations for required body water are based on the body's requirements for water in a normometabolic state at rest; estimated fluid requirements are then increased or decreased from these parameters based on increased or decreased water losses, such as with elevated body temperature or congestive heart failure. Daily maintenance fluid requirements are listed in Table 23.1.

Maintenance fluids contain both water and electrolytes and can be estimated from the child's age, body weight, degree of activity and body temperature. **Basal metabolic rate** (BMR) is derived from standard tables and adjusted for the child's activity, temperature and disease state. For example, for afebrile patients at rest, the maintenance water requirement is approximately 100 mL for each 418 kJ expended. Children with fluid losses or other alterations require adjustment of these basic needs to accommodate abnormal losses of both water and electrolytes as a result of a disease state. For example, insensible losses increase when basal expenditure increases by fever or hypermetabolic states. Hypometabolic states, such as hypothyroidism and hypothermia, decrease the BMR.

Changes in Fluid Volume Related to Growth

The percentage of TBW varies among individuals, and in adults and older children it is related primarily to the amount of body fat. Consequently, females, who have more body fat than males, and obese persons tend to have less water content in relation to weight.

The fetus is composed primarily of water, with little tissue substance. As the organism grows and develops, a progressive decrease occurs in TBW, with the fastest rate of decline taking place during fetal life. The changes in water content and distribution that occur with age reflect the changes that take place in the relative amounts of bone, muscle and fat making up the body. At maturity the percentage of TBW is somewhat higher in the male than in the female and is probably a result of the differences in body composition, particularly fat and muscle content (Fig 23.2).

Another important aspect of growth change as it corresponds to water distribution is related to the ICF and ECF compartments. In the fetus and prematurely born infant, the largest proportion of body water is contained in the ECF compartment. As growth and development proceed, the proportion within the ECF compartment decreases as the ICF and cell solids increase. The ECF diminishes rapidly from approximately 40% of body weight at birth to less than 30% at 1 year of age. The different effects on males and females become apparent at puberty.

Water Balance in Infants

Because of several characteristics, infants and young children have a greater need for water and are more vulnerable to alterations in fluid and electrolyte balance. Compared with older children and adults, they have a greater fluid intake and output relative to size. Water and electrolyte disturbances occur more frequently and more rapidly, and children adjust less promptly to these alterations.

The fluid compartments in the infant vary significantly from those in the adult, primarily because of an expanded extracellular compartment. The ECF compartment constitutes more than half of the TBW at birth and has a greater relative content of extracellular sodium and chloride. The infant loses a considerable amount of fluid in the first few days after birth and still maintains a larger amount of ECF than the adult until about 2 to 3 years of age. This contributes to greater and more rapid water loss during this age period.

Fluid losses create compartment deficits that reflect the duration of dehydration. In general, approximately 60% of fluid is lost from the ECF, and the remaining 40% comes from the ICF. The amount of fluid lost from the ECF increases with acute illness and decreases with chronic loss.

Fluid losses may be divided into insensible, urinary and faecal losses and vary with the patient's age. Approximately two-thirds of **insensible water losses** occurs through the skin, and the remaining one-third is lost through the respiratory tract. Environmental heat and humidity, skin integrity, body temperature and respiratory rate all influence insensible fluid loss. Infants and children have a much greater tendency to become highly febrile than do adults. Fever increases insensible water loss by approximately 7 mL/kg/24 hr for each 1°C rise in temperature above 37.2°C. Fever and increased surface area relative to volume both contribute to greater insensible fluid losses in young patients.

Body Surface Area. The infant's relatively greater **body surface area** (BSA) allows larger quantities of fluid to be lost through the skin. It is estimated that the BSA of the premature neonate is five times more, and that of the newborn is two or three times more, than that of the older child or adult. The proportionately longer gastrointestinal tract in infancy is also a source of relatively greater fluid loss, especially from diarrhoea.

Metabolic Rate. The rate of metabolism in infancy is significantly higher than in adulthood because of the larger BSA in relation to the mass of active tissue. Consequently, infants have a greater production of metabolic wastes that the kidneys must excrete. Any condition that increases metabolism causes greater heat production, with its concomitant insensible fluid loss and an increased need for water for excretion. The BMR in infants and children is higher to support cellular and tissue growth.

Kidney Function. The infant's kidneys are functionally immature at birth and are therefore inefficient in excreting waste products of metabolism. Of particular importance for fluid balance is the inability of the infant's kidneys to concentrate or dilute urine, to conserve or excrete sodium or to acidify urine. Therefore, the infant is less able to handle large quantities of solute-free water than is the older child and is more likely to become dehydrated when given concentrated formulas or overhydrated when given excessive free water or dilute formula.

Fluid Requirements. As a result of these characteristics, infants ingest and excrete a greater amount of fluid per kilogram of body weight than do older children. Because electrolytes are excreted with water and the infant has limited ability for conservation, maintenance requirements include both water and electrolytes. The daily exchange of ECF in the infant is much greater than that of older children, which leaves the infant little fluid volume reserve in dehydrated states. Fluid requirements depend on hydration status, size, environmental factors and underlying disease.

DISTURBANCES OF FLUID AND ELECTROLYTE BALANCE

Disturbances of fluids and their solute concentration are closely interrelated. Alterations in fluid volume affect the electrolyte component, and changes in electrolyte concentration influence fluid movement. Because intracellular water and electrolytes move to and from the ECF compartment, any imbalance in the ICF is reflected by an imbalance in the ECF. Disturbances in the ECF involve either an excess or a deficit of fluid or electrolytes. Of these, fluid loss occurs more frequently.

Sodium is the chief solute in ECF and the primary determinant of ECF volume. It is considered a unique electrolyte in that water balance determines sodium concentration; when water is lost and sodium concentration becomes elevated, compensatory mechanisms in the kidney stop ADH secretion so water is retained. The thirst mechanism (not fully functional in infants) is also stimulated so water is replaced, thus increasing the total body water content and returning sodium to a normal level (Elisha & Terry 2018, Greenbaum 2015). Sodium depletion in diarrhoea occurs in two ways: out of the body in stool and into the ICF compartment to replace potassium to maintain electrical equilibrium. Potassium is found primarily inside the cell (intracellular), but small amounts are also found in ECF.

Depletion of ECF, usually caused by gastroenteritis, is one of the most common problems encountered in infants and children. (See Chapter 25.) Until modern techniques for fluid replacement were perfected, gastroenteritis was one of the chief causes of infant mortality. Fluid and electrolyte problems related to specific diseases and their management are discussed throughout the book where appropriate. The major fluid disturbances, their usual causes and clinical manifestations are listed in Table 23.2; the most common fluid disturbances, dehydration and oedema, are elaborated further in the following sections. Problems of fluid and electrolyte disturbance always involve both water and electrolytes; therefore, replacement includes administration of both, calculated on the basis of ongoing processes and laboratory serum electrolyte values.

Dehydration

Dehydration is a common body fluid disturbance encountered in the nursing care of infants and young children; it occurs whenever the total output of fluid exceeds the total intake, regardless of the underlying cause. Dehydration is also commonly referred to as volume depletion. Although dehydration can result from lack of oral intake (especially in elevated environmental temperatures), more often it is a result of abnormal losses, such as those that occur in vomiting or diarrhoea, when oral intake only partially compensates for the abnormal losses. Other significant causes of dehydration are diabetic ketoacidosis and extensive burns.

In early dehydration (during the first 2 days), fluid loss is derived from both the ECF and the ICF because the increased osmolality of the diminished ECF volume causes fluid from the ICF compartment to move into the ECF compartment. As dehydration becomes chronic, the cellular losses become greater.

Types of Dehydration

Because sodium is the primary osmotic force that controls fluid movement between the major fluid compartments, dehydration is often described according to plasma sodium concentrations (e.g. isonatraemic, hyponatraemic or hypernatraemic). Other osmotic forces, however, such as glucose in diabetic ketoacidosis and protein in nephrotic syndrome, may also play a dominant role. Consequently, dehydration is conventionally classified as isotonic, hypotonic or hypertonic.

Isotonic (isosmotic or isonatraemic) dehydration occurs in conditions in which electrolyte and water deficits are present in approximately balanced proportions. This is the primary form of dehydration occurring in children. The observable fluid losses are not necessarily isotonic, but losses from other avenues make adjustments so that the sum of all losses, or the net loss, is isotonic. Because no osmotic force is present to cause a redistribution of water between the ICF and ECF, the major loss is sustained from the ECF compartment. This significantly reduces the plasma volume and thus the circulating blood volume, with its effect on the skin, muscles and kidneys. Shock is the greatest threat to life in isotonic dehydration, and the child with isotonic dehydration displays symptoms characteristic of hypovolaemic shock. Plasma sodium remains within normal limits, between 130 and 145 mmol/L (Friedman et al 2015, Government of Western Australia Child and Adolescent Health Service 2018, The Royal Children's Hospital Melbourne [RCHM] 2019).

Hypotonic (hypoosmotic or hyponatraemic) dehydration occurs when the electrolyte deficit exceeds the water deficit. Because ICF is more concentrated than ECF in hypotonic dehydration, water

TABLE 23.2 Disturbances of Fluid and Electrolyte Balance

Mechanisms and Situations	Manifestations	Management and Nursing Care
	WATER DEPLETION	
Failure to absorb or reabsorb water Complete or sudden cessation of intake or prolonged diminished intake: • neglect of intake by self or caregiver—confused, psychotic, unconscious or helpless • loss from gastrointestinal tract—vomiting, diarrhoea, nasogastric suction, fistula Disturbed body fluid chemistry: inappropriate ADH secretion Excessive renal excretion: glycosuria (diabetes) Loss through skin or lungs: • excessive perspiration or evaporation—febrile states, hyperventilation, increased ambient temperature, increased activity (basal metabolic rate) • impaired skin integrity—transudate from injuries • haemorrhage Iatrogenic: • overzealous use of diuretics • improper perioperative fluid replacement • use of radiant warmer or phototherapy	General symptoms dependent to some extent on proportion of electrolytes lost with water Thirst Variable temperature—increased (infection) Dry skin and mucous membranes Poor skin turgor Poor perfusion (decreased pulse, slowed capillary refill time) Weight loss Fatigue Diminished urinary output Irritability and lethargy Tachycardia Tachypnoea Altered level of consciousness, disorientation Laboratory findings: • high urine specific gravity • increased haematocrit • variable serum electrolytes • variable urine volume • increased BUN • increased serum osmolality	Provide replacement of fluid losses commensurate with volume depletion. Provide maintenance fluids and electrolytes. Determine and correct cause of water depletion. Measure fluid intake and output. Monitor vital signs. Monitor urine specific gravity. Monitor body weight. Monitor serum electrolytes.
	WATER EXCESS	
Water intake in excess of output: • excessive oral intake • hypotonic fluid overload • plain water enemas Failure to excrete water in presence of normal intake: • kidney disease • congestive heart failure • malnutrition	Oedema: • generalised • pulmonary (moist rales or crackles) • intracutaneous (noted especially in loose areolar tissue) Elevated central venous pressure Hepatomegaly Slow, bounding pulse Weight gain Lethargy Increased spinal fluid pressure Central nervous system manifestations (seizures, coma) Laboratory findings: • low urine specific gravity • decreased serum electrolytes • decreased haematocrit • variable urine volume	Limit fluid intake. Administer diuretics. Monitor vital signs. Monitor neurological signs as necessary. Determine and treat cause of water excess. Analyse serum electrolytes frequently. Implement seizure precautions.
	SODIUM DEPLETION (HYPONATRAEMIA)	
Prolonged low-sodium diet Decreased sodium intake Fever Excess sweating Increased water intake without electrolytes Tachypnoea (infants) Cystic fibrosis Burns and wounds Vomiting, diarrhoea, nasogastric suction, fistulas Adrenal insufficiency Renal disease Diabetic ketoacidosis (DKA) Malnutrition	Associated with water loss: • same as with water loss—dehydration, weakness, dizziness, nausea, abdominal cramps, apprehension • mild—apathy, weakness, nausea, weak pulse • moderate—decreased BP, lethargy Laboratory findings: • sodium concentration < 130 mEq/L (may be normal if volume loss) • urine specific gravity depends on water deficit or excess	Determine and treat cause of sodium deficit. Administer IV fluids with appropriate saline concentration. Monitor fluid intake and output.

TABLE 23.2 Disturbances of Fluid and Electrolyte Balance—cont'd

Mechanisms and Situations	Manifestations	Management and Nursing Care
	SODIUM EXCESS (HYPERNATRAEMIA)	
High salt intake—enteral or IV Renal disease Fever Insufficient breast milk intake in neonate (dehydration hypernatraemia) High insensible water loss: • increased temperature • increased humidity • hyperventilation • diabetes insipidus • hyperglycaemia	Intense thirst Dry, sticky mucous membranes Flushed skin Temperature possibly increased Hoarseness Oliguria Nausea and vomiting Possible progression to disorientation, convulsions, muscle twitching, nuchal rigidity, lethargy at rest, hyperirritability when aroused Laboratory findings: • serum sodium concentration ≤ 150 mEq/L • high plasma volume • alkalosis	Determine and treat cause of sodium excess. Administer IV fluids as prescribed. Measure fluid intake and output. Monitor laboratory data. Monitor neurological status. Ensure adequate intake of breast milk and provide lactation assistance with new mother–baby pair before hospital discharge.
	POTASSIUM DEPLETION (HYPOKALAEMIA)	
Starvation Clinical conditions associated with poor food intake Malabsorption IV fluid without added potassium Gastrointestinal losses—diarrhoea, vomiting, fistulas, nasogastric suction Diuresis Administration of diuretics Administration of corticosteroids Diuretic phase of nephrotic syndrome Healing stage of burns Potassium-losing nephritis Hyperglycaemic diuresis (e.g. diabetes mellitus) Familial periodic paralysis IV administration of insulin in DKA Alkalosis	Muscle weakness, cramping, stiffness, paralysis, hyporeflexia Hypotension Cardiac arrhythmias, gallop rhythm Tachycardia or bradycardia Ileus Apathy, drowsiness Irritability Fatigue Laboratory findings: • decreased serum potassium concentration ≥ 3.5 mEq/L • abnormal ECG—notched or flattened T waves, decreased ST segment, premature ventricular contractions	Determine and treat cause of potassium deficit. Monitor vital signs, including ECG. Administer supplemental potassium. Assess for adequate renal output before administration. For IV replacement, administer potassium slowly. Always monitor ECG for IV bolus potassium replacement. For oral intake, offer high-potassium fluids and foods. Evaluate acid–base status.
	POTASSIUM EXCESS (HYPERKALAEMIA)	
Renal disease Renal failure Adrenal insufficiency (Addison disease) Associated with metabolic acidosis Too-rapid administration of IV potassium chloride Transfusion with old donor blood Severe dehydration Crushing injuries Burns Haemolysis Dehydration Potassium-sparing diuretics Increased intake of potassium (e.g. salt substitutes)	Muscle weakness, flaccid paralysis Twitching Hyperreflexia Bradycardia Ventricular fibrillation and cardiac arrest Oliguria Apnoea—respiratory arrest Laboratory findings: • high serum potassium concentration ≤ 5.5 mEq/L • variable urine volume • flat P wave on ECG, peaked T waves, widened QRS complex, increased PR interval	Determine and treat cause of potassium excess. Monitor vital signs, including ECG. Administer exchange resin, if prescribed. Administer IV fluids as prescribed. Administer IV insulin (if ordered) to facilitate movement of potassium into cells. Monitor potassium levels. Evaluate acid–base status.
	CALCIUM DEPLETION (HYPOCALCAEMIA)	
Inadequate dietary calcium Vitamin D deficiency Rapid transit through gastrointestinal tract Advanced renal insufficiency Administration of diuretics Hypoparathyroidism Alkalosis Calcium trapped in diseased tissues Increased serum protein (albumin) Cow's milk—tetany of the newborn (inappropriate calcium/phosphorus ratio in whole milk for newborn) Exchange transfusion with citrated blood Inadequate parenteral administration in diseased status	Neuromuscular irritability Tingling of nose, ears, fingertips, toes Tetany Laryngospasm Generalised convulsions May be changes in clotting Positive Chvostek and Trousseau signs Hypotension Cardiac arrest Laboratory findings: • decreased serum calcium concentration (8.8–10.8 mEq/L) or increased serum protein levels • prolonged QT interval	Determine and treat cause of calcium deficit. Administer oral calcium supplements as prescribed; administer IV slowly and diluted. Monitor IV site; calcium may cause vascular irritation. Monitor serum calcium, vitamin D and parathyroid levels. Monitor serum protein levels. Avoid cow's milk in infants younger than 12 months.

Continued

TABLE 23.2 Disturbances of Fluid and Electrolyte Balance—cont'd

Mechanisms and Situations	Manifestations	Management and Nursing Care
	CALCIUM EXCESS (HYPERCALCAEMIA)	
Acidosis Prolonged immobilisation Conditions associated with increased bone catabolism Hypoproteinaemia Kidney disease Hypervitaminosis D Hyperparathyroidism Hyperthyroidism Excessive IV or oral administration	Constipation Weakness, fatigue Nausea, vomiting Anorexia Dry mouth (thirst) Muscle hypotonicity Bradycardia or cardiac arrest Increased calcium concentration in urine, causing formation of kidney stones Laboratory findings: • increased serum calcium levels or decreased serum protein levels • prolonged QRS complex or PR interval, shortened QT interval	Determine and treat cause of calcium excess. Monitor serum calcium levels. Monitor ECG.

ADH, Antidiuretic hormone; *ECG*, electrocardiogram; *IV*, intravenous.

transfers from the ECF to the ICF to establish osmotic equilibrium. This movement further increases the ECF volume loss, and shock is a frequent result. Because there is a greater proportional loss of ECF in hypotonic dehydration, the physical signs tend to be more severe with smaller fluid losses than in isotonic or hypertonic dehydration. Plasma sodium concentrations are typically less than 135 mmol/L (Farrell 2017, Government of Western Australia Child and Adolescent Health Service 2018).

Hypertonic (hyperosmotic or hypernatraemic) dehydration results from water loss in excess of electrolyte loss and is usually caused by a proportionately larger loss of water or a larger intake of electrolytes. This type of dehydration is the most dangerous and requires much more specific fluid therapy. This sometimes occurs in infants with diarrhoea who are given fluids by mouth that contain large amounts of solute or in children receiving high-protein nasogastric tube feedings that place an excessive solute load on the kidneys. This type of dehydration can be a result of other causes such as excessive administration of intravenous (IV) saline, diabetes insipidus, heat stroke and increased insensible water loss which can occur as a result of extensive burns or excessive hyperventilation (Farrell 2017). In hypertonic dehydration, fluid shifts from the lesser concentration of the ICF to the ECF. Plasma sodium concentration is greater than 145 mmol/L (Farrell 2017).

Because the ECF volume is proportionately larger, hypertonic dehydration consists of a greater degree of water loss for the same intensity of physical signs. Shock is less apparent in hypotonic dehydration. However, neurological disturbances, such as seizures, are more likely to occur. Cerebral changes are serious and may result in permanent damage. These include disturbance of consciousness, poor ability to focus attention, lethargy, increased muscle tone with hyperreflexia, and hyperirritability to stimuli (e.g. tactile, auditory, bright lights).

Degree of Dehydration

A determination of the type and degree of dehydration is necessary to develop an effective plan of therapy. The degree of dehydration has been described as a percentage of body weight dehydrated: mild, 3%; moderate, 5%; and severe, more than 10% (Carson et al 2016, Greenbaum 2015). Water constitutes only 60% to 70% of the infant's weight. However, adipose tissue contains little water and is highly variable in individual infants and children. A more accurate means of describing dehydration is to reflect acute fluid loss (timeframe of ≥ 48 hours) in millilitres per kilogram of body weight. For example, a loss of 50 mL/kg is considered to be a mild fluid loss, whereas a loss of 100 mL/kg produces severe dehydration.

Weight is the most important determinant of the per cent of total body fluid loss in infants and younger children. However, often the pre-illness weight is unknown. Other predictors of fluid loss include a changing level of consciousness (irritability to lethargy), altered response to stimuli, decreased skin elasticity and turgor, prolonged capillary refill (> 2 seconds), increased heart rate and sunken eyes and fontanels.

Clinical signs provide clues to the extent of dehydration (Table 23.3). The earliest detectable sign is usually tachycardia, followed by dry skin and mucous membranes, sunken fontanels, signs of circulatory failure (coolness and mottling of extremities), loss of skin elasticity and prolonged capillary filling time (see Table 23.4 for clinical manifestations of dehydration and Fig 23.3 for signs of dehydration). There is evidence that the clinical signs of abnormal capillary refill, abnormal skin turgor and abnormal respiratory pattern are the most useful in predicting dehydration of 5% or more in children (Carson et al 2017).

Compensatory mechanisms attempt to maintain fluid volume by adjusting to these losses. Interstitial fluid moves into the vascular compartment to maintain the blood volume in response to haemoconcentration and hypovolaemia, and vasoconstriction of peripheral arterioles helps maintain pumping pressure. When fluid losses exceed the body's ability to sustain blood volume and blood pressure, circulation is seriously compromised and the blood pressure falls. This results in tissue hypoxia with accumulation of lactic acid, pyruvate and other acid metabolites, which contribute to the development of metabolic acidosis.

Renal compensation is impaired by reduced blood flow through the kidneys, and little urine is formed. Increased serum osmolality stimulates the secretion of **antidiuretic hormone** (ADH) to conserve fluid and initiates the renin–angiotensin mechanisms in the kidney, causing further vasoconstriction. Aldosterone is released to promote sodium retention and conserve water in the kidneys. If dehydration increases in severity, urine formation is greatly diminished and metabolites and hydrogen ions that are normally excreted by this route are retained.

Shock, a common manifestation of severe depletion of ECF volume, is preceded by tachycardia and signs of poor perfusion and tissue oxygenation (by pulse oximeter readings). Peripheral circulation is poor as a result of reduced blood volume; therefore, the skin is cool and mottled with decreased capillary filling. Impaired kidney circulation often leads to **oliguria** and **azotaemia**. Although low blood pressure may accompany other symptoms of shock, in infants and young children it

TABLE 23.3 Evaluating Extent of Dehydration

	LEVEL OF DEHYDRATION		
Clinical Signs	**Mild**	**Moderate**	**Severe**
Weight loss—infants	3%–5%	6%–9%	≤ 10%
Weight loss—children	3%–4%	6%–8%	10%
Pulse	Normal	Slightly increased	Very increased
Respiratory rate	Normal	Slight tachypnoea (rapid)	Hyperpnoea (deep and rapid)
Blood pressure	Normal	Normal to orthostatic (> 10 mmHg change)	Orthostatic to shock
Behaviour	Normal	Irritable, more thirsty	Hyperirritable to lethargic
Thirst	Slight	Moderate	Intense
Mucous membranes*	Normal (moist)	Dry	Parched
Tears	Present	Decreased	Absent, sunken eyes
Anterior fontanel	Normal	Normal to sunken	Sunken
External jugular vein	Visible when supine	Not visible except with supraclavicular pressure	Not visible even with supraclavicular pressure
Skin*	Capillary refill > 2 sec	Slowed capillary refill (2–4 sec [decreased turgor])	Very delayed capillary refill (> 4 sec) and tenting; skin cool, acrocyanotic or mottled
Urine	Decreased	Oliguria	Oliguria or anuria

*These signs are less prominent in patients who have hypernatraemia.
Data from Jospe, N., & Forbes, G. (1996). Fluids and electrolytes—clinical aspects. Paediatrics in Review, 17(11), 395–403; and Steiner, M. J., DeWalt, D. A., & Byerly, J. S. (2004). Is this child dehydrated? Journal of the American Medical Association, 291(22), 2746–2754.

TABLE 23.4 Clinical Manifestations of Dehydration

Manifestation	**Isotonic (Loss of Water and Salt)**	**Hypotonic (Loss of Salt in Excess of Water)**	**Hypertonic (Loss of Water in Excess of Salt)**
Skin			
• Colour	Grey	Grey	Grey
• Temperature	Cold	Cold	Cold or hot
• Turgor	Poor	Very poor	Fair
• Feel	Dry	Clammy	Thickened, doughy
Mucous membranes	Dry	Slightly moist	Parched
Tearing and salivation	Absent	Absent	Absent
Eyeball	Sunken	Sunken	Sunken
Fontanel	Sunken	Sunken	Sunken
Body temperature	Subnormal or elevated	Subnormal or elevated	Subnormal or elevated
Pulse	Rapid	Very rapid	Moderately rapid
Respirations	Rapid	Rapid	Rapid
Behaviour	Irritable to lethargic	Lethargic or comatose; convulsions	Marked lethargy with extreme hyperirritability on stimulation

is usually a late sign and may herald the onset of cardiovascular collapse (Schlapbach et al 2015).

In the examination of an infant or younger child, one of the most important determinants of the extent of dehydration is body weight because this can assist in determining the percentage of total body fluid lost; however, because the pre-illness weight is often unknown, clinical manifestations must be evaluated (see Research Focus box). Important clinical manifestations include changing sensorium (irritability to lethargy); decreased response to stimuli; integumentary changes (decreased elasticity and turgor); prolonged capillary refill; increased heart rate; sunken eyes; and, in infants, sunken fontanels. Using multiple predictors increases the sensitivity of assessing the fluid deficit, and studies have shown a reasonably high degree of agreement between experienced observers in assessment of the level of dehydration. Objective signs of dehydration are present at a fluid deficit of less than 5%.

RESEARCH FOCUS

Paediatric Dehydration

In past reviews of paediatric dehydration assessment, the best three individual examination signs for assessing dehydration were prolonged capillary refill time (> 2 seconds), abnormal skin turgor and abnormal respiratory pattern (Emond 2009). A recent meta-analysis of nine studies of over 1000 children revealed that clinical dehydration assessment scales provide some improved diagnostic accuracy, but it is still suboptimal. Current evidence from this review did not support the routine use of ultrasound or urinalysis to determine dehydration severity (Freedman et al 2015). There is some evidence to support serum urea and creatinine as markers for dehydration along with bicarbonate that is consistently decreased in moderate to severe dehydration (Hoxha et al 2014, Whitney et al 2016).

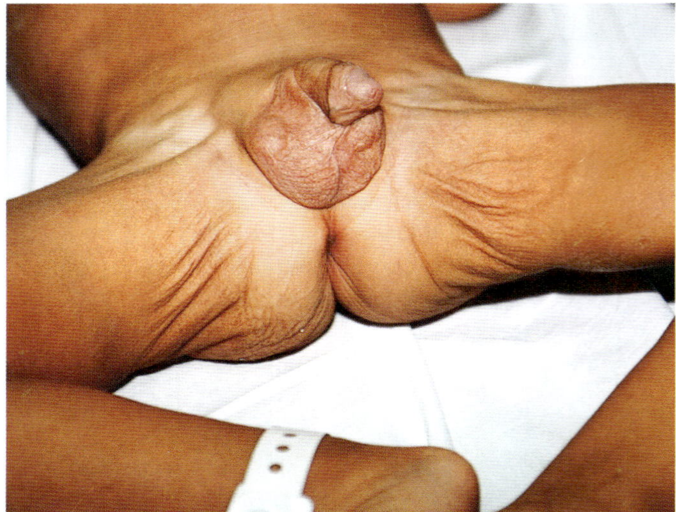

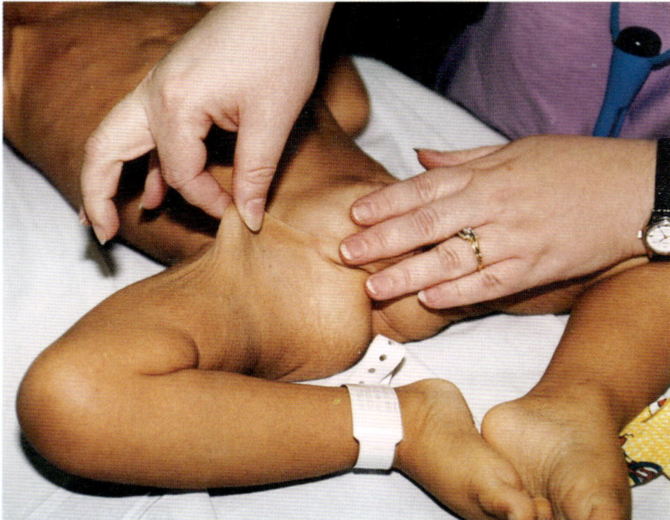

Fig 23.3 Loss of skin elasticity because of dehydration.

Therapeutic Management

Medical management is directed at correcting the fluid imbalance and treating the underlying cause. When the child is alert, awake and not in danger, correction of dehydration may be attempted with oral fluid administration. Most cases of dehydration are mild and can be managed at home by this method. Several commercial rehydration fluids are available for use (see Table 25.4). Oral rehydration management consists of replacement of fluid loss over 4 to 6 hours, replacement of continuing losses and provision for maintenance fluid requirements. In general, the mildly/moderately dehydrated child may be given 0.5 mL/kg every 5 minutes of **oral rehydration solution (ORS)** (RCHM 2020). The child with fluid losses from diarrhoea may be given an additional 10 mL/kg for each stool (Greenbaum 2015). Amounts and rates are determined from body weight and severity of dehydration and are increased if rehydration is incomplete or if excess losses continue, until the child is well hydrated and the basic problem is under control.

The child may not be thirsty even though dehydrated and may refuse oral fluids initially for fear of continued emesis (if occurring) or because of decreased strength, oral stomatitis or thrush. In such children rehydration may proceed by administering 2 to 5 mL of ORS by a syringe or small medication cup every 2 to 3 minutes until the child is able to tolerate larger amounts; if the child has emesis, administering small amounts (5 mL) of ORS every 5 minutes or so may help overcome fluid deficit, and the emesis will often lessen over time (Hendrickson et al 2017). Administration of antiemetics is not recommended due to high risk of side effects, so only a single dose of ondansetron should be administered (RCHM 2020). Oral rehydration therapy (ORT) is effective for treating mild or moderate dehydration in children, is less expensive and involves fewer complications than therapy (Carson et al 2016, Kleinman & Greer 2014). ORSs enhance and promote the reabsorption of sodium and water. These solutions greatly reduce vomiting and the need for IV infusions (Hendrickson et al 2017). ORSs, including lower-osmolarity ORS (240 mmol/L) such as Hydralyte and Gastrolyte, are available in Australia and New Zealand as commercially prepared solutions and are successful in treating the majority of infants with dehydration. See the Quality Patient Outcomes box. (Also see Diarrhoea, Chapter 25, for a complete discussion of fluid replacement therapy for dehydration.)

QUALITY PATIENT OUTCOMES

Fluid Volume Deficit

- Moist mucous membranes
- Sodium and potassium within normal limits
- Voiding (> 1 mL/kg/hr)
- Capillary refill of 2 seconds or less
- Skin turgor brisk
- Fluid intake and output balanced

Parenteral Fluid Therapy. Parenteral fluid therapy is initiated whenever the child is unable to ingest sufficient amounts of fluid and electrolytes to meet ongoing daily physiological losses, replace previous deficits and replace ongoing abnormal losses. Patients who usually require IV fluids are those with severe dehydration, those with uncontrollable vomiting, those who are unable to drink for any reason (e.g. extreme fatigue, coma) or those with severe gastric distension.

Because dehydration (volume depletion) constitutes a great threat to life, the first priority is the restoration of circulation by rapid expansion of the ECF volume to treat or prevent shock. IV administration of fluid begins immediately, although the exact nature of the dehydration and the serum electrolyte values are not known. The solution selected is based on what is known regarding the probable type and cause of the dehydration. This usually involves an isotonic solution such as 0.9% sodium chloride or Ringer's lactated solution, both of which are close to the body's serum osmolality of 285 to 300 mOsm/kg and do not contain glucose (which is contraindicated in the early treatment stages of rehydration, but especially in diabetic ketoacidosis). It is recommended that the fluid for rehydration should contain glucose as children with dehydration tend to be at a high risk for hypoglycaemia (RCHM 2020).

Parenteral rehydration therapy has three phases. The initial therapy is used to expand ECF volume quickly and to improve circulatory and renal function. During initial therapy, an isotonic electrolyte solution is used at a rate of 20 mL/kg, given as an IV bolus over 5 to 10 minutes and repeated as necessary after assessment of the child's response to therapy with repeat boluses of 10 to 20 mL/kg until reversal of signs of shock then maintenance IV therapy commenced (RCHM 2020). In a meta-analysis of 10 randomised clinical trials, isotonic fluids were found safer than hypotonic fluids in preventing severe hyponatraemia following administration (Shukla et al 2016, Wang et al 2014). Subsequent therapy is used to replace deficits, meet maintenance water and electrolyte requirements and catch up with ongoing losses. Water and sodium requirements for the deficit, maintenance and ongoing losses are calculated at 8-hour intervals, taking into consideration the amount of fluids given with the initial boluses and the amount administered during the first 24-hour period. With improved circulation during this phase, water and electrolyte deficits can be evaluated and acid–base status can be corrected either directly through the administration of fluids or indirectly through improved renal function. Potassium is withheld until kidney function is restored and assessed and circulation has improved.

The final phase of therapy allows the patient to return to normal and begin oral feedings, with a gradual correction of total body deficits. The potassium loss in ICF is replaced slowly by way of the ECF. The body fat and protein stores are replaced through diet. If the child is unable to eat or if feeding aggravates a chronic condition, IV maintenance fluids are provided.

Although the initial phase of fluid replacement is rapid in both isotonic and hypotonic dehydration, it is contraindicated in hypertonic dehydration because of the risk of water intoxication, especially in the brain cells, specifically the central pontine cells. Central pontine myelinolysis may occur with an overcorrection of fluid deficit and an overly rapid correction of serum sodium concentration (Greenbaum 2015). There is an apparent lag time for sodium to reach a steady state when diffusing in and out of brain cells, whereas water diffuses almost instantaneously. Consequently, rapid administration of fluid will cause equally rapid diffusion of water into the dehydrated brain cells, causing marked cerebral oedema. Because ECF volume is maintained relatively well in hypertonic as opposed to the other types of dehydration, shock is not a usual manifestation.

Water Intoxication

Water intoxication, or water overload, refers to hyponatraemia as a result of excessive intake of water and is observed less often than dehydration. However, it is important that nurses and others who care for children are alert to this possibility in certain situations. Children who ingest excessive amounts of electrolyte-free water develop a concurrent decrease in serum sodium accompanied by central nervous system (CNS) symptoms. It is important to note that water intoxication can lead to coma, brain damage and even death; therefore, water intoxication needs to be protected because children are at risk of this due to immature kidneys. There is a large urinary output, and because water moves into the brain more rapidly than sodium moves out, the child may also exhibit irritability, somnolence, headache, vomiting, diarrhoea or generalised seizures. The affected child usually appears well hydrated but may be oedematous or even dehydrated.

Fluid intoxication can occur during acute IV water overloading, too-rapid dialysis, tap water enemas, feeding of incorrectly mixed infant formula, or excess water ingestion, or with too-rapid reduction of glucose levels in diabetic ketoacidosis (Greenbaum 2015). Patients with CNS infections occasionally retain excessive amounts of water. Administration of inappropriate hypotonic solutions (e.g. 0.45% sodium chloride) may cause a rapid reduction in sodium and result in symptoms of water overload.

A number of clinicians have reported water intoxication in infants after swimming lessons, in waterbirths with excessive enema administration and with gastric lavage (Rodgers & Wilson 2017). Although they hold their breath, some infants apparently swallow a large amount of water during repeated submersion. Anticipatory guidance to parents should include a discussion of swimming instruction and advice to stop a lesson if the child swallows unusual amounts of water or exhibits any symptoms of hyponatraemia.

Oedema

Oedema represents an abnormal accumulation of fluid within the interstitial tissue and subsequent tissue expansion and develops when a defect in the normal cardiovascular circulation or a failure in the lymphatic drainage to remove the increased amounts occurs. The processes responsible for fluid removal include venous hydrostatic pressure, oncotic pressure of intravascular and interstitial spaces, an intact semipermeable capillary wall, tissue tension and lymphatic flow.

Mechanisms of Oedema Formation

A defect of any of the homeostatic mechanisms maintaining fluid balance can cause accumulation of interstitial fluid. Disequilibrium results from anything that: (1) alters the retention of sodium, such as renal disease or hormonal influences; (2) affects the formation or destruction of plasma proteins, such as starvation or liver disease; or (3) alters membrane permeability, such as minimal change nephrotic syndrome or trauma.

Oedema may be localised to a small or large area, such as that occurring in urticaria, infection and pulmonary congestion, or it can be generalised, as in the hypoproteinemia of the nephrotic syndrome and starvation. A severe, generalised accumulation of great amounts of fluid in all body tissues is termed **anasarca**.

Increased Venous Pressure. The colloidal osmotic pressure of the plasma proteins draws fluid back into the vascular system as long as this force is greater than the venous hydrostatic pressure. However, when the venous pressure increases, fluid tends to be retained in the interstitial spaces. This can occur when an individual remains in the same position for a long time, such as swollen ankles and feet after standing or sitting for long periods. Constrictive dressings or restraints applied too tightly to extremities will obstruct venous return, increase venous and capillary pressure and cause oedema. The most graphic pathological illustrations are pulmonary oedema caused by pulmonary circulation overload in cardiac defects with a left-to-right shunt and ascites caused by portal hypertension. Oedema from any cause is increased in dependent areas because of this added factor of increased venous hydrostatic pressure and the gravitational effects in these areas.

Capillary Permeability. Damage to capillary walls or alteration in their permeability permits exudation of plasma protein into the interstitial space. Most often this occurs as local oedema, such as that manifested in inflammatory and hypersensitivity reactions. Capillary damage from burns allows extensive exudation of protein-rich fluid into the interstitial spaces to compound oedema formation.

Diminished Plasma Proteins. A fall in plasma protein levels hampers the osmotic pull back into the vessels. Consequently, fluid remains in the interstitial spaces. Although other factors play a role, such as hydrostatic pressure of both the arterial vascular system and the tissues and sodium concentration, significantly low protein levels (< 4.5 mg/dL) are associated with oedema. Examples of this are the massive albumin losses of the minimal change nephrotic syndrome, diminished serum protein from insufficient dietary protein and (sometimes) haemodilution of plasma proteins from IV fluid administration in chronic dehydration.

Lymphatic Obstruction. Obstruction of lymph flow creates oedema high in protein content. This occurs infrequently in childhood but can result from trauma to the lymphatic glands or from removal of lymph nodes.

Tissue Tension. Tissue hydrostatic pressure is ordinarily of little consequence. However, it plays a significant role in determining distribution of oedema fluid in certain pathological conditions. Loose tissues allow a greater amount of fluid accumulation than tissues that are tightly bound by dense fibrous bands in which tissue pressure rapidly increases to limit further extravasation of fluid. Oedema appears earlier and more readily in loose structures such as those in the periorbital and genital tissues. The alveolar structure of lung tissue is probably a contributing factor in pulmonary oedema, as well as in increased hydrostatic pressure in the pulmonary vessels.

Other Factors in Oedema Formation. Any factor that causes sodium retention by the kidneys will produce or augment oedema formation. This includes stimulation of the renin–angiotensin–aldosterone mechanisms for sodium reabsorption created by the diminished plasma volume in oedema, which resulted from primary causes. The salt-retaining property of steroids is responsible for the oedema associated with their administration.

Several types of oedema exist, all of which can provide a palpable swelling of the interstitial space that is either localised or generalised. These include the following:

- peripheral oedema, or localised or generalised palpable swelling of the interstitial space
- **ascites**, or the accumulation of fluid in the abdominal cavity (usually associated with renal or liver abnormalities)
- pulmonary oedema, which occurs when interstitial volume increases
- cerebral oedema, which is a particularly threatening form of oedema caused by trauma, infection or other aetiological factors, including vascular overload or injudicious IV administration of hypotonic solutions
- overall fluid gain, especially seen in patients with kidney disease.

Assessment

Generalised oedema resulting from any of the previously listed types is manifested by swelling in the extremities, face, perineum and torso. Loss of normal skin creases may be assessed. Daily weights are more sensitive indicators of water gain or loss and should be obtained. Abdominal girth measurement changes may also be an indicator of oedema in children. Pitting oedema may occur and can be assessed by pressing the fingertip against a bony prominence for 5 seconds. If the tissue rebounds immediately on removing the finger, the patient does not have pitting oedema.

Therapeutic Management

The primary goal in the management of oedema is treatment of the underlying disease process, which is discussed elsewhere in relation to the specific disorder. However, an essential aspect in the management of any fluid overload is early recognition, in which nurses play a vital role. The management of oedema is discussed throughout the text with specific conditions. See the Nursing Care Considerations box.

NURSING CARE CONSIDERATIONS

Fluid Volume Excess

- Fluid intake and output balanced
- No oedema
- No weight gain
- No respiratory distress related to fluid volume excess

NURSING RESPONSIBILITIES IN FLUID AND ELECTROLYTE DISTURBANCES

Nursing observation and intervention are essential to the detection and therapeutic management of disturbances in fluid and electrolyte balance. Imbalances may be precipitated by a variety of circumstances, and the balance may be so precarious, especially in newborns and infants, that changes can take place in a very short time. Therefore, an important nursing responsibility is anticipation and perceptive observation for any signs of imbalance, particularly in those situations and conditions in which imbalance is likely to occur. Conditions in which changes can develop with surprising rapidity in young children include: diarrhoea; vomiting; sweating; fever; disorders such as type 1 diabetes, bowel surgery, renal disease and cardiac anomalies; administration of certain drugs such as diuretics and steroids; and trauma, such as major surgery, burns and other extensive injury.

Assessment

Whether the child is at home, in the practitioner's office or clinic or in the hospital, nursing assessment is an essential part of the nursing care plan. The assessment of suspected or potential fluid and electrolyte disturbance begins with the observation of general appearance. Ill children usually have drawn expressions, have dry mucous membranes and lips and 'look sick'. Loss of appetite is one of the first behaviours observed in most childhood illnesses, and the infant's or child's activity level is diminished from baseline or usual activities. The child is irritable, seeks the parent's comfort and attention and displays purposeless movements and inappropriate responses to people and familiar objects. In some cases the child may not protest advances by the healthcare worker and procedures such as taking vital signs or starting an IV infusion. These are signs that the child truly feels bad and that the condition is serious and immediate intervention is necessary. As the child's illness and level of dehydration become more severe, irritability progresses to lethargy and even unconsciousness.

History

The nurse can obtain much of the information regarding the child's behaviour from the parent or primary caregiver. In addition to initial observations, a good history is extremely valuable to the assessment. The amount and type of fluid intake and output (I&O) (especially abnormal output) are important. An accurate estimate of fluid losses is beyond the capacity of history givers, but rough estimates of excessive fluid losses or diminished output can usually be obtained from information such as the number and consistency of stools the child has passed in the past 24 hours, the number of times the child voided and the type and amount of food and fluid ingested or vomited. For an infant, ask about the number of wet nappies in the past 24 hours. Parents frequently omit this information from their discussion with the health professional. Having the parents' estimate the amount of urine in the nappy at each void is of little value because of the absorbent nappy material, which pulls fluids away from the child's skin. Encourage new parents of a newborn to record on a piece of paper the number of wet nappies and the times the infant has breastfed or bottle-fed.

A history of gradual weight gain and observations of any puffiness, especially in areas with less dense tissues (periorbital, scrotal), or 'clothes fitting tighter' offer early clues to oedema. A history of excessive water intake, especially when associated with diminished output, is important in assessing oedema and water intoxication.

Clinical Observations

Fever and infection can also produce tachycardia, the earliest manifestation of dehydration. Therefore, these are considered in the assessment of hydration status. Dry skin and mucous membranes (oral) usually appear early. A sunken fontanel is a useful observation if the status of the fontanel is known when the infant is healthy. Signs of circulatory failure usually indicate severe dehydration because compensatory mechanisms are able to sustain blood pressure in the low-normal range for some time. Loss of skin elasticity, generally manifested in children less than 2 years of age, is measured by the time it takes for pinched abdominal skin to recoil. This sign is also observed in undernourished children. Also, in hypertonic dehydration the skin has a smooth, velvety feel before it develops disturbed elasticity.

Assess capillary filling time by pinching a toe or a thumb or lightly pressing the abdominal skin and estimating the time it takes for the blood to return. Capillary filling time in mild dehydration is less than 2 seconds, increasing to more than 4 seconds in severe dehydration. The technique is effective in children of all ages. However, it can be altered in the presence of heart failure, which affects circulation time, and hypertonic dehydration, in which fluid loss is primarily intracellular. Additional clinical signs observed in children with dehydration include cool mottled extremities, sunken eyes, tachypnoea and changes in sensorium.

When caring for the acutely ill child, assess vital signs frequently and record weight frequently during the initial phase of therapy. It is important to use the same scale each time the child is weighed and to predetermine the weight of any equipment or devices that must remain attached during the weighing process, including arm boards, and any clothing the child might be wearing. Take routine weights at the same time each day. One of the nurse's most important roles in fluid and electrolyte disturbance is related to I&O. Accurate measurements are essential to the assessment of fluid balance. Measurements from all sources—including gastrointestinal and parenteral I&O from urine, stools, vomitus, fistulas, nasogastric suction, sweat and drainage from wounds—must be taken into consideration (see also Chapter 22).

Shock

Shock, or **circulatory failure**, is a complex clinical syndrome characterised by inadequate tissue perfusion to meet the metabolic demands of the body, resulting in cellular dysfunction and eventual organ failure. Although the causes are different, the physiological consequences are the same and include hypotension, tissue hypoxia and metabolic acidosis. Circulatory failure in children is a result of hypovolaemia, altered peripheral vascular resistance or pump failure.

Aetiology

The most common type of circulatory failure in infants and children is **hypovolaemic shock**, which follows a reduction in circulating blood volume related to blood loss (e.g. trauma, major bleeding), plasma losses (e.g. burns, peritonitis) or extracellular fluid losses (e.g. diarrhoea, dehydration) beyond the child's physiological ability to compensate. **Cardiogenic shock** results from impaired cardiac muscle function that leads to decreased cardiac output. This type of shock may be seen after cardiac surgery and in children with acute dysrhythmias, congestive heart failure, trauma or cardiomyopathy. **Distributive shock**, or vasogenic shock, results from a vascular abnormality that produces maldistribution of blood supply throughout the body. This classification includes: (1) neurogenic shock, characterised by massive vasodilation resulting from the loss of sympathetic nervous system tone, which can occur with spinal cord injuries; (2) anaphylactic shock, characterised by a hypersensitivity reaction that causes massive vasodilation and capillary leak and may occur with drug or latex allergy, insect stings or blood transfusion; and (3) septic shock, characterised by a decreased cardiac output and derangements in the peripheral circulation in response to a severe, overwhelming infection. **Obstructive shock** may resemble hypovolaemic shock but is caused by cardiac tamponade, tension pneumothorax, ductal-dependent congenital heart lesions or massive pulmonary embolism (Seckel & Lin 2020, Perkin et al 2013). The types of shock are described in Box 23.2. *Neurogenic shock* occurs in association with spinal cord injury and is discussed in Chapter 30.

BOX 23.2 Types of Shock

Hypovolaemic

Characteristics

- Reduction in size of vascular compartment
- Falling BP
- Poor capillary filling
- Low CVP

Most Frequent Causes

- Blood loss (haemorrhagic shock)—Trauma, gastrointestinal bleeding, intracranial haemorrhage
- Plasma loss—Increased capillary permeability associated with sepsis and acidosis, hypoproteinaemia, burns, peritonitis
- Extracellular fluid loss—Vomiting, diarrhoea, glycosuric diuresis, heatstroke

Distributive

Characteristics

- Reduction in peripheral vascular resistance
- Profound inadequacies in tissue perfusion
- Increased venous capacity and pooling
- Acute reduction in return blood flow to the heart
- Diminished cardiac output

Most Frequent Causes

- Anaphylaxis (anaphylactic shock)—Extreme allergy or hypersensitivity to a foreign substance
- Sepsis (septic shock, bacteraemic shock, endotoxic shock)—Overwhelming sepsis and circulating bacterial toxins
- Loss of neuronal control (neurogenic shock)—Interruption of neuronal transmission (spinal cord injury)
- Myocardial depression and peripheral dilation—Exposure to anaesthesia or ingestion of barbiturates, tranquillisers, opioids, antihypertensive agents or ganglionic blocking agents

Cardiogenic

Characteristic

- Decreased cardiac output

Most Frequent Causes

- After surgery for congenital heart disease
- Primary pump failure—Myocarditis, myocardial trauma, biochemical derangements, heart failure
- Dysrhythmias—Supraventricular tachycardia, atrioventricular block and ventricular dysrhythmias; secondary to myocarditis or biochemical abnormalities (occasionally)

Obstructive

Characteristic

- Mechanical obstruction of blood flow to or from the heart

Most Frequ`ent Causes

- Tension pneumothorax
- Cardiac tamponade
- Pulmonary embolism
- Congenital cardiac defects with left ventricular outflow tract obstruction (e.g. coarctation of the aorta, interrupted aortic arch, critical aortic stenosis)

BP, blood pressure; CVP, central venous pressure.

Source: Modified from Ralston, M., Hazinski, M. F., & Zaritsky, A. L. (Eds.). (2006). Pediatric advanced life support: Provider manual. Dallas, TX: American Heart Association; Perkin, R. M., de Caen, A. R., Berg, M. D., et al. (2013). Shock, cardiac arrest, and resuscitation. In M. F. Hazinski (Ed.), Nursing care of the critically ill child. St Louis, MO: Elsevier Mosby.

Pathophysiology

The circulatory system of the healthy child is able to transport oxygen and nutrients to meet the essential needs of body tissues and can respond to increased demands resulting from an elevated metabolic rate. The cardiac output and distribution to the various body tissues can change rapidly in response to intrinsic (myocardial and intravascular) or extrinsic (neuronal) control mechanisms. In shock states these mechanisms are altered or challenged.

Reduced blood flow, as in hypovolaemic shock, causes diminished venous return to the heart, low central venous pressure (CVP), low cardiac output and hypotension. The reduced intravascular volume triggers a chain of compensatory mechanisms. Fluid is mobilised from the extracellular fluid compartment. Vasomotor centres in the medulla are signalled, causing depressed vagal activity and increased sympathetic activity, which increase the force and rate of cardiac contraction and constrict the arterioles and veins, thereby increasing peripheral vascular resistance.

Simultaneously the lowered blood volume also leads to the release of large amounts of catecholamines, antidiuretic hormone, adrenocorticosteroids and aldosterone in an effort to conserve body fluids. The catecholamines augment the vasomotor activity to produce vasoconstriction and reduce blood flow to the skin, kidneys, muscles and splanchnic viscera in order to shunt the available blood to the brain and heart. Consequently, the skin feels cold and clammy, there is poor capillary filling and glomerular filtration and urinary output are significantly reduced.

Impaired perfusion to the peripheral tissues also produces metabolic alterations. Oxygen depletion causes the cells to revert to anaerobic glycolytic metabolism, forming pyruvic acid; pyruvic acid is then converted to lactic acid, producing lactic acidosis. The acidosis places an extra burden on the lungs as they attempt to compensate for the metabolic acidosis by increasing the respiratory rate. Impaired cellular uptake and metabolism of glucose create an early, transient hyperglycaemia. When plasma fluid is lost, haemoconcentration and diminished blood flow increase the viscosity of the blood and further impair perfusion.

Prolonged vasoconstriction results in fatigue, and the release of vasodilator substances such as histamine leads to vasodilation. Venules, which are less sensitive to vasodilator substances, remain constricted for a time. This causes massive pooling in the capillary and venular beds and transudation of plasma fluid into the tissues, which further depletes blood volume.

Complications of shock create further hazards. CNS hypoperfusion may eventually lead to cerebral oedema, cortical infarction or intraventricular haemorrhage. Renal hypoperfusion causes renal ischaemia with possible tubular or glomerular necrosis and renal vein thrombosis. Reduced blood flow to the lungs can interfere with surfactant secretion and result in shock lung or acute respiratory distress syndrome (ARDS). ARDS is characterised by sudden pulmonary congestion and atelectasis with formation of a hyaline membrane and subsequent lung tissue injury. (See Chapter 26.) Gastrointestinal (GI) tract bleeding and perforation are always a possibility following splanchnic ischaemia and necrosis of intestinal mucosa. Metabolic complications of shock may include hypoglycaemia, hypocalcaemia and other electrolyte disturbances.

Shock states characterised by vascular abnormalities (distributive shock) have a somewhat different pathophysiological pattern of haemodynamic collapse. In neurogenic shock, the sympathetic nervous system mechanisms that maintain vascular tone are interrupted, causing reduced vascular resistance and peripheral pooling of blood; with this increased vascular capacity there is loss of effective circulating blood volume. Septic shock produces a hyperdynamic state in which there is often an elevated plasma volume and reduced peripheral resistance that lead to widespread vasodilation. In many cases there is a high cardiac output caused by the vasodilation in infected tissues and elsewhere, plus a high metabolic rate resulting from the elevated body temperature. Degenerating tissues cause aggregation of red blood cells and sludging of the blood. Development of disseminated intravascular coagulation, triggered by either the degenerating tissue or bacterial toxins, consumes the clotting factors and produces widespread haemorrhages.

Clinical Manifestations

Shock can be regarded as a form of compensation for circulatory failure and, because of its progressive nature, can be divided into two stages or phases: **compensated** and **hypotensive** (previously referred to as decompensated). Cardiac arrest represents irreversible shock. At all stages the principal differentiating signs are the degree of tachycardia and perfusion to extremities, the level of consciousness and blood pressure (BP). Additional signs or modifications of these more universal signs may be present, depending on the type and cause of the shock. Initially, the child's ability to compensate is effective; therefore, early signs are subtle. As the shock state advances, signs are more obvious and indicate early decompensation (Table 23.5).

In early septic shock, there are chills, fever and vasodilation, with increased cardiac output that results in warm, flushed skin (hyperdynamic, or 'warm' shock). A later and ominous development is disseminated intravascular coagulation (see Chapter 28), the major haematological complication of septic shock. Anaphylactic shock is frequently accompanied by urticaria and angioneurotic oedema, which is life-threatening when it involves the respiratory passages (see Anaphylaxis, later in this chapter).

Compensated Shock. When vital organ function is maintained by intrinsic mechanisms and the child's ability to compensate is effective,

TABLE 23.5 Clinical Signs of Shock

Clinical Signs	Hypovolaemic Shock	Distributive Shock	Cardiogenic Shock	Obstructive Shock
Respiratory rate	Normal to increased	Normal to increased	Laboured	Laboured
Breath sounds	Normal	Normal (crackles may/may not be present)	Crackles, grunting	Crackles, grunting
Systolic blood pressure	Compensated-normal	Compensated-normal	Hypotensive-low	Hypotensive-low
Pulse pressure	Narrow	Variable	Narrow	Narrow
Heart rate	Tachycardia	Tachycardia	Tachycardia	
Peripheral pulses	Weak	Bounding or weak	Weak	
Skin	Pale, cool	Warm or cool	Pale, cool	
Capillary refill	Delayed (> 2 sec)	Variable	Delayed (> 2 sec)	
Urine output	Decreased (< 1 mL/kg/hr [<30 kg]; < 30–50 mL/kg/hr [> 30 kg])			
Level of consciousness	Irritable early	Late, lethargic		

Source: Data from Chameides, L., Samson, R., Schexnayder, S. M., et al. (Eds.). (2011). Pediatric advanced life support: Provider manual. Dallas, TX: American Heart Association. Part 6: Recognition of Shock (Figure 2, p. 83, Recognition of Shock Flowchart).

cardiac output and systemic arterial BP are usually normal or increased. However, blood flow is generally uneven or maldistributed in the microcirculation. Early clinical signs are subtle and include apprehension, irritability, normal BP, narrowing pulse pressure, thirst, pallor and diminished urinary output.

NURSING CARE CONSIDERATIONS

Unexplained mild tachycardia and a decrease in perfusion of the hands and feet are differentiating features of compensated shock.

Hypotensive (Decompensated) Shock. As shock progresses, perfusion in the microcirculation becomes marginal despite compensatory adjustments, and the signs are more obvious and indicate early decompensation. These signs are: tachypnoea; moderate metabolic acidosis; oliguria; and cool, pale extremities with decreased skin turgor and poor capillary filling. Hypotensive shock may be differentiated from compensated shock by evaluating BP; the child in hypotensive shock will have a low BP, but hypotension is a late finding. Another clinical sign of hypotensive shock is a change in level of consciousness as brain perfusion declines. The outcomes of circulatory failure that progress beyond the limits of compensation are tissue hypoxia, metabolic acidosis and eventual dysfunction of all organ systems.

NURSING CARE CONSIDERATIONS

In hypotensive shock, tachycardia is pronounced and pulse pressure (difference between systolic and diastolic BP) becomes narrowed. There is poor capillary filling, and the child exhibits confusion, sleepiness and decreased responsiveness.

As hypotensive shock progresses along a physiological continuum, clinical signs indicate a progression of circulatory damage. With the progression of shock there is damage to vital organs (e.g. the heart or brain) of such magnitude that the entire system is disrupted regardless of therapeutic intervention. There is pronounced systemic vasoconstriction and hypoxia of visceral and cutaneous circulations with hypotension, acidosis, lethargy or coma and oliguria or anuria. The child is totally obtunded. A thready and weak pulse, hypotension, periodic breathing or apnoea, anuria and stupor or coma are signs of impending cardiac arrest.

NURSING CARE CONSIDERATIONS

Hypotension is a late and poor prognostic sign of shock, so signs of shock must be recognised and appropriate interventions implemented before hypotension is evident.

Irreversible or **terminal shock** is the end point of the physiological continuum if interventions are not effective in reversing the effects of shock. Damage to vital organs, such as the heart or brain, is of such magnitude that the entire organism will be disrupted regardless of therapeutic intervention. Death occurs even if cardiovascular measurements return to normal levels with therapy.

Diagnostic Evaluation

The nurse can discern the cause of shock from the history and physical examination. The initial assessment should commence with primary survey (ABCDE: Airway, Breathing and Circulation, Disability and Exposure). The severity of shock is determined by measurement of vital signs, including neurological status, peripheral pulses, CVP, capillary refill and urine output. The history should include the events leading to the situation, onset and duration of the symptoms as well as the patient's health history and pre-hospital care/treatment provided (Seckel & Lin 2020). Laboratory tests that assist in assessment are blood gas measurements, pH and sometimes liver function tests. Coagulation tests are evaluated when there is evidence of bleeding, such as oozing from a venepuncture site, bleeding from any orifice or petechiae. Cultures of blood and other sites are indicated when there is a high suspicion of sepsis. Renal function tests are performed when impaired renal function is evident.

Therapeutic Management

Treatment of shock consists of three major components: oxygenation and ventilation, fluid administration and improvement of the pumping action of the heart (vasopressor support). The first priority is to establish an airway and administer oxygen. Once the airway is ensured, circulatory stabilisation is the major concern. Placement of one or more multilumen central lines, preferably above the diaphragm (to deliver drugs closer to the heart and limit tissue injury from caustic medications), is a priority in shock with the exception of mild shock or if there is immediate response to volume therapy (Hazinski et al 2019, Perkin et al 2013). These lines are needed for rapid volume replacement, administration of vasoactive drugs and haemodynamic monitoring (Hazinski et al 2019). However, if immediate IV access cannot be accomplished an intraosseous device should be inserted to administer medications and fluids (see Chapter 22).

Oxygenation and Ventilatory Support. Oxygen is the first drug to be administered to an infant or child in shock (Children's Health Queensland Hospital and Health Service 2019, Perkin et al 2013, World Health Organization 2016). The lung is very sensitive to shock. The decrease in or redistribution of blood flow to respiratory muscles plus the increased work of breathing can rapidly lead to respiratory failure. Critically ill patients are unable to maintain an adequate airway. To place the lung at rest and improve ventilation, endotracheal intubation is initiated early with positive-pressure ventilation and supplemental oxygen. Blood gases, oxygen saturation (using pulse oximetry) and pH are monitored frequently.

Increased extravascular lung fluid caused by oedema—both hydrostatic and permeable—contributes to the development of respiratory complications. Hydrostatic oedema occurs from the elevation of pulmonary microvascular pressure as a result of left ventricular dysfunction; permeable oedema occurs when damage to alveolar cell and pulmonary capillary epithelium causes fluid to leak into the interstitial space, resulting in ARDS. (See Chapter 26.) Direct therapy towards maintaining normal arterial blood gas measurements, normal acid–base balance and circulation, and make efforts to remove fluid and prevent its accumulation by increasing oncotic pressure and decreasing microvascular hydrostatic pressure. Promote elevated oncotic pressure by diuresis with frusemide or mannitol, colloid administration, or both.

Cardiovascular Support. In many cases rapid restoration of blood volume is the main therapy needed in the resuscitation of the child in shock. An isotonic crystalloid solution (0.9% normal saline or lactated Ringer's solution) is usually the first choice for fluid replacement. Crystalloid is given in IV boluses of 20 mL/kg over 5 to 20 minutes and repeated as necessary. Blood products may also be given if acute blood loss is the cause of hypovolaemia. The child's response is assessed after each bolus. An increase in BP and a decrease in heart rate indicate successful resuscitation. An increased cardiac output results in improved capillary circulation and skin colour. Colloids (protein-containing fluids) are often administered to children in shock; albumin is the most common. Because albumin is a protein solution, it remains in the vascular space much longer than crystalloid fluids. A smaller volume of albumin can be given to increase intravascular volume and support cardiac output; with crystalloid fluids, a larger volume is needed to achieve the same effect. Fresh-frozen plasma is used to correct coagulopathies, not as volume replacement.

For the critically ill child with shock and multisystem organ dysfunction, more aggressive monitoring is necessary. CVP measurements of right atrial pressure or pulmonary wedge pressure help guide fluid therapy. In children with persistent shock, place a pulmonary artery catheter for more accurate monitoring. Determination of arterial blood gases, haematocrit, serum electrolytes, glucose and calcium concentrations provides additional information concerning composition of circulating blood. Correction of acidosis, hypoxaemia and any metabolic derangements is mandatory.

Inotropic Support. Temporary pharmacological support may be required to enhance myocardial contractility, reverse metabolic or respiratory acidosis and maintain arterial pressure. The principal agents used to improve cardiac output and circulation are the exogenous catecholamines, administered by constant infusion pump. Dopamine is the preferred drug in most situations because it also improves renal perfusion. Other agents (e.g. dobutamine, milrinone and adrenaline) may be used to improve cardiac output, depending on the situation. Vasopressin has been used in adults to increase systemic vascular resistance and BP, but its use in paediatric shock may be limited to vasodilatory (warm) shock (Kawasaki 2017, Perkin et al 2013).

Metabolic acidosis is usually corrected with adequate tissue perfusion and improved renal function. This is accomplished with adequate ventilatory support, including oxygen, and restoration of blood volume and peripheral circulation. Calcium chloride may be administered to improve cardiac function and to offset the reduced ionised calcium associated with large amounts of albumin, whole blood or fresh-frozen plasma. Routine administration of calcium in a paediatric cardiac arrest is not recommended unless there is documented evidence of hypocalcaemia, hyperkalaemia, hypermagnesaemia or calcium channel blocker overdose (de Caen et al 2015). Diuretics, such as frusemide (Lasix), cause a reduction in ventricular filling pressures without changing cardiac output or heart rate and promote sodium and water excretion by the kidney in cases in which pulmonary congestion is a problem.

Nursing Care Management

The child in shock requires observation and care, preferably in an intensive care environment. The initial action in caring for the child in shock is ensuring adequate tissue oxygenation (see Nursing Care Considerations and Quality Patient Outcome boxes). The nurse should be prepared to administer oxygen by the appropriate route and to assist with any indicated intubation and ventilation procedures. Other procedures and activities that require immediate attention are establishing an IV line, estimating body weight (for calculating weight-based drug dosages), obtaining baseline vital signs, placing an indwelling urinary catheter, obtaining blood gas and other measurements and administering medications as indicated.

QUALITY PATIENT OUTCOMES

Shock

- Oxygen content of blood optimised
- Cardiac output improved
- Oxygen demand reduced
- Metabolic abnormalities corrected
- Type of shock identified and treated

NURSING CARE CONSIDERATIONS

Early clinical signs of shock include apprehension, irritability, normal BP, narrowing pulse pressure (difference between diastolic and systolic BP), thirst, pallor, diminished urinary output, unexplained mild tachycardia and decreased perfusion of the hands and feet.

The nurse's primary responsibilities are to monitor vital signs (systolic BP in particular), CVP, I&O, oxygenation status, cardiac output and mean arterial pressure and to perform a general assessment of the level of consciousness, circulatory perfusion and parenteral infusion sites. The nurse titrates IV medications according to patient responses and obtains vital signs every 15 minutes during the critical periods and thereafter as needed. Urinary output should be measured hourly; blood gases, lactate, haematocrit, pH and electrolytes should be monitored frequently to assess the child's status and the efficacy of therapy. Cardiorespiratory monitors are attached and monitored continuously. Oxygen saturation monitors provide continuous measurement of oxygenation, and a central venous (CvO_2) or mixed venous (SvO_2) oxygen saturation monitor may also be used. In the initial stages of acute shock, care of the child often requires a team of nurses due to the number of activities that must be carried out simultaneously.

Children may be sedated in the acute phase of shock, depending on the precipitating cause, the child's age and the ability to implement therapeutic interventions such as endotracheal intubation and placement of central venous and arterial lines for continuous monitoring of cardiopulmonary status. Parents will require additional reassurance that their child's comfort and pain needs are being adequately addressed. The acutely ill child requires close observation for complications related to immobilisation, including deep vein thrombosis prophylaxis, skin care, tissue oedema, muscle atrophy, constipation and bone demineralisation. (See Chapter 33, Immobilisation.) Special efforts are made to prevent skin breakdown and ventilator-associated pneumonia and to maintain adequate nutritional status in the child who must be on mechanical ventilation for a prolonged period.

Family Support

Throughout the intense activity, do not overlook the parents. A member of the staff, such as a nurse, social worker or clergy, may be

NURSING CARE CONSIDERATIONS

Shock

Ventilation

- Establish airway; be prepared for intubation.
- Administer 100% oxygen.

Fluid Administration

- Restore vascular volume.

Cardiovascular Support

- Administer inotropes and vasopressors.

General Support

- Keep child flat with legs raised above level of heart.
- Keep child warm and calm.
- Monitor and treat pain.

called to provide comfort and support. If the family is not at the hospital, someone should contact them at frequent intervals to inform them about what is being done and whether there is any improvement. Ideally, someone should remain with the parents to serve as a liaison between them and the intensive care team. However, this is not always feasible in such a critical situation. As soon as possible, the parents should be allowed to see the child.

Septic Shock

Sepsis and septic shock are caused by an infectious organism and the patient's immune, inflammatory and coagulation responses to the infecting organism (Hazinski et al 2019, Perkin et al 2013). Normally an infection triggers an inflammatory response in a local area, which results in vasodilation, increased capillary permeability and eventually elimination of the infectious agent. The widespread activation and systemic release of inflammatory mediators is called the **systemic inflammatory response syndrome (SIRS)** (Boehne et al 2017). Box 23.3 provides the exact definitions for SIRS, infection, sepsis and severe sepsis. SIRS can occur in response to both infectious and non-infectious (e.g. trauma, burns) causes. When caused by infection, it is called *sepsis*. Septic shock is sepsis with organ dysfunction and hypotension and SIRS in children with pneumonia should be identified early because they will need more intense monitoring and treatment (Frazier et al 2015). Most of the physiological effects of shock occur because the exaggerated immune response triggers more than 30 different mediators, which results in diffuse vasodilation, increased capillary permeability and maldistribution of blood flow. This impairs oxygen and nutrient delivery to the cells, resulting in cellular dysfunction. If the process continues, multiple organ dysfunction occurs and may result in death. Table 23.6 includes the age-specific vital signs and laboratory values reflective of septic shock in children.

The incidence of septic shock is increasing in children despite the advanced preventive and treatment measures (Children's Health Queensland Hospital and Health Service 2019), possibly as a result of greater numbers of immunosuppressed patients, more widespread use of invasive devices in the seriously ill, increased awareness of the diagnosis and a growing number of resistant microorganisms.

Three stages have been identified in septic shock. In early septic shock the patient has chills, fever and vasodilation with increased cardiac output, which results in warm, flushed skin that reflects vascular tone abnormalities and hyperdynamic, warm or hyperdynamic-compensated responses. BP and urinary output are normal. The patient has the best chance for survival in this stage. The second stage—the normodynamic, cool or hyperdynamic-decompensated stage—lasts only a few hours. The skin is cool, but pulses and BP are still normal. Urinary output diminishes and the mental state becomes depressed. With advancing

BOX 23.3 Definitions of Systemic Inflammatory Response Syndrome, Infection, Sepsis and Severe Sepsis

SIRS—The presence of at least two of the following four criteria, one of which must be abnormal temperature or leucocyte count.

- Core temperature of more than 38.5°C (101.3°F) or less than 36°C (96.8°F).
- Tachycardia, defined as a mean heart rate more than 2 SD above normal for age in the absence of external stimulus, chronic drugs or painful stimuli; or otherwise unexplained persistent elevation over a 0.5- to 4-hour period; or, for children younger than 1 year old: bradycardia, defined as a mean heart rate less than the 10th percentile for age in the absence of external vagal stimulus, β-blocker drugs or congenital heart disease; or otherwise unexplained persistent depression over a 0.5-hour period.
- Mean respiratory rate more than 2 SD above normal for age or mechanical ventilation for an acute process not related to underlying neuromuscular disease or the receipt of general anaesthesia.
- Leucocyte count elevated or depressed for age (not secondary to chemotherapy-induced leucopenia) or more than 10% immature neutrophils.

Infection—A suspected or proven (by positive culture, tissue stain or PCR test) infection caused by any pathogen; or a clinical syndrome associated with a high probability of infection. Evidence of infection includes positive findings on clinical examination, imaging or laboratory tests (e.g. white blood cells in a normally sterile body fluid, perforated viscus, chest radiograph consistent with pneumonia, petechial or purpuric rash or purpura fulminans).

Sepsis—SIRS in the presence of or as a result of suspected or proven infection.

Severe sepsis—Sepsis plus cardiovascular organ dysfunction or ARDS or two or more other organ dysfunctions.

ARDS, Acute respiratory distress syndrome; *PCR*, polymerase chain reaction; *SD*, standard deviations; *SIRS*, systemic inflammatory response syndrome.

Source: From Goldstein, B., Giroir, B., Randolph, A., et al. (2005). International Pediatric Sepsis Consensus Conference: Definitions for sepsis and organ dysfunction in pediatrics. Pediatric Critical Care Medicine, 6(1), 2–8; used with permission.

TABLE 23.6 Age-specific Vital Signs and Laboratory Variables in Septic Shock*

	HEART RATE (BEATS/MIN)				
Age Group	Tachycardia	Bradycardia	Respiratory Rate (Breaths/Min)	Leucocyte Count (Leucocytes × 10^3/mm^3)	Systolic BP (mmHg)
0 days to 1 week	> 180	< 100	> 50	> 34	< 65
1 week to 1 month	> 180	< 100	> 40	> 19.5 or < 5	< 75
1 month to 1 year	> 180	< 90	> 34	> 17.5 or < 5	< 100
2–5 years	> 140	N/A	> 22	> 15.5 or < 6	< 94
6–12 years	> 130	N/A	> 8	> 13.50 or < 4.5	< 105
13–< 18 years	> 110	N/A	> 4	> 11 or < 4.5	< 117

*Lower values for heart rate, leucocyte count and systolic BP are for 5th percentile, and upper values for heart rate, respiratory rate or leucocyte count are for 95th percentile.

N/A, Not applicable.

Source: Goldstein, B., Giroir, B., & Randolph, A. (2005). International pediatric sepsis consensus conference: Definitions for sepsis and organ dysfunction in pediatrics. Pediatric Critical Care Medicine, 6(1), 2–8; used with permission.

disease, certain signs of circulatory decompensation that deteriorate to signs of circulatory collapse are indistinguishable from late shock of any cause. In the hypodynamic, or cold, stage of shock, cardiovascular function progressively deteriorates, even with aggressive therapy. The patient has hypothermia, cold extremities, weak pulses, hypotension and oliguria or anuria. Patients are severely lethargic or comatose. Multiorgan failure is common. This is the most dangerous stage of shock.

Newer therapies are being developed to modify the host immune response by attempting to block various mediators, thereby interrupting the inflammatory cascade. Evidence-based management protocols for the management of adult and paediatric septic shock have recently been published (de Caen et al 2015, Dellinger et al 2013).

Nursing Care Management

Early identification of the symptoms of septic shock is critical to patient survival. A high index of suspicion is required in all critically ill patients who are at greater risk for sepsis because of multiple invasive lines and devices, poor nutrition and impaired immune function. Subtle alterations in tissue perfusion and unexplained tachypnoea and tachycardia often are early warning signs. Identification of the infectious agent and prompt treatment are also critical to patient survival. Patients should receive broad-spectrum antibiotics, and the nurse should remove the site of infection if possible (e.g. indwelling central lines). Patients should be managed in an intensive care unit (ICU) in which continuous monitoring and sophisticated cardiac and respiratory support are available. Multidisciplinary collaboration is essential in managing these critically ill patients.

NURSING CARE CONSIDERATIONS

To aid in early identification and management, nurses caring for children at risk for septic shock should be alert to early signs: fever, tachycardia and tachypnoea. It is important to follow guidelines and choose the appropriate age group, newborn or paediatric sepsis pathway (e.g. NSW Government's sepsis tools at https://www.cec.health.nsw.gov.au/keep-patients-safe/deteriorating-patient-program/sepsis/sepsis-tools).

BOX 23.4 Common Allergens Associated with Anaphylaxis

Drugs and Medical Products
- Antibiotics (penicillin, cephalosporins, aminoglycosides, amphotericin B)
- Analgesics (aspirin, indometacin)
- Local anaesthetics (lidocaine [lignocaine], procaine, bupivacaine)
- Chemotherapeutic agents (bleomycin, cisplatin, carboplatin, asparaginase (colaspase), etoposide)
- Antiepileptic drugs
- Diagnostic contrast media (sulfobromophthalein sodium dye, dehydrocholic acid, iodinated contrast media, iopanoic acid)
- Latex (gloves, urinary catheters)
- Blood products

Foods (see Chapter 11)
- Milk and milk products
- Nuts and seeds
- Legumes (peanuts, soybeans, beans, lentils)
- Eggs
- Seafood (fish, shellfish)
- Wheat
- Citrus fruits, strawberries
- Chocolate

Venoms
- Hymenopteran (bee, wasp)
- Snake
- Jellyfish
- Blue-ringed octopus
- Spider

Biological Agents
- Allergen extracts
- Antisera (snake, tetanus, diphtheria)
- Enzymes
- Hormones
- Immunoglobulin
- Blood and blood products

Anaphylaxis

Anaphylaxis is the acute clinical syndrome resulting from the interaction of an allergen and a patient who is hypersensitive. This antigen-antibody (immunoglobulin E [IgE]) reaction stimulates the release of chemical substances, primarily histamine, from mast cells (Moules 2019). Histamine release causes vasodilation and increases capillary permeability, allowing fluid to leak into the interstitial space. Severe reactions are immediate, often life-threatening and often involve multiple systems, primarily the cardiovascular, respiratory, GI and integumentary systems. Exposure to the antigen can be through ingestion, inhalation, skin contact or injection. Food allergy is the most common cause of anaphylaxis outside the hospital, whereas medication and latex allergies are more common in the hospital (Sampson et al 2016). The most common allergens are listed in Box 23.4.

Pathophysiology

An anaphylactic reaction occurs as a result of an interaction between an allergen and a pre-existing specific IgE. When the antigen enters the circulatory system, a generalised reaction rapidly occurs. Vasoactive amines (principally histamine or histamine-like substances) are released from mast cells and cause vasodilation, bronchoconstriction and increased capillary permeability. Consequently, there is increased venous capacity and pooling, reduced arterial pressure and rapid loss of fluid into interstitial spaces, causing a marked decrease in venous return to the heart.

Clinical Manifestations

The onset of clinical symptoms usually occurs within seconds or minutes of exposure to the antigen. The rapidity of the reaction is directly related to its intensity—the sooner the onset, the more severe the reaction. However, the onset may be delayed for as long as 2 hours. Typically the reaction is preceded by one or more prodromal signs and symptoms, including vague complaints of uneasiness or impending doom, restlessness, irritability, severe anxiety, headache, dizziness, paraesthesia and disorientation. The patient may lose consciousness.

Cutaneous signs of flushing and urticaria are common early signs followed by angio-oedema, most notable in the eyelids, lips, tongue, hands, feet and genitalia. Bronchiolar constriction may follow, causing narrowing of the airway; pulmonary oedema and haemorrhage also may occur. Laryngeal oedema with severe acute upper airway

BOX 23.5 Possible Manifestations of Anaphylactic Reaction

Cardiovascular
- Tachycardia
- Dysrhythmia
- Hypotension
- Relative hypovolaemia

Respiratory
- Rhinitis (sneezing, nasal itching, rhinorrhoea)
- Laryngeal oedema (stridor)
- Bronchospasm (cough, wheezing)

Gastrointestinal
- Nausea and vomiting
- Abdominal pain
- Diarrhoea

Cutaneous (Skin)*
- Diffuse flushing, feeling of warmth
- Urticaria (itching of skin and raised rash [hives])
- Angio-oedema (periorbital, perioral)

Central Nervous System, Other
- Sense of impending doom*
- Sometimes loss of consciousness*
- Headache*
- Seizures

*Early signs

obstruction may be life-threatening and requires rapid intervention. Shock occurs as a result of mediator-induced vasodilation, which causes capillary permeability and loss of intravascular fluid into the interstitial space. Sudden hypotension and impaired cardiac output with poor perfusion are seen. As outlined in Box 23.5, any or all of several reactions may affect one or more organ systems.

NURSING CARE CONSIDERATIONS

Penicillin allergy is associated with immediate onset (within 1 hour of administration) or accelerated onset (1 to 72 hours after administration) of skin eruption, especially an urticarial rash, or more serious symptoms such as laryngeal oedema or anaphylactic shock.

Therapeutic Management

Successful outcome of anaphylactic reactions depends on rapid recognition of their severity and prompt treatment. The goals of treatment are providing ventilation, restoring adequate circulation and preventing further exposure by identifying and removing the cause when possible.

A **biphasic reaction** may occur within 4 hours after symptoms have originally subsided, so it is important to monitor the child closely for this reaction (Pourmande et al 2018, Sampson et al 2016). Additional interventions such as fluid resuscitation, oxygen administration, beta-agonists, antihistamines and corticosteroids should be considered in the child who experiences a moderate to severe anaphylactic reaction.

If this is the initial anaphylactic reaction, it is especially important to identify the allergen and implement measures to prevent any future reaction. The patient should carry medical identification at all times. Desensitisation by a paediatric allergist may be recommended in certain cases.

Mild cutaneous reaction with no evidence of respiratory distress or cardiovascular compromise would be managed with antihistamines, such as diphenhydramine (Benadryl) or cetirizine. Moderate or severe distress presents a life-threatening emergency and requires immediate intervention (see also Food Sensitivity, Chapter 11).

Nursing Care Management

Major nursing responsibilities in anaphylaxis include anticipating which children are likely to develop a reaction, recognising the early signs and intervening appropriately. When an anaphylactic reaction is suspected, nursing responsibilities include immediate intervention and preparation for medical therapy. If emergency supplies such as adrenaline (epinephrine) are not immediately available, emergency medical services should be accessed. Ventilation is ensured by placing the child in a head-elevated position, unless contraindicated by hypotension, to facilitate breathing and administer oxygen. If the child is not breathing, cardiopulmonary resuscitation (CPR) is initiated and emergency medical services are summoned. (See Nursing Care Considerations box.)

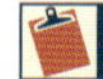

NURSING CARE CONSIDERATIONS

Anaphylaxis

- Early recognition of symptoms
- Airway patency maintained
- Adequate circulation restored and maintained
- Further exposure to allergic agent prevented

If the cause can be determined, implement measures to slow the spread of the offending substance. For example, discontinue an IV medication or contrast dye infusion. If the cause can be determined, measures are implemented to slow the spread of the offending substance. An IV infusion is established immediately. Emergency medications are given intravenously whenever possible; however, adrenaline (epinephrine) may be given intramuscularly. Vital signs and urinary output are monitored frequently. Medications are administered as prescribed, with regular assessment to monitor effectiveness and to detect signs of side effects of medication and fluid overload.

To prevent an anaphylactic reaction, parents are always asked about possible allergic responses to foods, medications, products such as latex and environmental conditions (see Chapter 32). These are displayed prominently on the patient's chart and an allergy alert wristband. Note the specific allergen and the type and severity of the reaction. Parents are excellent historians, especially when the child has displayed a dramatic reaction to a substance. Drugs, including related drugs (e.g. penicillin and nafcillin), that have produced a previous reaction are never given.

The child and the parents need as much reassurance as can be provided without giving false hope. Keep them informed of the child's progress, the reasons for the therapies and what they can reasonably expect. This is a frightening experience and one that the family will remember and make every effort to prevent from recurring. The use of a convenient and visible method of conveying medical information, such as a bracelet or necklace, is encouraged. For the child who is allergic to insect venom, prescribe the family an emergency kit to be kept with the child at all times (e.g. EpiPen or EpiPen Jr). Teach both the family and the child (if the child is old enough and is likely to be away from the family, such as at school) how to use the equipment.

Toxic Shock Syndrome

Toxic shock syndrome (TSS) is a relatively rare condition caused by the toxins produced by the *Staphylococcus* bacteria (Government of South Australia 2019, Ministry of Health New Zealand 2018). *S. aureus* is the most commonly found cause of TSS. First described in the late 1970s, TSS can cause acute multisystem organ failure and a clinical picture that resembles septic shock. TSS became well known in 1980 because of the striking relationship between the disease and tampon use. An aggressive health education campaign about the dangers of prolonged tampon use and a change in the chemical composition of tampons have markedly reduced the incidence of TSS in menstruating women. Cases of TSS have also been reported in men, older women and children.

Pathophysiology

Evidence from several sources suggests that TSS occurs secondary to infection with *S. aureus*—namely, toxic shock syndrome toxin–1 (TSST-1) (Gaensbauer & Todd 2016). Enterotoxin A and enterotoxin B may be associated with non-menstrual TSS (Gaensbauer & Todd 2016). The organism is believed to produce an epidermal toxin, but the precise mode of transmission is not known.

In approximately half the cases, TSS is seen in menstruating women and is usually associated with tampon use. The tampon may carry the organism from the fingers or vulva into the vagina during insertion, may traumatise the vaginal wall or may provide a favourable environment for growth of the organism. TSS has also been associated with other bacterial infections, such as sinusitis or pneumonia, catheter site infections, skin infections, postoperative wound infections and infection related to foreign bodies such as nasal packing or contraceptive diaphragms (Gaensbauer & Todd 2016).

Clinical Manifestations

The sudden development of high fever, vomiting and diarrhoea, profound hypotension, shock, oliguria and an erythematous macular rash with subsequent desquamation are characteristic manifestations of TSS. Other manifestations include headache, blurred vision, purulent conjunctivitis, abdominal guarding and purulent vaginal discharge.

Complications of TSS include respiratory distress, cardiac dysfunction, abnormal coagulation (particularly disseminated intravascular coagulation) and abnormal liver function. Impaired perfusion to the extremities may become severe, with eventual necrosis and loss of extremities.

Diagnostic Evaluation

A history of tampon use contributes to the diagnosis. Laboratory tests may include cultures from blood, vagina, cervix and discharge from any suspected source of infection. Other laboratory tests are those that facilitate the management of shock.

Therapeutic Management

The management of TSS is the same as management of shock of any cause. Because the disease is highly varied in intensity, therapy towards supportive care for mild cases should be directed to hospitalisation and for severe cases to intensive care. Appropriate parenteral antibiotics are usually administered after cultures are obtained. Preventing complications of impaired circulation demands constant observation and immediate therapeutic intervention for hypotension, pulmonary dysfunction, acidosis, haematological changes and renal impairment.

Nursing Care Management

Nursing care and observation of the acutely ill patient are the same as those described for shock of any cause. Because the disease is relatively rare, major nursing efforts should be directed towards prevention. The association between TSS and tampon use provides some direction for education. Avoiding the use of tampons offers the most certain preventive measure, although this approach is probably unacceptable to most adolescent girls, who prefer the freedom, comfort and inconspicuousness that tampons afford.

Adolescent girls who use tampons can be taught general hygiene measures, such as good hand washing, bathing/showering daily at a minimum and careful insertion to avoid vaginal abrasion. It is wise to modify their use, alternating with sanitary napkins—perhaps using the napkins during the night, when at home during the day and when flow is slight. Young girls are advised not to use superabsorbent tampons and not to leave any tampon in the body for more than 4 to 6 hours.

BURNS

Overview

Burn injuries are usually attributed to extreme heat sources but may also result from exposure to cold, chemicals, electricity or radiation. Most burns are relatively minor and do not require definitive medical treatment. However, burns involving a large body surface area, critical body parts or the paediatric or geriatric population often benefit from treatment in specialised burn centres. The New South Wales Health Agency for Clinical Innovation (NSW ACI 2019) has established criteria to guide decisions regarding the severity of injury and the need for transfer for specialised care.

Epidemiology and Aetiology

Burn injuries represent one of the most severe traumas a body can sustain. Ongoing efforts towards education, burn prevention, safer home and work environments and new methods of firefighting have significantly decreased burn injuries. Scald burns (e.g. hot water, grease, hot foods) are most common among young children, whereas flame burns are more prevalent among older children. The bathroom is the area where scald burns from tap water most often occur, and these injuries tend to be more severe covering a larger portion of the body. The death rate from fire and burn injury has declined by 53% from 1999 to 2013 (Safe Kids Worldwide 2015). Burns are one of the causes of unintentional injury and child injury death in Australia (Kidsafe Australia 2017). From 1 July 2016 to 30 June 2017, 3295 patients who had sustained burns were treated in the registered 17 specialist burn units in Australia and New Zealand (Burns Registry of Australia and New Zealand 2017). Thirty-three per cent of the paediatric cases were between ages 1 and 2 years (Burns Registry of Australia and New Zealand 2017).

According to Burns Registry of Australia and New Zealand (2017), 36% of burn injuries were due to scalds, while 33% and 17% of burns were due to flame burns and contact burns respectively. Careless smoking is associated with the majority of fatal house fires and is the most common cause of residential fire deaths. The use of heating sources is another common cause of house fires. The source of ignition is often a combustible material stored near the furnace or device, build-up of creosote in the chimney, spillage of fuel or use of the wrong fuel. Many of these fires result in multiple deaths and injuries, especially in rural areas. The majority of fatal house fires occur during the cold winter months with an incidence rate of 41% (Burns Registry of Australia and New Zealand 2017). The single most important element in the decrease in fire-related deaths is the use of smoke alarms (Coates et al 2019).

Flame burns involving flammable liquids account for approximately 30% of injuries seen in the paediatric population, especially in children over 8 years of age. The ignition of clothing is the second leading cause of burn admissions. Due to the high risk associated with nightwear, a legislation was developed and updated as a safety standard in Australia and New Zealand (Australian Government 2019). It is a legislative requirement for children's sleepwear to comply with the Australian/New Zealand Standard AS/NZS 1249:2014 Children's nightwear and limited daywear having reduced fire hazard (Australian Government 2019).

Chemical burns can cause extensive injury. The severity of injury is related to the chemical agent (e.g. acid, alkali or organic compound) and the duration of contact. The mechanism of injury differs from that in other burns in that there is a chemical disruption and alteration of the physical properties of the exposed body area. Noxious agents exist in many common household cleaning products used in the home. In addition to concern for localised damage, the potential for systemic toxicity must also be addressed. Of particular concern are the exposure of the eyes to chemical agents and the ingestion of caustic substances. Although radiation injuries are rare, the most common sources in paediatrics are related to radiation exposure from medical therapies and ultraviolet light.

Non-accidental injury, which is a leading cause of traumatic injury in children, is another source of burn injury. These sources that result in burn injuries most commonly occur in children 3 years of age and younger. In Australia and New Zealand, 93% of burns are due to non-intentional injury (Burns Registry of Australia and New Zealand 2017). With non-accidental burn injury, scald burns are the most common, followed by contact burns from hot objects. Non-accidental burn injury should be suspected if the burn distribution on the body is inconsistent with the reported incident, the injury is not consistent with the child's developmental level and there was a delay in seeking treatment. It is also important to explore any history of family instability and an inability to deal with stress in crisis situations. Laws now exist in all states requiring healthcare workers to mandatorily report any suspected child abuse.

The causative agent in all burns has important implications for the treatment and prognosis of the paediatric patient. The nurse uses knowledge of the pathophysiological processes of each type of injury in assessing the trauma and in planning, implementing and evaluating care. Psychosocial issues are also important considerations in planning for the optimum long-term outcome.

Burn Wound Characteristics

The child's physiological responses, therapy, prognosis and physical disposition are directly related to the amount of tissue destroyed; therefore, the severity of the burn injury is assessed on the basis of the percentage of BSA burned and the depth of the burn. Also important in determining the seriousness of injury are the location of the wounds, the child's age and general health, the causative agent, respiratory involvement and concomitant injuries.

Extent of Injury

The extent of the burn is expressed as a percentage of total body surface area (TBSA) injured and this is critical as it informs the treatment required for the injury (Victorian Adult Burns Service 2017). The child has different body proportions to the adult, resulting in an inaccurate estimation of injury if the standard adult rule of nines is used. The proportions of the child's trunk and arms are roughly the same as those of the adult. However, the infant's head and neck make up 18% of the TBSA and each lower extremity accounts for 14% of the TBSA. A modified rule of nines for the paediatric population proposes that for each year of life until greater than or equal to 8 years, 1% is deducted from the head and 0.5% is added to each leg and at 9 years 1% added to the perineum (NSW ACI 2019). After the age of 9 years, the proportions used are similar to those used in an adult. For small burns, the palmar surface involving the fingers and palm of the patient's hand can be used which is estimated to be 1% of the BSA (NSW ACI 2019). In the burn assessment, erythema must not be included to avoid inaccuracy in the assessment that could result in over-resuscitation or over-treatment (Victorian Adult Burns Service 2017). It is generally more efficient to use any of a variety of charts designed to assign body proportions to children of different ages (Fig 23.4).

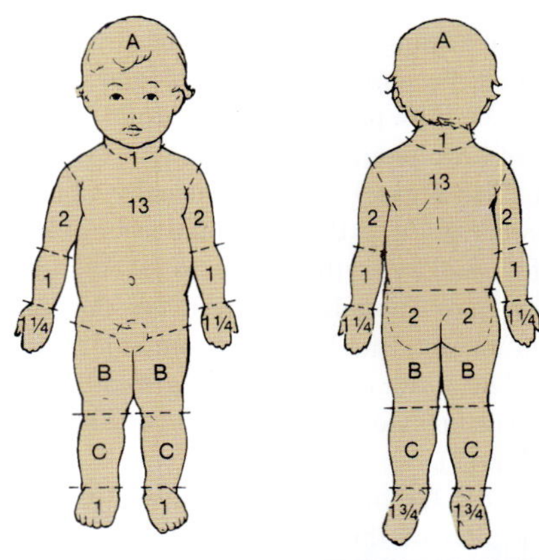

RELATIVE PERCENTAGES OF AREAS AFFECTED BY GROWTH

A

AREA	BIRTH	AGE 1 YR	AGE 5 YR
A = ½ of head	9½	8½	6½
B = ½ of one thigh	2¾	3¼	4
C = ½ of one leg	2½	2½	2¾

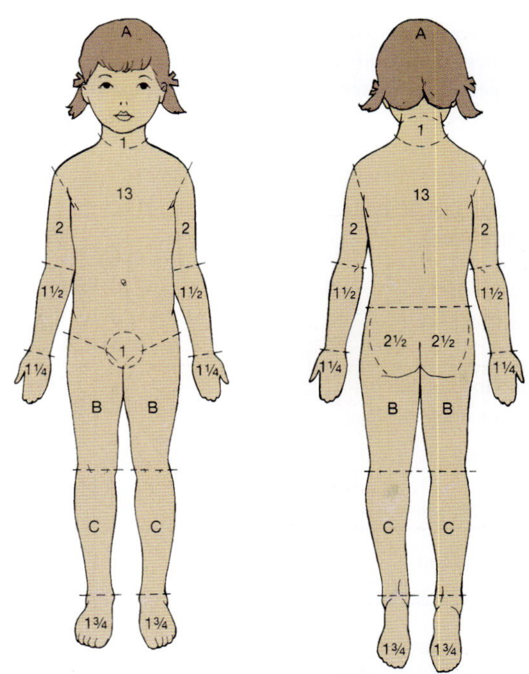

RELATIVE PERCENTAGES OF AREAS AFFECTED BY GROWTH

B

AREA	AGE 10 YR	AGE 15 YR	ADULT
A = ½ of head	5½	4½	3½
B = ½ of one thigh	4½	4½	4¾
C = ½ of one leg	3	3¼	3½

Fig 23.4 Charts for estimation of distribution of burns in children. (**A**) Children from birth to age 5 years. (**B**) Older children.

Depth of Injury

A thermal injury is a three-dimensional wound and is also assessed in relation to the depth of injury. Traditionally the terms *first, second, third and fourth degree* have been used to describe the depth of tissue injury. However, with the current emphasis on wound healing, this traditional terminology is being replaced by more descriptive terms related to the extent of destruction to the epithelialising elements of the skin. In general, first-degree burns are classified as superficial and second-degree burns as partial-thickness. Third- and fourth-degree wounds are classified as full-thickness wounds. Partial-thickness wounds are further classified as superficial or deep in relation to the time required for healing to occur and the functional and cosmetic results anticipated. Because both terminologies are often used interchangeably, they are both presented in Figure 23.5, which describes the characteristics of burn wounds.

Superficial (first-degree) burns are usually of minor significance. This type of injury involves the epidermal layer only. There is often a latent period followed by erythema due to vasodilation, tissue damage is minimum, the protective functions of the skin remain intact and systemic effects are rare. Pain is the predominant symptom and blisters do not form. The dead epidermis sloughs off and is replaced by regenerating keratinocytes within 3 or 4 days without scarring (Fredricks et al 2017).

Partial-thickness (second-degree) injuries involve the epidermis and varying degrees of the dermal layer where the skin barrier is disrupted. These wounds are painful, moist, red and blistered. Keratinocytes at the wound edge lose adhesion to each other, develop flexibility, migrate over the wound bed and proliferate (Horst et al 2017). With superficial partial-thickness burns, dermal elements are intact and the wound should heal in approximately 14 days with variable amounts of scarring. The wound is extremely sensitive to temperature changes, exposure to air and light touch. Although classified as second-degree or partial-thickness, deep dermal burns resemble full-thickness injuries in many respects, except the sweat glands and hair follicles remain intact. The burn may appear mottled, with pink, red or white areas exhibiting blisters and oedema formation (Fig 23.6). Systemic effects are similar to those encountered with full-thickness burns. Although these wounds heal spontaneously in approximately 21 days, they do so with extensive scarring.

Full-thickness (third-degree) burns are serious injuries that involve the entire epidermis and dermis and extend into the subcutaneous tissue. Thrombosed vessels can be seen beneath the surface of the wound, and nerve endings, sweat glands and hair follicles are destroyed. The burn varies in colour from red to tan, waxy white, brown or black and is distinguished by a dry, leathery appearance (Fig 23.7).

Fourth-degree burns are also full-thickness injuries and involve underlying structures such as muscle, fascia and bone. The wound appears dull and dry, and ligaments, tendons and bone may be exposed. Most often in the case of an extremity, it must be amputated due to the extensive damage and inability to repair the area. In some instances a plastic reconstruction procedure called a flap can be performed. A flap is where varying composites of different types of tissue components (e.g. skin, muscle, fat) with its blood supply intact are taken from one area of the person's body to cover the damaged area.

Severity of Injury

Burns are classified as major, moderate or minor, which is useful in determining the patient's disposition for treatment. Burn patients can usually be distinguished as: (1) those with a major burn injury that require the services and facilities of a specialised burn centre; (2) those with a moderate burn who may be treated in a hospital with expertise in burn care; and (3) those with minor injuries, who can be treated on an outpatient basis (Fig 23.8). The severity of the injury depends on the extent and depth of the burn, the causative agent, body area involved, patient's age and concomitant injuries and illnesses.

Certain areas of the body carry a higher risk of complications and therefore require specialised care. Burns of the hands and feet and across joints may not necessarily involve a large BSA, but injury and scar formation may interfere with normal growth and development. Specialised care is required to preserve maximum function. Burns to

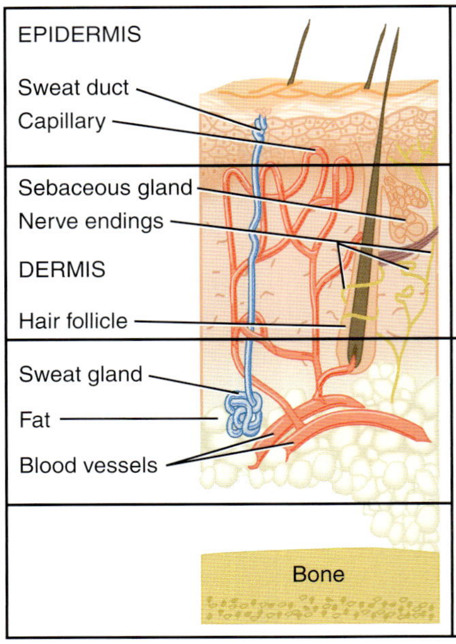

Skin layer	Burn	Degree	WOUND APPEARANCE	WOUND SENSATION	COURSE OF HEALING
EPIDERMIS; Sweat duct; Capillary	PARTIAL-THICKNESS BURN	1st-degree	Epidermis remains intact and without blisters Erythema; skin blanches with pressure	Painful	Discomfort lasts 48–72 hours. Desquamation occurs in 3–7 days.
Sebaceous gland; Nerve endings; DERMIS; Hair follicle	PARTIAL-THICKNESS BURN	2nd-degree	Wet, shiny, weeping surface Blisters Wound blanches with pressure	Painful Very sensitive to touch, air currents	Superficial partial-thickness burn heals in < 21 days. Deep partial-thickness burn requires > 21 days for healing. Healing rates vary with burn depth and presence/absence of infection.
Sweat gland; Fat; Blood vessels	FULL-THICKNESS BURN	3rd-degree	Colour variable (i.e. deep red, white, black, brown) Surface dry Thrombosed vessels visible No blanching	Insensate (↓ pinprick sensation)	Autografting is required for healing.
Bone	FULL-THICKNESS BURN	4th-degree	Colour variable Charring visible in deepest areas Extremity movement limited	Insensate	Amputation of extremities is likely. Autografting is required for healing.

Fig 23.5 Classification of burn depth according to depth of injury. (Source: Black, J. M. (2008]. Medical-surgical nursing: Clinical management for positive outcomes (8th ed.). Philadelphia, PA: Saunders.)

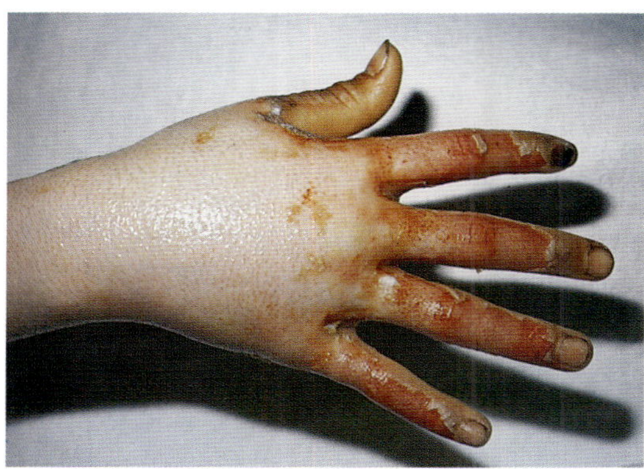

Fig 23.6 Deep partial-thickness burn.

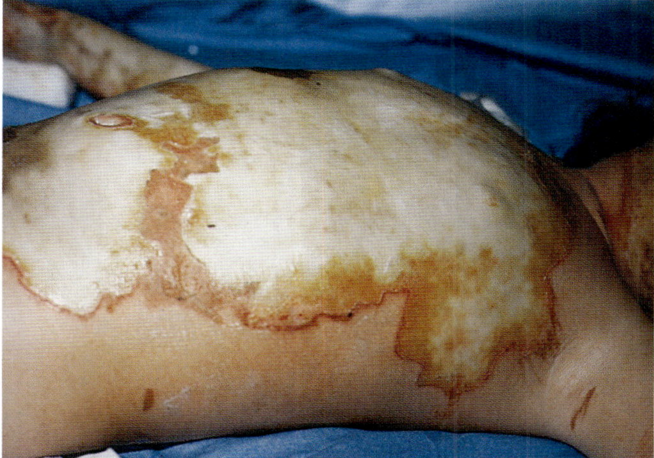

Fig 23.7 Full-thickness thermal injury.

the face and neck, along with a history of the injury occurring in an enclosed space, raise a high index of suspicion of inhalation injury. In addition, airway compromise and hypoxia may result from oedema formation and pulmonary injury. Damage to the delicate cartilage of the nose and ears can result in facial deformities. Perineal burns are prone to infection and maceration in all patients, especially in young children who are not toilet trained. Scar bands and contractures in the perineal area may interfere with hygiene and mobility.

Children younger than 2 years of age have a significantly higher mortality rate than older children with burns of a similar magnitude. The infant has minimum protein stores, which are rapidly depleted during burn shock; an immature immune response, which increases the risk of infection and sepsis; and a greater amount of body water in proportion to size that is intolerant of rapid fluid shifts. In addition, the child has not achieved mature renal function. This negatively affects the ability to retain sodium and water. These considerations, combined with the previously discussed fragility of the skin in the very young, increase the severity of injury.

Pathophysiology

A burn injury represents a catastrophic insult that involves all organ systems. Understanding the pathophysiology underlying thermal trauma is essential to provide appropriate nursing care to the paediatric burn victim.

Local Response

Damage to human skin by heat results in two types of injury: an immediate direct cellular response and a delayed response caused by dermal ischaemia. Irreversible cellular damage from protein denaturation occurs at temperatures exceeding 45°C. Three zones of injury demonstrate the evolution of local tissue damage (Fig 23.9). The unstable area of injured cells, which may survive under ideal conditions, is designated the zone of stasis. Progressive injury caused by dermal ischaemia may occur in this zone (Box 23.6).

Oedema Formation. Thermal injury to the vessels in the two outer zones results in increased capillary permeability. At the same time, vasodilation causes an increase in hydrostatic pressure within the capillaries. The increased hydrostatic pressure, combined with the increased capillary permeability, causes loss of water, protein and electrolytes from the circulating volume into the interstitial spaces.

To understand the physiological mechanism of the formation of burn oedema, an understanding of the microvascular fluid balance is necessary. Burn injury not only causes oedema at the site, but extravasated and sequestered fluid and protein also enter non-burned tissue. The directly injured cells have a damaged cell membrane that leads to an increase in sodium and potassium shift, resulting in cell swelling. Intracellular water and sodium increase. This process occurs not only in injured cells but also with those that are not directly heat injured. Oedema develops when the rate of fluid being filtered from the micro vessels exceeds that of the lymph flow. The oedema in the interstitial space develops rapidly over the first 8 to 12 hours following the injury and is dependent on the depth and extent of the burn injury (Rowan et al 2015).

Fluid Loss. Fluid transport across the microcirculatory wall in normal and pathological states is quantitatively described by the Landis-Starling equation. This equation describes the physical forces and physiological mechanisms that govern fluid transfer between vascular and extravascular compartments. Normal capillary barriers that separate the intravascular and interstitial compartments are disrupted, which results in severe depletion of plasma volume and an increase in extracellular fluid. This rapid and extensive fluid shift is manifested as hypovolaemia (Rae et al 2016).

Circulatory Status. Significant circulatory alterations take place in the zone of stasis located around the dead coagulated tissue. Heated red blood cells become spherical. These heat-damaged cells, together with haemoconcentration from fluid shifts, depressed cardiac output and tissue oedema, reduce the blood flow in the burned area, resulting in capillary stasis. Thrombi develop which further impedes circulation and produces tissue ischaemia and necrosis. Hyperviscosity and impaired blood flow are attributed to the release of substances such as thromboplastin and clot-activating factors from damaged cells. These substances cause the production of microemboli, platelet adhesion and aggregation and increased pain and oedema. Circulation in the area around partial-thickness wounds ceases immediately after injury but is usually restored within 24 to 48 hours. In full-thickness burns, however, the vascular supply is completely occluded, and no appreciable circulation is re-established until granulation takes place at the interface between burned and unburned skin.

Tissue Repair. With reasonable care, superficial partial-thickness injuries heal spontaneously and uneventfully through the generative capacity of the stratum germinativum and epithelial cells of the lining of skin appendages. Deep partial-thickness burns heal more slowly by regeneration from the epithelial lining of skin appendages, sweat glands and hair follicles. Infection, trauma or severe hypothermia easily converts a partial-thickness wound to a full-thickness injury, especially in the normally thinner skin of young children. Fluid loss and metabolic consequences may be considerable.

Cell destruction by coagulation necrosis occurs in full-thickness burns. Dead tissue and exudate convert to a thick, leathery eschar in 48 to 72 hours; the eschar liquefies and begins to separate in 12 to 21 days

Paediatric Burns Assessment Ruler

CONTACT DETAILS

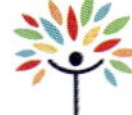

The Royal Children's Hospital Melbourne
Trauma Advice Line
(03) 9345 4701

Age: ____________

Sex: M○ F○

Height: ____________ cms

Weight: ____________ kgs

Date of Burn: / /

Mechanism of injury:
____

Associated injuries:
____

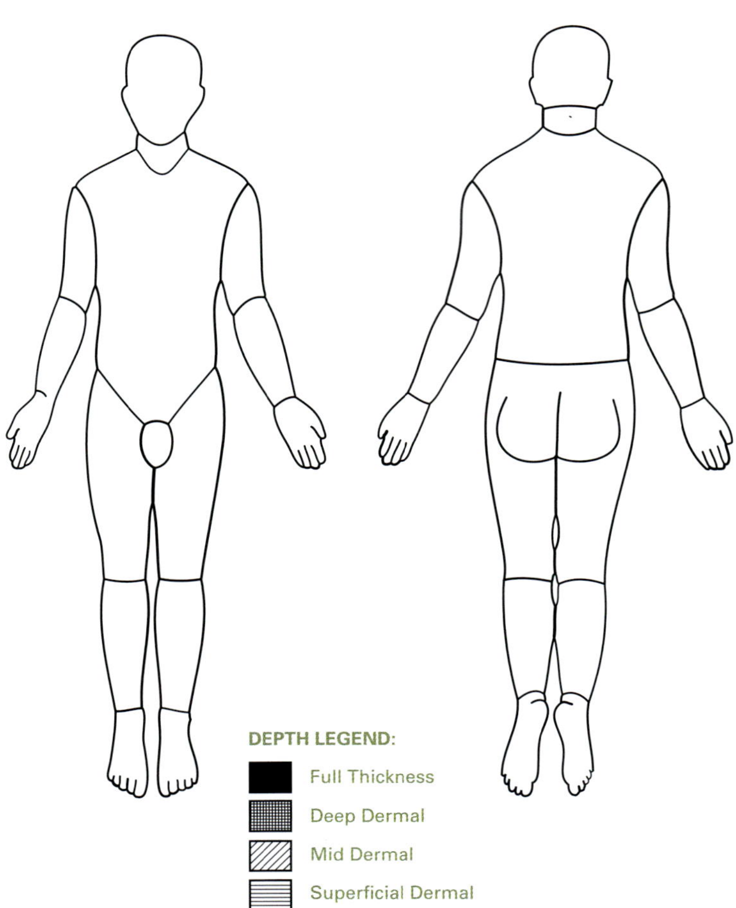

Estimated fluid (Parkland's)

4mls x TBSA% x Kg = mls/24hrs
Estimated Fluid required: ______mls
Total fluid since burn: ________mls

Maintenance fluids in children

Maintenance fluids should also be added over and above the Modified Parklands formula for children weighing less than 30kgs 5% Glucose and 1/2 Normal Saline used for maintenance fluid

Up to 10kgs 100ml/kg/day

10 – 20kgs
1000mls plus 50ml/kg/day for each kg over 10kgs

20 – 30 kgs
1500mlsplus 20ml/kg/day for each kg over 20 kgs

Oral fluids should be encouraged to supply maintenance fluids if the patient is stable and conscious, and no interventions are planned

Paediatric-Adult Rule of Nines expressed as a % of Body Surface Area

	1 yr	2 yr	3 yr	4 yr	5 yr	6 yr	7 yr	8 yr	9 yr	10 yr - Adult
Head	18	17	16	15	14	13	12	11	10	9
Trunk	18	18	18	18	18	18	18	18	18	18
Each arm	9	9	9	9	9	9	9	9	9	9
Each leg	14	14.5	15	15.5	16	16.5	17	17.5	18	18
Perineum										1

Chest+Abdo @ Front 18% / @ Back 18% Limbs are measured circumferentially

Last Updated: 08 May 2012

Fig 23.8 Paediatric Burns Assessment Ruler. (Source: Royal Children's Hospital, 2017. Paediatric Burns Assessment Ruler. https://www.vicburns.org.au/burn-assessment-overview/burn-tbsa/lund-browder/)

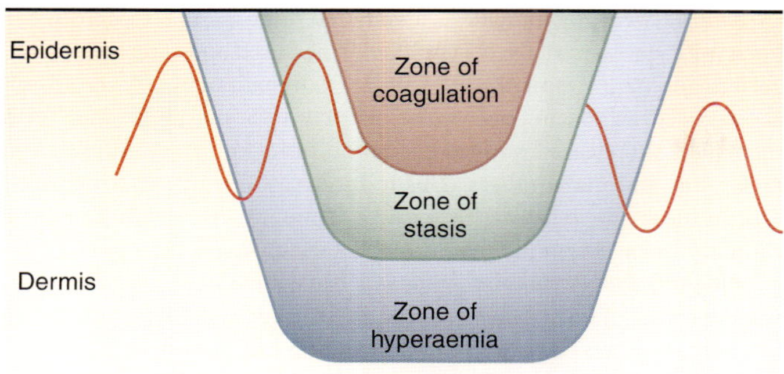

Fig 23.9 Zones of injury in burn. (Source: Townsend, C. M. (2007). Sabiston textbook of surgery (18th ed.). Philadelphia, PA: Saunders.)

BOX 23.6 Zones of Burn Injury

Zone of coagulation (necrosis)—Area beneath obviously destroyed tissue. Capillary flow has ceased and tissue destruction is irreversible; tissue is dead.

Zone of stasis—Area beneath and surrounding zone of coagulation; markedly reduced capillary flow; tissue severely damaged from heat but not coagulated. Tissue in this zone can be saved with prevention of further injury and with adequate perfusion.

Zone of hyperaemia—Area metabolically active; displays usual response to tissue injury.

if not surgically excised. This process is a result of autolysis, leucocyte digestion and disintegration of collagen fibres. The dead avascular tissue provides an ideal environment for bacterial growth. If tissue is not grafted, new granulation tissue forms on the wound bed. The wound heals slowly by granulation from the edges, with a high risk of infection and severe scarring. Full-thickness burns result in severe oedema with fluid and electrolyte shifts and extensive metabolic changes.

Systemic Responses

Cardiovascular System. The immediate postburn period is marked by dramatic alterations in circulation, known as **burn shock**. A precipitous drop in cardiac output precedes any change in circulating blood or plasma volumes. This initial decrease in cardiac output (approximately 50% of normal resting values) is attributed to a circulating myocardial depressant factor that is associated with severe burn injury and directly affects the contractility of the heart muscle. As a result of fluid losses through denuded skin, increased capillary permeability and vasodilation, the circulating volume decreases rapidly; cardiac output is reduced even further, usually levelling off at approximately 20% of normal resting values. After adequate fluid resuscitation, cardiac output spontaneously returns to normal in 24 to 36 hours. If fluid is not replaced, cardiac output continues to decrease, resulting in inadequate perfusion, organ dysfunction and ultimately death.

Capillary permeability with leakage of fluid takes place both in uninjured areas and in the burn wound. Together with the shrinkage of drying eschar, severe oedema caused by the rapid fluid shift to the interstitial spaces may produce a tourniquet effect, resulting in compartment syndrome. Compartments are composed of groups of muscles in the extremities and are surrounded by fibrous tissue. The inability of the fascia to expand in the presence of massive oedema increases the pressure in the compartment, compromising circulation and entrapping nerves. Treatment is required during the acute phase and consists of a surgical incision of the burned tissue (escharotomy)

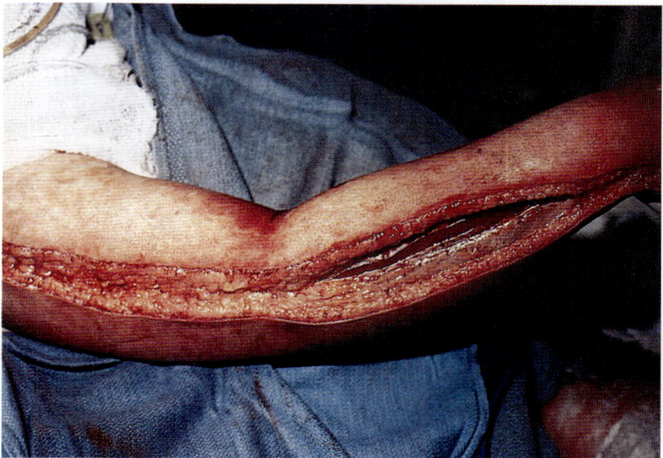

Fig 23.10 Escharotomy and fasciotomy in severely burned arm.

to restore distal circulation. If the escharotomy is not sufficient, an incision of the muscle sheath (fasciotomy) is performed (Fig 23.10).

Oedema fluid accumulates rapidly in the first 18 hours after injury and reaches a maximum in approximately 48 hours. Capillary permeability returns to normal, and fluid is reabsorbed, chiefly by way of the lymphatics. Reabsorption usually proceeds at the rate of fluid accumulation, although it may persist longer. Redistribution of fluid is often complex and unpredictable and is marked by diuresis.

In most children the cardiovascular system is able to withstand the demands placed on it, although shock is a prominent feature of large thermal injuries. Some children are prone to congestive heart failure and pulmonary oedema. In addition, peripheral circulation in infants is less efficient and more labile, which complicates the burn response and therapy in this age group.

Renal System. Children younger than 2 years of age lack the ability to concentrate urine because of the immaturity of their renal system and are therefore at an increased risk for dehydration. In addition, the child has a relatively larger TBSA in relation to weight than an adult. These issues, combined with limited physiological reserves, increase the fluid requirements for children during burn shock resuscitation and in compensating for evaporative water losses (Hazinski et al 2019). Loss of fluid from the intravascular compartment causes renal vasoconstriction that in turn leads to reduced renal plasma flow and depressed glomerular filtration. When adequate fluids are provided, the glomerular filtration rate returns to normal, and by the third or fourth postburn day, urinary output increases as oedema fluid is mobilised and eliminated. In the first few days, oliguria is more commonly the result of inadequate fluid replacement than of acute renal failure. If the child does not respond to treatment or if there is inadequate fluid resuscitation, acute renal failure may develop, with significant kidney damage.

Blood urea nitrogen (BUN) and creatinine levels are elevated as a result of tissue breakdown, decreased circulating volume and oliguria. Haematuria may also be evident from the haemolysis of red blood cells, and oliguria may develop as a consequence of the increased pigment load. Myoglobinuria is especially common after extensive electrical injury or burn injuries with deep muscle destruction. Cell destruction releases large amounts of myoglobin, which occludes the kidney tubules and places these victims, especially those of electrical trauma, at high risk for renal failure.

Gastrointestinal System. The GI system has been recognised as a target of systemic shock. After a burn injury, blood flow decreases to the GI system by a third even though cardiac output is maintained by resuscitation fluids. Ischaemia results and can produce ulcer formation, enterocolitis (severe enough to cause full-thickness necrosis) and even intestinal perforation. Poor perfusion to the kidney and the liver can ensue, resulting in organ dysfunction. The GI tract functions as a barrier to contain GI bacteria within it. Disruption of the GI mucosal integrity is possibly a focus for sepsis in the burn patient.

Depending on the proportion of burn size, atrophy of the GI tract mucosa can occur immediately after injury. The atrophy results in gut barrier dysfunction, leading to increased bacterial translocation and ultimately sepsis. Within hours after injury, enteral nutrition can be started safely. Implementing this practice assists in maintaining caloric goals and may also reduce infection for the burn patient. Intestinal motility returns as fluid losses are replaced unless irreversible necrosis of the bowel has occurred as a result of insufficient perfusion (Hazinski et al 2019).

The greatly accelerated metabolic rate in burn patients is supported by protein and lipid catabolism. The child has limited glycogen stores to provide energy, which therefore accelerates the protein and lipid breakdown. No other disease state produces as great a hypermetabolism as the burn injury. Therefore, protein breakdown in the muscle and also in other organs can lead to multiple organ dysfunction (Jeschke 2016). When the burn injury is extensive (> 50% of TBSA), energy needs may approach twice the predicted basal requirements.

The stress of injury places high demands on the body. Stress-invoked glycogen breakdown depletes the energy stores in 12 to 24 hours, after which the body resorts to glyconeogenesis for high-energy needs. Blood glucose levels may be elevated as a result of insulin resistance. Rapid protein breakdown and muscle wasting occur if sufficient protein replacement is not provided.

Body temperature reflects the net balance between heat production and heat loss. As a result of the accelerated metabolism, children with burn injuries typically exhibit an elevated body temperature, even in the absence of infection. The thermoregulatory response is activated and results in an elevation of core body temperature. Burn-injured patients strive for a core body temperature of about 38°C. Low or 'normal' temperature may indicate overwhelming sepsis or a fatigued physiological capability to maintain temperature and should be viewed with concern. Routine methods of heat conservation after a major burn injury are inadequate because of excessive heat loss through evaporation and convection (Hazinski et al 2019). Heat is lost as a result of the energy-consuming process of water evaporation from the damaged skin surface. The body tries to raise the core and skin temperature to offset heat losses secondary to evaporation through the burn eschar (Gauglitz et al 2012). Infants and young children are especially vulnerable because of the large surface area relative to metabolically active tissue. Burning destroys a lipid layer and converts skin that is normally impermeable to water to a state that transmits water vapour at least four times as rapidly as unburned skin. In partial-thickness burns this loss is greatest on the day of injury; in full-thickness burns it rises slowly at first and rapidly increases to reach a peak on approximately the fourth day after the burn. Evaporative losses continue until partial-thickness wounds are healed and full-thickness burns are grafted. Therefore, body stores of energy are rapidly depleted unless sufficient replacement is provided or losses are reduced.

Medications that affect metabolic rate may be used to prevent loss of body protein stores, thus protecting immunity, wound healing, muscle integrity and organ function. Oxandrolone is an anabolic steroid that works to maintain and restore muscle mass, increase weight gain and promote wound healing. Supplements of essential amino acids such as glutamine and arginine provide an anticatabolic effect, support wound healing, indirectly preserve lean body mass, improve immune function and provide an antioxidant quality (Quain & Khardori 2015).

Neuroendocrine System. As a systemic response to stress from the burn injury, adrenal activity is markedly increased and catecholamines, such as adrenaline (epinephrine) and noradrenaline (norepinephrine), are released, which initiates vasoconstriction. Soon after, other local mediators are released, such as histamine, bradykinin, serotonin, prostaglandins and many others. This induces vasodilation and increased cell permeability, resulting in local oedema and the development of capillary leakage, requiring fluid resuscitation (Rae et al 2016).

Anaemia and Metabolic Acidosis. The haematocrit is initially elevated because of haemoconcentration resulting from fluid shifts to the interstitial spaces, red blood cell destruction and increased blood viscosity. A combination of heat-damaged red blood cells, blood loss at the wound sites and dilution from resuscitation fluids results in anaemia for the burn patient (Fidkowski & Fuzaylov 2012). In addition, a reduced red blood cell half-life results from increased cell fragility. A significant loss of circulating red blood cell mass is predominantly associated with major burns.

Growth and Development. Children may demonstrate postburn growth restriction. Regular height and extremity assessments are necessary to detect subtle deformities until development is normalised.

Complications

Thermally injured children are subject to a number of serious complications, both from the wound and from systemic alterations resulting from the injury. The immediate threat to life is related to airway compromise and profound shock. During healing, infection—both local and systemic sepsis—is the primary complication. Mortality associated with thermal trauma in children increases with the severity of injury and decreases as age advances. In children older than 3 years, the mortality rate is similar to that of adults. Below this age, the rate of survival from the burn and its associated complications lessens considerably.

Pulmonary System. The impact of thermal injury on pulmonary function includes a full range of respiratory dysfunctions including inhalation injury, disruption of the oxygen supply to the body, aspiration of gastric contents, bacterial pneumonia, pulmonary oedema and insufficiency and emboli. In every age and burn size category, pneumonia is associated with a high risk of mortality and can cause a secondary insult leading to further toxic damage even days after the injury. Inhalation of carbonaceous debris impairs function of the cilia and results in a release of inflammatory mediators that are chemotactic to neutrophils and destroys alveolar-based macrophages, leading to a proliferation of bacteria (Nielson et al 2017).

The mortality rate of admitted patients due to smoke inhalation as a factor is 52% (Burns Registry of Australia and New Zealand 2017). Inhalation injuries result from trauma to the tracheobronchial tree after inhalation of the heated gases and toxic chemicals produced during combustion. Although direct thermal injury to the upper airway may occur, heat damage below the vocal cords is rare. Inspired heated air is cooled in the upper airway before reaching the trachea. Reflex closure of the cords and laryngeal spasm prevent full inhalation. Evidence of direct thermal injury to the upper airway includes burns of the face and lips, singed nasal hairs and laryngeal oedema. Clinical manifestation may be delayed as long as 24 to 48 hours (Rodgers et al 2017). Wheezing, increasing secretions, hoarseness, wet rales and carbonaceous secretions are signs of respiratory tract involvement. Upper airway obstruction is often associated with burn shock and fluid resuscitation. In such situations endotracheal intubation may be necessary to preserve a patent airway.

A common aetiological factor in respiratory failure in the paediatric population is bacterial pneumonia, which may be secondary to airway injury or contamination from intubation or may be acquired through haematogenous spread of bacteria. Early in the postburn period the largest percentage of pulmonary infections result from nosocomial exposure, immobility and abdominal distension. The haematogenous variety occurs later and is related to the septic burn wound or other foci, such as phlebitis at the site of an invasive IV line.

Wound Sepsis. Sepsis is a critical problem in the treatment of burns and is an ever-present threat after the shock phase. Initially, burn wounds are relatively pathogen free unless contaminated with potentially infectious material such as dirt or polluted water. However, dead tissue and exudate provide a fertile field for bacterial growth. On approximately the third postburn day, early colonisation of the wound surface by a preponderance of gram-positive organisms (primarily staphylococci) changes to predominantly gram-negative opportunistic organisms, particularly *Pseudomonas aeruginosa.* By the fifth postburn day, bacterial invasion is well under way beneath the surface of the burn wound.

Characteristics of the burn wound contribute to the proliferation of pathogenic organisms. Vascular supply to full-thickness burns is occluded immediately, and no appreciable blood is supplied to the area for approximately 3 weeks after the injury. In partial-thickness wounds the circulation to the injured area is suspended for 24 to 48 hours; circulation is then restored unless infection supervenes. Thrombosis from bacterial invasion will impair circulation sufficiently to convert partial-thickness wounds to full-thickness injuries. These large amounts of non-viable tissue also provide an excellent medium for the growth of microorganisms. Hence the burn wound serves as the site of primary invasion for instances of localised or generalised infection. Because the burned child is immunosuppressed for many weeks after the burn injury, maintaining the wound at low contamination levels by meticulous wound care and vigilance for signs of infection can decrease the frequency of septic episodes caused by wound flora (Rowan et al 2015).

Occlusion of the local blood supply impairs the delivery of both humoral and cellular defence mechanisms to the burned area. Initially there is a decrease in inflammatory and phagocytic cells to the wound, but the number of phagocytes gradually increases until they are present in abundance by the third postburn week, when granulation tissue is forming. Granulation tissue, with its rich blood supply, affords increasing resistance to infection. Organisms are normally a part of skin flora, so cultures with an organism concentration of $< 10^5$ bacteria/g tissue has been arbitrarily chosen as the level of burn wound invasion.

Microflora presence is influenced by the treatment modalities and choice of antibiotics. During the past 30 years there has been a reduction in the percentage of specific bacteria and fungi recovered from burn wounds. This reduction reflects improvements in patient management, nutritional support, aggressive excision and grafting of wounds, topical antimicrobial therapy and wound dressings. Sepsis, in burn injury, is a major complication and a significant factor in morbidity and mortality among paediatric patients (Tridente 2018).

NURSING CARE CONSIDERATIONS

Disorientation in the burned patient is one of the first signs of overwhelming sepsis. A spiking fever and diminished bowel sounds accompanied by paralytic ileus occur and progressively increase over 48 to 72 hours, after which the temperature falls to subnormal limits. Other factors suggesting sepsis include hyperglycaemia, insulin resistance, thrombocytopenia, abdominal distension, enteral feeding intolerance and diarrhoea. At this time the wound deteriorates, the white blood cell count is depressed and septic shock becomes manifest.

Gastrointestinal System. GI dysfunction is common after burn injury as evidenced by feeding intolerance, mucosa ulceration and bleeding, particularly in the stomach and duodenum. Within 72 hours of a major burn injury a significant number of patients may develop mucosal changes. This may progress to ulceration with septic episodes and hypoxaemia. Potential causes of stress ulcers in burn patients include mucosal ischaemia, increased acid production, increased acid back-diffusion, energy depletion, bile reflux and direct mucosal injury with placement of intraluminal tubes.

Excessive fluid volume and burns to the chest or abdomen decrease compliance and can contribute to a serious complication (increased intraabdominal pressure) that may have an underestimated incidence in burned individuals. Although children with increased intraabdominal pressure readings tended to be younger, larger TBSA injuries and full-thickness components were significantly associated with elevated pressures and can result in tissue ischaemia (Mondozzi et al 2018). Increased intraabdominal pressure has the potential to impair haemodynamics, renal function, hepatic malperfusion and pulmonary dysfunction. Despite maintaining cardiac output with fluid replacement, renal function remains impaired in the presence of increased intraabdominal pressure. A decompressive laparotomy is necessary to restore perfusion in children who have developed increased abdominal pressure.

Enteral feeding is one of the most important means of providing nutrition and has led to a decrease in mortality. Early enteral feeding often prevents some of these potential complications. Aggressive fluid resuscitation aids in maintaining adequate mucosal blood flow. Antacid and H_2 receptor antagonist therapy can effectively prevent ulceration of the stomach and duodenum.

Ileus is also a common complication after a burn injury. Sepsis, electrolyte imbalance, narcotics and renal failure are common causes. Patients experience abdominal distension and pain. Early enteral feeding again can assist in avoiding gastric ileus, which is an intestinal complication that can occur in severe burn injury (Victorian Adult Burns Management Service 2017).

Therapeutic Management

Emergency Care

The initial management of the burn patient begins at the scene of injury. The first priority is to stop the burning process. The child should then be transported immediately to the nearest medical facility for definitive treatment and evaluation for transfer to a burn centre. The child and the family will be extremely frightened and anxious; sensitivity to their emotional state provides reassurance during the transport process.

Stop the Burning Process. The chief aim of rescue in flame burns is to smother the fire, not fan it. Children tend to panic and run, which serves only to spread the flames and make assistance more difficult. Place the injured child in a horizontal position and roll in a blanket, rug or similar article, taking care to not cover the head and face because of the danger of inhaling toxic fumes. If nothing is available, the victim should lie down, cover the mouth with the hands and roll over slowly to extinguish the flames. Remaining in the vertical position may cause the hair to ignite or may lead to the inhalation of flames, heat or smoke.

Major burn injuries with large amounts of denuded skin should briefly be cooled with a single application of cool running water for 20 minutes within 3 hours following the burn injury (NSW ACI 2019). To prevent hypothermia, the rest of the body must be kept warm (NSW ACI 2019). Heat is rapidly lost from burned areas, and additional cooling leads to a drop in core body temperature and potential circulatory collapse. Continuous wet dressings or the application of ice promotes vasoconstriction because of cooling, resulting in impaired circulation to the burned area and increased tissue damage. Chemical burns present special circumstances and require flushing with copious amounts of water during transport to a medical facility. The use of neutralising agents on the skin is contraindicated because a chemical reaction is initiated and further injury may result. If the chemical is in powder form, the addition of water may spread the caustic agent. The powder should be brushed off if possible. If the chemical burn produces a blister, it is advisable to open the blister with a sterile object to remove any chemical present.

Assess the Victim's Condition. As soon as the flames are extinguished, assess the victim's condition. Airway, breathing and circulation are the priority concerns. Cardiopulmonary and cerebral emergencies are always a consideration after trauma. Cardiopulmonary complications may result from inhalation of toxic fumes and smoke, exposure to electric current, hypovolaemia and shock. Institute emergency measures as appropriate (e.g. CPR).

Cover the Burn. Cover the burn with a clean, dry dressing or cling wrap to prevent contamination and alleviate pain by eliminating air contact. Cover the child who has extensive burns to prevent hypothermia. No attempt should be made to treat the burn. Debridement of the burn at this time is unnecessary. The application of topical ointments, oils or other home remedies immediately post burn is contraindicated because these applications may intensify the burn.

Transport the Child to Medical Aid. Do not give the child with an extensive burn anything by mouth to avoid aspiration in the presence of paralytic ileus and upper airway oedema and to prevent water intoxication. The child is transported to the nearest medical facility. If this cannot be accomplished within a relatively short time, establish IV access if possible with a large-bore catheter. Oxygen, if available, is administered at 100%. Give a report of the initial assessment and any interventions implemented to the medical facility assuming responsibility for the child's care.

Provide Reassurance. Providing reassurance and psychological support to both the family and the child helps immeasurably during postinjury crisis. Reducing anxiety helps conserve the energy needed to cope with the physiological and emotional stress of a traumatic injury.

Management of Minor Burns

Treatment of burns classified as minor can usually be managed adequately on an outpatient basis when the caregiver is reliable and able to carry out instructions for care and observation. Patients with less than optimum circumstances may require close follow-up to ensure compliance with the treatment program.

Cleanse the burn with an approved solution such as normal saline or aqueous chlorhexidine 0.1% solution (NSW ACI 2019). Debridement of the burn includes removal of any embedded debris, devitalised tissue and chemicals. Removal of intact blisters remains controversial. Some authorities argue that blisters provide a barrier against infection as the fluid contained within the blisters is considered sterile (RCHM 2019); others maintain that blister fluid is an effective medium for the growth of microorganisms. In New South Wales, 'de-roofing (removal of skin and fluid)' is recommended in the management of minor burn blisters (NSW ACI 2019). Most practitioners favour covering the burn with an antimicrobial ointment to reduce the risk of infection and provide some pain relief. The dressing consists of a fine-mesh gauze placed over the ointment and a light wrap of gauze dressing that avoids interference with movement. This helps keep the burn clean and protect it from trauma. Instruct the caregiver to wash the burn, reapply the dressing and return the child to the office or clinic as directed for observation of signs of infection, progression of healing or any other related complications (e.g. ineffectiveness of pain medication, decreased appetite). The frequency of dressing changes can vary.

Some practitioners prefer an occlusive dressing, such as a hydrocolloid or a silver wound dressing, which is placed over the burn after cleansing. This method eliminates the discomfort associated with frequent dressing changes but impairs visualisation of the burn surface.

Management of Major Burns

When a child with extensive burns is admitted to the hospital burns unit for treatment, a variety of assessments are conducted and therapies initiated. Of these, the priority concerns include the establishment and maintenance of an adequate airway, initiation of fluid administration and evaluation and treatment of the burn. Although the order of implementation may vary from institution to institution and the condition of the child, a number of procedures and activities are generally initiated on admission. Some are carried out simultaneously (Box 23.7).

Other therapies, including nutritional support, positioning and splinting to prevent contractures, treatment of anaemia and hypoproteinaemia, psychosocial support and rehabilitative aspects of burn management, are initiated as appropriate throughout the course of treatment.

Establishment of An Adequate Airway. The first priority of care is airway maintenance. Thermal injuries to the face, nares and upper torso; a history of injury in an enclosed space; carbonaceous sputum; an examination of the oral and nasal membranes that reveals oedema, hyperaemia and blisters; and evidence of trauma to the upper respiratory passages all suggest inhalation of noxious agents or respiratory burns. If there is evidence of respiratory involvement, administer 100% oxygen and determine blood gas values, including carbon monoxide levels.

If the child exhibits changes in sensorium, air hunger, nasal flaring, grunting or other signs of respiratory distress insert an endotracheal tube to maintain the airway. When severe oedema of the face and neck is anticipated, perform intubation before swelling makes it difficult or

BOX 23.7 Major Burn Management

- Ascertain the adequacy of the airway, and provide oxygen, intubation and ventilatory support as indicated.
- Assess breathing rate and depth. Note any use of accessary muscles, nasal flaring or grunting which may indicate respiratory compromise.
- Insert a large-bore intravenous (IV) line, preferably through unburned skin, to deliver fluids at a sufficiently rapid rate to effect resuscitation.
- Remove clothing and jewellery, and examine for secondary trauma.
- Evaluate the burn wound, and determine the extent and depth of injury.
- Obtain an admission weight.
- Calculate fluid requirements, and establish the appropriate regimen.
- Obtain baseline laboratory studies.
- Provide IV medication for control of pain and anxiety only after adequate oxygenation is ensured and fluid resuscitation is initiated.
- Insert a nasogastric tube to empty stomach contents and maintain gastric decompression.
- Insert an indwelling Foley catheter to obtain specimens and monitor hourly output.
- Perform escharotomy or fasciotomy to the chest and extremities for constricting circumferential eschar, elevated compartment pressures or impaired circulation.
- Apply topical antimicrobials and dressings to the burn wounds.
- Obtain a history regarding the injury and other pertinent data.
- Administer appropriate tetanus prophylaxis.
- Prophylactic antibiotic administration is not recommended.

impossible. A controlled intubation is preferred to an emergency procedure. Intubation allows for the delivery of humidified oxygen, the removal of secretions from respiratory passages and the provision of ventilatory support.

Treatment may include bronchodilators (e.g. albuterol) to reduce bronchospasm. Bronchopulmonary hygiene to prevent atelectasis and pooling of secretions reduces the risk of pneumonia. Therapies include percussion and postural drainage, frequent position changes and suctioning to remove secretions. Placing the child in a semi-Fowler's position with high-flow oxygen and maximum humidity is often sufficient to relieve bronchospasm produced by trauma to the bronchial mucosa.

When full-thickness burns encircle the chest, constricting eschar may limit chest wall excursion. The child becomes increasingly difficult to ventilate. Escharotomy of the chest, where the eschar is incised through the fatty tissue, relieves this pressure and improves ventilation.

Fluid Replacement Therapy. The objectives of fluid therapy are compensation for water and sodium losses to the traumatised area and the interstitial spaces, replenishment of sodium deficits, restoration of circulating volume, provision of adequate perfusion, correction of acidosis and improvement of renal function. The volume of fluids should be just enough to provide adequate vital organ perfusion without producing unintentional (iatrogenic) pathological changes. Initiate treatment for burn shock in children with burns in excess of 15% of TBSA.

The composition of the fluid administered varies with the philosophy of the individual practitioner and may consist of an isotonic saline solution, a near-isotonic solution or even a hypertonic saline solution. Children's decreased tolerance to hypertonic solutions may result in hypernatraemia, hyperosmolality and intracellular dehydration. Many formulas have been proposed as guidelines for fluid administration after burn injury. The most commonly employed regimen is the Parkland formula. It is important to remember that any formula used during resuscitation serves only as a guideline; individual adjustments must be made based on the patient's response to therapy to avoid under or over resuscitation. Over-resuscitation can cause a condition called 'fluid creep' that can produce significant complications such as pulmonary oedema, ARDS, abdominal and extremity compartment syndrome and multiple organ dysfunction. Fluid replacement is maintained at a rate that provides an hourly urinary output of 1 mL/kg in children weighing less than 30 kg (Victorian Adult Burns Service 2017). For children who have burns of the perineum, it is recommended to insert an indwelling Foley catheter to reduce chances of wound contamination (Victorian Adult Burns Service 2017). Other parameters monitored during fluid resuscitation include vital signs, capillary refill and sensorium.

Some common reasons for patients to require fluids well in excess of the calculated volume include underestimation of burn size (particularly in paediatric patients), pulmonary injury that sequesters resuscitation fluid in the lung, electrical injury with greater tissue destruction than is visible and delay in the initiation of fluid resuscitation (Mondozzi et al 2018). Irreversible burn shock that persists despite aggressive fluid resuscitation remains a significant cause of death in the immediate postburn period.

NURSING CARE CONSIDERATIONS

Capillary refill, alterations in sensorium and urinary output are the most reliable indicators for assessing the adequacy of fluid resuscitation in burned children. BP can remain normotensive even in a state of hypovolaemia.

After the initial 24 to 48 hours, the capillary seal is restored. Fluid requirements decrease to a constant that persists until wound coverage is achieved. Colloid solutions such as albumin or plasma are useful to maintain plasma volume. Fluid balance may continue to be a problem throughout the course of treatment, especially during periods of increased evaporative loss from the burn wound. Approximately 48 to 72 hours after injury, interstitial fluid returns to the vascular compartment and diuresis occurs to eliminate excess fluids. During this phase, increasing intake to match urinary output can result in circulatory overload.

Nutrition. For 2 or 3 days immediately after injury, burn patients experience a hypometabolic phase when their metabolic rate and cardiac output decrease. Following this phase patients experience a hypermetabolic phase. This hypermetabolism is characterised by a hyperdynamic circulatory response with increased body temperature, oxygen and glucose consumption, carbon dioxide production, glycogenolysis, proteolysis and lipolysis. This response begins on the fifth postburn day and continues up to 9 months after the burn, causing erosion of lean body mass, muscle weakness, immunodepression and poor wound healing (Jeschke 2016). This hypermetabolism is thought to be directly and indirectly associated with poor outcomes after a burn and can lead to slow wound healing, loss of lean body mass and increased morbidity (Jeschke 2016). Nutritional support, particularly through enteral feedings and initiated early in the burn patient's course, has become more aggressive. The continuity of these feedings is important.

Some burn patients are able to eat. Encourage a high-protein, high-calorie diet as soon as possible after resolution of paralytic ileus. However, many have poor appetites and are unable to meet energy requirements solely by oral feeding. Most children with burns in excess of 25% TBSA require supplementation with tube feeding. An absence of bowel sounds does not preclude enteral nutrition. Because the small bowel maintains motility and absorptive capabilities, the placement of a small-bore feeding tube into the duodenum allows for the safe delivery of enteral nutrition during periods of paralytic ileus associated with trauma, sepsis and anaesthesia. A nasogastric tube that decompresses the stomach protects the patient from aspiration.

Use of total parenteral nutrition has essentially been replaced by enteral nutrition for both theoretical and practical reasons and only used for those children who are unable to tolerate enteral support due to risks. Enteral nutrition directly nourishes the bowel mucosa with nutrients (e.g. glutamine). Small amounts of these nutrients within the bowel lumen stimulate the function of intestinal cells and normal mucosa function. This may help preserve normal blood supply to the intestines. Maintaining intestinal integrity may reduce bacterial translocation and sepsis, as well as preserve immune function. Along with the hazards of central venous access, total parenteral nutrition appears to be associated with increased secretion of tumour necrosis factor and other proinflammatory mediators (Feng et al 2015).

Specific guidelines for vitamin and micronutrient supplementation for the burn patient have not been established. Although supplementation with a variety of micronutrients is common practice, limited research has been done in burn patients on the homeostasis of vitamins and trace elements after burn injury (Berger et al 2017).

Medication. Antibiotics are usually not administered prophylactically. The administration of systemic antibiotics to control wound colonisation is not indicated because decreased circulation to the injured area prevents delivery of the medication to areas of deepest injury. Surveillance cultures and monitoring of the clinical course provide the most reliable indicators of developing infection. Appropriate antibiotics can then be instituted to treat the identified organism. Group B streptococci cultured from the throat or wounds are particularly destructive to grafted tissue. Do not overlook otitis media as a source of fever in the paediatric population.

Pain management presents a significant challenge and provisions of some form of sedation and analgesia is necessary. Effective pain management can lead to better outcomes due to the reduction in physiological demands caused by stress on the body and a decrease in psychological disorders such as depression and posttraumatic stress (Meyer et al 2012). During the initial resuscitation period, IV administration of narcotics, along with anxiolytics, is required for baseline and procedural pain management. Morphine, fentanyl (Sublimaze) and midazolam Midazolam (Hypnovel) are the most commonly used agents (Singleton et al 2015). (See Pain Management, Chapter 5.)

Anaesthetic agents such as nitrous oxide, propofol and ketamine are also used to control procedural pain. A major drawback with nitrous oxide is that staff is exposed to the gas because it is self-administered by the patient. Propofol, a non-barbiturate hypnotic agent without analgesic activity, has advantages of rapid onset and little cumulative effect after extended infusion periods. It can cause depressed respiratory drive, loss of airway reflexes and hypertension. Propofol must be given in doses large enough to cause loss of consciousness to prevent response to painful procedures. Even though this drug has a 'black box' warning of increased morbidity when used for the paediatric population, it is perceived as effective and safe and ranks high in use (Singleton et al 2015). Ketamine has been widely used in burn patients and may preserve airway reflex; however, side effects may be noted, such as production of copious upper airway secretions, tachycardia and hypertension. Ketamine can produce post-administration hallucinations, particularly in adolescent boys. Repeated use may produce tolerance, so increased doses are required over time. To avoid volatile anaesthetics, a combination of midazolam and fentanyl can be given intravenously (Meyer et al 2012).

Management of the Burn Wound

After the initial period of shock and restoration of fluid balance, the primary concern is the burn wound. The primary goal for burn wound management is to close the burn as soon as possible (Rowan et al 2015). The objectives of burn wound management include prevention of infection, removal of devitalised tissue and closure of the wound. The application of dressings and topical antimicrobial therapy reduces pain by minimising air exposure.

Primary Excision. In children with large, full-thickness burn wounds, as soon as the patient is haemodynamically stable after initial resuscitation, a surgical intervention is required and usually an excision is performed which is followed by application of antimicrobial dressings (Quinn & Holland 2016). Because the burn wound is precipitating the exaggerated physiological response, many associated complications do not resolve until the eschar is excised and the wound is closed. One of the most effective therapies for decreasing mortality from major burn injuries is the early excision of the burn wound and its coverage by various techniques (Rowan et al 2015).

Wound Hygiene. Hydrotherapy is used to cleanse the burn and assist with separating eschar. This involves either showering (spraying off the burn) or immersion (soaking in a bath tub) at least once a day. There are variances from institution to institution on the particular method; however, immersion therapy is becoming less common and being replaced by shower hydrotherapy. Hydrotherapy helps cleanse not only the wound but the entire body and also aids in maintenance of range of motion. Partial-thickness burns require debridement of devitalised tissue to promote healing. Debridement is very painful and requires some type of analgesia and anxiolytic before the procedure. The water acts to loosen and remove sloughing tissue, exudate and topical medications. Mesh gauze entraps the exudative slough and is readily removed during hydrotherapy. Any loose tissue is carefully trimmed away before the burn is redressed (Fig 23.11).

Burn Wound Dressings. Dressing changes of the burn wound allow for inspection and cleansing of the burn and must be done according to the recommendation for the type of material used (e.g. Mepilex every 3 to 7 days, Acticoat every 3 to 4 days, Acticoat 7 every 7 days) (NSW ACI 2019). Dressing changes offer an opportunity to meticulously observe the burn for infection. The volume of draining and the physical condition of the dressing also dictate frequency of dressing change. Often burn dressings become saturated, soiled or dishevelled, indicating that additional dressing changes may be required (Hartford 2012).

Topical Antimicrobial Agents. Several methods are used for covering the burn wound (Box 23.8). All meet the objective of preparation for permanent wound coverage, and all use some type of topical agent. Before the development of effective topical agents for reducing the incidence of invasive organisms, wound sepsis was the major cause of mortality from burn injury. The goal is to minimise wound colonisation. A variety of specific agents are available; examples include silver sulfadiazine (Flamazine). Topical agents do not eliminate organisms from the wound but can effectively inhibit bacterial growth. To be effective, a topical application must be non-toxic, capable of diffusing through eschar, harmless to viable tissue, inexpensive and easy to

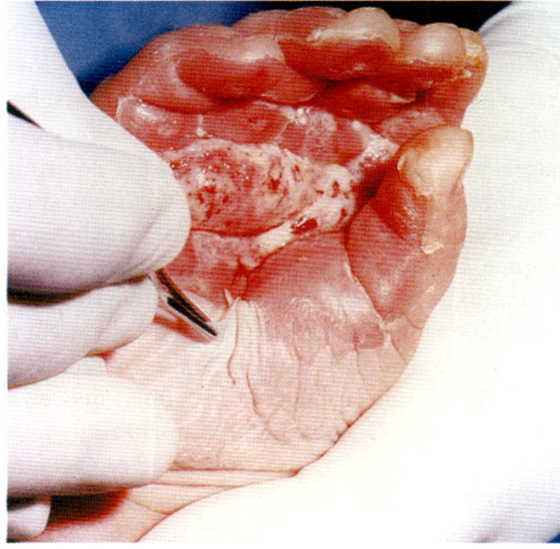

Fig 23.11 Dead skin and debris are carefully trimmed away before dressing is applied. (Source: Courtesy CR Boeckman Regional Burn Center, Akron, Ohio.)

BOX 23.8 Methods of Burn Wound Management

Exposure—Wounds are left open to air; crust forms on partial-thickness wounds and eschar forms on full-thickness burns.

Open—A thin layer of topical antimicrobial agent is applied directly to the wound surface, and the wound is left uncovered.

Modified—Antimicrobial is applied directly or impregnated into thin gauze and applied to the wound; gauze or net secures the area (see Fig 23.13).

Occlusive—Antimicrobial is impregnated in gauze or applied directly to the wound; multiple layers of bulky gauze are placed over the primary layer and secured with gauze or net. Occlusive methods may impede joint movement due to bulky gauze wraps. Advantages include reduction of evaporative heat loss from the wound, comfort and protection.

apply. It should not encourage the development of resistant strains of bacteria and should produce minimum electrolyte derangement.

Temporary Skin Substitutes. Permanent coverage of extensive burns is a prolonged process that requires repeated operations for debridement and grafting. Transient physiological wound closure is achieved by temporary skin substitutes, thereby helping control pain, absorb wound exudates and prevent wound desiccation (Rowan et al 2015). Temporary skin substitutes markedly reduce pain and facilitate movement of joints to retain range of motion.

Allograft (homograft) skin comes from human cadavers and is processed by commercial skin banks (Box 23.9). These skin banks screen donors for communicable diseases and track the skin much like blood transfusions. Allograft skin is particularly useful in the coverage of surgically excised, deep partial-thickness and full-thickness wounds in extensive burns when available donor sites are limited. Severe immunosuppression occurs in massively burned children, and the allograft becomes adherent (Fig 23.12). The allograft can remain in place until suitable donor sites become available. Typically rejection occurs approximately 14 days after application. The use of an allograft is limited by the availability of tissue banks and the supply of suitable donors.

BOX 23.9 Types of Skin Grafts

Temporary Grafts

Allografts (homografts)—Skin that is obtained from genetically different members of the same species who are free of disease.

Xenografts (heterografts)—Skin that is obtained from members of a different species, primarily pigskin.

Permanent Grafts

Autografts—Tissue obtained from undamaged areas of the patient's own body.

Isografts—Histocompatible tissue obtained from genetically identical individuals.

Methods of Applying Split-thickness Grafts

Sheet graft—A sheet of skin, removed from the donor site, is placed intact over the recipient site and sutured in place (see Fig 23.18 later in this chapter).

Mesh graft—A sheet of skin is removed from the donor site and passed through a mesher, which produces tiny slits in the skin. The meshing allows the expansion of the skin to cover 1.5 to 9 times the area of the sheet graft (see Fig 23.19 later in this chapter).

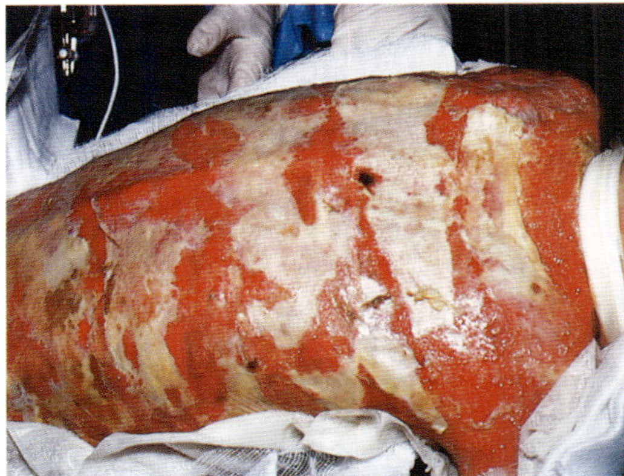

Fig 23.12 Adherent allograft applied to excised full-thickness wound.

Although various animal skins have been used to provide temporary coverage of wounds, only porcine xenograft is widely used today. Porcine xenograft does not vascularise, but it will adhere to a clean superficial burn and provide excellent pain control while the burn heals (Burkey 2016).

Synthetic Skin Coverings. A number of satisfactory skin substitutes are available for the management of partial-thickness burns. Ideally, the dressing should provide many of the properties of human skin: adherence, elasticity, durability and haemostasis. Synthetic skin substitutes are readily available, have varied shelf lives and are relatively expensive.

Synthetic dressings are composed of a variety of materials and can be used successfully in the management of superficial partial-thickness burns and donor sites. These dressings do not contain antimicrobial properties. Examples include a petrolatum dressing (Mepitel/Jelonet/Bactigras), a hydrocolloid dressing (DuoDERM) and transparent adhesive films (OpSite and Tegaderm). As with biological dressings, it is important that the burn is free of debris before applying the dressing. Body temperature elevation or evidence of purulence, erythema or cellulitis around the burn edges may indicate that the burn has become infected beneath the dressing. Prompt discontinuance of the synthetic dressing is indicated. All synthetic dressings are reputed to hasten burn wound healing and reduce discomfort.

Dermal Replacements. The development of products that replace or allows the dermis to regenerate has significantly improved burn wound healing and decreased scar formation. Acticoat or Acticoat 7 with or without IntraSite and Hyperfix is a two-layer product that can be applied to partial- and full-thickness burns. The inner layer is a porous matrix made of cross-linked fibres designed to induce better regeneration of the patient's normal tissue by acting as a scaffold. The outer layer is a soft silicone membrane that protects the wound from infection and holds moisture for 2 to 3 weeks acting like the skin's epidermis. The silicone layer is peeled off after the dermis is formed. The application of artificial skin does not replace the grafting procedure, but it prepares the burn wound to accept an ultrathin autograft. Advantages include faster healing of the burn wound when integrity of the dermis is restored, faster healing of donor sites with the use of ultrathin grafts and restoration of sweat glands and hair follicles. Integra must be observed for submembrane infection. A disadvantage is its high cost.

Permanent Skin Coverings. Permanent coverage of deep partial- and full-thickness burns is usually accomplished with a split-thickness skin graft. This graft consists of the epidermis and a portion of the dermis removed from an intact area of skin by a special instrument: the dermatome (Fig 23.13). If all the wounds cannot be grafted at once, there are priority areas for coverage: the face, hands, joint surfaces and neck. These preferential sites are chosen to hasten healing, establish function and improve the patient's sense of wellbeing.

With extensive burns it is often difficult to find enough viable skin to cover the wounds; therefore, available donor sites are used to the best advantage by special techniques. Box 23.9 describes the various types of split-thickness skin grafts. Sheet grafts (Fig 23.14) are used in areas where cosmetic results are most visible; mesh grafts (Fig 23.15) result in a less desirable cosmetic and functional outcome. Requirements for the successful vascularisation of any graft are listed in Box 23.10.

Until blood supply to the grafted skin is established, it is nourished by osmotic interchange with the recipient bed. Wound healing occurs as the area releases fibrin, which attaches the graft to the bed. The fibrin is infiltrated by leucocytes, fibroblasts and the capillary buds of the granulation tissue. This process begins within hours of grafting, and vascularisation is established after 3 days. Within 2 weeks the graft is attached to the recipient bed by connective tissue.

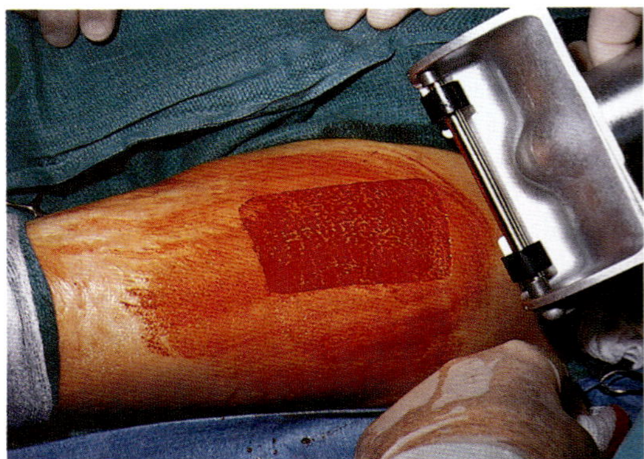

Fig 23.13 Removal of split-thickness skin graft with a dermatome.

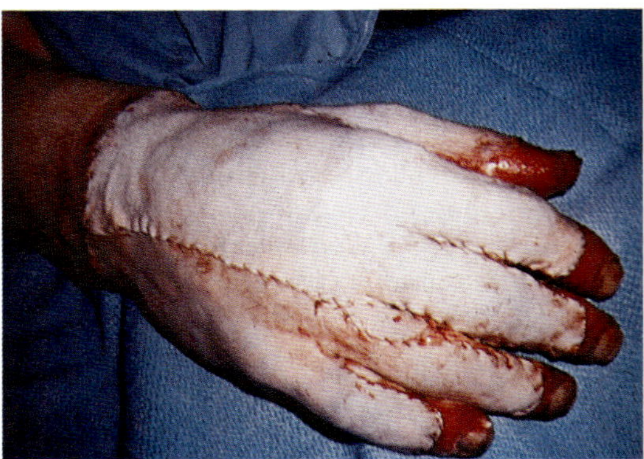

Fig 23.14 Sheet graft.

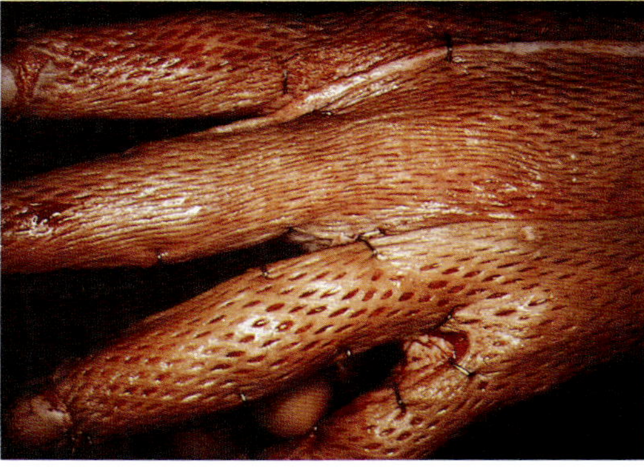

Fig 23.15 Mesh graft.

BOX 23.10 Requirements for a Successful Graft

- Sufficient nourishment until the new blood supply is established from the base of the recipient bed
- Primary tissue contact (e.g. actual contact between the surface of the graft and a recipient bed that is free of bacteria and necrotic skin)
- Avoidance of bleeding, haematoma formation and fluid accumulation beneath the graft
- Prevention of infection
- Prevention of mechanical trauma

Cultured Epithelium. For more than 30 years it has been possible to culture vast numbers of epithelial cells from a small skin biopsy, and this has led to the widespread use of cultured epithelial grafts to cover burns. Colonies of epithelial cells expand into broad sheets of undifferentiated epithelial cells. The resulting sheets are attached to a petrolatum gauze carrier to ease handling. Many of the imperfections associated with epithelial cell wound closure may be attributed to the lack of dermis. Despite scattered cases, application of cultured epithelial grafts onto dermal replacement products that have been vascularised can improve short- and long-term results (Brockmann et al 2018). High cost is a disadvantage of using both applications. (See Quality Patient Outcomes box.)

QUALITY PATIENT OUTCOMES

Acute Management of Burns

- Stable body temperature
- Adequate fluid replacement and urinary output
- Adequate nutrition and reduction of metabolic losses
- No evidence of acute complications
- Pain controlled
- Evidence of wound healing
- No evidence of contractures
- Adequate emotional support

Nursing Care Management

Nursing care of the paediatric burn patient represents a challenge to the nurse's knowledge of anatomy and physiology, the behavioural sciences and pathophysiology. Patient outcome after thermal injury is the result of the collaboration of an interprofessional burn team using a family-centred care approach. In addition to providing nursing care, the nurse functions as the patient care advocate to coordinate the efforts of the interprofessional burn team.

Because the care of burned children encompasses such a broad range of skills and foci, it has been divided into segments that correspond to the major phases of burn treatment. The acute phase, also referred to as the emergent or resuscitative phase, involves the first 24 to 48 hours. The management phase extends from the completion of adequate resuscitation through wound coverage. The rehabilitative phase begins once the majority of the wounds have healed and rehabilitation becomes the predominant focus of the care plan. This phase continues until all reconstructive procedures and corrective measures have been accomplished, which often extends over a period of months or years.

Acute Phase

The primary emphasis during the emergent phase is the treatment of burn shock and management of pulmonary status. Monitoring vital signs, output, fluid infusion and respiratory parameters are ongoing activities in the hours immediately after injury. IV infusion begins immediately and is regulated to maintain a urinary output of at least 1 mL/kg in children weighing less than 30 kg. Expect an output of 1 mL/kg/hr in children weighing more than 30 kg. Urinary output, vital signs, laboratory data and objective signs of adequate hydration guide the rate of fluid administration.

NURSING CARE CONSIDERATIONS

Early indicators for the adequacy of hydration are level of consciousness and capillary refill.

The nurse observes patients for changes in all parameters. They require constant observation and assessment, with special attention given to signs of respiratory, cardiac and renal complications. Alterations in electrolyte balance can produce clinical symptoms of confusion, weakness, cardiac irregularities and seizures. Changes in respiratory function and gas exchange are reflected clinically by restlessness, irritability, increased work of breathing and alterations in blood gas values. The loss of the skin's protective function exposes burned children to an increased risk of hypothermia.

Care of the burn wound is secondary to the more critical problems of respiratory and cardiac failure. When transfer to a special burn care facility is anticipated, it is important to cover the wounds with clean dry sheets and wrap the child in blankets to maintain body temperature during transfer. The burn can be evaluated and dressed after arrival at the burn centre. If no burn unit is available, the burn is cleansed and dressed in the emergency department.

Throughout the acute phase of care, do not overlook the psychosocial needs of the children and their families. The child is frightened, uncomfortable and often confused. Children may be isolated from familiar persons and surroundings, and the often overwhelming physical needs at this time are the primary focus of the staff and parents. In addition to feeling concern for their child, the parents experience guilt, which is related to the fact they did not or could not protect their child. Consistency in the information presented and the attitude of the staff creates a sense of familiarity and stability during the emergent phase.

Management and Rehabilitative Phases

After the patient's condition is stabilised, the management phase begins. The multidisciplinary team concentrates on preventing infections, closing the burn wound as quickly as possible and managing the numerous complications that may occur. Although the rehabilitative phase begins when permanent burn closure has been achieved, rehabilitation issues are identified on admission and are included in the care plan throughout the hospital course.

The management phase of burn care involves intensive nursing care, which is often difficult for the patient, family and nursing staff. Except for minor burn injuries, care should take place in a burn centre and involve a variety of disciplines, such as respiratory care, nutrition, physical therapy, occupational therapy, child life specialist and social services.

Comfort Management. The severe pain of the burn and resultant therapies, the anxiety generated by these experiences, sleep deprivation, itching related to healing and the conscious and unconscious interpretations of traumatic events contribute to the psychological reactions and behaviours commonly observed in children with burns. It is important to assess the individual experiences and needs of the burn-injured child. A common myth in paediatrics is that children do not feel pain as intensely as adults do. What may be more accurate is that children do not always express their pain in the same way as adults. Children may display pain through behaviours of fear, anxiety, agitation, anger, aggression, tantrums, depression, withdrawal and regression.

To reduce the anxiety associated with an unfamiliar environment and frightening treatments, it is important to offer thorough, age-appropriate explanations to the child before procedures. Compounding the pain is the child's interpretation of it and of the procedure; this is closely related to the child's developmental level. Children often feel anger, guilt and depression; as in all illnesses, they may also exhibit regressive behaviour. When children appear to accept pain with little or no response, psychological consultation is in order.

Care of the Burn Wound. Closing the burn is the primary goal of burn wound care. The nurse has a major responsibility for cleansing, debriding and applying topical medications and dressings to the burn. Because dressing removal is a painful procedure and causes anxiety, children should receive adequate analgesia along with anxiolytics before the scheduled dressing change. The nurse should administer medication so that the drug's peak effect coincides with the procedure. Children who have an understanding of the procedure to be performed and some perceived control demonstrate less maladaptive behaviour. Children respond well to participating in decisions and the actual procedure as their condition allows.

Outer dressings are removed; any dressings that have adhered to the burn are easier to remove by applying tepid water. Loose or easily detached tissue is also debrided during the cleansing process. Encourage children to participate in dressing removal. Giving them something constructive to do helps them focus on something other than the procedure. In providing coverage for the burn, it is important that all areas are clean, the medication is amply applied or dressing covers the entire burn, and that no two burned surfaces touch each other (e.g. fingers or toes, or ears touching the side of the head). If touching, the burned surfaces will heal together, causing deformity or dysfunction.

Topical medications are applied directly to the burn with a clean gloved hand or impregnated into fine-mesh gauze before application. Prepackaged dressings already come prepared. Apply the dressings to assist in exudate absorption, wound debridement and increased patient comfort. All dressings applied circumferentially should be wrapped in a distal-to-proximal manner. Apply the dressing with sufficient tension to remain in place without impairing circulation or limiting motion. A stable dressing is especially important when the child is ambulatory.

Another challenge for nurses is preventing graft loss. After a graft is applied in surgery, there is usually a period of immobility for the child. Positioning must be maintained in order to prevent graft loss from shearing forces of movement. Grafted joint areas may be splinted to maintain range of motion or prevent contracture formation, and this may cause discomfort. Dressings protect the grafts and must be monitored for increased drainage or odours that are signs of infection. The child must also be instructed not to pick under the dressings, which could result in graft loss or infection.

Burns that involve the eyelids require special care to prevent corneal ulceration. No solution other than saline should come in contact with the eyes during the cleansing process. Avoid vigorous debridement in this area of thin, delicate tissue. Assess the patient throughout the healing process for the ability to close the eyes. Inability to close the eyes because of contracture formation, administration of paralytic agents or corneal burns requires instilling ophthalmic ointment. Prophylactic antibiotic ointment is applied and padded if possible (Victorian Adult Burns Service 2017).

Universal precautions, including the use of personal protective equipment (PPE) and barrier techniques, should be followed when caring for all patients with thermal injuries. Frequent hand and forearm washing is the single most important element of the infection control program. Implement strict policies for cleaning the environment and patient care equipment to minimise the risk of cross-contamination. All visitors and members of other departments should be oriented to the infection control policies, including the importance of hand and forearm washing and use of PPE when needed. Screen all visitors for infection and contagious diseases before patient contact.

Nutrition. Oral feedings are common unless the child is intubated or paralytic ileus persists. Because children often lack an appetite, the nursing staff must patiently provide a great deal of encouragement and help. Consultation between the parents and dietitian helps determine food preferences. Children who are old enough should participate in meal planning.

Children who require enteral supplementation by tube feeding must be monitored on an ongoing basis for feeding intolerance and tube malposition. The nurse should monitor and record any indications of abdominal distension, diarrhoea or electrolyte and metabolic derangement. Accurate documentation of oral, parenteral and enteral nutritional intake is essential to evaluate the adequacy of nutritional support.

Prevention of Complications: Acute Care. The maintenance of body temperature is important to the child with burns. Reduction of heat loss is imperative to decrease energy demands and evaporative water loss. Ambient temperatures and humidity should be maintained at 28°C to 33°C and 80%, respectively, to control heat loss (Lee et al 2012). Large areas of the body should not be exposed simultaneously during dressing changes. Warmed solutions, linens, occlusive dressings, heat shields, a radiant warmer and warming blankets assist in preventing hypothermia. The optimum environment for the child with burns can be uncomfortable for persons attending the child.

The chief danger during acute care is infection—burn wound infection, generalised sepsis or bacterial pneumonia. The burn should be assessed for changes indicative of infection, which include conversion of a partial-thickness to a full-thickness burn injury, early eschar separation, subeschar haemorrhage, degeneration of granulation tissue, discolouration of unburned skin at the wound margins or green discolouration of subcutaneous fat (indicative of *Pseudomonas* and other gram-negative organisms). In addition to the signs of developing burn wound infection, the child with systemic sepsis may have a core temperature of more than 38.5°C or less than 36°C, tachycardia, tachypnoea and leucocytosis or leucopenia. Tachycardia and tachypnoea are common presenting symptoms in many paediatric diseases. Children with septic shock often maintain a normal BP until they are severely ill. Shock may occur long before hypotension in children and is a late sign leading to decompensated shock. Meticulous assessment should include signs of decreased perfusion (including decreased peripheral pulses), altered alertness, prolonged capillary refill (> 2 seconds), mottled or cool extremities or decreased urinary output.

Children are reluctant to move when doing so causes pain, and they are likely to assume a position of comfort. Unfortunately, the most comfortable position is flexion, which encourages the formation of contractures and loss of function. Ongoing efforts to prevent contractures include the positioning and splinting of involved extremities in extension, active and passive physical therapy and the encouragement of spontaneous movement when feasible. In addition to maintenance of proper body alignment, frequent position changes are important to improve bronchopulmonary hygiene and capillary perfusion to common pressure areas. Low-air loss beds are beneficial for the morbidly obese or for children with posterior grafts. Areas of particular concern for pressure area development in the paediatric population are the posterior scalp, heels and areas exposed to mechanical irritation from splints and dressings.

Prevention of Complications: Long-term Care. The rehabilitative phase of care begins once burn wound coverage has been achieved. Scar formation becomes a major problem as healing occurs (Fig 23.16). The scar tissue is metabolically active and highly vascular; collagen is deposited in an undefined pattern. Contractile properties of the scar tissue can result in disabling contractures, deformity and disfigurement. As long as the scar is raised, red and firm, it is considered active (Fig 23.17). Hypertrophic scarring typically reaches a peak approximately 4 to 6 months after burn wound healing, and most scars mature or become inactive in 1 to 2 years. The mature scar is characterised by pigmented colour, flattening and increased suppleness of the tissue (Fig 23.18).

Scar tissue has certain significant properties, particularly for growing children. Intense itching occurs in healing burn wounds and scar tissue until the scar is no longer active. Itching is usually treated with diphenhydramine and frequent applications of a fragrance-free moisturiser, such as Sorbolene. Massage therapy during the application of moisturisers is also beneficial to stretch scar tissue and help prevent contracture. Scar tissue has no sweat glands, and children with extensive scarring may experience difficulty during hot

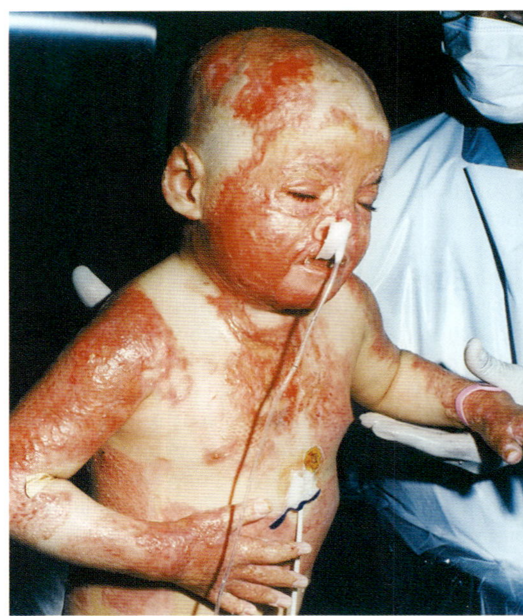

Fig 23.16 Extensive scars from flame burn. (Source: Courtesy CR Boeckman Regional Burn Center, Akron, Ohio.)

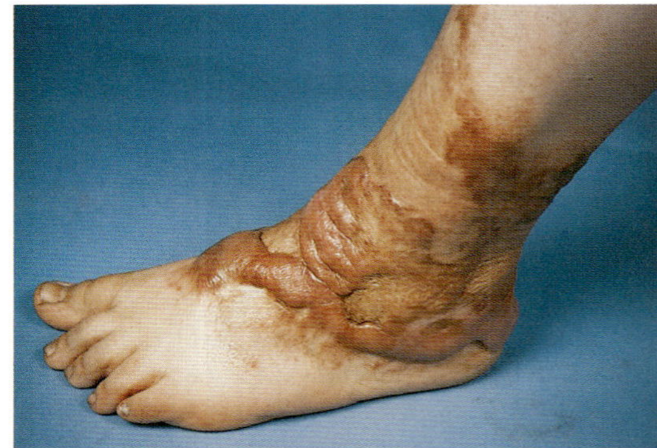

Fig 23.17 Hypertrophic immature scar.

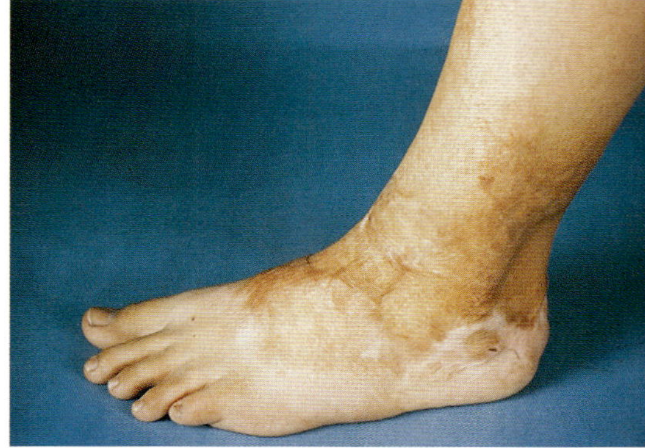

Fig 23.18 Flat, mature scar after pressure.

weather. Alert caregivers to this possibility and make sure they are prepared to institute alternative methods of cooling when necessary.

Scar tissue does not grow and expand like normal tissue, which may create difficulties, especially in functional areas such as the hands and over joints. Additional surgery is sometimes required to allow independent functioning in daily activities, to improve cosmetic appearance or to restore anatomical integrity. Reconstructive surgery employs various techniques, including local or distant flaps, full- or partial-thickness grafts, tissue expanders or pedicle flaps.

Psychosocial Support of the Child. Children should begin early to do as much for themselves as possible and to be active participants in their care. Loss of control and perceived helplessness may result in acting-out behaviours. Nurses should be sensitive to these feelings and allow the child the opportunity for choices and decision-making as the condition allows. At the same time, it is important to set boundaries and establish a daily schedule to provide a sense of predictability, security and control. During illness, children regress to a previous developmental level that allows them to deal with stress. As children begin to participate in their care, they gain in confidence and self-esteem. Fears and anxieties diminish with accomplishment and self-confidence. If the child demonstrates non-adherence in the rehabilitative phase, initiate a behaviour modification program to promote or reward the child's accomplishment in care.

Psychosocial Support of the Family. There is a growing recognition that trauma affects not only the victim but also those closest to the child. Severe trauma challenges the belief that the world is safe and predictable. Parents, caregivers and other family members are concerned about the child's survival, recovery and future potential. Recognising and respecting each family's strengths, differences and methods of coping allow the nurse to respond to their unique needs by implementing a family-centred approach to care. It is the family, particularly the parents or caregiver, who are the most significant persons in the child's life.

As in any emergency situation, all attention is focused on the child, and the parents or caregiver feel powerless and ineffectual. Most parents or caregivers feel overwhelming guilt, whether or not the guilt is justified. They feel responsible for the injury. These feelings may have a negative effect on the child's rehabilitation. For example, parents or caregivers may indulge the child and allow poor behaviour that affects physical and emotional recovery.

Caring for the Caregiver. Burn care is a complex and demanding specialty. Nurses who choose this field reap many rewards and endure many stresses. Ongoing support from peers, the multidisciplinary team and nursing management is important to assist burn nurses in caring for themselves so they can continue to render high-quality care to their patients.

Prevention of Burn Injury

Burn prevention is the responsibility of all members of the community. Nurses have an obligation to participate in educational efforts directed at parents, caregivers, children and others regarding the prevention of burn injuries and fire-related deaths. The best cure is prevention.

Infants and toddlers are most commonly injured by hot liquids in the kitchen and bathroom. These injuries often occur as a result of inadequate supervision of this curious and energetic age group. Target prevention efforts at parents and other caregivers; education includes the importance of adequate supervision and the establishment of safe play areas in the home. Hot liquids should be kept out of reach; tablecloths and dangling appliance cords are often pulled by toddlers, spilling hot grease and liquids on them. Electrical cords and outlets represent a potential risk to small children, who may chew on accessible cords and insert objects into outlets.

Established plumbing standards for newly constructed homes and residential units require antiscald technology and a maximum water heater temperature of 50°C (Australian Government 2013). By law, all newly installed hot water systems must comply with this regulation with the exception of early childhood centres, schools, aged care facilities or similar dwellings which are required to limit this to 45°C (Australian Government 2013). However, many hot water heaters remain set at levels well above the safe level. Small children are especially at risk for scald injuries from hot tap water because of their decreased reaction time and agility, their curiosity and the thermal sensitivity of their skin. Educate caregivers about never leaving a child in a bath without adult supervision. Caregivers should also test the water before placing a child in the bath tub or shower.

Future Research Needs

Many advances in burn prevention have reduced the occurrence of burn injury. Early excision and grafting of the burn wound, with control of infection, have improved survival rates for burn injury. Research in 2014 included areas in epidemiology, burn resuscitation, infection, critical care, nutrition and metabolism, pain management, rehabilitation, psychology, reconstruction, prevention and firefighter safety. A few examples of progress in research and the paediatric population resulted. It was found in the paediatric population that changes in fat metabolism, elevated fasting glucose and possible insulin resistance continue for months after the injury. Risk factors include age, percentage of burn injury and total body fat. In regard to increased body fat, it was found that this factor has a significant impact on a child's recovery from severe burn injury. Compared with non-obese paediatric burn patients, obese paediatric burn patients with comparable burn sizes suffered more pulmonary infections, required longer mechanical ventilation and sustained a lengthier ICU admission (Sen et al 2015). Areas for future research include multidisciplinary and holistic care needed to improve not only the physical recovery, but also the psychological recovery to treat this type of challenging trauma. Evidence for improvement of burn nursing care is best organised with research findings. Evidence-based practice integrates the nurse's clinical expertise with the best methods. It helps structure how to make accurate and timely decisions for care of the patient.

REFERENCES

Australian Government. (2019). Federal Register of Legislation: Consumer Goods (Children's Nightwear and limited daywear and Paper Patterns for Children's Nightwear) Amendment Safety Standard 2019. https://www.legislation.gov.au/Details/F2017L00452/Explanatory%20Statement/Text

Australian Government. (2013). Your home: Australia guide to environmentally sustainable homes: Hot water service. https://www.yourhome.gov.au/energy/hot-water-service

Berger, M. M., Sousse, L. E., Klein, G. L., et al. (2017). Micronutrient Homeostasis. In Herndon, D. N. (2017). Total Burn Care E-Book, (5th ed.). Elsevier Health Sciences.

Boehne, M., Sasse, M., Karch, A., et al. (2017). Systemic inflammatory response syndrome after paediatric congenital heart surgery: In cadence risk factors, and clinical outcome. Journal of Cardiac Surgery, 32, 116–125.

Brockmann, I., Ehrenpfordt, J., Sturmheit, T., et al. (2018). Skin-Derived Stem Cells for Wound Treatment Using Cultured Epidermal Autografts: Clinical Applications and Challenges. Stem Cells International, 1–9. https://doi.org/10.1155/2018/4623615

Burkey, B. & Davis, W. (2016). Porcine xenograft treatment of superficial partial-thickness burns in paediatric patients. Journal of Wound Care, 25, Sup 2, 1–10. https://doi.org/10.12968/jowc.2016.25.Sup2.S10

Burns Registry of Australia and New Zealand. (2017). Burns Registry of Australia and New Zealand, 2017: Annual Report. https://anzba.org.au/assets/BRANZ_AnnualReport_Year8_FINAL_V2.pdf

Carson, R. A., Mudd, S. S., & Madati, J. (2016). Clinical practice guideline for the treatment of paediatric acute gastroenteritis in the outpatient setting. Journal of Paediatric Health Care: Official Publication of National Association of Pediatric Nurse Associates & Practitioners, 30(6), 610–616.

Children's Health Queensland Hospital and Health Service. (2019). Queensland Paediatric Guideline: Emergency: Sepsis – Recognition and emergency management in children. https://www.childrens.health.qld.gov.au/wp-content/uploads/PDF/guidelines/CHQ-GDL-60010-Sepsis.pdf

Coates, L., Kaandorp, G., Harris, J., et al. (2019). Preventable residential fire fatalities: July 2003 to June 2017, Bushfire and Natural Hazards CRC. https://www.bnhcrc.com.au/sites/default/files/managed/downloads/preventable_residential_fire_fatalities_july_2003_to_june_2017_bushfire_and_natural_hazards_crc.pdf

de Caen, A. R., Berg, M. D., Chameides, L., et al. (2015). Pediatric advanced life support: 2015 American Heart Association guidelines for cardiopulmonary resuscitation and emergency cardiovascular care. Circulation, 132(Suppl. 2), S526–S542.

Dellinger, R. P., Levy, M. M., Rhodes, A., et al. (2013). Surviving sepsis campaign: International guidelines for management of severe sepsis and septic shock, 2012. Critical Care Medicine, 41(2), 580–637.

Elisha, S. & Terry, K. L. (2018). Neonatal Anesthesia. In Nagelhoult, J. J. & Elisha, S. (2018). Nurse anesthesia, (6th ed.). Missouri: Elsevier.

Emond, S. (2009). Dehydration in infants and young children. Annals of Emergency Medicine, 53(3), 395–397.

Farrell, M. (2017). Smeltzer & Bare's Textbook of Medical-Surgical Nursing, (4th Australian & New Zealand ed.). Sydney: Wolters Kluwer.

Feng Y., Tsai Y-H., Xiao W., et al. (2015). Loss of ADAM17-mediated tumor necrosis factor alpha signalling in intestinal cells attenuates mucosal atrophy in a mouse model of parenteral nutrition. Molecular and Cellular Biology, 35(21), 3604–3621.

Fidkowski, C., & Fuzaylov, G. (2012). Anesthesia for pediatric burn patients. In B. J. Phillips (Ed.), Pediatric burns. Amherst, MA: Cambria.

Frazier, S. B. N., Sepanski, R., Mangum, C., et al. (2015). Association of systemic inflammatory response syndrome with clinical outcomes of pediatric patients with pneumonia. Southern Medical Journal, 108(11), 665–669.

Fredricks, C. Yon, J. R. & Messer, T. A. (2017). Burns. In Myers, J. A., Bines, S. D., Milikan, K. W., et al. Rush University Medical Center Review of Surgery E-Book, (6th ed.). St Louis: Elsevier.

Freedman, S. B., Vandermeer, B., Milne, A., et al. (2015). Diagnosing clinically significant dehydration in children with acute gastroenteritis using noninvasive methods: A meta-analysis. Journal of Pediatrics, 166(4), 908–916.

Friedman, J. N., Beck, C. E., DeGroot, J., et al. (2015). Comparison of isotonic and hypotonic intravenous maintenance fluids: A randomized clinical trial. Pediatrics, 169(5), 445–451.

Gaensbauer, J. T., & Todd, J. K. (2016). Toxic shock syndrome. In R. M. Kliegman, B. F. Stanton, J. W. St Geme, et al. (Eds.), Nelson textbook of pediatrics (20th ed.). Philadelphia: Saunders.

Gauglitz, G. G., Finnerty, C. C., Herndon, D. N., et al. (2012). Modulation of the hypermetabolic response after burn. In D. N. Herndon (Ed.), Total burn care. Philadelphia: Saunders.

Government of South Australia. (2019). Toxic shock syndrome (TSS)—including symptoms, treatment and prevention. https://www.sahealth.sa.gov.au/wps/wcm/connect/public+content/sa+health+internet/conditions/infectious-+diseases/toxic+shock+syndrome/toxic+shock+syndrome+tss+-+including+symptoms+treatment+and+prevention

Government of Western Australia Child and Adolescent Health Service. (2018). Emergency department guidelines: hyponatraemia. https://pch.health.wa.gov.au/For-health-professionals/Emergency-Department-Guidelines/Hyponatraemia

Greenbaum, L. A. (2015). Electrolyte and acid-base disorders. In R. M. Kliegman, B. F. Stanton, J. W. St Geme, et al. (Eds.), Nelson textbook of pediatrics (20th ed.). Philadelphia: Saunders.

Hartford, C. E. (2012). Care of outpatient burns. In D. N. Herndon (Ed.), Total burn care. Philadelphia: Saunders.

Hazinski, M. F., Mondozzi, M. A., & Baker, R. A. U. (2019). Shock, Multiple Organ Dysfunction Syndrome, and Burns in Children. In McCance, K. L. & Huether, S. E. (2019). Pathophysiology: The Biologic Basis for Disease in Adults and Children (8th ed.). Missouri: Elsevier.

Hendrickson, M. A., Zaremba, J., Wey, A. R., et al. (2017). The use of a triage-based protocol for oral rehydration in a pediatric emergency department. Pediatric Emergency Care, pec-online.com.

Horst, B., Chouhan, G., Moiemen, N. S., et al. (2017). Advances in keratinocyte delivery in burn wound care. Advanced Drug Delivery Reviews, 123, 18–32. doi: 10.1016/j.addr.2017.06.012

Hoxha, T. F., Azemi, M., Avdiu, M., et al. (2014). The usefulness of clinical and laboratory parameters for predicting severity of dehydration in children with acute gastroenteritis. Medicinski Arhiv, 68(5), 304–307.

Jeschke, M. G. (2016). Postburn hypermetabolism: Past, present, and future. Journal of Burn Care and Research, 37(2), 86–96.

Kawasaki, T. (2017). Update on pediatric sepsis: a review. Journal of Intensive Care, 5(47), 1–12. DOI 10.1186/s40560-017-0240-1

Kidsafe Australia. (2017). Statistics. https://kidsafe.com.au/statistics-2/

Kleinman, R. E., & Greer, F. R. (2014). Pediatric nutrition (7th ed.). Elk Grove Village, IL: American Academy of Pediatrics.

Lee, J. O., Norbury, W. B., & Herndon, D. N. (2012). Special considerations of age: The pediatric burned patient. In D. N. Herndon (Ed.), Total burn care. Philadelphia: Saunders.

Meyer, W. J., Wiechman, S., Woodson, L., et al. (2012). Management of pain and other discomforts in burned patients. In D. N. Herndon (Ed.), Total burn care. Philadelphia: Saunders.

Ministry of Health New Zealand. (2018). Toxic shock syndrome. https://www.health.govt.nz/your-health/conditions-and-treatments/diseases-and-illnesses/toxic-shock-syndrome

Mondozzi, M. A., Baker, R. A. U. & Hockenberry, M. J. (2018). The child with fluid and electrolyte imbalance. In Hockenberry, M. J. & Wilson, D. (2018). Wong's Nursing Care of Infants and Children (11th ed.). Missouri: Elsevier.

Moules, P. (2019). Physiology and pathophysiology for emergency care. In Curtis, K., Ramsden, C., Shaban, R. Z., et al. (2019). Emergency and Trauma Care for Nurses and Paramedics (2nd ed.). Chatswood: Elsevier Australia.

New South Wales Agency for Clinical Innovation (NSW ACI). (2019). Clinical guidelines: Burn patient management. (4th edn). NSW Statewide Burn Injury Service. https://www.aci.health.nsw.gov.au/__data/assets/pdf_file/0009/250020/Burn-patient-management-guidelines.pdf

Nielson, C. B., Duethman, N. C., Howard, J. M., et al. (2017). Burns: Pathophysiology of systemic complications and current management. Journal of Burn Care and Research, 38(1), e469–e481. doi:10.1097/BCR.0000000000000355.

Perkin, R. M., de Caen, A. R., Berg, M. D., et al. (2013). Shock, cardiac arrest, and resuscitation. In M. F. Hazinski (Ed.), Nursing care of the critically ill child. St Louis, MO: Elsevier Mosby.

Pourmand, A., Robinson, C., Syed, W., et al. (2018). Biphasic anaphylaxis: A review of the literature and implications for emergency management. The American Journal of Emergency Medicine, 36(8), 1480–1485. https://doi.org/10.1016/j.ajem.2018.05.009

Quain, A. M. & Khardori, N. M. (2015). Nutrition in wound care management: a comprehensive overview. Wounds, 27(12), 327–335.

Quinn, L. & Holland, A. (2016). Burns trauma. In Curtis, K. & Ramsden, C. (2016). Emergency and trauma care (2nd ed.). Chatswood: Elsevier Australia.

Rae, L., Fidler, P., & Gibran, N. (2016). The physiologic basis of burn shock and need for aggressive fluid resuscitation. Critical Care Clinics, 32(4), 491–505.

Rodgers, C. C. & Wilson, K. (2017). The Child with Gastrointestinal Dysfunction. In Hockenberry, M. J. (2017). Wong's Essentials of Pediatric Nursing (10th ed.). Missouri: Elsevier.

Rodgers, C. C., Baker, R. U. & Mondozzi, M. A. (2017). Health Problems of Toddlers and Preschoolers. In Hockenberry, M. J., Wilson, D. & Rodgers, C. C. (2017). Wong's Essentials of Pediatric Nursing (8th ed.). Missouri: Elsevier.

Rowan, M. P., Cancio, L. C., Elster, E. A., et al. (2015). Burn wound healing and treatment: Review and advancements. Critical Care, 19, 243.

Safe Kids Worldwide (SKW). (2015). Burn and scalds safety. Washington, DC. http://www.safekids.org/fact-sheet/burns-and-fire-safety-fact-sheet-2015-pdf.

Sampson, H. A., Wang, J., & Sicherer, S. H. (2016). Anaphylaxis. In R. M. Kliegman, B. F. Stanton, J. W. St Geme, et al. (Eds.), Nelson textbook of pediatrics (20th ed.). Philadelphia: Saunders.

Schlapbach, L., Straney, L., Alexander, J., et al. (2015). Mortality related to invasive infections, sepsis, and septic shock in critically ill children in Australia and New Zealand, 2002–13: a multicentre retrospective cohort study. The Lancet Infectious Diseases, 15(1), 46–54. https://www-science-direct-com.ezproxy.csu.edu.au/science/article/pii/S1473309914710035

Seckel, M. A. & Lin, F. (2020). Nursing Management: Shock, systemic inflammatory response syndrome and multiple organ dysfunction syndrome. In Brown, D., Edwards, H., Buckley, T., et al. (2020). Lewis's Medical-Surgical Nursing ANZ (5th ed.). Sydney: Elsevier Australia.

Sen, S., Palmieri, T., & Greenhalgh, D. (2015). Review of burn research for year 2014. Journal of Burn Care and Research, 36(6), 587–594.

Shukla, S., Basu, S. & Moritz, M. L. (2016). Use of Hypotonic Maintenance Intravenous Fluids and Hospital-Acquired Hyponatremia Remain Common in Children Admitted to a General Pediatric Ward. Frontiers in Pediatrics, 4(90), 1–5. doi: 10.3389/fped.2016.00090

Singleton, A., Preston, R. J., & Cochran, A. (2015). Sedation and analgesia for critically ill pediatric burn patients: The current state of practice. Journal of Burn Care and Research, 36(3), 440–445.

The Royal Children's Hospital Melbourne (RCHM). (2019). Burns unit: Clinical information. https://www.rch.org.au/burns/clinical_information/

The Royal Children's Hospital Melbourne (RCHM). (2020). Clinical Practice Guidelines. Dehydration. Assessment. Management. Approach to rehydration. https://www.rch.org.au/clinicalguide/guideline_index/Dehydration/

Tridente, A. (2018). Sepsis 3 and the burns patient: do we need Sepsis 3.1? Scars, Burns & Healing, 4, 1–7.

Victorian Adult Burns Service. (2017). Burns management guidelines. http://www.vicburns.org.au/burn-assessment-overview/tips-and-pitfalls/

Wang, J., Xu, E., & Xiao, Y. (2014). Isotonic versus hypotonic maintenance IV fluids in hospitalized children: A meta-analysis. Pediatrics, 133(1), 105–113.

Whitney, R. E., Santucci, K., Hsiao, A., et al. (2016). Cost effectiveness of point-of-care testing for dehydration in the pediatric ED. The American Journal of Emergency Medicine, 34, 1573–1575.

World Health Organization. (2016). Updated Guideline: Paediatric emergency triage, assessment and treatment: Care of critically ill children. https://apps.who.int/iris/bitstream/handle/10665/204463/9789241510219_eng.pdf;jsessionid=7FDDFA4D1496A939CC979402B2098404?sequence=1

24

The Child with Renal Dysfunction

Lisa Speedie

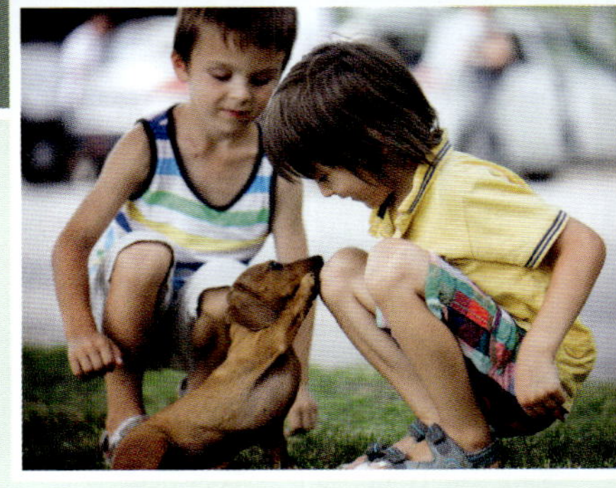

LEARNING OUTCOMES

- Describe renal dysfunction in the child
- Understand the impact of infection on renal function
- Be able to discuss acid–base balance and impact on care of the child and renal function
- Plan and implement the fluid regulation needs for a child with renal dysfunction
- Be able to fully assess a child with renal dysfunction and provide family-centred care to the child experiencing renal dysfunction

RENAL STRUCTURE AND FUNCTION

The kidney's primary responsibility is to maintain the composition and volume of the body fluids in equilibrium. To maintain this constant internal environment, the kidney must respond appropriately to alterations in the internal environment caused by variations in dietary intake and extra renal losses of water and solutes. This is accomplished by the formation of urine (the product of glomerular filtration), tubular reabsorption and tubular secretion. **Reabsorption** is the transport of a substance from the tubular lumen to the blood in surrounding vessels. **Secretion** is transport in the opposite direction (i.e. from the blood to the lumen). These processes are either active or passive. **Excretion** is the elimination of a substance from the body, in this case urine.

A secondary function of the kidney is the production of certain humoral substances. One such substance is an enzyme, erythropoietin-stimulating factor (or erythrogenin), which acts on a plasma globulin to form erythropoietin, which in turn stimulates erythropoiesis in the bone marrow. Its production increases in the presence of hypoxia and androgens. Few red blood cells form in the absence of erythropoietin, which accounts somewhat for the anaemia associated with advanced kidney disease. The kidney also secretes another enzyme, renin, in response to reduced blood volume, decreased blood pressure or increased secretion of catecholamines. Renin stimulates the production of the angiotensins, which produce arteriolar constriction and an elevation in blood pressure and stimulate the production of aldosterone by the adrenal cortex.

Renal Physiology

The structural and functional unit of the kidney is the **nephron**, which contains a complex system of tubules, arterioles, venules and capillaries (Fig 24.1A). The nephron consists of the Bowman capsule, which encloses a tuft of capillaries and is joined successively to the proximal convoluted tubule, the loop of Henle, the distal convoluted tubule and the straight or collecting duct (Fig 24.1B). Collecting tubules join larger ducts, and all the larger collecting ducts of one renal pyramid join to form a single duct that opens into a minor calyx. A number of calyces empty into one of several major calyces that converge into the renal pelvis. The renal pelvis narrows after it leaves the kidney and forms what then becomes a ureter, through which urine drains into the urinary bladder.

The blood supply to the kidneys constitutes approximately one fifth of the total cardiac output; therefore, profuse bleeding can accompany renal trauma. Because interstitial tissue is sparse, individual nephrons with their blood vessel component are closely packed together. A sizeable afferent arteriole, which separates into capillary loops that constitute the glomerular tuft, supplies each nephron. Blood leaves by a smaller efferent arteriole. From there the efferent arterioles branch into a peritubular capillary network and hairpin loops called the vasa recta, which parallel the loops of Henle and collecting ducts. The total surface area of the renal capillaries is approximately equal to the total surface area of the tubules.

The Bowman capsule is composed of two cellular layers that separate the blood from the glomerular filtrate: the capillary endothelium and a layer of tubular epithelial lining cells. Situated between these layers is the basal lamina, or basement membrane. This glomerular membrane is permeable because the capillary endothelium is fenestrated with pores, or fenestrae. Also, the outer surface of the glomerular epithelium consists of finger-like projections (pseudopodia, or podocytes) that cover the entire surface to form slits called slit pores. The basement membrane has no visible openings but behaves as though it contains pores or channels. Consequently, the glomerular filtrate (which has essentially the same composition as plasma except for the large protein molecules and cellular elements) passes through these three layers at a rapid rate. The structure of these layers becomes altered in kidney disease.

Glomerular Filtration

Filtration through the glomerular capillaries is governed by the same mechanism as filtration across other capillaries in the body (i.e. the size of the capillary bed, the permeability of the capillaries and the hydrostatic and osmotic pressure gradients across the capillaries). The filtration capacity of the glomerulus is the product of permeability of the glomerular capillaries and three pressure forces: glomerular hydrostatic pressure, colloidal osmotic (oncotic) pressure (COP) and intracapsular pressure.

Blood enters the nephron at a substantial pressure. This hydrostatic pressure forces plasma fluid and solutes through the capillary

PATHOPHYSIOLOGY REVIEW

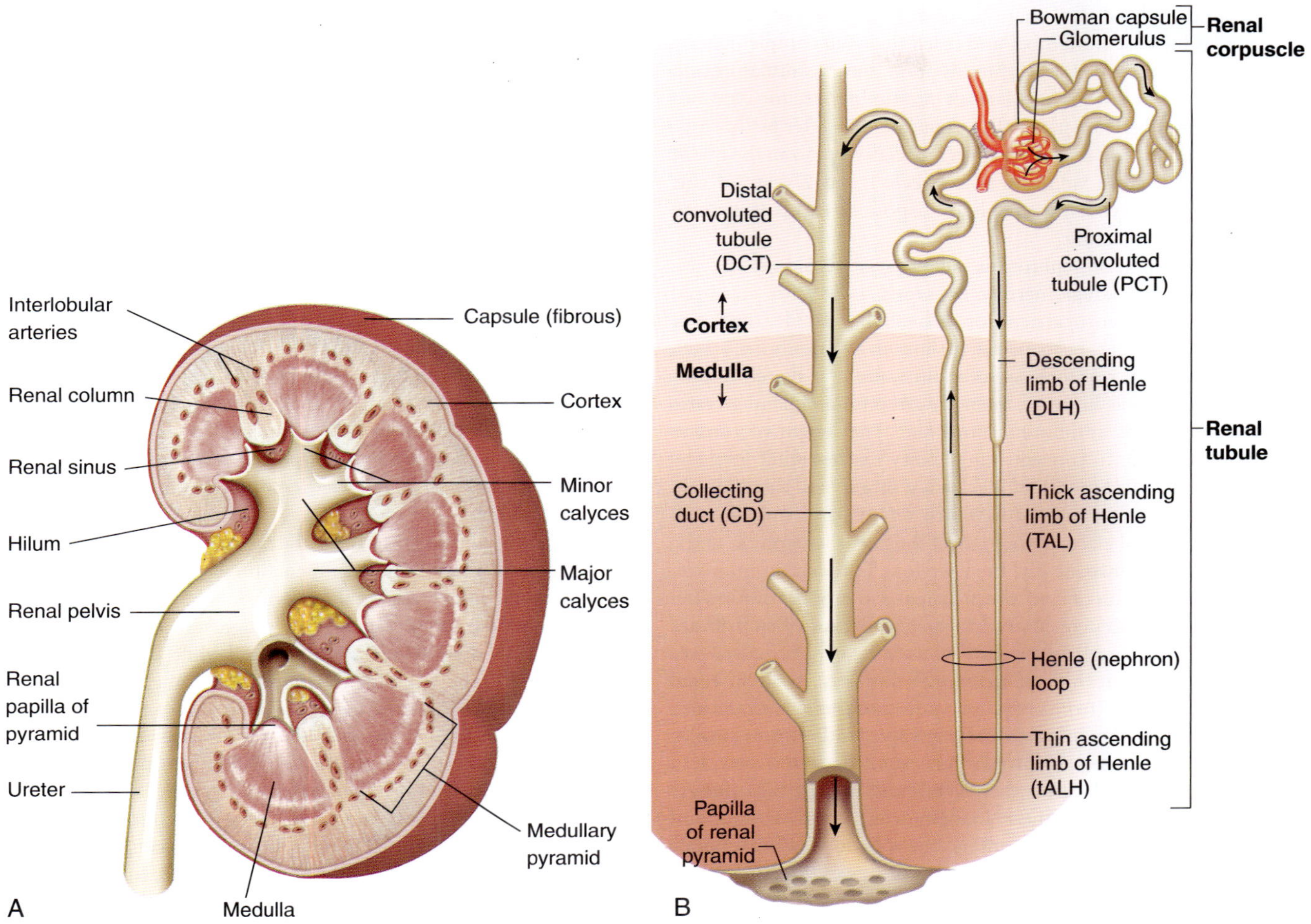

Fig 24.1 Pathophysiology review. (**A**) Kidney structure. (**B**) Components of the nephron. (Source: Patton, K. T., & Thibodeau, G. A. (2010). *Anatomy and physiology* (7th ed.). St Louis, MO: Mosby.)

membrane and into the unit's collecting apparatus. As this filtrate travels through the renal tubules, water and solutes are selectively reabsorbed back into the vascular compartment. That which is not reabsorbed is excreted as urine. Filtration takes place as long as hydrostatic pressure within the glomerular capillaries exceeds the opposing COP of the plasma proteins. If the pressure becomes equal through decreased hydrostatic pressure or decreased COP, no further filtration takes place. In a state of dehydration, more water is reabsorbed; when water intake is increased, more is excreted as urine. In conditions that produce osmotic diuresis (i.e. when large solutes, such as glucose, are filtered through the capillaries in such excessive amounts that they cannot be reabsorbed), the osmotic attraction of the solute causes less water to be reabsorbed, resulting in water being excreted in the urine with the solute.

Tubular Function

The function of the renal tubules is to modify the glomerular filtrate. Tubular cells may add more of a substance to the filtrate (tubular secretion), remove some or all of a substance from the filtrate (tubular reabsorption) or both. The reabsorption is selective and discriminating for substances essential to body processes and equilibrium, whereas non-essential substances are eliminated as waste. The substances are secreted or reabsorbed in the tubules by osmosis, passive movement down a chemical or electric gradient, or are actively transported against these gradients. These processes operate throughout the length of the tubules, but there are variations in the types, amounts and mechanisms by which substances are secreted or reabsorbed in the different tubular segments. The cellular characteristics of each segment are largely responsible for these variations (see Fig 24.1).

Active transport mechanisms move vital substances both inwards and outwards from the tubular filtrate. For example, the proximal tubule reabsorbs essential substances such as glucose, amino acids and sodium ions and returns them directly to the blood. Active transport mechanisms here, as elsewhere, have a limited capacity, or threshold, for moving the solute. When the maximum of the transport mechanism is reached, no more substance is reabsorbed and the remainder is excreted in the urine. For example, when blood glucose concentrations exceed their transport capacity, the surplus remains in the filtrate to be excreted in the urine (glycosuria). When two substances share a common transport mechanism, the first substance may be blocked by the addition of a second substance (selective inhibition). The effect of many therapeutic agents (e.g. diuretics) depends on this process.

Renal Development and Function in Early Infancy

Development of the kidney begins within the first weeks of embryonic life but is not completed until about the end of the first year after birth. The nephrons increase in number and reach their full complement by 34 to 46 weeks' gestation. However, at this point they are immature and less efficient than at later ages. Many of the tubular sections are not fully formed, and the glomeruli enlarge considerably after birth.

Glomerular filtration and absorption are relatively low in the infant and do not reach adult values until between 1 and 2 years of age. Consequently, the newborn is unable to dispose of excess water and solutes rapidly or efficiently.

The tubular length of nephrons is highly variable. Glomerular size is less variable. The juxtaglomerular nephrons show more advanced development than the cortical nephrons. The loop of Henle (the site of the urine-concentrating mechanism) is short in the newborn, which reduces the ability to reabsorb sodium and water and therefore produces very dilute urine; however, the newborn pituitary gland secretes adequate amounts of antidiuretic hormone. The length of tubules gradually increases until concentrating ability reaches adult levels by approximately the third month of life. Urea synthesis and excretion are slower during this time, and the newborn retains large quantities of nitrogen and essential electrolytes to meet the needs for growth in the first weeks of life. Consequently, the excretory burden is minimised. The lower concentration of urea, the principal end product of nitrogen metabolism, also reduces concentrating capacity because it contributes to the concentration mechanism.

Other characteristics of the newborn's kidneys result in renal function that differs from that of older children and adults. Newborn infants are unable to excrete a water load at rates similar to those of older persons. Hydrogen ion excretion is reduced, acid secretion is lower for the first year of life and plasma bicarbonate levels are low. Because of these inadequacies of the kidney and because of less efficient blood buffers, the newborn is more liable to develop severe metabolic acidosis. Sodium excretion is reduced in the immediate newborn period, and the kidneys are less able to adapt to sodium deficiencies and excesses. For example, an isotonic saline infusion may produce oedema because of impaired ability to eliminate excess sodium. Conversely, inadequate reabsorption of sodium from the tubules may increase sodium losses in disorders such as vomiting or diarrhoea. Moreover, infants have a diminished capacity to reabsorb glucose and, during the first few days, to produce ammonium ions.

The kidney functions during fetal life and produces urine that contributes to the amniotic fluid volume. The 24-hour urine volume is low at birth, rapidly increases in the neonatal period and steadily increases with normal growth. The kidneys continue to grow in size until body growth is complete in adolescence.

Renal Pelvis and Ureters: Structure and Function

The renal pelvis is a funnel-shaped structure that originates at the major calyces and terminates in the funnel-shaped ureter pelvic junction. The ureter is a thin mucomuscular tube that extends from the ureter pelvic to the ureter vesical junction in the base of the bladder.

The principal function of the renal pelvis and ureter is the transport of urine from the kidney to the bladder. Urine is moved via a process called **peristalsis**, whereby muscular movements originating in the renal pelvis propel a bolus of urine towards the urinary bladder for storage and eventual evacuation when the child urinates. The renal pelvis stores only a relatively small volume of urine (approximately 15 mL in adults) before a contraction is triggered that pushes the urine towards the bladder. The forward movement of urine from the kidney to the bladder is called **efflux**, whereas abnormal (or backward) urine movement is termed **reflux**. Aside from mechanical stretching, neurogenic and hormonal factors modulate ureteral peristalsis.

The ureterovesical junction joins the ureters and bladder. It is made up of three principal components: the lowest segment of the ureter, the trigone muscle and the adjacent bladder wall.

Urethrovesical Unit: Structure and Function

The urethrovesical unit consists of the bladder, urethra and pelvic muscles; it is also called the lower urinary tract. The urinary bladder is a muscle-lined sac that stores and empties itself of urine. In the infant the bladder lies entirely in the abdomen. The bladder assumes its place in the true pelvis shortly before puberty. This change in position is due to the maturation of the pelvic bone rather than migration of the bladder and urethra.

The bladder has two inlets (the ureteral orifices) and a single outlet (the urethral orifice). The base of the bladder is a relatively fixed, triangular area consisting of the bladder neck and trigone. In contrast, the body of the bladder is distensible, changing from a tetrahedron (four-sided shape) when relatively empty to a nearly spherical shape as the bladder fills.

One of the four layers of the bladder wall consists of smooth muscle bundles that promote bladder evacuation via micturition. Collectively this muscular tunic is called the **detrusor**. The muscular tunic of the bladder wall also contains **collagen**, a tough, non-elastic substance that maintains the integrity of the bladder wall while also preventing overdistension. Certain pathological factors, including denervation of the bladder and obstruction of the outlet, may cause an overabundance of collagen in the detrusor muscle. This causes a loss of bladder compliance (distensibility), abnormally high filling pressures and trabeculation (irregularity) of the bladder wall.

The urethra is a mucomuscular tube that connects the external meatus and the bladder. The male urethra originates at the bladder neck, piercing the prostate and pelvic floor before tunnelling through the posterior portion of the penis and terminating at the glans penis. The proximal portion of the urethra comprises the sphincter mechanism, whereas the distal portion serves as a conduit for the passage of urine or semen. The urethral meatus is a vertical slit located at the summit of the glans penis.

The female urethra follows a relatively short, straight course compared with the male. It originates at the bladder base and terminates at an external meatus located immediately superior to the vaginal orifice. The distal two-thirds of the female urethra are fused with the vaginal wall.

The primary responsibilities of the bladder are to store urine manufactured by the kidneys and to evacuate this urine at regular intervals via the process of micturition. During infancy the bladder is expected to empty spontaneously; by the fourth year of life (or earlier) the child is expected to gain control of detrusor and urethral sphincter function. Control of the urethrovesical unit is referred to as **urinary continence**. Continent individuals are expected to hold their urine for at least 2 hours while awake. During sleeping hours they may arise once to urinate, although many children and young adults sleep for 8 hours or more without interruption. Three factors—anatomical integrity of the lower urinary tract, detrusor control and competence of the urethral sphincter mechanism—must function normally for an individual to achieve and maintain continence.

Detrusor control requires successful integration of neurological structures in the brain, spinal cord and peripheral nervous systems. The brain influences bladder function via its inhibitory role on detrusor contractions. The stable detrusor contracts only when its owner gives permission and several areas of the brain work together to control detrusor stability. A pathological condition of one of these areas may produce detrusor overactivity, or the loss of control over detrusor contractions.

The spinal cord influences lower urinary tract function because it transmits messages between the brain and the target organ. Two areas in the spinal cord are particularly significant. The thoracolumbar cord (spinal levels T10–L2) influences bladder and urethral sphincter function. Sympathetic impulses from the brain travel to the bladder body and smooth muscle of the urethra, causing relaxation of the detrusor muscle and contraction of urethral smooth muscle. This combination of actions promotes bladder filling and storage of urine. The sacral spinal cord (spinal segments S2–S4) influences the bladder muscle, promoting micturition. Parasympathetic impulses travel from these nuclei, causing contraction of the detrusor muscle and indirectly promoting relaxation of smooth muscle in the urethra.

Two peripheral nerve plexuses directly influence control of the detrusor muscle. The pelvic plexus provides parasympathetic innervation to the bladder and urethra, and the inferior hypogastric plexus provides sympathetic innervation (Haley & Pillitteri 2016, Forster & Fraser 2018).

The final mechanism responsible for the attainment and maintenance of continence is the urethral sphincter mechanism. Traditionally two sphincters are described. The internal sphincter consists of the smooth muscle of the bladder and proximal urethra, and the external sphincter consists of the periurethral striated muscle. However, it is better to describe a single mechanism consisting of elements of compression and elements of tension.

Elements of compression are necessary for the urethra to form a watertight seal between episodes of urination. The softness (collapsibility) of the urethral wall is important for continence, particularly when a catheter alters urethral integrity. The mucus produced by the epithelium further enhances the watertight seal of the urethra. The mucus reduces surface tension, promoting collapse of the walls and sealing the microscopic fissures against urinary leakage.

The vascular cushion also acts as an element of compression (in addition to producing tension), contributing to urethral closure during physical stress. The vascular cushion, or network of the arterioles, venules and arteriovenous communications in the urethra promote urethral compression by transmitting pressure from the muscles surrounding the urethra and those intrinsic to its walls. The vascular cushion contributes to urethral closure pressure because it is filled with an incompressible fluid that has its own intrinsic pressure.

The elements of tension in the urethral sphincter mechanism consist of the vascular cushion, intrinsic smooth and skeletal muscles and periurethral striated muscle. These muscles are specially innervated to maintain the tension needed for urethral closure between episodes of micturition and to provide an extra measure of urethral tension, which is needed when significant physical exertion stresses sphincter closure. The pelvic muscles receive somatic innervation, which allows voluntary interruption of the urinary stream and provides added protection against precipitous rises in abdominal pressure (Haley & Pillitteri 2016, Forster & Fraser 2018).

Clinical Manifestations

As in most disorders of childhood, the incidence and type of kidney or urinary tract dysfunction change with the age and maturation of the child. In addition, the presenting complaints and the significance of these complaints vary with age. For example, a complaint of enuresis has greater significance at 8 years old than at 4 years old. In newborns, renal abnormalities may be associated with a number of other malformations; for example, obvious neural tube defects to the subtle abnormal shape or position of the outer ear. Faltering growth in children may be a sign of impaired renal function.

Many of the clinical manifestations of renal disease are common to a variety of childhood disorders, but their presence is an indication to obtain further information from the child's history, family history and laboratory studies as part of a complete physical examination. Important signs and symptoms that suggest possible renal or genitourinary tract disease in children at different ages are outlined in Box 24.1. Suspected renal disease can be further evaluated by means of laboratory tests, radiographic studies and renal biopsy.

BOX 24.1 Signs and Symptoms of Urinary Tract Disorders or Disease

Neonatal Period (Birth to 1 Month)

- Poor feeding
- Vomiting
- Failure to gain weight
- Rapid respiration (acidosis)
- Respiratory distress
- Spontaneous pneumothorax or pneumomediastinum
- Frequent urination
- Screaming on urination
- Poor urinary stream
- Jaundice
- Seizures
- Dehydration
- Other anomalies or stigmata
- Enlarged kidneys or bladder

Infancy (1 to 24 Months)

- Poor feeding
- Vomiting
- Failure to gain weight
- Excessive thirst
- Frequent urination
- Straining or screaming on urination
- Foul-smelling urine
- Pallor
- Fever
- Persistent nappy rash
- Seizures (with or without fever)
- Dehydration
- Enlarged kidneys or bladder

Childhood (2 to 14 Years)

- Poor appetite
- Vomiting
- Growth failure
- Excessive thirst
- Enuresis, incontinence, frequent urination
- Painful urination
- Swelling of face
- Seizures
- Pallor
- Fatigue
- Blood in urine
- Abdominal or back pain
- Oedema
- Hypertension
- Tetany

Laboratory Tests

Both urine and blood studies contribute vital information for the detection of renal problems. The single most important test is probably routine urinalysis. Specific urine and blood tests provide additional information. Other initial laboratory work up would also be electrolytes, urea, creatinine, calcium, magnesium, phosphorus, full blood examination (FBE) and if proteinuria on ward urinalysis, then a spot protein/creatinine ratio will be performed (The Royal Children's Hospital Melbourne [RCHM] 2009).

Glomerular filtration rate (GFR) is generally accepted as the best overall index of kidney function. Though the gold standard for measurement of GFR has been the filtration of the small carbohydrate inulin, this is not a practical test clinically. The kidney handles creatinine, an end product of protein metabolism in muscle, in a similar way so that its plasma concentration can be used to estimate GFR. Creatinine clearance tends to slightly overestimate GFR. Serum creatinine is a function of both creatinine excretion and production, so it varies, depending on muscle mass. Equations have been developed to estimate kidney function using serum creatinine and variables such as age, sex, race and body size. In the past, 12- or 24-hour urine collections have been used routinely to measure creatinine clearance, and therefore GFR, but studies have shown these difficult to obtain urine collections do not provide a better estimate of GFR than the equations (Webster et al 2017). In the case where a 24-hour urine collection is indicated, the nurse is responsible for assisting in obtaining a complete and accurate collection.

Table 24.1 outlines the major urine and blood tests. Radiological and other tests of urinary system function are described in Table 24.2: Blood tests of renal function are outlined in Table 24.3.

TABLE 24.1 Urine Tests of Renal Function

Test	Normal Range	Deviations	Significance of Deviations
PHYSICAL TESTS			
Volume	Age related Newborn: 30–60 mL Children: Bladder capacity (30 mL) = age (year) + 1	Polyuria	Osmotic factors (urinary glucose level in diabetes mellitus)
		Oliguria	Retention caused by obstructive disease Inadequate bladder emptying caused by neurogenic bladder or obstructive disorder
		Anuria	Obstruction of urinary tract; acute renal failure
Specific gravity	With normal fluid intake: 1.016–1.022 Newborn: 1.001–1.020 Others: 1.001–1.030	High	Dehydration Presence of protein or glucose Presence of radio-opaque contrast medium after radiological examinations
		Low	Excessive fluid intake Distal tubular dysfunction Insufficient antidiuretic hormone Diuresis
		Fixed at 1.010	Chronic glomerular disease
Osmolality	Newborn: 50–600 mOsm/L Thereafter: 50–1400 mOsm/L	High or low	Same as for specific gravity More sensitive index than specific gravity
Appearance	Clear pale yellow to deep gold	Cloudy	Contains sediment
		Cloudy reddish-pink to reddish-brown	Blood from trauma or disease Myoglobin after severe muscle destruction
		Light	Dilute
		Dark	Concentrated
		Red	Trauma
CHEMICAL TESTS			
pH	Newborn: 5–7 Thereafter: 4.8–7.8 Average: 6	Weak acid or neutral	If associated with metabolic acidosis, suggests tubular acidosis If associated with metabolic alkalosis, suggests potassium deficiency Urinary tract infection
		Alkaline	Metabolic alkalosis
Protein level	Absent	Present	Abnormal glomerular permeability (e.g. glomerular disease, changes in blood pressure) Most kidney disease Orthostatic in some individuals
Glucose level	Absent	Present	Diabetes mellitus Infusion of concentrated glucose-containing fluids Impaired tubular reabsorption
Ketone levels	Absent	Present	Conditions of acute metabolic demand (stress) Diabetic ketoacidosis
Leucocyte esterase	Absent	Present	Can identify both lysed and intact white blood cells via enzyme detection
Nitrites	Absent	Present	Most species of bacteria convert nitrates to nitrites in the urine

TABLE 24.1 Urine Tests of Renal Function—cont'd

Test	Normal Range	Deviations	Significance of Deviations
		MICROSCOPIC TESTS	
White blood cell count	< 1–2	> 5 polymorphonuclear leucocytes/field	Urinary tract inflammatory process
		Lymphocytes	Allograft rejection Malignancy
Red blood cell count	< 1–2	4–6/field in centrifuged specimen	Trauma Stones Glomerular injury Infection Neoplasms
Presence of bacteria	Absent to a few	> 100,000 organisms/mL in centrifuged specimen	Urinary tract infection
Presence of casts	Occasional	Granular casts	Tubular or glomerular disorders Degenerative process in advanced renal disease
		Cellular casts	Pyelonephritis
		White blood cell	Glomerulonephritis
		Red blood cell Hyaline casts	Proteinuria; usually transient

TABLE 24.2 Radiological and Other Tests of Urinary System Function

Test	Procedure	Purpose	Comments and Nursing Responsibilities
Urine culture and sensitivity	Collection of sterile specimen	Determines presence of pathogens and drugs to which they are sensitive	Send specimen to laboratory immediately after collection. Catheterisation, clean-catch or suprapubic specimen.
Renal bladder ultrasound	Transmission of ultrasonic waves through renal parenchyma, along ureteral course and over bladder	Allows visualisation of renal parenchyma, renal pelvis without exposure to external beam radiation or radioactive isotopes. Visualisation of dilated ureters and bladder wall also possible. Can show renal cysts and stones, though less sensitive than CT. Doppler ultrasonography can be used to evaluate renal vascular flow.	Non-invasive procedure.
Testicular (scrotal) ultrasound	Transmission of ultrasonic waves through scrotal contents and testis	Allows visualisation of scrotal contents, including testis. Testicular ultrasound used to identify masses and Doppler-enhanced ultrasound used to differentiate hyperaemia of epididymo-orchitis from ischaemia or torsion	Non-invasive procedure.
Plain film of the abdomen (KUB)	Flat plate x-ray film of abdomen and pelvis	Can identify certain types of stones that are calcium-containing as well as calculi or opaque foreign bodies in bladder (diagnostic choice for nephrolithiasis is non-contrast helical CT) Assess stool burden	Prepare for routine x-ray film.
VCUG	Contrast medium injected into bladder through urethral catheter until bladder is full; films taken before, during and after voiding	Visualises bladder outline and urethra, reveals reflux of urine into ureters. Provides information on bladder emptying. Used to diagnose PUV	Prepare child for catheterisation.

Continued

TABLE 24.2 Radiological and Other Tests of Urinary System Function—cont'd

Test	Procedure	Purpose	Comments and Nursing Responsibilities
Radionuclide (nuclear) cystogram	Radionuclide-containing fluid injected through urethral catheter until bladder is full; images generated before, during and after voiding	Alternative to voiding cystourethrography to evaluate reflux, although visualisation of anatomical details is relatively poor. Used in some institutions for follow-up of initial VCUG due to less radiation.	Prepare child for catheterisation.
Radioisotope imaging studies (renal scans)	Contrast medium injected intravenously; computer analysis to measure uptake or washout (excretion) for analysis of organ function	DMSA radioisotope to visualise renal scars and differential renal function; does not visualise ureters and bladder. MAG-3 radioisotope assesses obstruction and shows differential function between the two kidneys. DTPA is an alternative to MAG-3 but imaging is limited because it is only filtered at the glomerulus.	Insert or assist with insertion of IV. Monitor IV infusion. Urethral catheterisation may accompany MAG-3 or DTPA scan; prepare child for catheterisation when indicated.
MRI	Uses strong magnetic fields and radio waves to form images	MRI of kidneys used to evaluate renal mass. Magnetic resonance angiography used to evaluate renovascular hypertension and has reduced need for renal angiography. Magnetic resonance urogram used to detect specific urological abnormalities, such as ectopic ureter.	MRI often requires sedation in infants and children due to need to stay still, typically in an enclosed space. Follow NBM guidelines depending on timing of study. Assist with IV access if indicated. Magnetic devices or implants may be unsafe for MRI, including cochlear implants and permanent pacemakers.
CT	Narrow-beam x-rays and computer analysis provide precise reconstruction of area	Visualises vertical or horizontal cross-section of kidney Especially valuable to distinguish tumours, cysts and stones. Non-contrast helical CT is gold standard for radiological diagnosis of renal stone disease. Renal CT angiogram used to evaluate blood flow in hypertensive patients and is now used more commonly than renal arteriography.	Non-contrast scan is non-invasive. Contrast-enhanced CT scan preparation may require child be NBM for a few hours. With speed of newer scans, the need for sedation is decreased, but if required will also require NBM. Assist with IV access if needed. *Used selectively due to higher radiation exposure.*
Cystoscopy	Direct visualisation of bladder and lower urinary tract through small scope inserted via urethra	Investigation of bladder and lower tract lesions; visualises urethral openings, bladder wall, trigone and urethra	NBM orders per protocol, typically no solid food after midnight, liquids until 4–6 hours before procedure. Carry out preoperative preparations; cystoscopy is done under anaesthesia in children.
Renal biopsy	Removal of kidney tissue by open or percutaneous technique for study by light, electron or immunofluorescent microscopy	Yields histological and microscopic information about glomeruli and tubules; helps distinguish between types of nephritic syndromes Distinguishes other renal disorders	Nothing orally 4–6 hours before test. Premedicate as ordered. Prepare set-up for procedure. Assist with procedure. Take vital signs. Apply pressure to area with pressure dressing and, if feasible, a sandbag. Bed rest for 24 hours. Observe for abdominal pain, tenderness. Monitor intake and output. Surgical incision may be required in infants.
Urodynamics	Set of tests to measure bladder filling, storage and evacuation functions: Uroflowmetry—Test to determine efficiency of urination Cystometrography: Graphic comparison of bladder pressure as a function of volume Voiding pressure study: Comparison of detrusor contraction pressure, sphincter EMG and urinary flow	Determine characteristic of voiding dysfunction Used to identify type (cause) of incontinence or urinary retention Especially valuable for voiding dysfunction complicated by urinary tract infection, urinary retention or neurogenic bladder dysfunction	Prepare child for urinary catheterisation. The bladder will be filled with contrast, sterile water or saline solution. The child may experience fullness, coolness from the fluid and urine leakage during the study Insertion of rectal tube will produce feelings of rectal fullness or pressure. Insertion of needles may be required for sphincter EMG. (Institution specific, often use electrode patches.)

CT, Computed tomography; *DMSA,* dimercaptosuccinic acid; *DTPA,* diethylenetriamine pentaacetic acid; *EMG,* electromyography; *IV,* intravenous; *KUB,* kidney, ureters and bladder; *MAG-3,* mercaptoacetyltriglycine or mertiatide; *MRI,* magnetic resonance imaging; *NBM,* nil by mouth; *PUV,* posterior urethral valve; *VCUG,* voiding cystourethrogram.

TABLE 24.3 Blood Tests of Renal Function

Test	Normal Range (mg/dL)	Deviations	Significance of Deviations
Blood urea nitrogen (BUN)	Newborn: 4–18 Infant, child: 5–18	Elevated	Renal disease—Acute or chronic (the higher the BUN, the more severe the disease) Increased protein catabolism Dehydration Haemorrhage High protein intake Corticosteroid therapy
Uric acid	Child: 2.0–5.5	Increased	Severe renal disease
Creatinine	Infant: 0.2–0.4 Child: 0.3–0.7 Adolescent: 0.5–1.0	Increased	Severe renal impairment

Nursing Care Management

Nursing responsibilities in the assessment of renal disorders and diseases begin with observation of the child for any manifestations that might indicate dysfunction. The most significant ongoing assessments in children with renal conditions are accurate measurement and recording of weight and height, intake and output and blood pressure. (See Chapter 4.) These assessments are necessary not only for children with known renal dysfunction but also for those children at risk for developing renal complications (e.g. children in shock, postoperative patients).

In addition to the general manifestations of renal conditions, many conditions have specific characteristics that distinguish them from other disorders. These are discussed as appropriate throughout the chapter.

The nurse is generally responsible for preparing infants, children and parents for tests and collection of urine and (sometimes) blood specimens. (See Preparation for Diagnostic and Therapeutic Procedures, and Collection of Specimens, Chapter 22.) Nurses observe the characteristics of the urine collected, often perform any of a number of tests on urine specimens (e.g. urine specific gravity, protein, blood, glucose, ketones) and assist with more complex diagnostic tests. Nurses must be familiar with significant laboratory tests, their implications and pre-procedural care (RCHM n.d.).

GENITOURINARY TRACT DISORDERS

Urinary Tract Infection

Urinary tract infection (UTI) is a common and potentially serious problem in children. Caucasians, females and uncircumcised boys have the highest rates. Specifically, girls have a two-fold to four-fold higher prevalence than do circumcised boys. Uncircumcised males younger than 3 months old and females younger than 12 months old have the highest baseline prevalence of UTI (Schlager 2016, RCHM 2019a). UTI may involve the urethra and bladder (lower urinary tract) or the ureters, renal pelvis, calyces and renal parenchyma (upper urinary tract). Because of the difficulty in distinguishing upper from lower tract infection, particularly in young children, UTI is often broadly defined. Upper UTIs or kidney infection (pyelonephritis) tend to present with fever and may lead to renal scarring that may be associated with decreased kidney function, hypertension and renal disease over time. It is important to note that UTIs in neonates (infants $\leq$ 30 days of age) are often associated with congenital anomalies of the kidney and urinary tract (CAKUT) and resulting bacteraemia. The typical time of presentation of UTI in term infants is in the second or third week of life (Bonadio & Maida 2014).

Signs and symptoms of UTI can be non-specific in young children.

Collecting urine to exclude UTI is not required if there is another clear focus of fever and the child is not unwell. Urinary ward urinalysis is a useful screening test, but further laboratory microscopy results will complement the diagnosis. A single or combined result can confirm the UTI along with clinical presentation (RCHM 2019a).

Aetiology

A variety of organisms can be responsible for UTI. *Escherichia coli* remains the most common uropathogen overall, but the prevalence is higher in females (83%) than males (50%) (Buonocore et al 2018). Other gram-negative organisms associated with UTI include *Proteus mirabilis*, *Pseudomonas aeruginosa*, *Klebsiella* and *Enterobacter*. Gram-positive bacterial pathogens include *Enterococcus*, *Staphylococcus saprophyticus* and, rarely, *Staphylococcus aureus* (Schlager 2016). Viruses and fungi are uncommon causes of UTI in children. Most uropathogens originate in the gastrointestinal tract, migrate to the periurethral area and ascend to the bladder. A number of factors contribute to the development of UTI, including anatomical, physical and chemical conditions or properties of the host's urinary tract.

Pathogenesis and Host Factors. Evidence suggests that most UTIs after the newborn period result from ascending infection from uropathogens on the periurethral mucosa. A variety of virulence factors allow the bacteria to attach and ascend to the bladder and kidney. Host factors influence the risk of development of UTI and include urological abnormalities, genetic factors and functional abnormalities such as bowel bladder dysfunction.

After invasion by bacteria, the first line of defence in the lower urinary tract is complete evacuation by voiding. Inflammation in the bladder and urethral walls is apparent within 30 minutes of invasion by a bacterial pathogen. Polymorphonuclear leucocytes rapidly migrate to the bladder wall, which becomes completely injected within 2 hours. Complete evacuation of the bladder is particularly important for the eradication of bacteria from the urine. Urination not only helps remove bacteria and associated toxins contained in the urine but also allows more efficient destruction of the bacteria remaining on the thin film of urine that is adherent to the vesical wall.

Clinical Manifestations

The clinical manifestations of UTIs depend on the child's age. Infants and toddlers under 2 years of age have non-specific symptoms, such as fever, irritability, lethargy, poor feeding, vomiting and diarrhoea. Newborns may have fever, hypothermia, jaundice, tachypnoea or cyanosis, and they appear quite ill. The classic symptoms of UTI are often observed in children over 2 years of age. These include enuresis or daytime incontinence in the child who has been toilet trained, fever, foul-smelling urine, increased frequency of urination, dysuria or urgency. Symptoms of dysfunctional voiding are found in Box 24.2. Children may also complain of abdominal pain or costovertebral angle tenderness (flank pain). Some patients have haematuria or vomiting. Infants and young boys may develop obstructive-like symptoms, with dribbling of urine, straining with urination or a decrease in the force and size of the urinary stream. High fever and chills accompanied by flank pain, severe abdominal pain and leucocytosis suggest pyelonephritis. However, flank pain and tenderness may be the only indication of pyelonephritis on physical examination.

Manifestations in older children and adolescents are more specific. Symptoms of lower tract infections include frequency and painful

BOX 24.2 Symptoms of Dysfunctional Voiding

- Urinary tract infection without fever
- Changes in urinary frequency
- Constipation
- Squatting or holding to stay dry
- Daytime or night-time wetting
- Straining to void
- Urgency to void

urination of a small amount of turbulent urine that may be grossly bloody. Fever is usually absent or low grade. Upper tract infection is characterised by fever (> 38°C), chills and flank pain, often in addition to lower tract symptoms.

Many UTIs in children are asymptomatic or atypical in clinical presentation, and complaints may be unrelated to the urinary tract. Many are treated as respiratory or gastrointestinal tract infections. It is important to identify these children so treatment can be initiated. Significant renal scarring can occur, especially in infants and young children.

Diagnostic Evaluation

The diagnosis of UTI depends on a high degree of suspicion, evaluation of the history and physical examination and urinalysis and culture. Urine with a possible infection may appear cloudy, hazy or thick, with noticeable strands of mucus and pus; it also may have an unpleasant odour, even when fresh. Testing the child's urine is the only way to know for sure if they have a UTI. UTIs should not go untreated, as the infection can cause further problems with the kidneys. The child should see a doctor if they:

- develop any of the signs and symptoms of UTI
- are unwell with a fever without other obvious causes (RCHM 2018).

If a urinalysis obtained by a bag specimen is negative, that may be sufficient, but if it is positive, a specimen still needs to be obtained by catheterisation or suprapubic aspiration.

The most accurate tests of bacterial content are suprapubic aspiration (for children < 2 years of age) and properly performed bladder catheterisation (as long as the first few millilitres are excluded from collection). Care of a urine specimen obtained for culture is an important nursing responsibility related to diagnosis. The specimen must be fresh (< 1 hour after voiding with storage at room temperature or < 4 hours after voiding with refrigeration) to ensure sensitivity and specificity of the urinalysis and to prevent growth of organisms (RCHM 2019a) (see Translating Evidence into Practice box).

TRANSLATING EVIDENCE INTO PRACTICE

Urinary Specimen Collection in Infants and Children 2 to 24 Months with Suspected Urinary Tract Infection

Ask the Question

PICOT Question

In infants or children with a possible UTI, what is the preferred method for collecting a urine specimen?

Search for the Evidence

Search Strategies

Search criteria included English-language publications within the past 15 years and research-based articles on infants or children with signs or symptoms of UTI.

Databases Used

Cochrane Collaboration, Joanna Briggs Institute, National Guideline Clearinghouse (AHRQ), PubMed

Critically Analyse the Evidence

GRADE criteria: Evidence quality moderate; recommendation strong (LoBiondo-Wood et al 2018)

A review of the literature revealed several studies evaluating specimen collection techniques in infants and children. The Royal Children's Hospital Melbourne Renal Unit reaffirmed the clinical practice guideline for diagnosis and management of the initial UTI in febrile infants and children ages 2 to 24 months. There is a strong recommendation that a urine specimen should be obtained for culture and urinalysis before prescribing an antibiotic. The new guideline recommends that when the degree of illness warrants immediate antibiotic therapy, then urine specimens should be obtained through catheterisation or suprapubic aspiration (SPA) of urine (RCHM 2019a). When the degree of illness does not require immediate antibiotic therapy, a urine specimen evaluation within 1 hour of voiding can be evaluated for leucocyte esterase and nitrite using urine ward urinalysis testing (RCHM 2019a, Buonocore et al 2018). A systematic review comparing ward urinalysis testing and microscopy showed that ward urinalysis testing performed well for determining UTI in children over 2 years of age (Buonocore et al 2018). Ward urinalysis testing for leucocyte esterase or nitrite was not helpful when negative. For children younger than 2 years, microscopy showed the best diagnostic accuracy.

- Urine culture specimen in 452 children less than 2 years revealed contamination rates of 23% using clean-catch urine, 15% in catheter specimen urine and 1.3% in suprapubic aspirated urine. Authors recommend that when clean-catch specimens are necessary, the collection procedure needs to be optimised for all collections in this manner (Hamid et al 2020).
- An observational study of 700 infants less than 100 days old evaluated specimen collection via urinary catheterisation compared with a urine bag. Results showed that bag specimens sent for urine culture were more likely to have two organisms, non-pathogenic bacteria and ambiguous results. Although parents prefer the urine bag method of specimen collection, culture results are more accurate when specimens are collected via urinary catheterisation (Kaufman et al 2020).
- Eliacik and colleagues (2016) compared sensitivity and specificity of specimens collected via 'clean-void' bag technique versus specimens collected via urinary catheterisation to diagnose UTIs. The authors concluded that urine samples should be collected via catheterisation in infants less than 90 days old due to low sensitivity of bag specimens. Bag specimens are an acceptable method of collecting urine to screen for UTI but can miss up to 12% of UTIs.

Apply the Evidence: Nursing Implications

- Urine specimens should be collected by catheterisation or SPA in infants and children less than 2 years of age whose illness warrants immediate antibiotic therapy.
- When an infant or child less than 2 years of age is not assessed to appear ill and there is a low likelihood of UTI, a urine specimen can be obtained using the most convenient method for urinalysis. If the results are positive for leucocyte esterase or nitrite or there is microscopic evidence for leucocytes or bacteraemia, a urine specimen should be obtained through catheterisation or suprapubic aspirate.
- When a non-invasive method is used to obtain urine for UTI screening, meticulous methods for collection should be followed. The specimen should be evaluated within 1 hour of voiding.

Originally developed by Ashley R. Breland

Therapeutic Management

The main way of treating a UTI is with antibiotics, which can usually be taken by mouth as a tablet or syrup. Children who are very unwell may be admitted to hospital for antibiotics via intravenous (IV) therapy (RCHM 2018).

Antibiotic therapy depends on laboratory culture and sensitivity tests. Nonetheless, empiric therapy on the basis of the child's history and presenting symptoms may be necessary when fever or systemic illness complicates UTI. Common anti-infective agents used for UTI include the penicillins, sulfonamide (including trimethoprim-sulfamethoxazole), the cephalosporins and nitrofurantoin. All antibiotics may cause side effects or prove ineffective because of bacterial resistance (Table 24.4).

Historically, all children with a febrile UTI were evaluated for vesicoureteral reflux (VUR) because of concern of renal scarring with recurrent kidney infections (Schaeffer et al 2016).

Anatomical defects such as primary reflux or bladder neck obstruction may require surgical correction to prevent recurrent infection or may indicate the need for prophylactic antibiotics and careful follow-up monitoring. Follow-up is an important component of medical management because the relapse rate is high and recurrent infection tends to occur 1 to 2 months after termination of treatment. The aim of therapy and careful follow-up in such cases is to prevent morbidity and reduce the chance of renal scarring.

Prognosis. With prompt and adequate treatment at the time of diagnosis, the long-term prognosis for UTIs is usually excellent. Evidence shows that delay in treatment initiation of 72 hours or more increases risk of permanent renal scars after the first episode of febrile UTI (Karavanaki et al 2017, Shakih et al 2016). The hazard of progressive renal injury is greatest when infection occurs in young children (especially $<$ 2 years of age) and is associated with congenital renal malformations and reflux. Therefore, early diagnosis of children at risk is particularly important during infancy and toddlerhood.

TABLE 24.4 Common Side Effects of Urinary Anti-infective Agents

Drug	Side Effects	Nursing Interventions
Trimethoprim-sulfamethoxazole (Bactrim, Septrin)	Rash, urticaria, photosensitivity, nausea, bone marrow depression (long-term use)	Maintain adequate fluid intake. Advise parents and child to use sunscreen. May perform periodic blood counts in long-term use.
Amoxicillin (Amoxil, Alphamox)	Nausea, vomiting, diarrhoea	Refrigerate suspension; discard suspension after 14 days.
Nitrofurantoin (Macrodantin)	Nausea, pneumonitis or pulmonary fibrosis (long-term use)	Administer with food or milk.
Cefalexin (Keflex)	Nausea, diarrhoea	Administer with food or milk.
Ceftazidime (Fortum)	Renal toxicity	Keep child well hydrated.
Gentamicin (Genoptic, Septopal)	Renal toxicity, ototoxicity	Monitor urinary output, blood urea nitrogen, creatinine. Monitor serum levels, especially in infants.

Nursing Care Management

Objectives of nursing care include identification of children with UTI and education of parents and children regarding prevention and treatment of infection. Aside from the influence of renal abnormalities, girls between the ages of 2 and 6 years are in general a high-risk group. This is a common age for development of constipation and stool and urine withholding behaviours as children learn bowel and bladder control. Encouragement of good toilet habits and dietary intake of fluid and fibre can help avoid these problems. Parents should be aware of signs and symptoms of UTI, and a routine urinalysis should be performed if there are concerns. Nurses should instruct parents to observe for signs of UTI, which are not always as obvious as those of upper respiratory tract infection.

Because anti-infective drugs are indicated in the treatment of UTI, the nurse teaches the patient and parents the appropriate dosage and scheduling and provides suggestions for administration. Certain drugs are available in liquid form; others are available only in capsule or pill form. In general, capsules are separated and pills are crushed, with their contents mixed into a small volume of food, such as yoghurt or apple sauce, or chilled liquid to mask a disagreeable taste. Encourage brushing the teeth after administering medication at bedtime because there is often sugar in liquid formulations. Reinforce compliance with medication regimens and completion of therapy. Nurses may be instrumental in assisting parents with suggestions to help them incorporate medication administration into their routine, particularly when the child is on long-term urinary prophylaxis requiring daily medication.

Encourage adequate fluid intake for the prevention and treatment of UTI because this helps prevent risk factors such as constipation and urinary stasis. Fluid requirements are dependent on body size and fluid losses, but maintenance can be calculated based on the Holliday-Segar method, shown in Box 24.3. Using this formula, a 25-kg child should have 1600 mL (Haley & Pillitteri 2016). This formula is used for parenteral fluid replacement in children who are hospitalised. Fluid is also obtained from food, so this may be an overestimate of actual fluid intake. Have children avoid bladder irritants such as caffeinated or carbonated beverages. The child who is febrile and unable to drink liquids is given IV hydration until the fever resolves and oral liquids are tolerated.

Prevention. Prevention is the most important goal in both primary and recurrent infection. Most preventive measures are simple, ordinary hygienic habits that should be a routine part of daily care. Investigate any signs of intestinal parasites (e.g. scratching between the legs and around the anal area) and treat them appropriately. Advise sexually active adolescent girls to urinate as soon as possible after intercourse to flush out bacteria introduced during sex. Also teach parents and older children health practices that prevent UTI (Box 24.4).

Children who experience recurrent febrile UTIs or recurrent infections complicated by VUR may be given a suppressive or prophylactic antibiotic for a period of months or several years. The medication is commonly administered once a day; the patient and parents are typically advised to give the antibiotic before sleep because this represents the longest period without voiding. Commonly used antibiotics for urinary prophylaxis include gentamicin and benzylpenicillin.

BOX 24.3 Fluid Requirements in Children

Example: Determine fluid requirements for a 7-year-old child weighing 25 kg.
First 10 kg: 100 mL/kg/day × 10 kg = 1000 mL/day
Second 10 kg: 50 mL/kg/day × 10 kg = 500 mL/day
Each additional 1 kg: 20 mL/kg/day × 5 kg = 100 mL/day
Answer: 1600 mL/day

BOX 24.4 Preventing Measures for UTI

Factors Predisposing to Development	Measures of Prevention
Short female urethra close to vagina and anus	Perineal hygiene—wipe from front to back. Wear cotton panties rather than nylon.
Incomplete emptying and overdistension of bladder	Encourage toilet posture to relax the pelvic floor: knees separated and feet supported for girls. Avoid 'holding' urine; encourage child to void frequently, especially before a long trip or other circumstances in which toilet facilities are not available. Take time to relax and empty bladder completely with each void.

Gentamicin levels and renal function need to be checked prior to the third IV dose being administered if continuing with the gentamicin beyond 48 hours (RCHM 2019a).

Vesicoureteral Reflux

Vesicoureteral reflux (VUR) refers to the retrograde flow of urine from the bladder into the upper urinary tract. Reflux increases the chance for febrile UTI but does not cause it. When bladder pressure is high enough, refluxing urine can fill the ureter and renal pelvis. This is identified most often at peak bladder pressure during voiding, but it can occur as the bladder fills and remain after voiding, even draining down into the bladder, leaving residual urine until the next void. The International Classification System describes the degree of reflux from the bladder into upper genitourinary tract structures (Fig 24.2).

Primary reflux results from a congenital anomaly that affects the ureterovesical junction. Normally the ureter has a segment within the bladder wall that is compressed during a bladder contraction. This 'antireflux' mechanism does not work if that segment is shortened and not able to be compressed by the bladder muscle, allowing for backflow of urine. It is well recognised that children with UTI and VUR are at increased risk for pyelonephritis, as well as renal scarring (Garin 2019, Schlager 2016).

Secondary reflux occurs as a result of abnormally high pressure in the bladder, typically from anatomical (e.g. posterior urethral valves) or functional bladder obstruction (e.g. dysfunctional voiding or neurogenic bladder). It is a common finding in children with neurogenic bladder secondary to spina bifida. The severity of the bladder abnormality affects the degree of VUR, and treatment is typically focused on the underlying problem and not correction of the VUR in these cases.

Reflux with infection is the most common cause of pyelonephritis in children. There has been long-standing consensus that reflux of infected urine into the renal parenchyma results in renal scarring and predisposes to kidney disease. This belief has been increasingly questioned with the view that VUR is a sign of abnormal renal development that results in decreased formation of renal parenchyma, referred to as primary renal scarring. Current management is based on the premise that VUR is a risk factor for renal scarring because it allows bacteria to ascend from the bladder to the kidney and cause pyelonephritis. Because of the lack of conclusive evidence and the known association between VUR and renal scarring that can lead to chronic kidney disease, VUR is still regarded as a risk factor, and recommendations include performing an initial evaluation of renal status, growth and blood pressure on any child with VUR (Garin 2019, Schlager 2016).

Therapeutic Management

In most cases of VUR, conservative, non-operative therapy is effective in controlling infection. There is a high rate of spontaneous resolution over time. Factors associated with spontaneous resolution included diagnosis at less than 1 year of age, lower grades of VUR, prenatal hydronephrosis and unilateral reflux. The correlation of grade to rate of spontaneous resolution is 82%, 80%, 46%, 30% and 13% for grades I, II, III, IV and V, respectively (Garin 2019, Ripatti et al 2021). Other factors that may affect resolution rates are coexisting anomalies, voiding dysfunction, timing of reflux and gender (Kirsch et al 2014). Medical therapy consists of continuous antibiotic prophylaxis (CAP), based on the assumption that this will keep bacteria from multiplying and causing infection and that reflux of non-infected urine does not cause renal damage. The most common antibiotics used for this purpose are trimethoprim and sulfamethoxazole, trimethoprim or nitrofurantoin given once daily at bedtime. Amoxicillin is used in infants less than 2 months of age but is not otherwise used because of the increased likelihood of resistant organisms. Traditionally CAP has been used until documentation of resolution of VUR. This approach is being reconsidered, and the use of CAP is being individualised, with children often coming off after toilet training if they have no evidence of voiding dysfunction. Risks and benefits are discussed with parents with consideration of grade of reflux, rates of spontaneous resolution, elimination habits and family preferences. This long-term therapy requires medical supervision and reliable, cooperative parents who can be compliant with CAP recommendations and seek medical attention if there are symptoms suggestive of UTI or unexplained fever. Urine cultures are not recommended routinely but should be obtained if there are symptoms or unexplained fever because breakthrough infections can occur despite CAP (Bahat et al 2019).

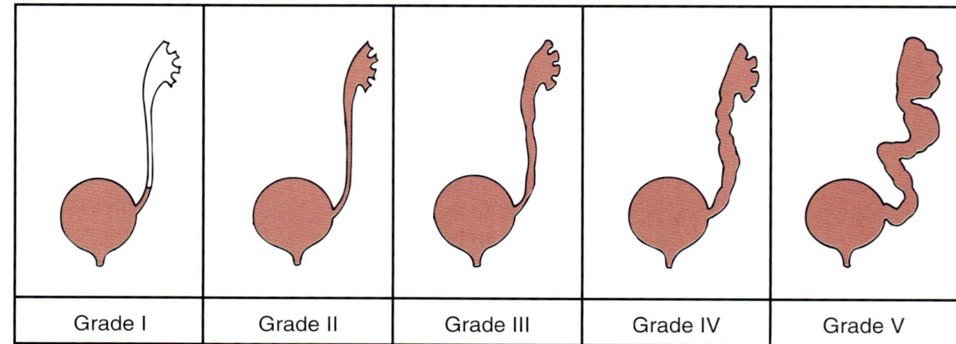

Fig 24.2 Grades of reflux. (Source: Retik, A. B., & Cukier, J. (Eds.). (1987). Pediatric urology. Baltimore, MD: Williams & Wilkins.)

Patients with prenatal hydronephrosis and asymptomatic VUR have been shown to be at a higher risk for the development of UTI resulting in the use of CAP. However, due to concerns about bacterial resistance and potential long-term side effects associated with the use of antibiotics, decisions about CAP use should be based on high-quality evidence (Leigh et al 2020).

Surgical management of VUR corrects the anatomy at the insertion of the refluxing ureter into the bladder and consists of open surgical correction with reimplantation of the ureter(s) or endoscopic correction. Surgical intervention is indicated in patients who are unlikely to resolve their reflux and are at risk for renal damage; including those with grade V reflux with scarring, grade V reflux over 6 years of age and children who fail medical therapy. Again, families play a role in the decision, in both their preferences and their ability to follow through with recommendations. For example a child with recurrent UTIs whose parents are not compliant with CAP may be a candidate for surgical correction regardless of the grade of reflux.

Renal ultrasonography is performed 1 month postoperatively to check for ureteral obstruction. The option of endoscopic correction is a minimally invasive alternative where injection of a bulking agent beneath the mucosa of the ureterovesical junction to change the angle of the ureter is performed during cystoscopy. The substance currently used is hyaluronic acid (Durolane), which has a success rate of upwards of 80%, depending on grade of reflux. There is no incision, and it is an outpatient procedure, whereas reimplantation requires a brief hospital stay.

Nursing Care Management

The primary nursing goal in children receiving medical therapy is encouraging compliance. Emphasise the importance of maintaining the medical regimen to parents and older children. The medications prescribed are usually well tolerated by children, but parents may need advice regarding encouraging children to take the medication. The methods described in Chapter 22 provide some guidelines for administration and encouraging compliance. The importance of hygiene and a frequent voiding schedule are also discussed. Parents need to know that breakthrough infections can occur despite CAP, so being aware of symptoms of UTI and seeking medical attention are critical.

GLOMERULAR DISEASE

Acute Glomerulonephritis

Acute glomerulonephritis (**AGN**) as a classification includes a number of distinct entities. It may be a primary event or a manifestation of a systemic disorder (Table 24.5), and the disease can range from mild to severe. The common features include oliguria, oedema, hypertension and circulatory congestion, haematuria and proteinuria. Many cases are postinfectious and have been associated with pneumococcal, streptococcal and viral infections. Postinfectious diseases are presumed to

TABLE 24.5 Renal Involvement Associated with Systemic Disease Process

Disease	Mechanism	Renal Manifestation	Comments
Systemic lupus erythematosus (SLE)	Deposition of autoantibody-antigen complexes in kidney	Variable degrees of haematuria and proteinuria More severe—Nephrotic syndrome, hypertension, renal insufficiency	Responsive to corticosteroid and antimetabolite therapy Renal failure most common cause of death from SLE Rare before adolescence but may occur in school-age children
Anaphylactoid (Schönlein-Henoch) purpura	Deposition of immunoglobulin (primarily IgA) in the glomerular mesangium	Haematuria (gross or microscopic) Less common—Oedema, hypertension, nephrotic syndrome with oliguria and hypertension, indicate severe involvement Rarely—Acute renal failure	Renal involvement in 20%–70% of cases Renal involvement most serious manifestation of the disease More common in children > 6 years old Immunosuppression medication may be beneficial in severe cases
Sickle cell disease	Infarction of renal vessels by sickle cells (especially medullary) Results in decreased circulation in vasa recta and impaired sodium and chloride ion reabsorption in collecting ducts	Haematuria Nephrotic syndrome Defective urine concentration Progressive glomerulonephritis	Irreversible with increasing age Severe urinary tract infections with bacteraemia not uncommon
Polyarteritis nodosa	Fibroid necrosis of arterial walls Large vessels—Patchy renal infarction Microscopic vessels—Necrotising glomerulitis	Proteinuria Haematuria Severe hypertension	Kidney function usually normal, but multiple renal infarcts may decrease renal function
Bacterial endocarditis	Focal or diffuse, immune-complex deposition related to chronic bacteraemia Some embolisation of glomeruli by bacteria and fibrin from endocardial vegetations	Proteinuria Haematuria	Renal involvement seen in approximately 50% of cases Renal involvement seldom of major significance
Prolonged bacteraemia (infected atrioventricular shunts)	Immune-complex deposition with exudation and cellular proliferation	Variable degrees of persistent nephrotic syndrome	Vigorous antibiotic therapy or removal of infected shunt required

IgA, Immunoglobulin A.

result from immune-complex formation and glomerular deposition, and the clinical presentations may be indistinguishable. Postinfectious glomerulonephritis exhibits a better clinical course than other acute proliferative glomerulonephritis.

Acute poststreptococcal glomerulonephritis (APSGN), also known as postinfectious glomerulonephritis, is the most common of the non-infectious renal diseases in childhood although the incidence in developed countries has declined over the past few decades (Demir & Caliskan 2020). APSGN can occur at any age but primarily affects early school-age children, with a median age of onset between 3 and 12 years (Dagan et al 2016). It is uncommon in children younger than 3 years of age.

Aetiology

It is generally accepted that APSGN is an immune-complex disease—that is, a reaction that occurs as a byproduct of an antecedent streptococcal infection with certain strains of the group A β-haemolytic streptococci, although other bacteria and viruses have also been implicated (VanDeVoorde 2015). Most streptococcal infections do not cause APSGN. A latent period of 1 to 2 weeks occurs between a streptococcal infection of the throat, or 3 to 6 weeks between a skin infection and the onset of clinical manifestations. The peak incidence of disease corresponds to the incidence of streptococcal infections. Disease secondary to streptococcal pharyngitis is more common in the winter or spring. However, when associated with pyoderma (principally impetigo), it may be more prevalent in late summer or early autumn, especially in warmer climates. Multiple cases tend to occur in families. Second attacks are rare.

Pathophysiology

The mechanism by which the reaction takes place is still speculative. One proposal to explain the pathological process is that the streptococcal infection is followed by the release of a membrane-like material from the specific organism into the circulation. Because it is antigenic, antibodies are formed and an immune-complex reaction occurs after the appropriate period. These immune complexes become trapped in the glomerular capillary loop.

The kidney itself appears normal or moderately enlarged, but microscopic examination reveals a diffuse proliferative and exudative process. Glomerular capillary loops are almost obliterated by swelling, and infiltration with polymorphonuclear leucocytes adds to the appearance of increased cellularity. Consequently, the glomeruli appear dense and lobulated. Examination with the electron microscope reveals discrete nodules or 'humps' in the basement membrane, which is identified as deposits of immune complexes. These deposits are not evident after approximately 6 weeks.

Endothelial cell proliferation and oedema occlude the capillary lumen of affected glomeruli, and the afferent arteriole is probably constricted by vasospasm, both of which significantly reduce the GFR. This occurs without a proportional decrease in renal blood flow and results in a reduced capacity to form filtrate from the glomerular plasma flow. Vascular and tubular changes are mild and non-specific; therefore, tubular function is less severely impaired.

The decreased filtration of plasma results in an excessive accumulation of water and retention of sodium. These cause expanded plasma and interstitial fluid volumes that lead to circulatory congestion, oedema and hypertension. It is unclear whether a decreased GFR, increased capillary permeability or vascular spasm is responsible for these various manifestations.

Clinical Manifestations

Typically, affected children are in good health until they experience the antecedent infection. In some instances there is no history of an infection, or it is described as only a mild cold. The onset of nephritis appears after a latent period. Because the child appears well during this time, parents may not recognise the association.

Initial signs of nephritic reaction include: puffiness of the face, especially around the eyes (periorbital oedema); anorexia; and the passage of cola-coloured urine. The oedema is more prominent in the face in the morning but spreads during the day to involve the extremities, genitalia and abdomen. The oedema is usually only moderate and may not be appreciated by someone unfamiliar with the child's normal appearance. The urine is cloudy, smoky brown or what parents describe as resembling tea or cola, and it is severely reduced in volume.

NURSING CARE CONSIDERATIONS

Evaluate a child who exhibits the following for possible AGN:

- periorbital, gonadal, abdominal or lower extremity oedema
- loss of appetite
- decreased urinary output
- cola- or tea-coloured urine
- antecedent streptococcal infection (other bacteria and viruses may also be responsible).

The child is pale, irritable and lethargic and appears unwell but seldom expresses specific complaints. Older children may complain of headaches, abdominal discomfort or dysuria. On examination there is usually a mild to moderate elevation in blood pressure compared with normal values for age, although severe hypertension may be present. Occasionally a child will have an onset with severe symptoms such as seizures from hypertensive encephalopathy, pulmonary and circulatory congestion, or haematuria in the absence of hypertension and oedema. Table 24.6 compares APSGN and minimal change nephrotic syndrome (MCNS).

TABLE 24.6 Comparison of Poststreptococcal Glomerulonephritis and Nephrotic Syndrome

Manifestations	Acute Poststreptococcal Glomerulonephritis	Minimal Change Nephrotic Syndrome
Streptococcal antibody titres	Elevated	Normal
Blood pressure	Elevated	Normal or decreased
Oedema	Primarily periorbital and peripheral	Generalised, severe
Circulatory congestion	Common	Absent
Proteinuria	Mild to moderate	Massive
Haematuria	Gross or microscopic	Microscopic or none
Red blood cell casts	Present	Absent
Azotaemia	Present	Absent
Serum potassium levels	Normal or increased	Normal
Serum protein levels	Minimum reduction	Markedly decreased
Serum lipid levels	Normal	Elevated
Peak age at onset (year)	5–7	2–3

Clinical Course. The acute oedematous phase of glomerulonephritis usually persists from 4 to 10 days but may persist for 2 or 3 weeks, during which time the child remains listless, anorexic and apathetic. The weight fluctuates, the urine remains smoky brown and the blood pressure may suddenly reach dangerously high levels at any time during this phase.

The first sign of improvement is an increase in urinary output with a corresponding decrease in body weight as oedema resolves. With diuresis the child begins to feel better, the appetite improves and the blood pressure decreases to normal. Gross haematuria diminishes, however microscopic haematuria and proteinuria may persist for months to years (Dagan et al 2016). Renal function and hypocomplementaemia usually normalise by 8 weeks.

Prognosis. Almost all children correctly diagnosed as having APSGN recover completely, and specific immunity is conferred so that subsequent recurrences are uncommon (Kim 2016). Deaths from complications can occur but fortunately are rare. A few children may develop chronic kidney disease.

Complications. The major complications that may develop during the acute phase of glomerulonephritis are hypertensive encephalopathy, acute cardiac decompensation and acute kidney injury (AKI). Normally, cerebral blood flow responds to acute arterial hypertension by vasoconstriction. However, acute and severe hypertension may cause this protective autoregulation of cerebral blood flow to fail, leading to hyperperfusion of the brain and cerebral oedema. The premonitory signs of encephalopathy are headache, dizziness, abdominal discomfort and vomiting. If the condition progresses, there may be transient loss of vision or hemiparesis, disorientation and generalised tonic-clonic seizures.

Hypervolaemia, not cardiac failure, causes cardiac decompensation during the acute oedematous phase of nephritis. However, signs of circulatory congestion are evident. The heart is enlarged, and increased pulmonary vascular markings are evident on x-ray examination. Increased pulmonary capillary permeability is also believed to be an important factor in the development of pulmonary oedema. AKI with persistent oliguria or anuria is an uncommon complication but one that requires an appropriate treatment regimen.

Diagnostic Evaluation

Urinalysis during the acute phase characteristically shows haematuria, proteinuria and increased specific gravity. Proteinuria generally parallels the haematuria but is not usually the massive proteinuria seen in nephrotic syndrome. Gross discolouration of urine reflects its red blood cell and haemoglobin content. Microscopic examination of the sediment shows many red blood cells, leucocytes, epithelial cells and granular and red blood cell casts. Bacteria are not seen, and urine cultures are negative.

Cultures of the pharynx are positive for streptococci in only a few cases, and the numbers are not significantly greater than the normal carrier incidence in many communities. Positive cultures help establish a diagnosis. Cultures should be obtained from other household members, and persons positive for group A streptococci should receive a course of antistreptococcal therapy.

Unless the disease has progressed to renal failure, the blood examination reveals normal electrolyte (sodium, potassium and chloride ions) and carbon dioxide levels. Azotaemia resulting from impaired glomerular filtration is reflected in elevated blood urea nitrogen (BUN) and creatinine levels in at least 50% of cases. When proteinuria is heavy, there may be changes associated with nephrotic syndrome (i.e. transient hypoproteinaemia and hyperlipidaemia).

Of more importance for clinical serological diagnosis is measurement of the C3 serum complement level. The serum C3 level is decreased initially but returns to normal within 8 to 10 weeks after onset of the glomerulonephritis. Other studies include a chest x-ray examination, which shows characteristic generalised cardiac enlargement, pulmonary congestion and pleural effusion during the oedematous phase of acute disease. Renal biopsy for diagnostic purposes is seldom required but may be useful in the diagnosis of atypical cases.

Therapeutic Management

No specific treatment is available for APSGN. Recovery is spontaneous and uneventful in most cases. Management consists of general supportive measures and early recognition and treatment of complications. Children who have normal blood pressure and a satisfactory urinary output can generally be treated at home but must be closely monitored. Those with substantial oedema, hypertension, gross haematuria or significant oliguria are often hospitalised because of the unpredictability of complications. Short hospitalisation may be necessary in uncomplicated cases; prolonged hospitalisation is required only for children with severely impaired renal function.

General Measures. Bed rest is not necessary during the acute phase because ambulation does not seem to have an adverse effect on the course of the disease. Because they are generally listless and experience fatigue and malaise, most children voluntarily restrict their activities during the most active phase of the disease.

Fluid Balance. Regular measurement of vital signs, body weight and intake and output is essential to monitor the disease's progress and detect complications that may appear at any time during the course of the disease. A record of daily weight is the most useful means to assess fluid balance and should be kept for children treated at home and for those who are hospitalised. Sodium and water restriction is useful when the output is significantly reduced ($<$ 2 to 3 dL/24 hr). In these children the water allowed is equivalent to the calculated insensible loss plus the volume of urine excreted.

Diuretics are of limited value when severe renal failure is present because little sodium reaches the distal tubules as a result of the reduced filtration rate. However, when renal failure is not severe, diuretic therapy (usually frusemide [Lasix]) is helpful if significant oedema and fluid overload are present. Rarely, children with APSGN develop AKI with oliguria that significantly alters the fluid and electrolyte balance. These children require careful management that may include peritoneal dialysis (PD) or haemodialysis (HD).

Loss of glomerular filtration in children with severe forms of APSGN may produce electrolyte imbalances, especially hyperkalaemia, acidosis, hypocalcaemia and hyperphosphataemia. Management of these electrolyte disturbances is described under Acute Kidney Injury.

Hypertension. Acute hypertension must be anticipated and identified early. Blood pressure measurements are taken at least every 4 to 6 hours. Significant but not severe hypertension is controlled with thiazide or loop diuretics. Other antihypertensive drugs, such as calcium channel blockers, beta blockers or angiotensin-converting enzyme inhibitors, may be needed in severe cases.

Nutrition. Dietary restrictions depend on the stage and severity of the disease, especially the extent of oedema. A regular diet is permitted in uncomplicated cases, but sodium intake is usually limited (no salt is added to foods) for children with hypertension or oedema. Foods with substantial amounts of potassium are generally restricted during the period of oliguria. Protein restriction is reserved only for children with severe azotaemia resulting from prolonged oliguria. The loss of appetite associated with the disease usually limits the protein intake sufficiently.

Antibiotics. Antibiotic therapy is indicated only for those children with evidence of persistent streptococcal infections. Antibiotics do not alter the course of the disease but are often recommended to prevent transmission of nephritogenic streptococci to other family members. Authorities are divided on the use of prophylactic antimicrobials for other family members.

Nursing Care Management. Nursing care of the child with glomerulonephritis involves careful assessment of the disease status, with regular monitoring of vital signs (including frequent measurement of blood pressure), fluid balance and behaviour. Vital signs provide clues to the severity of the disease and early signs of complications. The nurse carefully measures them and records and reports any abnormalities. The nurse notes the volume and character of urine and weighs the child daily. Assessment of the child's appearance for signs of cerebral complications is an important nursing function because the severity of the acute phase is variable and unpredictable. The child with oedema, hypertension and gross haematuria may be subject to complications, and anticipatory preparations are important nursing care responsibilities.

For most children a regular diet is allowed but should contain no added salt. Foods high in sodium and salted treats are eliminated, and the nurse should advise parents and friends against bringing items such as potato chips or corn chips. However, the total amount of salt ingested is usually less than prescribed because of poor appetite. Fluid restriction, if prescribed, is more difficult; the amount permitted should be evenly divided throughout the waking hours and served in small cups to give the illusion of larger servings. Meal preparation and service require special attention because the child has a poor appetite and is indifferent to meals during the acute phase. Collaboration with parents and the dietitian and special consideration for food preferences will facilitate meal planning.

Chronic or Progressive Glomerulonephritis

The majority of cases of renal glomerular disease are AGN, MCNS and glomerulonephritis associated with systemic diseases. These pose relatively few problems of diagnosis, and their natural course is fairly predictable. Some result in a prolonged course and a poor ultimate prognosis. They are defined by correlating the clinical manifestations, pathological conditions and natural course of the individual diseases.

Chronic glomerulonephritis (CGN) describes a variety of different disease processes that may be distinguished from one another by renal biopsy. These include membranoproliferative glomerulonephritis (MPGN), membranous glomerulonephritis, focal segmental glomerulosclerosis (FSGS) and immunoglobulin A nephropathy (IgA nephropathy). In CGN tissue damage and progression to fibrosis are related to the immune response that brings about inflammation, failure to activate glomerular repair and excessive fibrogenic activity. *Rapidly progressive glomerulonephritis* is the term used to describe an acute illness with severe, acute onset that causes rapidly progressive deterioration of renal function in weeks to months. Renal biopsy of these patients shows a variety of diseases, with the common feature of greater than 50% glomerular crescents found in the biopsy section.

Pathophysiology

In most cases of CGN, immunological mechanisms can be implicated either through direct attack on the kidney or secondary to the accumulation of immune complexes in the glomerular filter or fibrin deposition from previously damaged glomeruli. Either can contribute to further glomerular damage and can initiate chronic changes in the glomerular structure (Rheault & Wenderfer 2018). In many cases there is no history of an acute glomerular disease. In other cases CGN may represent one of a succession of exacerbations of a preexisting disease. CGN that is not associated with other diseases may go undetected for years and be relatively asymptomatic until kidney destruction produces marked reduction in renal function. Consequently, the disease is more common in adolescents than in younger children. Renal insufficiency with all its manifestations occurs as the ultimate event.

Clinical Manifestations

Early in the disease, clinical symptoms may be limited to proteinuria or microscopic haematuria detected on a routine examination. Laboratory findings may indicate decreased renal function. Nephrotic range proteinuria may be present. Symptoms vary based on the cause for the CGN but may include hypertension, oedema, intermittent gross haematuria and other manifestations of chronic kidney disease.

Diagnostic Evaluation

Laboratory findings may include proteinuria, with casts and red and white blood cells. Elevated BUN, creatinine and uric acid levels are evidence of decreased renal function. Electrolyte alterations include metabolic acidosis, elevated potassium, elevated phosphorus and decreased calcium levels. The renal insufficiency may extend from 5 to 15 years and even longer, or rapid deterioration may progress to end-stage renal disease (ESRD).

Therapeutic Management

Early in the course of the disease, treatment is appropriate to the underlying disease and is largely symptomatic in most cases. Nursing efforts should be directed towards providing optimum conditions for the child's physical, psychological and social development. As few restrictions as feasible should be imposed, and the child should be allowed to live as normal a life as possible for as long as possible. Some forms of CGN are treated with corticosteroids or cytotoxic agents. Marked hypertension is controlled with antihypertensive agents, and anaemia may require recombinant erythropoietin and iron supplements. Ultimately, dialysis or transplantation may be needed to restore relatively good health; however, these alternatives are reserved until renal failure is far advanced.

Nursing Care Management

The problems of CGN and those encountered in chronic renal insufficiency from any cause are discussed under Renal Failure.

Nephrotic Syndrome

Nephrotic syndrome is the most common presentation of glomerular injury in children. It is defined as massive proteinuria, hypoalbuminaemia, hyperlipidaemia and oedema and is a clinical manifestation of a large number of distinct glomerular disorders in which increased glomerular permeability to plasma protein results in massive urinary protein loss. After a description of the three major forms of nephrotic syndrome, the remainder of the discussion is devoted to minimal change disease (also known as idiopathic nephrosis, minimal lesion nephrosis, nil disease, childhood nephrosis, lipoid nephrosis or uncomplicated nephrosis).

Types of Nephrotic Syndrome

Nephrotic syndrome can be classified as primary, when the syndrome is restricted to glomerular injury, or secondary, when it develops as part of a systemic illness. Although it may have several different histological variations, the most common form of the primary disease is MCNS. A congenital form is also recognised.

Minimal Change Nephrotic Syndrome. Approximately 80% of cases of nephrotic syndrome in children result from MCNS. MCNS can be seen at any age but is predominantly a disease of the preschool child. Diagnosis of MCNS is rare in children younger than 6 months of age, uncommon in infants younger than 1 year of age and unusual after the age of 8 years (RCHM 2019b).

A non-specific illness, usually a viral upper respiratory tract infection, often precedes the manifestations by 4 to 8 days but is considered to be a precipitating factor rather than a cause.

Secondary Nephrotic Syndrome. Nephrotic syndrome may occur after or in association with glomerular damage of known or presumed cause. Prominent among causes of glomerular damage is AGN or CGN. Less commonly, secondary nephrotic syndrome occurs during the course of collagen vascular diseases (such as disseminated lupus erythematosus or anaphylactoid purpura) or as a result of toxicity to drugs (such as trimethadione and heavy metals), stings or venom. Nephrotic syndrome is the major presenting symptom of renal disease in paediatric patients with acquired immunodeficiency syndrome. Rare causes are sickle cell disease, hepatitis, malaria, cyanotic heart disease, tuberculosis, infected ventriculojugular shunts, renal vein thrombosis or malignancies.

Congenital Nephrotic Syndrome–Finnish Type. A recessive gene on an autosome causes the hereditary form of nephrotic syndrome. Infants who have congenital nephrotic syndrome–Finnish type are small for gestational age, and proteinuria and oedema manifest within the first few days to months of age. The disease does not respond to the usual therapy. Death in the first year or two of life is possible if the infant does not receive treatment, including IV administration of albumin, nutritional support, dialysis or a kidney transplant (Spahiu et al 2016).

Pathophysiology

The pathogenesis of MCNS is not completely understood. A metabolic, biochemical or physiochemical disturbance in the basement membrane of the glomeruli may lead to increased permeability to protein, but the causes and mechanisms are only speculative.

The glomerular membrane, which is normally impermeable to albumin and other large proteins, becomes permeable to proteins, especially albumin, that leak through the membrane and are lost in urine (hyperalbuminuria). This reduces the serum albumin level (hypoalbuminaemia), which decreases the COP in the capillaries. As a result, the hydrostatic pressure exceeds the pull of the COP, and fluid accumulates in the interstitial spaces and body cavities, particularly the abdominal cavity (ascites). The shift of fluid from the plasma to the interstitial spaces reduces the vascular fluid volume (hypovolaemia), which in turn stimulates the renin-angiotensin system and the secretion of antidiuretic hormone and aldosterone. Tubular reabsorption of sodium and water increases in an attempt to increase intravascular volume. The elevation of serum cholesterol, phospholipids and triglycerides is not fully understood. The sequence of events in nephrotic syndrome is shown in Figure 24.3.

Clinical Manifestations

A previously well child begins to gain weight, which progresses over a period of days or weeks. Puffiness of the face, especially around the eyes, is apparent on arising in the morning but subsides during the day, when swelling of the abdomen, genitalia and lower extremities is more prominent. Generalised oedema (anasarca) may develop gradually or rapidly. Oedema of the intestinal mucosa may cause diarrhoea, loss of appetite and poor intestinal absorption. The volume of urine is decreased, and it appears darkly opalescent and frothy.

The child often has extreme skin pallor and may experience skin breakdown during periods of severe oedema. The child may be irritable and more easily fatigued or lethargic but does not appear seriously

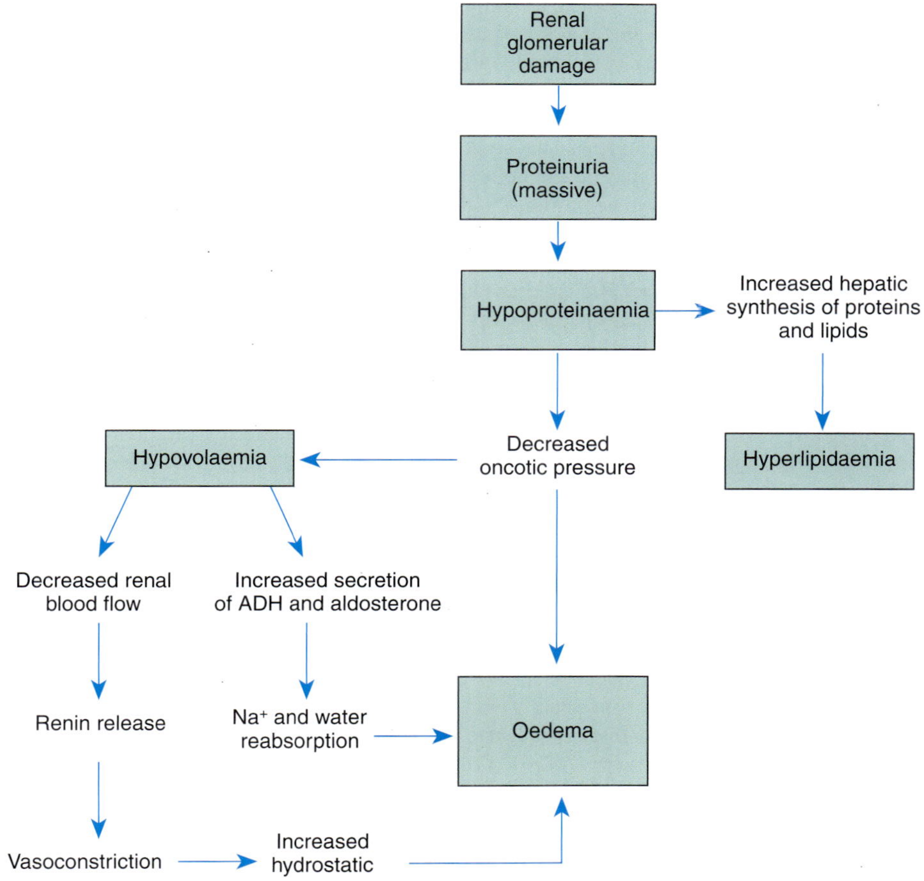

Fig 24.3 Sequence of events in nephrotic syndrome (ADH, *Antidiuretic hormone.*)

ill. Weight loss from poor appetite and loss of protein is not uncommon, although it is often obscured by oedema. Changes in the nails appear as white (Muehrcke) lines parallel to the lunula, which are caused by prolonged hypoalbuminaemia. The blood pressure is usually normal or slightly decreased. The child is more susceptible to infection, especially cellulitis, pneumonia, peritonitis or sepsis.

In rare cases children with MCNS have significant or persistent hypertension, gross or persistent haematuria or significant or persistent azotaemia (i.e. increased nitrogenous products in the blood).

Diagnostic Evaluation

The diagnosis of MCNS in children is based on the history and clinical manifestations (e.g. oedema, proteinuria, hypoalbuminaemia and hypercholesterolaemia in the absence of significant haematuria and hypertension). Massive proteinuria is reflected in urinary excretion of protein that often reaches levels in excess of 2 g/m^2 of body surface/day, with relatively greater clearance of low-molecular-weight proteins. Hyaline casts from high protein levels and sluggish flow and oval fat bodies, as well as a few red blood cells, can be found in the urine of most affected children, although there is seldom gross haematuria. Specific gravity is high and proportionate to the amount of protein concentration. If hypovolaemia is not significant and the child is well hydrated, the GFR is usually normal.

Total serum protein concentrations are reduced, with the albumin fractions significantly reduced ($<$ 2 g/dL) and plasma lipids elevated. Serum cholesterol may be as high as 450 to 1500 mg/dL. Haemoglobin and haematocrit are usually normal or elevated, and the platelet count is high (500,000 to 1,000,000/mm^3) as a result of haemoconcentration. Serum sodium concentration is usually low, approximately 130 to 135 mEq/L. Total calcium levels are low due to albumin binding, so ionised calcium is a more reliable measure of calcium levels.

If renal biopsy is performed, it provides information regarding the glomerular status and type of nephrotic syndrome, the likely response to drugs and the probable course of the disease. Under the microscope the foot processes of the basement membrane appear fused in a child with MCNS. The major focuses in differential diagnosis are to establish the oedema as renal in origin and to distinguish MCNS from other glomerulopathies with nephrotic syndrome as a manifestation.

Therapeutic Management

Medical management consists of both immunosuppressive and nonimmunosuppressive measures. The primary objective is to reduce the excretion of urinary protein and maintain protein-free urine. Additional objectives include prevention or treatment of acute infection, control of oedema, establishment of good nutrition and readjustment of any disturbed metabolic processes. Children with severe symptoms may be hospitalised for assessment and observation for evidence of infection, response to therapy and parental education.

General Measures. General treatment is principally supportive. During the oedema phase the child is often limited to quiet activities. Acute and intercurrent infections are treated with appropriate antibiotics, and providers make efforts to minimise the risk of infection. In addition to the usual vaccinations, children with nephrotic syndrome should receive the pneumococcal conjugate vaccine. Live vaccines should not be given while the child is on steroid therapy (Banerjee et al 2016).

Diet. The child in remission maintains a regular diet. However, salt is restricted during periods of massive oedema and while on corticosteroid therapy; no salt is added at the table, and foods with very high salt content are excluded. Although a low-sodium diet will not remove oedema, its rate of increase may be reduced. Water is seldom restricted. A diet generous in protein is logical, but there is no evidence that it is beneficial or alters the outcome of the disease. The presence of azotaemia and renal failure is a contraindication for high protein intake.

Corticosteroid Therapy. The response of most affected children to corticosteroids has established these drugs as the primary therapeutic agents in the management of nephrotic syndrome. Corticosteroid therapy begins as soon as the diagnosis has been determined and is administered orally in a dosage of 60 mg/m^2/day (with a maximum dose of 60 mg/day). Prednisone is the steroid of choice. The drug is continued daily for 4 weeks and then reduced to 40 mg/m^2 on alternate days for 10 days and then commence on 10 mg/m^2/day on alternate days for another 10 days, ceasing after completing this regimen (RCHM 2019b).

Studies suggest that the duration of steroid treatment for the initial episode should be at least 3 months. The course of the disease is fairly predictable. There is little change during the first few days of therapy. In most patients, diuresis occurs as the urinary protein excretion diminishes within 7 to 21 days after the initiation of steroid therapy. Other clinical manifestations stabilise or return to normal shortly thereafter. Approximately 90% of patients will achieve remission during the initial course of prednisone treatment. If the child has not responded to therapy within 28 days of daily steroid administration, the likelihood of subsequent response diminishes.

Children with MCNS are often described according to their response to corticosteroid therapy (Box 24.5). Children with MCNS typically relapse one to three times per year. Steroid-dependent children tend to have frequent relapses over many years and receive large amounts of steroids, which results in cushingoid features and may cause growth abnormalities. They may also require supportive treatment (e.g. diuretics, diet). Steroid-resistant children are thought to have a high risk of developing chronic kidney disease (Lombel et al 2013).

Diuretics. Oral diuretics may have a blunted effectiveness in treating the oedema of nephrotic syndrome (Ellis 2016). Loop diuretics, usually frusemide, are sometimes useful in cases in which oedema interferes with respiration or ambulation or there is hypertension or significant oedema in the scrotum or labia. In addition, plasma expanders such as salt-poor human albumin may be administered to severely oedematous children requiring prompt control; however, they must be administered frequently because the glomeruli are readily permeable to albumin in the acute stage (RCHM 2019b).

Prognosis. The prognosis for ultimate recovery in most cases is good. For children who respond to steroid therapy the tendency to relapse decreases with time. With early detection and prompt implementation of therapy to eradicate proteinuria, progressive basement membrane damage is minimised so that renal function is usually normal or near normal when the tendency for relapses is past. It is estimated that approximately 80% of affected children have this favourable prognosis, although more than 20% will continue to have relapses in adulthood (Hjorten et al 2016).

BOX 24.5 Classification of Nephrotic Syndrome According to Steroid Response

Steroid sensitive—Responds to steroids; relapses may occur after illness

Frequent relapse—Two or more relapses within 6 months of initial response; four or more relapses within a 12-month period

Steroid dependent—Two consecutive relapses while on steroid therapy or within 2 weeks of steroid cessation

Steroid resistant—Does not enter remission after 4 weeks of prednisone therapy

Source: Modified from Bagga, A., & Mantan, M. (2005). Nephrotic syndrome in children. Indian Journal of Medical Research, 122, 13–28.

Nursing Care Management

Daily monitoring of intake and output is an important nursing function. Strict and accurate measurement is essential but may be difficult in very young children. In these cases the nurse can measure for output by methods such as weighing nappies. Other methods of monitoring progress include examination of the urine for albumin, daily weight and measurement of abdominal girth. Assessment of oedema, such as increased or decreased swelling around the eyes and dependent areas, the degree of pitting (if noted) and colour and texture of the skin, is part of nursing care. The nurse monitors vital signs to detect any early signs of complications such as shock or an infectious process.

Loss of appetite that accompanies active nephrosis creates a perplexing problem for nurses. During this time the combined efforts of the nurse, dietitian, parents and child are necessary to formulate a nutritionally adequate and attractive diet. Small, frequent meals may be best tolerated. Salt and fluids are restricted during the oedema phase. (See Feeding the Sick Child, Chapter 22.)

Family Support and Home Care. Most children are treated at home during relapses unless the oedema and proteinuria are severe. Teach parents to detect signs of relapse and to notify the healthcare provider if they occur. Nurses should instruct parents in urine testing for albumin, administration of medications and general care. Urine is usually tested daily for albumin while the child is receiving medicine for nephrotic syndrome or if the child has an illness, and twice a week during remission. Salt is restricted to no additional salt during relapse and steroid therapy, but a regular diet is suitable for the child in remission. Social isolation may be a problem for these children. Isolation is related to frequent hospitalisation or confinement during relapse, the risk of infection that may precipitate an exacerbation, lack of energy and the child's reluctance to face friends at home or school because of the changes in appearance resulting from the disease or the medication. Both the parents and the child need someone to listen to their complaints, to assist them in coping with both short- and long-term problems associated with the disease and to find solutions to their problems. Continuous support of the child and family is one of the major nursing considerations.

RENAL TUBULAR DISORDERS

Disorders of renal tubular function include a variety of conditions involving one or more abnormalities in specific mechanisms of tubular transport or reabsorption. Glomerular function is normal or mildly impaired. Eventually more widespread kidney destruction with renal failure may occur. In some cases the dysfunction has little, if any, effect on renal function. These disorders may be permanent or transient and may originate as primary defects or arise as a secondary effect of metabolic disease or exogenous toxins. Renal tubular disorders may be congenital (usually displaying characteristic patterns of genetic transmission), appear without evidence of hereditary transmission or be acquired as a result of known or unknown causes.

Unlike the classic manifestations of glomerular diseases, oedema and hypertension are absent and the BUN level and routine urinalysis are usually normal. Tubular proteinuria may be demonstrated. Manifestations of tubular disorders are primarily metabolic disturbances or deficiencies, such as faltering growth, metabolic bone disease or persistent acidosis. The variety of these disorders is extensive, and the incidence is rare.

Tubular Function

The function of the proximal tubules is the reabsorption of substances from the glomerular filtrate, including sodium, potassium, chloride, bicarbonate, glucose, phosphate and amino acids. A number of disorders feature impairment of reabsorption of one or more filtrate constituents, and most involve defects in the transport mechanisms for these substances. Impaired tubular reabsorption of any specific substance causes that substance to appear in the urine, sometimes with reduced levels in the blood. Examples include bicarbonate and phosphate.

The primary functions of the distal renal tubules are: acidification of urine; potassium secretion; and selective and differential reabsorption of sodium, chloride and water, which determines the final urinary concentration. Because the contribution of the distal tubule to urine composition depends in part on the volume and composition of the filtrate from the proximal tubule, the net contribution of the distal tubule is related to proximal tubular function and glomerular filtration.

Renal Tubular Acidosis

Renal tubular acidosis (RTA) is a syndrome of sustained metabolic acidosis in which there is impaired reabsorption of bicarbonate or excretion of net hydrogen ion but in which glomerular function is normal. On the basis of underlying pathophysiology, RTA is divided into proximal RTA and distal RTA. Proximal RTA results from a defect in bicarbonate reabsorption, whereas distal RTA results from an inability to establish an adequate gradient of pH between blood and tubular fluid. A number of genetic abnormalities have been identified for all types of primary RTA (Santos et al 2015).

Proximal Tubular Acidosis (Type II)

Impaired bicarbonate reabsorption in the proximal tubule causes proximal tubular acidosis. It may occur as an isolated defect (primary), but more often it appears in association with other proximal tubular disorders (secondary). As a result of a depressed renal threshold, bicarbonate reabsorption in the proximal tubule is incomplete, causing the plasma concentration of bicarbonate to stabilise at a lower level than normal. This results in a hyperchloraemic metabolic acidosis. There is no impairment of distal tubular integrity or, in most cases, of the distal acidifying mechanism.

A more complex abnormality in the proximal tubules is Fanconi's syndrome, in which transport mechanisms are damaged by the accumulation of toxic metabolites or the tubular epithelium is damaged by heavy metals such as lead, cadmium or platinum. Fanconi's syndrome can be part of a number of hereditary diseases, be acquired or be idiopathic (with a cause that is not identifiable). The major clinical manifestation and presenting symptom of Fanconi's syndrome is growth failure. Tachypnoea from hyperchloraemic metabolic acidosis is also evident. Dehydration, vomiting, episodic fever, nephrolithiasis secondary to hypercalciuria, muscle weakness or paralysis as a result of hypokalaemia, and episodes of severe life-threatening acidaemia (sometimes triggered by a concurrent infection) may also be seen. The disorder may be transient or permanent.

Distal Tubular Acidosis (Type I)

Distal tubular acidosis is caused by the kidney's inability to establish a normal pH gradient between tubular cells and tubular contents. The most characteristic feature is the inability to produce a urinary pH below 6.0 despite the presence of severe metabolic acidosis.

Distal tubular acidosis usually occurs as a primary, isolated defect but may also occur in association with other diseases or disorders (Gomez et al 2016). Most secondary causes are rare. The primary disorder is usually considered to be a hereditary defect with a variable degree of expression and a greater penetrance in females. After the age of 2 years, the child usually has growth failure, often with a history of vomiting, polyuria, dehydration, anorexia and faltering growth.

Evidence of bone demineralisation may be present, along with the occasional formation of renal calculi in older children.

The inability to secrete hydrogen ions causes an accumulation of the ions in the body, which soon depletes the available hydrogen buffer and produces a sustained acidosis. Acidosis slows normal somatic growth, and demineralisation of bone occurs as bone salts are mobilised to buffer the excessive hydrogen ions. Increased serum levels of both calcium and phosphorus contribute to the development of stones within the renal system. Both sodium and potassium are secreted in larger amounts. Serum potassium levels are depleted as the distal tubules excrete large amounts of potassium ions in an attempt to conserve sodium because hydrogen ions are unable to participate in the exchange. Hyponatraemia stimulates increased aldosterone secretion, which further aggravates the hypokalaemia. With the depletion of bicarbonate ions, more chloride is reabsorbed in the proximal tubule to create a hyperchloraemia.

Prognosis. The primary disorder is usually permanent. However, secondary effects on growth and stone formation can be avoided with early diagnosis and therapy. When the disorder occurs as a secondary complication and renal damage is prevented, the prognosis is good (Gil-Peña et al 2014).

Therapeutic Management

Treatment of both proximal and distal disorders consists of the administration of sufficient bicarbonate or citrate to: balance metabolically produced hydrogen ions; maintain the plasma bicarbonate level within normal range; and correct associated electrolyte disorders, especially hypokalaemia. Proximal disorders require large volumes of bicarbonate to compensate for urinary losses; in distal disorders the alkali required to maintain a normal plasma concentration is low. Most authorities favour a mixture of sodium and potassium bicarbonate (or citrate) to prevent deficiencies of either cation. The citrate solutions are usually more easily tolerated than bicarbonate solutions.

Nursing Care Management

Nursing goals include recognising the possibility of RTA in children who fail to thrive or who display other symptoms suggestive of the disorders and referring these children for medical evaluation. Helping parents understand the importance of adhering to the medication plan as a long-term goal is essential. Children who must continue the medication indefinitely need to learn the importance of taking the medications as soon as they are old enough to assume responsibility for their own care.

Nephrogenic Diabetes Insipidus

Nephrogenic diabetes insipidus (NDI) is the major disorder associated with a defect in the ability to concentrate urine. In this disorder the distal tubules and collecting ducts are insensitive to the action of antidiuretic hormone or its exogenous counterpart, vasopressin. Although several inheritance patterns have been identified, more than 90% of patients have an X-linked defect of the vasopressin receptor (Bichet & Bockenhauer 2016). The disease is more variable in female carriers of the defective gene, who may exhibit only a mild defect in urine-concentrating ability. The differential diagnosis for NDI should include chronic obstructive renal disorders, sickle cell disease, renal tuberculosis and other renal disorders that may cause high urinary output with failure of the kidney to respond to vasopressin.

Clinical Manifestations and Diagnostic Evaluation

NDI is manifested in the newborn period by vomiting, unexplained fever, faltering growth and severe recurrent dehydration with hypernatraemia. The passage of copious amounts of dilute urine, which produces severe dehydration and hypoelectrolytaemia, is a serious threat to life during this period and may be responsible for the high incidence of cognitive impairment and motor restriction found in affected persons. Growth restriction is probably related to diminished food intake and poor general health because of uncontrolled polydipsia. Diagnosis is suspected on the basis of the patient and family history and confirmed by a urine osmolality value consistently below that of plasma. Lack of response to vasopressin administration rules out other causes.

Therapeutic Management

Therapy involves provision of adequate volumes of water to compensate for urinary losses and minimisation of urine output through diet and medication. As a result of an insatiable thirst, most of the child's time is spent drinking and voiding, with decreased time for activity and stimulation. These children may go to great lengths to satisfy their thirst. Supplemental potassium may be required to prevent hypokalaemia as a result of thiazide therapy. Normal growth and a normal life span are possible if the disease is recognised early and treatment is instituted and maintained.

Nursing Care Management

Nursing goals for children with NDI and their families are to recognise signs of the disorder early and assist them in coping with the long-term inconvenience of the continual thirst and elimination problems. Families need to learn to administer medications and help with diet planning for those on sodium restriction and needing supplemental potassium. The problem of ensuring adequate hydration is lifelong, and families need to adapt to away-from-home fluid needs and avoid activities that contribute to dehydration when fluids may not be available. Genetic counselling is recommended.

MISCELLANEOUS RENAL DISORDERS

Familial Nephritis (Alport's Syndrome)

Alport's syndrome (AS) is a hereditary disease characterised by high-tone sensorineural deafness, ocular disorders and chronic kidney disease caused by mutations in type IV collagen. Most people with AS have the X-linked form of the condition. Less common are autosomal recessive and dominant forms.

Haematuria presents during infancy in affected boys. Gross haematuria may be associated with acute respiratory tract infections. Proteinuria and progressive renal failure begin in childhood. The progression rate to end-stage kidney disease depends on the form of AS. Females may have only microhaematuria or progress to ESRD, again depending on the form of the condition they have (Savige et al 2016).

Treatment is symptomatic and supportive. Dialysis and kidney transplantation are ultimate therapeutic measures for ESRD. Hearing loss and ocular disorders should receive appropriate attention, and families should be counselled regarding the genetic implications of the disease.

Unexplained Proteinuria

Often apparently healthy children with no suggestion of renal disease demonstrate proteinuria on routine urinalysis. The percentage of children with unexplained proteinuria ranges from 1% at 6 years of age to 11% at puberty, reaching a maximum prevalence at age 13 in girls and age 16 in boys.

Unexplained proteinuria can be categorised as transient (inconstant), persistent, or orthostatic or postural. Transient proteinuria is a common finding with no known cause but sometimes increases with febrile illness, exercise or dehydration. Persistent proteinuria usually signifies renal disease. Orthostatic proteinuria is seen in 3% to 5% of adolescents and young adults; although proteinuria is evident in both the recumbent and the erect position, it is quantitatively greater in the erect position. The cause is unknown, but minor glomerular changes occur in many instances. The condition is benign and generally resolves over time.

In cases of unexplained proteinuria, it is important to confirm or exclude renal disease with appropriate diagnostic tests. Repeated examination for proteinuria, an orthostatic test, urine culture and (if proteinuria is persistent) more definitive tests—including 24-hour protein excretion, renal ultrasound and renal scan—are indicated.

Renal Trauma

Serious injuries of the genitourinary tract are not uncommon in the paediatric age group, with a peak incidence between ages 10 and 20 years. Despite their relatively protected location, the kidneys in children are more mobile than they are in adults and the outer borders are less well protected. They are separated from the skin surface by only 2 to 3 cm in young children. This results in an increased risk of renal trauma in children as opposed to adults.

Most injuries are of the non-penetrating or blunt type and usually involve falls, recreational motor vehicles such as dirt bikes, bicycle accidents and motor vehicle crashes (Dangle et al 2016). Penetrating trauma (e.g. stab wound) is much less common in children. Some children have preexisting renal abnormalities, particularly congenital anomalies associated with mild to moderate hydronephrosis that were unrecognised before the injury.

The nurse should suspect renal injury in children who complain of flank pain and have abrasions or contusions on the overlying skin. Haematuria is present, but the amount of blood in the urine is not a reliable indicator of the seriousness of the injury. Many relatively insignificant injuries are associated with grossly bloody urine, whereas some of the most severe injuries are found in children with only microscopic haematuria.

Renal rupture involves the actual splitting open of the kidney capsule, causing extravasation of blood or a mixture of blood and urine into the surrounding retroperitoneal space. Renal vascular injury, although unusual, requires immediate recognition and surgical intervention. Because the volume-per-minute blood flow through the kidney is greater (25% of cardiac output) than to any other abdominal organ, injury to the kidney may result in a rapid loss of blood.

Active children may or may not have a history of unusual trauma. Abdominal or flank pain and tenderness are caused by bleeding around the kidney and may or may not be associated with fever. Clots passing down the ureter may cause pain similar to that of renal colic, and dysuria is common. Patients with more severe injuries may complain of nausea or abdominal pain. There may be a palpable abdominal mass caused by loss of blood or urine into the retroperitoneum. The fibrous capsule enclosing the kidney prevents expansion of a haematoma; therefore, exsanguination and shock are seldom observed, even in severe renal trauma.

Diagnosis is made on the basis of IV pyelography, angiography or retrograde pyelography. Unsuspected hydronephrosis often is first detected as a result of traumatic injury.

Therapeutic Management

Severe injury requires close observation in the hospital intensive care unit and blood replacement if there is severe internal or external bleeding. In most cases bleeding subsides spontaneously. Surgical exploration is indicated if there are multiple injuries, extravasation of blood around the kidneys or disruption of the major vessels or the collecting system. Children with less severe injuries, such as contusions only, are placed on bed rest. They should remain on bed rest for 3 days after cessation of gross bleeding because the substance released from injured renal tissue (urinary urokinase) has strongly fibrinolytic properties that may precipitate serious bleeding. The prognosis depends on the nature and extent of the injury.

Nursing Care Management

Nursing management is directed towards recognising and assisting in the diagnosis of renal injury. Care of both the child and the family is primarily supportive. The nurse implements all the concepts related to emergency hospitalisation and care. (See Chapter 22.) Postsurgical care, if indicated, is the same as for any other surgical patient. Recommendations for children with a solitary kidney participating in sports are varied. Each child should be individually assessed and advised on the need for protective equipment before engaging in contact, collision or limited contact activities (Psooy 2014).

Renal Failure

Renal failure is the inability of the kidneys to excrete waste material, concentrate urine and conserve electrolytes. The disorder can be acute or chronic and affects most of the systems in the body. Two terms that are often used in relation to renal failure need some clarification: **azotaemia** is the accumulation of nitrogenous waste within the blood, whereas **uraemia** is a more advanced condition in which retention of nitrogenous products produces toxic symptoms. Azotaemia is not life-threatening, whereas uraemia is a serious condition that often involves other body systems.

Acute Kidney Injury

Acute kidney injury (AKI) is said to exist when the kidneys suddenly are unable to appropriately regulate the volume and composition of urine in response to food and fluid intake and the needs of the organism. The principal feature is oligoanuria associated with azotaemia, acidosis and diverse electrolyte disturbances. AKI is not common in childhood. The outcome depends on the cause, associated findings and prompt recognition and treatment.

Aetiology

AKI can develop as a result of a large number of related or unrelated clinical conditions: poor renal perfusion, acute renal injury or the final expression of chronic renal disease. The most common cause in children is transient renal failure resulting from dehydration or other causes of poor perfusion that respond to restoration of fluid volume. Causes of AKI are usually classified as prerenal, intrinsic renal and postrenal. Severe or long-standing prerenal or postrenal causes can produce severe secondary renal damage.

Prerenal Causes. Prerenal causes of AKI are most common in children and are related to the reduction of renal perfusion in an anatomically and physiologically normal kidney and collecting system. Dehydration secondary to diarrhoeal disease or persistent vomiting is the most common cause of prerenal failure in infants and children. Surgical shock and trauma (including burns) are also common causes. Hypovolaemia and decreased renal perfusion cause a decreased GFR and stimulate the secretion of renin, aldosterone and antidiuretic hormone, which further diminish urine flow. Extended and severe hypoperfusion (secondary to procedures such as cardiac surgery) can produce cortical or tubular necrosis. Increasing awareness of the potential for the development of AKI allows for earlier detection and treatment should it occur (Jefferies & Devarajan 2016). In general, the azotaemia that accompanies this type of renal failure is rapidly reversible with prompt attention to expansion of the extracellular fluid volume. Prerenal failure is often difficult to distinguish from tubular or cortical necrosis. Renal artery stenosis, altered peripheral vascular resistance related to sepsis and hepatorenal syndrome are less common causes.

Intrinsic Renal Causes. Intrinsic renal causes of AKI constitute the largest group that requires extended management. These include diseases and nephrotoxic agents that damage the glomeruli, tubules or renal vasculature. Glomerular disease is the most common cause of glomerular damage, whereas tubular destruction is more often caused by ischaemia or nephrotoxins. Vascular damage is an uncommon cause of renal failure in childhood. The type and extent of damage determine the degree and duration of renal insufficiency, and it is difficult to predict in any given case whether acute necrosis will develop.

Postrenal Causes. AKI resulting from obstructive uropathy is uncommon in children except during the first year of life. Relief of the obstruction can restore renal function. The degree of recovery depends on the duration of the renal failure.

Pathophysiology

AKI is usually reversible, but the deviations of physiological function can be extreme, and mortality in the paediatric age group is still high. There is severe reduction in the GFR, an elevated BUN level and decreased tubular reabsorption of sodium from the proximal tubule. Consequently, there is increased concentration of sodium in the distal tubule, which causes stimulation of the renin mechanism. The local action of angiotensin causes vasoconstriction of the afferent arteriole, which further reduces glomerular filtration and prevents urinary losses of sodium. There is a significant reduction in renal blood flow.

The pathological conditions that produce AKI caused by glomerulonephritis, HUS and other renal disorders are discussed in relation to those disease processes. The necrotic processes within the nephron can be cortical, tubular or both.

Cortical Necrosis. Complete cortical necrosis usually results from severe ischaemia, infection or intravascular coagulation and represents a severe cause of AKI. In the paediatric age group this occurs most commonly during the neonatal period as a result of hypoxia and shock. When cortical destruction is incomplete, some recovery of renal function may occur.

Tubular Necrosis. Damage to the renal tubules can be broadly classified as secondary to renal ischaemia and associated with the ingestion or inhalation of substances toxic to the kidneys. Renal tubules are particularly vulnerable to a wide variety of toxic agents that produce vasoconstriction and to focal patches of ischaemia that cause a necrosis of the tubular epithelium down to, but not including, the basement membrane. A lesion produced by sustained reduction in renal blood flow also involves the basement membrane, which may become fragmented and ruptured to the extent that the continuity of tubular structure is disrupted. The lesions may affect any segment of the tubules, appearing at irregular intervals along with normal segments throughout the kidney.

Reepithelialisation in the areas with intact basement membrane heals tubular lesions. Such healing is unable to take place in areas in which the basement membrane has been disrupted; connective tissue grows through the ruptured membrane, thus preventing reestablishment of tubular integrity. Individual cells within the nephron, but not the entire nephron, are capable of regeneration.

Clinical Course. The clinical course of the child with AKI is variable and depends on the cause. In reversible AKI there is a period of severe oliguria, or a low-output phase, followed by an abrupt onset of diuresis, or a high-output phase; this phase is followed by a gradual return to, or towards, normal urine volumes. The length of the oliguric phase in older children and adolescents is 10 to 14 days but is highly variable at all ages depending on the cause of the AKI. The onset of the diuretic phase appears unexpectedly, and over several days it proceeds in stepwise fashion from very low to above-normal urine volumes. During the oliguric phase, manifestations of uraemia are present but may also be accompanied by other clinical disorders that make assessment difficult, such as infection, anoxia and shock.

Clinical Manifestations

In many instances of AKI the infant or child is already critically ill with the precipitating disorder, and the explanation for development of oliguria may or may not be readily apparent. The underlying illness often overshadows the renal failure and often assumes the priority of care (e.g. the patient who is in shock from endotoxaemia, the infant who is severely dehydrated from gastroenteritis or a child who is subject to seizures as a result of hypertensive encephalopathy associated with AGN).

The prime manifestation of AKI is oliguria, generally a urinary output of less than 1 mL/kg/hr. Anuria (no urinary output in 24 hours) is uncommon, except in obstructive disorders. Other symptoms related to AKI include oedema, drowsiness, circulatory congestion and cardiac arrhythmia from hyperkalaemia. Seizures may be caused by hyponatraemia or hypocalcaemia and tachypnoea from metabolic acidosis. With continued oliguria, biochemical abnormalities can develop rapidly, and circulatory and central nervous system manifestations appear.

Diagnostic Evaluation

When a previously well child develops AKI without obvious cause, a careful history is obtained to reveal symptoms that may be related to: glomerulonephritis; obstructive uropathy; or exposure to nephrotoxic chemicals, such as ingestion of heavy metals or inhalation of carbon tetrachloride or other organic solvents or drugs (e.g. methicillin, sulfonamides, NSAIDs, neomycin, polymyxin and kanamycin). Laboratory data reflect the kidney dysfunction: hyperkalaemia, hyponatraemia, metabolic acidosis, hypocalcaemia, anaemia or azotaemia (Table 24.7).

Therapeutic Management

The most effective management of AKI is prevention. The development of AKI is a known risk in certain situations. This should be anticipated and recognised, and adequate therapy should be implemented (e.g. fluid therapy for children with hypovolaemia in conditions such as dehydration, burns and haemorrhage). Nephrotoxic drugs should be used with caution or avoided in children with renal disease, and all personnel should be knowledgeable about precautions related to their administration. For example, a generous fluid intake is needed for children receiving antimetabolite drugs and after radiotherapy.

The treatment of AKI is directed towards treatment of the underlying cause, management of the complications of renal failure and provision of supportive therapy within the constraints imposed by the renal failure. Treatment of poor perfusion resulting from dehydration consists of volume restoration as described in the treatment of dehydration. (See Chapter 23.) If oliguria persists after restoration of fluid volume or if the renal failure is caused by intrinsic renal damage, the physiological and biochemical abnormalities that have resulted from kidney dysfunction must be corrected or controlled. Central venous pressure monitoring is usually implemented.

Initially a catheter is inserted to rule out urine retention, to collect available urine for electrolytes and analysis and to monitor the results of diuretic administration. The catheter may or may not be removed. Some clinicians believe that it serves little purpose during the oliguric phase and predisposes the patient to bladder infections. Others maintain a catheter for hourly urine measurements.

TABLE 24.7 Laboratory Findings Associated with Acute Renal Failure

Clinical Problem	Mechanism	Clinical Considerations
Azotaemia	Ongoing protein catabolism	Lower rate of production in neonates and persons with depleted protein stores
Elevated blood urea nitrogen levels	Significantly decreased excretion	Increased in situations involving large amounts of necrotic tissue or extravasated blood
Elevated plasma creatinine levels	Continued production Significantly decreased excretion	Production less affected by other factors More sensitive measure of intensity of azotaemia Low in neonate because of small muscle mass relative to size
Metabolic acidosis	Continued endogenous acid production Significantly decreased excretion Depletion of extracellular and intracellular fluid buffers	Compensatory hyperventilation Opisthotonos Major threat to life
Hyponatraemia	Dilution of extracellular fluid Decreased excretion of water	May develop cerebral signs
Hyperkalaemia	Ongoing protein catabolism Decreased excretion compounded by metabolic acidosis	Most important electrolyte to be considered in acute renal failure May contribute to cardiac arrhythmia With electrocardiogram changes, major threat to life Loss may be from gastrointestinal tract
Hypocalcaemia	Associated with metabolic acidosis and hyperphosphataemia	During alkali therapy, may cause tetany

Fluid and Calories. The amount of exogenous water provided should not exceed the amount needed to maintain zero water balance. It is calculated on the basis of estimated endogenous water formation and losses from sensible (primarily gastrointestinal) and insensible sources. No allotment is calculated for urine as long as oliguria persists.

The child with AKI has a tendency to develop water intoxication and hyponatraemia, both of which make it difficult to provide calories in sufficient amounts to meet the child's needs and reduce tissue catabolism, metabolic acidosis, hyperkalaemia and uraemia. If the child is able to tolerate oral foods, concentrated food sources that are high in carbohydrates and fat but low in protein, potassium and sodium may be provided. However, many children have functional disturbances of the gastrointestinal tract, such as nausea and vomiting. Therefore, the IV route is generally preferred, and nourishment usually consists of essential amino acids or a combination of essential and non-essential amino acids administered by the central venous route.

Control of water balance in these patients requires careful monitoring of feedback information, such as accurate intake and output, body weight and electrolyte measurements. In general, during the oliguric phase, no sodium, chloride or potassium is given unless there are other large, ongoing losses. Regular measurement of plasma electrolytes, pH, BUN and creatinine levels is required to assess the adequacy of fluid therapy and to anticipate complications that require specific treatment.

Hyperkalaemia. An elevated serum potassium level is the most immediate threat to the life of the child with AKI. Potassium ions are not being excreted, while at the same time the release of potassium from cells is accelerated by acidosis, stress and tissue breakdown in cases associated with internal bleeding or trauma. Because cardiac arrhythmia and cardiac arrest may result, electrocardiograms (ECGs) and serum potassium ion levels are monitored regularly. Hyperkalaemia can be minimised and sometimes avoided by eliminating potassium from all food and fluids, by reducing tissue catabolism and by correcting acidosis.

Several measures are available to reduce the serum potassium concentration, and the priority of implementation is usually based on the rapidity with which the measures are effective. Temporary measures that produce a rapid but transient effect are as follows.

- Calcium gluconate administered intravenously over 2 to 4 minutes with continuous ECG monitoring exerts a protective effect on cardiac conduction.
- Sodium bicarbonate administered intravenously over 30 to 60 minutes elevates the serum pH to cause a transient shift of extracellular fluid potassium into the intracellular fluid. However, there is a risk of hypocalcaemia, tetany and fluid overload.
- Glucose and insulin administered intravenously accelerate glycogen synthesis, causing glucose and potassium to move into the cells. Insulin facilitates the entry of glucose into cells.

These effects produce only transient protection by redistributing existing potassium stores; they do not remove potassium from the body. However, they provide relief while more definitive but slower-acting measures are being implemented. Potassium can be removed by either of two methods.

1. Administration of a cation exchange resin such as sodium polystyrene sulfonate (Resonium A), 1 g/kg, administered orally or rectally, to bind potassium and remove it from the body. This requires time to be effective, and a sodium ion is exchanged for each potassium ion. This increased sodium concentration adds to the body fluids, which may contribute to fluid overload, hypertension and cardiac failure.
2. Dialysis or continuous haemofiltration (see p. 581). Haemodialysis is efficient but requires specialised facilities. Peritoneal dialysis is simpler and can be carried out in almost any hospital setting. Indications for dialysis in AKI are continued oliguria associated with any of the following:
   - severe, persistent acidosis
   - inability to reduce serum potassium levels to a safe range with other methods
   - clinical uraemic syndrome consisting of nausea and vomiting, drowsiness and progression to coma
   - circulatory overload, hypertension and evidence of cardiac failure.

The optimal timing for initiation of renal replacement therapy is controversial. One strategy is to institute renal replacement therapy within hours of the diagnosis of severe AKI being made, regardless of other symptoms. Another strategy is to delay renal replacement therapy until any of the previously listed symptoms presents. Differences in mortality have not been demonstrated between the two approaches (Gaudry et al 2016).

Hypertension. Hypertension is a common and serious complication of AKI, and blood pressure determinations are taken at least every 4 to 6 hours to detect it early. The most common cause of hypertension in AKI is overexpansion of the extracellular fluid and plasma volume, together with activation of the renin-angiotensin system. The goal of therapy is to prevent hypertensive encephalopathy and avoid overtaxing the cardiovascular system.

When there is a threat of encephalopathy, labetalol (a beta and alpha blocker) may be administered intravenously as bolus infusions or a continuous drip. Sodium nitroprusside may be given but requires close monitoring. For less urgent situations, hydralazine, clonidine or verapamil may be given intravenously. Oral drugs used for acute hypertension include nifedipine, captopril, minoxidil, hydralazine, propranolol or frusemide.

Other Complications. Other complications that may occur with AKI are anaemia, seizures and coma, cardiac failure and pulmonary oedema. Anaemia is commonly associated with AKI, but transfusion is not recommended unless the haemoglobin level drops below 6 g/dL. Transfusions consist of fresh, packed red blood cells given slowly to reduce the likelihood of increasing blood volume, hypertension and hyperkalaemia.

Seizures occur often when renal failure progresses to uraemia and are also related to hypertension, hyponatraemia and hypocalcaemia. Treatment is directed towards the specific cause when known. More obscure causes are managed with antiepileptic drugs.

Cardiac failure with pulmonary oedema is almost always associated with hypervolaemia. Treatment is directed towards reduction of fluid volume, with water and sodium restriction and administration of diuretics. Digitalis is ineffective and can be hazardous.

Diuretic, or High-output, Phase. When the output begins to increase, either spontaneously or in response to diuretic therapy, the nurse should monitor the intake of fluid, potassium and sodium, and provide adequate replacement to prevent depletion and its consequences. In some cases the high-output phase is mild and lasts only a few days; in others enormous amounts of electrolyte-rich urine are passed.

Prognosis. The prognosis of AKI depends largely on the nature and severity of the causative factor or precipitating event and the promptness and competence of management. The mortality rate is less than 20%. The outcome is least favourable in children with rapidly progressive nephritis and cortical necrosis. Children in whom AKI is a result of HUS or AGN may recover completely, but residual renal impairment or hypertension is more often the rule. Complete recovery is usually expected in children whose renal failure is a result of dehydration, nephrotoxins or ischaemia. AKI after cardiac surgery has a less favourable prognosis. It is often impossible to assess the extent of recovery for several months. (See Quality Patient Outcomes box.)

QUALITY PATIENT OUTCOMES

Acute Kidney Injury

- Underlying cause of AKI identified and treated
- Water balance maintained
- Hypertension controlled
- Electrolyte balance maintained
- Diet maintains calories while minimising tissue catabolism, metabolic acidosis, hyperkalaemia and uraemia

Nursing Care Management

Nursing care of the infant or child with AKI involves addressing the underlying cause plus carefully observing and managing the renal status. The major goals are: reestablishment of renal function (with emphasis on providing an adequate caloric intake to minimise reduction of protein stores); prevention of complications; and monitoring of fluid balance, laboratory data and physical manifestations. The probability of dialysis or continuous haemofiltration is high, and the nurse must anticipate the availability of the necessary equipment. Because the child requires intensive observation and often specialised equipment, the usual disposition is admission to an intensive care unit where equipment and trained personnel are available.

The major nursing tasks in the care of the infant or child with AKI are monitoring and assessing fluid and electrolyte balance. Limiting fluid intake requires ingenuity on the part of caregivers to cope with the child who is thirsty. One strategy involves rationing the daily intake with small amounts of fluid served in containers that give the impression of larger volumes. Older children who understand the rationale of fluid limits can help determine how their daily ration should be distributed.

Meeting nutritional needs is sometimes a problem because the child may be nauseated and because getting the child to eat concentrated foods without fluids may be difficult. When nourishment is provided by the IV route, careful monitoring is essential to prevent fluid overload. This can become a major challenge in the face of nutritional requirements and administration of IV medications. The IV drugs being used may be nephrotoxic, which can require a specified volume of solution for delivery. In some instances blood products must also be delivered. Preventing fluid overload while delivering medications and calories requires concerted collaboration. In addition, nursing measures such as maintaining an optimum thermal environment, reducing any elevation of body temperature and reducing restlessness and anxiety are used to decrease the rate of tissue catabolism.

The nurse must be continually alert for behaviour changes that indicate the onset of complications. Infection from reduced resistance, anaemia and general morbidity is a constant threat. Fluid overload and electrolyte disturbances can precipitate cardiovascular complications such as hypertension and cardiac failure. Fluid and electrolyte imbalances, acidosis and accumulation of nitrogenous waste products can produce neurological involvement manifested by coma, seizures or alterations in sensorium.

Although children with AKI are usually quite ill and voluntarily diminish their activity, infants may become restless and irritable, and children are often anxious and frightened. Frequent, painful and stress-producing treatments and tests must be performed. A supportive, empathetic nurse can provide comfort and stability in a threatening and unnatural environment.

Family Support. Providing support and reassurance to parents is among the major nursing responsibilities. The seriousness and emergency nature of AKI are stressful to parents, and most feel some degree of guilt regarding the child's condition, especially when the illness is the result of ingestion of a toxic substance, dehydration or a genetic disease. They need reassurance and an empathetic listener. They also need to be kept informed of the child's progress and provided explanations regarding the therapeutic regimen. The equipment and the child's behaviour are sometimes frightening and anxiety provoking. Nurses can do much to help parents comprehend and deal with the stresses of the situation.

Chronic Kidney Disease

The kidneys are able to maintain the chemical composition of fluids within normal limits until more than 50% of functional renal capacity is destroyed by disease or injury. Chronic kidney disease (CKD) occurs when the diseased kidneys can no longer maintain the normal chemical structure of body fluids under normal conditions. Progressive deterioration over months or years produces a variety of clinical and biochemical disturbances that conclude in the clinical syndrome known as uraemia. The final stage of CKD, ESRD, is irreversible. Treatment with dialysis or transplantation is required when the GFR decreases below 10% to 15% of normal. The pattern of renal dysfunction is remarkably uniform no matter what disease process initiates the advanced disease.

Aetiology

A variety of diseases and disorders can result in CKD. The most common causes of CKD before age 5 years are congenital renal and urinary tract malformations (particularly renal hypoplasia and dysplasia and obstructive uropathy) and VUR. Glomerular and hereditary renal diseases predominate in children 5 to 15 years of age. The glomerular diseases that most commonly lead to CKD are chronic pyelonephritis, CGN and glomerulonephropathy associated with systemic diseases such as anaphylactoid purpura and lupus erythematosus. Hereditary nephritis, congenital nephrotic syndrome, Alport's syndrome, polycystic kidney and several other hereditary disorders result in renal failure in childhood. Renal vascular disorders such as HUS, vascular thrombosis or cortical necrosis are less common causes (Francis et al 2019).

Pathophysiology

Early in the course of progressive nephron destruction, the child remains asymptomatic with only minimum biochemical abnormalities. Unless its presence is detected in the process of routine assessment, signs and symptoms that indicate advanced renal damage often emerge only late in the course of the disease. Midway in the disease process, as increasing numbers of nephrons are totally destroyed, and most others are damaged to varying degrees; the few that remain intact are hypertrophied but functional. These few normal nephrons are able to make sufficient adjustments to stresses to maintain reasonable degrees of fluid and electrolyte balance. Definitive biochemical examination at this time reveals restricted tolerance to excesses or restrictions. As the disease progresses to the end stage because of severe reduction in the number of functioning nephrons, the kidneys are no longer able to maintain fluid and electrolyte balance, and the features of uraemia appear.

The following sections briefly summarise the pathophysiology of specific biochemical abnormalities.

Retention of Waste Products. Serum creatinine and BUN levels are utilised to evaluate renal function. Creatinine is a waste product of muscle catabolism. Because muscle mass is relatively stable, creatinine production is also stable. Most creatinine is filtered out by the kidneys and expelled in the urine. BUN (a byproduct of protein breakdown) levels also increase as kidney function declines. BUN is a less precise marker than creatinine as it is not produced at a stable rate and can be influenced by protein intake, hydration status and other factors (Lopez-Giacoman & Madero 2015).

Water and Sodium Retention. The damaged kidneys are able to maintain sodium and water balance under normal circumstances, although the few remaining functional nephrons are required to increase their rate of filtration and reabsorption in proportion to their numbers. The limitations of this capacity become apparent under stress. The nature of abnormalities in adjustment depends on the underlying renal disease. Infants and small children with kidney dysplasia or urinary obstructive disease tend to excrete large volumes of dilute urine low in sodium content. Children with glomerular disease tend to retain both sodium and water as a result of a greater reduction of glomerular filtration than of tubular reabsorption. Children with defective sodium reabsorption from tubular disease tend to lose sodium, with a corresponding osmotic water loss. Consequently, sodium excesses may cause oedema and hypertension, whereas sodium deprivation can result in hypovolaemia and circulatory failure. Only in ESRD is markedly reduced glomerular filtration inadequate to handle normal amounts of sodium and water. Retention of these substances leads to oedema and vascular congestion.

Hyperkalaemia. Dangerous hyperkalaemia is uncommon in CKD until the end stage. However, the kidneys are unable to adjust readily to increased ingestion of potassium, and they require a longer period to rid the body of this excess.

Acidosis. A sustained metabolic acidosis is characteristic of CKD; it results from the damaged kidney's inability to excrete a normal load of metabolic acids generated by normal metabolic processes. There is reduced capacity of the distal tubules to produce ammonia and impaired reabsorption of bicarbonate. Despite continuous hydrogen ion retention and bicarbonate loss, the plasma pH is maintained at a level compatible with life by other buffering mechanisms, particularly the bone salt (see the following sections).

Calcium and Phosphorus Disturbances. Calcium and phosphorus homeostasis are affected by CKD. Profound and complex disturbances in the metabolism of these substances result in significant bone demineralisation and impaired growth. This appears to be related to several factors (Box 24.6). These complex disturbances in calcium, phosphorus and bone metabolism produce: growth arrest or delay; bone pain; and deformities known as renal osteodystrophy, sometimes called renal rickets, because the disorganisation of bone growth and demineralisation are similar to that caused by vitamin D–resistant rickets.

Anaemia. A consistent feature of CKD is anaemia, which appears to result from several factors (Box 24.7).

Growth Disturbance. One of the most striking effects of CKD in childhood, and one that can have profound psychological and social consequences for the developing child, is delayed growth. The cause is poorly understood but may be related to nutritional and biochemical factors (Box 24.8).

Sexual maturation may be delayed or may not occur in children with CKD, and secondary amenorrhoea commonly develops in girls

BOX 24.6 Factors Related to Bone Demineralisation in Chronic Renal Failure

- In a state of acidosis there is dissolution of the alkaline salts of bone, which serve as buffers, and the release of phosphorus and calcium into the bloodstream.
- Reduced glomerular filtration and excretion of inorganic phosphate lead to an elevation of plasma phosphate with a concomitant decrease in serum calcium.
- Decreased serum calcium concentration stimulates the secretion of parathyroid hormone, which results in reabsorption of calcium from bones. Under normal circumstances parathyroid hormone inhibits the tubular reabsorption of phosphates.
- Diseased kidneys are unable to complete the synthesis of vitamin D to its most active form, 1,25-dihydroxycholecalciferol, which is necessary for the absorption of calcium from the gastrointestinal tract and deposition of calcium in bone. This acquired resistance to vitamin D decreases calcium absorption, permits retention of phosphorus and contributes to secondary hyperparathyroidism.

BOX 24.7 Causes of Anaemia in Chronic Renal Failure

- Shortened life span of red blood cells caused by some extracorpuscular factor associated with the uraemic state
- Impaired red blood cell production resulting from decreased production of erythropoietin
- Blood loss related to increased tendency to bleed, associated with a prolonged bleeding time, probably related to impaired platelet function and laboratory blood samples
- Hyperparathyroidism
- Hypersplenism, which may be related to silicone deposition (from dialysis blood lines) and granuloma formation in the spleen
- Diseases related to haemolytic anaemia, such as systemic lupus erythematosus and sickle cell disease

BOX 24.8 Probable Causes of Growth Failure in Chronic Renal Failure

- Renal osteodystrophy
- Poor nutrition associated with dietary restrictions (especially protein) and loss of appetite
- Biochemical abnormalities associated with renal failure, such as sustained acidosis or renal sodium wasting
- Hypertension
- Corticosteroid treatment
- Tissue resistance to growth hormone
- Trace mineral and vitamin deficiencies

past puberty. CKD can also cause sexual dysfunction by creating imbalances in gonadal hormone levels. Decreased testosterone levels impair spermatogenesis in males; decreased oestrogen, luteinising hormone and progesterone cause anovulation and menstrual irregularities (usually amenorrhoea) in females. Autonomic neuropathy and anaemia are also factors that can alter sexual function.

Other Disturbances. Children with CKD are more susceptible to infection, especially pneumonia, UTI and septicaemia, although the reason for this is not entirely clear. Hyperventilation, a manifestation of the respiratory compensatory mechanism for metabolic acidosis, and pulmonary oedema may contribute to upper respiratory tract infection. These children become extraordinarily sensitive to changes in vascular volume that may cause, in addition to pulmonary overload, cerebral symptoms and circulatory manifestations such as hypertension and cardiac failure.

Numerous neurological manifestations appear with advanced renal failure, although no specific toxin or biochemical defect has been identified. However, disturbances in enzyme function, disturbances in water and electrolyte balance, altered calcium ion concentration, hypertension and accumulation of various 'uraemic toxins' have been implicated.

Clinical Manifestations

The first symptom of CKD may be loss of normal energy and increased fatigue on exertion. For example, the child may prefer quiet, passive activities rather than participation in more active games and outdoor play. The child is usually somewhat pale, but the change is often so subtle that it may not be evident to parents or others. Blood pressure is sometimes elevated. Growth is affected early in the development of CKD, and falling behind on the growth chart is often the first measurable sign.

Other manifestations may appear as the disease progresses. The child does not eat as well (especially breakfast), shows less interest in normal activities such as schoolwork or play, and has a decreased or increased urinary output and a compensatory intake of fluid. For example, a child who has achieved bladder control may wet the bed at night. Pallor becomes more evident as the skin develops a characteristic sallow, muddy appearance as a result of anaemia and deposition of urochrome pigment in the skin. The child may complain of headache, muscle cramps and nausea. Other signs and symptoms include weight loss, facial puffiness, malaise, bone or joint pain, growth abnormalities, dryness or itching of the skin, bruised skin and sometimes sensory or motor loss. Amenorrhoea is common in adolescent girls.

Therapy is generally initiated before the appearance of the uraemic symptoms, although on some occasions the symptoms may be observed. Manifestations of untreated uraemia reflect the progressive nature of the homeostatic disturbances and general toxicity. Gastrointestinal symptoms include loss of appetite, nausea and vomiting. Bleeding tendencies are apparent in bruises, bloody diarrhoeal stools, stomatitis and bleeding from the lips and mouth. Intractable itching occurs, probably related to a number of factors, including dry skin and hyperparathyroidism (Wojtowicz-Prus et al 2016, Becherucci et al 2016). Deposits of urea crystals may appear on the skin as uraemic frost but are seldom seen because of the availability of dialysis and transplantation. There may be an unpleasant uraemic odour to the breath. Respirations become deeper as a result of metabolic acidosis, and circulatory overload is manifested by hypertension, congestive heart failure and pulmonary oedema. Progressive confusion, dulling of the sensorium and ultimately coma are signs of neurological involvement. Other signs may include tremors, muscular twitching and seizures.

Diagnostic Evaluation

The diagnosis of CKD is usually suspected on the basis of any of a number of clinical manifestations, a history of prior renal disease or biochemical findings. The onset is usually gradual, and the initial signs and symptoms are vague and non-specific. Laboratory and other diagnostic tools and tests are of value in assessing the extent of renal damage, biochemical disturbances and related physical dysfunction. Often, they can help establish the nature of the underlying disease and differentiate between other disease processes and the pathological consequences of renal dysfunction.

Therapeutic Management

Classification of CKD as stage 1 (GFR $\geq$ 90) through stage 5 (GFR $<$ 15 or dialysis) helps with evaluation and management decisions (The Sydney Children's Hospital Network n.d.). The goals of management are to maximise effective renal function, maintain body fluid and electrolyte balance within acceptable limits, treat systemic complications and promote as active and normal a life as possible for the child for as long as possible. This becomes increasingly difficult as the disease progresses towards end stage. Therapeutic measures designed to relieve one manifestation may negatively affect another. For example, antihypertensive agents may further impair renal function.

Activity. Allow children unrestricted activity and to set their own limits regarding rest and extent of exertion. Encourage them to attend school. If the effort is too great, home tutoring can be arranged.

Diet. Regulation of diet has been seen as the most effective means, short of dialysis, for reducing the quantity of materials that require renal excretion. The goal of the diet in renal failure is to provide sufficient calories and protein for growth while minimising the excretory demands made on the kidney, to limit metabolic bone disease (osteodystrophy) and to minimise fluid and electrolyte disturbances. Dietary protein intake is limited to the recommended dietary allowance (RDA) for the child's age. Restriction of protein intake below the RDA is believed to negatively affect growth and neurodevelopment. Dietary phosphorus may need to be restricted. Remember that any attempt to restrict dietary intake in children potentially restricts caloric intake and can limit growth.

Potassium is not restricted as long as creatinine clearance remains at acceptable limits (30 to 35 mL/min). However, restrictions are instituted for patients with oliguria or anuria. Restrictions of any or all of these minerals may be imposed in later stages or at any time in which factors cause abnormal serum concentrations.

Osteodystrophy. Measures directed at prevention or correction of the calcium/phosphorus imbalance are reduction of dietary phosphorus, administration of a phosphorus-binding agent, provision of supplemental calcium, control of acidosis and administration of an active and/or inactive form of vitamin D.

The reduction of protein and milk intake can control dietary phosphorus. Oral administration of phosphorus-binding agents, which combine with the phosphorus to decrease gastrointestinal absorption and thus the serum levels of phosphate, can further reduce phosphorus levels.

Acidosis. Pharmacological treatment of acidosis is initiated early in children who have chronic renal insufficiency. In addition to reducing the formation of metabolic acids by avoiding excessive dietary protein intake, alkalising agents such as sodium bicarbonate or a combination of sodium and potassium citrate alleviate acidosis.

Anaemia. Because the anaemia associated with renal failure is related to decreased production of erythropoietin, it usually cannot be successfully managed with haematinic agents. Provide sufficient sources of folic acid and iron in the diet, although this is difficult when protein sources are restricted. Inadequate intake and iron losses that may occur are managed by supplemental iron, usually ferrous sulfate. Providing adequate sources of ascorbic acid at the same time that iron-rich foods or supplements are given enhances the absorption.

Hypertension. Hypertension of advanced renal disease may be managed initially by cautious use of a low-sodium diet, fluid restriction and perhaps diuretics such as thiazides or frusemide. Strict restriction of sodium intake may be necessary in patients with oliguria.

Nursing Care Management

The child with CKD has a life maintained by drugs and artificial means, and the multiple stresses placed on these children and their families are often overwhelming. Progressive deterioration of renal function occurs at varying rates. As the affected child progresses from renal insufficiency to uraemia and then to dialysis or transplantation, the need for supportive nursing care is intensified. Team effort is more important than ever and involves coordination of personnel from medicine, nursing, social services, child life, physical and occupational therapy, dietetics and psychological or psychiatric specialties.

RENAL REPLACEMENT THERAPY

Technological advances in the care of children with AKI and CKD provide several renal replacement therapies for maintaining excretory function in acute disease and for prolonging life in those with CKD stage 5. The primary modalities are haemodialysis, peritoneal dialysis, haemofiltration and transplantation.

Dialysis is the process of separating colloids and crystalline substances in solution by the difference in their rate of diffusion through a semipermeable membrane. Three processes accomplish this movement across the membrane: osmosis, diffusion and ultrafiltration

BOX 24.9 Processes of Fluid and Electrolyte Movement

Osmosis—Passive movement of water from a solution of lower concentration to a solution of higher concentration of particles

Diffusion—Random movement of particles from an area of greater concentration to an area of lower concentration

Ultrafiltration—Process by which plasma water is removed because of a pressure gradient between the blood and dialysate compartments

(Box 24.9). Methods of dialysis currently available for clinical management of renal failure are as follows:

- haemodialysis, in which blood is circulated outside the body through artificial cellophane membranes that permit a similar passage of water and solutes
- peritoneal dialysis, wherein the abdominal cavity acts as a semipermeable membrane through which water and solutes of small molecular size move by osmosis and diffusion according to their respective concentrations on either side of the membrane
- haemofiltration, in which blood filtrate is circulated outside the body by hydrostatic pressure exerted across a semipermeable membrane and replaced (simultaneously) by electrolyte solution.

The choice of whether to use haemodialysis, peritoneal dialysis or haemofiltration depends on the nature of the renal failure (acute versus chronic) and the cause of the renal failure. Haemodialysis is more efficient than peritoneal dialysis but is technically more difficult in infants and very young children. In these children haemofiltration may be a viable substitute for dialysis. As a rule, dialysis is reserved for children who are in end-stage renal failure because it requires creation of an access and special equipment. It may be used acutely for conditions such as severe metabolic acidosis, accidental poisoning, chronic heart failure with fluid overload, hyperkalaemia, severe hypernatraemia, severe hyperphosphataemia and tumour lysis syndrome.

The absolute indications for dialysis are: life-threatening electrolyte abnormalities; severe volume overload; and bilateral neoplastic disease or bilateral nephrectomies performed for various reasons, including intractable hypertension. Although each child is assessed on an individual basis, indications for instituting dialysis in CKD are biochemical abnormalities, including elevated BUN, acidosis, severe hyperphosphataemia and elevated potassium. Other indications include deteriorating central nervous system function or congestive heart failure that is unresponsive to other therapy. Growth failure, severe osteodystrophy, insufficient caloric intake and an inability to carry out normal activities are sometimes criteria for dialysis.

Haemodialysis

Haemodialysis is the preferred dialytic method for children with acute conditions such as life-threatening hyperkalaemia or poisoning with dialysable compounds. Protein loss is less extensive than with peritoneal dialysis. However, haemodialysis is technically difficult in small children less than 20 kg because their delicately balanced cardiovascular dynamics may be upset by the rapid changes in blood volume and systemic blood pressure that may occur with this method. In addition, it may be difficult to place vascular access for haemodialysis in small children.

Haemodialysis is the preferred form of dialysis for certain family situations in which any one person is unable to take the time and responsibility to perform the procedures at home. It is best suited to children who live close to the dialysis centre because they must come to the centre as often as three or more times a week for treatments. Children who are not good candidates for peritoneal dialysis because of family non-compliance, recurrent peritoneal infections or unstable living conditions are treated with haemodialysis.

Procedure

Haemodialysis requires special dialysis equipment: the haemodialyser, or so-called artificial kidney haemodialysers. Paediatric dialysis can be safely carried out when the total dialysis circuit volume does not exceed 10% of the child's estimated blood volume.

Haemodialysis also requires one of three means of blood access: grafts, fistulas or external access devices. An arteriovenous fistula is an access in which a vein and artery are connected surgically. The preferred site is the radial artery and a forearm vein. The creation of a subcutaneous (internal) arteriovenous fistula by anastomosing a segment of the radial artery and brachiocephalic vein produces dilation and thickening of the superficial vessels of the forearm to provide easy access for repeated venepuncture. Fewer complications and less restriction of activity are observed with the use of a fistula. If vessels are inadequate for an autogenous fistula, a synthetic graft may be placed in the arm or thigh with either a loop or straight configuration. Both the graft and the fistula require needle insertion at each dialysis session. For short-term external vascular access, percutaneous catheters are inserted in the femoral or internal jugular veins, even in very small children.

The length of a haemodialysis treatment, the blood flow rate and dialyser characteristics contribute to adequacy of treatment. The current target level for adequacy is a Kt/V (clearance × time/volume) of 1.4 or higher. Dietary limitations are necessary in chronic dialysis to avoid biochemical complications. Fluid and sodium are restricted to prevent fluid overload and its associated symptoms of hypertension, cerebral manifestations and congestive heart failure. Potassium is restricted to prevent complications related to hyperkalaemia; phosphorus restriction helps prevent parathyroid hyperactivity and its attendant risk of abnormal calcification in soft tissues. Adequate protein intake is necessary to maximise growth potential. Fluid limitations are determined by residual urinary output and the need to limit intradialytic weight gain.

Seizures during or after haemodialysis are now uncommon. With the current practice of haemodialysis, cerebral oedema caused by alterations in osmolality in the brain when the BUN level is lowered rapidly (associated with dialysis disequilibrium syndrome) is rare.

Home Haemodialysis

With appropriate cannulisation and proper training and education of both the child and the parents, haemodialysis can be performed at home. Benefits include less absence from school, more flexibility with dialysis timing and improved quality of life (Hothi et al 2016, Sinha et al 2018). Home haemodialysis is especially advantageous for children that live a great distance from the dialysis centre. Parents of children on home haemodialysis must know how to operate the equipment, connect the unit to the vascular access and assess the child's status.

Nursing Care Management

Initiating a haemodialysis regimen is a traumatic and anxiety-provoking experience for most children. After surgery for implantation of the graft, fistula or long-term external access device, the initial experience with the haemodialysis machine and its implication can be frightening. After weeks, months or years of haemodialysis, the parents and the child feel anxiety associated with the prognosis and continued pressures of the treatment. The relentless need for treatment interferes with family plans and activities, including school. Graft and fistula problems are a common source of aggravation. Most families and children on haemodialysis look to kidney transplantation as a desirable alternative to long-term treatment.

Peritoneal Dialysis

For acute conditions, peritoneal dialysis is quick, relatively easy to learn, safe to perform and requires minimum equipment with specially trained nurses. Peritoneal dialysis is a slow, gentle process that decreases the stress on body organs that can occur with the rapid chemical and volume changes of haemodialysis. The procedure is indicated for neonates, children with severe cardiovascular disease or those who are poor risks for vascular access.

Procedure

In acute situations peritoneal dialysis catheter insertion may be accomplished at the bedside; catheters for long-term use are placed surgically in the operating room with the patient under anaesthesia. A catheter is inserted through the anterior abdominal wall, and the catheter cuff is sutured into place. Chronic peritoneal dialysis catheters are tunnelled through a subcutaneous tract before exiting the skin in a manner similar to implantation of central venous access devices.

In peritoneal dialysis each pass or cycle is characterised by inflow time, dwell time and drain time. The length of each portion of the cycle is part of the dialysis prescription. The dwell time and type of solution used varies according to the goals of the treatment (i.e. removal of water, solute, electrolyte or all of these). The procedure is usually continued until renal function is restored, waste products are reduced or (in prolonged need) the patient is switched to a form of chronic peritoneal dialysis, such as continuous ambulatory peritoneal dialysis (CAPD) or continuous cycling peritoneal dialysis (CCPD). An acute peritoneal dialysis catheter may remain in place for several weeks, provided that all who enter the system adhere to aseptic technique.

Home Dialysis

The development of satisfactory methods for CAPD and its alternative, CCPD, has provided additional means for managing ESRD at home. CCPD is a modification of CAPD and intermittent peritoneal dialysis. The dialysis exchange is usually performed at night using a peritoneal dialysis machine that warms the dialysis fluid and automates the cycles of inflow of dialysis fluid and outflow of dialysate. As with CAPD, the CCPD system is opened during the day but is opened only twice as opposed to multiple times. Night-time dialysis allows the child more freedom during the day and relieves parents of the need to perform multiple exchanges.

Complications. CAPD and CCPD are currently considered the methods of choice for most children who require dialysis because they are easier to initiate and maintain than haemodialysis. Peritonitis is the major complication of home peritoneal dialysis. The patients are treated intraperitoneally with antibiotics, and some may require catheter replacement. Although the risk of infection is continuously present, most practitioners believe it is not great enough to discourage the use of these methods.

However, other complications have been noted in patients on home peritoneal dialysis. Tunnel infections are evidenced by swelling, warmth and tenderness along the subcutaneous catheter tract; such infections are managed with administration of antibiotics or catheter replacement. Peritoneal leaks and ventral hernias caused by the sustained intraabdominal pressure that develops within the peritoneum have also been found in a significant number of children. Few of these patients respond to a reduction in dialysis solution volume, and many require surgical intervention.

Nursing Care Management

The availability of home dialysis has offered a greater degree of freedom for persons undergoing long-term dialysis. It eliminates the need for a residence convenient to a dialysis unit and for frequent trips to the unit, except for monthly evaluations.

The family must learn how to take vital signs before and after the dialysis and how to interpret the significance of blood pressure and temperature variations. They need to know how to vary the composition of the dialysis solution to compensate for variations in the vital signs and to maintain an accurate record of all aspects of the treatment.

Continuous Venovenous Haemofiltration

A third type of 'dialysis' or renal replacement therapy used primarily in acute care settings is continuous venovenous haemofiltration (CVVH). This type of therapy uses specialised equipment (e.g. haemofilter, blood pump, tubing connected to a vascular access) to ultrafiltrate blood continuously at a very slow rate. With this procedure, fluid balance may be achieved within 24 to 48 hours after initiation. Continuous venovenous haemodialysis (CVVHD) is used to remove excess fluid from patients with severe oliguric fluid overload.

CVVHD is an ideal form of renal replacement therapy for children with fluid overload from surgical procedures (e.g. cardiovascular surgery) who do not have severe biochemical abnormalities. It is commonly used for critically ill children who require volume-expanding fluids such as hyperalimentation solution, albumin or packed red cells It creates space for the infusion of these replacement solutions in fluid-sensitive patients. CVVHD has proved to be a highly successful alternative form of dialysis for critically ill children who might not survive the rapid volume changes that occur with haemodialysis and peritoneal dialysis (Sinha et al 2018).

Transplantation

Kidney transplantation is the preferred means of renal replacement therapy in the paediatric age group. Although peritoneal dialysis and haemodialysis are life preserving and are able to be carried out in the home in a large number of cases, neither method is compatible with a normal lifestyle. Transplantation, on the other hand, offers the opportunity for a relatively normal life.

Kidneys for transplant are available from two sources: a living donor, usually a parent, grandparent or sibling; or a deceased donor, wherein the family of a dead or brain-dead patient consents to donation of a healthy kidney.

Children who have ESRD secondary to malignancy must be cancer free for a specified time before transplantation (depending on the type of malignancy). Generalised infection must be eradicated before attempted transplantation, and the recipient should have adequate bladder capacity. Some children may have bladder augmentation or other genitourinary surgery as preparation for transplantation. Children with abnormal urinary tracts may be subject to more post-transplant urological complications and infection than they would be otherwise (Becherucci et al 2016).

Procedure

The kidney graft is placed in the extraperitoneal space, usually the anterior iliac fossa; the renal artery is anastomosed to the internal iliac or hypogastric artery; the renal vein is anastomosed to the hypogastric vein; and the ureter is implanted into the bladder or anastomosed to the recipient's ureter. Small children receiving a large donor kidney may require placement within the abdomen with vessel anastomoses to the aorta and inferior vena cava. Unless there is medical contraindication, the recipient's failed kidneys are left in place. Severe hypertension, neoplasm, large and continuous protein losses and persistent severe VUR are the usual reasons for nephrectomy.

The primary goal in transplantation is the long-term survival of the grafted tissue. The means by which this is attempted include securing tissues that are antigenically similar to that of the recipient and suppressing the recipient's immune mechanism.

Selection of Donor Tissue

The source of a donor kidney is either a live person or a deceased donor. The closer the genetic relationship between the donor and the recipient, the better the possibility of long-term survival. The only truly compatible tissue match is that between identical twin siblings. The next best possible match is a sibling, followed by a parent or grandparent. In some states the use of siblings is impossible until the possible donor is of age to give consent for removal of a kidney. Unrelated donors are least likely to be compatible. Careful immunological studies are carried out to determine the donor whose kidney is least likely to be rejected by the recipient.

Suppression of the Immune Response

After the best possible tissue match is obtained for a transplant, suppressing the recipient's immune response can significantly lengthen the survival time. The immunosuppressant therapy of choice varies by institution. A combination of prednisone, tacrolimus and mycophenolate is commonly used. Other therapies include antilymphocyte globulin or monoclonal antibodies, administered intravenously either for induction or rescue from rejection.

The administration of these drugs is not without hazard. The major problem encountered with non-specific immunosuppression is that it not only suppresses the immune response to the grafted tissue but also suppresses the body's capacity to respond to other antigenic stimuli. Consequently, the child is vulnerable to overwhelming infections.

Prednisone is an immunosuppressant and anti-inflammatory agent that acts to stabilise cell walls, reduce migration of white blood cells into the inflamed area and inhibit deposition of fibrin and collagen. It also depresses T cells, B cells and phagocytes. A number of complications from corticosteroid therapy are cause for concern. Interference with linear growth has led many centres to use alternate-day administration in an effort to improve growth rates and to decrease other long-term side effects such as cataracts, fluid and sodium retention, hypertension, gastric ulcer and obesity. Researchers are studying steroid-free and early steroid withdrawal treatment protocols with the goal of minimising side effects without compromising graft survival (Haller et al 2016, Francis et al 2019).

Rejection

Rejection of a transplanted kidney is the most common cause of transplant failure. Rejection can be one of three types: hyperacute, acute or chronic. Hyperacute rejection is irreversible, develops immediately or within a few hours after revascularisation and is related to circulating antibodies preformed in the recipient against the donor tissue antigens.

Acute rejection usually occurs between the first few days and months after transplantation but may occur years later, especially if the patient becomes poorly compliant with immunosuppressant medications. Both biochemical and clinical abnormalities are evidence of rejection. The most common finding is an elevated serum creatinine and BUN. Fever, which is usually accompanied by swelling and tenderness over the graft, hypertension and diminished urinary output may occur.

NURSING CARE CONSIDERATIONS

The child with a kidney transplant who exhibits any of the following should be evaluated immediately for possible rejection:

- fever
- swelling and tenderness over graft area
- diminished urinary output
- elevated blood pressure
- elevated serum creatinine.

Slow, gradual deterioration of renal function that typically begins 6 months or more after transplantation characterises chronic rejection. Elevations of serum creatinine, proteinuria or haematuria are signs of rejection. In addition, the rejection may have symptomatology indistinguishable from that of the original kidney disease. No present therapy can halt the process, which inevitably leads to loss of the implanted kidney.

Prognosis

Predictors of graft survival for children include age at transplantation, pretransplantation dialysis, early rejection and race. Infections, cancer/malignancy and cardiovascular causes are the most life-threatening problems after transplantation (Holmberg & Jalanko 2016, Francis et al 2019). Long-term graft survival is not guaranteed, and many children require a second or third transplant. Successful kidney transplantation does improve rehabilitation of children with kidney failure, both educationally and psychologically.

Nursing Care Management

The possibility of kidney transplantation often comes as a hope for relief from the rigours of dialysis or the restriction of a conservative management regimen. Most children and families respond well to a kidney transplant. Children with successful kidney transplants are usually able to resume life activities similar to those of their unaffected peers. The rehabilitation of children with kidney transplants is influenced primarily by their pattern of functioning before becoming ill. It is important to remember that transplantation is a treatment that has a far less negative impact on the child's normal life activities than dialysis, although multiple medications and clinic visits remain a part of their life. Stresses remain for the child and family in relation to the uncertainty of the future, the child's health and wellbeing, social isolation and financial burdens.

A variety of serious emotional and psychological conflicts may arise as a consequence of donor selection, including ambivalence of donors faced with surgery and relinquishing a kidney, feelings of guilt if one should prove to be unacceptable as a donor and the emotional impact of having a live relative–donated kidney rejected by the recipient. This especially can result in guilt feelings when a parent is the donor.

The child recipient responds in various ways to a kidney transplant. The concept of having a foreign body, especially a deceased donor kidney, inside their own body is sometimes disturbing to children. They often speculate about the age, sex, personality and physical characteristics of the donor. They may fear that the kidney will wear out if it came from an older person. Some children are distressed to find that their donor kidney came from a person of the opposite sex. Corticosteroid therapy, necessary in kidney transplants, creates undesirable side effects (e.g. growth failure, obesity, characteristics of Cushing's syndrome, acne and hirsutism) that are often a source of emotional and social problems for older children. Gum hyperplasia, brittle fingernails and hair breakage can also occur.

Patient Education

Providing patient education is a critical role for nursing staff. The nurse must be aware of the potential side effects of every medication the child is taking and provide appropriate surveillance and education. Children who are concerned about changes in their body due to the immunosuppressant medications may stop taking them. Surveillance for the development of a number of conditions, including the BK polyomavirus, lymphoproliferative disease, diabetes mellitus, hypertension, dyslipidaemias and skin changes, is required (Holmberg & Jalanko 2016). Education for minimising the risk of developing these and other conditions is necessary.

NURSING CARE CONSIDERATIONS

Medication Non-compliance After Kidney Transplant

The most common reason for poor medication adherence in childhood kidney transplant recipients is dislike of undesirable side effects. The cosmetic implications of the side effects can be overwhelming, especially to adolescent girls. Deliberate discontinuation of the drugs is most common in teenage girls. Poor medication knowledge, number of medications and length of time since transplant can negatively affect medication adherence (Loghman-Adham 2003). (See Compliance, Chapter 22.)

DEFECTS OF THE GENITOURINARY TRACT

Phimosis

Phimosis is a narrowing or stenosis of the preputial opening of the foreskin that prevents retraction of the foreskin over the glans penis. It is a normal finding in infants and young boys and usually disappears as the child grows and the distal prepuce dilates. Occasionally the narrowing obstructs the flow of urine, resulting in a dribbling stream or even ballooning of the foreskin with accumulated urine during voiding.

Balanitis is an inflammation or infection of the phimotic foreskin, which occurs occasionally and is managed as any other inflammation or infection. Phimosis is often treated effectively by application of steroid cream twice a day for 1 month, with the option for surgical treatment with circumcision in severe cases.

Nursing Care Management

Proper hygiene of the phimotic foreskin in infants and young boys consists of external cleansing during routine bathing. The foreskin should not be forcibly retracted because it may create scarring that can prevent future retraction. Furthermore, retraction of the tight foreskin can result in paraphimosis, a condition in which the retracted foreskin cannot be replaced in its normal position over the glans. This causes oedema and venous congestion created by constriction by the tight band of foreskin—a urological emergency that requires immediate evaluation.

Hydrocele

Hydrocele is the presence of peritoneal fluid in the scrotum between the parietal and visceral layers of the tunica vaginalis and is the most common cause of painless scrotal swelling in children and adolescents, along with non-incarcerated inguinal hernia. Hydroceles may be communicating or non-communicating. A communicating hydrocele usually develops when the processus vaginalis does not close during development, allowing for communication with the peritoneum. Non-communicating hydroceles have no connection to the peritoneum with fluid coming from the mesothelial lining of the tunica vaginalis. Hydroceles are common in newborns and often resolve spontaneously, usually by 12 months of age. In older children, non-communicating hydroceles may be idiopathic or a result of trauma, epididymitis, orchitis, testicular torsion, torsion of the appendix testis or appendix epididymis or tumour (RCHM 2020).

Communicating hydroceles may change in size during the day or with straining, whereas non-communicating hydroceles are not reducible and so do not change in size with crying or straining. Surgical repair is indicated for communicating hydroceles persisting past 1 year of age because of the increased risk of development of an incarcerated inguinal hernia. Idiopathic hydroceles are repaired if symptomatic and reactive hydroceles usually resolve with treatment of the underlying cause, such as epididymitis.

Nursing Care Management

Surgical treatment is an outpatient procedure. Advise parents that there is often temporary swelling and discolouration of the scrotum that resolves spontaneously. Straddle toys are avoided for 2 to 4 weeks and strenuous activities in older boys may be avoided for 1 month. If a dressing is used, it is removed in 2 to 3 days and typically the child may bathe in 3 days.

Cryptorchidism

Cryptorchidism is failure of one or both testes to descend normally through the inguinal canal into the scrotum. Absence of testes within the scrotum can be a result of undescended (cryptorchid) testes, retractile testes or absent testes. There is also the potential for ascending testes, where testes were in the scrotum in early childhood and then 'ascended', also known as acquired undescended testes. Undescended testes can be located in the abdomen, the inguinal canal, the upper scrotum or, rarely, in an ectopic location outside of the normal pathway of descent.

Spontaneous descent is probable during the first 6 months of life; if persistent after 6 months, probability of spontaneous descent decreases. After this time, surgical intervention will most likely be required when further assessments are conducted to rule out other possible causes.

Pathophysiology

Testicular development is influenced by a number of genes, but the dominant one is located on the Y chromosome. This gene stimulates the medullary sex cords of the embryonic gonad to differentiate into secretory Sertoli cells. Beginning around week 7, these cells secrete a glycoprotein, müllerian inhibiting substance that leads to development of a male genital system. Testicular descent is a critical element of the development of the male genital system. This descent occurs in two phases; the first is dominated by müllerian inhibiting substance and the second phase by testosterone. Between weeks 8 and 15 a cordlike structure, the gubernaculum, extends from the developing testis (located in the lower abdomen) to the labioscrotal swelling. The fetus grows, but the length of this gubernaculum remains relatively fixed, anchoring the testis to the developing inguinal canal (transabdominal migration) in preparation for the second phase of descent. This second phase begins around weeks 25 to 30 and is characterised by shrinkage of the gubernaculum under the influence of testosterone, causing the testis to migrate down the inguinal canal and into a scrotal position (transinguinal migration). Descent is also characterised by protrusion of peritoneum, the processus vaginalis that closes before birth.

Several processes may slow or arrest testicular descent, including endocrine abnormalities affecting the hypothalamic–pituitary–testicular axis, denervation of the genitofemoral nerve, traction of the gubernaculum, abnormal development of the epididymis or preterm birth. Congenital hernias and abnormal testes often accompany cryptorchid testes, and they are at risk for subsequent torsion.

An ectopic testis emerges outside the inguinal ring into the perineum or femoral area, or lies in a transverse scrotal or prepenile location. The most common site is the superficial inguinal pouch. Ectopia is postulated to occur because of obstruction of the scrotal inlet, scarring (fibrosis) of the gubernaculum or other mechanical anomalies.

Absent testis may be due to agenesis or atrophy from loss of blood supply secondary to prenatal testicular torsion. This has been termed the *vanishing testis syndrome* or *testicular regression syndrome*. **Anorchism** is absence of both testes and may be associated with genotypical and phenotypical abnormalities such as congenital adrenal hyperplasia (CAH). A newborn with a male phallus and bilateral non-palpable testes may be a genetic female with CAH. Failure to diagnose CAH can result in life-threatening electrolyte imbalances. Disorders of sexual development or other abnormalities should also be considered, especially if there are also noted abnormalities of the phallus such as severe hypospadias or micropenis (Kolon et al 2014).

Associated conditions and complications resulting from undescended testes include inguinal hernia, testicular torsion, testicular trauma, subfertility and testicular cancer. Surgical repositioning of the testes may reduce but not prevent the potential long-term issues of infertility and testis cancer (Kolon et al 2014).

Retractile testes can be found at any level within the path of testicular descent, but they are most commonly identified in the groin. Fortunately, they are not truly cryptorchid. Instead, they are introverted to an inguinal or abdominal position because of an overactive cremasteric reflex. The cremasteric reflex, observed as withdrawal of the testis above the scrotum and into the inguinal canal in response to various stimuli, including exposure to cool temperatures, is active during infancy and peaks around age 4 to 5 years. Unlike the cryptorchid testis, the retractile testis can be gently moved into the scrotum without residual tension and does not require treatment. Retractile testes can become ascending testes and require annual monitoring.

Clinical Manifestations

A non-palpable testis is typically observed by the parent or detected during routine physical examination. If one testis is not palpable, the affected hemiscrotum will appear smaller than the other. With bilateral non-palpable testes, both hemiscrota appear small. In the case of retractile testes, the parents may report intermittently observing the testes in the scrotum, interspersed with periods when they cannot be visualised or palpated. Frequently, the retractile testis will be observed in the scrotum when the child is in a warm bath.

Diagnostic Evaluation

It is important to differentiate the true undescended testis from the more common retractile testis. Retractile testes can be 'milked' or pushed back into the scrotum, but truly undescended ones cannot. For examination, the examiner can obviate the cremasteric reflex by placing the child in a cross legged position or by applying firm finger pressure on the external ring before palpating the abdomen or genitalia. (See Fig 4.37.)

Therapeutic Management. Current evidence-based recommendations state that if spontaneous testicular descent does not occur by 6 months of age in congenital undescended testes, that surgical correction should be performed within the next year (Kolon et al 2014). **Orchiopexy** is the procedure for repositioning undescended testes that are palpable and is performed through an inguinal or scrotal incision.

The timing of the surgery is important, as it is in any genital surgery. Orchiopexy is usually performed between 6 and 24 months of age in the case of congenital cryptorchidism. Fewer psychological effects and a higher rate of fertility may be achieved when repair takes place at an early age. Having both testes in the scrotum by school age prevents psychological problems related to body image and peer group embarrassment because the empty scrotum is smaller in size and altered in shape.

Nursing Care Management

Postoperative nursing care is directed towards preventing infection and instructing parents in home care of the child, including pain control. Infection is prevented by carefully cleansing the operative site of stool and urine. Observation of the wound for complications and activity restrictions are discussed. The child should avoid vigorous sports activities and use of toys that are straddled for 2 weeks postoperatively.

Hypospadias

Hypospadias is a congenital anomaly of the male urethra that results in abnormal ventral placement of the urethral opening on the underside of the penis, ranging from the glans to the perineum (Fig 24.6). It is one of the most common congenital anomalies with an incidence reported. Both genetic and environmental factors have been associated with hypospadias. Severity of hypospadias is based on the position of the urethral opening and the degree of **chordee**, or ventral curvature of the penis. The more distant the opening from the normal position at the tip of the glans and the more marked curvature increases the severity and the need for more extensive surgical correction. In mild cases the meatus is just below the tip of the penis. In the most severe malformations the meatus is located on the perineum between the halves of the scrotum (bifid scrotum). In addition, the foreskin is usually absent ventrally and, when combined with chordee, gives the organ a hooded and crooked appearance. In severe cases the altered appearance may leave the infant's gender in doubt at birth because of the perineal position of the meatus and small penis. In any case of ambiguous genitalia, additional evaluation is essential. Cryptorchidism is present in about 10% of infants with hypospadias and increases with more proximal hypospadias with the meatus at the scrotum or perineum. There is an increased risk of disorders of sex development in patients with severe hypospadias, both with and without cryptorchidism.

Surgical Correction

The principal objectives of surgical correction are: (1) to enhance the child's ability to void in the standing position with a straight stream; (2) to improve the physical appearance of the genitalia for psychological reasons; and (3) to preserve a sexually adequate organ. The choice of surgical procedure is affected primarily by the severity of the defect and the presence of associated anomalies. Numerous techniques are utilised in repair of hypospadias and are performed under general anaesthesia typically as an outpatient procedure.

The preferred time for surgical repair is 6 to 12 months of age, before the child has developed body image. Occasionally a short course of testosterone is administered preoperatively to achieve additional penile size to facilitate the surgery.

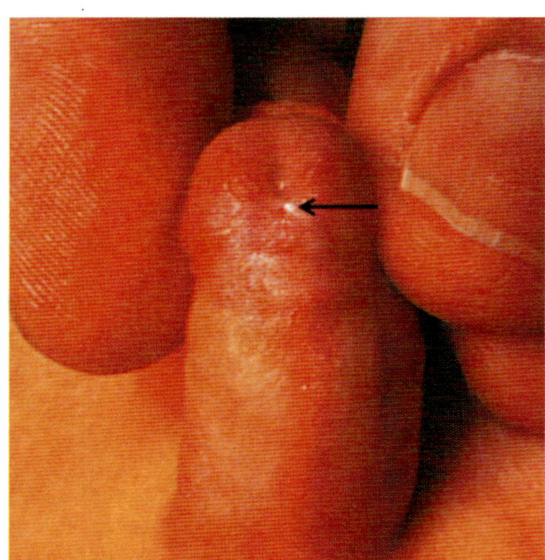

Fig 24.4 Distal hypospadias with a stenotic meatus *(arrow)* located on the glans with no chordee. (Source: Holcomb, G. W., Murphy, J. P., & Ostlie, D. J. (2014). Ashcraft's pediatric surgery (6th ed.). Philadelphia, PA: Elsevier.)

Nursing Care Management

Neonatal circumcision should be avoided in hypospadias where there is incomplete foreskin because this is not conducive to a safe clamp or Plastibell circumcision. In severe cases, the foreskin may be used in reconstruction. In mild hypospadias, the foreskin is not incomplete and the abnormality may not be noted until after circumcision. This does not affect future successful reconstruction if it is needed. In most cases, the appearance after reconstruction will be of a circumcised normal penis.

Hypospadias repair may require some type of urinary diversion with a silicone stent or feeding tube to promote optimum healing and to maintain the position and patency of the newly formed urethra.

Epispadias and Exstrophy Complex

Bladder exstrophy is a severe defect involving the musculoskeletal system and the urinary, reproductive and, in some cases, the intestinal tract. It is one of three anomalies that define the exstrophy-epispadias complex (EEC). **Epispadias** is the least severe of the complex and is due to failure of the urethra to close normally, resulting in an exposed or open dorsal urethra. Bladder exstrophy is a more severe defect characterised by an open, 'inside-out' bladder with the inner surface exposed and the dorsal urethra (epispadias) on the lower abdominal wall (Figs 24.5 and 24.6). Classic bladder exstrophy typically includes

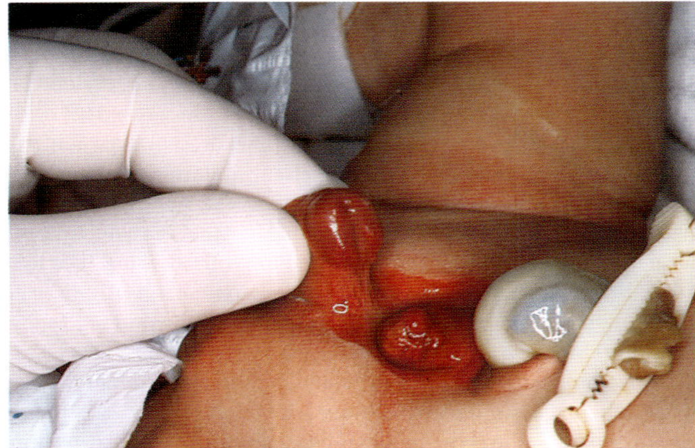

Fig 24.5 Newborn with bladder exstrophy and epispadias. (Source: Courtesy Tim Yankee, St Francis Hospital, Tulsa, Oklahoma.)

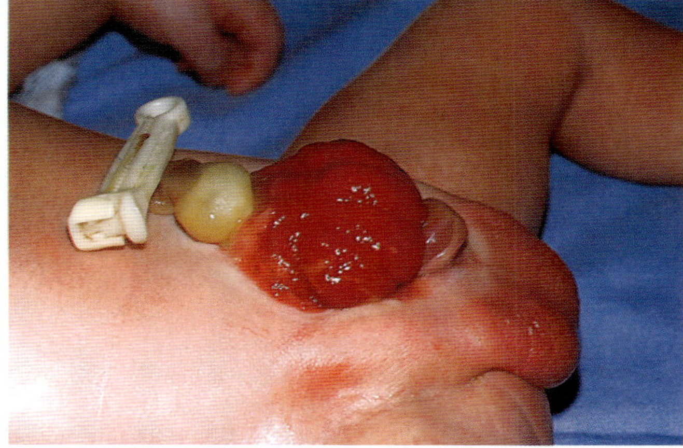

Fig 24.6 Exstrophy of bladder. (Source: Courtesy H. Gil Rushton, MD, Children's National Medical Center, Washington, DC.)

findings of diastasis (separation) of the symphysis pubis (pelvic bone), low set umbilicus, anteriorly displaced anus, defects of the genitalia and inguinal hernia. The third and most severe defect is **cloacal exstrophy**, which includes both bladder exstrophy and exstrophy of the large intestine (hindgut) through an abdominal wall defect. In addition, there is anal atresia, omphalocele, hypoplasia of the colon, anomalous genitalia and often spinal dysraphism. There may be abnormalities of one or both kidneys.

Pathophysiology

The pathogenesis of bladder exstrophy appears to be due to a complex embryological defect in abdominal wall development. The extent of the defect and the stage of development when the rupture occurs affect the extent the anomaly will be seen within the EEC.

In males with bladder exstrophy, the defect of the genitalia includes epispadias and upward curvature of a shortened penis and may include other abnormalities, such as undescended testes and inguinal hernias. In females, there is epispadias, a bifid clitoris and small labia minora. The vagina is shortened compared with normal. In cloacal exstrophy patients, there are often more severe anomalies, such as bifid or duplicated uterus, split clitoris, completely separated labia and a duplicate or absent vagina in females. Males may have a split penis and scrotum or a short, flat penis with hypospadias. In either sex, separation of the pubic bones is generally corrected by pelvic osteotomy, particularly if there is extreme diastasis, as this increases the likelihood of successful bladder closure. In bladder exstrophy patients, the upper urinary tract is usually normal. Fertility is possible in females but decreased in males, possibly because of semen abnormalities, abnormal ejaculation or a combination of both. Assisted reproductive techniques remain a viable option for patients with infertility. Recent studies indicate good long-term outcomes on erectile and general sexual function in both men and women with epispadias and bladder exstrophy (Suominen et al 2015).

Therapeutic Management

The objectives of treatment are: (1) preservation of renal function; (2) attainment of urinary control; (3) adequate reconstructive repair for acceptable appearance; (4) prevention of UTIs; and (5) preservation of optimum external genitalia with continence and sexual function. There are two surgical approaches currently utilised to correct bladder exstrophy. One is termed *modern staged repair of bladder exstrophy* (MSRBE), typically involving three surgeries beginning with closure of the bladder and abdominal wall. Complete primary repair of bladder exstrophy (CPRBE) is a single stage surgical closure combining closure of the bladder, abdominal wall, partial tightening of the bladder neck and, in some cases, bilateral ureteral reimplantation to correct reflux. Often, pelvic osteotomies are performed at the time of primary closure to deepen the flattened pelvis, close the pubic diastasis and release tension on the abdominal wall to improve success of primary closure (Inouye et al 2014).

Nursing Care Management

In bladder exstrophy the everted bladder appears bright red through the abdominal opening. It is important to prevent trauma to the exposed mucosa. After delivery of an infant with bladder exstrophy, the umbilical cord is clamped with the usual plastic clamp, but the clamp is exchanged for a soft umbilical tape or silk suture material to limit trauma to the exposed bladder. The bladder is covered with plastic wrap or a transparent adhesive dressing for protection. Specifics of care reflect surgeon preference.

Nursing care after the complete primary repair is focused on pain management and maintenance of immobilisation. Around the clock IV pain medications are important for several days after surgery as keeping the infant quiet is important to success of the bladder closure. This is extremely important in these cases, as achieving a successful initial closure is one of the best indicators for a good prognosis long term. Nasogastric tube decompression may be used to prevent abdominal distension. Dehiscence may occur postoperatively, and signs of suture separation or wound problems are promptly reported to the practitioner. Immobilisation of the pelvis with traction for 2 to 4 weeks is typical even if osteotomies are not performed. The child is kept supine and lifted to assess skin with sufficient help to manage lines and keep the patient in good alignment. Prevention of skin breakdown is important and adhesive foam dressings over pressure areas such as the sacrum or heels or where skin comes in contact with equipment may be helpful.

Postoperative nursing care after bladder neck reconstruction and antireflux surgery (ureteral reimplantation) includes routine wound care and careful monitoring of urinary output from the bladder and ureteral drainage tubes. The nurse should ensure the catheters are intact and are not twisted or kinked.

Children who fail to attain continence after bladder neck reconstruction may require further surgical intervention including bladder augmentation or bladder removal with a continent diversion.

Family Support and Home Care. Bladder exstrophy and other disorders of the EEC are significant congenital abnormalities that require lifelong care by a team of specialists. Improvement in surgical techniques has helped achieve better outcomes, specifically that of the goal of continence. Parental stress is significant, and support services may be helpful. Patients may also benefit from psychological support as adjustment problems are common, particularly in adolescents. Parents should receive teaching and practice on care of the infant or child at home and have access to resources to call if there are questions. Allowing time for the parent to voice concerns can facilitate evaluation of their understanding and help direct discharge needs.

When the infant is discharged with an unrepaired defect, plastic wrap is placed over the defect to prevent irritation of the exposed bladder from abrasive nappies. Current practice typically allows for the bladder to be immersed in water for a bath, cleansed with mild soap and rinsed with clean water. With these complex patients, post op care is individualised and may vary with physician preference. UTIs are common in these patients and parents learn to recognise the signs of UTI and to report a suspected infection to the practitioner.

DISORDERS OF SEX DEVELOPMENT

Infants born with a discrepancy between external genitalia, gonadal and chromosomal sex are currently referred to as having a **disorder of sex development (DSD)**. The presentation at birth may be a genital appearance that does not permit gender declaration and this is termed **ambiguous genitalia**. These may include bilateral cryptorchidism, perineal hypospadias with bifid scrotum, clitoromegaly, posterior labial fusion, phenotypical female appearance with a palpable gonad, and hypospadias and unilateral non-palpable gonad. Also included in the DSD category are infants with discordant genitalia and sex chromosomes. Turner syndrome (45, XO) and Klinefelter syndrome (47, XXY) are also DSDs that do not present with ambiguous genitalia.

Pathophysiology

Normal sexual differentiation starts at 7 weeks' gestation when fetuses with a Y chromosome begin developing testes. Early on both female (XX) and male (XY) fetuses have a similar reproductive structure. Multiple genes contribute to this process and mutations in these genes can lead to various DSDs. Congenital malformation of the genitalia are most frequently because of androgen deficiency in XY individuals and androgen excess in XX patient, though in many cases no endocrine aetiology can be found (Grinspon & Rey 2014).

Initial evaluation includes karyotype and assessment of adrenal and gonadal function, and this information can be used to categorise the infant into one of three categories:

- virilised XX (XX DSD)
- undervirilised XY (XY DSD)
- mixed sex chromosome pattern.

Therapeutic Management

The most common cause of ambiguous genitalia is **congenital adrenal hyperplasia (CAH)**, which can lead to life-threatening salt-wasting adrenal insufficiency in the first weeks of life. Laboratory testing includes a measurement of 17-hydroxyprogesterone in addition to karyotype with immediate probe for SRY (sex-determining region on the Y chromosome). Serum electrolytes are monitored as signs and symptoms of adrenal insufficiency may include hypoglycaemia, hypovolaemia, hyponatraemia, hyperkalaemia, vomiting and diarrhoea. Fluids and electrolytes need to be replaced urgently. Additional laboratory testing may be indicated, as well as pelvic and abdominal ultrasonography to evaluate for gonads, uterus and vagina.

Family Support

The birth of a child with ambiguous genitalia has been termed a psychosocial emergency for the family. They require support because the answers to a seemingly simple question as to what gender their child is requires evaluation and time. Involvement in an interdisciplinary team that may include endocrinology, urology, genetics, surgeons, in addition to nurses and social workers can make clear communication challenging and the nurse may be instrumental in coordinating family meetings with the team.

The infant and child with DSD pose very complex and controversial management questions, including sex assignment and potential genital surgery.

Obstructive Uropathy

Congenital urinary obstruction may be best defined as urinary flow impairment that has limited or may potentially limit normal renal development (Peters 2016). Urinary obstruction in children includes a wide spectrum and is one of the most common conditions affecting the urinary tract. Obstruction can be congenital or acquired, unilateral or bilateral, and complete or incomplete (Fig 24.7). Prenatal ultrasound has allowed for diagnosis of potential obstructive conditions before birth. **Hydronephrosis**, which is a dilation of the renal pelvis, with or without dilation of the calyces, is a common finding on fetal ultrasound and may be due to a transient dilation of the collecting system, upper or lower urinary tract obstruction or non-obstructive processes such as vesicoureteral reflux, megaureter and prune belly syndrome. It is important to realise that not all hydronephrosis represents obstruction. The most common causes of hydronephrosis are transient hydronephrosis, ureteropelvic junction obstruction (UPJO) and vesicoureteral reflux.

Bilateral involvement increases the risk of significant renal abnormality and impaired renal function. Obstruction may occur at any level of the urinary tract, causing dilation above the obstruction. For example, when the bladder outlet is obstructed, the bladder, kidneys and both ureters may become distended. When both ureter and renal pelvis are distended, it is termed **hydroureteronephrosis**. If there is obstruction at the ureterovesical junction (UVJ), the ureter and renal pelvis of that side will be dilated and the contralateral (opposite) side may remain normal in appearance and function. Similarly, if the

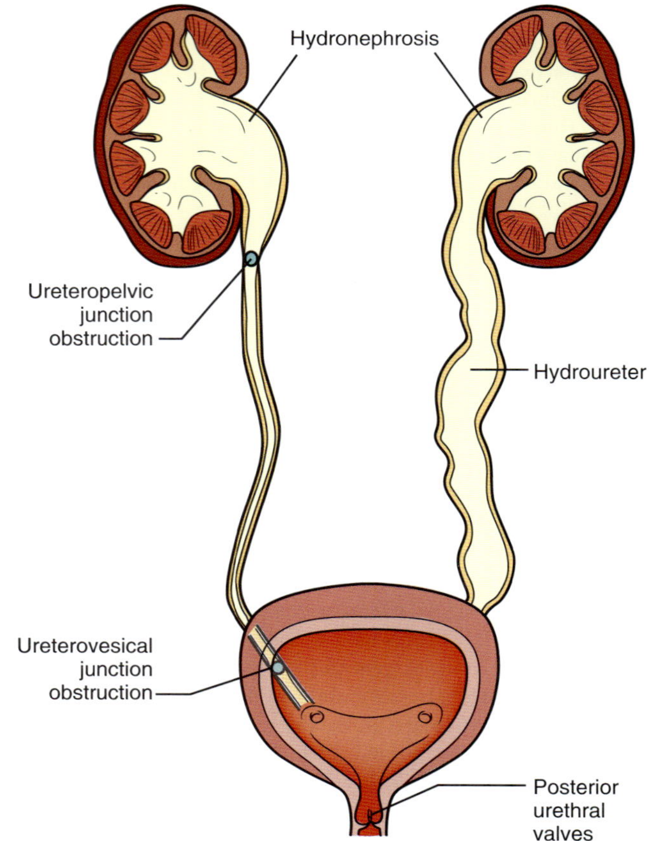

Fig 24.7 Major sites of urinary tract obstruction.

ureteropelvic junction (UPJ) becomes obstructed, the renal pelvis and calyces will become dilated. The ureteropelvic junction is the most common site of obstruction. Less common causes of obstruction include congenital megaureter, which is an enlarged ureter that may or may not be obstructed and also may or may not reflux. A **ureterocele** is an abnormality of ureteral development where the distal end of the ureter is dilated, forming a bulge that is usually in the bladder (intravesical) or partially extending beyond the bladder neck (ectopic). Though rare, urethral obstruction can result from a prolapsed ureterocele. Ureteroceles are commonly associated with the upper pole of a duplex system and if not detected by prenatal ultrasound, commonly present with urinary tract infection in the first few months of life.

Obstruction is the single largest entity leading to renal insufficiency in boys younger than 1 year and is the largest single cause of renal failure requiring transplantation (Peters 2016). Posterior urethral valves are obstructing membranes in the urethra that occur only in boys and are the most common cause of bladder outlet obstruction. Because the blockage is low, it affects everything 'upstream' and causes the bladder to become thick-walled, as well as causing bilateral hydroureteronephrosis. **Oligohydramnios** (low amniotic fluid volume) occurs because most of the amniotic fluid volume depends on fetal urine production and thus is an indicator of poor renal function or bilaterally obstructed kidneys. Severe oligohydramnios also affects lung development in the fetus and resulting pulmonary hypoplasia with poor postnatal outcomes. Although valves can be treated with ablation, there is commonly some degree of renal damage that decreases the renal reserve, affecting long-term function and resulting in renal insufficiency and renal failure when the child 'outgrows' his kidney function. The obstruction also may result in significant bladder dysfunction, referred to as 'valve bladder syndrome'.

Pathophysiology

The effects of obstruction on the developing kidney depend on when it occurs and the severity of obstruction. Because it occurs when the kidney is forming, it is very different from an acquired obstruction of a mature kidney. Obstruction during development alters the growth regulation, tissue differentiation and function. These changes can result in poorly functioning renal tissue called **dysplasia**. There may also be progression of renal dysfunction. Two forms of progressive renal dysfunction include an uncorrected partial obstruction, such as a UPJ obstruction; and a previously obstructed but corrected obstruction with some degree of renal damage, such as posterior urethral valves (PUVs). Structural alterations caused by obstruction are evident in significant hydronephrosis as a distortion in normal architecture and relative alterations in the amount of renal tissue elements. Subtle changes are functionally important and include fibrosis and increased interstitial tissue, as well as abnormal tubules and glomeruli (Peters 2016).

The pathophysiological changes produced by obstruction are influenced by the location and severity of the blockage and by the presence of complicating factors, such as infection. With obstruction, or in the event of a solitary kidney, compensatory renal growth occurs in the contralateral kidney. This is from cellular hypertrophy (enlargement) rather than hyperplasia or increase in nephrons (Meldrum 2016). The detrusor muscle of the bladder is also affected by obstruction of the bladder outlet and becomes thickened and trabeculated, with compromise in effectiveness and function.

Clinical Manifestations

The clinical manifestations of obstructive uropathy depend on the location of the obstructing lesion, its severity and the underlying cause. The most common presentation is the finding of abnormalities, typically hydronephrosis, on fetal ultrasound. If not diagnosed in utero, an infant may be noted to have an abdominal mass or develop UTI. Congenital obstruction is often asymptomatic, as in the case of the most common obstruction of the upper urinary tract, UPJO. In older children with UPJO, abdominal or flank pain, often with chronic nausea, is more common. Urinary tract infections or haematuria are more common presentations of ureterocele or megaureter. Maternal oligohydramnios may signal a significant obstruction or renal problem in the developing fetus. This can lead to respiratory distress due to pulmonary hypoplasia and is life-threatening. Although PUVs are diagnosed prenatally in most cases, respiratory distress, sepsis, abdominal distension, not voiding in the first 48 hours of life and renal failure can be manifestations. Depending on the spectrum of this disease, it may not be diagnosed until voiding problems are persistent later in childhood (Becherucci et al 2016).

Urolithiasis, formation of calculi (stones) in the urinary tract, has increased in children in recent years and can cause obstruction of the renal pelvis or ureter. It is associated with underlying metabolic conditions and urinary tract malformation. Stones can produce a characteristic pain called **renal colic,** which is more common in adolescents than young children. This pain is characterised by discomfort in the flank, lower back or lower abdomen. The discomfort is typically intense and it is not relieved by changes in position.

Obstruction of the bladder produces lower urinary tract symptoms. These symptoms are closely related to those produced by other dysfunctional voiding conditions, including detrusor overactivity and urinary retention. Symptoms include poor force of urinary stream, intermittency of voided stream, feelings of incomplete bladder emptying and post void dribbling. In addition, children with obstruction of the bladder or urethra may experience frequency of urination, nocturia, nocturnal enuresis, urgency and urge incontinence.

Diagnostic Evaluation

Imaging studies are used to assess for obstruction. Ultrasonography is the initial test to assess kidneys, including size, hydronephrosis, dilated ureters, bladder wall and bladder emptying. Stones may be visualised on ultrasound, although a plain film of the abdomen can show certain types of stones. Non-contrast helical computed tomography is the gold standard for diagnosis of stones, but is used selectively due to the greater radiation exposure.

Therapeutic Management. The management of obstructive uropathy depends on the degree of the obstruction and the likelihood that renal function will be compromised unless aggressive intervention is undertaken. For example, UPJ obstruction causing hydronephrosis in the neonate may or may not require surgical intervention. In contrast, PUV obstruction requires aggressive intervention to optimise renal function.

With the wide spectrum of obstructive changes, criteria for intervention remain somewhat controversial. Careful monitoring with intervention when indicated is more common in some of the conditions that in previous years would have always warranted surgery. In the case of severe obstructive uropathy with renal insufficiency, intervention is needed. The most common example of this is PUV, where primary valve ablation is done endoscopically to relieve the obstruction. In some cases, often in a premature infant with a very small urethra, a cutaneous vesicostomy is performed to allow urine to drain from the bladder via an incontinent stoma from the dome of the bladder to the abdominal wall and into the nappy. In some cases, transient diversion of the upper urinary tract is indicated, with ureterostomies brought out to the skin or nephrostomy tubes for temporary drainage. There is a trend towards non-operative management of megaureter, depending on the type and symptoms. If there are recurrent UTIs, pyelonephritis, persistent flank pain or haematuria, surgical correction is warranted. The procedure involves excision of the distal stenotic ureter with tapering and reimplantation into the bladder.

Permanent urinary diversion may involve a continent urinary diversion that incorporates a segment of bowel or ureter to increase bladder capacity (bladder augmentation), if needed, and creation of a stoma that allows the bladder to be emptied by placing a catheter through the stoma into the bladder. In contrast to transient diversions, this procedure is reserved for older children and requires ongoing intermittent catheterisation.

Prognosis. The prognosis depends on the type of obstruction, the degree of irreversible renal damage, whether renal dysplasia is present, the age at diagnosis and the severity of complications. Despite improvements in corrective surgery, some patients develop renal failure, which may evolve over a highly variable period that can extend into adulthood. Careful follow-up care should extend throughout childhood and adolescence, especially when any degree of renal insufficiency is present.

Nursing Care Management

Nursing goals in urinary tract obstruction include helping identify cases, assisting with diagnostic procedures and caring for children with complications. Preparing parents and children for procedures, especially urinary diversion procedures, is a major nursing responsibility. (See Preparation for Diagnostic and Therapeutic Procedures, Chapter 22.)

Parents and children need emotional support and counselling during the potentially lengthy management of these disorders. Parents are the primary caregivers during infancy and early childhood, when most reparative surgery is performed. They need assistance in learning to manage the care of the child and in detecting subtle signs of UTI or complications of procedures.

Non-compliance with care can be risky and is not uncommon when adolescents assert their independence and try to be 'like everyone else' and skip catheterisations and medications. Those with progressive renal deterioration may face the prospect of dialysis or transplantation and the emotional turmoil that accompanies these procedures.

REFERENCES

Banerjee, S., Dissanayake, P. V., & Abeyagunawardena, A. S. (2016). Vaccinations in children on immunosuppressive medications for renal disease. Pediatric Nephrology (Berlin, Germany), 31(9), 1437–1448.

Becherucci, F., Roperto, R., Materassi, M., et al. (2016). Chronic kidney disease in children. Oxford University Press. Clinical kidney journal, 9(4), 583–591.

Bichet, D. G., & Bockenhauer, D. (2016). Genetic forms of nephrogenic diabetes insipidus (NDI): Vasopressin receptor defect (X-linked) and aquaporin defect (autosomal recessive and dominant). Best Practice and Research. Clinical Endocrinology and Metabolism, 30(2), 263–276.

Bonadio, W., & Maida, G. (2014). Urinary tract infection in outpatient febrile infants younger than 30 days of age: A 10-year evaluation. The Pediatric Infectious Disease Journal, 33(4), 342–344.

Buonocore, G., Bracci, R. & Weindling, M. (2018). Neonatology A Practical Approach to Neonatal Diseases. 2nd ed. Champaign, IL: Springer International Publishing.

Dagan, R., Cleper, R., Davidovits, M., et al. (2016). Post-infectious glomerulonephritis in pediatric patients over two decades: Severity-associated features. The Israel Medical Association Journal, 18(6), 336–340.

Dangle, P. P., Fuller, T. W., Gaines, B., et al. (2016). Evolving mechanisms of injury and management of pediatric blunt renal trauma–20 years of experience. Urology, 90, 159–163.

Demir, E. & Caliskan, Y. (2020). Variations of type IV collagen-encoding genes in patients with histological diagnosis of focal segmental glomerulosclerosis. Pediatric Nephrology, 35(6), 927–936.

Eliacik, K., Kanik, A., Yavascan, O., et al. (2016). A Comparison of Bladder Catheterization and Suprapubic Aspiration Methods for Urine Sample Collection from Infants with a Suspected Urinary Tract Infection. SAGE Publications: Clinical pediatrics, 55(9), 819–824.

Ellis, D. (2016). Pathophysiology, evaluation and management of oedema in childhood nephrotic syndrome. Frontiers in Pediatrics, 3, 111.

Forster, E. & Fraser, J. (2018). Paediatric nursing skills for Australian nurses. Cambridge: Cambridge University Press, 2018.

Francis, A., Didsbury, M., van Zwieten, A., et al. (2019). Quality of life of children and adolescents with chronic kidney disease: a cross-sectional study. Archives of Disease in Childhood, 104(2), 134–140.

Garin, E. (2019). Primary vesicoureteral reflux; what have we learnt from the recently published randomized, controlled trials? Pediatric Nephrology, 34(9), 1513–1519.

Gaudry, S., Hajage, D., Schortgen, F., et al. (2016). Initiation strategies for renal-replacement therapy in the intensive care unit. New England Journal of Medicine, 375(2), 122–133.

Gil-Peña, H., Mejía, N., & Santos, F. (2014). Renal tubular acidosis. The Journal of Pediatrics, 164(4), 691–697.

Gomez, J., Gil-Peña, H., Santos, F., et al. (2016). Primary distal renal tubular acidosis: Novel findings in patients study by next-generation sequencing. Pediatric Research, 79, 496–501.

Grinspon, R. P., & Rey, R. A. (2014). When hormone defects cannot explain it: Malformative disorders of sex development. Birth Defects Research. Part C, Embryo Today: Reviews, 102(4), 359–373.

Haley, C. & Pillitteri, A. (2016). Pillitteri's child and family health nursing in Australia and New Zealand. Second edition. North Ryde, NSW: Wolters Kluwer, 2016

Haller, M. C., Royuela, A., Nagler, E. V., et al. (2016). Steroid avoidance or withdrawal for kidney transplant recipients (Review). Cochrane Database of Systematic Reviews (8), CD005632, http://onlinelibrary.wiley.com/doi/10.1002/14651858.CD005632.pub3/full.

Hamid, M. Afroz, R., Ahmed, U., et al. (2020). Collecting the golden water: Quality assessment on approach of diagnosing urinary tract infections in 0 to 36 months old children. Paediatrics & Child Health, 25(7), 419–424.

Hjorten, R., Anwar, Z., & Reidy, K. J. (2016). Long-term outcomes of childhood onset nephrotic syndrome. Frontiers in Pediatrics, 4, 53.

Holmberg, C., & Jalanko, H. (2016). Long-term effects of paediatric kidney transplantation. Nature Reviews. Nephrology, 12(5), 301–311.

Hothi, D. K., Stronach, L., & Sinnott, K. (2016). Home hemodialysis in children. Hemodialysis International, 20(3), 349–357.

Inouye, B. M., Tourchi, A., Di Carlo, H. N., et al. (2014). Modern management of the exstrophy-epispadias complex. Surgery Research and Practice, 2014, 58764.

Jefferies, J. L., & Devarajan, P. (2016). Early detection of acute kidney injury after pediatric cardiac surgery. Progress in Pediatric Cardiology, 41, 9–16.

Karavanaki, K. A., Soldatou, A., Koufadaki, A. M., et al. (2017). Delayed treatment of the first febrile urinary tract infection in early childhood increased the risk of renal scarring. Acta Paediatrica, 106, 149–154.

Kaufman, J., Knight, A. J., Bryant, P., et al. (2020). Liquid gold: the cost-effectiveness of urine sample collection methods for young precontinent children. Archives of Disease in Childhood, 105(3), 253–259.

Kim, K. H. (2016). Clinical manifestation patterns and trends in poststreptococcal glomerulonephritis. Child Kidney Disease, 20(1), 6–10.

Kirsch, A. J., Arlen, A. M., Leong, T., et al. (2014). Vesicoureteral reflux index (VURx): A novel tool to predict primary reflux improvement and resolution in children less than 2 years of age. Journal of Pediatric Urology, 10(6), 1249–1254.

Kolon, T. F., Herndon, C. D. A., Baker, L. A., et al. (2014). Evaluation and treatment of cryptorchidism: AUA guideline. Journal of Urology, 192, 337–345.

Leigh, J., Rickard, M., Sanger, S., et al. (2020). Antibiotic prophylaxis for prevention of urinary tract infections in the first year of life in children with vesicoureteral reflux diagnosed in the workup of antenatal hydronephrosis: a systematic review. Pediatric Nephrology, 35(9), 1639–1646. DOI: 10.1007/s00467-020-04568-6

LoBiondo-Wood, G. & Haber, J. (2018). Nursing research: methods and critical appraisal for evidence-based practice. 9th edition., St Louis, Missouri.

Loghman-Adham, M. (2003). Medication noncompliance in patients with chronic disease: Issues in dialysis and renal transplantation. The American Journal of Managed Care, 9(2), 155–171.

Lombel, R. M., Hodson, E. M., & Gipson, D. S. (2013). Treatment of steroid-resistant nephrotic syndrome in children: New guidelines from KDIGO. Pediatric Nephrology (Berlin, Germany), 28(3), 409–414.

Lopez-Giacoman, S., & Madero, M. (2015). Biomarkers in chronic kidney disease, from kidney function to kidney damage. World Journal of Nephrology, 4(1), 57–73.

Meldrum, K. K. (2016). Pathophysiology of urinary tract obstruction. In A. J. Wein, L. R. Kavoussi, A. W. Partin, et al. (Eds.), Campbell-Walsh Urology. Philadelphia: Elsevier.

Peters, C. A. (2016). Congenital urinary obstruction: Pathophysiology. In A. J. Wein, L. R. Kavoussi, A. W. Partin, et al. (Eds.), Campbell-Walsh Urology. Philadelphia: Elsevier.

Psooy, K. (2014). Sports and the solitary kidney: What parents of a young child with a solitary kidney should know. Canadian Urological Association Journal, 8(7–8), 233–235.

Ripatti, P., Soderlund, S., Ramo, J., et al. (2019). Polygenic hyperlipidemias and coronary artery disease risk. Journal of the American College of Cardiology, 73, 1690.

Santos, F., Ordóñez, F. A., Claramunt-Taberner, D., et al. (2015). Clinical and laboratory approaches in the diagnosis of renal tubular acidosis. Pediatric Nephrology (Berlin, Germany), 30(12), 2099–2107.

Savige, J., Colville, D., Rheault, M., et al. (2016). Alport syndrome in women and girls. Clinical Journal of the American Society of Nephrology: CJASN, 11(9), 1713–1720.

Schaeffer, A. J., Greenfield, S. P., Ivanova, A., et al. (2016). Reliability of grading of vesicoureteral reflux and other findings on voiding cystourethrography. Journal of Pediatric Urology, http://dx.doi.org/10.1016/j.jpurol.2016.06.020.

Schlager, T. A. (2016). Urinary tract infections in infants and children. Microbiology Spectrum, 4(5), UTI-0022.

Shakih, N., Mattoo, T. K., Keren, R., et al. (2016). Early antibiotic treatment for pediatric febrile urinary tract infection and renal scarring. Journal of the American Medical Association Pediatrics, 170(9), 848–854.

Sinha, R., Sinha, R., Sethi, S., et al. (2018). Prolonged intermittent renal replacement therapy in children. Pediatric Nephrology, 33(8), 1283–1296.

Spahiu, L., Merovci, B., Jashari, H., et al. (2016). Congenital nephrotic syndrome-Finnish type. Medical Archives (Sarajevo, Bosnia and Herzegovina), 70(3), 232–234.

Suominen, J. S., Santtila, P., & Taskinen, S. (2015). Sexual function in patients operated for bladder exstrophy and epispadias. Journal of Urology, 194(1), 195–199.

The Royal Children's Hospital (RCHM). (n.d.). Clinical Practice Guidelines. Metabolic disorders. https://www.rch.org.au/clinicalguide/guideline_index/Metabolic_disorders/

The Royal Children's Hospital Melbourne (RCHM). (2009). Chronic Renal Failure. Initial work-up. August. https://www.rch.org.au/kidsconnect/prereferral_guidelines/Chronic_Renal_Failure/#initial-work-up

The Royal Children's Hospital Melbourne (RCHM). (2018). Kids Health Information. Urinary Tract Infection (UTI). March. https://www.rch.org.au/kidsinfo/fact_sheets/Urinary_tract_infection_UTI/

The Royal Children's Hospital Melbourne (RCHM). (2019a). Clinical Practice Guidelines. Urinary Tract infection. July. https://www.rch.org.au/clinicalguide/guideline_index/Urinary_tract_infection/

The Royal Children's Hospital Melbourne (RCHM). (2019b). Clinical Practice Guidelines. Nephrotic Syndrome. Assessment and Management. November. https://www.rch.org.au/clinicalguide/guideline_index/Nephrotic_syndrome/

The Royal Children's Hospital Melbourne (RCHM). (2020). Clinical Practice Guidelines. Acute scrotal pain or swelling. Management. July. https://www.rch.org.au/clinicalguide/guideline_index/Acute_scrotal_pain_or_swelling

The Sydney Children's Hospital Network. (n.d.). Fact sheets. Nephrology (kidney diseases and disorders) at The Children's Hospital at Westmead. Urology. https://www.schn.health.nsw.gov.au/find-a-service/health-medical-services/nephrology-kidney-diseases-and-disorders/chw

VanDeVoorde, R. G. (2015). Acute poststreptococcal glomerulonephritis: The most common acute glomerulonephritis. Pediatrics in Review, 36(1), 3–13.

Webster, A. C., Nagler, E. V., Morton, R. L., et al. (2017). Chronic kidney disease. Lancet, 389(10075), 1238–1252.

Wojtowicz-Prus, E., Kili -Pstrusi ska, K., Reich, A., et al. (2016). Chronic kidney disease-associated pruritus in children. Acta Dermato-Venereologica, 96(7), 938–942.

25

The Child with Gastrointestinal Dysfunction

Lisa Speedie

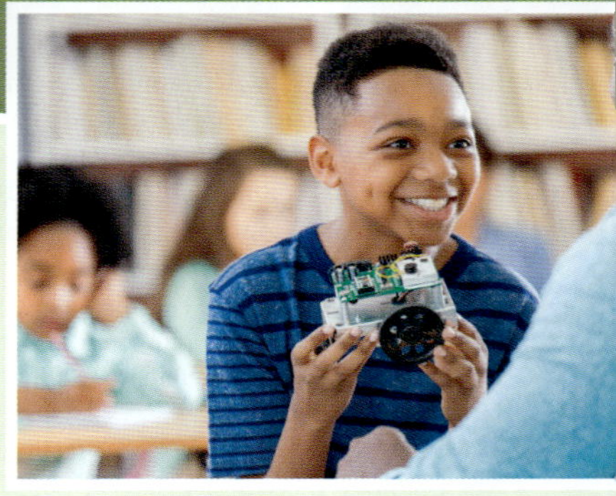

LEARNING OUTCOMES

- Demonstrate the assessments required for a child with a gastrointestinal disorder
- Describe the normal fluid and electrolyte requirements for children and adolescents
- Describe and care for inflammation of the gastrointestinal system in children and adolescents
- Care for infection of the gastrointestinal system and provide nursing and family-centred care to meet the needs of children and families
- Provide family-centred care and patient education in relation to gastrointestinal disorders and nursing care.

GASTROINTESTINAL STRUCTURE AND FUNCTION

The primary function of the gastrointestinal (GI) tract is the digestion and absorption of nutrients. The GI tract also has secretory, barrier, endocrine and immunological functions (Box 25.1). The extensive surface area of the GI tract and its digestive function represent the major means of exchange between the human organism and the environment. Thus any dysfunction of the GI tract can cause significant problems with the exchange of fluids, electrolytes and nutrients.

Development of the Gastrointestinal Tract

The development of the GI tract (from mouth to anus) occurs in several stages from conception through to birth. The GI tract may be divided into three parts in intrauterine life: foregut (oesophagus, stomach and proximal duodenum), midgut (distal duodenum, jejunum, ileum, caecum and proximal colon) and hindgut (distal colon and rectum). The salivary glands, liver, gallbladder and pancreas are outgrowths of the foregut and midgut.

The oesophagus develops from the foregut and can be identified by 4 weeks' gestation. It elongates rapidly after the fourth week to a length of approximately 10 cm at term. The stomach also develops from the primitive foregut and can be identified by the fourth week of gestation. It continues to develop in the second trimester. From the fifth week of gestation until term, the intestine lengthens a thousand-fold.

The third trimester is the period of most extensive and rapid growth of the gut. At full term, the small intestine is approximately 250 to 300 cm and will grow to approximately 2 to 4 m in the adult. The large intestine develops from the midgut and the hindgut and is approximately 30 to 50 cm at term.

At term the mechanical functions of digestion are relatively immature. Swallowing is an automatic reflex action for the first 3 months, and the infant has no voluntary control over swallowing until the striated muscles in the throat establish their cerebral connections. This begins at approximately 6 weeks of age. By 6 months the infant is capable of swallowing, holding food in the mouth or spitting it out at will. The mechanism of sucking is also a reflexive activity in the newborn, and the muscular action of the tongue has a typical forward thrust. With neural and muscular development, the infant gradually acquires the ability to perform the coordinated muscular action typical of the adult type of swallowing. (See Chapter 10.)

The stomach, which lies horizontally, is round until the child is approximately 2 years of age. It then gradually elongates until approximately 7 years of age, when it assumes the shape and anatomical position of the adult stomach. This anatomical placement of the stomach in infancy influences positioning practices during and after feeding. At birth the stomach capacity is small, but it increases rapidly with age.

The frequency and character of stools are affected by the rate of peristalsis and the nature of ingested food. The frequent, yellow stools of the neonate gradually assume a more adult regularity and character in the infant. When compared with the older child, the capacity of the infant's stomach is smaller, but the emptying time is faster. Both the stomach capacity and the emptying time have implications for the amount and frequency of feedings during infancy.

The secretory cells of the GI tract are believed to be functional at birth. However, because most of the digestive enzymes depend on a specific pH, their efficiency may be impaired. The newborn produces only small amounts of saliva, which contains the starch-splitting enzyme amylase. Therefore its primary purpose at this time is to moisten the mouth and throat. By the end of the second year, the salivary glands have increased in size about five times to reach their full size and function.

Digestion

Three processes—digestion, absorption and metabolism—are necessary for the body to convert nutrients into forms it can use. Nutrients are composed of six major substances: carbohydrates, proteins, fats, vitamins, minerals and water. Digestion is the initial preparation of food for use by the body. Two basic activities are involved: mechanical or muscular activity producing GI motility (movement); and chemical or enzymatic activity resulting from GI secretions.

Once a bolus of food has entered the stomach, the lower oesophageal sphincter (LES) contracts to prevent food from refluxing (returning)

BOX 25.1 Functions of the Gastrointestinal Tract

- Process and absorb nutrients necessary to maintain metabolic processes and to support growth and development.
- Perform an excretory function for both digestive residue and other waste products that pour into the intestine from the blood or are excreted in the bile.
- Provide detoxification while other routes of elimination (e.g. kidneys, liver, skin) are still immature.
- Participate in maintaining fluid and electrolyte balance in infancy.
- Serve a lymphoid function by providing a barrier to bacteria, viruses and parasites. The liver also processes antigens and produces immunoglobulins.

into the oesophagus. The stomach stores, mixes and empties the food during digestion. The gastric glands secrete enzymes, hydrochloric acid and mucus, which mix with the food to continue the process of digestion. The enzyme pepsin, formed from pepsinogen, begins the breakdown of whole proteins into polypeptides. Hydrochloric acid, secreted by the parietal cells, aids in the digestion of proteins. The hormone gastrin is released in the stomach in response to food. Gastrin stimulates the parietal cells to produce more hydrochloric acid. When the pH is very low, a feedback mechanism stops secretion of gastrin to prevent excessive acid formation. The mucus serves primarily to form a protective barrier between the acid and the gastric mucosa.

Partially digested food and watery secretions (**chyme**) are delivered to the small intestine. Up to this time, most of the digestion has been mechanical. The major part of chemical digestion, as well as several types of movement that aid in mechanical digestion, occurs in the small intestine. The small intestine secretes a large number of enzymes, each of which is specific for one of the fundamental types of nutrients. The mucosa of the small intestine secretes disaccharidases (maltase, lactase and sucrase) that convert maltose, lactose and sucrose to monosaccharides (glucose, fructose and galactose). Aminopeptidase and dipeptidase convert polypeptides to smaller peptides and amino acids.

Secretions from the liver and pancreas complete the process of chemical digestion. The pancreas produces insulin (a hormone necessary for the metabolism of carbohydrates, fats and proteins) and several enzymes that digest nutrients. Amylase converts starch to disaccharides. Trypsin and chymotrypsin convert proteins and polypeptides to smaller polypeptides. Lipase converts fats to glycerides and fatty acids. These pancreatic enzymes become active only after the inactive forms are secreted into the small intestine. For example, the enzyme enterokinase, secreted by the intestinal mucosal glands, is necessary for trypsinogen to be converted into trypsin. Otherwise, activated enzymes would digest the pancreas and pancreatic duct.

Another important aid in digestion and absorption in the small intestine is bile. Bile is produced in the liver and stored by the gallbladder. When fat enters the small intestine, the hormone cholecystokinin, which stimulates the gallbladder to release bile, is secreted by the intestinal mucosal glands. **Bile**, an emulsifying agent for fats that facilitates the digestion of fats by lipase, is necessary for the absorption of the fat-soluble vitamins A, D, E and K. Absence of bile causes increased amounts of ingested fat to appear in the faeces (steatorrhoea), as well as a deficiency of these vitamins.

Absorption

After digestion of the food is complete, the simplified nutrient end products—monosaccharides (glucose, fructose and galactose) from carbohydrates, fatty acids and glycerides from fats, and small peptides and amino acids from proteins—are ready for absorption. Vitamins and minerals are also released as a result of digestion. Water and electrolytes contribute to the fluid food mass that is finally absorbed.

The principal site for absorption of nutrients in the GI tract is the small intestine. The wall of the GI tract consists of folds and projections that are progressively smaller (Fig 25.1). These mucosal folds, villi and microvilli increase the inner surface area approximately 600 times over the outer serosa, yielding an extremely large surface for absorption.

The mucosal folds are elevated folds along the mucosa. The villi can be seen by light microscope and are small, finger-like projections covering the mucosal folds. The villi increase the surface area further. Each villus has a vascular supply, including venous and arterial capillaries and lacteals (lymphatic vessels in the small intestine that contain the substance chyle). The microvilli, numerous minute projections on the surface of each villus (visible by electron microscope), form the brush border.

The small intestine has several mechanisms of absorption, including passive diffusion, carrier-mediated diffusion, active energy-driven transport and engulfment. Passive diffusion (osmosis) occurs across the epithelial membrane in the direction from higher concentration to lower concentration. Carrier-mediated diffusion occurs as molecules are carried across the epithelial cells of microvilli by a molecule that serves as a vehicle. Large molecules must be combined with a smaller molecule to pass from a greater pressure gradient to a lesser one. For example, vitamin B_{12} requires intrinsic factor to be carried into the intestinal circulation.

In active energy-driven transport, nutrients require energy to be absorbed and to cross the intestinal epithelial membrane. This mechanism is referred to as a *pump*. The pump transports molecules across the membrane by means of energy supplied by the cell's metabolism. The sodium pump, which transports glucose, is an example of this mechanism.

Engulfment, or pinocytosis, is the process that allows large macromolecules to be absorbed by the epithelial cells of the villi. The epithelial cell engulfs the macromolecule and opens to allow the particle to enter the interior of the cell. The particle then enters the capillary blood. This mechanism transports some whole proteins and fat droplets.

After absorption by these mechanisms, the end products of carbohydrates and proteins are absorbed into the intestinal capillaries and enter the portal blood circulation of the liver, where further metabolic conversion occurs. The transfer of the end products of fat digestion is unique in that the fat molecules pass between the cells of the intestinal mucosa and into the lacteals of the villi. From there, they enter the larger lymph vessels and then the portal blood flow at the thoracic duct. Exceptions include the medium- and short-chain fatty acids, which can be absorbed directly into the blood circulation of the villi. Most of the fats commonly consumed are long-chain fatty acids, which are transported by way of the lacteals.

Fat-soluble vitamins are absorbed with digested fats in the presence of bile. Water-soluble vitamins, vitamin B complex and vitamin C are absorbed in the small intestine. Absorption of vitamin B_{12} takes place only in the ileum. The majority of water and electrolyte absorption also takes place in the small intestine.

The large intestine completes the process of absorption and functions primarily to absorb sodium and additional water. The remainder of the products of digestion passes into the large intestine through the ileocaecal valve. The muscular activity of the large intestine propels the mass forward. Most of the water and sodium are absorbed into the bloodstream in the proximal half of the colon. The colonic bacteria synthesise vitamin K, vitamin B_{12} and some of the vitamin B complex. Bacteria also affect the colour and odour of the stool and gas

PATHOPHYSIOLOGY REVIEW

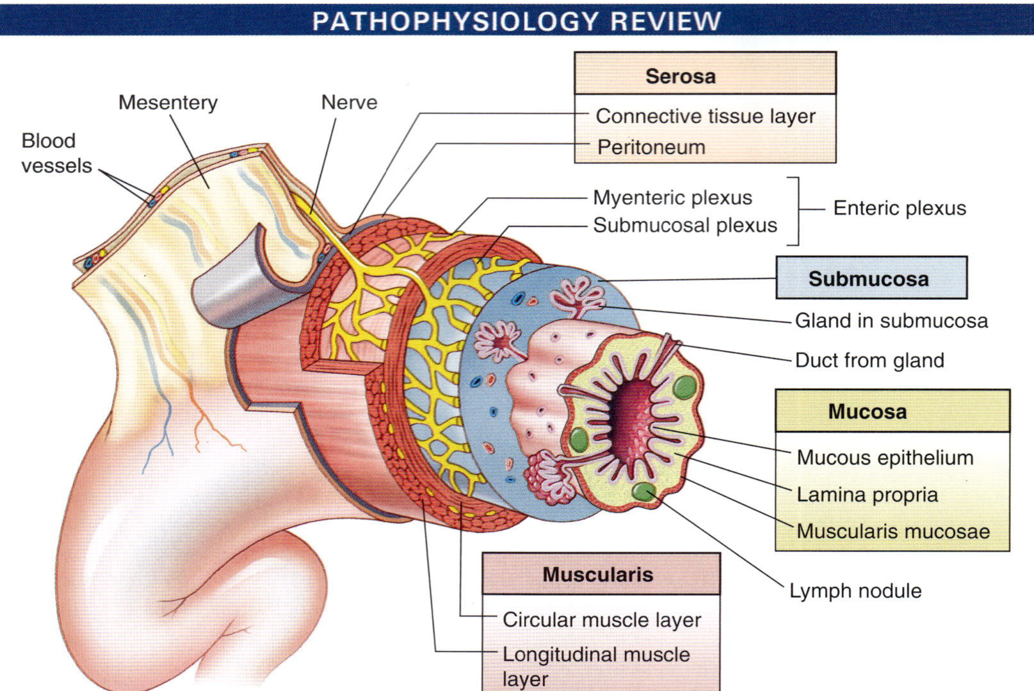

Fig 25.1 Wall of the gastrointestinal (GI) tract. The wall of the GI tract is made up of four layers with a network of nerves between the layers. Shown here is a generalised diagram of a segment of the GI tract. Note that the serosa is continuous with a fold of serous membrane called a *mesentery.* Note also that digestive glands may empty their products into the lumen of the GI tract by way of ducts. (Source; Patton, K. T., & Thibodeau, G. A. (2010). Anatomy and physiology (7th ed.). St Louis, MO: Mosby.)

formation. The odour is primarily caused by products of bacterial action and depends on the type of colonic flora and ingested food. Defects in digestion or absorption notably alter the odour and appearance of faeces. Colour is the result of bilirubin end products converted by bacteria to urobilinogen and then oxidised to urobilin (stercobilin). The faeces that are excreted consist of undigested residue, water, bacteria and mucus. Defecation occurs when the internal and external anal sphincters relax after distension of the rectum by faeces.

Assessment of Gastrointestinal Function

The most common consequences of GI disease in children include malabsorption, fluid and electrolyte disturbances, malnutrition and poor growth. (See Dehydration, Chapter 23, and Types of Diarrhoea later). A thorough GI assessment includes history questions, general observations, clinical examination and specific tests and procedures. The most important basic nursing assessments include measurement of intake and output, height and weight, abdominal examination and simple stool and urine tests.

Numerous clinical manifestations provide clues to specific GI problems (Box 25.2). Some cases involve only one manifestation, whereas others may involve several signs and symptoms as part of the disease complex or syndrome.

A number of tests assess GI function (Table 25.1). Nurses are often responsible for collecting specimens. (See Collection of Specimens, Chapter 22.)

GASTROINTESTINAL DISORDERS

Diarrhoea

Diarrhoea is a symptom that results from disorders involving digestive, absorptive and secretory functions. Diarrhoea is caused by abnormal intestinal water and electrolyte transport. Worldwide, there are an estimated 1.7 billion episodes of diarrhoea each year (Leung et al 2016).

Diarrhoea does not present as a health concern in the New Zealand Maternity Clinical Indicators 2018 report (Ministry of Health 2020) or in the Wai 2575 Māori Health Trends Report 2019 (Ministry of Health 2019). There is a decline in mortality and morbidity due to diarrhoea in Australia, particularly in rural and remote regions and within Aboriginal and Torres Strait Islander children in the last 10 years due to improvement in social determinants of health and access to healthcare via telehealth (Australian Institute of Health and Welfare [AIHW] 2018a).

Diarrhoea is caused by abnormal intestinal water and electrolyte transport. The transport of fluid and electrolytes in the developing GI tract is related to the child's age. The intestinal mucosa of the young infant is more permeable to water than that of an older child. Therefore, in young infants with increased intestinal luminal osmolality caused by diarrhoea, more fluid and electrolytes are lost than in older children (Box 25.3). Diarrhoea results from several pathophysiological processes.

Types of Diarrhoea

Diarrhoeal disturbances involve the stomach and intestines (gastroenteritis), the small intestine (enteritis), the colon (colitis) or the colon and intestines (enterocolitis). Diarrhoea is classified as acute or chronic.

Acute diarrhoea is defined as a sudden increase in frequency and a change in consistency of stools, often caused by an infectious agent in the GI tract (Box 25.4). It may be associated with upper respiratory or urinary tract infections, antibiotic therapy or laxative use. Acute diarrhoea is usually self-limited (4 days' duration) and subsides

BOX 25.2 Clinical Manifestations of Gastrointestinal Dysfunction in Children

Abdominal distension—Protuberant contour of the abdomen that may be caused by delayed gastric emptying, accumulation of gas or stool, inflammation or obstruction

Abdominal pain—Pain associated with the abdomen that may be localised or diffuse, acute or chronic; often caused by inflammation, obstruction or haemorrhage

Constipation—Passage of firm or hard stools or infrequent passage of stool with associated symptoms such as difficulty expelling the stools, blood-streaked stools and abdominal discomfort

Diarrhoea—Increase in the number of stools with increased water content as a result of alterations of water and electrolyte transport by the gastrointestinal (GI) tract; may be acute or chronic

Dysfunctional swallowing—Impaired swallowing resulting from central nervous system defects or structural defects of the oral cavity, pharynx, or oesophagus; can cause feeding problems or aspiration

Dysphagia—Difficulty swallowing caused by abnormalities in the neuromuscular function of the pharynx or upper oesophageal sphincter or by disorders of the oesophagus

Encopresis—Overflow of incontinent stool causing soiling; often caused by faecal retention or impaction

Faltering growth, failure to thrive—Deceleration from established growth pattern or consistently remaining below the 5th percentile for height and weight on standard growth charts; sometimes accompanied by developmental delays

Fever—Common manifestation of illness in children with GI disorders; usually associated with dehydration, infection or inflammation

Gastrointestinal bleeding—Bleeding from an upper or lower GI source; may be acute or chronic

Haematemesis—Vomiting of bright red blood or denatured blood that results from bleeding in the upper GI tract or from swallowed blood from the nose or oropharynx

Haematochezia—Passage of bright red blood per rectum, usually indicating lower GI tract bleeding

Hypoactive, hyperactive or absent bowel sounds—Evidence of intestinal motility problems that may be caused by inflammation or obstruction

Jaundice—Yellow colouration of the skin and sclerae associated with liver dysfunction

Melaena—Passage of dark-coloured, tarry stools caused by denatured blood, suggesting upper GI tract bleeding or bleeding from the right colon

Nausea—Unpleasant sensation vaguely referred to the throat or abdomen with an inclination to vomit

Projectile vomiting—Vomiting accompanied by vigorous peristaltic waves; typically associated with pyloric stenosis or pylorospasm

Vomiting or regurgitation—Passive transfer of gastric contents into the oesophagus or mouth

Vomiting—Forceful ejection of gastric contents; involves a complex process under central nervous system control that causes salivation, pallor, sweating and tachycardia; usually accompanied by nausea

without specific treatment. Acute infectious diarrhoea (infectious gastroenteritis) is caused by a variety of viral, bacterial and parasitic pathogens (Table 25.2).

Chronic diarrhoea is an increase in stool frequency and increased water content with duration of more than 14 days. It is often caused by chronic conditions such as malabsorption syndromes, inflammatory bowel disease (IBD), immunodeficiency, food allergy, lactose intolerance or chronic non-specific diarrhoea, or as a result of inadequate management of acute diarrhoea.

Intractable diarrhoea of infancy is a syndrome that occurs in the first few months of life, persists for longer than 2 weeks with no recognised pathogens and is refractory to treatment. The most common cause is acute infectious diarrhoea that was not managed adequately.

Chronic non-specific diarrhoea (CNSD), also known as *irritable colon of childhood* and *toddlers' diarrhoea*, is a common cause of chronic diarrhoea in children 6 to 54 months of age. These children have loose stools, often with undigested food particles, and diarrhoea lasting longer than 2 weeks' duration. Children with CNSD grow normally and have no evidence of malnutrition, no blood in their stool and no enteric infection. Poor dietary habits and food sensitivities have been linked to chronic diarrhoea. The excessive intake of juices and artificial sweeteners such as sorbitol, a substance found in many commercially prepared beverages and foods, may be a factor. Box 25.5 lists other factors that predispose patients to chronic diarrhoea.

Aetiology

Most pathogens that cause diarrhoea are spread by the faecal-oral route through contaminated food or water or are spread from person to person where there is close contact (e.g. day care centres). Lack of clean water, crowding, poor hygiene, nutritional deficiency and poor sanitation are major risk factors, especially for bacterial or parasitic pathogens. Infants are often more susceptible to frequent and severe bouts of diarrhoea because their immune system has not been exposed to many pathogens and has not acquired protective antibodies (Box 25.6). Worldwide, the most common causes of acute gastroenteritis are infectious agents, viruses, bacteria and parasites.

Rotavirus is the most important cause of serious gastroenteritis among children, with 28% of all cases causing fatality (Lamberti et al 2016). The virus is spread through the faecal-oral route or by person-to-person contact, and almost all children are infected with rotavirus at least once by the age of 5 years (Bass 2016).

Rotavirus is a common cause of severe gastroenteritis in infants and young children (AIHW 2018b). There were 426 hospital admissions for rotavirus in Australia in 2016. Almost half of these admissions were children under the age of 5 years. The main reason for the decline in admissions has been due to the introduction of the rotavirus vaccination on the National Immunisation Program in 2007. Hospitalisations in other age groups have also decreased, which has led to some suggestion that rotavirus vaccines may also provide some protective benefits for the population overall. Between 1997 and 2016, rotavirus was responsible for 16 deaths in Australia. All deaths were either in children aged 0–4 years or people aged over 70 years (AIHW 2018b).

Salmonella, Campylobacter and *Cryptosporidiosis* organisms are the most frequently isolated bacterial pathogens. These organisms are gram-negative bacteria and can be contracted through raw or undercooked food, contaminated food or water or through the faecal-oral route.

Pathophysiology

Invasion of the GI tract by pathogens results in increased intestinal secretion as a result of enterotoxins, cytotoxic mediators or decreased intestinal absorption secondary to intestinal damage or inflammation. Enteric pathogens attach to the mucosal cells and form a cuplike pedestal on which the bacteria rest. The pathogenesis of the diarrhoea depends on whether the organism remains attached to the cell surface,

TABLE 25.1 **Gastrointestinal Diagnostic Procedures**

Test	Description	Purpose	Comments
Stool examination	Gross, microscopic and chemical examination of stool specimen	To detect normal and abnormal constituents	Explain process for collecting samples. Fresh specimen is optimum.
Ova and parasites (O&P)	Microscopic examination of stool contents for parasites or their eggs	To aid in diagnosis of parasitic infections	Requires several fresh specimens placed in special preservative. Obtaining three samples improves probability of detection of organism.
Bacterial culture	Sample contents grown on culture medium	To detect bacterial pathogens in stool	Fresh specimen is important to improve probability of detection of organism. Serological tests determine presence of bacterial toxins.
Stool assay for vital pathogens	Enzyme-linked immunosorbent assay (ELISA)	To detect viral pathogens in stool	Standard ELISA test is available for detection of rotavirus and adenovirus.
Giardia antigen	ELISA	To detect presence of *Giardia* organisms	This is more sensitive than single stool for O&P.
Reducing substances	Unabsorbed sugars measured in stool (glucose, fructose, lactose, galactose and pentose)	To detect elevated levels of reducing substances in stool, which are abnormal and suggest carbohydrate malabsorption	This requires random fresh stool specimen delivered immediately to laboratory. Fermentation by bacteria can give false low level if stool is not tested immediately.
Occult blood guaiac test	Stool smeared on guaiac-impregnated paper, and 2 drops of developing solution added to reverse side; blue colour indicates haemoglobin	To detect presence of blood in stool	This is an easily and quickly measured screening test. Small amounts of blood (e.g. from bleeding mouth, gums, nose) may give positive results.
HELICOBACTER PYLORI TESTING			
Serology test	Blood test for antibody to *H. pylori* (anti-Hg IgG)	To assess for exposure to *H. pylori*	This test does not determine whether infection is acute or chronic.
C urea breath test	Collection of breath after ingestion of isotopic urea with either carbon 14 or carbon 13; measures labelled carbon dioxide in expired air	To determine if there is active infection with *H. pylori* in the stomach	This is one of the most accurate methods to determine *H. pylori* infection in children age 2 years or older. Carbon 13 is non-radioactive (preferred), and carbon 14 has low level of radioactivity.
RADIOGRAPHY			
Plain films	Anteroposterior and lateral radiographs of abdomen and pelvis	To detect foreign body or mass, reveal bowel gas patterns and detect obstruction or perforation in GI tract	Prepare family and child for study. No special physical preparation is required.
Contrast studies—upper GI and lower GI series	Radio-opaque media (barium or water-soluble contrast) or air swallowed or administered as enema	To assess structure and function of GI tract and to detect luminal defects, or masses	Barium enema sometimes requires cleansing enemas and oral cathartics before procedure. Contrast material may be given by nasogastric (NG) or gastrostomy tube. Contrast enemas may reduce intussusception. Prepare family and child for swallowing contrast media, NG tube insertion or enema. Encourage fluids after procedure.
Ultrasonography (sonography)	Measures and records reflection of pulsed or continuous high-frequency sound waves	To locate, measure and delineate abdominal organs	Prepare family and child for study. This is non-invasive, with no radiation involved. Doppler studies demonstrate presence and direction of blood flow; often require IV contrast material.
Computed tomography (CT)	Pinpoint x-ray directed on horizontal or vertical plane to provide series of 'cuts' or 'slices' that are fed into computer and assembled in image displays on video screen and transferred to permanent record	To visualise horizontal and vertical cross-section of abdomen at any axis To distinguish density of various tissue structure of organs To detect blunt trauma to internal organs and masses	Prepare family and child for study. CT is usually non-invasive, but may require oral or IV contrast material and may require sedation.
Magnetic resonance imaging (MRI)	Images formed by reemission of radio signals by atomic nuclei stimulated in magnetic field	To visualise internal body structures in any plane; permits soft tissue discrimination unavailable with many techniques	Prepare family and child for procedure. MRI is usually non-invasive, but may require oral or IV contrast material. MRI may require sedation for lengthy procedure. Patient remains NBM 3 to 4 hours before study; patient is immobilised and test takes a long time. MRI does not expose patient to ionising radiation. No magnetic material can be present in scanner.

TABLE 25.1 Gastrointestinal Diagnostic Procedures—cont'd

Test	Description	Purpose	Comments
		MANOMETRY	
Oesophagus	Multilumen catheter inserted into oesophagus, and water perfusion or solid state sensed by transducer and recorded	To evaluate dysphagia, oesophageal spasm, achalasia, dysmotility	Teach and prepare child and family before procedure. Patient remains NBM 6 to 8 hours before procedure. Patient cooperation is required.
		BIOPSY	
Liver	Removal of small piece of living tissue for microscopic examination by needle or surgically General sedation or local anaesthesia used	To evaluate for biliary obstruction, hepatitis, metabolic disease To assess response to treatment interventions	Teach and prepare patient and family before procedure. Preliminary laboratory studies are needed. Liver biopsy is contraindicated with prolonged bleeding or clotting times, anaemia, infection or obstructive jaundice.
Oesophagus, stomach, intestine	Small sample of mucosal tissue taken for microscopic evaluation	To evaluate for infection, inflammation, mucosal abnormalities	Teach and prepare patient and family before procedure. This biopsy requires conscious or general sedation. It is usually obtained with endoscopy.
		ENDOSCOPY	
Upper GI, colonoscopy, flexible sigmoidoscopy, anoscopy	Endoscope introduced into area to be examined Endoscope has flexible-tip light source and aspiration and instrument channel	To directly visualise GI tract to evaluate abnormalities, detect lesions, obtain biopsies To perform therapeutic procedures—polypectomies, removal of foreign bodies, sclerotherapy of oesophageal varices, placement of feeding tubes or percutaneous catheters	Teach and prepare patient and family before procedure. Patient remains NBM 4–8 hours before procedure. Lower GI requires bowel cleansing. Patient requires conscious or general sedation.
Breath hydrogen test	Non-invasive study to assess for carbohydrate intolerance Hydrogen generated in colon by bacterial fermentation of undigested carbohydrates and then absorbed into blood, where it diffuses into expired air via lungs	To evaluate for bacterial overgrowth, lactase or sucrase-isomaltase deficiency To evaluate for malabsorption or bacterial overgrowth by detecting rise in expired hydrogen after oral loading with specific carbohydrate	Teach and prepare patient and family before procedure. Patient remains NBM 12 hours before test. Previous night's dinner should consist of meat, rice and water; avoid other starches. Antibiotics may reduce hydrogen levels.
d-xylose absorption test	d-Xylose solution administered orally; serum levels of d-xylose measured at 30, 60, 90 and 120 minutes Urine collected for total of 5 hours to measure d-xylose excretion	To evaluate absorptive capacity of small intestinal mucosa To diagnose small bowel malabsorption caused by coeliac disease	Teach and prepare patient and family before procedure. Patient remains NBM 4–8 hours before test. Test is used less often, largely replaced by endoscopic biopsies to evaluate for villous atrophy.
Hepatobiliary scintigraphy	Nuclear medicine study Radiopharmaceutical administered intravenously, then sequential images of liver, biliary system and bowel obtained	To evaluate conditions of liver and biliary tract abnormalities and gallbladder disease To aid in diagnosis and monitoring of these conditions, such as biliary atresia	Prepare family and child for study. Images may be obtained for up to 24 hours if excretion is delayed.

GOR, Gastroesophageal reflux; *GI*, gastrointestinal; *NBM*, nil by mouth.

resulting in a secretory toxin (non-invasive, toxin-producing, non-inflammatory-type diarrhoea) or penetrates the mucosa (systemic diarrhoea). Non-inflammatory diarrhoea is the most common diarrhoeal illness, resulting from the action of enterotoxin that is released after attachment to the mucosa. The most serious and immediate physiological disturbances associated with severe diarrhoeal disease are dehydration, acid–base imbalance with acidosis and shock that occurs when dehydration progresses to the point that circulatory status is seriously impaired.

Diagnostic evaluation

Evaluation of the child with acute gastroenteritis begins with a careful history that seeks to discover the possible cause of diarrhoea, to assess the severity of symptoms and the risk of complications and to elicit information about current symptoms indicating other treatable illnesses that could be causing the diarrhoea. The history should include questions about recent travel, exposure to untreated drinking or washing water sources, contact with animals or birds, day care centre attendance, recent treatment with antibiotics or recent diet changes. History

BOX 25.3 Consequences of Fluid and Electrolyte Loss

Dehydration

- Voluminous losses of fluid in frequent, watery stools
- Losses when there is also vomiting
- Reduced fluid intake resulting from nausea or anorexia
- Increased insensible losses from fever, hyperpnoea and, sometimes, high environmental temperature
- Continued (although diminished) obligatory renal losses

Electrolyte Imbalance

- Losses of sodium, chloride, potassium and, in some cases, bicarbonate
- Inadequate replacement of electrolytes when hypotonic or hypertonic solutions are used

Metabolic Acidosis

- Increased absorption of short-chain fatty acids produced in the colon from bacterial fermentation of unabsorbed dietary carbohydrates
- Accumulation of lactic acid from tissue hypoxia secondary to hypovolaemia
- Loss of bicarbonate in stools
- Ketosis from fat metabolism when glycogen stores are depleted in untreated diarrhoeal dehydration or inadequate carbohydrate intake; may result in malnutrition

BOX 25.4 Causes of Acute Diarrhoea

Infection and Parasitic Infestation

Bacteria—*Salmonella, Shigella, Campylobacter, Escherichia coli, Yersinia, Aeromonas, Clostridium difficile, Staphylococcus aureus*

Viruses—Rotavirus, norovirus, small and round viruses, adenovirus, pestivirus, astrovirus, parvovirus

Parasites—*Giardia lamblia, Cryptosporidium, Cystoisospora belli, Microsporidia, Strongyloides, Entamoeba histolytica*

Associated Conditions

- Upper respiratory tract infections
- Urinary tract infections
- Otitis media

Dietary Causes

- Overfeeding
- Introduction of new foods
- Reinstituting milk too soon after diarrhoeal episode
- Osmotic diarrhoea from excess sugar in formula or juice
- Excessive ingestion of sorbitol or fructose

Medications

- Antibiotics
- Laxatives

Toxic Causes

Ingestion of:

- heavy metals (arsenic, lead, mercury)
- organic phosphates

Functional Causes

- Irritable bowel syndrome

Other Causes

- Pseudomembranous enterocolitis
- Hirschsprung's enterocolitis

questions should also explore the presence of other symptoms such as fever and vomiting, frequency and character of stools (e.g. watery, bloody), urinary output, dietary habits and recent food intake.

Extensive laboratory evaluation is not indicated in children who have uncomplicated diarrhoea and no evidence of dehydration because most diarrhoeal illnesses are self-limiting. Laboratory tests are indicated for children who are severely dehydrated and receiving intravenous (IV) therapy. Watery, explosive stools suggest glucose intolerance; foul-smelling, greasy, bulky stools suggest fat malabsorption. Diarrhoea that develops after the introduction of cow's milk, fruits or cereal may be related to enzyme deficiency or protein intolerance. Neutrophils or red blood cells in the stool indicate bacterial gastroenteritis or IBD. The presence of eosinophils suggests protein intolerance or parasitic infection. Gross blood or occult blood may indicate pathogens such as *Shigella*, *Campylobacter* or haemorrhagic *Escherichia coli* strains. Stool culture testing and/or viral testing is recommended for any infant or child who presents with bloody diarrhoea, watery diarrhoea with or without being febrile (rotavirus) and persistent diarrhoea and/or vomiting. It is also recommended for infants who present unwell to collect a stool specimen due to spikes in *Campylobacter* (The Royal Children's Hospital Melbourne [RCHM] 2020b). For travellers presenting with prolonged symptoms $>$ 10 days or for the immunocompromised patient who is febrile it is also recommended that stool cultures are collected (RCHM 2020b).

Determine urine specific gravity if dehydration is suspected. Obtain a full blood count, serum electrolytes, creatinine and blood urea nitrogen (BUN) in the child who has moderate to severe dehydration or who requires hospitalisation. The haemoglobin, haematocrit, creatinine and BUN levels are usually elevated in acute diarrhoea and should normalise with rehydration.

Therapeutic Management

The major goals in the management of acute diarrhoea include assessment of fluid and electrolyte imbalance, rehydration, maintenance fluid therapy and reintroduction of an adequate diet. Treat infants and children with acute diarrhoea and dehydration first with **oral rehydration therapy (ORT)**. ORT is one of the major worldwide healthcare advances. It is more effective, safer, less painful and less costly than IV rehydration. **Oral rehydration solutions (ORSs)** enhance and promote the reabsorption of sodium and water. These solutions greatly reduce vomiting, duration of illness and the need for IV infusions (Dekate et al 2013). Oral rehydration solutions (ORSs) enhance and promote the reabsorption of sodium and water. Refer to Box 25.7 for further information.

Early reintroduction of nutrients is desirable and has gained more widespread acceptance. Continued feeding or early reintroduction of a normal diet after rehydration has no adverse effects and actually lessens the severity and duration of the illness and improves weight gain when compared with the gradual reintroduction of foods (Bhutta 2016). Infants who are breastfeeding should continue to do so, and ORS should be used to replace ongoing losses in these infants. Formula-fed infants should resume their formula; if it is not tolerated, a lactose-free formula may be used for a few days. In toddlers there is no contraindication to continuing soft or pureed foods. In older children a regular diet, including milk, can generally be offered after rehydration has been achieved. In cases of severe dehydration and shock, IV fluids are initiated whenever the child is unable to ingest sufficient amounts of fluid

TABLE 25.2 **Infectious Causes of Acute Diarrhoea**

Agents	Pathology	Characteristics	Comments
		VIRAL	
Rotavirus Incubation—48 hours Diagnosis—EIA	Faecal-oral transmission 8 groups (A–H)—Most group A virus replicates in mature villus epithelial cells of small intestine; leads to (1) imbalance in ratio of intestinal fluid absorption to secretion and (2) malabsorption of complex carbohydrates	Mild to moderate fever Vomiting followed by onset of watery stools Fever and vomiting generally abate in approximately 2 days, but diarrhoea persists 5–7 days	Most common cause of diarrhoea in children < 5 years old; infants 6–12 months old most vulnerable; affects all ages; usually milder in children > 3 years old Immunocompromised children at greater risk for complications Peak occurrences in winter months Important cause of nosocomial infections
Norovirus Incubation—12–48 hours Diagnosis—PCR assays	Faecal-oral; contaminated water Pathology similar to that of rotavirus; affects villus epithelial cells of small intestine, leading to (1) imbalance in ratio of intestinal fluid absorption to secretion and (2) malabsorption of complex carbohydrates	Abdominal cramps, nausea, vomiting, malaise, low-grade fever, watery diarrhoea without blood; duration 2–3 days; tends to resemble so-called food poisoning symptoms with nausea predominating	Affects all ages Multiple strains often named for the location of outbreak (e.g. Norwalk, Sapporo, Snow Mountain, Montgomery)
		BACTERIAL	
Escherichia coli Incubation—3–4 days; variable depending on strain Diagnosis—Sorbitol MacConkey (SMAC) agar positive for blood, but faecal leucocytes absent or rare	*E. coli* strains produce diarrhoea as result of enterotoxin production, adherence or invasion (enterotoxigenic-producing *E. coli*, enterohaemorrhagic *E. coli*, enteroaggregative *E. coli*)	Watery diarrhoea 1 to 2 days, then severe abdominal cramping and bloody diarrhoea Can progress to haemolytic uraemic syndrome	Food-borne pathogen Traveller's diarrhoea Cause of nursery epidemics Symptomatic treatment Antibiotics may worsen course Avoid antimotility agents and opioids
***Salmonella* groups** (non-typhoidal) Gram-negative rods, non-encapsulated non-sporulating Incubation—6–72 hours Diagnosis—Gram stain, stool culture	Invasion of mucosa in the small and large intestine, oedema of the lamina propria, focal acute inflammation with disruption of the mucosa and micro-abscesses	Nausea, vomiting, colicky abdominal pain, bloody diarrhoea, fever; symptoms variable (mild to severe) May have headache and cerebral manifestations (e.g. drowsiness confusion, meningismus, seizures) Infants may be afebrile and non-toxic May result in life-threatening septicaemia and meningitis Nausea and vomiting typically of short duration; diarrhoea may persist as long as 2–3 weeks Typically shed virus for average of 5 weeks; cases reported up to 1 year	Incidence highest in summer months; food-borne outbreaks common Usually transmitted person to person but may transmit via undercooked meats or poultry; about half the cases caused by poultry and poultry products In children, related to pets (e.g. dogs, cats) Communicable as long as organisms are excreted Antibiotics not recommended in uncomplicated cases Antimotility agents also not recommended—prolong transit time and carrier state
Salmonella typhi Produces enteric fever—systemic syndrome Incubation—usually 7–14 days, but could be 3–30 days, depending on size of inoculum Diagnosis—positive blood cultures; also sometimes positive stool and urine cultures Late stage—positive bone marrow culture	Bloodstream invasion; after ingestion, organism attaches to microvilli of ileal brush borders and bacteria invade the intestinal epithelium via Peyer's patches Next, organism is transported to intestinal lymph nodes and enters bloodstream via thoracic ducts, and circulating organism reaches reticuloendothelial cells, causing bacteraemia	Manifestations dependent on age Abdominal pain, diarrhoea, nausea, vomiting, high fever, lethargy Must be treated with antibiotics	Incidence much lower in developed countries Ingestion of foods and water contaminated with human faeces is most common mode of transmission Congenital and intrapartum transmission possible
***Shigella* groups** Gram-negative non-motile anaerobic bacilli Incubation—1–7 days Diagnosis—stool culture loaded with polymorphonuclear leucocytes	Enterotoxins—invade the epithelium with superficial mucosal ulcerations	Children appear sick Symptoms begin with fever, fatigue, anorexia Crampy abdominal pain preceding watery or bloody diarrhoea Symptoms usually subside in 5–10 days	Most cases in children younger than 9 years old, with about one-third of cases in children ages 1–4 weeks old Antibiotics shorten illness and lower mortality All patients at risk for dehydration Acute symptoms may persist for ≤ 1 week

Continued

TABLE 25.2 **Infectious Causes of Acute Diarrhoea—cont'd**

Agents	Pathology	Characteristics	Comments
			Antidiarrhoeal medications not recommended because they may predispose patient to toxic megacolon
Campylobacter jejuni Microaerophilic, motile, gram-negative bacilli Incubation—1–7 days Ability to cause illness appears dose related Diagnosis—stool culture, sometimes blood culture Commonly found in GI tract of wild or domestic animals	Not fully understood, possibly (1) adherence to intestinal mucosa by toxin, (2) invasion of the mucosa in the terminal ileum and colon, (3) translocation in which the organisms penetrate the mucosa and replicate in the lamina propria	Fever, abdominal pain, diarrhoea that can be bloody, vomiting Watery, profuse, foul-smelling diarrhoea Clinically similar to infection by *Salmonella* or *Shigella* organisms Faecal-oral transmission	Most infections in humans relate to consumption of contaminated foods or water, such as undercooked meats, particularly chicken Also acquired from contaminated household pets (e.g. dogs, cats) Bimodal peaks in infants < 1 year old and again at ages 15–29 years old Antibiotics do not prolong the carriage of bacteria and may eliminate organism more quickly Ceftazidime may be used if severe with caution in children over 4 years IV. Antimotility agents not recommended because they tend to prolong symptoms
Vibrio cholerae Gram-negative, motile, curved bacillus living in bodies of salt water Incubation—1–3 days Diagnosis—stool culture	Enters via oral route in contaminated food or water; if survives acid stomach environment, travels to the small intestine, adheres to the mucosa and produces toxin	Onset abrupt; vomiting, watery diarrhoea without cramping or tenesmus Dehydration can occur quickly	More prevalent in developing countries Rehydration most important treatment Antibiotics can shorten diarrhoea Despite continued efforts, still no vaccine
Clostridium difficile Gram-positive anaerobic bacillus with the ability to produce spores Diagnosis—by detecting *C. difficile* toxin in stool culture	Produces two important toxins (A and B) Toxin binds to the enterocyte surface receptor, resulting in alteration permeability, protein synthesis and direct cytotoxicity	Mostly mild watery diarrhoea lasting a few days Some prolonged diarrhoea and illness May cause pseudomembranous colitis Some individuals extremely ill with high fever, leucocytosis, hypoalbuminaemia	Associated with alteration of normal intestinal flora by antibiotics Adults tend to have more severe symptoms than children Treatment with antibiotics (metronidazole) in mildly to moderately symptomatic patients; for non-responders, give vancomycin Resistant strains have developed Relapse common
Clostridium perfringens Anaerobic, gram-positive, spore-producing bacilli Incubation—8–24 hours	Toxins produced in the intestine after ingestion of organism	Acute onset—watery diarrhoea, crampy abdominal pain Fever, nausea and vomiting are rare Duration of illness usually 24 hours	Transmitted by contaminated food products, most often meats and poultry Usually self-limiting and medical intervention not needed Oral rehydration usually sufficient Antibiotics serve no purpose and should not be used
Clostridium botulinum Gram-positive anaerobic spore-producing bacilli Incubation—12–26 hours (range, 6 hours to 8 days) Diagnosis—To detect toxin, submit blood and stool culture to special laboratory (usually state health department)	Botulism caused by binding of toxin to the neuromuscular junction	Clinical presentation related to age and the strain of the botulism GI—abdominal pain, cramping and diarrhoea Other strains—respiratory compromise, CNS symptoms	Transmitted in contaminated food products Can be acquired via wound infection Treatment is supportive care and neutralisation of the toxin
Staphylococcus organisms Gram-positive, non-motile, aerobic or facultative anaerobic bacteria Incubation—generally short, 1–8 hours Diagnosis—identify organism in food, blood, pus, aspirate	Direct tissue invasion and production of toxin	Clinical presentation dependent on site of entry In food poisoning, profuse diarrhoea, nausea and vomiting	Transmitted in inadequately cooked or refrigerated foods Self-limiting Symptomatic treatment

CNS, Central nervous system; *EIA*, enzyme immunoassay; *ELISA*, enzyme-linked immunosorbent assay; *GI*, gastrointestinal; *PCR*, polymerase chain reaction.

BOX 25.5 Factors That Predispose to Diarrhoea

Age—As a rule, the younger the child, the greater the susceptibility and the more severe the diarrhoea. Diarrhoea occurs more commonly in infancy, is a lesser threat in early childhood and usually constitutes only a minor problem in older children.

Impaired health—Malnourished or immunocompromised children are more susceptible and tend to have more severe diarrhoea.

Environment—Diarrhoea occurs with greater frequency where there is crowding, substandard sanitation, poor facilities for preparation and refrigeration of food and generally inadequate healthcare education. The frequency of diarrhoea in infancy is closely related to the ingestion of contaminated milk; breastfed infants have a lower incidence of diarrhoea.

BOX 25.6 Causes of Chronic Diarrhoea

Malabsorptive Causes
- Coeliac disease
- Pancreatic insufficiency (cystic fibrosis, chronic pancreatitis, Shwachman syndrome)
- Short bowel syndrome
- Lactose intolerance
- Congenital enzyme deficiency (sucrase-isomaltase deficiency)

Allergic Causes
- Allergic gastroenteropathy
- Eosinophilic gastroenteritis

Immunodeficiency
- Acquired hypoglobulinaemia
- Wiskott-Aldrich syndrome
- Agammaglobulinaemia
- Severe combined immunodeficiency disease
- Thymic hypoplasia
- Selective immunoglobulin A deficiency
- Human immunodeficiency virus or acquired immunodeficiency syndrome

Inflammatory Bowel Disease
- Ulcerative colitis
- Crohn's disease

Endocrine Causes
- Hyperthyroidism
- Congenital adrenal hyperplasia
- Addison's disease

Motility Disorders
- Hirschsprung's disease
- Intestinal pseudo-obstruction

Parasitic Infestations
- *Ascaris* organisms
- *Giardia* organisms

Other Causes
- Radiation enteritis
- Protein-losing enteropathy (Ménétrier's disease, intestinal lymphangiectasia)
- Abdominal tumours

BOX 25.7 Fluid Replacement Recommendations

Oral Fluids for Gastroenteritis
- Most children with mild/no dehydration can be discharged without a trial of fluids after appropriate advice and follow-up arranged.
- **Aim for 10 to 20 mL/kg fluid over 1 hour of ORS;** give frequent small amounts.
- Significant ongoing GI losses (frequent vomiting or profuse diarrhoea) minimises the chance of success at home.
- Consider early NGT rehydration in these children.

Nasogastric Rehydration (NGTR)
- Nasogastric rehydration is a safe and effective way of rehydrating most children with moderate dehydration, even if the child is vomiting. It is preferred over the IV route.
- **Most children stop vomiting after NGT fluids are started.** If vomiting continues, consider ondansetron and slow NG fluids temporarily.
- Use ORS (e.g. Gastrolyte, Hydralyte).
- **This is not applicable to children with dehydration from respiratory illnesses (e.g. bronchiolitis or with hypernatraemia who require a tailored rehydration plan)**

Rapid Nasogastric Rehydration
- 25 mL/kg/hr for 4 hours
- Suitable for the majority of patients with gastroenteritis and **moderate dehydration** (see indications for 'slower' NGR and indications for IV rehydration below; **avoid in infants < 6 months**)

Source: The Royal Children's Hospital (2020) Clinical Practice Guidelines. Gastroenteritis. Assessment and Management. https://www.rch.org.au/clinicalguide/guideline_index/Gastroenteritis/

and electrolytes to: (1) meet ongoing daily physiological losses; (2) replace previous deficits; and (3) replace ongoing abnormal losses. Patients who usually require IV fluids are those with severe dehydration, uncontrollable vomiting, inability to drink for any reason (e.g. extreme fatigue, coma) and severe gastric distension.

Select the IV solution on the basis of what is known regarding the probable type and cause of the dehydration. The type of fluid normally used is a saline solution containing 5% glucose in water. Although the initial phase of fluid replacement is rapid in both isotonic and hypotonic dehydration, rapid replacement is contraindicated in hypertonic dehydration because of the risk of water intoxication (RCHM 2020a).

After the severe effects of dehydration are under control, begin specific diagnostic and therapeutic measures to detect and treat the cause of the diarrhoea. Because of the self-limiting nature of vomiting and its tendency to improve when dehydration is corrected, the use of antiemetic agents is usually not needed; however, ondansetron has few side effects and may be administered if vomiting persists and interferes with ORT (Bhutta 2016).

The use of antibiotic therapy in children with acute gastroenteritis is controversial. Antibiotics may shorten the course of some diarrhoeal illnesses (e.g. those caused by *Shigella* organisms). However, most bacterial diarrhoeas are self-limiting, and the diarrhoea often resolves before the causative organism can be determined. Antibiotics may prolong the carrier period for bacteria such as *Salmonella*. Antibiotics may be considered, however, in patients who are less than 3 months of age or on immunosuppressive medication, or who have clinical signs of shock, severe malnutrition, dysentery, suspected cholera or suspected giardiasis (Wen et al 2017). (See Intestinal Parasitic Diseases, Chapter 6.)

Nursing Care Management

The management of most cases of acute diarrhoea takes place in the home with education of the caregiver. Teach caregivers to monitor for signs of dehydration (especially the number of wet nappies or voidings) and the amount of fluids taken by mouth, and to assess the frequency and amount of stool losses. Education relating to ORT, including the administration of maintenance fluids and replacement of ongoing losses, is important. ORS should be administered in small quantities at frequent intervals. Vomiting is not a contraindication to ORT unless it is severe. Information concerning the introduction of a normal diet is essential. Parents need to know that a slightly higher stool output initially occurs with continuation of a normal diet and with ongoing replacement of stool losses. The benefits of a better nutritional outcome with fewer complications and a shorter duration of illness outweigh the potential increase in stool frequency. Address parents' concerns to ensure adherence to the treatment plan.

If the child with acute diarrhoea and dehydration is hospitalised, the nurse must obtain an accurate weight and carefully monitor intake and output. The child may be placed on parenteral fluid therapy with nil by mouth (NBM) for 12 to 48 hours. Monitoring the IV infusion is an important nursing function. The nurse must ensure that the correct fluid and electrolyte concentration is infused, that the flow rate is adjusted to deliver the desired volume in a given time and that the IV site is maintained.

Accurate measurement of output is essential to determine whether renal blood flow is sufficient to permit the addition of potassium to the IV fluids. The nurse is responsible for examination of stools and collection of specimens for laboratory examination. (See Collection of Specimens, Chapter 22.)

Constipation

Constipation is an alteration in the frequency, consistency or ease of passing stool. It is defined as unsatisfactory defecation due to infrequent stools, difficult stool passage or perceived incomplete defecation (Bruce et al 2016). Constipation is an alteration in the frequency, consistency or ease of passing stool. The frequency of bowel movements varies by age, but children 4 years and older can be diagnosed with constipation if they have less than three stools per week (Poddar 2016). Constipation is often associated with painful bowel movements, blood-streaked or retained stool, abdominal pain, lack of appetite and stool incontinence (i.e. soiling) (Bruce et al 2016). Having extremely long intervals between defecation is **obstipation**. Constipation with faecal soiling is **encopresis**.

The majority of children have **idiopathic** or **functional constipation** because no underlying cause can be identified. Chronic constipation may occur as a result of environmental or psychosocial factors, or a combination of both. Transient illness, withholding and avoidance secondary to painful or negative experiences with stooling, and dietary intake with decreased fluid and fibre all play a role in the aetiology of constipation.

Newborn Period

Normally, newborn infants pass a first meconium stool within 24 to 36 hours of birth. Any newborn that does not do so should be assessed for evidence of intestinal atresia or stenosis, Hirschsprung's disease (HD), hypothyroidism, meconium plug or meconium ileus. A **meconium plug** is caused by meconium that has reduced water content and is usually evacuated after digital examination but may require irrigations with a hypertonic solution or contrast medium. **Meconium ileus**, the initial manifestation of cystic fibrosis, is the luminal obstruction of the distal small intestine by abnormal meconium. Treatment is the same as for a meconium plug; early surgical intervention may be needed to evacuate the small intestine.

Infancy

The onset of constipation frequently occurs during infancy and may result from organic causes such as HD, hypothyroidism and strictures. It is important to differentiate these conditions from functional constipation. Constipation in infancy is often related to dietary practices. It is less common in breastfed infants, who have softer stools than bottle-fed infants. Breastfed infants may also have decreased stools because of more complete use of breast milk with little residue.

Childhood

Most constipation in early childhood is due to environmental changes or normal development when a child begins to attain control over bodily functions. A child who has experienced discomfort during bowel movements may deliberately try to withhold stool. Over time, the rectum accommodates to the accumulation of stool and the urge to defecate passes. When the bowel contents are ultimately evacuated, the accumulated faeces are passed with pain, thus reinforcing the desire to withhold stool.

Constipation in school-age children may represent an ongoing problem or a first-time event. The onset of constipation at this age is often the result of environmental changes, stresses and changes in toileting patterns. A common cause of new-onset constipation at school entry is fear of using the school bathrooms, which are noted for their lack of privacy. Early and hurried departure for school immediately after breakfast may also impede bathroom use.

Therapeutic Management

Treatment of constipation depends on the cause and duration of symptoms. A complete history and physical examination are essential to determine appropriate management. It may be necessary to facilitate passage of the obstruction by irrigation with a hypertonic solution or water-soluble enema. If the constipation is due to HD, surgical treatment may include resection of the intestine and saline irrigations.

Management of the infant should include education of the parents concerning normal bowel habits. Short, transient periods of constipation usually require no intervention. Mild constipation usually resolves as solid food is introduced into the diet. Stool softeners such as malt extract or lactulose may be used for hard stools or anal fissures.

The management of simple constipation consists of a plan to promote regular bowel movements. Often this is as simple as changing the diet to provide more fibre and fluids, eliminating foods known to be constipating and establishing a bowel routine that allows for regular passage of stool. Stool-softening agents may also be helpful.

Management of chronic constipation requires an organised and ongoing approach. It is important for families to realise that it usually requires months or years to resolve, and relapse is common. The goals for management include restoring regular evacuation of stool, shrinking the distended rectum to its normal size and promoting a regular toileting routine.

Nursing Care Management

Unfortunately, constipation tends to be self-perpetuating. A child who has difficulty or discomfort when attempting to evacuate the bowels has a tendency to retain the bowel contents, and thus constipation becomes a chronic problem. Nursing assessment begins with a history of bowel habits; diet; events that may be associated with the onset of constipation; drugs or other substances that the child may be taking; and the consistency, colour, frequency and other characteristics of the stool. If there is no evidence of a pathological condition that requires further investigation, the nurse's major task is to educate the parents regarding normal stool patterns and to participate in the education and treatment of the child.

Parents need reassurance concerning the prognosis for establishing normal bowel habits. Many parents are concerned about constipation and view the condition as dangerous. Families need thorough instructions about the treatment plan. If the child needs enemas or medication, give the family the appropriate instructions. It is important to discuss attitudes and expectations regarding toilet habits and the treatment plan.

Vomiting

Vomiting is the forceful ejection of gastric contents through the mouth. It is a well-defined, complex, coordinated process that is under central nervous system control and is often accompanied by nausea and retching. In contrast, regurgitation is a simpler, more passive and effortless phenomenon. Vomiting has many causes, including acute infectious diseases, increased intracranial pressure, toxic ingestions, food intolerances and allergies, mechanical obstruction of the GI tract, adrenal insufficiency, nephrological disease, pregnancy and psychogenic problems (Sreedharan & Liacouras 2016). Vomiting is common in childhood, is usually self-limiting and requires no specific treatment. However, complications can occur in children, including acute fluid volume loss (dehydration) and electrolyte disturbances, malnutrition, aspiration and Mallory-Weiss syndrome (small tears in the distal oesophageal mucosa).

Aetiology

The child's age, pattern of vomiting and duration of symptoms help determine the cause. The colour and consistency of the emesis vary according to the cause. Green, bilious vomiting suggests bowel obstruction. Curdled stomach contents, mucus or fatty foods that are vomited several hours after ingestion suggest poor gastric emptying or high intestinal obstruction. Gastric irritation by certain medicines, foods or toxic substances may cause vomiting. Forceful vomiting is associated with pyloric stenosis.

Associated symptoms also help identify the cause. Fever and diarrhoea accompanying vomiting suggest an infection. Constipation associated with vomiting suggests an anatomical or functional obstruction. Localised abdominal pain and vomiting often occur with appendicitis, pancreatitis or peptic ulcer disease. A change in the level of consciousness or a headache associated with vomiting indicates a central nervous system or metabolic disorder.

Pathophysiology

The act of vomiting, including nausea and retching, is under the control of the central nervous system. Two areas of the medulla are involved as the vomiting centre. The medullary centre is also activated by impulses from a second centre, the chemoreceptor trigger zone, which is located in the floor of the fourth ventricle (Table 25.3). **Nausea** is a sensation that may be induced by visceral, labyrinthine (inner ear) or emotional stimuli. It is characterised by the desire to vomit, with discomfort felt in the throat or abdomen. Nausea is often associated with autonomic symptoms such as salivation, pallor, sweating and tachycardia. Retching may occur with or without vomiting. **Retching** involves a series of spasmodic movements during inspiration, creating a negative intrathoracic pressure and contraction of the abdominal muscles. Projectile vomiting is preceded and accompanied by vigorous peristaltic waves.

Vomiting is a well-recognised response to psychological stress. During stress, adrenaline levels rise and may stimulate the chemoreceptor trigger zone. Nausea and vomiting are likely to be a protective mechanism to remove toxins from the system. Vomiting may follow GI infection or toxic ingestion, or it can be a learned behavioural response.

TABLE 25.3 Symptoms and Signs Associated with Possible Diagnoses of Vomiting

Nature of Vomiting	Differential Diagnoses
Bilious	GIT obstruction
Blood	Swallowed blood (e.g. epistaxis, or in neonate from maternal blood due to delivery or nipple trauma) Upper GI haemorrhage
Projectile	Pyloric stenosis
Early morning vomiting	Raised ICP
ASSOCIATED SIGNS AND SYMPTOMS	
Evidence of diarrhoea	Gastroenteritis
Fever or systemic illness	Infection or sepsis
Abdominal distension and tenderness, 'tinkling'/absence of bowel sounds	GIT obstruction
Headache	Migraine Intracranial pathology (i.e. raised ICP) Infection
Rectal bleeding	Gastroenteritis Colitis Intussusception Meckel's diverticulum
OTHER	
Previous history of head injury/NAI	Intracranial bleeding
Previous history of previous GIT obstruction or surgery	GIT obstruction
Other factors such as toxin ingestion/drug use, eating disorder, pregnancy	

GIT, gastrointestinal; *ICP*, intracranial pressure; *NAI*, non-accidental head injury.
Source: The Royal Children's Hospital Melbourne. (2020). Clinical Practice Guidelines. Vomiting. Assessment, History. Symptoms and signs associated with possible diagnoses. https://www.rch.org.au/clinicalguide/guideline_index/Vomiting/

Diagnostic Evaluation

The diagnostic evaluation includes a thorough history and physical examination. The description of the vomitus; relationship to meals or specific foods; behaviour; and presence of pain, constipation, diarrhoea or jaundice are important components of the history. Physical examination should include an assessment of the hydration status and an abdominal examination.

Further evaluation may include analysis of urine for protein or blood, serum electrolytes and radiographic studies. A plain radiograph of the chest or abdomen or ultrasonography may reveal anatomical abnormalities. Brain scans are used when tumours are considered. Endoscopy of the upper GI tract may be a valuable diagnostic procedure if the provider suspects oesophagitis. Self-induced vomiting and rumination may be a self-stimulation or gratification activity.

Therapeutic Management

Management is directed towards detection and treatment of the cause of the vomiting and prevention of complications, such as dehydration and malnutrition. Vomiting is often a symptom of a common infectious illness that is self-limiting and resolves with no specific treatment. Further investigation is indicated if there is dehydration, progressively severe vomiting or persistent vomiting for more than 24 hours, or if the history and physical examination fail to suggest a diagnosis. If vomiting leads to dehydration, oral rehydration or parenteral fluids may be required.

Antiemetic drugs may be indicated when the child is not able to tolerate anything orally or in the cases of postoperative vomiting, chemotherapy-induced vomiting, cyclic vomiting syndrome or acute motion sickness (Sreedharan & Liacouras 2016). Adverse effects with earlier-generation antiemetics (such as promethazine and metoclopramide) include somnolence, nervousness, irritability and dystonic reactions, and they should not be routinely administered to children (Tiziani 2020). Ondansetron (Zofran) is an antiemetic with limited adverse effects and is beneficial when the child is not able to tolerate anything orally or in the case of postoperative vomiting, chemotherapy-induced vomiting, cyclic vomiting syndrome or acute motion sickness (Sreedharan & Liacouras 2016).

Nursing Care Management

The major emphasis of nursing care of the vomiting infant or child is on observation and reporting of vomiting behaviour and associated symptoms and on the implementation of measures to reduce the vomiting. Accurate assessment of the type of vomiting, appearance of the emesis and the child's behaviour in association with the vomiting greatly aids in establishing a diagnosis.

TRANSLATING EVIDENCE INTO PRACTICE

Use of Antiemetics in Children with Acute Gastroenteritis

Ask the Question

In children with acute gastroenteritis (AGE), should antiemetics be used?

Search for the Evidence

Search Strategies

Search criteria included English-language publications within the period 2011 to 2017, research-based articles (level 3 or higher) regarding antiemetic use among children with AGE.

Databases Used

PubMed/Medline, CINAHL, Cochrane, National Guideline Clearinghouse (AHRQ), American Academy of Pediatrics, National Institute of Health and Clinical Excellence, European Society for Paediatric Gastroenterology, Hepatology and Nutrition, Joanna Briggs Institute

Critically Analyse the Evidence

GRADE criteria: Evidence quality moderate; recommendation strong (Balshem et al 2011)

A review of the literature revealed two systematic reviews and three randomised control trials from 2011 to 2017 that evaluated the use of antiemetics in the treatment of children with AGE.

- A Cochrane review in 2011 revealed 7 randomised controlled trials (1020 patients) evaluating the safety and efficacy of antiemetics to treat gastroenteritis-induced vomiting in children (Fedorowicz et al 2011). Ondansetron was found more effective than placebo in studies evaluating hospital admission rates, need for IV rehydration therapy and resolution of vomiting. When comparing placebo, dimenhydrinate was found more effective in one study, and metoclopramide was more effective in another single study.
- A systematic review from 1980 to 2012 revealed 10 studies (1479 participants) evaluating the evidence of safety and effectiveness of antiemetics (dexamethasone, dimenhydrinate, granisetron, metoclopramide and ondansetron) for gastroenteritis-induced vomiting in children and adolescents (Carter & Fedorowicz 2012). There is clear evidence from nine studies that ondansetron is more effective than placebo in resolving vomiting, reducing the need for IV rehydration therapy and reducing the hospital admission rate. A single study showed a reduction in mean vomiting days among children receiving dimenhydrinate versus placebo and among granisetron versus placebo. Studies of metoclopramide were underpowered, and a single study of dexamethasone versus placebo showed no statistically significant difference in vomiting.
- A group of 144 children diagnosed with acute gastroenteritis were randomised to receive dimenhydrinate or placebo in a paediatric emergency department (Gouin et al 2012). No statistically significant difference regarding the frequency of vomiting was noted between the two groups.
- A group of 76 children diagnosed with acute gastroenteritis were randomised to receive an orally disintegrating ondansetron tablet or domperidone suspension (dosing based on body weight), then evaluated for vomiting for the next 24 hours (Rerksuppaphol & Rerksuppaphol 2013). Sixty-two per cent of patients in the ondansetron group and 44% of patients in the domperidone group had no vomiting after treatment, although no statistically significant difference was noted ($p = 0.16$).
- Another study randomised 356 children to receive ondansetron ($n = 119$) versus domperidone ($n = 119$) versus placebo ($n = 118$) for treatment of acute gastroenteritis who failed oral rehydration in an emergency department (Marchetti et al 2016). Fourteen children (12%) needed IV rehydration in the ondansetron group compared with 30 children (25%) in the domperidone and 34 (29%) children in the placebo group.

Apply the Evidence: Nursing Implications

Ondansetron reduces the duration of vomiting in children with AGE and ondansetron and domperidone relieves the incidence of vomiting in children with AGE. There is limited evidence for dimenhydrinate and metoclopramide, and no evidence for other antiemetics in children with AGE who are vomiting. The number of children requiring IV rehydration and hospital admission for AGE is reduced with administration of ondansetron.

References

Balshem, H., Hefland, M., Schunemann, H. J., et al. (2011). GRADE guidelines: Rating the quality of evidence. Journal of Clinical Epidemiology, 64(4), 401–406.

Carter, B., & Fedorowicz, Z. (2012). Antiemetic treatment for acute gastroenteritis in children: An updated Cochrane systematic review with meta-analysis and mixed treatment comparison in a Bayesian framework. BMJ Open, 2, 1–11.

Fedorowicz, Z., Jagannath, V. A., & Carter, B. (2011). Antiemetics for reducing vomiting related to acute gastroenteritis in children and adolescents. Cochrane Database of Systematic Reviews, (9), CD005506.

Gouin, S., Vo, T., Roy, M., et al. (2012). Oral dimenhydrinate versus placebo in children with gastroenteritis: A randomized controlled trial. Pediatrics, 129, 1050–1055.

Marchetti, F., Bonati, M., Maestro, A., et al. (2016). Oral ondansetron versus domperidone for acute gastroenteritis in pediatric emergency departments: Multicenter double blind randomized controlled trial. PLoS ONE, 11(11), e0165441.

Rerksuppaphol, S., & Rerksuppaphol, L. (2013). Randomized study of ondansetron versus domperidone in the treatment of children with acute gastroenteritis. Journal of Clinical Medicine Research, 5(6), 460–466.

The cause of the vomiting determines the nursing intervention. When the vomiting is a manifestation of improper feeding methods, establishing proper techniques through teaching and example ordinarily corrects the situation. If the vomiting is a probable sign of GI obstruction, the nurse usually withholds food or implements special feeding techniques. The nurse should direct efforts towards maintaining hydration and preventing dehydration in a vomiting child.

The thirst mechanism is the most sensitive guide to fluid needs, and ad libitum administration of a glucose-electrolyte solution to an alert child restores water and electrolytes satisfactorily. It is important to include carbohydrates to spare body protein and to avoid ketosis resulting from exhaustion of glycogen stores. Small, frequent feedings of fluids or foods are preferable and more effective. Once vomiting has abated, offer more liberal amounts of fluids, followed by gradual resumption of the regular diet.

INGESTION OF FOREIGN SUBSTANCES

Children are prone to ingesting foreign substances because they frequently put their hands or other objects or substances in their mouth. Infants and small children in particular instinctively explore items with the mouth. Older children often place items in their mouth and accidentally swallow them. Rarely, a child deliberately swallows unusual objects or substances. Hands come into contact with dirt and contaminated objects that may contain lead, bacteria or parasites.

Pica

Pica is an eating disorder characterised by the compulsive and excessive ingestion of both food and non-food substances for at least 1 month (Katz et al 2016). Food picas include the excessive eating of ordinary foods or unprepared food substances. Non-food picas include the ingestion of substances such as clay, soil, stones and hair. Pica is more common in children, women (especially during pregnancy), individuals who have autism or cognitive impairment, and those with anaemia or chronic renal failure. In some cultures pica is an accepted practice based on the presumed nutritional or therapeutic properties or on religious or superstitious beliefs.

There are several theories on the cause of pica, including psychological theories (compulsive neurosis) and nutritional theories (craving caused by a nutrient deficiency). Pica is clearly associated with both iron and zinc deficiencies, although controversy exists regarding whether pica is the cause or the result of the deficiency. Pica has also been reported as the presenting symptom in children with coeliac disease thought to be caused by iron deficiency. Pica for dirt (geophagia) is the principal risk factor for visceral larva migrans (a common parasite in children and adults) (Katz et al 2016).

In some instances pica is relatively harmless. However, when the ingested substance contains a toxic ingredient the consequences can be serious. Other significant consequences of pica include intestinal obstruction or perforation, dental injury and malnutrition (Katz et al 2016).

The nurse can detect pica by the history, physical examination and radiological studies. However, it is often unrecognised, and children may deny any unusual eating behaviours. The nurse should consider pica when children known to be at risk for this condition develop abdominal pain, other GI symptoms or anaemia. Children exhibiting signs of this disorder should be evaluated, and if a potentially harmful substance is involved, it should be removed from the child's environment. Nursing education regarding the dangers of pica, especially lead, and assistance in helping families remove the substance are important.

Foreign Bodies

Foreign body ingestion is a preventable cause of mortality and morbidity in children. Most foreign body ingestions occur in children younger than 3 years old, with the peak incidence between 10 and 24 months of age (Laya et al 2017). The predisposition is due to the tendency to explore by placing objects in their mouth, immature swallowing coordination and inability to adequately chew certain foods due to lack of molars (Laya et al 2017). Nuts and seeds are the most commonly aspirated foods, but other items include coins, whole grapes and metal or plastic objects/small toys.

Where the foreign bodies are retained depends on the GI tract's size, shape, diameter and motility. Foreign bodies tend to become impacted at normally narrow sites of the GI tract. Pathological narrowing of the intestine or intestinal stomas can also be a cause of foreign body obstruction. Foreign bodies in the stomach or intestine usually pass on their own. However, if they do become impacted, this generally occurs in the oesophagus; other common sites include the ileocaecal valve, pylorus, duodenum or appendix.

Signs and Symptoms

A history of choking followed by an acute episode of vigorous coughing is the most common presentation of foreign body ingestion. Initial signs and symptoms also may include dyspnoea and wheezing. Aspirated foreign bodies that lodge in the larynx or trachea cause stridor. When these are in the large bronchi, crepitation and wheezes can be found. Wheezes and crepitation can be heard in both lungs, but unilateral findings have a higher specificity for foreign body aspiration (Khan & Orenstein 2016a).

Complications

Foreign bodies are generally classified as sharp or dull, pointed or blunt, and toxic or non-toxic. Some foreign bodies are ingested and may be excreted without complications, but other foreign bodies, especially those that are pointed, toxic or aspirated, require immediate treatment. Complications from foreign bodies include pneumonia, perforation, obstruction, pneumothorax and pneumomediastinum (Berdan & Sato 2017). Foreign bodies should be immediately removed if the child is in severe distress and unable to swallow secretions. Disc batteries are a medical emergency because the composition of the batteries can cause damage to the mucosa within 1 hour of aspiration/ingestion (Khan & Orstein 2016a). Single battery/magnet ingestion can be monitored closely with conservative management, but ingestion of multiple batteries/magnets has a high risk of complications and they must be removed promptly. Sharp objects (e.g. straight pins, needles, straightened paper clips) need to be removed without delay if lodged in the oesophagus.

Diagnostic Evaluation

As mentioned, there may be no signs or symptoms, but some children come to the medical practitioner for evaluation because of problems. The nurse should perform a complete history and physical examination. Assess the airway and breathing first. Findings on the chest evaluation might include inspiratory stridor or expiratory wheezing. Findings on an abdominal examination could be hypoactive or absent bowel sounds. The physical examination might demonstrate swelling, erythema or crepitus suggestive of oesophageal perforation.

Assessment often involves radiological evaluation. A plain x-ray film of the neck, chest and abdomen may be ordered.

Therapeutic Management

Intervention is urgent when a child has sharp objects, magnets or button batteries lodged in the oesophagus because of the risk of perforation or acid burns (Berdan & Sato 2017). Urgent intervention is also important anytime the airway is compromised. If the child is asymptomatic and the foreign body does not carry an emergent risk, it is reasonable to wait 24 hours to see if it will pass. Foreign objects should not be allowed to remain in the oesophagus for more than 24 hours because of the potential for complications such as erosion, perforation or formation of fistulas.

Nursing Care Management

The primary nursing intervention is prevention of foreign body ingestion through family teaching. All children who are old enough to understand are taught not to put anything in their mouth except food. Infants and young children who cannot follow such advice must have their environment protected.

Prevention includes supervision and ongoing education as the child matures.

Once an object is swallowed, parents need guidelines on seeking treatment (see Nursing Care Considerations box). When no treatment is advised and the object is left to pass spontaneously, parents should examine all stools for verification that the object has passed safely through the GI tract, usually within 3 or 4 days.

NURSING CARE CONSIDERATIONS

Foreign Body Ingestion

Seek medical treatment immediately if:

- any sharp or large object or a battery was ingested
- there are signs that the object may have been aspirated (i.e. coughing, choking, inability to speak or difficulty breathing) (see Chapter 26)
- there are signs of gastrointestinal perforation (i.e. chest or abdominal pain; evidence of bleeding in vomitus, stool, haematocrit or vital signs)
- there are signs that the object may be lodged in the oesophagus (i.e. increased salivation, drooling, gagging or difficulty swallowing)
- there are signs that the object may be lodged in the pharynx (i.e. discomfort in the throat or chest—more likely with a fish or chicken bone or large piece of meat).

Seek medical advice even if the object is smooth and small (usually less than the size of a five-cent piece).

If no treatment is advised, check the stool for passage of the object; do not give laxatives.

DISORDERS OF MOTILITY

Hirschsprung's Disease (Congenital Aganglionic Megacolon)

Hirschsprung's disease (HD) is a congenital anomaly that results in mechanical obstruction from inadequate motility of part of the intestine. It accounts for about a quarter of all cases of neonatal intestinal obstruction. The incidence is 1 in 5000 live births (Fiorino & Liacouras 2016). It is four times more common in males than in females and follows a familial pattern in a small number of cases.

Pathophysiology

The pathology of HD relates to the absence of ganglion cells in the affected areas of the intestine, resulting in a loss of the rectosphincteric reflex and an abnormal microenvironment of the cells of the affected intestine. The term *congenital aganglionic megacolon* describes the primary defect, which is the absence of ganglion cells in the myenteric plexus of Auerbach and the submucosal plexus of Meissner (Fig 25.2).

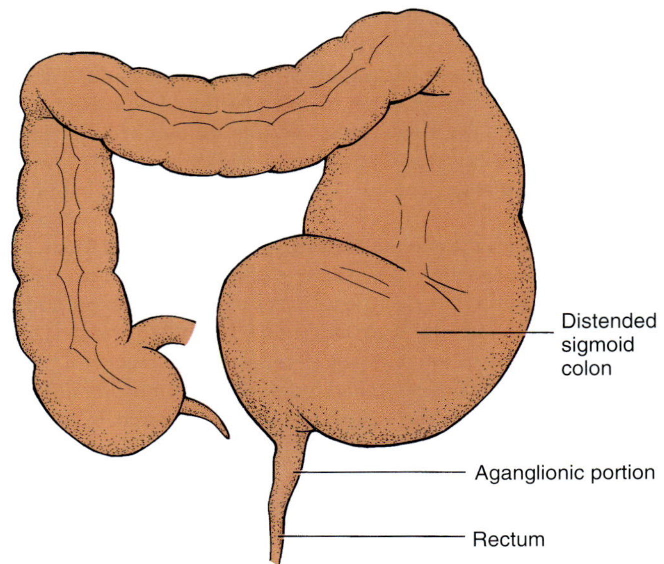

Fig 25.2 Hirschsprung's disease.

The absence of ganglion cells in the affected bowel results in a lack of enteric nervous system stimulation, which decreases the internal sphincter's ability to relax. Unopposed sympathetic stimulation of the intestine results in increased intestinal tone. In addition to the contraction of the abnormal bowel and the resulting lack of peristalsis, there is a loss of the rectosphincteric reflex. Normally, when a stool bolus enters the rectum, the internal sphincter relaxes and the stool is evacuated. In HD, the internal sphincter does not relax. In about 80% of the cases, the aganglionic segment includes only the rectum and some portion of the distal colon, termed *short-segment disease* (Fiorino & Liacouras 2016). However, the entire colon or part of the small intestine may be involved; this is considered *long-segment HD*. Occasionally, skip segments or total intestinal aganglionosis may occur. Approximately 15% have long-segment disease, and 5% have total intestinal aganglionosis (Fiorino & Liacouras 2016).

Clinical Manifestations

Most children with HD are diagnosed in the first few months of life. Clinical manifestations vary according to the age when symptoms are recognised and the presence of complications, such as enterocolitis (Box 25.8). A neonate usually is seen with a distended abdomen, feeding intolerance with bilious vomiting and a delay in the passage of meconium. Typically, 99% of term infants pass meconium in the first 48 hours of life, whereas few infants with HD do so (Fiorino & Liacouras 2016).

Diagnostic Evaluation

In the neonate the diagnosis is suspected on the basis of clinical signs of intestinal obstruction or failure to pass meconium. In infants and children the history is an important part of diagnosis and typically includes a chronic pattern of constipation. On examination the rectum is empty of faeces, the internal sphincter is tight and leakage of liquid stool and accumulated gas may occur if the aganglionic segment is short. A contrast enema often demonstrates the transition zone between the dilated proximal colon (megacolon) and the aganglionic distal segment. However, this typical megacolon and narrow distal segment may not develop until age 2 months or later.

BOX 25.8 Clinical Manifestations of Hirschsprung's Disease

Newborn Period

Failure to pass meconium within 24 to 48 hours after birth
Refusal to feed
Bilious vomiting
Abdominal distension

Infancy

Failure to thrive
Constipation
Abdominal distension
Episodes of diarrhoea and vomiting
Signs of enterocolitis

- Explosive, watery diarrhoea
- Fever
- Appears significantly ill

Childhood

Constipation
Ribbonlike, foul-smelling stools
Abdominal distension
Visible peristalsis
Easily palpable faecal mass
Undernourished, anaemic appearance

To confirm the diagnosis, rectal biopsy is performed either surgically to obtain a full-thickness biopsy specimen or by suction biopsy for histological evidence of the absence of ganglion cells. A non-invasive procedure that may be used is anorectal manometry, in which a catheter with a balloon attached is inserted into the rectum. The test records the reflex pressure response of the internal anal sphincter to distension of the balloon. A normal response is relaxation of the internal sphincter, followed by a contraction of the external sphincter. In HD the external sphincter contracts normally but the internal sphincter fails to relax.

Therapeutic Management

The majority of children with HD require surgery rather than medical therapy. Once the child is stabilised with fluid and electrolyte replacement and has received colonic cleansing if appropriate with enemas, if needed, surgery is performed, usually with a high rate of success. Surgical management consists primarily of the removal of the aganglionic portion of the bowel to relieve obstruction, restore normal motility and preserve the function of the external anal sphincter.

Nursing Care Management

The nursing concerns depend on the child's age and the type of treatment. If the disorder is diagnosed during the neonatal period, the main objectives are to help the parents adjust to a congenital defect in their child, foster infant–parent bonding, prepare the parents for the medical-surgical intervention and prepare the parents to assume the care of the child after surgery.

The child's preoperative care depends on the age and clinical condition. A child who is malnourished may not be able to withstand surgery until his or her physical status improves. Often this involves symptomatic treatment with enemas and a low-fibre, high-calorie, high-protein diet. Physical preoperative preparation includes the same measures that are common to any surgery. (See Surgical Procedures, Chapter 22.) In the newborn, whose bowel is presumed sterile, no additional preparation is necessary. Enterocolitis is the most serious complication of HD. Emergent preoperative care includes frequent monitoring of vital signs and blood pressure for signs of shock; monitoring fluid and electrolyte replacements, as well as plasma or other blood derivatives; and observing for symptoms of bowel perforation, such as fever, increasing abdominal distension, vomiting, increased tenderness, irritability, dyspnoea and cyanosis.

Because progressive distension of the abdomen is a serious sign, the nurse measures abdominal circumference with a paper tape measure, usually at the level of the umbilicus or at the widest part of the abdomen. The point of measurement is marked with a pen to ensure reliability of subsequent measurements. Abdominal measurement can be obtained with the vital sign measurements and is recorded in serial order so that any change is obvious.

Postoperative care is the same as that for any child or infant with abdominal surgery. (See Surgical Procedures, Chapter 22.) The nurse involves the parents in the care of the child, allowing them to help with feedings and observe for signs of wound infection or irregular passage of stool. After surgery, parents need instruction concerning the development of complications such as enterocolitis, faecal incontinence and obstruction. Some children will require daily anal dilations in the postoperative period to avoid anastomotic strictures. Although less common, a diverting colostomy may be performed in some children with HD. Parents are taught how to care for the colostomy and how to provide meticulous skin care to prevent skin breakdown; the assistance of a wound and skin care specialist is essential for optimal follow-up and consistent skin care.

In general the prognosis for the infant or child with HD is positive and most live a normal life. In a few cases problems with faecal incontinence may persist. A long-term study of children with HD for 1 to 19 years reported satisfying bowel control among 53% of the sample, soiling with 13%, constipation among 6% and abdominal distension with 26% (Muller et al 2016).

Gastro-oesophageal Reflux

Gastro-oesophageal reflux (GOR) is defined as the transfer of gastric contents into the oesophagus. This phenomenon is physiological, occurring throughout the day, most frequently after meals and at night; therefore, it is important to differentiate GOR from **gastro-oesophageal reflux disease (GORD)**. GORD represents symptoms or tissue damage that results from GOR. The peak incidence of GOR occurs at 4 months of age and generally resolves spontaneously in most infants by 1 year of age (Mousa & Hassan 2017). GOR becomes a disease when complications such as faltering growth, respiratory problems or dysphagia develop.

Certain conditions predispose children to a high prevalence of GORD, including neurological impairment, chronic respiratory disorders, oesophageal atresia and obesity (Mousa & Hassan 2017). Sandifer's syndrome is an uncommon condition, usually occurring in young children, that is characterised by repetitive stretching and arching of the head and neck that can be mistaken for a seizure. This manoeuvre is likely to represent a physiological neuromuscular response attempting to prevent acid refluxate from reaching the upper portion of the oesophagus (Khan & Orenstein 2016b).

Infants who are prone to develop GOR include premature infants and infants with bronchopulmonary dysplasia. Children who have had tracheo-oesophageal or oesophageal atresia repairs, neurological disorders, scoliosis, asthma, cystic fibrosis or cerebral palsy are also prone to develop GOR.

Pathophysiology

Although the pathogenesis of GOR is multifactorial, its primary causative mechanism is likely to involve inappropriate transient relaxation of the LES. Factors that increase abdominal pressure (e.g. coughing and sneezing, scoliosis and overeating) may contribute to GOR. Oesophageal symptoms are caused by inflammation from the acid in the gastric refluxate, whereas reactive airway disease may result from stimulation of airway reflexes by the acid refluxate.

Clinical Manifestations

During infancy the most common clinical manifestation of GOR is passive regurgitation. Regurgitation generally resolves spontaneously in most infants by 12 months and almost all infants by 24 months (Khan & Orenstein 2016b). Clinical manifestations of GOR are listed in Box 25.9. GOR is one of the causes of apparent life-threatening events and has also been associated with chronic respiratory disorders, including reactive airway disease, recurrent stridor, chronic cough and recurrent pneumonia in infants. Oesophagitis can also cause discomfort in the chest area, which may be manifested as unusual irritability or poor intake of nutrients. Poor weight gain and poor growth may occur in a child with an insufficient intake of nutrients or with a large amount of regurgitation.

For preschool children GOR may occur with intermittent vomiting. Older children tend to initially come to the medical practitioner with a more adult-like pattern of heartburn, regurgitation and reswallowing. GORD may cause severe inflammation, chronic blood loss with anaemia and haematemesis, hypoproteinaemia or melaena. If the inflammation goes untreated, scarring and strictures may form.

GOR is common in children with asthma, but recurrent pneumonia caused by GOR is uncommon except in children with neurological impairments. Hoarseness has also been associated with GOR in children.

BOX 25.9 Clinical Manifestations and Complications of Gastro-oesophageal Reflux

Symptoms in Infants
- Vomiting, regurgitation, recurrent vomiting (may be forceful)
- Excessive crying, irritability, arching of the back, stiffening
- Poor weight gain
- Respiratory problems (e.g. cough, wheeze, stridor, gagging, choking with feedings)
- Feeding refusal

Symptoms in Children
- Heartburn
- Abdominal pain
- Chronic cough, hoarse voice
- Dysphagia
- Asthma
- Recurrent vomiting

Complications
- Oesophagitis
- Oesophageal stricture
- Laryngitis
- Recurrent pneumonia
- Anaemia
- Barrett's oesophagus

Source: Adapted from Lightdale, J. R., Gremse, D. A., & Section on Gastroenterology, Hepatology, and Nutrition. (2013). Gastroesophageal reflux: Management guidance for the pediatrician. Pediatrics, 131(5), e1684–e1695.

Diagnostic Evaluation

The history and physical examination are usually sufficiently reliable to establish the diagnosis of GOR. An upper GI series is helpful in evaluating the presence of anatomical abnormalities (e.g. pyloric stenosis, malrotation, annular pancreas, hiatal hernia, oesophageal stricture). Endoscopy with biopsy may be helpful to assess the presence and severity of oesophagitis, strictures and Barrett's oesophagus and to exclude other disorders such as Crohn's disease. Scintigraphy detects radioactive substances in the oesophagus after a feeding of the compound and assesses gastric emptying. It can differentiate between aspiration of gastric contents from reflux and aspiration from poor oropharyngeal muscle coordination.

Therapeutic Management

Therapeutic management of GOR depends on its severity. No therapy is needed for the infant who is thriving and has no respiratory complications. Lifestyle modifications in children (e.g. weight control if indicated; small, more frequent meals) and feeding manoeuvres in infants (e.g. thickened feedings; upright positioning) can help as well.

Elevating the head of the bed and weight loss, if applicable, can reduce GOR symptoms. Prone positioning of infants also decreases episodes of GOR; however, due to the risk of sudden unexpected death in infancy, all infants should sleep in the supine position (Khan & Orenstein 2016b).

Pharmacological therapy may be used to treat infants and children with GORD. Surgical management of GOR is reserved for children with severe complications such as recurrent aspiration pneumonia, apnoea, severe oesophagitis or faltering growth and for children who have failed to respond to medical therapy.

Prognosis. The majority of infants with GOR have a mild problem that generally improves by 12 to 18 months of age and requires only conservative lifestyle changes or medical therapy. If GOR is severe and remains unsuccessfully treated, multiple complications can occur. Oesophageal strictures caused by persistent oesophagitis with scarring are one of the most significant complications. Recurrent respiratory distress with aspiration pneumonia, another serious complication, is an indication for surgery.

Nursing Care Management

Nursing care is directed at identifying children with symptoms suggestive of GOR; educating parents regarding home care, including feeding, positioning and medications when indicated; and caring for the child undergoing surgical intervention. For the majority of infants, parental reassurance of the benign nature of the condition and its relationship to physiological maturity is the most important intervention.

Irritable Bowel Syndrome

Irritable bowel syndrome (IBS) is classified as a functional GI disorder. IBS occurs more frequently in adolescents than children, 22% to 35% versus 6% to 14%, respectively (Giannetti et al 2017). Children with IBS often have alternating diarrhoea and constipation, flatulence, bloating or a feeling of abdominal distension, lower abdominal pain, a feeling of urgency when needing to defecate and a feeling of incomplete evacuation of the bowel. Abdominal pain should be present for at least 4 days per month over the last 2 months plus a change in either frequency or appearance of stool (Chopra et al 2017). IBS has been identified as a cause of recurrent abdominal pain in 68% of children (Giannetti et al 2017).

The cause of IBS is not clear, but it is believed to involve a combination of genetic and environmental factors. Strong predictors for the development of IBS in a child include having a mother, father or twin with IBS (Kridler & Kamat 2016). In addition, children with IBS have been noted to be less confident in their ability to deal with daily stress and have higher prevalence of anxiety, depression, introverted personalities and difficulty sleeping (Kridler & Kamat 2016). The intestinal microbiome is the focus of IBS research to evaluate whether inflammation may trigger nerves in the gut to cause IBS symptoms (Chopra et al 2017, Kridler & Kamat 2016).

Therapeutic Management

There is no cure for IBS, so management involves controlling the child's symptoms. The long-range goal of treatment is development of regular bowel habits and relief of symptoms. Management depends on whether IBS is constipation or diarrhoea predominant. Constipation-predominant IBS is managed by increasing fibre with diet changes and supplements, whereas diarrhoea-predominant IBS is managed with diet changes and, PPIs (Chopra et al 2017, Kridler & Kamat 2016). A recent Cochrane systematic review found evidence suggesting that probiotics are effective in relieving recurrent abdominal pain (Newlove-Delgado et al 2017).

Nursing Care Management

The primary nursing goal is family support and education. The disorder is stressful to children and parents. The nurse can help by providing support and reassurance that, although the symptoms are difficult to deal with, the disorder is not generally a threat to the child's health.

INFLAMMATORY CONDITIONS

Acute Appendicitis

Appendicitis, inflammation of the **vermiform appendix** (blind sac at the end of the caecum), is the most common cause of emergency abdominal surgery in childhood. The peak incidence of appendicitis is between 12 and 18 years, with boys affected slightly more often than girls (Aiken & Oldham 2016a). Classically, the first symptom of appendicitis is periumbilical pain, followed by nausea, right lower quadrant pain and, later, vomiting with fever (Rentea et al 2017). Perforation occurs in up to 82% of children under 5 years of age, and is likely to be as a result of an inability to verbalise their symptoms (Aiken & Oldham 2016a). Perforation of the appendix can occur within approximately 48 hours of the initial complaint of pain (Aiken & Oldham 2016a). Complications from appendiceal perforation include major abscess, phlegmon, enterocutaneous fistula, peritonitis and partial bowel obstruction. A **phlegmon** is an acute suppurative inflammation of subcutaneous connective tissue that spreads (RCHM 2019).

Aetiology

The cause of appendicitis is obstruction of the lumen of the appendix, usually by hardened faecal material (faecalith). Swollen lymphoid tissue, frequently occurring after a viral infection, can also obstruct the appendix. Another rare cause of obstruction is a parasite such as *Enterobius vermicularis,* or pinworms, which can obstruct the appendiceal lumen.

Pathophysiology

With acute obstruction, the outflow of mucus secretions is blocked and pressure builds within the lumen, resulting in compression of blood vessels. The resulting ischaemia is followed by ulceration of the epithelial lining and bacterial invasion. Subsequent necrosis causes perforation or rupture with faecal and bacterial contamination of the peritoneal cavity. The resulting inflammation spreads rapidly throughout the abdomen (**peritonitis**), especially in young children, who are unable to localise infection. Progressive peritoneal inflammation results in functional intestinal obstruction of the small bowel (**ileus**) because intense GI reflexes severely inhibit bowel motility. Because the peritoneum represents a major portion of total body surface, the loss of extracellular fluid to the peritoneal cavity leads to electrolyte imbalance and hypovolaemic shock.

BOX 25.10 Clinical Manifestations of Appendicitis

- Right lower quadrant abdominal pain
- Fever
- Rigid abdomen
- Decreased or absent bowel sounds
- Vomiting (typically follows onset of pain)
- Constipation or diarrhoea
- Anorexia
- Tachycardia
- Rapid, shallow breathing
- Pallor
- Lethargy
- Irritability
- Stooped posture

Clinical Manifestations. The first symptom of appendicitis is usually colicky, cramping, abdominal pain located around the umbilicus (Box 25.10). **Referred pain** is the term used for this vague periumbilical localisation. The midgut shares the same T10 dermatome, so pain is often perceived to be coming from this area. Generally, this pain progresses and becomes constant. The most important physical finding is focal abdominal tenderness. As the inflammation progresses to involve the serosa of the appendix and the peritoneum of the abdominal wall, the pain may shift to the right lower quadrant. **McBurney's point**, located two-thirds the distance along a line between the umbilicus and the anterosuperior iliac spine, is the most common point of tenderness. Localised peritoneal signs may occur with gentle percussion or manoeuvres such as heel strike or shaking the bed. Other helpful findings are Rovsing's sign, tenderness in the right lower quadrant that occurs during palpation or percussion of other abdominal quadrants; obturator sign, pain with flexion and internal rotation of the right hip; psoas sign, pain with left side with right hip extension; and Dunphy's sign, pain with coughing (Rentea et al 2017). Rebound tenderness—pain on deep palpation with sudden release—may be present, but it is not a finding specific to appendicitis (Aiken & Oldham 2016a). Nausea, vomiting and anorexia typically occur after the pain starts. Diarrhoea, as well as other common signs of childhood illness such as upper respiratory tract congestion, poor feeding, lethargy or irritability, may accompany appendicitis.

The child may not be able to walk well and may complain of pain in the right hip caused by inflammation in the psoas or iliopsoas muscles. Low-grade fever (38°C) may occur with the initial presentation; however, the absence of fever does not exclude appendicitis. Because of the great variability in the presentation and location of appendicitis, any child with focal tenderness, regardless of the location, should be considered to potentially have acute appendicitis (see Nursing Care Considerations box).

NURSING CARE CONSIDERATIONS

Acute Appendicitis

Abdominal pain is a common complaint among school-age children, but in some cases it may indicate acute appendicitis. Nurses in clinics should be familiar with the 'typical' pattern of symptoms in acute appendicitis and how to assess and evaluate an acute abdomen. Nurses also need to educate others on the importance of early referral to the health team for further assessment. Early referral to the health team or facility may make the difference between an uncomplicated appendectomy and a delayed diagnosis of a perforated appendix with peritonitis.

NURSING CARE CONSIDERATIONS

Signs of peritonitis in addition to fever usually include sudden relief from pain after perforation; subsequent increase in pain, which is usually diffuse and accompanied by rigid guarding of the abdomen; progressive abdominal distension; tachycardia; rapid, shallow breathing as the child refrains from using abdominal muscles; pallor; chills; irritability; and restlessness.

Diagnostic Evaluation

Diagnosis is not always straightforward. Fever, vomiting, abdominal pain and an elevated white blood cell count are associated with appendicitis but are also seen in IBD, pelvic inflammatory disease, gastroenteritis, urinary tract infection, right lower lobe pneumonia, mesenteric adenitis, Meckel's diverticulum and intussusception. Prolonged symptoms and delayed diagnosis often occur in younger children, in whom the risk of perforation is greatest because of their inability to verbalise their complaints.

The diagnosis is based primarily on the history and physical examination (see Box 25.10). Pain, the cardinal feature, is initially generalised (usually periumbilical). However, it usually descends to the lower right quadrant. The most intense site of pain may be at McBurney's point. Rebound tenderness is not a reliable sign and is extremely painful to the child. Referred pain, elicited by light percussion around the perimeter of the abdomen, indicates peritoneal irritation. Movement, such as riding over bumps in a car or on a gurney, aggravates the pain. In addition to pain, significant clinical manifestations include fever, a change in behaviour, anorexia and vomiting.

Laboratory studies usually include a full blood count (FBC); urinalysis (to rule out a urinary tract infection); and, in adolescent females, serum human chorionic gonadotropin (to rule out an ectopic pregnancy). A white blood cell count greater than 10,000/mm^3 and an elevated C-reactive protein (CRP) are common but are not necessarily specific for appendicitis. An elevated percentage of bands (often referred to as 'a left shift') may indicate an inflammatory process. CRP is an acute-phase reactant that rises within 12 hours of the onset of infection.

Ultrasound is the imaging technique of choice in diagnosing appendicitis, although a computed tomography (CT) scan may be used. Ultrasound is considered positive in the presence of enlarged appendiceal diameter; appendiceal wall thickening; and periappendiceal inflammatory changes, including fat streaks, phlegmon, fluid collection and extraluminal gas (Aiken & Oldham 2016a). The accuracy of imaging for diagnosing appendicitis is 95% (Rentea et al 2017).

Therapeutic Management

The treatment for appendicitis before perforation is surgical removal of the appendix (appendectomy). Usually antibiotics are administered preoperatively. IV fluids and electrolytes are often required before surgery, especially if the child is dehydrated as a result of the marked anorexia characteristic of appendicitis.

Ruptured Appendix. Management of the child diagnosed with peritonitis caused by a ruptured appendix often begins preoperatively with IV administration of fluid and electrolytes, systemic antibiotics and nasogastric (NG) suction. Postoperative management includes IV fluids, continued administration of antibiotics and NG suction for abdominal decompression until intestinal activity returns.

Prognosis. Complications are uncommon after a simple appendectomy, and recovery is usually rapid and complete. The mortality rate from perforating appendicitis has improved from nearly certain death a century ago to less than 1% at the present time (Rentea et al 2017). Complications, however, including wound infection and intraabdominal abscess, are not uncommon. Early recognition of the illness is important to prevent complications.

Nursing Care Management

Because successful treatment of appendicitis is based on prompt recognition of the disorder, an important nursing objective is to assist in establishing a diagnosis. Because abdominal pain is a common childhood complaint, the nurse needs to make some preliminary assessment of the severity of the pain. (See Chapter 5.)

Palpating the abdomen should be delayed until all other assessments have been made. Instruct the child to point with one finger to the site of the abdominal pain. Rebound tenderness may be present but is not always a sufficiently reliable test in children. Light palpation will satisfactorily elicit pain without causing excessive trauma (see Nursing Care Considerations box). Ask the child with mild pain to lift the heels and drop them to the floor two or three times, to hop on one foot or to 'puff out' or 'pull in' the abdomen to check for tenderness without more painful probing. Chapter 4 discusses other techniques for assessment of the abdomen.

Postoperatively the child is maintained on IV fluids and antibiotics and is allowed nothing by mouth. The child also remains on low, intermittent gastric decompression until there is evidence of return of intestinal motility. Listening for bowel sounds and observing for other signs of bowel activity (such as passage of stool) are part of the routine assessment.

Meckel's Diverticulum

Meckel's diverticulum is a remnant of the fetal omphalomesenteric duct, which connects the yolk sac with the primitive midgut during fetal life (Kennedy & Liacouras 2016a). Normally the structure is obliterated between the fifth and seventh week of gestation, when the placenta replaces the yolk sac as the source of nutrition for the fetus. Failure of obliteration may result in an omphalomesenteric fistula (a fibrous band connecting the small intestine to the umbilicus), umbilical cyst, vitelline duct remnant, mesodiverticular bands and Meckel's diverticula (Bagade & Khanna 2015).

Meckel's diverticulum is a true diverticulum because it arises from the antimesenteric border of the small intestine and includes all layers of the intestinal wall. Meckel's diverticulum is often referred to by the 'rule of 2s' because it occurs in 2% of the population, has a 2:1 male-to-female ratio, is located within 2 feet of the ileocaecal valve, is commonly 2 cm in diameter and 2 inches in length, contains 2 types of ectopic tissue (pancreatic and gastric) and is more common before age 2 (Kennedy & Liacouras 2016a).

Pathophysiology

Bleeding, obstruction or inflammation causes the symptomatic complications of Meckel's diverticulum (Lin et al 2017). Bleeding, which is the most common problem in children, is caused by peptic ulceration or perforation because of the unbuffered acidic secretion. Several mechanisms may cause obstruction such as intussusception or entanglement of the small intestine.

Clinical Manifestations

Signs and symptoms are based on the specific pathological process such as inflammation, bleeding or intestinal obstruction (Box 25.11) The most common clinical presentation is rectal bleeding caused by ulceration at the junction of the ectopic gastric mucosa and normal ileal mucosa. The bleeding is usually painless and may be dramatic and occur as bright red or currant jelly–like stools, or it may occur intermittently and appear as tarry stools. The bleeding may be significant enough to cause hypotension. Volvulus and intussusception are common obstructive mechanisms in children with Meckel's diverticulum, and these children present with symptoms of abdominal pain, distension, nausea and vomiting (Kennedy & Liacouras 2016a).

Diagnostic Evaluation

Diagnosis is usually based on the history, physical examination and radiographic studies. Meckel's diverticulum is often a diagnostic challenge. A technetium-99 pertechnetate scan (Meckel scan) is the most effective diagnostic testing, especially for a bleeding diverticulum, with sensitivity ranging from 80% to 90% and a specificity of 95% (Lin et al 2017). Laboratory studies such as a FBC and a basic metabolic panel are usually part of the general work-up to rule out any bleeding disorder and to evaluate for dehydration.

Therapeutic Management

The standard treatment for symptomatic Meckel's diverticulum is surgical removal. In instances in which severe haemorrhage increases the surgical risk, medical intervention to correct hypovolaemic shock (e.g. blood replacement, IV fluids and oxygen) may be necessary. Antibiotics may be used preoperatively to control infection. If intestinal obstruction has occurred, appropriate preoperative measures are used to correct fluid and electrolyte imbalances and prevent abdominal distension.

Prognosis. If symptomatic Meckel's diverticulum is diagnosed and treated early, full recovery is likely. Because of the potential for surgical complications, resection of asymptomatic Meckel's diverticulum remains controversial.

BOX 25.11 Clinical Manifestations of Meckel's Diverticulum

Abdominal Pain
- Similar to appendicitis
- May be vague and recurrent

Bloody Stools
- Painless
- Bright or dark red with mucus (currant jelly–like stool)
- In infants, bleeding sometimes accompanied by pain

Occasional
- Severe anaemia
- Shock

Nursing Care Management

Nursing objectives are the same as for any child undergoing surgery. (See Chapter 22.) When intestinal bleeding is present, specific preoperative considerations include frequent monitoring of vital signs and blood pressure, keeping the child on bed rest and recording the approximate amount of blood lost in stools.

Postoperatively the child requires IV fluids and an NG tube for decompression and evacuation of gastric secretions. Because the onset of illness is usually rapid, psychological support is important, as in other acute conditions, such as appendicitis. It is important to remember that massive rectal bleeding is usually traumatic to both the child and the parents and may significantly affect their emotional reaction to hospitalisation and surgery.

Inflammatory Bowel Disease

Inflammatory bowel disease (IBD) should not be confused with IBS. *IBD* is a term used to refer to three major forms of chronic intestinal inflammation: Crohn's disease (CD), ulcerative colitis (UC) and inflammatory bowel disease unspecified (IBDU). CD and UC have similar epidemiological, immunological and clinical features, but they are distinct disorders. The diagnosis of IBDU is used for patients with colonic disease, but their features are not specific to UC or CD; it is very rare (Conrad & Rosh 2017).

Both CD and UC tend to be more aggressive if the onset occurs in childhood (Conrad & Rosh 2017). Exacerbations and remissions without complete resolution of symptoms are also characteristics of IBD.

Aetiology

Despite decades of research, the aetiology of IBD is not completely understood and there is no known cure. There is evidence to indicate a multifactorial aetiology. Genetic, environmental and microbial factors are associated with IBD, and research focuses on genetic associations and theories of defective immunoregulation of the inflammatory response to bacteria or viruses in the GI tract (Rosen et al 2017). Genome-wide studies have confirmed at least 150 genes that increase the risk for IBD in individuals (Rosen et al 2017). Furthermore, children who immigrate from developing countries to Western countries show an incidence of IBD similar to that of Western populations, confirming an environmental factor with the disease (Rosen et al 2017). Finally, most individuals have 10 trillion bacteria and fungi in their intestinal microbiome, but children and adults with IBD have small diversity of intestinal bacterial species with an overrepresentation and underrepresentation of some species (Rosen et al 2017).

Pathophysiology. The inflammation found with UC is limited to the colon and rectum, with the distal colon and rectum the most severely affected. Inflammation affects the mucosa and submucosa and involves continuous segments along the length of the bowel with varying degrees of ulceration, bleeding and oedema. Thickening of the bowel wall and fibrosis are unusual, but long-standing disease can result in shortening of the colon and strictures. Toxic megacolon is the most dangerous form of severe colitis.

The chronic inflammatory process of CD involves any part of the GI tract from the mouth to the anus but most often affects the terminal ileum. The disease involves all layers of the bowel wall (transmural) in a discontinuous fashion, meaning that between areas of intact mucosa, there are areas of affected mucosa (skip lesions). The inflammation may result in: ulcerations; fibrosis; adhesions; stiffening of the bowel wall; stricture formation; and fistulas to other loops of bowel, bladder, vagina or skin.

Clinical Signs and Symptoms

Children with UC may experience mild, moderate or severe symptoms, depending on the extent of mucosal inflammation and systemic symptoms. UC often manifests with the insidious onset of diarrhoea, possibly with haematochezia, and usually without fever or weight loss. The course of the disease may remain mild with intermittent exacerbations. Some children and adolescents are seen with grossly bloody diarrhoea, cramps, urgency with defecation, mild anaemia, fever, anorexia, weight loss and moderate signs of systemic illness. Severe UC is characterised by frequent bloody stools, abdominal pain, significant anaemia, fever and weight loss. Extraintestinal manifestations are not common in UC. Enlarged lymph nodes (lymphadenopathy), arthritis and the skin lesions of erythema nodosum may be present.

Common presenting manifestations of CD include diarrhoea, abdominal pain with cramps, fever and weight loss. Extraintestinal manifestations, including aphthous ulcers, peripheral arthritis, erythema nodosum, digital clubbing, renal stones and gallstones, are more common with CD than UC (Grossman & Baldassano 2016). Growth failure and delayed sexual maturation are often present for several years before overt GI symptoms are present (Conrad & Rosh 2017). Both malabsorption and anorexia are factors that contribute to the growth problems that are prevalent in CD. Children with CD may have perianal disease, including tags, fissures, fistulas or abscesses (Rosen et al 2017). The effects of UC and CD are listed in Figure 25.3. Table 25.4 provides a comparison of UC and CD.

TABLE 25.4 Clinical Manifestations of Inflammatory Bowel Diseases

Characteristics	Ulcerative Colitis	Crohn's Disease
Rectal bleeding	Common	Uncommon
Diarrhoea	Often severe	Moderate to severe
Pain	Less frequent	Common
Anorexia	Mild or moderate	May be severe
Weight loss	Moderate	May be severe
Growth restriction	Usually mild	May be severe
Anal and perianal lesions	Rare	Common
Fistulas and strictures	Rare	Common
Rashes	Mild	Mild
Joint pain	Mild to moderate	Mild to moderate

Diagnostic Evaluation

The diagnosis of UC and CD comes from the history, physical examination, laboratory evaluation and other diagnostic procedures. Laboratory tests include a FBC to evaluate anaemia and an erythrocyte sedimentation rate (ESR) or CRP to assess the systemic reaction to the inflammatory process. The ESR or CRP may be elevated, indicating a systemic response to an inflammatory process. Levels of total protein, albumin, iron, zinc, magnesium, vitamin B_{12} and fat-soluble vitamins may be low in children with CD. Stools are examined for blood, leucocytes and infectious organisms. A serological panel is often used in combination with clinical findings to diagnose IBD and to differentiate between CD and UC.

In patients with CD, an upper GI series with small bowel follow-through assists in assessing the existence, location and extent of disease. Upper endoscopy and colonoscopy with biopsies are an integral part of diagnosing IBD (Rosen et al 2017). Endoscopy allows direct visualisation of the surface of the GI tract so that the extent of inflammation and narrowing can be evaluated. CT and ultrasound also may be used to identify bowel wall inflammation, intraabdominal abscesses and fistulas. Colonoscopy can confirm the diagnosis and evaluate the extent of the disease. Discrete ulcers are commonly seen in patients

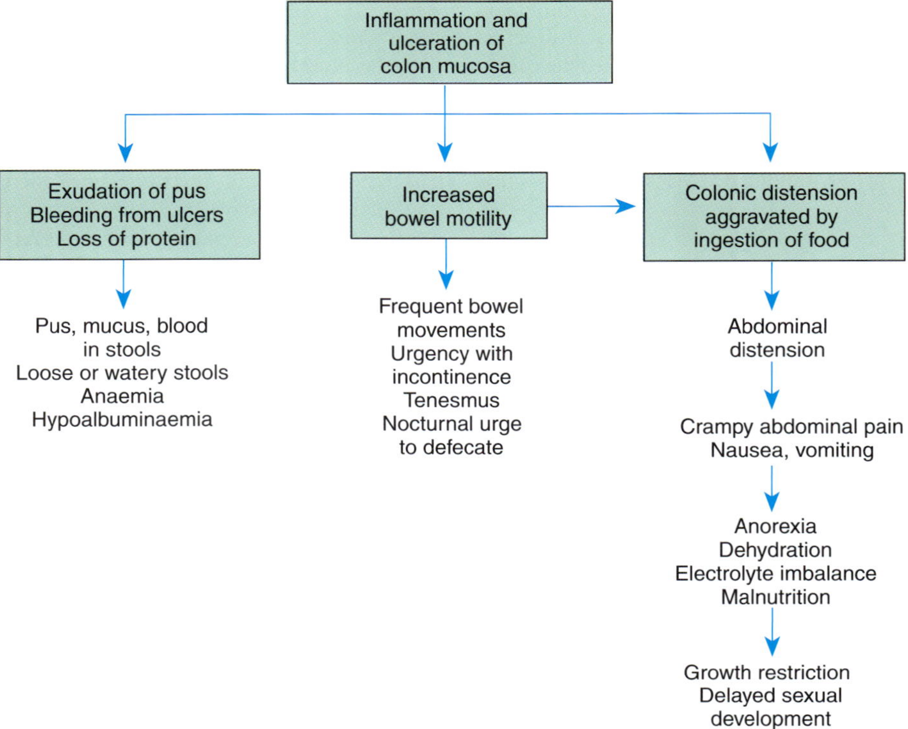

Fig 25.3 Effects of ulcerative colitis or Crohn's disease.

with CD, whereas micro-ulcers and diffuse abnormalities and inflammation are seen in patients with UC (Grossman & Baldassano 2016). CD lesions may pierce the walls of the small intestine and colon, creating tracts called *fistulas* between the intestine and adjacent structures such as the bladder, anus, vagina or skin.

Therapeutic Management

The natural history of the disease continues to be unpredictable and characterised by recurrent flare-ups that can severely impair patients' physical and social functioning (Grossman & Baldassano 2016). The goals of therapy are to control the inflammatory process to reduce or eliminate the symptoms, obtain long-term remission, promote normal growth and development and allow as normal a lifestyle as possible. Treatment is individualised and managed according to the type and the severity of the disease, its location and the response to therapy. CD is more disabling, has more serious complications and is often less amenable to medical and surgical treatment than is UC. Because UC is confined to the colon, a colectomy may cure UC.

Medical Treatment. The goal of any treatment regimen is first to induce remission of acute symptoms and then to maintain remission over time. 5-Aminosalicylates (5-ASAs) are effective in the induction and maintenance of remission in mild to moderate UC. Mesalazine, olsalazine and balsalazide are preferred over sulfasalazine because of reduced side effects (e.g. headache, nausea, vomiting, neutropenia and oligospermia). Suppository and enema preparations of Mesalazine are used to treat left-sided colitis. These drugs decrease inflammation by inhibiting prostaglandin synthesis. 5-ASAs can be used to induce remission in mild CD.

Corticosteroids, such as prednisone and prednisolone, are indicated in induction therapy in children with moderate to severe UC and CD. These drugs inhibit the production of adhesion molecules, cytokines and leukotrienes. Although these drugs reduce the acute symptoms of IBD, they are not commonly used for maintenance therapy because of their long-term side effects including growth suppression (adrenal suppression), weight gain and decreased bone density (Rosen et al 2017). High doses of IV corticosteroids may be administered in acute episodes and tapered according to clinical response.

Immunomodulators are used to induce and maintain remission in children with IBD who are steroid resistant or steroid dependent and in treating chronic draining fistulas. They block the synthesis of purine, thus inhibiting the ability of deoxyribonucleic acid (DNA) and ribonucleic acid (RNA) to hinder lymphocyte function, especially that of T cells. Side effects include infection, pancreatitis, hepatitis, bone marrow toxicity, arthralgia and malignancy. Methotrexate is also useful in inducing and maintaining remission in CD patients who are unresponsive to standard therapies. Patients on immunomodulating medications require regular monitoring of their FBC and differential to assess for changes that reflect suppression of the immune system because many of the side effects can be prevented or managed by dose reduction or discontinuation of medication.

Antibiotics, such as metronidazole and ciprofloxacin, may be used as an adjunctive therapy to treat complications such as perianal disease or small bowel bacterial overgrowth in CD. Side effects of these drugs are peripheral neuropathy, nausea and a metallic taste.

Biological therapies act to regulate inflammatory and anti-inflammatory cytokines. The use of anti–tumour necrosis factor-alpha (TNF-alpha) agents such as infliximab and adalimumab decrease active inflammation and are effective in healing the intestinal mucosal lining and perianal fistulas and have even improved linear growth in children (Grossman & Baldassano 2016, Rosen et al 2017). These agents are now being used as front-line therapy in children with CD with severe deep mucosal ulcerations, perianal fistulas or growth failure (Rosen et al 2017).

Nutritional Support. Nutritional support is important in the treatment of IBD. Growth failure is a common serious complication, especially in CD. Growth failure is characterised by weight loss, alteration in body composition, restricted height and delayed sexual maturation. Malnutrition causes the growth failure and its aetiology is multifactorial. Malnutrition occurs as a result of inadequate dietary intake, excessive GI losses, malabsorption, drug-nutrient interaction and increased nutritional requirements. Inadequate dietary intake occurs with anorexia and episodes of increased disease activity. Excessive loss of nutrients (e.g. protein, blood, electrolytes and minerals) occur secondary to intestinal inflammation and diarrhoea. Carbohydrate, lactose, fat, vitamin and mineral malabsorption, as well as vitamin B_{12} and folic acid deficiencies, occur with disease episodes and with drug administration and when the terminal ileum is resected. Finally, nutritional requirements are increased with inflammation, fever, fistulas and periods of rapid growth (e.g. adolescence).

The goals of nutritional support include correction of nutrient deficits and replacement of ongoing losses, provision of adequate energy and protein for healing and provision of adequate nutrients to promote normal growth. Nutritional support includes both enteral and parenteral nutrition. A well-balanced, high-protein, high-calorie diet is recommended for children whose symptoms do not prohibit an adequate oral intake. There is little evidence that avoiding specific foods influences the severity of the disease. Supplementation with multivitamins, iron and folic acid is recommended.

Total parenteral nutrition (TPN) has also improved nutritional status in patients with IBD. Short-term remissions have been achieved after TPN, although complete bowel rest has not reduced inflammation or added to the benefits of improved nutrition by TPN. Nutritional support is less likely to induce a remission in UC than in CD. Improvement of nutritional status is important, however, in preventing deterioration of the patient's health status and in preparing the patient for surgery.

Surgical Treatment. Surgery is indicated for UC when medical and nutritional therapies fail to prevent complications. Surgical options include a **subtotal colectomy** and **ileostomy** that leaves a rectal stump as a blind pouch.

Prognosis. IBD is a chronic disease. Relatively long periods of quiescent disease may follow exacerbations. The outcome is influenced by the regions and severity of involvement, as well as by appropriate therapeutic management. Malnutrition, growth failure and bleeding are serious complications. The overall prognosis for UC is good.

The development of colorectal cancer (CRC) is a long-term complication of IBD. Because the risk for CRC occurs 8 to 10 years after diagnosis, surveillance colonoscopy with multiple biopsies should begin approximately 7 to 10 years after diagnosis of UC or CD (Rosen et al 2017). In CD, surgical removal of the affected colon does not prevent cancer from developing elsewhere in the GI tract.

Nursing Care Management

The nursing considerations in the management of IBD extend beyond the immediate period of hospitalisation. These interventions involve continued guidance of families in terms of: (1) managing diet; (2) coping with factors that increase stress and emotional lability; (3) adjusting to a disease of remissions and exacerbations; and (4) when indicated, preparing the child and parents for the possibility of diversionary bowel surgery.

The importance of continued drug therapy despite remission of symptoms must be stressed to the child and family members. Failure to adhere to the pharmacological regimen can result in exacerbation of the disease. (See Compliance, Chapter 22.) Unfortunately, exacerbation of IBD can occur even if the child and family are compliant with the treatment regimen; this is difficult for the child and family to cope with.

Emotional Support. The nurse should attend to the emotional components of the disease and assess any sources of stress. Frequently, the nurse can help children adjust to problems of growth restriction, delayed sexual maturation, dietary restrictions, feelings of being 'different' or 'sickly', inability to compete with peers and necessary absence from school during exacerbations of the illness.

If a permanent colectomy-ileostomy is required, the nurse can teach the child and family how to care for the ileostomy. The nurse can also emphasise the positive aspects of the surgery, particularly accelerated growth and sexual development, permanent recovery and the normality of life despite bowel diversion.

Peptic Ulcer Disease

Peptic ulcer disease (PUD) is a chronic condition that affects the stomach or duodenum. Ulcers are described as gastric or duodenal and as primary or secondary. A **gastric ulcer** involves the mucosa of the stomach; a **duodenal ulcer** involves the pylorus or duodenum. Most **primary ulcers** are idiopathic or associated with *Helicobacter pylori* infection and tend to be chronic, occurring more frequently in the duodenum (Blanchard & Czinn 2016). **Secondary ulcers** result from the stress of a severe underlying disease or injury (e.g. severe burns, sepsis, increased intracranial pressure, severe trauma, multisystem organ failure) and are more frequently gastric with an acute onset (Blanchard & Czinn 2016).

Aetiology

The exact cause of PUD is unknown, although infectious, genetic and environmental factors are important. There is an increased familial incidence, likely due to *H. pylori*, which is known to cluster in families (Blanchard & Czinn 2016). *H. pylori* is a microaerophilic, gram-negative, slow-growing, spiral-shaped and flagellated bacterium known to colonise the gastric mucosa in about half of the population of the world (Blanchard & Czinn 2016). *H. pylori* synthesises the enzyme urease, which hydrolyses urea to form ammonia and carbon dioxide. Ammonia then absorbs acid to form ammonium, thus raising the gastric pH. *H. pylori* may cause ulcers by weakening the gastric mucosal barrier and allowing acid to damage the mucosa. It is believed that it is acquired via the faecal-oral route, and this hypothesis is supported by finding viable *H. pylori* in faeces.

In addition to ulcerogenic drugs, both alcohol and smoking contribute to ulcer formation. There is no conclusive evidence to implicate particular foods, such as caffeine-containing beverages or spicy foods, but polyunsaturated fats and fibre may play a role in ulcer formation. Psychological factors may play a role in the development of PUD, and stressful life events, dependency, passiveness and hostility have all been implicated as contributing factors.

Pathophysiology

Most likely, the pathology is due to an imbalance between the destructive (cytotoxic) factors and defensive (cytoprotective) factors in the GI tract. The toxic mechanisms include acid, pepsin, medications such as aspirin and non-steroidal anti-inflammatory drugs (NSAIDs), bile acids and infection with *H. pylori.* The defensive factors include the mucus layer, local bicarbonate secretion, epithelial cell renewal and mucosal blood flow. Prostaglandins play a role in mucosal defence because they stimulate both mucus and alkali secretion. The primary mechanism that prevents the development of peptic ulcer is the secretion of mucus by the epithelial and mucus glands throughout the stomach. The thick mucus layer acts to diffuse acid from the lumen to the gastric mucosal surface, thus protecting the gastric epithelium. The stomach and the duodenum produce bicarbonate, decreasing acidity on the epithelial cells and thereby minimising the effects of the low pH. When abnormalities in the protective barrier exist, the mucosa is vulnerable to damage by acid and pepsin. Exogenous factors, such as aspirin and NSAIDs, cause gastric ulcers by inhibition of prostaglandin synthesis.

Zollinger-Ellison syndrome is rare but may occur in children who have multiple, large or recurrent ulcers. This syndrome is characterised by hypersecretion of gastric acid, intractable ulcer disease and intestinal malabsorption caused by a gastrin-secreting tumour of the pancreas. The pathogenesis, manifestations and complications of PUD are outlined in Figure 25.4.

Clinical Manifestations

The clinical manifestations of PUD vary according to the child's age and the ulcer's location. Common clinical manifestations include: chronic abdominal pain, especially when the stomach is empty, such as during the night or early morning; recurrent vomiting; haematemesis; melaena; chronic anaemia; and abdominal tenderness (Box 25.12).

Diagnostic Evaluation

Diagnosis is based on the history of symptoms, physical examination and diagnostic testing. The focus is on symptoms such as epigastric abdominal pain, nocturnal pain, oral regurgitation, heartburn, weight loss, haematemesis and melaena. History should include questions relating to the use of potentially causative substances such as NSAIDs, corticosteroids, alcohol and tobacco. Frequently a history of epigastric and periumbilical pain accompanies PUD. However, children often find it difficult to describe the location of their pain and frequently indicate the location by moving their hand in a circular movement all around the stomach area. Asking the child to take one finger and point to the area where it hurts the most often helps identify the location of the pain. Pain may also be elicited during the examination with palpation.

Laboratory studies may include: a FBC to detect anaemia, stool analysis for occult blood, liver function tests (LFTs), ESR or CRP to evaluate IBD; amylase and lipase to evaluate pancreatitis; and gastric acid measurements to identify hypersecretion. Stool analysis is performed to rule out infection. Polyclonal and monoclonal stool antigen tests are an accurate, non-invasive method both for the initial diagnosis of *H. pylori* and for the confirmation of its eradication after treatment (Yang 2016). A ^{13}C urea breath test measures bacterial colonisation in the gastric mucosa and can be used as an additional non-invasive test to determine the presence of antibodies to *H. pylori.*

An upper GI series is the most reliable way to detect and diagnose PUD in children (Blanchard & Czinn 2016). Direct visualisation of the gastric and duodenal mucosa helps identify specific lesions and biopsy specimens can determine the presence of *H. pylori.*

Therapeutic Management

The major goals of therapy for children with PUD are to relieve discomfort, promote healing, prevent complications and prevent recurrence. Management is primarily medical and consists of administration of medications to treat the infection and to reduce or neutralise gastric acid secretion. Antacids are beneficial medications to neutralise gastric acid. Histamine (H_2) receptor antagonists (antisecretory drugs—PPIs) act to suppress gastric acid production. These medications have few side effects and act to inhibit the hydrogen ion pump in the parietal cells, thus blocking the production of acid. Many of the recommended medications have not been well studied in children; they are used in clinical practice to treat ulcers, GOR, oesophagitis

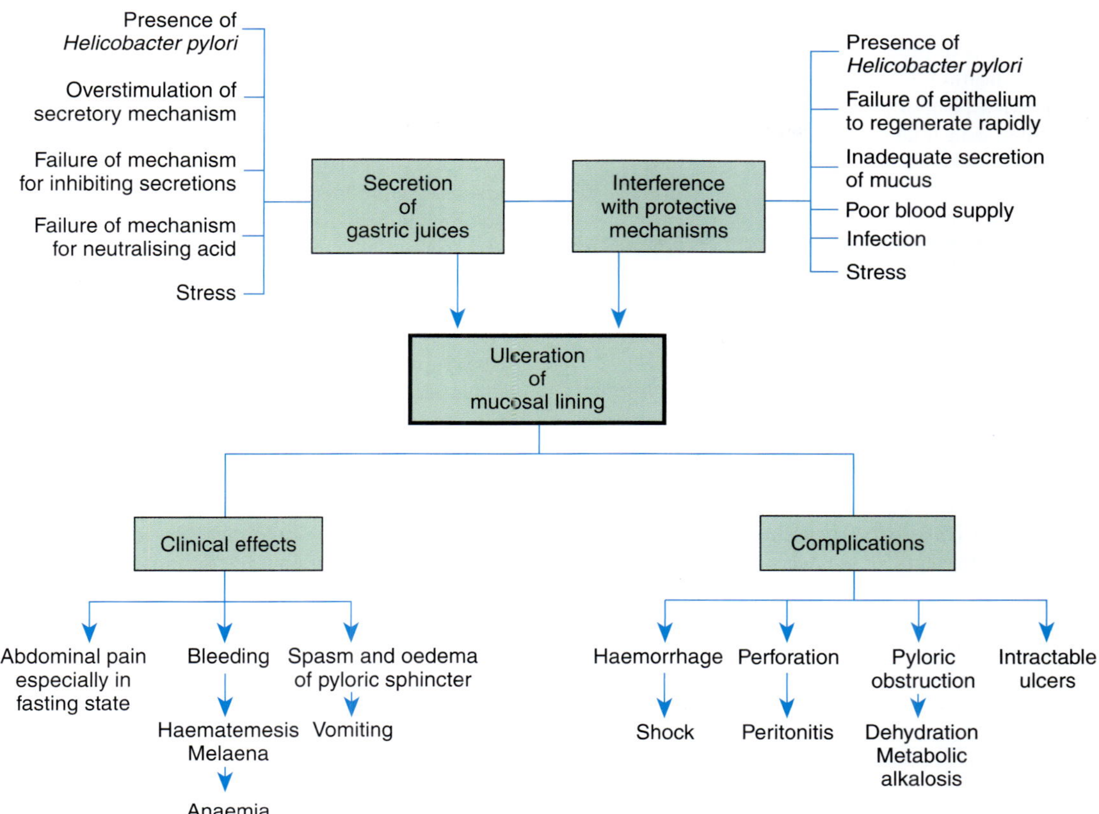

Fig 25.4 Possible causes and effects of peptic ulcer.

BOX 25.12 Characteristics of Peptic Ulcers

Neonates

- Usually gastric and secondary ulcers
- Commonly a history of prematurity, respiratory distress, sepsis, hypoglycaemia or an intraventricular haemorrhage
- Perforation possibly leading to massive bleeding

Infants to 2-year-old Children

- Most likely to have a secondary ulcer located equally in the stomach or duodenum
- Primary ulcers less common and usually located in stomach
- Likely to be noticed in relation to illness, surgery or trauma
- Haematemesis, melena or perforation

2- to 6-year-old Children

- Primary or secondary ulcers
- Located equally in stomach and duodenum
- Perforation more likely in secondary ulcers
- Periumbilical pain, poor eating, vomiting, irritability, night-time wakening, haematemesis, melaena

Children Over 6 Years

- Usually primary and most often duodenal ulcers
- More typical of adult type
- Chance of recurrence greater
- Often associated with *Helicobacter pylori*
- Epigastric pain or vague abdominal pain
- Night-time wakening, haematemesis, melaena and anaemia possible

and gastritis and appear to be well tolerated with infrequent side effects (e.g. headache, diarrhoea, nausea) (Blanchard & Czinn 2016).

Endoscopy is the gold standard for diagnosis for this condition, however due to this being not possible in many cases and an invasive procedure, treatment may go ahead without this procedure taking place. The goal of treatment is to eradicate the cause of the ulcer if any, triple antibiotic are ideal, being Amoxicillin, Clarithromycin, and Omeprazole. Australian therapeutic guidelines recommend the regime be given no less than 7 days and the international recommendations at up to 14 days. The inclusion of bismuth salts may sometimes be used after first line treatment with antibiotics.

Children with an acute ulcer who have developed complications, such as massive haemorrhage, require emergency care. The administration of IV fluids, blood or plasma depends on the amount of blood loss. Replacement with whole blood or packed cells may be necessary for significant loss.

Surgical intervention may be required for complications such as haemorrhage, perforation or gastric outlet obstruction. Ligation of the source of bleeding or closure of a perforation is performed. A vagotomy and pyloroplasty may be indicated in children with bleeding ulcers despite aggressive medical treatment (Patel et al 2015).

Prognosis. The long-term prognosis for PUD is variable. Many ulcers are successfully treated with medical therapy; however, primary duodenal peptic ulcers often recur. Complications such as GI bleeding can occur and extend into adult life. The effect of maintenance drug therapy on long-term morbidity remains to be established with further studies.

Nursing Care Management

The primary nursing goal is to promote healing of the ulcer through compliance with the medication regimen. If an analgesic-antipyretic is needed, paracetamol, not aspirin or NSAIDs, is used. Critically ill neonates, infants and children in intensive care units should receive H_2 blockers to prevent stress ulcers.

NURSING CARE CONSIDERATIONS

H_2 Blockers

Critically ill children receiving IV H_2 blockers should have their gastric pH values checked at frequent intervals.

OBSTRUCTIVE DISORDERS

Obstruction in the GI tract occurs when the passage of nutrients and secretions is impeded by a constricted or occluded lumen or when there is impaired motility (**paralytic ileus**). Obstructions may be congenital or acquired. Congenital obstructions, such as oesophageal or intestinal atresias, imperforate anus and meconium ileus, usually appear in the neonatal period. Other obstructions of congenital aetiology (e.g. malrotation, HD, pyloric stenosis, volvulus, incarcerated hernia and Meckel's diverticulum) appear after the first few weeks of life. Intestinal obstruction from acquired causes such as intussusception and tumours may occur in infancy or childhood.

Acute intestinal obstruction is commonly characterised by abdominal pain, nausea, vomiting, abdominal distension and a change in stooling patterns (Box 25.13). Pain is caused by intermittent muscular contractions proximal to the obstruction as the bowel attempts to move luminal contents along the normal path. It may also be due to severe abdominal distension, which results from accumulation of gas and fluid above the level of the obstruction. As abdominal distension progresses, the abdomen may become extremely tender, rigid and firm.

When abdominal contents continue to accumulate, nausea and vomiting occur. Vomiting of gastric contents is often the first sign of a high obstruction, such as obstruction of the pylorus, and vomiting of bile-stained material is a sign of obstruction of the small intestine.

BOX 25.13 Clinical Manifestations of Mechanical (Paralytic) Intestinal Obstruction

Colicky abdominal pain—From peristalsis attempting to overcome the obstruction
Abdominal distension—As a result of accumulation of gas and fluid above the level of the obstruction
Vomiting—Often the earliest sign of a high obstruction; a later sign of lower obstruction (may be bilious or feculent)
Constipation and obstipation—Early signs of low obstructions; later signs of higher obstructions
Dehydration—From losses of large quantities of fluid and electrolytes into the intestine
Rigid and boardlike abdomen—From increased distension
Bowel sounds—Gradually diminish and cease
Respiratory distress—Occurs as the diaphragm is pushed up into the pleural cavity
Shock—Caused by plasma volume diminishing as fluids and electrolytes are lost from the bloodstream into the intestinal lumen
Sepsis—Caused by bacterial proliferation with invasion into the circulation

Persistent vomiting can lead to dehydration and electrolyte disturbances. Constipation and obstipation (prolonged absence of defecation) are early signs of low obstructions and later signs of higher obstructions. In acute conditions such as intussusception, the clinical manifestations are apparent within a few hours of the onset of the disorder. In other conditions such as hypertrophic pyloric stenosis the signs and symptoms may have a more gradual onset. Bowel sounds may initially be hyperactive, then diminish or cease. Respiratory distress may occur when the diaphragm is pushed up into the pleural cavity as a result of severe abdominal distension.

Hypertrophic Pyloric Stenosis

Hypertrophic pyloric stenosis (HPS) occurs when the circumferential muscle of the pyloric sphincter becomes thickened, resulting in elongation and narrowing of the pyloric canal. This produces an outlet obstruction and compensatory dilation, hypertrophy and hyperperistalsis of the stomach. This condition usually develops in the first few weeks of life, causing non-bilious vomiting, which occurs after a feeding; projectile vomiting may develop and the infant is fussy and hungry after vomiting. If the condition is not diagnosed early, dehydration, metabolic alkalosis and faltering growth may occur. The precise aetiology of HPS is not known. Boys are affected four to six times more frequently than girls (Hunter & Liacouras 2016).

Pathophysiology

The circular muscle of the pylorus thickens as a result of hypertrophy. This produces severe narrowing of the pyloric canal between the stomach and the duodenum. Consequently, the lumen at this point is partially obstructed. Over time, inflammation and oedema further reduce the size of the opening, resulting in complete obstruction. The hypertrophied pylorus may be palpable as an olive-like mass in the upper abdomen (Fig 25.5).

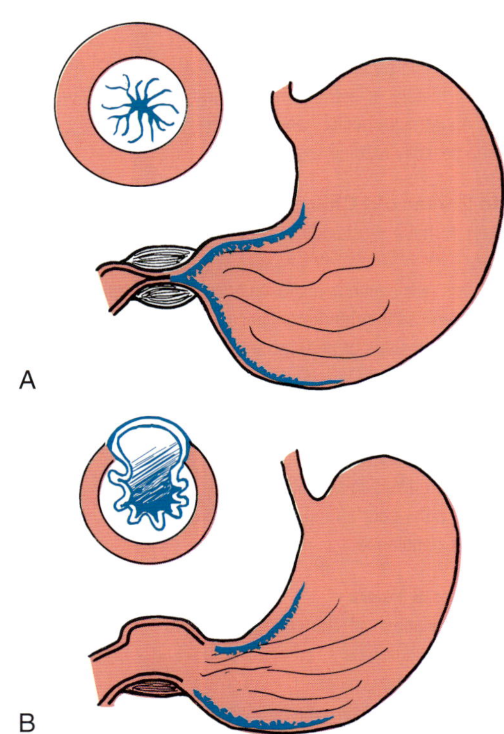

Fig 25.5 Hypertrophic pyloric stenosis. (**A**) Enlarged muscular tumour nearly obliterates pyloric canal. (**B**) Longitudinal surgical division of muscle down to submucosa establishes adequate passageway.

Pyloric stenosis is not a congenital disorder. It is believed that local innervation may be involved in the pathogenesis. In most cases, HPS is an isolated lesion; however, it may be associated with intestinal malrotation, oesophageal and duodenal atresia and anorectal anomalies.

Clinical Manifestations

Infants with HPS have non-bilious vomiting in the early stages (Box 25.14). Vomiting usually begins at 3 weeks of age but can start as early as 1 week and as late as 5 months. Vomiting usually occurs 30 to 60 minutes after feeding and becomes projectile as the obstruction progresses. Initially the infant is hungry and irritable, but prolonged vomiting may lead to dehydration, weight loss and faltering growth. Gastric peristalsis may be visible on examination, and the olive-shaped mass in the epigastrium just to the right of the umbilicus may be palpated (see Fig 25.5A).

Diagnostic Evaluation

The diagnosis of HPS is often made after the history and physical examination. The olive-like mass is most easily palpated when the stomach is empty, the infant is quiet and the abdominal muscles are relaxed. If the diagnosis is inconclusive from the history and physical examination, ultrasonography will demonstrate an elongated mass surrounding a long pyloric canal. If ultrasonography does not demonstrate a hypertrophied pylorus, upper GI radiography should be done to rule out other causes of vomiting.

If the condition is not diagnosed early, laboratory findings reflect the metabolic alterations created by moderate to severe depletion of both water and electrolytes from extensive and prolonged vomiting. There are decreased serum levels of both sodium and potassium, although these may be masked by the haemoconcentration from extracellular fluid depletion. Of greater diagnostic value are a decrease in serum chloride levels and increases in pH and bicarbonate (carbon dioxide content), indicative of metabolic alkalosis. The blood urea nitrogen will be elevated as evidence of dehydration. However, in those cases diagnosed early, laboratory findings may not be significant.

Therapeutic Management

Surgical relief of the pyloric obstruction by pyloromyotomy is the standard therapy for this disorder. Preoperatively the infant must be rehydrated and metabolic alkalosis corrected with parenteral fluid and electrolyte administration. Replacement fluid therapy usually delays surgery for 24 to 48 hours. The stomach is decompressed with an NG tube if the infant continues with vomiting. In infants with no evidence of fluid and electrolyte imbalance, surgery is performed without delay.

Prognosis. The prognosis for infants and small children with HPS is excellent when the diagnosis is confirmed early, and the mortality rate is low (0% to 0.5%). A small percentage of children with HPS will have GOR.

BOX 25.14 Clinical Manifestations of Hypertrophic Pyloric Stenosis

- Projectile vomiting
  - May be ejected 1 to 1.2 m from the child when in a side-lying position to 30 to 50 cm or more when in a back-lying position
  - Usually occurs shortly after a feeding, but may not occur for several hours
  - May follow each feeding or appear intermittently
  - Non-bilious vomitus that may be blood tinged
- Infant hungry, avid nurser; eagerly accepts a second feeding after vomiting episode
- No evidence of pain or discomfort except that of chronic hunger
- Poor weight gain
- Signs of dehydration
- Distended upper abdomen
- Readily palpable olive-shaped tumour in the epigastrium just to the right of the umbilicus
- Visible gastric peristaltic waves that move from left to right across the epigastrium

Nursing Care Management

Nursing care involves primarily observation for clinical features that help establish the diagnosis, careful regulation of fluid therapy and reestablishment of normal feeding patterns. Nurses must be alert to signs of HPS in infants and refer them for medical evaluation.

Preoperatively, the emphasis is on restoring hydration and electrolyte balance. The infant is kept NBM and given IV fluids with glucose and electrolytes based on serum electrolyte values and clinical appearance.

Postoperative vomiting is common, and most infants, even with successful surgery, exhibit some vomiting during the first 24 to 48 hours. IV fluids are administered until the infant is taking and retaining adequate amounts by mouth. Appropriate analgesics should be given around the clock because pain is continuous. The surgical incision(s) is inspected for drainage or erythema, and any signs of infection are reported to the surgeon. A surgical adhesive may be used for incision closure, and parents are instructed regarding the care of the incision and any dressings before discharge.

Intussusception

Intussusception is the most common cause of intestinal obstruction in children between 3 months and 6 years old (Carroll et al 2017). Intussusception is more common in males than in females and is more common in children younger than 2 years old. Although specific intestinal lesions occur in a small percentage of the children, generally the cause is not known. Only 12.5% to 25% of intussusception cases have a pathological lead point, such as a polyp, lymphoma or Meckel's diverticulum (Carroll et al 2017). The idiopathic cases may be caused by hypertrophy of intestinal lymphoid tissue secondary to viral infection.

Pathophysiology

Intussusception occurs when a proximal segment of the bowel telescopes into a more distal segment, pulling the mesentery with it. The mesentery is compressed and angled, resulting in lymphatic and venous obstruction. As the oedema from the obstruction increases, pressure within the area of intussusception increases. When the pressure equals the arterial pressure, arterial blood flow stops, resulting in ischaemia and the pouring of mucus into the intestine. Venous engorgement also leads to leaking of blood and mucus into the intestinal lumen, forming the classic currant jelly–like stools. The most common site is the ileocaecal valve (ileocolic), where the ileum invaginates into the caecum and then further into the colon (Fig 25.6). Other forms include ileoileal (i.e. one part of the ileum invaginates into another section of the ileum) and colocolic (i.e. one part of the colon invaginates into another area of the colon) intussusceptions, usually in the area of the hepatic or splenic flexure or at some point along the transverse colon.

Clinical Manifestations

Intussusception usually manifests with the sudden onset of crampy abdominal pain, inconsolable crying and a drawing up of the knees to the chest in an otherwise healthy child (Box 25.15). Between episodes the child appears normal. As the obstruction progresses, bilious vomiting may occur and lethargy increases. The classic triad of intussusception symptoms (abdominal pain, abdominal mass, bloody stools) is present

PATHOPHYSIOLOGY REVIEW

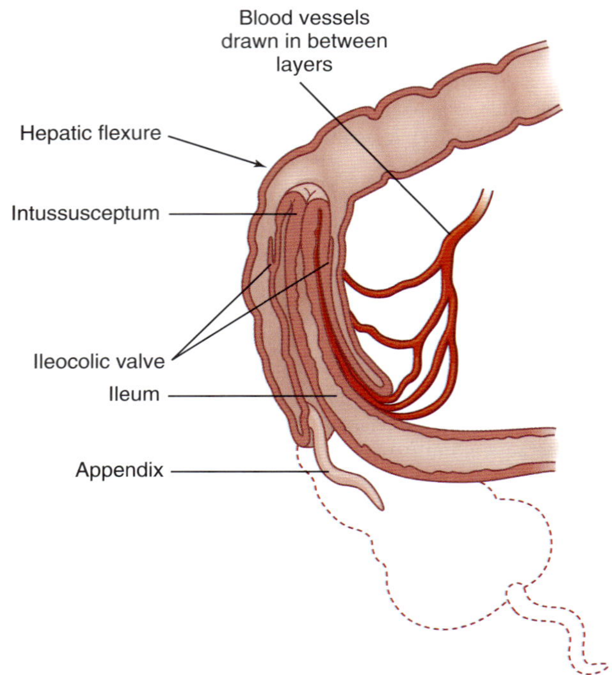

Fig 25.6 Ileocaecal valve (ileocolic) intussusception.

BOX 25.15 Clinical Manifestations of Intussusception

- Sudden acute abdominal pain
- Child screaming and drawing the knees up to the chest
- Child appearing normal and comfortable between episodes of pain
- Vomiting
- Lethargy
- Passage of red, currant jelly–like stools (stool mixed with blood and mucus)
- Tender, distended abdomen
- Palpable sausage-shaped mass in upper right quadrant
- Empty lower right quadrant (Dance's sign)
- Eventual fever, prostration and other signs of peritonitis

in less than 30% of children (Kennedy & Liacouras 2016b). A more chronic case may be presented, characterised by diarrhoea, anorexia, weight loss, occasional vomiting and periodic pain. Because intussusception is potentially life-threatening, be aware of such signs and closely observe, and refer these children for further medical evaluation. With atypical cases, lethargy may be the primary symptom. If the distal bowel remains distended, necrosis and perforation are possible.

Diagnostic Evaluation

Frequently, subjective findings lead to the diagnosis. However, definitive diagnosis is based on ultrasonography that reveals a characteristic heterogenous mass and a 'bull's-eye'.

Therapeutic Management

Conservative treatment consists of radiologist-guided pneumoenema (gas enema) or ultrasound-guided hydrostatic enema, the advantage of the latter being that no ionising radiation is needed (Kennedy & Liacouras 2016b). Recurrence of intussusception after conservative treatment is rare; however, this procedure should not be attempted with prolonged intussusception, signs of shock, peritoneal irritation or intestinal perforation (Kennedy & Liacouras 2016b).

IV fluids, NG decompression and antibiotic therapy may be used before hydrostatic reduction is attempted. If these procedures are not successful, the child may require surgical intervention. Surgery involves manually reducing the invagination and, when indicated, resecting any non-viable intestine.

Prognosis. Non-operative reduction is successful in the majority of stable cases. Gas enema is slightly more successful with reduction compared to a hydrostatic enema (83% versus 70%, respectively) (Carroll et al 2017). Surgery is required for patients in whom the reduction is unsuccessful or for patients who are unstable. With early diagnosis and treatment, serious complications and death are uncommon.

Nursing Care Management

The nurse can help establish a diagnosis by listening to the parent's description of the child's physical and behavioural symptoms. It is not unusual for parents to state that they thought something was seriously wrong before others shared their concerns. The description of the child's severe colicky abdominal pain combined with vomiting is a significant sign of intussusception.

Malrotation and Volvulus

Malrotation of the intestine is caused by the abnormal rotation of the intestine around the superior mesenteric artery during embryological development. Malrotation may manifest in utero or at any age, but the majority of patients (80%) present in the first month of life (Carroll et al 2017). Infants may have intermittent bilious vomiting, recurrent abdominal pain, distension or lower GI bleeding. Malrotation is the most serious type of intestinal obstruction because if the intestine undergoes complete volvulus (i.e. the intestine twisting around itself), compromise of the blood supply will result in intestinal necrosis, peritonitis, perforation and death.

Diagnostic Evaluation

It is imperative that malrotation and volvulus be diagnosed promptly and surgical treatment instituted quickly. In addition to a history and physical, a plain abdominal radiograph and lateral decubitus view are obtained; bowel distension will be present proximal to the distension on plain radiograph, and a lateral view will demonstrate air-fluid levels in the distended bowel (Bales & Liacouras 2016). An upper GI series is the most accurate imaging study (Carroll et al 2017).

Therapeutic Management

Surgery is indicated to remove the affected area. Because of the extensive nature of some lesions, short bowel syndrome (SBS) is a postoperative complication.

Nursing Care Management

Preoperatively the nursing care is the same as that provided to an infant or child with intestinal obstruction. IV fluids, NG decompression and systemic antibiotics are implemented. In the rapidly deteriorating infant, fluid volume resuscitation and vasopressors may be required for preoperative stabilisation. Postoperatively, the nursing care is similar to that provided to the infant or child who has undergone abdominal surgery.

MALABSORPTION SYNDROMES

Chronic diarrhoea and malabsorption of nutrients characterise malabsorption syndromes. An important complication of malabsorption syndromes in children is faltering growth. Most cases are classified according to the location of the supposed anatomical or biochemical defect. The term **coeliac disease** is often used to describe a symptom complex with four characteristics: (1) steatorrhoea (fatty, foul, frothy, bulky stools); (2) general malnutrition; (3) abdominal distension; and (4) secondary vitamin deficiencies.

Digestive defects are conditions in which the enzymes necessary for digestion are diminished or absent, such as: (1) cystic fibrosis, in which pancreatic enzymes are absent; (2) biliary or liver disease, in which bile flow is affected; or (3) lactase deficiency, in which there is congenital or secondary lactose intolerance.

Absorptive defects are conditions in which the intestinal mucosal transport system is impaired. This may occur because of a primary defect (e.g. coeliac disease) or secondary to inflammatory disease of the bowel that results in impaired absorption because bowel motility is accelerated (e.g. ulcerative colitis). Obstructive disorders (e.g. Hirschsprung's disease) also cause secondary malabsorption from enterocolitis.

Anatomical defects, such as extensive resection of the bowel or SBS, affect digestion by decreasing the transit time of substances and affect absorption by severely compromising the absorptive surface.

Coeliac Disease (Gluten-sensitive Enteropathy)

Coeliac disease, also known as *gluten-induced enteropathy, gluten-sensitive enteropathy* and *coeliac sprue,* is an autoimmune disorder triggered by the ingestion of gluten in genetically susceptible individuals (Fok et al 2016). The disorder results in permanent intestinal intolerance to dietary gluten, a protein present in wheat, barley and rye that causes damage to the villi in the small intestine. Children with unexplained iron deficiency anaemia, recurrent aphthous stomatitis, dental enamel defects, type 1 diabetes, Down syndrome, selective immunoglobulin A deficiency, autoimmune thyroid disease, Turner's syndrome or Williams syndrome are more susceptible to being diagnosed with the disease (Paul et al 2016).

Pathophysiology

Coeliac disease is characterised by villous atrophy in the small intestine in response to the protein gluten. When individuals are unable to digest the gliadin component of gluten, an accumulation of a toxic substance occurs that is damaging to the mucosal cells. Damage to the mucosa of the small intestine leads to villous atrophy, hyperplasia of the crypts and infiltration of the epithelial cells with lymphocytes. Villous atrophy leads to malabsorption due to the reduced absorptive surface area (see Fig 25.1).

Genetic predisposition is an essential factor in the development of coeliac disease. Membrane receptors involved in preferential antigen presentation to $CD4^+$ T cells play a crucial role in the immune response characteristic of coeliac disease. Children with genetic susceptibilities, namely *HLA-DQ2* or *HLA-DQ8*, are more susceptible to being diagnosed with coeliac disease (Lebwohl et al 2018).

Clinical Manifestations

Symptoms of coeliac disease appear when solid foods such as beans and pasta are introduced into the child's diet between the ages of 1 and 5 years (Box 25.16). There is usually an interval of several months between the introduction of gluten into the diet and the onset of symptoms. Intestinal symptoms are common in children diagnosed within the first 2 years of life. Other symptoms include faltering growth, chronic diarrhoea, abdominal distension and pain, muscle wasting, aphthous ulcers and fatigue.

BOX 25.16 Clinical Manifestations of Coeliac Disease

Impaired Fat Absorption

- Steatorrhoea (excessively large, pale, oily, frothy stools)
- Exceedingly foul-smelling stools

Impaired Nutrient Absorption

- Malnutrition
- Muscle wasting (especially prominent in legs and buttocks)
- Anaemia
- Anorexia
- Abdominal distension

Behavioural Changes

- Irritability
- Uncooperativeness
- Apathy

Coeliac Crisis*

- Acute, severe episodes of profuse watery diarrhoea and vomiting
- May be precipitated by:
  - infections (especially gastrointestinal)
  - prolonged fluid and electrolyte depletion
  - emotional disturbance

*In very young children

Diagnostic Evaluation

Gluten should not be excluded from the diet until the diagnostic evaluation is complete so proper identification can occur. The first step is a serological blood test for tissue transglutaminase and antiendomyseal antibodies in children 18 months of age or older (Branski et al 2016). Positive serological markers should be followed by an upper GI endoscopy with biopsy. The diagnosis of coeliac disease is based on a biopsy of the small intestine demonstrating the characteristic changes of mucosal inflammation, crypt hyperplasia and villous atrophy (Branski et al 2016).

Therapeutic Management

Treatment of coeliac disease consists primarily of dietary management. Although a gluten-free diet is prescribed, it is actually low in gluten because it is impossible to remove every source of this protein. Because gluten is found primarily in wheat and rye, but also in smaller quantities in barley and oats, these four foods are eliminated. Corn, rice and millet are substitute grain foods.

Children with untreated coeliac disease may have lactose intolerance, especially if their mucosal lesions are extensive. Lactose intolerance usually improves as the mucosa heals with gluten withdrawal. Specific nutritional deficiencies, such as iron, folic acid and fat-soluble vitamin deficiencies, are treated with appropriate supplements.

Prognosis. Coeliac disease is regarded as a chronic disease; its severity varies greatly among children. The most severe symptoms usually occur in early childhood and again in adult life. Most children who comply with dietary management are healthy and remain free of symptoms and complications; however, children should be evaluated annually for nutritional deficiencies, impaired growth, delayed puberty and reduced bone mineral density (Fok et al 2016).

Nursing Care Management

The main nursing consideration is helping the child adhere to the dietary regimen. Considerable time is involved in explaining the disease process to the child and parents, the specific role of gluten in aggravating the disorder and those foods that must be restricted. It is difficult to maintain a diet indefinitely when the child has no symptoms and temporary transgressions result in no difficulties. However, the majority of individuals who relax their diet will experience a relapse of their disease.

In addition to restricting gluten, other dietary alterations may be necessary. For example, in some children who have more severe mucosal damage, the digestion of disaccharides is impaired, especially in relation to lactose. Therefore these children often need a temporarily lactose-free diet, which necessitates eliminating all milk products. In general, dietary management includes a diet high in calories and proteins with simple carbohydrates such as fruits and vegetables, but low in fats. Because the bowel is inflamed as a result of the pathological processes in absorption, the child must avoid high-fibre foods such as nuts, raisins, raw vegetables and raw fruits with skin until inflammation has subsided.

It is important to stress long-range complications and to remind parents of the child's physical status before dietary treatment and the dramatic improvement after treatment. The nurse can be instrumental in allowing the child to express concerns and frustration while focusing on ways in which the child can still feel normal.

Short Bowel Syndrome

Short bowel syndrome (SBS) is a malabsorptive disorder that occurs as a result of decreased mucosal surface area, usually because of extensive resection of the small intestine. Malabsorption may be exacerbated by other factors, such as bacterial overgrowth and dysmotility. The most common congenital causes of SBS in children are short bowel syndrome, multiple atresias and gastroschisis; other causes resulting in bowel resection include necrotising volvulus, meconium peritonitis, Crohn's disease and trauma (Vanderhoof & Branski 2016).

The definition of SBS includes two important findings: (1) decreased intestinal surface area for absorption of fluid, electrolytes and nutrients; and (2) a need for parenteral nutrition (PN) (Martin et al 2017). The prognosis for infants with SBS has improved dramatically, but the mortality rate within 5 years after diagnosis remains at 27% to 37% (Martin et al 2017).

Therapeutic Management

The goals of therapy for infants and children with SBS include: (1) preserving as much length of bowel as possible during surgery; (2) maintaining optimum nutritional status, growth and development while intestinal adaptation occurs; (3) stimulating intestinal adaptation with enteral feeding; and (4) minimising complications related to the disease process and therapy (Vanderhoof & Branski 2016).

Nutritional Support. Nutritional support is the long-term focus of care for children with SBS. The initial phase of therapy includes PN as the primary source of nutrition. The second phase is the introduction of enteral feeding, which usually begins as soon as possible after surgery. Elemental formulas containing glucose, sucrose and glucose polymers, hydrolysed proteins and medium-chain triglycerides facilitate absorption. Usually these formulas are given by continuous infusion through an NG or gastrostomy tube. As the enteral feedings are advanced, the PN solution is decreased in terms of calories, amount of fluid and total hours of infusion per day. If enteral feedings are tolerated, oral feedings should be attempted to minimise oral aversion and preserve oral skills (Vanderhoof & Branski 2016).

The final phase of nutritional support occurs when growth and development are sustained. When PN is discontinued, there is a risk of nutritional deficiency secondary to malabsorption of fat-soluble vitamins (A, D, E and K) and trace minerals (iron, selenium, zinc). Serum vitamin and mineral levels should be monitored closely and supplemented enterally, if needed. Pharmacological agents have been used to reduce secretory losses. H_2 blockers, PPIs and octreotide inhibit gastric or pancreatic secretion.

Numerous complications are associated with SBS and long-term PN. Infectious, metabolic and technical complications can occur. Sepsis can occur after improper care of the catheter. The GI tract can also be a source of microbial seeding of the catheter. Bowel atrophy may foster increased intestinal permeability of bacteria. A lack of adequate sites for central lines may become a significant problem for the child in need of long-term PN. Hepatic dysfunction and cholestasis may also occur (Cohran et al 2017).

Bacterial overgrowth is likely to occur when the ileocaecal valve is absent or when stasis exists as a result of a partial obstruction or a dilated segment of bowel with poor motility. Alternating cycles of broad-spectrum antibiotics are used to reduce bacterial overgrowth. This treatment may also decrease the risk of bacterial translocation and subsequent central venous catheter infections. A high-fat and low-carbohydrate diet may be helpful in reducing bacterial overgrowth (Vanderhoof & Branski 2016). Other complications of bacterial overgrowth and malabsorption include metabolic acidosis and gastric hypersecretion.

Many surgical interventions, including intestinal valves, tapering enteroplasty or stricturoplasty, intestinal lengthening and interposed segments, have been used to slow intestinal transit, reduce bacterial overgrowth or increase mucosal surface area. Intestinal transplantation has been performed successfully in children. Children with a permanent dependence on PN or severe complications of long-term PN are candidates for transplantation.

Prognosis. The prognosis for infants with SBS has improved with advances in PN and with the understanding of the importance of intraluminal nutrition. Improved supportive care for the management of therapy-related problems and the development of more specific immunosuppressive medications for transplantation have all contributed to improved management. The prognosis depends in part on the length of the residual small intestine. An intact ileocaecal valve also improves the prognosis. Infants and children with SBS die from PN-related problems, such as fulminant sepsis or severe PN cholestasis.

Nursing Care Management

The most important components of nursing care are administration and monitoring of nutritional therapy. During PN therapy, care must be taken to minimise the risk of complications related to the central venous access device (i.e. catheter infections, occlusions, dislodgement or accidental removal). Care of the enteral feeding tubes and monitoring of enteral feeding tolerance are also important nursing responsibilities.

When hospitalisation is prolonged, the child's developmental and emotional needs must be met. This often requires special planning to promote normal family adjustment and adaptation of the hospital routines. Family members require psychosocial support and education to cope successfully with SBS.

Many infants with SBS have an intestinal ostomy performed at the time of the initial bowel resection. Routine ostomy care is another important nursing responsibility. Because infants and children with SBS have chronic diarrhoea, perineal skin irritation is often a problem after ostomy closure. Frequent nappy changes, gentle perineal cleansing and protective skin ointments help prevent skin breakdown.

Gastrointestinal Bleeding

GI bleeding in infants and children is an uncommon but potentially serious problem (Casciani et al 2017). Most actual or apparent instances of GI bleeding cause great anxiety for the parents or caregivers. Blood may be vomited or passed per rectum, but the origin of the blood may not be the GI tract. In the newborn, swallowed maternal blood at the time of delivery may account for some episodes of apparent GI bleeding. A bleeding site on the nipple of a nursing mother may lead to haem-positive stools in the breastfed infant. Finally, blood can be swallowed during epistaxis and then passed as haematemesis or melaena.

Once it has been established that the cause of bleeding is from a source in the GI tract, further investigation for the source and cause is undertaken. Upper GI bleeding is defined as bleeding from a site above the ligament of Treitz, which is attached to the duodenum at its junction with the jejunum. Lower GI bleeding comes from a source distal to the ligament of Treitz. Diagnostic studies such as endoscopy, scintigraphy and angiography have improved the ability to localise the site of bleeding.

Aetiology

The oesophagus is a common site of upper GI bleeding. Oesophagitis caused by GOR may lead to chronic and often occult blood loss. Oesophageal varices secondary to portal hypertension may cause massive bleeding. Peptic inflammation (gastritis and duodenitis) or ulceration is the most common cause of upper GI bleeding in children. Haemorrhagical gastritis may occur in the newborn infant after a difficult delivery or asphyxia. In this circumstance gastric perforation is a serious complication that requires emergent treatment. Less common causes of upper GI bleeding include bleeding disorders, vascular malformations, GI duplications, Mallory-Weiss syndrome (an oesophageal tear caused by protracted vomiting) and haematobilia (bleeding into biliary passages).

In lower GI bleeding, small amounts of bright red blood in the stool of a healthy child may be due to an anal fissure. Colonic polyps are another cause of passage of bright red blood per rectum in toddlers and older children. Bleeding associated with diarrhoea may indicate a serious problem. Enteric infections remain the leading cause, but the nurse should consider necrotising enterocolitis, haemolytic uraemic syndrome, IBD and food allergy. Other causes are intussusception with the passage of blood per rectum (see earlier in this chapter) or Meckel's diverticulum with the painless passage of currant jelly–like stools (see earlier in this chapter).

Pathophysiology

The GI tract has an extensive surface area and a rich vascular supply. Bleeding can occur anywhere along the GI tract from a vein, artery or vascular malformation. In an otherwise healthy newborn infant, haemophilia or inherited coagulation-factor deficits are rarely accompanied by bleeding unless other conditions are superimposed. Children with liver disease may also have deficient coagulation factors because of poor synthesis and malabsorption of vitamin K, which is a risk factor for GI bleeding.

Portal hypertension may lead to GI bleeding because the formation of portosystemic shunts can result in dilated venous channels in vulnerable locations such as the oesophagus and stomach. These dilated venous channels (varices) may bleed, causing severe GI haemorrhage.

Diagnostic Evaluation

The diagnosis of GI bleeding is often made on the basis of the history and physical examination. Haematemesis is the vomiting of bright red blood or denatured blood that looks like coffee grounds, usually representing an upper GI source of bleeding. Haematochezia is the passage of bright red blood per rectum, indicating lower GI bleeding. This blood may precede or follow a bowel movement or be mixed with or coat the stool. Bright red blood that coats the stool may be due to a hard bowel movement, haemorrhoids or anal fissures. Blood mixed with stool indicates a bleeding source proximal to the rectum. Blood passed alone after a bowel movement is most likely to be due to bleeding in the perianal or rectal area, possibly caused by a polyp. Blood with mucus in the stool indicates an inflammatory or infectious condition, and currant jelly–like stools indicate vascular compromise, such as intussusception. Melaena is the passage of black, tarry stools that contain denatured (digested) blood and suggests an upper GI source of bleeding. Occasionally, bright red blood may be passed per rectum from an upper GI source of bleeding when the bleeding is massive. It is important to test emesis or stool for occult blood to differentiate true bleeding from the ingestion of food containing food colouring. In older children, false-positive stool tests for occult blood can also occur with the ingestion of red meats and iron preparations.

Laboratory studies are determined on the basis of the history and physical examination. In many instances, a FBC with platelet quantification, prothrombin, partial thromboplastin and coagulation studies will be done. Children who have acute illness, fever and joint pain in addition to GI bleeding need an ESR and stool studies with culture to evaluate for enteric pathogens, ova and parasites and *C. difficile*. When IBD is suspected, a metabolic panel to determine total protein and albumin may be added to a FBC, ESR and LFTs. The child with massive painless rectal bleeding may require a nuclear medicine scan to rule out Meckel's diverticulum. If there is evidence of portal hypertension or chronic liver disease, LFTs, liver imaging studies and a liver biopsy may be necessary. A barium enema is performed if intussusception is suspected.

Imaging studies help differentiate among several suspected diagnoses. CT of the sinuses helps localise bleeding that is coming from the nasopharynx or sinuses. A chest radiograph may distinguish haemoptysis related to cystic fibrosis, bronchiectasis or other chronic lung conditions from haematemesis. Angiography can be used to identify the source of bleeding and to allow embolisation or vasopressin infusion for treatment. Endoscopy is the diagnostic method chosen when the source of bleeding is thought to be secondary to gastritis, oesophagitis, PUD, colitis or polyps. Endoscopic examinations also permit visualisation of the intestinal mucosa and collection of biopsy specimens and cultures.

Therapeutic Management

Treatment of GI bleeding in children depends on its severity and cause. The first step in management of acute GI bleeding is to assess the magnitude of blood loss and restore the child's haemodynamic stability. Severe bleeding necessitates hospitalisation. IV fluids (normal saline or lactated Ringer's solution) are administered rapidly. Oxygen therapy is indicated if the bleeding is severe. Transfusion of blood products may be required if the blood loss is significant, and any existing coagulopathy should be corrected.

Upper GI mucosal lesions are usually treated with prophylatic PPI's and beta-blockers or PPIs (e.g. omeprazole, lansoprazole, pantoprazole or esomeprazole) and antacids to reduce acidity and promote mucosal healing. Variceal haemorrhage can be treated with peripheral vasopressin infusion and endoscopic sclerotherapy to hasten tissue fibrosis. Balloon tamponade to place pressure on the bleeding area may be performed as a temporary measure until endoscopic sclerotherapy can be done.

Therapy for lower GI bleeding is directed towards the primary underlying condition. The treatment may include medical or surgical management. Surgery may be required if the bleeding is severe despite aggressive medical intervention.

Nursing Care Management

The infant or child with acute and severe GI bleeding requires emergency care. Initial management includes assessment of the magnitude of bleeding and haemodynamic status and assistance with resuscitation efforts (see Critical Thinking Case Study box).

CRITICAL THINKING CASE STUDY

Haematemesis

A 6-month-old infant is seen in the emergency department. The parents brought the infant to the hospital because he vomited up formula with blood streaks. In the emergency department the infant has tachypnoea, tachycardia and a fever of 39°C. A chest x-ray film shows pneumonia. The infant is admitted to the hospital to receive antibiotics and for observation. Several hours after admission to the inpatient unit, the mother calls the nurse when the infant vomits a large amount of bright red blood. The infant is pale and lethargic. Which of the following should *not* be included in the initial nursing actions?

1. Call for assistance and estimate the amount of blood loss.
2. Obtain vital signs and monitor capillary refill, skin colour and behaviour.
3. Prepare to pass a nasogastric tube, obtain blood for laboratory analyses and start an IV line.
4. Test stool for blood (haematest or haemoccult).

Questions

1. Evidence—Are there sufficient data to support your decision?
2. Assumptions—Describe some underlying assumptions about the following:
   a. haematemesis in an infant
   b. the diagnosis of haematemesis.
3. What are the priorities for this child at this time?
4. What are the nursing actions that need to be implemented?

Answers are available at http://evolve.elsevier.com/AU/Speedie/ncic/

HEPATIC DISORDERS

The liver is a vital organ whose functions can be divided into several groups: (1) vascular functions of storing and filtering blood; (2) secretory function of producing bile; (3) metabolism of carbohydrate, protein and fat; (4) synthesis of blood-clotting components and storage of iron and vitamins (A, D, B_{12} and K); and (5) detoxification and excretion of certain drugs and metabolic substances. Many disorders, including biliary atresia, hepatitis and cirrhosis, can cause liver dysfunction in children.

Acute Hepatitis

Hepatitis is an acute or chronic inflammation of the liver that can result from infectious or non-infectious reasons. Viruses such as hepatitis viruses, Epstein-Barr virus (EBV) and cytomegalovirus (CMV) are common causes of many types of hepatitis. Other causes of hepatitis are non-viral (e.g. abscess, amoebiasis), autoimmune, metabolic, drug induced, anatomical (e.g. choledochal duct cyst and biliary atresia), haemodynamic (e.g. shock, congestive heart failure) and idiopathic (e.g. sclerosing cholangitis and Reye's syndrome). Determining the cause of acute or chronic hepatitis is important in determining the treatment and prognosis for the child. Epidemiological features and serological testing are used to differentiate the causes. Table 25.5 compares the features of hepatitis A, B and C viruses.

Hepatitis A Virus

Hepatitis A virus (HAV) is spread directly or indirectly by the faecal-oral route by ingestion of contaminated foods, direct exposure to

TABLE 25.5 Comparison of Hepatitis Types A, B and C

Characteristics	Type A	Type B	Type C
Incubation period	15 to 50 days, average 28 days	45 to 160 days, average 120 days	2 to 24 weeks, average 7 to 9 weeks
Period of communicability	Believed to be latter half of incubation period to first week after onset of clinical illness	Variable Virus in blood or other body fluids during late incubation period and acute stage of disease; may persist in carrier state for years to lifetime	Begins before onset of symptoms May persist in carrier state for years
Mode of transmission	Principal route—Faecal-oral Rarely—Parenteral	Principal route—Parenteral Less frequent route—oral, sexual, any body fluid Perinatal transfer—Transplacental blood (last trimester), at delivery or during breastfeeding, especially if mother has cracked nipples	Principal route—parenteral Non-parenteral spread possible
Clinical features			
• Onset	Usually rapid, acute	More insidious	Usually insidious
• Fever	Common and early	Less frequent	Less frequent
• Anorexia	Common	Mild to moderate	Mild to moderate
• Nausea and vomiting	Common	Sometimes present	Mild to moderate
• Rash	Rare	Common	Sometimes present
• Arthralgia	Rare	Common	Rare
• Pruritus	Rare	Sometimes present	Sometimes present
• Jaundice	Present (many cases anicteric)	Present	Present
Immunity	Present after one attack; no crossover to type B or C	Present after one attack; no crossover to type A or C	Present after one attack; no crossover to type A or B
Carrier state	No	Yes	Yes
Chronic infection	No	Yes	Yes

HAV, hepatitis A virus; *HBV*, hepatitis B virus.

infected faecal material or close contact with an infected person. The virus is particularly prevalent in developing countries with poor living conditions, inadequate sanitation, crowding and poor personal hygiene practices. Before the introduction of the hepatitis A vaccination program for children (funded by the National Immunisation Program), hepatitis A was quite prevalent in the Indigenous communities; this has decreased significantly due to the introduction of the program (Australian Technical Advisory Group on Immunisation [ATAGI] 2020).

The spread of HAV has been associated with improper food handling and high-risk areas such as households with infected persons, residential centres for people with a disability and day care centres. The average incubation period is about 21 days (Jensen & Balistreri 2016). Faecal shedding of the virus can occur for 2 weeks before and for 1 week after the onset of jaundice. During this time, although the individual is asymptomatic, the virus is most likely to be transmitted. Infants with HAV infection are likely to be asymptomatic (anicteric hepatitis). Children often have diarrhoea, and their symptoms are frequently attributed to gastroenteritis. Younger children rarely develop jaundice; however, 70% of older children and adults infected with HAV develop clinical signs with icteric hepatitis that typically lasts 7 to 14 days (Jensen & Balistreri 2016). The prognosis of HAV infection is usually good, and complications are rare.

Hepatitis B Virus

Hepatitis B virus (HBV) can be an acute or chronic infection, ranging from an asymptomatic, limited infection to fatal, fulminant (rapid and severe) hepatitis (Jensen & Balistreri 2016). There are no environmental or animal reservoirs for HBV. Humans are the main source of infections. HBV may be transmitted parenterally, percutaneously or transmucosally. Hepatitis B surface antigen (HBsAg) has been found in all body fluids, including faeces, bile, breast milk, sweat, tears, vaginal secretions and urine, but only blood, semen and saliva have been found to contain infectious HBV particles. HBV infection from human bites has been documented, but transmission from faeces has not. HBV has been acquired after blood transfusion, but the likelihood of this has been reduced through blood product–screening procedures. Adults whose occupations are associated with considerable exposure to blood or blood products, such as healthcare workers, are at an increased risk of contracting HBV.

Most HBV infections in children are acquired perinatally. Transmission from mother to infant during the perinatal period (i.e. blood exposure during delivery) results in chronic infection in up to 90% of infants if the mother is positive for HBsAg and HBeAg (Jensen & Balistreri 2016). HBsAg has been inconsistently detected in breast milk, but no increased risk of transmission has been found and breastfeeding is currently recommended after infant immunisation (Jensen & Balistreri 2016). Infants and children who are not infected during the perinatal period remain at high risk for acquiring person-to-person transmission from their mother. Australia is categorised as low-prevalence country for HBV, less than 2% of the population. Again this has been due to the introduction of the vaccination within the National Immunisation Childhood Schedule and also due to the introduction of the adolescent Catch-up program for high-risk groups (National Centre for Immunisation Research and Surveillance 2015).

Hepatitis C Virus

Hepatitis C virus (HCV) is transmitted parenterally through exposure to blood and blood products from HCV-infected persons, whereas perinatal transmission is the most common mode of transmission among children (Jensen & Balistreri 2016). This is known as vertical transmission and is thought to occur in utero or during delivery. Within Australia, of 100 babies born to mothers who have HCV, approximately 5 to 7 of those babies will obtain the virus (The Sydney Children's Hospital Network n.d.). It is slightly lower in New Zealand but the data is difficult to obtain for overall population for New Zealand as it is broken into cultural groups.

For children the clinical course is variable and there is an incubation period for HCV ranging from 2 to 24 weeks, with an average of 7 to 9 weeks (Jensen & Balistreri 2016). The presentation for many children may be asymptomatic, but HCV can lead to a chronic condition and can cause cirrhosis and hepatocellular carcinoma. Approximately 85% of individuals infected with HCV develop chronic disease (Jensen & Balistreri 2016).

Hepatitis D virus

Hepatitis D virus (HDV) rarely occurs in children and must occur in individuals already infected with HBV (Jensen & Balistreri 2016). HDV is a defective RNA virus that requires the helper function of HBV. The incubation period is 2 to 8 weeks, but with coinfection of HBV the incubation period is similar to an HBV infection (Jensen & Balistreri 2016). HDV infection occurs through blood and sexual contact and commonly occurs among drug abusers, individuals with haemophilia and persons immigrating from endemic areas.

Hepatitis E virus

Hepatitis E virus (HEV) was formerly known as non-A, non-B hepatitis. Transmission may occur through the faecal-oral route or from contaminated water. The incubation period ranges from 15 to 60 days, with an average of 40 days (Jensen & Balistreri 2016). This illness is uncommon in children, does not cause chronic liver disease, is not a chronic condition and has no carrier state. However, it can be a devastating disease among pregnant women, with an unusually high fatality rate.

Pathophysiology

Pathological changes occur primarily in the parenchymal cells of the liver and result in: variable degrees of swelling; infiltration of liver cells by mononuclear cells; and subsequent degeneration, necrosis and fibrosis. Structural changes within the hepatocyte account for altered liver functions, such as impaired bile excretion, elevated transaminase levels and decreased albumin synthesis. The disorder may be self-limiting, with regeneration of liver cells without scarring, leading to a complete recovery. However, some forms of hepatitis do not result in complete return of liver function. These include fulminant hepatitis, which is characterised by a severe, acute course with massive destruction of the liver tissue causing liver failure and high mortality risk within 1 to 2 weeks; and subacute or chronic active hepatitis, which is characterised by progressive liver destruction, uncertain regeneration, scarring and potential cirrhosis.

The progression of liver disease is characterised pathologically by four stages: (1) stage one is characterised by mononuclear inflammatory cells surrounding small bile ducts; (2) in stage two there is proliferation of small bile ductules; (3) stage three is characterised by fibrosis or scarring; and (4) stage four is cirrhosis.

Clinical Manifestations

The clinical manifestations and course of uncomplicated acute viral hepatitis are similar for most of the hepatitis viruses. Usually the prodromal, or anicteric, phase (absence of jaundice) lasts 5 to 7 days. Anorexia, malaise, lethargy and easy fatiguability are the most common symptoms. Fever may be present, especially in adolescents. Nausea, vomiting and epigastric or right upper quadrant abdominal pain or tenderness may occur. Arthralgia and skin rashes may occur and are more likely in children with hepatitis B than those with hepatitis A. The transaminases, rather than the bilirubin, are often elevated in acute hepatitis, and hepatomegaly may be present. Some mild cases of acute viral hepatitis do not cause symptoms or can be mistaken for influenza.

In young children most of the prodromal symptoms disappear with the onset of jaundice, or the icteric phase. Many children with acute viral hepatitis, however, never develop jaundice. If jaundice occurs, it is often accompanied by dark urine and pale stools. Pruritus may accompany jaundice and can be bothersome for children.

Children with chronic active hepatitis may be asymptomatic but more commonly have non-specific symptoms of malaise, fatigue, lethargy, weight loss or vague abdominal pain. Hepatomegaly may be present, and the transaminases are often very high, with mild to severe hyperbilirubinaemia.

Fulminant hepatitis is due primarily to HBV or HCV. Many children with fulminant hepatitis develop characteristic clinical symptoms and rapidly develop manifestations of liver failure, including encephalopathy, coagulation defects, ascites, deepening jaundice and an increasing white blood cell count. Changes in mental status or personality indicate impending liver failure. Although children with acute hepatitis may have hepatomegaly, a rapid decrease in the size of the liver (indicating loss of tissue due to necrosis) is a serious sign of fulminant hepatitis. Complications of fulminant hepatitis include GI bleeding, sepsis, renal failure and disseminated coagulopathy.

Diagnostic Evaluation

Diagnosis is based on the history, physical examination and serological markers for hepatitis A, B and C. No LFT is specific for hepatitis, but serum aspartate aminotransferase (AST) and serum alanine aminotransferase (ALT) levels are markedly elevated. Serum bilirubin levels peak 5 to 10 days after clinical jaundice appears. Histological evidence from liver biopsy may be required to establish the diagnosis and to assess the severity of the liver disease. Serological markers indicate the antibodies or antigens formed in response to the specific virus and confirm the diagnosis. Serum immunological tests are not available to detect HAV antigen, but there are two HAV antibody tests: anti-HAV immunoglobulin G (IgG) and immunoglobulin M (IgM). Anti-HAV antibodies are present at the onset of the disease and persist for life. A positive anti-HAV antibody test can indicate acute infection, immunity from past infection, passive antibody acquisition (e.g. from transfusion, serum immunoglobulin infusion) or immunisation. To diagnose an acute or recent HAV infection, a positive anti-HAV IgM test that is present with the onset of the disease and that persists for only 2 or 3 days is required.

Diagnosis of hepatitis B is confirmed by the detection of various hepatitis virus antigens and the antibodies that are produced in response to the infection. These antibodies and antigens and their significance include the following.

- **HBsAg**—Hepatitis B surface antigen (found on the surface of the virus), indicating ongoing infection or carrier state
- **Anti-HBs**—Antibody to surface antigen HBsAg, indicating resolving or past infection
- **HBcAg**—Hepatitis B core antigen (found on the inner core of the virus), detected only in the liver
- **Anti-HBc**—Antibody to core antigen HBcAg, indicating ongoing or past infection
- **HBeAg**—Hepatitis B antigen (another component of the HBV core), indicating active infection
- **Anti-HBe**—Antibody to HBeAg, indicating resolving or past infection
- **IgM anti-HBc**—IgM antibody to core antigen

The history of all patients should include questions to seek evidence of: (1) contact with a person known to have hepatitis, especially a family member; (2) unsafe sanitation practices, such as contaminated drinking water; (3) ingestion of certain foods, such as oysters (especially from polluted water); (4) multiple blood transfusions; (5) ingestion of hepatotoxic drugs, such as salicylates, sulfonamides, antineoplastic agents, paracetamol and anticonvulsants; and (6) parenteral administration of illicit drugs or sexual contact with a person who uses these drugs.

Therapeutic Management

The goals of management include early detection, support and monitoring of the disease, recognition of chronic liver disease and prevention of spread of the disease. Special high-protein, high-carbohydrate, low-fat diets are generally not of value. The use of corticosteroids alone or with immunosuppressive drugs is not advocated in the treatment of chronic viral hepatitis. However, steroids have been used to treat chronic autoimmune hepatitis. Hospitalisation is required in the event of coagulopathy or fulminant hepatitis.

Prevention. Proper handwashing and standard precautions prevent the spread of viral hepatitis. Prophylactic use of standard immune globulin is effective in preventing hepatitis A in situations of pre-exposure (such as anticipated travel to areas where HAV is prevalent) or within 2 weeks of exposure.

Hepatitis B immune globulin (HBIg) is effective in preventing HBV infection after one-time exposures such as accidental needle punctures or other contact of contaminated material with mucous membranes and should be given to newborns whose mothers are HBsAg positive. HBIg is prepared from plasma that contains high titres of antibodies against HBV. HBIg should be given within 72 hours of exposure.

Prognosis. The prognosis for children with hepatitis is variable and depends on the type of virus and the child's age and immunocompetency. Infants are more likely than older children to develop chronic hepatitis.

Nursing Care Management

Nursing objectives depend largely on the severity of the hepatitis, the medical treatment and factors influencing the control and transmission of the disease. Encourage a well-balanced diet and a schedule of rest and activity adjusted to the child's condition. Caution parents about administering any medication to the child because normal doses of many drugs may become dangerous because of the liver's inability to detoxify and excrete them.

Standard precautions are followed when children are hospitalised. However, these children are not usually isolated in a separate room unless they are faecally incontinent or their toys and other personal items are likely to become contaminated with faeces. Discourage children from sharing their toys.

Biliary Atresia

Biliary atresia (BA), or extrahepatic biliary atresia (EHBA), is a progressive inflammatory process that causes both intrahepatic and extrahepatic bile duct fibrosis, resulting in eventual ductal obstruction. The incidence of BA is approximately 1 in 10,000 to 15,000 live births (Hassan & Balistreri 2016). Associated malformations include polysplenia and malrotation of the intestine. BA, if untreated, usually leads to cirrhosis, liver failure and death.

Pathophysiology

The exact cause of BA is unknown, although immune- or infection-mediated mechanisms may be responsible for the progressive process that results in complete obliteration of the bile ducts. BA is not seen in the fetus, the stillborn or the newborn infant. This suggests that BA is acquired late in gestation or in the perinatal period and is manifested a few weeks after birth.

Congenital infections have been implicated as a cause of hepatocellular damage leading to BA, yet no specific agent is identified in every case. Immune-mediated bile duct injury from viral exposure and immaturity of the neonatal immune system may play a role in the destruction of bile ducts and development of EHBA. Other potential causes include an early first trimester insult to the developing bile ducts or a postnatal viral insult (Hassan & Balistreri 2016). Early in the course of the disease, the intrahepatic ducts are patent from the interlobular ductules to the porta hepatis. The size of these structures is variable and is correlated with the infant's age and with bile excretion after surgical treatment. These structures are present in most affected infants under 2 months of age but gradually disappear over the next few months and by 4 months are completely replaced by fibrous tissue.

The degree of involvement of the extrahepatic biliary ducts is also variable. The majority of cases of BA (85%) have a complete obliteration of the extrahepatic biliary tree at or above the porta hepatis (Hassan & Balistreri 2016). But some infants have a patent proximal portion of the extrahepatic duct or patency of the gallbladder, cystic duct and common bile duct. Microscopic examination of the liver tissue reveals cholestasis with absent or diminished bile duct proliferation and fibrosis.

Clinical Manifestations

Many infants with BA are full term and appear healthy at birth. If **jaundice** persists beyond 2 weeks of age, especially if the direct (conjugated) serum bilirubin is elevated, the nurse should suspect BA. The urine may be dark, and the stools often become progressively acholic or grey, indicating absence of bile pigment. Hepatomegaly is present early in the course of the disease, and the liver is firm on palpation.

Diagnostic Evaluation

Early diagnosis is critical to the child with EHBA; the outcome in children surgically treated before 2 months of age is much better than in patients with delayed treatment. The diagnosis of BA is suspected on the basis of the history, physical findings and laboratory studies. Laboratory tests include a FBC, bilirubin levels and liver function studies. Additional laboratory analyses, including alpha$_1$-antitrypsin level, TORCH titres and other intrauterine infections (see Maternal Infections, Chapter 9), hepatitis serology and urine cytomegalovirus, may be indicated to rule out other conditions that cause cholestasis and jaundice. An abdominal ultrasound is usually performed to identify potential causes of extrahepatic obstruction, such as a choledochal cyst. The patency of the extrahepatic biliary system is demonstrated by a nuclear scintiscan using technetium 99m iminodiacetic acid (^{99m}Tc-IDA, or HIDA; **HIDA scan**). If there is no evidence of radioactive material excreted into the duodenum, BA is the most probable diagnosis. Because the nuclear scan may take up to 5 days for the results, a percutaneous liver biopsy is probably the most useful method of diagnosing BA (Govindarajan 2016). The definitive diagnosis of BA is further established during an exploratory laparotomy and an intraoperative cholangiogram that demonstrates complete obstruction at some level of the biliary tree.

Therapeutic Management

Medical management of BA is primarily supportive. It includes nutritional support with infant formulas that contain medium-chain triglycerides and essential fatty acids. Supplementation with fat-soluble vitamins (A, D, E and K); a multivitamin; and minerals, including iron, zinc and selenium, is usually required. Aggressive nutritional support in the form of continuous gastrostomy feedings or TPN may be indicated for moderate to severe growth failure; the enteral solution should be low in sodium. Phenobarbitone may be prescribed after hepatic portoenterostomy to stimulate bile flow, and ursodeoxycholic acid may be used to decrease cholestasis and the intense pruritus from jaundice. In cases of advanced liver dysfunction, management is the same as in infants with cirrhosis.

The primary surgical treatment of BA is hepatic portoenterostomy (**Kasai procedure**), in which a segment of intestine is anastomosed to the resected porta hepatis to attempt bile drainage (Fig 25.7). A Roux-en-Y jejunal limb is then anastomosed to the porta hepatis (a Y-shaped anastomosis performed to provide bile drainage without reflux). Complications after portoenterostomy include ascending cholangitis, cirrhosis, portal hypertension and GI bleeding. Prophylactic antibiotics are given after the Kasai procedure to minimise the risk of ascending cholangitis. After the Kasai procedure approximately one-third of infants become jaundice free and regain normal liver function. Another one-third of infants demonstrate liver damage; however, they may be supported by medical and nutritional interventions. A final third require liver transplantation. Liver transplantation is required for children who cannot regain bile flow and for those with end-stage liver disease or severe portal hypertension. Complications after liver transplantation include obstruction and bile leaks at the biliary anastomosis, portal hypertension, haemorrhage, infection and rejection. Immunosuppressive drugs are required after transplantation.

Prognosis. Untreated BA results in progressive cirrhosis and death in most children by 3 years of age (Govindarajan 2016). The Kasai procedure improves the prognosis but is not a cure. There is only 20% survival in patients 20 years after the Kasai procedure and only 10% survival in patients 30 years after the procedure (Govindarajan 2016).

The advances in surgical techniques for liver transplantation and the development of immunosuppressive and antifungal drugs have

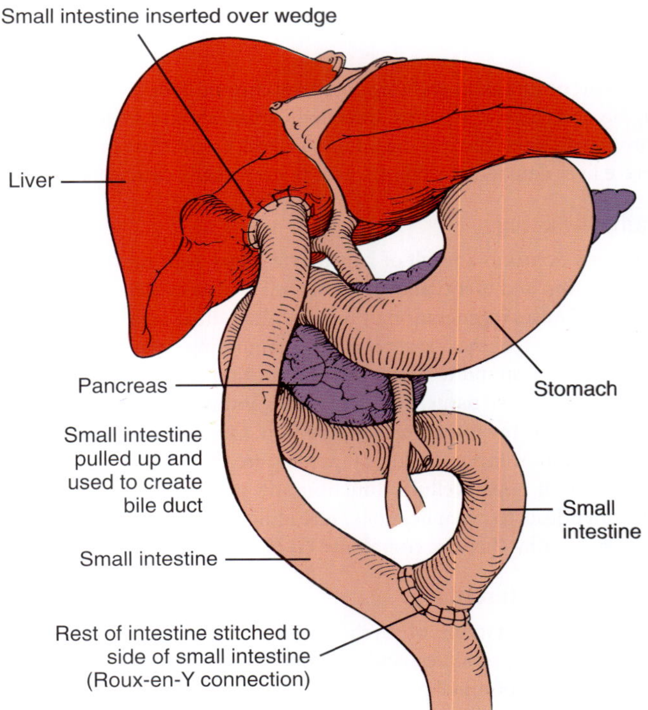

Fig 25.7 Biliary atresia—Kasai procedure.

significantly improved the success of transplantation. Surgical techniques and immunosuppression have contributed to survival rates of 83% to 91% in children who underwent transplant (Yanagi et al 2017). The major obstacle remains the shortage of suitable infant donors.

Liver disease progresses in infants with delayed diagnosis or in children in whom surgery has failed to provide adequate bile drainage. Cirrhosis and splenomegaly occur with hypoalbuminaemia, ascites and coagulopathy. Malabsorption of fat and fat-soluble vitamins and malnutrition result in severe growth failure. Retained bile salts and cholesterol further contribute to **pruritus** (itching) and xanthomas, often requiring the administration of **ursodeoxycholic acid**. The severity of pruritus intensifies as the jaundice progresses as the result of disease advancement.

Nursing Care Management

There are many important nursing interventions for the child with BA. The nurse should educate family members regarding all aspects of the treatment plan and the rationale for therapy. Immediately after a hepatic portoenterostomy, nursing care is similar to that after any major abdominal surgery. If an interrupted jejunal conduit has been performed, the family needs to learn how to care for the two stomas and how to refeed the bile after feedings. Teaching includes the proper administration of medications. Administration of nutritional therapy, including special formulas, vitamin and mineral supplements, gastrostomy feedings or PN, is an essential nursing responsibility. Growth failure in such infants is common, and increased metabolic needs combined with ascites, pruritus and nutritional anorexia constitute a challenge for care. The nurse teaches caregivers how to monitor and administer nutritional therapy in the home. Pruritus may be a significant problem that is addressed by drug therapy or comfort measures such as baths in colloidal oatmeal compounds and trimming of fingernails. The risk of complications of BA, such as cholangitis, portal hypertension, GI bleeding and ascites, should be explained to the caregivers.

These children and their families require special psychosocial support. The uncertain prognosis, discomfort and waiting for transplantation can produce considerable stress. (See Cirrhosis.)

Cirrhosis

Cirrhosis occurs as an end stage of many chronic liver diseases, including BA and chronic hepatitis. Infectious, autoimmune, toxic injury and chronic diseases such as haemophilia and cystic fibrosis can cause severe liver damage. A cirrhotic liver is irreversibly damaged.

Pathophysiology

Cirrhosis occurs as a result of hepatocyte injury with necrosis, fibrosis, regeneration and eventual degeneration. The diminished parenchymal cell mass causes regeneration of tissue with nodular areas of proliferating hepatocytes that stretch the surrounding connective tissue. Hepatocytes respond to injury with deposition of collagen that forms fibrous connective tissue. This scar tissue and nodular areas of regeneration impair the intrahepatic blood flow. Ongoing necrosis and self-perpetuation of this pathological process are the result of cirrhosis.

Failure of hepatocellular function and portal hypertension occur and often lead to complications, including ascites, severe cholestasis, encephalopathy (hepatic coma) and GI bleeding.

Clinical Manifestations

Clinical manifestations of cirrhosis include jaundice, poor growth, anorexia, muscle weakness and lethargy. Ascites, oedema, GI bleeding, anaemia and abdominal pain may be present in children with impaired intrahepatic blood flow. Pulmonary function may be impaired because of pressure against the diaphragm due to hepatosplenomegaly and ascites. Dyspnoea and cyanosis may occur, especially on exertion. Intrapulmonary arteriovenous shunts may develop, which can also cause hypoxaemia. Spider angiomas and prominent blood vessels on the upper torso are often present.

Diagnostic Evaluation

The diagnosis of cirrhosis is based on: (1) the history, especially in regard to prior liver disease, such as hepatitis; (2) physical examination, particularly hepatosplenomegaly; (3) laboratory evaluation, especially LFTs, such as bilirubin and transaminases, ammonia, albumin, cholesterol and prothrombin time; and (4) liver biopsy for characteristic changes. Doppler ultrasonography of the liver and spleen is useful to confirm ascites, to evaluate the blood flow through the liver and spleen and to determine the patency and size of the portal vein if liver transplantation is considered.

NURSING CARE CONSIDERATIONS

The most common complication from percutaneous liver biopsy is internal bleeding. Vital signs and laboratory values, especially haematocrit, should be monitored for evidence of haemorrhage and shock.

Therapeutic Management

Unfortunately, there is no successful treatment to arrest the progression of cirrhosis. The goals of management include monitoring liver function and managing specific complications such as oesophageal varices and malnutrition. Assessment of the child's degree of liver dysfunction is important so that the child can be evaluated for transplantation at the appropriate time.

Nutritional support is an important therapy for children with cirrhosis and malnutrition. Supplements of fat-soluble vitamins are often required, and mineral supplements may be indicated. In some instances aggressive nutritional support in the form of enteral feeding or PN may be necessary.

Oesophageal and gastric varices can be a life-threatening complication of portal hypertension. Acute haemorrhage is managed with IV fluids, blood products, vitamin K (if needed to correct coagulopathy) and gastric lavage. If acute haemorrhage persists, the most common secondary approach is endoscopic sclerotherapy or endoscopic banding ligation (Choudhary et al 2016). Balloon tamponade with a Sengstaken-Blakemore tube may be indicated for the unstable patient with acute haemorrhage (Choudhary et al 2016). Ascites is managed by sodium and fluid restrictions and diuretics. Severe ascites with respiratory compromise is managed with albumin infusions or by paracentesis.

Although the full mechanism of hepatic encephalopathy is unknown, failure of the damaged liver to remove endogenous toxins, such as ammonia, plays a role. Treatment is directed at limiting the ammonia formation and absorption that occur in the bowel, especially with the drugs neomycin and lactulose. Because ammonia is formed in the bowel by the action of bacteria on ingested protein, lactulose reduces the number of intestinal bacteria so less ammonia is produced. The fermentation of lactulose by colonic bacteria produces short-chain fatty acids, which lower the colonic pH, thereby inhibiting bacterial metabolism. This decreases the formation of ammonia from bacterial metabolism of protein.

Prognosis. The success of liver transplantation has revolutionised the approach to liver cirrhosis. Liver failure and cirrhosis are indications for transplantation. Careful monitoring of the child's condition and quality of life is necessary to evaluate the need for and timing of transplantation.

Nursing Care Management

Several factors influence nursing care of the child with cirrhosis, including the cause of the cirrhosis, the severity of complications and the prognosis. The prognosis is often poor unless successful liver transplantation occurs. Therefore, nursing care of this child is similar to that for any child with a life-threatening illness. (See Chapter 19.)

STRUCTURAL DEFECTS

Congenital defects of the GI tract can involve any portion from the mouth to the anus. Most are apparent at birth or shortly thereafter and are anomalies in which normal growth ceased at a crucial stage of embryonic development, leaving the structure in an embryonic form or only partially completed. The result may be atresia, malposition, non-closure or any number of variations.

Atresia is absence of a normal opening or normally patent lumen. Atresia at any point along the length of the GI tract creates an obstruction to the normal progress of nutrients and secretions. The most common anomalies requiring surgical intervention are atresias of the oesophagus, intestine and anus. The congenital defects considered in this chapter include abnormalities of the lip, palate, trachea, oesophagus and anus.

Oesophageal Atresia and Tracheo-oesophageal Fistula

Congenital oesophageal atresia (OA) and tracheo-oesophogeal fistula (TOF) are rare malformations that represent a failure of the oesophagus to develop as a continuous passage and a failure of the trachea and oesophagus to separate into distinct structures. These defects may occur as separate entities or in combination, and without early diagnosis and treatment they pose a serious threat to the infant's wellbeing.

Approximately 50% of the cases of OA/TOF are a component of VATER or VACTERL association, acronyms used to describe associated anomalies (VATER for **V**ertebral defects, imperforate **A**nus, **T**racheo-oesophageal fistula, and **R**adial and **R**enal dysplasia; and VACTERL for **V**ertebral, **A**nal, **C**ardiac, **T**racheal, o**E**sophageal, **R**enal and **L**imb) (Khan & Orenstein 2016c). Cardiac anomalies may also occur with OA/TOF; therefore all patients should undergo a work-up for associated anomalies.

Pathophysiology

The oesophagus develops from the first segment of the embryonic gut. During the fourth and fifth weeks of gestation, the foregut normally lengthens and separates longitudinally. Each longitudinal portion fuses to form two parallel channels (the oesophagus and the trachea) that are joined only at the larynx. Anomalies involving the trachea and oesophagus are caused by defective separation, incomplete fusion of the tracheal folds after this separation or altered cellular growth during embryonic development.

The most commonly encountered form of OA and TOF (80% to 90% of cases) is one in which the proximal oesophageal segment terminates in a blind pouch and the distal segment is connected to the trachea or primary bronchus by a short fistula at or near the tracheal bifurcation (Fig 25.8C). The second most common type (7% to 8%) consists of a blind pouch at each end, widely separated and with no communication to the trachea (Fig 25.8A). An H-type OA refers to an otherwise normal trachea and oesophagus connected by a fistula (4% to 5%) (Fig 25.8E). Extremely rare anomalies involve a fistula from the trachea to the upper oesophageal segment (0.8%) (Fig 25.8B) or to both the upper and the lower segments (0.7% to 6%) (Fig 25.8D).

Clinical Manifestations

The presence of OA is suspected in a newborn with frothy saliva in the mouth and nose, drooling, choking and coughing. Respiratory distress may be mild or significant, depending on the type of defect and the infant's gestational age. If fed, the infant may swallow normally but suddenly cough and gag, with return of fluid through the nose and mouth. The infant may become cyanotic and apnoeic because of aspiration of breastmilk or saliva.

In the infant who has OA with a distal TOF (type C), the stomach becomes distended with air, and thoracic and abdominal compressions (especially during crying) cause the gastric contents to be regurgitated through the fistula and into the trachea, producing a chemical pneumonitis. When the upper segment of the oesophagus opens directly into the trachea (types B and D), the infant is in danger of aspirating any swallowed material. Cyanosis or choking during feeding may be the only symptom of type H fistula (see Fig 25.8E). The child with this type of OA may not manifest symptoms until later in life when he or she shows signs of chronic respiratory problems, recurrent pneumonia and GOR (Khan & Orenstein 2016c).

Diagnostic Evaluation

Although the diagnosis is established on the basis of clinical signs and symptoms, the exact type of anomaly is determined by radiographic studies. A radio-opaque catheter is inserted into the hypopharynx and advanced until it encounters an obstruction. Chest radiographs are taken to ascertain oesophageal patency or the presence and level of a blind pouch. Films that show air in the stomach indicate a connection

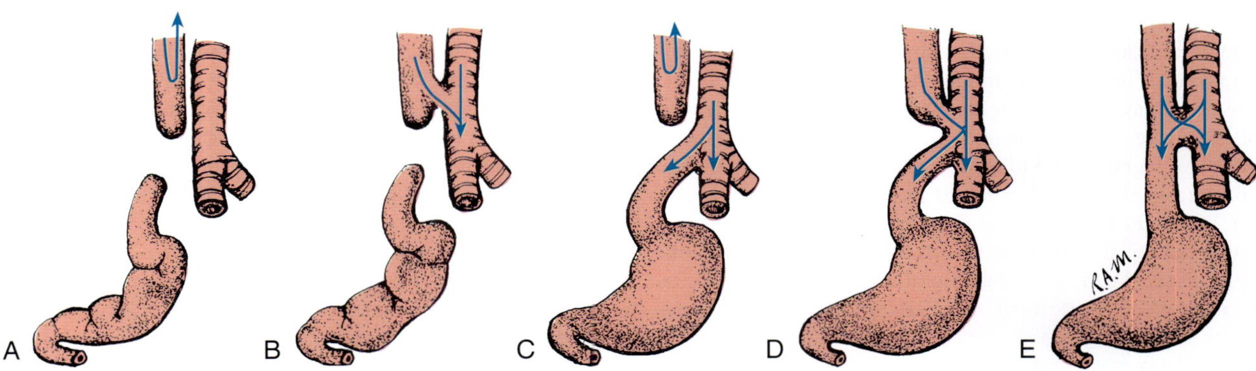

Fig 25.8 (**A–E**) Five most common types of oesophageal atresia and tracheo-oesophageal fistula. (See text for discussion.)

between the trachea and the distal oesophagus in types C, D and E. Complete absence of air in the stomach is seen in types A and B. Occasionally, fistulas are not patent, which makes their presence more difficult to diagnose. A careful bronchoscopic examination may be performed in an attempt to visualise the fistula.

The presence of **polyhydramnios** (accumulation of 2000 mL of amniotic fluid) prenatally is a clue to the possibility of OA in the unborn infant, especially with defect type A, B or C. With these types of OA/TOF, amniotic fluid normally swallowed by the fetus is unable to reach the GI tract to be absorbed and excreted by the kidneys. The result is an abnormal accumulation of amniotic fluid, or polyhydramnios.

Therapeutic Management

The treatment of OA and TOF includes maintenance of a patent airway, prevention of pneumonia, gastric or blind pouch decompression, supportive therapy and surgical repair of the anomaly.

When OA with a TOF is suspected, the infant is immediately deprived of oral intake, IV fluids are initiated and the infant is positioned to facilitate drainage of secretions and decrease the likelihood of aspiration. Accumulated secretions are suctioned frequently from the mouth and pharynx. A double-lumen catheter should be placed into the upper oesophageal pouch and attached to intermittent or continuous low suction. The infant's head is kept upright to facilitate removal of fluid collected in the pouch and to prevent aspiration of gastric contents. Broad-spectrum antibiotic therapy is often instituted if there is a concern about aspiration of gastric contents.

Most malformations can be corrected surgically in one operation or in two or more staged procedures. The success depends on early diagnosis before complications occur and on the presence and severity of associated anomalies and illness factors, including preterm birth. With measures instituted to prevent aspiration pneumonia and to ensure adequate hydration and nutrition, surgery may be postponed to allow for more effective treatment of pneumonia and physiological stabilisation so that the infant can better withstand the complex surgery. The delay also offers an opportunity for further evaluation and assessment to rule out any associated anomalies and to optimise respiratory support.

Thoracoscopic repair of OA/TOF is being used successfully, thus negating the need for a thoracotomy and minimising associated postoperative complications and morbidities (Khan & Orenstein 2016c). The surgery consists of a thoracotomy with division and ligation of the TOF and an end-to-end or end-to-side anastomosis of the oesophagus. A chest tube may be inserted to drain intrapleural air and fluid. For infants who are not stable enough to undergo definitive repair or those with a lengthy gap (> 3 to 4 cm) between the proximal and distal oesophagus, a staged operation is preferred that involves gastrostomy, ligation of the TOF and constant drainage of the oesophageal pouch (Khan & Orenstein 2016c). A delayed oesophageal anastomosis is usually attempted after several weeks to months.

A primary anastomosis may be impossible because of insufficient length of the two segments of oesophagus. This occurs if the distance between the two segments is 3 to 4 cm (approximately three vertebral bodies) or greater; this is often referred to as *long-gap OA* (Khan & Orenstein 2016c). In these cases an oesophageal replacement procedure using a part of the colon or gastric tube interposition may be necessary to bridge the missing oesophageal segment. Further surgical techniques may be performed later to facilitate oesophageal lengthening.

Tracheomalacia may occur as a result of weakness in the tracheal wall that exists when a dilated proximal pouch compresses the trachea early in fetal life. It may also occur as a result of inadequate intratracheal pressure causing abnormal tracheal development. Clinical signs of tracheomalacia include barking cough, stridor, wheezing, recurrent respiratory tract infections, cyanosis and sometimes apnoea.

Prognosis. The survival rate is nearly 100% in otherwise healthy children. Most deaths are the result of extreme prematurity or other lethal associated anomalies.

Potential complications after the surgical repair of OA and TOF depend on the type of defect and surgical correction. Complications of repair include an anastomotic leak, strictures caused by tension or ischaemia, oesophageal motility disorders causing dysphagia, respiratory compromise, scoliosis, chest wall deformity and GOR. Anastomotic oesophageal strictures may cause dysphagia, choking and respiratory distress. The strictures are often treated with routine oesophageal dilation. Feeding difficulties are often present for months or years after surgery, and the infant must be monitored closely to ensure adequate weight gain, growth and development. In some cases laparoscopic fundoplication may be required. At times the infant must be fed via gastrostomy or jejunostomy to provide adequate caloric intake.

Nursing Care Management

Nursing responsibility for detection of this serious malformation begins immediately after birth. For the infant with the classic signs and symptoms of OA (see Nursing Care Considerations) the major concern is the establishment of a patent airway and prevention of further respiratory compromise. Cyanosis is usually a result of laryngeal spasm caused by overflow of saliva into the larynx from the proximal oesophageal pouch or aspiration; it normally resolves after removal of the secretions from the oropharynx by suctioning. The passage of a small-gauge orogastric (OG) feeding tube via the mouth into the stomach during the initial nursing physical assessment is helpful to determine the presence of OA or other obstructive defects.

NURSING CARE CONSIDERATIONS

Any infant who has an excessive amount of frothy saliva in the mouth or difficulty with secretions and unexplained episodes of apnoea, cyanosis or oxygen desaturation should be suspected of having an OA/TOF and referred immediately for medical evaluation.

Preoperative Care. The nurse carefully suctions the mouth and nasopharynx and places the infant in an optimum position to facilitate drainage and avoid aspiration. The most desirable position for a newborn who is suspected of having the typical OA with a TOF (e.g. type C) is supine (or sometimes prone) with the head elevated on an inclined plane of at least 30 degrees. This positioning minimises the reflux of gastric secretions at the distal oesophagus into the trachea and bronchi, especially when intraabdominal pressure is elevated.

It is imperative to immediately remove any secretions that can be aspirated. Until surgery the blind pouch is kept empty by intermittent or continuous suction through an indwelling double-lumen catheter passed orally or nasally to the end of the pouch. In some cases a percutaneous gastrostomy tube is inserted and left open so that any air entering the stomach through the fistula can escape, thus minimising the danger of gastric contents being regurgitated into the trachea. The gastrostomy tube is emptied by gravity drainage. Feedings through the gastrostomy tube and irrigations with fluid are contraindicated before surgery in the infant with a distal TOF.

Nursing interventions include respiratory assessment, airway management, thermoregulation, fluid and electrolyte management and parenteral nutritional support.

Often the infant must be transferred to a hospital with a specialised care unit and paediatric surgical team. The nurse advises the parents of the infant's condition and provides them with necessary support and information.

Postoperative Care. Postoperative care for these infants is the same as for any high-risk newborn. Adequate thermoregulation is provided, the double-lumen NG catheter is attached to low-suction or gravity drainage, PN is provided and the gastrostomy tube (if applicable) is returned to gravity drainage until feedings are tolerated. If a thoracotomy is performed and a chest tube is inserted, attention to the appropriate function of the closed drainage system is imperative. Pain management in the postoperative period is important even if only a thoracoscopic approach is used. In the first 24 to 36 hours the nurse should provide pain management for the neonate just as for an adult undergoing a similar procedure. Tracheal suction should only be done using a premeasured catheter and with extreme caution to avoid injury to the suture line.

If tolerated, gastrostomy feedings may be initiated and continued until the oesophageal anastomosis is healed. Before oral feedings are initiated and the chest tube (if applicable) is removed, a contrast study or oesophagram will verify the integrity of the oesophageal anastomosis.

The nurse must carefully observe the initial attempt at oral feeding to make certain the infant is able to swallow without choking. Oral feedings are begun with sterile water, followed by frequent small feedings of breast milk or formula. Until the infant is able to take a sufficient amount by mouth, oral intake may need to be supplemented by bolus or continuous gastrostomy feedings. Ordinarily infants are not discharged until they can take oral fluids well. The gastrostomy tube may be removed before discharge or maintained for supplemental feedings at home.

Special Problems. Upper respiratory tract complications are a threat to life in both the preoperative and the postoperative periods. In addition to pneumonia, the infants are in constant danger of respiratory distress resulting from atelectasis, pneumothorax and laryngeal oedema. Any persistent respiratory difficulty after removal of secretions must be reported to the surgeon immediately. The infant should be monitored for anastomotic leaks and signs of infection such as purulent chest tube drainage, an increased white blood cell count and temperature instability.

For the infant who requires oesophageal replacement, non-nutritive sucking should be provided with a soother. Infants who are on NBM status for an extended period and have not received oral stimulation frequently have difficulty eating by mouth after corrective surgery and may develop oral hypersensitivity and feeding aversion. They require patient, firm guidance in learning the techniques of taking food into the mouth and swallowing after repair. A referral to a multidisciplinary feeding behaviour team may be necessary.

One of the difficulties in TOF is the immediate transfer of the sick infant to the intensive care unit and sometimes lengthy hospitalisation. Parent–infant bonding is facilitated by encouraging parents to visit the infant, participate in his or her care when appropriate and express their feelings regarding the infant's condition. The nurse in the intensive care unit should assume responsibility for ensuring that the parents are fully informed of the infant's progress.

Family Support, Discharge Planning and Home Care. Some infants with OA/TOF may require periodic oesophageal dilations on an outpatient basis. Discharge education should include instructions about feeding techniques in the child with a repaired oesophagus, including a semi-upright feeding position, small feedings and observation for adequacy of swallowing (e.g. regurgitation, cyanosis, choking). Tracheomalacia is often a complication; parents are educated about the signs and symptoms of this condition, which include a barking cough, stridor, wheezing, recurrent respiratory tract infections, cyanosis and sometimes apnoea. GOR may also occur when feedings resume and may contribute to reactive airway disease with wheezing and laboured respirations as the prominent clinical manifestations. Problems with thriving and gaining weight may occur in the first 5 years of life in the child with OA/TOF, especially if the infant is born preterm. The nurse should be alert to the achievement of developmental milestones that indicate a need for early intervention and multidisciplinary referral.

Preparing parents for discharge of their infant involves teaching the techniques that will be continued at home. The parents learn signs of respiratory difficulty and of oesophageal stricture (e.g. poor feeding, choking, dysphagia, drooling, regurgitating undigested food) and GOR.

Parents must be aware of feeding restrictions. Remind parents that it is particularly important to guard against the infant swallowing foreign objects. They should cut solid food into small pieces, teach the child to chew thoroughly, give frequent sips of liquid to help swallow food and avoid foods such as whole hot dogs or large pieces of meat that may become lodged in the oesophagus. (See Safety Promotion and Injury Prevention, Chapter 10.)

Discharge planning should include attainment of needed equipment and home nursing services to assist with ongoing assessment of the child and continuity of care.

Abdominal Wall Defects

Gastroschisis and omphalocele are two of the more common forms of congenital abdominal wall defects. Gastroschisis occurs in varying incidences worldwide from about 3 to 4 in 10,000 births, and omphalocele occurs in approximately 1 to 2 in 10,000 live births (St Louis et al 2017). Numerous reports cite an increase in the incidence of gastroschisis, although the cause of this increased incidence is unknown (St Louis et al 2017). An omphalocele occurs when the abdominal contents herniate through the umbilical ring (hernia of the umbilical cord), usually with an intact peritoneal sac, whereas gastroschisis occurs when the herniation of intestine is lateral to the umbilical ring. This herniation is usually to the right of the umbilicus, and a peritoneal sac is not present.

Omphalocele

Omphalocele is related to a true failure of embryonic development. It occurs when there is failure of the caudal or lateral infolding of the abdominal wall at approximately the third week of gestation. With the deficiency in the abdominal wall, the bowel is unable to complete its return to the abdomen between the 10th and 12th weeks of gestation.

The omphalocele is usually covered only by a translucent peritoneal sac (Fig 25.9). The sac may contain only a small portion of the bowel or most of the bowel and other abdominal viscera, such as the liver. If the sac ruptures, the abdominal contents become exposed. Omphalocele often is associated with other anomalies (50% to 70% incidence of anomalies) including: cardiac, neurological, skeletal and genitourinary (GU) anomalies; imperforate anus; ileal atresia; and bladder exstrophy. Omphalocele is also associated with trisomies 18, Beckwith-Wiedemann syndrome, congenital heart disease, Meckel's diverticulum, inguinal hernias, renal or limb deformities and closed gastroschisis (Watanabe et al 2017).

A small omphalocele may go undetected at first glance and appear as a bulge in the umbilical cord. It is therefore imperative to inspect an unusually large umbilical cord for omphalocele before clamping to prevent possible damage to bowel tissue. (See Care of the Umbilicus, Chapter 7.)

Initial management after delivery includes inspection of the defect and any associated anomalies. If the bowel covering is intact, a non-adherent dressing is placed over the defect to prevent injury; if the

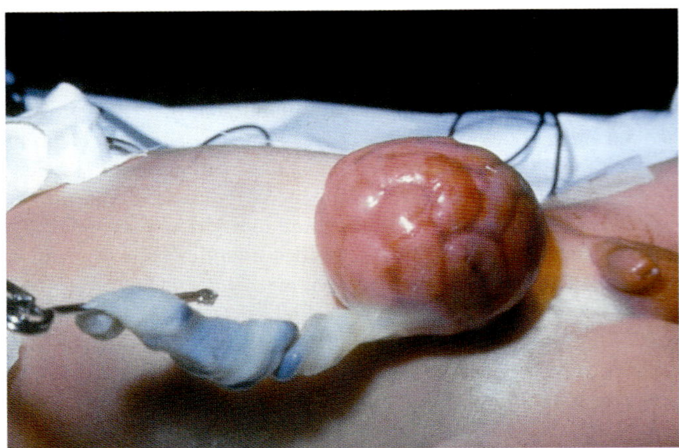

Fig 25.9 Omphalocele in membranous sac.

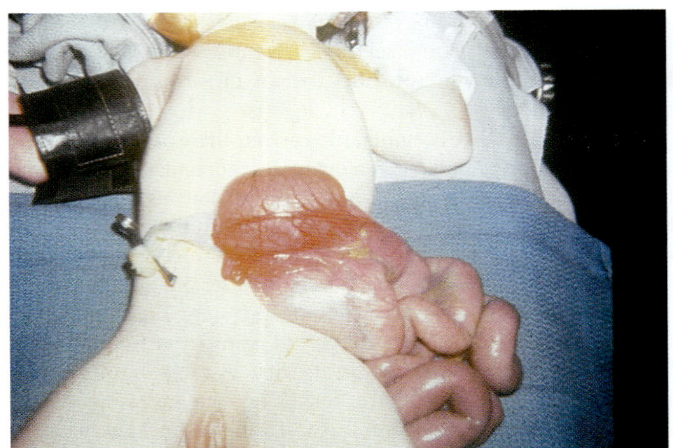

Fig 25.10 Gastroschisis with exposed bowel (uncovered for photo purposes only).

bowel is exposed, the exposed abdominal contents and membranes are covered with a bowel bag or moist dressings and a plastic drape to prevent excessive fluid loss, drying and temperature instability. IV fluids and antibiotics are administered, and a further evaluation for other associated anomalies is completed. Placement of a Silastic double-lumen catheter (NG-OG) is performed to accomplish gastric bowel decompression.

After initial medical management and stabilisation, several surgical options may be carried out, depending on the size of the defect, associated medical problems and surgeon preference. Primary closure of the omphalocele is one option if the defect is small. The sac is resected, contents are reduced into the abdominal cavity and an attempt is made to close the abdominal fascia with sutures. The abdominal wall may need to be stretched. If an intestinal atresia exists, a bowel resection may be performed, possibly involving a diverting stoma.

When primary closure of the defect is not possible because of the small size of the abdominal cavity or an extremely large omphalocele, staged reduction is accomplished. One non-operative approach with a large omphalocele is to treat the omphalocele sac with a topical substance such as silver sulfadiazine to enhance epithelialisation of the membrane (Ledbetter 2012). Additional reduction of the defect may be used by applying a compression dressing or elastic bandage. This process may take up to 12 months and the infant can be started on regular feedings; parents can be taught to apply the topical ointment or dressings at home (Ledbetter 2012). Another approach involves closure with skin flaps from the lateral abdominal wall. In the event that the sac has been disrupted, a silo mesh may be used to house the omphalocele as described in the care of the gastroschisis.

Postoperatively these infants may require mechanical ventilation and PN. Intraabdominal compression may prevent effective respiration and restrict blood flow to the lower extremities and abdominal organs. Feedings may resume once adequate bowel function is established. Postoperatively the infant is monitored for complications seen with abdominal surgery, including infection, evisceration, intestinal volvulus, obstruction and a ventral hernia.

Long-term complications include GOR, faltering growth, ventral hernia and feeding issues if the infant has been on NBM status for a lengthy period. Additional complications may occur related to the presence of associated conditions such as Beckwith-Wiedemann syndrome.

Gastroschisis

Gastroschisis occurs when the bowel herniates through a defect in the abdominal wall to the right of the umbilical cord and through the rectus muscle (Fig 25.10). There is no membrane covering the exposed bowel. Controversy exists regarding the aetiology of gastroschisis. It has been suggested that at some point between the bowel's stay in the umbilical cord and the completion of fixation, a tear occurs at the base of the umbilical cord, allowing the intestine to herniate. The gap between the cord and the tear is filled in by skin, giving the appearance of a defect in the abdominal wall to the right of the umbilical cord. The base of the defect is narrow, and the lack of membranes results in thickening and foreshortening of the bowel. Gastroschisis is usually not associated with other major congenital anomalies (10% to 20% incidence of associated anomalies); however, jejunoileal atresia, ischaemic enteritis and malrotation may occur as a result of the defect itself. Gastroschisis has been classified as simple and complicated; those within the latter category may involve bowel atresia, perforation, ischaemia or necrosis (Lakshminarayanan & Lakhoo 2014). Prenatal management of gastroschisis is evolving with emphasis on protection of the bowel from the effects of amniotic fluid, but there is no evidence-based consensus on prenatal management at this time.

Initial management involves covering the exposed bowel with a transparent plastic bowel bag or loose, moist dressings. If the opening in the abdominal cavity through which the bowel is protruding is small and strangulation of the bowel is possible, the abdominal opening is enlarged at the bedside. IV fluids and antibiotics are administered, and a double-lumen NG tube is inserted for bowel decompression. Fluid replacement for gastroschisis is increased two-fold to three-fold because of large losses from the exposed viscera.

Adequate thermoregulation and fluid management are extremely important for both omphalocele and gastroschisis. During surgery the abdominal wall is stretched and the mass of bowel is replaced in the abdomen. If primary closure is not possible, a prefabricated, spring-loaded Silastic silo is placed over the unprotected bowel in labour and delivery or in the neonatal intensive care unit shortly after birth to protect the bowel and decrease fluid loss; primary surgical closure is attempted at a later date once the bowel is reduced. The silo is reduced over several days or weeks, at which time it is removed surgically and the defect is closed. Infection is a concern during this period.

Infants with gastroschisis have traditionally been operated on within 24 hours of birth because of temperature instability, risk of infection in the unprotected bowel and fluid loss. Studies have shown that outcomes vary in regards to early surgical closure versus silo management and later surgical closure; some outcomes are heavily dependent on the amount of bowel to be replaced into the abdominal cavity and subsequent intraabdominal pressure with primary closure.

However, simple gastroschisis when the bowel is in good condition is usually treated with immediate closure (Lakshminarayanan & Lakhoo 2014).

Postoperatively most infants require mechanical ventilation because of respiratory distress secondary to increased abdominal pressure. Pain management is imperative, especially in the first 72 hours. Morphine and fentanyl are effective opioid analgesics. Many infants also require prolonged nutritional support (parenteral and enteral) because of poor bowel function. Prolonged PN may cause liver failure. Exposure of the bowel to amniotic fluid in utero predisposes the infant to prolonged paralytic ileus and hypomotility. Other complications include infection, transient renal impairment, intestinal obstruction, vena cava compression and a subsequent decrease in blood flow to the lower extremities.

Prognosis

Advanced surgical techniques, improved PN delivery systems and better medical management have improved the prognosis for the newborn with an abdominal wall defect. Survival estimates for infants with gastroschisis range from 96% for simple gastroschisis to 89% for complex gastroschisis (Lakshminarayanan & Lakhoo 2014). Because many newborns with omphalocele often have serious associated congenital anomalies, the prognosis for survival of such infants is often not as predictable or as positive as it is for those with gastroschisis (Watanabe et al 2017).

Nursing Care Management

Nursing care is similar to that for any high-risk infant. Infection is a constant threat before surgery, and careful positioning and handling are necessary to prevent rupture of the omphalocele sac or herniated bowel, or disturbance of the Silastic material used for gradual silo reduction. Viscera should be protected with moist dressings or a silo as described previously. Heat and fluid loss from the exposed viscera are major concerns in the preoperative period. Therefore thermoregulation and attention to adequate fluid volume are critical. Fluid replacement is vital and must compensate for losses. The GI tract is decompressed via an NG tube before surgery to aid in bowel reduction.

Postoperative care includes monitoring for signs of complications and assessment of bowel function; pain management with an opioid is also important in the recovery of the infant. Parenteral nutritional support may be necessary when ileus persists. It may require several days or weeks for normal bowel function to return and before full feedings can be achieved. Infants with a prolonged bowel recovery phase are prime candidates for the development of feeding resistance; therefore consultation with a feeding specialist in the early postoperative period is recommended to enhance feeding success. Associated long-term problems with gastroschisis include bowel adhesions, bowel obstruction, necrotising enterocolitis, PN-related cholestasis and poor weight gain (Lakshminarayanan & Lakhoo 2014).

Family Support, Discharge Planning and Home Care. Because these abdominal defects are visible and may be shocking to parents, immediate emotional support at the time of birth is essential. The family needs a brief explanation of the defect and reassurance that their child is in no immediate danger (unless circumstances are different). After the parents have had time to interact with their newborn, inform them about the surgical treatment and postoperative care.

HERNIAS

A **hernia** is a protrusion of a portion of an organ or organs through an abnormal opening. The danger of herniation arises when the protrusion is constricted, impairing circulation, or when the protrusion interferes with the function or development of other structures. The herniations discussed in this section are those that protrude through the diaphragm, the abdominal wall or the inguinal canal.

Umbilical Hernia

The **umbilical hernia** is a common hernia observed in infants. It occurs when fusion of the umbilical ring is incomplete at the point where the umbilical vessels exit the abdominal wall. It affects low-birth-weight and preterm infants more often than full-term infants. An umbilical hernia usually is an isolated defect, but it may be associated with other congenital anomalies, such as Down syndrome (trisomy 21) and trisomies 13 and 18. The size of the defect is variable, and the protrusion is more prominent when the infant is crying (Fig 25.11). **Incarceration**, in which the hernia is constricted and cannot be reduced manually, is rare. Hernias usually resolve spontaneously by 3 to 5 years of age. If the hernia persists beyond this age, it is usually surgically corrected on an elective basis.

Nursing Care Management

The appearance of an umbilical hernia may be disconcerting to parents. Therefore they need reassurance that the defect usually is not harmful. Taping or strapping the abdomen to flatten the protrusion does not aid in resolution and can produce skin irritation.

Nursing care of the child with an umbilical hernia repair is essentially the same as that for other minor GI surgery. The procedure may be performed on an outpatient basis. Observe the child for complications related to a haematoma or infection. The child may resume a normal diet and activity postoperatively; however, strenuous activity or play is restricted for 2 to 3 weeks.

Inguinal Hernia

Inguinal hernias account for approximately 80% of all childhood hernias and occur more frequently in boys than in girls (approximately 6:1). An incidence of 0.8% to 5% is reported in term newborns and up to 30% in low-birth-weight and preterm infants (Abdulhai et al 2017).

Pathophysiology

Inguinal hernia comes from persistence of all or part of the processus vaginalis, the tube of peritoneum that precedes the testicle through the inguinal canal into the scrotum (in boys) or the round ligament into the labia (in girls), during the eighth month of gestation. After descent of the testicle, the proximal portion of the processus vaginalis normally atrophies and closes, whereas the distal portion forms the tunica

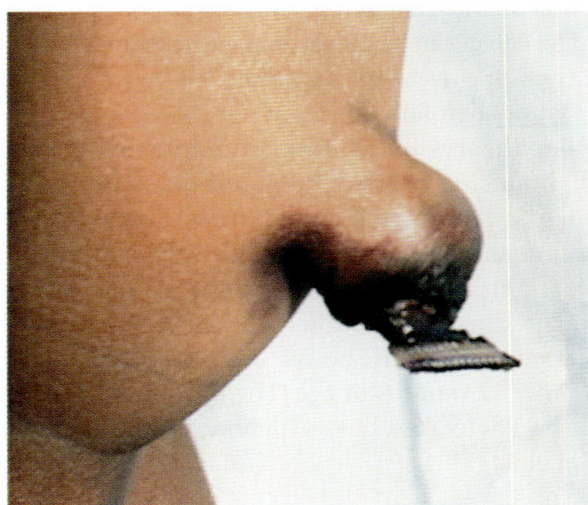

Fig 25.11 Newborn with umbilical hernia. (Source: Zitelli, B. J., & Davis, H. W. (2007). Atlas of pediatric physical diagnosis (5th ed.). St Louis, MO: Mosby.)

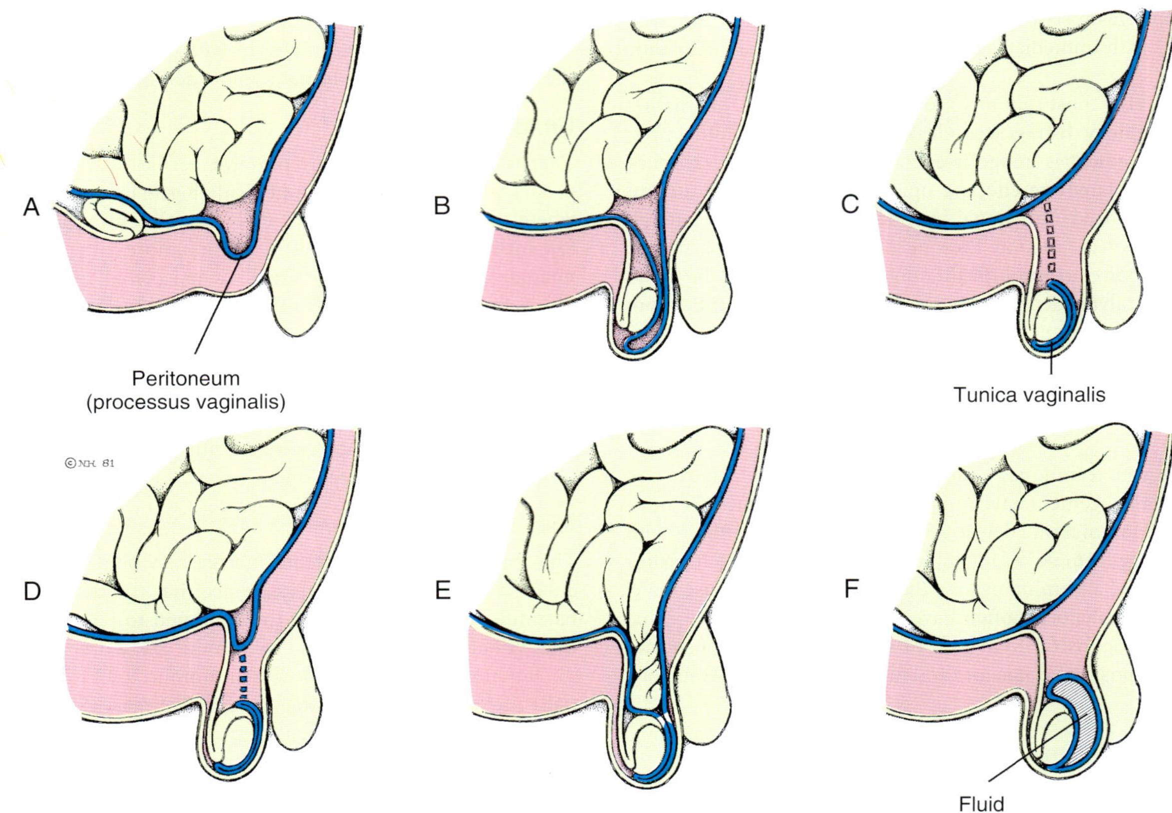

Fig 25.12 Development of inguinal hernias. (**A**) and (**B**) Prenatal migration of processus vaginalis. (**C**) Normal. (**D**) Partially obliterated processus vaginalis. (**E**) Hernia. (**F**) Hydrocele.

vaginalis, which envelops the testicle in the scrotum. When the upper portion fails to atrophy, the abdominal fluid or an abdominal structure (e.g. bowel, ovary, fallopian tubes) can be forced into it, creating a palpable bulge or mass. The persistent sac may end at any point along the inguinal canal; it may stop at the inguinal ring or extend all the way into the scrotum or labia (Fig 25.12).

Clinical Manifestations

This common defect is usually asymptomatic unless the abdominal contents are forced into the patent sac. Most often it appears as a painless inguinal swelling that varies in size. It disappears during periods of rest or is reducible by gentle compression. It appears when the infant cries or strains or when the older child strains, coughs or stands for a long time. The defect can be palpated as a thickening of the cord in the groin, and the silk glove sign can be elicited by rubbing together the sides of the empty hernial sac.

Sometimes the herniated loop of intestine becomes partially obstructed, producing variable symptoms that may include irritability, tenderness, anorexia, abdominal distension and difficulty defecating. Occasionally the loop of bowel becomes **incarcerated** (irreducible) or strangulated (loss of blood supply), with symptoms of complete intestinal obstruction that, if left untreated, will progress to strangulation and necrotic bowel. Incarceration occurs more often in infants under 12 months of age. The incidence of incarceration is reported to be 3% to 16% but as high as 30% in premature infants (Abdulhai et al 2017).

Therapeutic Management

The treatment for hernias is prompt, elective surgical repair in the healthy child as soon as the defect is diagnosed. However, an incarcerated hernia requires emergent surgical care. Because there was believed to be a significant incidence of bilateral involvement, many surgeons advocated exploration of both sides; however, this practice has gained disfavour due to complications occurring with open exploration (Aiken & Oldham 2016b). Laparoscopic exploration of the contralateral side may be performed without risk of injury to the vas deferens (Aiken & Oldham 2016b).

Nursing Care Management

Prompt recognition of an inguinal hernia is imperative. The hernia may first be noticed when the infant is crying or straining to stool (Valsalva manoeuvre). Nursing care of the infant or child with an inguinal hernia involves preoperative preparation of the infant and appropriate explanation to the parents of the child's expected postoperative status. Most hernia repairs can be managed on an outpatient basis. The preterm infant usually has hernia repair several days before discharge. The former preterm infant diagnosed after discharge is admitted the day of surgery and, after repair, is observed for 12 to 24 hours for apnoea and bradycardia.

Postoperatively the incision is kept clean and dry, and the infant's pain is managed appropriately.

Femoral Hernia

Femoral hernias are rare in children, with a reported incidence of less than 1% (Abdulhai et al 2017). The incidence is higher in girls than in boys. The hernia may manifest as a recurrent hernia after inguinal hernia repair. Initial symptoms are swelling in the groin area associated with severe abdominal pain and cramping. Treatment and management are the same as for inguinal hernia. Incarceration and strangulation are frequent complications.

BOX 25.17 Classification of Anorectal Malformations

Male Defects
- Perineal fistula
- Rectourethral bulbar fistula
- Rectourethral prostatic fistula
- Rectovesicular (bladder neck) fistula
- Imperforate anus without fistula
- Rectal atresia

Female Defects
- Perineal fistula
- Rectovestibular fistula
- Imperforate anus without fistula
- Rectal atresia
- Rectovaginal fistula
- Cloaca

Source: Gangopadhyay, A. N., & Pandey, V. (2015). Anorectal malformations. Journal of Indian Association of Pediatric Surgeons, 20(1), 10–15.

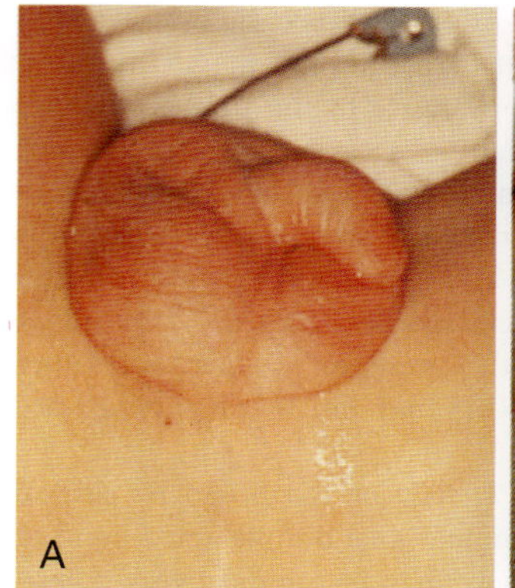

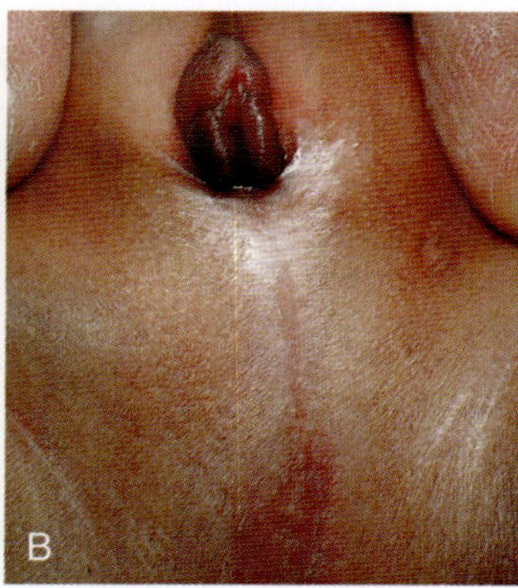

Fig 25.14 (**A**) No visible external opening is consistent with high imperforate anus defect; absence of intergluteal cleft is also common. (**B**) Imperforate anus in female, commonly associated with cloacal anomaly, which manifests as a single perineal opening on perineum. (Source: Zitelli, B. J., & Davis, H. W. (2007). Atlas of pediatric physical diagnosis (5th ed.). St Louis, MO: Mosby.)

Anorectal Malformations

Anorectal malformations (ARMs) are among the more common congenital malformations caused by abnormal development, with an incidence of approximately 1 in 3000 births (Akay & Klein 2016). These malformations may range from simple imperforate anus to other associated complex anomalies of GU and pelvic organs, which may require extensive treatment for faecal, urinary and sexual function. Anorectal malformations may occur in isolation or as a part of the VACTERL association (see earlier in this chapter). These anomalies are classified according to the newborn's gender and abnormal anatomical features, including GU defects (Box 25.17). More than half of all ARMs are associated with other anomalies.

Rectal atresia and stenosis occur when the anal opening appears normal, there is a midline intergluteal groove and usually no fistula exists between the rectum and urinary tract. **Rectal atresia** is a complete obstruction (inability to pass stool) and requires immediate surgical intervention. **Rectal stenosis** may not become apparent until later in infancy when the infant has a history of difficult stooling, abdominal distension and ribbonlike stools. A **persistent cloaca** is a complex anorectal malformation in which the rectum, vagina and urethra drain into a common channel opening into the perineum (Fig 25.13A).

Imperforate anus includes several forms of malformation without an obvious opening (Fig 25.14). Frequently a fistula (an abnormal communication) leads from the distal rectum to the perineum or GU system (see Fig 25.13B and C). The fistula may be evidenced when meconium is evacuated through the vaginal opening, the perineum below the vagina, the male urethra or the perineum under the scrotum. The presence of meconium on the perineum does not indicate anal patency. A fistula may not be apparent at birth, but as peristalsis increases, meconium is forced through the fistula into the urethra or onto the newborn's perineum.

Pathophysiology

During embryonic development the cloaca becomes the common channel for the developing urinary, genital and rectal systems. The cloaca is divided at the sixth week of gestation into an anterior urogenital sinus and a posterior intestinal channel by the urorectal septum. After the lateral folds join the urorectal septum, separation of the urinary and rectal segments takes place. Further differentiation results in the anterior GU system and the posterior anorectal channel. An interruption of this development leads to incomplete migration of the rectum to its normal perineal position.

Diagnostic Evaluation

The diagnosis of an anorectal malformation is based on the physical finding of an absent anal opening. Other symptoms may include abdominal distension, vomiting, absence of meconium passage or

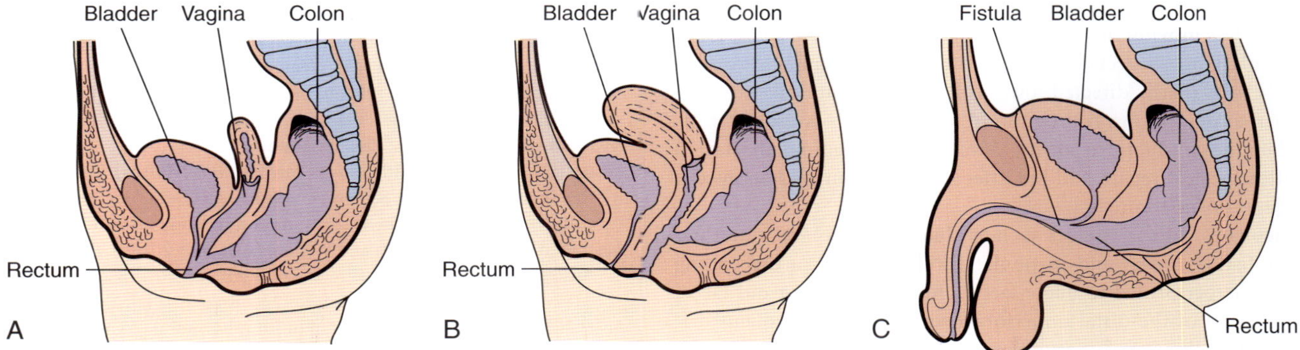

Fig 25.13 Anorectal malformations. (**A**) Typical cloaca (female). (**B**) Low rectovaginal fistula (female). (**C**) Rectourethral bulbar fistula (male).

presence of meconium in the urine. Additional physical findings with an anorectal malformation are a flat perineum and the absence of a midline intergluteal groove. The appearance of the perineum alone does not accurately predict the extent of the defect and associated anomalies. GU and spinal-vertebral anomalies associated with anorectal malformations should be considered when an anomaly is noted. OA with or without TOF, cardiac defects and spinal or vertebral anomalies may occur in association with anorectal malformations, and the infant should be carefully evaluated for the presence of these and other anomalies. Although rare, some ARMs may not be diagnosed until later in infancy or early childhood.

A perineal fistula (see Box 25.17) may be diagnosed by clinical observation. The presence of a prominent anal dimple and a band of skin tissue commonly known as a bucket handle is indicative of a perineal fistula. Abdominal and pelvic ultrasonography is performed to further evaluate the infant's anatomical malformation.

Therapeutic Management

The primary management of anorectal malformations is surgical. Once the defect is identified, steps need to be taken to rule out associated life-threatening defects, which need immediate surgical intervention. Provided no immediate life-threatening problems exist, the newborn is stabilised and kept NBM for further evaluation. IV fluids are provided to maintain glucose and fluid and electrolyte balance. Current recommendation is that surgery be delayed at least 24 hours to properly evaluate for the presence of a fistula and possibly other anomalies (Akay & Klein 2016).

Prognosis. The long-term prognosis depends on such factors as the type of defect, anatomy of the sacrum and vertebrae, quality of muscles and the success of the surgery.

The presence of a flat or 'rocker' bottom and no midline groove usually carries a poor prognosis for bowel continence because of associated neurological, muscular and anatomical problems. When the internal anal sphincter is absent, incontinence is a common long-term problem. These children may achieve socially acceptable continence over time with the aid of a bowel management program. Other potential complications after surgical treatment of anorectal anomalies include strictures, recurrent rectourinary fistula, mucosal prolapse and constipation.

Nursing Care Management

The first nursing responsibility is assisting in identification of anorectal malformations. A newborn who does not pass stool within 24 hours after birth or has meconium that appears at a location other than the anal opening requires further assessment. Preoperative care includes diagnostic evaluation, GI decompression, bowel preparation and IV fluids.

For the newborn with a perineal fistula, an **anoplasty** is performed, which involves moving the fistula opening to the centre of the sphincter and enlarging the rectal opening. Postoperative nursing care after anoplasty is primarily directed towards healing the surgical site without other complications. A program of anal dilations is usually initiated when the child returns for the 2-week check. Feedings are started soon after surgical repair, and breastfeeding is encouraged because it causes less constipation.

In neonates with anomalies such as **cloaca** (female), rectourethral prostatic fistula (male) and vestibular fistula (female), a descending colostomy is performed to allow faecal elimination and avoid faecal contamination of the distal imperforate section and subsequent urinary tract infection in infants with urorectal fistulas. With a colostomy, postoperative nursing care is directed towards maintaining appropriate skin care at the stoma sites (both distal and proximal), managing postoperative pain and administering IV fluids and antibiotics. Postoperative NG decompression may be required with laparotomy, and nursing care focuses on maintenance of appropriate drainage. (See Chapter 22 for colostomy care.)

Posterior sagittal anorectoplasty (PSARP) is a common surgical procedure for the repair of anorectal malformations in infants approximately 1 to 2 months after the initial colostomy. Preoperative PSARP care often involves irrigation of the distal stoma to prevent faecal contamination of the operative site. During this time parents must be given accurate yet simple information regarding the infant's appearance postoperatively and expectations as to their level of involvement in the child's care.

In the PSARP procedure the repair is made via a posterior midline sacral approach to dissect the different muscle groups involved without damaging strategic innervation of pelvic structures so optimum postoperative bowel continence is achieved. A laparotomy may be required if the rectum is unidentifiable by the posterior approach. Additional management after successful repair involves a program of anal dilations, colostomy closure and a bowel management program.

Parents are instructed in perineal and wound care or care of the colostomy as needed. Anal dilations may be necessary for some infants. Parents should observe stooling patterns and observe for signs of anal stricture or complications. Information on dietary modifications and administration of medications is included in counselling. Nurses have a vital role in helping families of a child with anorectal malformations provide optimum care so bowel management is successful and quality of life enhanced for the child and family.

Family Support, Discharge Planning and Home Care. Long-term follow-up care is essential for children with complex malformations. Parents need reassurance when a colostomy is performed regarding the child's appearance and their ability to care for the child at home.

After the definitive pull-through procedure, toilet training may be delayed. Complete continence is seldom achieved at the usual age of 2 to 3 years. Bowel habit training, bowel management irrigation programs, diet modification and administration of stool softeners or fibre help children improve bowel function and social continence. Some children never achieve bowel continence and must rely on daily bowel irrigations. Support and reassurance during the slow progression to normal, socially acceptable function are essential.

REFERENCES

Abdulhai, S. A., Glenn, I. C., & Ponsky, T. A. (2017). Incarcerated pediatric hernias. The Surgical Clinics of North America, 97(1), 129–145.

Akay, B., & Klein, M. D. (2016). Surgical conditions of the anus and rectum. In R. M. Kliegman, B. F. Stanton, J. W. St Geme, et al. (Eds.), Nelson textbook of pediatrics (20th ed.). Philadelphia: Elsevier/Saunders.

Aiken, J. J., & Oldham, K. T. (2016a). Acute appendicitis. In R. M. Kliegman, B. F. Stanton, J. W. St Geme, et al. (Eds.), Nelson textbook of pediatrics (20th ed.). Philadelphia: Elsevier/Saunders.

Aiken, J. J., & Oldham, K. T. (2016b). Inguinal hernias. In R. M. Kliegman, B. F. Stanton, J. W. St Geme, et al. (Eds.), Nelson textbook of pediatrics (20th ed.). Philadelphia: Elsevier/Saunders.

Australian Institute of Health and Welfare (AIHW). (2018a) Children's Headline Indicators. 18 September. https://www.aihw.gov.au/reports/children-youth/childrens-headline-indicators/contents/2-infant-mortality

Australian Institute of Health and Welfare (AIHW). (2018b). Rotavirus in Australia. Quick facts. https://www.aihw.gov.au/getmedia/a6a24843-1516-4487-8260-59cb2174e843/aihw-phe-236_Rotavirus.pdf.aspx

Australian Technical Advisory Group on Immunisation (ATAGI). (2020). Hepatitis A. Australian Immunisation Handbook. Australian Government Department of Health. Canberra. 3 June. https://immunisationhandbook.health.gov.au/vaccine-preventable-diseases/hepatitis-a

Bagade, S., & Khanna, G. (2015). Imaging of omphalomesenteric duct remnants and related pathologies in children. Current Problems in Diagnostic Radiology, 44(3), 246–255.

Bales, C., & Liacouras, C. A. (2016). Intestinal atresia, stenosis, and malrotation. In R. M. Kliegman, B. F. Stanton, J. W. St Geme, et al. (Eds.), Nelson textbook of pediatrics (20th ed.). Philadelphia: Elsevier/Saunders.

Bass, D. M. (2016). Rotaviruses, caliciviruses, and astroviruses. In R. M. Kliegman, B. F. Stanton, J. W. St Geme, et al. (Eds.), Nelson textbook of pediatrics (20th ed.). Philadelphia: Elsevier/Saunders.

Berdan, E. A., & Sato, T. T. (2017). Pediatric airway and oesophageal foreign bodies. The Surgical Clinics of North America, 97(1), 85–91.

Bhutta, Z. A. (2016). Acute gastroenteritis in children. In R. M. Kliegman, B. F. Stanton, J. W. St Geme, et al. (Eds.), Nelson textbook of pediatrics (20th ed.). Philadelphia: Saunders/Elsevier.

Blanchard, S. S., & Czinn, S. J. (2016). Peptic ulcer disease in children. In R. M. Kliegman, B. F. Stanton, J. W. St Geme, et al. (Eds.), Nelson textbook of pediatrics (20th ed.). Philadelphia: Elsevier/Saunders.

Branski, D., Troncone, R., & Fasano, A. (2016). Celiac disease. In R. M. Kliegman, B. F. Stanton, J. W. St Geme, et al. (Eds.), Nelson textbook of pediatrics (20th ed.). Philadelphia: Elsevier/Saunders.

Bruce, J. S., Bruce, C. S., Short, H., et al. (2016). Childhood constipation: Recognition, management and the role of the nurse. British Journal of Nursing (Mark Allen Publishing), 25(22), 1231–1242.

Carroll, A. G., Kavanagh, R. G., Ni Leidhin, C., et al. (2017). Comparative effectiveness of imaging modalities for the diagnosis and treatment of intussusception: A critically appraised topic. Academic Radiology, 24(5), 521–529.

Casciani, E., Nardo, G. D., Chin, S., et al. (2017). MR enterography in paediatric patients with obscure gastrointestinal bleeding. European Journal of Radiology, 93, 209–216.

Chopra, J., Patel, N., Basude, D., et al. (2017). Abdominal pain-related functional gastrointestinal disorders in children. British Journal of Nursing (Mark Allen Publishing), 26(11), 624–631.

Choudhary, N. S., Puri, R., Saigal, S., et al. (2016). Innovative approach of using oesophageal stent for refractory post-band ligation oesophageal ulcer bleed following liver donor liver transplantation. Journal of Clinical and Experimental Hepatology, 6(2), 149–150.

Cohran, V. C., Prozialeck, J. D., & Cole, C. R. (2017). Redefining short bowel syndrome in the 21st century. Pediatric Research, 81(4), 540–549.

Conrad, M. A., & Rosh, J. R. (2017). Pediatric inflammatory bowel disease. Pediatric Clinics of North America, 64(3), 577–591.

Dekate, P., Jayashree, M., & Singhi, S. (2013). Management of acute diarrhea in emergency room. Indian Journal of Pediatrics, 80(3), 235–246.

Fiorino, K., & Liacouras, C. A. (2016). Congenital aganglionic megacolon (Hirschprung disease). In R. M. Kliegman, B. F. Stanton, J. W. St Geme, et al. (Eds.), Nelson textbook of pediatrics (20th ed.). Philadelphia: Elsevier/Saunders.

Fok, C. Y., Holland, K. S., Gil-Zaragozano, E., et al. (2016). The role of nurses and dieticians in managing paediatric coeliac disease. British Journal of Nursing (Mark Allen Publishing), 25(8), 449–455.

Giannetti, E., Maglione, M., Sciorio, E., et al. (2017). Do children just grow out of irritable bowel syndrome? The Journal of Pediatrics, 183, 122–126.

Govindarajan, K . K. (2016). Biliary atresia: Where do we stand now? World Journal of Hepatology, 8(36), 1593–1601.

Grossman, A. B., & Baldassano, R. N. (2016). Chronic ulcerative colitis. In R. M. Kliegman, B. F. Stanton, J. W. St Geme, et al. (Eds.), Nelson textbook of pediatrics (20th ed.). Philadelphia: Elsevier/Saunders.

Hassan, H. H., & Balistreri, W. F. (2016). Cholestasis. In R. M. Kliegman, B. F. Stanton, J . W. St Geme, et al. (Eds.), Nelson textbook of pediatrics (20th ed.). Philadelphia: Saunders/Elsevier.

Hunter, A. K., & Liacouras, C. A. (2016). Pyloric stenosis and other congenital anomalies of the stomach. In R. M. Kliegman, B. F. Stanton, J. W. St Geme, et al. (Eds.), Nelson textbook of pediatrics (20th ed.). Philadelphia: Elsevier/Saunders.

Jensen, M. K., & Balistreri, W. F. (2016). Viral hepatitis. In R. M. Kliegman, B. F. Stanton, J. W. St Geme, et al. (Eds.), Nelson textbook of pediatrics (20th ed.). Philadelphia: Elsevier/Saunders.

Katz, E. R., Kitts, R. L., & DeMaso, D. R. (2016). Pica. In R. M. Kliegman, B. F. Stanton, J. W. St Geme, et al. (Eds.), Nelson textbook of pediatrics (20th ed.). Philadelphia: Elsevier/Saunders.

Kennedy, M., & Liacouras, C. A. (2016a). Intestinal duplications, Meckel diverticulum, and other remnants of the omphalomesenteric duct. In R. M. Kliegman, B. F. Stanton, J. W. St Geme, et al. (Eds.), Nelson textbook of pediatrics (20th ed.). Philadelphia: Elsevier/Saunders.

Kennedy, M., & Liacouras, C. A. (2016b). Intussusception. In R. M. Kliegman, B. F. Stanton, J. W. St Geme, et al. (Eds.), Nelson textbook of pediatrics (20th ed.). Philadelphia: Elsevier/Saunders.

Khan, S., & Orenstein, S. R. (2016a). Ingestions. In R. M. Kliegman, B. F. Stanton, J. W. St Geme, et al. (Eds.), Nelson textbook of pediatrics (20th ed.). Philadelphia: Elsevier/Saunders.

Khan, S., & Orenstein, S. R. (2016b). Gastroesophageal reflux disease. In R. M. Kliegman, B. F. Stanton, J. W. St Geme, et al. (Eds.), Nelson textbook of pediatrics (20th ed.). Philadelphia: Elsevier/Saunders.

Khan, S., & Orenstein, S. R. (2016c). Esophageal atresia and tracheoesophageal fistula. In R. M. Kliegman, B. F. Stanton, J. W. St Geme, et al. (Eds.), Nelson textbook of pediatrics (20th ed.). Philadelphia: Elsevier/Saunders.

Kridler, J., & Kamat, D. (2016). Irritable bowel syndrome: A review for general pediatricians. Pediatric Annals, 45(1), e30–e33.

Lakshminarayanan, B., & Lakhoo, K. (2014). Abdominal wall defects. Early Human Development, 90(12), 917–920.

Lamberti, L. M., Ashraf, S., Walker, C. L., et al. (2016). A systematic review of the effect of rotavirus vaccination on diarrhea outcomes among children younger than 5 years. The Pediatric Infectious Disease Journal, 35(9), 992–998.

Laya, B. F., Restrepo, R., & Lee, E. Y. (2017). Practical imaging evaluation of foreign bodies in children: An update. Radiologic Clinics of North America, 55(4), 845–867.

Lebwohl, B., Sanders, D. S., & Green, P. H. R. (2018). Coeliac disease, Lancet 391(10115), 70–81.

Ledbetter, D. J. (2012). Congenital abdominal wall defects and reconstruction in pediatric surgery: Gastroschesis and omphalocele. The Surgical Clinics of North America, 92(3), 713–727.

Leung, D. T., Chisti, M. J., & Pavia, A. T. (2016). Prevention and control of childhood pneumonia and diarrhoea. Pediatric Clinics of North America, 63(1), 67–79.

Lin, X. K., Huang, X. Z., Bao, X. Z., et al. (2017). Clinical characteristics of Meckel diverticulum in children: A retrospective review of a 15-year single-center experience. Medicine, 96(32), e7760.

Martin, L. Y., Ladd, M. R., Werts, A., et al. (2017). Tissue engineering for the treatment of short bowel syndrome in children. Pediatric Research, 83(1–2), 249–257.

Muller, C. O., Rossignol, G., Montalva, L., et al. (2016). Long-term outcome of laparoscopic Duhamel procedure for extended Hirschsprung's disease. Journal of Laparoendoscopic and Advanced Surgical Techniques. Part A, 26(12), 1032–1035.

Ministry of Health. (2019). Wai 2575 Māori Health Trends Report. Wellington: Ministry of Health. 30 October. https://www.health.govt.nz/publication/wai-2575-maori-health-trends-report

Ministry of Health. (2020). New Zealand Maternity Clinical Indicators 2018. 12 October. https://www.health.govt.nz/publication/new-zealand-maternity-clinical-indicators-2018

Mousa, H., & Hassan, M. (2017). Gastroesophageal reflux disease. Pediatric Clinics of North America, 64(3), 487–505.

National Centre for Immunisation Research and Surveillance. (2015). FactSheet: Hepatitis B. July. NCIRS: Sydney. https://www.tri.edu.au/filething/get/45769/hepatitis-B-vaccination-fact-sheet.pdf

Newlove-Delgado, T. V., Martin, A. E., Abbott, R. A., et al. (2017). Dietary interventions for recurrent abdominal pain in childhood. Cochrane Database of Systematic Review, (3), CD010972.

Patel, R., Bommayya, N., Choudhry, M., et al. (2015). Bleeding duodenal ulcer in a healthy infant presenting with rectal bleeding and requiring surgical treatment. Journal of Pediatric Surgical Special, 9, 38–40.

Paul, S. P., McVeigh, L., Gil-Zaragozano, E., et al. (2016). Diagnosis and nursing management of coeliac disease in children. Nursing Children and Young People, 28(1), 18–24.

Poddar, U. (2016). Approach to constipation in children. Indian Pediatrics, 53(4), 319–327.
Rentea, R. M., Peter, D., & Snyder, C. L. (2017). Pediatric appendicitis: State of the art review. Pediatric Surgery International, 33(3), 269–283.
Rosen, M. J., Dhawan, A., & Saeed, S. A. (2017). Inflammatory bowel disease in children and adolescents. JAMA Pediatrics, 169(11), 1053–1060.
Sreedharan, R., & Liacouras, C. A. (2016). Major symptoms and signs of digestive tract disorders. In R. M. Kliegman, B. F. Stanton, J. W. St Geme, et al. (Eds.), Nelson textbook of pediatrics (20th ed.). Philadelphia: Elsevier/Saunders.
St Louis, A. M., Kim, K., Browne, M. L., et al. (2017). Prevalence trends of selected major birth defects: A multi-state population-based retrospective study, United States, 1999 to 2007. Birth Defects Research, 109(18), 1442–1450.
The Royal Children's Hospital Melbourne (RCHM). (2019). Abdominal pain—acute. Clinical Practice Guidelines. https://www.rch.org.au/clinicalguide/guideline_index/Abdominal_Pain_-_Acute/
The Royal Children's Hospital Melbourne (RCHM). (2020a). Intravenous fluids. Management. Clinical Practice Guidelines. October. https://www.rch.org.au/clinicalguide/guideline_index/Intravenous_fluids/
The Royal Children's Hospital Melbourne (RCHM). (2020b). Gastroenteritis. Management. Clinical Practice Guidelines. December. https://www.rch.org.au/clinicalguide/guideline_index/Gastroenteritis/
The Sydney Children's Hospital Network. (n.d.). Hepatitis C virus infection in children. https://www.schn.health.nsw.gov.au/fact-sheets/hepatitis-c-virus-infection-in-children
Tiziani, A. (2020). Havard's Nursing Guide to Drugs. 10th Ed. Elsevier. Chatswood, Australia.
Vanderhoof, J. A., & Branski, D. (2016). Short bowel syndrome. In R. M. Kliegman, B. F. Stanton, J. W. St Geme, et al. (Eds.), Nelson textbook of pediatrics (20th ed.). Philadelphia: Elsevier/Saunders.
Watanabe, S., Suzuki, T., Hara, F., et al. (2017). Omphalocele and gastroschisis in newborns: Over 16 years of experience from a single clinic. Journal of Neonatal Surgery, 6(2), 27.
Wen, S. C., Best, E., & Nourse, C. (2017). Non-typhoidal Salmonella infections in children: Review of literature and recommendations for management. Journal of Paediatrics and Child Health, 53(10), 936–941.
Yanagi, Y., Matsuura, T., Hayashida, M., et al. (2017). Bowel perforation after liver transplantation for biliary atresia: A retrospective study of care in the transition from childhood to adulthood. Pediatric Surgery International, 33(2), 155–163.
Yang, H. R. (2016). Updates on the diagnosis of Helicobacter pylori infection in children: What are the differences between adults and children? Pediatric Gastroenterology, Hepatology & Nutrition, 19(2), 96–103.

SECTION XI Childhood Oxygenation Problems

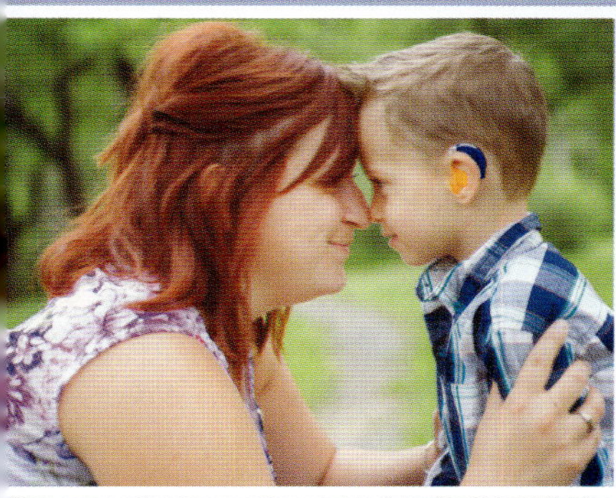

26

The Child with Respiratory Dysfunction

Kylie Smith and Felicity Radford

LEARNING OUTCOMES

- Develop an understanding of the significant differences in the child's respiratory system compared to an adult
- Develop an understanding of an appropriate and correct respiratory assessment in children
- Develop knowledge of different respiratory conditions/diseases affecting children
- Understand the importance of involving parents/carers in a child's treatments and education
- Understand the importance of cultural beliefs in a child's treatment
- Gain an understanding of the impact on treatment availability for rural and remote children and families

INTRODUCTION

Normal and adequate respiratory function in infants and children can be affected by a number of illnesses and conditions. Many are acute (short in duration) and may not require significant medical intervention (they may be treated at home or with brief hospitalisation), while other factors are chronic (lifelong), requiring ongoing treatments, therapies and support/services for the infant/child and their family.

Appropriate and timely treatments are essential for the child and their family. As health professionals we need to ensure that the child receives the right care at the right time and is supported by the correct services. Access to services is a major barrier. Many rural and remote communities have little or no services within their communities, thus increasing the need for travel to major centres for ongoing treatments, access to specialists and follow-up care.

CULTURAL CONSIDERATIONS

Australia and New Zealand have many different and diverse cultural groups. Consideration is essential when assessing and commencing medical treatments. Many cultures still believe in and utilise their traditional medicines/treatments.

In both countries, medical professionals need to understand the history of our Indigenous populations; that is, Aboriginal and Torres Strait Islander peoples and the M ori people. Many still live a traditional lifestyle. Cultural beliefs and at times, lack of trust in the medical system, can affect the abilities of families to seek ongoing medical treatments. Many Indigenous people prefer that their medical treatments occur as close to their home as possible, as family and the family support network remain a major factor in their culture.

RESPIRATORY TRACT STRUCTURE

The thoracic cavity, located in the bony framework provided by the ribs, vertebrae and sternum, consists of three major sections: the three-lobed lung on the right; the two-lobed lung on the left; and the mediastinum, or the space between the lungs. The mediastinum contains the oesophagus, trachea, large blood vessels and heart. Smooth parietal pleura line the entire thoracic cavity and adhere to the ribs and superior surface of the diaphragm. Each lung is encased in a separate visceral pleural sac that, when inflated, lies against the parietal pleura. Normally the two pleural membranes are separated by only enough fluid to lubricate the surface for painless movement during filling and emptying of the lungs.

The two cone-shaped lungs consist of the bronchi, bronchioles and innumerable small air sacs, or alveoli. Through these thin-walled sacs, gas exchange occurs by simple diffusion between the inspired air and the bloodstream. The amount of gas exchanged depends on many factors, including the amount and composition of air inhaled, thickness of the alveolar wall, adequacy of circulation to the alveoli and substances within the alveoli that either prevent their inflation (e.g. surface-active surfactant) or prevent gas exchange (e.g. fluids).

With age, changes take place in the air passages that increase the respiratory surface area. The major changes are in the number and size of alveoli and in the increased branching of terminal bronchioles. Although the number of conducting airways is complete early in fetal life, the air sacs are shallow with wide necks and have few shared walls, or septa, at birth. This promotes patency but limits surface area for gas exchange. The alveoli are large with thick septa that have little elastic recoil (not unlike the emphysemic lung). During the first year, bronchioles continue to branch, and the globular alveoli formed earlier in the terminal units rapidly increase in number with each generation. These alveoli partition and divide existing alveoli to form smaller lobular units separated by thinner septa, thus enlarging the area available for gas exchange.

Alveoli increase steadily in number, but it is unclear when septal division ceases and an increase in size begins. It appears to occur sometime during middle childhood, although evidence indicates that an increase in the number of alveoli for each terminal airway takes place at puberty. Approximately nine times more alveoli are present at age 12 years than at birth. In later stages of growth, the structures lengthen and enlarge. In addition, collateral pathways of ventilation develop, including pores through alveolar walls and possibly pathways between bronchioles.

Respiratory Function

Respiratory movements are first evident at approximately 20 weeks' gestation, and throughout fetal life amniotic fluid is exchanged in the alveoli. In the neonate the respiratory rate is rapid to meet the needs of a high metabolism. During growth the respiratory rate steadily decreases until it levels off at maturity. The volume of air inhaled increases with the growth of the lungs and is closely related to body size. In addition, a qualitative difference exists in expired air at different ages. During growth the amount of oxygen in the expired air gradually decreases and the amount of carbon dioxide increases.

Ventilation, the exchange of gases in the lungs, results from changes in pressure gradients created by changes in the size of the thoracic cavity. Contraction of the diaphragm and external intercostal muscles increases the size of the thorax and decreases the intrathoracic pressure. As a result, air moves from the atmosphere, which has a higher pressure, into the lungs, which have a lower pressure. The principles of artificial or mechanical ventilation are based on this concept. Mechanical (artificial) respiratory devices increase the pressure entering the air passages (positive pressure breathing devices) or lowers the pressure around the body (negative pressure ventilator).

The two primary forces that affect the mechanics of breathing are compliance and resistance. Compliance is a measure of chest wall and lung distensibility. It represents the relative ease with which the chest and lungs expand with increasing volume and then collapse away from the pleural wall with decreasing volume (elastic recoil). The two major factors determining compliance are alveolar surface tension, which is lowered by **surfactant**, a lipoprotein at the air–fluid interface that allows alveolar expansion and prevents alveolar collapse, and elastic recoil, the tendency of the lungs to return to the resting state after inspiration (a passive process that requires no muscular effort). Other factors influencing compliance include the degree of tissue hydration, lung blood volume, surface forces at the air–fluid interface, and chest or lung tissue pathological state (e.g. fibres of elastin or collagen). Factors that interfere with compliance and recoil increase the work of breathing.

Compliance is normally high in the newborn and infant because of a more pliant (flexible) rib cage. This greater compliance causes the rib cage to be easily distorted with increased negative pressure in the pleural cavity or when factors inhibit the stabilising action of the intercostal muscles. As the child grows, chest wall compliance decreases and elastic recoil increases; therefore, ventilation becomes progressively more efficient. In pathological states an increase in compliance indicates that the lungs or chest wall is abnormally easy to inflate and has lost some elastic recoil, such as in asthma. A decrease in compliance indicates that the lungs or chest wall is abnormally stiff or difficult to inflate.

Any condition that decreases or increases compliance or increases airway resistance results in increased work of breathing (e.g. increased respiratory rate, retractions, nasal flaring and use of accessory muscles). When respiratory muscle fatigue develops, respiratory failure can occur. Resistance is determined primarily by airway size. The body must overcome three sources of resistance during breathing: tissue resistance in the chest wall (about 20% resistance); tissue resistance in the lungs (about 15% resistance); and, most important, flow resistance in the airways (which often increases with respiratory disease). The four factors determining resistance are flow rate velocity, gas viscosity, length of airway and airway diameter. If any of the first three variables increases, resistance to airflow also increases. If airway diameter decreases, resistance increases exponentially.

The diameter of the airways and thus the airflow are determined by the balance of forces that tend to widen or narrow the airways. One of these is neural regulation of bronchial smooth muscles mediated through autonomic nerves. Sympathetic impulses relax the airways, and parasympathetic impulses constrict them. Reflex constriction occurs in response to irritating inhalants such as dust, smoke or sulfur dioxide; arterial hypoxaemia and hypercapnia; cold air; and some drugs, such as acetylcholine and histamine. Other factors that alter airway size are peribronchial pressure, which tends to narrow the airways, and intraluminal pressure, which tends to keep the airways open. For example, forced expiration causes increased peribronchial pressure and thus narrowing of the airways; a positive pressure breathing apparatus increases intraluminal pressure, keeping the airways open.

DEFENCES OF THE RESPIRATORY TRACT

The respiratory tract has several anatomic and biochemical characteristics that provide natural defences against the many biological and inanimate agents that can damage respiratory tissues. Intact defences help repel and resist the impact of injurious agents; factors that reduce the integrity of these mechanisms increase the vulnerability of these tissues to invasion and disease. Respiratory tract defences include the following.

- **Lymphoid tissues**—Faucial, lingual and pharyngeal tonsils (adenoids) and other pharyngeal lymphoid tissues form a protective circle around the entrance to the respiratory tract. These help localise and contain invading organisms so they can be destroyed by the body's humoral defence mechanisms.
- **Mucous blanket**—The epithelium of the respiratory tract secretes sticky mucus to which airborne organisms adhere.
- **Ciliary action**—The mucus secreted by the columnar epithelium of the respiratory tract is kept flowing, carrying microorganisms and other foreign agents away from the lungs to be coughed or swallowed.
- **Epiglottis**—The epiglottis and the epiglottis reflex protect the respiratory tract from invading material, including infectious exudate from the upper tract, and prevent such material from being aspirated into the lower tract.
- **Cough**—The expulsive force of the cough reflex propels foreign material out of the lower tract.
- **Position changes**—Changes in body position encourage drainage of tracheobronchial passages.
- **Lymphatics**—Lymphatics draining the terminal bronchi and bronchioles remove invading organisms, which are filtered and destroyed in the regional lymph nodes.
- **Humoral defences**—Organisms and other foreign material are removed or destroyed by phagocytes, enzymes and immunoglobulins, especially immunoglobulin A, secreted by the bronchial epithelium.

Some children have conditions (e.g. chronic asthma, cystic fibrosis and the various immunodeficiency disorders) that predispose them to infection as a result of interference with the efficiency of these mechanisms. Frequent, intense exposure to organisms that accompany conditions of crowding or continual exposure to irritating substances in the air results in breakdown of healthy defences. Concurrent illness, malnutrition or fatigue reduces the efficiency of natural defences. Drying of the mucous membranes also inhibits the activity of humoral defences, such as immunoglobulins.

ASSESSMENT OF RESPIRATORY FUNCTION

Physical Assessment

Information about the child's respiratory status is obtained from observations of physical signs and behaviour. However, to make a useful assessment, the nurse must know what to look for and how to interpret findings. (See Physical Examination, Chapter 4.) Auscultation of the lung fields is helpful in identifying specific pathological conditions, in assessing the child's responses to treatment and when determining airway patency. Palpation and percussion provide information regarding areas of pain and tissue density. Chapter 4 describes breath sounds and their terminology.

Respiration

The nurse should assess the configuration of the chest and the pattern of respiratory movement, including rate, regularity, symmetry of movements, depth, effort expended in respiration and use of accessory muscles of respiration. To determine deviations, the nurse must know the normal type and rate of respiration in relation to the child's size and age. (See inside cover.) Respirations (ventilations) are best determined when the child is sleeping or quietly awake. They should be counted for 1 full minute with the child's chest exposed (as practicable) while the child is unaware because an alteration in breathing rate may occur.

Tachypnoea (rapid respirations) often occurs with excitement, exertion, elevated temperature, severe anaemia, metabolic acidosis and respiratory alkalosis. By observing changes in respiratory rate, the nurse can evaluate the child's progress.

Alterations in the depth of respirations—too deep (**hyperpnoea**) or too shallow (**hypopnoea**)—are often recognised as abnormal only in the extremes. Hyperpnoea is noted with fever, severe anaemia, respiratory acidosis that accompanies disorders (such as diabetic ketoacidosis or diarrhoea) and respiratory alkalosis (associated with psychosis, central nervous system (CNS) disturbances). Hypoventilation may occur with metabolic alkalosis. Hypoventilation in preterm infants may occur as a result of pulmonary immaturity, absence of adequate substrate to support respiratory muscle activity, neurological insult and neurological immaturity.

Associated Observations

Recession, or a sinking in of soft tissues relative to the cartilaginous and bony thorax, may occur in some pulmonary disorders. In disease states (particularly in severe airway obstruction), recession becomes extreme. Subcostal recession, observed anteriorly at the lower costal margins, indicates a flattened diaphragm because it not only lowers the floor of the thorax but also pulls on the rib cage in response to a greater than normal decrease in intrathoracic pressure. In severe airway obstruction, recessions extend to the supraclavicular areas and the suprasternal notch.

Nasal flaring is a sign of respiratory distress and a significant finding in an infant. The enlargement of the nostrils helps reduce nasal resistance and maintains airway patency. Nasal flaring may be intermittent or continuous and should be described as mild, moderate or severe.

Head bobbing in a sleeping or exhausted infant is a sign of dyspnoea. The infant's head, bobs forward with each inspiration. This is caused by neck flexion resulting from contraction of the scalene and sternocleidomastoid muscles.

Noisy breathing such as 'snoring' is frequently associated with hypertrophied adenoidal tissue, choanal obstruction, polyps or a foreign body in the nasal passages (i.e. mucus).

Stridor, a high-pitched, noisy respiration, is usually an indication of narrowing of the upper airway, either as a result of oedema and inflammation or in association with an upper airway obstruction, often from mucus secretions or possibly from a foreign object. Stridor may be inspiratory or expiratory. Common causes in children include croup, epiglottitis, foreign body or tracheitis.

Grunting is frequently a sign of pain in older children, suggestive of acute pneumonia or pleural involvement. It is also observed in pulmonary oedema and is a characteristic of respiratory distress in newborns and infants. It is the body's attempt at more efficient respirations. Grunting serves to increase end-respiratory pressure and thus prolong the period of oxygen and carbon dioxide exchange across the alveolo-capillary membrane.

Wheezing is a continuous musical sound originating from vibrations in narrowed airways. Wheezing is primarily heard on expiration. Infants may have wheezing as a result of increased airway resistance and a compliant chest wall. Older children often have wheezing with a lower respiratory tract infection as a result of inflammation, bronchospasm and accumulated secretions.

Colour changes of the skin, especially mottling, pallor and cyanosis, are important. Except for the peripheral bluish discolouration (acrocyanosis) resulting from circulatory stasis in the newborn or the mottling resulting from a cool environment, mottling and cyanosis are significant and usually indicate cardiopulmonary disease.

Chest pain may be a complaint of older children and may have a variety of causes, both pulmonary and non-pulmonary. It may be caused by disease of any of the chest structures. Most pleural pain is related to respiration; therefore, respiratory movements are shallow and rapid and may be accompanied by grunting, especially in the younger patient.

Clubbing, or proliferation of tissue about the terminal phalanges, accompanies a variety of conditions, frequently those associated with chronic hypoxia, primarily cardiac defects and chronic pulmonary disease (e.g. cystic fibrosis). Although clubbing often worsens with lung disease, it does not accurately reflect disease progression. **Cough** is often associated with respiratory disease, although it may suggest other disorders. It serves as a protective mechanism and an indicator of irritation. Some types of cough are characteristic of specific diseases. For example, a severe cough is associated with measles and cystic fibrosis, and the paroxysmal cough accompanied by an inspiratory 'whoop' is typical of pertussis in infants and small children. A harsh barking, non-productive cough is part of the symptomatology of croup and foreign body aspiration. Because there are no cough receptors in the alveoli, a cough may be absent in a child with pneumonia in the early stages of the disease but is a common feature during active pneumonia and recovery.

Diagnostic Procedures

Several procedures are available for assessing respiratory function and diagnosing respiratory disease. All these procedures require preparation and support of the child and the family to ensure cooperation and accurate results.

Pulmonary Function Tests

Non-invasive pulmonary mechanics are often measured (e.g. spirometry/pneumotachography), These tests are useful to evaluate the severity and course of a disease and to study the effects of treatment; however, they have limitations due to different diseases having the same functional abnormalities.

Radiology and Other Diagnostic Procedures

Radiography/imaging is used frequently in diagnostic evaluation of children. Lead shields, correctly placed and consistently applied to areas not needed for diagnostic purposes (radiosensitive areas such as the patient's immature gonads and thyroid glands) are essential; this includes staff and parents/carers. Play and modification of methodology effectively reduce the trauma sometimes associated with the procedure, gain the child's cooperation and reduce the anxiety of the child and parent/caregiver.

Blood Gas Determination

Blood gas measurements are sensitive indicators of change in respiratory status in acutely ill patients. They provide valuable information regarding lung function, lung adequacy and tissue perfusion and are essential for monitoring conditions involving hypoxaemia, carbon dioxide retention and pH. For the acutely ill patient, this information also guides decisions regarding therapeutic interventions, such as: (1) positioning the child for maximum ventilation; (2) administering oxygen, continuous positive airway pressure (CPAP) or bilevel positive airway pressure (BiPAP); (3) modifying chest physiotherapy (CPT); or (4) adjusting mechanical ventilator settings.

Arterial blood gas (ABG) sampling helps evaluate gas exchange and oxygenation and may be performed on blood from an artery or a capillary. An accurate ABG or capillary blood gas (CBG) requires unclotted blood using a heparinised blood gas syringe or capillary tube. Air bubbles in the sample may alter the blood gas concentration. Depending on the laboratory facilities, as little as 0.1 mL may be sufficient in small infants.

Although ABG values are similar for children and adults, newborns can have slightly lower values and still be considered normal. For example, normal pH values for a newborn range from 7.26 to 7.29, the average PaO_2 is 70 mmHg, the average $PaCO_2$ is 33 mmHg and the average bicarbonate is 20 mEq/L. ABG values also depend on the concentration of oxygen the child is breathing. The arterial PaO_2 should rise in proportion to the oxygen concentration being inhaled. Therefore, when evaluating ABG values, consider the percentage of oxygen administered (if any), the child's body temperature (as little as 1°C can alter the blood gas values 5% to 8%) and the presence of anxiety (if children hyperventilate, $PaCO_2$ may be reduced) or crying (can cause breath holding, resulting in decreased PaO_2).

One approach to determine a simple acid–base disturbance is as follows.

- Evaluate the pH to determine whether acidemia or alkalemia is present.
- Evaluate the PCO_2 to determine whether the imbalance is respiratory.
- Evaluate the bicarbonate levels to determine whether the imbalance is metabolic.

Non-invasive Monitoring

Pulse oximetry provides a continuous or intermittent non-invasive method of determining oxyhaemoglobin saturation (SpO_2). Applying the sensor correctly is essential for accurate SpO_2 measurements, the sensor must identify every pulse beat to calculate the SpO_2, movement can interfere with accurate reading. Some devices synchronise the oxygen saturation reading with the heartbeat, thereby reducing the interference caused by motion. Sensors are not placed on extremities used for blood pressure monitoring or with indwelling arterial catheters because pulsatile blood flow can be affected. It is recommended that the probe site be changed according to manufacturer guidelines and local policies.

Sensory probes should be covered to reduce interference from ambient light (i.e. phototherapy, overhead lights, etc.). Skin and nails should be clean (i.e. no nail polish, ink, etc.). Secure the sensor with self-adhering tape (e.g. Elastoplast) to an infant's foot, hand or wrist and to a child's fingers or toes. Socks may be applied over the foot to help secure the sensor; the foot should be checked frequently for colour, temperature and pulses.

Elevated levels of carboxyhaemoglobin, methaemoglobin and fetal haemoglobin affect the accuracy of the device because it can only distinguish between oxyhaemoglobin and deoxyhaemoglobin; therefore, the child with carbon monoxide poisoning may have a normal SpO_2 reading but an abnormal (low) PaO_2. Oximetry is insensitive to hyperoxia because haemoglobin approaches 100% saturation for all PaO_2 readings above approximately 100 mmHg, which is a potentially dangerous situation for the preterm infant at risk for developing oxidative stress. Oxidative stress may lead to complications such as bronchopulmonary dysplasia and retinopathy of prematurity. Therefore, the preterm infant being monitored with oximetry should have a range of upper and lower limits identified, such as 90% to 93%, and a protocol should be established for decreasing oxygen when saturations are high.

Another non-invasive method is **transcutaneous monitoring** (TCM), which provides continuous monitoring of transcutaneous partial pressure of oxygen in arterial blood ($tcPaO_2$) and, with some devices, of carbon dioxide in arterial blood ($tcPaCO_2$). An electrode is attached to the warmed skin to facilitate arterialisation of cutaneous capillaries. The site of the electrode must be changed every 3 to 4 hours (or more frequently according to skin status) to avoid burning the skin, and the machine must be calibrated with every site change. This monitoring is used in neonatal intensive care units, but it may not reflect an accurate PaO_2 in infants with impaired local circulation.

End-tidal carbon dioxide monitoring ($ETCO_2$) measures exhaled carbon dioxide non-invasively. Capnometry provides a numeric display, and capnography provides a graph over time. Continuous capnometry is available in many bedside physiological monitors, as well as standalone monitors. $ETCO_2$ differs from pulse oximetry in that it is more sensitive to the mechanics of ventilation rather than oxygenation. Hypoxic episodes can be prevented through the early detection of hypoventilation, apnoea or airway obstruction.

$ETCO_2$ monitoring is obtained by measuring exhaled CO_2 and provides real-time evidence of ventilation. The use of capnography provides a non-invasive method for measuring the partial pressure of CO_2 during inspiration and expiration; the $ETCO_2$ waveform (capnograph) provides information about expired CO_2, as well as any underlying physiological conditions or disease processes. Measurement of PCO_2 at end expiration ($P_{ET}CO_2$) approximates alveolar PCO_2 in patients with normal lungs and pulmonary blood flow. $ETCO_2$ can be monitored with or without an artificial airway in place. A sudden decrease in $ETCO_2$ in an intubated patient may indicate endotracheal tube obstruction, extubation, oesophageal malposition or a leak or disruption in the system. In a non-intubated patient, a decrease in $ETCO_2$ may be indicative of hypoventilation, sepsis or malignant hypothermia.

Children who are experiencing an asthma exacerbation, receiving procedural sedation or are mechanically ventilated may have $ETCO_2$ monitoring. Although $ETCO_2$ monitoring is not a substitute for ABGs, it does have the advantage of providing ventilation information continuously and non-invasively. Normal $ETCO_2$ values are 30 to 43 mmHg, which is slightly lower than normal arterial PCO_2 of 35 to 45 mmHg. During cardiopulmonary resuscitation (CPR), $ETCO_2$

values consistently below 15 mmHg indicate ineffective compressions or excessive ventilation. Changes in waveform and numeric display follow changes in ventilation by a very few seconds and precede changes in respiratory rate, skin colour and pulse oximetry values.

When there is a change in the $ETCO_2$ value or waveform, assess the patient quickly for adequate airway, breathing and circulation. Sedated patients may be hypoventilating and need stimulation. Intubated patients may need suctioning, may have self-extubated or dislodged the tube or may have equipment failure or disconnection. Asthmatic patients may be deteriorating. Problems with the $ETCO_2$ monitoring system can include a kink in the sample line or disconnection. In general, check the patient first and then the equipment.

$ETCO_2$ monitoring may not be readily available in rural and remote facilities.

GENERAL ASPECTS OF RESPIRATORY TRACT INFECTIONS

Infections of the respiratory tract are described according to the areas of involvement. The upper respiratory tract, or upper airway, consists of the oronasopharynx, pharynx, larynx and upper part of the trachea. The lower respiratory tract consists of the lower trachea, bronchi, bronchioles and alveoli. The bronchi and bronchioles are the reactive portion of the lower respiratory tract because they have smooth muscle content and the ability to constrict. Respiratory tract infections spread from one structure to another because of the contiguous nature of the mucous membrane lining the entire tract. Consequently, infections of the respiratory tract involve several areas rather than a single structure, although the effect on one may predominate in any given illness.

Aetiology and Characteristics

Respiratory tract infections account for the majority of acute illnesses in children. The age of the child, season, living conditions and preexisting medical problems influence the cause and course of these infections.

Infectious Agents

The respiratory tract is subject to a wide variety of infective organisms. Most infections are caused by viruses, particularly respiratory syncytial virus (RSV), rhinovirus, non-polio enteroviruses (coxsackievirus A and B), parainfluenza virus, influenza virus, adenoviruses, human metapneumovirus and more recently coronavirus (COVID-19). Other agents involved in primary or secondary invasion include group A β-haemolytic streptococci (GABHS), *Bordetella pertussis*, staphylococci, *Haemophilus influenzae*, *Chlamydia trachomatis*, *Mycoplasma* organisms and pneumococci.

Age

Healthy full-term infants younger than 3 months are presumed to have a lower infection rate because of the protective function of maternal antibodies. However, infants are susceptible to respiratory infections, such as pertussis, during this time. The infection rate increases from 3 to 6 months old, which is the period between the disappearance of maternal antibodies and the infant's own antibody production. The viral infection rate continues to remain high during the toddler and preschool years. By 5 years old, viral respiratory tract infections are less frequent, but the incidence of *Mycoplasma pneumoniae* and GABHS infections increases. The amount of lymphoid tissue increases throughout middle childhood, and repeated exposure to organisms confers increasing immunity as children grow older.

Some viral and bacterial agents produce a mild illness in older children but cause severe lower respiratory tract illness or croup in infants. For example, RSV causes a relatively harmless tracheobronchitis in childhood but is a serious disease in infancy.

Size

Anatomic differences influence the response to respiratory tract infections. The diameter of the airways is smaller in young children and subject to considerable narrowing from oedematous mucous membranes and increased production of secretions. In addition, the distance between structures within the tract is shorter in the young child. Therefore, organisms move more rapidly down the respiratory tract for more extensive involvement. The relatively short and open eustachian tube in infants and young children allows pathogens easy access to the middle ear.

Resistance

The ability to resist pathogens depends on several factors. Deficiencies of the immune system place the child at risk for infection. Other conditions that decrease resistance are malnutrition, anaemia and fatigue. Conditions that weaken defences of the respiratory tract and predispose a child to infection include allergies (e.g. allergic rhinitis), bronchopulmonary dysplasia (BPD), asthma, history of RSV infection, cardiac anomalies that cause pulmonary congestion, and cystic fibrosis (CF). Day care attendance and exposure to second-hand smoke also increases the likelihood of infection.

Seasonal Variations

The most common respiratory tract pathogens appear in epidemics during the winter and spring months, but mycoplasmal infections occur more often in autumn and early winter. Infection-related asthma (e.g. asthmatic bronchitis) occurs more frequently during cold weather. Winter and spring are typically RSV season, when children are indoors in close contact and more likely to spread the disease to one another.

Clinical Manifestations

Infants and young children, especially those between 6 months and 3 years of age, react more severely to acute respiratory tract infection than do older children. Young children display a number of generalised signs and symptoms and local manifestations that differ from those seen in older children and adults. Signs and symptoms associated with respiratory tract illnesses are outlined in Box 26.1. Box 26.2 lists components for assessing respiratory function.

Nursing Care of the Child with a Respiratory Tract Infection

Assessment

Assessment of the respiratory system follows the guidelines described in Chapter 4 (for nose, mouth and throat, chest and lungs). The assessment should include heart rate, respiratory rate, depth, rhythm and respiratory effort, oxygenation, hydration status, body temperature, level of consciousness, activity level and level of comfort. Special attention is given to the observations outlined in Box 26.1 and the components in Box 26.2.

NURSING CARE CONSIDERATIONS

A non-invasive pulse oximeter (oxygen saturation) measurement should be performed on *all* children with a respiratory illness as part of the routine physical assessment.

BOX 26.1 Signs and Symptoms Associated with Respiratory Tract Infections in Infants and Small Children

Fever

May be absent in neonates (< 28 days)
Greatest at ages 6 months to 3 years
Temperature may reach 39.5°C to 40.5°C even with mild infections
Often appears as first sign of infection
May leave child listless and irritable or somewhat euphoric and more active than normal, temporarily; leads some children to talk with unaccustomed rapidity
Tendency to develop high temperatures with infection in certain families
May precipitate febrile seizures (see Chapter 30)

Meningismus

Meningeal signs without infection of the meninges
Occurs with abrupt onset of fever
Accompanied by:
- headache
- pain and stiffness in the back and neck
- presence of Kernig's and Brudzinski's signs

Subsides as the temperature drops

Anorexia

Common with most childhood illnesses
Frequently the initial evidence of illness
Persists to a greater or lesser degree throughout febrile stage of illness; often extends into convalescence

Vomiting

Occurs readily in small children with illness
A clue to the onset of infection
May precede other signs by several hours
Usually short lived but may persist during the illness
Is frequent cause of dehydration

Diarrhoea

Usually mild, transient diarrhoea, but may become severe
Often accompanies viral respiratory tract infections

Abdominal Pain

Common complaint
Sometimes indistinguishable from pain of appendicitis in older child
May be caused by mesenteric lymphadenitis
May represent referred pain (e.g. chest pain associated with pneumonia)
May be related to muscle spasms from vomiting, especially in nervous, tense children

Nasal Blockage

Small nasal passages of infants easily blocked by mucosal swelling and exudation
Can interfere with respiration and feeding in infants
May contribute to the development of otitis media and sinusitis

Nasal Discharge

Common feature
May be thin and watery (rhinorrhoea) or thick and purulent
Depends on the type and stage of infection
Associated with itching
May irritate upper lip and skin surrounding the nose

Cough

Common feature
May be evident only during the acute phase
May persist several months after a disease

Respiratory Sounds

Sounds associated with respiratory disease:
- cough
- hoarseness
- grunting
- stridor
- wheezing

Findings on auscultation:
- wheezing
- crackles
- absence of air movement

Sore Throat

Frequent complaint of older children
Young children (unable to describe symptoms) may not complain even when highly inflamed
Increased drooling noted by parents
Refusal by child to take oral fluids or solids

Ease Respiratory Efforts

Many acute respiratory tract infections are mild and cause few symptoms. Although children may feel uncomfortable and have a stuffy nose and some mucosal swelling, acute respiratory distress occurs infrequently. Interventions delivered at home are usually sufficient to relieve minor discomfort and ease respiratory efforts. However, in some cases, the infant or child may require hospitalisation for observation and therapy.

Promote Rest

Children who have an acute febrile illness should be encouraged to rest and engage in quiet activities. Most children limit activities when febrile and increase activity as the fever subsides.

Promote Comfort

Older children are usually able to manage nasal secretions with little difficulty. Instruct parents in the correct administration of nose drops or throat gargles, if ordered. For very young infants, who normally breathe through their noses, removing nasal secretions will be helpful in clearing nasal passages to promote feeding. Two to three drops of saline can be put into each nostril and a bulb syringe used to suction secretions out.

Infection Control

Perform careful handwashing (the Five Moments for Hand Hygiene) and wear appropriate personal protective equipment (PPE) when caring for children with respiratory tract infections. This could include gown, gloves, mask and eye goggles or face shield. Children and families should use a tissue or their elbow when they cough or sneeze. Children with respiratory tract infections should not share drinking cups, eating utensils, washcloths or towels. To decrease contamination with respiratory viruses, wash hands frequently and do not touch eyes or nose with hands.

BOX 26.2 Components for Assessing Respiratory Function

Pattern of Respirations

Rate—Rapid (tachypnoea), normal or slow for the particular child.

Depth—Normal depth, too shallow (hypopnoea), too deep (hyperpnoea); usually estimated from the amplitude of thoracic and abdominal excursion (age dependent).

Ease—Effortless, laboured (dyspnoea), orthopnoea, associated with intercostal or substernal recession (inspiratory 'sinking in' of soft tissues in relation to the cartilaginous and bony thorax), pulsus paradoxus (blood pressure falling with inspiration and rising with expiration), nasal flaring, head bobbing (head of sleeping child bobbing forward in synchrony with each inspiration), grunting or wheezing.

Laboured breathing—Continuous, intermittent, becoming steadily worse, sudden onset, at rest or on exertion, associated with wheezing, grunting, associated with chest pain.

Rhythm—Variation in rate and depth of respirations.

Other Observations

Oxygenation—Pulse oximetry skin colour.

Evidence of infection—Check for elevated temperature; enlarged cervical lymph nodes; inflamed mucous membranes; and purulent discharges from the nose, ears or lungs (sputum).

Cough—Observe the characteristics of the cough (if present): when the cough is heard (e.g. night only, on arising), the nature of the cough (paroxysmal with or without wheeze, 'croupy' or 'brassy'), frequency of the cough, association with swallowing or other activity, character of the cough (moist or dry), productivity.

Wheeze—Note whether it is expiratory or inspiratory, high pitched or musical, prolonged, slowly progressive or sudden, associated with laboured breathing.

Cyanosis—Note distribution (peripheral, perioral, facial, trunk as well as face), degree, duration, association with activity.

Chest pain—Older children may complain of this. Note location and circumstances: localised or generalised; referred to base of neck or abdomen; dull or sharp; deep or superficial; associated with rapid, shallow respirations or grunting.

Sputum—Older children may provide sputum sample by coughing, whereas young children may need use of bulb suction or gastric lavage in early morning to provide a sample. Note volume, colour, viscosity and odour.

Bad breath—May be associated with some throat and lung infections.

Observe child—Level of activity and level of comfort.

Affected children should be kept away from school, day care and social events to minimise spread of infection.

Reduce Body Temperature

If the child has a significantly elevated temperature, controlling the fever is important to ensure comfort. Nurses should verify that family members have a working thermometer and know how to take a child's temperature (i.e. under 2 years old via axillary thermometer) and read the thermometer accurately.

If the practitioner has prescribed an antipyretic such as ibuprofen (for infants and children 6 months and older) or paracetamol (from > 1 month of age unless directed by a practitioner), parents may need help administering the drug. Most parents can read the label and calculate the desired dose, but some may require careful instruction. It is important to emphasise accuracy in both the amount of drug given and the time intervals for drug administration to avoid cumulative effects (i.e. overdosing the child). Encourage cool oral liquids to reduce the temperature and minimise the chances of dehydration (see Controlling Elevated Temperatures, Chapter 22.)

NURSING CARE CONSIDERATIONS

Parents are cautioned regarding over-the-counter combination 'cold' remedies because these often include paracetamol. Careful calculation of both the paracetamol given separately and the paracetamol in combination medications is necessary to avoid an overdose.

Promote Hydration

Dehydration is a potential complication when children have respiratory tract infections and are febrile or anorexic, especially when vomiting or diarrhoea is present. Infants are especially prone to fluid and electrolyte deficits when they have a respiratory illness because a rapid respiratory rate that accompanies such illnesses precludes adequate fluid intake. In addition, the presence of fever increases the total body fluid turnover in infants. If the infant has nasal secretions, this further prevents adequate respiratory effort by blocking the narrow nasal passages when the infant reclines to bottle-feed or breastfeed and ceases the compensatory mouth-breathing effort, thus causing the child to limit intake of fluids. Parents encourage adequate fluid intake by offering small amounts of fluids frequently. High-calorie or thick fruit juices may not be tolerated if the child is also vomiting and has diarrhoea. Oral rehydration solutions, such as Hydralyte or Gastrolyte, are beneficial for infants and young children, and water or iceblocks may be appropriate for older children. Fluids with caffeine (tea, coffee) are avoided because these may act as diuretics and promote fluid loss. Fluids with a high sugar content (e.g. soft drinks and sports drinks) are not recommended as they can increase dehydration (The Royal Children's Hospital Melbourne [RCHM] 2018a). Infants who are breastfeeding should continue to be breastfed because human milk confers some degree of protection from infection (see Chapter 7). Fluids should not be forced, and children should not be awakened to take fluids unless advised by the treating medical practitioner. Forcing fluids may create the same difficulties as urging unwanted food (discussed later). Gentle persuasion with preferred beverages is usually successful. (See Chapter 23 for instructions on oral hydration.)

A nasogastric tube may be placed to provide enteral hydration using Hydralyte or Gastrolyte, or for infants expressed breast milk (EBM) or formula. Intravenous (IV) fluids may be required short term to re-establish hydration if the child is dehydrated and not drinking.

To assess their child's level of hydration (see Chapter 23), advise parents/carers/family to observe the frequency of voiding/wet nappies and to notify the nurse or practitioner if there is insufficient voiding.

NURSING CARE CONSIDERATIONS

Counting the number of wet nappies in a 24-hour period is a satisfactory method of assessing output in non-hospitalised infants and toddlers who are not acutely ill. Otherwise, urinary output should be approximately 0.5 to 1 mL/kg/hr in a child who weighs less than 30 kg and 30 mL/hr for children 30 kg and larger. The practitioner should be notified if the urine output is low.

Observe for Deterioration. Signs of clinical deterioration include increasing respiratory distress, increasing respiratory rate, increasing heart rate, worsening hypoxia, poor perfusion, reduced level of consciousness, and lethargy. Medical advice is to be sought if the child's condition deteriorates by escalating concerns to the medical/treating team.

Provide Nutrition

In the acute period of the illness, maintaining hydration with encouragement of fluids is of greatest importance.

Loss of appetite is characteristic of children with acute infections. In most cases children can be permitted to determine their own need for food. Urging foods on anorexic children may precipitate nausea and vomiting and cause an aversion to feeding that can extend into the convalescent period and beyond. Many children show no decrease in appetite, and others respond well to foods such as jelly, iceblocks, custards and yoghurts (see Feeding the Sick Child, Chapter 22.)

Provide Family Support and Home Care

Young children with respiratory tract infections may be irritable and difficult to comfort. Therefore, the family needs support, encouragement and practical suggestions concerning comfort measures and administration of medication.

In addition to antipyretics and nose drops, the child may require antibiotic therapy. Parents of children receiving oral antibiotics need to understand the importance of administering the medication regularly and continuing it for the prescribed length of time, regardless of whether the child appears ill. Parents are cautioned against giving the child any medications that are not approved by the practitioner or prescribed for another child. (See Chapter 22 for administration of medications and teaching parents.) Do not administer adult-prescribed/intended medications to children unless advised to do so by a practitioner.

UPPER RESPIRATORY TRACT INFECTIONS (URTI)

Acute Viral Nasopharyngitis

A number of viruses, usually rhinoviruses, RSV, adenovirus, influenza virus and parainfluenza virus, cause acute nasopharyngitis (the equivalent of the 'common cold').

Clinical Manifestations

Symptoms of nasopharyngitis are more severe in infants and children than in adults. Fever is common, especially in young children. Older children may have low-grade fevers, which appear early in the illness. In children 3 months to 3 years, fevers occur suddenly and are associated with irritability, restlessness, decreased appetite and fluid intake and decreased activity. Nasal inflammation may lead to obstruction of passages, producing open-mouth breathing. Vomiting and diarrhoea may also be present.

The initial symptoms in older children are dryness and irritation of nasal passages and the pharynx, followed by chilling sensations, muscular aches, an irritating nasal discharge and, occasionally, coughing or sneezing. Nasal inflammation may lead to obstruction. Continual wiping away of secretions causes skin irritation to nares.

The disease is self-limiting and symptoms last 10 to 14 days with a peak on day 2 to 3 of illness. Occasionally fever recurs and a child (particularly an infant) might experience otitis media (OM), usually early or after the initial phase of nasopharyngitis is past. Pneumonia is less frequent but may be observed in some infants.

Therapeutic Management

Children with nasopharyngitis are managed at home. There is no specific treatment, and effective vaccines are not available. Antipyretics may be prescribed for fever and discomfort. (See Chapter 22 for management of fever.) Fluids and rest are recommended.

Decongestants result in vasoconstriction of the nasal mucosa and are available orally and topically as nose drops, but there is little evidence to show efficacy in children. Spray bottles and bottles of nose drops should be used only for one child and only for one illness because they become easily contaminated with bacteria or viruses. Side effects can include nosebleeds, drying of the nasal membranes and rebound nasal congestion. To avoid rebound congestion, nose drops or sprays should not be administered for more than 3 days. Because these drugs affect all vascular beds, they should be given with caution to children with diabetes.

Over-the-counter cough suppressants and cough and cold medications are not routinely recommended, have not been proven to be effective in children, should not be given to children under 6 years of age and may pose health risks (Clarke 2017). A cough is normal when the airway is irritated, and suppressing it may result in adverse outcomes. Products containing pseudoephedrine, dextromethorphan or codeine or alcohol can cause confusion, hyperexcitability, dizziness, nausea and sedation. They should not be administered to young children and must be stored securely away.

Antihistamines are largely ineffective in the treatment of nasopharyngitis. These drugs have a weak atropine-like effect that dries secretions, but they can cause drowsiness or, paradoxically, have a stimulatory effect on children. There is no support for the usefulness of expectorants, and antibiotics are usually not indicated.

Prevention. Nasopharyngitis is so widespread in the general population that it is impossible to prevent. The best methods for preventing transmission of these viruses are frequent handwashing and avoiding touching one's eyes, nose and mouth. Children are more susceptible to colds because they have not yet developed resistance to many types of viruses. Very young infants are subject to relatively serious complications; therefore, they should be protected from exposure.

Nursing Care Management

A cold is often the parents' first introduction to an illness in their infants. Most discomfort of nasopharyngitis is related to the nasal obstruction, especially in small infants. Elevating the head of the bed or cot mattress assists with drainage of secretions. Saline nose drops and gentle suction with a bulb syringe, particularly before feeding, are useful.

Maintaining adequate fluid intake is essential during any infectious process. A child's appetite is often diminished for several days, so it is important to offer frequent small amounts of oral fluids to prevent dehydration.

Because nasopharyngitis is spread from secretions, the best means for prevention is avoiding contact with affected persons. This goal is difficult when large numbers of people are confined in a small area for a long time, such as day care centres and classrooms. Family members with a cold should try to 'keep it to themselves' by carefully disposing of tissues and not sharing towels, glasses or eating utensils. They should also cover the mouth and nose with tissues when coughing or sneezing and wash hands thoroughly after nose blowing or sneezing. The most frequent carriers of infection are the human hands, which deposit viruses on doorknobs, taps and other everyday objects. Children should wash their hands thoroughly or use hand sanitiser before touching their nose, mouth or eyes.

Family Support. Support and reassurance are important elements of care for families of young children with recurrent upper respiratory tract infections (URTIs). Because URTIs are so frequent in children less than 3 years of age, families may feel they are on an endless roller coaster of illness. Reassure them that frequent colds are a normal part of childhood, there are hundreds of viruses that cause them and that by 5 years of age most children will have developed immunity to many viruses. Parents who work outside the home should expect to take time off to care for ill children during the autumn and winter months.

Parents should know the signs of respiratory complications and should notify a health professional if any signs of complications appear, if signs of dehydration are present or if the child does not improve within 2 or 3 days (Box 26.3).

Acute Streptococcal Pharyngitis

Group A β-haemolytic streptococci (GABHS) infection of the upper airway (strep throat) is not in itself a serious disease, but affected children are at risk for serious sequelae: acute rheumatic fever, an inflammatory disease of the heart, joints and CNS (see Chapter 27), and acute glomerulonephritis, an acute kidney infection (see Chapter 24). Permanent damage can result from these sequelae, especially acute rheumatic fever. GABHS may also cause skin manifestations, including impetigo, contagiosa and carbuncle.

Scarlet fever may also occur as a result of a strain of group A streptococcus. The clinical manifestations of scarlet fever include pharyngitis and a characteristic erythematous sandpaper-like rash; otherwise scarlet fever shares the same clinical manifestations as those mentioned for GABHS, and treatment and sequelae are the same.

Clinical Manifestations

GABHS infection is generally a relatively brief illness that varies in severity from subclinical (no symptoms) to severe toxicity. The onset is often abrupt and characterised by pharyngitis, headache, fever and abdominal pain. The tonsils and pharynx may be inflamed and covered with exudate (Fig 26.1) which usually appears by the second day of illness. However, streptococcal infections should be suspected in children over the age of 2 years who have pharyngitis even if no exudate is present.

BOX 26.3 Early Evidence of Respiratory Complications

Parents are instructed to notify the health professional if they note any of the following:

- evidence of earache
- respirations faster than 50 to 60 beats/min and/or difficulty breathing
- persistent fever over 38.5°C
- listlessness and restlessness
- increasing irritability with or without fever
- persistent cough for 2 days or more
- wheezing
- non-blanching rash
- refusal to drink and decreased urine output.

Source: The Royal Children's Hospital Melbourne (RCHM). (2019). Viral illness fact sheet. Retrieved from https://www.rch.org.au/kidsinfo/fact_sheets/Viral_illnesses/

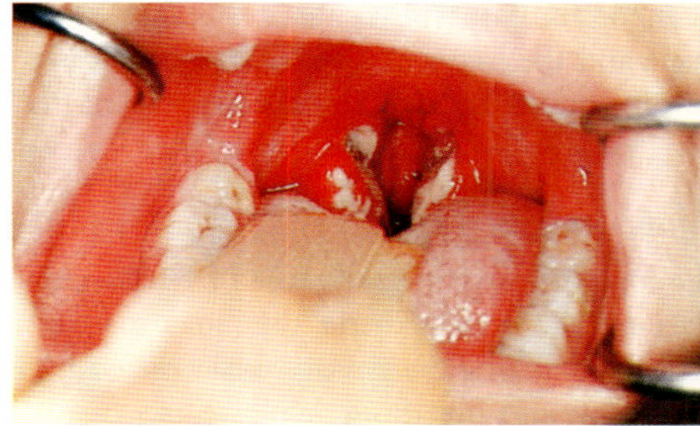

Fig 26.1 Tonsillitis and pharyngitis. (Source: Courtesy Dr. Edward L. Applebaum, Head, Department of Otolaryngology, University of Illinois Medical Center, Chicago.)

Anterior cervical lymphadenopathy usually occurs early, and the nodes are often tender. Pain can be relatively mild to severe enough to make swallowing difficult. Clinical manifestations usually subside in 3 to 5 days unless complicated by sinusitis or parapharyngeal, peritonsillar or retropharyngeal abscess. Non-suppurative complications may appear after the onset of GABHS—acute nephritis in about 10 days and rheumatic fever in an average of 18 days.

Children who are GABHS carriers may have a positive throat culture but often experience a coincidental viral illness. Although antibiotic administration is not indicated for most GABHS carriers, some conditions require antibiotic therapy (i.e. high-risk groups such as Aboriginal and Torres Strait Islander peoples, M ori and Pacific Islander peoples and people with a personal or family history of rheumatic fever or rheumatic heart disease) (RCHM 2019a). Transmission to others from a carrier is reportedly minimal.

Diagnostic Evaluation

Some children normally harbour streptococci in their throats; however, a positive culture or antigen test is not always conclusive evidence of active disease. Most streptococcal infections are short-term illnesses, and antibody (antistreptolysin O) responses appear later than symptoms and are useful only for retrospective diagnosis. Throat swabs are not recommended except in high-risk groups (RCHM 2019a) (Table 26.1).

Therapeutic Management

If streptococcal sore throat infection is present, particularly in high-risk groups, antibiotics may be prescribed to control the acute local manifestations and eliminate organisms that might remain to initiate rheumatic fever symptoms (Table 26.2).

Nursing Care Management

The nurse often obtains a throat swab for culture and instructs the parents about administering the antibiotic and analgesics as prescribed. Some children may prefer quiet activities during the acute phase of the illness, whereas others may limit activity only if the temperature is elevated. Cold or warm compresses to the neck may provide relief. In children old enough to cooperate, warm saline gargles offer some relief of throat discomfort. Pain may interfere with oral intake, and the child should not be forced to eat. Instead, encourage cool liquids or ice chips, which are usually more acceptable than solids.

Special emphasis is placed on correctly administering oral medication and completing the course of antibiotic therapy. (See Administration of Medication, and Compliance, Chapter 22.) If an antibiotic injection is required, it must be administered deep into a large muscle mass (e.g. the vastus lateralis or ventrogluteal muscle). Parents need to be aware of the residual tenderness. Local applications of heat are helpful in relieving discomfort. (For other atraumatic strategies to reduce

TABLE 26.1 Evaluation of Child with Suspected GABHS

When to Consider Checking for GABHS	When Suspicion of GABHS is Considered Low
Acute onset of sore throat	Children under 3 years
Exudate on pharynx	Children with symptoms more suggestive of viral cause (e.g. nasal discharge, conjunctivitis, hoarse, cough, diarrhoea, mouth ulcers, stomatitis)
Fever	
Enlarged anterior cervical lymph node	
History of exposure to GABHS	

GABHS, Group A β-haemolytic streptococcus.

TABLE 26.2 Paediatric Antibiotic Therapy for High-risk Groups with GABHS

Antibiotic therapy for suspected group A streptococcal pharyngitis is recommended only for high risk groups:

Antibiotic	Route	Dose	Duration
Phenoxymethylpenicillin	PO	< 20 kg: 250 mg two times daily ≥ 20 kg: 500 mg two times daily	10 days
Amoxicillin	PO	50 mg/kg once daily (max 1 g)*	10 days
POOR COMPLIANCE OR ORAL THERAPY NOT TOLERATED			
Benzathine Penicillin	IM	< 20 kg: 450 mg (600,000 U) ≥ 20 kg: 900 mg (1,200,000 U)	Single dose
HYPERSENSITIVITY TO PENICILLINS (EXCLUDE IMMEDIATE HYPERSENSITIVITY)			
Cefalexin	PO	25 mg/kg twice daily (max 1 g)	10 days
Anaphylaxis to beta-lactams			
Azithromycin	PO	Children: 12 mg/kg once daily (max 500 mg) Adults: 500 mg once daily	5 days

*Second line therapy for improved compliance

Source: The Royal Children's Hospital Melbourne (RCHM). (2019a). Sore Throat Clinical Practice Guidelines 2019. Retrieved from https://www.rch.org.au/clinicalguide/guideline_index/Sore_throat/

injection pain; see Administration of Medication: Intramuscular Administration, Chapter 22.) If the child continues to be febrile, has not improved within 24 to 48 hours or appears toxic, further evaluation by the healthcare provider is important.

Prevention. No immunisation is available for prevention of streptococcal disease. The organism is spread by close contact with affected persons—direct projection of large droplets or physical transfer of respiratory secretions containing the organism. Children with streptococcal infection are non-infectious to others 24 hours after initiation of antibiotic therapy. It is generally recommended that children not return to school or day care until they have been taking antibiotics for a full 24-hour period.

Nurses should remind children with a streptococcal throat infection to discard their toothbrush and replace it with a new one after they have been taking antibiotics for 24 hours. Orthodontic appliances must be washed thoroughly because they may harbour organisms. Parents are cautioned to prevent other household members, especially if immunocompromised, from having close contact with the sick child and avoid sharing towels, drinking or eating items.

Tonsillitis

The tonsils are masses of lymphoid tissue located in the pharyngeal cavity. The tonsils filter and protect the respiratory and alimentary tracts from invasion by pathogenic organisms. They also play a role in antibody formation. Although the size of tonsils varies, children generally have larger tonsils than adolescents or adults. This difference is thought to be a protective mechanism because young children are especially susceptible to URTIs.

Pathophysiology

Several pairs of tonsils are part of a mass of lymphoid tissue encircling the nasopharynx and oropharynx, known as Waldeyer's tonsillar ring (Fig 26.2). The palatine, or faucial, tonsils are located on either side of the oropharynx, behind and below the pillars of the fauces (opening from the mouth). A surface of the palatine tonsils is usually visible during oral examination. The **palatine tonsils** are those removed during tonsillectomy. The pharyngeal tonsils, also known as the **adenoids**, are located above the palatine tonsils on the posterior wall of the nasopharynx. Their proximity to the nares and eustachian tubes causes difficulties in instances of inflammation. The lingual tonsils are located at the base of the tongue. The tubal tonsils, found near the Posterior nasopharyngeal opening of the eustachian tubes, are not part of Waldeyer's tonsillar ring.

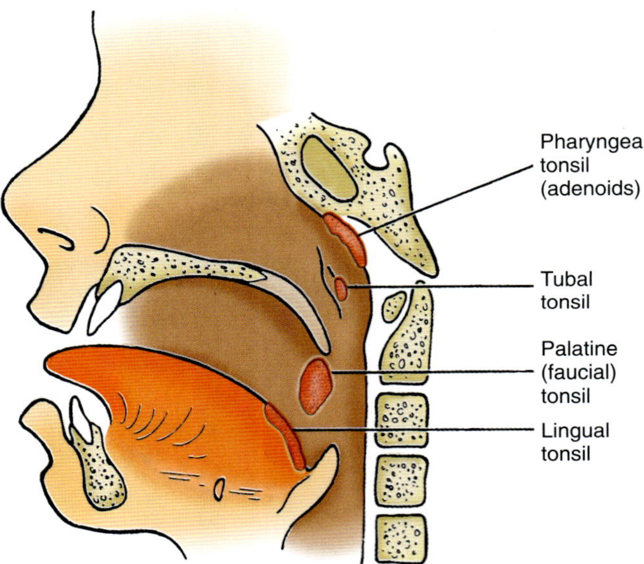

Fig 26.2 Location of various tonsillar masses.

Aetiology

Tonsillitis often occurs with pharyngitis. Because of the abundant lymphoid tissue and the frequency of URTIs, tonsillitis is a common cause of illness in young children. The causative agent may be viral or bacterial.

Clinical Manifestations

The manifestations of tonsillitis are caused by inflammation. As the palatine tonsils enlarge from oedema, they may meet in the midline (kissing tonsils), obstructing the passage of air or food. The child has difficulty swallowing and breathing. When enlargement of the adenoids occurs, the space behind the posterior nares may become blocked, making it difficult or impossible for air to pass from the nose to the throat. As a result, the child breathes through the mouth.

Chronic enlargement of the tonsils and adenoids may result in obstruction of breathing during sleep.

If mouth breathing is continuous, the mucous membranes of the oropharynx become dry and irritated. There may be an offensive mouth odour and impaired senses of taste and smell. Because air cannot be trapped for proper speech sounds, the voice has a nasal and muffled quality. A persistent cough is also common. Because of the proximity of the adenoids to the eustachian tubes, this passageway is frequently blocked by swollen adenoids, interfering with normal drainage and frequently resulting in OM or difficulty hearing.

Therapeutic Management

Medical Treatment. Because the illness is self-limiting, treatment of viral pharyngitis is symptomatic. Throat cultures positive for GABHS infection require antibiotic treatment. It is important to differentiate between viral and streptococcal infection in febrile, exudative tonsillitis. Because the majority of infections are of viral origin, early rapid tests can eliminate unnecessary antibiotic administration.

Surgical Treatment. Surgical treatment of chronic tonsillitis is controversial. Except in documented cases of recurrent, frequent streptococcal infection or a history of development of a peritonsillar abscess, tonsillectomy is not indicated in the child who has recurrent pharyngitis.

Tonsillectomy (surgical removal of the palatine tonsils) may be indicated for massive hypertrophy that results in difficulty breathing or eating. Indications include chronic and recurrent tonsillitis, enlargement causing OSA and snoring, chronic cryptic tonsillitis, unusual enlargement or appearance (i.e. tumour) (The Sydney Children's Hospital Network [SCHN] 2017). One episode of tonsillitis consists of a sore throat plus at least one of the following: temperature greater than 38.5°C, cervical adenopathy (> 2 cm or tender nodes), exudate on the tonsils or positive culture for GABHS.

Adenoidectomy (the surgical removal of the adenoids) is recommended for children who have hypertrophied adenoids that obstruct nasal breathing causing OSA and snoring.

For some children the effectiveness of tonsillectomy or adenoidectomy is modest and may not justify the risk of surgery. In practice, most providers rely on individualised decision-making and do not subscribe to an absolute set of eligibility criteria for these surgical procedures.

Contraindications to either tonsillectomy or adenoidectomy are: (1) cleft palate because both tonsils help minimise escape of air during speech; (2) acute infections at the time of surgery because the locally inflamed tissues increase the risk of bleeding; and (3) uncontrolled systemic diseases or blood dyscrasias.

Generally, removal of the tonsils should not occur until after 3 or 4 years of age because of the problem of excessive blood loss in young children and the possibility of regrowth or hypertrophy of lymphoid tissue. The tubal and lingual tonsils often enlarge to compensate for the lost lymphoid tissue, resulting in continued pharyngeal and eustachian tube obstruction.

Nursing Care Management

Nursing care of the child with tonsillitis involves providing comfort and minimising activities or interventions that precipitate bleeding. A normal diet is generally preferred, as tolerated by the child (SCHN 2016). Analgesic-antipyretic drugs such as paracetamol are useful to promote comfort. Often opioids are needed to reduce pain for the child to drink, such as oxycodone (Endone). Prescriptions for these medications may be given on discharge. Analgesics should be given routinely every 4 to 6 hours while symptoms persist, usually for the first 4 to 5 days and as symptomatic. Postoperatively, codeine and Painstop are not to be used (SCHN 2017).

If surgery is needed, the child requires the same psychological preparation and physical care as for any procedure. (See Chapter 22.) The following discussion focuses on specific nursing care for tonsillectomy and adenoidectomy (T&A), although both procedures may not be performed.

The nurse takes a complete history, with special notation of any bleeding tendencies because the operative site is highly vascular. Baseline vital signs are important for postoperative monitoring and observation. Signs of any URTI are noted and reported, and bleeding and clotting times may be obtained, if history indicates/warrants this. During physical assessment the presence of any loose teeth is noted. (See Surgical Procedures, Chapter 22.)

After the surgery, until they are fully awake, children are positioned to facilitate drainage of secretions. Suctioning is performed carefully to avoid trauma to the oropharynx. When alert, children may prefer sitting up. They are discouraged from coughing frequently, clearing their throat, blowing their nose or any activities that could aggravate the operative site.

Some secretions, particularly dried blood from surgery, are common. Inspect all secretions and vomitus for evidence of fresh bleeding (some blood-tinged mucus is expected). Dark brown (old) blood is usually present in the emesis, as well as in the nose and between the teeth. If parents are not prepared for this, they may be frightened at a time when they need to be calm and reassuring.

The throat is very sore after surgery. Most children experience moderate pain after a T&A and need pain medication at regular intervals for at least the first 24 to 48 hours. Liquid analgesics are given as tolerated. If not tolerated, analgesics may need to be given intravenously. Antiemetics such as ondansetron (Zofran) may be administered postoperatively.

Food and fluid are recommended when children are able to swallow them and are alert with no signs of haemorrhage. Cool water, crushed ice, ice blocks or diluted fruit juice is given; fluids with a red or brown colour are generally avoided to distinguish fresh or old blood in emesis from the ingested liquid. Straws should be avoided because they may damage the surgical site and cause subsequent bleeding. Citrus juice may cause discomfort and is usually poorly tolerated. Children are encouraged to eat all foods as tolerated: cool, warm, soft and firm.

NURSING CARE CONSIDERATIONS

The most obvious early sign of bleeding is the child's continuous swallowing of the trickling blood. Closely observe the child, noting the frequency of swallowing. If continuous bleeding is suspected, notify the surgeon immediately.

Postoperative haemorrhage is unusual but can occur. The nurse observes the throat directly for evidence of bleeding, using a good source of light and, if necessary, carefully inserting a tongue depressor. Other signs of haemorrhage are tachycardia, pallor, frequent clearing of the throat or swallowing by a younger child, and vomiting of bright red blood. Restlessness, an indication of haemorrhage, may be difficult to differentiate from general discomfort after surgery. Decreasing blood pressure is a much later sign of shock. A cream-coloured membrane is often visible on the tonsillar bed postoperatively for 5 to 10 days post-surgery; reassure parents this is an expected finding.

Surgery may be required to cauterise or ligate a bleeding vessel. Airway obstruction may also occur as a result of oedema or accumulated secretions and is indicated by signs of respiratory distress, such as stridor, drooling, restlessness, agitation, increasing respiratory rate and progressive cyanosis. Suction equipment and oxygen should be available after tonsillectomy.

Family Support and Home Care. Discharge instructions include: (1) avoiding foods that are irritating or highly seasoned; (2) avoiding the use of gargles or vigorous toothbrushing; (3) discouraging the child from coughing or clearing the throat or putting objects in the mouth; (4) using analgesics and opioids for pain as prescribed; and (5) limiting activity to decrease the potential for bleeding (i.e. quieter activities if possible). Haemorrhage may occur up to 10 days after surgery as a result of tissue sloughing from the healing process. Any sign of bleeding warrants immediate medical attention. Objectionable mouth odour and slight ear pain with a low-grade fever are common for a few days postoperatively. However, persistent severe earache, fever or cough requires medical evaluation. Most children are ready to resume normal activity within 1 to 2 weeks after the operation.

Most children are admitted to a same-day surgery or ambulatory surgery unit and discharged home after a recovery period. Rural and remote areas may require an overnight admission due to distance from medical assistance if postoperative complications occur. T&A often represents the first hospitalisation experience for the child and family. Because the surgery is usually an elective procedure, there is ample opportunity to prepare both children and parents for this event. Both need reassurance about what to expect at the time of admission, before and after surgery, and at discharge. Children are informed about postoperative discomfort and reassured that they will be able to talk. Some children believe the procedure will immediately 'make the throat all better' and are dismayed to find that it still hurts after the surgery.

Glandular Fever (Infectious Mononucleosis)

Glandular fever is an acute, self-limiting infectious disease that is common among young people under 25 years old. Symptoms include fever, exudative pharyngitis with petechiae, lymphadenopathy, hepatosplenomegaly and an increase in atypical lymphocytes. The course is usually mild but occasionally can be severe or accompanied by serious complications (rare).

Aetiology and Pathophysiology

The Epstein-Barr virus (EBV) is the principal cause of glandular fever. It appears in both sporadic and epidemic forms, but the sporadic cases are more common. The virus is believed to be transmitted by direct contact with oral secretions (close personal contact is needed to transmit the virus), blood transfusion or transplantation. It is mildly contagious, and the period of communicability is unknown. The incubation period after exposure is estimated to be 1 to 2 months (Monzr & Al Maliki 2020).

Clinical Manifestations

Symptoms of glandular fever can appear 10 days to 6 weeks after exposure and may be acute or insidious. The common presenting symptoms vary greatly in type, severity and duration. The characteristics of the disease are malaise, sore throat and fever with generalised lymphadenopathy and splenomegaly that may persist for several months. Often the symptoms appear insidiously with fatigue, lack of energy and sore throat. The child's chief complaint is difficulty in maintaining the usual level of activity. This is often attributed to lack of sleep or a URTI. In many instances the manifestations never arouse enough concern to bring the affected individual to medical attention. The clinical manifestations of glandular fever are usually less severe (often subclinical or unapparent), and the recovery phase is shorter in younger children than in older children and young adults. Many young children do not develop all the expected clinical and laboratory findings. Often an insidious symptom is the only or the presenting symptom.

A skin rash that involves a discrete macular eruption is present in some cases and is often associated with the administration of ampicillin or amoxicillin (Jenson 2016). Other symptoms include headache, epistaxis and a severe sore throat. The tonsils may be enlarged, reddened and sometimes covered with a diphtheria-like membrane. In some cases airway compromise may occur with tonsillar swelling. In about half the cases the spleen is enlarged to 2 to 3 cm below the costal margin (Jenson 2016). The extensive mononuclear infiltration produces symptoms related to any body tissue, and the clinical picture can resemble that of many conditions, including neurological manifestations and cardiac involvement.

Diagnostic Evaluation

The diagnosis is established on the basis of clinical manifestations, increase in atypical leucocytes in a peripheral blood smear and a positive monospot (EBV) test. Differential diagnosis depends on the clinical symptoms present. For example, the pharyngitis may simulate symptoms of diphtheria and streptococcal pharyngitis. Lymphadenopathy, fever, malaise, CNS manifestations and skin eruptions may be similar to symptoms seen in a variety of conditions. The leucocyte count may be normal or low, but usually lymphocytic leucocytosis develops.

The spot test (monospot) is a slide test of high specificity for the diagnosis of glandular fever. It is rapid, sensitive, inexpensive and easy to perform, and it has the advantage that it can detect significant agglutinins at lower levels, thus permitting earlier diagnosis. If the blood agglutinates, forming fragments or clumps, the test is positive for the infection.

Therapeutic Management

No specific treatment exists for glandular fever. A mild analgesic is usually sufficient to relieve the bothersome symptoms of headache, fever and malaise. Rest is encouraged for fatigue but is not imposed for any specified time. Affected children and adolescents should regulate activities according to their own tolerance unless complicating factors are present. If the spleen is enlarged, contact and collision sports are discouraged until it resolves (Monzr & Malik 2020).

A short course of corticosteroids may assist in decreasing some of the complications (e.g. airway obstruction) of the illness. Administration of ampicillin or amoxicillin frequently precipitates a maculopapular rash in affected persons (80% of cases); therefore, their use may be contraindicated. Gargles, warm drinks, analgesic or anaesthetic lozenges, or analgesics, including opioids, can relieve a sore throat.

Prognosis. The course of glandular fever is self-limiting and usually uncomplicated. Contrary to popular belief, glandular fever is not necessarily a difficult, prolonged or disabling disease and the prognosis is generally good. Acute symptoms usually disappear within 7 to 10 days, and the persistent fatigue subsides within 2 to 4 weeks. A number of affected children or adolescents may need to restrict activities for 2 to 3 months; the disease rarely extends for longer periods. The child is encouraged to maintain limited activities to prevent deconditioning.

Complications are uncommon but can be serious and require appropriate management. Neurological complications occur in some outbreaks and vary in severity and outcome. These include seizures, ataxia, aseptic meningitis, encephalitis, optic neuritis, cranial nerve palsies and perceptual distortions of shapes, spatial relationships and sizes. Other complications include pneumonitis, orchitis, myocarditis, transverse myelitis, haemolytic anaemia, agranulocytosis, thrombocytopenia, haemophagocytic lymphohistiocytosis and ruptured spleen. Some evidence indicates a depressed cellular immune reactivity during the course of the disease and for some time afterward. Thus it is best to avoid live vaccines until several months after recovery. The Epstein-Barr virus can replicate in B-lymphocytes, resulting in T-lymphocyte growth, and lymphomas can occur.

Nursing Care Management

Direct nursing responsibilities towards providing comfort measures to relieve the symptoms and helping affected children, adolescents and their families determine appropriate activities for the stage of the disease and their interests. Airway assessment for impending obstruction during the acute phase of the illness is imperative. The adolescent with glandular fever may not be able to swallow secretions and may be in considerable pain. The child or adolescent is encouraged to increase clear fluid intake and decrease solid foods that may exacerbate the pain. In addition, the nurse should encourage the affected individual to curtail activities that are strenuous until splenomegaly is resolved. Pain medications in elixir form such as paracetamol and ibuprofen may be required during the acute phase so the adolescent can swallow liquids. Make every effort to prevent a secondary infection by counselling the adolescent to limit exposure to persons outside the family, especially during the acute phase of illness.

NURSING CARE CONSIDERATIONS

Advise the family to seek medical evaluation of the child or adolescent if

- breathing becomes difficult
- severe abdominal pain develops
- sore throat pain is so severe that the child is unable to eat or drink
- respiratory stridor is observed.

Influenza

Influenza (the 'flu') is caused by the orthomyxoviruses and classified into three distinct groups: types A and B, which cause epidemic disease (and are included in the vaccine), and type C, which causes milder illness and is not included in the vaccine. The viruses undergo significant changes from time to time. Major changes that occur at intervals of usually 5 to 10 years are called **antigenic shift**; minor variations within the same subtypes, **antigenic drift**, occur almost annually. Consequently, antigenic drift can alter the virus sufficiently to result in susceptibility of individuals to a type for which they were previously immunised or infected.

The disease is spread from one individual to another by direct contact (large-droplet infection) usually occurring during talking, sneezing or coughing or by articles recently contaminated by nasopharyngeal secretions. There is no predilection for a specific age group, but attack rates are highest in young children who have not had previous contact with a strain, as well as patients with chronic medical conditions (e.g. diabetes, asthma) and pregnant women. It is frequently most severe in infants and older adults. During epidemics, infection among school-age children is believed to be a major source of transmission in a community. Influenza is more common during the winter months.

The disease has a 1- to 4-day incubation period (average of 2 days), and affected persons are most infectious for 24 hours before and 5 to 7 days after the onset of symptoms (ATAGI 2018). The virus has a peculiar affinity for epithelial cells of the respiratory tract mucosa, where it destroys ciliated epithelium with metaplastic hyperplasia of the tracheal and bronchial epithelium with associated oedema. The alveoli may also become distended with a hyaline-like material. The viruses can be isolated from nasopharyngeal secretions early after the onset of infection, and serological tests identify the type by complement fixation or the subgroups by haemagglutination inhibition. Outbreaks in the community can last many weeks.

H1N1 (swine flu) is a subtype of influenza type A. In 2009 a pandemic of H1N1 caused significant morbidity and mortality. In Australia, from May 2009 to November 2010 there were 44,403 confirmed cases with 213 deaths (ATAGI, 2018). A **pandemic** is defined by the World Health Organization (WHO) as the spread of a new disease to which the population has little or no immunity and that spreads rapidly from human to human. The H1N1 vaccine has been included in the seasonal influenza vaccination since the 2011–2012 season.

Clinical Manifestations

The manifestations of influenza may be subclinical, mild, moderate or severe. In most cases, there is a dry cough and a tendency towards hoarseness. A sudden onset of fever and chills is accompanied by flushed face, photophobia, myalgia, sore throat, headaches, hyperesthesia and sometimes prostration. Children may have vomiting or diarrhoea. Subglottal croup is common, especially in infants. The symptoms last 4 or 5 days. Complications include severe viral pneumonia (often haemorrhagic), febrile seizures, encephalitis, encephalopathy, dehydration and secondary bacterial infections, such as myocarditis, OM, sinusitis or pneumonia. Diagnosis is confirmed by analysing nasopharyngeal secretions for viral culture or rapid detection testing. Influenza A and B can be rapidly detected by direct fluorescent antibody and indirect immunofluorescent antibody staining.

Therapeutic Management

Uncomplicated influenza in children usually requires only symptomatic treatment: paracetamol or ibuprofen for fever and sufficient fluids to maintain hydration. Oseltamivir, zanamivir and peramivir are recommended to treat influenza for patients at high risk of complications from the flu (RCHM 2019b). A small number of influenza strains are resistant to oseltamivir (Tamiflu).

Oseltamivir (Tamiflu), usually first-line therapy, is a neuroaminidase inhibitor that may be administered orally for 5 days to decrease the flu symptoms. The medication can be used for infants and children of any age and is effective for types A and B influenza (RCHM 2019b). As with other antiviral drugs, for best results the medication should be started within 2 days of the onset of symptoms. Children should not receive aspirin because of its possible link with Reye syndrome.

Prevention. The influenza vaccine is recommended annually for everybody greater than 6 months of age (ATAGI 2020). It is administered yearly because different strains of influenza are used each year in the manufacture of the vaccine. It is safe and effective provided the antigens in the vaccine correlate with the circulating influenza viruses. (See Immunisations, Chapter 6.)

Nursing Care Management

Nursing care is the same as for any child with a URTI, including helping the family implement measures to relieve symptoms. Prolonged fever or appearance of fever during early convalescence is a sign of secondary bacterial infection and should be reported to the practitioner for antibiotic therapy. In addition to the measures mentioned previously, nursing care of the child with influenza includes educating the parents regarding the prevention of the spread of the disease to other individuals, especially those who are at higher risk for complications, and educating the parents about the use of antiviral medications.

Coronavirus (COVID-19)

COVID-19 (SARS-CoV-2) is a coronavirus belonging to the β-coronavirus cluster (Sun et al 2020). Coronaviruses cause a wide range of illness, ranging from the common cold to severe, fatal illness. Three coronaviruses causing severe illness in humans have emerged in the past 20 years: the virus causing SARS, which emerged in China in 2002; the virus causing Middle East respiratory syndrome (MERS), which emerged in the Arabian peninsula in 2012; and the virus causing COVID-19 (Ramussen & Thompson 2020). The World Health Organization declared coronavirus disease 2019 (COVID-19), the disease caused by SARS-CoV-2, a pandemic health emergency in 2020 (WHO 2020).

Common manifestations of COVID-19 include fever, dry cough, and fatigue accompanied by other respiratory symptoms such as nasal congestion and runny nose. Gastrointestinal symptoms include nausea, vomiting and diarrhoea. In a systematic review of paediatric cases of COVID-19, Castagnoli and colleagues (2020) found most children and adolescents who were infected by COVID-19 (i.e. tested positive by nasopharyngeal swab) presented with mild symptoms, had a good prognosis and recovered within 1 to 2 weeks after disease onset. Cases of paediatric death from COVID-19 were not reported in the 0 to 9 years age range (Castagnoli et al 2020).

Transmission of COVID-19 is thought to be primarily through respiratory droplets formed when a person with an infection coughs or sneezes, which can be inhaled by contacts within close range (within 1.5 metres), who then become infected. The median incubation period is 5 days (range 2 to 14 days). Children mainly acquire SARS-CoV-2 infection from their family members but seem to experience less severe COVID-19 than adults (Rasmussen & Thompson 2020). Despite the low frequency of illness and death from COVID-19 in children, it is important to remain vigilant about infection in children as they could be infected but asymptomatic, suggesting transmission to others could be possible (Sun et al 2020).

Treatment for COVID-19 in children is supportive (see Nursing Care of the Child with a Respiratory Tract Infection, Acute Respiratory Distress Syndrome and Acute Lung Injury in this chapter). In a pandemic, the best way to deal with the COVID-19 is to control the sources of infection. Strategies include: early diagnoses, reporting, isolation and supportive treatments; timely release of epidemic information; and maintenance of social orders. In Australia and New Zealand this has involved staged lockdowns. For individuals, protective measures, including improving personal hygiene, wearing medical masks, adequate rest and keeping rooms well ventilated can effectively prevent COVID-19 (Sun et al 2020). Nurses must be aware of and adhere to COVID-19 policies and protocols and COVID-19 safety plans within their workplace.

Vaccines for COVID-19 are not approved for children in Australia or New Zealand at the time of writing.

Otitis Media

Otitis media (OM) is the presence of fluid in the middle ear along with acute signs of illness and symptoms of middle ear inflammation (Venekamp et al 2017). It is one of the most prevalent illnesses of early childhood. Its incidence is highest in the winter months. Many cases of bacterial OM are preceded by a viral respiratory tract infection. The two viruses most likely to precipitate OM are RSV and influenza. Most episodes of *acute otitis media* (AOM) occur in the first 24 months of life, but the incidence decreases with age, except for a small increase at age 5 or 6 years when children enter school. OM occurs infrequently in children older than 7 years of age. Children who have siblings or parents with a history of chronic OM have a higher incidence of OM. Out-of-home day care is a significant risk factor for OM.

Children living in households with many members are more likely to have OM than those living with fewer persons. Passive smoking increases the risk of persistent middle ear effusion by enhancing attachment of the pathogens that cause otitis to the respiratory epithelium in the middle ear space, prolonging the inflammatory response and impeding drainage through the eustachian tube (Kerschner & Preciado 2016). Family socioeconomic status is another important risk factor for the occurrence of OM (Kerschner & Preciado 2016).

A relationship has been observed between the incidence of OM and infant feeding methods. Infants fed breast milk have a lower incidence of OM compared with formula-fed infants. Breastfeeding may protect infants against respiratory viruses and allergy because it contains secretory immunoglobulin A, which limits the exposure of the eustachian tube and middle ear mucosa to microbial pathogens and foreign proteins. Reflux of milk up the eustachian tubes is less likely in breastfed infants because of the semivertical positioning during breastfeeding compared with bottle-feeding. Breastfeeding should be encouraged for at least 6 months (Korvel-Hanquist et al 2017).

Aetiology

AOM is frequently caused by *Streptococcus pneumoniae*, *H. influenzae* and *Moraxella catarrhalis*. The two viruses most likely to precipitate OM are RSV and influenza, although the adenoviruses, human metapneumoviruses and picornaviruses (rhinovirus and enterovirus) also cause a significant number of URTIs and OM. The aetiology of the non-infectious type is unknown, although it is frequently the result of blocked eustachian tubes from the oedema of URTIs, allergic rhinitis or hypertrophic adenoids. *Chronic OM* is frequently an extension of an acute episode.

Pathophysiology

OM is primarily a result of a dysfunctioning eustachian tube. The eustachian tube is part of a contiguous system composed of the nares, nasopharynx, eustachian tube, middle ear, and mastoid antrum and air cells. Mechanical or functional obstruction of the eustachian tube causes accumulation of secretions in the middle ear. Infection or allergy can cause intrinsic (within) obstruction. Extrinsic (outside) obstruction is usually a result of enlarged adenoids or nasopharyngeal tumours. Eustachian tube obstruction results in negative middle ear pressure and, if persistent, produces a transudative middle ear effusion. Sustained negative pressure and impaired ciliary transport within the tube inhibit drainage. When the passage is not totally obstructed, contamination of the middle ear can take place by reflux, aspiration or insufflation during crying, sneezing, nose blowing and swallowing when the nose is obstructed. Several factors predispose infants and young children to development of OM (Box 26.4 and Fig 26.3).

Complications. The consequences of prolonged middle ear disorders can be either functional or structural. The principal functional

BOX 26.4 Factors Predisposing Children to Development of Otitis Media

- The eustachian tubes are short, wide and straight and lie in a relatively horizontal plane (see Fig 26.3).
- The cartilage lining is undeveloped, making the tubes more distensible and therefore more likely to open inappropriately.
- The normally abundant pharyngeal lymphoid tissue readily obstructs the eustachian tube openings in the nasopharynx.
- Immature humoral defence mechanisms increase the risk of infection.
- The usual lying-down position of infants favours the pooling of fluid, such as formula or exudate, in the pharyngeal cavity.

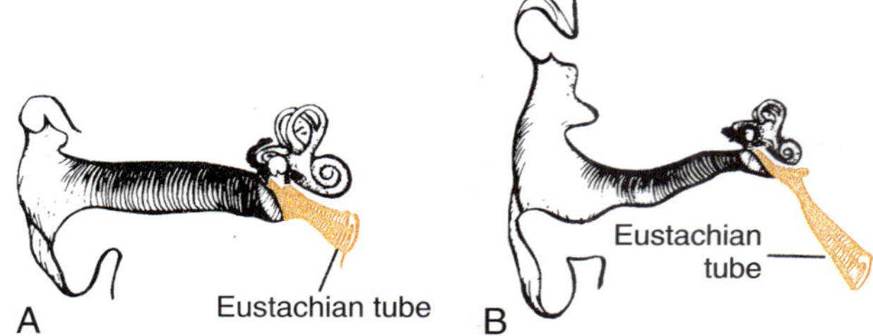

Fig 26.3 Comparison of anatomic position of eustachian tube in a child (**A**) and an adult (**B**). Eustachian tube is shorter, wider, straighter and more horizontal in a child than in an adult.

consequence is hearing loss, although loss in most children is conductive in nature and mild in severity. The causes of hearing loss are negative middle ear pressure, effusion in the middle ear, involvement of the eighth cranial nerve and structural damage to the tympanic membrane. However, the most feared consequence of hearing loss is its adverse effect on development of speech, language and cognition. Children who have prolonged periods of middle ear effusion have poorer performance on speech and language tests than those who have few or no middle ear diseases.

Structural complications or sequelae involve primarily the tympanic membrane. Tympanic membrane retraction or retraction pockets occur in areas of low tensile strength or atrophic segments of the drum head when continued negative middle ear pressure draws the tympanic membrane inward. This retraction may result in impaired sound transmission, perforation of the thinned-out areas or infection in the pockets and, later, cholesteatoma (abnormal skin growth).

Tympanosclerosis (eardrum scarring) is the deposition of hyaline material into the fibrous layer of the tympanic membrane. It often occurs in children with inflammatory middle ear disease or those with repeated tympanoplasty tube placement. Eardrum perforation is a common complication in AOM and often accompanies chronic disease. Persistent perforation is a complication of tympanostomy tube placement. Surgery is required to close some perforations.

Adhesive OM (glue ear) is a thickening of the mucous membrane by proliferation of fibrous tissue that can cause fixation of the ossicles with a resultant hearing loss. Chronic suppurative OM, an inflammation of the middle ear and mastoid, is evidenced by perforation and discharge (otorrhea) for up to 6 weeks' duration. Labyrinthitis, infection of the inner ear, and mastoiditis, infection of the mastoid sinus, are rare since the advent of antibiotic therapy. Meningitis and other suppurative intracranial conditions are possible complications of extension of infection from the middle ear or mastoid. However, these complications occur infrequently when adequate antibiotic therapy is implemented. Vestibular dysfunction or labyrinthitis may result in impaired balance and motor problems.

Cholesteatoma is the least common but most potentially dangerous sequela of OME. A cholesteatoma forms when the keratinising, stratified, squamous epithelial cell lining desquamates to form scales that accumulate within the middle ear space. As it enlarges, the cholesteatoma erodes all structures it encounters, especially bone, destroying the ossicles and gaining entry to the inner ear and meninges. Clinical signs are a foul-smelling, greyish-yellow discharge; sometimes pain; and permanent, progressive hearing loss. Treatment is surgical excision of the entire cholesteatoma.

Clinical Manifestations

As purulent fluid accumulates in the small space of the middle ear chamber, pain results from the pressure on surrounding structures. Infants become irritable and can indicate their discomfort by holding or pulling at their ears and rolling their head from side to side. Young children usually verbally complain of the pain. A temperature as high as 40°C is common, and postauricular and cervical lymph glands may be enlarged. Rhinorrhoea, vomiting, diarrhoea and signs of concurrent respiratory tract or pharyngeal infection may also be present. Loss of appetite typically occurs, and sucking or chewing tends to aggravate the pain. In children with OME, exudate accumulates and pressure increases, with the potential for tympanic membrane rupture. As a result of rupture, there is immediate relief of pain, a gradual decrease in temperature and the presence of purulent discharge in the external auditory canal.

Severe pain or fever is usually absent in OME, and the child may not appear ill. Instead there is a feeling of 'fullness' in the ear, a popping sensation during swallowing and a feeling of 'motion' in the ear if air is present above the level of fluid. Because chronic serous OM is the most frequent cause of conductive hearing loss in young children, audiometry may reveal deficient hearing.

Diagnostic Evaluation

Careful assessment of tympanic membrane mobility with a pneumatic otoscope is essential to differentiate AOM from OME (Box 26.5) (Kerschner & Preciado 2016). If an accumulation of cerumen prevents adequate visualisation of the tympanic membrane, the cerumen should be removed before inspection of the membrane. A diagnosis of AOM is made with moderate to severe bulging of the tympanic membrane, acute onset of ear drainage not due to acute otitis externa, mild bulging of the tympanic membrane with onset of pain occurring less than 48 hours and intense erythema of the tympanic membrane (Kerschner & Preciado 2016). An immobile tympanic membrane or an orange-coloured membrane indicates OME. In OME these symptoms may be absent, and other non-specific symptoms such as rhinitis, cough or diarrhoea are often present.

Several tests provide an assessment of mobility of the tympanic membrane. Chapter 4 discusses otoscopy and tympanometry. Acoustic reflectometry measures the level of sound transmitted and reflected from the middle ear to a microphone located in a probe tip placed against the ear canal opening and directed towards the tympanic membrane. The information provides a measure of canal length and presence of effusion. The greater the cancellation of transmitted sound by reflected sound, the greater the probability of middle ear effusion.

Therapeutic Management: Acute Otitis Media

Treatment for AOM is one of the most common reasons for antibiotic use in the ambulatory setting. However, recent concerns about drug-resistant strains have led infectious disease authorities to recommend careful and judicious use of antibiotics for treatment of this illness. The use of antibiotics should be avoided and in most cases AOM resolves spontaneously (RCHM 2018b).

Supportive care or symptomatic treatment of AOM includes treating the fever and pain. For fever or discomfort associated with OM, analgesic-antipyretic drugs such as paracetamol or ibuprofen (ibuprofen only

BOX 26.5 Standard Terminology for Otitis Media

Acute otitis media (AOM)—An inflammation of the middle ear space with a rapid onset of the signs and symptoms of acute infection—namely, fever and otalgia (ear pain)

Otitis media (OM)—An inflammation of the middle ear without reference to aetiology or pathogenesis

Otitis media with effusion (OME)—Fluid in the middle ear space without symptoms of acute infection

if over 6 months of age) may be given. Topical pain relief is recommended by external application of heat or cold. Antibiotic ear drops have no value in treating AOM. Decongestants and antihistamines are not recommended for children with ear infections (RCHM 2018b).

Myringotomy, a surgical incision of the eardrum, may be necessary to alleviate the severe pain of AOM. A myringotomy is also performed to drain infected middle ear fluid in the presence of complications (e.g. mastoiditis, labyrinthitis or facial paralysis) or to allow purulent middle ear fluid to drain into the ear canal for culture. A minimally invasive laser-assisted myringotomy procedure may be performed in outpatient settings. Rural areas do not currently have access to laser-assisted myringotomy. These procedures should only be performed by ear, nose and throat (ENT) specialists.

Therapeutic Management: Recurrent Acute Otitis Media

Therapy for recurrent AOM includes surgery. Chemoprophylaxis is no longer recommended because of the cost of therapy, potential adverse effects of therapy (e.g. allergic reaction, gastrointestinal [GI] upset) and most importantly contribution to bacterial resistance (Kerschner & Preciado 2016). Tympanostomy tube placement may be indicated with chronic OM (three episodes in 6 months or four episodes in 1 year, with one episode during the preceding 6 months) (Kerschner & Preciado 2016). Tympanostomy tubes are pressure equalisation devices (grommets) that facilitate drainage and ventilation of the middle ear.

Therapeutic Management: Otitis Media with Effusion (OME)

In some children, residual middle ear effusions remain after episodes of AOM. Management options for OM with residual effusion include observation, antibiotics alone or a combination of antibiotic and corticosteroid therapy. Antibiotics are not routinely required for treatment of OME (RCHM 2018b). Hearing testing is performed in children who have OME for 3 months or more.

Some children have fluid that persists in the middle ear for weeks or months. OME is frequently associated with mild to moderate hearing impairment. The major goal of therapy is to establish and maintain an aerated middle ear that is free of fluid with a normal mucosa and ultimately to achieve normal hearing.

Placement of grommets is recommended after a total of 3 to 6 months of bilateral effusion with a bilateral hearing deficit (Kerschner & Preciado 2016). This therapy allows for mechanical drainage of the fluid, which promotes healing of the membrane and prevents scar formation and loss of elasticity. The primary objective is to allow the eustachian tube a period of recovery while the surgically placed tube performs its functions. The surgery is relatively benign; however, sometimes the tubes become plugged, and they often require reinsertion. Complications of repeated or long-term tube placement are tympanosclerosis, localised or diffuse atrophy of the membrane, persistent perforation or, rarely, cholesteatoma. Myringotomy with or without insertion of PE tubes should *not* be performed for initial management of OME but may be recommended for children who have recurrent episodes of OME with a long cumulative duration. A recent meta-analysis concluded that tympanostomy tubes had a significant improvement in hearing and a decrease in the incidence of AOM compared with watchful waiting (Steele et al 2017).

Tonsillectomy, either alone or with adenoidectomy, is not considered an effective treatment of OME. Steroids are not recommended for treatment of OME in children of any age.

Prevention

Routine immunisation with the pneumococcal vaccine has reduced the incidence of AOM in some infants and children, especially those with frequent episodes of AOM (ATAGI 2018).

Parents are encouraged to reduce risk factors for AOM by breastfeeding infants for at least the first 6 months of life, avoiding propping the formula bottle, decreasing or discontinuing pacifier use after 6 months, and preventing exposure to tobacco smoke (Kerschner & Preciado 2016).

Prognosis

Most cases of OM resolve without any residual effects. However, varying degrees of hearing loss can occur. Although conductive hearing loss is most often associated with OM, sensorineural hearing loss may also be present, especially in severe forms of chronic or recurrent OM because of the passage of toxic products from fluids into the cochlea through the tympanic membrane. The longer the fluid is present, the greater the sensorineural hearing loss. Children who are prone to OM should be referred to a paediatric otolaryngologist and possibly a paediatric allergist for identification and treatment of the cause of their eustachian tube dysfunction. They should also be referred to a speech and language pathologist for primary prevention counselling. In addition, the child should ideally be monitored by an audiologist to evaluate the adequacy of hearing.

Large rural centres may have paediatricians who specialise in allergy testing; however, most children will need referral to metropolitan facilities.

Nursing Care Management

Nursing objectives for the child with AOM include relieving pain, facilitating drainage when possible, preventing complications or recurrence, educating the family in care of the child and providing support to the child and family.

Analgesics are helpful to reduce severe earache, as well as control fever (ibuprofen and paracetamol). Ibuprofen has a longer duration of action (about 6 to 8 hours) and is especially beneficial for night-time comfort but should not be used in children under 6 months of age unless directed by a general practitioner. The application of heat over the ear while the child lies on the affected side may reduce pain in some children but may aggravate discomfort in others. This position also facilitates drainage of the exudate if the eardrum has ruptured or if myringotomy was performed.

If the ear is draining, the external canal may be cleaned with sterile cotton swabs, as directed by the provider. If ear wicks or lightly rolled sterile gauze packs are placed in the ear after surgical treatment, they should be loose enough to allow accumulated drainage to flow out of the ear; otherwise the infection may be transferred to the mastoid process. Parents should keep these wicks dry during shampoos or baths. Occasionally drainage is so profuse that the pinna and surrounding skin become excoriated from exudate. Frequent cleansing and application of various moisture barriers (as per instructions from the treating team) can prevent or treat this.

Preventing recurrence requires adequate parent education regarding antibiotic therapy. Because the symptoms of pain and fever usually subside within 24 to 48 hours, nurses must emphasise that although the child may appear well, the infection is not completely eradicated until all the prescribed medication is taken. It is important to stress the potential complications of OM, especially hearing loss, which can be prevented with adequate treatment and follow-up care. (See Administration of Medication, and Compliance, Chapter 22.)

Grommets may be indicated to allow ventilation into the middle ear to equalise middle ear pressure. Most children's hearing improves right after surgery and ear drainage is common up to 1 week after insertion. The grommets are eventually pushed out of the eardrum usually 8 to 18 months after tube placement. Parents should be aware of the appearance of a grommet (usually a tiny plastic spool-shaped tube) so they can recognise it if it falls out. Give reassurance to parents/carers that this is normal and requires no immediate intervention, although they should notify their practitioner (e.g. ENT surgeon).

Healthcare providers offer recommendations for water precautions after grommet insertion. While grommets are in place, no bath or swimming pool water should enter the ears (i.e. use earplugs/swimming cap etc.) (SCHN 2017). After 2 weeks children may shower without earplugs/special water precautions.

Reducing the chances of OM is possible with simple measures, such as sitting or holding an infant upright for feedings. Propping bottles is discouraged to avoid pooling of milk while the child is in the supine position and to encourage human contact during feeding. Eliminating tobacco smoke and known allergens is also recommended. Forceful nose blowing during a URTI is discouraged to avoid forcing organisms to ascend through the eustachian tube. Early detection of middle ear effusion is essential in prevention of complications. Infants and preschool children should be screened for effusion, and all schoolchildren, especially those with learning disabilities, should be tested for middle ear effusion. Frequent audiological evaluations, medical consultation and education of parents and children are advised when middle ear effusion is detected.

Acute Otitis Externa

AOE is commonly caused by *Pseudomonas aeruginosa* or *Staphylococcus aureus* but may include other pathogens such as aspergillus and candidal species. Ordinarily the external ear canal is protected by a waxy, water-repellent coating composed of highly viscid secretions of the sebaceous glands and the watery, pigmented secretions of apocrine glands, in combination with exfoliated surface cells. Inflammation occurs when this environment is altered by swimming, bathing or increased environmental humidity; by infection, dermatoses or insufficient cerumen; or by trauma from a foreign body (FB) or a finger. The ear canal becomes irritated and maceration takes place. It is commonly referred to as swimmer's ear.

The predominant symptom of external ear infection is ear pain accentuated by manipulation of the pinna, especially pressure on the tragus. The pain often appears to be out of proportion to the degree of inflammation. Conductive hearing loss may be present as a result of the oedema, secretions and accumulation of debris within the canal. Oedema, erythema, a cheesy green-blue-grey discharge and tenderness appear as the infection progresses. The external canal may be so tender and swollen that visualisation is difficult. There may be a fever. In advanced cases the pain is intense, constant and aggravated by jaw motion or ear manipulation.

Therapeutic objectives include relief of pain, oedema and itching, as well as restoration of normal flora, cerumen and canal epithelium. Analgesics are prescribed for pain. A gauze wick may be inserted if oedema is present to facilitate the medication (if ordered or required as per the treating team) reaching the site of inflammation. The wick is removed after swelling and pain have subsided, but the drops are continued for at least 3 days after relief of pain. The best management for external ear inflammation is prevention.

Nursing Care Management

Nurses can teach parents or patients simple steps to prevent recurrent infections. Children should limit their stay in the water to less than an hour, if possible, and ears should dry completely (1 to 2 hours) before entering the water again.

Educate children not to pick at the ears or 'probe' the ear with any object (i.e. cotton buds, fingers, etc.) as this may injure or infect the ear canal.

CROUP SYNDROMES

Croup is a common respiratory disease of childhood. Croup is a general term applied to a group of symptoms characterised by hoarseness, a resonant cough described as 'barking' or 'croupy', varying degrees of inspiratory stridor and varying degrees of respiratory distress resulting from swelling or obstruction in the region of the larynx and subglottic airway. Acute infections of the larynx are of greater importance in infants and small children than they are in older children because of the increased incidence in children in this age group and the smaller diameter of the airway, which renders it subject to significantly greater narrowing with the same degree of inflammation (Fig 26.4).

The number of croup cases increases in the late autumn through early winter months. It occurs primarily in children 6 months to 6 years of age (RCHM 2019c). Hospitalisation may be necessary for some children with croup, and a small percentage of hospitalised children require positive airway pressure or intubation.

Croup syndromes affect to varying degrees the larynx, trachea and bronchi. However, laryngeal involvement often dominates the clinical picture because of the severe effects on the voice and breathing. Croup syndromes are usually described according to the primary anatomic area affected (i.e. epiglottitis [or supraglottitis], laryngitis, laryngotracheobronchitis [LTB] and tracheitis). In general, LTB tends to occur in very young children, whereas epiglottitis is more characteristic of older children. Table 26.3 provides a comparison of croup syndromes.

Because croup is one of the most benign conditions causing upper airway obstruction, it is vitally important to correctly identify it and distinguish the type of croup syndrome or condition (i.e. spasmodic croup or LTB as opposed to a potentially life-threatening condition such as epiglottitis, bacterial tracheitis, FB aspiration or a peritonsillar abscess). The key differences between LTB and epiglottitis are the absence of cough, the presence of dysphagia and the high degree of toxicity in children with epiglottitis. Children with epiglottitis usually look worse than they sound, in contrast to children with LTB, who sound worse than they look.

Acute Epiglottitis

Acute epiglottitis, or acute supraglottitis, is a medical emergency and requires immediate medical attention. It is a serious obstructive inflammatory process that occurs principally in children between 2 and 5 years of age but can occur from infancy to adulthood. The obstruction is supraglottic, as opposed to the subglottic obstruction of laryngitis. The causative agent is usually *H. influenzae.* LTB and

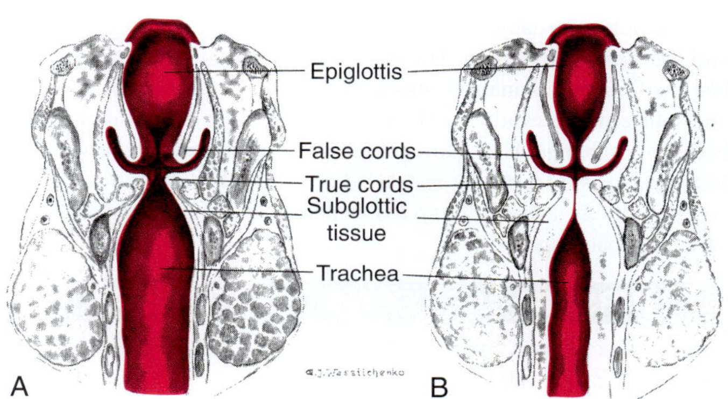

Fig 26.4 (**A**) Normal larynx. (**B**) Obstruction and narrowing resulting from oedema of croup.

TABLE 26.3 Comparison of Croup Syndromes

	Acute Epiglottitis	Acute LTB	Acute Spasmodic Laryngitis	Acute Tracheitis
Age group affected	2–5 years but varies	Infant or child < 5 years	1–3 years	1 months to 6 years
Etiological agent	Bacterial	Viral	Viral with allergic component	Viral or bacterial with allergic component
Onset	Rapidly progressive	Slowly progressive	Sudden; at night	Moderately progressive
Major symptoms	Dysphagia Stridor aggravated when supine Drooling High fever Toxic appearance Rapid pulse and respirations	URTI Stridor Brassy cough Hoarseness Dyspnoea Restlessness Irritability Low-grade fever Non-toxic appearance	URTI Croupy cough Stridor Hoarseness Dyspnoea Restlessness Symptoms awakening child Symptoms disappearing during day Tendency to recur	URTI Croupy cough Purulent secretions High fever No response to LTB therapy
Treatment	Airway protection, possible intubation, tracheotomy Humidified oxygen Fluids Antibiotics Reassurance	Corticosteroids Fluids Reassurance Nebulised adrenaline (possible short-term improvement)	Reassurance	Antibiotics Fluids

LTB, Laryngotracheobronchitis; *URTI,* upper respiratory tract infection.

epiglottitis do not occur together. Epiglottitis (non-infectious) may also be caused by ingestion of caustic agents, smoke inhalation or foreign bodies (O'Neal 2017).

Clinical Manifestations

The onset of epiglottitis is abrupt, less often preceded by cold symptoms and more often by a sore throat. It can rapidly progress to severe respiratory distress. The child usually goes to bed asymptomatic to awaken later complaining of sore throat and pain on swallowing. The child has a fever and appears sicker than clinical findings suggest. The child insists on sitting upright and leaning forward (tripod position), with the chin thrust out, mouth open and tongue protruding. Drooling of saliva is common because of the difficulty or pain on swallowing and excessive secretions.

NURSING CARE CONSIDERATIONS

Three clinical observations that are predictive of epiglottitis are absence of spontaneous cough, presence of drooling and agitation.

The child is irritable and extremely restless and has an apprehensive and frightened expression. The voice is thick and muffled, with a frog-like croaking sound on inspiration. The child is not hoarse. Suprasternal and substernal recession may be visible. Slow, quiet breathing provides better air exchange. The sallow colour of mild hypoxia may progress to frank cyanosis if treatment is delayed. The throat is red and inflamed, and a distinctive, large, cherry-red, oedematous epiglottis is visible on careful throat inspection.

NURSING CARE CONSIDERATIONS

Throat inspection should only be performed when resuscitation equipment and suction are immediately available at the child's bedside, and when immediate endotracheal intubation or an emergency tracheotomy can be performed if needed.

Therapeutic Management

Epiglottitis may develop suddenly, with respiratory obstruction appearing rapidly. Progressive obstruction leads to hypoxia, hypercapnia and acidosis, followed by decreased muscular tone, reduced level of consciousness and, when obstruction becomes more or less complete, sudden death.

A lateral neck x-ray of the soft tissues is indicated for diagnosis. Experienced medical staff with advanced airway management skills should accompany the child. For a young child who is likely to become more agitated by the procedure, it is preferable that the child remain on the parent's lap if content there during transportation and in the examination area during portable imaging.

Endotracheal intubation is usually considered for the child with epiglottitis with severe respiratory distress. Nasotracheal intubation is sometimes preferred. It is recommended that the intubation or any invasive procedure, such as starting an IV infusion, be performed in a resuscitation bay where emergency airway maintenance can be easily and quickly accomplished. For patients who are not intubated, humidified oxygen is administered as necessary either via mask in older children or as blow-over in younger children to avoid further agitation. Whether or not there is an artificial airway, the child requires intensive observation by experienced personnel. The epiglottal swelling usually decreases after 24 hours of antibiotic therapy, and the epiglottis is near normal by the third day. It is recommended that diagnostic tests and invasive procedures be postponed on the child with suspected epiglottitis until an airway has been established.

Children with suspected bacterial epiglottitis are given antibiotics intravenously, followed by oral administration to complete a 7- to 10-day course. Ceftriaxone/cefotaxime are generally the first antibiotics started. A blood culture and epiglottic culture for intubated patients should be considered before antibiotic administration. The use of corticosteroids for reducing oedema may be beneficial during the early hours of treatment.

Prevention. It is recommended that all children receive the *H. influenzae* type B conjugate vaccine as part of the National Immunisation

Program Schedule (ATAGI 2018, Ministry of Health 2020b) Since administration of the vaccine has become a routine part of the immunisation schedule, the incidence of epiglottitis has declined. The disease now tends to be caused by viral agents. (See Immunisations, Chapter 6.)

Nursing Care Management

Epiglottitis is a serious and frightening disease for the child, family and health professionals. It is important to act quickly but calmly and provide support without unduly increasing anxiety. The child is allowed to remain in the position that provides the most comfort and security, parents remain with the child and parental reassurance is provided. Droplet isolation precautions are indicated for 24 hours after initiation of effective antibiotic therapy to control the spread of respiratory organisms. Prophylactic antibiotic treatment of household and other contacts may be indicated. Continuous monitoring of cardiorespiratory status, including pulse oximetry (or blood gases if the patient is intubated), is an important part of nursing observations, and the IV infusion is maintained. (See Chapter 22.)

Acute Laryngitis

Acute infectious laryngitis is a common illness in older children and adolescents. Infants and smaller children experience more generalised involvement. (See next section on LTB.) Viruses are the usual causative agents, and the principal complaint is hoarseness, which may be accompanied by other upper respiratory symptoms (e.g. coryza, sore throat, cough, nasal congestion) and systemic manifestations (e.g. fever, headache, myalgia, malaise). Other complaints vary with the infecting virus. For example, adenoviruses and influenza viruses are responsible for more systemic involvement; parainfluenza virus, rhinoviruses and RSV cause more mild illness.

Therapeutic and Nursing Care Management

The disease is almost always self-limiting without long-term sequelae. Treatment is supportive with fluids and humidified oxygen.

Acute Laryngotracheobronchitis (Croup)

Acute *laryngotracheobronchitis* (LTB) is the most common type of croup experienced by children admitted for hospitalisation and primarily affects children 6 months to 3 years old. Organisms responsible for LTB are the parainfluenza virus types 1, followed by parainfluenza virus types 2 and 3, adenoviruses, RSV and *M. pneumoniae.* Less common causative organisms include influenza A and B, rhinoviruses, enteroviruses, herpes simplex virus, *Staphylococcus aureus, Streptococcus pyogenes* and *Streptococcus pneumoniae.* The illness is usually preceded by a URTI, which gradually descends to adjacent structures. It is characterised by the gradual onset of low-grade fever, and the parents often report that the child went to bed and later awoke with a barky, hoarse cough and at times inspiratory stridor. Symptoms are typically worse at night, and agitation and crying tend to exacerbate the symptoms.

Inflammation of the mucosa lining the larynx and trachea causes a narrowing of the airway. When the airway is significantly narrowed, the child struggles to inhale air past the obstruction and into the lungs, producing the characteristic inspiratory stridor and suprasternal recession. Other classic manifestations include cough and hoarseness. Respiratory distress in infants and toddlers may be manifested by nasal flaring, intercostal retractions, tachypnoea and continuous stridor. The degree of respiratory distress varies; hypoxia and decreased oxygen saturations are observed primarily when the obstruction is severe enough to prevent adequate ventilation and CO_2 removal. This can lead to respiratory acidosis and respiratory failure.

Therapeutic Management

The major objective in medical management of infectious LTB is maintaining an airway and providing for adequate respiratory exchange. Children with mild croup (no stridor at rest) are managed at home or observed in ED in the rural and remote settings. Parents need to learn the signs of respiratory distress so that they can call professional help when required. Children whose symptoms progressively get worse should receive medical attention immediately.

Nebulised adrenaline is administered as quickly as possible for moderate to severe cases. The beta-adrenergic effects cause mucosal vasoconstriction and subsequent decreased subglottic oedema. The onset of action is rapid. Peak effect is observed in less than 2 hours. Always follow local clinical practice guidelines for treatment course and duration. (See Fig 26.5 for the Royal Children's Hospital Melbourne's flow chart.) Close observation of patients receiving nebulised adrenaline is critical to detect the reappearance of symptoms, monitor the response to therapy and note any deterioration in respiratory status. The patient who has received nebulised adrenaline for croup should be observed for 3 to 4 hours for any visible signs of respiratory distress (RCHM 2019c).

The use of corticosteroids is beneficial because the anti-inflammatory effects decrease subglottic oedema. Oral steroids (dexamethasone or prednisolone) have proven effective in the treatment of croup and are considered standard treatement for this condition. IV or IM dexamethasone may be given to children who are unable to tolerate oral dosing. The onset of action is clinically detectable as early as 6 hours after administration, with continued improvement over a period of 12 to 24 hours.

Supplemental humidified oxygen may be needed if hypoxaemic. On occasion, intubation and ventilation may be required when airway obstruction becomes more severe. If in a rural or remote area, the intubated child would require aeromedical transport to a tertiary hospital.

It is essential to allow children with mild croup to continue to drink fluids they like and to encourage parents to use comforting measures with their child (e.g. holding, rocking, walking, singing, reading books). If the child is unable to take oral fluids, IV fluid therapy may be indicated.

Nursing Care Management

The most important nursing function in the care of children with LTB is continuous, vigilant observation. The child should be on continuous cardiorespiratory monitoring and nursed in a bed that is closely monitored by staff. Frequent and accurate assessment of respiratory status is essential. Changes in therapy are frequently based on nurses' observations and assessment of a child's status, response to therapy and tolerance of procedures. The trend away from early intubation of children with LTB emphasises the importance of nursing observation and the ability to recognise impending respiratory failure so that intubation can be implemented without delay. Intubation equipment and bag and valve mask equipment should be readily accessible (at the child's bedside) and taken with the child during transport to other areas (e.g. in rural/remote areas, emergency medical transport service involvement and transfer to a tertiary centre for paediatric intensive care if intubation and further observation are required). Paediatric Broselow (or similarly colour-coded emergency trolleys) Emergency Trolleys are available in most paediatric units and EDs throughout Australia and New Zealand. A croup scoring system may be used to determine severity of symptoms.

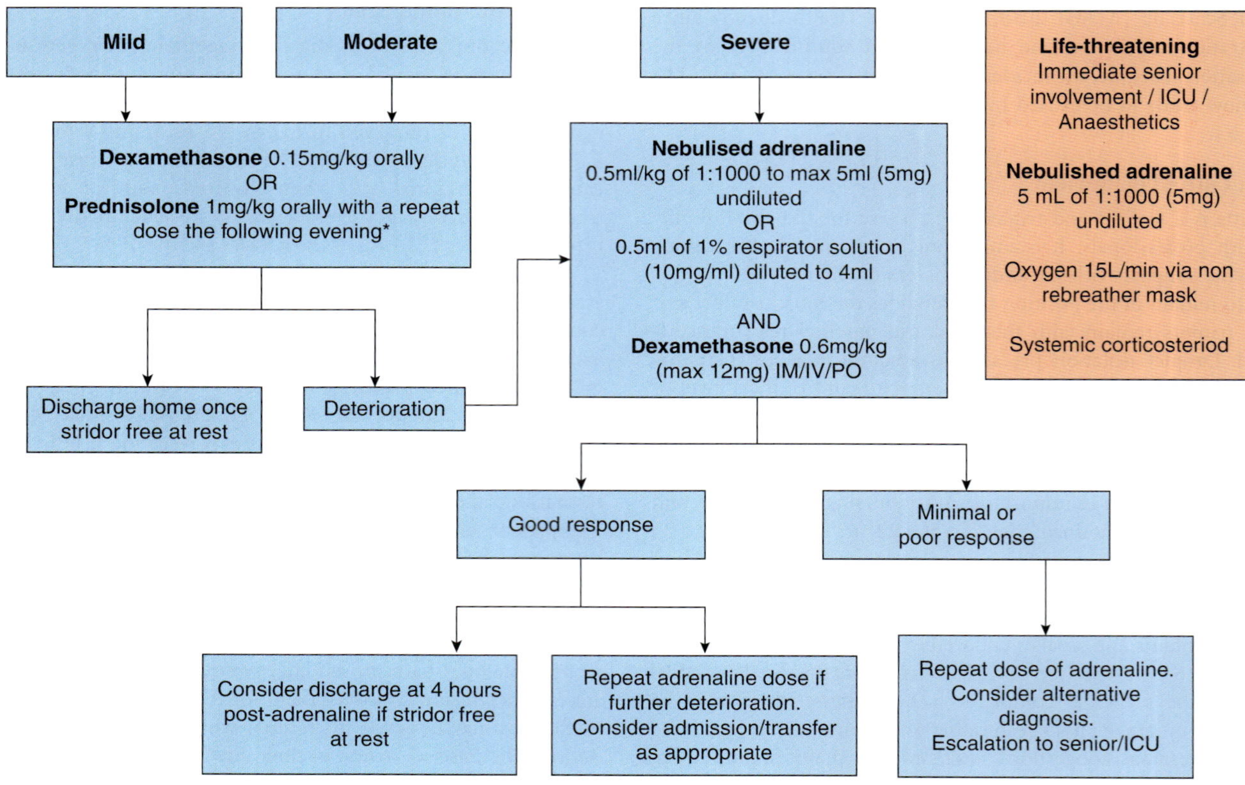

Fig 26.5 Croup management. (Source: The Royal Children's Hospital Melbourne (RCHM). (2019c). Croup (laryngotracheoBronchitis. Retrieved from: https://www.rch.org.au/clinicalguide/)

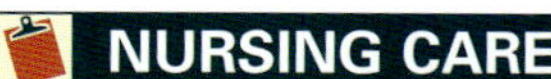

NURSING CARE CONSIDERATIONS

Early signs of impending airway obstruction include increased pulse and respiratory rate; substernal, suprasternal and intercostal recession; nasal flaring; and increased restlessness.

To conserve energy, children are given every opportunity to rest. Infants or small children find that being placed on a face mask, coughing, having laryngeal spasms and needing IV therapy are additional sources of distress. Infants and small children prefer sitting upright, and most want to be held. Blow-over oxygen therapy can be administered by a parent while the child is being held. Children need the security of the parent's presence. Crying increases respiratory distress and hypoxia; the nurse needs to assess a child's individual tolerance for these therapies. An extremely fussy child may do better when held in the parent's lap with blow-over oxygen using a face mask directed towards the child's face.

The rapid progression of croup, the alarming sound of the cough and stridor and the child's apprehensive behaviour and ill appearance combine to create a frightening experience for the parents. They need reassurance regarding the child's progress and an explanation of treatments. The family should be encouraged to remain with the child as much as possible, especially when this decreases the child's distress.

Fortunately, as the crisis subsides and the child responds to therapy, breathing becomes easier and recovery is generally prompt. Home care after discharge includes monitoring for worsening symptoms, continued humidity, adequate hydration and nourishment. Encourage parents to ask questions about home care and preparation for discharge.

Acute Spasmodic Laryngitis

Acute spasmodic laryngitis (spasmodic croup, 'midnight croup' or 'twilight croup') is distinct from laryngitis and LTB and characterised by paroxysmal attacks of laryngeal obstruction that occur chiefly at night. Signs of inflammation are absent or mild, and there is often a history of previous attacks lasting for 2 to 5 days, followed by an uneventful recovery. It usually affects children ages 1 to 3 years old. Some children appear to be predisposed to the condition; allergy and psychogenic factors contribute to some cases.

The child goes to bed well or with some mild respiratory symptoms but awakes suddenly with the characteristic barking, metallic cough, hoarseness, noisy inspiration and restlessness. The child appears anxious and frightened. However, there is no fever, the episode subsides in a few hours and the child appears well the next day with the exception of slight hoarseness.

Therapeutic and Nursing Care Management

Children with spasmodic croup can be managed at home. Warm mist provided by steam from hot running water in a closed bathroom may be helpful. Parents are usually advised to have the child sleep in humidified air until the cough has subsided to prevent subsequent episodes. Children with moderately severe symptoms may be hospitalised for observation and therapy with adrenaline, as for LTB. Patients may respond to corticosteroid therapy. The disease is usually self-limiting.

Bacterial Tracheitis

Bacterial tracheitis, an infection of the mucosa and soft tissues of the upper trachea, is a distinct entity with features of both croup and epiglottitis. The disease occurs typically at a mean age between 5 and 7 years and may cause severe airway obstruction (Roosevelt 2016). It is believed to be a complication of LTB or other viral upper respiratory infections, and although *Staphylococcus aureus* is the most frequent bacterial organism responsible, *M. catarrhalis*, *S. pneumoniae*, *S. pyogenes*, alpha-haemolytic streptococci and *H. influenzae* have also been implicated. Causes of bacterial tracheitis are often polymicrobial. Viruses such as influenza A and B, RSV, parainfluenza, measles and enteroviruses have been associated with bacterial tracheitis (Brashers & Huether 2019).

Anteroposterior or lateral neck x-rays show narrowing (Steeple sign), and infiltrates may be seen. An endoscopy of the airway performed in the operating room or intensive care unit (ICU) is usually indicated to remove secretions and obtain cultures.

Many of the manifestations of bacterial tracheitis are similar to those of LTB but are unresponsive to LTB therapy. There is a history of previous URTI with croupy cough, stridor unaffected by position, toxicity, absence of drooling, respiratory distress and high fever. A prominent manifestation is the production of thick, purulent tracheal secretions. Respiratory difficulties are secondary to these copious secretions. If not treated, children with this condition quickly develop a life-threatening respiratory failure and/or acute respiratory distress syndrome (ARDS) (Brashers & Huether 2019).

Therapeutic and Nursing Care Management

Bacterial tracheitis requires vigorous management with antipyretics, fluid status and antibiotics (10-day course). A trial of inhaled bronchodilators may be performed but is generally not beneficial. Many children require endotracheal intubation and mechanical ventilation; patients are closely monitored for impending respiratory failure if not intubated. Early recognition to prevent life-threatening airway obstruction is essential.

INFECTIONS OF THE LOWER AIRWAYS

The reactive portion of the lower respiratory tract includes the bronchi and bronchioles in children. Cartilaginous support of the large airways is not fully developed until adolescence. Consequently, the smooth muscle in these structures represents a major factor in constriction of the airway, particularly in the bronchioles—the portion that extends from the bronchi to the alveoli. Table 26.4 compares some of the major features of bronchial and bronchiolar infections.

Bronchitis

Bronchitis (sometimes referred to as tracheobronchitis) is an inflammation of the large airways (trachea and bronchi) that is frequently associated with a URTI. Viral agents are the primary cause of the disease, including influenza A and B, parainfluenza, coronavirus, rhinovirus, RSV and human metapneumovirus. The condition is characterised by a dry, hacking and non-productive cough that is worse at night, lasting more than 5 days but can persist for 1 to 3 weeks.

Bronchitis is a mild, self-limiting disease that requires only symptomatic treatment, including analgesics, antipyretics and humidity. Most patients recover uneventfully in 5 to 10 days. Adolescents with chronic bronchitis (> 3 months) should be screened for tobacco or marijuana use. Chronic bronchitis can be associated with underlying conditions such as CF and bronchiectasis.

Respiratory Syncytial Virus (RSV) and Bronchiolitis

Bronchiolitis is an acute viral infection with maximum effect at the bronchiolar level. The infection occurs primarily in winter and spring. Most cases of bronchiolitis are caused by RSV, adenoviruses, parainfluenza viruses and human metapneumovirus, but RSV is the most common cause. Approximately 13,500 Australian infants had bronchiolitis in 2018 (O'Brien et al 2018). Occasionally, *M. pneumoniae* has been associated with bronchiolitis in children. RSV occurs less frequently in breastfed infants, and more frequently in children who live

TABLE 26.4 Comparison of Conditions Affecting the Bronchi

	Asthma	Bronchitis	Bronchiolitis
Description	Exaggerated response of bronchi to a trigger such as URTI, dander, cold air, exercise bronchospasm, exudation and oedema of bronchi	Usually occurs in association with URTI Seldom an isolated entity	Most common infectious disease of lower airways Maximum obstructive impact at bronchiolar level
Age group affected	Infancy to adolescence or adulthood	First 4 years of life	Usually children 2–12 months of age; rare after age 2 years Peak incidence approximately age 6 months
Etiological agents	Most often viruses such as RSV in infants but may be any of a variety of URTI pathogens	Usually viral Other agents (e.g. bacteria, fungi, allergic disorders, airborne irritants) can trigger symptoms	Viruses, predominantly RSV; also adenoviruses, parainfluenza viruses, human metapneumovirus and *Mycoplasma pneumoniae*
Predominant characteristics	Wheezing, cough, laboured respirations	Persistent dry, hacking cough (worse at night) becoming productive in 2–3 days	Laboured respirations, poor feeding, cough, tachypnoea, recession, flaring nares, emphysema, increased nasal mucus, wheezing, may have fever
Treatment	Inhaled corticosteroids, bronchodilators, leukotriene modifiers, allergen and control of triggers		Provide supplemental oxygen if saturations ≤ 90%; bronchodilators (optional) Suction nasopharynx Ensure adequate fluid intake Maintain adequate oxygenation

RSV, Respiratory syncytial virus; *URTI,* upper respiratory tract infection

in crowded conditions. RSV infection is the most frequent cause of hospitalisation in children less than 2 years old. In addition, severe RSV infections in the first year of life represent a significant risk factor for the development of asthma that can persist into adulthood (Smith et al 2017). The precise link between RSV and asthma is unknown. It is important to note that not all infants and children with RSV will develop a bronchiolitis. Occasionally, infants with RSV may have a concurrent viral or bacterial infection (e.g. OM, pertussis). Subsequent reinfections are common but they are usually less severe (Jardins & Burton 2020a).

Aetiology

RSV is a paramyxovirus containing a single strand of RNA and is part of the Paramyxoviridae family. RSV strains have two major subgroups: A and B. More children develop bronchiolitis and pneumonia from RSV subgroup A infections than from subgroup B infections during major outbreaks. The disease usually begins in the autumn, reaches a peak during the winter and then decreases during the spring. Children who are preterm, have cyanotic or complicated congenital heart disease (CHD), have chronic lung disease or are immunosuppressed often have more severe illness.

Pathophysiology

RSV infection affects the epithelial cells of the respiratory tract. The ciliated cells swell, protrude into the lumen and lose their cilia. The infection produces a fusion of the infected cell membrane with cell membranes of adjacent epithelial cells, thus forming a giant cell with multiple nuclei. At the cellular level this fusion results in multinucleated masses of protoplasm, or syncytia.

The bronchiolar mucosa swells, and lumina are subsequently filled with mucus and exudate. The walls of the bronchi and bronchioles are infiltrated with inflammatory cells, and peribronchiolar interstitial pneumonitis is usually present. Because luminal epithelial cells are shed into the bronchioles when they die, the lumina are frequently obstructed, particularly on expiration. The varying degrees of obstruction produced in small air passages lead to hyperinflation, obstructive emphysema resulting from partial obstruction and patchy areas of atelectasis. Dilation of bronchial passages on inspiration allows sufficient space for intake of air, but narrowing of the passages on expiration prevents air from leaving the lungs. Thus air is trapped distal to the obstruction and causes progressive overinflation (emphysema).

Transmission

The transmission of RSV is predominantly through direct contact with respiratory secretions, mainly as a result of inoculation from hand to eye, nose or other mucous membranes. It can also occur by direct inoculation by large-particle aerosols or by self-inoculation from contaminated objects. RSV in secretions can survive for several hours on countertops, gloves, paper tissues and cloth, and for 30 minutes on skin; it remains infectious when transferred from hands or objects. There is no documentation of distant spread of RSV by small-particle aerosols (airborne transmission). The incubation period is 2 to 8 days, but viral shedding can last 3 to 4 weeks.

Clinical Manifestations

The younger the infant, the greater the likelihood that severe lower respiratory tract disease requiring hospitalisation will occur. The peak incidence for RSV is less than 3 months of age, but can occur at all ages. Higher rates occur in children who attend day care (either home or centre based). The severity of RSV tends to diminish with age and repeated infections.

Symptoms such as rhinorrhoea and low-grade fever often appear first. In time, a cough may develop. If the disease progresses, it becomes a lower respiratory tract infection and manifests typical symptoms (Box 26.6). Once the lower airway is involved, classic manifestations include signs of altered air exchange, such as wheezing, recession, crackles, dyspnoea, tachypnoea and diminished breath sounds. Bronchiolitis peaks on day 3 to 5 (Pedra & Stark 2017). Pneumonia may occur in conjunction with bronchiolitis.

Diagnostic Evaluation

Because RSV infection may be manifested as a URTI, it is often difficult to identify the specific etiological agent by clinical criteria alone. The most difficult distinction is between RSV and asthma because both conditions involve the lower airway and have similar symptoms.

Routine testing for specific viruses is no longer recommended because bronchiolitis may be caused by many viruses (Smith et al 2017). Routine x-rays are also not indicated (Smith et al 2017). If identification is necessary, rapid RSV antigen detection are performed on nasopharyngeal secretions (nasopharyngeal aspirate [NPA]). The more traditional viral culture is becoming obsolete because it takes several days to get a result (RCHM 2017).

Other simultaneous viral or bacterial infections may occur with RSV. The infant should be carefully evaluated for the presence of urinary tract infection, meningitis and bacteraemia; antibiotics are prescribed only for a coexisting bacterial infection.

Therapeutic Management

Most children with bronchiolitis can be managed at home. Uncomplicated cases of bronchiolitis are treated symptomatically with adequate fluid intake, airway maintenance and medications if required. Hospitalisation is usually recommended for children with respiratory distress or those with poor feeding, lethargy, dehydration, moderate to severe respiratory distress, apnoea or hypoxaemia. Other reasons for hospitalisation include complicating conditions, such as underlying lung or heart disease (e.g. prematurity), or caregiver inability to provide adequate care during illness.

BOX 26.6 Signs and Symptoms of Respiratory Syncytial Virus

Initial

- Rhinorrhoea
- Pharyngitis
- Coughing, sneezing
- Wheezing
- Possible ear or eye infection
- Intermittent fever

With Progression of Illness

- Increased coughing and wheezing
- Fever
- Tachypnoea and recession
- Refusal to nurse or bottle-feed
- Copious secretions

Severe Illness

- Tachypnoea $>$ 70 breaths/min
- Listlessness
- Apnoeic spells
- Poor air exchange; poor breath sounds
- Cyanosis

Each state has their own recommendations regarding acceptable monitoring. For example, New South Wales Health recommends saturations > 92% with continuous monitoring if severe, while the Royal Children's Hospital Melbourne recommends > 90% with continuous monitoring if severe (Agency for Clinical Innovation [ACI] 2018a, RCHM 2017). Heated, humidified high-flow nasal cannula therapy (HHFNC) has been increasingly used for hospitalised infants and young children with bronchiolitis. High flow allows extra humidity blended with oxygen administration and CPAP to be administered. The practitioner indicates the flow rate and percentage of the oxygen therapy. High flow improves functional residual capacity, reducing the work of breathing. A nasogastric tube should be inserted and placed on free drainage to vent air from the stomach. If respiratory acidosis is present CPAP, BiPAP or intubation may be required. Some rural facilities do not have the resources to do CPAP or BiPAP and the intubated infant/child will need to be cared for in metropolitan facilities.

Routine chest percussion and drainage is not recommended (RCHM 2017, ACI 2018a). Infants with abundant nasal secretions benefit from regular saline drops and suctioning, especially before feeding. Nasal aspiration of the external nares using an aspirator may be sufficient to remove most secretions. Nasopharyngeal suctioning is traumatic to the airways but can be considered if there are signs of respiratory distress or deoxygenation.

Fluids by mouth may be contraindicated because of tachypnoea, increased work of breathing, weakness and fatigue. Therefore, nasogastric fluids may be required, unless respiratory distress increases, then IV fluids may be necessary until the acute stage of the disease has passed.

Clinical assessments, non-invasive oxygen monitoring and, in severe cases, blood gas values guide therapy. Medical therapy for bronchiolitis is primarily supportive and aimed at decreasing airway hyperresonance and inflammation, and promoting adequate fluid intake. Bronchodilators, corticosteroids and nebulised hypertonic saline are not recommended and are rarely beneficial (ACI 2018a, RCHM 2017).

Antibiotics are not part of the treatment of RSV unless there is a coexisting bacterial infection such as OM or pneumonia. Additional treatment recommendations are to encourage breastfeeding, avoid passive tobacco smoke exposure and promote preventive measures, including handwashing and isolation from non-infectious children.

In Australia and New Zealand, palivizumab is available for prevention of RSV. It is a humanised monoclonal antibody that is given once every 30 days (15 mg/kg/dose) throughout the RSV season (up to 5 doses). It is usually given as an IM injection. Candidates for this drug include the following (RCHM 2018d):

- preterm infants (< 32 weeks' gestation) with or without chronic lung disease or congenital heart disease
- infants with haemodynamically significant congenital heart disease
- children with anatomic pulmonary abnormalities or neuromuscular disorders
- immunocompromised children assessed on an individual basis.

Some children acquire the illness despite palivizumab prophylaxis.

MEDICATION SAFETY

Palivizumab Administration

The lyophilised powder form of palivizumab should be administered immediately after being reconstituted with sterile water because it is preservative free.

QUALITY PATIENT OUTCOMES

Bronchiolitis

- Oxygen saturation 90% to 92% or higher
- Respiratory rate less than 60 breaths/min
- Adequate oral fluid intake/hydration levels

Nursing Care Management

Children admitted to the hospital with suspected RSV infection need to be isolated from non-infected children; once pathology results are reviewed, infants with RSV can be cared for in the same room. Contact and standard precautions are used with hospitalised patients and some institutions use droplet precautions in addition. Handwashing is essential to reduce spread of the illness—nurses need to follow the Five Moments for Hand Hygiene. Nurses assigned to children with RSV are not to care for other patients who are considered high risk. Staff must be careful to avoid touching the nasal mucosa or conjunctiva. Restricting visitors can assist in reducing the potential spread of RSV.

Infants with RSV infection often have copious nasal secretions, making breathing, breast feeding or bottle-feeding difficult. This causes concerns that the child will lose weight or stop feeding altogether. Encourage breastfeeding mothers to express their breast milk and store appropriately for later use. (See Chapter 7.) Parents should learn how to instil normal saline drops into the nares and suction the mucus with a bulb syringe before feeds and before bedtime so the child may eat and rest better; unfortunately, no medications appropriate for infants can help with these symptoms. To address the issue of decreased fluid intake, parents may offer small amounts of fluids, 5 to 10 mL at a time, with a medication/oral syringe every 10 minutes or so. Infants may cough or vomit as the secretions settle in the stomach and make them prone to emesis (vomiting) of such secretions.

The nurse aims additional interventions at monitoring oxygenation with pulse oximetry when clinically indicated, monitoring fluid intake (oral/nasogastric/IV) and output, monitoring for fever and administering antipyretics, and providing information for the parent regarding the infant's condition and treatments/care. Inform the parents that the infant's cough may persist for a few weeks.

In remote areas, infants/children requiring hospitalisation should be transferred to a paediatric unit at rural/base hospital. In rural settings, the critically ill infant with RSV may need to be transferred to a tertiary hospital for admission to a paediatric ICU for continuous monitoring of respiratory status, cardiac output and maintenance of adequate systemic pressure. IV fluids, antibiotics, high-flow nasal prong oxygen, positive airway pressure or mechanical ventilation, and inotropes may be required if the child is unstable. Parents and family members need emotional support and information regarding the child's status during this crisis.

The unpredictability of the infant's individual response to the disease compounds parental anxiety. However, in most cases the infant recovers quickly from the disease and resumes normal daily activities, including fluid intake.

Pneumonia

Pneumonia, an inflammation of the pulmonary parenchyma, is common in childhood, occurring more frequently in infancy and early childhood. Clinically, pneumonia may occur either as a primary disease or as a complication of another illness.

Pneumonia can be classified according to morphology, etiological agent or clinical form. Although morphological classification is typically used (Box 26.7), the most useful classification is based on the etiological agent (i.e. viral, bacterial, mycoplasmal or aspiration of

BOX 26.7 Types of Pneumonia

Bronchopneumonia—Begins in the terminal bronchioles, which become clogged with mucopurulent exudate to form consolidated patches in nearby lobules; also called *lobular pneumonia*.

Interstitial pneumonia—Inflammatory process more or less confined within the alveolar walls (interstitium) and the peribronchial and interlobular tissues.

Lobar pneumonia—All or a large segment of one or more pulmonary lobes is involved. When both lungs are affected, it is known as *bilateral* or *double pneumonia*.

foreign substances). The causative agent is usually introduced into the lungs through inhalation or from the bloodstream. Pneumonia may be caused by histomycosis, coccidioidomycosis and other fungi. Other terms that describe pneumonias are *haemorrhagic*, *fibrinous* and *necrotising*. **Pneumonitis** is a localised acute inflammation of the lung without the toxaemia associated with lobar pneumonia.

The clinical manifestations of pneumonia vary depending on the etiological agent, the child's age, the child's systemic reaction to the infection, the extent of the lesions, any underlying conditions and the degree of bronchial and bronchiolar obstruction. The clinical history, the child's age, the general health history, the physical examination, radiography and the laboratory examination can help identify the etiological agent. Many organisms can cause pneumonia, and they vary according to the age of the child. Examples include: *Chlamydia trachomatis* in $<$ 3 months of age, RSV and streptococcus in $<$ 5 year olds and *Mycoplasma* and *Chlamydia pneumoniae* in $>$ 5 year olds (ACI 2018b).

Viral Pneumonia

Viral pneumonias occur more frequently than bacterial pneumonias and are seen in children of all age groups. They are often associated with viral URTIs, and the pathological changes involve interstitial pneumonitis with inflammation of the mucosa and the walls of bronchi and bronchioles. There could also be parenchymal involvement. There are few clinical symptoms to distinguish among the responsible organisms, and only laboratory examination can differentiate among specific viruses.

Clinical Manifestations

The onset may be acute or insidious, and symptoms vary from mild fever, slight cough and malaise to high fever, severe cough and fatigue. Early in the illness, the cough is likely to be unproductive or productive of small amounts of whitish sputum. Radiography reveals diffuse or patchy infiltration with a peribronchial distribution.

Therapeutic and Nursing Care Management

The prognosis is generally good, although viral infections of the respiratory tract render the affected child more susceptible to secondary bacterial invasion. Treatment is usually symptomatic and includes measures to promote oxygenation and comfort, such as humidified oxygen administration, chest percussion and postural drainage, antipyretics for fever management, monitoring fluid intake and family support.

Primary Atypical Pneumonia

Atypical pneumonia refers to pneumonia that is caused by pathogens other than the traditionally most common and readily cultured bacteria (e.g. *S. pneumoniae*). In the category of atypical pneumonias, *M. pneumoniae* is the most common bacterial pathogen of **community-acquired pneumonia** in school-aged children (ACI 2018b). Community-acquired methicillin-resistant *Staphylococcus aureus* (CA-MRSA) has become prevalent in certain areas. Community-acquired pneumonia occurs principally in the autumn and winter months and is more prevalent in crowded living conditions. Most affected persons recover from acute illness at home in 7 to 10 days with symptomatic treatment, followed by 1 week of convalescence. The incubation period is 2 to 3 weeks, but the cough may last several weeks.

Clinical Manifestations

The onset may be sudden or insidious and is usually accompanied by general systemic symptoms, including fever, chills (in older children), headache, malaise, anorexia and muscle pain (myalgia). These symptoms are followed by rhinitis, sore throat and a dry, hacking cough. The cough, initially non-productive, produces seromucoid sputum that later becomes mucopurulent or blood streaked. The degree of fever varies widely, from several days to 2 weeks. Dyspnoea occurs infrequently.

Chest imaging reveals evidence of pneumonia before physical signs are apparent. There may be fine crepitant crackles over various areas of the lung fields, but consolidation is usually not demonstrated. The pathological process consists of interstitial round cell infiltration and oedema of alveolar septa and varying distribution of areas of inflammation, necrosis and ulceration of the mucosal lining of bronchi and bronchioles. Areas of consolidation and emphysema are present.

Therapeutic and Nursing Care Management

Most affected persons recover from acute illness in 7 to 10 days with symptomatic treatment, followed by a week of convalescence. Hospitalisation is rarely necessary. Erythromycin, azithromycin and clarithromycin are the primary oral antibiotics used for treating atypical pneumonia.

Bacterial Pneumonia

Bacterial pneumonia is often a serious infection. The pathogenetic mechanisms involved are often aspiration or haematogenous dissemination. The cause varies, depending on the child's age, underlying illness and degree of immunosuppression or immunocompetence.

Aetiology and Epidemiology

S. pneumoniae is the most common bacterial pathogen responsible for community-acquired pneumonia in both children and adults. Other bacteria that cause pneumonia in children are group A streptococci, *S. aureus*, *M. catarrhalis*, *M. pneumoniae* and *C. pneumoniae*.

Beyond the neonatal period, bacterial pneumonias display distinct clinical patterns that facilitate their differentiation from other forms of pneumonia. The onset of illness is abrupt and generally follows a viral infection that disturbs the natural defence mechanisms of the upper respiratory tract. In the 3-month to 5-year age group, *S. pneumoniae*, *M. catarrhalis* and group A streptococci are common causes. *H. influenzae* type B is causing fewer infections because of the Hib vaccine. *S. aureus* pneumonia is also now rarely seen in infants and toddlers.

Clinical Manifestations

The child with bacterial pneumonia usually appears ill. Symptoms include fever, malaise, rapid and shallow respirations, cough and chest pain. The older child may complain of headache, chills, abdominal pain, chest pain or meningeal symptoms (**meningism**) (Box 26.8). Respiratory distress may or may not be present. In some cases the only finding is an increased respiratory rate. The pain of pneumonia may be referred to the abdomen and confused with appendicitis.

BOX 26.8 General Signs of Pneumonia

Fever—Usually quite high
Respiratory signs
- Cough: unproductive to productive with whitish sputum
- Tachypnoea
- Breath sounds: rhonchi or fine crackles
- Dullness with percussion
- Chest pain
- Recession
- Nasal flaring
- Pallor to cyanosis (depends on severity)

Chest x-ray—Diffuse or patchy infiltration, with peribronchial distribution
Behaviour—Irritable, restless, lethargic
Gastrointestinal signs—Anorexia, vomiting, diarrhoea, abdominal pain

Infants and young children develop more severe symptoms than older children. Cyanosis and apnoea are common, and the parent may report the infant's activity and eating pattern was decreased for a few days. Additional clinical manifestations in infants include abrupt fever, vomiting, diarrhoea and abdominal distention. Because pneumonia in newborns carries a high morbidity and mortality rate, bacterial infection should be suspected in all neonates with respiratory symptoms.

Initially, the cough is usually hacking and non-productive, and breath sounds are diminished or heard as scattered crackles. When consolidation is present, breath sounds may be tubular in quality with no adventitious noises. As the infection resolves, coarse crackles and wheezing are heard, and the cough becomes productive with purulent sputum.

Staphylococcal pneumonia is rare but particularly progressive and must be treated aggressively. The onset is rapid, with rapid deterioration. Conjunctivitis and furuncles are signs of a probable staphylococcal infection.

Diagnostic Evaluation

The key to a preliminary diagnosis is finding pulmonary infiltrates on chest imaging, usually revealing lobar consolidation and, in some severe cases, pleural effusion. Laboratory studies include Gram stain and culture of sputum in older children, nasopharyngeal specimens, blood cultures and, on occasion, lung aspiration and biopsy. The white blood cell count may be elevated, but it may be normal for infants with staphylococcal disease. Children with streptococcal disease usually have an elevated antistreptolysin O titre. The infant or child with recurrent pneumonia should be further evaluated for CF or an immunodeficiency disease. Diagnostic evaluation should include ruling out aspiration pneumonia as a potential cause.

Therapeutic Management

Antimicrobial therapy has significantly reduced the morbidity and mortality from bacterial pneumonia (see Fig 26.6).

Most older children with pneumonia can be treated at home, especially if the condition is recognised and treatment initiated early. Antibiotic therapy, rest, liberal oral intake of fluids and administration of antipyretics for fever are the principal therapeutic measures. Hospitalisation is indicated when **pleural effusion** or **empyema** accompanies the disease, when compliance with therapy is estimated to be poor, when there are chronic illnesses such as congenital heart disease or bronchopulmonary dysplasia, and it may be indicated in infants less than 3 months old. Other indicators for hospitalisation include dehydration, respiratory distress (moderate to severe), hypoxaemia, failure of outpatient therapy or the presence of secondary comorbidities that generally result in a more severe infection (immunocompromised, cardiac disease, pulmonary disease).

Prognosis

The prognosis for pneumonia is generally good, with rapid recovery when it is recognised and treated early. The course of staphylococcal pneumonia is generally prolonged. The prognosis varies with the length of the illness before treatment, although early recognition and treatment are usually beneficial.

Prevention

In Australia and New Zealand the use of the pneumococcal conjugate vaccine is recommended for infants and children as part of the national immunisation program schedules for both Indigenous and non-Indigenous infants and children (AGDH 2020, Ministry of Health 2020b). (See Immunisations, Chapter 6.)

Complications. At present the classic features and clinical course of pneumonia are rarely seen because of early and vigorous antibiotic and supportive therapy. However, some children, especially infants, with staphylococcal pneumonia develop empyema, pyopneumothorax or tension pneumothorax (Fig 26.7). AOM and pleural effusion are common in children with pneumococcal pneumonia (Box 26.9).

When fluid is either suspected or identified by x-ray in the pleural cavity, a needle aspiration or thoracentesis may be performed. Non-purulent effusions do not require surgical drainage.

In metropolitan hospitals (not most rural/remote settings), continuous closed chest drainage may be instituted with a complicated pleural effusion. Closed drainage is continued until drainage fluid is free of pathogens, which rarely requires more than 5 to 7 days. If a large amount of purulent drainage is obtained, an appropriate antibiotic can be instilled into the pleural space; chest drainage is stopped for about an hour after instillation. Rarely, a thoracotomy with debridement of infected lung tissue is needed.

Additional therapies for empyema may involve instillation of intrapleural fibrinolytics such as urokinase or streptokinase or video-assisted thoracoscopy (SA Health 2019, Voss et al 2017). These may preclude the need for open debridement and thoracotomy.

Thoracentesis. Dyspnoea resulting from pressure from fluid accumulation in the pleural cavity requires removal by thoracentesis. Thoracentesis involves insertion of a needle percutaneously into the pleural space to remove pleural fluid and can be performed to obtain fluid for culture or to instil antibiotics directly into the pleural cavity. Adequate pain management is imperative.

Nursing Care Management

Nursing care of the child with pneumonia is primarily supportive and symptomatic but necessitates thorough respiratory assessment and administration of supplemental oxygen (as required) and antibiotics. The child's respiratory rate and effort, oxygenation, general disposition and level of activity are frequently assessed. To prevent dehydration, fluids are frequently administered intravenously during the acute phase. A nasogastric tube may be placed to provide hydration and antibiotics if oral intake is poor and if there is no IV access.

Nursing care of the child with a chest tube requires close attention to respiratory status, as noted previously. The chest tube and drainage device used are monitored for proper function (i.e. drainage is not impeded, vacuum setting is correct, tubing is free of kinks, dressing covering chest tube insertion site is intact, water seal is maintained [if used], drainage tube is below the chest tube entry site and chest tube remains in place). Movement in bed and ambulation with a chest tube

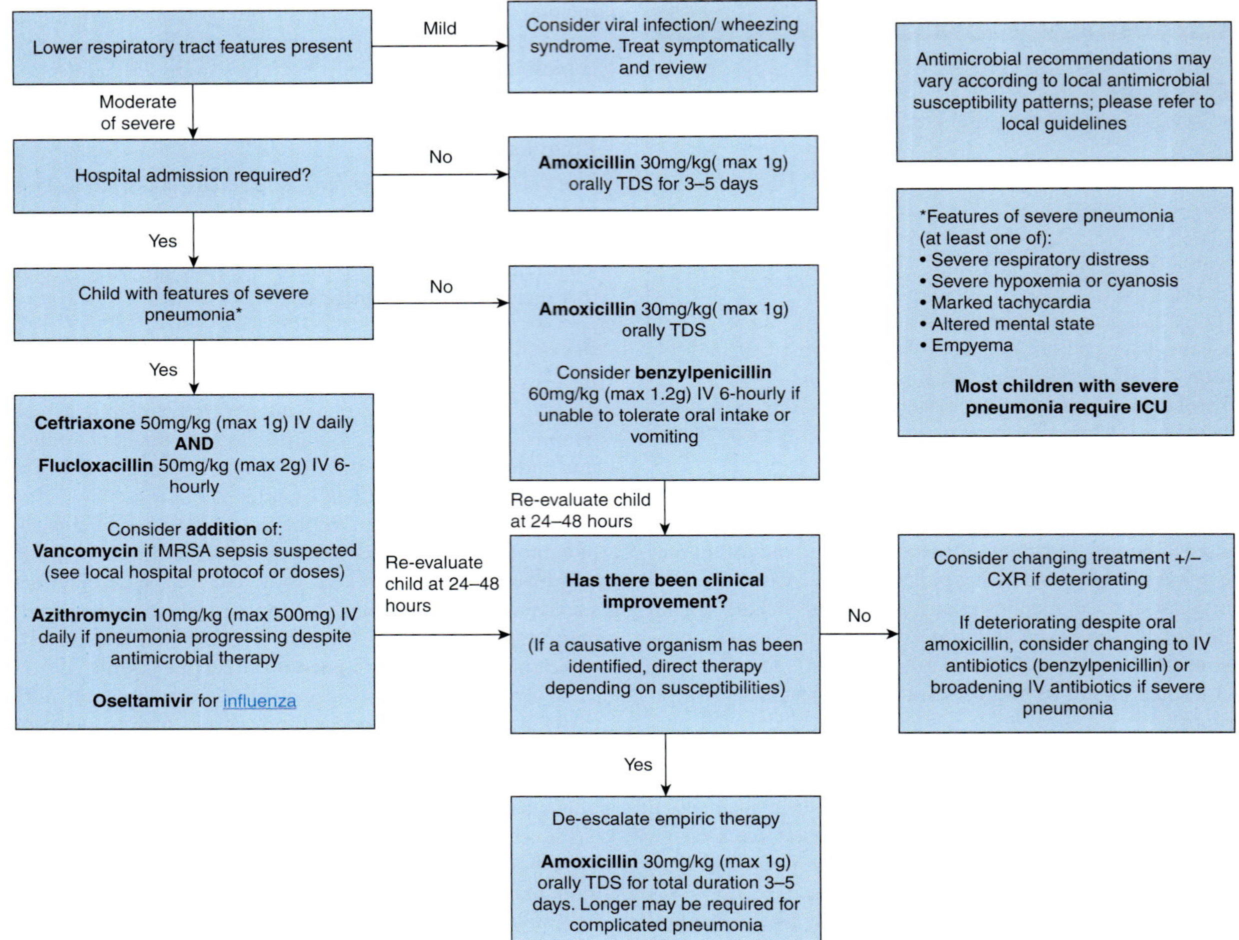

Fig 26.6 Flow chart for treatment of community-acquired pneumonia. (Source: The Royal Children's Hospital Melbourne (RCHM) (2020). Community-acquired pneumonia. Clinical Practice Guidelines. February. Retrieved from: https://www.rch.org.au/clinicalguide/guideline_index/Community_acquired_pneumonia/)

are encouraged according to the child's respiratory status, but children require frequent doses of analgesics such as paracetamol and ibuprofen because having a chest tube in place can be painful.

If needed, supplemental oxygen may be administered by nasal cannula/prongs, face mask or blow-over. Children are usually more comfortable in a semi-erect position but should be allowed to determine the position of comfort. Lying on the affected side ('good lung up') splints the chest on that side and reduces pleural rubbing that often causes discomfort. Fever is controlled by cooling the environment and administering antipyretic drugs as prescribed.

Vital signs and oxygenation are monitored to assess the progress of the disease and to detect early signs of complications. Children with ineffectual cough or those with difficulty handling secretions, especially infants, may require suctioning to maintain a patent airway. Older children can usually handle secretions without assistance. Postural drainage, chest percussion and nebulised bronchodilator therapy may be prescribed, depending on the child's condition. However, there is a lack of empirical support about the benefit of chest percussion in children with community-acquired pneumonia.

The nurse educates the family about observing for worsening symptoms, completing antibiotic therapy if prescribed, using antipyretics, encouraging oral fluids and not being concerned if the child has a poor appetite for a few days.

Neonatal Pneumonia

Pneumonia in the immediate neonatal period is different from other types of pneumonia described. If infection occurs within 3 to 5 days of birth, the pathogen is usually obtained from the mother transplacentally, or through aspiration of infected amniotic fluid intrauterine, or during or after birth. Group B haemolytic streptococcus may be present in the mother's vagina and asymptomatic but can cause a serious pneumonia to a newborn.

C. trachomatis, an intracellular microorganism similar to gram-negative bacteria, is responsible for one of the most common sexually transmitted infections. Chlamydial pneumonia is usually an afebrile illness; infants often become symptomatic before 8 weeks of age. It is characterised by a persistent cough, tachypnoea and sometimes rales. Imaging shows non-specific abnormalities. Oral azithromycin given for 3 days is the treatment of choice; alternatively, erythromycin base or ethylsuccinate is administered for 14 days (Batteiger & Tan 2020, John Hunter Children's Hospital 2018).

Herpes simplex virus (HSV) may also be transmitted at the time of birth and can result in fatal pneumonia (Speer 2017). Other viral or fungal infections can be transmitted intrauterine. Early symptoms of neonatal pneumonia can be non-specific but may include respiratory distress. IV aciclovir is started if HSV infection is suspected. A 10- to 14-day treatment course is usually indicated (Speer 2017).

PATHOPHYSIOLOGY REVIEW

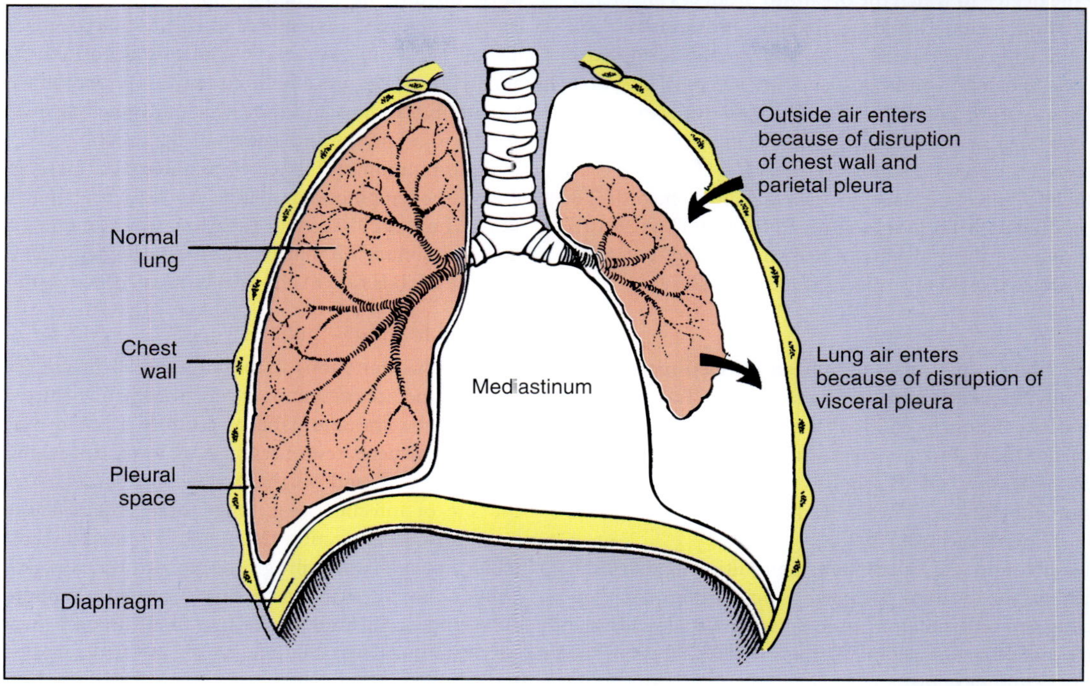

Fig 26.7 Pneumothorax. Air in the pleural space causes the lung to collapse around the hilus and may push mediastinal contents (heart and great vessels) towards the other lung. (Source: McDonald, V.M., Maltby, S. & Penola, D. (2019). Alterations of pulmonary function across the life span. In Understanding Pathophysiology, ANZ Edition (3rd ed.), Elsevier.)

BOX 26.9 Pneumothorax

Pneumothorax occurs when air accumulates in the pleural space; this air increases intrapleural pressure, making it more difficult to expand the affected lung. This leads to the clinical manifestations of chest pain, dyspnoea and often back pain, laboured respirations, tachycardia and decreased oxygen saturation. In neonates and infants on mechanical ventilation the first clinical signs of a pneumothorax are oxygen desaturation and hypotension. The three major types of pneumothorax are tension, spontaneous and traumatic. The definitive diagnosis of pneumothorax is a chest imaging. The emergent treatment involves needle aspiration of the air within the pleural space; subsequently a chest tube to closed drainage is usually inserted to prevent the reaccumulation of air.

Pleural effusion occurs when there is an excessive accumulation of fluid in the pleural space. The diagnosis is made by chest imaging, and the treatment involves evacuation of the fluid by needle aspiration followed by insertion of a chest tube to closed drainage.

OTHER INFECTIONS OF THE RESPIRATORY TRACT

Pertussis (Whooping Cough)

Pertussis, or whooping cough, is an acute respiratory tract infection caused by *Bordetella pertussis* that occurs primarily in children younger than 4 years of age who have not been immunised. It is highly contagious and is particularly threatening in young infants, who have a higher morbidity and mortality rate. Infants less than 6 months of age may not come in to the practitioner with the typical cough; in this age group, apnoea is a common presenting manifestation. Likewise, older children often manifest the disease with a persistent cough and the absence of the characteristic whoop. (See Table 6.2 for signs, symptoms and management of pertussis.) It presents as a URTI, and cough symptoms develop. The cough can be mild but is generally more severe in unimmunised children. It persists 6 to 10 weeks and can result in encephalopathy, seizures, pneumonia, rib fractures (adolescents), bleeding into the conjunctiva or even death (infants). The incubation period is 7 to 10 days but can be as long as 21 days (SCHN 2016b). The incidence is highest in the summer and autumn months, and a single attack confers lifetime immunity.

Pertussis is diagnosed via culture or polymerase chain reaction assay using nasopharyngeal secretions. Most children can be cared for at home on oral antibiotics (e.g. azithromycin, clarithromycin). Antibiotics in the early stage may result in a milder form of the infection, but they also limit its spread to others. Household members, high-risk individuals (immunodeficiency, pregnancy, chronic lung conditions, infants or those who care for infants) and close contacts (within 1 m of a person who has symptoms) may be treated to prevent them from developing the infection (SCHN 2016b).

Tuberculosis

Tuberculosis (TB) infections and mortality from TB have been declining since 1990 (WHO 2017). However, it is one of the leading causes of death worldwide. In 2015 approximately 1 million children developed TB infection and 170,000 children died from the disease (WHO 2017). In Australia and New Zealand, the incidence of TB is low, with the majority of cases occurring in overseas-born people; New South Wales has the highest number of cases (Al Yazid et al 2019).

Aetiology

TB is caused by *Mycobacterium tuberculosis*, an acid-fast bacillus not readily decolourised by acids after staining. Children are susceptible to the human *(M. tuberculosis)* and the bovine *(Mycobacterium bovis)* organisms.

Although the causative agent for TB is the tubercle bacillus, other factors influence the degree to which the organism produces an altered state in the host. These include heredity, malnutrition, immunodeficiency (HIV, immunosuppressive medications), intravenous drug/alcohol abuse, smoking, medical conditions and intercurrent infection (World Health Organization [WHO] 2019). The risk is increased for individuals who are born in another country, have a parent who was born in another country or who use tobacco (WHO 2017).

Children with HIV infection have an increased incidence of TB disease, and all children with TB should be tested for HIV (Box 26.10). TB is the leading cause of the mortality of persons infected with HIV. All contacts of an affected child are examined for the disease.

Pathophysiology

The source of infection in children is usually an infected member of the household or any frequent visitor to the household. Transmission of *M. tuberculosis* occurs when the child inhales microdroplets (usually 1 to 5 mm in size) into the respiratory tract after someone has coughed or sneezed. When the *M. tuberculosis* droplet is inhaled, it passes down the bronchial tree, implants in either a bronchiole or alveolus and starts to multiply (Ellner & Jacobson 2020).

Epithelial cells surround and encapsulate the multiplying bacilli in an attempt to ward off the invading organisms, thus forming the typical tubercle. During the inflammatory process, some bacilli leave the focal area and are carried to the regional lymph nodes that drain the area; as a result, the child develops a fever. The tuberculin skin test is positive, and chest imaging findings may or may not be evident.

Extension of the primary lesion at the original site causes progressive tissue destruction as it spreads within the lung, discharges material from foci to other areas of the lungs (e.g. bronchi or pleura) or produces pneumonia. Erosion of blood vessels by the primary lesion can cause widespread dissemination of the tubercle bacillus to near and distant sites (miliary TB). Organisms deposited in the upper lung zones, bones, kidneys and brain may find favourable environments for growth, but organs and tissue such as bone marrow, liver and spleen appear to inhibit multiplication of the bacilli.

Extrapulmonary TB may be manifested as meningitis or inflammation of the lymph nodes, middle ear, mastoid, bones, joints and on the skin (Thomas 2017). With the exception of meningitis, treatment for extrapulmonary TB may be the same drug regimen as for pulmonary TB. Renal TB is rare in children but may occur in adolescents.

BOX 26.10 Factors Affecting Resistance to Tuberculosis

Heredity

- No evidence of hereditary tendency
- Evidence that resistance to infection may be genetically transmitted

Age

- Diminished resistance to infection in infancy
    - Delay in development of acquired immunity
    - Diminished capacity to resist extension of infective process
- Increased tendency to develop disease during puberty and adolescence
    - New infection superimposed on a previous one
    - Increased contacts
    - Indigenous reinfection stimulated by metabolic changes or suboptimum diets during a period of rapid growth

Stress States

- Temporary stressful circumstances (e.g. injury or illness, malnutrition, emotional distress, chronic fatigue) increasing susceptibility to infection
- Increased secretion of adrenal steroids suppressing protective inflammatory response and permitting infection to spread
- Therapeutic administration of corticosteroids (similar effect)

Nutrition

- Active disease inversely proportional to state of nutrition
- Excellent nutrition essential to young children's recovery from disease

Intercurrent Infection

- Infectious diseases (especially human immunodeficiency virus, measles, pertussis) activating latent tuberculosis
- Non-compliance with therapy

Clinical Manifestations

Clinical manifestations of pulmonary TB in children are extremely variable and are present in approximately one-third of cases. The disease may be asymptomatic or produce a broad range of symptoms, including general responses such as fever, cough, night sweats, chills, delayed growth and weight loss or more specific symptoms related to the site of infection (e.g. lungs, bone, brain, kidneys) within 1 to 6 months after infection (WHO 2019). Lung disease may or may not include cough (which progresses slowly over weeks to months), aching pain and tightness in the chest and (rarely) haemoptysis.

As increasing amounts of lung tissue become involved, the respiratory rate increases, the lung on the affected side does not expand as well as the other, auscultation reveals diminished breath sounds and crackles, and there is dullness to percussion. In children (usually infants) who are unable to contain the spread of infection, the fever persists; the generalised symptoms are present; and the patient develops pallor, anaemia, weakness and weight loss.

Diagnostic Evaluation

Diagnosis is based on information derived from physical examination, history, reaction to a tuberculin test, organism cultures and radiographic examinations. In addition, it must be determined whether the lesion is in the active, quiescent or healed stage.

In Australia and New Zealand, screening programs focus on contacts of notified cases and people at risk of TB infection (i.e. refugees, some Aboriginal and Torres Strait Islander/M ori communities etc.) (ATAGI 2020, Ministry of Health 2020a).

The Xpert MTB/RIF rapid molecular test performed on sputum is used to diagnose TB and determine Rifampin resistance. Results are available in less than 2 hours, and are endorsed by the WHO. The test is a nucleic acid amplification that can diagnose multidrug resistant TB (WHO 2019) Reporting of confirmed cases of TB is mandatory in both Australia and New Zealand.

Tuberculin Skin Test. The **tuberculin skin test (TST)** is the most common test used to determine whether a child has been infected with the tubercle bacillus. A primary infection initiates a hypersensitivity reaction to the protein fraction of the tubercle bacillus, which can be detected 2 to 10 weeks after the infection. Bacille Calmette-Guerin (BCG) immunisation can result in a positive TST. The TST should not take place within 6 weeks of administration of a live vaccine (e.g. MMR 11) (RCHM 2018e).

The tuberculin is injected intradermally in the volar or dorsal aspect of the forearm. A wheal 6 to 10 mm in diameter should form between the layers of the skin when the solution is injected properly. If the wheal does not form, the procedure is repeated. The reaction to the skin test is determined in 48 to 72 hours; reactions occurring after 72 hours should be measured and considered to be the result. The size of the transverse diameter of induration, not the erythema, is measured.

A positive TST reaction indicates that the person has been infected and has developed sensitivity to the protein of the tubercle bacillus; it does not, however, confirm the presence of active disease. Once individuals react positively, they will always react positively. Any negative reaction does not exclude active disease because false negatives can occur due to immunosuppression or certain medications. A clinical examination and a chest x-ray are recommended if the child has a positive TST reaction.

A negative reaction does not exclude the presence of latent tuberculosis infection or active disease. Children with immunosuppression, concurrent viral infection (e.g. measles, varicella, influenza), HIV, disseminated TB disease and recent TB infection may have decreased TST reactivity. Several factors can produce false-negative results. Prompt radiographic evaluation of all children with a positive TST is recommended.

A finding of **latent tuberculosis infection (LTBI)** indicates infection in a person who has a positive TST, no physical findings of disease and normal chest imaging findings. A diagnosis of LTBI or TB disease in a young child represents a public health sentinel event indicating recent transmission of the *M. tuberculosis* organism (RCHM 2018e) The term *tuberculosis disease* is used when a child has clinical symptoms or imaging manifestations caused by the *M. tuberculosis* organism.

Bacteriological Examination. A definitive diagnosis is made by demonstrating the presence of mycobacteria in culture. The organism is identified from microscopic examination of properly prepared and stained smears from early-morning gastric washings or from sputum, pleural fluid, urine, spinal fluid, draining lymph nodes and other body fluids. Induced sputum and gastric lavage sputum specimens are often obtained for culture from children who are unable to expectorate a sputum specimen.

Immunological Testing. The QuantiFERON-TB Gold and T-SPOT TB are tests of interferon quantification (interferon gamma release assay [IGRA]). They are not recommended as first-line screening in younger children; however, they may be performed on asymptomatic children (RCHM 2018e). These tests cannot determine latent infection but children with a positive IGRA test are considered to be infected with the *M. tuberculosis* bacterium.

Radiographic Studies. Imaging may be normal or may show lymphadenopathy, pleural effusion or cavitary TB. However, the lesions of numerous chronic intrathoracic diseases resemble tuberculous lesions; therefore, chest radiography is not diagnostic by itself.

Therapeutic Management

Medical management of tuberculous lesions in children consists of adequate nutrition, antimicrobial therapy, general supportive measures, prevention of unnecessary exposure to other infections that further compromise the body's defences, prevention of reinfection and sometimes surgical procedures.

A child with LTBI is treated with antimicrobial drugs to decrease the risk of acquiring active TB disease in the years after the initial acquisition and to reduce the lifelong chance of developing TB disease. The recommended drug regimen for LTBI in children and adolescents includes a daily dose of isoniazid for 6 months (10 mg/kg, maximum 300 mg) daily. Isoniazid is usually well tolerated in children. If intolerant to isoniazid-Rifampicin (10 mg/kg, maximum 600 mg) daily can be given for 4 months OR Rifampicin and isoniazid daily for 3 months (RCHM 2018e).

Pulmonary and Extrapulmonary Tuberculosis. For the child with clinically active pulmonary and extrapulmonary TB, the goal is to achieve sterilisation of the tuberculous lesion. A combination of isoniazid, pyrazinamide, rifampicin and ethambutol daily or twice weekly for 2 months is recommended, followed by isoniazid and rifampicin for 4 months. Intermittent medication regimens (i.e. 3 times per week) may be considered after the initial 2 months of treatment (Daniel et al 2019). Alternative treatment regimens may be used when managed by a TB specialist.

Tuberculosis Meningitis. The same antimicrobial medications are used in the treatment of TB meningitis, but the duration is different. For *M. tuberculosis,* a 2-month treatment with isoniazid, pyrazinamide, rifampicin and ethionamide or ethambutol daily, followed by a 10-month course of isoniazid and rifampicin, 12 months in total, is recommended. The duration of therapy is also longer for patients who have HIV infection or who have cavitary lesions or positive sputum analysis after 2 months of antimicrobial therapy (Daniel et al 2019).

When drug resistance is suspected, other antimicrobials are added to the therapeutic regimen until drug susceptibility results are available. It is not within the scope of this text to outline the treatment regimen for multiple drug–resistant and extensively drug–resistant TB.

Surgical procedures may be required to remove the source of infection in tissues that are inaccessible to antimicrobial therapy or that are destroyed by the disease. Orthopaedic procedures for correction of bone deformities, bronchoscopy for removal of a tuberculous granulomatous polyp or resection of a portion of a diseased lung may also be performed.

Prognosis. Most children recover from primary TB infection and may be unaware of its presence. However, very young children have a higher incidence of disseminated disease. It is a serious disease during the first 2 years of life and in children infected with HIV. Except in cases of tuberculous meningitis, death seldom occurs in treated children. Antibiotic therapy has decreased mortality and haematogenous spread from primary lesions.

Prevention. The only certain means to prevent TB is to avoid contact with the tubercle bacillus. Maintaining an optimum state of health with adequate nutrition and avoiding debilitating infections promote natural resistance but do not prevent infection.

Pasteurisation of milk and routine testing and elimination of diseased cattle have helped to eradicate/decrease bovine TB, in Australia and New Zealand. Infants and children should be given only pasteurised milk from TB-free cattle.

A source of concern is that the infected child or family members may spread the disease when visiting in the hospital. Most children with TB, especially under 10 years of age, are not contagious and can be hospitalised on an open unit if they are receiving therapy. Children with no cough and a negative sputum smear can also be cared for without isolation. Children and adolescents with infectious pulmonary TB (i.e. those whose sputum smears show acid-fast bacilli) should be on isolation precautions until effective therapy has been initiated, their sputum smears show a diminishing number of organisms and their cough is improving. Ideally, they should be cared for in an airborne isolation (negative pressure) room (Australian Government, National Health and Medical Research Council 2019). Staff should be fitted for appropriately sized P-2 or higher-level particulate-filtering respirator.

Masks are indicated when children are coughing and not reliably covering their mouths. Family members should be managed with airborne precautions when visiting until they are demonstrated not to have infectious TB.

Limited immunity can be produced by administration of BCG. The freshly prepared vaccine, injected intradermally, produces definite, although incomplete, protection against TB (ranging from 50% to 80%). In most instances, positive tuberculin reactions develop after inoculation. The BCG is a very painful vaccination.

Nursing Care Management

Hospitalisation for TB is seldom necessary. Only children with the more serious forms of the disease are placed in the hospital. The major nursing care of children with TB involves nurses in ambulatory settings: outpatient departments, schools and community health services.

Asymptomatic children can lead an essentially unrestricted life. They can and should attend school (or day care) once they have started therapy and clinical symptoms have been reduced. Older children are restricted from vigorous activities such as competitive games and contact sports during the active stage of primary TB. They should also continue the regular immunisation schedule and maintain optimum health with proper diet, adequate rest and avoidance of infection. Nurses assume several roles in management of the disease, including helping the family understand the rationale for diagnostic procedures, assisting with radiology examinations, performing and interpreting skin tests correctly (potentially not performed by nurses at every facility), obtaining specimens for laboratory examination and educating about the antimicrobial regimen.

Sputum specimens are difficult or impossible to obtain from an infant or young child because they swallow any mucus coughed from the lower respiratory tract. The best means for obtaining material for smears or culture is by gastric washing (i.e. aspiration of lavaged contents from the fasting stomach with a nasogastric tube). The procedure is carried out and the specimen obtained early in the morning before the customary breakfast time.

Ambulatory Care. Nursing supervision of the child at home involves teaching the parents and child about the disease and its ramifications. Historically the disease has been regarded with fear, and numerous misconceptions need to be addressed. Reducing parental anxieties helps them deal with the illness more constructively and collaborate more effectively in planning the child's continued care. Because the success of therapy depends on compliance with drug therapy, instruct the parents regarding the importance of giving the medication as often and as long as it is ordered. (See Compliance, Chapter 22.) Promoting optimum general health and preventing intercurrent infections and reinfections with the tubercle bacillus are important.

Case Finding. Case finding and follow-up of known contacts are important, and TB cases are notifiable diseases in Australia and New Zealand (AGDH 2020, Ministry of Health 2020a). Every case of TB identified in the community involves nurses in follow-up of known contacts—individuals from whom the affected person may have acquired the disease and persons who may have been exposed to the diseased individual. Early diagnosis affords a means for early protection or treatment and prevents further spread of the disease.

RESPIRATORY DISTURBANCE CAUSED BY NON-INFECTIOUS IRRITANTS

Foreign Body Ingestion and Aspiration

Foreign body (FB) aspiration is a life-threatening event due to potential airway obstruction and inability to adequately oxygenate the body. Small children characteristically explore objects with their hands and mouth and are prone to place FBs into the air passages (nose and mouth). They also place objects such as beads, paper clips, plastic toys, small magnets or food items in the nose or mouth, which can easily be aspirated into the trachea. Small items may also be placed into the external ear canal (i.e. small rocks, pebbles, beads, etc.).

When such objects are placed into the nose or mouth, they can be aspirated into the airway, causing subsequent obstruction. Ingestion or aspiration of an FB can occur at any age but is most common in older infants and children ages 1 to 3 years. Severity depends on the location, type of object aspirated and extent of obstruction. For example, dry vegetable matter, such as a seed, nut, piece of carrot or popcorn, that does not dissolve and that may swell when moistened creates a particularly difficult problem. The high fat content of potato chips and peanuts may cause the added risk of lipoid pneumonia. 'Fun foods' such as hard lollies and hot dogs are among the worst offenders. Offending foods include nuts, hot dogs, round lollies, peanuts and other types of nuts, grapes, biscuits, pieces of meat, carrots, apples, peas, celery, popcorn, fruit and vegetable seeds, cherry pits, chewing gum and peanut butter. Round foods are the most frequent offenders. Other items include plastic or glass beads, button or disc batteries, burst latex balloons, pen or marker caps and coins. Objects such as small lithium or cadmium batteries may cause oesophageal or tracheal corrosion. Magnets can trap tissue/mucosa in between them, which can result in necrosis of that area. Aspiration of certain medications can cause inflammation and stenosis.

A sharp or irritating object produces irritation and oedema. A round, pliable object that does not readily break apart is more likely to occlude an airway than an object with a different shape. A small object may cause little if any pathological change, whereas an object of sufficient size to obstruct a passage can produce various changes, including atelectasis, emphysema, inflammation and abscess.

Pathophysiology

Most inhaled FBs lodge in a mainstem or lobar bronchus, a few find their way into more distal portions of the lung field and the remaining FBs lodge in the trachea. They also may shift over time so symptoms can change. The site is determined by the object's size, weight and configuration. For example, heavy objects such as bullets, coins and nails are more likely to drop into the dependent portions of the tracheobronchial tree. The object may remain in the same location or move in the airway. It can be coughed from a smaller to a larger airway and reaspirated in a different passage—or it might be ejected forcefully into the mouth and subsequently swallowed.

Signs of obstruction caused by an FB in a bronchus are explained by the same mechanisms that control the flow of fluids in pipes (Fig 26.8). During normal respiration the calibre of bronchi and bronchioles becomes larger during inspiration and smaller during expiration. When a small object partially obstructs a passage, air passes around the obstruction during both inspiration and expiration (bypass valve). In this type of obstruction a wheeze is heard. A somewhat larger obstruction will allow air to enter the distal portion when bronchioles enlarge during inspiration, but when they diminish in calibre during expiration, the lumen becomes occluded and air becomes trapped distal to the obstruction (check valve). This type of obstruction produces obstructive hyperinflation. When there is complete blockage of the bronchus by an FB or by the FB and swollen mucosa, air is unable to move in either direction (stop valve) and the air distal to the obstruction is absorbed, leaving an area of obstruction atelectasis. The right bronchus, with its shorter length and straighter angle, is the usual site of bronchial obstruction.

Clinical Manifestations

Initially, a FB in the air passages produces choking, gagging or coughing, but symptoms depend on the site of obstruction and on the interval between aspiration and presentation. Up to half of all children with FB ingestion may be asymptomatic. Laryngotracheal obstruction most commonly causes dyspnoea, cough, stridor and hoarseness because of a decreased air entry. Cyanosis may also occur if the obstruction becomes worse. Bronchial obstruction usually produces cough (frequently paroxysmal), wheezing, asymmetric breath sounds, decreased

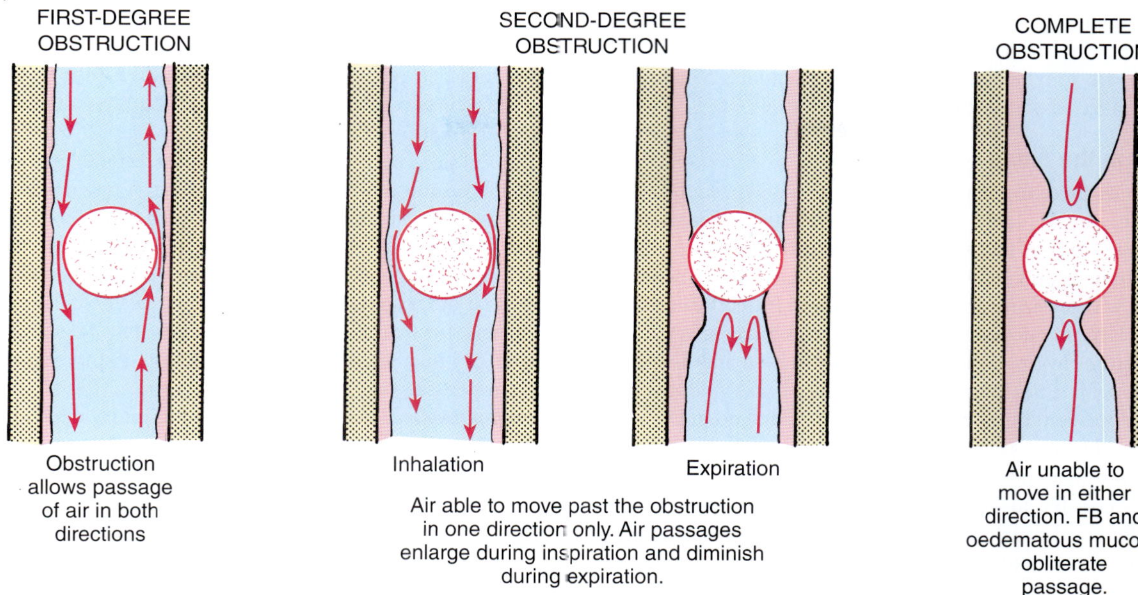

Fig 26.8 Mechanisms of airway obstruction by foreign body.

airway entry and dyspnoea. In some cases, a FB obstruction may be mistaken for croup or asthma.

If the obstruction progresses, the child's face may become livid and sometimes the child becomes unconscious and dies of asphyxiation if the object is not removed. If obstruction is partial, hours, days or even weeks may pass without symptoms after the initial period. Secondary symptoms are related to the anatomic area in which the FB is lodged and are usually caused by a persistent respiratory tract infection located distal to the obstruction. A history of recurrent intractable pneumonia is reason to consider a FB in an airway. Often, by the time secondary symptoms appear, the parents have forgotten the initial episode of coughing and gagging. The most common symptoms observed in children brought to medical attention are stridor, wheezing, sternal recession and cough. When an object is lodged in the larynx, the child is unable to speak or breathe.

Diagnostic Evaluation

The diagnosis of FB obstruction is usually suspected on the basis of the history and physical signs. Imaging reveals opaque FBs but is of limited value in localising vegetable matter and some plastic items. Up to half of children with tracheal foreign bodies have a normal chest x-ray. Bronchoscopy is required for a definitive diagnosis and removal of objects in the larynx and trachea.

Fluoroscopic examination is valuable in detecting FBs in the bronchi. On fluoroscopy, a check-valve–obstructed lung remains expanded, the diaphragm remains low and fixed on the obstructed side and the heart and mediastinum shift to the unobstructed side during expiration. In a stop-valve obstruction, the heart and mediastinum are drawn to the obstructed side and remain there during both inspiration and expiration. The diaphragm on the obstructed side remains high, whereas that on the unobstructed side moves normally.

The mainstay of diagnosis and management of foreign bodies is endoscopy and bronchoscopy. If there is doubt about the presence of a FB, these procedures can be diagnostic and therapeutic.

Therapeutic Management

FB aspiration may result in life-threatening airway obstruction, especially in infants because of the small diameters of their airways. Current recommendations for the emergency treatment of the choking child include the use of back blows and chest thrusts. A FB is rarely coughed up spontaneously; therefore, it must be removed by endoscopy or bronchoscopy. Removal of the FB must be done as soon as possible because the progressive local inflammatory process triggered by the foreign material hampers removal. In addition, a chemical pneumonia soon develops, and vegetable matter begins to macerate within a few days, further complicating its removal.

Nursing Care Management

A major role of nurses is to recognise the signs of FB aspiration and implement immediate measures to relieve the obstruction. All persons working with children should be prepared to deal effectively with aspiration of a FB. Choking on food or other material should not be fatal. Two simple procedures—back blows and chest thrust, which can be used by both health professionals and lay persons—can save lives. It is the nurse's obligation to learn these techniques and teach them to parents and other groups. To aid a child who is choking, nurses need to recognise the signs of distress. Not every child who gags or coughs while eating is truly choking.

NURSING CARE CONSIDERATIONS

The child in distress: (1) cannot speak; (2) becomes cyanotic; and (3) collapses. These three signs indicate that the child is truly choking and requires immediate and quick action. The child can die within 4 minutes. Follow-up care after the FB is removed includes monitoring for respiratory distress and educating the parents.

Prevention

Small children should not be allowed access to small objects that they might place in their nose or mouth. Anticipatory guidance for parents of small children is essential. Nurses are in a position to teach prevention in a variety of settings. They can educate parents singly or in groups about hazards of aspiration in relation to the developmental level of their children and encourage them to teach their children safety. Caution parents about behaviours that their children might imitate (e.g. holding foreign objects, such as pins, nails and toothpicks, in their lips or mouth). Education can also be provided to ancillary health staff, day care providers and babysitters. (Chapters 10 and 12 discuss prevention based on the child's age.)

Foreign Body in the Nose

Children sometimes place foreign objects, such as food (peanuts are a favourite), crayons, small plastic toys, pieces of plastic, beans, beads, erasers, wads of paper, peas and small stones, into their nose. A FB is suspected when there is unilateral nasal discharge that is foul smelling, local obstruction with sneezing, mild discomfort and (rarely) pain. The irritation produces local mucosal swelling if the items increase in size as they absorb moisture (hygroscopic). Signs of obstruction and discomfort may increase with time. Infection usually follows, as evidenced by foul breath and a purulent or bloody discharge from one nostril.

Although the object is usually situated anteriorly, unskilled attempts at removal may move it further posteriorly. Removal should occur as soon as possible to prevent the risk of aspiration and local tissue necrosis. Removal usually occurs easily with forceps, suction or inflation of a balloon catheter behind the obstruction. In some cases mild sedation may be necessary.

NURSING CARE CONSIDERATIONS

Parental report of a small child swallowing an item or placing it into the nose requires careful evaluation of the child's airway, even if the child is asymptomatic. The child may insert an object in the nose that may not be visible, but during play or other activities the object may be aspirated into the trachea, causing obstruction and distress.

Aspiration Pneumonia

Aspiration pneumonia occurs when food, secretions, vomitus, medications, inert materials, volatile compounds, hydrocarbons (e.g. kerosene, petrol, solvents, lighter fluid, furniture polish and mineral oil) or liquids enter the lung and cause inflammation and a chemical pneumonitis. Many conditions increase the risk of aspiration (Box 26.11). Aspiration of fluid or food substances is particularly hazardous in the child who has difficulty swallowing or is unable to swallow because of paralysis, weakness, debility, congenital anomalies such as cleft palate or tracheoesophageal fistula, or absent cough reflex (unconsciousness), or if the child is force-fed, especially while crying or breathing rapidly.

BOX 26.11 Conditions that Increase Risk of Aspiration

Altered Level of Consciousness
- Central nervous system injury or disease (e.g. meningitis, seizures, paralysis, trauma, poisoning, toxic ingestion)
- Sedation
- General anaesthesia

Dysphagia
- Oesophageal dysmotility
- Neurological deficit
- Gastroesophageal reflux

Mechanical Disruption of Defensive Barriers
- Endotracheal tube
- Tracheostomy
- Feeding tube (orogastric or nasogastric)
- Persistent vomiting

Source: Modified from Patient Education: Aspiration Pneumonia, Pediatric. (2020). Elsevier Interactive Patient Education.

Clinical signs of the aspiration of oral secretions may not be distinguishable from other forms of acute bacterial pneumonia. For example, if vegetable matter has been aspirated, manifestations may not appear for several weeks after the event. Classic symptoms include an increasing cough or fever, foul-smelling sputum, deteriorating chest x-rays and other signs of lower airway involvement. These deviations may persist for weeks, while the child starts to feel better. The irritated mucosa can be a site for bacterial infection. Aspiration can result in death from asphyxia.

Pathogenesis. The severity of the lung injury depends on the pH of the aspirated material, the presence of bacteria and the volatility and viscosity of the substance. Irritation from aspiration during swallowing, vomiting or gastric lavage may also cause pulmonary involvement. Pathological changes include: signs of inflammation (e.g. oedema, hyperaemia, infiltration of polymorphonuclear cells); vascular thrombosis and haemorrhage; and necrosis of bronchial, bronchiolar and alveolar tissues. Other reactions are bronchospasm, atelectasis, emphysema, pulmonary haemorrhage, necrosis, surfactant impairment and pulmonary oedema. Aspiration of inert fluids may not produce a chemical or bacterial pneumonia, but these fluids can decrease lung compliance and cause hypoxaemia.

Clinical Manifestations. Acid aspiration may produce immediate pulmonary symptoms that worsen over the first 24 hours. Coughing and vomiting, which occur almost immediately after ingestion, contribute to the aspiration. CNS symptoms include agitation, restlessness, confusion, drowsiness and coma. The temperature is elevated (37.8°C to 40°C).

After swallowing, coughing and choking, the child becomes short of breath, and older children complain of dyspnoea. There are varying degrees of cyanosis, tachycardia, tachypnoea, nasal flaring and recession. Intercostal recession, grunting, cough and fever may appear within 30 minutes or be delayed for a few hours. Localised areas of dullness are felt on percussion, and moderately intense wheezes and crackles are heard. Severe injury causes haemoptysis, pulmonary oedema, severe cyanosis and death within 24 hours of aspiration.

Therapeutic Management. Inducing the child to vomit is contraindicated because of the renewed danger of aspiration. Bronchitis or pneumonia usually develops early (within the first 24 hours) but may be delayed. Recovery from pulmonary involvement occurs in most instances despite a severe clinical course. Treatment is the same as for any lower respiratory tract inflammation and consists of high humidity, supplemental oxygen, hydration and treatment of any secondary infection. Endotracheal intubation may be required if the child develops respiratory failure.

Hydrocarbon Aspiration Pneumonia

Children frequently develop pneumonia secondary to the ingestion of various forms of hydrocarbons (e.g. petrol, motor oil, lamp oil, lighter fluid, mineral spirits), which are commonly found in the home or garages. Petroleum distillates are generally impure substances contaminated with heavy metals or other toxic chemicals that cause systemic, as well as local, effects.

Hydrocarbons are usually packaged in attractive containers, and some have a pleasant aroma; consequently, they are frequently ingested accidentally by young children. On average, children swallow less than 30 mL (often about 3 to 4 mL). They begin coughing severely and do not ingest any more of the contents. Although CNS abnormalities,

GI irritation, cardiomyopathy and renal toxicity can occur, the most serious complication is pneumonitis. Distillates that have high volatility (evaporate quickly), decreased viscosity (thinner solution) and low surface tension are more likely to be aspirated and produce respiratory complications. Decreased viscosity enhances penetration into distal airways. Lower surface tension facilitates spread over a larger area of lung surface. Consequently, ingestion of lighter fluid, kerosene or petrol is more likely to cause a pathological condition than substances that have high viscosity (e.g. petroleum jelly, tar or lubricating oil).

Even in small amounts, hydrocarbons spread over the surface of tissues and the lungs and interfere with gas exchange. They are readily absorbed by the GI tract and excreted by the lungs.

Lipoid Pneumonia

Oily substances aspirated into the respiratory passages initially cause an interstitial proliferative inflammation that may include an exudative pneumonia. The next stage involves a diffuse, chronic, proliferative fibrosis that is often complicated by acute bronchopneumonia. The final stage features multiple localised nodules or tumour-like paraffinomas. There are no characteristic manifestations. Cough is usually present, and dyspnoea occurs in severe cases. Secondary bronchopneumonia is common. The outcome depends on the extent of pulmonary damage, the general condition of the infant or child and discontinuation of the oily inhalation. No specific treatment exists.

Powder Inhalation

A significant number of infants suffer talcum powder aspiration. Commercial talcum powder is predominantly a mixture of talc (hydrous magnesium silicate) and other silicates. Severe respiratory distress occurs immediately as a result of an inflammatory reaction in small bronchioles initiated by deep inhalation of the extremely light powder.

Nursing Care Management

Care of the child with aspiration pneumonia is the same as that described for the child with pneumonia from other causes. However, the major focus of nursing care is on *prevention* of aspiration. Proper feeding techniques should be carried out for weak, debilitated and uncooperative children, and measures should be taken to prevent aspiration of any material that might enter the nasopharynx. Nasogastric tubes used for feedings are checked before the initiation of bolus feedings; continuous nasogastric tube feedings are also evaluated periodically for proper tube placement. The child should be maintained with the head elevated during feeding and for 30 minutes after it, if possible.

Children who are at risk for swallowing difficulties as a result of illness, physical debilitation, anaesthesia or sedation are kept nil-by-mouth until they can properly swallow fluids effectively. An evaluation by an occupational therapist or speech therapist may be indicated to assess ability to swallow effectively. The child who is at risk for vomiting and is incapable of protecting the airway should be positioned in a side-lying position.

Oily nose drops and oil-based medications are not ideal for infants and small children. Solvents, lighter fluid and other hydrocarbon substances should be kept away from older infants and small children, who are likely to put anything in their mouth and who may be attracted by the slightly sweet smell. Talcum powder is not necessary for newborn hygiene and should be avoided.

Pulmonary Oedema

Pulmonary oedema (PE) is the movement of excess fluid into the alveoli and interstitium of the lungs caused by extravasation from the pulmonary vasculature (Mazor & Green 2016). It can cause respiratory compromise, which can be life-threatening. The two main types of PE are cardiogenic and non-cardiogenic.

Cardiogenic (hydrostatic, haemodynamic) PE is caused by an increase in pulmonary capillary pressure because of an increase in pulmonary venous pressure. It can be caused by excessive IV fluid administration, renal failure, left ventricular failure, heart valve disorder (e.g. aortic regurgitation, aortic stenosis, mitral regurgitation), myocardial ischaemia, myocarditis, acute tachydysrhythmia or coronary artery disease (Powell et al 2016). Non-cardiogenic PE is caused by various conditions that result in increased pulmonary capillary permeability. Some subtypes of non-cardiogenic PE include permeability PE (caused by ARDS or acute lung injury [ALI]), high-altitude PE (caused by rapid ascension to heights above 3500 metres) or neurogenic PE (after CNS insult, such as seizures, head injury or cerebral haemorrhage). Some less-common forms of PE are: reperfusion PE (after removal of thromboemboli from the lung or a lung transplant); re-expansion PE (caused by rapid re-expansion of a collapsed lung); or PE that results from opiate overdose (methadone or heroin), salicylate toxicity (chronic), aspiration (FB inhalation), inhalation injuries, submersion injury, pulmonary embolism, viral infections or pulmonary veno-occlusive disease. Other causes include traumatic injury, organ dysfunction caused by sepsis, multiorgan failure, alcoholism or substance abuse, pregnancy (eclampsia), chronic renal impairment, malnutrition, hypertension or a blood transfusion (transfusion-related ALI).

Pathophysiology

Fluid flows from the pulmonary vasculature into the alveolar interstitial space and then returns to the systemic circulation in a normal lung. Movement of this fluid is controlled by the net difference between hydrostatic and osmotic pressures and the permeability of the capillary membrane (Mazor & Green 2016). Increased pulmonary hydrostatic pressure or increased permeability of the vascular membrane results in movement of fluid into the alveoli and interstitium of the lung. The pulmonary lymph system normally drains away any fluid from the alveoli, but when the amount of fluid present in the alveoli exceeds lymph drainage, PE occurs.

Symptoms include extreme shortness of breath, cyanosis, tachypnoea, diminished breath sounds, anxiety, agitation, confusion, diaphoresis, orthopnoea, respiratory crackles, expiratory wheezing (in young infants), heart murmur, third heart sound (S_3) gallop, cool peripheries, jugular venous distention, nocturnal dyspnoea, cough, pink frothy sputum (if severe), tachycardia, hypertension or hypotension (if caused by left ventricle dysfunction).

Therapeutic Management

Management of PE depends on the cause but can include oxygen therapy, peak end-expiratory pressure (PEEP) via CPAP, and intubation with ventilatory support if respiratory failure occurs. If ventricular failure is the cause, medications such as diuretics, digoxin, positive inotropes and vasodilators (nitroglycerin) may be started, and the child may be placed on a fluid and sodium restriction. Morphine may be prescribed to relieve dyspnoea. The primary goal of management is to determine why PE occurred and treat the underlying condition.

Nursing Care Management

Nursing care of the child with PE is similar to that for any other acute respiratory condition. Pulse oximetry is monitored, and vital signs are observed closely for any deterioration. The nurse should note changes in SaO_2, $ETCO_2$ and ABG values. An ongoing assessment of the child's cardiopulmonary status is needed by checking lung sounds and observing respiratory rate, rhythm, depth and effort. Oxygen, medications and other respiratory treatments are administered as prescribed. Close monitoring of intake and output, electrolytes and comfort is important. The child should be monitored for restlessness, anxiety and air hunger. Placing the child in a high-Fowler position may help with lung expansion. Because this position places pressure on bony prominences in the sacrum and hips, pressure areas must be relieved at intervals. Most of the care of PE occurs in the ICU, which is anxiety provoking for the child and family. They should be given the opportunity to express their fears and anxieties and to ask questions. (For other nursing care activities, see the following section on ARDS and ALI.)

Acute Respiratory Distress Syndrome and Acute Lung Injury

Acute respiratory distress syndrome (ARDS) and *acute lung injury* (ALI) are potentially life-threatening inflammatory lung conditions that may occur in children and adults. They are caused by direct injury to the lungs or by systemic insults that lead indirectly to lung injury with subsequent hypoxaemia and respiratory failure due to non-cardiogenic pulmonary oedema. Sepsis, trauma, viral pneumonia, aspiration, fat emboli, drug overdose, reperfusion injury after lung transplantation, smoke inhalation and submersion injury, among others, have been associated with ARDS and ALI. Both are characterised by respiratory distress and hypoxaemia that occur within 72 hours of a serious injury or surgery in a person with previously normal lungs. ALI involves a spectrum of inflammatory disease responses to a precipitating event, with ARDS being the more severe form of ALI.

Animation—Bag Ventilation

According to the Pediatric Lung Injury Consensus Conference (PALICC) definition, paediatric acute respiratory distress syndrome (PARDS) occurs within 1 week of a known clinical insult or new or worsening respiratory symptoms; is characterised by bilateral/unilateral opacities on chest imaging not fully explained by effusions, lobar/lung collapse or nodules; and manifests as respiratory failure not fully explained by cardiac failure or fluid overload. Hypoxaemia is expressed using oxygen index (OI) ($FiO_2 \times$ mean airway pressure $\times 100/PaO_2$) and oxygen saturation (OSI) ($FiO_2 \times$ mean airway pressure $\times 100/SpO_2$) (Orloff et al 2019) (see Table 26.5).

Pathologically, the hallmark of PARDS is increased permeability of the alveolar-capillary membrane that results in pulmonary oedema (Fig 26.9). During the acute phase of ARDS, inflammatory mediators cause damage to the membrane, with consequent increase in pulmonary capillary permeability and the development of interstitial oedema. Later stages are characterised by pneumocyte and fibrin infiltration of the alveoli, with the start of either the healing process or fibrosis. When fibrosis occurs, the child may demonstrate respiratory distress and the need for mechanical ventilation. In PARDS, the lungs become stiff as a result of surfactant inactivation; gas diffusion is impaired; and eventually, bronchiolar mucosal swelling and congestive atelectasis occur. The net effect is decreased functional residual capacity, pulmonary hypertension and increased intrapulmonary right-to-left shunting of blood. Surfactant secretion is reduced, and the atelectasis and fluid-filled alveoli provide an excellent medium for bacterial growth. Hypoxaemia or increased work of breathing may require ventilatory support.

The child with PARDS may first demonstrate only symptoms caused by an injury or infection, but as the condition deteriorates, tachypnoea, increasing respiratory effort, cyanosis and decreasing oxygen saturation occur. The hypoxaemia may be refractory to oxygen administration.

TABLE 26.5 PARDS Severity Classification

OI	< 4 with O_2 supplementation required to keep $SpO_2 > 88\%$	$4 \leq 8$	$8 \leq 16$	≥ 16
OSI	< 5 with O_2 supplementation required to keep $SpO_2 > 88\%$	$5 \leq 7.5$	$7.5 \leq 12.3$	≥ 12.3

Source: Orloff, KE, Turner, DA and Rehder, KJ. June 2019. Pediatric Allergy Immunology and Pulmonary. Vol 32, Issue 2, 35-44. Retrieved from: https://www.liebertpub.com/doi/full/10.1089/ped.2019.0999

Therapeutic Management

Treatment involves supportive measures to ensure adequate oxygenation and pulmonary perfusion, treatment of infection (or the precipitating cause), maintenance of adequate cardiac output and vascular volume, hydration, adequate nutritional support, comfort measures, prevention of complications such as GI ulceration and aspiration, and psychological support. Specific treatment should be directed against the underlying cause (e.g. antibiotics and source control for infection).

Definitive therapy is directed towards improvement of oxygenation. The use of endotracheal intubation, PEEP and low tidal volume may be required to ensure maximum oxygen delivery by increasing functional residual capacity, reducing intrapulmonary shunting and reducing pulmonary fluid. Inappropriate use of mechanical ventilation may worsen the lung injury, resulting in volutrauma, barotrauma, atelectrauma and biotrauma to the injured lungs. Ventilation with low tidal volume (6 mL/kg of ideal body weight) has been associated with lower mortality rates in children with ALI (Wong et al 2017). Other supportive strategies include use of the prone position, pharmacological neuromuscular blockade to facilitate ventilation, administration of inhaled nitric oxide or prostaglandins and high-frequency oscillatory ventilation. The evidence to support these therapies is variable and evolving. Extracorporeal membrane oxygenation (ECMO) should be considered in cases of severe ARDS when the cause of respiratory failure is believed to be reversible or if the child is likely to be suitable for consideration for lung transplantation (Orloff et al 2019).

Fluid administration to maintain adequate intravascular volume and end-organ perfusion must be balanced against the desire to decrease lung fluid to improve oxygenation. The provision of adequate nutrition, maintenance of patient comfort and prevention of complications such as GI ulceration are essential. Psychological support of the patient and family is also important.

Prognosis. The prognosis for patients with ARDS is improving. Nonetheless, the mortality rate remains high and is approximately 24% in children (Orloff et al 2019). The precipitating disorder influences the outcome; the worst prognosis is associated with uncontrolled sepsis, bone marrow transplantation, cancer and multisystem involvement with hepatic failure. Children who recover may have persistent pulmonary function test abnormalities, cough and exertional dyspnoea.

Nursing Care Management

The child with PARDS is cared for in the ICU during the acute stages of illness. Nursing care involves close monitoring of oxygenation and respiratory status, as well as assessment of cardiac output, perfusion, fluid and electrolyte balance, and renal function (urinary output). Blood gas analysis, acid–base status and pulse oximetry are important evaluation tools. Most children with PARDS require invasive monitoring via

PATHOPHYSIOLOGY REVIEW

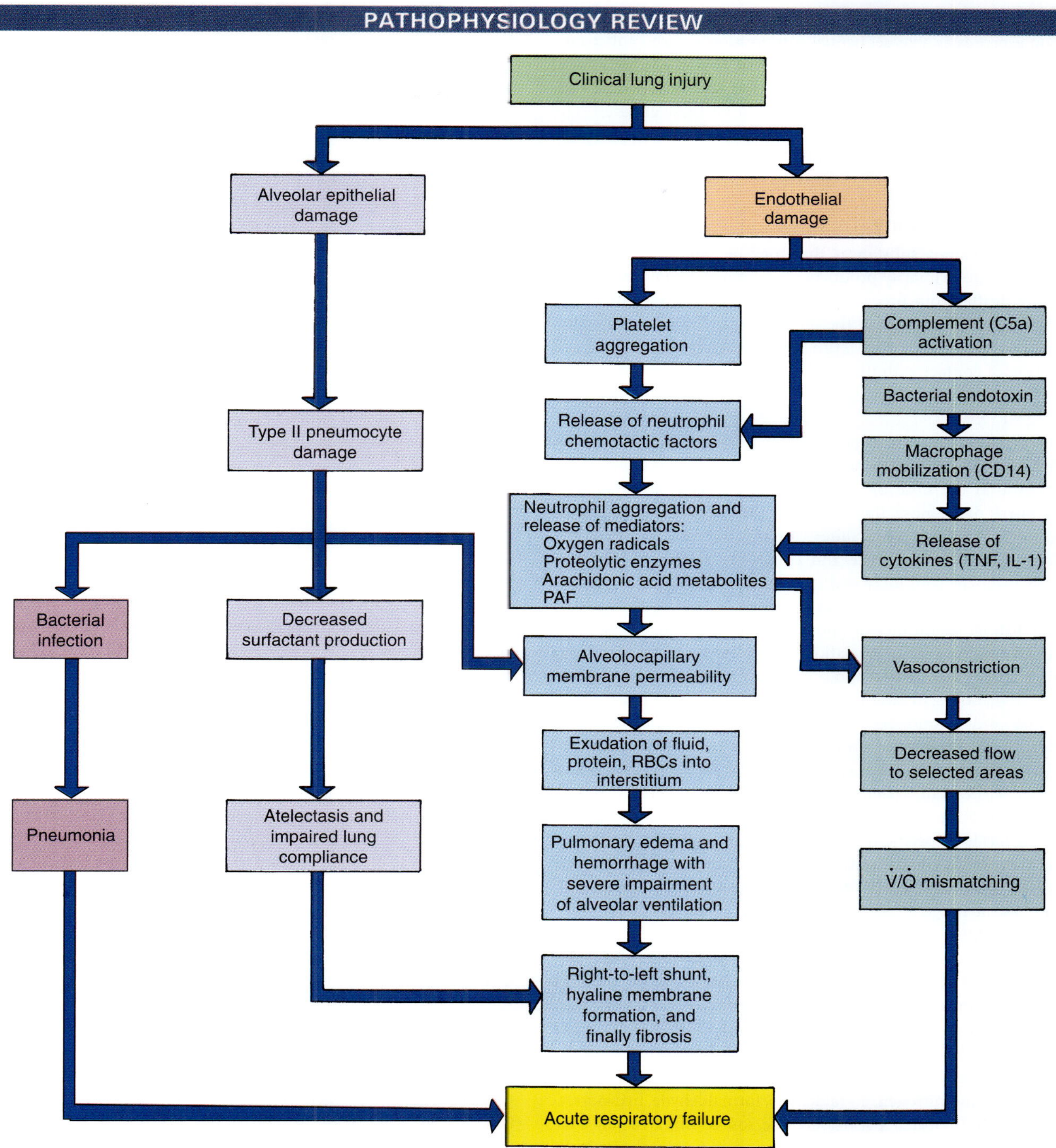

Fig 26.9 Pathogenesis of acute respiratory distress syndrome. (*IL-1, Interleukin-1; PAF, platelet-activating factor; RBCs, red blood cells; TNF, tumour necrosis factor; V/Q, ventilation-perfusion.)* (Source: Sauls, J. L. (2017). Acute respiratory failure. In Introduction to Critical Care Nursing (7th ed.), Elsevier.)

arterial and central venous catheters. Diuretics may be administered to reduce pulmonary fluid, and vasodilators to decrease pulmonary vascular pressure. Nutritional support is often required. Nursing management also includes monitoring the effects of the numerous parenteral fluids and drugs used to stabilise the child and monitoring for changes in the child's haemodynamic status. Preventing superimposed ventilator-associated pneumonia (VAP), nursing care includes elevation of the head of the bed to between 30 and 45 degrees (crib at 20 degrees) unless contraindicated and frequent oral care at least every 2 to 4 hours, suction as per the child's needs and avoiding reintubation (SCH 2017). The risk of pressure ulcers is greater with the head of the bed in an elevated position, and this must be balanced with the risk of VAP. Careful and ongoing skin assessment and pressure area observation are essential. The multidisciplinary care team performs a daily assessment of readiness to wean or liberate from mechanical ventilation. The child must also be assessed for risk of deep-vein thrombosis, and appropriate prophylactic strategies must be initiated (e.g. passive range of motion exercises as able, sequential compression devices, anticoagulant therapy and early ambulation). Respiratory distress is a frightening situation for both the child and the parents, and attention to their psychological needs is a major element in the care of these children. The child is often sedated during the acute phase of the illness, and weaning from sedation requires close monitoring and interventions to promote comfort.

Smoke Inhalation Injury

A number of noxious substances that may be inhaled are toxic to humans. They are primarily products of incomplete combustion and cause more deaths from fires than flame injuries. The severity of the injury depends on the nature of the substances generated by the material being burned, whether the victim is confined in a closed space and the duration of contact with the smoke.

General Aspects

Possible inhalation injury is suspected when there is a history of flames or smoke in a closed space, whether or not burns are present. Sooty material around the nose or in the sputum; singed nasal hairs; or mucosal burns of the nose, lips, mouth or throat are all signs that the affected person requires observation for possible pulmonary injury from inhalants. A hoarse voice and cough are further evidence of airway involvement, and increased inspiratory and expiratory stridor indicates severe damage to the upper passages.

Three distinct syndromes of pulmonary complications may occur in the child suffering from inhalation injury: early carbon monoxide poisoning, airway obstruction and pulmonary oedema; PARDS occurring at 24 to 48 hours, or later in some cases; and late complications of pneumonia and pulmonary emboli (Antoon & Donovan 2016). Strangulation may also occur from the cervical eschar secondary to a severe burn. Smoke inhalation causes three different types of injury: heat, local chemical and systemic.

Heat Injury. Heat causes thermal injury to the upper airway, but because air has low specific heat, the injury goes no further than the upper airway. Reflex closure of the glottis prevents injury to the lower airway. Heat may reach the middle airway occasionally, but it rarely penetrates to the lungs.

Chemical Injury. The combustion of materials such as clothing, furniture and floor coverings can generate a wide variety of gases. Acids, alkalis and their precursors in smoke can produce chemical burns. These substances can be carried deep into the respiratory tract, including the lower respiratory tract, in the form of insoluble gases. Soluble gases tend to dissolve in the upper respiratory tract.

Synthetic materials are especially toxic, producing gases such as oxides of sulfur and nitrogen, acetaldehyde, formaldehyde, hydrocyanic acid and chlorine. Heated plastics are the source of extremely toxic vapours, including chlorine and hydrochloric acid from polyvinylchloride, and hydrocarbons, aldehydes, ketones and acids from polyethylene. Irritant gases such as nitrous oxide or carbon dioxide combine with water in the lungs to form corrosive acids. Aldehydes cause denaturation of proteins, cellular damage and oedema of pulmonary tissues. Chemical burns to the airways are similar to burns on the skin, except they are painless because the tracheobronchial tree is relatively insensitive to pain.

Inhalation of small amounts of noxious irritants produces alveolar and bronchiolar damage that can lead to obstructive bronchiolitis. Severe exposure causes further injury, including alveolocapillary damage with haemorrhage, necrotising bronchiolitis, inhibited secretion of surfactant and formation of hyaline membranes, all manifestations of PARDS.

Systemic Injury. Systemic injury occurs from gases that are non-toxic to the airways (e.g. carbon monoxide, hydrogen cyanide). They can result in injury and death by interfering with or inhibiting cellular respiration. Carbon monoxide (CO) is a colourless, odourless, tasteless gas with an affinity for haemoglobin 230 times greater than that of oxygen. CO is produced by incomplete combustion of carbon or carbonaceous material such as wood or charcoal. When CO enters the bloodstream, it readily binds with haemoglobin to form carboxyhaemoglobin (COHb). Because CO combines more readily and is released less readily than oxygen, very low levels of tissue oxygen must be reached before appreciable amounts of oxygen are released from the haemoglobin. Therefore, tissue hypoxia reaches dangerous levels before oxygen is available to meet tissue needs.

> **NURSING CARE CONSIDERATIONS**
>
> With carbon monoxide poisoning, the oxygen saturation (SpO_2) obtained by pulse oximetry will be normal because the device measures only oxygenated and deoxygenated haemoglobin; it does not measure dysfunctional haemoglobin, such as COHb.

Accidental CO poisoning is most often a result of exposure to fumes from heaters or smoke from structural fires. Poorly ventilated recreational vehicles, improperly operated or maintained gas lamps or stoves and cooking in underventilated areas with charcoal grills are also frequent causes. Intentional CO poisoning may occur in an attempted suicide in a vehicle parked in a closed garage for a long period. Accidental CO poisoning may also occur in a vehicle with inadequate vented exhaust that leaks into the vehicle's passenger (or closed truck bed) compartment.

The signs and symptoms of CO poisoning are secondary to tissue hypoxia and vary with the level of COHb. Younger children may display symptoms before older children and adults after exposure due to their increased oxygen use and respiratory rate. Mild manifestations include headache, visual disturbances, irritability and nausea, whereas more severe intoxication causes confusion, hallucinations, ataxia and coma. CO may increase cerebral blood flow, increase cerebral capillary permeability and increase cerebrospinal fluid pressure, all of which contribute to the CNS signs observed. The bright, cherry-red lips and skin often described are less common than pallor and cyanosis. Patients who have significant exposure to CO can develop a delayed neurological deficit, which can occur 3 to 240 days after initial exposure and can last up to a year.

Therapeutic Management

The treatment of children with smoke toxicity is largely symptomatic. The most widely accepted treatment is placing the child on humidified 100% oxygen as quickly as possible and monitoring for signs of respiratory distress and impending failure. Baseline blood gases and COHb levels are drawn. Arterial oxygen partial pressure may be within normal limits unless there is marked respiratory depression. If CO poisoning is confirmed, 100% oxygen is continued until COHb levels fall to the non-toxic range of about 10%. CO is removed by the lung circulation due to oxygen combining competitively with haemoglobin and displacing the CO.

Respiratory distress may occur early in the course of smoke inhalation as a result of hypoxia, or patients who are breathing well on admission may suddenly develop respiratory distress. Therefore, endotracheal intubation equipment should be readily available. Transient oedema of the airways can occur at any level in the tracheobronchial tree. Assessment and localisation of the obstruction should be accomplished before severe swelling of the head, neck or oropharynx occurs. Intubation is often necessary when: (1) severe burns in the area of the nose, mouth and face increase the likelihood of developing oropharyngeal oedema and obstruction; (2) vocal cord oedema causes obstruction; (3) the patient has difficulty handling secretions; and (4) progressive respiratory distress requires artificial ventilation. Controversy surrounds tracheotomy, but many prefer this procedure when the obstruction is proximal to the larynx and reserve nasotracheal intubation for lower tract involvement. An electrocardiogram should be considered with significant exposure to rule out myocardial ischaemia.

Pulmonary care may be facilitated by bronchodilators, inhaled corticosteroids, humidification and Chest Physiotherapy (CPT) to enhance the removal of necrotic material, minimise bronchoconstriction and avoid atelectasis. Bronchoscopy may be needed to clear heavy secretions.

CO is excreted primarily through the lungs. Treatment of CO intoxication with 100% oxygen via non-rebreathing face mask reduces the COHb level by one-half in 40 to 60 minutes. Hyperbaric oxygen therapy (HBOT) may be required for severe carbon monoxide poisoning (COHb level > 25% in children, end-organ ischaemia, loss of consciousness) to dissolve additional oxygen from COHb in the blood (Kostic 2016). HBOT significantly decreases the half-life of COHb compared with 100% oxygen treatment alone.

Nursing Care Management

Nursing care of the child with inhalation injury is the same as that for any child with respiratory distress. The initial goal is to maintain a patent airway and effective ventilation status; endotracheal intubation may be required early, depending on the patient's respiratory status and the progression of airway and pulmonary oedema. (See also Respiratory Failure, later in this chapter.) In the acute phase, the nurse should monitor vital signs, oxygenation, work of breathing and other respiratory assessments frequently. The administration of nebulised bronchodilators, humidified oxygen and inhaled corticosteroids is often part of the nursing care. Chest percussion and postural drainage are often required. Fluid requirements for children experiencing inhalation injury are greater than for those with surface burns alone, and IV fluids are generally prescribed. However, one concern is the development of pulmonary oedema; therefore, accurate monitoring of intake and output is essential.

In addition to the observation and management of the physical aspects of inhalation injury, the nurse also deals with the psychological needs of a frightened child and distraught parents. Parents need support, reassurance and information about their child's condition, treatment and progress. The nurse can also provide anticipatory guidance and educate families on prevention of inhalation injuries and the importance of CO detectors in the home.

Environmental Tobacco Exposure

Numerous investigations indicate that parental or family smoking is an important cause of morbidity in children. Children exposed to passive or environmental tobacco smoke have an increased number of respiratory illnesses, increased respiratory symptoms (e.g. cough, sputum and wheezing) and reduced performance on pulmonary function tests. AOM and OME are also increased in children who have smoking family members. Indoor exposure to tobacco smoke has been linked to asthma in children (Makadia et al 2017). Among children with asthma, there is an association between parental/family member cigarette smoking and asthma exacerbations, trips to the ED, medication use and impaired recovery after hospitalisation for acute asthma. Children and infants exposed to second-hand smoke experience more wheezing episodes. Maternal cigarette smoking is associated with: increased respiratory symptoms and illnesses in children; decreased fetal growth; increased deliveries of low-birth-weight, preterm and stillborn infants; and a greater incidence of sudden infant death syndrome (SIDS). Antenatal maternal smoking is a significant risk factor for SIDS (Friedmann et al 2017). The risk for diagnosis of early-onset asthma in the first 3 years of life is associated with in utero exposure to maternal smoking.

State, federal and local governments have enacted legislation prohibiting smoking in public places and workplaces. Children experience more second-hand smoke exposure in the home setting than anywhere else. The impact of tobacco smoke also contributes to an increase in childhood deaths attributed to residential fires in households where adults smoke. The financial impact of second-hand smoke exposure is significant.

Electronic cigarettes have increased in popularity among adults as well as adolescents. Regular use of electronic cigarettes has increased tenfold among high-school students (12 to 17 year olds), from 2.1% in 2013 to 6.2% in 2016 (Greenhalgh & Scollo 2018). This increase may be due to adolescents' belief that electronic cigarettes are less harmful and less addictive than cigarettes (Amrock et al 2016). Although these products are advertised as being safe because they are smokeless, the battery-powered cigarettes still contain nicotine and other chemicals. Recent studies have shown toxic effects on the pulmonary system, including altered airways, increased oxidative stress, interference in lung development and impaired immune defence against bacterial and viral pathogens (Chun et al 2017). Electronic cigarettes can also increase the risk for cancer (Canistro et al 2017).

Second-hand smoke consists of passive smoke exposure emitted from a tobacco product. The amount of passive smoke exposure in infants and children is directly related to the number of smokers in a household.

In recent years, concern has grown regarding 'third-hand' tobacco exposure—the tobacco toxins that remain in the environment long after the smoker has stopped smoking (Campbell et al 2017). Such toxins may be found in cars, homes, clothing and hands.

Nursing Care Management

Passive smoke exposure during childhood may also contribute to the development of bronchopulmonary dysplasia in adulthood, and some have attributed infertility in adults to exposure to second-hand smoke as children. Nurses and other healthcare professionals need to include assessments of passive smoke exposure in all children, especially those with respiratory illnesses. In families where smokers refuse to quit, house rules should be established for reducing smoke in the child's environment, such as smoking outside of the home, wearing removable clothing while smoking and not smoking in vehicles. Nurses should also inform caregivers of the health hazards of children's exposure to tobacco smoke; set an example for children and families; and become advocates for 'no smoking' ordinances in public places, prohibition of advertising tobacco products in the media and inclusion of health warnings of sidestream smoke on tobacco products. Nurses have an important role in offering tobacco smoking cessation counselling and in teaching such classes in the community at large. The role of the nurse in promoting smoking cessation among adolescents is discussed in Chapter 18.

STRUCTURAL DEFECTS

Congenital Diaphragmatic Hernia

Congenital diaphragmatic hernia (CDH) results when the diaphragm does not form completely, resulting in an opening between the thorax and the abdominal cavity (Fig 26.10). The diaphragm forms at 4 to 8 weeks of gestation when two membranes close together to separate the abdominal and thoracic cavities. The most common type of CDH (90%) is a left posterolateral defect, also known as a Bochdalek hernia because the herniation occurs through the foramen of Bochdalek. The less common type is the hernia of Morgagni, which is more anterior and often not detected until adulthood. With the Bochdalek hernia, the intestines and other abdominal structures, such as the stomach, liver or bowel, can enter the thoracic cavity, compressing the lung. Lung hypoplasia may occur on the affected side and to a lesser degree on the contralateral side. Ventilation is further compromised by hypoplasia and compression of the lung, including the airways and blood vessels. In addition to the anatomic defect, pulmonary hypoplasia and pulmonary hypertension have also been recently recognised as components in the pathology of CDH.

This serious defect requires prompt recognition (usually in utero) and aggressive treatment to reduce its high mortality risk. The incidence of CDH is approximately 1 in 2000 to 5000 live births, females are affected twice as often as males and it occurs more commonly on the left side (Maheshwari & Carlo 2016). Associated anomalies have occurred in 10% to 20% of cases, and CDH is observed in several chromosomal syndromes.

Clinical Manifestations

The most common manifestation of CDH is acute respiratory distress in the newborn. Infants with a CDH may be dyspnoeic and cyanotic and have a scaphoid abdomen (because of abdominal contents in the chest). Cardiac output is impaired, and the infant exhibits signs and symptoms of shock. Some infants with small defects may not exhibit respiratory symptoms until later in infancy.

Diagnostic Evaluation

Prenatal diagnosis of CDH as early as 24 weeks' gestation is possible. The three main features detected by ultrasound that confirm the diagnosis are polyhydramnios, mediastinal shift and loops of bowel in the chest cavity. In severe cases fetal hydrops is evident. Low maternal serum alpha-fetoprotein levels are seen in cases of CDH; however, the finding is not specific for this anomaly.

Antenatal diagnosis of CDH has the advantages of: counselling the family regarding pregnancy alternatives and potential problems of the neonatal period (especially if other syndromes or chromosomal abnormalities are present); continuing the pregnancy and further management, including possible antenatal treatment; and transporting the fetus with a CDH in utero to a tertiary centre for management. A multidisciplinary team of neonatologists, neonatal nurses, respiratory therapists and paediatric surgeons can intervene early in the acute phase to improve the infant's chances for survival and a positive outcome. After birth, the diagnosis of CDH may depend on the type of hernia present. In the majority of cases the diagnosis is suspected on the basis of the clinical manifestations and is confirmed by a chest x-ray. The chest x-ray shows fluid- and air-filled loops of intestine in the affected side of the chest. The mediastinum may be shifted to the unaffected side, and auscultation may reveal decreased breath sounds on the affected side. The presence or absence of liver herniation is a predictive indicator of postnatal survivability, as well as lung-to-head ratio and fetal lung volume (Oluyomi-Obi et al 2017).

Therapeutic Management

Fetal Surgery. Fetoscopic endoluminal tracheal occlusion has been performed in cases of severe CDH to expand the lungs and push the abdominal contents back into the abdomen, thus producing larger, functional lungs.

After Birth. The severity of symptoms depends on the size of the defect in the diaphragm, how much of the abdominal contents are present in the chest, the size of the lungs and at what stage of gestation the herniation occurred. Many infants with a CDH have respiratory distress and require immediate respiratory assistance, which includes endotracheal intubation and GI decompression with a double-lumen catheter to decompress the stomach and reduce compression of the lung. At birth, bag and mask ventilation is contraindicated to prevent air from entering the stomach and especially the intestines, further compromising pulmonary function. When the newborn cries at birth, air is swallowed and the bowel becomes inflated, so its presence in the chest cavity can further compromise lung function. Close attention to the infant's acid–base status is imperative in the management and prevention of pulmonary hypertension. Low ventilatory positive pressure and the lowest mean airway pressure possible, combined with rapid ventilatory rates (80 to 120 breaths/min), may reduce the incidence of pulmonary leaks from overinflation of the unaffected lung. ECMO may also be indicated after birth if severe.

An umbilical arterial catheter will help monitor postductal arterial oxygen tension (PaO_2) and allow infusion of IV fluids, glucose and electrolytes. Bicarbonate-containing IV fluids may be administered to maintain a pH between 7.5 and 7.6 to prevent acidosis. A transcutaneous oxygen pressure monitor or pulse oximeter may be placed preductally (right hand) and postductally (left hand, arm or either foot) to monitor the amount of ductal shunting through the patent ductus arteriosus. Ductal shunting of deoxygenated blood occurs when pressure in the pulmonary artery is equal to or less than peripheral blood pressure. If pulmonary hypertension is severe with decreased pulmonary venous return, right atrial pressure will be greater than left atrial pressure, resulting in right-to-left shunting of blood through the foramen ovale. The net results of these events cause further hypoxia, hypercarbia and acidosis. (See Persistent Pulmonary Hypertension of the Newborn, Chapter 9.) Echocardiography is performed to determine any cardiac anomalies, as well as to detect any pulmonary hypertension and ductal shunting. Survival rates are lower with underlying cardiac disease, such as hypoplastic left heart syndrome.

Close attention to the infant's thermoregulatory status (maintaining a neutral thermal environment), glucose requirements and acid–base status during the acute phase is a priority of care. Ventilatory management should be individualised on the basis of the infant's response and requirements.

Surfactant replacement therapy may also be used to stabilise neonates with CDH, but outcomes have not demonstrated an overall advantage in relation to ECMO requirements and mortality rate (Chandrasekharan et al 2017). The use of inhaled nitric oxide to relieve pulmonary hypertension of CDH has also been used in some cases, with mixed results (Maheshwari & Carlo 2016).

Another strategy that has demonstrated considerable success in the management of CDH is the use of permissive hypercapnia wherein hyperventilation is not employed in order to reduce iatrogenic lung injury and barotrauma. Preductal SpO_2 is maintained at 85 to 90, PCO_2 is ignored and metabolic acidosis is corrected with buffers instead of hyperventilation. Using lung-protective ventilation (gentle ventilation) strategies aimed at decreasing mean inflation pressures ($<$ 25 cm H_2O) and avoiding hyperventilation have demonstrated better overall outcomes and have significantly decreased pulmonary complications such as pneumothorax (Minter & Walker 2018).

Operative treatment involves returning the abdominal organs to the abdomen and repairing the diaphragmatic defect. The timing of surgical repair may vary. With milder symptoms, such as no pulmonary hypertension or pulmonary hypoplasia, surgical correction occurs 2 to 3 days after birth. Most repairs occur 5 to 10 days after birth in the absence of severe pulmonary hypoplasia and pulmonary hypertension.

Postoperative management involves continuation of ventilatory therapy, monitoring of acid–base balance and allowing slight hypercapnia. In addition, gastric decompression, thermoregulation, sedation and maintenance of adequate cardiac output and peripheral perfusion are continued. If the infant is too unstable for surgical repair, ECMO is considered.

Prognosis. CDH is a complex problem of pulmonary hypoplasia, immature lungs and other associated problems. The overall mortality rates for CDH are decreasing, as the pathophysiology is better understood in relation to current treatment modalities. Current data suggest overall survival rates of 70% to 92%; however, survival rates vary according to CDH severity and associated conditions such as oesophageal atresia and cardiac anomalies (Burgos et al 2017). Surgical repair of the defect alone does not resolve the infant's problems related to organ immaturity. Long-term complications of CDH include chronic lung disease, gastroesophageal reflux, feeding problems, recurrent diaphragmatic herniation, pneumonia, failure to grow, sensorineural hearing loss, scoliosis and impaired motor and cognitive function.

Nursing Care Management

Assessment of the infant at birth is an integral component of nursing care. Prompt recognition of neonatal respiratory distress, cyanosis, a scaphoid abdomen and a possible mediastinal shift would alert the nurse to investigate possible causes of these symptoms. Any one or a combination of these signs may signal the presence of CDH. A newborn in respiratory distress at birth who does not initially respond to resuscitation is further evaluated for CDH; endotracheal intubation is an option for providing adequate oxygenation until CDH is ruled out. If CDH is diagnosed prenatally and the infant is in distress, endotracheal intubation is required to prevent further accumulation of air in the stomach and intestines and subsequent respiratory compromise.

NURSING CARE CONSIDERATIONS

Any newborn infant with a scaphoid abdomen, moderate to severe respiratory distress, decreased breath sounds unilaterally and a history of polyhydramnios should be suspected of having a CDH. Ventilation should not be given with bag and mask to prevent further intestinal air and subsequent respiratory compromise.

Preoperative care involves prompt recognition, resuscitation and stabilisation of the infant, including ventilatory support, blood gas monitoring, fluid volume maintenance and administration of IV fluids and electrolytes. Gastric decompression is achieved with a double-lumen tube, and the infant is observed for signs of impaired cardiac output, acidosis and hypoxemia.

Postoperative care includes the routine observations discussed in the care of the high-risk infant. Close observation to detect signs of respiratory distress, fluid and electrolyte imbalances, mediastinal shift, pulmonary air leak and infection. Hypovolaemia as a result of third spacing of intravascular fluids may occur. The nurse should also pay attention to skin care because these infants often experience prolonged sedation, an increase in skin moisture, tubes and drains coming in contact with the skin, altered nutrition and altered haemodynamics, all of which place the infant at risk for skin breakdown.

Nursing care of the infant with a CDH is also aimed at reducing noxious stimulation either from care activities such as routine suctioning or from environmental factors such as environmental noise. Measures that further reduce infant stress, such as management of pain, should be a routine aspect of care for the infant with a CDH.

Because of the serious nature of the condition and the urgency of treatment, the parents are in great need of ongoing support and education regarding postoperative care. The infant with a CDH may require long-term hospitalisation and care. As soon as medically possible, the parents should be involved in the daily care of their child, and every effort must be made to promote bonding.

Pierre Robin Sequence

Pierre Robin sequence (PRS), which is also known as Pierre Robin syndrome, is a defect characterised by mandibular hypoplasia, retroposition of the tongue and mandible, and cleft palate, which often results in airway obstruction, respiratory distress and feeding problems. The condition has an incidence of 1 in 8500 live births and is often associated with other congenital anomalies (Ren et al 2017). The tongue may be large (glossoptosis) and frequently falls over the neonate's airway, causing occlusion and respiratory distress. In severe upper airway obstruction, a tracheostomy and a feeding tube may be required. From a lateral view the infant's lower jaw can be seen to be positioned posterior (micrognathia) to the upper jaw. PRS may be diagnosed in the nursery when the infant has apnoea and cyanosis, due primarily to the upper airway obstruction. The neonate is positioned to facilitate an open airway (ideally not supine), and the practitioner is notified immediately.

A tongue-lip adhesion is a common surgical procedure that repositions the tongue anteriorly (Ren et al 2017). A nasal trumpet may be indicated to maintain an open airway, but ultimately, surgical distraction of the mandible is required. There are usually no associated neurocognitive defects in isolated PRS.

Nursing care is aimed at early recognition of the infant with PRS, positioning to maintain an open airway and providing parents with information and reassurance.

Choanal Atresia

Choanal atresia, the most common congenital anomaly of the nose, is a bony and/or membranous septum located between the nose and the pharynx. The atresia may be unilateral or bilateral. Because most infants are preferential nasal breathers, bilateral choanal atresia may be associated with apnoea and cyanosis when the infant is at rest. When the infant cries, he or she breathes in through the mouth and pinks up. Unilateral choanal atresia may not be associated with apnoea. Inability to pass a suction catheter through the nose into the pharynx or cyanosis without obvious respiratory distress usually leads to its detection. Nearly half of the infants with choanal atresia have other anomalies (CHARGE syndrome, Treacher Collins syndrome and Tessier syndrome). Surgical correction is required.

LONG-TERM RESPIRATORY DYSFUNCTION

Allergic Rhinitis

Allergic rhinitis affects as many as 20% to 40% of the paediatric population and is associated with numerous airway disorders, including asthma, OME and chronic sinusitis (Milgrom & Sicherer 2016). Seasonal allergic rhinitis (also known as hay fever) usually follows a spring-autumn pattern and is caused by tree, grass and weed pollens. Seasonal allergic rhinitis usually does not develop until the individual has been sensitised by two or more pollen seasons. Year-round or perennial allergic rhinitis is more common and is triggered by household inhaled allergens such as feathers, household dust, animal dander, air pollutants and moulds. The risk for allergic rhinitis is increased in infants exposed to tobacco smoke, heavy exposure to indoor allergens and delivery by caesarean section if there is a family history of allergies or asthma (Milgrom & Sicherer 2016). However, early exposure to dogs and cats appears to be a protective factor (Milgrom & Sicherer 2016).

Pathophysiology

Allergic rhinitis requires two conditions: a familial predisposition to develop allergy and exposure of a sensitised person to the allergen. Inhalation of microscopic airborne particles enter the upper respiratory tract and bind to submucosal mast cells in the respiratory tract epithelium.

In the allergic child, symptoms are mediated by immunoglobulin E (IgE), which is produced by the child's B-lymphocytes. The IgE molecules on the cell surfaces trigger the rapid release of mast cell mediators (e.g. histamine, prostaglandins and leukotrienes), as well as the slower synthesis of cell interactive compounds called cytokines; this action is often called the **early-phase response**. Histamine, a potent vasodilator, acts directly on local receptors to produce vasodilation, mucosal oedema and increased production of mucus. The cytokines summon cells to the area and are responsible for the slower **late-phase allergic** reaction of inflammation and destruction of the mucosal surface, which progresses to chronic nasal obstruction. The late-phase response typically occurs 4 to 8 hours after antigen exposure as a result of the migration of neutrophils, basophils, eosinophils, macrophages and T-lymphocytes into the nasal mucosa (Milgrom & Sicherer 2016). Repeated exposure of these sensitised membranes to specific aeroallergens results in clinical allergic disease. Allergic rhinitis is rare in children under 2 years of age because repeated exposure to the allergen is needed to develop the allergy.

Clinical Manifestations

Children who have allergic rhinitis have a history of watery rhinorrhoea, nasal obstruction, sneezing, itchy throat or nasal pruritus. Symptoms may be chronic, recurrent or acute and include itching of the nose, eyes, palate, pharynx and conjunctiva. The nasal stuffiness sometimes progresses to partial or total obstruction of airflow, and mucus secretion with postnasal drainage can occur. Nasal itching is troublesome, and the affected child attempts to alleviate the symptoms by rubbing the nose. The presence of nasal itching helps identify allergic rhinitis from other types of rhinitis. Other symptoms include throat clearing, irritability, snoring during sleep, fatigue, malaise, headache and poor school performance.

On physical examination, children may display dark circles beneath their eyes, or 'allergic shiners', secondary to obstruction of normal outflow from regional lymphatics and veins. If the nasal obstruction is severe, the child becomes an obligate mouth breather and is seen with an open mouth, or 'allergic gape'. Facial findings include a horizontal nasal crease across the lower third of the nose caused by frequent rubbing induced by the nasal pruritus, and Dennie-Morgan lines, or extra wrinkles below the lower eyelids. The child may develop facial tics and mannerisms in an attempt to avoid scratching the nose. Examination of the child's nose often reveals a pale, boggy nasal mucosa with enlarged nasal turbinates.

Symptoms that appear during peak periods include tearing and soreness of the eyes and gelatinous conjunctival discharge in the morning, irritability, fatigue, depression and loss of appetite.

When the nurse suspects allergic rhinitis, it is important to obtain information regarding clinical signs of related disorders, including middle ear disease, ear pain, delayed speech or language development, chronic cough, wheezing, exercise intolerance, eczema or urticaria. It is also important to ask about any family history of allergies and to obtain information about specific triggers or environmental changes that may have precipitated an episode of rhinitis, such as seasonal pollens, feathers, mould, pets, fungi, dust mites, cockroaches, rodents, cigarette smoking or the use of a woodburning stove. Chronic rhinitis with significant nasal obstruction can lead to various abnormalities in growth and in physical, psychosocial and intellectual development. It can also lead to social stigmatisation related to ongoing symptoms.

Diagnostic Evaluation

Diagnosis of allergic rhinitis is based on a thorough history and physical examination. Because allergic rhinitis is often associated with atopic dermatitis or asthma, examination of the skin and chest is indicated. Diagnostic tests include blood examination for total IgE and elevated eosinophils, skin tests and various challenge tests.

Skin testing is a useful adjunct in establishing a definitive diagnosis for allergic rhinitis. Skin testing involves a small prick on the skin (with a sterile lancet) made through a drop of the allergen extract (usually on the arm or back), performed by a practitioner educated in allergy treatment. After a suitable time (15 to 20 minutes), the size of the resultant wheal and flare reaction is measured to assess the patient's sensitivity. The magnitude of the wheal and flare response correlates roughly with the severity of symptoms produced by natural exposure to the same allergen. However, a positive skin test does not always indicate the presence of clinical reactivity. Before skin testing occurs, the patient should withhold medications for 3 to 7 days such as montelukast (Singulair, antihistamines, antihistamine nasal sprays, corticosteroids, decongestants, antidepressants, cold remedies and antacids) to prevent false-negative results (Australasian Society of Clinical Immunology and Allergy [ASCIA] 2019a).

Skin testing and immunotherapy (see discussion later in this chapter) are generally safe procedures, but they are not without risk. Severe and even fatal reactions can occur within a short time, depending on the type of extract used and individual sensitivity.

NURSING CARE CONSIDERATIONS

The onset of a reaction is often insidious. Mild initial symptoms may include local pruritus, pallor, flushing, cyanosis, shortness of breath, dyspnoea, cough, malaise or abdominal pain. Later developments include hypotension, airway obstruction, chest pain, ventricular fibrillation and loss of consciousness. Nurses need to recognise these symptoms and be able to initiate emergency treatment.

Therapeutic Management

Therapy is directed towards avoidance of offending allergens and the use of medication and immunotherapy (hyposensitisation or desensitisation). Avoidance measures involve removing allergens from the environment and are usually effective for allergies to foods, drugs and animals. If a patient is unable to avoid allergens, symptoms can be controlled with medication, but treatment should be individualised. For mild symptoms or intermittent symptoms with exposure to a known allergen, a second-generation oral antihistamine such as cetirizine or loratadine is recommended. An antihistamine (azelastine), glucocorticoid (fluticasone) or sodium cromoglycate nasal spray could also be considered. If the allergic rhinitis symptoms are more persistent, the glucocorticoid nasal sprays are first-line treatment and may even be used in combination sprays with an antihistamine twice daily.

Topical nasal corticosteroids are safe and effective therapies and are more effective than oral antihistamines for symptom relief. Inhaled corticosteroids are administered with the nasal tip pointing away from the nasal septum (cartilage) to prevent nasal perforation (a rare but reported complication). Experts have expressed concerns in relation to possible decreased linear growth in children who take intranasal corticosteroids. Side effects are minimal, with occasional nasal irritation, epistaxis and changes in smell or taste.

Antihistamines reduce sneezing, rhinorrhoea and nasal itching but have less effect on nasal stuffiness than nasal corticosteroids. Antihistamines act by inhibiting the effects of histamine by binding to H_1 receptors. Classic first-generation antihistamines such as diphenhydramine (Benadryl) and chlorpheniramine may produce undesirable side effects such as dry mouth, urinary retention, constipation and sedation or restlessness that results in impaired school performance. The second-generation antihistamines such as loratadine (Claratyne) and cetirizine

(Zyrtec) are approved for use in children 12 months and older (Milgrom & Sicherer 2016). Azelastine is a topically active antihistamine available in nasal spray for children over 5 years old. These drugs are non-sedating and have few cardiovascular adverse effects.

Oral/nasal decongestants are not recommenced and, if used, should only be for short courses.

Sodium cromoglycate is a mast cell stabiliser, more useful for episodic treatment and is effective in preventing both the early and the late responses to antigen by preventing release of histamine and other inflammatory mediators. It can also be used before expected exposure to an allergen, such as a pet. Ipratropium bromide (Atrovent), available as a nasal spray, may be used for serious rhinorrhoea but should be limited to less than 5 days per month to avoid rebound nasal congestion (Milgrom & Sicherer 2016).

The leukotriene modifier, montelukast, is approved for patients 2 years or older with perennial allergic rhinitis and asthma. This class of drugs inhibits mucosal oedema and mucus production and decreases bronchoconstriction. Montelukast may cause neuropsychiatric side effects (e.g. agitation, sleep disturbance and depression) (Therapeutic Goods Administration [TGA] 2018).

Allergen immunotherapy may be necessary if drug therapy and avoidance of allergens are ineffective in controlling symptoms or if drugs evoke undesirable side effects. Before allergen immunotherapy is begun, a positive skin test reaction to the allergen should be confirmed. Allergen immunotherapy is used to desensitise the child to the allergen over time and can be accomplished by sublingual administration (tablets, sprays or drops) or by subcutaneous injection of the allergen (ASCIA 2019b). Allergen immunotherapy is performed using increasing doses of allergen extracts. This process is usually for 3 to 5 years and generally for children over 5 years of age allergen immunotherapy is most effective in reducing symptoms caused by seasonal pollen-related allergy (see also Food Sensitivity, Chapter 11).

Nursing Care Management

An important aspect in nursing care of the child with allergic rhinitis is to counsel the parents and patient about the causes of the condition, or triggers, and assist in the implementation of steps to avoid the triggers. Environmental modification in the home is important.

Another important aspect of caring for the child with allergic rhinitis is preparation for skin tests and allergen immunotherapy injections. These procedures are a source of stress and discomfort for many children. Young children, in particular, cannot understand how uncomfortable injections that must be given regularly over a long period will make them feel better. The use of a vapocoolant spray and distraction can be considered with these procedures. All children who receive skin tests need an explanation of the procedure.

Children with allergic rhinitis and their family members need specific and detailed information relating to their medications. Having poorly controlled allergies can result in poor sleep, fatigue, decreased cognitive functioning and a decreased quality of life. In the case of seasonal rhinitis, antihistamines or topical anti-inflammatory medications are often started approximately 2 weeks before the allergy season begins. Phone or mailed reminders to families to start their medications are helpful in preventing lower respiratory tract complications of allergic rhinitis. In addition, some nasal sprays may not reach their maximum effect or improve symptoms until a week after they are started. First-generation antihistamines that have sedation as a side effect should not be given to teenagers who are driving, and children should be cautioned to avoid hazardous activities such as bicycling or skating if drowsiness occurs; these are often best taken at night to minimise daytime drowsiness. Teachers and parents should monitor children receiving sedating antihistamines for any changes in learning or cognitive functioning in school. Follow-up monitoring is essential to be sure children do not exceed the correct dosage and that correct administration procedures are followed, especially with inhaled medications.

Asthma

Asthma is a chronic inflammatory disorder of the airways characterised by recurring symptoms, airway obstruction and bronchial hyperresponsiveness (National Asthma Council Australia 2019). In susceptible children, inflammation causes recurrent episodes of wheezing, breathlessness, chest tightness and cough, especially at night or in the early morning. These asthma episodes are associated with airflow limitation or obstruction that is reversible either spontaneously or with treatment. The inflammation also causes an increase in bronchial hyperresponsiveness to a variety of stimuli. Asthma is the most common chronic disease of childhood, the primary cause of school absences. One in 9 (over 2.5 million) Australians and 1 in 7 (over 597,000) New Zealanders have asthma (National Asthma Council Australia 2019, Asthma + Respiratory Foundation NZ 2020). Although the onset of asthma may occur at any age, 80% to 90% of children have their first symptoms before 4 or 5 years of age.

Based on the symptom indicators of disease severity, asthma is classified into four categories: intermittent, mild persistent, moderate persistent and severe persistent. Symptoms increase in frequency or intensity until the last category of severe persistent asthma (Box 26.12). These categories provide a stepwise approach to the pharmacological management, environmental control and educational interventions needed for each category. Therapy and management should be reviewed every 1 to 6 months and should be individualised to the patient. In addition to pharmacological management, environmental control and educational interventions are essential at each step (National Asthma Council Australia 2019).

Aetiology

Studies of children with asthma indicate that allergy influences both the persistence and the severity of the disease. In fact, **atopy**, or the genetic predisposition for the development of an IgE-mediated response to common aeroallergens, is the strongest identifiable predisposing factor for developing asthma (Jardins & Burton 2020b). Although allergens play an important role in asthma, 20% to 40% of children with asthma have no evidence of allergic disease. The allergic reaction in the airways is significant because it can cause an immediate reaction, with obstruction, and it can precipitate a late bronchial obstructive reaction several hours after the initial exposure. This delayed bronchial response is associated with an increase in the airway hyperresponsiveness to non-immunological stimuli and can persist for several weeks or more after a single allergen exposure.

In addition to allergens, other substances and conditions can serve as triggers that may exacerbate asthma. Asthma is a complex disorder involving biochemical, genetic, immunologic, environmental, infectious, endocrine and psychological factors. Evidence shows that viral respiratory tract infections may have a significant role in the development and expression of asthma (Jardins & Burton 2020b).

Risk factors for asthma include the following:

- atopy (includes a history of allergies or atopic dermatitis)
- heredity (e.g. parent/sibling with asthma)
- gender (boys are affected more frequently than girls until adolescence, when the trend reverses)
- smoking or exposure to second-hand smoke
- maternal smoking during pregnancy
- ethnicity
- low birth weight
- being overweight.

BOX 26.12 Asthma Severity Classification in Children

Good Control	Partial Control	Poor Control
All of: • Daytime symptoms† ≤ 2 days per week (lasting only a few minutes and rapidly relieved by rapid-acting bronchodilator) • No limitation of activities‡: • No symptoms§ during night or when wakes up • Need for SABA reliever# ≤ 2 days per week	Any of: • Daytime symptoms† > 2 days per week (lasting only a few minutes and rapidly relieved by rapid-acting bronchodilator) • Any limitation of activities* • Any symptoms during night or when wakes up†† • Need for SABA reliever# > 2 days per week	Either of: • Daytime symptoms† > 2 days per week (lasting from minutes to hours or recurring, and partially or fully relieved by SABA reliever) • ≥ 3 features of partial control within the same week

SABA: short-acting beta2 agonist
†e.g. wheezing or breathing problems
‡child is fully active; runs and plays without symptoms
§including no coughing during sleep
#not including doses taken prophylactically before exercise. (Record this separately and take into account when assessing management.)
*e.g. wheeze or breathlessness during exercise, vigorous play or laughing
††e.g. waking with symptoms of wheezing or breathing problems
Notes: Recent asthma control is based on symptoms over the previous 4 weeks. Each child's risk factors for future asthma outcomes should also be assessed and taken into account in management.
Source: National Asthma Council Australia. (2021). Assessing symptoms and control in children 6 years and over. National Asthma Handbook. https://www.asthmahandbook.org.au/management/children/6-years-and-over/initial-assessment

Pathophysiology

There is general agreement that inflammation contributes to heightened airway reactivity in asthma. Multiple mechanisms contribute to airway inflammation, involving a number of different pathways. It is unlikely that asthma is caused by either a single cell or a single inflammatory mediator. Rather, it appears that asthma results from complex interactions among inflammatory cells, mediators and the cells and tissues present in the airways (Fig 26.11) (Liu et al 2016). However, recognition of the importance of inflammation has made the use of anti-inflammatory agents, such as steroids, a key component of asthma therapy.

Another important component of asthma is bronchospasm and obstruction. The mechanisms responsible for the obstructive symptoms in asthma (Fig 26.12) include inflammatory response to stimuli; airway oedema and accumulation and secretion of mucus; spasm of the smooth muscle of the bronchi and bronchioles, which decreases the calibre of the bronchioles; and airway remodelling, which causes cellular changes (Jardins & Burton 2020b).

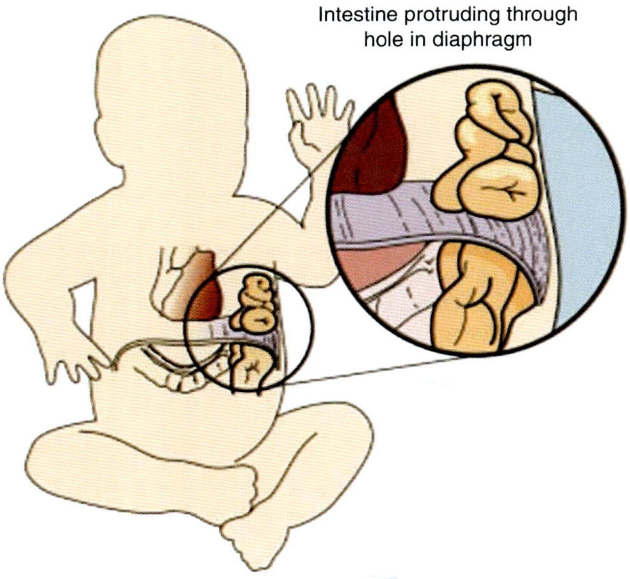

Fig 26.10 Diaphragmatic hernia. (Source: Ball, J. W., Dains, J. E., Flynn, J. A., et al. (2019). Chest and Lungs. In Seidel's Guide to Physical Examination (9th ed), Elsevier.)

Airflow is determined by the size of the airway lumen, degree of bronchial wall oedema, mucus production, smooth muscle contraction and muscle hypertrophy. Bronchial constriction is a normal reaction to foreign stimuli, but in the child with asthma it is abnormally severe, producing impaired respiratory function. The smooth muscle arranged in spiral bundles around the airway causes narrowing and shortening of the airway, which significantly increases airway resistance to airflow.

Because the bronchi normally dilate and elongate during inspiration and contract and shorten on expiration, the respiratory difficulty is more pronounced during the expiratory phase of respiration.

Increased resistance in the airway causes forced expiration through the narrowed lumen. The volume of air trapped in the lungs increases as airways are functionally closed at a point between the alveoli and the lobar bronchi. This trapping of gas forces the individual to breathe at higher and higher lung volumes. Consequently, the person with asthma fights to inspire sufficient air. This expenditure of effort for breathing causes fatigue, decreased respiratory effectiveness and increased oxygen consumption. The inspiration occurring at higher lung volumes hyperinflates the alveoli and reduces the effectiveness of the cough. As the severity of obstruction increases, there is reduced alveolar ventilation with carbon dioxide retention, hypoxaemia, respiratory acidosis and eventually respiratory failure. Chronic inflammation may also cause permanent damage (airway remodelling) to airway structures and is difficult to successfully treat with current therapies.

Exacerbations are episodes of progressively worsening shortness of breath, cough, wheezing or chest tightness, or some combination of these changes. A decrease in expiratory airflow is also characteristic. Airways narrow because of bronchospasm, mucosal oedema and mucus plugging, with air being trapped behind occluded or narrowed airways. Functional residual capacity rises because the child is breathing close to total lung capacity; hyperinflation enables the child to keep the airways open and permits gas exchange to occur. Hypoxaemia can occur during such episodes because of the mismatching of ventilation and perfusion. This is seen with increasing carbon dioxide tension and decreasing oxygen tension levels.

Allergies and Asthma

Having an allergy is the strongest epidemiological risk factor for chronic asthma morbidity and mortality. Many substances in the

PATHOPHYSIOLOGY REVIEW

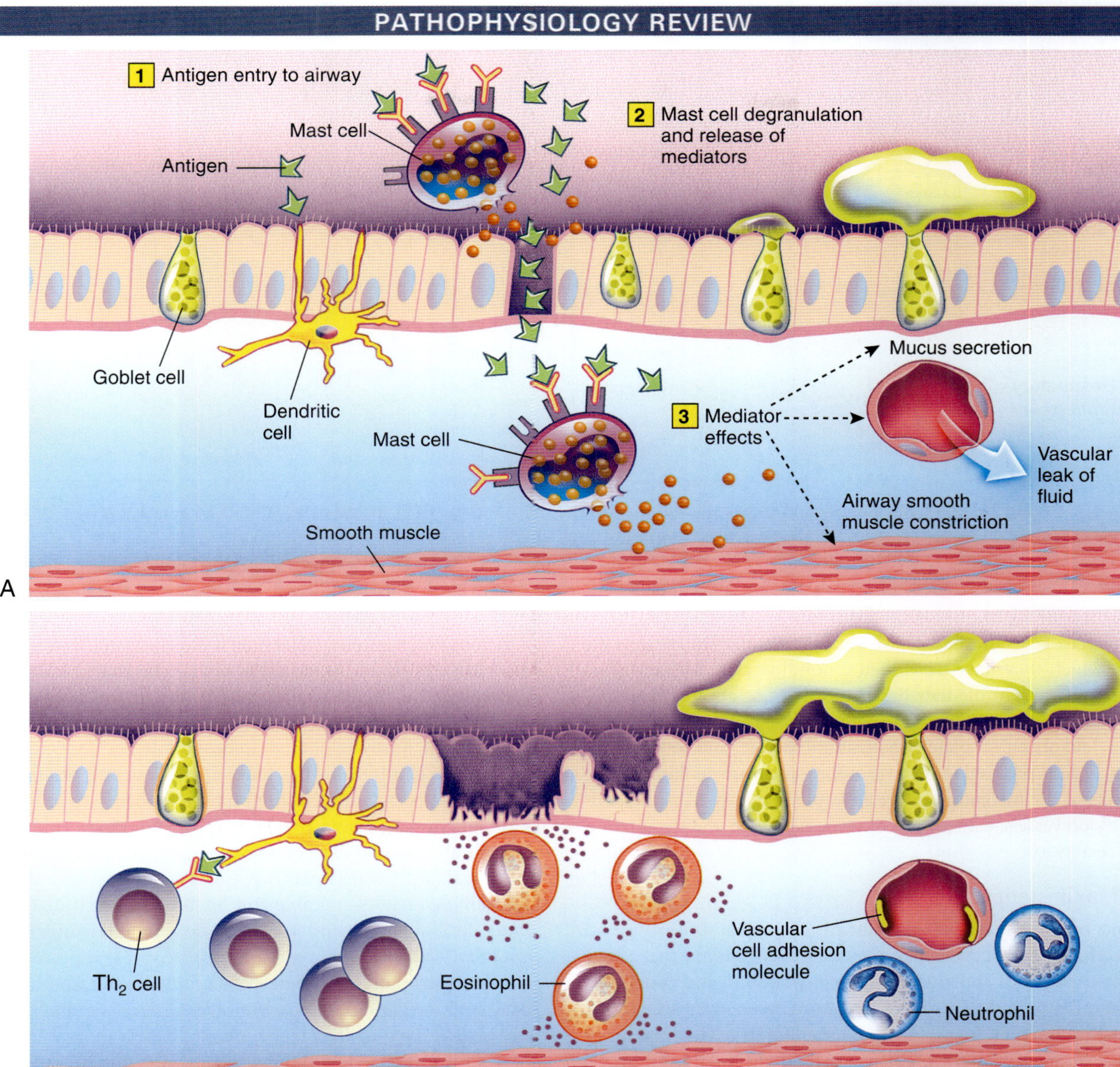

Fig 26.11 Asthmatic responses. (**A**) In the early asthmatic response, inhaled antigen (1) binds to preformed immunoglobulin E (IgE) on mast cells. Mast cells degranulate (2) and release mediators such as histamine, leukotrienes, prostaglandin D_2, platelet-activating factor and others. Acute inflammation opens intercellular tight junctions, allowing antigen to penetrate and activate submucosal mast cells. Secreted mediators (3) induce active bronchospasm, oedema and mucus secretion. Inflammatory responses are set in motion by chemotactic factors and upregulation of adhesion molecules (not shown). At the same time, as shown on the left, antigen may be received by dendritic cells that process and later present it, either in regional lymph nodes to naive (Tho) T-lymphocytes or locally to memory Th_2 cells in the airway mucosa (see **B**). (**B**) In the late asthmatic response, areas of epithelial damage are caused at least in part by toxicity of eosinophil products (major basic protein, eosinophilic cationic protein, eosinophil-derived neurotoxin and eosinophil peroxidase). Many inflammatory cells have been recruited by chemokines and upregulation of vascular cell adhesion molecules. Local T-lymphocytes display a predominant Th_2 cytokine profile. They produce interleukin-4 (IL-4) and IL-13, which promote switching of B cells to favour IgE production, and IL-3, IL-5, and granulocyte-macrophage colony–stimulating factor, which encourage eosinophil differentiation and survival. (Source: McDonald, V. M., Maltby, S. & Penola, D. (2019). Alterations of Pulmonary Function across the life span. In Understanding Pathophysiology, ANZ Edition (3rd ed), Elsevier).)

environment can induce an asthmatic response, but the most significant are those that are antigenic (i.e. that evoke the immune response). The antigen (or foreign substance) is deposited on the respiratory mucosa, where lysozymes immediately digest its outer coating, releasing fragments of foreign protein that initiate the immune sequence.

The antibody (immunoglobulin) most active in allergic disorders, including asthma, is IgE, located primarily in skin and mucous membranes.

IgE mediates the immediate hypersensitive reaction in the bronchial mucosa that leads to specific tissue binding. IgE attaches to

PATHOPHYSIOLOGY REVIEW

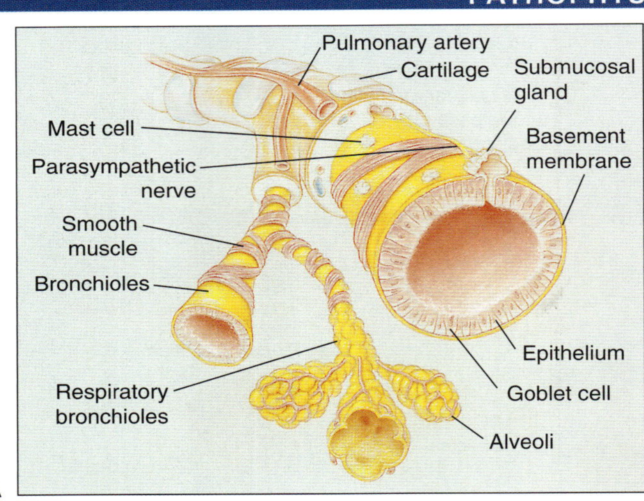

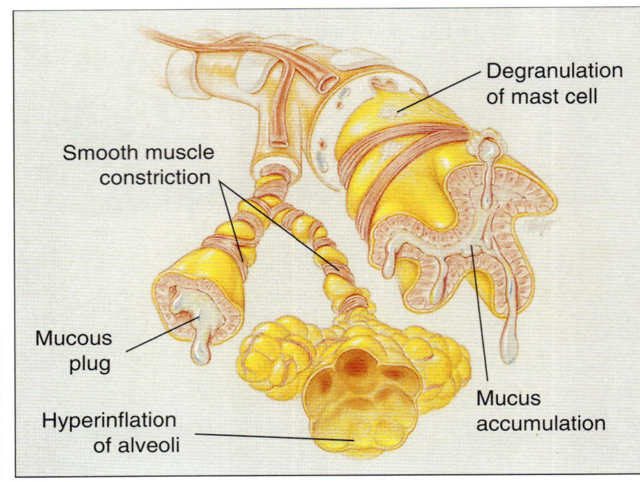

Fig 26.12 Airway obstruction caused by asthma. (**A**) The normal lung. (**B**) Bronchial asthma: thick mucus, mucosal oedema and smooth muscle spasm causing obstruction of small airways; breathing becomes laboured and expiration is difficult. (Source: McDonald, V. M., Maltby, S. & Penola, D. (2019). Alterations of Pulmonary Function across the life span. In Understanding Pathophysiology, ANZ Edition (3rd ed), Elsevier).

surfaces of mast cells and basophils, where it reacts with the specific antigen to which they have developed a bonding capacity. Antigenic substances trigger an immediate hypersensitivity reaction with subsequent release of chemical mediators from mast cells and basophils: histamine; leukotrienes; platelet-activating factor; and other substances, including prostaglandins, serotonin and various kinins. The major effects of the mediators in the airways are increased permeability of the blood vessels, contraction of smooth muscle and stimulation of mucus secretion.

Clinical Manifestations

The classic manifestations of asthma are dyspnoea, wheezing and coughing. However, children may experience symptoms that range from acute episodes of shortness of breath, wheezing and cough followed by a quiet period to a relatively continuous pattern of chronic symptoms that fluctuate in severity. Older children may complain of chest tightness and an intermittent generalised chest pain. An attack may develop gradually or appear abruptly and may be preceded by a URTI. Symptoms are often worse at night or during exercise. The child's age is often a significant factor because the first attack frequently occurs between ages 3 and 8 years. In infancy, an exacerbation usually follows a respiratory tract infection. Bronchoconstriction in response to an allergen can have an immediate, histamine type of pattern or a late response with airway hypersensitivity lasting for days, weeks or months. A second wave of symptoms can occur 6 to 8 hours after the initial antigen exposure.

Children may experience a prodromal itching localised at the front of the neck or over the upper part of the back. An asthmatic episode usually begins with children feeling uncomfortable or irritable and increasingly restless. They may also complain of having a headache, feeling tired or feeling tightness in the chest. Respiratory symptoms include a hacking, paroxysmal, irritative and non-productive cough caused by bronchial oedema. Accumulated secretions, acting as a foreign body, stimulate the cough. As the secretions become more profuse, the cough becomes rattling and productive of frothy, clear, gelatinous sputum. Bronchial spasm and mucosal oedema reduce the size of the bronchial lumen, and the bronchi may be occluded by mucus plugs.

A common symptom of asthma is coughing in the absence of respiratory tract infection, especially at night. This may disrupt sleep, leading to excessive fatigue during the day and poor school performance. Wheezing may be mild or discernible only on auscultation at the end of expiration, or severe enough to be audible.

Younger children have a tendency to assume the tripod sitting position, whereas older children have a tendency to sit upright with shoulders hunched over, hands on the bed or chair, and arms braced to facilitate the use of accessory muscles of respiration. The child may speak with short, panting, broken phrases. Infants and small children are restless, irritable and unable to be comforted. If hypoxaemia develops, the child may become agitated, confused and more irritable.

Infants may display supraclavicular, intercostal, suprasternal, subcostal and sternal retractions. However, clinical symptoms of asthma may be less obvious in infancy; infants have a more pliant (flexible) chest so a prolonged expiratory phase may not be easy to observe. Wheezing may occur in infants with respiratory tract infections, cardiac defects and aspiration pneumonia.

Examination of the chest reveals hyperresonance on percussion. Breath sounds are coarse and loud, with sonorous crackles throughout the lung fields. Expiration is prolonged. Coarse rhonchi can be heard, as well as generalised inspiratory and expiratory wheezing that becomes more high pitched as obstruction progresses. With minimum obstruction, wheezing may be mild (discernible only on auscultation at the end of expiration) or even absent.

With severe spasm or obstruction, breath sounds and crackles may be inaudible. Cough is ineffective despite repeated hacking manoeuvres. This represents a lack of air movement and may be misinterpreted as improvement by unknowing examiners.

NURSING CARE CONSIDERATIONS

Shortness of breath with air movement in the chest restricted to the point of absent breath sounds accompanied by a sudden rise in respiratory rate is an ominous sign indicating respiratory failure and imminent asphyxia.

Children with chronic asthma develop generalised vascularisation, mucosal thickening and hypertrophy of the mucous glands and fibres of the bronchial musculature. With repeated episodes the thoracic cavity becomes fixed in a hyperaerated state (barrel chest), with a depressed diaphragm, elevated shoulders and increased use of accessory muscles of respiration.

Diagnostic Evaluation

The diagnosis is determined primarily on the basis of clinical manifestations, history, physical examination and to a lesser extent laboratory tests. Generally, chronic cough in the absence of infection or diffuse wheezing during the expiratory phase of respiration is sufficient to establish a diagnosis.

Pulmonary function tests (PFTs) provide an objective method of evaluating the presence and degree of lung disease and the response to therapy. Spirometry can generally be performed reliably on children by the age of 6 years and includes either the traditional and simple mechanical spirometer.

Bronchoprovocation testing (i.e. direct exposure of the mucous membranes to a suspected antigen in increasing concentrations) helps identify inhaled allergens in children over 8 years of age. Exposure to methacholine (methacholine challenge), histamine or cold or dry air may be performed to assess airway responsiveness or reactivity. Exercise challenges may be used to identify children with exercise-induced bronchospasm (EIB) (National Asthma Council Australia [NACA] 2019). Although these tests are highly specific and sensitive, they place the child at risk for an asthmatic episode and should be done under close observation in a paediatric respiratory clinic.

The **peak expiratory flow rate** (PEFR) can be measured using a peak expiratory flow meter (PEFM). The PEFR is the maximum flow of air that can be forcefully exhaled in 1 second and is measured in litres per minute. Monitoring PEFR generally starts when a child reaches 12 years (NACA 2019).

Skin testing is useful in identifying specific allergens, and those obtained by the puncture technique correlate better than intracutaneous tests with symptoms and measurements of specific IgE antibody. Identifying allergens which trigger a child's asthma may be an important part of managing their asthma (NACA 2019). Frontal and lateral chest x-rays show infiltrates and hyperexpansion of the airways, with the anteroposterior diameter on physical examination indicating an increased diameter (suggestive of barrel chest) and is not generally recommended in asthma diagnosis. Imaging may assist in ruling out a respiratory tract infection.

Therapeutic Management: General

The overall goals of asthma management are to maintain normal activity levels, maintain normal pulmonary function, prevent chronic symptoms and recurrent exacerbations, provide optimal drug therapy with minimal or no adverse effects, and assist the child in living as normal and happy a life as possible. This includes facilitating the child's social adjustments in the family, school and community and normal participation in recreational activities and sports. General management includes (NACA 2019) the following.

- Regular contact with the healthcare practitioner is necessary to control symptoms and prevent exacerbations.
- Prevention of exacerbations includes avoiding triggers, avoiding allergens and using medications as needed.
- Therapy includes efforts to reduce underlying inflammation and relieve or prevent symptomatic airway narrowing.
- Therapy includes patient and family education, environmental control, pharmacological management and the use of objective measures to monitor the severity of disease and guide the course of therapy.

Allergen Control. Non-pharmacological therapy is aimed at the prevention and reduction of exposure to airborne allergens and irritants. House dust mites and other components of house dust are frequent agents identified in children who are allergic to inhalants. Additional sources of pollutants include particulate matter produced by tobacco smoke, burning wood, pesticides, lead, mould spores, damp environment and nitrogen dioxide (from burning fuels or vehicle emissions); these are believed to contribute to asthma morbidity in children and should be avoided or minimised (NACA 2019). Exposure to tobacco smoke is a significant contributing factor in the development and triggering of asthma in infants and children (Makadia et al 2017).

Skin testing can identify specific allergens, and steps can then be taken to eliminate or avoid them. Often, simply removing the offending environmental allergens or irritants (e.g. removing carpeting) decreases the frequency of asthma episodes. Dehumidifiers or air conditioners control non-specific factors, such as extremes of temperature, that trigger an episode. Avoiding known outdoor allergens such as tree, grass and weed pollen when these are high may reduce asthma exacerbations as well. Additional suggestions include the following.

- Cover pillows and mattresses with dustproof covers.
- Wash bedding in hot water once a week. Dry completely.
- Avoid using feather- or down-filled pillows and mattresses.
- Keep the child indoors while lawn is being mowed, bushes and trees are being trimmed or pollen count is high.
- Keep windows and doors closed during pollen season; use air conditioner if possible, when the weather is hot.
- The child should not be present during cleaning activities.
- Wet-mop bare floors weekly; wet-dust and clean the child's room weekly.
- Vacuum carpet and fabric-covered furniture every week to reduce dust build-up, using a high-efficiency particulate air filter.
- Limit or prevent the child's exposure to tobacco and wood smoke; do not allow cigarette smoking in the house or car; select day care centres, play areas and shopping centres that are smoke free.
- Use air conditioners with high-efficiency particulate air filters.
- Use indoor air purifiers with high-efficiency particulate air filters.
- Choose stuffed toys that can be washed in hot water. Dry completely before the child plays with the toy.

Drug Therapy. Pharmacological therapy is used to prevent and control asthma symptoms, reduce the frequency and severity of asthma exacerbations and reverse airflow obstruction. A stepwise approach is recommended based on the severity of the child's asthma. Because inflammation is considered an early and persistent feature of asthma, therapy is directed towards long-term suppression of inflammation.

Asthma medications are categorised into two general classes: (1) long-term control medications (preventive medications) to achieve and maintain control of inflammation; and (2) quick-relief medications (rescue medications) to treat symptoms and exacerbations.

Quick-relief and long-term medications are often used in combination. Inhaled corticosteroids, sodium cromoglycate and nedocromil, long-acting β_2-agonists, methylxanthines and leukotriene modifiers are used as long-term control medications. Short-acting β_2-agonists, anticholinergics and systemic corticosteroids are used as quick-relief (or rescue) medications. Bronchodilators that relax bronchial smooth muscle and dilate the airways include β_2-agonists, methylxanthines and anticholinergics that can be used as both quick-relief and long-term medications.

Many asthma medications are given by inhalation with a nebuliser or a **metered-dose inhaler (MDI)**. The MDI should always be attached to a spacer when an inhaled corticosteroid is administered to prevent

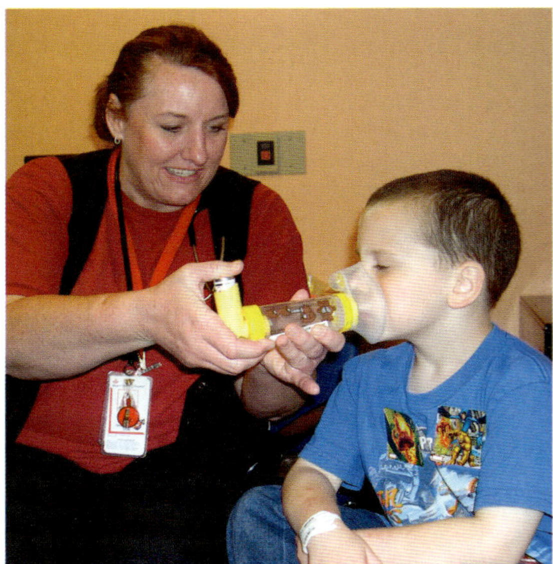

Fig 26.13 Child using metered-dose inhaler with AeroChamber and face mask.

yeast infections in the mouth. Spacers are also important for children who have difficulty coordinating or learning proper inhalation technique. The spacer should be equipped with a mask or a mouthpiece (Fig 26.13) (see Family-Centred Care box later in this chapter). The Diskus inhaler and the Turbuhaler are a dry powder inhaler. These devices are breath activated, and the child needs to inhale as quickly and as deeply as possible to use them effectively. The Diskhaler and Aerosoliser are similar, but with the Aerosoliser the medication must be loaded into the inhaler before use. Infants and young children who have difficulty using MDIs or other inhalers can receive their asthma medications via a **handheld nebuliser** (Fig 26.14). When this device is used, the premixed medication is nebulised with compressed air. Children should breathe normally with the mouth open to provide a direct route to the trachea.

Corticosteroids are anti-inflammatory drugs used to treat reversible airflow obstruction and control symptoms and reduce bronchial hyperresponsiveness in chronic asthma. Inhaled corticosteroids (ICSs) can be used as first-line therapy for chronic Asthmatics. Clinical studies of corticosteroids have indicated significant improvement of all asthma parameters, including decreases in symptoms, emergency visits, hospitalisations and medication requirements (Falk et al 2016).

Corticosteroids may be administered parenterally, orally or by inhalation. Oral medications are metabolised slowly, with an onset of action up to 3 hours after administration and peak effectiveness occurring within 6 to 12 hours. Oral systemic steroids may be given for short periods (e.g. 3- or 5-day 'bursts') to gain prompt control of inadequately controlled persistent asthma or to manage severe persistent asthma. These drugs should be given in the lowest effective dose. They have few side effects (cough, dysphonia and oral thrush), and there is evidence that they improve the long-term outcomes for children of all ages with mild or moderate persistent asthma. Evidence from clinical trials that monitored children for 6 years indicates that the use of ICSs at recommended dosages does not have long-term significant effects on growth, bone mineral density or suppression of the adrenal-pituitary axis (Falk et al 2016). However, practitioners should frequently monitor (at least every 3 to 6 months) the growth of children and adolescents taking corticosteroids to assess the systemic effects of these drugs and make appropriate reductions in dosages or changes to other types of asthma therapy when necessary. ICSs include budesonide and fluticasone.

β-adrenergic agonists (short acting) (primarily salbutamol and terbutaline) are used for treatment of acute exacerbations and for the prevention of EIB. These drugs bind with the β-receptors on the smooth muscle of airways, where they activate adenylate cyclase and convert adenosine monophosphate (AMP) to cyclic AMP (cAMP). The increased cAMP enhances binding of intracellular calcium to the cell membrane, reducing the availability of calcium and thus allowing

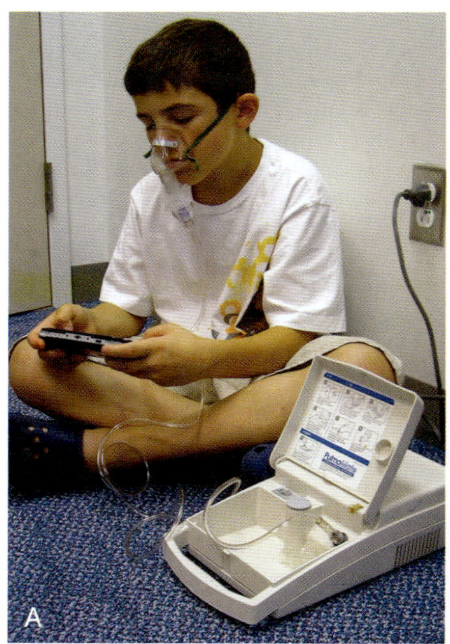

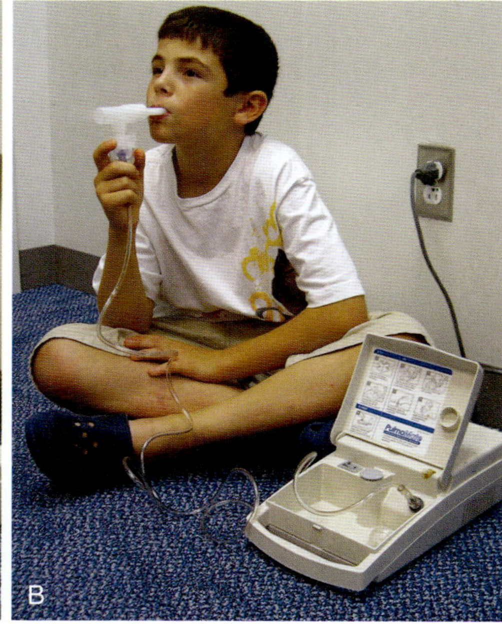

Fig 26.14 Child with asthma may take a nebulised aerosol treatment with (**A**) a mask or (**B**) a mouthpiece. (Source: Courtesy Texas Children's Hospital, Houston.)

smooth muscle to relax. Other effects of the drug help stabilise mast cells to prevent release of mediators. Most β-adrenergics used in asthma therapy affect predominantly the $β_2$-receptors, which help eliminate bronchospasm. $β_1$-adrenergic effects such as increased heart rate and GI disturbances have been minimised. There continues to be some discussion about the administration of $β_2$-agonists via an MDI versus a nebuliser. However, administration via an MDI and spacer is as effective to delivery of medication by a small-volume nebuliser in reversing bronchospasm (NACA 2019).

Long-acting $β_2$-agonists (LABAs) can be single-ingredient products (Serevent and Flixotide) or in combination products containing ICS (Seretide and Symbicort). The Australian Medicines Handbook (AMH) (2020) recommends use of a LABA with low- or medium-dosage inhaled corticosteroid to improve lung function and asthma symptoms, as well as reduce use of short-acting $β_2$-agonists. They are used in children over 6 years of age whose symptoms cannot be adequately controlled on asthma controller medications.

LABAs must be added to anti-inflammatory therapy and never as monotherapy (Liu et al 2016). Inhaled β-adrenergic agents should not be taken more than three or four times daily for acute symptoms without medical supervision. LABAs without ICS can increase the risk of severely worsening asthma symptoms, potentially leading to hospitalisations and death.

Cromones (sodium cromoglycate and nedocromil sodium) may be used as an alternative to ICS in children with persistent or frequent intermittent asthma. Cromones stabilise mast cell membranes; inhibit activation and release of mediators from eosinophil and epithelial cells; and inhibit the acute airway narrowing after exposure to exercise, to cold, dry air and the sulfur dioxide. It does not result in immediate relief of symptoms and has minimal side effects (occasional cough from inhalation of the powder formulation). It requires multiple daily dosing and can be used in children over 2 years of age (AMH 2020).

Leukotrienes are mediators of inflammation that cause increases in airway hyperresponsiveness. Leukotriene modifiers (such as montelukast sodium/Singulair) block inflammatory and bronchospasm effects. These drugs are not used to treat acute episodes but are given orally in combination with β-agonists and steroids to provide long-term control and prevent symptoms in mild persistent asthma. Montelukast is approved to treat asthma in children over 2 years of age. **Anticholinergics** (atropine and ipratropium) help relieve acute bronchospasm. However, these drugs have adverse side effects that include drying of respiratory secretions, blurred vision, and cardiac and CNS stimulation. The primary anticholinergic drug used is ipratropium, which does not cross the blood-brain barrier and therefore elicits no CNS effects (as does atropine). Ipratropium, when used in combination with salbutamol, has been effective during acute severe asthma in significantly improving lung function (Liu et al 2016).

Omalizumab (Xolair) is a monoclonal antibody that is used for patients with moderate to severe persistent allergic asthma whose asthma symptoms are not controlled by ICS. It blocks the binding of IgE to mast cells to inhibit the inflammation associated with asthma. Many patients with asthma are atopic and possess specific IgE antibodies to allergens responsible for airway inflammation. It has been approved for use in children 6 years and older. IgE levels are measured before beginning treatment. Dosage and frequency of administration of Xolair are dependent on the serum total IgE level and body weight. The drug is administered once or twice a month by subcutaneous injection. Efficacy of omalizumab is not immediate and takes 12 to 16 weeks. It is expensive, and there have been reported cases of severe immediate or delayed anaphylactic reactions (within 2 hours or > 24 hours). Recommendations include observing the child for 2 hours after the doses are administered (AMH 2020).

Some children with severe asthma and a history of severe life-threatening episodes may need a prescription for an EpiPen (subcutaneous injectable adrenaline).

Magnesium sulfate, a potent muscle relaxant that acts to decrease inflammation and improves pulmonary function and peak flow rate, may be used in paediatric patients treated in the ED or ICU with acute severe asthma. Studies on the use of intravenous magnesium sulfate offer significant benefits for children with acute asthma exacerbations (AMH 2020).

Antibiotics should not be used to treat acute asthma attacks except when a bacterial infection resulting from another condition such as pneumonia or sinusitis is present.

Breathing Exercises and Physical Training. These therapies help produce physical and mental relaxation, improve posture, strengthen respiratory musculature and develop more efficient patterns of breathing. For the motivated child, breathing exercises and controlled breathing help prevent overinflation and improve efficiency of the cough. However, these exercises are not recommended during acute exacerbations of asthma.

Hyposensitisation. The role of hyposensitisation in childhood asthma is somewhat controversial. In the past, *allergen immunotherapy* was used for seasonal allergies and when single substances were identified as the offending allergen. It is not recommended for allergens that can be eliminated, such as foods, drugs and animal dander.

Specific allergen immunotherapy can be considered when there is evidence of a relationship between asthma symptoms and unavoidable exposure to an allergen to which the patient is sensitive (NACA 2019).

Injection therapy is usually limited to clinically significant allergens. The initial dose of the offending allergen(s), based on the size of the skin reaction, is injected subcutaneously. The amount is increased at weekly intervals until a maximum tolerance is reached, after which a maintenance dose is given at 4-week intervals. This may be extended to 5- or 6-week intervals during the off-season for seasonal allergens. Successful treatment is continued for a minimum of 3 years and then stopped. If no symptoms appear, acquired immunity is assumed; if symptoms recur, treatment begins again. Hyposensitisation injections should be administered by specifically educated personnel and only with emergency equipment and medications readily available in the event of an anaphylactic reaction.

Exercise and Exercise-induced Bronchospasm

Exercise-induced bronchospasm (EIB) is an acute, reversible, usually self-terminating airway obstruction that develops during or after vigorous activity, reaches its peak 5 to 10 minutes after stopping the activity and usually stops in another 20 to 30 minutes. Patients with EIB have cough, shortness of breath, chest pain or tightness, wheezing and endurance problems during exercise.

The problem occurs rarely in activities that require short bursts of energy (e.g. baseball, sprints, gymnastics) and more commonly in those that involve endurance exercise (e.g. soccer, basketball, distance running). Swimming is well tolerated by children with EIB because they are breathing air fully saturated with moisture and because of the type of breathing required in swimming.

Exercise is advantageous for children with asthma and most children can participate in activities at school and in sports with minimal difficulty, provided their asthma is under control. Parents, teachers and practitioners often exclude children with asthma from exercise, and the children themselves are reluctant to participate because it may provoke an attack. However, doing so can seriously hamper peer interaction and physical health. Evaluate participation on an individual basis. Appropriate prophylactic treatment with salbutamol before exercise usually permits full participation in strenuous exertion.

Therapeutic Management: Specific

Children with asthma have exacerbations at varying intervals, with severity ranging from wheezing to life-threatening status asthmaticus (Table 26.6). Protocols have been developed for treating the child experiencing an asthmatic episode at home (asthma action plan) or in the ED (NACA 2019). Nurses should be aware of their institution's protocols and clinical guidelines.

Successful home management of acute asthma begins before symptoms develop. All patients and family members should learn how to monitor symptoms to recognise early signs of deterioration. All children should be given a written action plan to follow in the event of symptoms or an exacerbation. This plan should include information on how to adjust medications in response to signs and symptoms and when to seek medical help. Day care and school-age children should have a written action plan that is appropriate for the organisation's setting.

Status Asthmaticus. Status asthmaticus is a medical emergency that can result in respiratory failure and death if unrecognised and untreated. Children who continue to display respiratory distress despite vigorous therapeutic measures, especially the use of sympathomimetics (e.g. salbutamol, adrenaline), are in status asthmaticus. The condition may develop gradually or rapidly, often coincident with complicating conditions, such as pneumonia or a respiratory virus, which can influence the duration and treatment of the exacerbation.

NURSING CARE CONSIDERATIONS

The child with asthma who sweats profusely, remains sitting upright and refuses to lie down is in severe respiratory distress. Also, the child who suddenly becomes agitated, or the agitated child who suddenly becomes quiet, may be seriously hypoxic and requires immediate intervention.

Therapy for status asthmaticus is aimed at improving ventilation, decreasing airway resistance and relieving bronchospasm, correcting dehydration and acidosis, allaying child and parent anxiety related to the severity of the event, and treating any concurrent infection. Humidified oxygen is recommended and should be given to maintain an oxygen saturation greater than 90%. Inhaled salbutamol is recommended for all patients. Three treatments of salbutamol spaced 20 minutes apart are usually given as initial therapy (burst therapy), and continuous administration of salbutamol may be initiated. A systemic corticosteroid (oral, IV or IM) should also be given to decrease the effects of inflammation. An anticholinergic such as ipratropium bromide may be given. Anticholinergics have resulted in additional bronchodilation in patients with severe airflow obstruction. An IV infusion is often initiated to provide a means for hydration and to administer medications. Correction of dehydration, acidosis, hypoxia and electrolyte disturbance is guided by frequent determination of arterial pH, blood gases and serum electrolytes.

Additional therapies in acute asthma exacerbations may include the use of IV magnesium sulfate and IV aminophylline, a potent muscle relaxant that decreases inflammation and improves pulmonary function and peak flow rate among paediatric patients with moderate to severe asthma when treated in the ED or ICU.

A child suspected of having status asthmaticus is usually seen in the ED and is often admitted to a paediatric ICU (PICU) or transferred to a tertiary hospital with a PICU for close observation and continuous cardiorespiratory monitoring. A key component in the prevention of morbidity is helping the child, parents, teachers, coaches and other adults to recognise features of deteriorating respiratory status, use the correct rescue drugs effectively and immediately place the child with deteriorating respiratory status into the care of trained healthcare professionals instead of waiting to see if the asthma gets better on its own. For the child going into early status asthmaticus, immediate medical care is required to prevent irreversible respiratory failure and possible death.

Prognosis. Asthma-related deaths in Australia are declining, with 389 in 2018 compared to 964 in 1989 (NACA 2019). In New Zealand, asthma-related deaths have been variable, reaching its lowest rate

TABLE 26.6 Estimating Severity of Asthma Exacerbations

INITIAL SEVERITY ASSESSMENT TREAT IN THE HIGHEST CATEGORY IN WHICH ANY SYMPTOMS OCCURS			
Symptoms	Mild Likely to go home	Moderate Possible admission	Severe/Life Threatening Will be admitted
Oximetry in Air	>94%	90%–94%	<90%
Heart rate	Close to normal range for age	Mild-moderate Tachycardia for age	Marked tachycardia – beware bradycardia
Age appropriate ability to talk	Sentences or long vigorous cry	Phrases or Shortened Cry	Words/Weak Cry or Unable to Speak/Cry
Wheeze Intensity	Variable	Moderate to loud	Often quiet Life threatening – silent chest
Accessory Muscle Use	None or very mild	Mild to moderate	Moderate to Severe
Altered Consciousness	Alert Age Appropriate	Easily engaged Age appropriate	May be Agitated. Confused or Drowsy
Cyanosis in Air	None	None	May be Cyanosed
Treatment Options (Treatments to be considered)	↓	↓	Notify Consultant/Fellow **(ED, Medical or Respiratory)** ↓
Oxygen	To maintain $SpO_2 > 94\%$	To maintain $SpO_2 > 94\%$	To maintain $SpO_2 > 94\%$

Source: The Sydney Children's Hospital Network (SCHN). (2018). Asthma – Acute Management Practice Guideline. Retrieved from: https://www.schn.health.nsw.gov.au/_policies/pdf/2007-8358.pdf

2009/2010 before increasing to 87 in 2015 (Asthma + Respiratory Foundation NZ 2020). Asthma can generally be effectively controlled with appropriate medications, care and an asthma plan. There has been a significant increase in asthma-related ED visits and hospitalisations. Most asthma deaths in children occur in the home, school or community before lifesaving medical care can be administered.

Some children's asthma symptoms may improve at puberty, but up to two-thirds of children with asthma continue to have symptoms through puberty and into adulthood. The prognosis for control or disappearance of symptoms varies in children from those who have rare and infrequent attacks to those who are constantly wheezing or are subject to status asthmaticus. In general, when symptoms are severe and numerous, when symptoms have been present for a long time and when there is a family history of allergy, there is a greater likelihood of a poor prognosis. Risk factors that may predict persistence of symptoms into childhood (from infancy) include atopy, male gender, exposure to environmental tobacco and maternal history of asthma. Many children who outgrow their exacerbations continue to have airway hyperresponsiveness and cough as adults. Furthermore, airway hyperresponsiveness in adults appears to be associated with decreased lung function.

The adolescent age group appears to be the most vulnerable, with the greatest increase in mortality from the condition occurring in children 10 to 14 years of age. No reliable data exist to explain this increase. Factors that have been postulated include exposure of atopic persons to more allergens (particularly in large urban centres), change in severity of the disease, abuse of drug therapy (toxicity), failure of families and practitioners to recognise the severity of asthma, failure to take asthma controller medications daily and psychological factors such as denial and refusal to accept the disease. Risk factors for asthma deaths include early onset, frequent attacks, difficult-to-manage disease, adolescence, history of respiratory failure, psychological problems (refusal to take medications), dependency on or misuse of asthma drugs (high use), presence of physical stigmata (e.g. barrel chest, intercostal retractions) and abnormal PFTs.

Nursing Care Management

Acute Asthma Care. Children who are admitted to the hospital with acute asthma are ill, anxious and uncomfortable. The progression or resolution of status asthmaticus is variable. Continual observation and assessment are essential.

When β_2-agonists and corticosteroids are given, the child is monitored closely and continuously for relief of respiratory distress and signs of side effects or toxicity (e.g. tachycardia, restlessness, irritability, hyperactivity). Although food may not be well tolerated in the acute phase, the child may avoid upset stomach associated with corticosteroids by taking small amounts of a food, once the respiratory status has stabilised somewhat. Pulse oximetry is monitored along with rate and depth of breathing, auscultation of air movement, adventitious sounds and any signs of respiratory distress (e.g. nasal flaring, tachypnoea, recession). The child on supplemental oxygen requires intermittent or continuous oxygenation monitoring, depending on the severity of respiratory compromise and initial oxygenation status. The child in status asthmaticus should be placed on continuous cardiorespiratory (including blood pressure) and pulse oximetry monitoring.

If required, IV access is usually initiated once the child has been placed on oxygen. The child may respond well to topical anaesthesia for the procedure (e.g. EMLA). Oral fluid intake may be limited during the acute phase; IV fluid replacement may be required to provide adequate hydration. Endotracheal intubation equipment should be readily available. Medications administered intravenously are monitored for their desired effect and for any untoward effects.

Children with acute asthma are apprehensive and anxious, and they often hyperventilate as a result of the anxiety. Calm coaching to increase depth and slow rate of respirations while administering oxygen with a simple mask may alleviate the child's fears. The calm, efficient presence of a nurse helps reassure the child that he or she is safe and will be cared for during this stressful period. Assure children that they will not be left alone and that their parents are allowed to remain with them.

Parents need reassurance and want to be informed of their child's condition and therapies. They may believe that they have in some way contributed to the child's condition or could have prevented the episode. Reassurance regarding their efforts expended on the child's behalf and their parenting capabilities can help alleviate their stress. Efforts to reduce parental apprehension also reduce the child's distress. Anxiety is easily communicated to the child from parents and members of the staff.

General Care. The nursing care of the child with asthma begins with a review of the child's health history; the home, school and play environment; the parents' and child's attitudes about the child's condition; and a comprehensive physical assessment with focus on the respiratory system. Nursing care of children with asthma involves both acute and long-term care. Nurses who are involved with children in the home, hospital, school, outpatient clinic or practitioner's office play an important role in helping children and their families learn to live with the condition. The disease can be managed so that it does not require ED visits or hospitalisation and does not interfere with family life, physical activity or school attendance.

Physical assessment of asthma involves the same observations and techniques described in Chapter 4. In addition, the nurse notes and evaluates physical characteristics of chronic respiratory involvement, including chest configuration (e.g. barrel chest), posturing (tripod) and type of breathing. A history of the current and previous episodes and precipitating factors or events provides important information. An asthma scoring system may be used to determine severity of symptoms. The nursing assessment should include questions about night-time waking related to symptoms, frequency of use of the quick-acting bronchodilator, ability to participate in school or other activities, any medication side effects and other visits to a provider related to asthma symptoms.

Nurses perform a variety of vital functions in asthma care, including asthma education in the primary care setting and in schools and other community settings, care of the child with asthma in the acute care setting, ambulatory care and intensive care. Nurses also obtain information on how asthma affects the child's everyday activities and self-concept, the child's and family's adherence to the prescribed therapy and their personal treatment goals. Assess the child's and family's satisfaction with asthma control, the quality of care, their perception of the severity of the disease and their level of social support.

One of the major emphases of nursing care is outpatient management by the family. Parents are taught how to recognise and respond to symptoms of bronchospasm, maintain health and prevent complications, and promote normal activities. The child's asthma action plan should be reviewed periodically at least every 6 months in children with moderate to severe disease; precipitating factors, illness management and medication use should be discussed. The nurse determines any cultural or ethnic beliefs or practices that influence self-management and that may necessitate modifications in educational approaches to meet the family's needs.

Avoid Allergens. One goal of asthma management is avoidance of an acute exacerbation. The nurse educates the parent and child on how to modify the environment to reduce contact with the offending allergen(s). Caution the parents to avoid exposing a sensitive child to: excessive cold, wind or other extremes of weather; smoke; sprays; and other irritants. Parents should also eliminate from the diet any foods known to provoke symptoms.

Children with asthma may be sensitive to aspirin, non-steroidal anti-inflammatory drugs (NSAIDs) and tartrazine (yellow dye number 5, a common food colouring). Paracetamol is safe for children with asthma and is the analgesic of choice. Nurses should caution parents to use analgesic-antipyretic drugs for discomfort or fever and to read package labelling. Parents are taught to avoid administering aspirin to *any* child because of its association with Reye syndrome unless specifically recommended by and under the supervision of a health practitioner. Salicylate compounds are in other common medicines, which should be avoided.

Relieve Bronchospasm. Teach parents and older children to recognise early signs and symptoms of an impending attack so that it can be controlled before symptoms become distressing. Most children can recognise prodromal symptoms well before an attack (about 6 hours) and implement preventive therapy. Objective signs that parents may observe include rhinorrhoea, cough, low-grade fever, irritability, itching (especially in front of the neck and chest), apathy, anxiety, sleep disturbance, abdominal discomfort and loss of appetite.

Children who use a nebuliser, MDI, Diskus or Turbuhaler to deliver drugs need to learn how to use the device correctly. The MDI device, with the use of a spacer, delivers medication directly to the airways and slows down the delivery of those particles to assist with their inhalation (see Fig 26.15 and Family-Centred Care box). It is recommended for all patients who use MDIs because less medication is lost in the air and more enters the lungs.

All children and adults should use a spacer with MDI. These devices allow the parent or child to deliver the medication from the MDI into the spacer, from which the child then inhales the medication, while taking slow, steady breaths at his or her own pace. Spacers also help prevent yeast infections in the mouth when corticosteroids are inhaled via an MDI.

The nurse also needs to caution the child and parents about the adverse effects of prescribed drugs and the dangers of overuse of β_2-agonists. They should know that it is important to use these drugs when needed but not indiscriminately or as a substitute for avoiding the symptom-provoking allergen. Educate parents on how to read labels on prepared foods and snacks to determine the presence of allergens.

A written asthma action plan can significantly reduce the risk of asthma death (Liu et al 2016) (see Fig 26.16). Medications used for asthma exacerbations are also included in the asthma plan. This action plan should be used to make decisions about asthma management at home, day care and school.

Asthma action plans can be created by the treating medical team (doctor and nurse) or a GP. It is reviewed with the child and family, and copies are sent to the child's local practitioner and relevant services.

Maintain Health and Prevent Complications. The child should be protected from a respiratory tract infection that can trigger an exacerbation or aggravate the asthmatic state, especially in young children whose airways are mechanically smaller and more reactive. Annual influenza vaccinations are recommended for all children over 6 months. Vaccination against pneumococcal infection is part of the national immunisation program schedule, and children with asthma should be immunised, especially those on prolonged high-dose corticosteroids (ATAGI 2018). Equipment used for the child, such as nebulisers, must be kept absolutely clean to decrease the chances of contamination with bacteria and fungi.

FAMILY-CENTERED CARE

Use of a Metered-dose Inhaler

Steps for Checking How Much Medicine is in the Canister

1. If the canister is new, it is full.
2. Check product label to see how many inhalations should be in each canister.
3. The most accurate way to determine how many doses remain in a metered-dose inhaler (MDI) is to count and record each dose as it is used.
4. Many dry powder inhalers have a dose-counting device or dose indicator on the canister to let you know when the canister is empty.
5. Placing dry powder inhalers or MDIs with hydrofluoroalkanes in water will destroy these inhalers.

Steps for Using the Inhaler and Spacer with Mouthpiece

(Note: Follow the manufacturer's recommendation as to how to prime the spacer before first use.)

1. Remove the cap and hold inhaler upright.
2. Shake the inhaler.
3. Attach spacer, as appropriate.
4. Tilt the head back slightly and breathe out slowly.
5. With the inhaler in an upright position, insert the mouthpiece into the mouth, forming an airtight seal between the lips and the mouthpiece
6. At the end of a normal expiration, depress the top of the inhaler canister firmly to release the medication (into the spacer) and breathe in slowly (about 3 to 5 seconds). Relax the pressure on the top of the canister.
7. Breath normally for 4 breaths in and out between each puff (without breaking the seal on the mouthpiece).

Note: Inhaled dry powder such as budesonide (Pulmicort) requires a different inhalation technique. To use a dry powder inhaler, the base of the device is turned until a click is heard. It is important to close the mouth tightly around the mouthpiece of the inhaler and inhale rapidly.

Steps for Using the Inhaler with an AeroChamber or Spacer with Mask (see Fig 26.13)

The AeroChamber comes with a mask (small, medium and large sizes). (Note: Follow the manufacturer's recommendation as to how to prime the chamber before first use.)

1. Remove the cap and hold inhaler upright.
2. Shake the inhaler.
3. Attach AeroChamber.
4. Attach mask to spacer or AeroChamber
5. Apply AeroChamber mask to child's face and make sure there is a good seal.
6. Have child breathe slow, regular breaths. Depress the top of the inhaler canister firmly to release the medication (into the AeroChamber) as the child breathes slowly in and out. Relax the pressure on the top of the canister.
7. Hold the AeroChamber in place over the child's face until six breaths have been taken. Give one puff at a time.
8. If the seal over the child's face is broken before they have taken four breaths, repeat that puff.
9. Remove the inhaler and the AeroChamber.

The AeroChamber is washed weekly using soap and water to decrease chances of contamination; don't rinse and allow to air dry (NACA 2019).

Puffer vs puffer and spacer

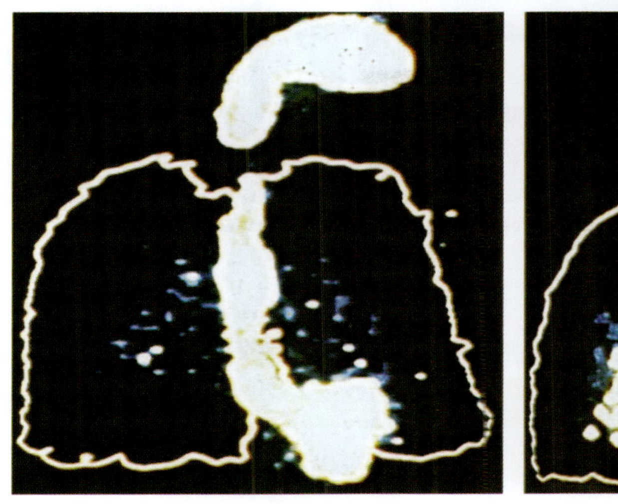

Puffer alone

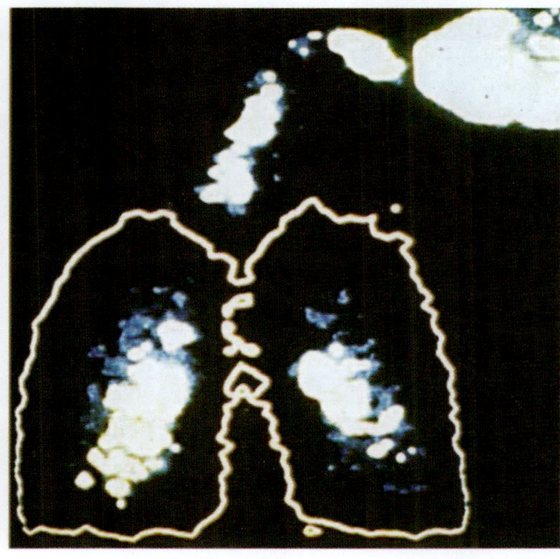

Puffer and spacer

Fig 26.15 Effectiveness of puffer versus puffer and spacer. (Source: Asthma Australia.)

Teach and encourage breathing exercises and controlled breathing for motivated children, and provide information concerning activities that promote diaphragmatic breathing, side expansion and improved mobility of the chest wall. Play techniques that can be used for younger children to extend their expiratory time and increase expiratory pressure include blowing cotton balls or a Ping-Pong ball on a table, blowing a pinwheel, blowing bubbles or preventing a tissue from falling by blowing it against the wall.

Promote Self-care and Normalisation. Self-care and asthma self-management programs are important in helping the child and family cope with asthma. Most asthma self-management programs for children convey several principles. First, asthma is a common disease that can be controlled with appropriate medication therapy, environmental control, education and management skills. Second, it is much easier to prevent than to treat an asthma episode; adherence to a therapeutic program is necessary to prevent exacerbations. Third, children with asthma can live full and active lives. Although a visit to the ED or hospital due to an asthma exacerbation is undesirable, it also presents an opportunity to assess the child's/family's current knowledge about asthma, its triggers, prevention and treatment to prevent future visits. The technique used for MDI and spacer or nebuliser administration should be observed and education provided when needed.

Self-contained programs and brochures for patient education are available from the National Asthma Council Australia (https://www.nationalasthma.org.au/) and the Asthma + Respiratory Foundation NZ (https://www.asthmafoundation.org.nz/).

Child and Family Support. The nurse working with children with asthma can provide support in a number of ways. Many children voice frustration because their exacerbations interfere with their daily activities and social lives. These children also need reassurance from the health team that they can learn to control and cope with their asthma and live a normal life. Be aware of children, especially adolescents, who demonstrate signs of depression and may not comply with therapy.

Children in disruptive family situations (e.g. divorce, separation, violence, custodial battles) may disregard their daily asthma medication regimen or may be at higher risk as a result of neglect by adults who are in charge of their care. Adolescents struggling with a sense of identity and body image often regard asthma as a condition that will 'go away', especially if there is a time lapse between symptoms, and may abandon the therapeutic regimen. They also have a sense of invincibility and may not recognise the future impact of poor adherence to their treatment regimen. In some cases adolescents find themselves in charge of other siblings in blended family situations and may ignore their own health needs. Referral for counselling and guidance is appropriate when the child's or adolescent's life is potentially in danger and the therapeutic regimen for asthma is abandoned due to other crises. Nurses and other caregivers are mandated reporters of medical neglect in these situations. Consideration needs to be given to children from different cultural/ethnic backgrounds, as cultural beliefs may interfere with appropriate management of asthma.

The short- and long-term adaptation of children with asthma often depends on the family's acceptance of the disorder. The task of living day to day with affected children involves the entire family. There are periodic crises and the ever-present threat of a crisis, requiring parental vigilance; sleepless nights; frequent trips to the practitioner, ED or hospital; and often overwhelming medical expenses. Throughout, these stresses encourage parents to promote as normal a life as possible for their children.

Cystic Fibrosis

Cystic fibrosis (CF) is a condition characterised by exocrine (or mucus-producing) gland dysfunction that produces multisystem involvement. CF is the most common lethal genetic illness among Caucasian children, adolescents and young adults. In Australia, 1 in 25 people are a carrier (generally asymptomatic) and 1 in 2500 babies born have CF (Cystic Fibrosis Australia 2017). In New Zealand, 1 in 25 people are carriers and 1 in 3500 babies born have CF (Cystic Fibrosis NZ 2019).

Aetiology

CF is inherited as an autosomal recessive trait. The affected child inherits the defective gene from both parents, with an overall incidence of 1 in 4 births if both parents carry the gene. The mutated gene responsible for CF is located on the long arm of chromosome 7. This gene codes a protein of 1480 amino acids called the **cystic fibrosis transmembrane regulator (CFTR)**. The CFTR protein is related to a family of membrane-bound glycoproteins. The glycoproteins constitute a cAMP-activated chloride channel and also regulate other chloride and sodium channels at the surfaces of the epithelial cells.

ASTHMA ACTION PLAN

Take this **ASTHMA ACTION PLAN** with you when you visit your doctor

NAME

DATE

NEXT ASTHMA CHECK-UP DUE

DOCTOR'S CONTACT DETAILS

EMERGENCY CONTACT DETAILS

Name

Phone

Relationship

WHEN WELL

Asthma under control (almost no symptoms)

ALWAYS CARRY YOUR RELIEVER WITH YOU

Your preventer is: .... (NAME & STRENGTH)

Take .... puffs/tablets .... times every day

☐ Use a spacer with your inhaler

Your reliever is: .... (NAME)

Take .... puffs ....

When: You have symptoms like wheezing, coughing or shortness of breath

☐ Use a spacer with your inhaler

Peak flow* (if used) above:

OTHER INSTRUCTIONS

(e.g. other medicines, trigger avoidance, what to do before exercise)

WHEN NOT WELL

Asthma getting worse (needing more reliever than usual, having more symptoms than usual, waking up with asthma, asthma is interfering with usual activities)

Keep taking preventer: .... (NAME & STRENGTH)

Take .... puffs/tablets .... times every day

☐ Use a spacer with your inhaler

Your reliever is: .... (NAME)

Take .... puffs ....

☐ Use a spacer with your inhaler

Peak flow* (if used) between .... and ....

OTHER INSTRUCTIONS ☐ Contact your doctor

(e.g. other medicines, when to stop taking extra medicines)

IF SYMPTOMS GET WORSE

Severe asthma flare-up/attack (needing reliever again within 3 hours, increasing difficulty breathing, waking often at night with asthma symptoms)

Keep taking preventer: .... (NAME & STRENGTH)

Take .... puffs/tablets .... times every day

☐ Use a spacer with your inhaler

Your reliever is: .... (NAME)

Take .... puffs ....

☐ Use a spacer with your inhaler

Peak flow* (if used) between .... and ....

OTHER INSTRUCTIONS ☑ **Contact your doctor today**

(e.g. other medicines, when to stop taking extra medicines)

Prednisolone/prednisone:

Take .... each morning for .... days

DANGER SIGNS

Asthma emergency (severe breathing problems, symptoms get worse very quickly, reliever has little or no effect)

DIAL 000 FOR AMBULANCE

Peak flow (if used) below:

Call an ambulance immediately

Say that this is an asthma emergency

Keep taking reliever as often as needed

☐ **Use your adrenaline autoinjector (EpiPen or Anapen)**

* Peak flow not recommended for children under 12 years.

NationalAsthma CouncilAustralia
leading the attack against asthma

nationalasthma.org.au

Fig 26.16 Asthma action plan. (Source: National Asthma Council Australia (2019). Asthma Action Plan. Retrieved from: https://www.nationalasthma.org.au/living-with-asthma/asthma-action-plans)

ASTHMA ACTION PLAN

what to look out for

WHEN WELL

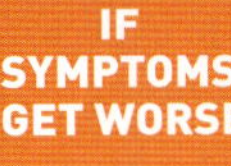

THIS MEANS:
- you have no night-time wheezing, coughing or chest tightness
- you only occasionally have wheezing, coughing or chest tightness during the day
- you need reliever medication only occasionally or before exercise
- you can do your usual activities without getting asthma symptoms

WHEN NOT WELL

THIS MEANS ANY ONE OF THESE:
- you have night-time wheezing, coughing or chest tightness
- you have morning asthma symptoms when you wake up
- you need to take your reliever more than usual
- your asthma is interfering with your usual activities

THIS IS AN ASTHMA FLARE-UP

IF SYMPTOMS GET WORSE

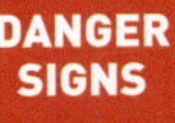

THIS MEANS:
- you have increasing wheezing, cough, chest tightness or shortness of breath
- you are waking often at night with asthma symptoms
- you need to use your reliever again within 3 hours

THIS IS A SEVERE ASTHMA ATTACK (SEVERE FLARE-UP)

DANGER SIGNS

THIS MEANS:
- your symptoms get worse very quickly
- you have severe shortness of breath, can't speak comfortably or lips look blue
- you get little or no relief from your reliever inhaler

CALL AN AMBULANCE IMMEDIATELY: DIAL 000
SAY THIS IS AN ASTHMA EMERGENCY

DIAL 000 FOR AMBULANCE

ASTHMA MEDICINES

PREVENTERS

Your preventer medicine reduces inflammation, swelling and mucus in the airways of your lungs. Preventers need to be taken **every day**, even when you are well.

Some preventer inhalers contain 2 medicines to help control your asthma (combination inhalers).

RELIEVERS

Your reliever medicine works quickly to make breathing easier by making the airways wider.

Always carry your reliever with you – it is essential for first aid. Do not use your preventer inhaler for quick relief of asthma symptoms unless your doctor has told you to do this.

To order more Asthma Action Plans visit the National Asthma Council website. A range of action plans are available on the website – please use the one that best suits your patient

nationalasthma.org.au

Developed by the National Asthma Council Australia and supported by GSK Australia.

National Asthma Council Australia retained editorial control. © 2015

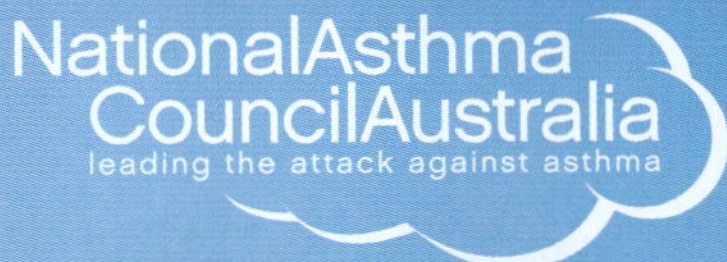

Fig 26.16, con'd

Functional expression of the CF defect reduces the ability of the epithelial cells in the airways and pancreas to transport chloride. Abnormal transport of sodium and chloride across the epithelium leads to increased viscosity of airway mucus, abnormal mucociliary clearance and lung disease. The severity of lung disease and presence of hepatic disease cannot be predicted by genotype, which suggests a major environmentally acquired component of organ system dysfunction or another gene that modifies the CF phenotype (Egan et al 2016).

The ΔF508 gene mutation is the most common alteration found in CF. It occurs in 70% of all known CF chromosomes and is closely related to pancreatic insufficiency. Most of the remaining cases of CF are explained by more than 1500 other mutations. CFTR may be divided into five classes based on the type of defect. Individuals in the first three classes have more severe pulmonary disease and pancreatic insufficiency, whereas those in classes 4 and 5 have milder pulmonary symptoms and better weight gain. However, experts emphasise that even within each class there is substantial phenotype variability (Egan et al 2016).

Pathophysiology

With the discovery of the CFTR gene, research is continuing to determine its multisystem effects on the body. Several clinical features characterise CF: increased viscosity of mucous gland secretions; a striking elevation of sweat electrolytes; an increase in several organic and enzymatic constituents of saliva; and abnormalities in autonomic nervous system function. Although both sodium and chloride are affected, the defect appears to be primarily a result of abnormal chloride movement; the CFTR appears to function as a chloride channel.

Children with CF demonstrate decreased pancreatic secretion of bicarbonate and chloride and an increase in sodium and chloride in both saliva and sweat. This last characteristic is the basis for the sweat chloride diagnostic test. The sweat electrolyte abnormality is present from birth, continues throughout life and is unrelated to the severity of the disease or the extent to which other organs are involved. The sodium and chloride content of sweat in 98% to 99% of children with CF is two to five times greater than that of children without CF and they taste 'salty' when kissed.

The primary factor, and the one responsible for many of the clinical manifestations of the disease, is mechanical obstruction caused by the increased viscosity of mucous gland secretions (Fig 26.17). Instead of forming a thin, freely flowing secretion, the mucous glands produce a thick, heavy mucoprotein that accumulates and dilates them. Small passages in organs such as the pancreas and bronchioles become obstructed as secretions precipitate or coagulate to form concretions in glands and ducts.

Because of the increased viscosity of bronchial mucus, there is greater resistance to ciliary action (probably secondary to infection and ciliary destruction), a slower flow rate of mucus and incomplete expectoration, which also contributes to the mucous obstruction. This retained mucus serves as an excellent medium for bacterial growth. Reduced oxygen–carbon dioxide exchange causes variable degrees of hypoxia, hypercapnia and acidosis. In severe, progressive lung involvement, compression of pulmonary blood vessels and progressive lung dysfunction frequently lead to pulmonary hypertension, cor pulmonale, respiratory failure and death.

Pulmonary complications are present in almost all children with CF, but the onset and extent of involvement are variable. Symptoms are produced by stagnation of mucus in the airways, with eventual bacterial colonisation leading to destruction of lung tissue. The abnormally viscous and tenacious secretions are difficult to expectorate and gradually obstruct the bronchi and bronchioles, causing scattered areas of

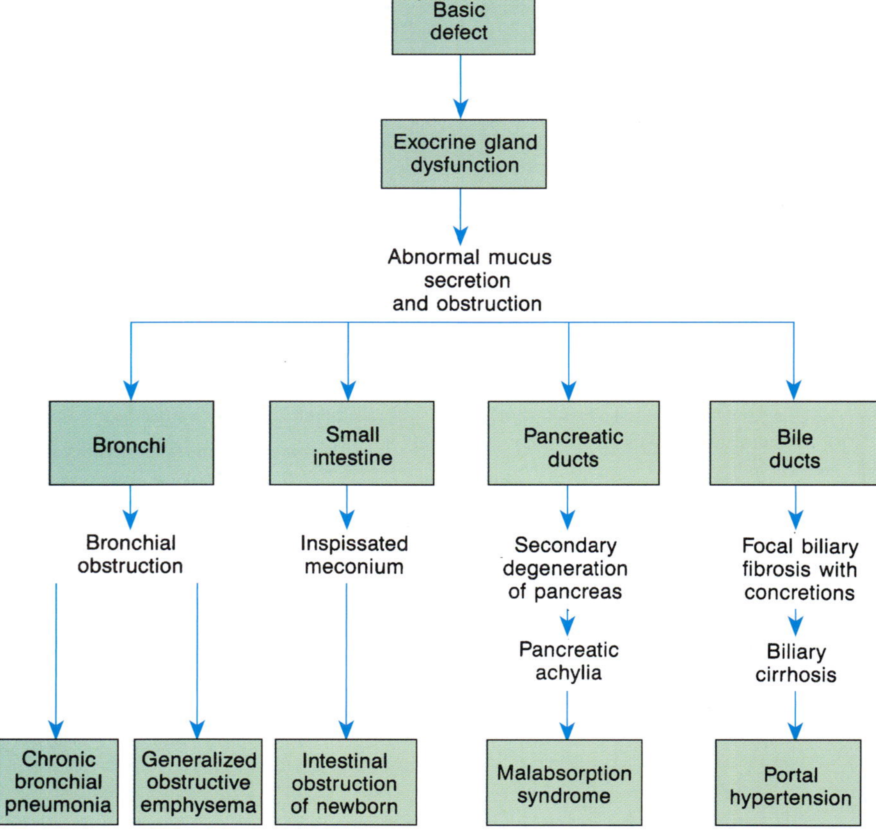

Fig 26.17 Various effects of exocrine gland dysfunction in cystic fibrosis.

bronchiectasis, atelectasis and hyperinflation. The stagnant mucus also provides an optimal environment for bacterial growth.

The most common pathogens are *P. aeruginosa*, *B. cepacia*, methicillin-resistant *S. aureus* (MRSA), *B. dolosa*, *S. aureus*, *H. influenzae*, *Escherichia coli* and *K. pneumoniae*. Children with CF who are chronically colonised with these organisms have poorer survival rates than children who are not colonised. Fungal colonisation with *Candida* or *Aspergillus* organisms in the respiratory tract is also common.

The pseudomonal strains are particularly pathogenic for children with CF because in most patients the alveolar macrophages cannot destroy *Pseudomonas* organisms. The pseudomonal strains also quickly develop resistance to most medications by developing mucoid strains and once a person with CF is colonised with these organisms, they are difficult to eradicate. *P. aeruginosa* infection is not specific for CF but occurs much more frequently in CF than in other diseases characterised by chronic airway obstruction.

B. cepacia is especially worrisome because this organism is extremely virulent, produces bacteraemia and has been associated with rapid pulmonary function deterioration and death in a significant number of CF patients. Methicillin-sensitive *S. aureus* is the most common organism to colonise the respiratory tract and likely to occur with coinfection of *P. aeruginosa*, *A. fumigatus* or *H. influenzae* (Sobin et al 2017).

Gradual progression of pulmonary disease follows chronic infection. Bronchial epithelium is destroyed, and infection spreads to peribronchial tissues, resulting in weakening of bronchial walls and peribronchial fibrosis. The pattern is chronic, progressive fibrosis with decreased oxygen–carbon dioxide exchange and a concurrent alteration in pulmonary vasculature. Chronic hypoxemia causes contraction and hypertrophy of medial muscle fibres in pulmonary arteries and arterioles, leading to pulmonary hypertension and eventual cor pulmonale. Pneumothorax may occur when peripheral bullae rupture; haemoptysis can occur with the erosion of bronchial arteries into a bronchus.

The paranasal sinuses are often filled with secretions and inflammatory products. Nasal and sinus polyps are common, sometimes resulting in bone erosion. Treatment for chronic sinusitis may involve oral antibiotics, decongestants, nasal saline lavage, nasal sinus washout under anaesthesia and nasal corticosteroids.

The extent of GI involvement varies. In the pancreas of many patients, thick secretions block the ducts, leading to cystic dilations of the acini (small lobes of the gland), which then undergo degeneration and progressive diffuse fibrosis. This event prevents essential pancreatic enzymes from reaching the duodenum, which causes marked impairment in the digestion and absorption of nutrients, particularly fats, proteins and, to a lesser degree, carbohydrates. Disturbed absorption is reflected in excessive stool fat (steatorrhoea) and foul smells from putrefied protein (azotorrhoea).

The endocrine function of the pancreas often remains unchanged because the islets of Langerhans are normal but may decrease in number as pancreatic fibrosis develops and progresses. The incidence of diabetes mellitus (cystic fibrosis–related diabetes [CFRD]) is greater in children with CF than in the general population, which may be caused by changes in pancreatic architecture and diminished blood supply over time. Consequently, with increased survival, and primarily in adolescents and adults, CFRD has been reported to be the most common complication associated with CF. Around 30% of people with CF develop diabetes by 30 years of age. It is associated with increased morbidity, and mortality. Severe insulin deficiency occurs as a result of β islet cell dysfunction, and severe insulin resistance may occur, especially during an acute illness. Consequently, CFRD has characteristics of both types 1 and 2 diabetes mellitus. Adequate insulin is needed to maintain a high nutritional status, and this correlates with optimal lung function.

In the liver, focal biliary obstruction and fibrosis are common and become more extensive with time, eventually giving rise to a distinctive type of multilobular biliary cirrhosis. Some children develop extensive liver involvement with fatty infiltration despite adequate nutrition. The gallbladder is small and contains a firm, gelatinous material that also fills the cystic duct. Findings similar to those in the pancreas are found in the salivary glands and contribute to a dry mouth and susceptibility to infection as a result of interference with salivation.

The reproductive systems of both males and females are adversely affected with CF. The glands of the uterine cervix are often filled with mucus, and copious amounts of mucus may block the cervical canal and prevent sperm entry. More than 95% of males with CF are sterile due to obliteration or atresia of the epididymis, vas deferens and seminal vesicles, resulting in decreased or absent sperm production (Egan et al 2016).

Clinical Manifestations

The clinical manifestations vary widely and change as the disease progresses. The most common symptoms are: (1) progressive chronic obstructive lung disease associated with infection; (2) maldigestion from exocrine pancreatic insufficiency; (3) growth failure from malabsorption and anorexia; and (4) diabetes symptoms of hyperglycaemia, polyuria, glycosuria and weight loss from pancreatic insufficiency. The usual pattern is one of faltering growth (previously failure to thrive), with an increased weight loss despite an increased appetite and gradual deterioration of the respiratory system. The diagnosis may not be readily apparent, especially when there is no familial evidence of CF. Some children display symptoms at birth. Others may not develop symptoms for weeks, months or years. Some show only mild forms of the disease, with limited impairment of digestion and respiratory problems, whereas others have severe malabsorption and life-threatening pulmonary complications. Although most affected children display both pulmonary and GI symptoms, a few have only enzyme deficiency without pulmonary disease and a few have only pulmonary disease without pancreatic insufficiency.

Respiratory Tract. Initial pulmonary manifestations are often wheezing respirations and a dry, non-productive cough. Eventually diffuse bronchial and bronchiolar obstruction leads to irregular aeration with progressive pulmonary disturbance and secondary infection. The most prominent and constant feature of pulmonary involvement is chronic cough. Dyspnoea increases, the cough often becomes paroxysmal and the mucoid impactions within the small air passages cause a generalised obstructive hyperinflation and patchy areas of atelectasis.

Progressive pulmonary involvement with hyperaeration of functioning alveoli produces the overinflated, barrel-shaped chest in which the anteroposterior diameter approaches the lateral diameter. Bronchiectasis cysts and subpleural blebs in the upper lobes occur in advanced disease and may rupture, causing pneumothorax. When ventilation and subsequent diffusion and gas exchange are significantly impaired, cyanosis and clubbing of the fingers and toes may occur. The child or adolescent has repeated episodes of bronchitis and bronchopneumonia and is subject to chronic nasal congestion, rhinitis, chronic sinusitis and nasal polyps. Ear, nose and throat surgeries are often needed.

Gastrointestinal Tract. The earliest postnatal manifestation of CF is **meconium ileus**, which occurs in 10% to 15% of newborns with the disease (Egan et al 2016). Thick, putty-like, tenacious, mucilaginous meconium blocks the lumen of the small intestine, usually at or near the ileocecal valve, which gives rise to signs of intestinal obstruction, including abdominal distention, vomiting, failure to pass stools and rapid development of dehydration with associated electrolyte imbalance. Thick intestinal secretions continue to be problematic throughout life. Children of all ages are subject to intestinal obstruction (distal ileum) from heavy or impacted faeces. Gumlike masses in the caecum can obstruct the bowel, causing pain, nausea and vomiting. This is referred to as *meconium ileus equivalent. Distal intestinal obstruction syndrome* is partial or complete intestinal obstruction that occurs in some children with CF.

As the disease progresses, obstruction of pancreatic ducts prevents digestive enzymes (e.g. trypsin, chymotrypsin, amylase, lipase) from being released into the duodenum, which prevents conversion of ingested food into compounds that can be absorbed by the intestinal mucosa. Consequently, the undigested food (chiefly unabsorbed fats and proteins) is excreted, increasing the bulk of faeces to two or three times the normal amount. The bulky nature of the stools may go unnoticed at first, but usually by 6 months of age the child passes large, loose stools with normal frequency or has chronic diarrhoea with unformed stools. As solid foods are added to the diet, the excessively large stools become frothy and extremely foul smelling (steatorrhoea).

Because so little is absorbed from the intestine, affected children have difficulty maintaining weight despite a healthy appetite and diet. Unable to compensate for the faecal losses, many children lose weight and exhibit marked wasting of tissues and growth failure. Faltering growth is common due to decreased absorption of nutrients, vitamins and fat; increased oxygen demands for pulmonary function; and delayed bone growth.

Infants with CF who have faltering growth frequently demonstrate hypoalbuminaemia resulting from diminished absorption of protein, which in severe cases causes generalised oedema. The abdomen is distended, the extremities are thin and the sallow skin droops from wasted buttocks. The impaired ability to absorb fats results in a deficiency of the fat-soluble vitamins A, D, E and K, which may cause bleeding problems if vitamin K deficiency is significant. Anaemia is a common complication. Many older children with CF have an increased prevalence of gastroesophageal reflux.

Another common GI complication is prolapse of the rectum, which occurs in infancy and early childhood and is related to large, bulky stools; malnutrition; and increased intraabdominal pressure secondary to paroxysmal cough. Appendicitis, intussusception and constipation may also occur more frequently in children with CF (Demeyer et al 2016).

Reproductive System. Delayed puberty in girls with CF is common even when their nutritional and clinical status is good. Women with CF who become pregnant have an increased incidence of premature labour and delivery and low birth weight in the infant. Favourable nutritional status and pulmonary function are positively correlated with favourable pregnancy outcomes.

Integumentary System. The chloride channel defect in sweat glands prevents reabsorption of sodium and chloride, which leaves the affected person at risk for abnormal salt loss, dehydration and hypochloremic and hyponatremic alkalosis during hyperthermic conditions. This is especially important to the infant because of limited fluid stores and the potential for inadequate sodium intake with most commercially prepared infant formulas. The disease is sometimes expressed in other ways (e.g. hyponatraemia caused by massive losses through sweat, especially in high environmental temperatures or febrile episodes).

Diagnostic Evaluation

Newer diagnostic methods make it possible to diagnose CF early in infancy so therapies can be implemented to increase the child's overall survival and quality of life. Newborn screening detects some CF; however, the sweat chloride test continues to be the definitive test (Cystic Fibrosis Australia 2017).

The quantitative **sweat chloride test** (pilocarpine iontophoresis) involves stimulating the production of sweat with a special device (involving stimulation with 3 mA electric current), collecting the sweat on filter paper and measuring the sweat electrolytes. The quantitative analysis requires a sufficient volume of sweat (> 75 mg). Two separate samples are collected to ensure the reliability of the test. Normally sweat chloride content is less than 40 mEq/L, with a mean of 18 mEq/L. A chloride concentration greater than 60 mEq/L is diagnostic of CF; in infants younger than 3 months, a sweat chloride concentration greater than 40 mEq/L is highly suggestive of CF. In some situations DNA testing may be indicated.

The presence of a mutation known to cause CF on the CFTR gene predicts with a high degree of certainty that the individual has CF; however, multiple CFTR mutations may also be present and detected with DNA assay. Chest imaging reveals characteristic patchy atelectasis and obstructive emphysema. PFTs are sensitive indices of lung function, providing evidence of abnormal small airway function in CF. Imaging, including contrast enema, are used for diagnosis of meconium ileus.

Other diagnostic tools that may aid in diagnosis include stool fat or enzyme analysis. Stool analysis requires a 72-hour sample with accurate recording of food intake during that time. In some cases, CF may go undiagnosed until the child is older and is seen with clinical manifestations that previously were not acute.

Screening

Early detection of CF is associated with better clinical outcomes and fewer hospitalisations. The newborn screening test consists of an immunoreactive trypsinogen analysis performed on a dried spot of blood, which may be followed by direct analysis of DNA for the presence of the ΔF508 mutation or other mutations on the same dried blood spot. Benefits of early screening and detection include earlier nutritional intervention and preservation of lung function for identified infants. Children who were identified and treated early in infancy with aggressive nutritional support had improved growth and cognitive function well into adolescence (Egan et al 2016).

Therapeutic Management

Improved survival among patients with CF during the past two decades is attributable largely to antibiotic therapy and improved nutritional and respiratory management. The goals of CF therapy are to prevent or minimise pulmonary complications, ensure adequate nutrition for growth, encourage appropriate physical activity and promote a reasonable quality of life for the child and the family. A multidisciplinary system approach is needed to accomplish these goals.

CFTR modulator therapies are available to patients who have specific mutations in the CFTR gene. In Australia there are two approved medications for this: Kalydeco, which is available for children ages 12 months and older, and Orkambi, which is available to children ages 2 years and older. The medications last 12 hours, so twice-daily dosing is required. These medications regulate the flow of sodium and fluids in cell linings in the affected organs, reducing the likelihood of the development of sticky mucus in organs.

Management of Pulmonary Problems. Management of pulmonary problems is directed towards prevention and treatment of pulmonary infection by improving ventilation, removing mucopurulent secretions and administering antimicrobial agents. Many children develop respiratory symptoms by 3 years of age. The large amounts and viscosity of respiratory secretions in children with CF contribute to the likelihood of respiratory tract infections. Recurrent pulmonary infections in the child with CF result in greater damage to the airways; small airways are destroyed, causing bronchiectasis.

Airway Clearance Therapy. Chest Physiotherapy (CPT) has been the cornerstone of airway clearance therapy (ACT) in the prevention of pulmonary infection for many years. Several other ACT strategies are now available to assist with removal of secretions, including percussion and postural drainage, positive expiratory therapy (PEP), active-cycle-of-breathing technique, autogenic drainage, oscillatory PEP, high-frequency chest compressions and exercise. The decision on which technique to use is based on the child and the family. Several techniques may be used, and they are usually adapted over time. It is important to foster adherence to ACTs from a young age. They are usually performed on average twice daily (on rising and in the evening) and more frequently if needed, especially during pulmonary infection. Percussion and postural drainage is especially useful for infants and young children but is often not adequate for older children.

PEP is performed by breathing out with a moderate force through a device. This creates resistance and a positive pressure in the airways, helping keep them open. It allows airflow to get around the mucus and moves it towards the larger airways, where it can be expectorated. Three devices that help accomplish this are PEP valves, flutters and acapellas. The PEP valve allows air to be inhaled through a one-way valve and blown out through a hole or resistance. The **Flutter mucous clearance device** is a small, handheld plastic pipe with a stainless-steel ball on the inside. An acapella provides high-frequency oscillation as well as PEP.

The active-cycle-of-breathing technique is a series of breathing techniques that help clear secretions. Examples include forced expiration, or 'huffing', with the glottis partially closed; thoracic expansion exercises; and relaxation and breathing control. Young children can be taught games with breathing that can develop into these techniques as they get older.

Autogenic drainage involves a variety of breathing techniques that the older child can use to force mucus in lower lobes up into the airways so it can be successfully expelled.

Patients with CF have been found to regress when conventional ACT is discontinued. Therefore, although it is time consuming for the child and family, it is an essential part of care.

Bronchodilator medication delivered in an aerosol opens bronchi for easier expectoration and is administered before ACTs when the patient exhibits evidence of reactive airway disease or wheezing. Another aerosolised medication is recombinant human deoxyribonuclease (DNase, known generically as dornase alfa [Pulmozyme]), which decreases the viscosity of mucus. It is well tolerated and has no major adverse effects; minor reactions are voice alterations and laryngitis. This medication, given once or twice daily via nebulisation, has resulted in improvements in spirometry, PFTs, dyspnoea scores and perceptions of wellbeing and has reduced the viscosity of sputum (Yang et al 2016).

Nebulised hypertonic saline (6%) has shown some effectiveness in improving airway hydration and increases mucus clearance in patients with CF; however, this treatment may cause bronchospasm. It is useful to use a bronchodilator before this treatment (Cystic Fibrosis Australia 2017).

Clinical trials are in progress to examine the effects of inhaled dry powdered mannitol (Bronchitol) for improving mucociliary clearance in CF by rehydrating the airway. Initial reports showed significant improvement in lung function and sputum (De Boeck et al 2017).

Physical exercise is an important adjunct to daily ACT. Exercise stimulates mucus excretion and provides a sense of wellbeing and increased self-esteem. Any aerobic exercise that the patient enjoys should be encouraged. The ultimate aim of exercise is to increase lung vital capacity, remove secretions, increase pulmonary blood flow and maintain healthy lung tissue for effective ventilation.

Colonisation with *P. aeruginosa* and *B. cepacia* signals progressive involvement. Although the bacteria are impossible to eradicate, they can be successfully controlled. Patients with CF metabolise antibiotics more rapidly than normal; therefore, drug dosage is often higher than would be expected. Depending on its sensitivity, *P. aeruginosa* is usually treated with either ceftazidime, ciprofloxacin or tobramycin. Antibiotic treatment of *B. cepacia* and *S. aureus* should be based on susceptibility and synergy testing. The duration of therapy depends on the patient's response, which is measured by clinical indicators, including cough, fatigue and exercise intolerance, in addition to tests such as PFTs, chest imaging and oxygen measurements.

The cystic fibrosis core principles of infection prevention and control advise that staff, people with CF and their families need regular and ongoing education that all patients with CF have some colonisation of the secretions in the respiratory tract. As a result, individuals with CF should separate from others with CF by at least 4 metres to reduce the chance of cross-infection and contact precautions are needed for all patients, regardless of what pathogens are present in their sputum (Cystic Fibrosis Australia 2017). Patients with CF are advised to wear a mask in common areas of healthcare facilities, but healthcare workers are not required to wear a mask routinely in the care of these patients, unless droplet precautions are requires (Cystic Fibrosis Clinical Network 2016).

Pulmonary infections are treated as soon as they are recognised. In patients with CF, characteristic signs of pulmonary infection—fever, tachypnoea and chest pain—may be absent. Therefore, a careful history and physical examination are essential. The presence of anorexia, weight loss and decreased activity alerts the practitioner to pulmonary infection and the need for an antibiotic regimen. Aerosolised tobramycin is beneficial for patients with frequent pulmonary exacerbations (Egan et al 2016). This medication is usually administered by jet or ultrasonic nebulisers after ACT is performed. This type of delivery system allows for direct antimicrobial application with little systemic absorption. It is not uncommon for the child with CF to be placed on as many as two or three antibiotics and one antifungal medication to treat coexisting pulmonary infections.

IV antibiotics may be administered at home as an alternative to hospitalisation (depending on local practices/programs available). The use of peripherally inserted central catheters (PICCs) for the administration of antibiotics in children with CF is a viable option with limited complications and fewer needle punctures to obtain blood specimens and to maintain often lengthy treatment with parenteral antibiotics. Alternatively, an implanted vascular access device offers the advantage of access for blood sampling and antibiotic infusion. Patients may receive antibiotic therapy at home and continue daily activities with minimum disruptions. Paediatric hospital in the home (HITH) programs may be offered in metropolitan areas and some rural areas that have paediatricians and paediatric units. However, when pulmonary function does not improve with outpatient management, hospitalisation may be recommended for continued antibiotic therapy and vigorous ACT. Some children with CF are hospitalised for IV antibiotic therapy and ACT periodically (a 'tune-up') to keep them well. Oxygen administration may be used for children with acute episodes but must be used cautiously because many children with CF have chronic carbon dioxide retention, and the unsupervised use of oxygen can be harmful. With repeated infection and inflammation, bronchial cysts and emphysema may develop. These cysts may rupture, resulting in a pneumothorax (see Box 26.9).

Blood streaking of the sputum is usually associated with increased pulmonary infection or advanced lung disease. Haemoptysis greater than 250 mL/24 hr for the older child (less for a younger child) indicates a potentially life-threatening event and needs to be treated immediately. Sometimes bleeding can be controlled with bed rest, IV antibiotics, replacement of acute blood loss, tranexamic acid and correction of any coagulation defects with vitamin K or fresh frozen plasma. If haemoptysis persists, the site of bleeding should be localised via bronchoscopy and cauterised or embolised. Children and adolescents with CF should be given the age-appropriate immunisations, including the annual influenza virus vaccine. Treatment of nasal polyps includes intranasal corticosteroids, oral antihistamines and decongestants. If these measures are ineffective, surgical interventions may be necessary. Patients with haemoptysis should not receive non-steroidal anti-inflammatory medications.

Long-term daily ibuprofen (NSAID) given in a dose sufficient to achieve a peak plasma concentration between 50 and 100 microgram/ml has been shown to slow the rate of decline in pulmonary function and to decrease the need for IV antibiotics in young patients with mild pulmonary involvement. Although this therapy is generally well tolerated, careful monitoring for adverse effects (GI bleeding) is essential.

Lung transplantation is a final therapeutic option for many CF patients with severe disease. Heart-lung and double-lung procedures have been successfully performed in children with advanced pulmonary vascular disease and hypoxia; however, whether such procedures significantly improve quality of life and survival rates in children with CF is debated in the current literature. The obstacles surrounding this technique are: availability of donated organs; complications from surgery; and recurrence of pulmonary infections and obstructive bronchiolitis, which decreases transplanted lung function. Some experts state that infections such as *B. cepacia,* diabetes and older age represent a negative factor for long-term survival after transplant (Egan et al 2016).

Management of Gastrointestinal Problems. The principal treatment for pancreatic insufficiency is replacement of pancreatic enzymes (i.e. Creon), which are administered with meals and snacks to ensure that digestive enzymes are mixed with food in the duodenum. Enteric-coated products prevent the neutralisation of enzymes by gastric acids, thus allowing activation to occur in the alkaline environment of the small bowel. The amount of enzymes depends on the severity of the insufficiency, the child's response to enzyme replacement and published guidelines. A dosing schedule is based on grams of consumed fat or body weight. To avoid overdosing, enzyme replacement should not exceed 2500 units lipase/kg/meal for children over 12 months of age (Egan et al 2016). The amount of enzyme is adjusted to achieve normal growth and a decrease in the number of stools to one or two per day. Pancreatic enzymes should be taken within 30 minutes of eating. The enteric-coated beads should not be chewed or crushed because destroying the enteric coating can lead to inactivation of the enzymes and excoriation of oral mucosa. The granule form (i.e. Creon Micro) is used with infants and young children. Enzymes are mixed into pureed fruit for small children. Enzyme dosing may need to be adjusted by the provider if abdominal side effect occurs such as flatus, pain, loose stools, bloating or steatorrhoea.

Because the uptake of fat-soluble vitamins is decreased, water-miscible forms of these vitamins (A, D, E and K) are given, along with multivitamins and the pancreatic enzymes. When high-fat foods are eaten, the child is encouraged to add extra enzymes.

Children with CF require a well-balanced, high-protein, high-caloric diet, with unrestricted fat (because of the impaired intestinal absorption). Improved nutrition in children with CF has been associated positively with improved lung function. To meet daily energy requirements, children with CF will need to consume 20% to 50% more than the recommended dietary intake (RDI) (Cystic Fibrosis Australia 2017). Persons with CF also require an intake of fat that is 35% to 40% of daily energy needs in comparison to the recommendation for the general population (20% to 30%) (Turck et al 2016).

Regular nutritional monitoring should be a standard part of the medical care of the child with CF and should occur every month from birth to 6 months, then every 2 months until 12 months of age; during the second year of life growth assessments should take place every 2 to 3 months and between 2 years of age and 18 years every 3 months (Turck et al 2016). The weight-for-length goal for growth in the first 2 years of life should be above the 50th percentile on WHO standard growth charts, and in children 2 to 18 years a body mass index (BMI) above the 50th percentile should be the goal for growth (Turck et al 2016). Breastfeeding with enzyme supplementation should be continued as long as possible and, when necessary, supplemented with a higher-calorie-per-mL formula to achieve adequate growth. For formula-fed infants, commercial cow's milk–based formulas may be adequate to achieve desired growth. There is no evidence to support the use of high-energy or hydrolysed formula (Turck et al 2016). Faltering growth, despite adequate nutritional support may indicate deterioration of pulmonary status. Data indicate that better forced expiratory volume in 1 second (FEV_1) status (≤ 80%) strongly correlates with BMI percentiles above the 50th percentile; therefore, as noted earlier, the target weight for children with CF ages 2 to 20 years should be ideally maintained above the 50th percentile (Turck et al 2016). Patients with CF may experience frequent anorexia as a result of the copious amounts of mucus produced and expectorated, persistent cough, effects of medications, fatigue and sleep disruption. They may be placed on oral nutritional supplements, night-time (or continuous) supplemental nasogastric/gastrostomy feedings or, rarely, parenteral alimentation in an effort to build up nutritional reserves if there has been a history of inability to maintain weight. An enzyme supplement is encouraged with enteric feedings; these may be given at the initiation of the infusion, at bedtime and at the conclusion of the feeding infusion.

Meconium ileus and meconium ileus equivalent, or total or partial intestinal obstruction, can occur at any age. Constipation is often the result of a combination of malabsorption (either from inadequate pancreatic enzyme dosage or a failure to take the enzymes), decreased intestinal motility and abnormally viscous intestinal secretions.

Rectal prolapse occurs in a small number of children with CF.

Children with CF often experience transient or chronic gastro-esophageal reflux, which should be treated with the appropriate histamine-receptor antagonist and GI motility drug, dietary modifications and an upright position after feedings or meals.

Management of Endocrine Problems. The management of CFRD is critical in the therapeutic treatment of the child with CF. CFRD presents a combination of insulin resistance and insulin deficiency, with unstable glucose homeostasis in the presence of acute lung infection and treatment. Children with CF may be at increased risk for glucose management problems as a result of decreased nutrient absorption, anorexia and severity of pulmonary illness. Diagnosis of CFRD is made using an oral glucose tolerance test. Children with CFRD require close monitoring of blood glucose, administration of insulin injections, diet and exercise management, and quarterly glycosylated haemoglobin (A1c) monitoring. The prevalence of CFRD increases with age, and there is increased morbidity and mortality among children with CFRD compared with those without (Castellani & Assael 2017). Microvascular complications such as retinopathy and nephropathy may occur in children and adolescents with CFRD (Egan et al 2016). However, ketoacidosis is reported to be rare in individuals with CFRD (Egan et al 2016).

Bone health is of concern in children and adults with CF. The pancreatic insufficiency of CF and chronic steroid use present potential risks for less than optimum bone growth in such children. Assessment of bone health by history and bone mass density evaluation should be considered in assessing the child's (≤ 8 years old) health status to detect and prevent osteoporosis or osteopenia.

Prognosis. The median survival age for CF patients is 38 years (Cystic Fibrosis Australia 2017). Despite considerable progress and a recent surge in new treatment modalities, CF remains a progressive and incurable disease. The pulmonary involvement ultimately determines the patient's outcome because pancreatic enzyme deficiency is less of a problem if adequate nutrition is ensured. With advances in technology, parents and adolescents are challenged to set future goals that may include university/TAFE, careers, social relationships and marriage. Concurrently they are faced with increasing morbidity and higher rates of CF complications as they grow older.

Nursing Care Management

Assessment of the child with CF involves comprehensive assessment of all affected systems, with special focus on pulmonary and GI systems Pulmonary assessment is the same as that described for asthma, with special attention to lung sounds, observation of cough and evidence of decreased activity or fatigue. GI assessment primarily involves observing the frequency and nature of the stools and abdominal distention. The observer is also alert to evidence of growth failure. Family members are interviewed to determine the child's eating and eliminating habits and confirm a history of frequent respiratory tract infections or bowel obstruction in infancy.

The nurse assesses the newborn for feeding and stooling patterns, which may indicate a potential problem such as meconium ileus. The nurse also participates in diagnostic testing such as the initial newborn screening.

Parents are often anxious and puzzled about the diagnostic tests and the possible implications of the test results. They need careful explanations of the disease, how it might affect their family and what they can do to provide the best possible care for their child. It is crucial to involve the parents in the follow-up for early diagnostic testing; the neonate may require several follow-up visits in the first few weeks of life if initial test results are not conclusive.

Hospital Care. Most patients with CF require hospitalisation only for treatment of pulmonary infection (exacerbation of their pulmonary symptoms), uncontrolled diabetes or a coexisting medical problem that cannot be treated on an outpatient basis. All patients with CF require contact isolation for their own protection and should wear a mask in communal areas of the hospital.

When the child with CF is hospitalised for diagnosis or treatment of pulmonary complications, aerosol therapy, chest percussion therapy and postural drainage are instituted or continued. The nurse may, at times, administer aerosol therapy, perform CPT and assist with ACTs. ACT should not be performed before or immediately after meals. Planning ACT so that it does not coincide with meals is difficult in the hospital situation but is essential to the effectiveness of this treatment. In rural and remote areas, physiotherapists provide ACT (if services are available).

Nursing assessments, including observation of respiratory pattern, work of breathing and lung auscultation, are vital. Non-invasive pulse oximetry provides valuable data about the patient's oxygenation status. Supplemental oxygen therapy may be administered to the child with mild or moderate respiratory distress. One of the nursing challenges in the care of the child with CF is encouraging compliance with the therapeutic regimen, which often involves taking a significant number of medications (pancreatic enzymes; vitamins A, D, E and K; oral antifungals for *Candida* infection; antihistamines; anti-inflammatory agents; and oral antibiotics). This may be overwhelming to the child. Factor in multiple inhaled bronchodilators, ACT and aerosol treatments, potential blood glucose monitoring and insulin administration, various other medications and increased mucus production during the acute phase, and it is not uncommon for the child with CF to rebel with this regimen and refuse some interventions. Gentle coaxing, positive reinforcement and frank negotiation may be required to enlist cooperation for effective medication compliance.

The child's sleep is disrupted frequently by hospital routines; therefore, nursing care should be flexible enough to allow him or her some quiet time without affecting vital care. In some cases a daily schedule of events, including medication administration, CPT, aerosolised therapy and dressing changes, may need to be mutually developed with the child and healthcare providers so that the child feels he or she has some control of the care.

The diet for the child with CF represents another challenge; careful planning with a paediatric dietitian and the child's input may help decrease the loss of appetite and weight loss that are often part of the condition. Age-appropriate nutrition education with specific nutritional goals for CF patients may increase compliance with prescribed enzyme therapy and nutritional supplements.

When dietary intake fails to meet the child's needs for growth, enteral feedings or supplements may be considered. These feedings may be administered via an enteric tube (nasogastric tube, gastrostomy or percutaneous endoscopic gastrostomy [PEG]) during the night to minimise the disruption of daily activities, including school.

The child needs support during the many treatments and tests that are a part of the hospitalisation, as the child soon associates hospitalisation with these stress-provoking procedures.

Depression, anxiety and disturbed self-image may occur in children and adolescents with CF. Older adolescents and young adults are especially prone to depression due to the realisation of the poor prognosis and unmet life expectations and goals.

Providing support to both the child and the family is essential. The progressive nature of the disease makes each illness requiring hospitalisation a potentially life-threatening event. Skilled nursing care and sympathetic attention to the emotional needs of the child and family help them cope with the stresses associated with repeated respiratory tract infections and hospitalisations.

Home Care. Most children and adolescents with CF can be managed at home. The goals of care include normalisation and daily activities, including school and peer involvement. The care plan should be flexible so that family activities are disrupted as little as possible.

Patients and family members need education about the preferred diet of nutritious meals with tolerated fat, increased protein and carbohydrate, and the administration of pancreatic enzymes and nutritional supplements.

One of the most important aspects of educating parents for home care is teaching ACTs. The number of times these therapies are performed each day is determined on an individual basis, and often parents readily learn to adjust the number and intensity of the treatments to the child's needs.

For pulmonary infection, home IV antibiotics may be appropriate and available in certain areas. Occasionally infusion through an ambulatory infusion pump may be beneficial/available. At-home administration is not always possible in rural and remote areas, due mostly to the limited availability of appropriately trained staff and clinical support.

For the child or adolescent with chronic sinusitis, daily or twice-daily nasal lavage may be helpful. Adolescents need instruction on performing this procedure themselves.

Families also need information about medications and possible side effects. Children receiving antibiotics may require serum drug levels and other routine blood tests to ensure therapeutic dosing.

Children and adolescents with CF should receive routine primary care with special attention to diet, growth and development and immunisations. Home palliative care for the child or adolescent with CF who is in the terminal stages may be carried out with the assistance of a hospice. There is limited availability of paediatric palliative/hospice care in rural and remote areas.

Family Support. The most challenging aspect of providing care for the family of a child or adolescent with CF is meeting the emotional needs of the child and family. The diagnosis, treatment and prognosis for CF are often associated with many problems and frustrations. The diagnosis can evoke feelings of guilt and self-recrimination in parents.

The long-range problems for an infant, child or adolescent with CF are those encountered in any chronic illness. (See Chapter 19.) Both the child and the family must make many adjustments, the success of which depends on their ability to cope and also on the quality and quantity of support they receive from outside sources. Combined efforts of a variety of health professionals are needed to provide the most comprehensive services to families.

The persistent need for treatment several times a day places tremendous strain on the family. Children often baulk at these treatments and the parents are in the position of insisting on adherence. The stress and anxiety related to this routine may produce feelings of resentment in both the child and the family members.

The affected child or adolescent may become resentful about the disease, its relentless routine of therapy and the necessary restrictions it places on activities and relationships. The child's activities are interrupted or built around treatments, medications and diet. This imposes hardships and influences his or her quality of life. The nurse should encourage the child to attend school and join age-appropriate peer groups to live as normally and productively as possible. Sports are often an important part of the child's and adolescent's life; interaction with peers is a valuable life experience, especially to adolescents. In addition, depression in CF patients has been associated with worse health outcomes, adherence and quality of life (Smith et al 2016). As the disease progresses, however, family stress should be expected and the patient may become angry and non-compliant. It is important for the nurse to recognise the family's changing needs and the grief they may experience as the CF worsens. Families should be made aware of resources for counselling. Patients need to be guided into activities that enable them to express anger, sorrow and fear without guilt.

The nurse can assist the family in contacting resources that provide help to families with affected children.

Transition to Adulthood. As life expectancy continues to rise for children and adolescents with CF, issues related to marriage, sexuality, childbearing and career choice become more pressing. Males must be informed at some point that they will often be unable to produce offspring. It is important that the distinction be made between sterility and impotence. Normal sexual relationships can be expected. Female patients may be able to bear children but should be informed of the possible harmful effects on the respiratory system created by the burden of pregnancy. They also need to know that their children will be carriers of the CF gene; therefore, genetic counselling for those planning on having children is essential. Adolescent females should be offered counselling concerning the use of oral contraceptives and other contraceptive options.

Adolescents with CF should take personal ownership and management of the illness to maximise their life's potential. Many adolescents and young persons with the illness enrol in university/TAFE and complete degrees by either distance learning or attending a local school. Young people should set life goals and live normal lives to the extent their illness allows. Adolescents who have had lung transplantation are encouraged to continue taking antirejection medications even though they may feel as though their respiratory status has improved to the point that these medications are no longer necessary.

Life as an independent adult should be encouraged for children with CF. From the time that children can take partial responsibility for their own care (e.g. ACT and taking pancreatic enzymes), independence and accountability should be fostered. Although the prognosis for these children has improved, many will need continued support as they cope with the demands of surviving with CF.

Anticipatory grieving and other aspects related to care of a child with a terminal illness are also part of nursing care. For example, it is important to prepare the child and family members for end-of-life decisions and care. Families may need information about specific interventions such as palliative care and treatments for pain and dyspnoea. (See Chapter 19.)

Obstructive Sleep Apnoea

Paediatric obstructive sleep-disordered breathing reportedly affects between 2% to 3% of all children (RCHM 2018c). Sleep-disordered breathing problems in this spectrum range from partial obstruction of the upper airway to continuous episodes of complete upper airway obstruction, with the most severe form being obstructive sleep apnoea (OSA) (Owens 2016).

Obstructive sleep apnoea is defined as a disorder of breathing during sleep with prolonged partial upper airway obstruction and/or complete obstruction that disrupts normal respiration during sleep and normal sleep patterns (RCHM 2018c). Adenotonsillar hypertrophy is a common cause of OSA, but tonsil size does not correlate with the degree of OSA (Owens 2016). Other causes of OSA include allergies associated with chronic rhinitis/nasal obstruction, craniofacial abnormalities, gastroesophageal reflux, nasal septal deviation and cleft palate repair (Owens 2016). OSA in children is a distinctly separate condition from OSA in adults with regard to aetiology, clinical manifestations and treatment. Common symptoms of OSA include nightly snoring, breathing pauses, choking or gasping on arousal, disturbed sleep patterns, secondary enuresis, daytime sleepiness and daytime neurobehavioral problems (Owens 2016). OSA is to be distinguished from primary snoring, which is snoring without obstructive apnoea or abnormalities in gas exchange. If left untreated, OSA may result in complications such as faltering growth, cor pulmonale, hypertension, poor attention span, behavioural problems (impulsiveness, hyperactivity, rebelliousness and aggression), attention-deficit/hyperactivity disorder, hypertension, cardiac ventricle dysfunction and death.

The diagnosis of OSA is made by an overnight sleep study (polysomnography), which provides evidence of sleep disturbance, respiratory pauses and changes in oxygenation. The six-channel polysomnography can be performed in children of all ages with videotaping and audiotaping. Polysomnography can distinguish between OSA and primary snoring (Owens 2016). Polysomnography is not available in rural and remote settings; children would need to attend metropolitan/tertiary facilities or sleep study facilities. Overnight oxygen saturations can be monitored in rural paediatric units.

Therapeutic Management

Adenotonsillectomy is now recommended as the first-line treatment of children with adenotonsillar hypertrophy (Owens 2016). Cure rates after adenotonsillectomy are reported to range between 80% and 90% in uncomplicated cases (RCHM 2018c). However, more recent evidence indicates that it may not be as effective in children with obesity (Boudewyns et al 2017).

CPAP and BiPAP (cycles between high and low pressure) may be helpful in older children with OSA whose condition persists after surgical intervention or in children who are not good candidates for surgical intervention. CPAP is a long-term therapy with frequent assessments to evaluate the required amount of pressure and the overall effectiveness of the intervention. Children from rural and remote areas would be required to attend a respiratory clinic and consultation with respiratory clinicians in tertiary setting. Many children resist wearing the CPAP or BiPAP devices. Gentle coaxing, patience, reassurance and gradually building up the duration of time on the therapies may help when possible.

Nursing Care Management

Nursing care of the child with OSA involves early detection by observation of the infant's or child's sleep patterns, active participation in the diagnostic polysomnography in tertiary facilities, observation of oxygenation and vital signs, application of CPAP when indicated and monitoring the patient's response to diagnostic therapy. Counselling families of children with OSA may involve dietary counselling for exercise programs and weight management, use of the CPAP or BiPAP equipment and direct postoperative care after the surgical intervention of tonsillectomy or adenoidectomy. The nurse can be instrumental in helping the child and family cope with the chronic illness diagnosis should intervention such as CPAP or BiPAP be required.

RESPIRATORY EMERGENCY

Respiratory Failure

Effective pulmonary gas exchange requires clear airways, normal lungs and chest wall, and adequate pulmonary circulation. Anything that affects these functions or their relationships can compromise respiration. In general, the term **respiratory insufficiency** is applied to two conditions: (1) when there is increased work of breathing but gas exchange function remains near normal; and (2) when normal blood gas tensions cannot be maintained and hypoxaemia and acidosis develop secondary to carbon dioxide retention. **Respiratory failure** is the inability of the respiratory apparatus to maintain adequate gas exchange. This process involves pulmonary dysfunction that generally results in impaired alveolar-capillary gas exchange, which can lead to hypoxaemia or hypercapnia. **Respiratory arrest** is the cessation of respiration. Respiratory failure is the most common cause of cardiopulmonary arrest in children.

Apnoea is generally defined as cessation of breathing for more than 20 seconds, or for a shorter period when associated with hypoxemia or bradycardia (RCHM 2019d). Apnoea can be: (1) central, in which both airflow and chest wall movement are absent; (2) obstructive, in which airflow is absent but chest wall motion is present; and (3) mixed, in which both central and obstructive components are present.

Respiratory dysfunction may have an abrupt or an insidious onset. Respiratory failure can occur as an emergency situation or may be preceded by gradual and progressive deterioration of respiratory function. Most clinical manifestations are non-specific and are affected by variations among individual patients and differences in the severity and duration of inadequate gas exchange.

Conditions that Predispose to Respiratory Failure

Respiratory disorders are classified according to three dominant functional abnormalities, although all three types may be present in the disease. In **obstructive lung disease** there is increased resistance to airflow in either the upper or the lower respiratory tract. Obstruction can result from anomalies (e.g. tracheomalacia, choanal atresia, vocal paralysis), aspiration (e.g. meconium, mucus, vomitus, FB), infection (e.g. pneumonia, pertussis, severe tonsillitis), tumours (e.g. haemangioma, cystic hygroma), anaphylaxis and laryngospasm from local irritation (e.g. intubation, drowning, aspiration).

In **restrictive lung disease**, impaired lung expansion results from loss of lung volume, decreased distensibility or chest wall disturbance. Causes of pulmonary restriction include respiratory distress syndrome, pneumonia, CF, pneumothorax, pulmonary oedema, pleural effusion, submersion injury, congenital diaphragmatic hernia, abdominal distention, muscular dystrophy, paralytic conditions (e.g. poliomyelitis, botulism) and severe structural obstructions such as severe scoliosis.

In **primary inefficient gas transfer** there is insufficient alveolar ventilation for carbon dioxide removal or impaired oxygenation of pulmonary capillary blood as a result of dysfunction of the respiratory control mechanism or a diffusion defect. Causes of respiratory centre depression include: cerebral trauma (e.g. birth injuries, shaken baby syndrome); intracranial tumours; CNS infection (e.g. meningitis, encephalitis); overdose with barbiturates, opioids or benzodiazepines; and severe asphyxia (e.g. hypercapnia, hypoxaemia). Pulmonary diffusion defects include: pulmonary oedema, fibrosis, embolism or hypertension; collagen disorders; *Pneumocystis carinii* pneumonia; anaemia; and haemorrhage.

Recognition of Respiratory Failure

Respiratory failure that occurs as a result of acute obstruction of a major airway or cardiac arrest is sudden and readily apparent. Gradual and more covert development of signs and symptoms is less easily recognised. Evaluation of respiratory adequacy is based on both clinical assessment and laboratory studies.

Unless respiratory arrest occurs suddenly, signs of hypoxaemia and hypercapnia are usually subtle in their development, becoming more obvious as respiratory failure progresses. The unknowing observer may attribute early signs such as mood changes and restlessness to other causes, and some signs can be altered by other factors. Clinical manifestations of respiratory failure are listed in Box 26.13.

In clinical situations in which impaired ventilation can be anticipated or clinical manifestations indicate impending hypoxaemia, serial measurements of blood gases should be obtained and monitored to detect impending respiratory failure and therapy should be implemented before respiratory acidosis becomes extreme.

Nursing Care Management

Nursing observation and judgment are vital to successful management of respiratory failure. The interventions used in the management of respiratory failure are often dramatic, requiring special skills and are frequently emergency procedures. If respiratory arrest occurs, the primary objectives are to recognise the situation and immediately initiate resuscitative measures

When the situation is not an arrest, the suspicion of respiratory failure is confirmed by assessment, and the severity is defined by capillary or arterial blood gas analysis. Interventions such as administering supplemental oxygen, opening the airway, positioning, stimulation, suctioning and early intubation may avert an arrest. When severity is established, an attempt is made to determine the underlying cause by thorough evaluation.

The principles of management are to: (1) maintain ventilation and maximise oxygen delivery; (2) correct hypoxaemia and hypercapnia; (3) treat the underlying cause; (4) minimise extrapulmonary organ failure; (5) apply specific and non-specific therapy to control oxygen demands; and (6) anticipate complications. Monitoring the patient's condition is critical.

Observation and Monitoring

The nurse monitors the child to anticipate respiratory failure, determine a course of action and assess the patient's response to treatment. Often the child is transferred to a paediatric ICU; rural and remote areas transfer children to larger hospitals if the child's conditions requires PICU care. The child is kept as comfortable as possible, and

BOX 26.13 Clinical Manifestations of Respiratory Failure

Cardinal Signs
- Restlessness
- Tachypnoea
- Tachycardia
- Diaphoresis

Early But Less Obvious Signs
- Mood changes, such as euphoria or depression
- Headache
- Altered depth and pattern of respirations (increased work of breathing)
- Hypertension
- Exertional dyspnoea
- Anorexia
- Increased cardiac output and urinary output
- Central nervous system symptoms (e.g. decreased efficiency, impaired judgment, anxiety, confusion, restlessness, irritability, depressed level of consciousness)
- Nasal flaring
- Recession expiratory grunting
- Wheezing or prolonged expiration

Signs of More Severe Hypoxia
- Hypotension
- Depressed respirations
- Diminished vision
- Bradycardia
- Arrhythmias
- Drowsiness/strong desire to sleep
- Cyanosis (peripheral or central)
- Stupor
- Coma
- Dyspnoea

observation is geared towards general appearance, responsiveness, pulse oximetry and vital signs. The child is positioned to allow maximum lung expansion and comfort, such as sitting upright or leaning forward (depending on respiratory status).

The nurse closely monitors the child's cardiac and respiratory status by observation and by electronic means. Because one goal of therapy is to control the body's oxygen demands, assessments of fever and pain should be frequent. Both conditions (as well as cold stress) can dramatically increase oxygen requirements, especially in younger children, and therefore increase respiratory effort. Measure oxygenation by the use of pulse oximetry or blood gas monitoring.

Family Support

Children who are in respiratory distress often relax after an airway is established (PICU at tertiary hospitals or EDs in rural/remote hospitals) and their respiratory effort is assisted. However, they are anxious and frightened when they are unable to communicate; therefore, it is important to effectively manage the child's anxiety. This may be accomplished initially with mild sedation until the child's ventilatory status has improved. It is also stressful to parents to watch their child's inability to vocalise and helplessness. It is important to talk to the child and parents to reassure them that the child's voice will return when the breathing tube (endotracheal tube or tracheostomy) is removed. Assistive communication devices should be offered as appropriate to age and development (e.g. electronic pads, paper and pen, picture boards).

Parents are often concerned about the (often) life-threatening implications generated by the need for the procedure and the possible long-term residual effects on the brain and on the child's psychological status. For families whose child had a respiratory arrest, support focuses on keeping the family informed of the child's status and helping them cope with a near-death experience or an actual death. (See Chapter 19.) Knowing that their child requires CPR is a frightening and often overwhelming experience for parents. Uncertainty regarding outcome—both mortality and morbidity—is a primary concern.

REFERENCES

Agency for Clinical Innovation (ACI) (2018a). Infants and Children—Acute Management of Bronchiolitis. New South Wales Government. 10 January. Retrieved from: https://www1.health.nsw.gov.au/pds/pages/doc.aspx?dn=GL2018_001

Agency for Clinical Innovation (ACI) (2018b). Infants and Children—Acute Management of Community Acquired Pneumonia (CAP) Guideline. New South Wales Government. Retrieved from: https://www1.health.nsw.gov.au/pds/ActivePDSDocuments/GL2018_007.pdf

Al Yazidi, L.S., Marais, B.J, Wickens, M., et al (2019). Overview of Paediatric Tuberculosis cases treated in The Sydney Children's Hospitals Network, Australia. A Journal of The Sax Institute. 29(2). Retrieved from: https://www.phrp.com.au/issues/july-2019-volume-29-issue-2/overview-of-paediatric-tuberculosis-cases-treated-in-the-sydney-childrens-hospitals-network-australia/

Amrock, S. M., Lee, L., & Weitzman, M. (2016). Perceptions of e-cigarettes and noncigarette tobacco products among US youth. Pediatrics, 138(5), e20154306.

Antoon, A. Y., & Donovan, M. K. (2016). Burn injuries. In R. M. Kliegman, B. F. Stanton, J. W. St Geme, et al. (Eds.), Nelson textbook of pediatrics (20th ed.). Philadelphia: Saunders.

Australasian Society of Clinical Immunology and Allergy (ASCIA). (2019a). Allergy Testing: Information for Patients, Consumers and Carers. Retrieved from: https://allergy.org.au/patients/information

Australasian Society of Clinical Immunology and Allergy (ASCIA). (2019b). Allergic Rhinitis (hay fever): Information for Patients, Consumers and Carers. Retrieved from: https://allergy.org.au/patients/information

Australian Government Department of Health (AGDH). (2020). National Immunisation Program Schedule. Retrieved from: https://www.health.gov.au/health-topics/immunisation/immunisation-throughout-life/national-immunisation-program-schedule#national-immunisation-program-schedule-from-1-july-2020

Australian Government, National Health and Medical Research Council, Australian Commission on safety and Quality in Healthcare, Australian Guidelines for the Prevention and Control of Infection in Healthcare 2019. Retrieved from: https://www.nhmrc.gov.au/about-us/publications/australian-guidelines-prevention-and-control-infection-healthcare-2019

Australian Medicines Handbook. (2020). Australian Medicines Handbook, Pty Ltd: Adelaide. Online version: https://amhonline.amh.net.au

Australian Technical Advisory Group on Immunisation (ATAGI) (2018). Australian Immunisation Handbook, Australian Government Department of Health, Canberra. Retrieved from: https://immunisationhandbook.health.gov.au/

Batteiger, B.E. & Tan, M. (2020). Chlamydia Trachomatis (Trachoma and Urogenital Infections). Mandell, Douglas and Bennett's Principles and Practice of Infectious Diseases, 9th edition. Elsevier

Boudewyns, A., Abel, F., Alexopoulos, E., et al. (2017). Adenotonsillectomy to treat obstructive sleep apnea: is it enough? Pediatric Pulmonology, 52(5), 699–709.

Brashers, V.L. & Huether, S.E. (2019). Alterations of Pulmonary Function in Children. In Pathophysiology: The Biologic Basics for disease in Adults and Children. 8th edition. Elsevier.

Burgos, C. M., Modee, A., Ost, E., et al. (2017). Addressing the causes of later mortality in infants with congenital diaphragmatic hernia. J Pediatric Surgery, 52(4), 526.

Campbell, MA, Ford, C. & Winstanley, MH. (2017) CH 4 The Health effects of secondhand smoke. 4.3 Thirdhand smoke. In Tobacco in Australia: facts and Issues. Melbourne, Cancer Council Victoria. Retrieved from: https://www.tobaccoinaustralia.org.au/chapter-4-secondhand/4-3-thirdhand-smoke

Canistro, D. Vivarelli, F. & Cirillo, S. et al. (2017) E-cigarettes induce toxicological effects that can raise the cancer risk, Scientific Reports, 7, 2028.Retrieved from: https://www.ncbi.nlm.nih.gov/pmc/articles/PMC5435699/

Castagnoli, R., Votto, M., Licari, A. (2020). Severe Acute Respiratory Syndrome Coronavirus 2 (SARS-CoV-2) Infection in Children and Adolescents A Systematic Review, JAMA Pediatr. 174(9) 882-889.

Castellani, C., & Assael, B. M. (2017). Cystic fibrosis: a clinical view. Cellular and Molecular Life Sciences, 74(1), 129–140.

Chandrasekharan, PK, Rawat, M. Madappa, R et al 2017. Congenital Diaphragmatic Hernia- a review. Maternal Health, Neonatology and Perinatology. 3:6. Retrieved from: https://www.ncbi.nlm.nih.gov/pmc/articles/PMC5356475/

Chun, L. F., Moazed, F., Calfee, C. S., et al. (2017). Pulmonary toxicity of e-cigarettes. American Journal of Physiology. Lung Cellular and Molecular Physiology, 313(2), L193–L206.

Clarke, K. E. N. (2017). Can I give my 5-year-old over-the-counter cough medicine? American Academy of Pediatrics, Retrieved from: http://www.kjkidmd.com/uploads/1/5/5/0/1550313/can_i_give_my_5-year-old_over-the-counter_cough_medicine__-_healthychildren.pdf

Cystic Fibrosis Australia (2017). What is CF? Retrieved from: https://www.cysticfibrosis.org.au/about-cf/what-is-cf

Cystic Fibrosis Clinical Network. (2016). Infection control practices for children and young people with Cystic Fibrosis. New Zealand Child and Youth Clinical Networks (NZCYCN). 26 October. Retrieved from: https://www.starship.org.nz/guidelines/infection-control-practices-4-children-and-young-people-with-cystic/

Cystic Fibrosis NZ (2019). What is CF? Retrieved from: https://www.cfnz.org.nz/about/what-is-cf/

Daniel BD, Grace GA & Natrajan M. 2019. Tuberculosis Meningitis in Children: Clinical Management and Outcome. Indian Journal of Medical Research. Aug 150(2):117-130.

De Boeck, K., Haarman, E., Hull, J., et al. (2017). Inhaled dry powder mannitol in children with cystic fibrosis: a randomised efficacy and safety trial. Journal of Cystic Fibrosis, 16(3), 380–387.

Demeyer, S., De Boeck, K., Witters, P., et al. (2016). Beyond pancreatic insufficiency and liver disease in cystic fibrosis. European Journal of Pediatrics, 175(7), 881–894.

Egan, M., Green, D. M., & Voynow, J. A. (2016). Cystic fibrosis. In R. M. Kliegman, B. F. Stanton, J. W. St Geme, et al. (Eds.), Nelson textbook of pediatrics (20th ed.). Philadelphia: Elsevier/Saunders.

Ellner, J.J, and Jacobson, K.R. (2020). Tuberculosis. In Goldman-Cecil Medicine. 26th edition: 308, 2000-2010e2. Elsevier

Falk, N. P., Hughes, S. W., & Rodgers, B. C. (2016). Medications for chronic asthma. American Family Physician, 94(6), 454–462.

Friedmann, I., Dahdouh, E. M., Kugler, P., et al. (2017). Maternal and obstetrical predictors of sudden infant death syndrome (SIDS). The Journal of Maternal-fetal and Neonatal Medicine, 30(19), 2315–2323.

Greenhaigh, EM, & Scollo, MN. (2018). Indepth 18B: Electronic cigarettes(e-cigarettes). In Tobacco in Australia: Facts and Issues. Melbourne, Cancer Council Victoria. Retrieved from: https://www.tobaccoinaustralia.org.au/chapter-18-harm-reduction/indepth-18b-e-cigarettes

Jardins, T.D. & Burton, G.G. (2020a). Respiratory Syncytial Virus Infection (Bronchiolitis), In clinical manifestations and assessment of respiratory Disease, (8th edition) Chapter 39, 550-558. Elsevier.

Jardins, TD & Burton, GG (2020b). Asthma. In- Clinical Manifestations and Assessment of respiratory Disease (8th edition). Chapter 14, 218-242. Elsevier.

Jenson, H. (2016). Epstein-Barr virus. In R. M. Kliegman, B. F. Stanton, J. W. St Geme, et al. (Eds.), Nelson textbook of pediatrics (20th ed.). Philadelphia: Elsevier/Saunders.

John Hunter Children's Hospital. (2018). NICU, Neonatal Medicines Formulary Group- Azithromycin-Neonatal Use Only (2018). Retrieved from: http://hnekidshealth.nsw.gov.au/site/nicuguidelines

Kerschner, J. E., & Preciado, D. (2016). Otitis media. In R. M. Kliegman, B. F. Stanton, J. W. St Geme, et al. (Eds.), Nelson textbook of pediatrics (20th ed.). Philadelphia: Elsevier/Saunders.

Korvel-Hanquist, A., Djurhuus, B. D., & Homoe, P. (2017). The effect of breastfeeding on childhood otitis media. Current Allergy and Asthma Reports, 17(7), 45.

Kostic, M. A. (2016). Poisonings. In R. M. Kliegman, B. F. Stanton, J. W. St Geme, et al. (Eds.), Nelson textbook of pediatrics (20th ed.). Philadelphia: Elsevier/Saunders.

Liu, A. H., Covar, R. A., Spahn, J. D., et al. (2016). Childhood asthma. In R. M. Kliegman, B. F. Stanton, J. W. St Geme, et al. (Eds.), Nelson textbook of pediatrics (20th ed.). Philadelphia: Saunders.

Maheshwari, A., & Carlo, W. A. (2016). Diaphragmatic hernia. In R. M. Kliegman, B. F. Stanton, J. W. St Geme, et al. (Eds.), Nelson textbook of pediatrics (20th ed.). Philadelphia: Elsevier/Saunders.

Makadia, L. D., Roper, P. F., Andrews, J. O., et al. (2017). Tobacco use and smoke exposure in children: new trends, harm, and strategies to improve health outcomes. Current Allergy and Asthma Reports, 17(8), 55.

Mazor, R., & Green, T. P. (2016). Pulmonary edema. In R. M. Kliegman, B. F. Stanton, J. W. St Geme, et al. (Eds.), Nelson textbook of pediatrics (20th ed.). Philadelphia: Elsevier/Saunders.

Milgrom, H., & Sicherer, S. H. (2016). Allergic rhinitis. In R. M. Kliegman, B. F. Stanton, J. W. St Geme, et al. (Eds.), Nelson textbook of pediatrics (20th ed.). Philadelphia: Elsevier/Saunders.

Minter, K. & Walker, K. (2018). Care of The Neonate with Surgical Condition. In: Neonatal Nursing in Australia and New Zealand. Chapter 19, 387-404, Elsevier.

Monzr, M & AL Malik, M.D. (2020). Epstein-Barr Virus Infection: 520-521. In Ferri's Clinical Advisor 2020, Elsevier.

Ministry of Health. (2020a). Immunisation Handbook. Wellington: Ministry ofHealth.https://www.health.govt.nz/publication/immunisation-handbook-2020

Ministry of Health. (2020b). New Zealand Immunisation Schedule. Wellington: Ministry of Health. https://www.health.govt.nz/our-work/preventative-health-wellness/immunisation/new-zealand-immunisation-schedule

National Asthma Council Australia (NACA) (2019). Retrieved from: https://www.nationalasthma.org.au/

O'Brien, S., Borland, M.L., Cotterell, E. et al (2018). Australasian Bronchiolitis Guideline. Journal of Paediatrics and Child Health. Volume 55, Issue 1, Jan 2019, Pages 42-53.

O'Neal, L.M (2017). Epiglottitis; Chapter 97: Page 403-406.el. Primary Care 5Th edition. Elsevier.

Oluyomi-Obi, T., Kuret, V., Puligandla, P., et al. (2017). Antenatal predictors of outcome in prenatally diagnosed congenital diaphragmatic hernia (CDH). Journal of Pediatric Surgery, 52(5), 881–888.

Orloff, KE, Turner, DA and Rehder, KJ. June 2019. Pediatric Allergy Immunology and Pulmonary. Vol 32, Issue 2, 35-44. Retrieved from: https://www.liebertpub.com/doi/full/10.1089/ped.2019.0999

Owens, J. A. (2016). Sleep medicine. In R. M. Kliegman, B. F. Stanton, J. W. St Geme, et al. (Eds.), Nelson textbook of pediatrics (20th ed.). Philadelphia: Elsevier/Saunders.

Pedra, P. A., & Stark, A. R.: Bronchiolitis in infants and children: Treatment outcome and prevention, In UpToDate, Mallory GB and Edwards MS (Ed), UpToDate, Waltham MA, 2017.

Powell, J., Graham, D., O'Reilly, S., et al. (2016). Acute pulmonary oedema. Nursing Standard, 39(23), 51–59.

Rasmussen, S. & Thompson, L. (2020). Coronavirus Disease 2019 and Children: What Pediatric Health Care Clinician Need to Know, JAMA Pediatr. 174 (8) 743-744.

Ren, X. C., Gao, Z. W., Li, Y. F., et al. (2017). The effects of clinical factors on airway outcomes of mandibular distraction osteogenesis in children with Pierre Robin sequence. International Journal of Oral and Maxillofacial Surgery, 46(7), 805–810.

Roosevelt, G. E. (2016). Acute inflammatory upper airway obstruction. In R. M. Kliegman, B. F. Stanton, J. W. St Geme, et al. (Eds.), Nelson textbook of pediatrics (20th ed.). Philadelphia: Elsevier/Saunders.

SA Health. (2019). South Australian Paediatric Clinical Practice Guidelines—Paediatric Empyema Excluding Neonates (2019). Government of

South Australia. Retrieved from: https://www.sahealth.sa.gov.au/wps/wcm/connect/public+content/sa+health+internet/about+us/publications+and+resources/policies+and+guidelines

Smith, B. A., Georgiopoulos, A. M., & Quittner, A. L. (2016). Maintaining mental health and function for the long run in cystic fibrosis. Pediatric Pulmonology, 51(S44), S71–S78.

Smith, D. K., Seales, S., & Budzik, C. (2017). Respiratory syncytial virus bronchiolitis in children. American Family Physician, 95(2), 94–99.

Sobin, L., Kawai, K., Irace, A. L., et al. (2017). Microbiology of the upper and lower airways in pediatric cystic fibrosis patients. Otolaryngology–Head and Neck Surgery: Official Journal of American Academy of Otolaryngology–Head and Neck Surgery, 157(2), 302–308.

Speer, M. E. (2017). Neonatal pneumonia. In J.A. Barcia-Prats and M.S. Edwards (Eds.), UpToDate.

Steele, D. W., Adam, G. P., Di, M., et al. (2017). Effectiveness of tympanostomy tubes for otitis media: a meta-analysis, Pediatrics epub ahead of print.

Sun, P., Lu, X., Xu, C., et al. (2020). Understanding of COVID-19 based on current evidence. Journal of Medical Virology. Retrieved from https://www.ncbi.nlm.nih.gov/pmc/articles/PMC7228250/

Therapeutic Goods Administration (TGA). (2018). Montelukast. Department of Health. 12 July. Retrieved from: https://www.tga.gov.au/alert/montelukast

The Royal Children's Hospital, Melbourne (RCHM) (2017). Clinical Practice Guidelines—Bronchiolitis. Retrieved from: https://www.rch.org.au/clinicalguide/guideline_index/Bronchiolitis

The Royal Children's Hospital Melbourne (RCHM). (2018a). Dehydration Fact Sheet. Retrieved from: https://www.rch.org.au/kidsinfo/fact_sheets/Dehydration/

The Royal Children's Hospital Melbourne (RCHM). (2018b). Acute Otitis Media Clinical Practice Guidelines 2018, Retrieved from: https://www.rch.org.au/clinicalguide/guideline_index/Acute_otitis_media/

The Royal Children's Hospital Melbourne (RCHM) (2018c). Obstructive sleep apnoea (OSA): factsheet. Retrieved from: https://www.rch.org.au/kidsinfo/fact_sheets/childhood_obstructive_sleep_apnoea_OSA/

The Royal Children's Hospital Melbourne (RCHM) (2018d). Palivizumab for at-risk Patients. Clinical Guidelines. Retrieved from: https://www.rch.org.au/clinicalguide/

The Royal Children's Hospital Melbourne (RCHM). (2018e). Tuberculosis Screening, Immigrant health Service. Retrieved from: https://www.rch.org.au/immigranthealth/

The Royal Children's Hospital Melbourne (RCHM). (2019a). Sore Throat Clinical Practice Guidelines 2019. Retrieved from https://www.rch.org.au/clinicalguide/

The Royal Children's Hospital Melbourne (RCHM) (2019b). Influenza Clinical Guidelines, retrieved from: https://www.rch.org.au/clinicalguide/

The Royal Children's Hospital Melbourne (RCHM). (2019c). Croup (laryngotracheoBronchitis. Retrieved from: https://www.rch.org.au/clinicalguide/

The Royal Children's Hospital Melbourne (RCHM). (2019d). Apnoea (Neonatal), Clinical Guidelines (nursing). Retrieved from: https://www.rch.org.au/rchcpg/hospital_clinical_guideline_index/Apnoea_Neonatal/

The Sydney Children's Hospital (SCH). 2017. Ventilated Patient: Patient Care in CICU-SCH Practice guideline. Retrieved from: https://www.schn.health.nsw.gov.au/our-policies/index/clinical

The Sydney Children's Hospital Network (SCHN). (2016a). Tonsillectomy Factsheet 2016. Retrieved from: https://www.schn.health.nsw.gov.au/our-policies/index/clinical

The Sydney Children's Hospital Network (SCHN). (2017). Ears, nose and throat: post operative management and care. Practice guideline. 6 January. https://www.schn.health.nsw.gov.au/our-policies/index/clinical

The Sydney Children's Hospital Network (SCHN). (2016b). Pertussis—Emergency Department Management Practice Guideline. Retrieved from: https://www.schn.health.nsw.gov.au/our-policies/index/clinical

Thomas, T.A. (2017). Tuberculosis in Children. Pediatric Clinics of North America, Volume 64, Issue 4. Pages 893-909. Full text article from clinicalkey. Elsevier.

Turck, D., Braegger, C. P., Colombo, C., et al. (2016). ESPEN-ESPGHAN-ECFS guidelines on nutrition care for infant, children, and adults with cystic fibrosis. Clinical Nutrition: Official Journal of the European Society of Parenteral and Enteral Nutrition, 35 (3), 557–577.

Venekamp, R. P., Damoiseaux, R. A., & Schilder, A. G. (2017). Acute otitis media in children. American Family Physician, 95(2), 109–110.

Voss, L., Hamill, J., Twiss, J, Stefanutti, S. (2017). Empyema Clinical Guidelines. Starship Child Health. 20 January. Retrieved from: https://www.starship.org.nz/guidelines/empyema/

Wong, J. J., Jit, M., Sultana, R., et al. (2017). Mortality in pediatric acute respiratory distress syndrome: a systematic review and meta-analysis. Journal of Intensive Care Medicine, epub ahead of print.

World Health Organization (WHO). (2017). TB: global tuberculosis report 2017. Retrieved from http://www.who.int/mediacentre/factsheets/fs104/en/.

World Health Organization (WHO). (2019). Tuberculosis Factsheet. Retrieved from: https://www.who.int/en/news-room/fact-sheets/detail/tuberculosis

World Health Organization (WHO). (2020). WHO Director-General's opening remarks at the media briefing on COVID-19: 11 March 2020. Retrievedfrom.https://www.who.int/dg/speeches/detail/who-director-general-s-opening-remarks-at-the-media-briefing-on-covid-19---11-march-2020

Yang, C., Chilvers, M., Montgomery, M., et al. (2016). Dornase alfa for cystic fibrosis. Cochrane Database of Systematic Review, (4), CD001127.

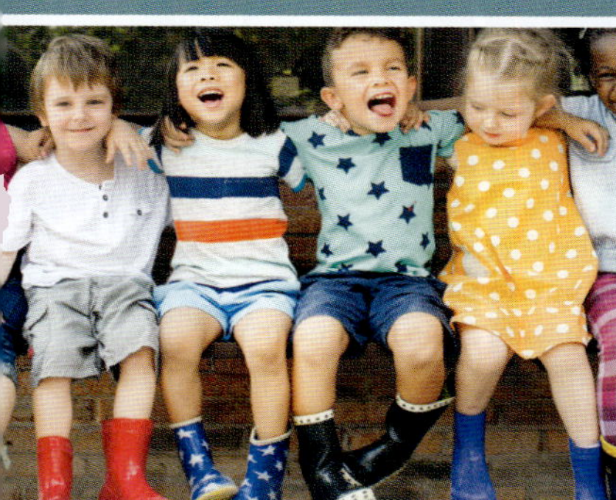

27

The Child with Cardiovascular Dysfunction

Lauren Kendrick

LEARNING OUTCOMES

- Develop an understanding of cardiac structure and the cardiovascular system
- Develop an understanding of common problems children experience with cardiovascular dysfunction
- Understand the complexities in assessment of children with cardiovascular dysfunction
- Understand the importance of family centred care of children with cardiovascular dysfunction

CARDIAC STRUCTURE AND FUNCTION

Cardiovascular disorders in children are divided into two major groups: congenital cardiac defects and acquired heart disorders. Congenital heart defects are anatomical abnormalities present at birth that result in abnormal cardiac function. The clinical consequences of congenital heart defects fall into two broad categories: heart failure (HF) and hypoxaemia. *Acquired cardiac disorders* refer to disease processes or abnormalities that occur after birth and can be seen in the normal heart or in the presence of congenital heart defects. They result from various factors, including infection, autoimmune responses, environmental factors and familial tendencies.

Understanding the effects of congenital and acquired heart defects requires knowledge of the normal heart's structure and function, including embryological development, fetal circulation and postnatal changes. Basic cardiac physiology is presented in this section; altered haemodynamics are discussed on p. 708.

Cardiac Development and Function

The heart is a muscular four-chambered organ whose primary purpose is to pump blood throughout the body. It is located slightly to the left of the sternum in the space between the two pleural cavities, called the **mediastinum**. The main mass of the heart is formed by the muscular tissue, the myocardium. Lining the inner surface of the myocardium is the endocardium, a thin layer of endothelial tissue. The heart also has its own special covering, a double-walled membrane called the **pericardium**. Between the two layers is a slight space (pericardial space), which is filled with a few drops of serous fluid (pericardial fluid). These layers provide for frictionless movement of the heart muscle.

The interior of the heart is divided into four chambers. The two upper chambers are called **atria**, and the two bottom chambers are called **ventricles**. The atria are divided into the right atrium (RA) and the left atrium (LA) by the atrial septum. The ventricles are divided into the right ventricle (RV) and the left ventricle (LV) by the ventricular septum. Located within the heart are four valves, whose main function is to prevent the backflow of blood. The tricuspid valve, so named because it has three leaflets, or cusps, of endocardial tissue projecting into the ventricles, is located between the RA and the RV. The mitral valve has two leaflets and is located between the LA and the LV. Together these two valves are often termed **atrioventricular (AV) valves**. The valve leaflets are attached to the heart muscle by several cordlike structures called **chordae tendineae**. The semilunar valves are located in the pulmonary artery (pulmonic valve) and the aorta (aortic valve). Heart sounds (S_1 and S_2) are related to the vibrations that result during closing of these valves. (See Chapter 4.)

Embryological Development

The heart and other components of the circulatory system (blood, blood vessels, lymph) begin to develop from the mesoderm during the fourth week of gestation and are completely formed by the eighth week.

During the third week, two endocardial tubes fuse to become the heart tube. As the tube elongates, it begins to coil to the right (dextro- or d-looping). This looping occurs by approximately the 28th day, when the heart begins to beat. Concentrations of mesenchymal cells enlarge and cause their lining (endocardium) to bulge into the heart lumen. These internal bulges are called *endocardial cushions* and eventually merge to divide the heart chambers. During the fifth week, the midcardiac tube grows rapidly and assumes a characteristic convoluted shape with identifiable structures. These structures ultimately give rise to the heart chambers and great vessels and include: (1) a common atrium; (2) a common ventricle; (3) the bulbus cordis, which eventually helps form the outflow tracts of the ventricles; (4) the sinus venosus, which develops into the inferior and superior vena cava and coronary sinus; and (5) the truncus arteriosus, which divides into the pulmonary artery and aorta and also gives rise to the aortic arch.

The atrial septum is formed by the growth of both the septum primum and the septum secundum at about the fourth week of fetal development. Overlapping of the septum primum and septum secundum before fusion occurs results in a temporary flap opening known as the foramen ovale. The ventricular septum develops from the joining of the muscular and membranous ventricular septa during the fourth to eighth weeks of growth (Fig 27.1). Congenital defects may result if disturbances occur in the formation of various structures during this partitioning process.

Fetal Circulation. The fetal circulation directs the maximum concentration of oxygenated blood to the most vital organ, the brain. During fetal life, the lungs are essentially non-functional, and the liver is only partially functional so the fetus needs less blood directed to these organs.

Blood carrying oxygen and nutritive materials from the placenta enters the fetal system through the umbilicus via the large umbilical vein (Fig 27.2A). The blood then travels to the liver, where it divides. Part of the blood enters the portal and hepatic circulation of the liver, and the remainder travels directly to the inferior vena cava (IVC) by way of the ductus venosus. Because of the higher pressure of blood entering the RA from the IVC, it is directed in a straight pathway across the RA and through the foramen ovale to the LA. In this way, the better-oxygenated blood enters the LA and LV to be pumped through the aorta to the head and upper extremities. Blood from the head and upper extremities entering the RA from the superior vena cava (SVC) is directed downwards through the tricuspid valve into the RV. From there it is pumped through the pulmonary artery, where the major portion is shunted to the descending aorta via the ductus arteriosus. A small amount flows to and from the non-functioning fetal lungs. Blood is returned to the placenta from the descending aorta through the two umbilical arteries.

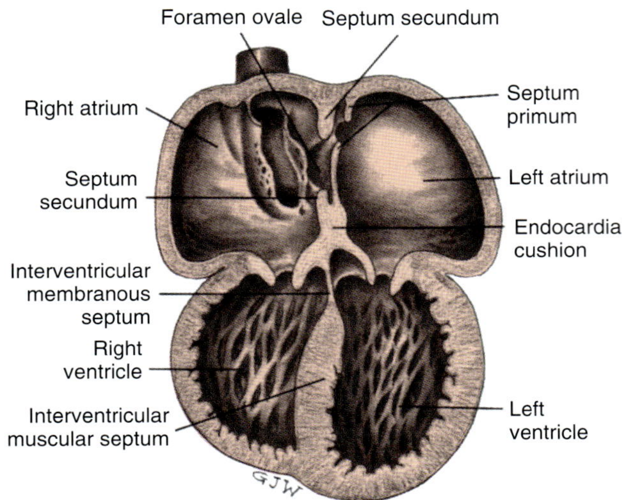

Fig 27.1 Septal development of the heart.

Before birth, the high pulmonary vascular resistance created by the collapsed fetal lung causes greater pressures in the right side of the heart and the pulmonary artery. At the same time, the free-flowing placental circulation and the ductus arteriosus produce a low systemic vascular resistance in the remainder of the fetal vascular system.

Postnatal Circulation. With the clamping of the umbilical cord and the expansion of the lungs at birth, the haemodynamics of the fetal vascular system undergoes pronounced and abrupt changes. The low-pressure placenta is removed from the circulation, the heart takes over pumping blood around the body and systemic vascular resistance starts to rise. With the postnatal rise in systemic vascular resistance, the LV walls become thicker than the walls of the RV, and the pressures on the left side of the heart rise. The lungs expand and take over oxygenation; the increased oxygen has a vasodilating effect on the pulmonary bed, causing a fall in pulmonary vascular resistance. Pressures on the right side of the heart decrease because the RV is pumping blood to the low-pressure pulmonary bed. The transition to a high-pressure systemic circulation and low-pressure pulmonary circulation (seen throughout life) usually takes 6 to 8 weeks.

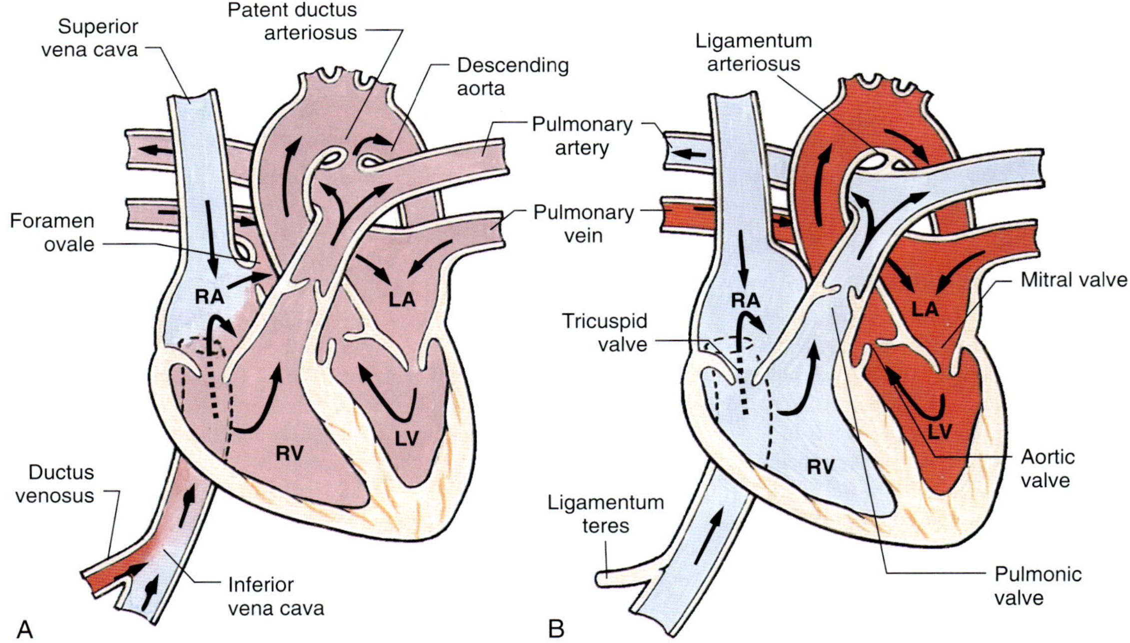

Fig 27.2 Changes in circulation at birth. (**A**) Prenatal circulation. (**B**) Postnatal circulation. Arrows indicate direction of blood flow. Although four pulmonary veins enter the LA, for simplicity this diagram shows only two. (*RA*, right atrium; *LA*, left atrium; *RV*, right ventricle; *LV*, left ventricle.)

The patent ductus arteriosus (PDA) starts to close within the first day after birth by constriction of smooth muscle in the vessel. Closure is influenced by oxygen levels, prostaglandin levels and maturity. The PDA in a preterm infant responds differently, with less responsiveness to oxygen and higher levels of prostaglandins, both of which can cause delayed ductal closure. The PDA usually closes completely by 2 to 3 weeks of age (Park 2014).

After birth, the normal adult blood flow patterns within the heart begin. Blood returning from the body via the SVC and IVC is received in the RA. It flows to the RV through the tricuspid valve. The RV pumps the blood through the pulmonic valve into the pulmonary artery and then to the lungs, where the blood becomes saturated with oxygen. The blood is then returned from the lungs via the pulmonary veins into the LA, where it flows through the mitral valve to the LV, and finally through the aortic valve to the aorta and into the systemic circulation (see Fig 27.2B).

The arterial system provides resistance to blood flow to maintain blood pressure (BP) and circulation. The venous system acts as a collecting system and a reservoir to accommodate changes in circulating blood volume. Both work together to provide equilibrium and maintain BP.

The heart muscle receives its blood supply through the coronary circulation during diastole. The right and left coronary arteries, which arise above the aortic valve, supply all of the myocardium. The heart is the first organ to receive blood with each heartbeat; the brain is next. These two organs depend most on adequate oxygen levels for normal function. Coronary veins collect the blood and return it to the RA directly or through the coronary sinus, which drains into the RA. The flow of blood throughout the systemic circulatory system is shown in Figure 27.3.

Conduction System. To maintain an orderly and effective pumping action, the heart has a specialised electrical conduction system. Electrical impulses generated within the heart initiate the mechanical contraction that leads to the circulation of blood. Although all myocardial cells are capable of developing an action potential and depolarising without external stimulation, certain specialised cells make up the heart's normal conduction system. These structures include the following:

- **sinoatrial (SA) node**, located within the RA wall near the opening of the SVC
- **AV node**, also located within the RA but near the lower end of the septum
- **AV bundle (bundle of His)**, which extends from the AV node along each side of the interventricular septum and then divides into right and left bundle branches
- **Purkinje fibres**, which extend from the AV bundle into the walls of the ventricles.

The SA node is normally the heart's pacemaker and initiates an impulse. The impulse spreads from the SA node throughout the atria to cause depolarisation. As the atria depolarise, impulses spread to the AV node to conduct to the ventricles. The AV node is the major pathway by which the impulses from the atria can be transmitted to the ventricles. The impulses then spread to the AV bundle and Purkinje fibres to cause simultaneous depolarisation of the ventricles.

A cardiac cycle is composed of sequential contraction (**systole**) and relaxation (**diastole**) of both the atria and the ventricles. First, the atria contract, ejecting blood into the relaxed ventricles. Then, as the atria relax, the ventricles contract to eject blood into the pulmonary artery and aorta. During diastole, blood enters the atria from the systemic and pulmonary veins, which completes one cardiac cycle. The coronary arteries fill in diastole.

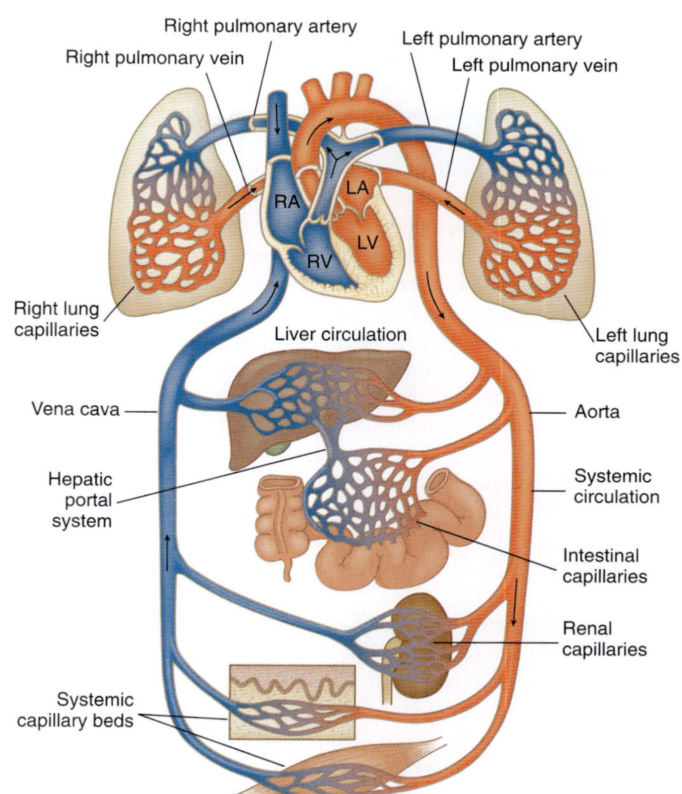

Fig 27.3 Diagram showing serially connected pulmonary and systemic circulatory systems and how to trace the flow of blood. Right heart chambers propel unoxygenated blood through the pulmonary circulation, and the left side of the heart propels oxygenated blood through the systemic circulation. (*RA*, right atrium; *LA*, left atrium; *RV*, right ventricle; *LV*, left ventricle. Source: McCance, K. L., & Huether, S. E. (2010). Pathophysiology: The biological basis for disease in adults and children (6th ed.). St Louis, MO: Mosby.)

Basic Cardiac Physiology

The heart is basically a complex pump, ejecting blood throughout the body. The heart and lungs function together to deliver oxygen to the tissues and remove waste products such as carbon dioxide. The primary function of the cardiopulmonary system is to provide effective oxygen transport to meet the body's metabolic needs. To perform this function, the heart must maintain an adequate cardiac output. By definition, **cardiac output** is the volume of blood ejected by the heart in 1 minute. This is calculated by multiplying the heart rate (number of beats per minute) by the stroke volume. Stroke volume is the amount of blood ejected by the heart in any one contraction. Three factors influence stroke volume: preload, afterload and contractility.

cardiac output = heart rate × stroke volume
↑
preload
afterload
contractility

The autonomic nervous system influences heart rate. The sympathetic fibres increase heart rate, and the parasympathetic fibres, acting through the vagus nerve, decrease heart rate. Levels of circulating catecholamines and other hormones also influence heart rate. Generally, an increase in heart rate increases cardiac output, and a decrease or irregularity in heart rate (bradycardia, dysrhythmia) impairs cardiac output. However, a very fast heart rate shortens diastole and impairs coronary artery perfusion, which causes eventual impairment of cardiac muscle function.

In simple terms, **preload** is the volume of blood returning to the heart, or the circulating blood volume. In physiological terms, preload refers to myocardial fibre length. If the amount of blood delivered to the heart increases, the myocardial fibres lengthen and a greater amount of blood is pumped out of the heart. The circulating blood volume is easiest to assess clinically using the central venous pressure (CVP).

Afterload refers to the resistance against which the ventricles must pump when ejecting blood (ventricular ejection). Conditions that make it more difficult for the heart to pump blood forwards into the circulation (e.g. severe hypertension) increase the afterload. Afterload is determined by several complex factors, primarily the relative resistances of the systemic circulation (systemic vascular resistance) and the pulmonary circulation (pulmonary vascular resistance). Clinically, in the absence of haemodynamic monitoring, measurement of arterial BP gives some indication of afterload. Higher BP indicates greater afterload.

Contractility refers to the efficiency of myocardial fibre shortening, or the ability of the cardiac muscle to act as an efficient pump. There is no simple bedside technique to assess contractility, although an echocardiogram may be useful. Contractility is often inferred in clinical practice. Assessments of peripheral tissue perfusion (pulses, warmth of extremities and capillary refill) and urinary output can be helpful. Decreased contractility is suspected if the extremities are cool with thready pulses and urinary output is diminished. Certain states are known to depress contractility (e.g. hypoxia, acidosis).

Adequate systemic perfusion depends on an appropriate heart rate, adequate circulating blood volume, efficient pump function, appropriate systemic and pulmonary vascular resistances, capillary permeability and tissue utilisation of oxygen. The body makes frequent adjustments in the various determinants of cardiac output to maintain a steady state. Cardiac output is often low in the early postoperative period after cardiac surgery.

Several clinical examples are useful to illustrate these principles. Starling's law (Frank-Starling curve) demonstrates that an increase in ventricular end-diastolic volume (caused by an increased preload) somewhat increases stroke volume. Because the myocardial fibres can stretch only to a certain point and still function effectively, any increase in volume beyond this point impairs cardiac output. When decreased cardiac output results from decreased preload (e.g. in hypovolaemia due to blood loss), treatment involves providing volume, with either intravenous (IV) fluids or blood products. If decreased cardiac output results from a dramatic increase in afterload (e.g. severe hypertension) that increases the myocardial workload, treatment involves reducing afterload with vasodilating drugs. Medications such as digoxin or IV inotropic agents such as dopamine or dobutamine enhance contractility. Adjustments in heart rate are the most common response to changes in cardiac output. The heart rate is slowest during sleep and can more than double with strenuous physical exercise.

Assessment of Cardiac Function

History

Taking an accurate health history is an important first step in assessing an infant or child for possible heart disease. Parents may have specific concerns, such as poor feeding or fast breathing in their infant or the inability of their 7 year old to keep up with his friends on the soccer field. Other parents may not realise that their child has a medical problem; the child may always have been pale and an unsettled baby.

Asking details about the mother's health history, pregnancy and birth history is important in assessing infants. Mothers with chronic health conditions, such as diabetes or lupus erythematosus, are more likely to have infants with heart disease. Some medications, such as phenytoin (Dilantin), are teratogenic to the fetus. Maternal alcohol use or illicit drug use increases the risk of congenital heart defects. Exposure to infection, such as rubella, early in pregnancy may result in congenital anomalies. Infants with low birth weight because of intrauterine growth restriction are more likely to have congenital anomalies. High-birth-weight infants, often offspring of diabetic mothers, also have an increased incidence of heart disease.

A detailed family history is also important. There is an increased incidence of congenital cardiac defects if either parent or a sibling has a heart defect. Some diseases, such as Marfan syndrome and hypertrophic cardiomyopathy, are hereditary. A family history of frequent fetal loss, sudden infant death and sudden death in adults may indicate heart disease. Congenital heart defects occur in many disorders such as Down syndrome and Turner's syndrome.

The health history of an infant should include details about feeding patterns, weight gain and development. Feeding difficulties accompanied by fatigue, rapid breathing and sweating with feeds and poor weight gain are common in infants with heart disease. The incidence of frequent respiratory infections and breathing problems should be noted. Parents should be asked about colour changes, particularly cyanosis or pallor.

With older children and adolescents, history taking should include questions about exercise tolerance and activities, oedema and respiratory problems, chest pain, palpitations and neurological problems such as fainting or headaches. Recent infections or toxic exposures may precede the development of heart diseases such as cardiomyopathy or rheumatic fever.

In all patients, a review of all other health problems and the presence of other congenital anomalies are important. All medications taken, including over-the-counter medications and herbal supplements, should be reviewed because prolonged or incorrect use of many medications can cause cardiac symptoms.

Physical Examination

Assessment of vital signs is helpful in screening patients for diseases of the cardiovascular system. A normal pulse rate varies with age. The younger the patient, the faster the rate. A heart rate that is abnormally fast (**tachycardia**) or abnormally slow (**bradycardia**) may indicate cardiac disease. It is important to note that an acceleration of the heart rate with inspiration is normal. A fast respiratory rate (**tachypnoea**) may indicate HF. Hypertension is diagnosed by serial BP measurements.

Several aspects of physical examination may yield evidence of heart disease. (See Chapter 4 for a general discussion of physical assessment of the heart.) During inspection, perform a general assessment of skin colour (particularly the presence of cyanosis), position of comfort and overall nutritional status. During palpation, establish the point of maximum intensity and the apical impulse because they may offer clues to the position of the heart. Note the presence of a thrill, a soft vibration over the heart that reflects the transmitted sound of a heart murmur. Assess the quality of chest activity ('active praecordium'), quality and symmetry of all pulses, warmth of extremities and presence or absence of oedema. Locating the hepatic and splenic borders for evidence of organ enlargement is also important.

Auscultation of heart sounds begins with assessment of heart rate and rhythm. The normal heart sounds S_1 and S_2 are auscultated, and the normal physiological splitting of S_2 is noted. This splitting is caused by the normal closure of the aortic valve before the pulmonic valve. The presence of additional heart sounds, such as a gallop or a murmur, is noted. Auscultation of lung sounds, in particular crackles, wheezing, grunting or decreased or absent breath sounds in some areas, is also important in the assessment of cardiovascular disease.

Murmurs are heart sounds that reflect the flow of blood within the heart. They may occur in either systole or diastole or in both (a continuous murmur). They may reflect blood flow through a normal heart (particularly during periods of increased cardiac output such as fever, anaemia or rapid growth) or indicate abnormalities within the heart or the great arteries. (See Chapter 4 for a more detailed discussion of heart murmurs.) About 80% of children have an innocent murmur of one type at some point during childhood (Park 2014). Innocent murmurs are present in infants and children with normal cardiac anatomy and heart function.

Tests of Cardiac Function

A variety of invasive and non-invasive tests may be employed in the diagnosis of heart disease. The more frequently conducted tests are described here.

Electrocardiography

Electrocardiography (ECG) measures the electrical activity of the heart displayed in graphic form and provides information on heart rate and rhythm, abnormal rhythms or conduction, ischaemic changes and other information (Fig 27.4). The normal ECG consists of the following.

- **P wave**—Represents the spread of the impulse over the atria (atrial depolarisation). The sinus node's electrical activity is not represented in the ECG.
- **P-R interval**—Represents the time that elapses from the beginning of atrial depolarisation to the beginning of ventricular depolarisation. It is termed P-R instead of P-Q because the Q wave is frequently absent.
- **QRS complex**—Represents ventricular depolarisation. It is actually composed of three separate waves—the Q, the R and the S—that result from the currents generated when the ventricles depolarise before their contraction.
- **T wave**—Represents ventricular repolarisation.
- **Q-T interval**—Represents ventricular depolarisation and repolarisation. This interval varies with heart rate; the faster the rate, the shorter the Q-T interval. Therefore, in children this interval is normally shorter than in adults.
- **ST segment**—Represents the time that the ventricles are in the absolute refractory period, the period between ventricular depolarisation and repolarisation.

An ECG is taken by placing leads or electrodes on the skin to transmit electrical impulses back to a recording machine. Usually the electrodes are attached to the extremities and chest with an adhesive, such as hydrogel. An electrolyte lubricant is placed between the skin and the lead to increase conductivity. Chest leads must be positioned correctly because even minor misplacement can cause considerable inaccuracy in the recording. The standard adult ECG is measured using 12 leads (6 limb leads and 6 chest leads). The standard paediatric ECG is measured using 15 leads, with leads added on the right side of the chest and on the left lateral chest area.

An ECG takes about 15 minutes to perform and the child must remain still while the tracing is done. Infants and young children may be unsettled with lead placement. The leads can be frightening and may pull at the skin when being placed and removed. Infants and young children may be more cooperative if they can rest in the parent's lap during the procedure.

ECG has been adapted for ambulatory use to diagnose and monitor patients with arrhythmias. Continuous ambulatory monitoring is done with a **Holter monitor**, a transistorised tape recorder attached to chest leads. Holter recording, often used when a child is having daily symptoms of a potential arrhythmia, records the heart rhythm continuously for 24 to 72 hours. The recording is then sent to a paediatric cardiologist to interpret. The child and the parents are instructed to keep a diary of activities so that any correlation between activity and

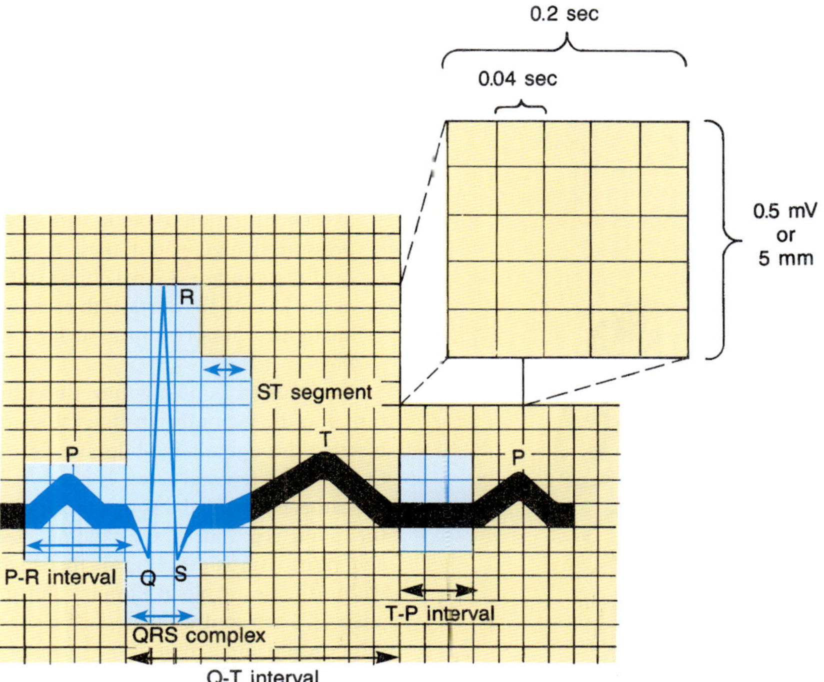

Fig 27.4 Normal electrocardiogram pattern. Inset *(upper right)* shows conventional time and voltage or amplitude (height) calibrations.

any rhythm event may be interpreted. For intermittent rhythm events, an **event monitor**, which can be used when a child feels an abnormal rhythm, is often used. **Implantable loop recorders** can be placed under the skin for months to capture infrequent symptoms. There are now smart phone applications that can detect some arrhythmias (Haberman et al 2015).

Bedside ECG cardiac monitoring is commonly used in paediatrics, especially in the care of children with heart disease. The bedside monitor provides valuable information about heart rate and rhythm through a graphic display of the ECG tracing and a digital display. An alarm can be set with parameters matched to individual patient requirements and will sound if the heart rate is above or below the set parameters. Gelfoam electrodes are commonly used and are placed on the right side of the chest (above the level of the heart) and on the left side of the chest; a ground electrode is placed on the abdomen (Fig 27.5). Electrodes should be changed every 1 or 2 days because they irritate the skin. Bedside monitors are an adjunct to patient care and should never be substituted for direct assessment and auscultation of heart sounds. The nurse should assess the patient, not the monitor.

Echocardiography

Echocardiography is one of the most frequently used procedures for detecting cardiac dysfunction in children. Echocardiography involves the use of ultra-high-frequency sound waves to produce an image of the heart's structure. A transducer placed directly on the chest wall delivers repetitive pulses of ultrasound and processes the returned signals (echoes).

Recent improvements in echocardiographic technology allow the diagnosis of most congenital heart defects by non-invasive echo imaging. Many defects are now diagnosed prenatally with fetal echocardiography, and the number of infants diagnosed with heart defects in utero is rising.

There are three types of transthoracic echocardiography. Motion-mode (M-mode) echocardiography provides a one-dimensional view of the heart and is useful in determining its size, the presence or absence of structures and their relationship to one another. Two-dimensional (2D), or cross-sectional, echocardiography provides information about spatial relationships between structures. Pulse, or continuous Doppler, echocardiography is generally used with 2D 'echo' to provide information about volume flow rate. Three-dimensional (3D) imaging is used primarily to assess valve anatomy and function.

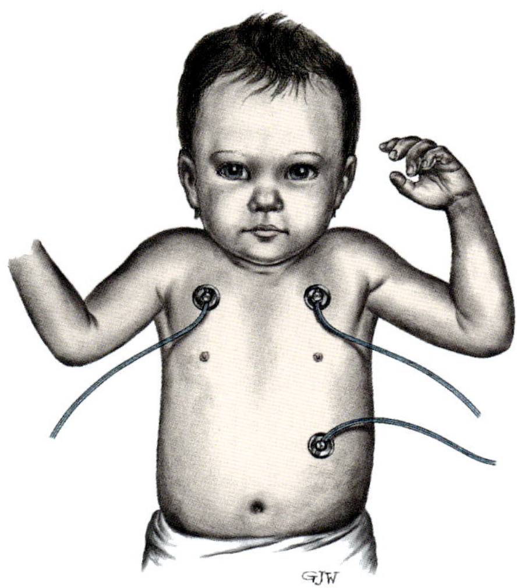

Fig 27.5 Electrode placement for standard chest lead II in cardiac monitoring.

Although the test is non-invasive, painless and associated with no known side effects, it can be stressful for children. The child must lie quietly for up to an hour for a full anatomical study. Lack of cooperation can limit the ability to obtain all the needed images. Infants and young children may need a mild sedative or anaesthesia. Older children benefit from preparation for the test; a play therapist could be beneficial in this preparation. The distraction of a movie or music is often helpful.

Transoesophageal echocardiography (TOE) is performed with the transducer passed into the oesophagus to an area behind the atria. It can provide information in cases in which it is difficult to obtain images using the transthoracic approach. In paediatrics, the most common use is in the operating room to assess the cardiac repair before the patient comes off cardiopulmonary bypass. Patients require IV sedation or general anaesthesia, and often intubation, for a TOE.

Cardiac Magnetic Resonance Imaging

Cardiac magnetic resonance imaging (MRI) uses magnetic field and pulses of radio wave energy to produce real-time 3D images of the intracardiac and extracardiac vascular structures and assessments of ventricular function. It is often used in older children and adolescents when more quantitative information (e.g. volume of ventricular chambers, measurement of valve regurgitation) is needed that cannot be obtained by echo or if echo imaging windows have become limited. The use of MRI has rapidly expanded in the last decade. Although MRI is non-invasive, it can take an hour or more and patients have to lie still inside the scanner. Children under age 7 years, patients with claustrophobia and those with developmental delays or other issues that limit cooperation will require anaesthesia, deep sedation or conscious sedation (depending on institutional preferences). Because the MRI is a magnet, patients with metal implants such as pacemakers, implantable cardioverter-defibrillators or cochlear implants cannot be scanned and all patients are carefully screened for safety compatibility.

CARDIAC CATHETERISATION

Cardiac catheterisation is an invasive diagnostic procedure, in which a radio-opaque catheter is inserted through a peripheral blood vessel into the heart. It is usually combined with angiography (angiocardiography), in which a radio-opaque contrast material is injected through the catheter and into the circulation. Cardiac catheterisation provides information regarding the following:

- oxygen saturation of blood within the chambers and great vessels
- pressure changes within these structures
- cardiac output or stroke volume (the amount of blood pumped out of the LV into the aorta with each contraction)
- anatomical abnormalities, such as septal defects or obstruction to flow.

The catheter is usually introduced through a percutaneous puncture into the femoral vein (the catheter is threaded over a guide wire inserted through a large-bore needle). Other blood vessels are sometimes used if femoral access is not possible. Once the vessel is entered, the catheter is guided through the heart with the aid of fluoroscopy. As the tubing is advanced, the child may feel pressure at the insertion site and vasospasm (fluttering) of the small vessels. Once the catheter is within the heart, blood samples and pressure readings are taken for analysis. Then contrast material may be injected and films taken of the dilution and circulation of the material.

Cardiac catheterisation may be performed for diagnostic, interventional or electrophysiological purposes (Table 27.1). The two types of **diagnostic cardiac catheterisation** are right-sided, or venous,

TABLE 27.1 Common Interventional Cardiac Catheterisation Procedures in Children and Adolescents

Intervention	Diagnosis
Balloon atrial septostomy	Transposition of the great vessels Other complex defects
Balloon dilation	Valvar pulmonary stenosis Branch pulmonary artery stenosis Congenital valvar aortic stenosis Rheumatic mitral stenosis Recurrent coarctation of the aorta
Stent placement	Pulmonary artery stenosis Coarctation of the aorta in adolescents
Coil occlusion	Small patent ductus arteriosus Collateral vessels in single-ventricle patients
Transcatheter device closure	Some atrial septal defects (secundum type) Larger patent ductus arteriosus Fenestrations after Fontan procedures
Transcatheter pulmonary valve replacement	Incompetent pulmonary valves after surgery to repair right ventricular outflow tract
Radiofrequency ablation	Some tachydysrhythmias

All patients are evaluated for suitability for a catheter-based intervention (age, size and location of defect, risk and benefits of procedure, etc.). Surgery may be indicated for some patients (Feltes et al 2011, Holzer & Hijazi 2016).

catheterisation, in which the catheter is introduced from a vein into the RA, and left-sided, or arterial, catheterisation, in which the catheter is threaded by way of a systemic artery retrograde into the aorta and LV, from a right-sided approach across the LA by means of a septal puncture, or through an existing abnormal septal opening. In children, the most common method is right-sided catheterisation because septal defects permit entry into the left side of the heart. The number of diagnostic catheterisations is decreasing as improvements in echocardiography and other non-invasive imaging methods allow more accurate non-invasive diagnosis.

Interventional cardiac catheterisation is the use of a catheter-delivered device to treat heart disease, such as use of a balloon catheter to dilate narrowed valves and vessels and catheter delivery of devices to close some simple defects. It has rapidly expanded in the last 30 years as new techniques, devices and applications have been developed. It has replaced surgical treatment for some congenital heart defects, such as isolated valvular pulmonary artery stenosis, and has become an alternative therapy for others, such as closing patent ductus arteriosus or atrial septal defects in some patients with favourable anatomy.

Electrophysiological studies are used to evaluate and treat dysrhythmias. Diagnostic electrophysiological catheterisation employs catheters with tiny electrodes that record the heart's electrical impulses directly from the conduction system. Interventional electrophysiological catheterisation uses radiofrequency ablation to destroy abnormal accessory pathways. Some pacemakers can be placed in the catheterisation laboratory.

Nursing Care Management. Cardiac catheterisation has become a routine procedure and may be done on an outpatient basis. Catheterisation is not without risks, however, especially in neonates and seriously ill infants and children. Patients are exposed to radiation, general anaesthesia for many cases and contrast materials and medications that can cause allergic reactions or renal insufficiency. Possible complications include acute haemorrhage from the entry site requiring transfusion (more likely with interventional procedures because larger catheters are used), loss of a pulse due to vascular injury in the catheterised extremity (usually transient, resulting from a clot, haematoma or intimal tear) and transient dysrhythmias (generally catheter induced). Serious complications such as valve damage, perforation of the heart, central nervous system (CNS) injury, stroke or death are rare (Feltes et al 2011).

Preprocedural care. A complete nursing assessment is necessary to ensure a safe procedure with minimum complications. This assessment should include accurate height (essential for correct catheter selection) and weight. Obtaining a history of allergic reactions is important because some of the contrast agents are iodine based. Specific attention to signs and symptoms of infection is crucial. Severe nappy rash may be a reason to cancel the procedure if femoral access is required. Because assessment of pedal pulses is important after catheterisation, the nurse should assess and mark the pulses (dorsalis pedis, posterior tibial) before the child goes to the catheterisation laboratory. Baseline oxygen saturation using pulse oximetry in children with cyanosis is also recorded.

Preparing the child and family for the procedure is the joint responsibility of the healthcare team. School-age children and adolescents benefit from a description of the catheterisation laboratory and a chronological explanation of the procedure, emphasising what they will see, feel and hear. They may bring earphones so that they can listen to music during the catheterisation procedure. Preparation materials such as picture books, electronic applications or tours of the catheterisation laboratory may be helpful. Preparation should be geared to the child's developmental level.

The child's caregivers often benefit from the same explanations. Additional information, such as the expected length of the catheterisation, description of the child's appearance after catheterisation and usual postprocedure care, should be outlined (also see the Prepare the Child and Family for Invasive Procedures section later in this chapter).

Methods of sedation vary among institutions and may include oral or IV medications (see Chapter 22). The child's age, heart defect, clinical status and type of catheterisation procedure planned are considered when sedation is determined. General anaesthesia is needed for most interventional procedures. Infants and patients with polycythaemia may need IV fluids to prevent dehydration and hypoglycaemia.

Postprocedural care. Patients may recover from the catheterisation procedure in a recovery unit or in their hospital rooms. Some may require care in the intensive care unit (ICU). Patients are placed on a cardiac monitor and a pulse oximeter for the first few hours after catheterisation.

The most important nursing assessments include the following:

- pulses, especially below the catheterisation site, for equality and symmetry (pulse distal to the site may be weaker for the first few hours after catheterisation but should gradually increase in strength)
- temperature and colour of the affected extremity because coolness or blanching may indicate arterial obstruction
- vital signs, which may be taken as frequently as every 15 minutes, with special emphasis on the heart rate, which is counted for 1 full minute for evidence of dysrhythmias or bradycardia
- BP, especially for hypotension, which may indicate haemorrhage from cardiac perforation or bleeding at the site of initial catheterisation
- dressing, for evidence of bleeding or haematoma formation in the femoral or antecubital area

- fluid intake, both IV and oral, to ensure adequate hydration (blood loss in the catheterisation laboratory, the child's pre-procedure nil by mouth status and diuretic actions of contrast material used during the procedure put the child at risk for hypovolaemia and dehydration).

Infants are particularly at risk for hypoglycaemia. They should receive glucose-containing IV fluids, and blood glucose levels should be checked.

Depending on hospital policy, the child may remain in bed with the affected extremity maintained straight for 4 to 6 hours after venous catheterisation and 6 to 8 hours after arterial catheterisation to facilitate healing of the cannulated vessel. If younger children have difficulty complying, they can be held in the parent's lap with the leg maintained in the correct position. The child's usual diet can be resumed as soon as tolerated, beginning with sips of clear liquids and advancing as the condition allows it. Generally there is only slight discomfort at the percutaneous site. Paracetamol or ibuprofen is usually adequate to treat pain. The catheterisation site is covered with an occlusive dressing to prevent bleeding and contamination that could cause infection. Home care instructions are listed in the Family-Centred Care box.

FAMILY-CENTRED CARE

After Cardiac Catheterisation

- Remove pressure dressing the day after catheterisation. Cover the site with an adhesive bandage strip for several days. Put a new bandage on every day for the next 2 days.
- Keep site clean and dry. Avoid baths for the first 3 days; older children may shower the first day after catheterisation.
- Observe site for redness, swelling, drainage and bleeding. Monitor the child for fever. Observe the catheter leg for coolness. Notify the practitioner if these occur.
- The child should avoid strenuous exercise for several days but may attend school.
- The child can resume regular diet without restrictions.
- Use paracetamol or ibuprofen for pain.
- Keep follow-up appointments per practitioner's instructions.

Congenital Heart Disease

A congenital heart defect can be a single defect in the septum, a heart valve or the arteries and veins, but it is often a combination of defects in one or more of these areas. The exact cause of most congenital cardiac diseases is unknown. Most are thought to be a result of multiple factors—a complex interaction of genetic and environmental influences. Some risk factors are known to be associated with increased incidence of congenital heart defects. Maternal risk factors include chronic illnesses such as diabetes or poorly controlled phenylketonuria, alcohol consumption and exposure to environmental toxins and infections (Department of Health [DoH] 2019). Family history of a cardiac defect in a parent or sibling increases the likelihood of a cardiac anomaly. The risk of congenital heart disease (CHD) increases if a first-degree relative (parent or sibling) is affected. The familial risk is higher with left-sided obstructive lesions (DoH 2019).

Congenital heart anomalies are often associated with chromosomal abnormalities, specific syndromes or congenital defects in other body systems. Down syndrome (trisomy 21) and trisomy 13 and 18 are highly correlated with congenital heart defects. Syndromes associated with heart defects include DiGeorge's syndrome, also known as 22q11 deletion syndrome (heart defects, poor immune system function, a cleft palate, complications related to low levels of calcium in the blood and delayed development with behavioural and emotional problems), Noonan's syndrome (pulmonic valve anomalies and cardiomyopathy), Williams syndrome (aortic and pulmonic stenosis) and Holt-Oram syndrome (upper limb anomalies and atrial septal defect). Extracardiac defects such as tracheo-oesophageal fistula, renal abnormalities and diaphragmatic hernia are seen in association with heart anomalies.

Altered Haemodynamics

The physiology of heart defects is defined by pressure gradients, blood flow and resistance within the circulation. Blood flows because of pressure gradients in different parts of the body and because of the heart's pumping action. Like any fluid, blood flows from an area of high pressure to one of low pressure and takes the path of least resistance. The rate of flow is directly proportional to the pressure gradient (i.e. the higher the pressure gradient, the greater the rate of flow) and inversely proportional to the resistance (i.e. the higher the resistance, the lower the rate of flow). However, increased resistance does not always decrease flow. If the proximal cardiac chamber can increase the driving pressure proportionally, flow can remain unchanged.

Normally the pressure on the right side of the heart is lower than that on the left side, and the resistance in the pulmonary circulation is less than that in the systemic circulation. Likewise, vessels entering or exiting these chambers have corresponding pressures (e.g. lower pressure in the pulmonary artery and higher pressure in the aorta). Therefore, if an abnormal connection exists between the heart chambers, such as a septal defect, blood flows from an area of higher pressure (left side) to one of lower pressure (right side). This directional flow of blood is termed a *left-to-right shunt*. If the opening is small, the amount of blood shunted to the atrium or ventricle may be minimal.

An understanding of saturations within the heart is also helpful in understanding CHD. The blood returning to the heart via the great veins (the SVC and the IVC) should have the lowest oxygen saturation because the tissues should have extracted oxygen, leaving the venous blood desaturated. Saturations in the RA, RV and pulmonary artery should be equal. Blood returning from the lungs to the heart through the pulmonary veins should be fully saturated, the most oxygen-rich blood in the body. Saturations on the left side of the heart should all be equal, with fully saturated blood entering the aorta and first supplying the heart muscle through the coronary arteries and then supplying the brain (Fig 27.6). Normally, saturated blood circulates separately from desaturated blood. Depending on the type of defect, saturated and desaturated blood may be mixed. The amount of mixed blood that reaches the systemic circulation is a significant feature of several cardiac anomalies, and varying degrees of hypoxaemia and cyanosis result.

Clinical Consequences of Congenital Heart Disease

Depending on the severity of the cardiac defect and the altered haemodynamics, two principal clinical consequences can occur: congestive heart failure (CHF) and hypoxaemia (DoH 2019). Defects that result in left-to-right shunting of blood cause symptoms of CHF. Defects that result in decreased pulmonary blood flow cause cyanosis. The conditions can occur alone or together. They can also occur both before surgical repair and after surgical intervention in some cases. Advanced HF, a situation in which HF persists despite surgical and medical interventions, is addressed later in this chapter. Pulmonary hypertension, an uncommon condition, may occur as a result of congenital heart defects and is included in this section. Pulmonary hypertension as a congenital condition is discussed later in this chapter. Nursing care plays a critical role in the early identification and supportive management of these conditions.

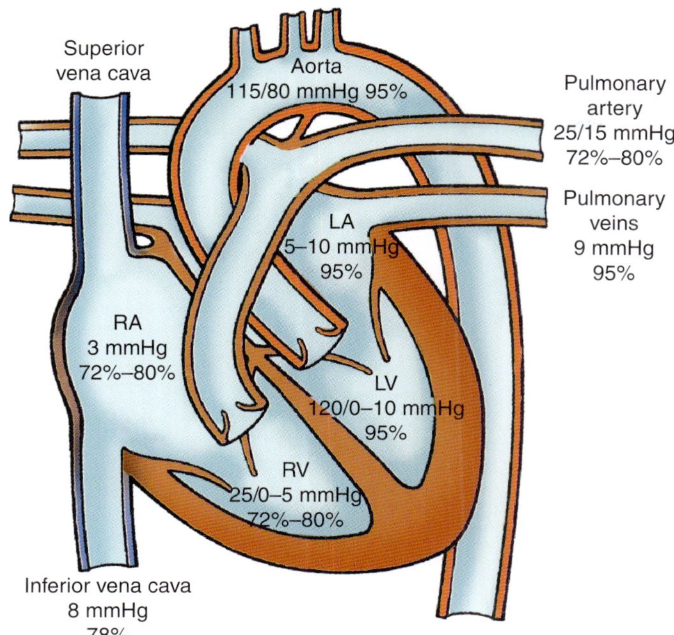

Fig 27.6 Normal chamber pressures (mmHg) and oxygen saturations (SaO_2) in cardiac chambers and great arteries. For simplicity, only two of the four pulmonary veins are shown. (*RA*, right atrium; *LA*, left atrium; *RV*, right ventricle; *LV*, left ventricle.)

Congestive Heart Failure

Congestive heart failure is the inability of the heart to pump an adequate amount of blood to the systemic circulation at normal filling pressures to meet the body's metabolic demands. It can be referred to as either *congestive heart failure* (CHF) or *heart failure* (HF). Causes of CHF can be classified in terms of the following changes:

- volume overload, especially with left-to-right shunts that may cause the RV to hypertrophy to compensate for the additional blood volume
- pressure overload, primarily resulting from obstructive lesions, such as valvular stenosis or coarctation of the aorta
- decreased contractility, primarily decreased contractility of the myocardium, caused by factors such as cardiomyopathy or myocardial ischaemia from severe anaemia or asphyxia; heart block; acidaemia; and low levels of potassium, glucose, calcium or magnesium
- high cardiac output demands, in which the body's need for oxygenated blood exceeds the heart's cardiac output (even though the volume may be normal), such as in sepsis, hyperthyroidism and severe anaemia.

The aetiology of HF varies according to the age of onset; CHF occurs in children with both CHD and normal cardiac structure. CHF occurs most frequently secondary to congenital heart defects in which structural abnormalities result in an increased volume load or increased pressure load on the ventricles. For example, septal defects can cause large left-to-right shunts, which result in a volume load on the RV. Obstruction to flow out of the LV, such as narrowing of the aorta (coarctation of the aorta), can cause increased pressure inside the ventricle. HF can also be a result of an excessive workload on a normal myocardium. Myocardial failure, in which the contractility of the heart muscle is impaired, can result from cardiomyopathy, drugs, electrolyte imbalances, dysrhythmias and other causes. Diseases in other organ systems, particularly the lungs, also can cause CHF. Obstructive changes in the lungs result in increased pulmonary vascular resistance, which increases the RV workload. In time, the right side of the heart has difficulty pumping blood forwards to the lungs, becomes dilated and hypertrophies; then signs and symptoms of right-sided heart failure are seen. *Cor pulmonale* is the term for CHF resulting from obstructive lung diseases such as cystic fibrosis or bronchopulmonary dysplasia.

Altered Haemodynamics

Theoretically, HF may be divided into two types: right-sided failure and left-sided failure. In right-sided failure, RV function is reduced. RV end-diastolic pressure rises, causing increased CVP and systemic venous engorgement. Systemic venous hypertension causes hepatomegaly and may cause oedema in the extremities. In left-sided failure, LV dysfunction occurs and LV end-diastolic pressure rises; the result is increased pressure in the LA and also in the pulmonary veins. The lungs become congested with blood, which leads to elevated pulmonary pressures and pulmonary oedema.

Although each type of HF produces different signs and symptoms, clinically it is unusual to observe solely right- or left-sided failure in children. Because each side of the heart depends on adequate functioning of the other side, failure of one chamber causes a reciprocal change in the opposite chamber.

Compensatory Mechanisms. The heart initially tries to meet the body's demand for increased cardiac output through several compensatory mechanisms called the **cardiac reserve**. These include hypertrophy and dilation of the cardiac muscle and stimulation of the sympathetic nervous system (Fig 27.7).

Hypertrophy and dilation of the cardiac muscle. In response to the need to increase cardiac output, the cardiac muscle hypertrophies, developing greater tension. It is able to generate increased pressure within the ventricle, pumping blood out of the heart at a higher pressure. Also, the cardiac muscle can dilate and increase the stretch of its fibres, which increases the force of contraction. However, both hypertrophy and dilation have potentially negative effects. Hypertrophy may result in decreased ventricular compliance over time. When compliance decreases, a higher filling pressure is required to produce the same stroke volume. The increased muscle mass impairs oxygenation to the heart muscle. Beyond a certain amount of dilation, the force of contraction decreases and the heart fails. (See discussion of Starling's law, p. 704.)

Stimulation of the sympathetic nervous system. When cardiac output begins to fall, stretch receptors and baroreceptors in the blood vessels stimulate the sympathetic nervous system, releasing catecholamines. Catecholamines increase the force and rate of myocardial contraction, as manifested by tachycardia. They cause peripheral vasoconstriction, which results in increased systemic vascular resistance; increased venous return; and reduced blood flow to the limbs, viscera and kidneys. Sympathetic cholinergic fibres cause sweating.

Although initially successful in increasing cardiac output, prolonged sympathetic stimulation also has negative effects. By shortening the diastolic period, tachycardia increases oxygen consumption by the heart muscle, eliminates the heart's resting phase and impairs coronary artery perfusion. A continued increase in systemic vascular resistance increases the afterload on the heart muscle, which requires extra work by the heart muscle and reduces systemic blood flow.

The renal system is particularly sensitive to reductions in blood flow and renal perfusion, which activate the renin-angiotensin-aldosterone mechanism. Renin-angiotensin secretion causes vasoconstriction and leads to an increase in aldosterone secretion, which causes retention of salt and water. Retention of salt and water causes an increase in preload. Although at first helpful to the failing heart, the sodium and water retention becomes excessive, resulting in signs of systemic venous congestion and fluid overload.

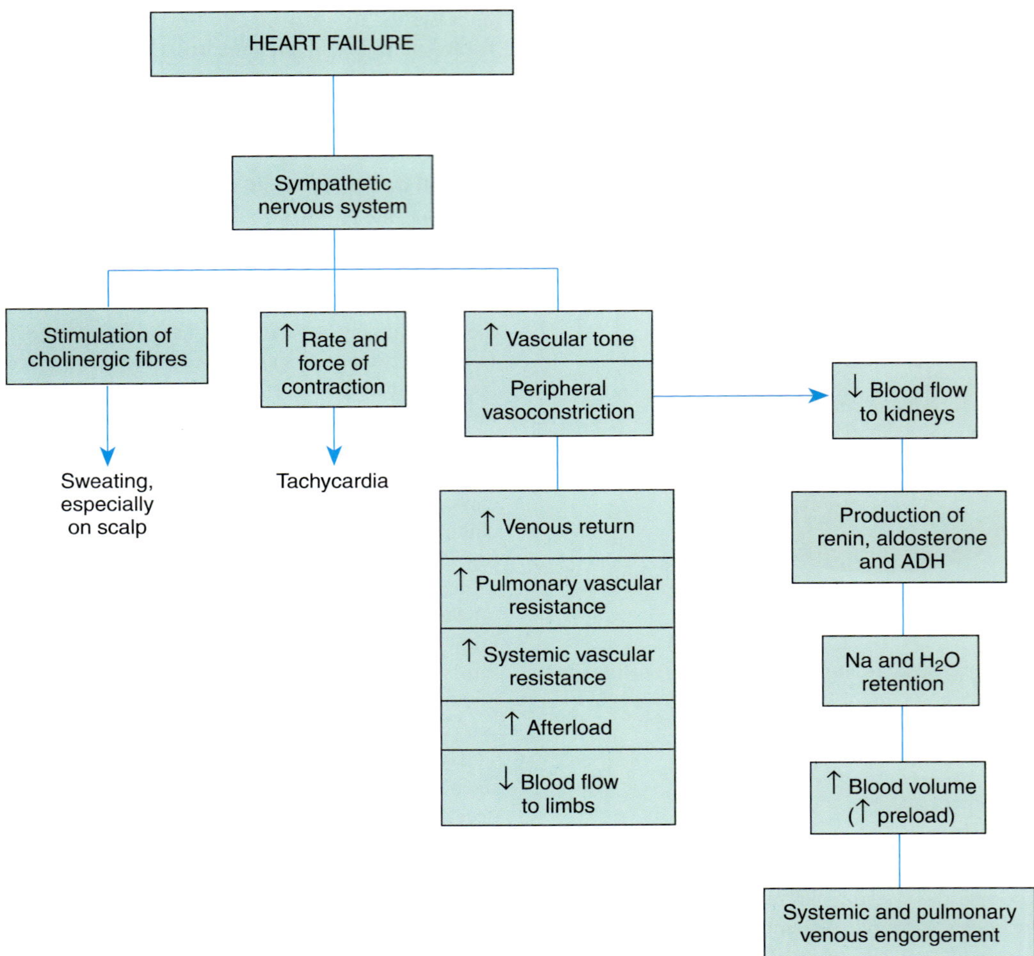

Fig 27.7 Pathophysiology of heart failure. (*ADH*, Antidiuretic hormone.)

Clinical Manifestations

As the capacity of the compensatory mechanisms is exceeded, the child exhibits signs of HF because of decreased myocardial contraction, increased preload and increased afterload. The signs and symptoms of CHF can be divided into three groups: (1) impaired myocardial function; (2) pulmonary congestion; and (3) systemic venous congestion (Box 27.1). Because these haemodynamic changes occur from different causes and at different times, the clinical presentation may vary among children.

Impaired Myocardial Function. One of the earliest signs of CHF is tachycardia (sleeping heart rate > 160 beats/min in infants) as a direct result of sympathetic stimulation. Heart rate is elevated even during rest but becomes extremely rapid with the slightest exertion. Ventricular dilation and excess preload result in extra heart sounds S_3 and S_4, referred to as **gallop rhythm**. Diaphoresis often occurs, especially on the head during exertion. Children are easily fatigued, have poor exercise tolerance and are often irritable. Decreased cardiac output results in poor perfusion, manifested by cold extremities, weak pulses, slow capillary refill, low BP and mottled skin. Extreme pallor or duskiness is an ominous sign.

Pulmonary Congestion. Tachypnoea (respiratory rate > 60 breaths/min in infants) occurs in response to decreased lung compliance (ability to expand). Tachypnoea can lead to hypoxaemia because oxygen does not reach the alveoli for gas exchange in adequate amounts with fast breathing rates. Mild cyanosis results from impaired gas exchange and is relieved by oxygen administration. Dyspnoea is caused by a decrease in the distensibility of the lungs. Inability to feed with resultant poor weight gain is primarily a result of tachypnoea and dyspnoea on exertion. Costal retractions occur as the pliable chest wall in the infant is drawn inwards during attempts to ventilate the non-compliant lungs. Initially dyspnoea may be evident only on exertion, but it may progress to the point that even slight activity results in laboured breathing. In infants dyspnoea at rest is a prominent sign and may be accompanied by flaring nares.

As the LV fails, blood volume and pressure increase in the LA, pulmonary veins and lungs. Eventually the pulmonary capillary pressure exceeds the plasma osmotic pressure, which forces fluid into the interstitial space and finally causes pulmonary oedema. Increased interstitial lung water also decreases the compliance of the lungs and increases the work of breathing.

Orthopnoea (dyspnoea in the recumbent position) is caused by increased blood flow to the heart and lungs from the extremities. It is relieved by sitting up because then blood pools in the lower extremities, which decreases venous return. In addition, this position decreases pressure from the abdominal organs on the diaphragm. In infants orthopnoea may be evident in the inability to lie supine and the desire to be held upright.

Oedema of the bronchial mucosa may produce wheezing from obstruction to airflow. Mucosal swelling and irritation result in a

BOX 27.1 Clinical Manifestations of Heart Failure

Impaired Myocardial Function
- Tachycardia
- Sweating (inappropriate)
- Decreased urinary output
- Fatigue
- Weakness
- Restlessness
- Anorexia
- Pale, cool extremities
- Weak peripheral pulses
- Decreased blood pressure
- Gallop rhythm
- Cardiomegaly

Pulmonary Congestion
- Tachypnoea
- Dyspnoea
- Retractions (infants)
- Flaring nares
- Exercise intolerance
- Cough, hoarseness
- Cyanosis
- Wheezing
- Grunting

Systemic Venous Congestion
- Weight gain
- Hepatomegaly
- Peripheral oedema, especially periorbital
- Ascites
- Neck vein distension (children)

persistent, dry, hacking cough. As pulmonary oedema increases, the cough may be productive due to increased secretions. Pressure on the laryngeal nerve results in hoarseness. A late sign of HF is gasping and grunting respirations.

Systemic Venous Congestion. Systemic venous congestion from right-sided failure results in increased pressure and pooling of blood in the venous circulation. Hepatomegaly occurs from pooling of blood in the portal circulation and transudation of fluid into the hepatic tissues. The liver may be tender on palpation, and its size is an indication of the course of HF.

Oedema develops as the sodium and water retention causes systemic vascular pressure to rise. The earliest sign is weight gain. However, as additional fluid accumulates, it leads to swelling of soft tissue that is dependent and favours the flow of gravity, such as the sacral area and scrotum (when recumbent) and loose periorbital tissues. In infants oedema is usually generalised and difficult to detect. Gross fluid accumulation may produce ascites and pleural effusions.

Distended neck and peripheral veins result from consistently elevated CVP. Normally neck and hand veins collapse when the head or hands are raised above the level of the heart because the blood drains by gravity back to the heart. When the venous pressure is high, however, it slows venous return, which causes the veins to remain distended. Distended neck veins are difficult to detect in the short, fat necks of infants and are usually observed only in older children.

Diagnostic Evaluation

Diagnosis is made on the basis of clinical symptoms such as tachypnoea and tachycardia at rest, dyspnoea, retractions, activity intolerance (especially during feeding in infants), weight gain caused by fluid retention and hepatomegaly. A chest x-ray film demonstrates cardiomegaly and increased pulmonary vascular markings due to increased pulmonary blood flow. Signs of ventricular hypertrophy appear on the ECG. Echocardiography is performed to determine the cause of HF, such as a congenital heart defect or poor ventricular function.

Therapeutic Management. The goals of treatment are to: (1) improve cardiac function (increase contractility and decrease afterload); (2) remove accumulated fluid and sodium (decrease preload and minimise fluid overload); (3) decrease cardiac demands; and (4) improve tissue oxygenation and decrease oxygen consumption. For most infants diagnosed with CHF the cause is a congenital heart defect. Infants are stabilised on medical therapy and then referred for surgical repair. Many children are being surgically repaired in the neonatal and early infancy stages before the onset of CHF symptoms. In infants who do manifest these symptoms, medical and nutrition management are optimised preoperatively. For children newly diagnosed with CHF, the cause may be worsening ventricular function after a previous cardiac repair, cardiomyopathy, arrhythmia or other condition. In addition to management of the CHF, the underlying cause is treated if possible.

Remove Accumulated Fluid and Sodium. Treatment to remove accumulated fluid and sodium consists of administration of diuretics, possible fluid restriction and possible sodium restriction. Diuretics are the mainstay of therapy to eliminate excess water and salt and to prevent reaccumulation.

Fluid restriction may be required in the acute stages of CHF and must be carefully calculated to avoid dehydrating the child, especially if cyanosis and significant polycythaemia are present. Infants rarely need fluid restriction because CHF makes feeding so difficult that they struggle to take maintenance fluids.

Sodium-restricted diets are used less often in children than in adults to control CHF because of their potential negative effects on the child's appetite and ultimate growth. If salt intake is restricted, the diet usually focuses on avoiding additional table salt and highly salted foods. Low-salt formulas are available but are used infrequently because infants need a normal sodium source to offset the sodium depletion of chronic diuretic therapy. Most infant formulas have slightly more sodium than does breast milk.

Improve Cardiac Function. Two groups of drugs are used to enhance myocardial function in CHF: digitalis glycosides (digoxin), which improve contractility, and angiotensin-converting enzyme (ACE) inhibitors, which reduce the afterload on the heart and thus make it easier for the heart to pump. Myocardial efficiency is improved through administration of digitalis glycosides. The beneficial effects are increased cardiac output, decreased heart size, decreased venous pressure and relief of oedema. In children, digoxin (Lanoxin) is used almost exclusively because of its more rapid onset of action and decreased risk of toxicity as a result of its relatively short half-life (days) compared with other digitalis preparations. Because digoxin has a very narrow margin of safety, the dosage must be calculated exactly. Premature infants are more sensitive to digoxin and require smaller dosages because their impaired renal excretion causes the drug to accumulate in the blood faster than in full-term infants and children.

Treatment consists of a digitalising dose, given intravenously or orally in divided doses over 24 hours to produce optimal cardiac effects, and a maintenance dose given orally twice a day to maintain blood levels. During digitalisation, the child is monitored by means of an ECG to observe for the desired effects (prolonged PR interval and reduced ventricular rate) and detect side effects, especially dysrhythmias.

NURSING CARE CONSIDERATIONS

A fall in the serum potassium level enhances the effects of digoxin, increasing the risk of digoxin toxicity. Increased serum potassium levels diminish digoxin's effect. Therefore, serum potassium levels (normal range, 3.5 to 5.5 mmol/L) must be carefully monitored.

Digoxin is the only oral inotropic agent generally available for infants and children. For patients with severe HF, IV inotropic agents such as dopamine or milrinone are used to improve contractility. They are generally given in ICU settings.

Reduce Afterload. Another group of drugs used in the treatment of HF is the ACE inhibitors. ACE inhibitors inhibit the normal function of the renin-angiotensin system in the kidney. The production of renin triggers the production of angiotensin I and angiotensin II, which causes vasoconstriction and aldosterone secretion. The ACE inhibitors block the conversion of angiotensin I to angiotensin II so that, instead of vasoconstriction, vasodilation occurs. Vasodilation results in decreased pulmonary and systemic vascular resistance, decreased BP, a reduction in afterload and decreased RA and LA pressures. It also reduces the secretion of aldosterone, which reduces preload by preventing volume expansion from fluid retention and decreases the risk of hypokalaemia. Renal blood flow is improved, which enhances diuresis. The principal side effects of ACE inhibitors are hypotension, renal dysfunction, hyperkalaemia and cough.

Decrease Cardiac Demands. To lessen the workload on the heart, metabolic needs are minimised by: (1) providing a neutral thermal environment to prevent cold stress in infants; (2) treating any existing infections; (3) reducing the effort of breathing (by placement in semi-Fowler's position); (4) using medication to sedate an irritable child; and (5) providing for rest and decreasing environmental stimuli.

Improve Tissue Oxygenation. All the preceding measures serve to increase tissue oxygenation, either by improving myocardial function or by lessening tissue oxygen demands. In addition, supplemental cool humidified oxygen may be administered to increase the amount of available oxygen during inspiration. Oxygen administration is especially helpful in patients with pulmonary oedema, intercurrent respiratory tract infections and increased pulmonary vascular resistance (oxygen is a vasodilator that decreases pulmonary vascular resistance).

Nasal cannula is used to deliver supplemental oxygen. They are ideal for long-term oxygen administration because the child can be ambulatory and can easily eat and drink. Humidification may be necessary to counteract the drying effect of oxygen.

Nursing Care Management

Infants or children with CHF may be acutely ill, and some may require intensive care until their symptoms improve. Expert nursing care is essential to reduce the cardiac demands that strain the failing heart muscle. During this time the child and family require emotional support; for some children, severe HF represents end-stage cardiac disease (see Advanced Heart Failure, later in this chapter). Although the objectives of nursing care are the same, interventions for infants often differ from interventions for older children. (See Quality Patient Outcomes box.)

QUALITY PATIENT OUTCOMES

Heart Failure

- Adequate cardiac output
- Decreased cardiac demands
- Improved respiratory function
- No evidence of fluid excess
- Adequate support and education

Minimise Fluid Overload. Diuresis assists in decreasing preload and minimising volume overload. When diuretics are given, the nurse records fluid intake and output and monitors body weight at the same time each day to evaluate the benefit of the drug. Because profound diuresis may cause dehydration and electrolyte imbalance (e.g. loss of sodium, potassium, chloride, bicarbonate), the nurse observes for signs indicating one of these complications, as well as signs and symptoms suggesting reactions to the drugs. Give diuretics early in the day to children who are toilet trained to avoid the need to urinate at night. If potassium-losing diuretics are given, the nurse encourages consumption of foods high in potassium, such as bananas, oranges, whole grains, legumes and leafy vegetables, and administers prescribed supplements.

Fluid restriction is rarely necessary in infants because of their difficulty in feeding. However, if fluids are restricted, the nurse plans fluid intake schedules for a 24-hour period, allowing for administration of most fluids during waking hours. With toddlers and preschoolers it is psychologically advantageous to give small amounts of liquid in small cups so that the containers appear full. Suitable containers are decorated medicine cups, small paper cups, doll-sized teacups and measuring cups. It is also important to avoid leaving extra fluids at the bedside because older children may help themselves to additional servings. Placing them in charge of recording fluid intake will help gain their cooperation.

If salt intake is to be limited, the nurse discusses food sources of sodium with the family and discourages their bringing salt-containing treats to the child. At mealtime check the child's tray to make sure the appropriate diet is provided.

Improve Cardiac Function. Digoxin is used to improve cardiac function. Digoxin is a potentially dangerous drug because the margin of safety between therapeutic, toxic and lethal doses is very narrow. Many toxic responses are extensions of its therapeutic effects. The nurse's responsibility in administering digoxin includes calculating and giving the correct dosage and observing for signs of toxicity. The child's apical pulse is always checked before administering digoxin. As a rule, the drug is not given if the pulse is below 90 to 110 beats/min in infants and young children or below 70 beats/min in older children (the cut-off point for adults is 60 beats/min). The nurse should also use judgment in evaluating the pulse rate. If it is significantly lower than the previous recording, the dose should be withheld until the practitioner is notified.

The apical rate is measured because a pulse deficit (radial pulse rate lower than apical) may be present with decreased cardiac output. The pulse is auscultated for 1 full minute to evaluate alterations in rhythm. If the child is monitored by ECG, a rhythm strip is obtained and attached to the chart for rate and rhythm analysis, such as abnormal lengthening of the P-R interval (> 50% increase over the predigitalisation interval) and dysrhythmias.

The most common signs of digoxin toxicity in infants and children are bradycardia (although other dysrhythmias may occur), anorexia, nausea and vomiting. Although vomiting should alert the nurse to observe for other evidence of cardiac toxicity, one episode of vomiting does not warrant cessation of the drug because vomiting from other causes frequently occurs, especially in infants. Vomiting associated with digoxin toxicity is often unrelated to feedings, and infants are usually less interested in feeding and show a recent decrease in oral intake. When in doubt regarding what caused the vomiting and whether another dose of digoxin should be given, the nurse should seek the practitioner's advice before administering the next dose. When concerned about possible digoxin toxicity, the nurse should check the digoxin drug level.

Other extracardiac signs of toxicity are neurological and visual disturbances, which are extremely difficult to identify in children and consequently are of little value in assessing toxicity in infants.

Because digoxin toxicity can occur from accidental overdose, great care must be taken in properly calculating and measuring the dosage. When converting milligrams to micrograms to millilitres, the nurse carefully checks the placement of the decimal point because an error causes a significant change in dosage. For example, 0.1 mg is 10 times the dosage of 0.01 mg.

If digoxin toxicity occurs, especially as a result of a drug overdose, withhold all subsequent doses. The nurse monitors the child closely for dysrhythmias, which are treated appropriately if they occur. Digoxin immune Fab fragment (Digibind) is used as an antidote to digoxin in cases of severe digitalis toxicity. Because of the long half-life of digoxin (18 to 35 hours in infants and children with normal renal function; longer in those with renal impairment and in premature infants and adults), it may be several days before the blood level returns to normal.

These same principles are taught to parents in preparation for the child's discharge, although the correct dose in millilitres is usually specified on the container, which reduces potential errors in calculation. The nurse observes the parent measuring the elixir in the dropper and stresses that the level mark is the meniscus of the fluid observed at eye level. Nurses should also advise parents of the signs of digoxin toxicity.

Reduce Afterload. For patients receiving ACE inhibitors for afterload reduction, the nurse should carefully monitor BP before and after dose administration, observe for symptoms of hypotension and notify the practitioner if BP is low. Monitor serum electrolyte levels. Because ACE inhibitors also block the action of aldosterone, they act as potassium-sparing agents. Most patients do not need potassium supplements or spironolactone while receiving these medications. Numerous medications affecting the kidney can potentiate renal dysfunction, so children taking multiple diuretics along with an ACE inhibitor require accurate measurement of urine output.

Decrease Cardiac Demands. The infant requires rest and conservation of energy for feeding. Make every effort to organise nursing activities to allow for uninterrupted periods of sleep. Whenever possible, encourage parents to stay with their infant to provide the holding, rocking and cuddling that help children sleep more soundly. To minimise disturbing the infant, changing bed linen and complete bathing are done only when necessary. Plan feeding to accommodate the infant's sleep and wake patterns. The child is fed when hungry, such as when sucking on fists, rather than when crying for a bottle because the stress of crying exhausts the limited energy supply. Because infants with HF tire easily and may sleep through feedings, smaller feedings every 3 hours may be helpful. Nasogastric tube feedings may be instituted to provide adequate nutrition and allow the infant to rest. Oral stimulation should still be encouraged during this time; giving a dummy or skin-to-skin cuddles (Fig 27.8) is a great way to decrease infant stress levels and to allow infant–parent attachment and bonding (Flacking et al 2012).

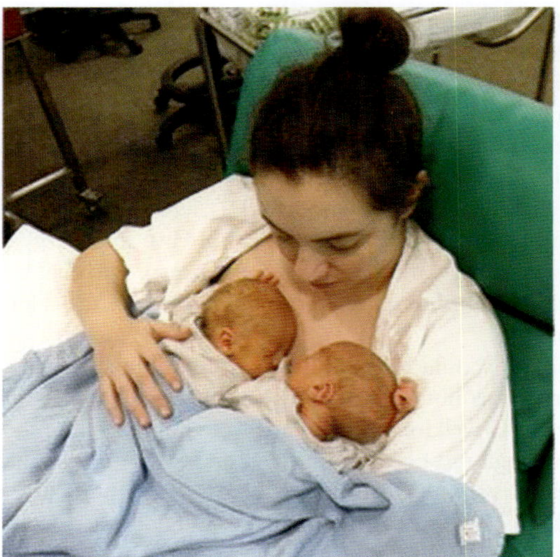

Fig 27.8 Skin-to-skin cuddles.

Older children need an explanation of what is happening to them to decrease anxiety about their illness and necessary treatments, such as cardiac monitoring, oxygen administration and medications. Outlining a plan for the day, preparing the child for tests and procedures, providing quiet activities and providing adequate rest periods are all helpful interventions with older children. Some infants and children require sedation during the acute phase of illness to allow them to rest.

Carefully monitor temperature for hyperthermia (a sign of infection) or hypothermia (loss of heat to ambient air). Report fevers because infection must be treated promptly. Fever increases oxygen demands and is poorly tolerated. If body temperature is low, keep the child warm with additional blankets or a radiant heater. Maintaining body temperature is important for children who are receiving cool, humidified oxygen and for children who tend to be diaphoretic, losing heat via evaporation.

Prevent skin breakdown from oedema with frequent change of position and the use of pressure-relieving or pressure-reducing mattresses or beds. The skin, especially over the sacrum, is checked for evidence of redness from pressure.

Reduce Respiratory Distress. Careful assessment, positioning and oxygen administration can reduce respiratory distress. Respirations are counted for 1 full minute during rest. Any evidence of increased respiratory distress is reported because this may indicate worsening HF. The infant or child is often given humidified supplemental oxygen via nasal cannula or mask. The child's response to oxygen therapy is carefully evaluated by noting: the respiratory rate; ease of respiration; colour; and especially oxygen saturations, as measured by oximetry.

Respiratory tract infections can exacerbate CHF and should be appropriately treated and prevented if possible. The child should be protected from persons with respiratory tract infections and should have a non-infectious roommate. Practise good handwashing technique before and after caring for any hospitalised child. Antibiotics may be given to combat respiratory tract infection. The nurse ensures that the drug is given at equal intervals over a 24-hour period to maintain high blood levels of the antibiotic.

Maintain Nutritional Status. Meeting the nutritional needs of infants with CHF or serious cardiac defects is a nursing challenge. The metabolic rate of these infants is greater because of poor cardiac function and increased heart and respiratory rates. Their caloric needs are greater than those of the average infant because of their increased metabolic rate, yet fatigue limits their ability to take in adequate calories. For a fragile infant with serious CHD, feeding is similar to exercise in an adult, and the infant often does not have the energy or cardiac reserve to do extra work. The nurse seeks measures to enable the infant to feed easily without excess fatigue and to increase the caloric density of the formula.

The infant should be well rested before feeding and fed soon after awakening so as not to expend energy on crying. A 3-hour feeding schedule works well for many infants. (Feeding every 2 hours does not provide enough rest between feedings, and a 4-hour schedule requires an increased volume of feeding, which many infants are unable to take.) The feeding schedule should be individualised to the infant's needs. Infants should be well supported and fed in a semi-upright position. The infant may need to rest frequently and may need to have the jaw and cheeks stroked to encourage sucking. Generally, giving an infant about half an hour to complete a feeding is reasonable. Prolonging the feeding time can exhaust the infant and decrease the rest period between feedings.

Infants with feeding difficulties are often gavage fed using a nasogastric tube to supplement oral feedings and ensure adequate caloric intake. If they are stressed and fatigued, in respiratory distress or tachypnoeic at 80 to 100 breaths/min, oral feedings may be withheld and all nutrition given by gavage feedings. Gavage feedings are usually a temporary measure until the infant's medical status improves and nutritional needs can be met through oral feedings. Some infants with severe CHF, neurological deficits or significant gastro-oesophageal reflux may need placement of a gastrostomy tube to allow adequate nutrition.

The caloric density of formulas is frequently increased by concentration and then the addition of Calogen (or, less commonly, corn oil or medium-chain triglycerides oil). Most commonly the goal is for infants to achieve 150 to 180 mL/kg/day with the supplement of a maximum of 30 kcal/kg/day from Calogen. Generally it is recommended that the child receives 1 kcal/kg/mL of infant formula. This allows the infant to obtain more calories despite intake of a smaller volume of formula. The caloric density of the formula must be increased slowly to prevent diarrhoea or formula intolerance. Encourage breastfeeding mothers to provide the infant with alternating feedings of breast milk and high-calorie formula. Some lactating mothers prefer to feed the child expressed breast milk that has been fortified with Poly-Joule to increase caloric intake. A diet plan specific to the individual infant's needs is calculated and prescribed by the dietitian in collaboration with the other healthcare personnel.

Support the Child and Family. HF is a serious complication of heart disease. Parents and older children are usually acutely aware of the critical nature of the condition. Because stress places additional demands on cardiac function, the nurse should focus on reducing anxiety through anticipatory preparation, frequent communication with the parents regarding the child's progress and constant reassurance that everything possible is being done.

Home care involves many of the same interventions discussed later in this chapter under Plan for Discharge and Home Care. The nurse teaches the family about the medications that need to be administered and alerts them to the signs of worsening HF that require medical attention, such as increased sweating, decreased urinary output or poor feeding. Compliance can be a major issue because patients are often prescribed multiple medications, and the medication regimen can change frequently. Facilitate the family's adherence to the medication schedule by adapting the schedule to their usual home routines, avoiding medication administration at night and providing charts or visual aids to help them remember when to give medications. (See Chapter 23.)

Hypoxaemia

Hypoxaemia refers to an arterial oxygen tension (or pressure, PaO_2) that is lower than normal and can be identified by measuring arterial oxygen saturation (SaO_2) or PaO_2 to detect decreased levels. Hypoxia is a reduction in tissue oxygenation that is caused by low SaO_2 and PaO_2 and results in impaired cellular processes. Cyanosis is a blue discolouration of the mucous membranes, skin and nail beds of the child with reduced oxygen saturation.

Altered Haemodynamics

Heart defects that cause hypoxaemia and cyanosis are those that allow desaturated venous blood (blue blood) to enter the systemic circulation without passing through the lungs. Three types of defect cause cyanosis in infants. The first involves severe obstruction to pulmonary blood flow and blood shunting from the right side to the left side of the heart, or right-to-left shunting. Tetralogy of Fallot is the most common example. The second is mixing of arterial and venous blood within the chambers of the heart itself; a single ventricle is an example. The third defect, transposition of the great arteries, presents a unique situation in which the pulmonary and systemic circulations are parallel rather than in sequence. Fully oxygenated blood returns to the lungs, and desaturated blood returns to the body. Newborns with transposition of the great arteries depend on intracardiac mixing from a patent foramen ovale, septal defect or ductus arteriosus to allow oxygenation.

Clinical Manifestations

Over time, two physiological changes occur in the body in response to chronic hypoxaemia: polycythaemia and clubbing. Persistent hypoxaemia stimulates erythropoiesis, which results in polycythaemia, an increased number of red blood cells. Theoretically a greater number of red blood cells increases the oxygen-carrying capacity of the blood. However, this increased red blood cell formation may result in anaemia if iron is not readily available for the formation of haemoglobin. In addition, polycythaemia increases the viscosity of the blood, and platelets and other coagulation factors tend to be crowded out. These haematological changes increase the likelihood of postoperative bleeding. Clubbing, a thickening and flattening of the tips of the fingers and toes, is thought to occur because of chronic tissue hypoxaemia and polycythaemia (Fig 27.9).

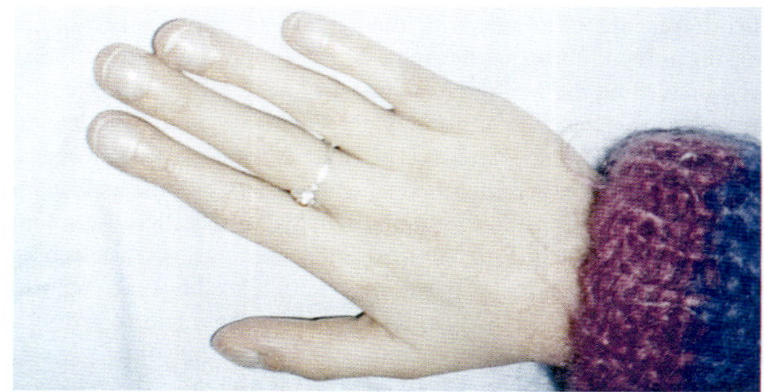

Fig 27.9 Clubbing of the fingers.

Infants with mild hypoxaemia may be asymptomatic except for cyanosis and exhibit near-normal growth and development. Those with more severe hypoxaemia may exhibit fatigue with feeding, poor weight gain, tachypnoea and dyspnoea. Children who are cyanotic from birth are generally smaller than their peers, exhibit poor weight gain, have dyspnoea on exertion, fatigue easily and have poor exercise tolerance.

Severe hypoxaemia resulting in tissue hypoxia is manifested by clinical deterioration and signs of poor perfusion. The infant is pale and dusky with increased cyanosis; cool to the touch with diminished pulses; and lethargic with signs of respiratory distress, including hyperpnoea and gasping respirations. Tissue hypoxia causes metabolic acidosis, which leads to hyperventilation and a rapidly worsening clinical course unless prompt treatment is instituted.

Hypercyanotic spells, also referred to as *blue spells* or *tet spells* because they are often seen in infants with tetralogy of Fallot, may occur in any child whose heart defect includes obstruction to pulmonary blood flow and communication between the ventricles. When sudden infundibular spasms decrease pulmonary blood flow there is an increase in right-to-left shunting (the proposed mechanism in tetralogy of Fallot), and the infant becomes acutely cyanotic and hyperpnoeic. This then leads to hypoxia. Hypoxia causes acidosis, which further increases pulmonary vascular resistance; this, in turn, further decreases pulmonary blood flow. Thus a vicious cycle ensues. Spells, rarely seen before 2 months of age, occur most frequently in the first year of life and more often in the morning, and they may be preceded by feeding, crying or defecation. Because profound hypoxaemia causes cerebral hypoxia, hypercyanotic spells require prompt assessment and treatment to prevent brain damage or possibly death.

Patients with persistent right-to-left shunts as a result of CHD are at risk for significant neurological complications. Polycythaemia and the resultant increased viscosity of the blood increase the risk of thromboembolic events. Small blood clots in the venous system reach the right side of the heart and can enter the systemic circulation and travel to the brain through the right-to-left shunt. The presence of poor ventricular function and atrial arrhythmias further increases the risk of cerebrovascular accidents (CVAs) or strokes. More common in patients with severe cyanosis, thromboembolic events may occur spontaneously but often follow an acute febrile illness, a hypoxic spell, cardiac catheterisation or cardiac surgery, including the Fontan procedure with fenestration. Patients who are cyanotic, especially those with systemic-to-pulmonary shunts, are at increased risk of bacterial endocarditis (BE; infective) (see p. 730).

Negative developmental consequences, particularly in the area of motor and cognitive development, may occur from chronic hypoxaemia. Fifty per cent of postnatal brain growth takes place in the first year of life, so chronic hypoxaemia, poor growth and poor nutrition during this period can have significant adverse effects. In addition, the risks of CVA; periods of profound cyanosis and hypoxia during hypercyanotic spells; and multiple surgeries, hospitalisations and cardiac catheterisations significantly increase the possibility of neurological insult, resulting in developmental delays. The desire to minimise these risks is an important factor in the trend towards early corrective surgical repair of cyanotic defects in infancy.

Diagnostic Evaluation

Cyanosis in the newborn can be a result of cardiac, pulmonary, metabolic or haematological disease, although cardiac and pulmonary causes occur most often. To distinguish between the two, a hyperoxia test may be helpful. The infant is placed in a 100% oxygen environment, and blood parameters are monitored. A PaO_2 of 100 mmHg or higher suggests lung disease, and a PaO_2 lower than 100 mmHg suggests cardiac disease (the problem is related to inadequate perfusion of the pulmonary bed) (Park 2014). An accurate history, a chest radiograph (demonstrating reduced pulmonary blood flow) and especially an echocardiogram contribute to the diagnosis of cyanotic heart disease.

Therapeutic Management

Newborns generally exhibit cyanosis within the first few days of life as the ductus arteriosus, which provided pulmonary blood flow, begins to close. Prostaglandin E_1, which causes vasodilation and smooth muscle relaxation and thus increases dilation and patency of the ductus arteriosus, is administered intravenously to re-establish pulmonary blood flow. The use of prostaglandins has been lifesaving for infants with ductus-dependent cardiac defects. The increase in oxygenation allows the infant's condition to be stabilised and a complete diagnostic evaluation to be performed before further treatment is needed.

Hypercyanotic spells occur suddenly, and prompt recognition and treatment are essential. In the hospital setting, spells are often seen during blood drawing or IV line insertion, when the child is highly agitated or after cardiac catheterisation. Placing an infant in the knee-chest position reduces the venous return from the legs (which is desaturated) and increases systemic vascular resistance, which diverts more blood into the pulmonary artery (Fig 27.10). Morphine, administered subcutaneously or through an existing IV line, is helpful in reducing infundibular spasm.

The cyanotic infant or child is well hydrated to keep the haematocrit and blood viscosity within acceptable limits to reduce the risk of CVA. Monitor the infant closely for anaemia because of the risk of CVAs and the reduced arterial oxygen-carrying capacity that occurs. Iron supplementation and possibly blood transfusion are used as needed.

Respiratory tract infections or reduced pulmonary function from any cause can worsen hypoxaemia in the cyanotic child. Adequate airway clearance, chest physiotherapy, administration of antibiotics and use of oxygen to improve arterial saturations are important interventions.

Surgical Intervention. Many cardiac causes of hypoxaemia can be repaired surgically and are described in the discussion of the particular cardiac defect (see Boxes 27.2 to 27.5 later in this chapter). However, some severely hypoxaemic newborns have cardiac defects, particularly those with single-ventricle anatomy, which are not amenable to

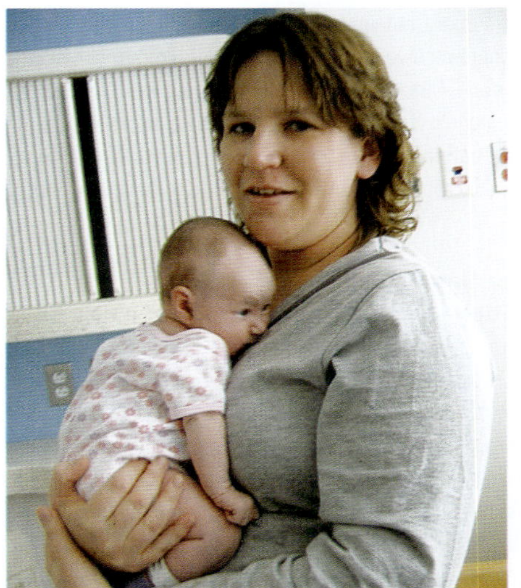

Fig 27.10 Infant held in the knee-chest position.

BOX 27.2 Defects with Increased Pulmonary Blood Flow

Atrial Septal Defect (see Fig 27.11A)

- **Description**—Abnormal opening between the atria, allowing blood from the higher-pressure left atrium to flow into the lower-pressure right atrium. There are three types of atrial septal defect (ASD).
    - *Ostium primum (ASD 1)*—Opening at lower end of septum; may be associated with mitral valve abnormalities
    - *Ostium secundum (ASD 2)*—Opening near centre of septum
    - *Sinus venosus defect*—Opening near junction of superior vena cava and right atrium; may be associated with partial anomalous pulmonary venous connection
- **Pathophysiology**—Because left atrial pressure slightly exceeds right atrial pressure, blood flows from the left to the right atrium, causing an increased flow of oxygenated blood into the right side of the heart. Despite the low pressure difference, a high rate of flow can still occur because of low pulmonary vascular resistance and the greater distensibility of the right atrium, which further reduces flow resistance. This volume is well tolerated by the right ventricle because it is delivered under much lower pressure than with a ventricular septal defect. Although there is right atrial and ventricular enlargement, cardiac failure is unusual in an uncomplicated ASD. Pulmonary vascular changes usually occur only after several decades if the defect is left unrepaired.
- **Clinical manifestations**—Patients may be asymptomatic. Spontaneous closure of ASDs are most likely to occur in younger patients and those with small defects (Vick & Bezold 2017). They may develop heart failure (HF), particularly in the third or fourth decade of life if the ASD goes undiagnosed, as the pulmonary artery pressure then begins to rise. There is a characteristic murmur. Patients are at risk for atrial dysrhythmias (probably caused by atrial enlargement and stretching of conduction fibres) and pulmonary vascular obstructive disease and emboli formation later in life from chronically increased pulmonary blood flow.
- **Surgical closure**—Surgical patch closure (pericardial patch or Dacron patch) is done for moderate to large defects. Open repair with cardiopulmonary bypass is usually performed before school age. In addition, the sinus venosus defect requires patch placement, so the anomalous right pulmonary venous return is directed to the left atrium with a baffle. The ASD 1 type may require mitral valve repair or, rarely, replacement of the mitral valve.
- **Transcatheter closure**—ASD 2 closure with a device during cardiac catheterisation is becoming commonplace and can be done as an outpatient procedure. The Amplatzer septal occluder is most commonly used. Smaller defects that have a rim around them for attachment of the device can be closed with a device; large, irregular defects without a rim require surgical closure. Successful closure in appropriately selected patients yields results similar to surgery but involves shorter hospital stays and fewer complications. Patients receive low-dose aspirin for 6 months (Moore et al 2013).
- **Prognosis**—Outcomes for both treatment options is very good. Limited data also suggest that the rates of procedural success may be comparable to or possibly better with surgery versus transcatheter closure, but that there may be an increased rate of reintervention associated with percutaneous closure.

Ventricular Septal Defect (see Fig 27.11B)

- **Description**—Abnormal opening between the ventricles. May be classified according to location: membranous (accounting for 80%) or muscular. May vary in size from a small pinhole to absence of the septum, which results in a common ventricle. Ventricular septal defects (VSDs) are frequently associated with other defects, such as pulmonic stenosis, transposition of the great vessels, patent ductus arteriosus, atrial defects and coarctation of the aorta. Many VSDs (20% to 60%) close spontaneously. Spontaneous closure is most likely to occur during the first year of life in children having small or moderate defects.
- **Pathophysiology**—Because of the higher pressure within the left ventricle and because the systemic arterial circulation offers more resistance than the pulmonary circulation, blood flows through the defect into the pulmonary artery. The increased blood volume is pumped into the lungs, which may eventually result in increased pulmonary vascular resistance. Increased pressure in the right ventricle as a result of left-to-right shunting and pulmonary resistance causes the muscle to hypertrophy. If the right ventricle is unable to accommodate the increased workload, the right atrium may also enlarge as it attempts to overcome the resistance offered by incomplete right ventricular emptying.
- **Clinical manifestations**—HF is common. There is a characteristic murmur.
- **Surgical treatment**
    - *Palliative*—Pulmonary artery banding (placement of a band around the main pulmonary artery to decrease pulmonary blood flow) may be done in infants with multiple muscular VSDs or complex anatomy. Improvements in surgical techniques and postoperative care make complete repair in infancy the preferred approach.
    - *Complete repair (procedure of choice)*—Small defects are repaired with sutures. Large defects usually require sewing a knitted Dacron patch over the opening. Cardiopulmonary bypass is used for both procedures. The approach for the repair is generally through the right atrium and the tricuspid valve. Postoperative complications include residual VSD and conduction disturbances.
- **Transcatheter closure**—Catheter closure of muscular, postoperative or fenestrated defects is also widely used in centres nationwide. Device closures of VSDs carry more risk than with ASDs. The most common complication noted in one study was complete atrioventricular (AV) block requiring pacemaker placement in 5.7% of the subjects (Butera et al 2007).
- **Prognosis**—Risks depend on the location of the defect, the number of defects, surgical versus transcatheter closure and the presence of other associated cardiac defects. Single membranous defects are associated with low mortality risk (< 2%); multiple muscular defects can carry a higher risk (Jacobs et al 2004).

Atrioventricular Canal Defect (see Fig 27.11C)

- **Description**—Also referred to as *AV septal defects* or *endocardial cushion defects*. Incomplete fusion of the endocardial cushions. Consists of a low ASD that is continuous with a high VSD and clefts of the mitral and tricuspid valves, which creates a large central AV valve that allows blood to flow between all four chambers of the heart. The directions and pathways of flow are determined by pulmonary and systemic resistance, left and right ventricular pressures and the compliance of each chamber, although flow is generally from left to right. It is the most common cardiac defect in children with Down syndrome.
- **Pathophysiology**—The alterations in haemodynamics depend on the severity of the defect and the child's pulmonary vascular resistance. Immediately after birth, while the newborn's pulmonary vascular resistance is high, there is minimum shunting of blood through the defect. Once this resistance falls, left-to-right shunting occurs and pulmonary blood flow increases. The resultant pulmonary vascular engorgement predisposes the child to development of HF.
- **Clinical manifestations**—Patients usually have moderate to severe HF. There is a characteristic murmur. There may be mild cyanosis that increases with crying. Patients are at high risk for developing pulmonary vascular obstructive disease.
- **Surgical treatment**
    - *Palliative*—Pulmonary artery banding is occasionally done in small infants with severe symptoms. Single-ventricle palliation is necessary for some infants who have a right or left ventricle dominant canal defect (see p. 721).

BOX 27.2 Defects with Increased Pulmonary Blood Flow—cont'd

- *Complete repair*—Surgical repair consists of patch closure of the septal defects and reconstruction of the AV valve tissue (either repair of the mitral valve cleft or fashioning of two AV valves). Postoperative complications include heart block, HF, mitral regurgitation, dysrhythmias and pulmonary hypertension.
- **Prognosis**—Operative mortality rate is generally low with patients who are younger (> 2.5 months) and smaller (< 3.5 kg) having worse outcomes (Jacobs et al 2004, St Louis et al 2014). A potential later problem is mitral regurgitation, which may require valve replacement.

Patent Ductus Arteriosus (see Fig 27.11D)

- **Description**—Failure of the fetal ductus arteriosus (artery connecting the aorta and pulmonary artery) to close within the first weeks of life. The continued patency of this vessel allows blood to flow from the higher-pressure aorta to the lower-pressure pulmonary artery, which causes a left-to-right shunt.
- **Pathophysiology**—The haemodynamic consequences of patent ductus arteriosus (PDA) depend on the size of the ductus and the pulmonary vascular resistance. At birth the resistance in the pulmonary and systemic circulations is almost identical, so the resistance in the aorta and pulmonary artery is equalised. As the systemic pressure comes to exceed the pulmonary pressure, blood begins to shunt from the aorta across the duct to the pulmonary artery (left-to-right shunt). The additional blood is recirculated through the lungs and returned to the left atrium and left ventricle. The effect of this altered circulation is increased workload on the left side of the heart, increased pulmonary vascular congestion and possibly resistance and potentially increased right ventricular pressure and hypertrophy.
- **Clinical manifestations**—The amount of shunting will determine the degree of clinical manifestations. There is a characteristic machinery-like murmur. Patients may be asymptomatic or show signs of HF. Moderate to large PDAs may present as left-sided volume overload or reversible pulmonary arterial hypertension.
- **Medical management**—Administration of indomethacin (prostaglandin inhibitor) has proved successful in closing a patent ductus in premature infants and some newborns.
- **Surgical treatment**—Surgical division or ligation of the patent vessel is performed via a left thoracotomy. In video-assisted thoracoscopic surgery, a thoracoscope and instruments are inserted through three small incisions on the left side of the chest to place a clip on the ductus. The surgical approach is dependent on the size and age of the patient.
- **Transcatheter treatment**—Coils to occlude the PDA are placed in the catheterisation laboratory in many centres. Premature or small infants (with small-diameter femoral arteries) and patients with large or unusual PDAs may require surgery.
- **Prognosis**—Both surgical and non-surgical procedures can be done at low risk with less than 1% mortality rate. PDA closure in very premature infants has a higher mortality rate because of the additional significant medical problems.

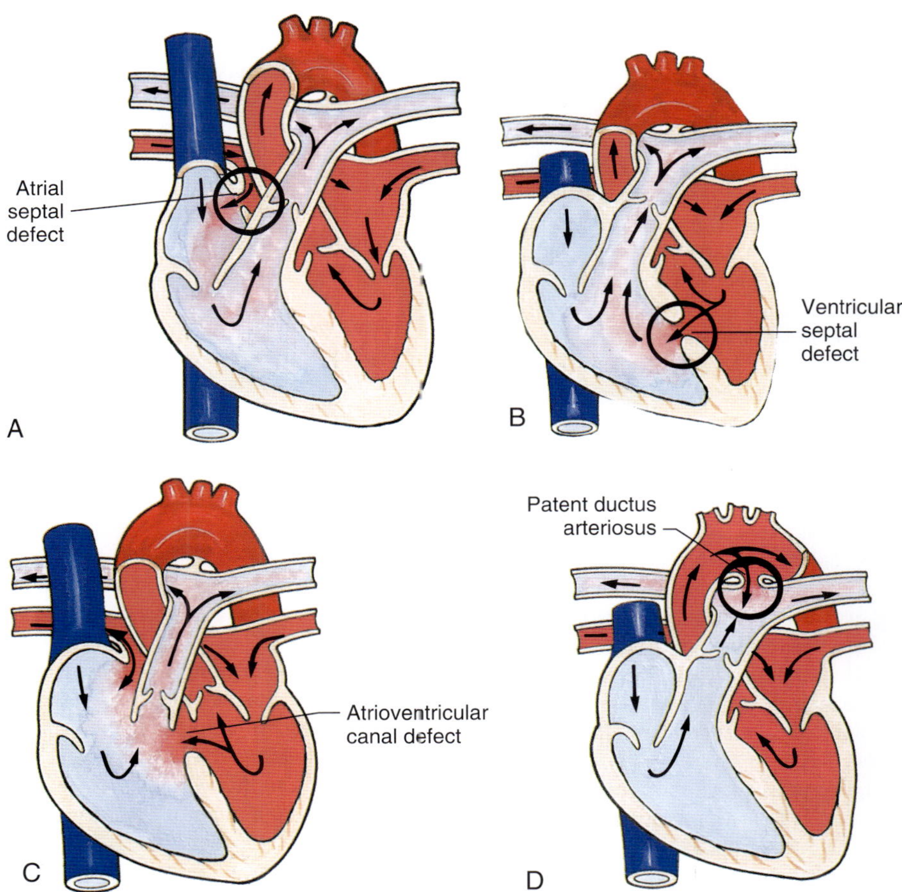

Fig 27.11 (**A**) Atrial septal defect. (**B**) Ventricular septal defect. (**C**) Atrioventricular canal defect. (**D**) Patent ductus arteriosus.

BOX 27.3 Obstructive Defects

Coarctation of the Aorta (see Fig 27.12A)

- **Description**—Localised narrowing near the insertion of the ductus arteriosus, which results in increased pressure proximal to the defect (head and upper extremities) and decreased pressure distal to the obstruction (body and lower extremities).
- **Pathophysiology**—The effect of a narrowing within the aorta is increased pressure proximal to the defect (upper extremities) and decreased pressure distal to it (lower extremities).
- **Clinical manifestations**—There may be high blood pressure and bounding pulses in the arms, weak or absent femoral pulses and cool lower extremities with lower blood pressure. There are signs of heart failure in infants. In infants with critical coarctation, the haemodynamic condition may deteriorate rapidly with severe acidosis and hypotension. Mechanical ventilation and inotropic support are often necessary before surgery. Older children may experience dizziness, headaches, fainting and epistaxis resulting from hypertension. Patients are at risk for hypertension, ruptured aorta, aortic aneurysm and stroke.
- **Surgical treatment**—Surgical repair is the treatment of choice for infants younger than 6 months of age and for patients with long-segment stenosis or complex anatomy. Repair is by either: (1) resection of the narrowed portion with an end-to-end anastomosis of the aorta or (2) enlargement of the section using a graft of prosthetic material or portion of the left subclavian artery. Because this defect is outside the heart and pericardium, cardiopulmonary bypass is not required, and a thoracotomy incision is used. Postoperative hypertension is treated with intravenous sodium nitroprusside, esmolol or milrinone, followed by oral medications, such as angiotensin-converting enzyme inhibitors or beta blockers. Residual permanent hypertension after repair of coarctation of the aorta (COA) seems to be related to age and time of repair. To prevent both hypertension at rest and exercise-provoked systemic hypertension after repair, elective surgery for COA is advised within the first 2 years of life. Percutaneous balloon angioplasty techniques have proved to be very effective in relieving residual postoperative coarctation gradients.
- **Transcatheter treatment**—Balloon angioplasty is a primary intervention for COA in older infants and children. In adolescents, stents may be placed in the aorta to maintain patency. The goal of the procedure is to achieve a reduction in gradient to less than 10%, or more than 90% relief of obstruction angiographically. Dilation and/or stent implantation for native or recurrent coarctation seems to immediately relieve obstruction in more than 90% of cases (Holzer et al 2008).
- **Prognosis**—There are low rates of morbidity, mortality and reintervention for infants and children who underwent COA repair via a left thoracotomy (Mery et al 2015). Major long-term complications include recoarctation, aortic aneurysm and systemic hypertension (Brown et al 2013).

Aortic Stenosis (see Fig 27.12B)

- **Description**—Narrowing or stricture of the aortic valve, causing resistance to blood flow in the left ventricle, decreased cardiac output, left ventricular hypertrophy and pulmonary vascular congestion. Valvular aortic stenosis (AS), the most common type, is usually caused by malformed cusps that result in a bicuspid rather than tricuspid valve or fusion of the cusps. Subvalvular stenosis is a stricture caused by a fibrous ring below a normal valve; supravalvular stenosis occurs infrequently. Valvular AS is a serious defect because: (1) the obstruction tends to be progressive; (2) sudden episodes of myocardial ischaemia, or low cardiac output, can result in sudden death; and (3) surgical repair rarely results in a normal valve. This is one of the rare instances in which strenuous physical activity may be curtailed because of the cardiac condition.
- **Pathophysiology**—A stricture in the aortic outflow tract causes resistance to ejection of blood from the left ventricle. The extra workload on the left ventricle causes hypertrophy. If left ventricular failure develops, left atrial pressure will increase; this causes increased pressure in the pulmonary veins, which results in pulmonary vascular congestion (pulmonary oedema).
- **Clinical manifestations**—Newborns with critical AS demonstrate signs of decreased cardiac output with faint pulses, hypotension, tachycardia and poor feeding. Children show signs of exercise intolerance, chest pain and dizziness when standing for a long period. There is a characteristic murmur. Patients are at risk for infective endocarditis, coronary insufficiency and ventricular dysfunction.

Valvular Aortic Stenosis

- **Surgical treatment**—Aortic valvotomy is performed under inflow occlusion. It is rarely used because balloon dilation in the catheterisation laboratory is the first-line procedure. Newborns with critical AS and small left-sided structures may undergo a stage 1 Norwood procedure (see Hypoplastic Left Heart Syndrome, page 721).
- **Prognosis**—Aortic valvotomy remains a palliative procedure and the patient may require further surgery to repair or even replace the aortic valve. An aortic homograft with a valve may also be used (extended aortic root replacement) or the pulmonic valve may be moved to the aortic position and replaced with a homograft valve (Ross procedure). If the obstruction is at the subvalvular region and results from narrowing of the left ventricular outflow tract with a small aortic valve annulus, a patch may be required to enlarge the entire left ventricular outflow tract and annulus and replace the aortic valve, an approach known as the Konno procedure. Patients that have obstruction at both the valvular and the subvalvular regions may undergo a combination of these two procedures, also called a Ross-Konno procedure.
- **Non-surgical treatment**—The narrowed valve is dilated using balloon angioplasty in the catheterisation laboratory. This procedure is usually the first intervention.
- **Prognosis**—Complications include aortic insufficiency or valvular regurgitation, tearing of the valve leaflets and loss of pulse in the catheterised limb.

Pulmonary Stenosis (see Fig 27.12C)

- **Description**—Narrowing at the entrance to the pulmonary artery. Resistance to blood flow causes right ventricular hypertrophy and decreased pulmonary blood flow. Pulmonary atresia is the extreme form of pulmonic stenosis (PS) in that there is total fusion of the commissures and no blood flows to the lungs. The right ventricle may be hypoplastic.
- **Pathophysiology**—When PS is present, resistance to blood flow causes right ventricular hypertrophy. If right ventricular failure develops, right atrial pressure increases and this may result in reopening of the foramen ovale, shunting of deoxygenated blood into the left atrium and systemic cyanosis. If PS is severe, HF occurs and systemic venous engorgement is noted. An associated defect such as a patent ductus arteriosus partially compensates for the obstruction by shunting blood from the aorta to the pulmonary artery and into the lungs.
- **Clinical manifestations**—Patients may be asymptomatic; some have mild cyanosis or HF. Progressive narrowing causes increased symptoms. Newborns with severe narrowing are cyanotic. There is a characteristic murmur. Cardiomegaly is evident on chest radiographic films. Patients are at risk for infective endocarditis.
- **Surgical treatment**—Need for surgical treatment is rare with widespread use of balloon angioplasty techniques, but in some cases pulmonary valvotomy with cardiopulmonary bypass is necessary.
- **Transcatheter treatment**—Balloon angioplasty in the cardiac catheterisation laboratory to dilate the valve. A catheter is inserted across the stenotic pulmonic valve into the pulmonary artery, and a balloon at the end of the catheter is inflated and rapidly passed through the narrowed opening. The procedure is associated with few complications and has proved to be highly effective. It is the treatment of choice for discrete PS in most centres and can be done safely in neonates.
- **Prognosis**—Risk is low for both surgical and transcatheter procedures; mortality rate is low, slightly higher in neonates. Both balloon dilation and surgical valvotomy leave the pulmonary valve incompetent because they involve opening the fused valve leaflets; however, these patients are clinically

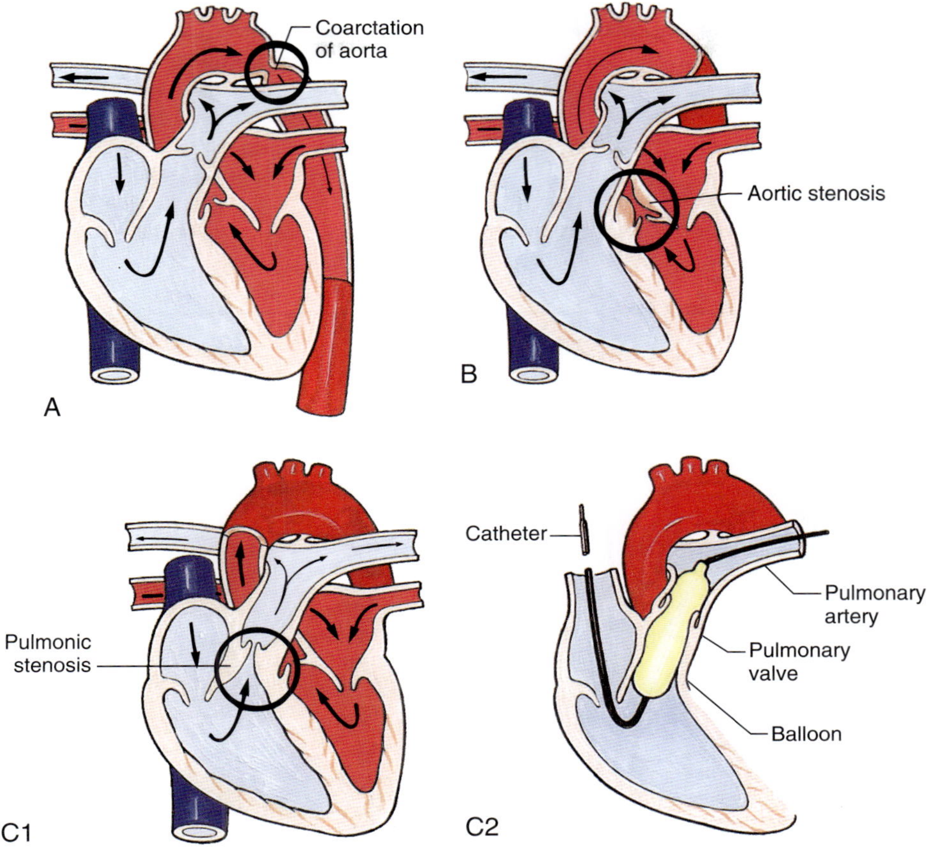

Fig 27.12 (**A**) Coarctation of the aorta. (**B**) Aortic stenosis. (**C**) Pulmonary stenosis.

BOX 27.4 Defects with Decreased Pulmonary Blood Flow

Tetralogy of Fallot (see Fig 27.13A)

- **Description**—The classic form includes four defects: (1) ventricular septal defect (VSD); (2) pulmonic stenosis; (3) overriding aorta; and (4) right ventricular hypertrophy.
- **Pathophysiology**—The alteration in haemodynamics varies widely, depending primarily on the degree of pulmonary stenosis, but also on the size of the VSD and the pulmonary and systemic resistance to flow. Because the VSD is usually large, pressures may be equal in the right and left ventricles. Therefore, the shunt direction depends on the difference between pulmonary and systemic vascular resistance. If pulmonary vascular resistance is higher than systemic resistance, the shunt is from right to left. If systemic resistance is higher than pulmonary resistance, the shunt is from left to right. Pulmonary stenosis decreases blood flow to the lungs and consequently the amount of oxygenated blood that returns to the left side of the heart. Depending on the position of the aorta, blood from both ventricles may be distributed systemically.
- **Clinical manifestations**—Some infants may be acutely cyanotic at birth; others have mild cyanosis that progresses over the first year of life as the pulmonary stenosis worsens. There is a characteristic murmur. There may be acute episodes of cyanosis and hypoxia, called *blue spells* or *tet spells*. Anoxic spells occur when the infant's oxygen requirements exceed the blood supply, usually during crying or after feeding. Patients are at risk for emboli, seizures and loss of consciousness or sudden death after an anoxic spell.
- **Surgical treatment**—Elective repair is usually performed in the first year of life. Indications for repair include increasing cyanosis and the development of hypercyanotic spells. Complete repair involves closure of the VSD and resection of the infundibular stenosis, with placement of a pericardial patch to enlarge the right ventricular outflow tract. In some repairs, the patch may extend across the pulmonic valve annulus (transannular patch), making the pulmonic valve incompetent. The procedure requires a median sternotomy and the use of cardiopulmonary bypass.
- **Prognosis**—The operative mortality rate for total correction of tetralogy of Fallot is less than 3% (Jacobs et al 2004). Long-term complications include chronic pulmonary regurgitation with right ventricular enlargement and decreased function requiring pulmonary valve replacement, residual right ventricular outflow tract obstruction, aortic root dilation and aortic valve insufficiency, arrhythmias and sudden cardiac death. Pulmonary valve replacement is performed either surgically or in the catheterisation laboratory using a transcatheter approach (Doyle et al 2016).

Tricuspid Atresia (see Fig 27.13B)

- **Description**—The tricuspid valve fails to develop; consequently, there is no communication from the right atrium to the right ventricle. Blood flows through an atrial septal defect (ASD) or a patent foramen ovale to the left side of the heart and through a VSD to the right ventricle and out to the lungs. The condition is often associated with pulmonary stenosis and transposition of the great arteries. There is complete mixing of deoxygenated and oxygenated blood in the left side of the heart, which results in systemic desaturation, and varying amounts of pulmonary obstruction, which causes decreased pulmonary blood flow.
- **Pathophysiology**—At birth the presence of a patent foramen ovale (or other atrial septal opening) is required to permit blood flow across the septum into the left atrium; the patent ductus arteriosus allows blood flow to the pulmonary artery into the lungs for oxygenation. A VSD allows a modest

Continued

BOX 27.4 Defects with Decreased Pulmonary Blood Flow—cont'd

amount of blood to enter the right ventricle and pulmonary artery for oxygenation. Pulmonary blood flow is often diminished.

- **Clinical manifestations**—Cyanosis is usually seen in the newborn period. There may be tachycardia and dyspnoea. Older children have signs of chronic hypoxaemia with clubbing.
- **Therapeutic management**—For the neonate whose pulmonary blood flow depends on the patency of the ductus arteriosus, a continuous infusion of prostaglandin E_1 is started at 0.1 microgram/kg/min until surgical intervention can be arranged.
- **Surgical treatment**—Patients with tricuspid atresia follow the staged surgical approach for single-ventricle anatomy (see p. 721) with the left ventricle becoming the ventricular pump.
- **Prognosis**—Surgical mortality rate is less than 5% (Jacobs et al 2004); the rate increases when the anatomy is more complex and other risk factors are present. Postoperative complications include dysrhythmias, systemic venous hypertension, pleural and pericardial effusions and ventricular dysfunction.

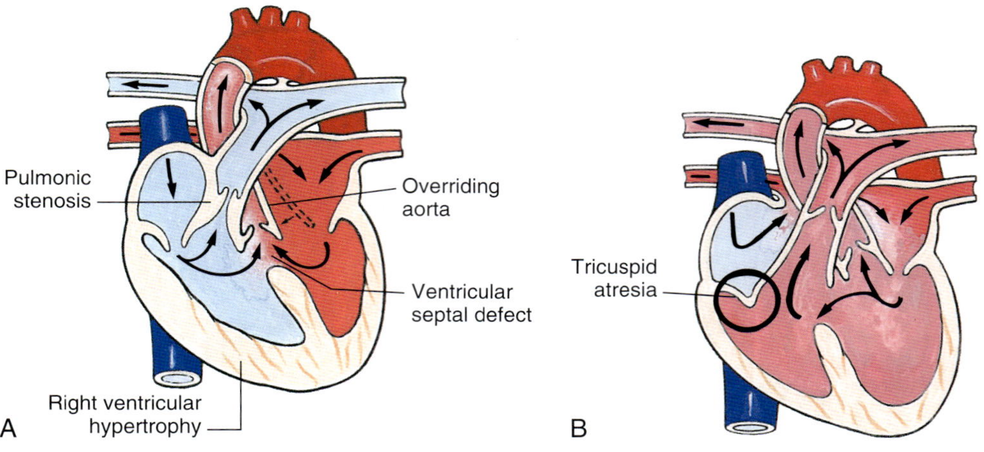

Fig 27.13 (**A**) Tetralogy of Fallot. (**B**) Tricuspid atresia.

BOX 27.5 Mixed Defects

Transposition of the Great Arteries or Transposition of the Great Vessels (see Fig 27.14A)

- **Description**—The pulmonary artery leaves the left ventricle, and the aorta exits from the right ventricle, with no communication between the systemic and pulmonary circulations.
- **Pathophysiology**—Associated defects such as septal defects or patent ductus arteriosus must be present to permit blood to enter the systemic circulation or the pulmonary circulation for mixing of saturated and desaturated blood. The most common defect associated with transposition of the great arteries is a patent foramen ovale. At birth there is also a patent ductus arteriosus, although in most instances this closes after the neonatal period. Another associated defect may be a ventricular septal defect (VSD). The presence of a VSD increases the risk of heart failure (HF) because it permits blood to flow from the right to the left ventricle, into the pulmonary artery and finally to the lungs. However, it also produces increased pulmonary blood flow under high pressure, which can result in high pulmonary vascular resistance.
- **Clinical manifestations**—Vary according to the type and size of the associated defects. Newborns with minimum communication are severely cyanotic and have depressed function at birth. Those with large septal defects or a patent ductus arteriosus may be less cyanotic but have symptoms of HF. Heart sounds vary according to the type of defect present. Cardiomegaly is usually evident a few weeks after birth.
- **Therapeutic management** (to provide intracardiac mixing)—Intravenous prostaglandin E_1 may be administered preoperatively to maintain ductal patency and ensure adequate systemic blood flow. During cardiac catheterisation or under echocardiographic guidance, a balloon atrial septostomy (Rashkind procedure) may also be performed to increase mixing by opening the atrial septum.
- **Surgical treatment**—An arterial switch operation (ASO; also called a Jatene procedure) is the procedure of choice performed in the first weeks of life. It involves transecting the great arteries and anastomosing the main pulmonary artery to the proximal aorta (just above the aortic valve) and anastomosing the ascending aorta to the proximal pulmonary artery. The coronary arteries are switched from the proximal aorta to the proximal pulmonary artery to create a new aorta. Reimplantation of the coronary arteries is critical to the infant's survival, and they must be reattached without torsion or kinking to provide the heart with its supply of oxygen. The advantage of the arterial switch procedure is the reestablishment of normal circulation, with the left ventricle acting as the systemic pump. Potential complications of the arterial switch include narrowing at the great artery anastomoses and coronary artery insufficiency.
  - *Intraatrial baffle repairs*—Intraatrial baffle repairs are rarely performed, although many adults survive today with repairs that were done more than 20 years ago. An intraatrial baffle is created to divert venous blood to the mitral valve and pulmonary venous blood to the tricuspid valve using the patient's atrial septum (Senning procedure) or a prosthetic material (Mustard procedure). A disadvantage is the continuing role of the right ventricle as the systemic pump and the late development of right ventricular failure and rhythm disturbances. Other potential postoperative complications include loss of normal sinus rhythm, baffle leaks and ventricular dysfunction.
  - *Rastelli procedure*—This procedure is the operative choice in infants with TGA, VSD and severe pulmonary stenosis. It involves closure of the VSD with a baffle so left ventricular blood is directed through the VSD into the aorta. The pulmonary valve is then closed, and a conduit is placed from the right ventricle to the pulmonary artery to create a physiologically normal circulation. Unfortunately, this procedure requires multiple conduit replacements as the child grows.

BOX 27.5 Mixed Defects—cont'd

- **Prognosis**—Outcomes after the ASO are quite good. There are some long-term complications, including neoaortic, pulmonary and coronary artery complications, but most patients maintain normal cardiovascular function and exercise capacity (Khairy et al 2013). Patients who undergo a Senning or Mustard procedure demonstrate diminished long-term survival rates and substantial morbidity (Cuypers et al 2014).

Total Anomalous Pulmonary Venous Connection (see Fig 27.14B)

- **Description**—Rare defect characterised by failure of the pulmonary veins to join the left atrium. Instead, the pulmonary veins are abnormally connected to the systemic venous circuit via the right atrium or various veins draining towards the right atrium, such as the superior vena cava. The abnormal attachment results in mixed blood being returned to the right atrium and shunted from the right to the left through an atrial septal defect (ASD). Total anomalous pulmonary venous connection (TAPVC; also called *total anomalous pulmonary venous return* or *total anomalous pulmonary venous drainage*) is classified according to the pulmonary venous point of attachment as follows.
  - *Supracardiac*—Attachment above the diaphragm, such as to the superior vena cava (most common form) but not directly to the heart (see Fig 27.14B)
  - *Cardiac*—Direct attachment to the heart, such as to the right atrium or coronary sinus
  - *Infradiaphragmatic*—Attachment below the diaphragm, such as to the inferior vena cava (most severe form)
- **Pathophysiology**—The right atrium receives all the blood that normally would flow into the left atrium. As a result, the right side of the heart hypertrophies, whereas the left side, especially the left atrium, may remain small. An associated ASD or patent foramen ovale allows systemic venous blood to shunt from the higher-pressure right atrium to the left atrium and into the left side of the heart. As a result, the oxygen saturation of the blood in both sides of the heart (and ultimately in the systemic arterial circulation) is the same. If the pulmonary blood flow is large, pulmonary venous return is also large, and the amount of saturated blood is relatively high. However, if there is obstruction to pulmonary venous drainage, pulmonary venous return is impeded, pulmonary venous pressure rises and pulmonary interstitial oedema develops and eventually contributes to HF. Infradiaphragmatic TAPVC is often associated with obstruction to pulmonary venous drainage and is a surgical emergency.
- **Clinical manifestations**—Most infants develop cyanosis early in life. The degree of cyanosis is inversely related to the amount of pulmonary blood flow—the more pulmonary blood, the less cyanosis. Children with unobstructed TAPVC may be asymptomatic until pulmonary vascular resistance decreases during infancy, increasing pulmonary blood flow, with resulting signs of HF. Cyanosis becomes worse with pulmonary vein obstruction; once obstruction occurs, the infant's condition usually deteriorates rapidly. Without intervention, cardiac failure progresses to death.
- **Surgical treatment**—Corrective repair is performed in early infancy. The surgical approach varies with the anatomical defect. In general, however, the common pulmonary vein is anastomosed to the back of the left atrium, the ASD is closed and the anomalous pulmonary venous connection is ligated. The cardiac type is most easily repaired; the infradiaphragmatic type carries the highest morbidity and mortality rates because of the higher incidence of pulmonary vein obstruction. Potential postoperative complications include: reobstruction; bleeding; dysrhythmias, particularly heart block; pulmonary artery hypertension; and persistent heart failure.
- **Prognosis**—Mortality rate for all types is less than 10% (Jacobs et al 2004) and is lowest for the cardiac type; morbidity increases with the presence of pulmonary vein obstruction.

Truncus Arteriosus (see Fig 27.14C)

- **Description**—Failure of normal septation and division of the embryonic bulbar trunk into the pulmonary artery and the aorta, which results in development of a single vessel that overrides both ventricles. Blood from both ventricles mixes in the common great artery, which leads to desaturation and hypoxaemia. Blood ejected from the heart flows preferentially to the lower-pressure pulmonary arteries, so pulmonary blood flow is increased and systemic blood flow is reduced. There are three types.
  - *Type I*—A single pulmonary trunk arises near the base of the truncus and divides into the left and right pulmonary arteries.
  - *Type II*—The left and right pulmonary arteries arise separately but in close proximity and at the same level from the back of the truncus.
  - *Type III*—The pulmonary arteries arise independently from the sides of the truncus.
- **Pathophysiology**—Blood ejected from the left and right ventricles enters the common trunk, so pulmonary and systemic circulations are mixed. Blood flow is distributed to the pulmonary and systemic circulations according to the relative resistances of each system. The amount of pulmonary blood flow depends on the size of the pulmonary arteries and the pulmonary vascular resistance. Generally, resistance to pulmonary blood flow is less than systemic vascular resistance, which results in preferential blood flow to the lungs. Pulmonary vascular disease develops at an early age in patients with truncus arteriosus.
- **Clinical manifestations**—Most infants are symptomatic with moderate to severe HF and variable cyanosis, poor growth and activity intolerance. There is a characteristic murmur. Thirty-five per cent of patients have 22q11 deletions (Goldmuntz & Lin 2008).
- **Surgical treatment**—Early repair is performed in the first month of life. It involves closing the VSD so that the truncus arteriosus receives the outflow from the left ventricle, excising the pulmonary arteries from the aorta and attaching them to the right ventricle using a right ventricle to pulmonary artery conduit and possible repair of the truncal valve. Postoperative complications include truncal valve insufficiency, persistent heart failure, bleeding, pulmonary artery hypertension, dysrhythmias and residual VSD. Because conduits are not living tissue, they will not grow along with the child and may also become narrowed with calcifications. One or more conduit replacements will be needed in childhood.
- **Prognosis**—Perioperative mortality rate is about 10%, with highest mortality rate in patients who required repair for both truncal valve and aortic arch interruption (Russell et al 2012). Long-term complications include truncal valve regurgitation and conduit stenosis.

Hypoplastic Left Heart Syndrome (HLHS) (see Fig 27.14D)

- **Description**—Underdevelopment of the left side of the heart with significant hypoplasia of the left ventricle including atresia, stenosis or hypoplasia of the aortic and/or mitral valves and hypoplasia of the ascending aorta and arch. Most blood from the left atrium flows across the patent foramen ovale to the right atrium, to the right ventricle and out the pulmonary artery. The descending aorta receives blood from the patent ductus arteriosus supplying systemic blood flow.
- **Pathophysiology**—An ASD or patent foramen ovale allows saturated blood from the left atrium to mix with desaturated blood from the right atrium and to flow through the right ventricle and out into the pulmonary artery. From the pulmonary artery, the blood flows both to the lungs and through the ductus arteriosus into the aorta and out to the body. The amount of blood flow to the pulmonary and systemic circulations depends on the relationship between the pulmonary and systemic vascular resistances. The coronary and cerebral vessels receive blood by retrograde flow through the hypoplastic ascending aorta.

Continued

BOX 27.5 Mixed Defects—cont'd

- **Clinical manifestations**—There is mild cyanosis and signs of HF until the patent ductus arteriosus closes, then progressive deterioration with cyanosis and decreased cardiac output, leading to cardiovascular collapse. The condition is usually fatal in the first months of life without intervention.
- **Therapeutic management**—Neonates require stabilisation with mechanical ventilation and inotropic support preoperatively. A prostaglandin E_1 infusion is needed to maintain ductal patency and ensure adequate systemic blood flow until surgical intervention can occur.
- **Surgical treatment**—Patients with HLHS follow the staged surgical approach for single-ventricle anatomy (see p. 721) with the right ventricle becoming the ventricular pump. Postoperative complications include dysrhythmias, systemic venous hypertension, pleural and pericardial effusions, thrombotic events and ventricular dysfunction.
- **Transplantation**—Heart transplantation in the newborn period is another option for these infants. Problems include the shortage of newborn organ donors, risk of rejection, long-term problems with chronic immunosuppression and infection.
- **Prognosis**—Thirty-five years ago a diagnosis of HLHS was uniformly fatal. Today, for children who survive to the age of 12 months, long-term survival is now approximately 90% (Alsoufi et al 2015, Siffel et al 2015). Improved outcomes have been associated with early diagnosis and repair and increased monitoring in the hospital and at home, particularly between the first- and second-stage. Long-term problems include worsening ventricular function, tricuspid regurgitation, recurrent aortic arch narrowing, dysrhythmias, thrombotic complications and developmental delays.

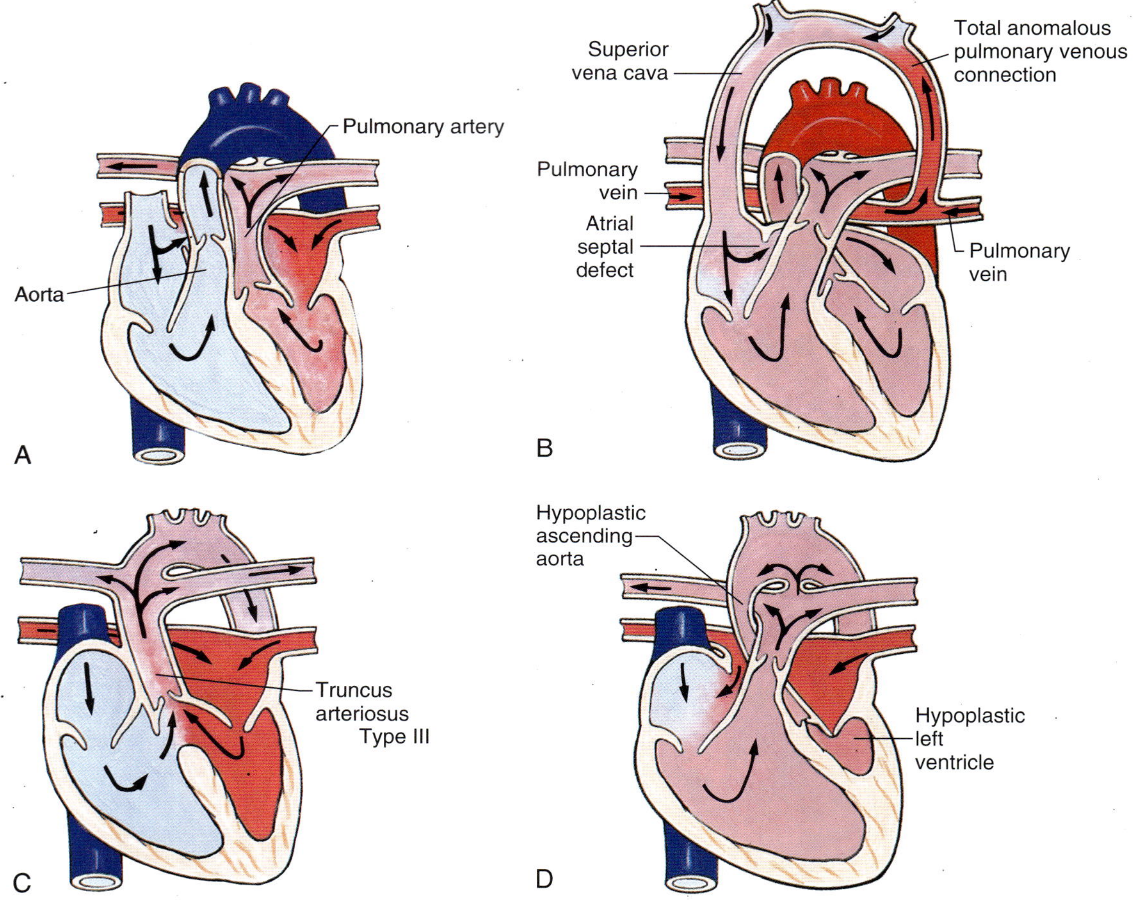

Fig 27.14 (**A**) Transposition of the great arteries or transposition of the great vessels. (**B**) Total anomalous pulmonary venous connection. (**C**) Truncus arteriosus. (**D**) Hypoplastic left heart syndrome (HLHS).

corrective repair and may undergo a palliative surgical procedure to establish a shunt. The shunt serves the same purpose as the ductus arteriosus: to increase blood flow to the lungs through a systemic artery to pulmonary artery connection. Table 27.2 outlines the most commonly performed shunt procedures today. More detailed discussion of surgical palliation for the infant with single-ventricle anatomy is on p. 721.

After a shunt procedure, assess the infant for signs of increased or decreased pulmonary blood flow. If the shunt is too small or has narrowed, the newborn may remain severely hypoxaemic, with oxygen saturations below 70%. Surgical revision of the shunt or placement of an additional shunt may be needed. In some patients, the shunt is too large, causing increased pulmonary blood flow resulting in signs and symptoms of HF and oxygen saturations above 85%. The infant may

TABLE 27.2 Selected Shunt Procedures for Children with Cardiac Defects

Shunt Type	Comments
Modified Blalock-Taussig shunt—Subclavian artery to pulmonary artery using Gore-Tex or Impra tube graft	Shunt flow sometimes excessive, requiring use of diuretics Possibility of thrombosis; aspirin usually prescribed postoperatively Easy to ligate at time of definitive correction Shunt size fixed and may become too small as child grows
Sano modification—Right ventricular to pulmonary artery conduit using Gore-Tex	Prevents diastolic run-off of systemic blood into the pulmonary arteries Provides a higher diastolic blood pressure and seemingly better coronary perfusion Used in place of the modified Blalock-Taussig shunt in the Norwood procedure
Bidirectional Glenn shunt (cavopulmonary anastomosis)—Superior vena cava to side of right pulmonary artery; blood flow to both lungs	Done as a second shunt; often used as a staging step to a Fontan procedure Can be incorporated into eventual modified Fontan procedure Relieves severe cyanosis and decreases volume overload on ventricle Carries risk of embolic events (mixing defect); aspirin often prescribed Pulmonary arteriovenous fistulas may occur months or years later, causing desaturation (uncommon finding)
Central shunt—Ascending aorta to main pulmonary artery using Gore-Tex graft	Length of shunt acts to restrict blood flow; symptoms of heart failure may occur; diuretic therapy may be required Uncommon; used when modified Blalock-Taussig shunt cannot be used Easy to insert and remove at time of repair Possibility of thrombosis; aspirin usually prescribed postoperatively

require diuretic therapy, afterload reduction and increased calories (see discussion of HF). Most surgeons place infants on low-dose aspirin therapy for several months to prevent platelet aggregation and subsequent narrowing of the shunt. Acute cyanosis and signs of tissue hypoxia may occur if the shunt is occluded and pulmonary blood flow is severely limited; shunt occlusion is a medical emergency. The presence of prosthetic material puts patients at risk for infective (bacterial) endocarditis.

Nursing Care Management

The general appearance of infants and children with significant cyanosis poses unique concerns. Blue lips and fingernails are obvious signs of the hidden cardiac defect. Clubbing and small, thin stature in older children further indicate severe heart disease. Body image concerns are important. Patients and families need a simple explanation of hypoxaemia and cyanosis and reassurance that cyanosis does not imply a lack of oxygen to the brain. Their questions and fears need to be addressed in a calm, supportive manner and positive aspects of their child's growth and development must be emphasised.

Dehydration must be prevented in hypoxaemic children because it increases the risk of stroke. Fluid status is carefully monitored through accurate intake and output and daily weight measurements. Maintenance fluid therapy is the minimum requirement; supplemental fluids should be readily available, and gavage feeding or IV hydration is given to children unable to take in adequate fluids orally. Fever, vomiting and diarrhoea can cause dehydration and require prompt treatment. Instruct parents in the importance of adequate fluid intake and measures to prevent dehydration.

Preventive measures and accurate assessment of respiratory infection are important nursing considerations. Any compromise in pulmonary function increases the infant's hypoxaemia. Good handwashing and protection from individuals with an obvious respiratory tract infection are important. Airway clearance, treatment with antibiotics or antiviral agents as indicated and delivery of supplemental oxygen to decrease hypoxaemia are necessary measures. Infants may need to be gavage fed or given parenteral nutrition if respiratory distress prevents oral feeding.

Classification of Congenital Heart Defects

Congenital heart defects have been classified into several categories. Traditionally a physical characteristic, cyanosis, has been used as the distinguishing feature, so the anomalies have been divided into acyanotic and cyanotic defects. In clinical practice this system is problematic because children with acyanotic defects may develop cyanosis. Also, more often, those with cyanotic defects may be pink and have more clinical signs of HF. Because of the complexity of many defects and the variability of their clinical manifestations, the cyanotic-acyanotic classification system has proven to be inadequate and misleading.

A more useful classification system is based on haemodynamic characteristics, or movements involved in the circulation of blood. The defining characteristic is blood flow patterns: (1) increased pulmonary blood flow; (2) decreased pulmonary blood flow; (3) obstruction to blood flow out of the heart; and (4) mixed blood flow, in which saturated and desaturated blood mix within the heart or great arteries. Figure 27.15 outlines both classification systems.

With the haemodynamic classification system, the clinical manifestations of each group are more uniform and predictable. Defects that allow blood flow from the high-pressure left side of the heart to the lower-pressure right side (left-to-right shunt) result in increased pulmonary blood flow and cause HF. Obstructive defects impede blood flow out of the ventricles; obstruction on the left side of the heart results in HF, whereas severe obstruction on the right side causes cyanosis. Defects that cause decreased pulmonary blood flow result in cyanosis. Mixed lesions present a variable clinical picture based on the degree of mixing and amount of pulmonary blood flow; hypoxaemia (with or without cyanosis) and HF usually occur together. (For more detailed explanations, see discussions of specific defects later in this chapter.)

More than 35 types of congenital heart defect have been identified, and some patients have multiple defects. Although some defects are common and fairly uniform, such as atrial septal defects or pulmonic stenosis, others are uncommon and highly variable, such as single-ventricle anomalies. The more common defects require no intervention or are treated with a single surgical intervention. Severe critical congenital heart defects often require multiple surgical and catheterisation interventions and lifelong management by a cardiologist. Severe defects include all cyanotic heart disease and other complex defects such as AV canal, critical aortic stenosis, critical coarctation of the aorta and complex ventricular septal defects. Most patients with these defects are identified during the newborn period or early infancy, are severely ill and require surgical treatment. The clinical presentation

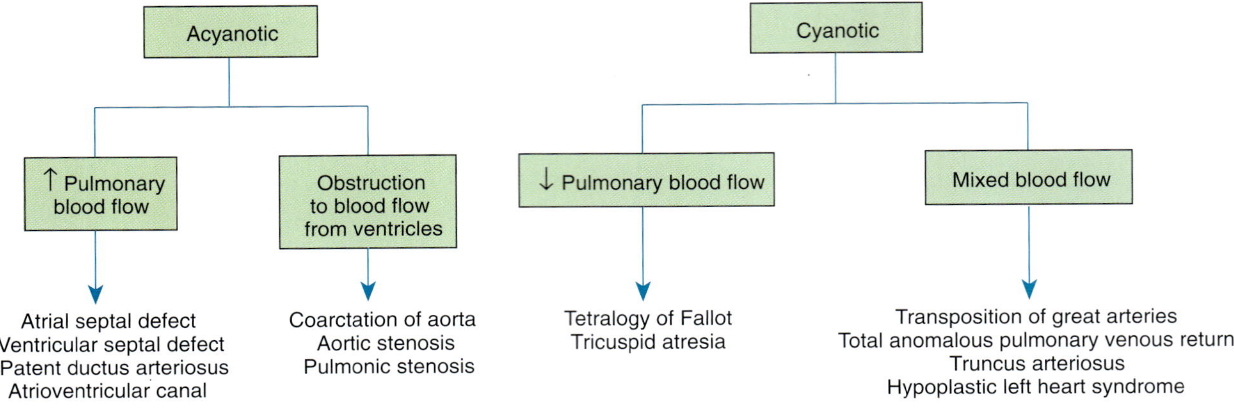

Fig 27.15 Comparison of acyanotic-cyanotic and haemodynamic classification systems for congenital heart disease.

and management of the most common defects are outlined in the following sections, Boxes 27.2 to 27.5, and Figs 27.11 to 27.14.

Nursing Care of the Child with Congenital Heart Disease and Their Family

When a child is born with a severe cardiac anomaly, parents face the immense psychological and physical tasks of adjusting to the birth of a child with special needs. Family issues and nursing interventions to support the family are similar to those described in Chapters 9 and 19. This section focuses primarily on: (1) educating the family about the disorder; (2) management of the illness at home; and (3) care and support of the child and his or her family during an invasive procedure such as catheterisation or surgery. For nursing care related specifically to the child with hypoxaemia and CHF, the reader should refer to earlier discussions of these topics.

Nursing care of the child with a congenital heart defect begins as soon as the diagnosis is suspected. The rate of prenatal diagnosis of CHD is variable, ranging from 28% to 33% in some centres to as high as 74% in other centres (Levy et al 2013, DoH 2019). As the rate of prenatal diagnosis increases, new demands are being placed on nurses to counsel and support families as they prepare for the birth of these infants. Once the infant is born, the unremitting stresses of care—physical exhaustion, financial costs, emotional upset, fear of death and concern for the child's future—are frequently not fully appreciated by those caring for the family. Even when the child's condition is stabilised or corrected, the family may need to make new adjustments in their lifestyle.

FAMILY-CENTRED CARE

Heart Beads—Documenting the Patient Story

Heart Beads is a program developed by nurses in the heart centre at the Children's Hospital at Westmead, Sydney. Heart Beads involved the families and children receiving unique beads to thread onto string to acknowledge each procedure or treatment associated with their cardiac condition. The program allowed the families and the staff to visually reflect and appreciate the journey of each child who has a cardiac condition. The program also allowed the children to feel a sense of achievement for their bravery and a way for more collaborative relationships between families and healthcare professionals (Dengler et al 2012).

Educate the Family About the Disorder

When parents learn of the heart defect, they are often initially in a period of shock, followed by high anxiety, especially fear of the child's death. Once parents are ready to hear about their child's heart condition, it is essential that they receive a clear explanation based on their level of understanding. A review of normal cardiac anatomy is helpful before explaining the anatomical defect. A simple diagram, pictures or a model of the heart can be most helpful in visualising the heart and the congenital defect. Parents appreciate receiving written information about the specific condition.* Healthcare professionals should take advantage of subsequent encounters with the family to assess parental understanding of the condition and clarify information as needed.

Different health personnel may convey the same information using different diagrams and medical terms. To prevent this from becoming a problem, the same type of diagram should be used by all, and the parents should write down any unclear terms or ask for clarification. Sometimes it is helpful to provide the family with a glossary of frequently used words for reference.

Parents often use multiple resources, particularly the Internet, to obtain information about their child's heart defect. Locating information can be easy with helpful information located at national organisations and large parent support groups.† Parents also find support through contacts with other parents and parent groups. Social media plays an important role for many families affected by congenital anomalies and offers a place for them to provide support, seek education and make friends with other families sharing similar experiences (Jacobs et al 2016). It is important for parents to realise that not all websites offer medically accurate information and that information from other parents may not be applicable to their own situation. Some children with rare, complex heart defects require individualised treatment plans, and general information on the internet or in books may not apply to them. Parents should talk to their healthcare team, in particular their cardiologist, about information they have received from other sources.

The nurse must give information to the child in a manner that is appropriate to the child's developmental age. As the child matures, the

*Heart Centre for Children, http://www.heartcentreforchildren.com.au, Royal Children's Hospital Melbourne Cardiology, https://www.rch.org.au/cardiology/parent_info/Parent_information/, HeartKids Australia, https://www.heartkids.org.au, HeartKids New Zealand https://heartkids.org.nz, Heart Foundation NZ, https://www.heartfoundation.org.nz, The Australian and New Zealand Fontan Registry, https://www.fontanregistry.com. Many major medical centres that perform paediatric heart surgery also have information on their websites.

level of information is revised to match the child's new cognitive level. Preschoolers need basic information about what they will experience more than what is actually occurring physiologically. School-age children benefit from a concrete explanation of the defect. Preadolescents and adolescents often appreciate a more detailed description of how the defect affects their heart. Children of all ages need to be able to express their feelings concerning the diagnosis.

Help the Family Manage the Illness at Home

Parents are the child's principal caregivers and need to develop a positive, supportive working relationship with the healthcare team. Because most children spend the majority of their time at home with occasional trips to the hospital, parents manage their child's illness on a daily basis. They monitor for signs of illness, give medications and treatments, bring their child to appointments, work with a variety of caregivers and alert the team to problems. Successful relationships are a partnership between parents and caregivers that is built on mutual trust and respect. Good communication between the family, the cardiology specialists and the primary care provider is essential. As children reach adolescence, they begin to take a larger role in managing their illness and making decisions about their care.

Parents should be aware of the symptoms of their child's cardiac condition and signs of worsening clinical status. They should know how to contact their child's cardiologist at all times and know what to do in an emergency. Parents of children who may develop CHF should be familiar with the symptoms (see Box 27.1) and know when to contact the practitioner. Parents of children with cyanosis should be informed about fluid management and hypercyanotic spells (see p. 715). Parents should have an information sheet with their child's diagnosis, significant treatments such as surgical procedures, allergies, other healthcare problems, current medications and healthcare providers' contact numbers available in case of emergencies and to share with other caregivers such as teachers, babysitters or day care providers.

The family also needs to be knowledgeable regarding the therapeutic management of the disorder and the role that surgery, other procedures, medications and a healthy lifestyle play in maintaining good health. Medications play a critical role in the management of some cardiac conditions such as arrhythmias and severe HF, in anticoagulation after implantation of artificial valves and in antirejection treatment after heart transplantation. Some patients must take multiple medications daily for life. Many medications can be dangerous if taken incorrectly and require close monitoring. Teach parents the correct procedure for giving medications and caution them to keep them in a safe area to prevent accidental ingestion.

Another area of parental concern is the child's level of physical activity. Most children do not need to restrict activity, and the best approach is to treat the child normally and allow self-limited activity. Exceptions primarily involve strenuous recreational and competitive sports in children with specific cardiac problems. Discuss activities and exercise restrictions with the child's cardiologist. Avoid deliberately attempting to prevent crying because it can establish a maladaptive parental pattern of relating to the infant.

Infants and children with congenital heart disease (CHD) require good nutrition. Breastfeeding is possible for many infants with CHD. Countering a common misconception that breastfeeding would not be possible for these infants because they would get tired or exhibit poor growth, Barbas and Kelleher (2004) found that breastfeeding could be successful with adequate support and education of the mother. Providing adequate nutrition to infants with HF or complex congenital defects is especially difficult due to their high caloric requirements and inability to suck effectively because of fatigue and tachypnoea. Instructing parents in feeding methods that decrease the work of the infant and giving high-calorie formula are important interventions.

Infants with heart disease should be immunised according to the current guidelines. Immunisation schedules may need to be modified around times of acute illness or surgical procedures (Smith 2001). Children with CHD are required to have an annual influenza vaccine and an additional pneumococcal vaccine (Prevenar 13) at 6 months of age or at diagnosis and pneumococcal polysaccharide vaccine (Pneumovax 23) at 4 years old according to the Australian Immunisation Handbook (Australian Technical Advisory Group on Immunisation [ATAGI] 2018) and New Zealand Immunisation Handbook (Ministry of Health 2020).

Infants and children who have serious heart disease are at risk for developmental delays (Majnemer et al 2009). There is growing interest in characterising and mitigating these outcomes through early identification and initiation of integrated developmental services. Multiple factors can influence neurodevelopmental outcomes, including genetics (e.g. chromosomal abnormalities and microdeletions), family background (e.g. parental intelligence quotient [IQ] and socioeconomic status), preoperative factors (including prematurity, cyanosis, shock), intraoperative factors (e.g. use of cardiopulmonary bypass, deep hypothermic circulatory arrest) and postoperative factors (e.g. haemodynamic instability, hypoxia, acidosis, cardiac arrest, stroke, ischaemic events).

Prepare the Child and Family for Invasive Procedures

Chapter 22 provides an extensive discussion of the principles for preparing children for invasive procedures. It is important that children and families are prepared for invasive cardiac procedures. Both the Heart Centre for Children at Westmead, Sydney and the cardiology department in the Royal Children's Hospital in Melbourne (RCHM) have a variety of online resources on their websites for families to access; however, these are all adult focused, which may not be useful to alleviate the anxiety of the child. One platform that is child focused is 'Howies Place' (https://www.rch.org.au/howie/) from RCHM which is an interactive website specifically for children. It features videos in which a puppet kangaroo prepares for cardiac surgery, explains cardiac defects and uses child friendly language to explain what will happen to the child while they are in hospital. This may be useful for children to navigate before they have their procedure as it is targeted at the child's developmental level and could increase the child's coping skills.

The expected outcomes for pre-procedure preparation include reducing anxiety, improving patient cooperation with procedures, enhancing recovery, developing trust with caregivers and improving long-term emotional and behavioural adjustment after procedures. Important factors to consider in planning preparation strategies are the child's cognitive developmental level, previous hospital experiences, temperament and coping style, the timing of the preparation and the involvement of the parents. The most beneficial preparation strategies usually combine information giving and training in coping skills such as conscious breathing exercises, distraction techniques, guided imagery and other behavioural interventions.

Handling preoperative and pre-catheterisation workups on an outpatient basis is common for most elective procedures. Children are then admitted on the morning of the procedure. Pre-procedure teaching is often done in the clinic setting or at home, and a tour of the ICU and the inpatient facilities may be added. Children of different ages and developmental levels require different amounts of information and different approaches. Young children should be prepared close in time to the event; older children and adolescents may benefit from teaching several weeks in advance. Include parents in the preparation session to support their child and learn about upcoming events.

The preoperative or pre-catheterisation preparation should include information on the environment, equipment and procedures that the child will encounter during and after the procedure. The nurse or play therapist can use many educational techniques, such as verbal and written information, hospital tours, preoperative classes, picture books or videos. Information about what the child will see, hear and feel should be included, especially for older children and adolescents. Some of the sensory experiences of being in an ICU or catheterisation laboratory include sights (e.g. monitors, many people, lots of equipment), sounds (e.g. beeping noises, alarms, voices) and sensations (e.g. lines and dressings, tape, feelings of discomfort, thirst). Familiar aspects of the environment, such as BP cuffs, stethoscopes or oximeter probes, are reviewed, and new equipment such as monitors, IV lines and oxygen masks are described. Comforting aspects of the environment are emphasised, such as play areas, chairs for parents and televisions. Many patients who will be sedated during catheterisation or receive narcotic pain relievers after surgery will have minimal recall of that period and will not need detailed information about the equipment or procedures used. Information should be specific to the planned procedure for each patient.

Discuss ways the child can cope with the experience and be helped to recover. For young children, bringing a familiar stuffed animal or comfort object with them will help relieve anxiety, whereas for older children bringing music with headphones to the catheterisation laboratory will help distract them during the procedure. Topics to discuss regarding recovery after catheterisation include the need to lie still to prevent bleeding at the catheter site, progression of the diet, pain control measures and monitoring methods. Review the importance of ambulation, coughing and deep breathing, and drinking and eating after surgery, and describe pain management and monitoring routines. Review simple coping strategies for use during painful procedures, including distraction techniques such as counting, blowing, singing or telling stories.

Children and their families should have a choice about an ICU tour. Exposure to the ICU environment can actually increase anxiety in some children, particularly young children, those with previous hospital experiences and those who are highly anxious (LeRoy et al 2003). If a visit to the recovery room and ICU is planned, it should take place when there is minimal activity in the area, when the parents can accompany the child and when the child is well rested. Usually the day before the procedure is ample time to allow the child to ask questions and to prevent undue fantasising about the experience. Protect the child from frightening sights in the unit. The child and parents are encouraged to ask questions and to explore further any equipment in the room, but they should not be pushed to assimilate more information than they are able.

Preoperative physical care differs little, if any, from that provided for any other surgery and is discussed in Chapter 22. Assure the child that the parents will be there when the child wakes up. Also allow the parents to accompany the child as far as possible to the operating suite. After all of the equipment and procedures have been explained, it is important to talk about 'getting well' and going home.

Provide Postoperative Care

Immediate postoperative care is usually provided by specially trained nurses in the ICU or cardiac specialty unit. Performing many of the procedures, specialised monitoring and observations related to vital functions requires advanced educational training (the reader should refer to critical care texts for further information). However, nurses caring for the child before surgery and during the convalescent period need to be familiar with the major principles of care.

Observe Vital Signs and Arterial and Venous Pressures. During the immediate postoperative period, record vital signs frequently, including BP, until the child's condition is stable. The heart rate and respirations are counted for 1 full minute, compared with the values on the ECG monitor. The heart rate is normally increased after surgery. The nurse observes cardiac rhythm and notifies the practitioner of any changes in regularity. Dysrhythmias may occur postoperatively secondary to administration of anaesthetics, acid–base and electrolyte imbalance, hypoxia, surgical intervention or trauma to conduction pathways.

At least hourly, auscultate the lungs for breath sounds. Diminished or absent breath sounds may indicate an area of atelectasis, pleural effusion or pneumothorax. All such cases require further assessment. Auscultation guides the nurse's selective use of postural drainage and percussion to those pulmonary lobes most in need. It also allows a more objective evaluation of effective ventilation.

Temperature changes are typical during the early postoperative period. Hypothermia is expected immediately after surgery due to hypothermia procedures, effects of anaesthesia and loss of body heat to the cool environment. During this period the child is kept warm to prevent additional heat loss. Infants may be placed under radiant heat warmers. During the next 24 to 48 hours the body temperature may rise to 37.8°C or slightly higher as part of the inflammatory response to tissue trauma. After this period an elevated temperature is most likely to be a sign of infection and warrants immediate investigation for probable cause.

Intraarterial monitoring of BP is almost always done after open-heart surgery. Residual vasoconstriction after cardiopulmonary bypass makes indirect BP readings less reliable, and intraarterial monitoring permits continuous rather than intermittent observation. A catheter is passed into the radial artery or the dorsalis pedis or posterior tibial artery. The other end is attached to an electronic monitoring system, which provides a continuous recording of the BP. The intraarterial line is maintained with a low-rate, constant infusion of heparinised saline to prevent clotting and the amount of irrigant is recorded as intake fluid. Continuous BP readings are compared with those taken indirectly using a sphygmomanometer or oscillometric device (Dinamap). A discrepancy between the two may indicate a change in peripheral vascular resistance, a malfunction in the electronic device or human error in using the wrong-size BP cuff. The nurse also observes for potential complications of intraarterial monitoring, such as arterial thrombosis, infection, air emboli or blood loss through the catheter. Prevention of each of these hazards is similar to care for any other type of infusion line.

Several IV lines are inserted preoperatively, including a peripheral IV to give fluids and medications and a CVP line that is usually inserted in a large vessel in the neck. Intracardiac monitoring lines are placed intraoperatively in the RA, LA or pulmonary artery. Intracardiac lines allow assessment of pressures inside the cardiac chambers, which give vital information on blood volume, cardiac output, ventricular function, pulmonary artery pressures and responses to drug therapy in the immediate postoperative period. The RA and CVP lines may also be used to infuse fluids and medications. LA lines and pulmonary artery lines are used with more complex repairs. Intracardiac lines are used only in the ICU, although CVP lines may remain for use as a central IV line outside the ICU. All lines must be cared for using strict aseptic technique to prevent infection. Patients must be carefully assessed for bleeding at the time of line removal. See critical care texts for a more complete discussion of intracardiac lines.

Maintain Respiratory Status. Infants usually require mechanical ventilation in the immediate postoperative period. Children may be extubated in the operating room or in the first few postoperative hours, especially if cardiopulmonary bypass was not required. Once extubated, humidified O_2 via nasal cannula or mask prevents drying of mucosa and helps bridge to room air. Encourage the child to turn and deep breathe at least hourly. When developmentally appropriate, encourage the use of incentive spirometry by blowing bubbles. Every means is employed to enhance ventilation and decrease pain, such as splinting of the operative site and use of analgesics.

For the intubated patient, suctioning is performed only as needed and is done carefully to avoid vagal stimulation (which can trigger cardiac dysrhythmias) and laryngospasm, especially in infants. Suctioning is intermittent and is maintained for no more than 5 seconds to prevent depleting the oxygen supply. Supplemental oxygen is administered with a manual resuscitation bag before and after the procedure to prevent hypoxia. The heart rate is monitored after suctioning to detect changes in rhythm or rate, especially bradycardia. The child should always be positioned facing the nurse to permit assessment of the child's colour and tolerance of the procedure.

Chest tubes are inserted into the pleural or mediastinal space during surgery or in the immediate postoperative period to remove pleural drainage and air. The chest tube is attached to a disposable water-seal drainage system. The underwater drainage prevents air from travelling up the tube into the pleural space and causing a pneumothorax. Nursing considerations include never interrupting water-seal drainage unless the chest tube is clamped, checking for tube patency (fluctuation in the water-seal chamber) and maintaining sterility.

Check drainage hourly for colour and quantity. Immediately postoperatively the drainage may be bright red, but afterwards it should be serous. The largest volume of drainage occurs in the first 12 to 24 hours, and drainage is greater after extensive heart surgery.

NURSING CARE CONSIDERATIONS

Chest tube drainage of more than 3 mL/kg/hr for more than 3 consecutive hours or 5 to 10 mL/kg in any 1 hour is excessive and may indicate postoperative haemorrhage. Notify the surgeon immediately because cardiac tamponade can develop rapidly and is life-threatening.

Chest x-rays are taken when the tubes are inserted to check their location and after they are removed to evaluate the inflation of the lungs. Chest tubes are usually removed on the first to third postoperative day when drainage has diminished.

Removal of chest tubes can be an uncomfortable, frightening experience. Warn children that they will feel a sharp, momentary pain. After the suture is cut, the tubes are quickly pulled out at the end of full inspiration in the extubated patient to prevent intake of air into the pleural cavity. (In the intubated patient, the tubes are pulled out on inspiration because the lungs are stented open with the positive pressure ventilation.) A purse-string suture (placed when the tubes were inserted) is pulled tight to close the opening. A petrolatum-covered gauze dressing is immediately applied over the wound and securely taped to the skin on all four sides so that an airtight seal is formed. The dressing is checked for signs of drainage and is removed the next day. Breath sounds are auscultated because pneumothorax is a possible complication of chest tube removal. A chest x-ray film is usually obtained after removal to assess for pneumothorax or pleural effusion.

NURSING CARE CONSIDERATIONS

Chest Tube Removal

Intravenous (IV) analgesics such as morphine sulfate (0.1 mg/kg), often in combination with midazolam, may be given before the procedure. Oral analgesics and sedatives are an alternative to IV medications. The use of a play therapist and distraction techniques may also be useful in decreasing anxiety at the time of chest drain removal. Distraction should not replace pain relief but used in combination with pain relief.

Always encourage parents to stay with their child if they wish to and support both the child and the parent during and after procedure (Fig 27.16).

Provide Maximum Rest. After heart surgery maximum rest should be provided to decrease the workload of the heart and to promote healing. Nursing care is planned according to the child's usual activity and sleep patterns. The simplest way to ensure individualised, efficient, high-quality care is to plan at the beginning of the shift the nursing procedures to be done. Identify periods of rest and discuss the schedule with the parents.

Provide Comfort. Heart surgery is both painful and frightening for children, and providing comfort is a primary nursing concern. Several incisions are used for heart surgery. A median sternotomy following the sternum down the centre of the chest is most common. A mini-sternotomy opens the lower sternum. A thoracotomy incision is most uncomfortable because it goes through muscle tissue. It allows access to the side of the chest through an incision that runs from under the arm around the back to the scapula.

Adequate pain control decreases postoperative complications such as atelectasis, pneumonia and deep vein thrombosis by improving coughing and ambulation. Pain level is now considered the fifth vital sign. Many pain assessment tools are available for infants and children of different ages. (See Measuring Pain in Children, Chapter 5.)

Continuous IV infusion of opioids, particularly morphine and fentanyl, is a safe and effective method of pain control. Patient-controlled analgesia may be used with children old enough to understand the concept. Children receiving opioid infusions for a prolonged period are weaned slowly from the medication to prevent withdrawal symptoms. Non-steroidal anti-inflammatory drugs (NSAIDs) such oral ibuprofen may provide relief of moderate postoperative pain.

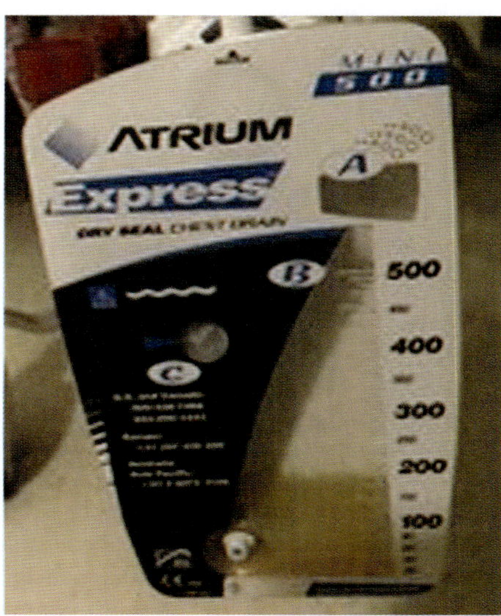

Fig 27.16 Chest drain.

Most patients need IV analgesics for pain control during the 24- to 48-hour postoperative period. After lines and tubes have been removed and when patients are tolerating oral fluids, pain may be controlled with oral narcotics such as oxycodone often combined with paracetamol or an oral NSAID such as ibuprofen, or with paracetamol alone. As noted earlier, thoracotomy incisions are usually more painful than sternotomies because the incision is through muscle. Paracetamol or ibuprofen alone is usually adequate for pain control after discharge.

In addition to providing pharmacological pain control, make every effort to minimise the discomfort of procedures by other means, such as by placing a firm pillow or favourite stuffed animal against the chest incision during coughing and performing treatments after pain medication is given, preferably at a time that coincides with the drug's peak effect. Employ non-pharmacological measures to lessen the perception of pain, and encourage parents to comfort their child as much as possible. (See Nursing Care Guidelines: Biobehavioural Strategies for Pain Management, Chapter 5.)

Monitor Fluids. Intake and output of all fluids must be accurately calculated. Intake is primarily IV fluids; however, the nurse also needs to keep a record of fluid used to flush the arterial, CVP and intracardiac lines or to dilute medications. Monitoring of output includes hourly recordings of urine (usually a Foley catheter is inserted and attached to a closed collecting device), drainage from chest and nasogastric tubes and blood drawn for analysis. Low cardiac output is common after open-heart surgery and is characterised by low urine output. This places the patient at a higher risk for renal failure.

During open-heart surgery, the cardiopulmonary pump is primed with a large volume of fluid (usually electrolyte solution), which may greatly dilute the patient's blood. The large amount of fluid also diffuses into the interstitial spaces, causing total-body oedema and pulmonary oedema. Patients return from the operating room with fluid overload. Fluids are restricted to less than maintenance level during the first postoperative day, and drugs are used to promote diuresis. A return to maintenance fluid levels then occurs over the next few days. Electrolyte levels are closely monitored because electrolyte imbalances, especially hypokalaemia, are a common result of diuresis and fluid shifts, and electrolytes may need replacement.

Fluid requirements are based on the child's weight and body surface area. Weights are obtained daily at the same time of day. Oral fluids are usually withheld until the child is extubated. Patients begin taking clear liquids when bowel sounds are heard and advance slowly to a regular diet. Nausea and vomiting are common in the first few days after surgery; they are a likely side effect of anaesthesia and analgesics, it is important to provide antiemetics as appropriate. Providing adequate nutrition, ideally by oral intake, becomes important by the fourth or fifth postoperative day. Consider nasogastric tube feedings or parenteral nutrition for patients who are unable to tolerate oral feedings.

Plan for Progressive Activity. Fatigue and weakness are common after heart surgery. However, moderate activity is essential to prevent pulmonary and vascular complications. Initially, turning, coughing and deep breathing are sufficient to promote respiratory expansion. Passive range-of-motion exercises, especially to the lower extremities, are instituted to prevent venous stasis.

A progressive schedule of ambulation and activity is planned, based on the child's preoperative activity patterns and postoperative cardiovascular and pulmonary function. Provide the child with toys to encourage movement. It is important to plan the activity at times when the child is well rested, is comfortable (usually has had analgesic medication) and is not scheduled for any strenuous procedure or treatment immediately afterwards.

Once extubated, ambulation is initiated early. Patients progress from sitting on the edge of the bed and dangling the legs to standing up and to sitting in a chair or in a carer's lap while being assisted and assessed by the nursing staff. Carefully monitor the heart rate, oxygen saturation and respirations to assess the degree of cardiac demand imposed by each activity. Tachycardia, dyspnoea, cyanosis, desaturation, progressive fatigue or dysrhythmias indicate the need to limit further energy expenditure.

Observe for Complications of Heart Surgery. Several complications can occur after heart surgery, most of which are related to open-heart surgery and the use of cardiopulmonary bypass. Many of the procedures discussed in the preceding paragraphs are aimed at preventing these problems. Only those that have not already been discussed are included here. A serious complication, infective endocarditis (bacterial), is discussed on p. 730.

Cardiac changes. Preoperatively the workload of the heart is increased because of the abnormal haemodynamics caused by the congenital defect. In the initial postoperative period the heart is under increased stress because of the effects of surgery and the use of the heart-lung machine. In some cases cardiac function can actually be worse in the early postoperative period despite repair of the congenital defect. HF, hypoxia, low cardiac output, dysrhythmias and tamponade are all potential postoperative problems.

HF may occur postoperatively because of excessive pulmonary blood flow or fluid overload (see p. 709 for assessment and management of HF). Hypoxia may occur because of inadequate pulmonary blood flow or because of respiratory problems. Rapid assessment of the causes of hypoxia and appropriate interventions to improve ventilation and perfusion are vital because hypoxia can rapidly lead to acidosis, which can impair ventricular function.

Low cardiac output syndrome and decreased peripheral perfusion can occur from hypothermia or inability of the LV to maintain systemic circulation. It affects up to 25% of infants and young children after cardiac surgery (Hoffman et al 2003). The most important signs of adequate peripheral perfusion are rapid capillary refill, good skin colour, warm extremities and strong pulses. Indications of low cardiac output are similar to signs of shock (i.e. decreased BP, decreased pulse pressure, cool extremities, metabolic acidosis and oliguria). Low cardiac output states are aggressively treated with IV inotropic medications such as dopamine, dobutamine, adrenaline and milrinone. Milrinone, widely used in paediatrics, has also been shown to prevent low cardiac output syndrome (Hoffman et al 2003). If maximum medical therapy is failing, cardiac assist methods such as extracorporeal membrane oxygenation or a ventricular assist device may be used.

Dysrhythmias are common in the early postoperative period and can result from electrolyte imbalance, especially hypokalaemia and surgical intervention to the septum or myocardium. The heart rate and rhythm are carefully monitored by observing the ECG pattern and by counting the apical pulse for 1 full minute. In some children, a faster than normal rate may be required to maintain an adequate cardiac output in the postoperative period, and a slower than normal rhythm can impair cardiac output. Epicardial pacing wires may be inserted during surgery for managing cardiac dysrhythmias postoperatively.

Cardiac tamponade is compression of the heart by blood and other effusion (clots) in the pericardial sac, which severely restricts the normal heart movement. Signs include rising and equalising RA and LA filling pressures, narrowing pulse pressure, tachycardia, dyspnoea, apprehension and an abrupt stop to chest tube drainage from mediastinal tubes. The nurse immediately reports any evidence of this potentially fatal complication. An echocardiogram confirms the diagnosis. Treatment consists of prompt pericardiocentesis to remove the blood or fluid. If active haemorrhage and coagulopathy are present, steps are taken to enhance blood clotting.

Pulmonary changes. Areas of atelectasis are common immediately after surgery as a result of deflation of the lung during cardiopulmonary bypass. Other pulmonary complications include pneumothorax, especially caused by faulty chest tubes; pulmonary oedema from increased pulmonary blood flow or HF; and pleural effusion caused by persistent venous congestion. Signs of pneumothorax are persistent decreased breath sounds, sudden dyspnoea, tachycardia, rapid shallow respirations, cyanosis and sometimes sharp chest pain. Signs of pulmonary oedema are tachypnoea, rales, wheezing, moist dyspnoeic respirations, tachycardia, cyanosis and restlessness. Signs and symptoms of pleural effusions include increased respiratory rate, vomiting, decreased breath sounds, fatigue, irritability and decreased oxygen saturation. Chest radiography is important in the accurate diagnosis of pulmonary complications and is done frequently postoperatively.

Neurological changes. Neurological complications such as seizures, strokes, cerebral oedema and hypoxic or ischaemic brain injury are uncommon after open-heart surgery but can be devastating when they occur. Nurses are alert to the possibility of neurological symptoms and perform ongoing neurological assessments, including evaluation of the equality of strength and reflexes in both extremities for evidence of paralysis; pupil size, equality, reaction to light and accommodation; and the child's orientation to the environment. The nurse also observes for focal or generalised seizure activity. Any evidence of cerebral damage is reported immediately. Further neurological evaluation and management are needed for all abnormalities.

Seizures are the most common neurological condition, seen most often in infants. Longer periods of deep hypothermic cardiopulmonary bypass (> 40 minutes), sometimes needed in complex repairs on neonates, have been associated with an increased risk of seizure activity and later developmental delays (Wypij et al 2003). Significant improvements in cardiopulmonary bypass techniques, arterial filters and a better understanding of neuroprotection during heart surgery have resulted in a reduced incidence of seizures and better neurodevelopmental outcomes (Menasche et al 2002). Continuous postoperative EEG monitoring also has identified subclinical seizures that previously may not have been discovered without this monitoring. Neonates post cardiac surgery should be monitored with continuous EEG monitoring (BrainZ) especially if cardiac bypass was used (Gist et al 2019).

Infection. All patients are at risk for infections postoperatively; especially vulnerable are infants, those with poor cardiac function and those who require multiple invasive lines and procedures for a prolonged period. Prophylactic antibiotics are given for the first 1 or 2 days. All dressings are applied and changed using aseptic technique. Good handwashing, careful use of aseptic technique when placing and accessing lines and close attention to surgical wounds are all important to prevent infection. Monitor patients closely for fever and signs of infection. Monitor all IV sites for signs of infection or phlebitis. Appropriate treatment is instituted if an infection is identified.

Haematological changes. While passing through the heart-lung machine, blood is exposed to substantial trauma because of mechanical action and direct contact with oxygen, foreign substances and massive doses of anticoagulants. The result of mechanical trauma is red blood cell haemolysis and potential renal tubular necrosis. Heparinisation of the blood during extracorporeal circulation can result in clotting abnormalities from decreased thrombin and prothrombin levels, decreased levels of platelets and altered platelet aggregation. Because blood-clotting mechanisms are affected, signs of haemorrhage, especially bleeding from the chest tubes and a fall in arterial and venous pressures, are important observations.

Haemolysis of red blood cells leads to blood loss and anaemia, which may require packed red blood cell transfusion. The nurse monitors results of full blood counts to identify the severity of the haemolysis. Urine is tested for blood. If transfusions are required, the child is closely observed for signs of reaction and fluid overload. The need to measure urinary output hourly has already been discussed.

Normally the filter and bubble trap on the heart-lung machine remove air emboli, tiny clots, fat debris and organisms from the arterialised (oxygenated) blood before its return to the body. However, the entry of impure blood into the systemic circulation can cause fat embolism, thromboembolism and infection anywhere in the body and, most importantly, in the brain.

Postpericardiotomy syndrome. The postpericardiotomy syndrome of fever, leucocytosis, pericardial friction rub or pericardial and pleural effusion can occur any time the pericardium is opened, either in the immediate postoperative period or after surgery, typically around days 7 to 21. The cause is unknown, although aetiological theories include viral infection, autoimmune response to myocardial tissue and a reaction to blood in the pericardium. The syndrome is self-limiting and is treated with rest, salicylates, NSAIDs and sometimes steroids. Pericardiocentesis or pleurocentesis may be needed to treat large effusions.

Provide Emotional Support

Children may become depressed after surgery. This is thought to be caused by preoperative anxiety, postoperative psychological and physiological stress and sensory overstimulation. Typically the child's disposition improves on leaving the ICU. (See Chapter 21.)

Children may also be angry and uncooperative after surgery as a response to the physical pain and to the loss of control imposed by the surgery and treatments. They need an opportunity to express feelings, either verbally or through activity. Nurses can praise children for their efforts to cooperate and should refrain from expecting too much courage or bravery. Children often regress in their behaviour during the stress of surgery and hospitalisation. Children also may express feelings of anger or rejection towards parents. The nurse must reassure parents that this is normal and that with continued support the anger will subside.

The nurse can support the parents by being available to provide information and explaining all the procedures to them. The first few postoperative days are particularly difficult because parents see their child in pain and realise the potential risks from surgery. They often are overwhelmed by the physical environment of the ICU and feel useless because they can do so little for their child. The nurse can minimise such feelings by: including parents in caregiving activities and comfort and play activities; providing information about the child's condition; and being sensitive to their emotional and physical needs. The use of social workers, peer support groups and ward grandparents all can provide parents and children with emotional support.

The importance of their presence in making the child feel more secure is stressed, even if they do not provide physical care.

Plan for Discharge and Home Care

Assessment of discharge needs should begin at admission so parents and healthcare providers have ample time to plan for a safe discharge and arrange for necessary equipment and supports. The family needs verbal and written instructions on medication, nutrition, activity restrictions, wound care, pain management and signs and symptoms of infection or complications. Other discussion topics may include return to school and work, special medication teaching for warfarin (Coumadin) or other drugs that require detailed home management, and infective endocarditis (subacute bacterial endocarditis [SBE]) prophylaxis. Referrals to community agencies may be necessary to assist parents in the transition from hospital to home and to reinforce the teaching (see Family-Centred Care box).

FAMILY-CENTRED CARE

Discharge Teaching After Cardiac Surgery

- Medication teaching
- Activity restrictions
- CPR training
- Diet and nutrition
- Wound care (include dressings, if any, suture removal, bathing)
- Infective endocarditis (bacterial) prophylaxis
- Follow-up appointments: cardiologist, primary care provider
- Contact information for community agencies as needed: visiting nurse service, early developmental intervention, home supply companies
- When to call the cardiologist or general paediatrician
- Signs and symptoms of postoperative problems
- Review of cardiac defect and surgical repair

Encourage parents to keep an updated summary of their child's diagnosis, surgical procedures, allergies, medications, healthcare providers with contact information and other health problems readily available for emergencies and to share this summary with school personnel, babysitters and others. Appropriate medical identification, such as a medical alert bracelet, is indicated for children with a pacemaker or a heart transplant and for those receiving anticoagulation therapy or antidysrhythmic medication.

The nurse also discusses common behaviour disturbances that may occur after discharge, such as nightmares, sleep disturbances, separation anxiety and overdependence. A supportive, consistent response is essential to allow the child to overcome the surgical experience. The child may work out feelings and fears through therapeutic play, and this should be encouraged.

Although surgical correction of heart defects has improved dramatically, it is still not possible to totally repair many complex anomalies. Some repairs require several operations over a period of years. For many children, repeat procedures are required to replace conduits or valves or to manage complications such as restenosis. Consequently, the long-term prognosis is uncertain, and full recovery is not always possible. For these families, close medical follow-up and continued emotional support are essential.

ACQUIRED CARDIOVASCULAR DISORDERS

Acquired cardiac disorders include disease processes or abnormalities that occur after birth and can be seen in the otherwise normal heart or in the presence of congenital heart defects. They occur for a variety of reasons, including infection, autoimmune response, environmental factors and familial tendencies. Nursing care often plays a critical role in the identification and supportive management of these cardiovascular disorders.

Infective Endocarditis

Infective endocarditis (IE) (also called *bacterial endocarditis* or *subacute bacterial endocarditis [SBE]* in the past) is an infection of the inner lining of the heart (endocardium), generally involving the valves. The incidence of IE is much less frequent in children than in adults but increasing in both groups (Gupta et al 2016). In the past, it was most often a result of bacteraemia in children with acquired or congenital anomalies of the heart or great vessels, particularly those with valvular abnormalities, prosthetic valves, shunts, recent cardiac surgery with invasive lines and rheumatic heart disease (RHD) with valve involvement. More recently, only half the cases were in children with underlying heart disease (Gupta et al 2016). The increased incidence of IE in children without cardiac abnormalities is likely to be related to the increased use of indwelling central lines to treat other serious diseases (Bragg & Alvarez 2014). The incidence of neonatal IE has also increased because of the increased use of indwelling lines and fewer than a third of the IE cases seen in neonates occur in those with CHD (Day et al 2009). Endocarditis can also occur without any known risk factors, commonly affecting the mitral or aortic valve.

The most common causative agents are *Streptococcus viridans* and *Staphylococcus aureus*. Gram-negative bacteria known as HACEK and fungi such as *Candida* and *Aspergillus* are also causes of IE (Baltimore et al 2015). Positive blood cultures are present in most patients; however, endocarditis can also be present despite negative blood cultures, especially if antibiotics have already been given. Culture-negative endocarditis has been reported in 5% to 10% of IE cases (Bragg & Alvarez 2014) and up to 30% in other studies (Gupta et al 2016).

Pathophysiology

Organisms may enter the bloodstream from any site of localised infection. Endocarditis may occur from routine exposure to bacteraemia associated with usual daily activities such as brushing teeth although it can also occur after procedures such as dental work, invasive procedures involving the gastrointestinal and genitourinary tracts, cardiac surgery, especially if synthetic material is used (valves, patches, conduits); or it may occur from long-term indwelling catheters. The microorganisms grow on the endocardium, forming vegetations (verrucae), deposits of fibrin and platelet thrombi. The lesion may invade adjacent tissues, such as the aortic and mitral valves, and may break off and embolise elsewhere, especially to the spleen, kidney and CNS.

Clinical Manifestations

The onset of symptoms is usually insidious, with unexplained low-grade, intermittent fever. Other common non-specific symptoms are malaise, anorexia, HF symptoms, arthralgias and weight loss (Baltimore et al 2015). IE should be considered in at-risk patients who have any of these symptoms. Patients can also present acutely with high fevers and rapidly declining health, requiring immediate hospitalisation and treatment.

The presentation in newborns and infants can be non-specific with signs of sepsis or HF. Feeding intolerance, respiratory distress, tachycardia and hypotension may be seen. Septic emboli are more common in infants resulting in infection outside the heart (osteomyelitis, meningitis, pneumonia) (Baltimore et al 2015).

The clinical findings of IE in children are seen in four areas: bacteraemia (or fungaemia), valvulitis, immunological responses and emboli (Baltimore et al 2015). A new murmur or a change in a previously existing one is frequently found as a result of damage to valves or perforation of the myocardium. Symptoms of HF may be present. Signs that result from embolus formation elsewhere in the body include splinter haemorrhages (thin black lines) under the nails, Osler nodes (red, painful intradermal nodes with white centres found on the pads of the phalanges), Janeway spots (painless haemorrhagical areas on the palms and soles), petechiae on the oral mucous membranes and splenomegaly, although all these signs are less common in children than in adults (Baltimore et al 2015).

Diagnostic Evaluation

Definitive diagnosis can be made after growth of the organism and identification of the causative agent in the blood. Several blood specimens (three are recommended) are drawn for culture to rule out contamination during venepuncture and dilution. Because the most common organisms causing IE, staphylococci and streptococci, are found on the skin, strict sterile technique is practised in obtaining cultures to avoid contamination. Obtaining an adequate blood volume for culture is also important. When an organism is identified, sensitivity studies are done to determine appropriate antibiotic therapy. Echocardiographic findings include new or increasing valvular insufficiency, vegetations, abscesses and decreased ventricular function. Vegetations cannot always be visualised with echo imaging. Other findings may support the diagnosis of IE, such as ECG changes (AV block), anaemia, an elevated erythrocyte sedimentation rate, leucocytosis, microscopic haematuria and radiographic evidence of cardiomegaly. A diagnosis of culture-negative endocarditis is made when the patient has echocardiographic or clinical evidence of IE but no organism can be cultured (Baltimore et al 2015).

The Duke criteria provide guidelines for the diagnosis of IE in adults and are useful in the diagnosis of childhood endocarditis as well These criteria divide signs and symptoms into major and minor criteria. IE can be diagnosed if the child has two major criteria, or one major and three minor, or five minor criteria. The two major criteria include positive blood culture results and echocardiographic evidence of endocardial involvement (vegetations or new valvular regurgitation). Minor criteria include: fever, predisposing risk factors of CHD, presence of a central venous line or IV drug use; vascular phenomena that include major arterial emboli, septic pulmonary infarcts, mycotic aneurysm, intracranial haemorrhage, conjunctival haemorrhage or Janeway lesions; and immunological phenomena such as glomerulonephritis, Osler's nodes, Roth spots and rheumatoid factor (Li et al 2000).

Therapeutic Management

Treatment for IE includes the administration of high-dose antibiotics given intravenously for 2 to 8 weeks to completely eradicate the infecting microorganism (Bragg & Alvarez 2014). Infectious disease specialists should be consulted to assist in determining the appropriate regimen for each patient. Blood cultures are performed periodically to evaluate the response to antibiotic therapy. Serial echocardiograms are done to evaluate for ventricular function, vegetations and valve damage. Cardiac surgery may be indicated to repair or replace damaged valves.

Early medical treatment for IE is successful in many patients. However, patients diagnosed late, patients with underlying heart disease or a clinical course complicated by HF, embolic events or significant valvular dysfunction, or IE caused by antibiotic-resistant organisms or fungi carry a mortality rate of 5% to 10% (Baltimore et al 2015). Infections with *Staphylococcus aureus* have a higher mortality rate in the modern era than those caused by streptococci (Gupta et al 2016). Non-fatal complications result from embolism to other structures, especially to the CNS (causing hemiplegia, aphasia, meningitis, convulsions), kidney (resulting in haematuria, proteinuria), spleen and bowel.

Prevention of Endocarditis

Prevention involves administration of prophylactic antibiotic therapy to high-risk patients before dental procedures that are associated with the risk of entry of organisms. Additional procedures that require prophylaxis (only in the high-risk group) include invasive procedures of the respiratory tract and procedures on infected skin or musculoskeletal tissue. Maintenance of excellent oral hygiene and prevention of oral disease is still of utmost importance, especially in children with CHD (Baltimore et al 2015).

Nursing Care Management

Nurses counsel parents of high-risk children concerning the signs and symptoms of endocarditis and the need for prophylactic antibiotic therapy before dental work. The family's dentist should be advised of the child's cardiac diagnosis as an added precaution to ensure preventive treatment. It is important that all children with congenital or acquired heart disease maintain the highest level of oral health to reduce the chance of bacteraemia from oral infections. (See Chapter 12.)

Parents should also have a high index of suspicion regarding potential infections. Without unduly alarming them, the nurse stresses that any unexplained fever, weight loss or change in behaviour (lethargy, malaise, anorexia) must be brought to the practitioner's attention. Children at risk (e.g. those with CHD) should have blood drawn for culture if they have a fever without an obvious source. Early diagnosis and treatment are important in preventing further cardiac damage, embolic complications and growth of resistant organisms. (See Quality Patient Outcomes box.)

> **QUALITY PATIENT OUTCOMES**
>
> ***Infective Endocarditis***
>
> - Prevention in high-risk patients with antibiotic prophylaxis
> - Early recognition and treatment

Treatment of endocarditis requires long-term parenteral drug therapy. In many cases, IV antibiotics may be administered at home via a peripherally inserted central catheter (PICC line) with nursing supervision. Nursing goals during this period are: (1) preparation of the child for IV infusion, usually with an intermittent-infusion device and several venepunctures for blood cultures; (2) observation for side effects of antibiotics, especially inflammation along venepuncture sites; (3) observation for complications, including embolism and HF; and (4) education regarding the importance of follow-up visits for cardiac evaluation, echocardiographic monitoring and blood cultures. Some children may need preparation for surgery and, later, postoperative care.

Acute Rheumatic Fever and Rheumatic Heart Disease

Acute rheumatic fever (ARF) is a result of an abnormal immune response to a group A streptococci (GAS) infection, usually pharyngitis, in a genetically susceptible host (Marijon et al 2012). It occurs most often in late school-age children and adolescents and is rare in adults. ARF is a self-limited illness that occurs after untreated pharyngitis and involves inflammation of connective tissues: the joints, skin, brain and heart. Cardiac valve damage, which is referred to as rheumatic heart disease (RHD), the most significant complication of ARF, occurs in more than half the cases. The mitral valve is most often affected (Maguire et al 2012, Pennock et al 2014).

To date, Aboriginal and Torres Strait Islander peoples and New Zealand Māori and Pacific Islanders have among the highest rates of ARF in the world and experience an inequitable burden of RHD. These groups experience considerable inequities across a wide range of social, educational and health outcomes compared with the general population (RHDAustralia [ARF/RHD writing group] 2020).

Table 27.3 identifies risk groups for ARF.

TABLE 27.3 Risk Groups for Primary Prevention of ARF

At high risk	Living in an ARF-endemic setting† Aboriginal and/or Torres Strait Islander peoples living in rural or remote settings Aboriginal and/or Torres Strait Islander peoples and Māori and/or Pacific Islander peoples living in metropolitan households affected by crowding and/or lower socioeconomic status Personal history of ARF/RHD and aged < 40 years
May be at high risk	Family or household recent history of ARF/RHD Household overcrowding (> 2 people per bedroom) or low socioeconomic status Migrant or refugee from low- or middle-income country and their children
Additional considerations which increase risk	Prior residence in a high ARF risk setting Frequent or recent travel to a high ARF risk setting Aged 5–20 years (the peak years for ARF)

†This refers to populations where community ARF/RHD rates are known to be high (e.g. ARF incidence > 30/100,000 per year in 5 to 14 year olds or RHD all-age prevalence > 2/1000).
Source: RHDAustralia (ARF/RHD writing group). (2020). The 2020 Australian guideline for prevention, diagnosis and management of acute rheumatic fever and rheumatic heart disease (3rd ed.). https://www.rhdaustralia.org.au/system/files/fileuploads/arf_rhd_guidelines_3rd_edition_web_updated.pdf

Aetiology

Strong evidence supports a relationship between upper respiratory tract infection with GAS and subsequent development of ARF (usually within 2 to 6 weeks). Prevention or treatment of GAS infection prevents ARF. If the GAS infection is untreated, antibodies are produced to fight the infection, which can also act against the heart valves causing damage. If children have one strep infection, they are at greater risk for repeated infections and recurrent infections cause the cumulative valve damage of RHD.

Pathophysiology and Clinical Manifestations

ARF is the result of an immune response after infection with GAS, which can be asymptomatic and often go untreated. The diagnosis is based on a set of diagnostic criteria first described by Dr T. Duckett Jones in 1944 and known as the Jones criteria. Endorsed by the American Heart Association and the World Heart Federation, the most recent revision was completed in 2015 and added evidence supporting the use of Doppler echocardiogram in the diagnosis of carditis (Gewitz et al 2015). Minor changes made in the recent 2020 Australian guideline for prevention, diagnosis and management of acute rheumatic fever and rheumatic heart disease (3rd edition) aligns with the 2015 revised Jones criteria (RHDAustralia [ARF/RHD writing group] 2020) (Box 27.6). RHDAustralia has developed a free app for use on iPhone, iPad and Android devices to support the Australian health workforce with the clinical aspects of ARF and RHD. The app includes a summary of key information from the 2020 Australian guideline and an ARF diagnosis calculator.

The most significant manifestation of ARF is carditis. Carditis is the only manifestation of ARF that leads to permanent damage. In the acute illness, clinical signs and symptoms reflect valvulitis, myocarditis and pericarditis. Clinically, rheumatic carditis is most commonly associated with the left-sided valves, especially the mitral valve. The classic presentation of carditis was the auscultation of a new regurgitant murmur. Increasingly, as echocardiography is more available in the developing world, ARF and RHD is diagnosed by echo Doppler before the murmur is present. It is now recommended that echocardiograms be performed in all suspected and confirmed cases of ARF (Gewitz et al 2015). Patients with valve involvement may experience progressive valvular damage as time passes.

The second major manifestation is polyarthritis caused by oedema, inflammation and effusions in joint tissue. Joint manifestations usually accompany the acute febrile period, most often in the first 1 to 2 weeks; however, they can persist for 4 weeks in untreated patients.

The other manifestations, erythema marginatum and subcutaneous nodules, are uncommon but are highly specific for ARF.

BOX 27.6 Clinical Manifestations of Acute Rheumatic Fever

Major Manifestations

- Polyarthritis
  - Swollen, hot, red and very painful joint
  - Migratory: affects one joint for 1 to 2 days, then another is affected
  - Large joints most commonly affected: knees, elbows, hips, shoulders, wrists
- Chorea (also called Sydenham's chorea)
  - Sudden aimless irregular movements of extremities, exacerbated by stress
  - Profound muscle weakness
  - Facial grimaces and speech disturbances
  - More common in females particularly in adolescence
  - Common symptom for Aboriginal and Torres Strait Islander children
- Carditis (seen in 50% to 70% of cases)
  - New murmur of valve regurgitation (mitral valve most common)
  - Cardiac enlargement
  - Cardiac decompensation
  - Pericardial friction rub
  - Echo Doppler evidence of cardiac involvement
  - Tachycardia out of proportion to fever
  - Chest pain
  - Muffled heart sounds
  - Prolonged PR interval on electrocardiogram
- Subcutaneous nodules
  - Non-tender swelling over bony prominences
  - May persist for many weeks and then resolve
  - More common in Māori and Pacific Islander children
- Erythema marginatum
  - Pink rash with pale centre and wavy, well-demarcated borders
  - Seen on trunk and extremities
  - More prominent with heat, blanches with pressure
  - Non-pruritic

Minor Manifestations

- Arthralgias
- Fever (greater than 38.5°C)
- ESR above 60 mm and/or CRP greater than 3 mg/dL
- Prolonged PR interval

CRP, C-reactive protein; *ESR,* erythrocyte sedimentation rate.
Source: Adapted from RHDAustralia (ARF/RHD writing group). (2020). The 2020 Australian guideline for prevention, diagnosis and management of acute rheumatic fever and rheumatic heart disease (3rd ed.). https://www.rhdaustralia.org.au/system/files/fileuploads/arf_rhd_guidelines_3rd_edition_web_updated.pdf

In addition to these major manifestations, minor manifestations that may support the diagnosis include arthralgia and fever, which may be low grade and which often spikes in the late afternoon. Laboratory findings reflect an inflammatory process. Other vague signs and symptoms include unexplained epistaxis, abdominal pain that may be severe enough to simulate appendicitis, weakness, fatigue, pallor, anorexia and weight loss.

Diagnostic Evaluation

No single symptom or laboratory test can provide a definitive diagnosis of ARF. Rather, the diagnosis is based on the diagnostic Jones criteria, which were updated in 2015 (Gewitz et al 2015) and aligned with Australian and New Zealand guidelines in 2020 (RHDAustralia [ARF/RHD writing group] 2020). Clinical and laboratory findings are divided into major and minor manifestations shown previously in Box 27.6. Patients must have two major manifestations or one major and two minor manifestations for diagnosis. Some recurrent episodes of ARF in high-risk populations may only have three minor manifestations (RHDAustralia [ARF/RHD writing group] 2020). Age of the patient (5 to 15 years) and preceding sore throat are also important diagnostic clues.

Laboratory tests are done to confirm the clinical diagnosis. Rapid antigen detection test and a throat culture are done to assess for GAS colonisation. Streptolysin O is a streptococcal extracellular product that produces lysis of the red blood cells. Antistreptolysin O (ASLO) titres measure the concentration of antibodies formed in the blood against this product. Normally, the titres begin to rise about 7 days after onset of the infection and reach maximum levels in 4 to 6 weeks. Therefore, a rising titre demonstrated by at least two ASLO tests is the most reliable evidence of recent streptococcal infection. Elevated titres are seen in at least 80% of patients with ARF (Steer & Gibofsky 2017). Tests to assess for inflammation include a full blood count, erythrocyte sedimentation rate (ESR) and C-reactive protein levels (CRP). An electrocardiogram is done to assess for a prolonged PR interval. A chest radiograph is done to assess cardiomegaly and signs of cardiac involvement. An echocardiogram with Doppler to confirm the presence of carditis is done in all patients, even those without clinical signs of carditis. Echo Doppler has been found to be more sensitive than auscultatory findings of a new murmur in identifying cardiac valve dysfunction (Gewitz et al 2015). In high-risk populations, a lower threshold for fever (38°C) and lower inflammatory markers (ESR above 30, CRP above 3) are considered diagnostic (RHDAustralia [ARF/RHD writing group] 2020).

Therapeutic Management

Primary prevention involves prompt diagnosis and treatment of strep throat infections so that ARF does not occur. For children with ARF, treatment includes antibiotics, anti-inflammatory therapy and supportive care and management of HF in some. Antibiotics are given to treat the GAS infection and begin long-term prophylactic treatment to prevent future infections. Penicillin is the drug of choice. Salicylates are used to control the inflammatory process, especially in the joints, and reduce the fever and discomfort. The diagnosis must be confirmed before aspirin therapy is started so clinical signs are not masked by the therapy. Administration of prednisone may be indicated in patients with pericarditis or HF and in patients who do not respond to aspirin therapy. Neither salicylates nor prednisone has been shown to affect cardiac sequelae.

Supportive care involves initial bed rest during the acute illness and then quiet activities as symptoms subside. Good nutrition is important. Care for children with significant carditis includes HF therapies such as supplemental oxygen, diuretics, fluid and salt restriction, digoxin or ACE inhibitors. Children with chorea with motor impairment must be protected from injury and eliminate physical and emotional stress, which can exacerbate their symptoms.

Children who have had ARF are susceptible to recurrent infections that are likely to result in RHD and further damage to the heart valves. Prophylactic treatment against recurrence of ARF (secondary prevention) is started after the acute therapy. The treatment of choice is intramuscular injections of benzathine penicillin G every 28 days because it is most effective. Alternative therapy includes oral doses of penicillin or erythromycin twice a day. The duration of secondary prophylaxis is based on the presence of residual heart disease. If ARF occurs without carditis, prophylaxis is recommended for 5 years or until age 21 years, whichever is longer. In patients with carditis, 10 years is recommended or until 21 years old. In patients with RHD, prophylaxis can continue until the age of 40 years and may be indicated indefinitely depending on the individual's risk (Heart Foundation of New Zealand 2014).

Patients with significant cardiac valve damage will need ongoing medical management for HF. They are also at risk for atrial fibrillation and embolic events. Management of RHD may require surgical valve repair or replacement. Valve replacement with a mechanical valve requires lifelong anticoagulation with warfarin.

Nursing Care Management

The objective of nursing care is, firstly, prevention. Clinicians need to be aware that untreated or undertreated strep throat infections can cause ARF. Rapid strep tests or throat cultures should be done and prompt treatment with antibiotics and follow-up is important. Parents need to be clear that all the antibiotic medicine must be finished. Repeat strep pharyngitis infections may have fewer symptoms or be asymptomatic and trigger ARF or cause further valve damage so a high index of suspicion is important. All patients with ARF receive antibiotic prophylaxis to prevent future infections.

For the child with ARF, nursing care goals include: (1) encouraging compliance with drug regimens; (2) facilitating recovery from the illness; and (3) providing emotional support. Nurses play an important role in secondary prevention by educating parents about ARF and RHD and working with patients and families to ensure follow-up with antibiotic prophylaxis. Because compliance is a major concern in long-term drug therapy, every effort is made to encourage adherence to the therapeutic plan (see Compliance, Chapter 22). A community-based approach including healthcare facilities, Aboriginal healthcare liaisons, schools and families with excellent communication among them and a personalised approach has been most successful in gaining compliance with years of antibiotic medications (Bono-Neri 2016).

Dedicated health teams that deliver secondary prophylaxis have been most successful (Remond et al 2016). The Australian federal government, in partnership with experts and members of the Aboriginal and Torres Strait Islander populations, have launched the rheumatic heart disease strategy. This advisory committee provides high-level strategic advice to government agencies as well as many healthcare initiatives and online education programs for healthcare professionals working with communities with a high incidence of RHD. The strategy also provides information on the RHD register which improves case detection and compliance to secondary prophylaxis for healthcare workers as well as developing electronic applications for patients that can help provide reminders when the next injection is due (Remond et al 2012).

Interventions for ARF are primarily concerned with providing rest, adequate nutrition and management of cardiac symptoms or chorea. HF management may entail multiple medications, oxygen, fluid restrictions and careful education about home care management. One of the most disturbing manifestations of ARF is chorea. The onset is gradual and may occur weeks to months after the illness. Sometimes mistaken for nervousness, clumsiness or inattentiveness, it is usually a source of great frustration to the child because the movements, incoordination and weakness severely limit physical ability. It is important that parents and teachers are aware of the involuntary, sudden nature of the movements and that the movements are transitory and will eventually disappear. Safety precautions to protect the child from harm or falls are instituted.

Children with RHD will need lifelong follow-up, education and management of HF and monitoring for progressive valve disease. If surgery is required, preparation for the procedure is provided. An important aspect of postoperative care is education about anticoagulation medications and follow-up. (See Quality Patient Outcomes box.)

QUALITY PATIENT OUTCOMES

Acute Rheumatic Fever

- Group A beta-haemolytic streptococcus tonsillopharyngitis identified and treated
- Early recognition and treatment to prevent cardiac valve damage
- Recurrence prevented with prophylaxis compliance

Cultural Considerations:

ARF and RHD has a large burden of disease in the Indigenous people of Australia, People of Pacific nations and the Māori people. It is important that nurses treating these populations do so within a culturally safe environment. The Australian Commission on Safety and Quality in Healthcare have targets specifically improving cultural safety and cultural competence in healthcare agencies. Some recommendations that should be adopted are:

- culture should be the at the centre of all care
- all forms of racism are harmful and not to be tolerated
- cultural awareness alone is not enough to produce change: the journey to cultural safe care includes cultural sensitivity and self-reflection as an important part to providing appropriate care (McKivett et al 2019).

Kawasaki Disease

Kawasaki disease (KD) is an acute systemic vasculitis of unknown cause. The illness is self-limiting and resolves in 6 to 8 weeks. Without treatment, however, approximately 20% to 25% of children develop cardiac sequelae. Damage to the coronary arteries (the blood vessels that supply the heart muscle) is the most common sequelae and involves dilation of the coronary arteries and/or coronary artery aneurysm formation. Infants younger than 1 year of age are at the greatest risk for heart involvement. Children older than 5 years of age are also at increased risk of developing coronary sequelae, perhaps because KD is often not suspected in older children, which may lead to delayed diagnosis and treatment. KD has become a leading cause of acquired heart disease in children in Australia and New Zealand.

The aetiology of KD remains unconfirmed. Although KD is not spread by person-to-person contact, several factors support an infectious cause or trigger. KD is often seen in geographic and seasonal outbreaks, with more cases reported in the late winter and early spring. KD is also a paediatric illness, which suggests the development of passive immunity. Some experts believe that the illness may represent a final common pathway triggered by an infectious agent or more than one potential agent. Genetic studies are ongoing in order to ascertain why some children are more likely to get KD than others (i.e. the possibility that the illness represents a final common pathway in a genetically susceptible host).

Pathophysiology

KD involves widespread inflammation of the small and medium-sized blood vessels with the coronary arteries being the most susceptible to damage. During the acute stage of the illness there is progressive inflammation of the small vessels (capillaries, venules, arterioles) along with pancarditis. This inflammation is reflected in the clinical signs and symptoms and in laboratory test results. Inflammatory markers (CRP level and ESR) are elevated in the acute illness. The vasculitis can progress to the medium-sized muscular arteries, potentially damaging the walls of the vessels and leading to the formation of coronary artery aneurysms in some children. Initial evidence of enlargement of the coronary arteries by echocardiogram can be detected as early as day 7 of illness. Affected vessels can continue to enlarge for several weeks and generally reach their largest diameter approximately 4 to 6 weeks from the onset of fever. Longer duration of fever is associated with the development of aneurysms (Wilder et al 2007). Aneurysms of the peripheral vessels (axillary, brachial, iliac, cervical and renal arteries) can occur, although this is rare and usually is seen only in children who have the large/giant coronary aneurysms. In the acute phase, myocarditis (inflammation of the myocardium) is common. Decreased LV function may be evident on echocardiogram; however, the majority of children do not have clinical signs of HF. Ventricular function usually improves after the administration of IV immune globulin (IVIg). Occasionally, however, a child will present with severe ventricular dysfunction and/or cardiogenic shock. The systemic inflammation gradually subsides and eventually ceases with normalisation of inflammatory markers 6 to 8 weeks from the onset of fever.

Over time, aneurysmal vessels try to heal through multiplication of cells in the vessels in an attempt to restore a 'normal' lumen diameter. This process is called myointimal proliferation. The smaller the initial dilation, the more likely the vessel lumen diameter will regress to a normal size. However, even if the lumen size is restored, the affected vessel may not be completely normal. The walls of these vessels are thicker and may be subject to scarring and calcification (potentially causing stenosis), especially at the distal ends of the aneurysm in patients with large/giant aneurysms.

Almost all of the morbidity and mortality resulting from KD are due to cardiac complications and mainly occur in patients who have giant aneurysms. Coronary thrombosis may result from sluggish blood flow in a dilated or aneurysmal vessel. Over the years, in patients with large aneurysms, stenosis and scarring may lead to impeded blood flow, which can result in myocardial ischaemia or infarction.

Clinical Manifestations

The course of KD can be divided into three phases: acute, subacute and convalescent. The acute phase begins with an abrupt onset of high fever that is unresponsive to antibiotics and antipyretics. Over the first week or so, the diagnostic symptoms become evident. The bulbar conjunctivae of the eyes become reddened, with clearing around the iris (limbal sparing). The eyes are generally dry, without significant drainage. Inflammation of the pharynx and the oral mucosa develops, with red, cracked lips and the characteristic 'strawberry tongue' (i.e. the normal coating of the tongue sloughs off, leaving the large papillae exposed, so the tongue resembles a strawberry). The rash of KD differs from child to child but is never vesicular and is most often accentuated in the perineum. Often the groin area may desquamate early in the illness. The child's hands and feet become oedematous, and the palms and soles become erythematous. The child may have cervical lymphadenopathy (usually unilateral ≤ 1.5 cm). The node is not usually very tender or red. To meet 'classic' criteria, children have prolonged fever (≤ 4 days) along with four out of five of the diagnostic criteria. During the acute stage, the child is typically very irritable and inconsolable. This behaviour may continue for several weeks and is often one of the last features to improve. Approximately one-third of patients develop a temporary arthritis beginning in the small joints. Cardiac manifestations during this period may include myocarditis, decreased LV function, pericardial effusion and mitral regurgitation. Generally, these findings are subclinical, but occasionally children with poor ventricular function present with symptoms of cardiogenic shock. On physical examination, the child may be tachycardic with a gallop rhythm. The coronary arteries may begin to show enlargement during this phase.

The subacute phase begins with resolution of the fever and lasts until all outward clinical signs of KD have disappeared. If changes in the coronary arteries occur, enlargement or dilation is generally evident by echocardiography during the second week of illness. Damaged vessels can continue to enlarge and reach their maximum diameter approximately 4 to 6 weeks from the onset of illness. Thrombocytosis and hypercoagulability in a child with expanding aneurysms and disrupted blood flow place him or her at risk for coronary thrombosis. During the subacute period, the child may develop periungual desquamation (peeling that begins under the fingertips and toes) of the hands and feet. A temporary arthritis may be evident during this phase and can affect the larger weight-bearing joints. Irritability persists during this period.

In the convalescent phase, the clinical signs of KD have mostly resolved, but the laboratory values may still be abnormal. Arthritis may continue into this stage. Coronary dimensions peak approximately 4 to 6 weeks from the onset of illness. The convalescent phase is complete when all laboratory values return to normal (6 to 8 weeks after onset). At the end of this stage, most parents report that the child appears to have returned to baseline in terms of temperament, energy and appetite.

Cardiac Involvement. The most serious complication of KD is the development of coronary artery aneurysms and the potential for myocardial infarction in children who have developed aneurysm formation. Any vessel that has a z-score ≥ 2.5 (standard deviations above the mean) is considered to be outside the normal range. A small aneurysm is defined as having a z-score of 2.5 to 5.0 and a medium aneurysm is defined as having a z-score of ≥ 5 to < 10, and an absolute dimension < 8 mm. Although giant aneurysms have traditionally been defined as those measuring greater than 8 mm in diameter, recent data suggest that coronary dimensions should be standardised for body mass index (BMI) using z-scores (standard deviations above/below mean). The rationale for this relates to the theory that an 8-mm vessel in a 4 month old is relatively larger than an 8-mm vessel in a 12 year old. As would be expected, blood flow is extremely abnormal in large/giant aneurysms, placing these patients at highest risk for thrombus formation. Myocardial ischaemia can result from thrombotic occlusion or stenotic occlusion of a coronary aneurysm. Symptoms of acute myocardial infarction in young children can be subtle and may include abdominal pain, vomiting, restlessness, inconsolable crying, pallor and shock. Complaints of actual chest pain or pressure are more typical in older children (Kato et al 1986).

Diagnostic Evaluation. Currently no specific diagnostic test exists for KD. Therefore, the diagnosis is established on the basis of clinical findings and associated laboratory results that support the diagnosis. The clinical criteria in Box 27.7 should be used as guidelines. Many children with KD do not meet standard diagnostic criteria, and infants often have an incomplete presentation. It is therefore important to consider KD as a possible diagnosis in any infant or child with prolonged elevated temperature that is unresponsive to antibiotics and is not attributable to another cause.

BOX 27.7 Clinical Criteria for Diagnosis of Kawasaki Disease

- Fever for at least 5 days
- Presence of at least four of the five following symptoms:
  - Changes in extremities
  - *Acute*—Erythema of palms and soles, oedema of hands and feet
  - *Subacute*—Periungual peeling of fingers and toes in second and third week
  - Polymorphous exanthem
  - Bilateral bulbar conjunctival injection without exudate
  - Erythema and cracking of lips, strawberry tongue and/or erythema of oral and pharyngeal mucosae
  - Cervical lymphadenopathy (node > 1.5 cm in diameter), usually unilateral
- Patients with fever for at least 5 days and fewer than four symptoms described above can be diagnosed as having Kawasaki disease when coronary artery abnormalities are detected by two-dimensional echocardiography or angiography. When four or more principal features are present, the diagnosis of Kawasaki disease can be made on day 4 of illness. In very rare occurrences, with an experienced clinician, diagnoses can be made on day 3.

Note: These criteria should be used as a guideline; however, not all of the symptoms need to be present at once. In addition, atypical or incomplete Kawasaki disease should be considered in patients with some features, prolonged fever and no alternative diagnosis.

Associated laboratory findings, when combined with clinical data, can be helpful in making the diagnosis of KD. The typical child with KD is somewhat anaemic and has a leucocytosis with a 'shift to the left' (increased immature white blood cells) during the acute phase. Thrombocytosis with hypercoagulability becomes evident in the subacute phase with peak platelet counts occurring approximately 3 weeks after the onset of fever. An elevated ESR and CRP level reflect ongoing inflammation and can persist for 6 to 8 weeks. The ESR can be further elevated by the administration of IVIg; therefore, it is better to measure the CRP level as an indicator of inflammation after IVIg administration. Microscopic urinalysis reveals a sterile pyuria with mononuclear cells that will not be evident with a regular dipstick test because the white blood cells are not polymorphonuclear neutrophils. Transient elevation of liver enzymes may occur during the acute phase, reflecting inflammation of the liver. Examination of cerebrospinal fluid may show aseptic meningitis (presence of inflammatory cells). Albumin levels may be lower than normal, particularly in the sickest children (Newburger et al 2016). Some children experience a temporary arthritis during the illness that resolves over time. Both small and large joints may be affected in the short term. A rare sequela can be sensorineural hearing loss. If decreased hearing is suspected, the child should undergo audiological testing.

Echocardiograms are used to monitor myocardial function and coronary artery dimensions. A baseline echocardiogram is obtained at the time of diagnosis to evaluate coronary size and ventricular and valvar function. Common findings on echocardiogram during the acute phase may include pericardial effusions, mitral regurgitation and decreased ventricular function. Follow-up echocardiograms should be performed within 1 to 2 weeks after diagnosis and again 4 to 6 weeks after treatment. More frequent echocardiograms to assess coronary dimensions are indicated in patients who have continued fever, those who require retreatment with IVIg and those with coronary dilation on baseline or other studies. In these patients, echocardiograms may be performed twice a week until coronary dimensions stabilise.

Therapeutic Management

The standard treatment of KD includes high-dose IVIg along with salicylate therapy. High-dose IVIg has been shown to reduce the duration of fever and the incidence of coronary artery abnormalities when given within the first 10 days of illness and optimally within the first 7 days. A single large infusion of 2 g/kg over 8 to 12 hours is recommended (McCrindle et al 2017). Approximately 10% to 20% of children continue to have fever after the initial treatment with IVIg and may be candidates for retreatment or adjunctive therapies (Tremoulet et al 2008). In addition, patients with coronary dilation or aneurysm formation are candidates for additional treatment focused on decreasing inflammation. Retreatment with a second dose of IVIg is often given for patients with persistent or recrudescent fever without other cause 36 hours after the completion of the initial dose of IVIg. Additional therapies such as steroids and infliximab (Remicade) have also been used after IVIg failure. The use of other agents such as cyclosporine or cyclophosphamide and other anti-inflammatory drugs may be considered in the sickest patients with developing aneurysms (McCrindle et al 2017). However, the best therapy for this group of high-risk patients is still unknown and warrants continued research.

Aspirin is given initially in an anti-inflammatory/antipyretic dosage (ranging from moderate to high dose, 30 to 50 mg/kg/day or 80 to 100 mg/kg/day) divided every 6 hours to control fever and symptoms of inflammation. Practice as to dose preference varies between institutions. It is important to note that the administration of moderate- or high-dose aspirin has not been shown to make a difference in the incidence of coronary artery sequelae. Once fever has subsided, the aspirin dosage is decreased to an antiplatelet dosage (3 to 5 mg/kg/day). Low-dose aspirin therapy is continued in patients without echocardiographic evidence of coronary abnormalities until the platelet count has returned to normal (4 to 6 weeks). If the child develops coronary abnormalities, low-dose (antiplatelet) salicylate therapy is continued. Additional anticoagulation therapy, such as warfarin administration, is indicated in children with medium or large/giant coronary enlargement, respectively.

Prognosis. The vast majority of children with KD recover fully after treatment without cardiovascular sequelae. When cardiovascular complications occur, however, serious morbidity may result. Death occurs very rarely (< 0.1% to 0.2%) and is almost always a result of ischaemia caused by coronary thrombosis or stenosis. The long-term prognosis for a particular child depends on whether or not a child develops coronary enlargement and, if so, the extent of the coronary damage (i.e. how large the enlargement is). Children with coronary abnormalities are followed closely. Long-term testing may include periodic ECGs, echocardiography, stress testing (stress echoes and/or myocardial perfusion scans) at rest and during exercise, and cardiac computed tomography angiogram (CTA) and/or MRI. The frequency and type of testing depends on individual risk, as well the availability of various testing modalities at the individual centres (Baker & Newburger 2008, Newburger et al 2004). Although echocardiography is sensitive in visualising coronary dilation in the proximal coronaries, it does not detect stenoses of the coronary arteries. Cardiac catheterisation or cardiac CTA may be performed to obtain a more complete picture of the full coronary system in children who still have significant abnormalities 6 months to 1 year after illness onset. In addition, these tests may be indicated in situations in which stenosis or thrombosis and/or myocardial ischaemia is suspected from the results of non-invasive testing. Both of these modalities can visualise the proximal and distal vessels, and decisions as to the best imaging technique are made on an individual basis.

Children without coronary artery aneurysms have now been followed for more than 40 years in Japan and the United States and do not show an increased incidence of accelerated atherosclerosis or premature heart disease. Recent studies have suggested that peripheral vessels are not stiffer in patients who have had KD without aneurysms and those children have an excellent long-term prognosis (McCrindle et al 2017). Nonetheless, it is recommended that children who have had KD have as few other risk factors for coronary disease as possible. Cholesterol levels and BP should be monitored as per the general population guidelines, and children should be encouraged to lead a heart-healthy lifestyle in terms of diet, exercise and avoidance of smoking. Children without coronary enlargement may be discharged from cardiology follow-up between 1 month and 1 year after initial onset, depending on practice variations (McCrindle et al 2017).

Nursing Care Management

The nursing care of children with KD can be challenging. Inpatient care focuses on symptomatic relief, emotional support, diagnostic assistance, medication administration and education of the child and family. (See Quality Patient Outcomes box.)

QUALITY PATIENT OUTCOMES

Kawasaki Disease

- Early diagnosis and treatment
- Prevention of cardiovascular complications

In the initial phase of illness, the nurse must monitor the child's cardiac status carefully. Intake and output and daily weight measurements are recorded. The child may be reluctant to eat and may be partially dehydrated. IV fluids need to be administered with care because of the usual finding of myocarditis. The child should be assessed frequently for signs of HF, including decreased urinary output, gallop rhythm, tachycardia and respiratory distress. Close cardiac monitoring is indicated during the infusion of IVIg (because of the large fluid load), particularly in children younger than 1 year of age, and in any child with cardiac symptoms. Sedation is generally required before echocardiography in children younger than 2½ to 3 years of age because the child must remain still in order to obtain adequate visualisation of the coronary arteries, cardiac structures and function.

Nursing care for patients with KD is focused primarily on symptomatic relief. To minimise skin discomfort, application of cool cloths and unscented lotions and use of soft, loose clothing are helpful. During the acute phase, mouth care, including application of lubricating ointment to the lips, is important for the mucosal inflammation. The nurse should offer clear liquids and soft foods and monitor temperature carefully. It is important to document temperature just before aspirin administration because fever reflects ongoing inflammation and may indicate the need for further treatment. If the temperature is very high, paracetamol may be given in addition to high-dose aspirin. If arthritis develops, passive range-of-motion exercises may help maintain mobility and can be done most easily during the child's bath.

The administration of IVIg should follow the same guidelines as for administration of any blood product, with frequent monitoring of vital signs. Patients must be watched for allergic reactions and are often premedicated with an antihistamine. The nurse must monitor cardiac status because of the large fluid volume being administered to patients who may have subclinical myocarditis or diminished LV function. Check patency of the IV line because extravasation can result in tissue damage. Hypercoagulability and venous fragility often make it difficult to maintain IV access in children with KD.

Patient irritability is perhaps the most challenging problem for parents of children with KD. These children need to be placed in a quiet environment that promotes adequate rest. Their parents need to be supported in their efforts to comfort an often inconsolable child. They may need time away from their child, and nurses can often provide respite care for the family. Parents need to understand that irritability is a hallmark of KD and that they need not feel guilty or embarrassed about their child's behaviour.

Discharge Teaching. Parents need accurate information about the usual course of KD, including the importance of follow-up monitoring and the circumstances under which they should contact their practitioner. Irritability is likely to persist for up to 2 months after the onset of symptoms. Peeling of the hands and feet is painless and occurs primarily in the second and third weeks. Arthritis, especially of the larger weight-bearing joints, may persist for several weeks. Affected children are typically most stiff in the mornings, during cold weather and after naps. Passive range-of-motion exercises while having a bath are often helpful in increasing flexibility. Although the arthritis in KD is always temporary, it can be severe and may interfere with walking. (Note: Other high-dose NSAIDs should not be given with high-dose salicylates, and the use of NSAIDs may interfere with the antiplatelet effects of low-dose aspirin.)

Most importantly, parents should be educated about the potential for recrudescent illness after discharge. Persistent or recrudescent fever 36 hours after IVIg completion should prompt re-evaluation and possible additional treatments. Instruct the parents to take the child's temperature daily after discharge and to contact their clinician if the child has a fever.

Parents should be instructed about the administration of salicylates. It is rare to give high-dose aspirin for a prolonged length of time in this era. However, if the child is receiving high dosages, parents should be aware of the signs of aspirin toxicity: ringing in the ears (tinnitus), headache, dizziness and confusion. The main side effect of low-dose aspirin is easy bruising. In addition, aspirin should be temporarily discontinued and the practitioner notified if the child is exposed to chickenpox or influenza because of the drug's possible association with Reye's syndrome.

All parents should understand the unlikely but real possibility of myocardial infarction and the signs and symptoms of cardiac ischaemia in a child. At the time of hospital discharge, the final cardiac sequelae are often evolving, as changes in the coronary arteries occur over the first 4 to 6 weeks after the onset of KD. Because coronary artery changes take place over the initial 4 to 6 weeks after illness onset, it is important that follow-up planning includes an echocardiogram and cardiology appointment approximately 1 to 2 weeks after hospital discharge and again in 4 to 6 weeks. More frequent echocardiograms are indicated for patients with coronary dilation or aneurysm formation and may include twice-weekly echocardiograms until vessel dimensions stabilise (McCrindle et al 2017). If the child has developed coronary artery aneurysms, parents should be taught cardiopulmonary resuscitation.

Finally, children with coronary abnormalities may require indefinite antiplatelet therapy with low-dose aspirin or other anticoagulants. In such cases children should avoid contact sports and have yearly influenza vaccines. The administration of measles-mumps-rubella vaccine should be delayed for 11 months after the administration of IVIg because the body might not produce the appropriate number of antibodies. In addition, the varicella vaccine should not be given for at least 11 months after IVIg therapy (Kimberlin et al 2015).

Systemic Hypertension

Hypertension is the most common cause of CVA and is a major contributor to atherosclerotic disease in adults. Traditionally, primary hypertension has been considered a disease of older adults. However, in recent years there has been increasing evidence that primary hypertension does occur in children and adolescents, posing long-term health risks. End-organ effects can be seen in young children as a result of chronic hypertension.

The National High Blood Pressure Education Program (NHBPEP) (2004) working group defines the diagnosis of hypertension for children ages 1 to 13 years old as follows.

- *Elevated blood pressure* is defined as a systolic or diastolic BP that falls at or above the 90th percentile for age and height but is under the 95th percentile or 120/80 mmHg to less than the 95th percentile (whichever is lower).
- Stage 1 hypertension is classified as BPs that fall persistently at or above the 95th percentile to less than the 95th percentile + 12 mmHg or 130/80 to 139/89 (whichever is lower).
- Stage 2 hypertension is defined as BPs that are persistently at or above the 95th percentile plus 12 mmHg or ≥ 140/90.

For children ≥ 13 years old, the following definitions are currently used:

- Elevated BP is defined simply as 120 to 129/< 80 mmHg.
- Stage 1 hypertension is defined as 130 to 139/80 to 89 mmHg.
- Stage 2 hypertension is defined as ≥ 140/90 mmHg.

White-coat hypertension is diagnosed when the patient's BP is higher than the 95th percentile in the clinician's office but falls under the 95th percentile outside of this setting.

Aetiology

Hypertension in young children, compared with older adolescents and adults, was thought to occur more commonly secondary to a structural abnormality or an underlying pathological process. However, the results of screening programs of relatively healthy children have challenged this view. When secondary hypertension is diagnosed, the most common causes in young children is renal disease, followed by cardiovascular, endocrine or some neurological disorders. In older children/adolescents, stress/anxiety and/or effects from pharmacological agents may play a role (Mattoo 2017). As a rule, the younger the child and the more severe the hypertension, the more likely it is to be due to a secondary cause. The conditions associated with secondary hypertension in children and adolescents are listed in Box 27.8.

The causes of primary or idiopathic hypertension are undetermined. There is evidence that both genetic and environmental factors play a role. The incidence of hypertension is greater in children with a family history of hypertension. Indigenous children in Australia and Māori children in New Zealand have a higher incidence of hypertension than children of different ethnicities. The New Zealand Health survey 2016–17 found that 50% of Māori adults were obese and childhood obesity of 2 to 14 year olds was at 33% (Ministry of Health 2017). Obesity greatly increases risk of developing childhood hypertension.

Environmental factors that contribute to the risk of developing hypertension may include obesity, salt ingestion, smoking, lead exposure, medications, rural isolation and socioeconomic disadvantage.

Clinical Manifestations

Clinical manifestations associated with hypertension depend largely on the underlying cause and the degree of hypertension. Adolescents and older children with significant hypertension may complain of frequent headaches, dizziness or changes in vision. In infants or young children who cannot communicate symptoms, observation of behaviour may provide clues, although gross behavioural changes may not be apparent until complications are present. Parents of infants and small children who have been treated for hypertension report that their child had previously been irritable and often indulged in an abnormal degree of head banging or rubbing.

BOX 27.8 Conditions Associated with Secondary Hypertension in Children

Renal Disorders

- Congenital defects
  - Polycystic kidney, ectopic kidney, horseshoe kidney
  - Obstructive anomalies
  - Hydronephrosis
- Renal tumour
  - Wilms tumour
  - Renovascular tumour
- Abnormalities of renal arteries
- Renal vein thrombosis
- Acquired disorders
  - Glomerulonephritis—acute or chronic
  - Pyelonephritis
  - Nephritis associated with collagen disease

Cardiovascular Disease

- Coarctation of aorta
- Arteriovenous fistula
- Aortic or mitral insufficiency

Metabolic and Endocrine Diseases

- Adrenal tumours
  - Adenoma
  - Phaeochromocytoma
  - Neuroblastoma
- Cushing's syndrome
- Adrenogenital syndrome
- Hyperthyroidism
- Aldosteronism
- Hypercalcaemia
- Diabetes mellitus

Neurological Disorders

- Space-occupying lesions of the cranium (increased intracranial pressure)
  - Tumours, cysts, haematoma
  - Cerebral oedema
  - Encephalitis (including Guillain-Barré and Reye's syndromes)

Miscellaneous Causes

- Drugs (corticosteroids, oral contraceptives, pressor agents, stimulant drugs, amphetamines)
- Burns
- Genitourinary surgery
- Trauma (e.g. stretching of femoral nerve with leg traction)
- Insect bites (e.g. scorpion)
- Intravascular overload (blood, fluid)
- Hypernatraemia
- Toxaemia of pregnancy
- Heavy metal poisoning
- Liquorice

Source: Mattoo, T. K. (2017). Evaluation of hypertension in children and adolescents. UpToDate. https://www.uptodate.com/contents/evaluation-of-hypertension-in-children-and-adolescents.

Diagnostic Evaluation

It is clear from the increasing numbers of cases of hypertension and prehypertension being identified in children and adolescents that a BP determination should be a routine part of annual assessment. Current guidelines recommend BP ascertainment in all children older than 3 years of age and earlier in children with individual risk factors or health conditions. Measure BP in children of any age if they are diagnosed as having or are suspected of having coarctation of the aorta, unexplained HF, unexplained heart murmurs, prematurity, unexplained seizures or other neurological signs, an abdominal mass or masses, oedema, ascites, evidence of renal failure, hypernatraemia, faltering growth, possible obstructive sleep apnoea, respiratory distress, hyperlipidaemia or unexplained headaches. Because hypertension is strongly associated with obesity, a BMI should be calculated for each child at the routine physical examination.

Before initiating a workup for hypertension, BP should be measured several times in the sitting position. If BP readings are in the elevated range, they should be repeated at three separate times. Automated BPs should be taken several times, the first one discarded and the next three averaged. Ideally, elevated automated BP readings should be repeated by auscultation. *Note:* BP norms are based on auscultated pressures. To obtain an accurate reading, take care to quiet the child or relax the adolescent while the measurement is recorded to avoid false readings. The chief cause of falsely elevated BP readings is the use of improperly fitting, narrow cuffs. Therefore, attention to correct measurement technique is essential. (See Blood Pressure, Chapter 4.) Note that a child who is large for his or her age may normally have a higher BP than a child who is of average size. Upper and lower extremity BP in the supine position should always be assessed when hypertension is suspected, along with the presence of femoral pulses because of the possibility of secondary hypertensions from undiagnosed coarctation of the aorta. Twenty-four-hour BP (ambulatory BP [AMBP]) monitoring devices detect changes in pressure throughout the day and night, and thus may give a more realistic picture. These devices are especially helpful in diagnosing white-coat hypertension and can be used with older children or adolescents, who are able to tolerate being attached to an ambulatory monitor (Flynn et al 2014). To be the least intrusive, it is recommended that the 24-hour BP monitor be worn on the non-dominant arm. The child or parent should keep a log during AMBP monitoring to document level of activity or, at a minimum, sleeping and waking times. AMBP monitors should document readings at least hourly and ideally more often (every 20 minutes).

Evaluation of the child with high BP includes a thorough assessment of lifestyle and additional risk factors, detection of potential secondary causes and documentation of the presence or absence of end-organ effects. For children whose BP falls in the elevated range, weight management and lifestyle modifications (e.g. regular moderate to vigorous exercise, DASH diet [see later discussion], stress reduction, adequate sleep and avoidance of smoking) should be reviewed and BPs should be repeated in 6 months. Upper and lower BPs (right arm, left arm and one leg) should be measured if a patient continues to have elevated BPs at the 6-month check with reinforcement of lifestyle counselling. If auscultated BP is still elevated at three separate visits in 12 months, an AMBP should be obtained (if child old enough to cooperate) and further testing should be done. The workup occurs more quickly in patients with stage 1 or 2 hypertension. Lifestyle modification is recommended for all. In addition, in patients with stage 1 hypertension, BP is rechecked by auscultation in 1 to 2 weeks (with upper and lower BPs) and again at 3 months. If still elevated, AMBP is obtained and further diagnostic workup is indicated with possible specialty referral and initiation of treatment. For stage 2 hypertension, upper and lower BP should be checked immediately, with repeat BP measurements within 1 week or referral to a specialist promptly (within 1 week). If still high, AMBP and diagnostic evaluation should begin and treatment initiated. In severe cases of very high BP the patient should be referred to an emergency department for immediate

TABLE 27.4 Childhood Hypertension Evaluation

Diagnostic Procedures or Tests	Rationale	Indications
Thorough history, including the following: • detailed past medical history • family history • lifestyle factors: diet, exercise, smoking, alcohol, drugs • assess sleep habits	Help focus further evaluation	All patients with elevated BP or higher
Laboratory evaluation: • electrolytes, blood urea nitrogen, creatinine, urinalysis, fasting lipid panel	Identify concerns for secondary causes	Children with the following: • persistent elevated BP after 1 year • stage 1 hypertension over 3 visits in 3 months • stage 2 hypertension for 2 visits in 1 week or sooner depending on severity
HbA_{1C} AST, ALT	Screening for diabetes, fatty liver	Obese children/adolescents with persistently elevated or stage 1 or 2 BP (in addition to above laboratory evaluation)
Renal ultrasonography	Assess renal size, Doppler gradient, congenital anomaly	Children $\leq$ 6 years old Children > 8 years old if suspected of having renovascular hypertension
Full blood count	Identify anaemia, chronic renal disease	Patients with abnormal renal function
Polysomnography	Identify sleep disorder associated with hypertension	Children with history of loud, frequent snoring
Drug screen	Identify substances that cause hypertension	Children with history suggestive of possible contribution by substances or drugs
Echocardiography	Identify left ventricular hypertrophy, LV geometry, rule out coarctation	Assess before considering medication; if normal, reassess yearly in patients with stage 2 hypertension or incompletely treated stage 1; in abnormal, reassess every 6–12 months; obtain in all patients with BP gradient (upper to lower)
ADDITIONAL EVALUATION AS INDICATED		
Magnetic resonance angiography or computed tomography Arteriography	Identify renovascular disease	Patients suspected of having renal artery stenosis
Ambulatory BP monitoring	Identify white-coat hypertension, abnormal diurnal BP pattern, BP load	Children > 5 years old in whom white-coat hypertension is suspected and those for whom other information on BP pattern is needed after elevated BP for $\geq$ 1 year or stage 1 after 3 clinic visits; in addition, obtain for surveillance on patients with high-risk conditions such as repaired coarctation
Plasma and urine catecholamine levels	Identify catecholamine-mediated hypertension	If concern for catecholamine excess based on family history, patient history or physical examination (flushing, palpitations, headache, sweating), abdominal mass
Plasma and urine steroid levels	Identify steroid-mediated hypertension	If concern for congenital adrenal hyperplasia
Plasma renin level Plasma aldosterone	Identify low renin level or elevated aldosterone	If concern for mineralocorticoid-related disease

ALT, Alanine aminotransferase; *AST,* aspartate aminotransferase; *BP,* blood pressure; *HbA_{1C},* haemoglobin A_{1C}; *LV,* left ventricle.
Source: Modified from Flynn, J. T., Kaelber, D. C., Baker-Smith, C. M., et al & Subcommittee on Screening and Management of High Blood Pressure in Children. (2017). Clinical practice guideline for screening and management of high blood pressure in children and adolescents. Pediatrics, 140(3), e20171904.

evaluation. Table 27.4 outlines the recommended work-up for patients with persistent elevated BP or stage 1 or 2 hypertension (Flynn et al 2017).

The nurse should take a careful medical history of the child or adolescent, including perinatal and all past medical history and current medications, drug use (particularly stimulant drugs) or smoking. In addition, the nurse should obtain a thorough family history to screen for other relatives with hypertension or other cardiovascular risk factors, including age of onset in first- or second-degree relatives. Psychosocial history including stressors should be documented, as well as lifestyle habits (diet, physical activity, sleep habits, smoking, alcohol, drugs).

Therapeutic Management

Therapy for secondary hypertension involves diagnosis and treatment of the underlying cause. In those cases amenable to surgical repair, the nature of the condition, the type of surgery and the child's age are all important considerations. Children or adolescents with consistently elevated BP readings from no known cause (primary or idiopathic hypertension) or those with secondary hypertension not amenable to surgical correction may be treated with a combination of non-pharmacological and pharmacological interventions.

Dietary practices and lifestyle changes are important in the control of hypertension for both children and adults and should be instituted first, except in severe cases. In salt-sensitive children, high salt intake increases the risk of hypertension for those genetically predisposed and aggravates existing hypertension unless salt intake is limited. The DASH diet provides a lower-salt diet that has been associated with improvement in BP and is thought to be beneficial for all patients with hypertension. *DASH* stands for *D*ietary *A*pproaches to *S*top *H*ypertension. The DASH diet consists of vegetables, fruits, whole grains and low-fat dairy products, and it is low in sugar and salt.

Because obesity and hypertension are closely related, a weight-reduction program is recommended for overweight youngsters. Regular aerobic exercise augments weight reduction and improves BP measurements. Ideally, children should be counselled to obtain 3 to 5 days of moderate or vigorous exercise (30 to 60 minutes each time). The exercise regimen is most effective if it can be individualised to the child's interest. It is helpful to quantify how much time is spent in sedentary activities (e.g. overall screen time) compared with how much time daily is spent in aerobic activities. Regular sleep habits are important. In addition, stress reduction strategies may be beneficial and may include biofeedback, yoga and relaxation. Smoking should be avoided.

Drug therapy is initiated with caution in children. Because the long-term effects of antihypertensive agents on children are not known, drug treatment of asymptomatic children with mild or borderline hypertension is not recommended. However, antihypertensive drug therapy is indicated for treating those patients who have significant elevations of BP despite non-pharmacological intervention. This includes children and adolescents with persistent hypertension (stage 1 or higher), symptomatic hypertension, secondary hypertension, end-organ evidence of hypertension (e.g. increased LV mass) and/or significant additional risk factors, such as diabetes.

Pharmacological intervention needs to be tailored to meet the needs of the individual child and is determined by the hypotensive effect produced and the appearance of any side effects. For example, ACE inhibitors and angiotensin receptor blockers have been effective in children with diabetes or certain renal diagnoses, whereas beta blockers and calcium channel blockers are often used by children with a history of migraine headaches. The goal of treatment is to use the lowest dose of medication to achieve a normotensive state throughout the day without accompanying side effects. For many antihypertensive drugs, minimal data are available regarding side effects in children. Therefore, the nurse should consider any behavioural or physical changes that occur after institution of therapy as possible side effects and should revise therapy as needed.

Nursing Care Management

The nurse is a valuable link in the delivery of healthcare for hypertension in the paediatric age group. Active in detection, diagnosis and therapy in any setting—hospital, school, clinic, private office, public health service and private practice—nurses are frequently the primary contact in well-child care and follow-up clinics. They are often the liaison between the family and the healthcare services. (See Quality Patient Outcomes box.)

QUALITY PATIENT OUTCOMES

Hypertension

- Underlying cause of hypertension identified
- Blood pressure control maintained
- Dietary practices (DASH diet) and lifestyle changes (regular exercise, no smoking, optimise BMI) effectively used to control hypertension
- Compliance with medication regimen, if prescribed

DASH, Dietary approaches to stop hypertension.

Nursing counselling and guidance of affected children can be challenging. Education aimed at understanding hypertension and its implications over the life span is essential in promoting patient and family compliance with both non-pharmacological and pharmacological therapies. (See Compliance, Chapter 22.)

Home BP and 24-hour ambulatory BP measurement can facilitate surveillance in children with chronic hypertension and can also provide documentation of the effectiveness of therapy. A family member can be instructed in how to take and record accurate BP measurements, which can decrease the number of trips to a healthcare facility. Parameters should be reviewed and should include instructions on when to contact the practitioner regarding elevated values. When this option is not feasible, the school nurse can often be a valuable resource in monitoring BP.

The nurse plays an important role in assessing individual families and providing targeted information regarding non-pharmacological modes of intervention, such as reviewing the DASH diet, weight loss, smoking cessation and exercise programs. If extensive dietary counselling is required, the child should be referred to a registered dietitian with expertise in working with children and adolescents. Exercise regimens should be individualised. Children and young adolescents generally prefer team sports rather than individual training, which they may view as a burden rather than an enjoyable activity. If peers and family members can participate in any of the management strategies, the child is more likely to comply with the plan. In recent years, many health-related exercise applications (apps) have become available for computers, phones and handheld devices. These apps may be of interest for children/adolescents who prefer to exercise at home and/or use technology. It also gives the child/adolescent some autonomy in deciding what type of activity to do.

If drug therapy is prescribed, the nurse needs to provide information to the family regarding the reasons for drug therapy, how the drug works, frequency of BP monitoring and possible side effects of the medication. Explain that the drug needs to be taken consistently to achieve any prolonged control of BP. Stress the need for close follow-up, especially because antihypertensive therapy can sometimes be safely decreased or discontinued if BP remains under control over time.

Learning needs vary greatly depending on developmental levels and individual differences. Some children and families require a great deal of support, education and guidance, whereas others need only education and periodic follow-up. A positive approach is essential; negative feedback will only alienate the family. Exploring the reasons for difficulty in compliance can often provide realistic alternatives. Continued education, support and reinforcement for positive behaviour are major nursing responsibilities.

Dyslipidaemia (Abnormal Lipid Metabolism)

Hyperlipidaemia is a general term for excessive lipids (fat and fatlike substances). *Dyslipidaemia* refers to all disorders of lipid metabolism resulting in abnormalities in the lipid profile that can include elevated total cholesterol, low-density lipoprotein (LDL) cholesterol or triglycerides, and/or low levels of high-density lipoprotein (HDL) cholesterol. Dyslipidaemia plays an important role in producing atherosclerosis (build-up of fatty plaques in the arteries), which eventually can lead to coronary artery disease (CAD), the leading cause of morbidity and mortality in the adult population in Australia and New Zealand. The risk of premature CAD has been shown to increase with elevated plasma concentrations of total cholesterol and LDL cholesterol and with low levels of HDL cholesterol. Elevated non-HDL cholesterol (LDL + very-low-density lipoprotein [VLDL]) is also associated with an increased incidence of atherosclerosis. In adults, interventions that decrease LDL levels and increase HDL levels have been shown to lower the risk for CAD. In addition to abnormal cholesterol levels, known risk factors correlating with the development CAD include the following:

- positive family history of elevated cholesterol and/or early heart disease
- cigarette smoking
- obesity
- sedentary lifestyle
- nutritional factors
- older age
- male gender
- hypertension
- type 1 or type 2 diabetes.

In addition to these risk factors, the American Heart Association has categorised patients with certain comorbid conditions as higher risk. These include the following (Kavey et al 2006):

- chronic inflammatory diseases
- cancer survivors
- transplant patients
- CHD
- coronary artery aneurysms from KD.

Higher levels of total cholesterol, LDL cholesterol and non-HDL cholesterol and low levels of HDL cholesterol are associated with more severe atherosclerosis. Lipid values show trends from childhood to adulthood, particularly in children with the most severely abnormal lipid values (Zachariah & de Ferranti 2013). These children with elevated lipids are more likely to become adults with elevated lipids. In addition, recent studies support a relationship between the presence of risk factors in young people and subclinical markers of atherosclerosis (Kusters et al 2014), supporting the rationale for universal screening and management of lipid levels and cardiovascular risk factors (National Heart, Lung, and Blood Institute 2011). The benefits of statin therapy are well documented in the adult population in the reduction of CAD. The goal of lipid screening is to identify children and adolescents with familial hyperlipidaemia (FH) and/or other types of dyslipidaemias early in life so that treatment can begin in those patients at increased risk.

FH is a genetic defect that causes significant elevation of LDL cholesterol and is associated in an increased risk of premature CAD. Homozygous FH is very rare (1 in 1 million) and is known to cause CAD during childhood. This condition is usually diagnosed in the first year or two of life by the appearance of xanthomas on the skin. Treatment options are limited as these patients do not have the LDL receptors necessary to respond to statin therapy. Patients with this rare condition may require more invasive treatments, such as plasmapheresis, to control LDL levels. New medications are being trialled in this population. In contrast to homozygous FH, the incidence of heterozygous FH is much more common (with a reported incidence of 1 in 200 to 500 people). Untreated heterozygous FH results in elevated LDL cholesterol (> 160 to 190 mg/dL) and is associated with a significant increase in early coronary disease in young to middle adult years, supporting the recommendation for early screening and interventions aimed at lowering LDL cholesterol (Watts et al 2014).

Lifestyle modification comprises the first-line of treatment for the vast majority of patients with dyslipidaemia. In addition to lifestyle, patients with heterozygous FH generally require lipid-lowering medications (statin therapy) to attain adequate LDL reduction.

Box 27.9 provides the definitions of cholesterol.

> **BOX 27.9 What is Cholesterol?**
>
> Cholesterol, a fatlike steroid alcohol, is part of the lipoprotein complex in plasma that is essential for cellular metabolism. Triglycerides, natural fats synthesised from carbohydrates, are used for energy. Both are major lipids transported on lipoproteins, a combination of lipids and proteins, which include the following.
>
> - **Chylomicrons**—Produced in the intestine in response to the intake of dietary fat. These are the principal transporters of dietary fat (triglycerides) from the intestine to the blood and ultimately to the fatty tissue. Chylomicrons are usually not present in the blood after a 12- to 14-hour fast.
> - **Very-low-density lipoproteins (VLDLs)**—Contain high concentrations of triglycerides, moderate concentrations of cholesterol and little protein.
> - **Low-density lipoproteins (LDLs)**—Contain low concentrations of triglycerides, high levels of cholesterol and moderate levels of protein. The end product of VLDL synthesis, LDLs are the major carriers of cholesterol to the cells. Cells use cholesterol for synthesis of membranes and steroid production. Elevated levels of circulating LDL are a strong risk factor for cardiovascular disease.
> - **High-density lipoproteins (HDLs)**—Contain very low concentrations of triglycerides, relatively little cholesterol and high levels of protein. HDLs transport free cholesterol to the liver for secretion in the bile. High levels of HDL are thought to protect against cardiovascular disease, whereas low levels of HDLs are considered an independent risk factor.
>
> The cholesterol profile includes the following:
>
> $$\text{total cholesterol} = \text{LDL} + \text{HDL} + \text{VLDL}$$
>
> Levels of total cholesterol, triglycerides and HDL cholesterol are measured directly via a blood test. In the fasting state, LDL concentration is calculated using the following formula:
>
> $$\text{LDL} = \text{total cholesterol} - (\text{HDL} + [\text{triglycerides}/5])$$
>
> A calculated LDL is considered accurate as long as the fasting triglyceride level is below 350 to 400 mg/dL. If triglycerides are higher than this, LDL cholesterol can be measured directly using a more specialised test.

Diagnostic Evaluation/Screening

The diagnosis of dyslipidaemia is based on analysis of blood. A blood specimen for determination of a full lipid profile should ideally be drawn after a 12-hour fast. However, a non-HDL cholesterol value (total cholesterol minus HDL cholesterol) can be obtained in the non-fasting state. It is important to note that lipid values can be affected by significant febrile illnesses, and therefore lipids should not be measured within 3 weeks of a febrile illness. Average lipid values vary by age and gender, with HDL values decreasing in males as they go through puberty. Total cholesterol and LDL cholesterol may also decrease during puberty. Children/adolescents are considered to have elevated cholesterol if their total cholesterol value is over 200 mg/dL and/or their LDL cholesterol value is over 130 mg/dL or if their non-HDL cholesterol is over 145 mg/dL. Higher HDL values are desirable. HDL values below 40 mg/dL are considered to be low with an average HDL being approximately 55 mg/dL. Triglycerides should be less than 100 mg/dL in young children (under 10) and less than 130 mg/dL in older children and adolescents. It is common to see elevated triglycerides in the setting of elevated BMI. Triglyceride values respond well to dietary modifications, particularly a low-glycaemic diet.

In Australia and New Zealand, universal screening is not routine practice. Screening is currently recommended for cholesterol abnormalities in older children (10 to 12 years) with a positive family history of dyslipidaemia, premature CAD or other risk factors such as obesity, kidney disease or congenital heart disease (Ayer & Sholler 2012).

Therapeutic Management

Regardless of the cause of high cholesterol (genetic or lifestyle factors, or a combination), the treatment of high cholesterol levels in paediatrics begins with lifestyle modification. Lifestyle habits, including diet, exercise patterns and smoking—all known to be risk factors for cardiovascular disease—are normally established at a young age. The Ministry of Health in New Zealand and the Australian dietary guidelines recommend a heart-healthy diet for all children, with dietary counselling recommended for those children with known elevated cholesterol values (Innes-Hughes et al 2012). Dietary management is tailored to the individual patient, depending on his or her specific dyslipidaemia. A heart-healthy diet focuses on a balanced intake of nutrients for children over 2 years of age, favouring low-fat dairy products, avoiding trans fats, decreasing saturated fats and reducing sweetened beverages and simple sugars. The recommended diet for all children and adolescents is one that is rich in fruits and vegetables and whole grains.

For families to understand the recommendations for lifestyle modification, it is important to schedule enough time in the visit to provide accurate dietary information to families, as food labelling can be confusing. Without counselling, patients tend to replace foods high in fat with foods low in fat but high in simple sugars, which can raise triglyceride values, decrease the effectiveness of nutritional interventions and provide wasted calories.

Current research favours a 'Mediterranean'-type diet. Whole grains, fruits and vegetables form the foundation of this diet. In addition, this diet favours the use of monounsaturated fats, such as nuts, fish, avocadoes, olive oil and canola oil, which have beneficial effects on HDL cholesterol values.

For patients with elevated LDL cholesterol, total fat should be limited to 30% of calories. In addition, children with abnormal LDL cholesterol levels are advised to reduce saturated fat intake to 7% to 10% of calories and dietary cholesterol intake to less than 300 mg/day. Dietary recommendations can be confusing, and individualised guidelines should ideally be provided by a certified dietitian with expertise in lipid management for children and adolescents.

HDL cholesterol responds to an increase in monounsaturated fats such as those mentioned previously. Avoidance of smoking and increased physical exercise also raise HDL values and should be encouraged.

If triglyceride levels are elevated, specific dietary recommendations include a low-glycaemic diet, decreasing the intake of foods high in simple carbohydrates such as white flour, white rice, white bread, white pasta, sugary cereals, juice and soft drink. Weight management should be addressed if the child has an elevated BMI. In addition to food choice, portion size may also be an issue for these children, and the 'plate method' is often recommended (½ fruits and vegetables, ¼ protein and ¼ complex carbohydrates).

Dietary supplements such as plant stanols reduce LDL and may be beneficial in lowering LDL cholesterol. Data are mixed as to the benefit of fibre supplementation. Many clinicians favour obtaining fibre from natural dietary sources—whole grains, fruits and vegetables—rather than from supplements.

Population recommendations intended to decrease cardiovascular risk have been in place for several decades, yet the incidence of childhood obesity in Australia and New Zealand has increased significantly during this time period. Education and programs aimed at decreasing this trend and increasing heart-healthy living (e.g. diet and exercise, avoidance of smoking) are extremely important to decrease cardiovascular risk for the next generation. Assessment of BMI, targeted nutritional and lifestyle education, referral to programs geared to achieving weight loss if indicated and follow-up of abnormal parameters should be an integral part of every well-child visit. Moderate or vigorous exercise of at least 300 minutes per week is recommended for children and adolescents. The use of screen time for computers, video games, television and phones has increased sedentary time periods in this population. Ideally, recreational screen time should be limited to less than 2 hours daily, and physical exercise should be encouraged instead. However, technology can also be used in a positive way: there are many applications for devices that provide exercise classes online and are readily available for use at home. In addition, patients can use devices to track lifestyle (diet, exercise, sleep). These options may be appealing to young people and should be incorporated into counselling.

Dietary changes alone can decrease LDL values 10% to 15%; however, it is quite likely that despite lifestyle changes, children with severe genetic hypercholesterolaemia such as FH and those with individual risk factors will ultimately meet the recommendations for the use of lipid-lowering medication (McCrindle et al 2007).

The most common medications include the class of drugs known as 'statins' or hydroxymethylglutaryl–coenzyme A (HMG-CoA) reductase inhibitors. Some of the more common statins include atorvastatin, simvastatin, rosuvastatin and pravastatin. In young children, some clinicians may use bile acid–resin binders such as cholestyramine (Questran) and colestipol (Colestid) before beginning statin therapy. Nicotinic acid can help raise HDL cholesterol but is rarely used in paediatrics because of symptoms of flushing and documentation of elevated liver transaminases. Fish oil supplementation may be helpful in situations with very high triglyceride levels.

Pharmacological Intervention

The recent National Heart, Lung, and Blood Institute guidelines recommend waiting until age 10 years to consider lipid-lowering medication unless the child has severe individual risk factors or homozygous hyperlipidaemia, in which case medication may be indicated earlier (National Heart, Lung, and Blood Institute 2011, Zachariah & de Ferranti 2013). The current guidelines recommend the initiation of lipid-lowering medications if, after 6 months of lifestyle modification, cholesterol values are still elevated.

The target level for LDL-C in childhood is aimed at the 95th percentile or less than 130 mg/dL and ideally less than 110 mg/dL, which is the 75th percentile. Clinicians start at the lowest dose of medication initially, increasing as required to obtain goal LDL values. Certain individual risk factors, such as diabetes, hypertension, history of childhood cancer, inflammatory disorders, transplant or coronary artery aneurysms from KD, lower the threshold for pharmacological intervention and lower the LDL goal as well.

HMG-CoA reductase inhibitors (statins) continue to be the most effective medication for lipid lowering. Before initiation of statin therapy, baseline liver function tests (alanine aminotransferase [ALT]) and creatine kinase (CK) levels are generally obtained. Clinical practice varies but ALT, along with a fasting lipid profile, is generally repeated approximately 1 to 2 months after the initiation of therapy and with any dosage changes. Once the patient is taking a stable dosage, laboratory tests are repeated at 6- to 12-month intervals, depending on the individual practice. Some clinicians measure CK in routine follow-up, whereas others only measure this parameter in the setting of clinical complaints of muscle aches. Side effects may include elevation of liver transaminase levels but are generally well tolerated in an otherwise healthy child/adolescent. Potential side effects should be reviewed with patients/families, including rhabdomyolysis. This is a very rare occurrence, particularly in young people, but when it happens, it is serious and can cause renal failure. Patients should be instructed to discontinue the medication and contact their clinician if they experience the new onset of muscle aches or dark brown urine. In addition, female patients need to be educated that statins are considered teratogenic and cannot be taken during pregnancy. Oral contraceptives may be given in conjunction with lipid-lowering medication; however, they may increase lipid values, potentially necessitating modification of the statin dose.

Bile acid–resin binders act by binding bile acids in the intestinal lumen. Because they are not absorbed by the intestine, they do not produce systemic toxicity and are safe for children. Cholestyramine and colestipol are both powders that are mixed with water or juice just before ingestion. Many patients cannot tolerate resin binders because the powder has a gritty texture and does not dissolve completely in liquid. Colestid also comes in a tablet form but the tablet is quite large. Side effects may include constipation, abdominal pain, gastrointestinal bloating, flatulence and nausea.

Patients who take resin binders should be instructed to take one multivitamin supplement daily because bile acid–binding agents may interfere with the absorption of fat-soluble vitamins. Because they can interfere with absorption of other medications, any other medications should be given at least 1 hour before or 6 hours after the bile acid–binding agent is ingested. The results of a full blood count, chloride and folate levels, and serum concentrations of vitamins A, D and E should be evaluated yearly.

Nursing Care Management

Nurses play an important role in the screening, education and support of children with hyperlipidaemia and their families. When a child is referred to a preventive cardiology or lipid clinic, it is essential that the family be adequately prepared for the visit. Generally the parents/child will be asked to keep some type of dietary history before this visit. Families are instructed to keep their child fasting for at least 12 hours before blood tests. Therefore, it is important to schedule the blood test early in the morning. At the visit, a complete individual and family health history is taken. The family history should include both biological parents and all first- and second-degree relatives. Questions are asked about the presence of early heart disease, hypertension, CVAs, sudden death, hyperlipidaemia, diabetes, metabolic syndrome and endocrine abnormalities. Nurses may also uncover risk factors when obtaining a health history for other purposes in their general practice. It is therefore important that nurses be familiar with current screening practices and with the availability of resources for children with concerning family histories.

At the visit, parents and extended families are informed about cholesterol and hyperlipidaemia. This education should include a brief introduction to the different lipoprotein categories, including cholesterol, HDL, LDL and triglycerides. In addition, behavioural risk factors for heart disease, such as smoking and lack of exercise, are reviewed. For management to be effective, parents, as well as the child (particularly older children), should understand the rationale for dietary and pharmacological intervention in the prevention of future cardiovascular disease.

Nutritional education is an important part of the treatment of any child or teenager with high cholesterol. Ideally, dietary counselling should be provided by a dietitian with expertise in paediatric lipid disorders/management. Dietary compliance may become an issue of control and a source of great stress for many families. Children with high cholesterol levels should not be viewed as having a disease. Rather, the positive aspects of healthy eating, regular exercise and avoiding smoking are emphasised. Basic dietary changes are encouraged for the whole family so the affected child is not singled out. The focus is positive, with emphasis on making healthy dietary choices, such as substituting chicken and fish for sausages and processed meats. Children can learn to participate in food preparation and decision-making. (See Cultural Considerations box.)

CULTURAL CONSIDERATIONS

Cultural Food Differences

Cultural differences must be considered and recommendations individualised. Substitution rather than elimination needs to be emphasised. Visual aids are often helpful, especially for children (e.g. 1 can of cola = 10 teaspoons of sugar). For example, the Australian Health survey from the Australian Bureau of Statistics showed that 50% of Aboriginal and Torres Strait Islander people aged 2 years and older consumed sugar-sweetened drinks daily, compared to 34% of non-Indigenous people (Avery et al 2017). The Rethink Sugary Drink initiative is a partnership between health and community organisations to give recommendations and health promotion around the overconsumption of sugar-sweetened beverages.

Diets should be flexible and individually tailored by a dietitian experienced in combining recommendations that meet both the nutritional demands of the growing child and lipid modifications. Parents are encouraged to participate in dietary and educational sessions, ask questions and share ideas and experiences.

Parents often feel guilty about the hereditary component of hyperlipidaemia. Many of these same parents are frustrated if diet alone is not making a significant enough difference in their child's lipid profile. However, it is important to discuss the fact that a dietary approach alone is often not sufficient, especially for children with FH who have LDL values greater than the 95th percentile.

If pharmacological therapy is recommended, parents and patients should receive counselling as to the rationale, current knowledge of benefit, dosage and possible side effects of the drug. Medication schedules should remain flexible and should not interfere with the child's daily activities. Follow-up phone calls by the nurse between visits allow parents to discuss their concerns and ask any questions that may have arisen.

Cardiac Dysrhythmias

Dysrhythmias, or abnormal heart rhythms, can occur in children with structurally normal hearts, as features of some congenital heart defects and in patients after surgical repair of congenital heart defects. They occur in patients with cardiomyopathy and cardiac tumours. They can occur secondary to metabolic and electrolyte imbalances. Childhood dysrhythmias can have a genetic or familial aetiology. Dysrhythmias can be classified in several ways, such as by heart rate characteristics (bradycardia and tachycardia) or by the origin of the dysrhythmia in the atria or ventricles. Most are due to abnormalities in impulse generation in the RA or to abnormalities in the conduction pathways.

Some dysrhythmias are well tolerated and self-limiting. Others may cause decreased cardiac output with associated symptoms. Some dysrhythmias can cause sudden death. Treatment depends on the cause of the dysrhythmia and its severity. Underlying causes are treated if possible (as with electrolyte imbalances). Some dysrhythmias (such as bradycardia caused by congenital heart block) are well tolerated and may not require treatment for many years. Others may require medications, radiofrequency ablation or pacemaker placement. Some can be difficult to treat and require multiple therapies.

Many advances have been made in the diagnosis and treatment of paediatric dysrhythmias. Improvements in technology have allowed better diagnosis, the development of ablation techniques and the expansion of pacemaker capabilities. New antidysrhythmic medications have proven safe and effective in children. Radiofrequency ablation has offered a cure for some dysrhythmias. Paediatric electrophysiology has become a highly specialised field, and the student is referred to more detailed sources for an in-depth discussion. The following sections describe diagnostic studies and provide a general discussion of the most common tachycardia (supraventricular tachycardia) and the most common bradycardia (complete heart block) that require treatment in the paediatric population.

Diagnostic Evaluation

Before diagnosing an infant or child with an abnormal heart rate, nurses must be familiar with the standards for normal heart rate in the particular age group. Heart rate patterns considered normal for a particular child can vary tremendously. An initial nursing responsibility is recognition of an abnormal heartbeat, in either rate or rhythm. When a dysrhythmia is suspected, the apical rate is counted for 1 full minute and compared with the radial rate, which may be lower because not all of the apical beats are felt. Consistently high or low heart rates should be regarded as suspicious. Accurate nursing assessment is essential. The patient should be placed on a cardiac monitor with recording capabilities. A 12-lead ECG yields more information than the monitor recording and should be taken as soon as possible. Recent advances in bedside telemetry allow storage of ECG tracings for later analysis.

Several advances in the diagnosis of cardiac dysrhythmias have greatly improved the understanding and treatment of these conditions in children. The basic diagnostic procedure is the ECG, including 24-hour Holter monitoring. However, more definitive procedures include both non-invasive and invasive techniques.

Electrophysiological cardiac catheterisation allows identification of conduction disturbances and immediate investigation of drugs that may control the dysrhythmia. Electrode catheters are introduced intravenously and directed towards the right side of the heart. The heart is then selectively stimulated to induce dysrhythmias. Once a dysrhythmia occurs, different antidysrhythmic drugs are administered intravenously to monitor which pharmacological agent is most successful in terminating the dysrhythmia.

Another procedure that may be employed is transoesophageal recording. An electrode catheter is passed to the lower oesophagus and, when in position at a point proximal to the heart, is used to stimulate and record dysrhythmias.

The onset and diagnosis of a cardiac dysrhythmia are frightening experiences for parents and older children. Sometimes the dysrhythmia rapidly leads to HF and a medical crisis. In this situation parents need much support to express their feelings and to understand the diagnosis and its treatment. Often parents and children have an unspoken fear of potential death even if the dysrhythmia is benign, and repeated explanations are needed to relieve anxiety.

Bradydysrhythmias. Sinus bradycardia in children can be due to the influence of the autonomic nervous system, as with hypervagal tone, or can be in response to hypoxia and hypotension. Once the infant receives adequate oxygenation and any acidosis is eliminated, the heart rate often returns to baseline. Sinus bradycardias are also known to develop after atrial repairs involving atrial suture lines such as in the Fontan procedure.

Complete AV block is also referred to as *complete heart block* (Fig 27.17). This can be either congenital (occurring in children with structurally normal hearts) or acquired after surgery to repair cardiac defects. AV blocks are most often related to oedema around the conduction system and resolve without treatment. Temporary epicardial wires are placed in most patients at surgery; if a rhythm disturbance occurs, temporary pacing can be employed. Just before discharge the health practitioner removes the wires by pulling slowly and deliberately down on them from the site of insertion.

A permanent pacemaker may be needed in some children, such as those with postsurgical AV block or, less frequently, congenital AV block. The pacemaker takes over or assists in the heart's conduction function. The surgical implantation of a pacemaker is usually a low-risk procedure. Once the wire has been introduced, a small incision is made and a pocket is formed under the muscle to house and protect the generator. The generator is placed under the abdominal muscle in infants and young children and in the upper chest below the clavicle in older children and adolescents. Depending on patient size and cardiac anatomy, some pacemakers can be placed transvenously in the catheterisation laboratory, rather than in the operating room. Continuous ECG monitoring is necessary during the recovery phase to assess pacemaker function. The nurse should be aware of the programmed rate and expected individual generator variations. A baseline ECG and chest x-ray film are obtained for future comparison. The pacemaker pocket site is monitored for signs of infection. Analgesics are given for pain.

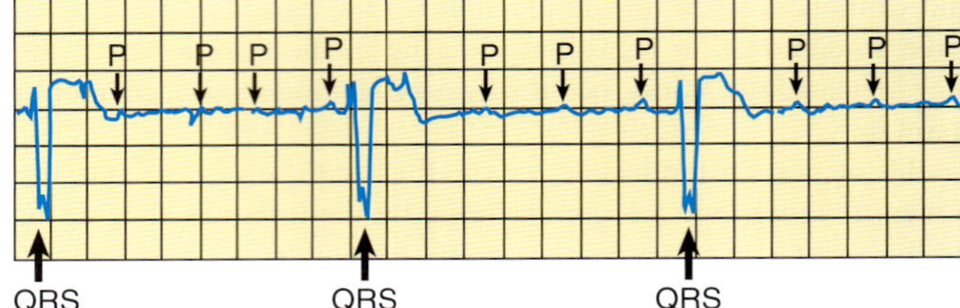

Fig 27.17 Complete heart block. Note slow rhythm and several P waves not followed by a QRS complex.

Pacemaker functions have become dramatically more sophisticated; pacemakers can control heart rate according to activity, cardiac output and respirations. In addition, some models can be programmed for overdrive pacing or cardioversion when the generator detects accelerated rates beyond established normal values.

When a pacemaker is implanted, the education of the parents and child includes an explanation of the device, a description of the component parts, an explanation of the surgical procedure and discharge teaching. The pacemaker is made up of two basic parts: the pulse generator and the lead. The pulse generator is composed of the battery and the electronic circuitry. The function is to produce the electrical impulse sent to the heart and to receive and respond to signals produced by the heart. The lead is an insulated, flexible wire that conducts the electrical impulse from the pulse generator to the heart. Two types of leads are available: transvenous and epicardial. The child's size and the heart's structure determine which lead is more appropriate. Transvenous leads are inserted into a large vein, often the subclavian, and advanced into the right side of the heart. Placement is secured by engaging a small corkscrew or fishhook attachment at the end of the lead into the endocardium. Epicardial leads are attached directly to the epicardial layer of the heart. Parents should be aware of which type of lead is in place in their child.

Discharge teaching includes information about the signs and symptoms of infection, general wound care and activity restrictions. Parents, and patients if they are old enough, should learn to take the pulse and should know the settings of the pacemaker. If the patient's low rate is set at 80 beats/min and the heart rate is only 68 beats/min, there is a possible problem with the pacemaker that needs to be investigated. Instructions for telephone transmission of ECG readings are also given. Telephone connections can be used to transmit ECG data and also to monitor battery life and pacemaker function. The pacemaker generator has to be replaced periodically because of battery depletion. Children with pacemakers should wear a medical alert device, and their parents should have a paper identification card with specific pacemaker data in case of an emergency. Cardiopulmonary resuscitation instruction is suggested for parents.

Tachydysrhythmias. Sinus tachycardia (abnormally fast heart rate) secondary to fever, anxiety, pain, anaemia, dehydration or any other aetiological factor requiring increased cardiac output should be ruled out first before diagnosing it as pathological. Supraventricular tachycardia (SVT), the most common tachydysrhythmia found in children, refers to a rapid regular heart rate of 200 to 300 beats/min (Fig 27.18). The two most common forms of SVT are atrioventricular re-entrant tachycardia (AVRT), including the Wolff-Parkinson-White (WPW) syndrome, and atrioventricular nodal re-entrant tachycardia (AVNRT). The more common form, AVRT, occurs in about 73% of the population (Ko et al 1992). The rapid rhythm originates above the ventricle and is most commonly caused by a re-entry mechanism that involves an accessory pathway or the AV conduction system. The onset and termination of SVT are abrupt. The QRS complex is usually narrow (in contrast with ventricular tachycardia, in which the QRS complexes are typically wide), and the P waves are often absent. Infants and young children with SVT may be unable to compensate for the rapid heart rate, and the clinical course can progress to HF. Important signs in the infant and young child are poor feeding, extreme irritability and pallor. Older children may experience palpitations, dizziness, chest pain, diaphoresis and syncope.

The treatment of SVT depends on the degree of compromise imposed by the dysrhythmia. In some instances, vagal manoeuvres, such as applying ice to the face, massaging the carotid artery (on one side of the neck only) or having an older child perform a Valsalva manoeuvre (e.g. exhaling against a closed glottis, blowing on the thumb as if it were a trumpet for 30 to 60 seconds) can reverse the SVT. When vagal manoeuvres fail, adenosine may be used to end the episode of SVT by impairing AV node conduction. IV adenosine is the first-line pharmacological measure for termination of SVT in infants and children in the emergency setting. Adenosine must be given by rapid IV push with a saline bolus immediately after the drug. Incrementally increasing doses given about 2 minutes apart may be needed. The desired effect usually occurs in 10 to 20 seconds. Synchronised shock with a defibrillator is also used for cardioversion for patients who are haemodynamically unstable with a tachyarrhythmia such as SVT with a palpable pulse, or electively in patients with haemodynamically stable SVT, under the direction of a paediatric cardiologist.

Traditional first-line medical management of chronic SVT is a beta blocker or digoxin. Digoxin should not be used in patients with WPW syndrome because it can accelerate conduction across the accessory pathway in this particular group of patients. Choice of beta blockers is based on age, using propranolol, a shorter-acting agent for infants, and atenolol, a longer-acting beta blocker for older children. More aggressive pharmacological treatment with amiodarone or flecainide may be needed for those with more severe symptoms or recurrence of SVT.

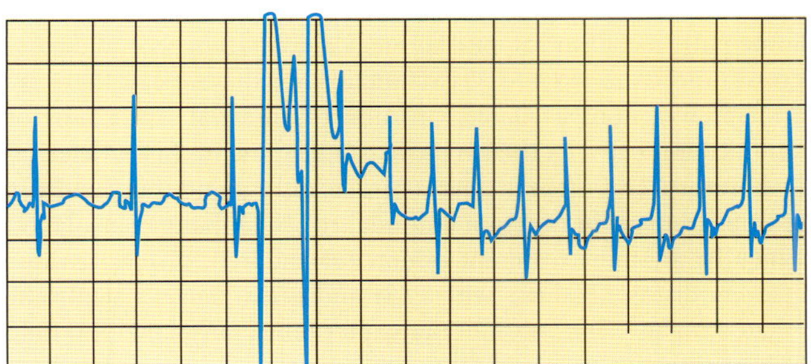

Fig 27.18 Supraventricular tachycardia (SVT). Note normal sinus rhythm (three PQRST complexes) on the left and abrupt onset of a very fast rhythm (SVT) on the right.

If cardiac output is significantly compromised or signs of HF exist, oesophageal overdrive pacing or synchronised cardioversion can be employed in the intensive care setting. Transoesophageal atrial overdrive pacing is accomplished through placement of a protected lead into the oesophagus, behind the LA of the heart. The lead is then attached to a stimulator capable of pacing at very rapid rates to interrupt the tachydysrhythmia. Synchronised cardioversion is the timed delivery of a preset amount of energy through the chest wall in an attempt to re-establish an organised rhythm. Sedation is needed for both procedures. Cardioversion should never be performed on a conscious patient.

Radiofrequency ablation has become first-line therapy for some types of SVT. The procedure is done in the cardiac electrophysiology catheterisation laboratory and begins with mapping of the conduction system to identify the dysrhythmia focus. A catheter delivering radiofrequency current is directed at the site, and the identified area is heated to destroy the tissue in the area. Success rates vary but can be as high as 90% (Dubin 2016). A successful ablation is curative, and antidysrhythmic medications can be discontinued.

Another procedure, cryoablation, is also used in treatment of SVT, particularly the AVNRT form. Liquid nitrous oxide is used to cool a catheter to subfreezing temperatures, which then destroys the tissue of target by freezing. This procedure also takes place in the cardiac electrophysiology catheterisation laboratory.

Preparation is similar to that for cardiac catheterisation and other electrophysiological studies. The risks and benefits of ablation need to be reviewed. These are lengthy procedures, often 6 to 8 hours, and sedation or general anaesthesia is required. Postprocedure care is similar to that for cardiac catheterisation, with the addition of careful dysrhythmia monitoring. Patients and their families often have great hope for a cure and are disappointed if the ablation is unsuccessful.

A primary focus of nursing care is education of the family regarding the symptoms of SVT and the treatment. SVT may occur again despite therapy. After the first episode of SVT, parents should learn to take a radial pulse for 1 full minute. If medication is prescribed, instructions regarding accurate dosage and the importance of administering the correct dose at specified intervals are stressed.

Pulmonary Hypertension

Pulmonary hypertension (PH) is a pulmonary vascular disease associated with diverse cardiac, lung and systemic diseases, as well as familial and idiopathic aetiologies. The pulmonary arteries are described as having vascular narrowing due to decreased vascular growth and surface area and intraluminal obstruction, and they undergo structural remodelling of the vessel wall (Abman & Ivy 2011). It is defined by a mean pulmonary arterial pressure (mPAP) $\geq$ 25 mmHg in children over 3 months of age and is categorised based on the World Health Organization classification system (Table 27.5). In the paediatric population, there are three causes of PH: (1) increased pulmonary venous pressures (e.g. mitral stenosis, LV non-compliance); (2) posttricuspid cardiac shunts (e.g. large ventricular septal defect, large PDA); and (3) small PAs, that is, too few or too narrow (e.g. idiopathic pulmonary arterial hypertension, persistent PH of the newborn, connective tissue disorders, hypoxia, drugs, toxins). There is no cure for PH and there is significant morbidity and mortality. Advancements in therapeutic management in the last 10 to 15 years, however, are helping to slow the progression of the disease and improve quality of life.

TABLE 27.5 World Health Organization Classification of Pulmonary Hypertension (Nice)

1. Pulmonary arterial hypertension (PAH)
   1. Idiopathic pulmonary arterial hypertension (IPAH)
   2. Heritable
   3. Drug and toxin induced
   4. Associated pulmonary arterial hypertension (APAH; pulmonary arterial hypertension associated with other disease, e.g. connective tissue disorder, human immunodeficiency virus, portal hypertension, congenital heart disease, schistosomiasis)
      - 1′. Pulmonary veno-occlusive disease (PVOD)
      - 1″. Persistent pulmonary hypertension of the newborn (PPHN)
2. Pulmonary hypertension (PH) due to left-sided heart disease (e.g. left ventricular dysfunction, mitral valve disease)
3. PH due to lung disease or hypoxaemia (e.g. chronic obstructive pulmonary disease)
4. Chronic thromboembolic disease
5. Unclear multifactorial mechanisms

Source: Adapted from Simonneau, G., Gatzoulis, M. A., Adatia, I., et al. (2013). Updated clinical classification of pulmonary hypertension. Journal of the American College of Cardiology, 62(25 Suppl), D34–D41.

Pathophysiology

No one knows what causes the pathological changes for PH, but the pathophysiology is likely to be multifactorial. Proliferative vasculopathy of the small pulmonary arterioles characterised by hypertrophy and hyperplasia of the intima, as well as smooth muscle contraction, contribute to increasing pulmonary vascular resistance. High pulmonary vascular resistance causes progressive right-sided HF, low cardiac output and high mortality rates.

Although seen less often today due to early surgical intervention, congenital heart defects with a large left-to-right shunt (such as a ventricular septal defect, PDA or complete AV canal), which cause increased pulmonary blood flow, may result in PH. If these defects are not repaired early, the high pulmonary flow will cause changes in the pulmonary artery vessels and the vessels will lose their elasticity. This causes increased resistance in the pulmonary bed and results in eventual right-sided HF because the heart cannot pump against the greater resistance. The flow of blood becomes right to left, and cyanosis is seen. This is known as Eisenmenger syndrome. Because of surgical repair of these defects early in life, this occurs infrequently now.

Clinical Manifestations

The clinical manifestations include dyspnoea with exercise, chest pain and syncope. Dyspnoea is the most common symptom and is caused by impaired oxygen delivery. Chest pain is the result of coronary ischaemia in the RV from severe hypertrophy. Syncope reflects a limited cardiac output, leading to decreased cerebral blood flow. Right-sided heart dysfunction is steadily progressive as the pulmonary vessels become obstructed and the pulmonary artery pressure increases. The RV hypertrophies in an attempt to maintain a normal cardiac output. With time and continued increases in pulmonary vascular resistance, the cardiac output decreases. When signs of right-sided HF with systemic venous congestion and oedema are evident, the prognosis is poor.

Diagnostic Evaluation

Initial evaluation consists of physical examination, chest radiography, ECG, echocardiography and cardiac catheterisation (Abman et al 2015). An extensive workup is needed to better characterise the causes, associated factors, haemodynamics and disease severity. It includes evaluation of cardiac and pulmonary function, coagulation tests, collagen vascular evaluation, sleep study and other studies. Right-sided cardiac catheterisation is essential to evaluate the degree of PH and the response to vasodilator therapy. Oxygen, nitric oxide and prostacyclin may all be used during the catheterisation to assess the ability of various therapies to reduce pulmonary artery pressure. Exercise capacity, as assessed by the 6-minute walk test, is predictive of disease severity.

Therapeutic Management

Paediatric PH guidelines in tertiary centres in both Australia and New Zealand outline treatment recommendations for conditions specific to the paediatric population such as persistent PH of the newborn, congenital diaphragmatic hernia and CHD. Some useful links to this information are as follows.

- Persistent pulmonary hypertension guideline: https://www.starship.org.nz/guidelines/persistent-pulmonary-hypertension-of-the-newborn/
- Congenital diaphragmatic hernia guideline: https://www.starship.org.nz/guidelines/congenital-diaphragmatic-hernia-postnatal-management-in-picu
- Paediatric pulmonary arterial hypertension: https://www.starship.org.nz/guidelines/paediatric-pulmonary-arterial-hypertension-guideline

The discussion here focuses on pharmacotherapy, supportive therapy and, briefly, invasive interventions.

There are three classes of drugs that are used extensively in the treatment of paediatric PH: PDE5 inhibitors (sildenafil, tadalafil), endothelin receptor antagonists (bosentan, ambrisentan), and prostanoids or PGI_2 analogues (epoprostenol, treprostinil). Vasoconstriction is a primary component of PH and these drugs work on different aspects to promote vasodilation and smooth muscle relaxation. For patients who are responsive to inhaled nitric oxide (iNO) or vasodilator drug testing during cardiac catheterisation, oral calcium channel blockers (nifedipine and diltiazem) have been successful and are the treatment of choice. Choice of treatment is determined by the severity of the disease, and all of these medications carry adverse effects.

In general, situations that may exacerbate the disease and cause hypoxia are avoided. Exercise prescriptions are specific to each patient. Patients should avoid high altitudes because of the relative hypoxia, and some patients have moved to sea level to slow the progress of the disease. Supplemental oxygen is commonly used to relieve hypoxia, especially at night while sleeping. Patients with pulmonary arterial hypertension (PAH) are at risk for thromboembolic events. Anticoagulation therapy has been shown to increase survival in adults. Many patients are treated with warfarin to prevent pulmonary embolism, which can be fatal. Digoxin and diuretics are often used to treat right-sided HF.

Some patients fail to respond to medical management and disease progression leads to severe RV dysfunction. In these cases, there are two potential options available. Creation of an atrial septostomy or communication between the two atria can be done in the catheterisation laboratory. This often increases cardiac output and thus results in some improvement in function and quality of life. Lung transplantation may be another treatment option for children, primarily those with severe disease. Patients with PAH and Eisenmenger's syndrome have had a higher early mortality rate after lung transplantation than other lung transplant patients.

Nursing Care Management

The diagnosis of PH is devastating for the child and family. There is no known cure, and the treatments require significant lifestyle changes and commitment on the part of patient and family to make them successful. Anxiety, depression and fear of the future are common. Patients and families require extensive education about the disease and its management. They need emotional support to cope with a poor prognosis and make decisions about treatment options.

The medical treatment is complex and involves different medications and therapies. Families are often referred to a specialised centre that has experience in the management of PH. This may involve travel far from home with associated emotional and financial hardships The patient and family must cope with the symptoms of the disease and the side effects of the treatment. Dealing with a continuous IV infusion or continuous oxygen administration requires a major adjustment in lifestyle to accommodate the therapy. The prostacyclin infusion cannot be interrupted at any time because symptoms can worsen and cause acute pulmonary hypertensive crisis, which can be fatal. Backup systems must be in place at all times. The patient and family must make a commitment to adhere to a complex regimen of preparing the infusion, maintaining the equipment and maintaining sterility of the central line. Treatments are expensive, so insurance coverage and financial issues are critical. Nurses have an important role in educating and preparing families to perform these complex therapies. Discharge planning involves many team members and outside agencies. The nurse has a pivotal role in coordinating the child's care in the hospital and the transition to home.

Cardiomyopathy

Cardiomyopathy refers to abnormalities of the myocardium in which the cardiac muscles' ability to contract or relax is impaired. Cardiomyopathies are relatively rare in children. Possible causes include familial or genetic factors, infection, deficiency states, metabolic abnormalities and collagen vascular diseases. Most cardiomyopathies in children are considered primary or idiopathic disorders, in which the cause is unknown and the cardiac dysfunction is not associated with systemic disease. Abnormalities of the cardiac myocyte and essential cellular functions underlie the clinical manifestations of organ dysfunction. Some of the known causes of secondary cardiomyopathy are toxicity from anthracyclines (e.g. the antineoplastic agents doxorubicin [Adriamycin]), haemochromatosis (from excessive iron storage), Duchenne's muscular dystrophy, KD, collagen diseases and thyroid dysfunction.

Cardiomyopathies can be divided into three broad clinical categories according to the type of abnormal structure and dysfunction present: dilated cardiomyopathy, hypertrophic cardiomyopathy and restrictive cardiomyopathy. Dilated cardiomyopathy is characterised by ventricular dilation and greatly decreased contractility, which result in symptoms of HF. This is the most common type of cardiomyopathy in children. Its cause is often unknown, although carnitine deficiency, metabolic diseases, drug toxicities, dysrhythmias and infection causing myocarditis should be considered. The clinical findings are of HF with tachycardia, dyspnoea, hepatosplenomegaly, fatigue and poor growth. Dysrhythmias may be present and may be more difficult to control with worsening HF. Chest radiography demonstrates cardiomegaly and congested lung fields. The echocardiogram demonstrates poor ventricular contractility, dilated LV and reduced shortening and ejection fraction. Cardiac catheterisation with endomyocardial biopsy is usually performed for diagnosis and identification of a possible infectious cause.

Hypertrophic cardiomyopathy is characterised by an increase in heart muscle mass without an increase in cavity size. It usually occurs in the LV and is associated with abnormal diastolic filling. Mutations of several genes that encode proteins of the cardiac sarcomere have been identified. The expression of clinical disease varies greatly among patients. Infants of diabetic mothers may have a hypertrophic cardiomyopathy that resolves with time. Clinical symptoms usually appear in the school-age period or adolescence and may include anginal chest pain, dysrhythmias and syncope. Sudden death is possible. One study confirmed that unexplained syncope in the childhood age group (< 18 years of age) with known hypertrophic cardiomyopathy had a 60% cumulative risk of sudden death within 5 years of the syncopal event (Spirito et al 2009). Presentation in infancy includes signs of HF and carries a poor prognosis. Chest radiography shows a mildly enlarged heart. The ECG demonstrates LV hypertrophy, often with ST-T changes. The echocardiogram is most helpful and demonstrates asymmetrical septal hypertrophy and an increase in LV wall thickness, with a small LV cavity.

Restrictive cardiomyopathy, rare in children, involves a restriction to ventricular filling caused by endocardial or myocardial disease or both. RA or LA enlargement or both, apparent on the ECG, are often seen. The chest radiograph shows an enlarged heart. The echocardiogram reveals atrial dilation. Systolic function, the ability of the heart to squeeze, is often normal or mildly impaired, whereas diastolic function, the ability of the heart to relax, is very abnormal. Patients are at risk for embolic events and the development of PH. Symptoms are dizziness, exercise intolerance and dry cough and can progress to those of HF (see p. 709).

Therapeutic Management

Treatment is directed at correcting the underlying cause whenever feasible. In most affected children, however, this is not possible, and treatment is aimed at managing HF (see p. 709) and dysrhythmias. Administration of digoxin and diuretics and aggressive use of afterload-reduction agents have been found to be helpful in managing symptoms in those with dilated cardiomyopathy. Carvedilol (Coreg), a beta blocker, is the newest medication to be added to the treatment of some children with chronic HF. The alpha- and beta-adrenergic receptors are blocked, causing decreased heart rate, decreased BP and vasodilation. In addition, beta blockers have antiarrhythmic effects, coronary artery vasodilatory effects and negative chronotropic effects (Moffett & Chang 2006). Carvedilol is used in compensated HF, not in the acute diagnostic or decompensated HF phase (Rossano & Shaddy 2014). Practice guidelines for the management of HF in children have been outlined and provide an in-depth review of available therapies (Rosenthal et al 2004). Digoxin and inotropic agents are usually not helpful in the other forms of cardiomyopathy because increasing the force of contraction may exacerbate the muscular obstruction and actually impair ventricular ejection. Beta blockers such as propranolol or calcium channel blockers such as verapamil have been used to reduce LV outflow obstruction and improve diastolic filling in those with hypertrophic cardiomyopathy.

Careful monitoring and effective treatment of dysrhythmias are essential. The placement of an implantable defibrillator should be considered for patients at high risk of sudden death due to ventricular arrhythmias. Anticoagulants may be given to reduce the risk of thromboembolism, a complication of the sluggish circulation through the heart.

Advanced Heart Failure

Heart failure is a syndrome that results from ventricular dysfunction, volume overload or pressure overload and is a complex disorder that can result from structural or functional abnormalities. In children, it leads to characteristic signs and symptoms such as poor growth, feeding difficulties, respiratory distress, exercise intolerance and fatigue. For the paediatric population, a four-tiered standard classification system, the Ross Heart Failure Classification System, stratifies the levels of HF based on these signs and symptoms from Level I (no limitations or symptoms) to the most advanced HF, Level IV (symptomatic at rest with tachypnoea, retractions, grunting or diaphoresis) (Francis et al 2010, Ross 2012). Interventions and therapies are advanced if patients progress to higher levels of HF.

Cardiac resynchronisation therapy (CRT) using biventricular pacing is an effective treatment in adult patients with HF and is beginning to be applied in the paediatric population. With pharmacological therapies discussed earlier, CRT has the potential to improve cardiac function in this group of patients. The causes for HF in the young are more varied and often include patients with a single ventricle, making CRT more challenging. Initial studies of CRT in this population demonstrate improved outcomes in those with adequate follow-up (Cecchin et al 2009, Dubin et al 2005).

For worsening HF and signs of poor perfusion, severely ill children may benefit from mechanical ventilation, oxygen administration, IV inotropic support and IV administration of afterload-reduction agents such as milrinone. Mechanical support devices such as extracorporeal membrane oxygenation or ventricular assist devices may be used in patients with progressive decline in cardiac status. Extracorporeal membrane oxygenation is employed primarily for infants and younger patients. Its use is limited to several weeks or less because of complications such as bleeding and infection. Ventricular assist devices, currently standard for older children and adolescents and becoming more readily available for infants and younger children, can be used for longer periods (Cassidy et al 2013). Risks include infection and embolic complications. Both devices can be used as a bridge to heart transplantation to allow more time to wait for a donor organ. Heart transplantation may be a treatment option for patients who have worsening symptoms despite maximum medical therapy (see below).

Nursing Care Management

Because of the poor prognosis for many children with cardiomyopathy, nursing care is consistent with that for any child with a life-threatening disorder (see Chapter 19). One of the most difficult adjustments for the child may be the realisation of failing health and the need for restricted activity, especially if the child is a normally active youngster. Include the child in decisions regarding activity and allow him or her to discuss feelings, particularly if the disease follows a progressive and fatal course. Once symptoms of HF or dysrhythmias develop, implement the same nursing care as discussed on p. 709. If cardiac transplantation is being considered, the child and family have great needs in terms of psychological preparation and postoperative care. The nurse plays an important role in assessing the family's understanding of the procedure and long-term consequences. Children of school age and older should be fully informed to give their consent to the procedure (see Informed Consent, Chapter 22).

Heart Transplantation

Heart transplantation has become a treatment option for infants and children with worsening HF and a limited life expectancy despite maximum medical and surgical management. Indications for cardiac transplantation in children are cardiomyopathy and end-stage CHD. It is also an option for patients with some forms of complex congenital cardiac defects, such as hypoplastic left heart syndrome, for which conventional surgical approaches have a high mortality risk or they have experienced severe complications such as valve regurgitation, ventricular dysfunction or dysrhythmias.

The heart transplant procedure may be orthotopic or heterotopic. **Orthotopic** heart transplantation refers to removal of the recipient's own heart and implantation of a new heart from a donor who has experienced brain death but whose heart is healthy. The donor and recipient are matched by weight. In **heterotopic** heart transplantation, the recipient's own heart is left in place and a new heart is implanted to act as an additional pump or 'piggyback' heart; this type of transplantation is rarely done in children.

Before transplantation, potential recipients undergo a careful cardiac evaluation to determine whether any other medical or surgical options could improve the patient's cardiac status. Other organ systems are assessed to identify problems that might preclude or increase the risk of transplantation. A psychosocial evaluation of the patient and family is done to assess family function, support systems and ability to comply with the complex medical regimen after the transplant. Support services to help the family successfully care for their child are provided when possible. Parents and older adolescents need extensive education about the risks and benefits of transplantation so they can make an informed decision.

In Australia patients are listed on a national computer network organised by the DonateLife Agency and the relevant donation specialist coordinator in each state to match donors and recipients. All heart transplants that are undertaken in Australia and New Zealand are reported to the Australian and New Zealand Cardiothoracic Organ Transplant Registry. This registry allows for nationally uniform eligibility criteria and national allocation protocols as well as data collection from all transplant sites across Australia and New Zealand (Dwyer et al 2017).

The waitlist mortality rate remains high, particularly in the smallest children. Progress in suitable ventricular assist devices for use in children as a bridge to transplantation has made outcomes to survival for cardiac transplantation more successful (Blume et al 2006). A review of medical records was performed from 1988 to January 2010 at Australia's National Paediatric Heart Transplant Centre at the RCHM. The results showed that of the 139 children accepted onto the heart transplant list during the study, 93 children went on to have heart transplantation surgery. Waitlist mortality was 32% and survival post-transplant was 90% at 1 year and 68% at 10 years, which shows that results of paediatric heart transplant are comparable to international results despite the low organ donation rate and the limitations of a small population that is geographically large (Alexander et al 2014).

In addition, ABO-incompatible heart transplants are being performed successfully in the younger population (Urschel et al 2021).

The posttransplantation course is complex. Overall causes of death within the Pediatric Heart Transplant Study (PHTS) dataset include rejection (8%), infection (12%), early graft failure (10%), sudden cardiac death (9%) and myocardial infarction (8%), as well as smaller numbers of multisystem causes. Although heart function is greatly improved or normal after transplantation, the risk of rejection is serious. The leading cause of death in the first 3 years after heart transplantation is rejection, with the greatest risk in the first 6 months. Rejection of the heart is diagnosed primarily by endomyocardial biopsy in children. Serial echocardiograms are often used in infants to reduce the need for invasive biopsies. Immunosuppressants must be taken for life and have many systemic side effects. Induction followed by double-drug therapy for immunosuppression with a calcineurin inhibitor (tacrolimus) and mycophenolate mofetil is most commonly used in paediatric patients. Steroids are used with induction at the time of transplant and are commonly discontinued with induction or weaned off over several months unless the patient is highly sensitised at the time of transplant.

Potential long-term problems that may limit survival include: coronary artery disease, often termed *chronic rejection*; renal dysfunction; lymphoma; and infection. In the short term, after successful transplantation, children are able to return to full participation in age-appropriate activities and appear to adapt well to their new lifestyle.

Transplantation is not a cure because patients must live with the lifetime consequences of chronic immunosuppression. It is to be expected that paediatric patients will require a second heart transplant in their lifetime.

Nursing Care Management

Nursing care after transplantation is complex, demanding careful attention to both the physical needs of the child and the emotional needs of the child and family. Successfully caring for a child after heart transplantation requires the expertise and dedication of many members of the healthcare team. Nurses play vital roles in assessment, coordination of care, psychosocial support and patient and family education. The nurse must monitor the heart transplant recipient carefully for signs of rejection, infection and the side effects of the immunosuppressant medications. Optimising long-term health includes managing cholesterol levels, participating in routine exercise, refraining from smoking, aggressively controlling BP and optimising bone health. The nurse also needs to assess the patient's and family's psychosocial wellbeing to identify issues such as increased family stress, depression, substance abuse and school problems. Non-compliance with an intense medication regimen, especially during adolescence, can lead to serious medical problems and can be fatal. Some patients and families need psychiatric support, and many patients need supportive services for learning problems. Chapter 24 discusses immunosuppressants and their nursing implications in relation to renal transplantation. Chapter 29 reviews care of the immunosuppressed child. Chapter 19 presents psychosocial concerns and appropriate interventions for the child with a life-threatening disorder.

The first 6 months to 1 year after transplantation are most intense because the risk of complications is greatest and the patient and family are adjusting to a new lifestyle. Parents of heart transplant recipients also have a high incidence of posttraumatic stress symptoms, and the transplant team should routinely assess the parent's or caretaker's psychological functioning (Farley et al 2007). The healthcare team monitors patients closely, with frequent visits and laboratory tests. Care is usually shared between local healthcare providers and the transplant centre. Many patients are able to return to school and other age-appropriate activities within 2 to 3 months after the transplant.

REFERENCES

Abman, S. H., Hansmann, G., Archer, S. L., et al. (2015). Pediatric pulmonary hypertension: Guidelines from the American Heart Association and American Thoracic Society. Circulation, 132(21), 2037–2099.

Abman, S. H., & Ivy, D. D. (2011). Recent progress in understanding pediatric pulmonary hypertension. Current Opinion in Pediatrics, 23(3), 298–304.

Alexander, P. M. A., Swager, A., Lee, K. J., et al. (2014). Paediatric heart transplantation in Australia comes of age: 21 years of experience in a national centre. Internal Medicine Journal, 44(12a), 1223–1231. http://doi.org/10.1111/imj.12567

Alsoufi, B., Mori, M., Gillespie, S., et al. (2015). Impact of patient characteristics and anatomy on results of Norwood operation for Hypoplastic Left Heart Syndrome. The Annals of Thoracic Surgery, 100(2), 591–598.

Australian Technical Advisory Group on Immunisation (ATAGI). (2018). Australian Immunisation Handbook, Australian Government Department of Health, Canberra. http://immunisationhandbook.health.gov.au.

Avery, J. C., Bowden, J. A., Dono, J., et al. (2017). Sugar-sweetened beverage consumption, correlates and interventions among Australian Aboriginal and Torres Strait Islander communities: A scoping review protocol. BMJ Open, 7(7). http://doi.org/10.1136/bmjopen-2017-016431

Ayer, J., & Sholler, G. F. (2012). Cardiovascular risk factors in Australian children: hypertension and lipid abnormalities. Australian Prescriber, *35*(2), 51–55. http://doi.org/10.18773/austprescr.2012.024

Baker, A. L., & Newburger, J. W. (2008). Kawasaki disease. Circulation, 118, e110–e112.

Baltimore, R. S., Gewitz, M., Baddour, L. M., et al. (2015). Infective endocarditis in childhood: 2015 update. Scientific statement from the American Heart Association. Circulation, 132, 1487–1515.

Barbas, K. H., & Kelleher, D. K. (2004). Breastfeeding success among infants with congenital heart disease. Pediatric Nursing, 30, 285–289.

Blume, E. D., Naftel, D. C., Bastardi, H. J., et al. (2006). Outcomes of children bridged to heart transplantation with ventricular assist devices: A multi-institutional study. Circulation, 113, 2313–2319.

Bono-Neri, F. (2016). Acute rheumatic fever: Global persistence of a preventable disease. Journal of Pediatric Health Care, 31(3), 275–284.

Bragg, L., & Alvarez, A. (2014). Endocarditis. Pediatrics in Review, 35(4), 162–167.

Brown, M. L., Burkhart, H. M., Connolly, H. M., et al. (2013). Coarctation of the aorta: Lifelong surveillance is mandatory following surgical repair. Journal of the American College of Cardiology, 62(11), 1020–1025.

Butera, G., Carminati, M., Chessa, M., et al. (2007). Transcatheter closure of perimembranous ventricular septal defects: Early and long-term results. Journal of the American College of Cardiology, 50(12), 1189–1195.

Cassidy, J., Dominguez, T., Haynes, S., et al. (2013). A longer waiting game: Bridging children to heart transplant with the Berlin Heart EXCOR device—the United Kingdom experience. The Journal of Heart and Lung Transplantation, 32(11), 1101–1106.

Cecchin, F., Frangini, P. A., Brown, D. W., et al. (2009). Cardiac resynchronization therapy (and multisite pacing) in pediatrics and congenital heart disease: Five years experience in a single institution. Journal of Cardiovascular Electrophysiology, 20(1), 58–65.

Cuypers, J. A., Eindhoven, J. A., Slager, M. A., et al. (2014). The natural and unnatural history of the Mustard procedure: Long-term outcome up to 40 years. European Heart Journal, 35(25), 1666–1674.

Day, M. D., Gauvreau, K., Shulman, S., et al. (2009). Characteristics of children hospitalized with infective endocarditis. Circulation, 119(6), 865–870.

Dengler, K. A., Wilson, V., Redshaw, S., et al. (2012). Appreciation of a Child's Journey: Implementation of a Cardiac Action Research Project. Nursing Research and Practice, 2012, 145030. http://doi.org/10.1155/2012/145030

Department of Health (DoH). (2019). National strategic action plan for childhood heart disease. Beyond the heart: transforming care. Australian Government. February. https://www.heartkids.org.au/page/192/standards-of-care

Doyle, T., Kavanaugh-McHugh, A., & Fish, F. A. (2016). Management and outcome of tetralogy of Fallot. UpToDate. https://www.uptodate.com/contents/management-and-outcome-of-tetralogy-of-fallot.

Dubin, A. M. (2016). Management of supraventricular tachycardia in children. UpToDate. https://www.uptodate.com/contents/management-of-supraventricular-tachycardia-in-children.

Dubin, A. M., Janousek, J., Rhee, E., et al. (2005). Resynchronization therapy in pediatric and congenital heart disease patients. Journal of the American College of Cardiology, 46(12), 2277–2283.

Dwyer, M. K., Clark, J. C., Macdonald, A. K., et al. (2017). Gender Equity in Transplantation: A Report from the Women in Transplantation Workshop of The Transplantation Society of Australia and New Zealand. Transplantation, 101(10), 2266–2270. doi:10.1097/TP.0000000000001900

Farley, L. M., DeMaso, D. R., D'Angelo, E., et al. (2007). Parenting stress and parental post-traumatic stress disorder in families after pediatric heart transplantation. The Journal of Heart and Lung Transplantation, 2, 120–126.

Feltes, T. F., Bacha, E., Beekman, R. H., et al. (2011). Indications for cardiac catheterisation and intervention in pediatric cardiac disease: A scientific statement from the American Heart Association. Circulation, 123, 2607–2652.

Flacking, R., Lehtonen, L., Thomson, G., et al. (2012). Closeness and separation in neonatal intensive care. Acta Paediatrica, *101*(10), 1032–1037. https://doi.org/10.1111/j.1651-2227.2012.02787.x

Flynn, J. T., Daniels, S. R., Hayman, L. L., et al. (2014). Update: Ambulatory blood pressure monitoring in children and adolescents: A scientific statement from the American Heart Association. Hypertension, 63(5), 1116–1135.

Flynn, J. T., Kaelber, D. C., Baker-Smith, C. M., et al & Subcommittee on Screening and Management of High Blood Pressure in Children. (2017). Clinical practice guideline for screening and management of high blood pressure in children and adolescents. Pediatrics, 140(3), e20171904.

Francis, G. S., Greenberg, B. H., Hsu, D. T., et al. (2010). ACCF/AHA/ACP/HFSA/ISHLT 2010 Clinical competence statement on management of patients with advanced heart failure and cardiac transplant: A report of the ACCF/AHA/ACP Task Force on Clinical Competence and Training. Journal of the American College of Cardiology, 56(5), 424–453.

Gewitz, M. H., Baltimore, R. S., Tani, L. Y., et al. (2015). Revision of the Jones Criteria for the diagnosis of acute rheumatic fever in the era of Doppler echocardiography: A scientific statement from the American Heart Association. Circulation, 131, 1806–1818.

Gist, K., Blinder, J., Bailly, D., et al. (2019). Neonatal and Paediatric Heart and Renal Outcomes Network: design of a multi-centre retrospective cohort study. Cardiology in the Young, 29(4), 511–518. https://doi.org/10.1017/S1047951119000210

Goldmuntz, E., & Lin, A. (2008). Genetics of congenital heart defects. In H. D. Allen, D. J. Driscoll, R. E. Shaddy, et al. (Eds.), Moss and Adams' Heart Disease in Infants, Children, and Adolescents (7th ed.). Philadelphia, PA: Lippincott Williams & Wilkins.

Gupta, S., Sakhuja, A., McGrath, E., et al. (2016). Trends, microbiology, and outcomes of infective endocarditis in children during 2000 to 2010 in the United States. Congenital Heart Disease, 12(2), 196–201.

Haberman, Z. C., Jahn, R. J., Bose, R., et al. (2015). Wireless Smartphone ECG enables large scale screening in diverse populations. Journal of Cardiovascular Electrophysiology, 26(5), 520–526.

Heart Foundation of New Zealand. (2014). New Zealand Guidelines for Rheumatic Fever: Diagnosis, Management and Secondary Prevention of Acute Rheumatic Fever and Rheumatic Heart Disease. https://assets.heartfoundation.org.nz/documents/shop/marketing/non-stock-resources/diagnosis-management-rheumatic-fever-guideline.pdf?

Henderson, H. T., Canter, C. E., Mahle, W. T., et al. (2012). ABO-incompatible heart transplantation: Analysis of the Pediatric Heart Transplant Study (PHTS) database. The Journal of Heart and Lung Transplantation, 31(2), 173–179.

Hoffman, T. M., Wernovsky, G., Atz, A. M., et al. (2003). Efficacy and safety of milrinone in preventing low cardiac output syndrome in infants and children after corrective surgery for congenital heart disease. Circulation, 107, 996–1002.

Holzer, R. J., Chisolm, J. L., Hill, S. L., et al. (2008). Stenting complex aortic arch obstructions. Catheterisation and Cardiovascular Interventions, 71(3), 375–382.

Holzer, R. J., & Hijazi, Z. M. (2016). Transcatheter pulmonary valve replacement: State of the art. Catheterisation and Cardiovascular Interventions, 87(1), 117–128.

Innes-Hughes, C., Hebden, L., King, L., et al. (2012). Green and amber foods: the nutritional content of food and beverages registered for sale in New South Wales school canteens with Healthy Kids Association. (Report). Nutrition & Dietetics: The Journal of the Dietitians Association of Australia, *69*(2), 111–118.

Jacobs, R., Boyd, L., Brennan, K., et al. (2016). The importance of social media for patients and families affected by congenital anomalies: A Facebook cross-sectional analysis and user survey. Journal of Pediatric Surgery, 51, 1766–1771.

Jacobs, J. P., Mavroudis, C., Jacobs, M. L., et al. (2004). Lessons learned from the data analysis of the second harvest (1998-2001) of the Society of Thoracic Surgeons (STS) Congenital Heart Surgery Database. European Journal of Cardio-thoracic Surgery, 26(1), 18–37.

Kato, H., Ichinose, E., & Kawasaki, T. (1986). Myocardial infarction in Kawasaki disease: Clinical analysis in 195 cases. The Journal of Pediatrics, 108(6), 923–927.

Kavey, R. W., Allada, V., Daniels, S. R., et al. (2006). Cardiovascular risk reduction in high-risk pediatric patients: A scientific statement for the American Heart Association expert panel on population and prevention science. Circulation, 114, 2710–2738.

Khairy, P., Clair, M., Fernandes, S. M., et al. (2013). Cardiovascular outcomes after the arterial switch operation for D-transposition of the great arteries. Circulation, 127(3), 331–339.

Kimberlin, D. W., Long, S. S., Brady, M. T., et al. (2015). Kawasaki disease. In 2015 Red Book: Report of the committee on infectious diseases (30th ed.). Elk Grove Village, IL: American Academy of Pediatrics.

Ko, J. K., Deal, B. J., Strasburger, J. F., et al. (1992). Supraventricular tachycardia mechanisms and their age. American Journal of Cardiology, 69(12), 1028.

Kusters, D. M., Wiegman, A., Kastelein, J. J., et al. (2014). Carotid-intima thickness in children with familial hypercholesterolemia. Circulation Research, 114, 307–310.

LeRoy, S. S., Elixson, E. M., O'Brien, P., et al. (2003). Recommendations for preparing children and adolescents for invasive cardiac procedures: A statement from the American Heart Association Pediatric Nursing Subcommittee of the Council on Cardiovascular Nursing in collaboration with the Council on Cardiovascular Diseases of the Young. Circulation, 108, 2550–2564.

Levy, D. J., Pretorius, D. H., Rothman, A., et al. (2013). Improved prenatal detection of congenital heart disease in an integrated health care system. Pediatric Cardiology, 34(3), 670–679.

Li, J. S., Sexton, D. J., Mick, N., et al. (2000). Proposed modifications to the Duke criteria for the diagnosis of infective endocarditis. Clinical Infectious Diseases, 30(4), 633–638.

Maguire, G. P., Carapetis, J. R., Walsh, W. F., et al. (2012). The future of acute rheumatic fever and rheumatic heart disease in Australia. Medical Journal of Australia, *197*(3), 133–134. https://doi.org/10.5694/mja12.10980

Majnemer, A., Limperopoulos, C., Shevell, M. I., et al. (2009). A new look at outcomes of infants with congenital heart disease. Pediatric Neurology, 40, 197–204.

Marijon, E., Mirabel, M., Celermajer, D. S., et al. (2012). Rheumatic heart disease. Lancet, 379, 953–964.

Mattoo, T. K. (2017). Evaluation of hypertension in children and adolescents, UpToDate. https://www.uptodate.com/contents/evaluation-of-hypertension-in-children-and-adolescents.

McCrindle, B. W., Rowley, A. H., Newburger, J. W., et al. (2017). Diagnosis, treatment, and long-term management of Kawasaki Disease: A scientific statement of health professionals from the American Heart Association. Circulation, 135, 1379–1381.

McCrindle, B. W., Urbina, E. M., Dennison, B. A., et al. (2007). Drug Therapy of High-Risk Lipid Abnormalities in Children and Adolescents, Circulation, 115(14), 1948–1967.

McKivett, A., Paul, D., & Hudson, N. (2019). Healing conversations: developing a practical framework for clinical communication between Aboriginal communities and healthcare practitioners. Journal of Immigrant and Minority Health, 21(3), 596–605. doi:10.1007/s10903-018-0793-7

Menasche, C. C., DuPlessis, A. J., Wessel, D. L., et al. (2002). Current incidence of acute neurological complications after open heart operations in children. The Annals of Thoracic Surgery, 73, 1752–1758.

Mery, C. M., Guzmán-Pruneda, F. A., Trost, J. G., et al. (2015). Contemporary results of aortic coarctation repair through left thoracotomy. The Annals of Thoracic Surgery, 100(3), 1039–1046.

Ministry of Health (2020). Immunisation Handbook. Wellington: Ministry of Health. https://www.health.govt.nz/our-work/immunisation-handbook-2020/

Ministry of Health. (2017). Annual Update of Key Results 2016/17: New Zealand Health Survey. https://www.health.govt.nz/publication/annual-update-key-results-2016-17-new-zealand-health-survey

Moffett, B. S., & Chang, A. C. (2006). Future pharmacologic agents for treatment of heart failure in children. Pediatric Cardiology, 27, 533–551.

Moore, J., Hegde, S., El-Said, H., et al. (2013). Transcatheter device closure of atrial septal defects: A safety review. JACC. Cardiovascular Interventions, 6(5), 433–442.

National Heart, Lung, and Blood Institute. (2011). Expert panel on integrated guidelines for cardiovascular health and risk reduction in children and adolescents: Summary report. Pediatrics, 128(Suppl. 5), S213–S256.

National High Blood Pressure Education Program (NHBPEP) Working Group on High Blood Pressure in Children and Adolescents. (2004). The Fourth Report on the Diagnosis, Evaluation, and Treatment of High Blood Pressure in Children and Adolescents. Pediatrics. 114(2), 555–576.

Newburger, J. W., de Ferranti, S. D., & Fulton, D. R. (2016). Cardiovascular sequelae of Kawasaki disease. UpToDate. http://www.uptodate.com/contents/cardiovascular-sequelae-of-kawasaki-disease.

Newburger, J. W., Takahashi, M., Gerber, M. A., et al. (2004). Diagnosis, treatment, and long-term management of Kawasaki disease: A statement for health professionals from the Committee on Rheumatic Fever, Endocarditis, and Kawasaki Disease, Council on Cardiovascular Disease in the Young, American Heart Association. Circulation, 110(17), 2747–2771.

Park, M. K. (2014). Pediatric cardiology for practitioners (6th ed.). Philadelphia, PA: Elsevier/Saunders.

Pennock, V., Bell, A., Moxon, T., et al. (2014). Retrospective epidemiology of acute rheumatic fever: a 10-year review in the Waikato District Health Board area of New Zealand. The New Zealand Medical Journal (Online), 127(1393), 26–37.

Pincus, M. (2016). Management of digoxin toxicity. Australian Prescriber, 39(1), 18–20. https://doi.org/10.18773/austprescr.2016.006

Remond, M. G., Coyle, M. E., Mills, J. E., et al. (2016). Approaches to improving adherence to secondary prophylaxis for rheumatic fever and rheumatic heart disease: A literature review with global perspective. Cardiology in Review, 24(2), 94–98.

Remond, M., Wheaton, G., Walsh, W., et al. (2012). Acute rheumatic fever and rheumatic heart disease-priorities in prevention, diagnosis and management. A Report of the CSANZ Indigenous Cardiovascular Health Conference, Alice Springs 2011. Heart Lung and Circulation, 21(10), 632–638. doi:10.1016/j.hlc.2012.05.006

RHDAustralia (ARF/RHD writing group). (2020). The 2020 Australian guideline for prevention, diagnosis and management of acute rheumatic fever and rheumatic heart disease (3rd ed.). https://www.rhdaustralia.org.au/system/files/fileuploads/arf_rhd_guidelines_3rd_edition_web_updated.pdf

Rosenthal, D., Chrisant, M. R., Edens, E., et al. (2004). International Society for Heart and Lung Transplantation: Practice guidelines for management of heart failure in children. The Journal of Heart and Lung Transplantation, 23, 1313–1333.

Ross, R. D. (2012). The Ross classification for heart failure in children after 25 years: A review and age stratified revision. Pediatric Cardiology, 33, 1295.

Rossano, J. W., & Shaddy, R. E. (2014). Heart failure in children: Aetiology and treatment. The Journal of Pediatrics, 165(2), 228–233.

Russell, H. M., Pasquali, S. K., Jacobs, J. P., et al. (2012). Outcomes of repair of common arterial trunk with truncal valve surgery: A review of the Society of Thoracic Surgeons congenital heart surgery database. The Annals of Thoracic Surgery, 93(1), 164–169.

Siffel, C., Riehle-Colarusso, T., Oster, M. E., et al. (2015). Survival of children with hypoplastic left heart syndrome. Pediatrics, 136(4), e864–e870.

Smith, P. A. (2001). Primary care in children with congenital heart disease. Journal of Pediatric Nursing, 16, 308–319.

Spirito, P., Autore, C., Rapezzi, C., et al. (2009). Syncope and risk of sudden death in hypertrophic cardiomyopathy. Circulation, 1109, 1703–1710.

St Louis, J. D., Jodhka, U., Jacobs, J. P., et al. (2014). Contemporary outcomes of complete atrioventricular septal defect repair: Analysis of the Society of Thoracic Surgeons congenital heart surgery database. The Journal of Thoracic and Cardiovascular Surgery, 148(6), 2526–2531.

Steer, A., & Gibofsky, A. (2017). Acute rheumatic fever: clinical manifestations and diagnosis. UpToDate. https://www.uptodate.com/contents/acute-rheumatic-fever-clinical-manifestations-and-diagnosis.

Tremoulet, A. H., Best, B. M., Song, S., et al. (2008). Resistance to intravenous immunoglobulin in children with Kawasaki disease. The Journal of Pediatrics, 153(1), 117–121.

Urschel, S. (2021). Clinical outcomes of children receiving ABO-incompatible versus ABO-compatible heart transplantation: a multicentre cohort study. The Lancet Child & Adolescent Health. https://doi.org/10.1016/S2352-4642(21)00023-7

Vick, G. W., & Bezold, L. I. (2017). Classification of atrial septal defects (ASDs), and clinical features and diagnosis of isolated ASDs in children, UpToDate. http://www.uptodate.com/contents/classification-of-atrial-septal-defects-asds-and-clinical-features-and-diagnosis-of-isolated-asds-in-children.

Watts, G. F., Gidding, S., Wierzbicki, A. S., et al. (2014). Integrated guidance on the care of familial hypercholesterolemia from the International FH Foundation. Journal of Clinical Lipidology, 8(2), 148–172.

Wilder, M. S., Palinkas, L. A., Kao, A. S., et al. (2007). Delayed diagnosis by physicians contributes to the development of coronary artery aneurysms in children with Kawasaki syndrome. Pediatric Infectious Disease, 26(3), 256–260.

Wypij, D., Newberger, J. W., Rappaport, L. A., et al. (2003). The effect of duration of deep hypothermic circulatory arrest in infant heart surgery on late neurodevelopment: The Boston Circulatory Arrest Trial. The Journal of Thoracic and Cardiovascular Surgery, 126, 1397–1403.

Zachariah, J. P., & de Ferranti, S. D. (2013). NHLBI integrated pediatric guidelines: Battle for a future free of cardiovascular disease. Future Cardiology, 9(1), 13–22.

28

The Child with Haematological or Immunological Dysfunction

Julia Laing

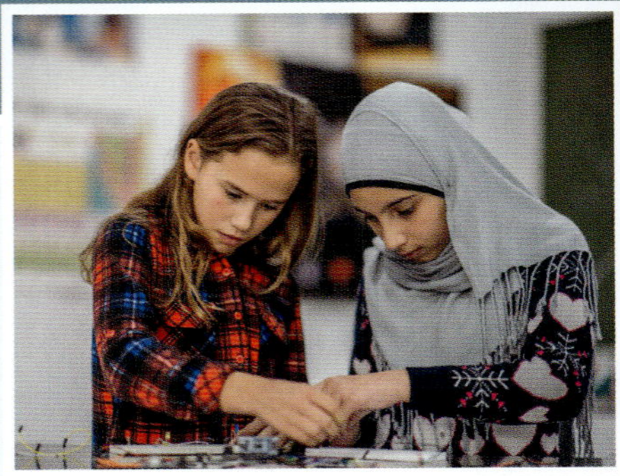

LEARNING OBJECTIVES

- To gain an understanding of some common disorders of the blood and immune system prevalent in children, including the pathophysiology, some possible causes, treatment and key nursing management issues

THE HAEMATOLOGICAL SYSTEM AND ITS FUNCTION

Origin of Formed Elements

Blood is composed of a fluid portion called plasma and a cellular portion known as the formed elements of the blood. The two components are approximately equal in volume. Plasma is about 90% water and 10% solutes. The principal solutes are albumin, electrolytes and proteins. Among the proteins are clotting factors, globulins, circulating antibodies and fibrinogen. The cellular elements sequentially develop into mature red blood cells (RBCs, erythrocytes), white blood cells (WBCs, leucocytes) and platelets (thrombocytes).

The major haematopoietic (blood-forming) organs of the body are the red bone marrow (myeloid tissue) and the lymphatic system, which consists of lymph (fluid), lymphatic vessels and lymphoid structures (the lymph nodes, spleen, thymus and tonsils). Although the lymphatic system plays an important role in regulating blood cells, the lymph vessels and fluids do not produce cells. The lymph nodes regulate the manufacture of WBCs. The spleen and liver are the primary organs for haematopoiesis in the young fetus and for cell removal in postnatal life. **Macrophages** (formerly called *reticular cells*) are cells of mesodermal origin that are widely dispersed in the lining of the vascular and lymph channels. Macrophages form a network and are capable of **phagocytosis** (ingestion and digestion of foreign substances); formation of immune bodies; and differentiation into other cells, such as haemocytoblasts, myeloblasts and lymphoblasts.

All of the formed elements of the blood, except to some extent the agranulocytes, are produced in myeloid tissue during postnatal life. During embryonic development the mesenchyme, spleen, liver, thymus and yolk sac serve as additional sites of blood cell formation. In individuals with certain blood disorders, these sites, particularly the spleen, can be stimulated to produce blood cells and constitute extramedullary haematopoiesis. In infants and young children all of the bone contains red marrow (so-called because of its colour from the formation of erythrocytes), but as bone growth ceases near the end of adolescence, only the ribs, sternum, vertebrae and pelvis continue to produce blood cells. The remainder of the bone marrow becomes yellow from deposition of fat. However, in conditions of increased demand for blood cells, the yellow marrow can revert to red marrow and become another haematopoietic source.

Although the progressive development of each blood cell is fairly well delineated, there is considerable controversy regarding the origin of the blood cell. One of the most widely held theories (monophyletic theory) is that each blood cell originates from a primordial (primitive) cell called a blast, or totipotential stem cell, which has the ability to self-replicate and transform into all the blood components.

The second-generation stem cell, called the pluripotent stem cell, is committed to produce erythroblast, myeloblast, monoblast, lymphoblast or megakaryoblast. The blast cells sequentially develop into mature RBCs (erythrocytes), WBCs (leucocytes), platelets (thrombocytes) and other cells (such as mast cells and macrophages) (see Fig 28.1).

Red Blood Cells (Erythrocytes)

The erythrocyte is formed from the haemocytoblast in the red bone marrow. The pluripotential stem cell forms the proerythroblast. The initial cell of this series has a deep blue–staining (basophilic) cytoplasm and therefore is called a basophilic erythroblast. The chief change in the erythroblast is accumulation of haemoglobin in the cytoplasm. As the basophilic material decreases and the amount of haemoglobin increases, the cell comes to be called a polychromatic erythroblast, which describes its mixture of staining properties. At the same time that the nucleus decreases in size, the basophilic material disappears, so the cell is uniformly stained by eosin dye—hence the name *orthochromatic erythroblast* or *normoblast.* Finally, the normoblast completely loses its nucleus by a process of extrusion as it squeezes through the pores of the membrane into the capillary. Because of the loss of its nucleus, the cell caves in on both sides, which gives the mature erythrocyte its characteristic appearance as a biconcave disc. During each of these stages the different cells continue to undergo mitosis so that increasingly greater numbers of cells are produced. Because the mature RBC does not have a nucleus, it is unable to multiply.

The reticulocyte is the last stage of development before the mature erythrocyte. Reticulocytes are slightly larger than erythrocytes and their presence indicates active RBC production (**erythropoiesis**). Ordinarily the total proportion of circulating reticulocytes is between

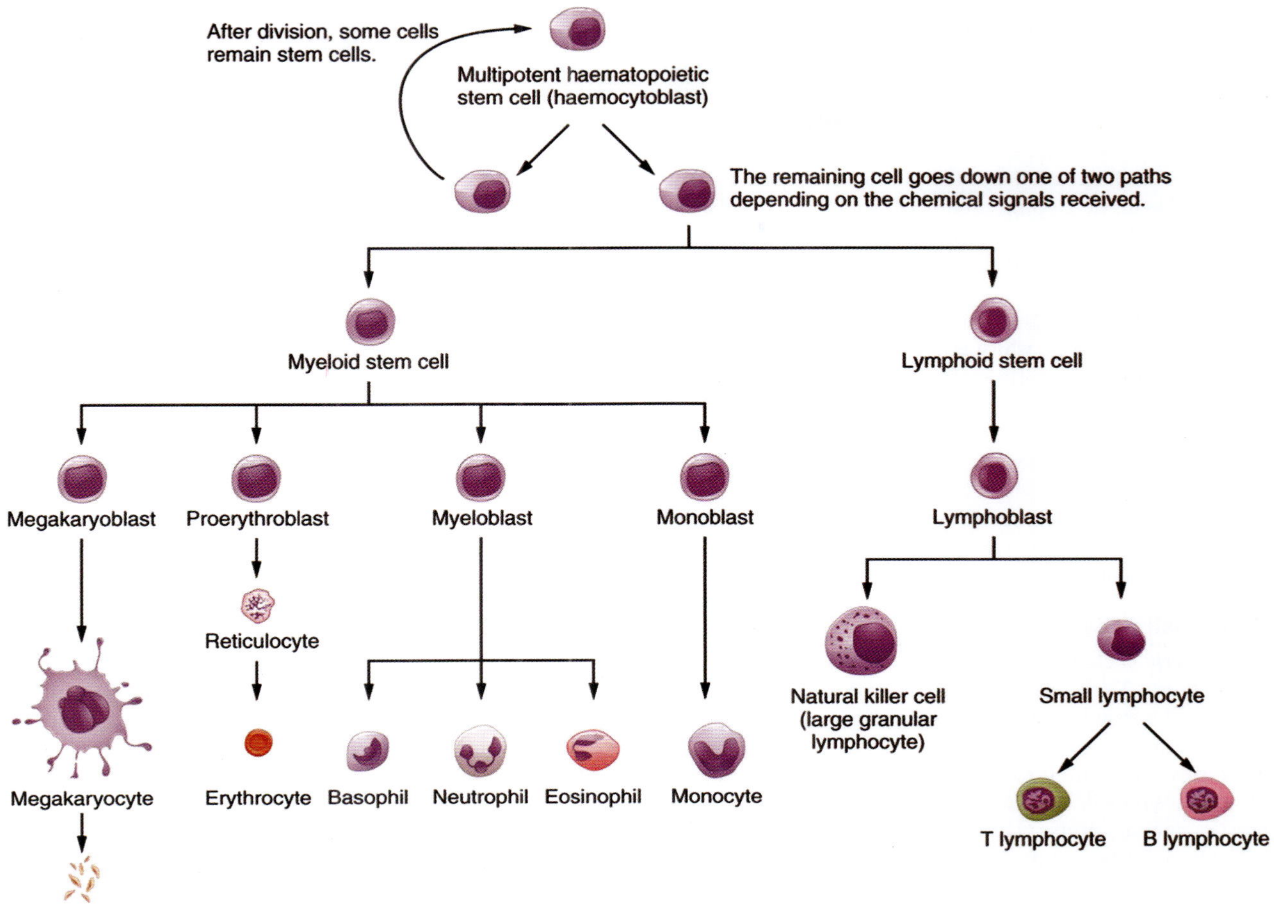

Fig 28.1 Blood cell maturation. (Source: https://courses.lumenlearning.com/suny-ap2/chapter/production-of-the-formed-elements/)

0.5% and 1.5%. The reticulocyte, or 'retic', count is a simple laboratory test frequently used to indirectly analyse haematopoiesis.

Regulation of Erythrocyte Production. The usual life span of the mature erythrocyte is 120 days. Apparently, as RBCs grow old, their membranes become fragile and eventually rupture. The contents of the cell fragment as they circulate through the blood vessels and are phagocytised by the macrophages in the spleen, liver and bone marrow. The haemoglobin is broken down into the iron-containing pigment haemosiderin and the bile pigments biliverdin and bilirubin. Most of the iron is reused by the bone marrow for production of new RBCs or stored in the liver and other tissues for future use. The bile pigments are excreted by the liver in bile.

Normally there is a homeostatic balance between RBC production and destruction. This balance ensures adequate tissue oxygenation and a blood viscosity that allows the blood to flow freely through the vessels. The basic regulator of erythrocyte production is tissue oxygenation and renal production of erythropoietin (also called erythropoietic stimulating factor). In states of tissue hypoxia, the kidney releases erythropoietin into the bloodstream. As a result the bone marrow is stimulated to produce new RBCs. The major activity seems to be an increase in both maturation rate and mitosis at all stages of erythrocyte production but primarily at the stem cell level.

During this rapid increase in RBC production, the circulating erythrocytes may not be totally mature. Consequently, the number of reticulocytes may increase dramatically (as high as 30% or more of the total RBC count). Even normoblasts or nucleated RBCs may appear in the blood. A failure of this rise in erythrocyte and reticulocyte count to occur may indicate bone marrow failure.

Once tissue oxygenation is adequate, the production of erythropoietin ceases. Thus tissue oxygen requirements control both the stimulation and the termination of erythrocyte production. Note that the basic regulatory mechanism is the ability of RBCs to transport oxygen to the tissues in response to their needs, not the circulating numbers of erythrocytes. Oxygen transport depends on both the number of circulating RBCs and the amount of normal haemoglobin in the cell. This explains why **polycythaemia** (increase in the number of erythrocytes) occurs in conditions characterised by prolonged tissue hypoxia, such as cyanotic heart defects. (See Chapter 27.) If the circulating numbers of erythrocytes controlled erythropoietin release, this feedback mechanism would maintain erythrocyte production at a constant level (4.5 to 5.5 million/mm^3 of blood) regardless of existing tissue hypoxia.

Functions of Erythrocytes. The major function of RBCs is to transport haemoglobin, which in turn carries oxygen to all cells of the body. However, erythrocytes have other significant functions: they contain carbonic anhydrase, an enzyme that catalyses the reaction between carbon dioxide and water, which allows large quantities of carbon dioxide to react with blood for transportation to the lungs, and the haemoglobin, a protein, serves as an acid–base buffer, which, in combination with carbon dioxide, maintains the blood pH at a constant level.

Haemoglobin

Haemoglobin is a complex molecule composed of four globin chains. The type of haemoglobin in the cells depends on both the stage of life and the presence of any abnormalities in the genes that regulate the production of haemoglobin. Fetal haemoglobin, composed of two alpha and two gamma chains, has a greater affinity for oxygen and is best suited to the fetal environment. During the latter part of pregnancy, the fetus begins developing adult haemoglobin (two alpha and two beta chains). When a defect in haemoglobin synthesis is present (e.g. sickle cell disease [SCD] or thalassaemia), fetal haemoglobin may be produced into adulthood.

Several tests offer important information about haemoglobin (Table 28.1). The haematocrit, which is approximately three times the concentration of haemoglobin (in grams per decilitre), indicates the percentage volume of circulating packed RBCs in the total blood. Under normal conditions, haemoglobin and the haematocrit are in a fixed relationship with each other and vary according to the child's age and sex (Lerner 2016).

RBC indices are based on ratios of packed RBC volume, haemoglobin concentration and RBC count, and they are a useful way of designating different types of anaemias (Fig 28.1).

White Blood Cells (Leucocytes)

The term *leucocyte* encompasses a number of cells with similar yet distinct functions. They are divided into two major classes—granulocytes and agranulocytes—based on the presence or absence, respectively, of granules within the cytoplasm of the cells.

Granulocytes. There are three types of granulocytes: neutrophils, basophils and eosinophils. The name of each of these refers to the characteristic staining property of the granule during laboratory analysis. Neutrophils stain neutral to the dyes, whereas basophils stain purple to the basic methylene blue dye, and eosinophils take on a red colour from acidic eosin dye. Because the nuclei of neutrophils have two or more lobules that are connected by fine chromatin strands, the term **polymorphonuclear leucocytes** (cells with many-formed nuclei), or simply *polys,* or *segs* (segmented or mature neutrophils) and *bands* (immature neutrophils with the nuclei connected) may be used collectively to refer to the neutrophils.

The granulocytes, like erythrocytes, are produced in the bone marrow. For this reason, these cells are sometimes referred to as *myelogenous leucocytes.* These cells, in theory, originate from primitive stem cells, which develop into myeloblasts. The genesis of neutrophils, basophils and eosinophils is similar to the stages observed during erythrocyte production. The differentiation of myeloblasts into various mature WBCs is primarily a result of specialisation within the cytoplasm and degeneration of the nucleus. Unlike erythrocytes, however, all WBCs are nucleated.

Accelerated production of immature granulocytes leads to increased numbers of bands in the peripheral circulation (referred to as a shift to the left in the full blood count [FBC]), which is indicative of a bacterial infection. The absolute neutrophil count (ANC) reflects the body's ability to handle bacterial infections. If the ANC is less than 500/mm^3, a severe risk of infection is present.

Agranulocytes. The agranulocytes include two cell types: monocytes and lymphocytes. Characteristically these cells do not develop granules, and the nuclei are not lobulated. They originate in various lymphogenous organs, and for this reason they are sometimes referred to as **lymphogenous leucocytes.** However, because stem cells and reticular cells are capable of differentiating into monocytes or lymphocytes, the origin of these cells is frequently designated as the *lymphomyeloid complex,* which includes bone marrow, lymph nodes, spleen, liver, thymus, subepithelial lymphoid tissue (tonsils, vermiform appendix and intestinal lymphoid tissues) and connective tissues (mesenchymal cells of the reticuloendothelial system).

The monocytes follow the same sequence of development from the stem cell as the granulocytes. The monocytes in turn have the ability to exit the vessels and develop into macrophages, large cells that are highly effective phagocytes. Kupffer cells are macrophages located in the liver. Histiocytes are macrophages in the connective tissue. These names are remnants of the old reticular endothelial system designations.

Lymphocytopoiesis (lymphocyte formation) takes place anywhere in the lymphomyeloid complex. Lymphocytes develop from blast (stem) cells. The lymphocyte has the potential to develop into other cells, such as T-cells or B-cells (see p. 753).

Regulation of Leucocyte Production. The exact life span of the leucocytes is not as clearly defined as that of the erythrocytes because they exist in the circulation primarily for transport to extravascular areas, where they reside in reservoirs or where they are needed to resist infection. Therefore, their survival rate is described in terms of three phases: (1) the haematopoietic phase, extending from the development of the blast cell to the delivery of the mature leucocyte into the circulation; (2) the intravascular phase, the period within the circulation; and (3) the extravascular phase, the time spent in the viscera or tissues.

Granulocytes have a half-life of 6 to 8 hours in the blood and, after entering the tissues, die over a period of 4 to 5 days. Agranulocytes live for an extended period because they remain in inflamed tissue areas longer than the granulocytes. Monocytes wander back and forth between the blood and tissues and are capable of becoming macrophages; their half-life in the blood is 8 to 10 hours, but their half-life in the tissue is 60 to 90 days.

The regulation of leucocytes is based on the body's need for them. Tissue damage from bacterial or viral agents promotes leucocyte circulation and production. However, **leucocytosis** (increase in leucocytes) results from tissue destruction from almost any source, such as haemorrhage, neoplastic disease, toxicity, operative procedures, chemical and thermal injury and tissue ischaemia.

The leucocytes probably die as a result of their activity at the site of injury and are phagocytised by other newly formed WBCs. Effective control of the inflammatory process with subsequent tissue recovery most likely results in feedback to the bone marrow and causes lymphogenous organs to cease increased production of WBCs.

Functions of Leucocytes. Although all of the leucocytes play some role in the immune process, each of the WBCs has a specific role. Neutrophils and monocytes are effective phagocytes and as a result are primarily involved in inflammatory reactions. **Neutrophilia** (increased numbers of neutrophils) is most evident in an acute inflammation, whereas **monocytosis** (increased numbers of monocytes) is more evident in chronic conditions. The reason is that as the affected area becomes acidic from tissue necrosis, neutrophils, which prefer a neutral environment, become less efficient, and monocytes, which become macrophages, become more powerful. These cells also increase in number during chronic inflammation. The other functions of lymphocytes in terms of the immune process are discussed on p. 778.

The function of eosinophils is still not completely known. They seem to have parasiticidal properties because they can selectively destroy parasites. They may also function in the immediate type of allergic or anaphylactic hypersensitivity reaction because **eosinophilia** (increased numbers of eosinophils) is well documented in such conditions. Eosinophils also are thought to release a substance called profibrinolysin, which, when activated to form fibrinolysin, digests fibrin and thereby helps dissolve a clot.

The function of basophils is also not completely understood, although **basophilia** (increased numbers of basophils) occurs during

TABLE 28.1 **Tests Performed as Part of a Full Blood Count**

Test (Average Value)	Description, Comments
Red blood cell (RBC) count (4.5–5.5 million/mm³)	Number of RBCs/mm³ of blood
	Indirectly estimates Hgb content of blood
	Reflects function of bone marrow
Haemoglobin (Hgb) determination (11.5–15.5 g/L)	Amount of Hgb (g)/L of whole blood
	Total blood Hgb primarily depends on number of circulating RBCs but also on amount of Hgb in each cell
Haematocrit (Hct) (35%–45%)	Per cent volume of packed RBCs in whole blood
	Indirectly measures Hgb content
	Is approximately three times Hgb content
RBC volume distribution width (RDW) (13.4% ± 1.2%)	Average size of RBCs
	Differentiates some types of anaemia
Reticulocyte count (0.5%–1.5% erythrocytes)	Per cent reticulocytes in RBCs
	Index of production of mature RBCs by bone marrow
	Decreased count indicates depressed bone marrow function
	Increased count indicates erythrogenesis in response to some stimulus
	When reticulocyte count is extremely high, other forms of immature RBCs (normoblasts, even erythroblasts) may be present
	Indirectly estimates hypochromic anaemia
	Usually elevated in patients with chronic haemolytic anaemia
WBC count (4.5–13.5 × 10³ cells/mm³)	Number of WBCs/mm³ of blood
	Total number of WBCs less important than differential count
Differential WBC count	Inspection and quantification of WBC types present in peripheral blood
	Values are expressed as percentages; to obtain absolute number of any type of WBC, multiply its respective percentage by total number of WBCs
Neutrophils (polys) (54%–62%) (3–5.8 × 10³ cells/mm³)	Primary defence in bacterial infection; capable of phagocytising and killing bacteria
Bands (3%–5%) (0.15–0.4 × 10³ cells/mm³)	Immature neutrophil
	Increased numbers in bacterial infection
	Also capable of phagocytosis and killing
Eosinophils (1%–3%) (0.05–0.25 × 10³ cells/mm³)	Named for their staining characteristics with eosin dye
	Increased in allergic disorders, parasitic diseases, certain neoplasms and other diseases
Basophils (0.075%) (0.015–0.030 × 10³ cells/mm³)	Named for their characteristic basophilic stippling
	Contain histamine, heparin and serotonin; believed to cause increased blood flow to injured tissues while preventing excessive clotting
Lymphocytes (25%–33%) (1.5–3.0 × 10³ cells/mm³)	Involved in development of antibody and delayed hypersensitivity
Monocytes (3%–7%)	Large phagocytic cells that are involved in early stage of inflammatory reaction
ANC (> 1000/mm³)	Per cent neutrophils/bands times WBC count
	Indicates body's capability to handle bacterial infections
Platelet count (150–400 × 10³/mm³)	Number of platelets/mm³ of blood
	Cellular fragments that are necessary for clotting to occur
Stained peripheral blood smear	Visual estimation of amount of Hgb in RBCs and overall size, shape and structure of RBCs
	Various staining properties of RBC structures may be evidence of immature forms of erythrocytes
	Shows variation in size and shape of RBCs: microcytic, macrocytic, poikilocytic (variable shapes)

ANC, Absolute neutrophil count; *Hct*, haematocrit; *Hgb*, haemoglobin; *MCH*, mean corpuscular haemoglobin; *MCHC*, mean corpuscular haemoglobin concentration; *MCV*, mean corpuscular volume; *RBC*, red blood cell; *WBC*, white blood cell.

the healing phase of inflammation and during prolonged inflammation. Basophils in the blood exit the vessels and become mast cells in the tissue. They are responsible for histamine release, which results in increased permeability of the vessels to allow WBCs to exit the vessels at the site of injury.

Platelets

Platelets are actually small fragments of megakaryocytes. They are smaller than blood cells, do not possess a cellular structure and consist of a clear substance containing granules. Platelets originate from part of the myelogenous group of WBCs. Platelets are formed when the megakaryocytic membrane invaginates, fuses within the cell to separate the cytoplasm and then fragments.

Regulation of Platelet Production. The life span of platelets is estimated as 8 to 10 days. Apparently, the body regulates platelet levels to maintain a fairly constant level (between 150,000 and 400,000/mm^3). Platelet production is probably regulated by a hormone, thrombopoietin, but the source and mode of action of this substance are unknown. Old platelets are most likely removed by the liver and spleen.

Function of Platelets. The term **thrombocyte** means 'clot' *(thrombo)* and 'cell' *(cyte)* and accurately describes the main function of platelets. When there is a break in the continuity of a blood vessel, the platelets, which are normally flat and round or oval, come in contact with the wet vessel surface and dramatically change their shape to become swollen spheres with long, irregular projections called pseudopodia (false feet). As a result, the platelets begin to adhere to the wet endothelium and to one another. The first platelets at the site of injury release substances that attract other thrombocytes to the area. This causes a layering of platelets, which eventually forms a plug. This plug is large enough to partially or totally occlude the opening in the vessel wall but small enough to allow blood flow to continue unimpaired through the vessel.

In small vessel tears the platelet plug is sufficient to produce haemostasis, and additional blood coagulation is not necessary. When platelet counts are low, however, these numerous small ruptures, which occur continually in the body as a result of general functioning, are not repaired. Consequently, small haemorrhagic areas called **petechiae** form under the skin. They are similar in appearance to reddish freckles or tiny spiderwebs.

Platelets also influence haemostasis by releasing a substance called serotonin at the site of injury. Serotonin is a vasoconstrictor that produces vascular spasm to decrease the blood flow to the injured area.

Assessment of Haematological Function

Several tests assess haematological function, and additional procedures can identify the cause of the dysfunction. The following discussion is limited to a description of the most common and one of the most valuable tests, the FBC. Other procedures, such as those related to iron, coagulation and immune status, are discussed throughout the chapter as appropriate.

The history and physical examination are essential to the identification of haematological dysfunction, and the nurse is often the first person to suspect a problem based on information from these sources. Comments by the parent regarding the child's lack of energy, food diary showing decreased sources of iron, frequent infections and bleeding that is difficult to control offer clues to the more common disorders affecting the blood. A careful physical appraisal can reveal findings such as persistent fatigue, pallor, petechiae or bruising that may indicate minor or serious haematological conditions. Nurses need to be aware of the clinical manifestations of blood diseases to assist in recognising symptoms and establishing a diagnosis.

RED BLOOD CELL DISORDERS

Anaemia

Anaemia is a reduction in RBCs mass and/or haemoglobin concentration compared with normal values for age (Brugnara et al 2015, Lerner 2016). The anaemias are the most common haematological disorders of infancy and childhood and are not diseases but manifestations of underlying pathological processes (see Fig 28.2).

Classification

The anaemias can be classified using two basic approaches: aetiology as manifested by erythrocyte or haemoglobin depletion and morphology, the characteristic changes in RBC size, shape and colour.

Although the morphological classification is useful in the laboratory evaluation of anaemia, the aetiology provides direction for planning nursing care. For example, anaemia with reduced haemoglobin concentration may be caused by a dietary depletion of iron, and the principal intervention is replenishing iron stores.

The main causes of anaemia are inadequate production of RBCs or RBC components, increased destruction of RBCs and excessive loss of RBCs through haemorrhage. Each of these factors affects the amount of haemoglobin that is available to carry oxygen to the cells.

Pathophysiology and Clinical Manifestations

The basic physiological defect caused by anaemia is a decrease in the oxygen-carrying capacity of blood and consequently a reduction in the amount of oxygen available to the cells. When the anaemia has developed slowly, the child usually adapts to the declining haemoglobin level. Most children seem to have a remarkable ability to function well despite low levels of haemoglobin. Also, compensatory mechanisms such as a shift in the oxyhaemoglobin dissociation curve may delay the development of any obvious signs.

When the haemoglobin level falls sufficiently to produce clinical manifestations, the signs and symptoms (e.g. weakness, fatigue and a waxy pallor in severe anaemia) are due to tissue hypoxia (Box 28.1). Cyanosis, which results from an increased quantity of deoxygenated haemoglobin in arterial blood, is typically not evident. Anaemia is caused by decreased levels of haemoglobin or RBCs, not inadequate oxygen saturation of existing haemoglobin.

Central nervous system manifestations include headache, dizziness, light-headedness, irritability, slowed thought processes, decreased attention span, apathy and depression. Growth retardation resulting from decreased cellular metabolism, and coexisting anorexia is a common finding in chronic severe anaemia. It is frequently accompanied by delayed sexual maturation in the older child.

The effects of anaemia on the circulatory system can be profound. A reduction in haemoglobin concentration that results in decreased oxygen-carrying capacity of the blood is associated with a compensatory increase in heart rate and cardiac output (see Box 28.1). Initially this greater cardiac output compensates for the lower oxygen-carrying capacity of the blood because blood replenished with oxygen returns to the tissues at a faster than normal rate. The increased circulation and turbulence within the heart may produce a heart murmur. Because the cardiac workload increases during exercise, infection or emotional stress, cardiac failure may occur.

Acute or chronic haemorrhage results in loss of plasma and all formed elements of the blood. After acute haemorrhage the body replaces plasma within 1 to 3 days, maintaining blood volume. However, this results in a low concentration of RBCs, which are gradually replaced within 3 to 4 weeks. During this period there is usually a normocytic normochromic anaemia, provided that iron stores are sufficient for haemoglobin synthesis.

In chronic blood loss the actual number of RBCs may be normal because of continuous replacement. However, insufficient iron is available to form haemoglobin as quickly as it is lost. As a result, erythrocytes are usually microcytic and hypochromic.

Diagnostic Evaluation

In general, anaemia may be suspected from findings on the history and physical examination, such as lack of energy, easy fatiguability and pallor. Unless the anaemia is severe, however, another clue to the

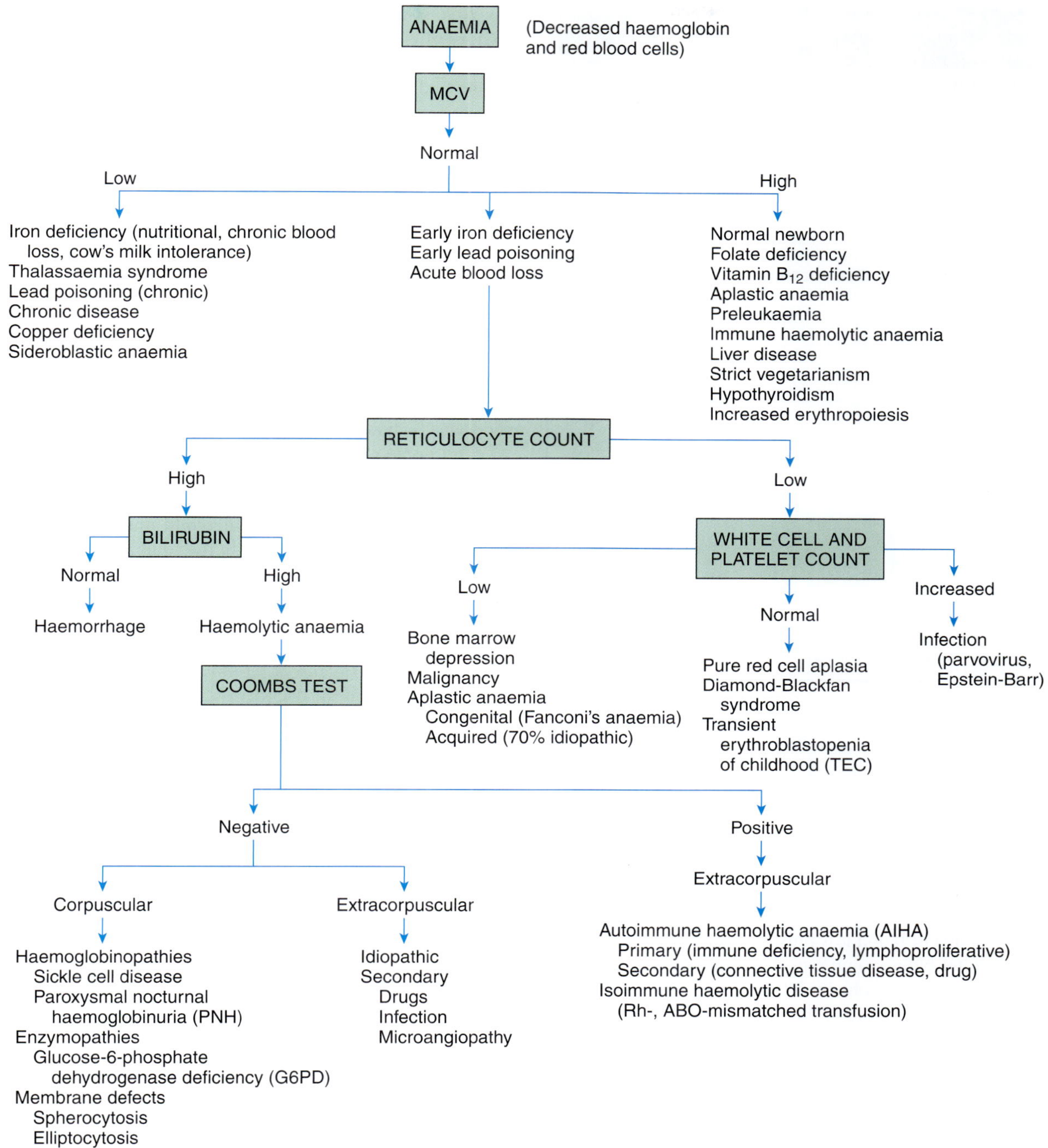

Fig 28.2 Approach to the diagnosis of anaemia by MCV and reticulocyte count. (Source: Modified data from Brugnara, C., Oski, F. A., & Nathan, D. G. (2015). Diagnostic approach to the anemic patient. In S. H. Orkin, D. E. Fisher, D. Ginsburg, et al. (Eds.), Nathan and Oski's hematology of infancy and childhood (8th ed.). Philadelphia, PA: Saunders; Lanzkowsky, P. (2016). Classification and diagnosis of anemia in children. In P. Lanzkowsky, J. M. Lipton, & J. D. Fish: Lanzkowsky's manual of pediatric hematology and oncology (6th ed.). San Diego, CA: Elsevier; Lerner, N. (2016). The anemias. In R. M. Kliegman, B. F. Stanton, J. W. St. Geme III, et al (Eds.), Nelson textbook of pediatrics (20th ed.). Philadelphia, PA: Elsevier.)

disorder may be alterations in the FBC, such as decreased numbers of RBCs and decreased haemoglobin and haematocrit levels.

Various findings of the FBC are also significant, such as increased reticulocyte levels, which indicate the body's response to an increased demand for RBCs. A peripheral smear may demonstrate significant changes in the shape of RBCs, such as sickled cells. Tests to measure the amount of haemoglobin in a single cell are helpful in determining the cause of the anaemia. Sometimes a bone marrow aspiration may be necessary to evaluate the body's ability to produce normal cells. For example, in leukaemia the bone marrow is hyperplastic (producing increased numbers of cells), whereas in aplastic anaemia (see Aplastic Anaemia, later in this chapter) the bone marrow is hypoplastic (producing decreased numbers of cells) or aplastic (producing no cells).

BOX 28.1 Signs and Symptoms of Anaemia

Decreased Red Blood Cell Production
- Pallor
- Tachycardia
- Fatigue, headache
- Muscle weakness
- Systolic heart murmur
- Frontal bossing

Increased Red Blood Cell Destruction
- Icteric sclera, jaundice
- Fatigue, headache
- Tachycardia
- Dark urine
- Splenomegaly
- Hepatomegaly
- Low blood pressure (late sign of shock)

Increased Red Blood Cell Loss
- Pallor
- Fatigue, headache
- Muscle weakness
- Cool skin
- Tachycardia
- Decreased peripheral pulses
- Low blood pressure (late sign of shock)

Tests for haematological function do not always reflect the immediate changes occurring in the blood. For example, in acute massive haemorrhage the haemoglobin and haematocrit values may not be reliable because the plasma volume may not increase for several hours. Without the haemodilution caused by the re-expansion of the vascular space, the haemoglobin and haematocrit may be close to normal, and the RBC loss may not be apparent. Consequently, assessing the quantity of blood loss in a seriously ill child may be difficult. The estimated volume of blood loss must be analysed in conjunction with the child's total blood volume to determine the percentage of blood loss. Blood specimens obtained from central lines may more accurately reflect the patient's status than specimens obtained from an extremity because of the vasoconstriction of the peripheral vasculature. Decreased blood pressure changes are a late sign because of the compensatory mechanisms.

Therapeutic Management

The objective of medical management is to reverse the anaemia by treating the underlying cause. In nutritional anaemias the specific deficiency is corrected. In blood loss from acute haemorrhage, RBC transfusion may be given. In patients with severe anaemia, supportive medical care may include oxygen therapy, bed rest and replacement of intravascular volume with intravenous (IV) fluids. In addition to these general measures, the nurse may implement more specific interventions, depending on the cause. The next sections discuss these interventions.

Nursing Care Management

The physical examination yields valuable evidence regarding the severity of the anaemia and some indication of its possible cause (see Fig 28.1 and Box 28.1). In interviewing the family, the nurse should pay careful attention to the following areas: (1) nutrition, especially if the child is lactose intolerant or has inadequate intake of iron; (2) past history of chronic, recurrent infection; (3) eating habits, particularly pica (consumption of non-nutritive substances such as dirt, starch, lead-based paint chips, paper); (4) bowel habits and presence of frank blood in stools or black, tarry stools as a result of chronic blood loss; and (5) familial history of hereditary diseases, such as SCD or thalassaemia.

The nurse should also be aware of the importance of taking a thorough history to obtain pertinent information that may aid in identifying the cause of the anaemia. For example, statements such as 'My child drinks a lot of milk' or 'My teenager is on a liquid or vegetarian diet' are clues to possible iron deficiency.

Prepare the Child and Family for Laboratory Tests. Several blood tests may be ordered sequentially. Therefore, the child may undergo multiple finger or heel sticks or venepunctures enduring repeated puncture trauma. These invasive procedures may be better tolerated with the application of a topical anaesthetic such as EMLA (a eutectic mixture of lidocaine [lignocaine] and prilocaine) before needle punctures.

The nurse can support the child in preparing for the tests by: (1) explaining the significance of each test, particularly why the tests are not all done at one time; (2) encouraging parent(s) or another supportive person to be with the child during the procedure; and (3) allowing the child to play with the equipment on a doll or to participate in the actual procedure (e.g. by holding the bandaid).

Older children may appreciate the opportunity to observe the blood cells under a microscope or in photographs. This experience is especially important if a serious blood disorder, such as aplastic anaemia, is suspected because it serves as a foundation for explaining the pathophysiology of the disorder.

Bone marrow aspiration is not a routine haematological test but is essential for definitive diagnosis of the certain anaemias such as severe aplastic anaemia. Bone marrow aspiration is usually done under a short general anaesthetic. (Chapter 22 presents information on preparing the child.)

Assess the child's level of tolerance for activities of daily living and play, and make adjustments to allow as much self-care as possible without undue exertion. During periods of rest the nurse measures vital signs and observes behaviour to establish a baseline of non-exertion energy expenditure. During periods of activity the nurse repeats these measurements and observations to compare them with resting values.

Prevent Complications

Children with anaemia are prone to infection because tissue hypoxia causes cellular dysfunction, and the disturbed metabolic processes weaken the host's defences against foreign agents. Infection also worsens the anaemia by increasing metabolic needs and, in instances of chronic infection, also interferes with erythropoiesis and shortens the survival time of RBCs. Take all of the usual precautions to prevent infection, such as practising thorough handwashing, selecting an appropriate room in a non-infectious area and maintaining adequate nutrition. The nurse also observes for signs of infection, particularly temperature elevation and leucocytosis. However, an elevated WBC count sometimes occurs in anaemia without the presence of systemic or local infection.

Drawing multiple blood samples may present a problem with cumulative blood loss and necessitate blood replacement. This situation occurs most often in infants with severe anaemia. To prevent this situation, blood may be withdrawn through a continuous IV line and replaced after the exact amount needed has been tested and discarded. As a precaution, keep a record of the volume of blood withdrawn. Using micro-methods of testing whenever possible minimises the amount of blood required for the test. The nurse needs to observe for cumulative effects of blood loss, particularly signs of shock and increased hypoxia, and to explain to parents the necessity for taking multiple blood samples and the reason for blood replacement.

The main complication of anaemia is cardiac decompensation, which can result from excessive demands on the heart due to increased metabolic needs or cardiac overload. The nurse should observe for signs and symptoms of heart failure such as tachycardia, dyspnoea, moist respirations, cough and sweating. Obviously, preventing heart failure by minimising hypoxia and closely monitoring IV infusions is of first priority. Packed RBCs are usually administered to prevent circulatory hypervolemia. When blood transfusions are required in severe anaemia to increase the haemoglobin level, follow all of the usual precautions for administering blood and observe for signs of transfusion reactions.

Blood Transfusion Therapy

Technological advances in blood banking and transfusion medicine allow the administration of only the blood component needed by the child, such as packed RBCs in anaemia or platelets for bleeding disorders (Table 28.2). Regardless of the blood component administered, the nurse must be aware of the possibility of transfusion reactions.

Although haemolytic reactions are rare, ABO incompatibility remains the most common cause of death from blood transfusion, and human error is usually responsible (e.g. administration of blood of the wrong type to the patient or mislabelling of a blood product) (Pahuja et al 2017, Strauss 2016). Blood is usually matched between the donor and recipient for blood group (A, B, AB or O) and Rh factor (positive or negative). However, AB-type RBCs can be transfused into individuals with blood types A, B and AB, and Rh-negative RBCs can be given to Rh-positive individuals.

TABLE 28.2 Nursing Administration of Blood Components

Component and Indications	Nursing Administration
Packed red blood cells (PRBCs) Symptomatic anaemia Renal or liver disease Haemolysis Decreased erythropoiesis Splenic or liver sequestration	1. Assess for PRBC reaction (e.g. pruritus, rash, cough, fever). 2. Administer using a microaggreagate filter via an infusion pump at the prescribed rate over 2-4 hours. Do not use the tubing to infuse more than 1 unit of blood. 3. Monitor vital signs as per clinical guidelines usually before transfusion, 15 minutes after initiation, hourly during transfusion and on completion of transfusion. 4. Do not refrigerate blood in the ward/clinical unit. Use only the blood bank refrigerator. 5. Ensure that each unit is infused ≤ 4 hours. If a longer infusion time is needed, the unit must be divided in the blood bank. 6. Do not infuse solutions other than normal saline in the line with RBCs.
Fresh frozen plasma (FFP) Deficiencies of plasma clotting factors in bleeding patients (e.g. disseminated intravascular coagulation [DIC]); liver failure; vitamin K deficiency with bleeding; or replacement of antithrombin III (ATIII), protein C or protein S	1. Assess for FFP reaction (e.g. pain, bleeding, swelling). 2. Administer using a microaggrate filter at the prescribed rate. 3. Monitor prothrombin time (PT) and partial thromboplastin time (PPT) before and after FFP infusion. 4. Monitor levels of other coagulation factors (e.g. fibrinogen, fibrin split products, D-dimer, ATIII, protein C and protein S).
Platelets (plt) Active haemorrhage, DIC Thrombocytopenia with bleeding or if indicated by clinical status	1. Assess for plt reaction (e.g. pruritus, rash, fever, bleeding). 2. Administer using 170-mm microaggrate filter via IV push or over an hour or as fast as the patient can tolerate. 3. Monitor vital signs before transfusion, 15 minutes after initiation and at the end of infusion. 4. Obtain postplatelet count 60 minutes to 24 hours after infusion.
Factor VIII (plasma derived or recombinant) Haemophilia A Acquired factor VIII deficiency	1. Assess adverse reaction (e.g. hives, itchy wheals with redness, tightness in chest, wheezing, low blood pressure or dyspnoea). Notify healthcare provider immediately if symptoms are present. 2. Use reconstituted factor within 3 hours of mixing. 3. Inject reconstituted factor intravenously over 2–5 minutes.
Factor IX (plasma derived or recombinant) Haemophilia B	
FEIBA (factor eight inhibitor bypass activity), plasma derived Haemophilia A or B with inhibitors (antibodies)	
Factor VIIa (recombinant) Haemophilia A or B with inhibitors	

DIC, Disseminated intravascular coagulation; *HIV,* human immunodeficiency virus; *RBC,* red blood cell.

In addition to nursing precautions and responsibilities, other general guidelines that apply to all transfusions include the following.

- Take vital signs, including blood pressure, before administering blood to establish baseline data for intratransfusion and posttransfusion comparison: 15 minutes after initiation, hourly while blood is infusing and on completion of the transfusion.
- Check the blood type and group of the recipient against the donor's, regardless of the blood product used.
- Administer the first 50 mL of blood or initial 20% of volume (whichever is smaller) slowly and stay with the child.
- Administer with normal saline in a piggyback set-up or have normal saline available.
- Administer blood through an appropriate filter to eliminate particles in the blood and prevent the precipitation of formed elements; gently shake the container frequently.
- Use blood within 30 minutes of its arrival from the blood bank. If it is not used, return it to the blood bank; do not store it in a regular unit refrigerator.
- Infuse a unit of blood (or the specified amount) within 4 hours. If the infusion will exceed this time, have the blood divided into appropriate-size quantities by the blood bank, with the unused portion refrigerated under controlled conditions.
- If a reaction of any type is suspected, stop the transfusion, take vital signs, maintain a patent IV line with normal saline and new tubing, notify the practitioner and do not restart the transfusion until the child's condition has been medically evaluated.

ANAEMIA CAUSED BY NUTRITIONAL DEFICIENCIES

Iron Deficiency Anaemia (IDA)

Anaemia caused by an inadequate supply or loss of iron is the most prevalent nutritional disorder worldwide and the most preventable mineral disturbance. Over the past decade, the prevalence of IDA has declined during infancy. The reduced prevalence of IDA in infants has been partly attributed to promotion of iron-fortified formula instead of cow's milk during the first year of life in conjunction with the widespread promotion and use of nutritional supplements for breastfeeding mothers (Fleming 2015, Sills 2016). Adolescents are also at risk for iron deficiency because of their rapid growth rate, menses, poor eating habits, obesity and strenuous activities (Fleming 2015, Sills 2016). However, iron deficiency both with and without anaemia still remains to be a relatively common health problem, especially among at-risk children (Fleming 2015, Mahoney 2017, Miller 2013).

In Australia, the prevalence of anaemia in children under the age of 5 years is about 8%, corresponding to over 100,000 preschool children (National Blood Authority [NBA] 2017).

The prevalence of IDA in children from remote Indigenous communities is high. A retrospective cohort study found that 68% of Indigenous infants from remote northern Australia were anaemic (Bar-Zeeve et al 2013). The Early Childhood Nutrition and Anaemia Prevention Project found that nearly 90% of Indigenous infants and young children were anaemic at least once between 6 months and 2 years of age (Anqunio et al 2013). M ori and Pacific Islander children are also at risk of IDA (Starship 2016). Factors that put children at risk of developing IDA include maternal iron deficiency, late or insufficient introduction of iron-rich solids, increased iron requirements, poor intestinal iron absorption and increased loss of iron due to blood loss (NBA 2017).

Aetiology

IDA can be caused by any number of factors that decrease the supply of iron, impair its absorption, increase the body's need for iron or affect the synthesis of haemoglobin (Box 28.2). Although the clinical manifestations and diagnostic evaluation are similar regardless of the cause, the therapeutic and nursing care management depends on the specific reason for the iron deficiency. The following discussion is limited to IDA resulting from inadequate iron in the diet.

At birth the full-term infant has approximately a 0.5 g supply of iron, and an average of 0.8 mg of iron must be absorbed each day during the first 15 years of life (NBA 2017, Sills 2016). During the last trimester of pregnancy, iron is transferred from the mother to the fetus at the rate of 4 mg/day. Most of the iron is stored in the circulating haemoglobin of the erythrocytes, and the remainder is deposited in the liver, spleen and bone marrow. Along with maternal iron supplements, delayed umbilical clamping for 1 to 3 minutes can improve iron status and reduce the risk of iron deficiency in the newborn (Anderson et al 2014, Mercer et al 2017, Miller 2013, Sills 2016). Maternally derived iron stores are adequate for the first 5 to 6 months in the full-term infant but for only about 2 to 3 months in premature infants or infants of multiple births. If dietary sources of iron are not supplied to meet the infant's growth demands after depletion of fetal iron stores, IDA results. Physiological anaemia should not be confused with IDA resulting from nutritional causes.

Vegetarian or vegan diets have been associated with nutritional deficiencies. Some infants and toddlers who have been fed vegan or

BOX 28.2 Causes of Iron Deficiency Anaemia

Inadequate Supply of Iron

Deficient Dietary Intake

- Rapid growth rate
- Excessive milk intake, delayed addition of solid foods
- Poor general eating habits
- Exclusive breastfeeding of infant after 6 months of age

Inadequate Iron Stores at Birth

- Low birth weight, prematurity, multiple births
- Severe iron deficiency in mother (haemoglobin level < 9 g/dL)
- Fetal blood loss at or before delivery

Impaired Iron Absorption

Presence of Iron Inhibitors

- Phytates, phosphates or oxalates
- Gastric alkalinity

Malabsorption Disorders

- Lactose intolerance
- Inflammatory bowel disease

Chronic Diarrhoea

Blood Loss

- Acute or chronic haemorrhage
- Parasitic infestation

Excessive Demands for Iron Required for Growth

- Prematurity
- Adolescence
- Pregnancy

vegetarian diets may have had severe protein-energy malnutrition, as well as deficiencies of iron, vitamin B_{12} and vitamin D. Unrefined cereals contain substances that modify the absorption of minerals such as zinc, calcium and iron. Individuals consuming strict vegetarian diets that include a large amount of unrefined cereals could be at a greater risk of rickets, vitamin B_{12} and folate deficiency and IDA (Camaschella 2015, Renda & Fischer 2009).

Pathophysiology

Iron is required for the production of haemoglobin. One molecule of haemoglobin consists of protein (globin) combined with four molecules of a pigmented compound (haem). Each molecule of haem contains one atom of iron. When iron stores are deficient, the production of haemoglobin is reduced. Consequently, the main effect of iron deficiency is decreased haemoglobin level and reduced oxygen-carrying capacity of the blood.

Clinical Manifestations

The clinical manifestations are directly attributable to the reduction in the amount of oxygen available to the tissues and resemble those seen in any type of anaemia. Usually the signs are insidious and obscure, and the severity is directly related to the duration of the dietary deficiency.

Although infants with IDA tend to be underweight, many are overweight because of excessive milk ingestion (known as *milk baby*). These children become anaemic for two reasons: milk, a poor source of iron, is given almost to the exclusion of solid foods, and increased faecal loss of blood occurs in 50% of iron deficient infants fed cow's milk. This asymptomatic loss of haemoglobin causes iron deficiency (Griebler et al 2015, Sills 2016). Although chubby, these infants are pale (sometimes porcelain-like), usually demonstrate poor muscle development and are prone to infection.

Although the mechanism is unknown, IDA enhances the leakage of plasma proteins, which causes oedema; growth restriction; and decreased serum concentration of the proteins albumin, gamma globulin and transferrin (a protein that binds iron and transports it through the plasma). Other manifestations of iron deficiency include irritability, tachycardia, fatigue, glossitis, angular stomatitis and koilonychia (concave or 'spoon' fingernails). The association between IDA and impaired neurocognitive function (e.g. attention span, memory, alertness, learning and behavioural problems) in both infants and adolescents has been established, but the mechanism by which IDA impairs neurological function is unknown (Fleming 2015, Sills 2016).

Diagnostic Evaluation

Laboratory tests that measure or describe haemoglobin, the morphological changes in the RBC and iron concentration are usually performed (see Table 28.1). The RBC count may be normal, borderline or moderately reduced in the child with IDA. Typically, the nearly normal number of erythrocytes is strikingly out of proportion to the low haemoglobin concentration. For infants 1 year of age, a mean corpuscular volume (MCV) below 70 femtolitres (fL) is considered diagnostic. In children from 1 to 10 years of age, an MCV value of 70 fL plus the child's age in years is a quick calculation of the lower limit of normal.

The reticulocyte count is usually normal or slightly reduced because of decreased stores of iron (see Table 28.1). However, in severe anaemia, when tissue hypoxia elicits an erythropoietic response, the reticulocyte count may be elevated to 3% or 4%. The level of erythrocyte protoporphyrin, the immediate precursor of haem, becomes elevated in RBCs whenever haem synthesis is disturbed.

In terms of differential diagnosis, a stool analysis for occult blood (guaiac test) is commonly performed to confirm or rule out the possibility of chronic faecal blood loss, especially from milk intolerance or structural anomalies such as diverticulitis.

Iron Studies. In addition to tests that indirectly indicate the level of iron by revealing the effects of iron deficiency on the RBCs, several other tests are usually performed that more directly measure the amount of circulating iron. The serum iron concentration (SIC) is the amount of circulating iron and is normally about 70 microgram/dL in infants and slightly higher in older children. Lower limits of SIC vary not only with age but also with the time of day; they are highest in the morning, when the test should be performed.

The **total iron-binding capacity (TIBC)** is the amount of transferrin (iron-binding globulin) which is necessary for the transport of iron in the bloodstream. When combined with transferrin, the iron is loosely bound to the globulin molecule so that it can be released easily to tissue cells anywhere in the body. In IDA TIBC is elevated above the normal range of 350 microgram/dL (6 months to 2 years) or 450 microgram/dL (children > 2 years and adults). The elevated TIBC represents the body's compensatory mechanism to absorb more iron from exogenous sources than normal during states of deficiency. Transferrin saturation is calculated by dividing the SIC by the TIBC and multiplying the result by 100 to express the value as a percentage. A transferrin saturation of 10% suggests anaemia.

These biochemical tests (ferritin, TIBC, SIC) are acute phase reactants, which means in an inflammatory setting a positive acute phase reactant may overestimate iron stores (Fleming 2015, Sills 2016). It has been recommended that the ferritin level be used simultaneously with measurement of C-reactive protein (CRP) to identify false-negative results associated with inflammation (Baker et al 2010, Sills 2016). Other tests not affected by inflammation that are available in some clinical laboratories are the serum transferrin receptor (validated only in adults as elevated in iron deficiency) and reticulocyte haemoglobin content used in all ages, which has been used to accurately assess iron status (Baker et al 2010, DeLoughery 2014, Fleming 2015, Sills 2016).

Therapeutic Management

Prevention is the primary goal and is achieved through optimum nutrition and appropriate iron supplementation. After the diagnosis of IDA is made, therapeutic management focuses on increasing the amount of supplemental iron the child receives. This is usually done through dietary counselling and the administration of oral iron supplements. For infants and neonates see Table 28.3. In formula-fed infants the most convenient and best sources of supplemental iron are iron-fortified commercial formula and iron-fortified infant cereal (Baker et al 2010, NBA 2017). Iron-fortified formula provides a relatively constant and predictable amount of iron and is not associated with an increased incidence of gastrointestinal (GI) symptoms, such as colic, diarrhoea or constipation. Infants younger than 12 months old should *not* be given fresh cow's milk because it may increase the risk of GI blood loss occurring from exposure to a heat-labile protein in cow's milk or cow's milk–induced GI mucosal damage resulting from a lack of cytochrome iron (haem protein) (Kett 2012, Subramaniam & Girish 2015). If GI bleeding is suspected, several stool analyses for occult blood known as *guaiac tests* are performed to identify any intermittent blood loss.

If the addition of iron-rich foods to the diet does not provide sufficient supplemental quantities of the mineral, oral iron supplements are prescribed. Ferrous iron is more readily absorbed than ferric iron and results in higher haemoglobin levels. Ingested iron is absorbed largely from the duodenum, and absorption is facilitated by an acid environment. Children normally absorb an average of 10% to 20% of the iron in oral supplements, but during periods of iron deficiency they absorb an additional 5% to 10%. Ideally the daily dose of iron

TABLE 28.3 Iron Requirements in Neonates and Infants

Age	Iron requirement	Feeding	Supplementation
Term; 0–6 months	AI 0.2 mg per day	Breast milk Iron-fortified formula	Not routinely required
Term; 6–12 months	RDI 11 mg per day	Breast milk then iron-rich foods Formula then iron-rich foods	Not routinely required
Preterm (< 32 weeks) or low birth weight infants; from 1–12 months	2–3 mg per day provided as either of the feeding options given in the next column	Iron-fortified formula with iron-rich foods from appropriate age	1–2 mg/kg/day of elemental iron until adequate daily iron intake ~6–12 months (corrected for gestation)
		Breast milk, with iron-rich foods from appropriate age	2–3 mg/kg/day of elemental iron until adequate daily iron intake ~6–12 months (corrected for gestation)

AI, adequate intake; *RDI*, recommended daily intake
Source: National Blood Authority Australia (NBA). (2017). Paediatric and Neonatal Iron Deficiency Anaemia Guide. Canberra.

should be given in two or three divided doses between meals. Ascorbic acid (vitamin C) appears to facilitate absorption of iron and may be given as vitamin C–enriched foods and juices with the iron preparation. Side effects of oral iron therapy include nausea, gastric irritation, diarrhoea or constipation, and anorexia, but these occur infrequently, especially in infants. If the iron produces vomiting and diarrhoea, it should be administered with meals and in gradually increasing doses.

The response to oral iron therapy is reflected in a peak increase in the reticulocyte count by the fifth to tenth day of administration. After the reticulocyte rise, the haemoglobin and haematocrit levels and RBC count increase (Sills 2016).

If the haemoglobin level fails to rise after 1 month of oral therapy, it is important to assess non-compliance, persistent bleeding, iron malabsorption, improper iron administration or other causes of anaemia. Parenteral (IV or intramuscular) iron administration is safe and effective but is painful, expensive and occasionally associated with regional lymphadenopathy, transient arthralgias or serious allergic reaction (Bregman & Goodnough 2014, Fleming 2015). Therefore, parenteral iron administration is reserved for children who have iron malabsorption, chronic haemoglobinuria or intolerance to oral preparations. The deep intramuscular injection route for iron administration is discouraged because it is painful and may leak into the subcutaneous tissue causing skin discolouration at the injection site. Careful observation with IV iron administration is required because of the risk of anaphylaxis, so a test dose is recommended before use. Transfusions are indicated for the most severe anaemia and in cases of serious infection, cardiac dysfunction or surgical emergency when anaesthesia is required. Packed RBCs (2 to 3 mL/kg), not whole blood, are used to minimise the chance of circulatory overload. Supplemental oxygen is administered when tissue hypoxia is severe.

As macrocytic anaemias, both folate and vitamin B_{12} deficiencies result in defective ribonucleic acid (RNA) and deoxyribonucleic acid (DNA) synthesis (Carmel et al 2015, Lerner 2016). Folate deficiency is a common micronutrient disorder that is caused by inadequate diet, overcooking of vegetables with loss of folates and/or malabsorption. The deficiency is treated with correctly prepared and intake of folate-enriched foods and/or 1 mg of folate daily (Carmel et al 2015, Smith 2012).

Vitamin B_{12} deficiency commonly develops when the gastric mucosa fails to secrete sufficient intrinsic factor, which is essential for absorption of vitamin B_{12}. Deprived of vitamin B_{12}, the bone marrow produces fewer but macrocytic RBCs. The erythrocytes are usually immature and, because of their extremely fragile cell membranes, are rapidly destroyed during circulation. Treatment initially involves the administration of a 100 microgram or higher dose of vitamin B_{12} parenteral therapy for several days, followed by injections of 500 or 1000 microgram of vitamin B_{12} every 1 to 2 months. Researchers compared oral and parenteral vitamin B_{12} therapy and found that they yielded comparable benefits (Chan et al 2016, Smith 2012, Vidal-Alaball et al 2016).

Prognosis. Prognosis for a child with IDA, folate deficiency or vitamin B_{12} deficiency is very good. There is evidence that if the anaemia is severe and long-standing, diminished cognitive function, behavioural changes, delayed infant growth and development, decreased exercise tolerance and impaired immune function may develop (Angulo-Barroso et al 2016, Fleming 2015). However, there is a lack of convincing evidence that iron treatment of young children with IDA or non-anaemic iron deficiency has an effect on psychomotor development or cognitive function (Abdullah et al 2015, McDonagh et al 2015, Thompson et al 2013, Wang et al 2013).

Nursing Care Management

A primary nursing objective is to prevent nutritional anaemia through family education. Nurses need to be aware of recommendations regarding iron supplementation during infancy and appropriate sources of dietary iron. The nurse should encourage parents to limit the quantity of milk, to use iron-fortified infant formulas and to introduce solid foods. Sources of each of these nutrients and the role they play in preventing deficiencies need to be discussed with the family, especially the person responsible for feeding the infant. It should be stressed with the family that the iron medication must continue for 2 to 3 months after blood values normalise to replenish the body's iron stores.

Instructing parents regarding proper administration of oral iron supplements is an essential nursing responsibility. Several factors, such as stomach acidity, affect the absorption of iron (see Quality Patient Outcomes box).

QUALITY PATIENT OUTCOMES

Iron Deficiency Anaemia

- Early recognition of signs and symptoms of IDA
- Appropriate quantity of milk, use of iron-fortified infant formula and introduction of solid foods
- Adherence to oral iron supplement and appropriate administration
- Haemoglobin increase within 1 month and anaemia resolved within 6 months

An adequate dosage of oral iron turns the stools a tarry green or black colour. The nurse advises parents of this normally expected change and enquires about its occurrence on follow-up visits.

Absence of the greenish-black stool may be a clue to poor compliance. If compliance is an issue, make every effort to institute strategies to improve adherence to the medication regimen, such as administering the drug once a day at the most convenient time. (See Compliance, Chapter 22.)

Oral iron supplements are available in liquid or tablet form. Liquid preparations may temporarily stain the teeth. If possible, take the medication through a straw or give it through a syringe or medicine dropper placed towards the back of the mouth. Brushing the teeth after administration of the drug lessens the discolouration.

Counselling families whose children are anaemic is often a difficult and challenging task. Meal planning must be based on the family's budget, cultural pattern and food preferences (see Cultural Considerations box). Often this requires more than a brief discussion with the mother or usual caregiver about foods high in iron. For teaching to be effective, the nurse may need to offer recipes, assist in planning a shopping list and investigate food prices for economy. Because the physical effects of anaemia are insidious, parents may not consider their child ill and consequently may view the medication and diet changes as unnecessary. Emphasising the physical and behavioural improvements and what effect the improved diet will have on the child's development and the health of all family members may encourage parents to adhere to the treatment plan.

ANAEMIAS CAUSED BY INCREASED DESTRUCTION OF RED BLOOD CELLS

Excessive destruction or haemolysis of erythrocytes can occur from a defect in the RBC (intracorpuscular defect) that shortens the life span of the cell so that production cannot keep pace with destruction. In sickle cell anaemia and thalassaemia, erythrocyte life spans are decreased because of a haemoglobin defect, whereas in spherocytosis erythrocyte life span is decreased due to a defective red cell membrane. Extracorpuscular factors are those conditions that cause haemolysis in otherwise normal RBCs. A classic example is blood group incompatibility, such as haemolytic disease of the newborn or incompatibility secondary to mismatched blood transfusion. Damage to a normal red cell may be caused by toxic drugs, burns, poisonings (such as from lead), infections (such as malaria) and splenic sequestration (hypersplenism).

Hereditary Spherocytosis

Hereditary spherocytosis (HS), a common haemolytic disorder, is caused by a defect in the proteins that form the RBC membrane (Lux 2015). It occurs in most ethnic groups, but it is primarily prevalent in persons of northern European heritage, with a reported incidence of 1 in 2000 to 3000 (DaCosta et al 2013, Lux 2015).

The condition is transmitted in an autosomal dominant pattern. However, 25% of cases are thought to represent new mutations or inheritance through an autosomal recessive mode or autosomal dominant mode with reduced penetrance (Bolton-Maggs et al 2011). The affected cells have a smaller surface area relative to their volume than normal RBCs so they become inflexible spheres known as **spherocytes**. The inflexibility of these cells makes it difficult for them to circulate through the spleen and leads to their early destruction.

Clinical manifestations vary widely from very mild to severe that includes anaemia, splenomegaly (usually modest and does not correlate with the severity of disease) and jaundice (most often scleral icterus). HS frequently manifests in the first 24 hours of the newborn's life as severe hyperbilirubinaemia. Folic acid supplementation should be given to these children to prevent deficiency due to the rapid cell turnover. Laboratory findings include a haemoglobin level between 70 and 100 g/L, a reticulocyte count of 6% to 20% (inversely correlated with haemoglobin level), high mean corpuscular haemoglobin concentration (MCHC) and an increase in osmotic fragility.

Aplastic crisis, which results in a sudden cessation of RBC production by the bone marrow, is a serious complication. Haemoglobin and haematocrit values drop rapidly, which results in severe anaemia. Transfusion support may be needed, and close monitoring of the child's cardiovascular status is necessary.

Splenectomy, a treatment for HS, is generally reserved for children older than 5 years of age with symptomatic anaemia. The splenectomy corrects the haemolysis but not the RBC defect. Occasionally splenectomy is performed in children younger than 5 years of age who are severely anaemic and are showing signs of failure to thrive. Children who are scheduled to undergo a splenectomy should be evaluated for the presence of gallstones before surgery. If gallstones are present, a cholecystectomy is performed at the time of splenectomy.

Because of the risk of life-threatening bacterial infection after splenectomy, these children are immunised with the pneumococcal, meningococcal and *Haemophilus influenzae* type b vaccines before surgery and receive prophylactic penicillin for several years after splenectomy. The parents should be instructed on the importance of seeking immediate medical attention if their child develops a fever of 38.5°C or higher as a common sign of infection or postsplenectomy sepsis (DaCosta et al 2013, Lux 2015). Given the lifelong increased risk of severe infection and thromboembolic complications in splenectomised children, partial splenectomy may be useful for selected patients with HS, with the goal of decreasing haemolysis while maintaining splenic phagocytic function (Lux 2015, Rosman et al 2017).

Sickle Cell Anaemia

Sickle cell anaemia (SCA) is one of a group of diseases collectively termed **haemoglobinopathies**, in which normal adult haemoglobin (haemoglobin A [HgbA]) is partly or completely replaced by abnormal sickle haemoglobin (HgbS). SCD refers to a group of hereditary disorders, all of which are related to the presence of HgbS. Although the name *SCD* is sometimes used to refer to SCA, this usage is incorrect. The correct terms for SCA are *HgbSS disease* and *homozygous sickle cell disease*. The most common forms of SCD are as follows.

- **SCA**—The homozygous form of the disease (HgbSS), in which valine, an amino acid, is substituted for glutamic acid at the sixth position of the beta chain.
- **Sickle cell C disease**—A heterozygous variant of SCD (HgbSC), characterised by the presence of both HgbS and haemoglobin C (HgbC), in which lysine is substituted for glutamic acid at the sixth position of the beta chain.
- **Sickle thalassaemia disease**—A combination of sickle cell trait and beta-thalassaemia trait. In the β^+ (beta plus) form, some normal adult haemoglobin can still be produced. In the β^0 (beta zero) form, there is no ability to produce normal adult haemoglobin.

SCD is one of the most common genetic diseases worldwide, affecting African Americans, Africans, Hispanics, Italians, Greeks, Iranians and Turks; and individuals of Arab, Caribbean and Asian Indian descent. The incidence of the disease varies in different geographic locations. Among African Americans, the incidence of sickle cell trait is about 8%, whereas among inhabitants of West Africa the frequency of sickle cell trait is reportedly as high as 40%. The high incidence of sickle cell trait in these individuals is believed to be a selective protection against malaria caused by endemic *Plasmodium falciparum* infection (McCavit 2012, Nussbaum et al 2016). The physiological basis for the influence of malaria on the sickle gene (so-called balanced polymorphism) is known but not well understood (Nussbaum et al 2016).

Mode of Transmission

The gene that determines the production of HgbS is situated on an autosome. When both parents have sickle cell trait, there is a 25% chance with each pregnancy of producing an offspring with SCA. Other forms of SCD occur through the union of two individuals who carry the heterozygous form of haemoglobin variants.

Basic Defect

The basic defect responsible for the sickling of erythrocytes is contained in the globin fraction of haemoglobin, which is composed of 574 amino acids. Under conditions of dehydration, acidosis, hypoxia and temperature elevation, the relatively insoluble HgbS changes its molecular structure to form long, slender crystals. These filamentous crystals cause distortion of the cell membrane, so the cell changes from a pliable disc to a crescent- or sickle-shaped RBC. The filamentous forms are associated with much greater viscosity than those with the normal holly leaf structure of HgbA.

In most instances the sickling response is reversible under conditions of adequate oxygenation and hydration. During this time the RBCs are indistinguishable from normal erythrocytes on peripheral examination. RBCs with HgbS can sickle and unsickle under appropriate conditions. After repeated cycles of sickling and unsickling, the RBCs become irreversibly sickled.

Although the defect is inherited, the sickling phenomenon is usually not apparent until later in infancy because of the presence of fetal haemoglobin (HgbF). The newborn with SCD is generally asymptomatic because of the protective effect of HgbF (60% to 80%), but this rapidly decreases during the first year, so the child is at risk for sickle cell–related complications (Ellison 2012, Heeney & Ware 2015).

Sickle Cell Trait. Persons with sickle cell trait have the same basic defect, but only about 35% to 45% of the total haemoglobin is HgbS. The remainder is HgbA. Normally these individuals are asymptomatic. Although complications are rare, they have been described in individuals with sickle cell trait. Non-painful gross haematuria is the major complication, seen primarily in the teenage and adult years. Under conditions of extreme or prolonged deoxygenation, such as riding in a non-pressurised aircraft or undergoing military training, splenic sequestration with profound anaemia can occur, resulting in death.

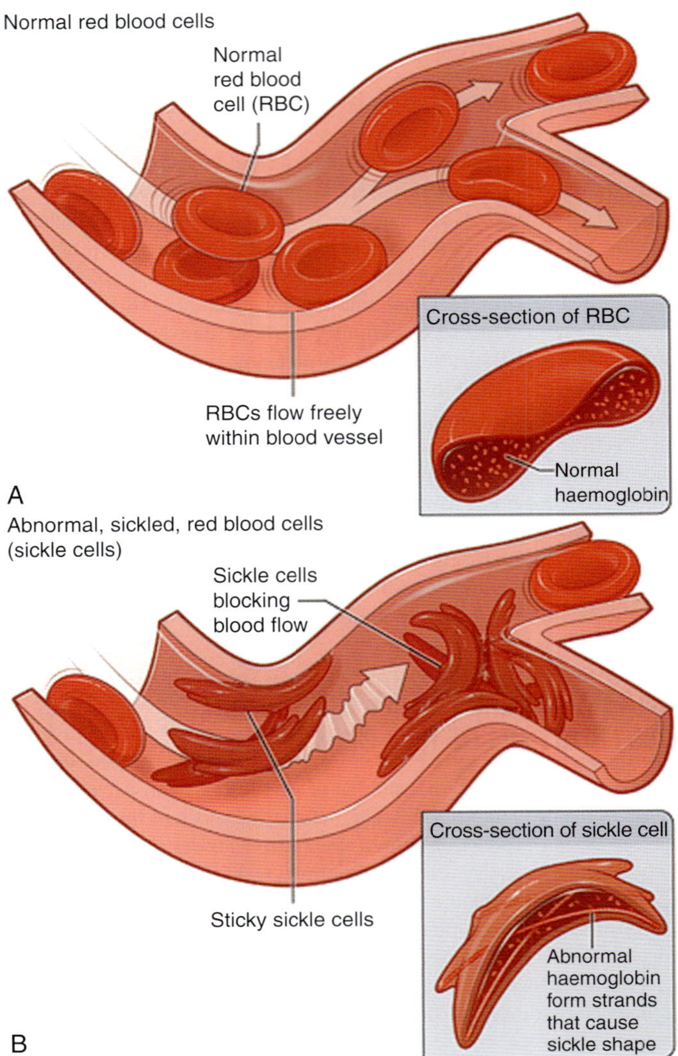

Fig 28.3 (**A**) Normal RBCs flowing freely in a blood vessel. The inset image shows a cross-section of a normal red blood cell with normal haemoglobin. (**B**) Abnormal, sickled RBCs clumping and blocking blood flow in a blood vessel. (Other cells also may play a role in this clumping process.) The inset image shows a cross-section of a sickle cell with abnormal haemoglobin. (Credit: National Heart, Lung, and Blood Institute. (2016). What is sickle cell anemia? August. Bethesda, MD: National Institutes of Health.)

Pathophysiology and Clinical Manifestations

The clinical manifestations of SCA are primarily the result of: (1) obstruction caused by the sickled RBCs; (2) vascular inflammation; and (3) increased RBC destruction. The abnormal adhesion, entanglement and enmeshing of rigid sickle-shaped cells accompanied by the inflammatory process intermittently blocks the microcirculation, causing vasoocclusion (Fig 28.3). The resultant absence of blood flow to adjacent tissues causes local hypoxia, which leads to tissue ischaemia and infarction (cellular death) (Box 28.3). Most of the complications seen in SCA can be traced to this process and its impact on various organs of the body (Fig 28.3).

Initially the spleen may become enlarged from congestion and engorgement with sickled cells. This repeated insult to the splenic sinuses results in infarction. The functioning cells are gradually replaced by fibrotic tissue until, by the age of 5 years, the spleen has decreased in size and has been totally replaced by a fibrous mass (functional asplenia). Without the spleen to filter bacteria and to promote the release of large numbers of phagocytic cells, these individuals are highly susceptible to infection.

The liver is also altered in form and function. Liver failure and necrosis are the result of severe impairment of hepatic blood flow from anaemia and capillary obstruction. Moderate hepatomegaly is common by the age of 1 year and usually persists throughout childhood and early adulthood. The rapid destruction of RBCs often results in the development of pigmented gallstones. Obstruction of the common bile duct by gallstones is uncommon; therefore, cholecystectomy is generally not recommended for asymptomatic patients. If recurrent episodes of right upper abdominal pain occur, cholecystectomy may be indicated.

Kidney abnormalities are probably the result of the same cycle of congestion of glomerular capillaries and tubular arterioles with sickle cells and haemosiderin, tissue necrosis and eventual scarring. The principal results of kidney ischaemia are haematuria, inability to concentrate urine, enuresis and occasionally nephrotic syndrome.

Bone changes include hyperplasia and congestion of the bone marrow, which result in osteoporosis, widening of the medullary spaces and thinning of the cortices. As a result of the weakening of bone, especially in the lumbar and thoracic regions, skeletal

BOX 28.3 Clinical Manifestations of Sickle Cell Anaemia

General
- Possible growth retardation
- Chronic anaemia (haemoglobin level of 6 to 9 g/dL)
- Possible delayed sexual maturation
- Marked susceptibility to sepsis

Vasoocclusive Crisis
- Pain in area(s) of involvement
- Manifestations related to ischaemia of involved areas:
  - **Extremities**—Painful swelling of hands and feet (sickle cell dactylitis, or hand-foot syndrome), painful joints
  - **Abdomen**—Severe pain resembling acute surgical condition
  - **Cerebrum**—Stroke, visual disturbances
  - **Chest**—Symptoms resembling pneumonia, protracted episodes of pulmonary disease
  - **Liver**—Obstructive jaundice, hepatic coma
  - **Kidney**—Haematuria
  - **Genitals**—Priapism (painful penile erection)

Sequestration Crisis
- Pooling of large amounts of blood
  - Hepatomegaly
  - Splenomegaly
  - Circulatory collapse

Effects of Chronic Vasoocclusive Phenomena
- **Heart**—Cardiomegaly, systolic murmurs
- **Lungs**—Altered pulmonary function, susceptibility to infections, pulmonary insufficiency
- **Kidneys**—Inability to concentrate urine, enuresis, progressive renal failure
- **Liver**—Hepatomegaly, cirrhosis, intrahepatic cholestasis
- **Spleen**—Splenomegaly, susceptibility to infection, functional reduction in splenic activity progressing to autosplenectomy
- **Eyes**—Intraocular abnormalities with visual disturbances, sometimes progressive retinal detachment and blindness
- **Extremities**—Avascular necrosis of hip or shoulder; skeletal deformities, especially lordosis and kyphosis; chronic leg ulcers; susceptibility to osteomyelitis
- **Central nervous system**—Hemiparesis, seizures

deformities, particularly lordosis and kyphosis, may occur. Because of chronic hypoxia, the bone becomes susceptible to osteomyelitis, frequently from *Salmonella* organisms. Aseptic necrosis of the femoral head from chronic ischaemia is an occasional problem.

Changes in the central nervous system are primarily vascular and result from the same cyclic reaction of occlusion, ischaemia and infarction. Stroke, or cerebrovascular accident, is a major complication occurring in approximately 11% of children with SCD before the ages of 18 to 20 years who present with focal neurological findings lasting greater than 24 hours and abnormal brain neuroimaging that can result in permanent paralysis or death (DeBaun et al 2016, Estcourt et al 2017). Silent cerebral infarct occurs in 20% of SCA children who lack focal neurological findings lasting greater than 24 hours and are diagnosed as an abnormality on magnetic resonance imaging (MRI) (DeBaun et al 2016, McCavit 2012). Any number of neurological symptoms can indicate a minor cerebral insult, such as headache, aphasia, weakness, convulsions, visual disturbances or unilateral hemiplegia. Loss of vision is usually the result of progressive retinopathy and retinal detachment. Cognitive impairment (e.g. developmental delays, poor or declining school performances) from SCA without any other overt signs tends to be associated with silent cerebral infarct (DeBaun et al 2012, Yawn et al 2014).

Heart problems are mainly attributable to the stress of chronic anaemia, which can eventually result in decompensation and failure. Cardiomegaly is visualised on chest radiographic examination (x-ray or echocardiogram), and a systolic flow murmur is frequently present as a consequence of the anaemia. An echocardiogram may be necessary to diagnose abnormal cardiac structure as it shows cardiomegaly, septal hypertrophy and impaired contractility (Heeney & Ware 2015).

Cardiac dysfunction with sickle-related pulmonary arterial restriction tends to cause pulmonary hypertension that is routinely screened and diagnosed in adult sickle cell patients using echocardiogram. However, screening asymptomatic children for pulmonary hypertension with echocardiogram for elevated pulmonary arterial pressure is controversial.

With the formation of sickled erythrocytes, mechanical fragility increases, which decreases the life span of the RBC. Haemolysis occurs both during intravascular circulation and as a result of stagnation of sickled cells in the congested spleen (see Fig 28.3). Although the body attempts to compensate through stimulated erythropoietic activity, as evidenced by a hyperplastic bone marrow, the rate of destruction exceeds the rate of production. A normocytic normochromic anaemia results. With increased haemolysis, haemosiderosis (increased storage of iron) is present in the liver, spleen, bone marrow, kidneys and lymph nodes.

Sickle Cell Crises. The clinical manifestations of SCA vary markedly in severity and frequency. The most acute symptoms of the disease occur during periods of exacerbation called *crises.* There are several types of episodic crises: vasoocclusive, acute splenic sequestration, aplastic, hyperhaemolytic, stroke, chest syndrome and infection related. The crises may occur individually or concomitantly with one or more other crises.

Vasoocclusive crisis (VOC), preferably called a *painful episode* or *event,* is the most common type of non–life-threatening crisis. It is characterised by ischaemia that causes mild to severe pain that may last from minutes to days. A child experiencing a VOC alone may have localised or generalised pain, acute abdominal pain from visceral hypoxia or gallstones, priapism (an unwanted painful penile erection) and arthralgia. The pain is often migratory, with the presence of a low-grade fever.

VOCs can result in a variety of skeletal problems. One of the more frequent is hand-and-foot syndrome (dactylitis), which occurs primarily in young children aged 6 months to 2 years. It is caused by infarction of short tubular bones and is characterised by pain and swelling of the soft tissue over the hands and feet. It usually resolves spontaneously within a couple of days to weeks. Localised swelling over joints with arthralgia can occur from erythrostasis with sickle cells.

Sequestration crisis is caused by the pooling of large quantities of blood, usually in the spleen and infrequently in the liver, which causes a decrease in blood volume and ultimately shock. The splenic crisis may be acute or chronic. The chronic manifestation is termed **hypersplenism**. The acute form occurs most commonly in children between 2 months and 5 years of age and may result in death from profound anaemia and cardiovascular collapse. Splenic sequestration has occurred in older children and adolescents with sickle cell C disease or sickle beta-thalassaemia.

Aplastic crisis is diminished RBC production, usually triggered by infection with a virus (especially the human parvovirus) or other organism. When it is superimposed on the rapid destruction of RBCs, a profound anaemia results. Packed RBC transfusion is occasionally required in children exhibiting signs and symptoms of congestive heart failure.

Megaloblastic anaemia is attributed to an excessive nutritional need for folic acid and/or vitamin B_{12} during periods of pronounced erythropoiesis. Because infection is not always antecedent to aplastic or hypoplastic crises, it is possible that folic acid deficiency is a causative agent.

Hyperhaemolytic crisis is an accelerated rate of RBC destruction characterised by anaemia, jaundice and reticulocytosis. This complication frequently suggests other coexisting conditions, such as viral illness; transfusion reactions to alloantibodies; or glucose-6-phosphate dehydrogenase (G6PD) deficiency, which is also common in people from African nations.

A cerebrovascular accident (CVA, stroke) is a sudden and severe complication, often with no related illnesses. Sickled cells block the major blood vessels in the brain, which results in cerebral infarction causing variable degrees of neurological impairment. Repeat CVA causes progressive brain damage in the majority of children who have already experienced one stroke and did not receive monthly transfusions because long-term red cell transfusions reduce the risk of CVA as supported by a moderate quality of evidence (DeBaun & Kirkham 2016, Estcourt et al 2017, Heeney & Ware 2015, Wang & Dwan 2013).

Another serious complication is acute chest syndrome (ACS), which is clinically similar to pneumonia. ACS is defined as a new pulmonary infiltrate on chest x-ray of a SCD patient that may be accompanied by chest pain, fever, cough, tachypnoea, wheezing and hypoxia (Dastgiri & Dolatkhah 2016, Heeney & Ware 2015, Meier & Miller 2012). Repeated episodes of chest syndrome may cause restrictive lung disease and pulmonary hypertension.

Overwhelming infection, especially with *Streptococcus pneumoniae* and *H. influenzae* type b as a result of defective splenic function, is the major cause of death in children with SCD under the age of 5 years. Repeated insults on the splenic sinuses by sickled cells result in impaired filtration and function, which allows the development of septicaemia and possibly subsequent death.

Diagnostic Evaluation

Although SCA is usually reported during the neonatal period and early part of infancy, it may not be recognised until the toddler or preschool period during a crisis precipitated by an acute upper respiratory tract or GI infection. However, early diagnosis (before 2 months of age) facilitates initiation of appropriate interventions to minimise complications. Several specific tests detect abnormal haemoglobin in the homozygous or heterozygous form of the disease.

Examination of a stained blood smear may reveal a few sickled RBCs. Because the erythrocyte assumes its normal discoid shape under adequate oxygenation, however, no sickled cells may be present even in the homozygous form of the disease. Whenever sickle cells are found, diagnostic test results are usually positive for SCA, not sickle cell trait.

Screening of Newborns. Universal screening of newborns for SCD has become standard globally (Kuznik et al 2016, Therrell et al 2015, McCavit 2012, McGann 2016, Meier & Miller 2012). The screening provides early identification of these children before complications develop. At birth, infants have up to 80% of HbF, which does not carry the defect. Because levels of HgbS are low at birth, Hgb electrophoresis or other tests that measure Hgb concentrations are indicated. Early diagnosis (before 2 months of age) facilitates parental education regarding the importance of maintaining current immunisations, taking prophylactic antibiotics, detecting splenomegaly and recognising of early signs of infection and other SCD complications.

Penicillin prophylaxis is started by 2 months of age, and parents are instructed to seek medical attention if their child develops a fever of 38.5°C or higher.

Therapeutic Management

The aims of therapy are to prevent the sickling phenomenon, which is responsible for the pathological sequelae, and to treat the medical emergency of sickle cell crisis. The successful achievement of these aims depends on prompt nursing interventions and medical therapies, child and family preventive measures and innovative treatment interventions.

Medical management of a crisis is directed at supportive, symptomatic and specific treatments. The main objectives are to provide: (1) bed rest to minimise energy expenditure and to improve oxygen utilisation; (2) hydration through oral and IV therapy; (3) electrolyte replacement because hypoxia results in metabolic acidosis, which also promotes sickling; (4) analgesia for severe pain from vasoocclusion; (5) blood replacement to treat anaemia and to reduce the viscosity of the sickled blood; and (6) antibiotic therapy to treat any existing infection.

Administration of pneumococcal, *H. influenzae* type b and meningococcal vaccines is recommended for these children because of their susceptibility to infection from functional asplenia. Oral penicillin prophylaxis is recommended by 2 months of age to reduce the chance of pneumococcal sepsis. The nurse assumes an important role in helping the family comply with a medication regimen and seek medical attention immediately when the child has a fever of 38.5°C or higher, an increase in spleen size or severe pallor (Heeney & Ware 2015, Yawn & John-Sowah 2015, Yawn et al 2014).

Oxygen therapy is of little therapeutic value unless the patient is hypoxic (Heeney & Ware 2015). Oxygen administration is usually not effective in reversing sickling or reducing pain because the oxygen is not able to reach the enmeshed sickled RBCs through the clogged vessels.

Another important component of care is the use of blood transfusions. An RBC transfusion is used in aplastic, hyperhaemolytic and splenic sequestration crises; in stroke prevention; and before general surgery. Exchange transfusion (erythrocytapheresis) is a successful, rapid method of reducing the number of circulating sickle cells and therefore slowing down the vicious circle of hypoxia, tissue ischaemia and injury. It is used in ACS and after a stroke to prevent recurrence and further tissue damage. Routine transfusions to maintain the haemoglobin value between 90 and 100 g/L in children with central nervous system disease can minimise the chances of further neurological problems.

The appropriate time for beginning treatment is controversial, but chelation is often initiated when the ferritin level is higher than 1000 nanogram/mL or after a year or more of monthly transfusions. Ferritin level is also an acute phase reactant that is recognised as an ineffective or inaccurate test to determine iron overload; however, it is widely used to monitor effectiveness of chelation (DeBaun et al 2016, Kahnooji et al 2016, Yawn & John-Sowah 2015).

In children with recurrent life-threatening splenic sequestration, splenectomy may be a lifesaving measure. However, the spleen usually atrophies on its own through progressive fibrotic changes (functional asplenia) by 6 years of age in children with SCA. Surgical splenectomy or autosplenectomy has several benefits because the spleen is the major site of sickling, sequestration and destruction of RBCs.

Prognosis. The prognosis varies, but most patients live into their fifth decade. The greatest risk is usually in children younger than 5 years of age, and the majority of deaths in these children are caused by overwhelming infection. As the child grows older, however, the crises may become less severe and less frequent, although death in early adulthood is not uncommon. Consequently, SCA is a chronic illness with a potentially terminal outcome. Physical and sexual maturation are delayed in adolescents with SCA. Although adults achieve normal height, typically below normal weight, and normal sexual function, the delay may present problems to the adolescent (Heeney & Ware 2015).

Individuals with SCD who have higher levels of HbF tend to have a milder disease with fewer complications than those with lower levels (Adewoyin 2015, Meier & Miller 2012). Hydroxyurea is a widely approved medication that increases the production of HbF, reduces endothelial adhesion of sickle cells, improves the sickle cell hydration and cell size, increases nitric oxide production (a vasodilator) and lowers leucocyte and reticulocyte counts (Nevitt et al 2017, Yawn et al 2014).

Nursing Care Management

Assessment of the child in sickle cell crisis includes all areas and systems that can be affected by circulatory obstruction, including: vital signs; neurological signs; vision; hearing; and the respiratory, GI, renal and musculoskeletal systems. It is also important to identify the location and intensity of pain.

Minimise Tissue Deoxygenation. Anything that increases cellular metabolism also results in tissue hypoxia. For the child, minimisation of tissue deoxygenation includes: (1) taking frequent rest breaks during physical activities; (2) avoiding contact sports if the spleen is enlarged because rupture will cause massive internal haemorrhage; (3) avoiding environments with low oxygen concentration, such as high altitudes or non-pressurised aeroplane flights; and (4) avoiding known sources of infection. If the child has even a mild infection, the parents must seek medical attention at once.

Promote Hydration. The nurse emphasises the importance of adequate hydration to prevent sickling and delay the vasoocclusion and hypoxia-ischaemia cycle.

Encourage children to drink by giving them a special cup, thermos or water bottle with a straw from which to drink throughout the day. The nurse advises parents to: take advantage of times of thirst, such as on awakening or after playing; serve frequent small portions; and leave the cup within easy reach for self-service. Flavoured iceblocks/icy poles and crushed ice drinks are sources of fluid commonly accepted by children.

Because the kidneys' ability to concentrate urine is impaired, the child is especially prone to dehydration. Dilute urine or urine of low specific gravity is no longer a valid sign of adequate hydration. Parents should observe for other indications of fluid loss, such as dry mucous membranes, dry nappies, weight loss and a sunken fontanel in infants. In addition, without the ability to conserve water by concentrating urine, the child is prone to dehydration from environmental factors, particularly overheating. The nurse alerts parents to the need for the child to wear proper indoor and outdoor clothing and avoid excessive exposure to the sun.

Increased fluid intake combined with impaired kidney function results in the problem of enuresis. Parents who are unaware of this fact could employ measures to discourage bedwetting, such as limiting fluids at night, and may resort to punishment and shaming to force bladder control. The nurse discusses this problem with the parents, stressing that the child's ability to concentrate urine is impaired. Reminding the child to urinate frequently during the day is helpful, and waking the child during the night may prove beneficial if the child's sleep patterns are not disturbed. Parents who are toilet training their toddlers should be aware of the more frequent pattern of urination and increased difficulty in learning control. Enuresis is treated as a complication of the disease to alleviate parental pressure on the child and to prevent any fluid restriction.

Minimise Crises. Because infection is the major cause of death due to the body's inability to resist infection, the nurse stresses to parents the importance of adequate nutrition, frequent medical supervision, proper handwashing and isolation from known sources of infection. Keep in mind that children also need to live a normal life.

Medication given by mouth can be as effective as IV medication when equianalgesic dosages are prescribed. The nurse should combine any pain management program with psychological support to help the child deal with the depression, anxiety and fear that accompany the disease. This includes regular visits with the child to discuss his or her concerns during the hospitalisation and positive reinforcement of adaptive coping skills, such as successful methods of dealing with the pain and compliance with treatment prescriptions. To reduce the negative connotation associated with the term crisis, it is best to say: 'pain episode'.

Frequently, heat to the affected area is soothing. Cold compresses are not applied to the area because doing so enhances vasoconstriction and occlusion. Bed rest is usually well tolerated during a crisis, although the actual rest obtained depends a great deal on pain alleviation and the use of organised schedules of nursing care. Although the objective of bed rest is to minimise oxygen consumption, some activity, particularly passive range-of-motion exercises, is beneficial to promote circulation. Usually the best course is to let children determine their activity tolerance.

Oxygen administration is not beneficial in vasoocclusive episodes unless hypoxaemia is present (Heeney & Ware 2015). It does not reverse sickled RBCs, and if used in a non-hypoxic patient, it decreases erythropoiesis. Because prolonged oxygen therapy can aggravate the anaemia, report any signs of lack of therapeutic benefit, such as restlessness, increased pallor and continued pain.

Record intake, especially of IV fluids, and output. The child's weight should be taken on admission because it serves as a baseline for evaluating hydration. Because diuresis can result in electrolyte loss, the nurse observes for signs of hypokalaemia and should be familiar with normal serum electrolyte values to report changes. Nurses also need to be aware of the signs of chest syndrome and stroke, both potentially fatal complications

QUALITY PATIENT OUTCOMES

Sickle Cell Disease

- Early recognition of signs and symptoms of SCA
- Tissue deoxygenation minimised
- Sickle cell crisis prevented or quickly managed
- Pain appropriately managed
- Stroke prevented
- Prophylactic penicillin regimen followed
- Hypoxia prevented when surgery is necessary
- Pneumococcal, *H. influenzae* type b and meningococcal vaccines administered

Encourage Screening and Genetic Counselling. Screening is recommended during the neonatal period because early diagnosis allows earlier, more prevention-oriented treatment, such as prophylactic antibiotic therapy and parent education about potential complications. The advantages of trait identification lie in selective reproduction of offspring not afflicted with HgbS.

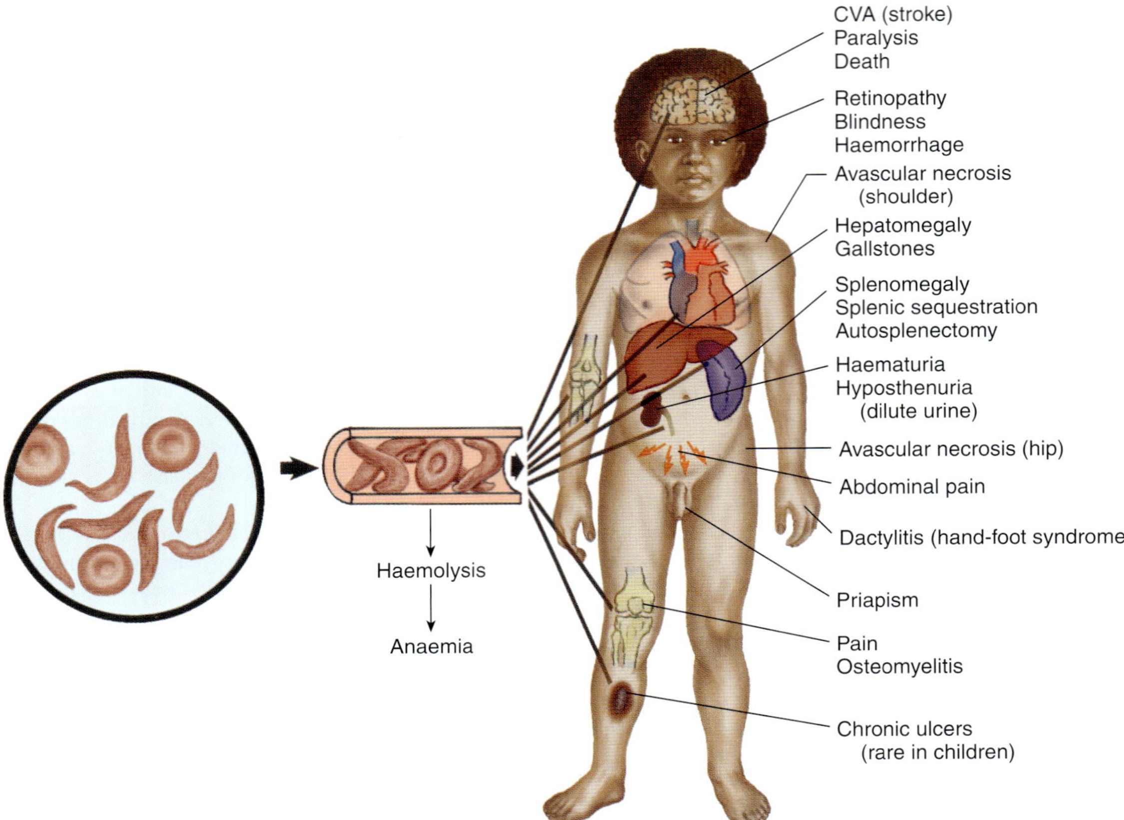

Fig 28.4 Effects of sickled RBCs on circulation with related complications. *(CVA, cerebrovascular accident.)*

Prenatal diagnosis is possible through amniocentesis or fetoscopy and fetal blood sampling during the sixteenth week of gestation. Analysis of amniotic cells for a DNA fragment associated with the gene responsible for sickled beta-globulin chain synthesis can be performed as early as the twelfth week with chorionic villi sampling. In the event the fetus is affected, the decision regarding termination of the pregnancy should be left to the couple.

Explain the Disease. Because SCA may be recognised in the young child, most of the nurse's counselling is directed at the parents. The nurse explains to parents the basic effect of tissue hypoxia on RBCs and the effect of sickling on the circulation (see Fig 28.4). Taking time to establish a sound basis of understanding regarding why certain measures are beneficial to the child encourages parents to practise them.

The nurse advises the parents to inform all treating practitioners of the child's condition. The use of a medical identification bracelet is another way of ensuring awareness of the disease.

Support the Family. Families need the opportunity to discuss their feelings regarding transmitting a potentially fatal, chronic illness to their child. Some parents are able to cope with this fact; some feel great guilt and remorse for giving their child the disease, whereas others regret not knowing that they carried the trait. For many parents, decision-making regarding subsequent pregnancies is fraught with doubt and ambivalence.

Beta-thalassaemia (β-thalassaemia or Cooley's Anaemia)

Worldwide, thalassaemia is a common monogenic disorder affecting as many as 15 million people (Yaish 2015). The term *thalassaemia* comes from the Greek word *thalassa,* meaning 'sea', and is applied to a variety of inherited blood disorders characterised by deficiencies in the rate of production of specific globin chains in haemoglobin. The name appropriately refers to people living near the Mediterranean Sea—namely, Italians, Greeks and Syrians, or to their descendants. Evidence suggests that the high incidence of the disorder among these groups is a result of selective advantage of the trait in protecting against malaria, as is postulated for SCD. The disorder has a wide geographical distribution, however, probably as a result of genetic migration through intermarriages or possibly as a result of spontaneous mutation.

The thalassaemias are classified according to the haemoglobin chain affected and the amount of the globin chain that is synthesised. The two major categories are alpha-thalassaemia and beta-thalassaemia. Thalassaemia is seen in various population groups in India, Asia, Africa and inhabitants of the Mediterranean and Middle Eastern regions, and the majority of births of affected individuals occur in these groups (Choudhry 2017, Higgs et al 2012).

Beta-thalassaemia is the most common of the thalassaemias and occurs in four forms: two heterozygous forms, *thalassaemia minor* (generally an asymptomatic silent carrier state) and *thalassaemia trait* (which produces a mild microcytic anaemia); *thalassaemia intermedia,* which may involve either homozygous or heterozygous abnormalities and is manifested as splenomegaly and moderate to severe anaemia; and a homozygous form, *thalassaemia major* (also known as Cooley's anaemia), which results in a severe anaemia that is not compatible with life without transfusion support.

Mode of Transmission

Thalassaemia is an autosomal recessive disorder with varying expressivity. Both parents must be carriers to produce a child with beta-thalassaemia major. The typical mode of transmission is between parents who are heterozygous for thalassaemia.

Pathophysiology and Clinical Manifestations

Normal postnatal HgbA is composed of two alpha and two beta polypeptide chains. In beta-thalassaemia there is a partial or complete deficiency in the synthesis of the beta chain of the haemoglobin molecule. Consequently, there is a compensatory increase in the synthesis of alpha chains, and gamma-chain production remains activated, which results in formation of defective haemoglobin. This unbalanced polypeptide unit is unstable; when it disintegrates, it damages the RBCs, which causes severe anaemia. To compensate for the haemolytic process, an overabundance of erythrocytes is formed unless transfusion therapy suppresses the bone marrow. Excess iron from packed RBC transfusions and from the rapid destruction of defective cells is stored in various organs (haemosiderosis).

The onset of clinical manifestations in thalassaemia major may be insidious and not recognised until late infancy or early toddlerhood (Box 28.4). The clinical effects of thalassaemia major are primarily attributable to defective synthesis of HgbA, structurally impaired RBCs and the shortened life span of the erythrocyte. The major consequences of thalassaemia are caused by the pathological condition, resultant chronic hypoxia and iron overload from the supportive treatment of multiple blood supplements (Fig 28.5 and Box 28.4).

Anaemia results from the body's inability to maintain a level of erythropoiesis equal with haemolysis. The bone marrow compensates by producing large numbers of immature cells, such as normoblasts and erythroblasts; large cells that are extremely thin and form bizarre shapes; and target cells, which have abnormal staining properties. As a result of the excessive production of abnormal RBCs, their life span is severely shortened.

BOX 28.4 Clinical Manifestations of Beta-thalassaemia

Anaemia (Before Diagnosis)

- Pallor
- Unexplained fever
- Poor feeding
- Enlarged spleen or liver

Progressive Anaemia

- Signs of chronic hypoxia
- Headache
- Praecordial and bone pain
- Decreased exercise tolerance
- Listlessness
- Anorexia

Other Features

- Small stature
- Delayed sexual maturation
- Bronzed, freckled complexion (if not receiving chelation therapy)

Bone Changes (Older Children if Untreated)

- Enlarged head
- Prominent frontal and parietal bosses
- Prominent malar eminences
- Flat or depressed bridge of the nose
- Enlarged maxilla
- Protrusion of the lip and upper central incisors and eventual malocclusion
- Generalised osteoporosis

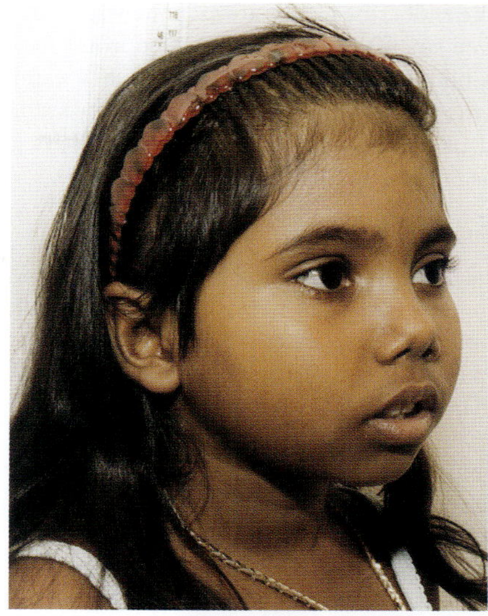

Fig 28.5 A young girl with beta-thalassaemia demonstrating mild frontal bossing of the right forehead and mild maxillary prominence. (Source: Courtesy James DeLeon, Texas Children's Hospital, Houston.)

Aplastic crises after infection, folic acid deficiencies from the demands of bone marrow hyperplasia and progressive haemolysis from repeated blood transfusions all worsen anaemia. The spleen becomes greatly enlarged as a result of extramedullary haematopoiesis (blood cell formation outside of the bone marrow), rapid destruction of the defective erythrocytes and, rarely, progressive fibrosis from haemochromatosis (excess iron storage). Splenomegaly may progress until the organ's very size interferes with the function of other abdominal organs and respiratory expansion.

With progressive anaemia, signs of chronic hypoxia—namely, headache, irritability, praecordial and bone pain, decreased exercise tolerance, listlessness and anorexia—may develop. Another common symptom in these children is frequent epistaxis, although the exact reason is unknown. Hyperuricaemia and gout from rapid cellular catabolism also occur.

Haemosiderosis refers to excess iron storage in various tissues of the body, especially the spleen, liver, lymph glands, heart and pancreas, but without associated tissue injury. **Haemochromatosis** refers to excess iron storage that results in cellular damage. It is not known how iron storage causes tissue destruction. Chronic hypoxia is believed to be an important contributing factor.

In thalassaemia, excess of haemosiderin, the iron-containing pigment from the breakdown of haemoglobin, results from decreased haemoglobin synthesis and increased haemolysis of transfused erythrocytes. Decreased production of haemoglobin results in an excess supply of available iron. In addition, the body probably responds to the anaemia by increasing the rate of GI absorption of dietary iron because ineffective erythropoiesis is a potent controlling factor in exogenous iron use. However, the primary source of additional iron is from the haemolysis of supplemental erythrocytes and the rapid destruction of defective RBCs. With the prophylactic use of intravenous and/or oral chelators to minimise excess iron storage, the characteristic changes in body structures from haemochromatosis have been greatly reduced.

Restricted growth and, especially, delayed sexual maturation are common findings. There is evidence that both may also be caused by pituitary failure, although the exact reasons for this are unclear, but the impaired growth is probably also related to haemochromatosis. It is possible that the endocrine glands are extremely sensitive to iron toxicity and that even small amounts of deposited iron can produce organ dysfunction. Children with severe disease usually exhibit significant growth retardation. The development of secondary sexual characteristics is delayed or absent in many adolescents (Chatterjee & Bajoria 2010, Nienhuis & Nathan 2012, Sankaran et al 2015).

Diagnostic Evaluation

Haematological studies reveal characteristic changes in the RBCs (e.g. microcytosis, hypochromia, anisocytosis, poikilocytosis, target cells and basophilic stippling of various stages). Low haemoglobin and haematocrit levels often occur in severe anaemia, although they are typically less pronounced than the reduction in the RBC count because of the proliferation of immature erythrocytes.

Haemoglobin electrophoresis confirms the diagnosis and is helpful in distinguishing the type and severity of the thalassaemia because it analyses the quantity and kind of haemoglobin variants found in the blood. In beta-thalassaemia, levels of HgbF and $HgbA_2$ (a type of normal adult haemoglobin) are elevated because neither depends on beta-chain polypeptides for synthesis.

Therapeutic Management

The objective of supportive therapy is to maintain sufficient haemoglobin levels to prevent bone marrow expansion and bony deformities and to provide sufficient RBCs to support growth and normal physical activity. Transfusions are the foundation of medical management, with a goal of maintaining the haemoglobin level above 95 g/L, an aim that may require transfusions as often as every 3 weeks. The advantages of this therapy include: (1) improved physical and psychological wellbeing because of the ability to participate in normal activities; (2) decreased cardiomegaly and hepatosplenomegaly; (3) fewer bone changes; (4) normal or near-normal growth and development until puberty; and (5) fewer infections.

One of the potential complications of frequent blood transfusions is iron overload (haemosiderosis). Each millilitre of packed RBCs contains 1 milligram of iron. Because the body has no effective means of eliminating the excess iron, the mineral is deposited in body tissues. To minimise the development of haemosiderosis and haemochromatosis in a thalassaemia major patient, the child could be started on iron-chelating treatment.

Significant liver fibrosis, cardiac dysfunction and growth impairment may be prevented if chelation therapy is adequate (Sankaran et al 2015). Therefore, adherence to an intensive schedule is required for substantial chelation therapy.

MRI is used to evaluate the iron content of the liver, heart and other organs and has become the method of choice for guiding iron-chelating therapy in combination with laboratory measurement of serum ferritin levels and, in certain circumstances, liver biopsy (Kahnooji et al 2016).

To reduce the requirement of blood transfusions in patients with thalassaemia, a few investigations and protocols reported that hydroxyurea may reduce the need for transfusions and recommended the need for well-designed randomised controlled trials to establish high-quality evidence (Ansari et al 2016, Foong et al 2016).

In some children with severe splenomegaly who require repeated transfusions, a splenectomy may be necessary to decrease the disabling effects of abdominal pressure and to increase the life span of supplemental RBCs. Over time the spleen may accelerate the rate of RBC destruction and therefore increase transfusion requirements. After a splenectomy, children generally require fewer transfusions, although the basic defect in haemoglobin synthesis remains unaffected. A major postsplenectomy complication is severe and overwhelming infection. Therefore, these children are often on prophylactic antibiotics with close medical supervision for many years and should receive the pneumococcal and meningococcal vaccines in addition to regularly scheduled immunisations.

Prognosis. Most children treated with blood transfusions and early chelation therapy have a remarkably improved life span as they survive well into adulthood (Higgs et al 2012, Sankaran et al 2015). The most common causes of death are heart disease, liver damage with cirrhosis, postsplenectomy sepsis and multiorgan failure secondary to haemochromatosis (Choudhry 2017, Sankaran et al 2015, Yaish 2015). The three adverse prognostic factors for event-free survival are presence of hepatomegaly (2 cm below costal margin), iron overload (serum ferritin greater than 1000 ng/mL) and portal fibrosis (Choudhry 2017). Children with the absence of these adverse prognostic factors have greater than 97% event-free survival (Choudhry 2017). A curative treatment for some children is haematopoietic stem cell transplantation (HSCT). Children younger than 16 years of age who undergo allogeneic HSCT have a high rate of complication-free survival; approximately 80% to 97% of these children are cured (DeBaun et al 2016, Issaragrisil & Kunacheewa 2016, Lucarelli et al 2012). Also, related cord-blood transplantation has a disease-free survival of about 90% (Higgs et al 2012, Issaragrisil & Kunacheewa 2016). Children without a matched donor may benefit from haploidentical family member transplant, which has shown encouraging results (Lucarelli et al 2012, Locatelli et al 2016). New approaches for correction of thalassaemia through the introduction of gene therapy strategies, including the use of lentiviral vectors, generation of pluripotent stem cells and gene targeting, are ongoing but continue to have concerns (Arlet et al 2016, Raja et al 2012, Sankaran et al 2015).

Nursing Care Management

The objectives of nursing care are to: (1) promote compliance with transfusion and chelation therapy; (2) assist the child in coping with the anxiety-provoking treatments and the effects of the illness; (3) foster the child's and family's adjustment to a chronic illness; and (4) observe for complications of multiple blood transfusions. Basic to each of these goals is explaining to parents and older children the defect responsible for the disorder, its effect on RBCs and the potential effects of untreated haemosiderosis (such as delayed growth and maturation and heart disease). Because this condition is prevalent among families of Mediterranean descent, the nurse may also enquire about the family's previous knowledge about thalassaemia. All families with a child with thalassaemia should be tested for the trait and referred for genetic counselling.

Support the Family. As with any chronic illness, the family's needs must be met for optimum adjustment to the stresses imposed by the disorder. (See Chapter 21.) Genetic counselling for the parents and fertile offspring is mandatory, and both prenatal diagnosis using amniocentesis or fetal blood sampling and screening for thalassaemia trait are available. There has been a marked decline in the number of new cases of thalassaemia worldwide. This may be a result of education and testing of parents.

Assist in Coping with the Effects of the Disorder. Body image alterations, decreased growth and sexual immaturity are frequently difficult adjustment problems for older children. These children feel different from their peers, and the delayed sexual development is a major issue for the maturing adolescent with an improved life expectancy. Adolescents need an opportunity to express their thoughts and feelings about these complex issues.

With frequent transfusion therapy there is less restriction on physical activity because of severe anaemia, and the nurse should encourage these children to pursue activities that they are able to tolerate. The frequency of treatment, however, can interfere with a normal lifestyle. To minimise disruptions and improve cooperation, the nurse can help arrange for blood transfusions and medical supervision at times that interfere least with the child's regular activities, especially school.

ANAEMIAS CAUSED BY IMPAIRED OR DECREASED PRODUCTION OF RED BLOOD CELLS

Impaired or decreased production of RBCs can occur as a result of either bone marrow failure or deficiency of essential nutrients. Bone marrow failure may be caused by: (1) replacement of bone marrow by fibrous tissue or by neoplastic cells, as in leukaemia; (2) depression of marrow activity by irradiation, chemicals or drugs; and (3) interference with bone marrow activity caused by systemic disorders such as severe infection, chronic renal disease, widespread malignancy (without marrow infiltration), collagen diseases or hypothyroidism. When depression of the haematological system is extensive, aplastic anaemia develops.

The reason systemic disorders affect erythrocyte production varies according to the condition. For example, in severe chronic infection there is evidence that depression of erythropoiesis is caused by a defect in the conversion of protoporphyrin into haemoglobin. In addition, there is some degree of haemolysis, although the exact mechanism is not known.

Aplastic Anaemia

Aplastic anaemia (AA) is a rare and life-threatening disorder that affects approximately 2 to 6 in 1 million children and adults each year (Hord 2016, Korthof et al 2013). AA refers to a condition in which production of the formed elements of the blood is simultaneously depressed. The peripheral blood smear demonstrates cytopenia, including at least two of the triad that consists of leucopenia, thrombocytopenia and profound anaemia. Hypoplastic anaemia is characterised by a profound depression of RBC formation but normal or slightly decreased production of WBCs and platelets. One type of hypoplastic anaemia is pure RBC aplasia, which can be congenital or acquired. The acquired defect in erythropoiesis is an autoimmune condition that occurs mostly in adults. The congenital condition (Diamond-Blackfan syndrome) is marked by complete or almost complete absence of all cells of the erythroid series with normal production of the other myeloid cells. Its treatment, which consists of transfusions, splenectomy and administration of corticosteroids, is similar to that for other diseases that result in profound anaemia. The prognosis varies, although long-term survival is possible. The principal causes of death are cardiac failure, hepatitis from transfusion therapy and sepsis. Haemosiderosis and haemochromatosis (see p. 1046) also affect vital tissues necessary for survival.

AA can be primary (congenital, or present at birth) or secondary (acquired). The best-known congenital disorder of which AA is an outstanding feature is Fanconi's anaemia syndrome, a rare hereditary disorder that is characterised by pancytopenia, hypoplasia of the bone marrow and patchy brown discolouration of the skin due to the deposition of melanin. It is associated with multiple congenital anomalies of the musculoskeletal and genitourinary systems. The syndrome appears to be inherited as an autosomal recessive trait with varying penetrance; therefore, affected siblings may demonstrate different combinations of defects.

Several factors contribute to the development of acquired hypoplastic anaemia; however, most of the cases are considered idiopathic (Box 28.5).

BOX 28.5 Common Causes of Acquired Aplastic Anaemia

- Human parvovirus infection, hepatitis or overwhelming infection
- Irradiation
- Immune disorders such as eosinophilic fasciitis and hypoimmunoglobulinaemia
- Drugs such as certain chemotherapeutic agents, anticonvulsants and antibiotics
- Industrial and household chemicals, including benzene and its derivatives, which are found in petroleum products, dyes, paint remover, shellac and lacquers
- Infiltration and replacement of myeloid elements, such as in leukaemia or the lymphomas

Therapeutic Management

The objectives of treatment are based on the recognition that the underlying disease process is failure of the bone marrow to carry out its haematopoietic functions. Therefore, therapy is directed at restoring function to the marrow and involves two main approaches: immunosuppressive therapy to counter the presumed immunological responses that prolong aplasia and replacement of the bone marrow through transplantation. Bone marrow transplantation is the treatment of choice for severe AA when an HLA-matched sibling donor exists.

Immunosuppressive therapy (IST) is an alternative preferred line of treatment for children with acquired AA who do not have a matched sibling bone marrow donor (Shimamura & Williams 2015). Antithymocyte globulin (ATG) or antilymphocyte globulin (ALG) is the principal drug treatment used for AA. The rationale for using ATG is based on the theory that AA may be a result of autoimmunity.

Because of the hypersensitivity response associated with ATG (i.e. fever, chills, myalgias), methylprednisolone is given intravenously to prevent these side effects. Growth factors, given parenterally, may be used to prevent neutropenic infection and enhance bone marrow production (Passweg & Marsh 2010).

NURSING CARE CONSIDERATIONS

The care of the child with AA is similar to the care of the child with leukaemia and includes preparing the child and family for the diagnostic and therapeutic procedures, preventing complications from the severe pancytopenia and emotionally supporting the family in the face of potentially fatal outcome.

Defects in Haemostasis

Haemostasis is the process that stops bleeding when a blood vessel is injured. Vascular and plasma clotting factors, as well as platelets, are required. A complex system of clotting, anticlotting and clot breakdown (**fibrinolysis**) mechanisms exists in equilibrium to ensure clot formation only in the presence of blood vessel injury and to limit the clotting process to the site of vessel wall injury. Dysfunction in these systems leads to bleeding or abnormal clotting.

Mechanisms Involved in Normal Haemostasis

Understanding the role that factor deficiencies play in promoting bleeding tendencies requires a review of the normal coagulation process of the blood. Although the coagulation process is complex, clotting depends on three main elements: vascular events, platelets and clotting factors.

Vascular Events

At the time and site of injury, several events occur to initiate haemostasis: local vasoconstriction, compression of the blood vessels by extravasated blood and release of von Willebrand factor by endothelial walls. Collagen present in exposed subendothelial cells acts as a site for platelet adhesion.

Platelets

Normally the platelets do not adhere to one another or to normal endothelium. However, when a blood vessel is injured, certain events take place. First, platelet adhesion occurs at the site of the injury, providing a plug. The platelets change shape, develop pseudopods and release a variety of chemicals to stimulate vasoconstriction and vessel repair and to activate and recruit more platelets to the injury site. Receptor sites are located on the platelets for fibrinogen and other adhesive proteins, which cause the platelets to stick together (**aggregation**). As the membranes of the platelets change, the phospholipids necessary for blood coagulation are exposed so that fibrin, which secures the platelet plugs to the site, can be produced. Finally, the clot compresses and is secured to the injury.

Defects in platelets and clotting factors are the most common causes of bleeding during childhood. The following discussion focuses on the major conditions that require nursing intervention.

Clotting Factors

The clotting factors (Fig 28.6) are activated in sequence to develop a fibrin clot. Two mechanisms exist that can generate prothrombin to produce thrombin.

1. **Intrinsic pathway**—Factor XII, high-molecular-weight kininogen (HMK, Fitzgerald factor) and prekallikrein (KAL, Fletcher factor) react on a negatively charged surface (contact activation reaction) to activate factor XI (PTA, plasma thromboplastin antecedent). The partial thromboplastin time measures abnormalities in the intrinsic pathway (abnormalities in factors I, II, V, VIII, IX, X, XII, HMK and KAL).
2. **Extrinsic pathway**—A lipoprotein tissue factor stimulates activation of factor VII. The prothrombin time measures abnormalities of the extrinsic pathway (abnormalities in factors I, II, V, VII and X).

Haemophilia

The term *haemophilia* refers to a group of bleeding disorders resulting from congenital deficiency, dysfunction or absence of specific coagulation proteins or factors (Di Paola et al 2015, Sharathkumar & Pipe 2008). Although the symptomatology is similar regardless of which clotting factor is deficient, the identification of specific factor deficiencies has allowed definitive treatment with replacement agents.

In about 80% of all cases of haemophilia, the inheritance pattern is demonstrated as X-linked recessive. (See Chapter 3.) The two most common forms of the disorder are factor VIII deficiency (haemophilia A, or classic haemophilia) and factor IX deficiency (haemophilia B, or Christmas disease). In Australia around 2900 people are diagnosed with varied severities of haemophilia (Haemophilia Foundation of Australia [HFA] 2020) while in New Zealand around 430 people have the condition (Haemophilia Foundation of New Zealand [HFNZ] 2020). Von Willebrand disease (vWD) is another hereditary bleeding disorder characterised by a deficiency, abnormality or absence of the protein called *von Willebrand factor (vWF)*. The following discussion is primarily concerned with factor VIII deficiency, which accounts for 80% to 85% of all cases.

Modes of Transmission

Haemophilia is transmitted as an X-linked recessive disorder, but only about 60% of affected children have a positive family history for the disease. Up to one-third of all haemophilia cases may be caused by a gene mutation. The most frequent pattern of transmission is through the union of an unaffected male with a trait-carrier female. Because the treatment of persons with haemophilia has improved, the results of a union between an affected male and a normal female or a carrier female must also be considered. For example, the chances are equal (e.g. 1 in 4) that an offspring of an affected male and a carrier female will be an affected son, an affected daughter, a carrier daughter or a normal son. Such parentage is one of the few ways in which a female inherits the disorder. Female carriers may have low levels of factor VIII and be symptomatic.

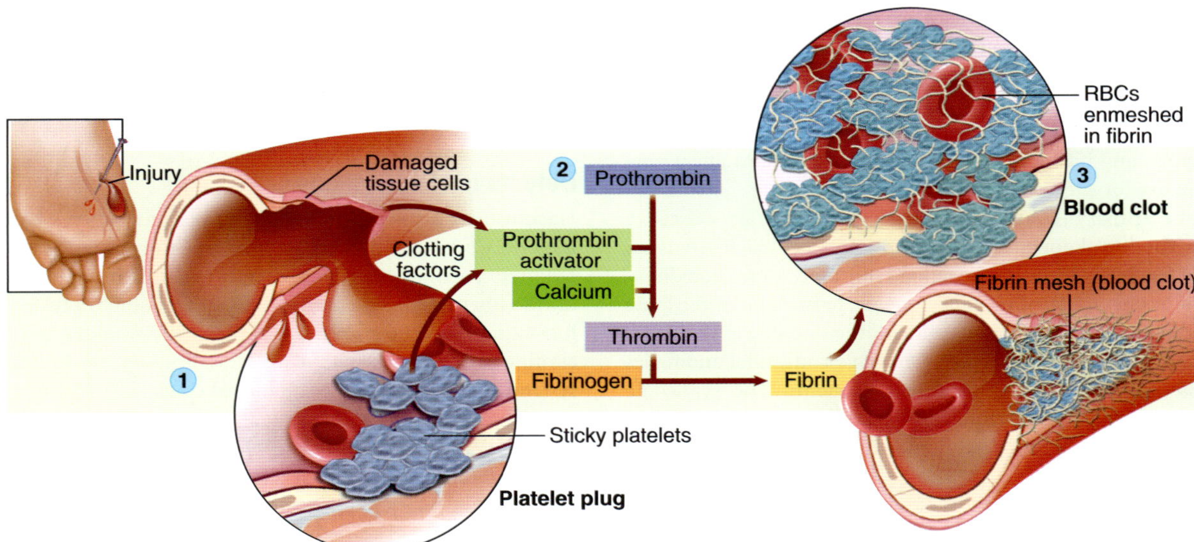

Fig 28.6 Blood clotting. The extremely complex clotting mechanism can be distilled into three basic steps: release of clotting factors from both injured tissue cells and sticky platelets at the injury site (which form a temporary platelet plug); series of chemical reactions that eventually result in the formation of thrombin; and formation of fibrin and trapping of RBCs to form a clot. (Source: Thibodeau, G. A., & Patton, K. T. (2010). The human body in health and disease (5th ed.). St Louis, MO: Mosby.)

Pathophysiology and Clinical Manifestations

The basic defect of haemophilia A is a deficiency of factor VIII (antihaemophilic factor). Factor VIII is produced by the liver and is necessary for the formation of thromboplastin in phase I of blood coagulation. The less factor VIII that is found in the blood, the more severe the disease.

A major feature of haemophilia is that its expression varies markedly with regard to the degree of bleeding severity. Haemophilia is generally classified into three groups according to the severity of the factor deficiency; 60% to 70% of children with haemophilia demonstrate the severe form of the disorder (Table 28.4).

The effect of haemophilia is prolonged bleeding anywhere from or in the body. With severe factor deficiencies, haemorrhage can occur as a result of minor trauma, such as after circumcision, during loss of deciduous teeth or as a result of a slight fall or bruise. In children with less severe deficiencies, however, the bleeding tendency may not be noted until the onset of walking.

Subcutaneous and intramuscular haemorrhages are common. Haemarthrosis, which refers to bleeding into the joint cavities, especially the knees, elbows and ankles, is the most frequent form of internal bleeding. Bony changes and crippling deformities occur after repeated bleeding episodes over several years. Early signs of haemarthrosis are a feeling of stiffness, tingling or ache in the affected joint, followed by a decrease in the ability to move the joint. Obvious signs and symptoms are warmth, redness, swelling and severe pain, with considerable loss of movement. Spontaneous haematuria is not uncommon. Epistaxis may occur but is not as frequent as other kinds of haemorrhage. Petechiae are uncommon in persons with haemophilia because repair of small haemorrhages depends on platelet function, not on blood-clotting mechanisms.

Bleeding into the tissue can occur anywhere but is serious if it occurs in the neck, mouth or thorax because the airway can become obstructed. Intracranial haemorrhage can have fatal consequences and is one of the major causes of death. Haemorrhage anywhere along the GI tract can lead to anaemia, and bleeding into the retroperitoneal cavity is especially hazardous because of the large space for blood to accumulate. Haematomas in the spinal cord can cause paralysis.

Diagnostic Evaluation

The diagnosis is usually made from a history of bleeding episodes, evidence of X-linked inheritance (only one-third of cases are new mutations), and laboratory findings. To understand the significance of various tests of haemostasis, it is helpful to recall the usual mechanisms to control bleeding (e.g. the function of platelets and clotting factors). The results of tests that measure platelet function, such as the bleeding time, are all normal in persons with haemophilia, whereas the results of tests that assess clotting factor function may be abnormal. The tests specific for haemophilia include factor VIII and IX assays, procedures normally done by specialised laboratories. Other tests are those that depend on specific factors for a reaction to occur, especially the partial thromboplastin time. Carrier detection is possible in classic haemophilia using DNA testing and is an important consideration in families in which female offspring may have inherited the trait.

TABLE 28.4 Clinical Severity of Haemophilia

Clinical Severity	Factor VIII Activity	Bleeding Tendency
Severe	< 1%	Spontaneous bleeding without trauma
Moderate	1%–5%	Bleeding with trauma
Mild	> 5%–40%	Bleeding with severe trauma or surgery

Therapeutic Management

The primary therapy for haemophilia is replacement of the missing clotting factor. The products currently available are factor VIII concentrates, either produced through genetic engineering (recombinant form) or derived from pooled plasma, which are reconstituted with sterile water immediately before use. A synthetic form of (antidiuretic hormone), desmopressin (1-deamino-8-D-arginine vasopressin (DDAVP)), is the treatment of choice in mild haemophilia and vWD (types I and IIA only) if the child shows an appropriate response. After desmopressin administration a threefold to fourfold rise in factor VIII activity should occur. Because the goal is to raise the factor VIII level at least 30%, patients with moderate factor VIII deficiency do not benefit. In addition, various therapies are employed when bleeding occurs or is anticipated.

Aggressive factor concentrate replacement therapy is initiated to prevent chronic crippling effects from joint bleeding. If replacement therapy begins immediately, local measures such as ice applications and splinting are seldom needed. Other drugs may be included in the therapy plan, depending on the source of the haemorrhage. Corticosteroids are given for haematuria, acute haemarthrosis and chronic synovitis. It is recommended that patients with haemophilia avoid aspirin and non-steroidal anti-inflammatory drugs (NSAIDs) because they inhibit platelet function (Australian Haemophilia Centre Directors' Organisation [AHCDO] 2016, Scott 2016a). However, NSAIDs such as ibuprofen are effective in relieving pain caused by synovitis and are occasionally used with caution (Hermans et al 2011, AHCDO 2016).

In some children with haemophilia, the factor replacement is seen by the body as a foreign protein when it is administered and the body produces an antibody (inhibitor) that destroys the factor. When individuals are resistant to first-line therapy, they are treated with one of two equally effective agents, recombinant activated factor VIIa or human activated prothrombin complex concentrate (Guelcher 2016, Matino et al 2015).

A regular program of exercise and physical therapy is an important aspect of management. If started early and continued throughout adulthood, planned, individualised physical activity strengthens muscles around joints and may decrease the number of spontaneous bleeding episodes.

Treatment without delay results in more rapid recovery and a decreased likelihood of complications; therefore, most children are treated at home. The family is taught how to perform venepuncture and how to administer factor VIII to children over 2 to 3 years of age. The child learns the procedure for self-administration at 8 to 12 years of age. Home treatment is highly successful, and the rewards, in addition to the immediacy, are less disruption of family life, fewer school or work days missed and enhancement of the child's self-esteem and independence. Although home treatment for haemophilia promotes freedom, flexibility and autonomy for the boys and the family, mothers or caregivers who usually provide the daily childcare may view the treatment experience as a burden (von der Lippe et al 2017). It is important for the health professionals to provide practical and emotional support for the caregivers of these boys.

Prophylactic therapy is periodic factor replacement for children with severe haemophilia to prevent bleeding complications, including arthropathy and spontaneous and life-threatening bleeding events (Di Paola et al 2015, Scott 2016a, von der Lippe et al 2017). Primary prophylaxis in patients with severe haemophilia has been practised for many years in developed countries and has proved to be effective in preventing naturopathy. In primary prophylaxis, factor VIII concentrate is infused on a regular basis before the onset of joint damage. Secondary prophylaxis involves the infusion of factor VIII concentrate on a regular basis after the child experiences his or her first joint bleed. The infusions are given every other day or three times a week for several weeks to promote healing. Episodic factor replacement may be a cost-effective alternative to primary prophylaxis, but prophylaxis decreases the development of joint disease compared with on-demand treatment (Manco-Johnson et al 2007). However, prompt appropriate treatment of haemorrhage and prophylactic therapy are key to excellent care and prevention of long-term morbidity in patients with haemophilia (Di Paola et al 2015, Lillicrap 2013).

Prognosis. The progress made in haemophilia care over the years has been striking. The institution of home infusion therapy and the use of safer, more effective factor concentrates, coupled with the establishment of comprehensive treatment centres and the adoption of prophylactic treatment regimens, have revolutionised the treatment and management of haemophilia (Di Paola et al 2015, Sharathkumar & Carcao 2011). Early recognition of joint and muscle bleeds is emphasised because immediate adequate treatment with clotting factor is possible using home infusion therapy. Early treatment has significantly reduced the morbidity formerly associated with haemophilia. The availability of comprehensive haemophilia treatment centres offers the child with haemophilia and the family a coordinated multidisciplinary approach to meeting their needs and improving the child's health and wellbeing.

Although there is no cure for haemophilia, its symptoms can be controlled and its potentially crippling deformities markedly reduced or even avoided. Today many children with haemophilia function with minimal or no joint damage. They have an average life expectancy and are normal in every aspect but one: they have a tendency to bleed, which is a significant inconvenience but not necessarily a life-threatening event.

Gene therapy may prove to be a treatment option in the future. Techniques are under development to introduce the factor VIII or IX genes into hepatocytes, fibroblasts, endothelial cells using adeno-associated viral vectors and other novel ideas for genetic correction (Branchford et al 2013, Nienhuis et al 2017, Walsh & Batt 2013). The scientific community remains undaunted in its attempt to make gene-addition therapy a 21st-century reality for patients with haemophilia A and B (Di Paola et al 2015, Lytle et al 2016, Nienhuis et al 2017).

Nursing Care Management

The earlier a bleeding episode is recognised, the more effectively it can be treated. Signs that indicate internal bleeding are especially important to recognise. Children are aware of internal bleeding and are reliable in telling the examiner the location of an internal bleed. In addition, the nurse maintains a high level of suspicion when a child with haemophilia shows signs such as headache, slurred speech, loss of consciousness (from cerebral bleeding), and black, tarry stools (from GI bleeding). (See Quality Patient Outcomes box.)

QUALITY PATIENT OUTCOMES

Haemophilia

- Early recognition of signs and symptoms of haemophilia
- Bleeding episodes prevented
- Bleeding episodes treated early with factor replacement
- Adherence to prophylactic factor replacement program when indicated
- Haemarthrosis prevented when possible with limited joint damage
- Exercise program and physical therapy ongoing

Prevent Bleeding. The goal of prevention of bleeding episodes is directed towards decreasing the risk of injury. Prevention of bleeding episodes is geared mostly towards appropriate exercises to strengthen muscles and joints and to allow age-appropriate activity. During infancy and toddlerhood, the normal acquisition of motor skills creates innumerable opportunities for falls, bruises and minor wounds. Restraining the child from mastering motor development can bring more serious long-term problems than allowing natural development. However, the environment should be made as safe as possible, with close supervision maintained during playtime to minimise incidental injuries.

For older children the family usually needs assistance in preparing the child for school. A nurse who knows the family can be instrumental in discussing the situation with the school nurse and in joint planning of an appropriate activity schedule. Because almost all individuals with haemophilia are boys, the physical limitations in regard to active sports may be a difficult adjustment, and activity restrictions must be tempered with sensitivity to the child's emotional and physical needs. Use of protective equipment, such as helmets, face masks, shin/wrist/forearm guards, kneepads and other equipment appropriate for the type of athletic activity, is encouraged to prevent injury. Children and adolescents with severe haemophilia can participate in non-contact sports such as swimming, golf, walking, jogging, fishing and bowling. Contact sports such as football, boxing, hockey, wrestling and rugby are strongly discouraged because the risk of injury outweighs the physical and psychosocial benefits of participating in these sports (Anderson & Forsyth 2017, Scott 2016a). However, studies have reported that the absolute increase in risk of bleeds associated with regular participation in high-impact athletic activities (e.g. basketball, football, hockey, gymnastics, karate, soccer, skateboarding) that is supported by adult coaching and supervision of school-age children with haemophilia who received routine prophylactic factor replacement is small and is accompanied with improved quality of life and joint health (Broderick et al 2012, Cuesta-Barriuso et al 2016).

To prevent oral bleeding, some readjustment in terms of dental hygiene may be needed to minimise trauma to the gums, such as using a water irrigating device, softening the toothbrush in warm water before brushing or using a sponge-tipped disposable toothbrush. A regular toothbrush should be soft-bristled and small. Adolescents also need to be advised of the dangers of shaving and using safety razors with blades and should use an electric shaver.

Because any trauma can lead to a bleeding episode, all persons caring for these children must be aware of their disorder. These children should wear medical identification, and older children should be encouraged to recognise situations in which disclosing their condition is important, such as during dental extractions or injections. Health personnel need to take special precautions to prevent the use of procedures that cause bleeding such as intramuscular injection. The subcutaneous route is substituted for intramuscular injection whenever possible. Venepunctures for blood samples are usually preferred by children. There is usually less bleeding after venepuncture than after finger or heel puncture. Neither aspirin nor any aspirin-containing compound should be used. Paracetamol is a suitable aspirin substitute, especially for use during control of pain at home.

Recognise and Control Bleeding. As noted, the earlier a bleeding episode is recognised, the more effectively it can be treated. Factor replacement therapy should be instituted according to established medical protocol, and supportive measures may be implemented, such as RICE, which is the mnemonic for **R**est, **I**ce, **C**ompression and **E**levation. When parents and older children are taught such measures beforehand, they can be prepared to initiate immediate treatment. However, such measures do not take the place of factor replacement.

Support the Family and Prepare for Home Care. Factor concentrates have greatly changed the outlook for these children by minimising the bleeding and allowing the child to live a normal, unrestricted life. Children are taught to take responsibility for their disease at an early age. They learn their limitations, preventive measures and self-administration of the factor replacement.

The needs of families who have children with haemophilia are best met through a comprehensive team approach of physicians (e.g. paediatrician, haematologist, orthopaedist), nurse practitioner or specialist nurse, social worker and physical therapist.

Parent-group discussions are beneficial in meeting the needs of similarly affected families. For example, with the improved prognosis for these children, adolescents with haemophilia and their parents face vocational and financial problems in addition to concern over future childbearing.

Von Willebrand Disease

Von Willebrand disease (vWD) is a hereditary bleeding disorder characterised by a deficiency of or defect in a protein called *von Willebrand factor* (vWF). The vWF protein contributes to the adherence of platelets to damaged endothelium and serves as a carrier protein for factor VIII (Flood & Scott 2016, Marcdante & Kliegman 2015, Neutze & Roque 2016). This results in prolonged bleeding time because platelets fail to adhere to the walls of the ruptured vessel to form a platelet plug. Even though bleeding time is insensitive to platelet function defects, it is still used by some centres. The platelet function analyser (PFA-100) is a rapid, accurate detection of platelet dysfunction and vWD used by many centres, but its results may be affected by some conditions (e.g. sepsis, pregnancy, certain medications) and therefore requires the need for further platelet aggregation testing (Flood & Scott 2016, Kehrel & Brodde 2013, Sarangi & Acharya 2017). The disease can cause mild, moderate or severe bleeding. Most cases of vWD are mild and require intervention only for dental and surgical procedures.

The most characteristic clinical feature of vWD is an increased tendency towards bleeding from mucous membranes. The most common symptom is frequent nosebleeds, followed by gingival bleeding, easy bruising and excessive menstrual bleeding (menorrhagia) in females. Unlike haemophilia, vWD affects both males and females because its inheritance shows an autosomal dominant pattern. However, the treatment and final outcome are similar in both disorders. Treatment of bleeding is with DDAVP and/or a specially concentrated clotting factor such as Humate-P. Currently, a recombinate vWD preparation is undergoing clinical trials (Flood & Scott 2016).

Nursing Care Management

The nursing goals are similar to those for haemophilia, with special considerations related to epistaxis. Nosebleeds are often a frightening experience for the child and parents. A calm, reassuring manner can alleviate anxiety and promote the child's cooperation. Because most of the nosebleeding originates in the anterior part of the nasal septum, bleeding can be controlled by applying pressure to the tip of the nose with the thumb and forefinger (see Nursing Care Considerations box). During this time the child breathes through the mouth. If local measures are not successful at stopping the bleeding, DDAVP is used to treat mild and moderate vWD (Ben-Ami & Revel-Vilk 2013, Marcdante & Kliegman 2015). DDAVP increases vWF and factor VIII secretion from storage in the endothelial cells (Castaman & Linari 2017, Flood & Scott 2016, Marcdante & Kliegman 2015).

NURSING CARE CONSIDERATIONS

Epistaxis

- Have child sit up with neck forward or erect (not lie down).
- Apply continuous pressure to tip of nose with thumb and forefinger for at least 10 minutes.
- Do not insert cotton or wadded tissue into nostril or blow nose because this may dislodge clot.
- Apply ice or cold cloth to bridge of nose if bleeding persists.
- Keep child calm and quiet.

For menorrhagia, factor replacement therapy or the administration of DDAVP may be beneficial on the first day of the menstrual cycle to lessen the flow. Teaching the adolescent methods to prevent embarrassing accidents during menstruation, such as using double sanitary pads, helps her adjust to the inconvenience.

Immune Thrombocytopenia (Idiopathic Thrombocytopenic Purpura)

Idiopathic or immune thrombocytopenic purpura (ITP), the formerly used term because purpura is an infrequent sign at presentation, is being referred to as immune thrombocytopenia by some expert sources (Rodeghiero et al 2009). ITP is an acquired haemorrhagical disorder that is characterised by thrombocytopenia (e.g. easy bruising, mucosal bleeding, petechiae, menorrhagia) and normal bone marrow with a normal or increased number of immature megakaryocytes and eosinophils. Although the causes are not known, it is understood that ITP involves the evolution of antibodies against multiple platelet antigens, leading to reduced platelet survival and impaired platelet production (McCrae 2011, Scott 2016b, Wilson 2015). ITP is the most common thrombocytopenia of childhood and usually presents 1 to 4 weeks after a viral illness, with the majority of cases in children younger than 10 years of age with peak incidence between ages 1 and 6 years (McCrae 2011, Scott 2016b, Wilson 2015).

The disease occurs in one of two forms: an acute, self-limiting course or a chronic course (> 12 months' duration). The acute form occurs most commonly after upper respiratory tract infections; after the childhood diseases of measles, rubella, mumps or chickenpox; or after infection with human parvovirus.

Clinical symptoms include petechiae, bruising, bleeding from mucous membranes and prolonged bleeding from abrasions. Symptomatic bleeding does not usually occur until the platelet count is lower than 20,000/mm^3. Fatal haemorrhages have been reported in less than 1% of all patients.

Diagnostic Evaluation

In ITP the platelet count is reduced to less than 20,000/mm^3; therefore, results of tests that depend on platelet function, such as the tourniquet test, bleeding time and clot retraction time, are abnormal. There is no definitive test that establishes a diagnosis of ITP; several tests are usually performed to rule out other disorders of which thrombocytopenia is a manifestation, such as systemic lupus erythematosus, lymphoma and leukaemia.

Therapeutic Management

Management of ITP is primarily supportive because the disease is self-limiting in the majority of cases. Activity is restricted at the onset while the platelet count is low and while active bleeding or progression of lesions is occurring. Treatment for acute presentation is symptomatic and has included prednisone, IV immune globulin (IVIg) and anti-D antibody. These are not curative therapies. Some experts suggest that no therapy is necessary for asymptomatic patients because there is no difference in the recovery time of platelet counts with and without treatment (Kuhne & Imbach 2013, Scott 2016b, Wilson 2015). Anti-D antibody is a plasma-derived immunoglobulin that causes a transient haemolytic anaemia in Rh(D)-positive patients with ITP. The platelet count usually increases approximately 48 hours after an infusion of anti-D antibody; therefore, it is not appropriate therapy for patients who are actively bleeding. The benefits of choosing anti-D antibody IV therapy over prednisone or IVIg are that anti-D antibody can be given in one dose over a period of 5 to 10 minutes, and it is significantly less expensive than IVIg. Historically patients who were treated with prednisone first underwent a bone marrow examination to rule out leukaemia, but this is now controversial because leukaemia rarely manifests with a low platelet count alone (Marcdante & Kliegman 2015, Wilson 2015). Therefore, the use of anti-D antibody and IVIg alleviates the need for a bone marrow examination. Before receiving the initial dose of anti-D antibody, patients must meet certain criteria.

Splenectomy is for patients who have chronic severe ITP that is not responsive to pharmacological management and have increased risk of severe haemorrhage. It is the only treatment associated with long-term remission for the majority of children with chronic ITP and therefore removes the risk of haemorrhage (Marcdante & Kliegman 2015, McCrae 2011, Wilson 2015). Before splenectomy is considered, it is generally recommended to wait until the child is older than 5 years of age because of the increased risk of bacterial infection. The child also receives penicillin prophylaxis after splenectomy. The appropriate length of prophylactic therapy is controversial, but in general a minimum of 3 years of therapy is recommended.

Prognosis. The majority of children with ITP have a self-limiting course without major complications. Some children develop chronic ITP and require ongoing therapy. A splenectomy may modify the disease process, and the child may be asymptomatic. Splenectomy is associated with a lifelong risk of overwhelming infection caused by encapsulated organisms, increased risk of thrombosis and the potential development of pulmonary hypertension in adulthood. As an alternative to splenectomy, rituximab has been used off-label (currently unapproved for treating ITP) in children to treat chronic ITP, with 30% to 40% of children obtaining a partial or complete remission (Scott 2016b).

Nursing Care Management

Nursing care is largely supportive and should include teaching regarding the possible side effects of therapy and restriction of contact sports while the child's platelet count is less than 50,000/mm^3 as some experts recommend (Kumar et al 2015). Children with ITP should not participate in any contact sports, bike riding, skateboarding, in-line skating, gymnastics, climbing or running. Parents are encouraged to engage their children in quiet activities and to prevent any injuries to the child's head (e.g. by having the child wear protective headgear). Instruct the parents to obtain prompt medical evaluation if the child sustains head or abdominal trauma. As with any condition with an uncertain outcome, the family needs emotional support.

OTHER HAEMATOLOGICAL DISORDERS

Neutropenia

Neutropenia is a reduction in the absolute number of circulating neutrophils and band forms in the blood that is below the normal level by age and race (Dale 2017, Dinauer et al 2015, Walkovich & Newburger 2016). Neutropenia is usually defined as an ANC of less than 1000/mm^3 in infants 2 weeks to 1 year of age or less than 1500/mm^3 in children older than 1 year of age. The ANC is calculated by multiplying the total WBC count by the percentage of neutrophils and bands in the differential count (see Table 28.1). When the ANC is less than 500/mm^3, it is defined as severe neutropenia with an increased risk of life-threatening infection (Celkan & Koc 2015, Walkovich & Newburger 2016). Several different types of neutropenia occur in children. This discussion focuses on the most common type: chronic benign neutropenia.

Diagnostic Evaluation

Chronic benign neutropenia generally represents disorders characterised by mild to moderate neutropenia that are not associated with an increase in infections and often have spontaneous remissions (Celkan & Koc 2015, Walkovich & Newburger 2016). Neutropenia is often detected as an incidental finding during the evaluation of a child with fever. The ANC is usually below 500/mm^3, and the only physical findings (if any) are those related to infection. Oral ulcerations and skin infections are the most common manifestation of chronic benign neutropenia. However, most children have no infections despite the markedly reduced ANC. Examination of bone marrow aspirates shows normal cellularity with absence of mature neutrophils. Antineutrophil antibodies are usually present, but their absence does not exclude the diagnosis.

Therapeutic Management

Therapy to increase the ANC is rarely required. Children who have recurrent or severe infections, however, may benefit from the administration of granulocyte colony-stimulating factor (G-CSF). G-CSFs are a naturally occurring group of glycoproteins.

Children with chronic benign neutropenia have normal cellular immunity; therefore, they should receive their routine childhood immunisations.

Nursing Care Management

The care of the child with neutropenia primarily focuses on educating the parents. Instruct parents to keep their child away from large indoor crowds (e.g. shopping centre on Saturday morning, movie theatres and day care centres) and individuals who are ill. Parents also need to seek medical attention if their child has a fever of 38.5°C or higher, or if skin lesions develop. Because G-CSF is administered parenterally only, parents need to know how to administer subcutaneous injections.

Support the Family. Neutropenia can have many effects on family life. Some parents must quit their jobs to avoid sending their child to day care. Provide financial counselling as indicated. Parents of children with neutropenia need a listening ear for their frustrations and continued reassurance that these children usually recover by the age of 4½ years.

Henoch-Schönlein Purpura

Henoch-Schönlein purpura (HSP), also referred to as allergic vasculitis, allergic purpura and anaphylactoid purpura, is a relatively common acquired disorder in children characterised by a non-thrombocytopenic purpura, arthritis, nephritis and abdominal pain.

The aetiology is unknown, but the disease often follows an upper respiratory tract infection, and allergy or drug sensitivity plays a role in some instances. The disease occurs in children ages 6 months to 16 years but more frequently in children ages 2 to 11 years. It is observed more often in Caucasian children than in those of other ethnicities and almost twice as often in boys than in girls.

Pathophysiology

The disease is characterised by inflammation of small blood vessels, and the manifestations observed are influenced by the size and distribution of the affected vessels. A generalised vasculitis of dermal capillaries (and to a lesser extent small arterioles and veins), causing extravasation of RBCs, produces the petechial skin lesions. Inflammation and haemorrhage may also occur in the GI tract, synovium, glomeruli and central nervous system.

Clinical Manifestations

The onset of the disease may be abrupt, with the simultaneous appearance of several manifestations, or gradual, with the sequential appearance of different manifestations. The primary feature, however, is a symmetric purpura that involves the buttocks and lower extremities but may extend to include the extensor surfaces of the upper extremities and, less commonly, the upper trunk and face. The rash may be associated with maculopapular lesions, urticaria and erythema. There is often marked oedema of the scalp, eyelids, lips, ears and dorsal surfaces of the hands and feet, especially in infants and younger children. In severe cases the skin may slough, leaving denuded areas that are similar in appearance and treatment to partial-thickness burns.

Arthritic effects are evident in two-thirds of affected children and range from asymptomatic swelling around a single joint to painful, tender swelling of several joints, most often the knees and ankles. The involvement is periarticular and resolves in a few days without permanent damage or deformity.

Two-thirds of affected children have GI involvement manifested by recurrent colicky midabdominal pain, often associated with nausea and vomiting. The stools contain gross or occult blood and mucus.

Renal involvement occurs in up to 50% of affected children and is potentially the most serious long-term complication. Initially the nephritis is manifested as blood, casts and protein in the urine. Although the majority of children with renal involvement recover completely, some develop chronic renal disease with eventual renal failure.

Diagnostic Evaluation

Diagnosis is usually established on the basis of the history and clinical manifestations. Laboratory tests are used to assess GI and renal involvement and to determine adequacy of haemostatic function. Tests for occult blood in the stool are performed. Increased levels of immunoglobulin A are a frequent finding.

Therapeutic Management

Management is primarily supportive, with close observation for signs of renal or GI involvement. Oedema, rash, malaise and arthralgia are usually managed with appropriate analgesics such as NSAIDs and mild sedation if necessary. Corticosteroids may be prescribed for relief of more severe oedema, arthralgia and colicky abdominal pain. The nephropathy requires careful monitoring of fluid and electrolyte balance, salt intake and blood pressure. Antihypertensive agents may be needed.

The majority of children recover without the need for hospitalisation, and in most instances a single acute episode clears spontaneously within a month. Others may have periodic recurrences for as long as 2 to 3 years before attaining permanent remission from symptoms. Rarely, death occurs from severe GI complications, acute renal failure or central nervous system involvement. Children with HSP nephritis should receive long-term follow-up because renal involvement is evident in 40% of the patients, many of whom exhibit severe proteinuria (Wilson 2015).

Nursing Care Management

Nursing care of the child hospitalised with HSP is primarily supportive, with vigilant observation for signs of complications. The nurse should measure vital signs and record them at regular intervals, obtain specimens for laboratory examination and administer medication as prescribed. Carefully observe urine and stools for fresh and occult blood.

If the child suffers from joint pain, proper positioning, careful movement and administration of analgesics, including opioids, helps reduce discomfort. More severe involvement, such as GI symptoms and nephritis, is managed as for any such disorder.

Concern about the unsightly appearance of the rash is common. Inform the child and parents that it is only a temporary phenomenon and that the child can wear clothing that helps hide the rash, such as a long-sleeved shirt or long pants. If the skin surface is denuded, treatment may involve debridement and dressing changes similar to that in the care of burns. (See Chapter 23.)

IMMUNOLOGICAL DEFICIENCY DISORDERS

A number of disorders can cause profound, often life-threatening, alterations in the body's immune system. The most serious are those conditions that completely depress immunity, such as severe combined immunodeficiency disease (SCID). However, the one disorder that generates the most anxiety in both the family and the community is human immunodeficiency virus (HIV) infection and the subsequent development of AIDS.

Several classifications of immune dysfunction exist. AIDS, SCID and Wiskott-Aldrich syndrome are disorders in which the body is unable to mount an immune response. The immune response can also be misdirected. In autoimmune disorders, antibodies, macrophages and lymphocytes attack healthy cells. Some such disorders and their target organs are myasthenia gravis (muscle cells), Graves' disease (thyroid cells) and type 1 diabetes (B-cells in the pancreas). AIDS, SCID and Wiskott-Aldrich syndrome are discussed here; the other disorders are covered elsewhere in this book.

Mechanisms Involved in Immunity

The function of the immune system is to differentiate 'self' from 'non-self' and to initiate a response to eliminate the 'non-self' or foreign substance, known as an antigen. All cells in the body have specific cell surface markers unique to the individual. These cell surface markers are known as the **major histocompatibility complex (MHC)**. Because the markers were first identified on human leucocytes, they are commonly referred to as **human leucocyte antigens (HLAs)**.

The body's protective mechanisms consist of complex, overlapping defence systems. Intact skin serves as the first line of protection for the body. Body secretions such as saliva, sweat and tears contain chemicals that can kill many organisms. The stomach contains acids that can destroy swallowed pathogens. Organisms trapped in the mucus of the nose and mouth are expelled by sneezing or coughing. If the foreign substance has penetrated these barriers, cellular elements are mobilised.

The immune system is composed of the primary lymphoid organs (thymus, bone marrow and probably liver) and the secondary lymphoid organs (lymph nodes, spleen and gut-associated lymphoid tissue). The immune system has two types of function: non-specific and specific. Non-specific immune defences are activated on exposure to any foreign substance but react similarly regardless of the type of antigen; they are unable to identify the antigen, except to know that it is 'non-self'. The principal activity of this system is phagocytosis, the process of ingesting and digesting foreign substances.

Specific Immune Mechanisms

Specific (adaptive) defences are those that have the ability to recognise the antigen and respond selectively. The components of adaptive immunity are humoral immunity and cell-mediated immunity. The cells responsible for these two forms of immunity are the lymphocytes, specifically B-lymphocytes and T-lymphocytes.

Humoral immunity involves antibody production and complement and is concerned with immune processes occurring outside the cells, such as on cell surfaces or in body fluids. The principal cell involved in antibody production is the B-lymphocyte, which is probably produced in the bone marrow. When challenged with an antigen, B-cells divide and differentiate into plasma cells. The plasma cells produce and secrete large quantities of antibodies specific to the antigen. Five classes of immunoglobulin (Ig) antibodies have been identified: IgG, IgM, IgA, IgD and IgE, each serving a specific function.

On initial exposure to an antigen, the B-lymphocyte system begins to produce antibody, predominantly IgM, which appears in 2 to 3 days. This process is referred to as the primary antibody response. With subsequent exposure to the antigen, a secondary antibody response occurs. Specific IgG antibodies are formed within 4 to 10 days. An example of the secondary response is the response that occurs with repeat administration of an immunisation agent, often called a booster. Memory B-cells allow the immune system to recognise the same antigen for months or years.

When antibody reacts with antigen, they bind to form an antigen–antibody complex. This binding serves several functions. Antibody aids in the phagocytosis of antigen by sensitising it in such a manner that it is more readily destroyed by phagocytes, a process known as opsonisation.

Antibody also activates or fixes complement, the second component of humoral immunity. The complement system is a series of proteins (C1 to C9) present in serum that results in a cascade of enzymatic actions and death of a viable antigen. After being activated by antibody, complement produces a chemotactic factor that summons T-lymphocytes and macrophages to the antigen site.

Cell-mediated immunity involves a variety of specific functions mediated by the T-lymphocyte and occurs within the cell. T-lymphocytes do not carry typical immunoglobulins on their surfaces as the B-cells do. Microscopically, T-cells appear identical, but they are functionally heterogeneous, and there are several subsets, including cytotoxic T-cells, helper T-cells and suppressor T-cells. T-cells may also be classified structurally by the distinctive molecules on their surfaces, known as cluster designations (CDs). Once mature, T-cells carry markers known as T2 (CD2), T3 (CD3), T5 (CD5) and T7 (CD7). Helper T-cells carry a T4 (CD4) marker and a suppressor, and cytotoxic T-cells carry a T8 (CD8) marker.

Specific functions of cell-mediated immunity include protection against most viral, fungal and protozoan infections and slow-growing bacterial infections, such as tuberculosis; rejection of incompatible grafts; mediation of cutaneous delayed hypersensitivity reactions, such as in tuberculin testing; and probably immune surveillance for malignant cells. In addition, T-lymphocytes also have regulatory functions within the immune system. For example, helper T-lymphocytes help B-lymphocytes and other types of T-cells to mount an optimum immune response. The cellular immune response is initiated when a T-lymphocyte is sensitised by antigen. In response to this contact, the T-cell releases numerous humoral factors called **lymphokines**, which eventually bring about the death of the antigen. Interferons are a group of proteins secreted by leucocytes and infected host cells that non-specifically inhibit viral replication, promote phagocytosis and stimulate the killer activity of sensitised lymphocytes.

Human Immunodeficiency Virus Infection and Acquired Immunodeficiency Syndrome

HIV infection and AIDS have generated intense investigation and constitute one of the world's most serious medical, public health and social challenges of our time (Grace 2015). Advances in research and major improvements in the treatment and management of HIV infection have stabilised the incidence of new HIV infections and AIDS globally, with disproportionate distribution of HIV infections and AIDS deaths occurring among people of sub-Saharan Africa (United Nations AIDS 2019). HIV is rare in children in Australia and New Zealand. It is estimated that in 2019 there were 29,000 people with HIV in Australia (AFAO 2020) and 3500 people in New Zealand (New Zealand AIDS Foundation [NZAF] 2020), with the majority of these cases attributed to sexual contact between men and injecting drug use (AFAO 2020, NZAF 2020).

Aetiology

HIV is a retrovirus that is the primary cause of AIDS. There are different strains of HIV. HIV-2 is prevalent in Africa, whereas HIV-1 is the more common form in Australia and New Zealand. Horizontal transmission of HIV occurs through intimate sexual contact or parenteral exposure to blood or body fluids containing visible blood. Perinatal (vertical) transmission occurs when an HIV-infected pregnant woman passes the infection to her infant. There is no evidence that casual contact between infected and uninfected individuals can spread the virus.

Children with HIV fall into two subpopulations: infants born to HIV-infected women and adolescents infected as a result of high-risk behaviours. Children in Australia who became infected with HIV in 1985 or earlier generally acquired the virus through contaminated blood products; these were mainly children with medical conditions that required multiple blood products for treatment (e.g. children with bleeding conditions like haemophilia and premature babies who needed blood cells for anaemia).

Since 1985, all blood products used in Australia and New Zealand have been screened for HIV and new HIV infections in Australia among children are the result of mother-to-child-transmission (MTCT)—an extremely rare event in this country since the discovery of effective MTCT prevention strategies (Miller et al 2013).

It has been recommended that all pregnant women be tested for HIV, and if positive treated with antiretroviral regimen, irrespective of viral load or CD4 count (Ishikawa et al 2016, Yogev & Chadwick 2016). Sexual contact is the leading source of exposure to HIV. In the young paediatric population this is an infrequent route of transmission. In contrast, sexual activity is a major cause of HIV infection in adolescents. Adolescents commonly take risks and experiment; participation in high-risk behaviours, including IV drug use and unsafe sexual practices, increases their risk of becoming infected with HIV.

Pathophysiology

HIV primarily infects a specific subset of T-lymphocytes, the $CD4^+$ T-cells, but it can also invade cells of the monocyte-macrophage lineage. The virus takes over the machinery of the $CD4^+$ lymphocyte, using it to replicate itself and rendering the $CD4^+$ cell dysfunctional. With suppression of cell-mediated immunity, the person is at risk for opportunistic infections. HIV also causes dysfunction of B-cells and antigen-presenting cells, which results in suppression of humoral immunity.

Although the course of HIV infection varies among individuals, a common progression of events has been recognised. Immediately after primary infection, there is dissemination of virus and seeding of lymphoid organs, along with a transient decrease in the number of $CD4^+$ lymphocytes in peripheral blood. An immune response follows, and the resulting level of plasma virus is generally maintained for years. A period of clinical latency ensues that may be longer than 10 years in adults. The $CD4^+$ lymphocyte count gradually decreases over time; at some point, physical symptoms appear. The count eventually reaches a critical level below which there is substantial risk of opportunistic illnesses, followed by death.

A more rapid progression of disease tends to occur in perinatally infected children. This is primarily due to the immaturity of the developing immune system. Rapid progression of HIV infection in infants and children is also correlated with higher viral burden and faster depletion of infected CD4 lymphocytes than in adults (Yogev & Chadwick 2016).

Clinical Manifestations

The majority of infants with perinatally acquired HIV infection are clinically normal at birth. Common clinical manifestations of HIV infection in children vary and include such signs as lymphadenopathy, hepatosplenomegaly and unexplained diarrhoea. Diarrhoea may be a result of pathogens or HIV itself due to malabsorption of carbohydrate, protein and fat (Yogev & Chadwick 2016). HIV-infected children often do not grow normally; they may be proportionally smaller in both length and weight for age.

Recurrent bacterial infections, parotitis, lymphoid interstitial pneumonitis (LIP) and early onset of progressive neurological deterioration are characteristic of children with HIV infection but are rarely seen in affected adults. Kaposi's sarcoma, one of the hallmarks of adult disease, is found in fewer than 1% of affected children.

Central nervous system abnormalities considered to be the direct effects of HIV infection occur in most children with AIDS. Secondary infections with opportunistic and common pathogens are infrequent in this population. Either global or specific neuropsychological deficits may occur at random intervals. Many affected children display evidence of developmental disability. Deficits in motor skills, communication and behavioural functioning are common. Expressive language (use of language) is more frequently impaired than receptive language (understanding of language).

Diagnostic Evaluation

For children 18 months of age and older, the HIV enzyme-linked immunosorbent assay (ELISA) and Western blot immunoassay are performed to determine HIV infection. In infants born to HIV-infected mothers, results of these assays are positive because of the presence of maternal antibodies derived transplacentally. Maternal antibodies may persist in the infant for up to 18 months. Therefore, other diagnostic tests are used, most commonly the HIV polymerase chain reaction (PCR) for detection of proviral DNA.

With the identification of HIV antigen, individuals may be diagnosed with HIV infection before development of symptoms.

Before testing, provide counselling to the parent or guardian, including an explanation of HIV infection, the reason for the test, implications of positive test results, confidentiality issues, risk reduction behaviours and beneficial effects of early intervention.

Therapeutic Management

The goals of therapy for HIV infection include slowing the growth of the virus, preventing and treating opportunistic infections and providing nutritional support and symptomatic treatment. Antiretroviral drugs work at various stages of the HIV life cycle to prevent reproduction of functional new virus particles. Antiretroviral therapy regimens are continually evolving. Although antiretroviral drugs are not a cure, they can delay progression of the disease (Yogev & Chadwick 2016). Antiretroviral therapy regimens and guidelines are continually evolving. Therapy is lifelong, making adherence difficult. Laboratory markers (e.g. $CD4^+$ lymphocyte count, viral load) assist in monitoring both disease progression and response to therapy.

Strict scheduling requirements, side effects and need for multiple medications, which at times are not very palatable, make it difficult for children and adolescents to take their medications at the right time and in proper coordination with their meals. Yet adhering to the medication schedule is critical to preventing the development of resistant forms of HIV (Yogev & Chadwick 2016). Clinical improvements include weight gain in children with previous growth retardation, decreased hepatosplenomegaly, improvement in symptoms of HIV-associated encephalopathy and improvement in immune system function.

Pneumocystis jiroveci pneumonia (PJP), formerly known as Pneumocystis carinii pneumonia (PCP), is the most common opportunistic infection in children infected with HIV. It occurs most frequently between 3 and 6 months of age, when HIV status may be unclear. All infants born to HIV-infected women should receive prophylaxis until HIV infection is reasonably excluded (Siberry 2014). For children older than 1 year of age, the need for prophylaxis depends on the presence of severe immunosuppression or a history of PJP. Trimethoprim-sulfamethoxazole is the agent of choice.

HIV infection often leads to marked failure to thrive and multiple nutritional deficiencies. Nutritional management may be difficult because of recurrent illness, diarrhoea and other physical problems. The nurse should implement intensive nutritional interventions if the child's growth begins to slow or weight begins to decrease. Children with opportunistic infections (e.g. *Pneumocystis* pneumonia), encephalopathy and regressing developmental milestones, or wasting syndrome have the worst prognosis, with 75% dying before 3 years of age (Yogev & Chadwick 2016).

Prognosis. Early recognition and improved medical care have changed HIV infection from a rapidly fatal disease to a chronic one. After the introduction of combination antiretroviral therapy, the numbers of new AIDS cases and deaths declined substantially.

Nursing Care Management

Education concerning the transmission and control of infectious diseases, including HIV infection, is essential for children with HIV infection and anyone involved in their care. The basic tenets of standard precautions should be presented in an age-appropriate manner, with careful consideration of the educational level of the individual. To reduce the incidence of opportunistic infections, parents and children should be counselled about: (1) the importance of good handwashing; (2) avoiding raw or undercooked food (*Salmonella*); (3) avoiding drinking or swimming in lake or river water or being in contact with young farm animals (*Cryptosporidium*); and (4) the risk of playing with pets (*Toxoplasma* and *Bartonella* from cats, *Salmonella* from reptiles) (Yogev & Chadwick 2016). Safety issues, including appropriate storage of special medications and equipment (e.g. needles and syringes), are emphasised.

Prevention is a key component of HIV education. Educating adolescents about HIV is essential in preventing HIV infection in this age group. Education should include information on the routes of transmission, the hazards of IV and other recreational drug use and the value of safe sex practices (AFAO 2020, NZAF 2020, Yogev & Chadwick 2016). Such education should be a part of anticipatory guidance provided to all adolescent patients. Nurses should also encourage adolescents at risk to undergo HIV counselling and testing. In addition to identifying infected teenagers and getting them into care, such counselling affords adolescents an opportunity to learn about, and possibly change, their risk behaviours. (See Quality Patient Outcomes box.)

QUALITY PATIENT OUTCOMES

Human Immunodeficiency Virus

- Early recognition of signs and symptoms of HIV
- HIV infection slowed or maintained
- Growth and development promoted
- No infectious complications or cancer development
- Adherence to antiretroviral therapy
- Prolonged survival
- Quality of life supported

The nurse's role in the care of the child with HIV is multifaceted. The nurse serves as educator, direct care provider, case manager and advocate. As with all children with chronic illnesses, these children have much involvement with the healthcare system. Clinic visits and hospitalisations may become frequent as the disease progresses. The physiological care of the child is directed at minimising exposure to infections; delaying the development of viral resistance; supplying nutritional support; providing comfort measures, including pain management; and assessing and recognising changes in status that may indicate new complications. The scope of nursing care changes with new symptoms, changes in treatment and disease progression. Psychological interventions vary with the unique circumstances of each child and family.

Common psychosocial concerns include disclosing the diagnosis to the child and anticipating the loss of a family member. Other stressors may include financial difficulties, HIV-associated stigma, attempts to keep the diagnosis a secret, infection of other family members and any losses associated with HIV. Mothers of these children who are also HIV infected often attend to the needs of their child first, neglecting their own health in the process. The nurse can encourage the mother to receive regular healthcare. Family members are often involved in the care of the child, particularly if the mother has symptomatic illness. The nurse is an integral part of the multidisciplinary team necessary for the successful management of the complex medical and social problems of these families.

REFERENCES

Abdullah, K., Thorpe, K. E., Mamak, E., et al. (2015). Optimizing early child development for young children with non-anemic iron deficiency in primary care practice setting (OptEC): Study protocol for a randomized controlled trial. Trials, 16, 132.

Adewoyin, A. S. (2015). Management of sickle cell disease: A review for physician education in Nigeria (Sub-Saharan Africa). Anemia, 791498 (21 pages).

Anderson, O., Domeliof, M., Anderson, D., et al. (2014). Effect of delayed vs early umbilical cord clamping on iron status and neurodevelopment at age 12 months: A randomized clinical trial. JAMA Pediatrics, 168(6), 547–554.

Anderson, A., & Forsyth, A. (2017). Playing it safe: bleeding disorders, sports and exercise. The National Hemophilia Foundation.

Angulo-Barroso, R. M., Li, M., Santos, D. C. C., et al. (2016). Iron supplementation in pregnancy or infancy and motor development: A randomized controlled trial. Pediatrics, 137(4), e20153547.

Aquino, D., Marley, J. V., Senior, K., et al. (2013). Early Childhood Nutrition and Anaemia Prevention Project: Executive summary. Darwin: The Fred Hollows Foundation, Indigenous Australia Program.

Ansari, S. H., Lassi, Z. S., Ali, S. M., et al. (2016). Hydroxyurea for β-thalassemia major. Cochrane Database of Systematic Reviews, (1), CD012064.

Arlet, J., Dussiot, M., Moura, I. C., et al. (2016). Novel players [beta]-thalassemia dyserythropoiesis and new therapeutic strategies. Current Opinion in Hematology, 23(3), 181–188.

Australian Confederation of AIDS Organisations (AFAO). (2020). HIV Statistics. https://www.afao.org.au/about-hiv/hiv-in-australia/

Australian Haemophilia Centre Directors' Organisation (AHCDO). (2016). Guidelines for the management of haemophilia in Australia. https://www.blood.gov.au/system/files/HaemophiliaGuidelines-interactive-updated-260317v2.pdf

Baker, R. D., Greer, F. R., & Committee on Nutrition. (2010). Diagnosis and prevention of iron deficiency and iron-deficiency anemia in infants and young children (0-3 years of age). Pediatrics, 126, 1040–1050.

Bar-Zeev, S. J., Kruske, S. G., Barclay, L. M., et al. (2013). Adherence to management guidelines for growth faltering and anaemia in remote dwelling Australian Aboriginal infants and barriers to health service delivery. BMC Health Services Research, 13(250), 1–12.

Ben-Ami, T., & Revel-Vilk, S. (2013). The use of DDAVP in children with bleeding disorders. Pediatric Blood and Cancer, 60, S41–S43.

Bolton-Maggs, P. H. B., Langer, J. C., Iolascon, A., et al. (2011). Guidelines for the diagnosis and management of hereditary spherocytosis—2011 update. British Journal of Haematology, 156, 37–49.

Branchford, B. R., Monahan, P. E., & Di Paola, J. (2013). New developments in the treatment of pediatric hemophilia and bleeding disorders. Current Opinion in Pediatrics, 25, 23–30.

Bregman, D. B., & Goodnough, L. T. (2014). Experience with intravenous ferric carboxymaltose in patients with iron deficiency anemia. Therapeutic Advances in Hematology, 5(2), 48–60.

Broderick, C. R., Herbert, R. D., Latimer, J., et al. (2012). Association between physical activity and risk of bleeding in children with hemophilia. The Journal of the American Medical Association, 308(14), 1452–1459.

Brugnara, C., Oski, F. A., & Nathan, D. G. (2015). Diagnostic approach to the anemic patient. In S. H. Orkin, D. E. Fisher, D. Ginsburg, et al. (Eds.), Nathan and Oski's hematology of infancy and childhood (8th ed.). Philadelphia: Saunders.

Camaschella, C. (2015). Iron-deficiency anemia. The New England Journal of Medicine, 372, 1832–1843.

Carmel, R., Watkins, D., & Rosenblatt, D. S. (2015). Megaloblastic anemia. In S. H. Orkin, D. E. Fisher, D. Ginsburg, et al. (Eds.), Nathan and Oski's hematology of infancy and childhood (8th ed.). Philadelphia: Saunders.

Castaman, G., & Linari, S. (2017). Diagnosis and treatment of von Willebrand Disease and rare bleeding disorders. Journal of Clinical Medicine, 6, 45.

Celkan, T., & Koc, B. S. (2015). Approach to the patient with neutropenia in childhood. Turkish Archives of Pediatrics, 50, 136–144.

Chan, C. Q. H., Low, L. L., & Lee, K. H. (2016). Oral vitamin B12 replacement for the treatment of pernicious anemia. Frontiers in Medicine, 3, 38.

Chatterjee, R., & Bajora, R. (2010). Critical appraisal of growth retardation and pubertal disturbances in thalassemia. Annals of the New York Academy of Sciences, 1202, 100–114.

Choudhry, V. P. (2017). Thalassemia minor and major: Current management. Indian Journal of Pediatrics, 84(8), 607–611.

Cuesta-Barriuso, R., Torres-Ortuno, A., Perez-Alenda, S., et al. (2016). Sporting activities and quality of life in children with hemophilia: An observational study. Pediatric Physical Therapy, 28, 453–459.

DaCosta, L., Galimand, J., Fenneteau, O., et al. (2013). Hereditary spherocytosis, elliptocytosis, and other red cell membrane disorders. Blood Reviews, 27, 167–178.

Dale, D. C. (2017). How I manage children with neutropenia. British Journal of Haematology, 178(3), 351–363.

Dastgiri, S., & Dolatkhah, R. (2016). Blood transfusions for treating acute chest syndrome in people with sickle cell disease. Cochrane Database of Systematic Reviews, (8), CD007843.

DeBaun, M. R., Armstrong, F. D., McKinstry, R. C., et al. (2012). Silent cerebral infarcts: A review on a prevalent and progressive cause of neurologic injury in sickle cell anemia. Blood, 17, 4587–4596.

DeBaun, M. R., Frei-Jones, M., & Vichinsky, E. (2016). Hemoglobinopathies. In R. M. Kliegman, B. F. Stanton, J. W. St. Geme, et al. (Eds.), Nelson textbook of pediatrics (20th ed.). Philadelphia: Elsevier.

DeBaun, M. R., & Kirkham, F. J. (2016). Central nervous system complications and management in sickle cell disease. Blood, 127(7), 829–838.
DeLoughery, T. G. (2014). Microcytic Anemia. The New England Journal of Medicine, 371, 1324–1331.
Dinauer, M. C., Newburger, P. E., & Borregaard, N. (2015). Phagocyte system and disorders of granulopoiesis and granulocyte function. In S. H. Orkin, D. E. Fisher, D. Ginsburg, et al. (Eds.), Nathan and Oski's hematology of infancy and childhood (8th ed.). Philadelphia: Elsevier Saunders.
Di Paola, J., Montgomery, R. R., Gill, J. C., et al. (2015). Hemophilia and von Willebrand disease. In S. H. Orkin, D. E. Fisher, D. Ginsburg, et al. (Eds.), Nathan and Oski's hematology of infancy and childhood (8th ed.). Philadelphia: Elsevier Saunders.
Ellison, A. M. (2012). Sickle cell disease: Advice on handling emergencies. Contemporary Pediatrics, 18–27.
Estcourt, L. J., Fortin, P. M., Hopewell, S., et al. (2017). Blood transfusion for preventing primary and secondary stroke in people with sickle cell disease. Cochrane Database of Systematic Reviews, (1), CD003146.
Fleming, M. D. (2015). Disorders of iron and copper metabolism, the sideroblastic anemias and lead toxicity. In S. H. Orkin, D. E. Fisher, D. Ginsburg, et al. (Eds.), Nathan and Oski's hematology of infancy and childhood (8th ed.). Philadelphia: Saunders.
Flood, V. H., & Scott, J. P. (2016). Von Willebrand disease. In R. M. Kliegman, B. F. Stanton, J. W. St. Geme III, et al. (Eds.), Nelson textbook of pediatrics (20th ed.). Philadelphia: Elsevier, Inc.
Foong, W. C., Ho, J. J., Loh, C. K., et al. (2016). Hydroxyurea for reducing blood transfusion in non-transfusion dependent beta thalassaemias. Cochrane Database of Systematic Reviews, (10), CD011579.
Grace, R. F. (2015). Hematologic manifestations of systemic diseases. In S. H. Orkin, D. E. Fisher, D. Ginsburg, et al. (Eds.), Nathan and Oski's hematology of infancy and childhood (8th ed.). Philadelphia: Saunders.
Griebler, U., Bruckmuller, M. U., Kien, C., et al. (2015). Health effects of cow's milk consumption in infants up to 3 years of age: A systematic review and meta-analysis. Public Heath Nutrition, 19(2), 293–307.
Guelcher, C. J. (2016). Evolution of the treatments for hemophilia. Journal of Infusion Nursing, 39(4), 218–224.
Haemophilia Foundation of Australia (HFA). (2020). Haemophilia Fast Facts. https://www.haemophilia.org.au/about-bleeding-disorders/fast-facts#splash-timed
Haemophilia Foundation of New Zealand (HFNZ). (2020). Haemophilia. http://www.haemophilia.org.nz/bleeding-disorders/haemophilia/
Heeney, M., & Ware, R. (2015). Sickle cell disease. In S. H. Orkin, D. E. Fisher, D. Ginsburg, et al. (Eds.), Nathan and Oski's hematology of infancy and childhood (8th ed.). Philadelphia: Saunders.
Hermans, C., De Moerloose, P., Fischer, K., et al. (2011). Management of acute haemarthrosis in haemophilia A without inhibitors: Literature review, European survey and recommendations. Haemophilia, 17, 383–392.
Higgs, D. R., Engel, J. D., & Stamatoyannopoulos, G. (2012). Thalassaemia. Lancet, 379, 373–383.
Hord, J. D. (2016). The acquired pancytopenias. In R. M. Kliegman, B. F. Stanton, J. W. St. Geme III, et al. (Eds.), Nelson textbook of pediatrics (20th ed.). Philadelphia: Elsevier Inc.
Issaragrisil, S., & Kunacheewa, C. (2016). Matched sibling donor hematopoietic stem cell transplantation for thalassemia. Current Opinion in Hematology, 23(6), 508–514.
Ishikawa, N., Dalal, S., Johnson, C., et al. (2016). Should HIV testing for all pregnant women continue? Cost-effectiveness of universal testing compared to focused approaches across high to very low HIV prevalence settings, JIAS 19, http://www.jiasociety.org/index.php/jas/article/view/21212.
Kahnooji, M., Rashidinejad, H. R., Yazdanpanah, M. S., et al. (2016). Myocardial iron load measured by cardiac magnetic resonance imaging to evaluate cardiac systolic function in thalassemia. ARYA Atherosclerosis, 12(5), 226–230.
Kehrel, B. E., & Brodde, M. F. (2013). State of the art in platelet function testing. Transfusion Medicine and Hemotherapy: Offizielles Organ der Deutschen Gesellschaft fur Transfusionsmedizin und Immunhamatologie, 40, 73–86.
Kett, J. C. (2012). Anemia in infancy. Pediatrics in Review, 33(4), 186–187.
Korthof, E. T., Bekassy, A. N., & Hussein, A. A. (2013). Management of acquired aplastic anemia in children. Bone Marrow Transplantation, 48(2), 191–195.
Kuhne, T., & Imbach, P. (2013). Management of children and adolescents with primary immune thrombocytopenia: Controversies and solutions. Vox Sanguinis, 104, 55–66.
Kumar, M., Lambert, M. P., Breakey, V., et al. (2015). Sports participation in children and adolescents with immune thrombocytopenia (ITP). Pediatric Blood and Cancer, 62, 2223–2225.
Kuznik, A., Habib, A. G., Munube, D., et al. (2016). Newborn screening and prophylactic intervention for sickle cell disease in 47 countries in sub-Saharan Africa: A cost-effectiveness analysis. BMC Health Service Research, 16(304), 1572–1576.
Lerner, N. (2016). The anemias. In R. M. Kliegman, B. F. Stanton, J. W. St. Geme III, et al (Eds.), Nelson textbook of pediatrics (20th ed.). Philadelphia: Elsevier Inc.
Lillicrap, D. (2013). The future of hemostasis management. Pediatric Blood and Cancer, 60(Suppl. 1), S447–S451.
Locatelli, F., Merli, P., & Strocchio, L. (2016). Transplantation for thalassemia major: Alternative donors. Current Opinion in Hematology, 23(6), 515–523.
Lucarelli, G., Isgro, A., Sodani, P., et al. (2012). Hematopoietic stem cell transplantation in thalassemia and sickle cell anemia. Cold Spring Harbor Perspectives in Medicine, 2(5), a011825. Published online April 4, 2012.
Lux, S. E. (2015). Disorders of the red cell membrane. In S. H. Orkin, D. E. Fisher, D. Ginsburg, et al. (Eds.), Nathan and Oski's hematology of infancy and childhood (8th ed.). Philadelphia: Saunders.
Lytle, A. M., Brown, H. C., Paik, N. Y., et al. (2016). Effects of FVIII immunity on hepatocyte and hematopoietic stem cell-directed gene therapy of murine hemophilia A, Molecular Therapy-Methods and Clinical Development. Molecular Therapy. Methods & Clinical Development, 10(3), 15056.
Mahoney, D. H. (2017). Iron deficiency in infants and young children: Screening, prevention, clinical manifestations, and diagnosis, UpToDate, http://www.uptodate.com.
Manco-Johnson, M. J., Abshire, T. C., Shapiro, A. D., et al. (2007). Prophylaxis versus episodic treatment to prevent joint disease in boys with severe hemophilia. The New England Journal of Medicine, 357, 535–544.
Marcdante, K. J., & Kliegman, R. M. (2015). Hemostatic Disorders. In K. J. Mardante & R. M. Kliegman (Eds.), Nelson essentials of pediatrics (20th ed.). Philadelphia: Elsevier Saunders.
Matino, D., Makris, M., Dwan, K., et al. (2015). Recombinant (non-human) factor VIIa clotting factor concentrates versus plasma concentrates for acute bleeds in people with haemophilia and inhibitors. Cochrane Database of Systematic Reviews, (12), CD004449.
McCavit, T. L. (2012). Sickle cell disease. Pediatrics in Review, 33, 195–206.
McCrae, K. (2011). Immune thrombocytopenia: No longer 'idiopathic'. Cleveland Clinic Journal of Medicine, 78(6), 358–373.
McDonagh, M. S., Blazina, I., Dana, T., et al. (2015). Screening and routine supplementation for iron deficiency anemia: A systematic review. Pediatrics, 135(4), 723–733.
McGann, P. T. (2016). Time to invest in sickle cell anemia as a global health priority. Pediatrics, 137(6), 210160348.
Meier, E. R., & Miller, J. L. (2012). Sickle cell disease in children. Drugs, 72, 895–906.
Mercer, J. S., Erickson-Owens, D. A., Collins, J., et al. (2017). Effects of delayed cord clamping on residual placental blood volume, hemoglobin and bilirubin levels in term infants: A randomized controlled trial. Journal of Perinatology, 37(3), 260–264.
Miller, J. L. (2013). Iron deficiency anemia: A common and curable disease. Cold Spring Harbor Perspectives in Medicine, 3(3), Published online April 23, 2013.
Miller, A., Ziegler, J. & Palasanthiran, P. (2013). Paediatric HIV in Australia: 30 years of a changing landscape. HIV Australia, 11(1).
National Blood Authority Australia (NBA). (2017). Paediatric and Neonatal Iron Deficiency Anaemia Guide. Canberra.
Neutze, D., & Roque, J. (2016). Clinical evaluation of bleeding and bruising in primary care. American Family Physician, 93(4), 279–286.
Nevitt, S. J., Jones, A. P., & Howard, J. (2017). Hydroxyurea (hydroxycarbamide) for sickle cell disease. The Cochrane Database of Systematic Reviews, (4), CD002202.

New Zealand AIDS Foundation (NZAF). (2020). HIV in New Zealand. https://www.nzaf.org.nz/awareness-and-prevention/hiv/hiv-in-nz/

Nienhuis, A. W., & Nathan, D. (2012). Pathophysiology and clinical manifestations of the β-thalassemias. Cold Spring Harbor Perspectives in Medicine, 2(12), a011726.

Nienhuis, A. W., Nathwani, A. C., & Davidoff, A. M. (2017). Gene therapy for hemophilia. Molecular Therapy, 25(5), 1163–1167.

Nussbaum, R. L., McInnes, R. R., & Willard, H. F. (2016). Genetic variation in populations. In R. L. Nussbaum, R. R. McInnes, & H. F. Willard (Eds.), Thompson and Thompson Genetics in Medicine (8th ed.). Philadelphia: Elsevier.

Pahuja, S., Puri, V., Mahajan, G., et al. (2017). Reporting adverse transfusion reactions: A retrospective study from tertiary care hospital from New Delhi, India. Asian Journal of Transfusion Science, 11(1), 6–12.

Passweg, J. R., & Marsh, J. C. W. (2010). Aplastic anemia: First-line treatment by immunosuppressive and sibling marrow transplantation. Hematology, 2010, 36–42.

Raja, J. V., Rachchh, M. A., & Gokani, R. H. (2012). Recent advances in gene therapy for thalassemia. Journal of Pharmacy & Bioallied Sciences, 4, 194–201.

Renda, M., & Fischer, P. (2009). Vegetarian diets in children and adolescents. Pediatrics in Review, 30, e1–e8.

Rodeghiero, F., Stasi, R., Gernsheimer, T., et al. (2009). Standardization of terminology, definitions and outcome criteria in immune thrombocytopenic purpura of adults and children: Report from an international working group. Blood, 113(11), 2386–2393.

Rosman, C. W. K., Broens, P. M. A., Trzpis, M., et al. (2017). A long-term follow-up study of subtotal splenectomy in children with hereditary spherocytosis. Pediatric Blood and Cancer, 64(10).

Sankaran, V. G., Nathan, D. G., & Orkin, S. H. (2015). The thalassemias. In S. H. Orkin, D. E. Fisher, D. Ginsburg, et al. (Eds.), Nathan and Oski's hematology of infancy and childhood (8th ed.). Philadelphia: Saunders.

Sarangi, S. N., & Acharya, S. S. (2017). Bleeding disorders in congenital syndromes. Pediatrics, 139(2).

Scott, J. P. (2016a). Platelet and blood vessel disorders. In R. M. Kliegman, B. F. Stanton, J. W. St. Geme, et al. (Eds.), Nelson textbook of pediatrics (20th ed.). Philadelphia: Elsevier.

Scott, J. P. (2016b). Hereditary clotting factor deficiencies: Factor VIII or factor IX deficiency (hemophilia A or B). In R. M. Kliegman, B. F. Stanton, J. W. St.Geme, et al. (Eds.), Nelson textbook of pediatrics (20th ed.). Philadelphia: Elsevier.

Sharathkumar, A. A., & Carcao, M. (2011). Clinical advances in hemophilia management. Pediatric Blood and Cancer, 57, 910–920.

Sharathkumar, A. A., & Pipe, S. W. (2008). Post-thrombotic syndrome in children: A single center experience. Journal of Pediatric Hematology, 30(4), 261–266.

Shimamura, A., & Williams, D. A. (2015). Aquired aplastic anemia and pure red cell aplasia. In S. H. Orkin, D. E. Fisher, D. Ginsburg, et al. (Eds.), Nathan and Oski's hematology of infancy and childhood (8th ed.). Philadelphia: Saunders.

Siberry, G. K. (2014). Preventing and managing HIV infection in infants, children, and adolescents in the United States. Pediatrics in Review, 35(7), 268–286.

Sills, R. (2016). Iron-deficiency anemia. In R. M. Kliegman, B. F. Stanton, J. W. St. Geme III, et al. (Eds.), Nelson textbook of pediatrics (20th ed.). Philadelphia: Elsevier.

Smith, A. (2012). Guide to evaluation and treatment of anaemia in general practice. Drug Review, 5, 25–42.

Starship. (2016). Iron Deficiency. https://www.starship.org.nz/guidelines/iron-deficiency/

Strauss, R. G. (2016). Risk of blood transfusions. In R. M. Kliegman, B. F. Stanton, J. W. St. Geme III, et al. (Eds.), Nelson textbook of pediatrics (20th ed.). Philadelphia: Elsevier.

Subramaniam, G., & Girish, M. (2015). Iron deficiency anemia in children. Indian Journal of Pediatrics, 82(6), 558–564.

Therrell, B. L., Padilla, C. D., Loeber, J. G., et al. (2015). Current status of newborn screening worldwide: 2015. Seminars in Perinatology, 39, 171–187.

Thompson, J., Biggs, B. A., & Pasricha, S. R. (2013). Effects of daily iron supplementation in 2- to 5-year-old children: Systematic review and meta-analysis. Pediatrics, 131, 739–753.

United Nations AIDS. (2019). AIDS info. https://aidsinfo.unaids.org/

Vidal-Alaball, J., Butler, C. C., Cannings-John, R., et al. (2016). Oral vitamin B12 versus intramuscular vitamin B12 for vitamin B12 deficiency. Cochrane Database of Systematic Review, (3), CD004655.

von der Lippe, C., Frich, J. C., Harris, A., et al. (2017). Treatment of hemophilia: A qualitative study of mothers' perspectives. Pediatric Blood and Cancer, 64, 121–127.

Walkovich, K., & Newburger, P. E. (2016). Leukopenia. In R. M. Kliegman, B. F. Stanton, J. W. St. Geme III, et al. (Eds.), Nelson textbook of pediatrics (20th ed.). Philadelphia: Elsevier.

Walsh, C. E., & Batt, K. M. (2013). Hemophilia clinical gene therapy: Brief review. Translational Research: The Journal of Laboratory and Clinical Medicine, 161, 307–312.

Wang, W. C., & Dwan, K. (2013). Blood transfusion for preventing primary and secondary stroke in people with sickle cell disease. Cochrane Database of Systematic Review, (11), CD003146.

Wang, B., Zhan, S., Gong, T., et al. (2013). Iron therapy for improving psychomotor development and cognitive function in children under the age of three with iron deficiency anaemia. Cochrane Database of Systematic Review, (6), CD001444, 1–50.

Wilson, D. B. (2015). Acquired platelet defects. In S. H. Orkin, D. E. Fisher, D. Ginsburg, et al. (Eds.), Nathan and Oski's hematology of infancy and childhood (8th ed.). Philadelphia: Saunders.

Yaish, H. M. (2015). Pediatric thalassemia, http://emedicine.medscape.com/article/958850-overview.

Yawn, B. P., Buchanan, G. R., Afenyl-Annan, A. N., et al. (2014). Management of sickle cell disease: Summary of the 2014 evidence-based report by expert panel members. JAMA: The Journal of the American Medical Association, 312(10), 1033–1048.

Yawn, B. P., & John-Sowah, J. (2015). Management of sickle cell disease: Recommendations from the 2014 expert panel report. American Family Physician, 92(12), 1069–1076.

Yogev, R., & Chadwick, E. G. (2016). Acquired immunodeficiency syndrome (human immunodeficiency virus). In R. M. Kliegman, B. F. Stanton, J. W. St. Geme III, et al. (Eds.), Nelson textbook of pediatrics (20th ed.). Philadelphia: Elsevier.

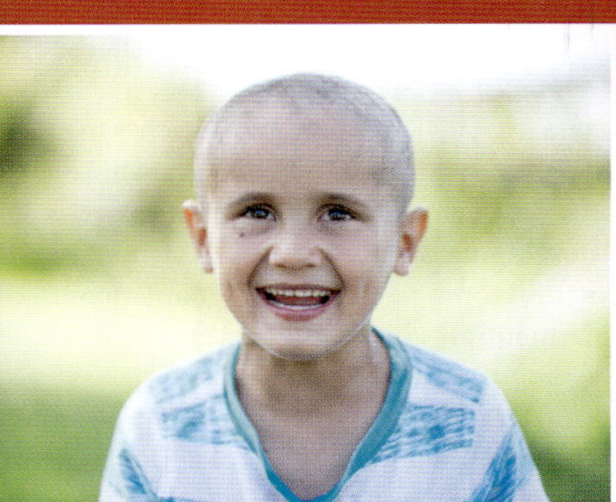

The Child with Cancer

Elyce Kenny

LEARNING OUTCOMES

- Understand the different types of cancers in children, their epidemiology and how they are treated.
- Discuss how and why childhood cancer are different from adult cancers.
- Discuss the role of clinical trials in childhood cancers.
- Understand the nursing role in caring for children and families diagnosed with childhood cancer.
- Outline the long-term effects of treatment for childhood cancer.

CANCER IN CHILDREN

Few situations in nursing exceed the challenges of caring for a child with cancer. Despite dramatic improvements in survival rates, the family's informational and support needs are great as they cope with a serious physical illness and the fear that the child will not be cured. Children's cancer is different in the methods and medicines used, due to the fact that there are no obvious behavioural preventions like giving up smoking that will prevent it from occurring. This difference also extends to research, where paediatric oncology is one of the few areas in which clinical research is expertly integrated with clinical care. It is for this reason that the survival rates of children diagnosed with cancer have increased so dramatically over the last 50 years. Despite this, any cancer treatment is a long, drawn-out and gruelling process for children and their family, and there are still those that will succumb to their disease or its side effects. Beyond the loss of young life, the burden of childhood cancer extends to the long-term adverse health effects that are experienced by a large proportion of survivors, as a result of their cancer and its treatment. Both treatment and these long-term effects will have a significant psychosocial impact on the child, their family and their siblings. Families must face financial strain, balancing work while caring for an acutely unwell child and the disruption of normal family and social routines (Australian and New Zealand Children's Haematology Oncology Group [ANZCHOG] 2020, Ballentine & NZCCR Working Group 2017, Youlden & Aitken 2019). Nurses should base support of patients and their families on the premise that effective communication promotes understanding and clarity. With informed, honest communication and compassionate care, fear diminishes, hope emerges and the cancer journey feels less overwhelming.

Epidemiology

Compared to the adult population, childhood cancer is rare and accounts for less than 1% of all cancers diagnosed each year. Despite this low incidence, it is still a significant health issue in Australia and New Zealand and accounts for almost a quarter of all the deaths recorded in this population. It is the second most common cause of childhood death behind injuries and accidents (Ballentine & NZCCR Working Group 2017, Youlden & Aitken 2019).

In Australia, 770 children were diagnosed with some form of childhood cancer between 2011 and 2015. Of those, 55% were boys and 45% were girls (Ballentine & NZCCR Working Group 2017, Youlden & Aitken 2019). In New Zealand, 762 children were diagnosed between 2010 and 2014. Approximately 50% of all children will be aged 4 or younger at the time of diagnosis (Ballentine & NZCCR Working Group 2017, Youlden & Aitken 2019).

The incidence of specific subtypes of childhood cancer varies according to age, sex and race/ethnicity. Leukaemias account for the largest number of diagnoses each year, with approximately 32% of children being diagnosed. This is closely followed by central nervous system tumours which account for approximately 25% of diagnoses each year. The incidence and mortality of childhood cancer in the Indigenous and Māori population was comparable to their non-Indigenous and non-Māori counterparts (Ballentine & NZCCR Working Group 2017, Youlden & Aitken 2019).

It has only been due to extensive clinical trials over the last few decades that there has been an increase in the percentage of children surviving a cancer diagnosis (Children's Oncology Group [COG] 2019c, European Society for Paediatric Oncology [SIOP Europe] 2020). The overall 5-year survival rate is approximately 84%, but this will vary depending on the type of cancer. A child diagnosed with acute lymphoblastic leukaemia has a 5-year survival rate of 92%, while a child diagnosed with a glioma has a 46% chance of surviving to 5 years post diagnosis (Ballentine & NZCCR Working Group 2017, Youlden & Aitken 2019).

But with greater percentages of children surviving their cancer treatment comes long-term side effects and an increased risk of secondary cancers. Childhood cancer survivors are five times more likely to be diagnosed with a secondary cancer later in life, compared to the rest of the population (Youlden & Aitken 2019).

RESEARCH FOCUS

Childhood Cancer Survival Rates

Childhood cancer survival has dramatically increased over the past five decades since chemotherapy was first given to children. In the 1960s, the overall survival rate of childhood cancer was 28% compared with 5-year survival rates that now exceed 80% (Scheurer et al 2016). Improvement in survival among the adolescent group has lagged behind younger age groups, although that is changing. The cancers demonstrating the greatest improvement in survival rates are acute lymphoblastic leukaemia, non-Hodgkin's lymphoma and Wilms tumour. A general definition of 'cure' in childhood cancer includes completion of all therapy, no clinical and radiological evidence of disease and a period of 5 years since diagnosis.

Aetiology

Often the first question asked by parents of children newly diagnosed with cancer is, 'How did my child get this, and did I do something to cause it?' Parents are also understandably concerned about whether their other children also will get cancer. In most cases we do not know why children get cancer. They are too young to have the same risk factors that affect adults. It is not caused by a bump on the head, or by anything the child or their parents did or did not do. Cancer cannot be passed from one child to another like a virus (Cancer Australia 2020, Murphy 2011). There are numerous hypotheses concerning what causes childhood cancer, but the most enduring theory is that genetic alteration results in the unregulated proliferation of cells. Significant advances have been made in our understanding of cell proliferation, programmed cell death (**apoptosis**), genes that activate tumour growth (**oncogenes**), genes that keep tumour growth in check (**tumour suppressor genes**) and changes in gene expression without gene alteration (**epigenetics**). Cancer is the result of multiple genetic events, but it is not necessarily hereditary. Overall, the incidence of cancers caused by direct inheritance is low, but much has been learned about cancer by studying its inherited forms.

In the early 1970s Alfred Knudson proposed the 'two-hit hypothesis'. This explanation of cancer inheritance is best illustrated in the inherited form of retinoblastoma. Like most genes, the retinoblastoma gene (*Rb1*) is normally present in two copies on each cell. *Rb1* is a tumour suppressor gene responsible for controlling cell growth. When just one of the gene copies is lost—the 'first hit'—the cell remains normal. However, if the second copy is lost—the 'second hit'—abnormal cell proliferation occurs and retinoblastoma develops (Knudson et al 1975). A child can inherit one altered copy of the retinoblastoma gene from either mother or father. When this happens, it takes only one more hit (e.g. an environmental exposure) for retinoblastoma to develop.

Chromosome abnormalities have been identified in many childhood malignancies and are important in the development of various types of cancer. Chromosome abnormalities can be confined to the tumour or can be present in all cells; the latter are called **germ-line mutations**. Chromosome abnormalities can be due to **translocations** (a rearrangement of information between two chromosomes) or **abnormal numbers** of chromosomes. Not only does our increased understanding of these chromosome abnormalities help us to accurately diagnose the malignancy, it is also key to guiding clinicians in the most appropriate treatment path.

Perhaps the most well-known inherited cancer predisposition syndrome is Li-Fraumeni syndrome, which is mainly due to constitutional (in all cells) mutation in the tumour suppressor gene, *p53*. This syndrome is characterised by early incidence of brain tumours, premenopausal breast cancer, soft tissue and bone sarcomas, leukaemias and lymphomas (Plon & Malkin 2016). Other genetic syndromes that can affect genes or chromosomes and are associated with a predisposition to cancer include Fanconi's anaemia, Bloom's syndrome, Beckwith-Wiedemann syndrome, neurofibromatosis type 1, ataxia-telangiectasia and Klinefelter's syndrome.

Children with immunodeficiencies, such as Wiskott-Aldrich syndrome or acquired immunodeficiency syndrome, or children whose immune system has been suppressed, such as after transplant procedures, are at a greater risk for developing various cancers. Of major concern is the increased risk of developing second malignant neoplasms (SMNs) after curative treatment for childhood cancer.

Risk Factors

Lifestyle-related behaviours are the main factors that increase the risk of cancer in adults, but as far as is now known, they have little to no effect on cancer in children. There is relatively little information to support a major environmental role in the development of childhood cancer. However, there are a few well-established risk factors, including exposure to ionising radiation, carcinogenic drugs, immunosuppressive therapy, certain viral infections (e.g. Epstein-Barr virus, human papillomavirus [HPV]), race/ethnicity, and genetic conditions or chromosomal abnormalities (Table 29.1) (Scheurer et al 2016).

Prevention. Knowledge of the risk factors that increase the likelihood of cancer holds the promise of prevention. Unfortunately, because few carcinogens are associated with cancer in children, there are no generally recognised preventive measures for childhood cancer.

Nevertheless, paediatric health professionals have another role in cancer prevention, namely educating parents and children about the hazards of known carcinogens associated with adult-type cancers. This is particularly true for the effects of cigarette smoking (and exposure to second-hand smoke) and excessive exposure to ultraviolet radiation (e.g. exposure to sunlight and tanning) because lung cancer is the leading cause of death from cancer in adults, and malignant melanoma is the leading cause of death from diseases of the skin. Children at higher risk for skin cancer are those with sun or tanning bed exposure; light-coloured eyes, complexion and hair; a history of sunburn; skin that burns, freckles and reddens easily; and certain types of moles (Cancer Australia 2020). Children and teens should have periodic health examinations by a healthcare professional, including a cervical screening test for females and testicular examination for males when developmentally appropriate (Department of Health 2020b). In addition, to prevent HPV-associated malignancies, HPV vaccine is recommended for routine vaccination at age 11 to 13 years, or as per the relevant vaccination schedule (Australian Technical Advisory Group on Immunisation [ATAGI] 2018, Ministry of Health 2020).

Diagnostic Evaluation

The evaluation of a child suspected of having cancer may take several days to complete. This is a very stressful time for families as they await results. The essential components of a comprehensive evaluation include complete history and review of symptoms, physical examination, laboratory tests, diagnostic imaging, diagnostic procedures (e.g. lumbar puncture [LP], bone marrow aspirate and biopsy) and surgical pathology depending on whether biopsy/surgical resection is performed.

Complete History

History of present illness—Onset of symptoms, severity and duration, alleviating or potentiating factors

History of previous illnesses and comorbidities—Allergies, communicable diseases, infections, medication history, previous

TABLE 29.1 Known Risk Factors for Childhood Cancers

Cancer Type	Risk Factors
Acute lymphoblastic leukaemia	Ionising radiation (primarily of historical importance) Race (i.e. Caucasian) Genetic conditions (i.e. Down syndrome, Bloom's syndrome and others) Birth weight more than 400 g
Acute myeloid leukaemia	Chemotherapeutic agents (i.e. alkylating agents and epipodophyllotoxins) Genetic conditions (i.e. Down syndrome and neurofibromatosis 1)
Brain tumours	Therapeutic radiation to the head Genetic conditions (i.e. neurofibromatosis 1, tuberous sclerosis and others)
Hodgkin's disease	Family history (i.e. monozygotic twins) Infections (i.e. Epstein-Barr virus)
Non-Hodgkin's lymphoma	Immunodeficiency (i.e. acquired and congenital immunodeficiency, immunosuppressive therapy) Infections (i.e. Epstein-Barr virus associated with Burkitt's lymphoma in African countries)
Osteosarcoma	Ionising radiation (i.e. cancer radiation therapy and high radium exposure) Chemotherapy (i.e. alkylating agents) Genetic conditions (i.e. Li-Fraumeni syndrome, hereditary retinoblastoma)
Ewing's sarcoma	Race (Caucasian)
Neuroblastoma	None known
Retinoblastoma	No known non-hereditary risk factors
Wilms tumour	Congenital anomalies (i.e. aniridia, Beckwith-Wiedemann syndrome, other congenital and genetic conditions)
Rhabdomyosarcoma	Congenital anomalies and genetic conditions (i.e. Li-Fraumeni syndrome and neurofibromatosis 1)
Hepatoblastoma	Genetic conditions (i.e. Beckwith-Wiedemann syndrome, hemihypertrophy, Gardner's syndrome, family history of adenomatous polyposis)
Malignant germ cell tumours	Cryptorchidism associated with testicular germ cell tumours

Source: Scheurer, M. E., Lupo, P. J., & Bondy, M. L. (2016). Epidemiology of childhood cancer. In P. A. Pizzo & D. G. Poplack (Eds.), Principles and practice of pediatric oncology (7th ed.). Philadelphia, PA: Lippincott.

hospitalisations or surgeries, exposure to blood products, immunisation status, comorbid conditions, disabilities

Family history—Complete family tree and note any family members with prior cases of cancer: type, age at diagnosis, treatment and outcome; any other significant family history

Present health status of family members—History of illness or disease in other family members

Developmental factors—Age milestones reached, recent regression in any milestones

Psychosocial factors—Religion; culture; ethnicity; language; identification as Aboriginal, Torres Strait Islander, Māori or Pacific Islander; employment and financial status; current family support structure; any family concerns

Review of Symptoms

- **Skin**—History of bruising or bleeding, lesions, lumps, open sores
- **Neurological**—Loss of developmental milestones, changes in behaviour, sensations or vision, altered consciousness, abnormal reflexes, headaches, seizure, history of trauma
- **Ear, nose and throat (ENT)**—History of trauma, infection, difficulty swallowing
- **Eyes**—Proptosis, pupil discolouration, unequal ocular movements
- **Heart**—History of murmur or congenital heart defect
- **Lungs**—History of infection, asthma or reactive airway disease, cough, wheezing, shortness of breath, dyspnoea
- **Gastrointestinal (GI)**—History of abdominal swelling, vomiting, pain (location, timing, exacerbating and alleviating factors), mass, change in bowel or bladder patterns
- **Musculoskeletal**—History of weakness in extremities, limited range of motion (impairment of function), tenderness or swelling, pain
- **Lymphatic**—History of enlarged lymph nodes, frequent infections
- **Haematological**—History of bruising, epistaxis or gum bleeding, pallor, fatigue, bloody or tarry-coloured stools

Physical Examination

See Physical Examination, Chapter 4.

- **General**—Orientation, general state of health
- **Skin**—Petechiae or ecchymosis, lesions or sores, presence of blood from gum or nose, colour of skin
- **Neurological**—Full neurological assessment (see Chapter 4), macrocephaly, bulging fontanel, altered consciousness or sensations, abnormal reflexes, unsteady gait, dysarthria.
- **ENT**—Evidence of infection
- **Eyes**—Intact ocular movements, pupil discolouration, limited peripheral vision, nystagmus, anisocoria, leucocoria
- **Heart**—Murmur or thrill, peripheral pulses, blood pressure, perfusion status
- **Lungs**—Evidence of infection, crackles or wheeze, decreased breath sounds, dyspnoea, tachypnoea, oxygen saturations
- **Abdomen**—Hepatosplenomegaly, mass, decreased bowel sounds, striae
- **Lymphatic**—Enlarged lymph nodes

Tests and Procedures

Due to complex and ever-changing nature of paediatric cancers and their treatments, many tests and procedures will be performed to detect, diagnose, stage and determine the treatment for the malignancy. This is because every child is different, and an accurate diagnosis needs to be determined to ensure that the best course of treatment can be commenced.

Laboratory Tests

Several laboratory tests must be performed to accurately diagnose and treat children with cancer. They are also important to help detect the extent of disease and also to closely monitor for side effects during therapy (PDQ Pediatric Treatment Editorial Board 2020, COG 2019b).

- Full blood count (FBC): haemoglobin, platelet, white cell count and differential
- Biochemistry including calcium, magnesium and phosphate
- Liver function tests: urate, LDH
- Coagulation studies including extended coagulation times
- Blood group and cross match
- Immunoglobulin status
- Urinalysis
- Stool sample

Consequently, regular blood chemistries and urinalysis are standard procedures throughout the course of the disease and its treatment.

Diagnostic Procedures and Imaging

There are many different procedures and images that can be utilised to help determine, detect, diagnose and stage cancers. The tests performed will be determined by the presenting symptoms and type of malignancy (Department of Health 2020a, PDQ Pediatric Treatment Editorial Board 2020, COG 2019b).

- Plain x-ray—A high-level energy beam that is projected through the body to produce an image. Used to look for abnormal masses, infections and broken bones.
- Computed tomography (CT) scan—A series of detailed pictures of areas inside the body are taken from many different angles. Looks at bones, soft tissue and blood vessels. Allows the exact size and location of tumours to be determined.
- Magnetic resonance imaging (MTI) scan—A procedure that uses a magnet and radio waves to make a series of detailed pictures of areas inside the body, especially soft tissue. Allows the exact size and location of tumours to be determined.
- Positron emission tomography (PET) scan—A procedure that helps to find malignant cells within the body. A small amount of radioactive glucose is injected into the child's vein, which is taken up by malignant cells. As the PET scanner rotates around the body, any areas of brightness indicate the presence of a malignant cell.
- Ultrasound—A procedure in which high-energy sound waves are bounced off internal tissues and organs to create a picture. Allows the exact size and location of tumours to be determined.
- Meta-iodobenzylguanidine (MIBG) scan—A series of detailed pictures of areas inside the body, useful for locating both bone and soft tissue tumours. A small amount of radioactive dye is injected into the child's vein through an IV. When the MIBG scan is combined with this tracer, it provides a way in which to identify primary and metastatic disease. Cells that have taken up this tracer will appear bright in the scan and indicate malignant cells.
- Lumbar puncture (LP)—Also called a spinal tap. A procedure in which a needle is inserted into the lower back in order to remove cerebrospinal fluid (CSF) to test for cancer cells or infection. The same procedure can be performed to instil intrathecal chemotherapy agents in the CSF as well as a part of the child's treatment protocol.
- Bone marrow biopsy—Performed using a large-bore needle, which is placed into the bone, allowing a small piece of spongy bone marrow to be removed. This bone marrow can then be tested for cancer cells, as well as treatment response.
- Biopsy—A small piece of tumour is removed and taken out of the body to be examined for malignant cells. It can be a closed or open biopsy.

Pathological and Molecular Evaluation

For most types of childhood cancer, a biopsy is necessary to establish the diagnosis. Besides determining what type of cancer the patient has, this tissue sample can also be sent for various biological studies that help diagnose the cancer and assist in defining the patient's risk category, also called 'risk stratification'. This, in turn, guides the treatment decision-making process and helps determine prognosis. This type of cytogenetic testing has made it possible to determine the cancer subtype, where the mutations in the cell genome can then be targeted with therapeutic interventions. Some of these tests include the following (Johnson 2018, PDQ Pediatric Treatment Editorial Board 2019).

- Fluorescence in situ hybridisation (FISH)—Identifies where a specific gene is located on a chromosome, how many copies of that gene are present and any chromosomal abnormalities. It is used to diagnose and guide treatment decisions.
- Polymerase chain reaction (PCR)—A laboratory technique sued to amplify DNA sequences, allowing the DNA to be viewed in detail. Changes in genes or chromosomes can then be detected, aiding in diagnosis.
- Minimum residual disease (MRD) testing—A term used to describe a very small number of cancer cells that can be found in the body before, during and after cancer treatment. This is a highly sensitive laboratory method that allows one cancer cell among 1 million cells to be found, and guides treatment planning and response.
- Immunophenotyping—Identifies cells based on the types of antigens present on the cell surface. It is used to diagnose, stage and monitor cancers of the blood system and other haematological disorders.
- Flow cytometry—A method in which blood, bone marrow or other tissue can be tested for the presence of tumour markers. Aids in the diagnosis and treatment plan for newly diagnosed children.
- Tumour marker test—This measures the presence, level or activity of specific proteins or genes in tissue, blood or bodily fluids for cancer activity. It is used to diagnose, select appropriate treatment pathway and evaluate response to an implemented treatment plan. A tumour that has a greater than normal level of tumour marker may respond to treatment that directly targets that marker.

For example, a bone marrow biopsy determines whether the patient has acute lymphoblastic leukaemia or acute myeloid leukaemia, and indicates the specific leukaemia subtype that is the basis for how aggressively it should be treated. Similarly, patients with neuroblastoma undergo a biopsy of the tumour to establish the diagnosis and to evaluate the tumour for amplification of an oncogene, *MYCN*, which is a prognostic factor considered for treatment. As more is learned about these cell changes in cancer, it is becoming possible to design therapies that target these abnormalities or block their effects; this is called **targeted therapy**, which is the basis of precision medicine.

Precision cancer treatment is based on matching the genetics/mutations of the child's cancer with appropriate targeted therapy. The tests mentioned previously allow therapies to be designed that target the cell abnormalities or block their effects, also known as targeted therapy. This tailoring of treatment to suit the individual patient, rather than using a 'one-size-fits-all' approach, stands to revolutionise the way childhood cancer is treated (Zero Childhood Cancer 2020).

Clinical Trials

Everything we know about how to cure children with cancer has been learned from research. Clinical trials are an integral part of treating children with cancer, and it is because of these trials that the survival rates have increased so dramatically over the last 50 years (SIOP Europe 2020, COG 2019c). During this time researchers have begun to unravel cancer's complexity and have a greater understanding of the biological and genetic changes that allow children's cancers to develop, grow and spread (SIOP Europe 2020, COG 2019c). Not only can clinical trials test new treatments, they can help to determine the best use of existing interventions. This has resulted in new standard treatments with fewer or reduced side effects.

Due to the small percentage of children diagnosed with cancer worldwide each year, paediatric oncology centres collaborate with other international bodies to conduct these clinical trials (COG 2019c). The Australian and New Zealand Children's Haematology Oncology Group (ANZCHOG) brings a range of clinical trials to our region which are both therapeutic and supportive in nature. The Children's Oncology Group (COG), based in the United States, is the largest paediatric clinical trials group, with more than 210 hospitals participating around the world (COG 2019c).

It is important to understand that clinical trials are standard practice in the treatment of cancer in children. Participation in these trials spans an average of 2 to 3 years and requires a lifetime of follow-up care (Murphy 2011, COG 2019c). Patients are families must have the opportunity to ask questions about proposed trial participation. It is up to each institution's clinical trial team to ensure informed consent is obtained. All clinical trials conducted in Australia and New Zealand are subject to approval of the appropriate governing body. This ensures that the trial is following good clinical practice, and that the rights and safety of the patient are maintained.

NURSING CARE CONSIDERATIONS

Informed Consent

Soon after diagnosis, a family conference will take place in which the treatment team will discussion all available treatment options with the patient and their family. It is up to the parents as to whether they would like their child involved in these discussions. In this meeting the child's diagnosis and the planned treatment will be discussed. Given that treatment relates to being involved in clinical trials, this can take some time to explain. The family is allowed to decline participation in a clinical trial, but treatment will still be offered in line with the current best practice. The information shared can be difficult and complex to understand. The patient and their family must be allowed ample opportunity to ask questions until they feel they are well informed about the planned care for their child (COG 2019a). Whenever informed consent is required, local intuitional policies should also be adhered to.

Treatment Modalities

Survival of children with cancer has greatly improved through the use of: (1) multimodal therapy consisting of surgery, chemotherapy/immunotherapy, blood or marrow transplant (now referred to as haematopoietic stem cell transplant [SCT]) and radiation therapy; (2) enrolment of large numbers of children in cooperative group clinical trials or protocols; and (3) improvements in supportive care.

Current efforts are aimed at increasing the survival of patients with high-risk malignancies, decreasing the acute and long-term side effects of treatment, and studying the biology and genomics of the diseases to better identify patients who are at different risk levels for disease recurrence and can therefore benefit from risk-adapted and targeted therapies.

Each type of cancer will be treated differently depending on its type, cytogenetics and stage, and each child will receive one or a combination of the following treatments. It isn't until the diagnosis is confirmed that an appropriate treatment path will be decided upon. At all times during this process the treating team should be in constant communication with the patient and their family. This is a very stressful time for families, and it is important that they understand what the treatment plan involves.

Surgery

The main goal of surgery, besides obtaining biopsies, is to remove the tumour and restore normal body functioning to the greatest extent possible. Surgery is most successful when the tumour is encapsulated and localised (confined to the site of origin). Surgery may be used for palliation when the cancer is regional (metastasised to an area adjacent to the original site) or advanced (widespread throughout the body). Generally, the best prognosis is directly related to early detection of the tumour because that facilitates surgical removal.

Because the majority of paediatric cancers respond well to chemotherapy, more conservative surgical excision is increasingly used in a variety of tumours in an attempt to preserve function and cosmesis. For example, in some types of bone cancer, such as osteosarcoma, patients are successfully treated with resection of the diseased portion of the bone rather than amputation.

Radiation Therapy. Radiation therapy is frequently used in the treatment of childhood cancer, usually in conjunction with chemotherapy or surgery. It can be used for curative purposes and for palliation to relieve symptoms by shrinking the size of the tumour. Recent advances in radiation therapy that allow the beam to be aimed precisely have optimised its beneficial effects and minimised many of the undesirable side effects by sparing normal tissue.

Ionising radiation is cytotoxic in at least three different ways: (1) damaging the pyrimidine bases cytosine, thymine and uracil needed for the synthesis of nucleic acids; (2) causing single-strand breaks in the DNA or ribonucleic acid (RNA) molecule; or (3) causing double helical-strand breaks in these molecules. Disturbing cellular metabolic and reproductive functions causes lethal or sublethal damage. *Lethal damage* refers to the death of the cell. *Sublethal damage* refers to injured cells that may subsequently be repaired. Many of the acute side effects are the result of lethal damage to radiosensitive tissue, particularly proliferating cells such as those of the bone marrow, gastrointestinal tract and hair follicles. Late effects (late-occurring or long-term effects) are usually the result of cell death.

The acute untoward reactions from radiation therapy depend primarily on the area being irradiated. Total body irradiation is associated with the most severe reactions and is employed to prepare the immune system for SCT. Table 29.2 summarises the acute effects of radiation therapy and nursing interventions that may be helpful in mitigating or preventing them.

Proton beam therapy is a new form of radiation that uses a highly precise beam to target the radiation directly at a tumour site, decreasing the risk of damage to healthy tissues, in turn reducing long-term side effects. This new and evolving treatment can be utilised in CNS tumours, lymphoma and some solid tumours.

Chemotherapy

Chemotherapy may be the primary form of treatment, or it may be an adjunct to surgery, radiation therapy or SCT. Either alone, or in combination, the aim of chemotherapy is to cure, control or palliate. Chemotherapy works by stopping or slowing the growth on cancer cells, and destroying rapidly dividing cells by interfering with the function and production of nucleic acids. Chemotherapy cannot discriminate between which is a cancer cell and which is not; therefore, healthy cells are also destroyed by chemotherapy. It is this damage to healthy cells that can cause side effects. There are many different terms that can be used to describe the role of chemotherapy agents in cancer therapy.

TABLE 29.2 **Early Side Effects of Radiotherapy**

Site	Effects	Nursing Interventions
Gastrointestinal tract	Nausea and vomiting	Give antiemetic on schedule around the clock. Measure amount of emesis to assess for dehydration.
	Anorexia	Encourage fluids and foods best tolerated, usually light, soft, small and frequent meals. Monitor weight.
	Mucosal ulceration	Use frequent mouth rinses and oral hygiene to prevent mucositis.
	Diarrhoea	Control with antispasmodics Observe for signs of dehydration.
Skin	Alopecia (occurs within 2 weeks; hair may regrow by 3–6 months)	Introduce idea of wig. Stress necessity of scalp hygiene and need for head covering in sun and cold weather.
	Dry or moist desquamation	Do not refer to skin change as a 'burn' (implies use of too much radiation). Avoid lotions and other creams to skin. Wash daily, using soap (e.g. Dove) sparingly. Do not remove skin marking for radiation fields. Avoid exposure to sun. For desquamation, consult practitioner for skin hygiene and care.
Head	Nausea and vomiting (from stimulation of vomiting centre in brain)	Same as for gastrointestinal tract.
	Alopecia	Same as for skin.
	Mucositis	Encourage regular dental care, fluoride treatments.
	Potential effects: • parotitis • sore throat • loss of taste • xerostomia (dry mouth)	Provide analgesics as needed to relieve discomfort Combat severe dryness of mouth with oral hygiene and liquid diet.
Urinary bladder	Rarely cystitis	Encourage liberal fluid intake and frequent voiding. Monitor for haematuria.
Bone marrow	Myelosuppression	Observe for fever (temperature > 38.0°C). Initiate workup for sepsis as ordered. Administer antibiotics as prescribed. Avoid use of suppositories, rectal temperatures. Institute bleeding precautions. Observe for signs of anaemia.

- Induction—Initial therapy with the aim of achieving significant reduction in the cancer cell count, ideally complete remission of the disease.
- Consolidation/intensification—Administered following induction to prolong overall survival.
- Adjuvant therapy—Chemotherapy agents used in conjunction with other treatment modalities (i.e. radiation, surgery, immunotherapy).
- Neo-adjuvant therapy—Use of chemotherapy agents to reduce the size/burden of disease before definitive treatment.
- Maintenance therapy—Prolonged, low-dose chemotherapy administered to increase duration of remission and achieve cure.
- Primary therapy—Chemotherapy agents used as the definitive therapy.
- Combination therapy—Using two of more chemotherapy agents to treat the disease.
- Myeloablative therapy—Treatment that prepares patients for haematopoietic SCT.
- Salvage therapy—Chemotherapy agents given after the failure of other treatments to control the disease or to provide palliation.

Chemotherapy can be given via a number of different routes (Murphy 2011):

- oral
- intravenous (IV)
- subcutaneous
- intrathecal
- intramuscular.

Although several drugs have been effective in treating different forms of cancer as single agents, the remarkable increase in survival rates has been the result of improved combination drug regimens. Combining drugs allows for optimum cell cycle destruction with minimum toxic effects and decreased resistance by the cancer cells to the agent. For example, a treatment regimen called VAC (vincristine, doxorubicin and cyclophosphamide) combines complementary cytotoxic effects with distinct side effects. Doxorubicin and cyclophosphamide are myelosuppressive, whereas vincristine is neurotoxic.

In addition to more effective combinations of drugs, several advances in the administration of chemotherapy have permitted continuous or intermittent intravenous (IV) administration without multiple venepunctures. The use of venous access devices (e.g. catheters and implantable infusion ports) has greatly facilitated safe and effective drug administration with minimum discomfort for the child. Continuous infusions over an extended period using syringe pumps have made possible the administration of certain drugs, such as cytarabine, in higher doses with less toxicity than when the drug is administered intermittently.

Chemotherapeutic agents can be classified according to their primary mechanism of action. Alkylating agents replace a hydrogen atom of a molecule by an alkyl group. The irreversible combination of alkyl groups with nucleotide chains, particularly DNA, causes unbalanced growth of unaffected cell constituents so that the cell eventually dies. These agents have a steep dose-response curve and, for this reason, can be used in high-dose therapy regimens. Examples of alkylating agents include cyclophosphamide, ifosfamide and cisplatin. Antimetabolites resemble essential metabolic elements needed for cell growth but are sufficiently altered in molecular structure to inhibit further synthesis of DNA or RNA; their maximum effect occurs in cells that are actively producing DNA. Examples of antimetabolites include methotrexate and mercaptopurine. Plant alkaloids arrest cells in metaphase (a phase of mitosis) by binding to microtubular protein needed for spindle formation. Examples include vincristine and vinblastine. Antitumour antibiotics are natural products that interfere with cell division by reacting with DNA in such a way as to prevent further replication of DNA and transcription of RNA. Examples include doxorubicin and daunorubicin.

Both adrenal and gonadal hormones have antineoplastic properties, although the precise mechanism of action is still unclear. In theory, adrenocorticosteroids bind with DNA and alter the transcription process. Although there are a number of cortisone preparations, dexamethasone and prednisone are most often used in cancer therapy.

Chemotherapy is given in cycles according to the treatment protocol that the child is on, which may or may not be a clinical trial. A cycle is a period of treatment followed by a period of no treatment. This rest period allows the child's body to recover after the chemotherapy. The length of this rest period is determined by the protocol and the child's response.

An understanding of the actions and side effects of these drugs is essential to nursing care of children with cancer. Unfortunately, almost all standard chemotherapy drugs are not selectively cytotoxic for malignant cells, and other cells with a high rate of proliferation, such as the bone marrow elements, hair, skin and epithelial cells of the gastrointestinal tract, are also affected. Frequently the problems related to the destruction of these normal cells require more nursing care than those related to the disease itself.

Central Venous Lines. Central venous lines are inserted in order to administer the required treatment. A central venous line is a semi-permanent line that allows treatment and supportive care to be administered into a large central vein, directly into the heart. There are two types of central venous lines.

- External—Broviac, Hickmann, peripherally inserted central catheter (PICC). There can be up to four access points in order to deliver different therapies at the same time.
- Internal—Called an infusaport, this is placed under the skin on the chest wall. A needle is inserted to access the infusaport and deliver therapy. They can have single or double ports. (See Fig 29.1.)

Nursing staff should ensure that infection control principles are maintained when accessing these lines due to the risk of infection and dislodgement. Children and families should also be educated on how to care for these lines when at home.

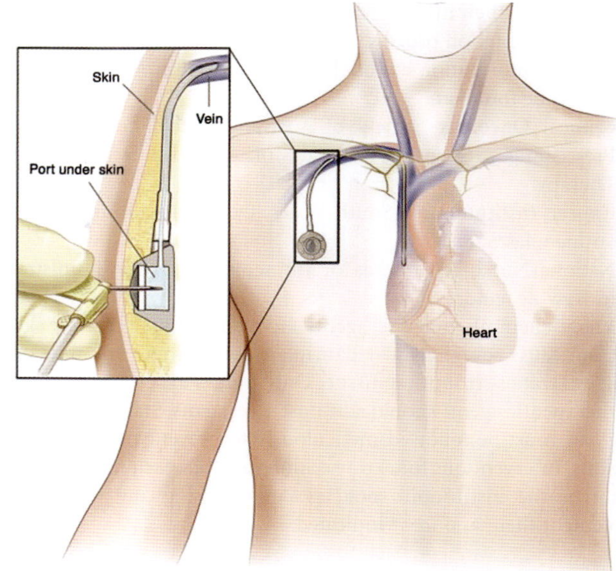

Fig 29.1 Infusaports are common central venous lines. (Source: Murphy, K. (2011). The Children's Oncology Group Family Handbook for Children with Cancer (2nd ed.). p. 73. https://www.childrensoncology-group.org/downloads/English_COG_Family_Handbook.pdf)

FAMILY-CENTRED CARE

Medication Safety—family Education

Patients and families should receive adequate education about the chemotherapy their child is receiving, as well as all supportive care. This information should be provided verbally, but written information should also be given as a reference. Medication diaries can be used to help parents track which medications need to be given when, especially when at home.

Administering and Handling Chemotherapeutic Agents. The complexity of the treatment plans designed to achieve maximal anti-cancer effect balanced against potential toxicity leaves minimal margin for error when administering anti-cancer therapy (Clinical Oncology Society of Australia [COSA] 2018). All staff involved in the management of cancer and its therapies must have the relevant knowledge, experience and skills and be competent to perform the task. These treatments have a high potential for harm; overdosaging can result in death, while underdosing can have significant implications for the management of the disease and patient outcome (COSA 2018).

Prescribing, dispensing and administration errors relating to anti-cancer treatment that result in patient harm are well documented (COSA 2018). These errors may occur due to procedural, technical or behavioural reasons and be a combination of human and system errors, producing an unintended harmful outcome (COSA 2018). Medication safety initiatives should target all stages of the treatment process and include all members of the multidisciplinary team. Success in reducing the incidence of errors is based on a multidisciplinary approach of those involved in the prescribing, dispensing and administration of treatment (COSA 2018).

All staff involved in the management of anti-cancer therapy must be competent to perform the required skills (COSA 2018). Each nurse should refer to their institution's local policy that will outline the training and accreditation process.

Further information about chemotherapy administration accreditation can be found at:

- Clinical Oncology Society of Australia, Guidelines for the Safe Prescribing, Dispensing and Administration of Systemic Cancer Therapy
- Cancer Institute New South Wales, eviQ-Safe administration of antineoplastic drugs
- National Nursing Standards for Antineoplastic Drug Administration in New Zealand.

Many chemotherapeutic agents are **vesicants** (sclerosing agents) that can cause severe cellular damage if even minute amounts of the drug infiltrate surrounding tissue. Only nurses experienced with chemotherapeutic agents should administer vesicants. Standards are available and must be followed meticulously to prevent tissue damage to patients. Interventions for extravasation vary, but each nurse should be aware of the institution's policies before giving any vesicant, and implement them at once if indicated.

NURSING CARE CONSIDERATIONS

Anti-cancer medications can easily extravasate from the blood vessel into the surrounding tissue. The infusion is stopped immediately if any sign of infiltration (e.g. pain, stinging, swelling or redness at needle site) occurs. Individual local institution policy should be followed in the event of possible extravasation. Further information can be found at https://www.eviq.org.au/clinical-resources/extravasation/157-extravasation-management

In addition to extravasation, a potentially fatal complication is anaphylaxis, especially from asparaginase (colaspase), bleomycin, cisplatin or etoposide. (See Anaphylaxis, Chapter 23.) Hypersensitivity reactions to these chemotherapeutic agents are characterised by urticaria, angiooedema, flushing, rashes, difficulty breathing, hypotension and nausea or vomiting. Nursing responsibilities include prevention, recognition and preparation for serious reactions. Prevention begins with a careful history of known allergies, and recognition includes education of the patient and family regarding signs and symptoms to report. If a reaction is suspected, the nurse discontinues the drug, flushes and maintains the IV line with saline and monitors the child's vital signs and subsequent responses.

NURSING CARE CONSIDERATIONS

When chemotherapy or immunotherapy agents with known anaphylactic potential are given, it is standard practice to observe the child for 1 hour after the infusion for signs of anaphylaxis (e.g. rash, urticaria, hypotension, wheezing, nausea, vomiting). Emergency equipment (especially blood pressure monitor, bag and valve mask and suction) and emergency drugs (especially oxygen, adrenaline, antihistamine and corticosteroids) must be readily available.

In addition to the many patient-focused responsibilities during chemotherapy administration, nurses must also use safeguards to protect themselves. Handling chemotherapeutic agents may present risks to handlers and to their offspring, although the exact degree of risk is not known. Staff who are pregnant, trying to conceive or breastfeeding should not handle chemotherapeutic agents. Basic nursing guidelines are in the Nursing Care Guidelines box.

NURSING CARE CONSIDERATIONS

Handling Chemotherapeutic Agents

- Aseptic technique should be maintained at all times—prevent physical contact with the drug.
- Drugs should be stored and handled as per institutional policy.
- Wear appropriate personal protective equipment (PPE): impervious gown, gloves and eye and respiratory protection.
- All hazardous waste, including contaminated waste and related equipment, should be sealed in appropriate secondary packaging and disposed of into the appropriate hazardous waste bin. Cytotoxic waste containers should be specifically labelled and disposed of as per relevant legislation (Fig 29.2).

Biological Therapy

Biological therapy, also called biotherapy, uses substances made from living organisms, derived from living organisms or laboratory-produced versions of these substances to treat cancer (Ceppi et al 2017). Biotherapies can be grouped into three main types: (1) those that do not target cancer cells directly, but stimulate the body's immune system to act against cancer cells, and are collectively referred to as immunotherapy or biological response modifier therapy; (2) those that use antibodies or segments of genetic material to target cancer cells directly; and (3) therapies that interfere with specific molecules involved in tumour growth and progression and are referred to as targeted therapies (Ceppi et al 2017).

Immunotherapy works by stimulating the activity of the immune system against cancer cells or by counteracting signals produced by cancer cells that suppress immune responses. Immunotherapy includes the use of monoclonal antibodies that attach to proteins on cancer cells so the immune system can find and destroy the cells. Other antibodies block pathways that allow cancer cells to escape the immune system; these are called checkpoint inhibitors. Non-specific immunotherapies include two types of cytokines: interferons and interleukins. Other immunotherapies include oncolytic virus therapy and chimeric antigen receptor (CAR) T-cell therapy. CAR T-cell therapy is being studied

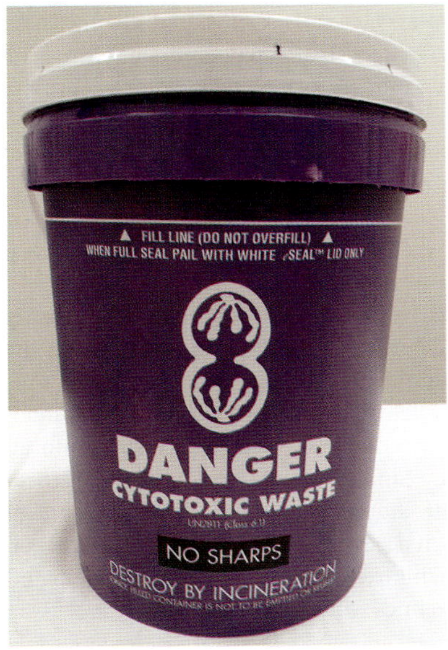

Fig 29.2 Cytotoxic disposal bin.

in childhood acute leukaemia that does not respond to traditional chemotherapy. Surveillance for and management of side effects of immunotherapy are critical nursing responsibilities. Side effects may range from mild to severe. For example, with CAR T-cell therapy, adverse events may include cytokine release syndrome, neurological symptoms, tumour lysis syndrome and graft-versus-host disease (Becze 2017).

Targeted therapies are substances that interfere with specific molecules involved in cancer. They are different from standard chemotherapy in two ways (Cancer Australia 2021): (1) they act on molecular targets, rather than affecting all rapidly dividing normal and malignant cells; and (2) they are selected or designed to affect their target, compared with chemotherapy drugs that were identified because they kill cells. Previously, targeted therapies have had limited use in paediatric patients but are now being evaluated in clinical trials. Careful monitoring of side effects is essential because the profile of adverse events may be different to that seen in adults, and because these agents may affect the process of growth and development in paediatric patients in unexpected ways (Gore et al 2013).

Haematopoietic Stem Cell Transplant

Another approach to the treatment of childhood cancer is transplantation of haematopoietic (blood-forming) stem cells. SCT restores stem cells in children who have diseases that require high doses of chemotherapy or radiation therapy and/or replacement of dysfunctional bone marrow. Blood-forming stem cells from bone marrow, peripheral blood or cord blood can be sources for SCT. The main types of SCT are **allogeneic**, where cells are obtained from a family member or volunteer donor, and **autologous**, where cells previously stored from the patient are given back to the patient by IV infusion. In either type of SCT, if it is successful, the newly transfused cells begin to produce functioning non-malignant blood cells. In essence, the recipient accepts a new blood-forming organ.

Children receiving an allogeneic SCT undergo a pretransplant conditioning regimen consisting of radiation therapy and/or high-dose chemotherapy to rid the body of malignant cells and suppress the immune system to prevent rejection of the transplanted marrow.

Once the preparatory regimen begins and the child's immune system is destroyed, there is no turning back. Unlike kidney transplantation, SCT does not have a 'rescue' procedure, such as dialysis, for supportive therapy. If the donor is a sibling, the expectation that his or her marrow will 'save' the brother or sister can be a concern, especially if the transplant fails. Parents often must leave home to stay at the transplant centre and encounter additional stressors such as arranging child care, taking leave from work and managing finances. If old enough to understand the risks, the patient faces the greatest stress, such as fear of SCT failure or life-threatening complications.

The selection process for a suitable donor and the potential complications in allogeneic transplantation are related to the human leucocyte antigen (HLA) system complex. Some of the major HLA antigens are A, B, C, D, DR and DQ. There is wide diversity for each of these HLA loci. For example, more than 20 different HLA-A antigens and more than 40 different HLA-B antigens can be inherited. The genes are inherited as a single unit, or haplotype. A child inherits one unit from each parent; thus a child and each parent have one identical and one non-identical haplotype. Because the possible haplotype combinations among siblings follow the laws of Mendelian genetics, there is a 1 in 4 chance that two siblings have identical haplotypes and are perfectly matched at the HLA loci.

The importance of HLA matching is to prevent the serious complication of graft-versus-host disease (GVHD) after allogeneic transplant. Because the child's immune system is essentially rendered non-functional, the recipient is unlikely to reject the bone marrow. However, the donor's marrow may contain antigens not matched to the recipient's antigens, which begin attacking body cells. The more closely the HLA systems match, the less likely GVHD is to develop. However, GVHD can occur even with a perfect HLA match because of unidentified and thus unmatched histocompatibility antigens (Gottschalk et al 2016).

Umbilical cord blood or haploidentical family donors (i.e. parents) are additional sources of haematopoietic stem cells for use in children with cancer (Gottschalk et al 2016). The benefit of using umbilical cord blood is the blood's relative immunodeficiency at birth, allowing for partially matched, unrelated cord blood transplants to be successful, with a lower risk of GVHD-related problems (Sarvaria et al 2017). A benefit of using a haploidentical family member is the immediate availability of the donor, which is especially important when children urgently need SCT.

Autologous Transplantation. Autologous transplants use the patient's own marrow that was collected from disease-free tissue, frozen and may have been treated to remove malignant cells. Peripheral blood stem cell transplant (PBSCT) is also used in children with cancer. This type of transplant differs in the way stem cells are collected. Most commonly, colony-stimulating factor (CSF) is first given to stimulate the production of many stem cells (Karakukcu & Unal 2015). Once the white blood cell count is high enough, the stem cells are collected by an apheresis machine. This machine filters out peripheral stem cells from whole blood and returns the remainder of the blood cells and plasma to the child. Stem cells have been collected without problems in even very small children weighing 20 kg or less (Gottschalk et al 2016). The peripheral stem cells are then frozen until the patient is ready for the PBSCT. Children with solid tumours such as neuroblastoma, Hodgkin's lymphoma, non-Hodgkin's lymphoma, rhabdomyosarcoma, Ewing's sarcoma and Wilms tumour have been treated with autologous transplants.

Complications of Therapy

Although great advances have been achieved through current modes of cancer therapy, the successes are not without consequences. Numerous acute side effects are commonly expected with chemotherapy/biotherapy and radiation therapy. Several other complications that are less frequent, but generally more serious, are described here.

Paediatric Oncological Emergencies

Tumour Lysis Syndrome. Life-threatening conditions may develop in children with cancer as a result of the malignancy and/or aggressive treatment modalities. Acute tumour lysis syndrome has hallmark metabolic abnormalities that are the direct result of rapid release of intracellular contents during the lysis of malignant cells. This typically occurs in patients with acute lymphoblastic leukaemia or Burkitt's lymphoma during the initial treatment period, but may occur spontaneously before onset of therapy. Tumour lysis syndrome also may occur in other malignancies that have a large tumour burden, are very sensitive to chemotherapy or have a rapid proliferative rate. The metabolic abnormalities of tumour lysis syndrome include hyperuricaemia, hypocalcaemia, hyperphosphataemia and hyperkalaemia. The crystallisation of uric acid that can occur with hyperuricaemia can lead to acute renal failure (Freedman et al 2016).

Risk factors for development of tumour lysis syndrome include high white blood cell count at diagnosis, large tumour burden, cancer cell sensitivity to chemotherapy and high proliferative rate. In addition to the described metabolic abnormalities, children may develop a spectrum of clinical symptoms, including flank pain, lethargy, nausea and vomiting, muscle cramps, pruritus, tetany and seizures.

Management of tumour lysis syndrome consists of early identification of patients at risk, prophylactic measures and early interventions. Patients at risk for tumour lysis syndrome should have serum chemistries and urine pH monitored frequently, strict recording of intake and output and aggressive administration of IV fluids that do not contain potassium (unless clinically indicated). Medications, such as allopurinol, that reduce uric acid formation and promote excretion of by-products of purine metabolism are often used. If tumour lysis syndrome occurs, IV hydration continues and the specific metabolic abnormalities are treated. Hyperuricaemia is now effectively treated with recombinant urate oxidase, or rasburicase. This medication converts uric acid to allantoin, which is more soluble in urine. Blood transfusions are sometimes necessary to reduce the metabolic consequences of massive tumour lysis, especially in children with a high tumour burden.

Hyperleucocytosis. Hyperleucocytosis, defined as a peripheral white blood cell count greater than 50×10^9/L, can lead to capillary obstruction, microinfarction and organ dysfunction. Children often experience respiratory distress and cyanosis. They also experience neurological changes, including altered level of consciousness, visual disturbances, agitation, confusion, ataxia and delirium. Management consists of rapid cytoreduction by chemotherapy, hydration, urinary alkalinisation and allopurinol. Leucapheresis or blood transfusion may be necessary.

Superior Vena Cava Syndrome. Space-occupying lesions located in the chest, especially from Hodgkin's disease and non-Hodgkin's lymphoma, may cause superior vena cava syndrome (SVCS), leading to airway compromise and potentially to respiratory failure. The second leading cause of SVCS is thrombotic complications of implantable IV devices, such as central venous catheters and port catheters (Freedman et al 2016).

Children are initially seen with cyanosis of the face, neck and upper chest; facial and upper extremity oedema; and distended neck and chest veins. They may be anxious and have dyspnoea, wheezing or a frequent cough from airway obstruction. Management consists of airway protection and alleviation of respiratory distress. Rapid treatment is initiated, and symptoms typically improve as the disease is effectively treated.

Spinal Cord Compression. Malignancies can invade or impinge on the spinal cord, causing acute symptoms of cord compression. Primary CNS tumours can originate or spread to the spinal cord. Other solid tumours, such as neuroblastoma or rhabdomyosarcoma, can metastasise to the spinal cord and cause compression. Back pain is a common initial manifestation, but other symptoms can include sensation change, extremity weakness, loss of bowel and bladder function and respiratory insufficiency. Careful physical examination is essential in early detection of symptoms, and MRI is the gold standard for diagnosis (Freedman et al 2016). Treatment may include high-dose steroids to reduce associated oedema and alleviate symptoms and rapid initiation of treatment such as emergent radiation or laminectomy if indicated.

Disseminated Intravascular Coagulation. Overwhelming infections in the immunocompromised child constitute an emergency situation. Sepsis from bacteria or fungus can result in numerous complications, including disseminated intravascular coagulation (DIC). Children with DIC form excessive microthrombi throughout the vascular system due to hyperactivation of the clotting cascade, downregulation of anticoagulants and impaired fibrinolysis, which leaves the child susceptible to haemorrhage. Life-threatening haemorrhage can occur from DIC with thrombocytopenia (platelet count of less than 20,000/mm^3) (Andrews et al 2016). Treatment is focused on identifying and treating the underlying cause, along with infusing heparin to minimise microthrombi and cryoprecipitate to replace fibrinogen.

NURSING CARE MANAGEMENT

This section presents an overview of general nursing concepts that apply to most childhood cancers. Specific nursing care for children with a particular type of cancer is discussed under each disease section later in this chapter. This discussion focuses on the physical aspects of care. In addition, refer to Chapter 21 for family-centred care and Chapter 19 for end of life care. (See Quality Patient Outcomes box.)

QUALITY PATIENT OUTCOMES

The Child with Cancer

- Child and family educated about disease and treatment
- Child and family safely perform self-care as appropriate
- Treatment administered on schedule with appropriate drug doses
- Side effects of treatment managed
- Treatment complications prevented
- Child and family strengths and coping skills supported
- Quality of life during treatment maintained
- Child and family adjusted to chronic illness
- Growth and development maintained during treatment
- Monitor late effects post treatment

Signs and Symptoms of Cancer in Children

Early detection is critical to starting treatment with the best prospect for eventual cure. Cancers in children are often difficult to recognise. Therefore, being alert to the persistence of possible signs and symptoms is essential (Box 29.1). This section discusses some of the more significant clues leading to a diagnosis of paediatric cancer.

Pain may be an early or late initial sign of cancer and requires a careful history of its onset, characteristics, location, intensity and alleviating factors. Pain may be generalised or present at a specific location. For example, bone pain occurs in approximately 20% of children with leukaemia. Pain, swelling and tenderness at the tumour site may be initial signs in solid tumours. In addition, a mass is a typical finding in children with solid tumours. An abdominal mass in a child must be evaluated for a malignancy, such as Wilms tumour or neuroblastoma.

Fever is a frequent occurrence during childhood and is caused by numerous illnesses, including cancer. The cause of fever in cancer patients is infection or the malignant process itself. This is often referred to as tumour-associated fever. The exact mechanism by which the malignancy causes a fever is not completely understood. Cytokines (e.g. interleukin, tumour necrosis factor) are known to be involved,

BOX 29.1 Possible Signs and Symptoms of Childhood Cancer

- Unusual mass or swelling
- Unexplained paleness and loss of energy
- Easy bruising
- Persistent, localised pain or limping
- Prolonged, unexplained fever or illness
- Frequent headaches, often with vomiting
- Sudden eye or vision changes
- Unexplained, rapid weight loss

Source: Data from American Cancer Society. (2016). Finding cancer in children. https://www.cancer.org/cancer/cancer-in-children/finding-childhood-cancers-early.html.

and are thought to be released either directly from tumour cells or from macrophages responding to tumour (Foggo & Cavenagh 2015).

A careful skin assessment will reveal signs of a low platelet count. Ecchymosis and petechiae are most commonly found on the child's extremities and under constricting parts of clothing like waistbands. Spontaneous gum or nose bleeding may occur when the platelet count falls below 20,000/mm^3.

The child with malignant invasion of the bone marrow often appears pale, with symptoms of lethargy, weight loss and malaise. These symptoms may be attributed to anaemia caused by the replacement of normal cells with malignant cells in the bone marrow. The nurse should assess for signs and symptoms of anaemia. (See Chapter 28.)

Swollen lymph nodes are another common finding in children. However, enlarged, firm lymph nodes in a child with fever for more than 1 week, a recent history of weight loss or an abnormal chest x-ray film may indicate a serious disease and should be evaluated further.

Recognising one sign is facilitated by the widespread use of mobile phone photography. Leucocoria or white eye reflex can be seen as a yellow 'glow' in the pupil, as opposed to the normal red pupillary reflex, in photographs. It can be a sign of retinoblastoma that needs prompt medical attention. Squinting, strabismus or swelling can indicate other solid tumours of the eye.

The child with a brain tumour develops signs and symptoms related to the area of the brain involved. The nurse's thorough physical assessment can indicate the likely area of tumour involvement.

Managing Side Effects of Treatment

Cancer care encompasses more than treatments aimed at eliminating the malignant cells. Because of the delicate balance between killing malignant cells and preserving functional cells, supportive therapy usually is needed during those times that serious damage occurs to normal body tissues. A major concern for the child receiving treatment for cancer is the risk for the development of complications secondary to the treatment.

NURSING CARE CONSIDERATIONS

Fertility Preservation

It can be difficult to predict the exact impact that cancer treatment will have on the long-term fertility of those children who have begun to go through puberty. These teenagers should be given the opportunity to discuss their options for preserving their fertility, prior to treatment commencing. Further information can be found at https://www.canteen.org.au/wp-content/uploads/2015/07/A-guide-to-fertility-for-young-people-with-cancer.pdf.

Infection

The nurse caring for the child with fever must be aware of the signs and symptoms of septic shock, as discussed in Chapter 23. The child with fever who has an absolute neutrophil count (ANC) lower than 500/mm^3 is at risk for the following:

- overwhelming infection
- malaise
- dehydration
- seizures (young infants and children)
- invasion of organisms producing secondary infections.

The child with fever is evaluated for potential sites of infection, such as from a needle puncture, mucosal ulceration, minor abrasion or skin tears (e.g. a hangnail). Although the body may not be able to produce an adequate inflammatory response to the infection and the usual clinical signs of infection may be partially expressed or absent, fever will occur. Therefore, the child's temperature is monitored closely. To identify the source of infection, the healthcare team takes blood, stool, urine and nasopharyngeal cultures and chest x-rays.

Once infection is suspected, broad-spectrum IV antibiotic therapy must be commenced within 60 minutes, before the organism is identified and may be continued for 7 to 10 days. If the child does not have a venous access device, an IV should be inserted to prevent the inconvenience and discomfort of multiple venepunctures in administering antibiotic therapy.

The organisms most lethal to these children are: (1) viruses, particularly varicella (chickenpox), herpes zoster, herpes simplex, respiratory syncytial virus, influenza and cytomegalovirus; (2) protozoan, *Toxoplasma gondii*; (3) fungi, especially *Pneumocystis jiroveci* (formally known as *carinii*) and *Candida albicans*; (4) gram-negative bacteria, such as *Pseudomonas aeruginosa, E. coli* and *Klebsiella* organisms; and (5) gram-positive bacteria, especially *Staphylococcus* and *Enterococcus* species (Ardura & Koh 2016).

Prophylaxis against *Pneumocystis* pneumonia, such as trimethoprim-sulfamethoxazole, is routinely given to most children during treatment for cancer (Ardura & Koh 2016). CSFs, a family of glycoprotein hormones that regulate the reproduction, maturation and function of blood cells, are now routinely used as supportive measures to prevent the side effects caused by low blood counts. CSFs promote stem cell proliferation and stimulate a more rapid maturation of the cells, allowing them to enter the bloodstream earlier. Granulocyte colony-stimulating factor (G-CSF; filgrastim [Neupogen], pegfilgrastim [Neulasta]) directs granulocyte development and can decrease the duration of neutropenia. This reduces the incidence and duration of infection in children receiving treatment for cancer. G-CSF is also being used to decrease the bone marrow recovery time after SCT (Ardura & Koh 2016). G-CSF is usually administered intravenously or subcutaneously 24 hours after chemotherapy is discontinued. The pegylated or long-acting form of G-CSF, pegfilgrastim, is given only once after completion of therapy and typically has its peak efficacy (highest white blood cell count) about 8 to 10 days after administration. During G-CSF therapy, children may experience bone pain, fever, rash, malaise and headaches.

Prevention of infection continues as a priority after discharge from the hospital. Some institutions allow the child to return to school when the ANC is above 500/mm^3. Other institutions place no restrictions on the child, regardless of the blood count. If the ANC falls below 500/mm^3, cautious isolation from crowded areas, such as shopping centres or subways, is advisable. At all times, family members should be encouraged to practise good hand washing to avoid introducing pathogens into the home, and they should know how to take a temperature and who to call in the event of fever.

Haemorrhage

Before the use of transfused platelets, haemorrhage was a leading cause of death in children with some types of cancer. Now most bleeding episodes can be prevented or controlled with judicious administration of platelet concentrates or platelet-rich plasma. The incidence of severe spontaneous internal haemorrhage varies, but usually does not occur until the platelet count is 20,000/mm^3 or less (Hockenberry et al 2016).

Because infection increases the tendency towards haemorrhage, and because bleeding sites become more easily infected, take special care to avoid performing skin punctures whenever possible. When performing finger pricks, venepunctures, intramuscular injections and bone marrow biopsies, employ aseptic technique with continued observation for bleeding. Meticulous mouth care is essential because gingival bleeding with resultant mucositis is a frequent problem. Because the rectal area is prone to ulceration from various drugs, hygiene is essential. To prevent additional trauma, avoid rectal temperatures and suppositories. Frequent turning and the use of a pressure-reducing mattress under bony prominences prevent development of pressure sores and decubital ulcers.

Platelet transfusions are generally reserved for active bleeding episodes that do not respond to local treatment and that may occur during induction or relapse therapy. Epistaxis and gingival bleeding are the most common. The nurse teaches parents and children measures to control nose bleeding. Applying pressure at the site without disturbing clot formation is the general rule. Platelet concentrates normally do not have to be cross-matched for blood group or type. However, because platelets contain specific antigen components similar to blood group factors, children who receive multiple transfusions may become sensitised to a platelet group other than their own. Therefore, platelets are cross-matched with the donor's blood components whenever possible.

Transfused platelets generally survive in the body for 1 to 3 days. The peak effect is reached in about 1 hour and decreased by half in 24 hours. After a transfusion, the nurse observes and records the approximate time when haemostasis of bleeding sites occurs. Delayed haemostasis is evidence of platelet destruction. For long-term patients, multiple transfusion therapy becomes progressively less effective.

During bleeding episodes the parents and child need much emotional support (see Critical Thinking Case Study box). The sight of oozing blood is upsetting. Often parents request a platelet transfusion, unaware of the necessity of trying local measures first. The nurse can help calm their anxiety by explaining the reason for delaying a platelet transfusion until absolutely necessary. Because compatible donors decrease the risk of antigen formation in the recipient, the nurse should encourage parents to locate suitable donors for eventual blood use.

Children at home who have low platelet counts (usually $< 100{,}000/mm^3$) should avoid activities that might cause injury or bleeding, such as riding bicycles or skateboards, skating, climbing trees or playground equipment, and contact sports such as football or soccer. Once the platelet count rises, these restrictions are not necessary. In addition, aspirin and aspirin-containing products are not used; for mild pain or significantly elevated temperature, paracetamol is substituted.

Anaemia

Initially anaemia may be profound if there is complete replacement of the bone marrow by cancer cells. During induction therapy, blood transfusions with packed red blood cells may be necessary to raise the haemoglobin to levels approaching 10 g/dl. The usual precautions in caring for the child are instituted. (See Chapter 28.)

Anaemia is also a consequence of drug-induced myelosuppression. Although not as severely affected as the white blood cells, erythrocyte production may be delayed. Because children have an amazing capacity to withstand low haemoglobin levels, the best approach is to allow the child to regulate activity with reasonable adult supervision. It may be necessary for the parents to alert the schoolteacher to the child's physical limitations, particularly in terms of strenuous activity.

Nausea and Vomiting

The nausea and vomiting that occur shortly after administration of several of the drugs and as a result of cranial or abdominal irradiation can be profound and debilitating. The advent of serotonin receptor blockers (5-hydroxytryptamine-3 or 5-HT_3 receptor antagonists) has greatly improved management of nausea and vomiting caused by chemotherapy and radiation therapy. The advantage of these agents over conventional drugs is that they produce no extrapyramidal side effects, such as difficulty speaking or swallowing, shuffle walk, slow movements, trembling, stiffness of the arms and legs or loss of balance. Published guidelines recommend 5-HT_3 antagonists and corticosteroids for children receiving highly or moderately emetogenic chemotherapy (Patel et al 2017). Aprepitant has also been found to be highly effective in managing those at high emetogenic risk.

Ondansetron is used as first-line treatment in most cases. Metoclopramide is a more effective antiemetic for acute nausea or vomiting. Unfortunately, the drug causes a number of side effects in children, particularly extrapyramidal reactions, such as muscle tremors or twitching, agitation, grimacing, dysarthria and oculogyric crisis (fixation of eyes in one position for minutes or hours). The prevention and treatment of nausea and vomiting related to chemotherapy treatment should be thought of prior to the commencement of each treatment cycle (Cancer Institute of New South Wales 2019).

The most beneficial regimen for antiemetic control has been the administration of the antiemetic before chemotherapy begins (30 minutes to 1 hour before) and regular (not as-needed) administration for at least 24 hours after chemotherapy. The goal is to prevent the child from ever experiencing nausea or vomiting because this can prevent the development of anticipatory symptoms (the conditioned response of developing nausea and vomiting before receiving the drug). Other non-pharmacological interventions (similar to those discussed for pain management in Chapter 5) can be useful in controlling posttherapy and anticipatory nausea and vomiting. Giving the antineoplastic drug with a mild sedative at bedtime is also helpful for some children, and there is evidence that night-time administration of drugs such as methotrexate and mercaptopurine may be more effective than morning administration.

Altered Nutrition

Altered nutrition is a common side effect of treatment. Continued assessment of the child's nutritional status, child's intake and energy expenditure must occur throughout treatment. The child's height, weight and head circumference (for children younger than 3 years old) must be measured routinely during visits to the hospital or clinic. Energy reserves should be evaluated with routine skinfold measurements. Biochemical assays such as serum prealbumin, transferrin and albumin may be helpful to evaluate nutritional status in some children, but a single assay should not be used alone for a nutritional evaluation (Lawson et al 2013). There are no specific criteria that mandate nutritional interventions in children undergoing cancer treatment. Instead each child should have an individualised nutritional care plan based on routine assessments. Most paediatric cancer treatment centres have a dietitian who can be consulted to develop the nutritional care plan and revise it as needed. Nutritional status is important to maintain because a compromised nutritional status can contribute to reduced tolerance to treatment, altered metabolism of chemotherapy drugs, prolonged episodes of neutropenia and increased risk for infection.

Supportive nutrition measures include oral supplements with high-protein and high-calorie foods. Ways to increase calories include using whole milk, adding tofu (high in protein) to most meals and serving full-fat yoghurt, ice-cream and milk instead on non-fat or low-fat items. Cooking with butter, putting sugar on cereal and making high-calorie snacks such as trail mix, peanut butter or dried fruit readily available for the child are other ways to increase calories. Enteral feeding may be necessary when children are unable to maintain the necessary calories to prevent weight loss. Parenteral hyperalimentation is used most frequently for children who have digestive problems, after surgery or with SCT. Chapter 22 discusses these interventions in more detail.

Despite such approaches, some children still do not eat. Theories to explain persistent anorexia include the following: (1) a physical effect related to the cancer that is non-specific; (2) a conditioned aversion to food from nausea and vomiting during treatment; (3) a response to stress in the environment, related to eating or to the child's condition; (4) a result of depression; and (5) a control mechanism when so much else has been imposed on the child. When loss of appetite and weight decline persists, the nurse should investigate the family situation to determine whether any of these variables are contributing to the problem, and discuss with the treatment team.

Mucosal Ulceration

One of the most distressing side effects of several drugs is gastrointestinal mucosal cell damage, which results in ulcers anywhere along the alimentary tract. Oral ulcers (stomatitis) are red, eroded, painful areas in the mouth or pharynx. (See Stomatitis, Chapter 6.) Similar lesions may extend along the oesophagus and occur in the rectal area. They greatly compound anorexia because eating is extremely uncomfortable.

Some helpful interventions when oral ulcers develop are feeding a bland, moist, soft diet; using a soft toothbrush; frequently rinsing the mouth with chlorhexidine mouthwash or sodium bicarbonate and salt mouth rinses; and administering local anaesthetics without alcohol (Chaveli-Lopez & Bagan-Sebastian 2016). Although local anaesthetics are effective in temporarily relieving the pain, many children dislike the taste and numb feeling they produce.

Administering mouth care is particularly difficult in infants and toddlers. A satisfactory method of cleaning the gums is to wrap a piece of gauze around a finger; soak it in saline or plain water; and swab the gums, palate and inner cheek surfaces with the finger. Children should perform mouth care routinely before and after any feeding and as often as every 2 to 4 hours to rid mucosal surfaces of debris, which becomes an excellent medium for bacterial and fungal growth if left undisturbed.

Dental hygiene can become a serious problem if the child wears an orthodontic appliance. The accumulated debris on braces is difficult to remove without vigorous brushing, and the appliance itself traumatises the gums. For this reason, sometimes braces are removed before starting chemotherapy treatment.

Difficulty eating is a major problem with stomatitis and may warrant hospitalisation if the child refuses fluids. The child usually chooses the foods that are best tolerated. Surprisingly, some children prefer salty foods to bland ones. Drinking can usually be encouraged if a straw is used to bypass the ulcerated oral mucosa. The nurse should encourage parents to relax any eating pressures because the anorexia accompanying stomatitis is well justified. In addition, because it is a temporary condition, once the ulcers heal, the child can resume good food habits. Ordinarily, severe mucosal ulceration indicates a need for decreased chemotherapy until complete healing takes place, usually within a week. Analgesics, including opioids, may be needed when treatment cannot be altered, such as during SCT.

If rectal ulcers develop, meticulous toilet hygiene, warm sitz baths after each bowel movement and an occlusive ointment applied to the ulcerated area promote healing; the use of stool softeners is necessary to prevent further discomfort. The child may avoid defecation to prevent discomfort; for this reason, parents should record bowel movements to keep track. Rectal temperatures and suppositories are always avoided because they may traumatise the area.

Neurological Problems

Vincristine, and to a lesser extent vinblastine, can cause various neurotoxic effects. One of the more common neurotoxic effects is severe constipation caused from decreased bowel innervation. Administration of opioids can further aggravate constipation. The nurse advises parents to record bowel movements and to notify the practitioner of a change in stool habits. Physical activity and stool softeners are helpful in preventing the problem, but laxatives, such as macrogol, are often necessary to stimulate evacuation. Dietary changes such as increased fibre may not be effective because the increased bulk tends to increase faecal distension and discomfort without producing the necessary mechanical stimulation.

Footdrop and weakness and numbness of the extremities may cause difficulty in walking or fine hand movement. The nurse should observe for these problems and warn parents of these side effects, which are reversible once the drug is stopped. Wearing high-top tennis shoes or using a footboard in bed may help preserve proper alignment. If weakness occurs while the child is attending school, temporary alteration of activity may be necessary.

Another neurotoxic effect is severe jaw pain. Analgesics may help relieve the discomfort. Children may avoid movement by not talking or chewing, although continuous chewing, such as with gum, may actually reduce the pain.

A neurological syndrome, postirradiation somnolence, may develop 5 to 8 weeks after CNS irradiation and last for 4 to 15 days. It is characterised by somnolence with or without fever, anorexia, and nausea and vomiting. Parents should be warned of the possibility of such symptoms and be encouraged to seek medical evaluation because somnolence may be an early indicator of long-term neurological sequelae after cranial irradiation.

Haemorrhagic Cystitis

Sterile haemorrhagic cystitis is a side effect of chemical irritation to the bladder from chemotherapy or radiation therapy. It can be prevented by: (1) a liberal oral or parenteral fluid intake (at least 1.5 times the recommended daily fluid requirement [2 L/m^2/day]); (2) frequent voiding immediately after feeling the urge, including immediately before bed, one night-time void and on arising; (3) administration of the drug early in the day to allow for sufficient fluids and frequent voiding; and (4) administration of mesna, a drug that inhibits the urotoxicity of cyclophosphamide and ifosfamide (Freedman et al 2016).

In most cases IV fluids are given before, during and after the drug to ensure adequate hydration, thereby eliminating the need for the child to drink large amounts of fluid. If oral home administration is prescribed, the family needs specific instructions on exactly how much fluid the child must have.

Alopecia. Hair loss is a side effect of several chemotherapeutic drugs and cranial irradiation. Not all children lose their hair during chemotherapy, and some children may experience thinning of the hair rather than baldness. However, retaining hair is the exception rather than the rule. It is better to warn children and parents of this side effect to allow them some time to adapt to hair loss.

The family should know that the hair falls out in clumps, causing patchy baldness. To lessen the trauma of seeing large amounts of hair on bed linen or clothing, the child can wear a disposable surgical cap to collect the shed hair during the period of greatest hair loss, or the hair can be cut short or the head shaved. Hair typically regrows in 3 to 6 months, and it is often a different colour and texture than before cancer treatment.

If the child chooses not to wear a wig, attention to some type of head covering is important, especially in cold or sunny climates. Scalp hygiene is also important. The scalp should be washed regularly as with any other body part.

Steroid Effects

Short-term steroid therapy produces physical changes and alterations in body image, which, although not clinically significant, can be extremely distressing to older children. One of these is cushingoid appearance. The child's face becomes rounded and puffy. Unlike hair loss, little can be done to camouflage this obvious change, although careful avoidance of salt and salt-containing foods can help reduce fluid accumulation. It is not unusual for other children to tease the child. It is helpful to reassure the child that, after cessation of the drug, the facial contours will return to normal. The use of loose-fitting clothes, such as warm-up outfits, can help camouflage the change in weight.

Children receiving steroid therapy look healthy. The moon face, red cheeks, supraclavicular fat pads, protuberant abdomen and fluid retention indicate weight gain. However, the actual weight gain resulting from increased muscle mass and subcutaneous tissue may be small. Therefore, the nurse should evaluate weight gain by observing the extremities and measuring skinfold thickness and arm circumference during steroid therapy to determine whether the weight gain is a result of increased dietary intake.

Shortly after beginning steroid therapy, children may experience mood changes, which range from feelings of wellbeing and euphoria to depression and irritability. If parents are unaware of these drug-induced changes, they may become unduly concerned. Therefore, the nurse should warn them of the reactions and encourage them to discuss the behavioural changes with each other and the child.

Nursing Care During Haematopoietic Stem Cell Transplantation

Because of the aggressive preconditioning therapy used to remove the marrow and the potential for complications while waiting for engraftment of transplanted stem cells, children undergoing SCT are usually hospitalised for several weeks. SCT patients must have numerous procedures performed, such as the insertion of a venous access device, administration of intensive chemotherapy and irradiation and strict infection precautions. During the period after transplantation and before the new marrow begins adequately replacing granulocytes, the child is extremely susceptible to infection and any infection can be life-threatening. In addition, many of the side effects previously discussed occur in the child undergoing SCT.

The most common complication in allogeneic transplants is acute GVHD, which can affect the skin, gastrointestinal tract and liver. The characteristics and severity of the manifestations vary according to the severity and area affected. Emphasis is now placed on the prevention of GVHD, using various agents such as a calcineurin inhibitor in conjunction with mycophenolate mofetil, methotrexate or sirolimus (Gottschalk et al 2016). Treatment involves the use of steroids or other immunosuppressive medications. However, this treatment further increases the risk of infection in the already susceptible patient. All blood products are irradiated to minimise the introduction of additional antigens.

Skin breakdown and delayed wound healing frequently occur in the patient undergoing SCT. Preventive interventions to minimise pressure on dependent areas of the skin include the use of pressure-relieving or pressure-reducing beds or mattresses and frequent movement. Measures to promote healing when breakdown occurs include frequent sitz baths to the perianal area and protective skin barriers, such as hydrocolloid dressings or occlusive ointments.

Throughout this long ordeal the family is worried about successful engraftment and possible fatal complications. An unfortunate post-transplant possibility is recurrence of the disease after engraftment. Consequently, nurses need to provide sensitive care and maintain a supportive attitude during the many crises that may arise. If the procedure is not successful, the care needed by these families is consistent with that required by the family of any child with a life-threatening disorder (see Chapter 19).

Preparation for Procedures

Children in particular need psychological preparation for the various treatment interventions, which often involve surgery, IV injections, bone marrow aspirations and LPs. The diagnostic procedures initially employed to confirm the diagnosis and those that are repeated to monitor treatment can be a source of discomfort and stress to the child and family. Even non-invasive procedures such as imaging and radiological tests are frightening to a young child. Some of these tests require the child to lie motionless for a prolonged time in a confined space with little or no communication. Consequently, infants and young children are usually sedated, and older children need an explanation of what to expect and reminders during the test of how much longer they must remain still. The same principles for preparing children for procedures that are discussed in Chapter 22 apply here, including the option of having parents stay with the child whenever possible. Children who undergo repeated tests need additional preparation and emotional support to manage their stress.

Two procedures, bone marrow studies and LPs, are so commonly performed in many types of childhood cancer that they deserve special consideration in preparing children. Both tests can be frightening to children because they are done behind the child's field of vision. Professionals caring for children with cancer recommend the use of developmentally appropriate support using both pharmacological and non-pharmacological approaches and sedation if required. These decisions should always be made in consultation with the child and their family.

Topical anaesthetics such as eutectic mixture of local anaesthetics (EMLA) and LMX4 creams are used as a local anaesthetic before intrusive procedures, including venepunctures, implanted port access, LP's (lumbar puncture) and subcutaneous or intramuscular injections (Hockenberry et al 2016). Deeper infiltration of the muscle and periosteum of the bone with buffered lidocaine (lignocaine) further reduces the pain from the large-bore aspiration or biopsy needle entering the bone.

For bone marrow studies, LP's (lumbar puncture) and other procedures, children of preschool age and older should be prepared beforehand. Bone marrow biopsies are usually performed under a general anaesthetic, while LP's (lumbar puncture) can be done under sedation if the child sedates well. Physical care after the procedures is minimal. A small pressure bandage is applied to the bone marrow puncture site, and an adhesive bandage is applied to the LP (lumbar puncture) site. No activity restriction is necessary after the bone marrow test, although the site is usually sore and the child may prefer to remain quiet. Recommendations after LP (lumbar puncture) vary. If medication was instilled, the child may be placed in a slight Trendelenburg position to facilitate circulation of the medicated spinal fluid.

Pain Management

Nurses must be knowledgeable about the basic pathophysiology of cancer pain and treatment-related side effects. The World Health Organization's three-step analgesic pain ladder should be incorporated into the approach to pain management for every child with cancer (Ullrich et al 2016). Nurses must acquire extensive knowledge of non-opioid and opioid analgesics, as well as non-pharmacological approaches used in paediatric pain management (see Chapter 5.) Interdisciplinary pain management teams are used in many paediatric cancer centres. These teams serve as consultants and provide expertise in the assessment and management of pain. The nurse often serves as the coordinator of care, playing a key role in cancer pain management and implementing the pain team's plan of care.

Pharmacological management of disease-related pain involves a variety of methods. It may take more than one trial of one type of medication to find the appropriate agent to manage a patient's pain. The route of administration must be considered as well. Providing 'pain relief' by administering painful intramuscular injections as an alternative to the IV route is not appropriate therapy because many oral preparations are now available with comparable efficacy. Furthermore, children may refuse needed pain medication if it involves an injection. Paracetamol, with or without codeine, oxycodone and morphine are commonly used agents in the management of disease-related pain (Fielding et al 2013). Appropriate dosing is imperative. Doses are titrated to increase the amount of analgesia and minimise side effects.

Health Promotion

Children with cancer require the same basic health supervision as do any children. Sometimes the overwhelming needs and demands placed on the family, coupled with the singular concern focused on the cancer by both family and healthcare professionals, result in a lack of attention to typical healthcare needs. Nurses should monitor the type of primary care the child receives, using guidelines for recommended medical supervision. Areas of particular concern are growth, physical and cognitive development and neurological status. Two other areas are also important: (1) dental care because of potential side effects from treatment; and (2) immunisations because of concern with live virus vaccines and immunosuppression.

Dental Care

Irradiation to the head and neck can cause a number of late complications (Landier et al 2016). Some are irreversible, such as facial asymmetry, but those affecting the teeth and gums (e.g. caries, periodontal disease) benefit from excellent oral hygiene, including regular use of systemic and topical fluoride and regular dental examinations and cleaning. (See Dental Health, Chapter 12.) Delayed or absent development of the permanent teeth can occur (Effinger et al 2014). Depending on the child's age, this can be a source of acute psychological distress, especially during early school-age years, when 'losing a tooth' is a status symbol. Children need to be aware of this possibility and need help to explain the delay to peers.

Daily toothbrushing and flossing are encouraged in children with granulocyte counts in excess of 500/mm^3 and platelet counts above 40,000/mm^3. Fluoride rinses are used as discussed in Chapter 12.

Immunisations

Viral replication after the administration of live vaccine for polio, measles, rubella and mumps can cause serious disease in immunocompromised children. The child receiving chemotherapy for cancer should not receive live, attenuated vaccines. Inactivated vaccines can be given to immunosuppressed children. Siblings and other family members can receive the live measles, mumps and rubella vaccine and the varicella vaccine without risk to the child who is immunosuppressed. Guidelines for immunisation of children receiving chemotherapy and SCT patients have been published (Ardura & Koh 2016).

An important indication for isolation is an outbreak of childhood communicable disease, especially chickenpox. Ideally the school nurse should work with the treating practitioner to decide the optimum time for school attendance. Parents should be taught to work with the school or day care staff to be sure they understand the risk to the child being treated for cancer and that they notify the parents immediately of any exposure. If the child has been exposed to the varicella virus, varicella-zoster immune globulin given within 96 hours may favourably alter the course of the disease. Antiviral agents, such as aciclovir, should be given if the child develops varicella. Without treatment, death from disseminated varicella can occur due to disease in the liver, lung and CNS (Ardura & Koh 2016). (See also Immunisations, Chapter 6.)

NURSING CARE CONSIDERATIONS

Children will need to be re-vaccinated at an appropriate time once treatment has finished. Most institutions have individual guidelines regarding vaccinations in a child undergoing immunosuppressive therapy. The nurse should be aware of these guidelines and educate patients and families about the need for and timing of immunisations.

Family Education

Nurses working with children who have cancer have a significant supportive role in helping the family understand the various therapies, preventing or managing expected side effects or toxicities and observing for late effects of treatment. Helping families learn what they need to know is a constant feature of the nursing role, especially in terms of new treatments, clinical trials, home care and transition to off-therapy and adult-focused healthcare. Nurses must stay well informed themselves to be able to help families learn as they establish a 'new normal' in their lives. Several excellent resources are available to use in family education available from cancer centres in major children's hospitals across Australia and New Zealand including:

- Children's Cancer Centre, The Royal Children's Hospital Melbourne (https://www.rch.org.au/ccc/)
- Cancer Centre for Children, The Children's Hospital at Westmead (http://cancercentreforchildren.org.au/)
- Starship's Blood and Cancer Centre (https://www.starship.org.nz/directory-of-services/blood-&-cancer-centre/).

Instruction regarding home care frequently involves teaching about medication schedules, observing for side effects or toxicities that require further evaluation, taking measures to prevent or manage these problems and caring for special devices such as central venous catheters. Medication adherence is an important issue because poor adherence to treatment regimens can result in disease relapse or serious medical complications (Gupta & Bhatia 2017). Every effort must be made to ensure that the family understands the importance of adhering to the prescribed treatment schedule and follow-up care. Finding methods to identify and minimise non-adherence is an active area of current research. (See Chapter 22.)

Many families use complementary and alternative medicine (CAM), primarily for symptom relief. CAM includes therapies that are not thought of as standard medical care. Complementary therapies are used along with standard medical treatment; alternative therapies are used instead of standard medical treatment. There are many different types of CAM therapy available. A few examples include dietary supplements, homeopathy and acupuncture. Most families using CAM therapies do not abandon standard care, but often they do not tell their medical practitioner about CAM use (McLean & Kemper 2016). Undisclosed use of alternative therapies may interfere with the effectiveness of the prescribed treatment. Reasons given by families for not communicating about their use of CAM therapies include anticipation of negative response from their medical practitioner, believing that medical practitioners do not need to know and that they are not asked (McLean & Kemper 2016).

Nurses are instrumental in building trusting relationships with families to facilitate discussion of concerns and questions openly with their medical practitioner who can guide them. To provide family education, nurses should familiarise themselves with reliable resources about CAM, so that they can counsel families about CAM therapies.

Completion of Therapy

Care does not end when the child completes therapy. With the increasing awareness of late effects, nurses have an important role in the assessment of the child for problems such as delayed growth, secondary malignancies and disturbances in body systems. The family needs to be aware of the importance of continued medical supervision, for both primary care and survivorship care. Other healthcare professionals caring for the child, such as school nurses, family doctors and dentists, should be informed of the child's cancer diagnosis. As children reach adulthood, transition services may be available in the treatment centre to help ease the transfer of primary care to adult healthcare professionals in the community. Adolescents/young adults may benefit from genetic counselling regarding cancers that are likely to be inherited. If the possibility of infertility exists, fertility options should be discussed for pubertal males and females before the start of treatment and readdressed during survivorship care. The Children's Oncology Group has developed guidelines for long-term follow-up care for paediatric cancer survivors. Nurses involved with these children should be familiar with these guidelines and use all opportunities to help patients and families access needed survivorship and transition care.

CANCERS OF BLOOD AND LYMPH SYSTEMS

Acute Leukaemias

Leukaemia is a broad term given to a group of malignant diseases of the bone marrow, blood and lymphatic system. In healthy children, the bone marrow makes blood stem cells that mature to become lymphoid or myeloid stem cells. Myeloid cells differentiate into red blood cells, platelets and white blood cells. Lymphoid stem cells become lymphoblasts that differentiate into B-lymphocytes, T-lymphocytes and natural killer cells (Leukaemia Foundation 2021). In acute leukaemias, immature cells predominate that cannot function effectively. Two types of leukaemia are seen most often in children: acute lymphoblastic leukaemia (ALL) and acute myeloid leukaemia (AML).

Acute Lymphoblastic Leukaemia

ALL is the most common form of childhood cancer, with 25% of children who are diagnosed with cancer each year in Australia and New Zealand being diagnosed with ALL. It occurs more often in boys than in girls, with the peak age of onset between 0 and 4 years old (Ballentine & NZCCR Working Group 2017, Youlden & Aitken 2019). Risk factors for ALL include prenatal exposure to x-rays, previous treatment with chemotherapy and certain genetic conditions (e.g. Down syndrome, Bloom's syndrome, Fanconi's anaemia) (Leukaemia Foundation 2021). Various chromosomal abnormalities also have been identified in leukaemic cells of children with ALL (Rabin et al 2016).

Clinical Staging and Prognosis. The standard accepted method to classify ALL is immunophenotyping in which panels of monoclonal antibodies are used to determine T-lineage, B-lineage and myeloid antigens (Rabin et al 2016). In addition, chromosomal number (ploidy) and structural rearrangements are evaluated using molecular genetic analyses. The most important prognostic factors in determining long-term survival for children with ALL (Table 29.3) include the child's age, initial white blood cell count, CNS involvement, testicular involvement, Down syndrome, sex, race and ethnicity, and nutritional status; leukaemic cell characteristics that affect prognosis include morphology, immunophenotype and cytogenetics/genomic alterations such as ploidy and structural rearrangements. ALL has demonstrated dramatic improvements in survival rates such that current long-term disease-free survival rates for children with ALL approach 90% in major paediatric cancer treatment centres (Ballentine & NZCCR Working Group 2017, Youlden & Aitken 2019).

Clinical Manifestations. The onset of leukaemia varies from acute to insidious. In most instances the child displays remarkably few symptoms. For example, leukaemia may be diagnosed when a minor infection, such as a cold, fails to completely disappear. The child continues to be pale, listless, irritable, febrile and anorexic. Parents often suspect some underlying problem when they observe the child's weight loss, petechiae, bruising without cause and continued complaints of bone and joint pain. At other times there may be an extended history of signs and symptoms mimicking such conditions as rheumatoid arthritis or mononucleosis. Sometimes leukaemia is an incidental finding on a routine physical examination or during treatment for an injury.

Signs and symptoms of ALL reflect infiltration of the bone marrow by non-functional leukaemic cells ('blasts'). The three main consequences of bone marrow infiltration are: (1) anaemia from decreased erythrocytes; (2) infection from neutropenia; and (3) bleeding from decreased platelet production. Approximately half of patients have an elevated white blood cell count at presentation (> 10,000/mm^3). Other signs and symptoms indicate leukaemic cell infiltration of other

TABLE 29.3 Selected Prognostic Factors for Acute Lymphoblastic Leukaemia

Factor	Criteria
Age	Favourable: > 1 year or ≤ 10 years at diagnosis.
Initial white blood cell count	Favourable: < 50,000/mm^3 (B-cell ALL; association not seen in T-cell ALL).
Sex	Favourable: Female.
Immunophenotype	Survival is better in B-cell ALL than in T-cell ALL. (Specific immunophenotypic markers are no longer used to determine prognosis, but are important as targets for therapeutic agents.)
Cytogenetics/genomic alterations	Favourable: high hyperdiploidy (50–65 chromosomes); *ETV6-RUNX1* gene fusion. Unfavourable: Philadelphia chromosome; *MLL* gene rearrangements; hypodiploidy; intrachromosomal amplification of *AML1* gene.
Treatment response	Favourable: rapid response to treatment (best prognosis associated with undetectable levels of minimal residual disease or at least < 10−4 at the end of standard induction).
Nutritional status	Unfavourable: malnutrition or obesity at diagnosis, and ongoing poor nutritional status throughout intensive postinduction treatment.

ALL, acute lymphoblastic leukaemia.

Source: Adapted from Rabin, K. R., Gramatges, M. M., Margolin, J. F., et al. (2016). Acute lymphoblastic leukaemia. In P. A. Pizzo & D. G. Poplack (Eds.), Principles and practice of pediatric oncology (7th ed.). Philadelphia, PA: Lippincott; National Institutes of Health, National Cancer Institute. (2017). Childhood acute lymphoblastic leukaemia treatment. https://www.cancer.gov/types/leukemia/hp/child-all-treatment-pdq.

organs; highly vascular organs, such as the spleen and liver, are most severely affected. Commonly seen are hepatosplenomegaly (68% of patients), splenomegaly (63%), fever (61%), lymphadenopathy (50%), bleeding (e.g. petechiae or purpura, 48%) and bone pain (23%) (Rabin et al 2016). Two important sites of extramedullary disease are the CNS and testes because they can serve as 'sanctuaries' for leukaemic cells that require specific therapy.

Diagnostic Evaluation. Leukaemia is usually suspected from the history, physical manifestations and a peripheral blood smear that contains leukaemic blasts, frequently in combination with low blood counts. The diagnostic evaluation includes a thorough history and physical examination, laboratory tests (FBC with differential, blood chemistries) and bone marrow aspiration/biopsy (cytogenetic analysis, immunophenotyping). Definitive diagnosis is based on analysis of the bone marrow sample. Typically the bone marrow of a child with ALL shows a monotonous infiltrate of blast cells. Once the diagnosis is confirmed, an LP is performed to determine whether there is any CNS involvement. Although only a small number of children have CNS involvement at diagnosis, they are usually asymptomatic.

Therapeutic Management. Treatment of ALL is based on risk groups defined by clinical and laboratory findings. Children with a higher risk of relapse/recurrence are treated with the most intensive therapy. Although specifics for various risk groups vary, treatment is generally divided into phases: induction, CNS preventive therapy/consolidation, interim maintenance, delayed intensification, maintenance or continuation therapy and remission.

Almost immediately after confirmation of the diagnosis, induction therapy begins and lasts for 4 to 5 weeks (Rabin et al 2016). The principal drugs are the corticosteroids (dexamethasone or prednisone), vincristine and asparaginase (colaspase), with or without an anthracycline. A complete remission is determined by the presence of less than 5% blast cells in the bone marrow and no detectable leukaemia in extramedullary sites.

Because many of the drugs also cause myelosuppression of normal blood elements, the period immediately after a remission can be critical. The body is defenceless against invading organisms (especially normal bacterial flora) and susceptible to spontaneous haemorrhage. Consequently, supportive therapy during this time is essential. Supportive care consists of transfusion support and use of antibacterial and antifungal agents.

CNS preventive therapy is based on the understanding that leukaemic cells could be present in the CNS where they are protected from many systemic chemotherapy drugs by the blood–brain barrier. For this reason, all children receive CNS prophylactic therapy. The combination of intrathecal chemotherapy (either methotrexate alone or in combination with cytarabine and hydrocortisone) plus CNS-directed systemic chemotherapy (dexamethasone, asparaginase (colaspase) and high-dose methotrexate with leucovorin rescue) is standard; cranial radiation may be used for children at highest risk for CNS relapse.

Past clinical trials have shown that postinduction therapy is needed to maintain remission. Treatment regimens vary, but all patients receive consolidation/intensification after achieving a complete remission. Most commonly used is the Berlin, Frankfurt, Münster (BFM) 'backbone' (a very intensive chemotherapy regimen from the International BFM Study Group that greatly increased ALL survival). This backbone includes consolidation with cyclophosphamide, cytarabine and mercaptopurine given initially, followed by interim maintenance with high-dose methotrexate with or without leucovorin rescue. Next, delayed intensification is given using drugs and schedules similar to those used in the induction and consolidation phases. This is followed by maintenance therapy with daily mercaptopurine and weekly low-dose methotrexate; vincristine and a corticosteroid may be given, as well as continued intrathecal therapy (Rabin et al 2016). A critical challenge during maintenance therapy is medication adherence because it has been shown that anything less than 95% adherence increases the risk of relapse (Bhatia et al 2015).

Although the optimum duration of therapy is not known, current practice is to continue treatment for 2 to 3 years. After cessation of therapy all children require regular medical follow-up to observe for relapse and late effects of treatment.

Acute Myeloid Leukaemia

AML accounts for 20% of all cases of childhood leukaemia in Australia and New Zealand, with approximately 188 new cases per million children each year (Ballentine & NZCCR Working Group 2017, Youlden & Aitken 2019). AML is associated with a variety of predisposition syndromes, including constitutional chromosome abnormalities, inherited single gene mutations and inherited cytopenias (Arceci & Meshinchi 2016). In addition, therapy-related AML can be caused by treatment with certain chemotherapeutic drugs and/or radiation therapy.

Clinical Staging and Prognosis. There is no established clinical staging system for AML; it is considered disseminated at diagnosis. The World Health Organization (WHO) classification system is used to categorise subtypes of AML. These subtypes have distinguishing chromosomal changes, as well as changes in morphology, histochemistry, immunophenotype and molecular characteristics; some specific subtypes are associated with prognosis (Arceci & Meshinchi 2016).

Favourable prognosis is associated with Down syndrome in children who are less than 4 years of age at diagnosis, no minimal residual disease (MRD) findings after initial therapy and certain cytogenetic and genetic abnormalities. Unfavourable prognosis is associated with an initial white blood cell count greater than 100,000/mm^3, presence of MRD after initial therapy and specific cytogenetic and genetic abnormalities (Arceci & Meshinchi 2016).

Progress in the management of AML has improved the 5-year survival rate of 75% (Ballentine & NZCCR Working Group 2017, Youlden & Aitken 2019). However, there is a wide range in outcome for different biological subtypes of AML, which needs to be taken into account when considering prognosis for an individual patient. Research is focused on improving the survival rates and defining risk groups to enable risk-adapted therapy.

Clinical Manifestations. Many signs and symptoms of AML are similar to those of ALL and reflect infiltration of the bone marrow or extramedullary sites by myeloblasts. Typical signs and symptoms include fever with or without an infection, night sweats, shortness of breath, weakness or fatigue, easy bruising/bleeding, petechiae, bone or joint pain and an eczema-like skin rash. In AML, painless lumps (leukaemia cutis) that may be blue or purple in colour may appear in the neck, underarm, abdomen, groin or elsewhere. Other painless lumps, blue-green in colour and called chloromas, may be found around the eyes.

Diagnostic Evaluation. With a few differences, the workup for AML is similar to that for ALL. Procedures and tests include physical examination and history, FBC with differential, blood chemistries, chest x-ray, bone marrow aspiration/biopsy, cytogenetic analysis, RT-PCR test, immunophenotyping, molecular testing and a lumbar puncture. A chloroma may be biopsied if present.

Therapeutic Management. Treatment for AML is generally more intense and of shorter duration than treatment for ALL. Chemotherapy is the main treatment modality for AML and is generally given in two phases: induction followed by post remission consolidation/intensification (Leukaemia Foundation 2019). For most subtypes of AML, maintenance therapy has not been shown to improve outcome and is therefore not used in most treatment regimens. Typically children are given two courses of induction chemotherapy and two courses of intensification. Standard remission induction consists of a three-drug regimen of cytarabine, daunorubicin and etoposide. CNS treatment with intrathecal medication is usually included in treatment regimens; CNS irradiation is not usually used in AML treatment. Once remission is achieved (no signs of leukaemia detected), SCT may be performed. Alternatively, intensive chemotherapy may be given and SCT reserved in case the AML relapses. Intensification chemotherapy usually consists of high-dose cytarabine with or without daunorubicin; intrathecal chemotherapy is given every 1 to 2 months during intensification. The following discussion elaborates on the pathological process and related clinical manifestations in the most susceptible organs of the body (Fig 29.3).

Nursing Care Management

Nursing care of the child with acute leukaemia, ALL or AML, is directly related to the regimen of therapy. Myelosuppression, drug toxicity and leukaemic infiltration cause secondary complications that necessitate supportive physical care. This discussion focuses on supportive interventions for the child with leukaemia and the family. General aspects of care appropriate for the child with leukaemia are discussed earlier under Nursing Care Management (p. 792).

Prepare the Family for Diagnostic and Therapeutic Procedures. From the time before diagnosis to cessation of therapy, children must undergo several tests, the most traumatic of which are bone marrow aspiration or biopsy and LP. Multiple fingerpricks and venepunctures for blood analysis and drug infusion are common occurrences for several years after the diagnosis. Therefore, children need an explanation of the rationale for each procedure, what can be expected and what they can do to help. (See Preparation for Diagnostic and Therapeutic Procedures, Chapter 22.)

Depending on the child's age, one way of beginning diagnostic preparation is to explain the tests, procedures and treatment plan. Using a drawing or letting the child look at a drop of blood under a microscope not only teaches but also fosters trust between the nurse and the child. It also allows the nurse to assess the child's level of understanding. An error many health professionals make is to overestimate children's knowledge about their bodies. For example, a bone marrow aspiration makes sense only when it is clarified that the centre of a bone contains the cells that later become 'working' blood cells or leukaemic cells.

Provide Continued Emotional Support. Nursing care of the child with leukaemia is based on typical problems the family confronts during the treatment phases and afterwards. Therefore, the nurse's role is one of continual support, guidance, clarification and clinical judgment. Parents need to know how to recognise symptoms that demand medical attention. Although some of the reactions discussed are expected, parents should still report them to their practitioner. Warning parents of their possible occurrence beforehand also allows

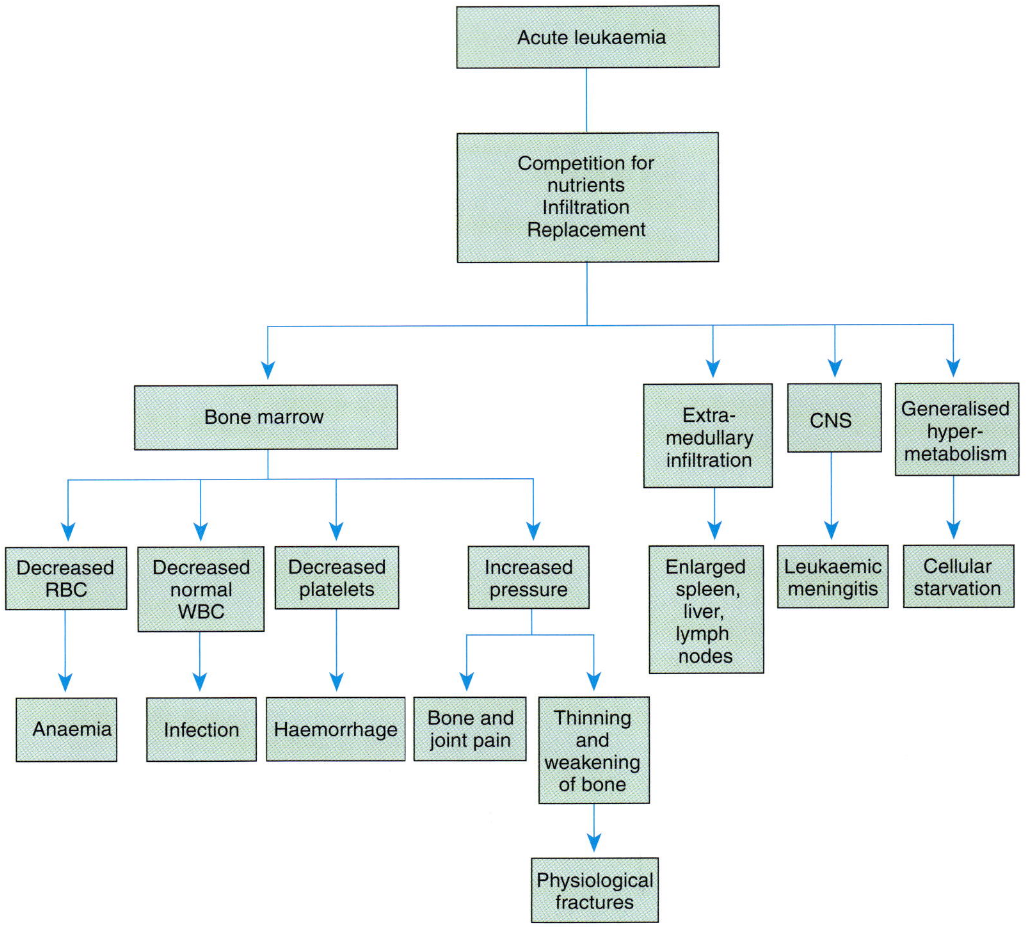

Fig 29.3 Principal sites of tissue involvement in leukaemia. (*CNS*, central nervous system; *RBC*, red blood cell; *WBC*, white blood cell.)

parents to prepare. At the same time, it reassures them that these reactions are not caused by a return of leukaemic cells.

The nurse must also use judgment in recognising which side effects are normal reactions and which indicate toxicity. Frequently it is the office or clinic nurse who screens such telephone calls and gives advice when appropriate. Usually nausea and vomiting are not indications for drug cessation. However, severe vomiting may require immediate intervention to prevent dehydration. Signs of infection, mucosal ulceration, haemorrhagic cystitis, peripheral neuropathy and constipation require medical evaluation.

Another aspect of continued emotional support involves prognosis. Leukaemia is not invariably fatal, but present statistics must be correctly interpreted. Although almost 90% of children with ALL live 5 years or longer, these are average estimates that apply to those children treated with the most successful protocols since diagnosis (Ballentine & NZCCR Working Group 2017, Youlden & Aitken 2019). For the high-risk child with ALL or the child with AML, the prognosis may be significantly poorer. Of those who do survive after completing therapy, some will relapse.

The nurse must be familiar with survival statistics to interpret them correctly to parents. At the same time, the nurse must realise that a realistic understanding of the chances for survival requires an adjustment period. During the initial diagnosis or when a relapse occurs, parents may find it difficult to hear the facts.

Statistics are numbers. Sometimes they bring hope, and at other times they bring despair. Although they are important in terms of research, better treatment and identification of high- or low-risk populations, they present a general picture of what to expect. The nurse who is working with family members must individualise the numbers to relate to the people. An understanding of each member's emotional needs, as well as competent care of physical ones, is essential to the positive, growth-promoting support of the family. Comprehensive emotional support for the family of a child with a chronic illness and of a child at end of life is described in Chapter 19.

Lymphomas

The lymphomas, a group of neoplastic diseases that arise from the lymphoid and haematopoietic systems, are divided into Hodgkin's disease and non-Hodgkin's lymphoma (NHL). These diseases are further subdivided according to tissue type and extent of disease. Approximately 10% of all cancer diagnoses in children will be for a type of lymphoma, with Hodgkin's lymphoma being slightly more common than NHL (Ballentine & NZCCR Working Group 2017, Youlden & Aitken 2019). Although Hodgkin's disease is extremely rare before 5 years of age, there is a striking increase in children ages 15 to 19 years, when it occurs with almost the same frequency as leukaemia. Epstein-Barr virus is thought to have a role in the causation of Hodgkin's lymphoma (Lymphoma Australia 2021a).

Hodgkin's Lymphoma

Hodgkin's lymphoma affects about 26 children per million children each year in Australia and New Zealand, with the peak incidence seen in the adolescent age group (Ballentine & NZCCR Working Group 2017, Youlden & Aitken 2019). Hodgkin's lymphoma has a childhood form, a young adult form and an older adult form. The malignancy originates in the lymphoid system and primarily involves the lymph nodes. It predictably metastasises to non-nodal or extra lymphatic sites, especially the spleen, liver, bone marrow, lungs and mediastinum (i.e. mass of tissues and organs separating the lungs, including the heart and its vessels, trachea, oesophagus, thymus and lymph nodes), although no tissue is exempt from involvement (Fig 29.4). It is classified according to four histological types: (1) lymphocytic predominance; (2) nodular sclerosis; (3) mixed cellularity; and (4) lymphocytic depletion.

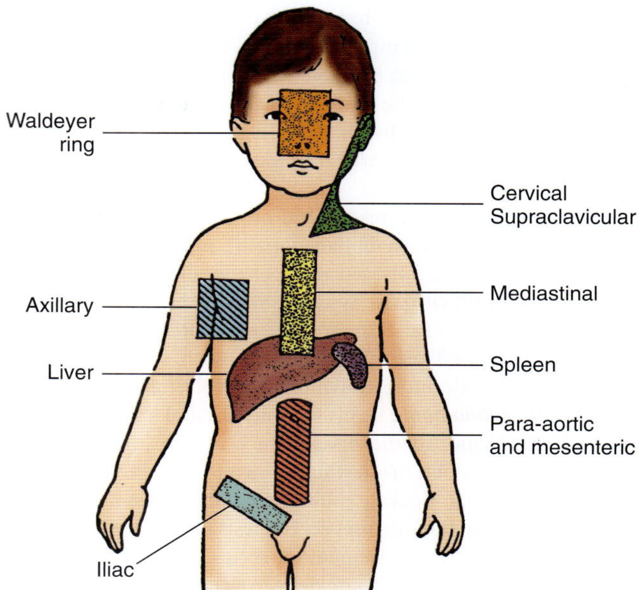

Fig 29.4 Main areas of lymphadenopathy and organ involvement in Hodgkin's disease.

Clinical Staging and Prognosis. Accurate staging of the extent of disease is the basis for treatment protocols and expected prognosis. More than one staging system exists; Box 29.2 shows the Ann Arbor Staging Classification.

Each stage is further subdivided into A, B, E, S or X. Stage A denotes absence of associated general symptoms. Stage B indicates presence of symptoms, such as night sweats, fever (38°C) or weight loss of 10% or more during the preceding 6 months. Stage E represents extra lymphatic disease beyond the contiguous nodal disease. Stage S indicates splenic involvement, and stage X indicates mediastinal bulky disease.

The prognosis for patients with Hodgkin's lymphoma has improved dramatically, largely as a result of systematic staging, risk group stratification and improved treatment protocols. The prognosis is excellent in children with localised disease. Overall survival rates for patients with Hodgkin's lymphoma are as high as 99%; however, the survival rate is dependent on histology and staging (Ballentine & NZCCR Working Group 2017, Youlden & Aitken 2019). Even in those with disseminated disease, long-term remissions are possible in more than half the patients. For relapses, complete remission may occur in 30% to 60% of patients undergoing autologous SCT (Metzger et al 2016).

BOX 29.2 Ann Arbor Staging of Hodgkin's Disease

Stage I—Lesions are limited to one lymph node area or only one additional extralymphatic site (I_E), such as the liver, lungs, kidney or intestines.

Stage II—Two or more lymph node regions on the same side of the diaphragm or one additional extralymphatic site or organ (II_E) on the same side of the diaphragm is involved.

Stage III—Lymph node regions on both sides of the diaphragm are involved with spread to one extralymphatic site (III_E), spleen (III_S) or both (III_{SE}).

Stage IV—Diffuse spread throughout the body to one or more extralymphatic sites with or without involvement of associated lymph nodes.

Clinical Manifestations. Hodgkin's lymphoma is characterised by painless enlargement of lymph nodes. The most common finding is enlarged, firm, non-tender, movable nodes in the supraclavicular or cervical area. In children the lymph node located near the left clavicle may be the first enlarged node, which is referred to as the sentinel node. Enlargement of axillary and inguinal lymph nodes is less frequent.

Other signs and symptoms depend on the extent and location of involvement. Mediastinal lymphadenopathy may cause a persistent, non-productive cough. Enlarged retroperitoneal nodes may produce unexplained abdominal pain. Systemic symptoms include low-grade or intermittent fever (Pel-Ebstein disease), anorexia, nausea, weight loss, night sweats and pruritus. Generally, such symptoms indicate advanced lymph node and extralymphatic involvement.

Diagnostic Evaluation. The history and physical examination often yield important clues to the disease, such as a history of systemic symptoms, presence of a mediastinal mass and enlargement of lymph nodes, spleen or liver. Because multiple organs can become involved, the diagnostic evaluation requires several tests to confirm the diagnosis and assess the extent of involvement for accurate staging. Tests include FBC, biochemistry profile (lactate dehydrogenase, albumin, renal and hepatic function studies, alkaline phosphatase), erythrocyte sedimentation rate, C-reactive protein and serum ferritin. Imaging tests include chest radiography, CT of neck and chest and CT or MRI of abdomen and pelvis (Metzger et al 2016).

A lymph node biopsy is essential to establish histological diagnosis and staging. The presence of Hodgkin and Reed-Sternberg cells is considered diagnostic of Hodgkin's disease because it is absent in the other lymphomas; however, it may occur in infectious mononucleosis. A bone marrow aspiration or biopsy also is usually performed.

Therapeutic Management. The primary treatment modalities for Hodgkin's lymphoma are chemotherapy and irradiation. The length and intensity of therapy are based on disease-related factors (e.g. stage, number of involved nodal regions, tumour bulk, B symptoms and early response); other factors that may be considered are age, sex and histology (Lymphoma Australia 2021a). The goal of treatment is cure; however, aggressive therapy increases the chances of complications that can seriously compromise quality of life. One of the major concerns with combined radiation and cytotoxic drug therapy is the risk of serious late effects in children with an excellent prognosis. Consequently, treatment that is risk-adapted and response-based aims to minimise long-term complications. Because of the diversity of approaches to treatment, the following is an overview of general principles that may not apply to all children.

Most newly diagnosed children are treated with risk-adapted chemotherapy alone or in combination with radiation therapy. Radiation may entail involved field radiation, extended field radiation (involved areas plus adjacent nodes) or total nodal irradiation (the entire axial lymph node system), depending on the extent of involvement. Various combinations of chemotherapy drugs may be used, based on the most effective combinations used in the past: MOPP (methotrexate, vincristine [Oncovin], procarbazine and prednisone) and ABVD (doxorubicin [Adriamycin], bleomycin, vinblastine and dacarbazine). Today, COPP (substituting cyclophosphamide for methotrexate) has generally replaced MOPP. In addition, etoposide has been included in chemotherapy regimens in place of alkylating agents to reduce gonadal toxicity (Lymphoma Australia 2021a).

Follow-up care of children who have completed therapy is essential to identify relapse and long-term complications. Children without a functioning spleen are at increased risk of infection; therefore, prophylactic antibiotics are administered for an indefinite period, and survivors are advised to seek immediate medical care if they develop symptoms of infection even if they are taking antibiotics. Also, pneumococcal, meningococcal and haemophilus influenzae type B (Hib) immunisations are recommended. (See Chapter 6.)

Nursing Care Management. Nursing care involves preparation for diagnostic and operative procedures, explanation of treatment side effects and child and family support. Once the child is hospitalised for suspected Hodgkin's lymphoma, a battery of diagnostic tests is ordered. The family and child need an explanation of why each test is performed because many of them, such as bone marrow aspiration and lymph node biopsy, are invasive procedures.

Explanations of chemotherapeutic reactions are based on the specific drug regimen. The most common side effects, such as nausea and vomiting, body image changes, neuropathy and mucosal ulceration, are discussed in the Nursing Care Management section. Involved field radiation results in few side effects, sometimes consisting only of a mild skin reaction. With extended field radiation to the chest and abdomen, nausea and vomiting, weight loss and mucosal ulceration (oesophagitis, gastric ulcers) are common. The usual measures for providing relief are discussed previously in this chapter and outlined in Table 29.2.

The most common side effect of extensive irradiation is malaise, which may result from damage to the thyroid gland, causing hypothyroidism. Lack of energy is particularly difficult for adolescents because it prevents them from keeping up with their peers. Sometimes adolescents push themselves to the point of physical exhaustion rather than admit fatigue and give in to their decreased activity tolerance. Parents should observe for such behaviour, such as extreme fatigue at the end of the day, falling asleep at the dinner table, inability to concentrate on homework or an increased susceptibility to infection. Regular bedtimes and periodic rest times are important for these children, especially during chemotherapy, when myelosuppression increases the risk of infection and debilitation. Before discharge (if the child has been hospitalised), the nurse should discuss a feasible school schedule with the parents and child. If alterations are necessary, such as elimination of strenuous physical education, they are discussed with the teacher, school nurse and principal. Follow-up care is essential to diagnose hypothyroidism early and institute thyroid replacement.

An area of concern for adolescents is the high risk of sterility from irradiation and chemotherapy. Both irradiation to the gonads and drugs, particularly procarbazine and alkylating agents, may lead to infertility. Younger patients with a greater complement of oocytes are more likely to retain ovarian function. Adolescents should be informed of these side effects, and any options for fertility preservation, early in the course of the diagnosis and treatment.

Although sexual function is not altered, the appearance of secondary sexual characteristics and menstruation may be delayed in the pubescent child. Delayed sexual maturation may be an extremely sensitive and painful area for children. (See Chapter 17.)

Non-Hodgkin's Lymphoma

There are approximately 24 cases per million children diagnosed with NHL each year in Australia and New Zealand (Ballentine & NZCCR Working Group 2017, Youlden & Aitken 2019). The aetiology of NHL is basically unknown, but possible risk factors include past cancer treatment, infection with Epstein-Barr virus or human immunodeficiency virus and inherited or acquired immunodeficiency (Lymphoma Australia 2021b).

Staging and Prognosis. NHL exhibits a variety of morphological, cytochemical and immunological features. Classification is based on immunophenotype, molecular biology and clinical response to treatment, with the majority of cases categorised as lymphoblastic, mature B-cell (including Burkitt's lymphoma) and anaplastic large cell lymphoma (Lymphoma Australia 2021b). Immunologically these cells are also classified as T-cells; B-cells (an example of which is Burkitt's lymphoma); or non-T-, non-B-cells, which lack specific immunological properties.

A favourable prognosis is defined by young age, low stage without mediastinal involvement, low tumour burden and good response to initial therapy (Allen et al 2016). The staging system used for Hodgkin's lymphoma is not used for NHL. Box 29.3 presents the most commonly used NHL staging system.

The use of aggressive combination chemotherapy has had a major impact on NHL survival rates in children. The most effective treatment regimens result in an 88% 5-year event-free survival rate, dependent on the extent of the disease at diagnosis (Ballentine & NZCCR Working Group 2017, Youlden & Aitken 2019).

Clinical Manifestations. Clinical manifestations depend on the anatomical site and extent of involvement. Many of the signs and symptoms seen in Hodgkin's lymphoma may be present in NHL, although it is rare for a single symptom to lead to the diagnosis. Rather, metastasis to the bone marrow or CNS may produce signs and symptoms typical of leukaemia. Lymphoid tumours compressing various organs may cause intestinal or airway obstruction, cranial nerve palsies or spinal paralysis.

Diagnostic Evaluation. Current recommendations for diagnostic evaluation and staging include: history and physical examination; blood chemistries; total body imaging (CT, PET, MRI); LP; bone marrow aspiration; and biopsy. Cancer cells are examined by immunophenotyping (immunohistochemistry, flow cytometry), cytogenetics and/or FISH (Lymphoma Australia 2021a).

Therapeutic Management. Because NHL is generally considered to be widespread at diagnosis, most children are treated with combination chemotherapy. The role of radiation is limited, although it may be used in children who do not have a complete response to chemotherapy (Lymphoma Australia 2021b). Treatment for NHL is based on histological subtype. Lymphoblastic lymphoma therapy is similar to leukaemia therapy; the protocols include induction, consolidation and maintenance phases, some with intrathecal chemotherapy with or without cranial-spinal radiation therapy. The most commonly used chemotherapy regimens for newly diagnosed lymphoblastic lymphoma include prednisone, dexamethasone, vincristine, daunorubicin, doxorubicin, pegaspargase, cyclophosphamide, cytarabine, methotrexate, mercaptopurine, 6-thioguanine and intrathecal treatments during maintenance. Newly diagnosed children with diffuse mature B-cell lymphoma are treated with surgery (stage I and II only) and chemotherapy; those with anaplastic large cell lymphoma are treated with surgery (stage I) and chemotherapy. These multiagent regimens are administered for 6 to 24 months.

Nursing Care Management. Nursing care of the child with NHL is similar to the care discussed under Nursing Care Management (p. 792). With intensive chemotherapy, nursing care is primarily directed towards managing the side effects of these agents.

BOX 29.3 St Jude Staging of Non-Hodgkin's Lymphoma

Stage I—Disease limited to one lymph node area or only one additional extralymphatic site (excluding thoracic or abdomen).

Stage II—Single tumour with regional lymph node involvement; two or more lymph node regions on the same side of the diaphragm; two single tumours with/without regional involvement on the same side of the diaphragm; or primary resectable gastrointestinal tumour with/without involvement of adjacent mesenteric nodes.

Stage III—Two single tumours on opposite sides of diaphragm; two nodal areas above/below the diaphragm; primary intrathoracic tumour or extensive intraabdominal disease; or paraspinal or epidural tumours.

Stage IV—Tumour has spread into central nervous system and/or bone marrow

NERVOUS SYSTEM TUMOURS

Brain Tumours

Tumours of the CNS are the most common solid tumour in children and account for approximately 25% of all childhood cancers, with on average 192 cases per million children per year children being diagnosed with a CNS tumour in Australia and New Zealand (Ballentine & NZCCR Working Group 2017, Youlden & Aitken 2019). Brain tumours in children have between a 46% and an 83% 5-year event-free survival rate. About 60% of the tumours are **infratentorial** (below the tentorium cerebelli), which means they occur in the posterior part of the brain, primarily in the cerebellum or brainstem. This anatomical distribution accounts for the frequency of symptoms resulting from increased intracranial pressure (ICP). The other tumours are **supratentorial** or lie within the midbrain structures. Fig 29.5 shows the major brain tumours of childhood.

Because brain tumours can arise from any cell within the cranium, it is possible to have tumours originating from the glial cells, nerve cells, neuroepithelium, cranial nerves, blood vessels, pineal gland and hypophysis. Within each of these structures, specific cells may be involved that provide a histological classification. For example, astrocytes, cells that form most of the supportive tissue for the neurons, may form astrocytomas, the most common glial tumour. Brain tumours may be benign or malignant, although what matters the most is location, given the vital functions the brain controls. A small percentage of childhood brain tumours is associated with genetic predisposition; examples include Li-Fraumeni syndrome and neurofibromatosis. Other known risk factors include cranial irradiation and immunosuppression (Parsons et al 2016). Genomic studies of brain tumours are an active area of research.

Clinical Manifestations

The signs and symptoms of brain tumours are directly related to their anatomical location, tumour size and to some extent the child's age. For instance, in infants whose sutures are still open, a bulging fontanel indicates hydrocephalus. Head circumference measurements allow for detection of increased head size. Even in older children, clinical manifestations may be non-specific. However, the most common symptoms of infratentorial brain tumours are headache, especially on awakening, and vomiting that is not related to feeding. Tumours in this area of the brain often obstruct the flow of cerebrospinal fluid, causing increased ICP and the symptoms mentioned earlier. In addition, patients may have symptoms related to the specific structure involved. Tumours of the cerebellum often cause nystagmus, ataxia, dysarthria and dysmetria. Supratentorial symptoms more commonly include seizures, personality or behavioural changes, visual disturbances and hemiparesis. Tumours involving the structures of the midbrain, including the hypothalamus and pituitary gland, may cause endocrinopathies such as diabetes insipidus, delayed or precocious puberty and growth failure. Table 29.4 shows the common presenting symptoms of brain tumours.

Diagnostic Evaluation

Diagnosis of a brain tumour is based on presenting clinical signs and diagnostic imaging. Because the signs and symptoms may be vague

PATHOPHYSIOLOGY REVIEW

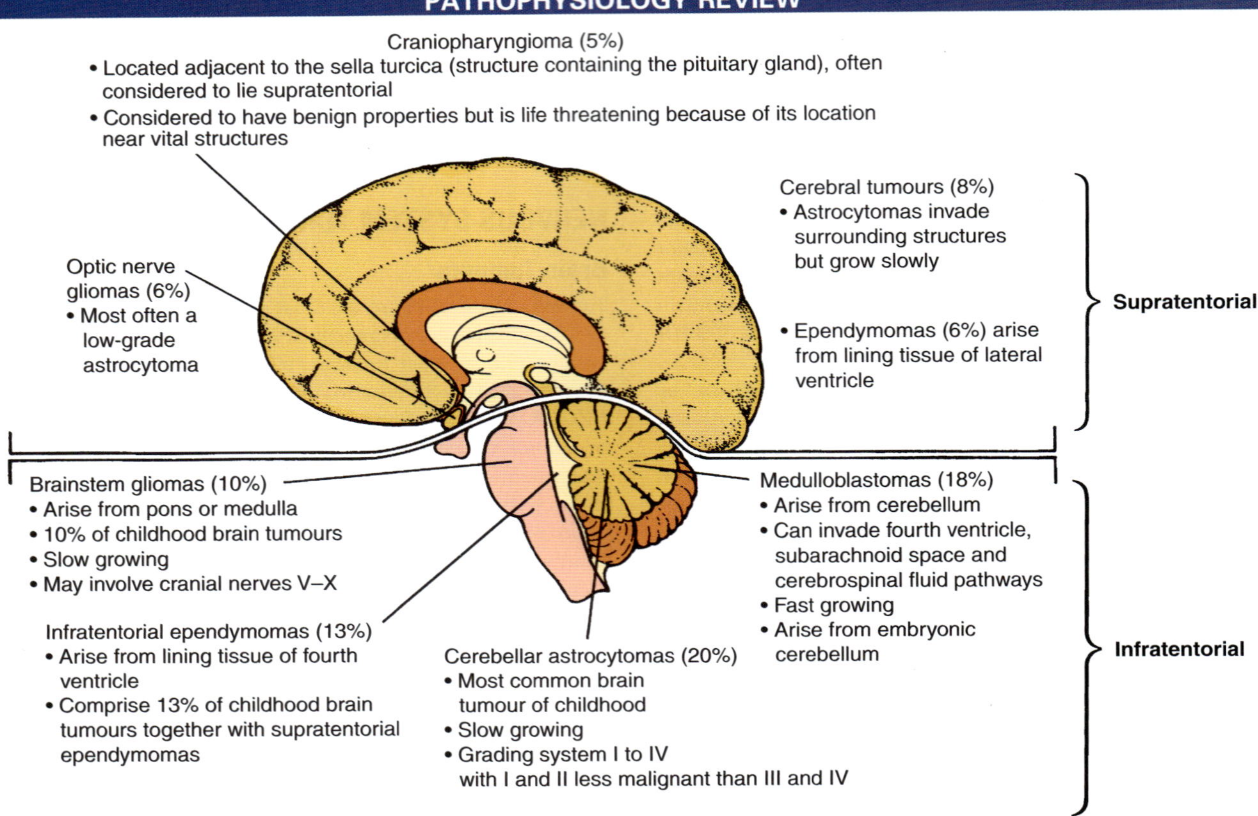

Fig 29.5 Location of brain tumours in children. (Source: McCance, K. L., & Huether, S. E. (2014). Pathophysiology: The biological basis for disease in adults and children (7th ed.). St Louis, MO: Elsevier.)

and easily overlooked, early diagnosis requires a high index of suspicion during history taking. A number of tests may be employed in the neurological evaluation (see Table 30.1), but the gold standard diagnostic procedure is MRI, which permits early diagnosis of brain tumours and assessment of tumour growth during or after treatment. Diffusion-weighted imaging, spectroscopy and perfusion imaging are other MRI tools used to investigate and diagnose tumour types (Poussaint et al 2015). The CT scan permits direct visualisation of the brain parenchyma, ventricles and surrounding subarachnoid space, and it is commonly used in urgent cases of suspected tumours when MRI is not available. Other tests may include an MRI of the spine and electroencephalography. In the presence of increased ICP, LP is avoided due to the danger of possible brainstem herniation after sudden release of pressure.

Definitive diagnosis is based on tissue specimens obtained during surgery. Occasionally, special techniques are required for determining the cell type. Because of the location of some brain tumours, such as brainstem tumours, a biopsy is not possible and the diagnosis is made by the findings of imaging alone.

Therapeutic Management

Treatment may involve the use of surgery, radiation therapy and chemotherapy. All three may or may not be used, depending on the type of tumour. The treatment of choice is total removal of the tumour without residual neurological damage. Patients with the most complete tumour removal have the greatest chance of survival. Several surgical advances have allowed the biopsy and removal of tumours in areas previously considered too dangerous for traditional operative techniques. Stereotactic surgery involves the use of CT and MRI in conjunction with other special computer techniques to reconstruct the tumour in three dimensions. With computer-assisted instruments, total resection of the tumour is sometimes possible. Stereotactic biopsy is performed with CT or MRI computer guidance for inserting the biopsy needle. This procedure has the benefit of a shorter hospital stay and a lower morbidity and mortality rate in comparison with an open craniotomy (Parsons et al 2016). Other procedures include the use of lasers to vaporise tumour tissue and brain mapping to determine the precise location of critical brain areas to avoid during surgery.

Radiation therapy is used to treat most tumours and to shrink the size of the tumour before attempting surgical removal. The use of chemotherapy has had an increasingly important role, either in combination with surgery and/or radiation, or alone. All three modes of therapy are associated with serious late effects. Surgery can cause injury to important areas of the brain, especially when the surgeon is attempting to remove invasive tumours. The long-term consequences of radiation therapy include tissue necrosis, subsequent malignancies, endocrine dysfunction and behavioural or intellectual deficits. For these reasons, the use of irradiation is deferred for as long as possible in young children. Chemotherapy may allow a delay or reduction in radiation therapy. Proton beam radiation therapy, available at some sites, is being studied to learn whether it offers greater efficacy and less long-term toxicity (Parsons et al 2016).

Nursing Care Management

Nursing care of the child with a brain tumour is similar regardless of the type of intracranial lesion. Because a brain tumour is potentially fatal, the reader is urged to incorporate the psychological interventions discussed in Chapter 19 with those elaborated on in this section.

TABLE 29.4 Clinical Manifestations and Assessment of Brain Tumours

Signs and Symptoms	Assessment
HEADACHE	
Recurrent and progressive In frontal or occipital areas Usually dull and throbbing Worse on arising, less during day Intensified by lowering head and straining, such as during bowel movement, coughing, sneezing	Record description of pain, location, severity and duration. Use pain rating scale to assess severity of pain. (See Chapter 5.) Note changes in relation to time of day and activity. Observe changes in behaviour in infants (e.g. persistent irritability, crying, head rolling).
VOMITING	
With or without nausea or feeding Progressively more projectile More severe in morning on arising Relieved by moving about and changing position	Record time, amount and relationship to feeding, nausea and activity.
NEUROMUSCULAR CHANGES	
Incoordination or clumsiness Loss of balance (e.g. use of wide-based stance, falling, tripping, banging into objects) Poor fine motor control Weakness Hyporeflexia or hyperreflexia Positive Babinski's sign Spasticity Paralysis	Test muscle strength, gait, coordination and reflexes. (See Chapter 4.)
BEHAVIOURAL CHANGES	
Irritability Decreased appetite Failure to thrive Fatigue (frequent naps) Lethargy Coma Bizarre behaviour (e.g. staring, automatic movements)	Observe behaviour regularly. Compare observations with parental reports of normal behavioural patterns. Monitor growth and food intake. Monitor activity and sleep.
CRANIAL NERVE NEUROPATHY	
Cranial nerve involvement varied according to tumour location Most common signs: • head tilt • visual defects (e.g. nystagmus, diplopia, strabismus, episodic 'greying out' of vision, visual field defect)	Assess cranial nerves, especially VII (facial), IX (glossopharyngeal), X (vagus), V (trigeminal, sensory roots) and VI (abducens). (See Chapter 4.) Assess visual acuity, binocularity and peripheral vision. (See Chapter 4.)
VITAL SIGN DISTURBANCES	
Decreased pulse and respiration Increased blood pressure Decreased pulse pressure Hypothermia or hyperthermia	Measure vital signs frequently. Monitor pulse and respirations for 1 full minute. Record pulse pressure (difference between systolic and diastolic blood pressure).
OTHER SIGNS	
Seizures Cranial enlargement* Tense, bulging fontanel at rest* Nuchal rigidity Papillo-oedema (oedema of optic nerve)	Record seizure activity. (See Chapter 30.) Measure head circumference daily (infant and young child). Perform funduscopic examination if skilled in procedure.

*Present only in infants and young children.

However, it is important to remember that many brain tumours are curable; some astrocytomas have a 5-year event-free survival rate of 83% (Ballentine & NZCCR Working Group 2017, Youlden & Aitken 2019). Despite the grave nature of some brain tumours, new and emerging therapies are bringing hope to the families of many paediatric brain tumour patients.

Assess for Signs and Symptoms. A child admitted to the hospital with neurological dysfunction is often suspected of having a brain tumour, even though the actual diagnosis is not yet confirmed. Establishing a baseline of data for comparing preoperative and postoperative changes is an essential step towards planning physical care and preventing complications. It also allows the nurse to assess the degree of physical incapacity and the family's emotional reaction to the diagnosis. For example, children with cerebellar astrocytoma may have displayed vague cerebellar symptoms for several years before a tumour is suspected. For these parents the revelation of a neoplasm may be as shocking as for those who witnessed a rapid deterioration in their child's abilities. Table 29.4 summarises common presenting signs and assessment procedures to document significant changes in the child's condition.

Prepare the Family for Diagnostic and Operative Procedures. The suspected diagnosis of a brain tumour is always a crisis. Although some tumours are removed with excellent results, the medical practitioner can rarely give definitive answers regarding prognosis until after surgery. Therefore parents, the child and other family members require much emotional support to face the diagnostic procedures and a craniotomy.

How the child is prepared for the diagnostic tests depends on the child's age and experience. Chapter 22 discusses preparing children for an MRI or a CT scan. Once surgery is scheduled, the child needs an explanation of what to expect. By the time most children are late preschoolers, they know that the head and brain are important parts of their body. It may be helpful to have children draw their concept of the brain to clarify misconceptions and base the explanation on their level of understanding. Although it may be tempting to justify the surgery by stating that removing the tumour will take away various symptoms, the nurse should refrain from emphasising this point too strenuously. Postsurgical headaches and cerebellar symptoms, such as ataxia, may be aggravated rather than improved. Surgery may not improve vision. With optic gliomas the child will be blind in one eye even if the tumour is fully resected. Finally, surgical removal of the mass may be impossible, and after surgery, functioning may temporarily deteriorate or result in permanent damage. Being honest before surgery most often makes honesty after the procedure easier because no false hopes were created.

It is best to deliver information in small amounts to let the child pursue additional answers. For example, some children ask about what happens when part of the tumour is left. An honest reply is that after surgery the medical practitioner will try to shrink the tumour with special x-rays and medicines. Delay a further explanation of irradiation or chemotherapy until a decision regarding these treatments is made.

The hair is usually shaved in the operating room just before surgery, or sometimes in the child's room, usually the night before surgery. When shaving is done with the child awake, the procedure is approached in a sensitive, positive way. If the child's hair is long, braid it so that the long swatch can be saved. Showing children how they look at different stages of the process helps them prepare for their changed appearance.

Once the hair is clipped short or shaved, give the child a cap or scarf to camouflage the baldness. Take every precaution to provide privacy during the procedure and to protect the child from teasing or ridicule by other children before surgery. Also emphasise that the hair will regrow shortly after surgery. Depending on the child's immediate adjustment to the hair loss, the nurse may introduce the idea of wearing a wig until the hair grows in, particularly if additional irradiation or chemotherapy is anticipated.

Also tell children about the size of the dressing. Usually the entire scalp is covered to maintain tight wound closure, even if a small incision is made. Infratentorial head dressings may be attached to the upper back and extend forwards to the neck to maintain slight extension and alignment as a precaution against wound rupture. Applying a similar dressing or 'special hat' to a doll is often a less traumatic way of demonstrating the physical appearance.

Children also need a brief explanation of how they will feel after surgery and where they will be. Ordinarily they will return to a special intensive care unit, which they may visit beforehand, depending on hospital policy. They should be aware that they may be sleepy for some time after surgery and that a headache is likely, which may last a few days.

Parents need similar explanations before surgery, especially in terms of special equipment used in the intensive care unit, dressings and their child's behaviour. For example, they should know that it is not unusual for the child to be lethargic for a few days after surgery. The nurse may wish to encourage less frequent visiting during this period so that parents can rest and be able to support their child when the child is awake.

The nurse should participate in preoperative conferences with the medical practitioner and parents. The nurse needs to know what information the parents have been given in order to provide further explanations or emotional support when necessary.

Prevent Postoperative Complications. After surgery the surgeon prescribes specific orders for taking vital signs, positioning, regulating fluids and administering medication. These vary somewhat, depending on the location of the craniotomy. The following are general principles of care for patients undergoing infratentorial or supratentorial surgery. Chapter 30 discusses additional aspects of care, such as care of the child with seizures and care of the unconscious child in terms of respiratory status and neurological assessment.

Assessment. Vital signs are taken as often as every 15 to 30 minutes until the patient is stable. Temperature measurement is particularly important because of hyperthermia resulting from surgical intervention in the hypothalamus or brainstem and from some types of general anaesthesia. To prepare for this reaction, a cooling blanket may be placed on the bed before the child returns to the unit, or it may be used when needed. Because the temperature control centres are affected and hypothermia can occur suddenly, the nurse monitors body temperature often when any cooling measures are employed.

The most likely types of infection are meningitis and respiratory tract infection. The probable cause of meningitis is wound contamination. The risk of respiratory tract infections is high because of the imposed immobility, danger of aspiration and possible respiratory depression from the brainstem. The usual precautions of deep breathing and turning as allowed are instituted. Regular respiratory assessments are performed to identify adventitious sounds or any areas of diminished or absent breath sounds. Blood pressure is also taken at frequent intervals. The deflated cuff is left on the arm between readings to allow for the least movement and disturbance of the child. Ocular signs are recorded at least every hour.

As soon as possible the nurse should begin testing reflexes, hand grip and functioning of the cranial nerves. Muscle strength is usually reduced after surgery because of general weakness but should improve daily. Ataxia may be significantly worse with cerebellar intervention, but it slowly improves. Oedema near the cranial nerves may depress important functions such as the gag, blink or swallowing reflex.

Neurological checks are an essential aspect of care and include pupillary reaction to light, level of consciousness, sleep patterns and response to stimuli. Although children may be comatose for a few days, once they regain consciousness there should be a steady increase in alertness. Regression to a lethargic, irritable state indicates increasing pressure, possibly caused by meningitis, haemorrhage or oedema.

Dressings are observed for evidence of drainage. If soiled, the dressing is not removed but reinforced with dry sterile gauze. The approximate amount of drainage is estimated and recorded.

Once the younger child is alert, the arms may need to be restrained to preserve the dressing. Even a child who has been cooperative before surgery must be closely supervised during the initial stages of regaining consciousness, when disorientation and restlessness are common. Elbow restraints are satisfactory to prevent the hands from reaching the head, although additional restraint may be necessary to preserve an infusion line and maintain a specific position.

Positioning. Correct positioning after surgery is critical to prevent pressure against the operative site, reduce ICP and avoid the danger of aspiration. If a large tumour was removed, the child is not placed on the operative side because the brain may suddenly shift to that cavity, causing trauma to the blood vessels, linings and the brain itself. The nurse confers with the surgeon to be certain of the correct position, including the degree of neck flexion. The first 24 to 48 hours after brain surgery are critical. If positioning is restricted, notice of this is posted above the head of the bed. When the child is turned, every precaution is used to prevent jarring or misalignment to prevent undue strain on the sutures. Two nurses, one supporting the head and the other the body, are needed. The use of a turning sheet may facilitate turning a heavy child.

The child with an infratentorial craniotomy is usually positioned flat and on either side. Pillows should be placed against the child's back, not head, to maintain the desired position. Ordinarily the head and neck are kept in midline with the body and slightly extended. After a supratentorial craniotomy the head is usually elevated above the heart to facilitate cerebrospinal fluid drainage and decrease excessive blood flow to the brain to prevent haemorrhage.

Fluid Regulation. With an infratentorial craniotomy the child is allowed nothing by mouth for at least 24 hours or longer if the gag and swallowing reflexes are depressed or the child is comatose. With a supratentorial procedure, feeding may be resumed soon after the child is alert, sometimes within 24 hours. Clear water is always started first because of the danger of aspiration. If the child vomits, stop oral liquids. Vomiting not only predisposes the child to aspiration but also increases ICP and the risk for incisional rupture.

IV fluids are continued until fluids are well tolerated by mouth. Because of cerebral oedema postoperatively and the danger of increased ICP, fluids are carefully monitored and usually infused less than the maintenance rate. If drugs, such as prophylactic antibiotics, are given intravenously the medication amount is calculated as part of the IV fluid. For example, if the child is to receive 20 mL/hr and the diluted drug is 5 mL, the IV solution is reduced to 15 mL for that hour.

A hypertonic solution such as mannitol may be necessary to remove excess fluid. These drugs cause rapid diuresis. After surgery the child may have a urine catheter in place. Urinary output is monitored after administration of these drugs to evaluate their effectiveness.

When able to take fluids, the child should be fed to conserve strength and minimise movement. If there is any sign of facial paralysis, the child is fed slowly to prevent choking or aspiration. Scrupulous mouth care is essential to prevent oral infection. Sometimes gavage feeding is necessary when body functions are too depressed to permit safe oral feedings or the child refuses to eat or drink. In the latter instance the nurse should employ every measure to encourage acceptance of fluids or solids. (See Chapter 22 for nursing interventions.)

Comfort Measures. Headache may be severe and is largely the result of cerebral oedema. Measures to relieve some of the discomfort include: providing a quiet, dimly lit environment; restricting visitors; preventing any sudden jarring movement, such as banging into the bed; and preventing an increase in ICP. The last is most effectively achieved by proper positioning and prevention of straining, such as during coughing, vomiting or defecating. The use of opioids, such as morphine, to relieve pain has been controversial because it is thought that they may mask signs of altered consciousness or depress respirations. However, opioids are considered safe because naloxone can be used to reverse opioid effects, such as sedation or respiratory depression. Paracetamol and codeine are also effective analgesics. Regardless of the drugs used, adequate dosage and regular administration are essential to provide optimum pain relief. (See Pain Assessment and Pain Management, Chapter 5.)

Monitor bowel movements to prevent constipation. Stool softeners may be given as soon as liquids are tolerated to facilitate easy passage of stool.

Brain oedema may severely depress the gag reflex, necessitating suctioning of oral secretions. Facial oedema may also be present, necessitating eye care if the lids remain partially open. Ice compresses applied to the eyes for short periods help relieve the oedema. A depressed blink reflex also predisposes the corneas to ulceration. Irrigating the eyes with saline drops and covering them with eye dressings are important steps in preventing this complication.

Support the Family. The family's informational and support needs are great when the diagnosis is a brain tumour, and are influenced by the extent of surgery, any neurological deficits, the prognosis and additional therapy. Because few definitive answers can be given before surgery, the surgeon's report is a significant finding that can vary from a completely benign, resected neoplasm to a highly malignant, invasive and only partially removed tumour. Although parents try to prepare themselves for a potentially fatal diagnosis, it is understandably a shock for them.

Ideally, a nurse who will be involved in the continuing care of this child should be with the family when the medical practitioner discusses the prognosis and plan of therapy. Although parents may hear only a fraction of what they are told, they can begin to put the future into perspective. Regardless of the future prospects, direct the parents' thinking towards helping the child recover and resume a normal life to his or her fullest potential. Providing the opportunity for the family to share their concerns and questions with other families who have a child with a brain tumour may help the family cope, and the nurse can direct them to resources.

It is also a time to encourage parents to verbalise their feelings about the diagnosis. Often they express guilt for attributing the insidious onset of symptoms, such as ataxia, visual difficulty or headache, to minor 'complaints' by the child. Parents may have punished their child for clumsiness, mistaking it for carelessness or for their declining performance in school. The nurse listens to such statements and emphasises the normality of the parents' reactions. Sometimes it may be helpful to start a discussion with a statement such as 'It is difficult to know when a child's complaints are significant because so often they are caused by minor ailments and you would never have imagined they were the result of a brain tumour'. The nurse avoids any comments that insinuate the parents should have sought medical advice sooner because such remarks only add to the parents' guilt feelings.

During this period the nurse should also discuss with parents what they plan to tell the child. If the child was prepared honestly, as described previously, the diagnosis can be expressed in a similar manner, such as 'The surgeon removed most of the tumour, and the rest will be treated with special drugs and x-ray treatments'. During recovery the child needs additional explanation about the treatment and the reason for residual neurological effects, such as ataxia or blindness. Hair loss is a normal concern for the child, and its regrowth will be delayed, depending on the length of therapy. This is an appropriate time to reintroduce the idea of a wig.

Promote Return to Optimum Functioning. The ultimate goal is a cured child who has optimum functioning. As soon as possible, the child should resume usual activities within tolerable limits, especially returning to school. Until the skull is completely healed, the child may need to wear a helmet when engaging in any active sport. This decision is made by the child's neurosurgeon. The school nurse and teacher should confer with the parents on activity restrictions, such as physical education, as well as the reactions of schoolmates to the child's appearance.

After discharge the family needs continuing medical and emotional support from health personnel. Children who are long-term survivors after treatment for a brain tumour require ongoing follow-up due to residual disabilities, such as short stature, cranial nerve palsies, sensory defects, motor abnormalities (especially ataxia), intellectual deficits, dysphagia, dysgraphia and behavioural problems (Parsons et al 2016).

The realm of all possible consequences after the diagnosis of a brain tumour is not discussed here. The reader is referred to other sections of the text that deal with possible outcomes, such as the paralysed, visually impaired or unconscious child or the child with a ventricular shunt, seizure disorder or meningitis. Numerous physical problems can occur with progression of the tumour that may necessitate additional procedures. For example, frequent vomiting, anorexia and nausea may require non-oral routes of feeding, such as gastrostomy or parenteral alimentation. Trials with chemotherapy may necessitate the use of central venous access devices. Whenever these procedures are instituted, the nurse may be responsible for teaching the family appropriate home care to allow the child the highest quality of life for the longest time. (See discussion of discharge planning and home care in Chapter 21.)

Neuroblastoma

Neuroblastoma is the most common extracranial childhood solid tumour and accounts for approximately 6% of new cancer diagnoses each year in Australia and New Zealand (Ballentine & NZCCR Working Group 2017, Youlden & Aitken 2019). It is a disease of infancy and early childhood, with the median age at diagnosis of about 19 months (Brodeur et al 2016). Neuroblastoma can occur in a hereditary form, and two genes that play a part in hereditary neuroblastoma have been identified, as have other genes that contribute to neuroblastoma predisposition (Brodeur et al 2016). Within the tumour cells, a hallmark is amplification of an oncogene, *MYCN*. Neuroblastomas originate from embryonic neural crest cells that normally give rise to the adrenal medulla and the sympathetic nervous system. Consequently, the majority of the tumours arise from the adrenal gland or from the retroperitoneal sympathetic chain.

Clinical Manifestations

The signs and symptoms of neuroblastoma depend on the location and extent of disease. The most common primary site is within the abdomen; other sites include the head and neck region, chest and pelvis. With abdominal tumours, the most common presenting sign is a firm, non-tender, irregular mass in the abdomen that crosses the midline (in contrast to Wilms tumour, which is usually confined to one side). Other signs related to abdominal location include pain or discomfort, vomiting, anorexia and respiratory compromise; compression of the kidney, ureter or bladder may cause urinary frequency or retention. Tumours in the thoracic or cervical region can involve dyspnoea, Horner syndrome (ptosis, miosis, anhidrosis), neck mass, stridor and dysphagia. Spinal cord and brain sites can present with neurological deficits, difficulty breathing, bladder and bowel dysfunction, paraparesis, paraplegia or seizures. Neuroblastoma that infiltrates the bone marrow can produce anaemia, thrombocytopenia and neutropenia. Tumours in the orbit/optic nerves can produce exophthalmos, periorbital ecchymosis and impaired vision. Tumours in bone can result in pain/limping. Metastases to the skin can appear as subcutaneous skin nodules, described as 'blueberry muffin lesions' due to their colour; this is usually only seen in infants.

Diagnostic Evaluation

Diagnostic evaluation is aimed at determining the primary site and extent of disease. Tumour imaging by CT or MRI is used to locate the primary tumour in neck, chest, abdomen and pelvis. Evaluation for metastases includes examination of the bone marrow with bilateral aspirates and biopsies and the bony skeleton with iodine-131 metaiodobenzylguanidine (I-MIBG) scanning.

Neuroblastomas, particularly those arising on the adrenal glands or from a sympathetic chain, excrete the catecholamines adrenaline and noradrenaline. Urinary excretion of catecholamine metabolites (vanillylmandelic acid [VMA] and homovanillic acid [HVA]) is measured before therapy; these markers can be used to monitor response to therapy and detection of relapse after therapy (National Institutes of Health 2017). Diagnosis is based on the presence of tumour cells in a biopsy of tumour tissue (biopsy also provides tissue for determining *MYCN* copy number [amplification] and other chromosomal/genetic tests) or the presence of tumour cells in bone marrow plus increased urinary catecholamine metabolites (National Institutes of Health 2017).

Staging and Prognosis

Neuroblastoma is a 'silent' tumour. In more than 70% of cases, diagnosis is made after metastasis occurs, with the first signs caused by involvement in a non-primary site, usually the lymph nodes, bone marrow, skeletal system or liver. The staging system in widespread use is the International Neuroblastoma Staging System, which is based on histology and extent of disease (Box 29.4). Newer staging systems that incorporate multiple other parameters are being used in clinical trials.

Factors that influence prognosis include age, site of primary tumour, tumour histology, regional lymph node involvement, response to treatment and biological features such as *MYCN* amplification (National Institutes of Health 2017). At 5 years after diagnosis, the survival rate for children with neuroblastoma is 76%; children with more advanced-stage disease will have a much lower chance of survival (Ballentine & NZCCR Working Group 2017, Youlden & Aitken 2019). Adrenal primary tumours are more often associated with unfavourable prognostic features, in contrast to thoracic tumours, which have fewer deaths and recurrences. Certain characteristics of neuroblastoma

BOX 29.4 Staging of Neuroblastoma by International Neuroblastoma Staging System

Stage 1—Localised tumour that is confined to the area of origin and complete gross excision; representative ipsilateral lymph nodes negative for tumour microscopically (nodes that are attached to and removed with the primary tumour may be positive)

Stage 2A—Unilateral tumour with incomplete gross resection; representative ipsilateral non-adherent lymph nodes and contralateral lymph nodes negative for tumour microscopically

Stage 2B—Unilateral tumour with or without complete gross excision, with ipsilateral non-adherent lymph nodes positive for tumour; enlarged contralateral lymph nodes must be negative microscopically

Stage 3—Tumour infiltrating across the midline, with or without regional lymph node involvement; or localised unilateral tumour with contralateral regional lymph node involvement; or midline tumour with bilateral lymph node involvement

Stage 4—Dissemination of tumour to distant lymph nodes, bone, bone marrow, liver, skin and/or other organs

Stage 4S—Localised primary tumour (as defined for stage 1, 2A or 2B) with dissemination limited to liver, skin or bone marrow but not to bone

tumour histology are prognostically favourable (e.g. cellular differentiation/maturation). Children who have metastatic disease in lymph nodes that cross the midline and are on the opposite side of the body from the primary tumour have a poorer prognosis. Poor response to treatment (e.g. persistence of neuroblastoma cells in bone marrow) predicts a poor prognosis. Neuroblastoma is one of the few tumours that demonstrate spontaneous regression (especially stage 4S), possibly as a result of maturation of the embryonic cell or development of an active immune system.

Therapeutic Management

Accurate clinical staging is important for establishing initial treatment. Therefore, the purpose of surgery is both to remove as much of the tumour as possible and to obtain biopsies. In stages 1 and 2, complete surgical removal of the tumour is the treatment of choice. If the tumours are large, partial resection is attempted, with a course of radiation therapy postoperatively to shrink the tumour in the hope of complete removal at a later date. Surgery is usually limited to biopsy in stages 3 and 4 because of extensive metastasis.

The precise role of radiation therapy is unclear. It does not appear to be of any benefit in children with stage 1 and 2 disease. It can be used with stage 3 disease, although it may not improve survival expectancy. Radiotherapy for paraspinal neuroblastoma is no longer recommended because the radiation therapy has long-term morbidity and chemotherapy is a safe and effective initial treatment modality (Brodeur et al 2016).

Chemotherapy is the mainstay of therapy for extensive local or disseminated disease. The drugs are administered in a variety of combinations according to specific protocols. In addition, the use of consolidative myeloablative therapy using autologous marrow or peripheral stem cells followed by 13-*cis*-retinoic acid has improved the outcome of patients with high-risk disease.

Nursing Care Management

Nursing care management is similar to that discussed under Nursing Care Management (p. 792), including psychological and physical preparation for diagnostic and operative procedures; prevention of postoperative complications for abdominal, thoracic or cranial surgery; and explanation of chemotherapy and radiation therapy and their side effects.

Because this tumour carries a poor prognosis for many children, the nurse evaluates and addresses the needs of the family in terms of coping with a life-threatening illness. (See Chapter 19.) Because of the high frequency of metastasis at the time of diagnosis, many parents suffer guilt for not having recognised signs earlier. Parents need skilled support in dealing with these feelings and expressing them to the appropriate members of the healthcare team.

BONE TUMOURS

General Considerations

Osteosarcoma and Ewing's sarcoma are the primary bone tumours that occur most often in young people. Although both are bone tumours, they are different in many ways. Osteosarcoma is the most common bone tumour in adolescents and young adults, with approximately 14 cases per million children being diagnosed each year in Australia and New Zealand (Ballentine & NZCCR Working Group 2017, Youlden & Aitken 2019). Ewing's sarcoma is slightly less common in New Zealand with four cases per million children being diagnosed each year, compared to 14 in Australia (Ballentine & NZCCR Working Group 2017, Youlden & Aitken 2019).

Clinical Manifestations

Most malignant bone tumours produce localised pain in the affected site, which may be severe or dull and may be attributed to trauma or the vague complaint of 'growing pains'. The pain is often relieved by a flexed position, which relaxes the muscles overlying the stretched periosteum. Frequently a bone tumour draws attention when the child limps, curtails physical activity or is unable to hold heavy objects. A palpable mass is also a common manifestation of bone tumours. Systemic symptoms (such as fever) and other clinical symptoms (such as spinal cord compression and respiratory distress) are more frequent in patients with Ewing's sarcoma.

Diagnostic Evaluation

Diagnosis begins with a thorough history and physical examination. A primary objective is to rule out causes such as trauma or infection. Careful questioning regarding pain is essential in attempting to determine the duration and rate of tumour growth. Physical assessment focuses on functional status of the affected area; signs of inflammation; size of the mass; and any systemic indication of generalised malignancy, such as anaemia, weight loss and frequent infection.

Definitive diagnosis is based on imaging studies, such as plain films and CT or MRI scan of the primary site, CT scan of the chest and radioisotope bone scans to evaluate metastasis and bone marrow examination in patients with Ewing's sarcoma. A needle or surgical biopsy is necessary to establish the diagnosis. Ewing's sarcoma most commonly involves the pelvis, long bones of the lower extremities and chest wall; imaging reveals involvement of the diaphysis with detachment of the periosteum from the bone (Codman triangle). In osteosarcoma, lesions are most commonly located in the metaphyseal region of the bone, often involving the long bones. Radial ossification in the soft tissue gives the tumour a 'sunburst' appearance on plain radiograph.

Prognosis

A better understanding of the biology of neoplastic growth has resulted in more aggressive treatment and improved prognosis. The natural history of osteosarcoma and Ewing's sarcoma suggests that multiple submicroscopic foci of metastatic disease are present at the time of diagnosis despite clinical evidence indicating only localised involvement. The lungs, distant bones and bone marrow are the most common sites for metastatic bone tumour disease. With current therapies that include surgery and chemotherapy for osteosarcoma and surgery, radiation therapy and chemotherapy for Ewing's sarcoma, the majority of patients with localised disease can be cured.

Osteosarcoma

Osteosarcoma occurs most often in adolescents and young adults, coinciding with the period of rapid bone growth (Gorlick et al 2016). It presumably arises from bone-forming mesenchyme, which gives rise to malignant osteoid tissue. Most primary tumour sites are in the diametaphyseal region (wider part of the shaft, adjacent to the epiphyseal growth plate) of long bones, especially in the lower extremities. More than half occur in the femur, particularly the distal portion, with the rest involving the humerus, tibia, pelvis, jaw and phalanges. Risk factors include ionising radiation exposure, genetic predisposition syndromes and a history of retinoblastoma, particularly the hereditary form (Gorlick et al 2016).

Therapeutic Management

Optimum treatment of osteosarcoma includes surgery and chemotherapy. The surgical approach consists of surgical biopsy followed by either limb salvage or amputation. To ensure local control, all gross and microscopic tumours must be resected. A limb salvage procedure has become the standard approach to surgical intervention and involves resection of the primary tumour with prosthetic replacement of the involved bone (Gorlick et al 2016). For example, with osteosarcoma of the distal femur, a total femur and joint replacement is performed. Frequently children undergoing a limb salvage procedure receive preoperative chemotherapy in an attempt to decrease the tumour size and make surgery more manageable (Gorlick et al 2016).

Chemotherapy plays a vital role in treatment of osteosarcoma. Cytotoxic drugs, such as high-dose methotrexate with folinic acid rescue, doxorubicin, cisplatin, ifosfamide and etoposide, may be administered singly or in combination and may be employed both before and after surgical resection of the tumour. When pulmonary metastases are found, thoracotomy and chemotherapy have resulted in prolonged survival and potential cure. These combined-modality approaches have significantly improved the prognosis in osteosarcoma to approximately 70% for patients with non-metastatic disease (Ballentine & NZCCR Working Group 2017, Youlden & Aitken 2019).

Nursing Care Management

Nursing care depends on the type of surgical approach. The family may or may not have more difficulty adjusting to an amputation than a limb salvage procedure. In either instance, preparation of the child and family is critical. Straightforward honesty is essential in gaining the child's cooperation and trust. The responsibility of telling the child is generally left to the medical practitioner, depending on the family's preference. If at all possible, the nurse should be present at the discussion or be aware of exactly what is said in order to follow-up with the child and family afterwards. The child should be told well before surgery to allow time to think about the diagnosis and consequent treatment and to ask questions.

Sometimes children have many questions about the prosthesis, limitations on physical ability and prognosis in terms of cure. At other times they react with silence or with a calm manner that belies their concern and fear. Either response must be accepted because it is part of grieving the loss of an aspect of their physical appearance and function. For those who desire information, it may be helpful to introduce them to another amputee or survivor with a limb salvage procedure before surgery or to show them pictures of the prosthesis. However, the nurse must be careful not to overwhelm children with information. A sound approach is to answer questions without offering additional information. For those who do not pursue additional information, the nurse expresses a willingness to talk.

The child is also informed of the need for chemotherapy and its side effects before surgery. Exercise caution about offering too much information at one time. When discussing hair loss, emphasise coping strategies, such as wearing a wig. Because bone tumours occur most often in adolescents and young adults, when appearance and peer acceptance are key developmental issues, it is not unusual for them to become angry over all the radical body alterations.

The child will require stump care, which is the same as for any amputee. A permanent prosthesis is typically fitted within 6 to 8 weeks. During hospitalisation the child begins physical therapy to become proficient in the use and care of the device.

Phantom limb pain may develop in 60% to 80% of patients after amputation. The exact pathophysiology is still unclear, but may include a combination of physical and psychological factors that need to be further clarified by research (Luo & Anderson 2016). This symptom is characterised by sensations such as tingling, itching and, more frequently, pain felt in the amputated limb. The child and family need to know that the sensations are real, not imagined. Although various pharmacological and non-pharmacological techniques have been used for phantom limb pain, none provide complete relief or are curative for phantom limb pain (Luo & Anderson 2016). A study of paediatric patients with cancer-related amputation found that 76% had phantom limb pain during the first year after amputation, but only 10% still had phantom limb pain more than 1 year after amputation (Burgoyne et al 2012). The nurse works with the institution's pain team to address the problem of phantom limb pain.

Discharge planning begins early in the postoperative period. Once the child has begun physical therapy, the nurse consults with the therapist and oncology team to evaluate the child's physical and emotional readiness to re-enter school. It is an opportune time to involve a community nurse in the child's home care. Every effort is made to promote normality and gradual resumption of realistic pre-amputation activities. Role playing in anticipation of such experiences is beneficial in preparing the child for the inevitable confrontation by others. Environmental barriers, such as stairs, are assessed in terms of accessibility in the school and home, especially because the child may need to use crutches or a wheelchair before complete healing and prosthetic competency are achieved.

The nurse encourages the child to select clothing that best camouflages the prosthesis, such as pants or long-sleeved shirts, if that is what they desire. Well-fitted prostheses are so natural looking that girls can usually wear sheer stockings without revealing the device. Emphasising feminine or masculine apparel helps the child regain a feeling of self-identity. Even during the postoperative period, encouraging the child to wear jeans and a T-shirt may distract attention from the deformity and focus it on familiar aspects of appearance.

The family and child need much support in adjusting not only to a life-threatening diagnosis but also to alteration in body form and function. Because loss of a limb entails a grieving process, those caring for the child need to recognise that the reactions of anger and depression are normal and necessary. Often parents view the anger as a direct affront to them for allowing the amputation to occur, or they see the depression as rejection. These are not personal attacks but the child's attempts to cope with a loss. Psychosocial support programs (or members of the healthcare team such as psychologists, social workers and child life specialists) at the institution may be particularly helpful in supporting the patient and family's strengths in coping.

Ewing's Sarcoma (Primitive Neuroectodermal Tumour of the Bone)

Ewing sarcomas, or the Ewing's sarcoma family of tumours, which includes primitive neuroectodermal tumour of the bone, are the second most common malignant bone tumour (after osteosarcoma) in childhood (Hawkins et al 2016). Ewing's sarcoma arises in the marrow spaces of the bone rather than from osseous tissue. The tumour originates in the shaft of long and trunk bones, most often affecting the pelvis, femur, tibia, fibula, humerus, ulna, vertebra, scapula, ribs and skull (Hawkins et al 2016).

Therapeutic Management

Limb salvage procedures may be feasible in extremity lesions, although amputation may be considered if the results of radiation therapy would render the extremity useless or deformed (e.g. from growth retardation in young children). The treatment of choice for the majority of localised lesions involves field radiation therapy and chemotherapy. The standard chemotherapy protocol includes vincristine, doxorubicin and cyclophosphamide alternating with ifosfamide, and etoposide. Approximately two-thirds of patients with localised Ewing's sarcoma can expect to be cured (Hawkins et al 2016). Improving survival, especially for patients with metastatic or recurrent disease, is a focus of ongoing research.

Nursing Care Management

Ewing's sarcoma differs from osteosarcoma because preservation of the affected limb is more likely. Families may accept the diagnosis with some relief in knowing that this type of bone cancer does not necessitate amputation. They need preparation for the various diagnostic tests, including bone marrow aspiration and surgical biopsy, and adequate explanation of the treatment regimen.

High-dose radiation therapy often causes a skin reaction of dry or moist desquamation followed by hyperpigmentation. The child should wear loose-fitting clothes over the irradiated area to minimise additional skin irritation. Because of increased sensitivity, the area should be protected from sunlight and sudden changes in temperature, such as from heating pads or ice packs. Encourage the child to use the extremity as tolerated. Occasionally the physiotherapist may plan an active exercise program to preserve maximum function.

The child needs the same considerations for adjusting to the effects of chemotherapy as any other patient with cancer. The drug regimen usually results in hair loss, severe nausea and vomiting, peripheral neuropathy and possible cardiotoxicity. Make every effort to outline a treatment plan that allows the child maximum resumption of a normal lifestyle and activities.

OTHER SOLID TUMOURS

In addition to the cancers already discussed, several other types of solid tumours may occur in children. Wilms tumour, rhabdomyosarcoma and retinoblastoma are unique in that they tend to be diagnosed early, typically before 5 years of age. Wilms tumour and retinoblastoma are also unusual in that they are among the few types of cancer that may occur in both hereditary and non-hereditary forms.

Wilms Tumour

Wilms tumour (nephroblastoma) is the most common kidney tumour of childhood with approximately 36 cases per million children diagnosed each year in New Zealand and Australia (Ballentine & NZCCR Working Group 2017, Youlden & Aitken 2019). The average age at diagnosis is 44 months in children with single kidney disease, but younger (31 months) in those with bilateral disease. Approximately 10% of children with Wilms tumour have congenital anomalies, some of which are associated with syndromes such as WAGR (Wilms tumour, aniridia, genitourinary anomalies and cognitive impairment) and Beckwith-Wiedemann syndrome (hemihypertrophy, macroglossia, omphalocele and visceromegaly). A number of genes and chromosomal alterations have been implicated in the biology of Wilms tumour. The incidence of bilateral involvement is higher in children with genetic predisposition syndromes.

Clinical Manifestations

The most common presenting sign is swelling or mass within the abdomen; pain is present in about 40% of patients (Fernandez et al 2016). The mass is characteristically firm, non-tender, confined to one side and deep within the flank. If it is on the right side, it may be difficult to distinguish from the liver, although, unlike that organ, it does not move with respiration. The mass usually is discovered during routine bathing or dressing of the child.

Other clinical manifestations may result from compression by the tumour mass, metabolic alterations secondary to the tumour or metastases. Haematuria occurs in less than 25% of children with Wilms tumour. Anaemia, usually secondary to haemorrhage within the tumour, results in pallor, anorexia and lethargy. Hypertension, probably caused by secretion of excess amounts of renin by the tumour, occurs occasionally. Other effects of malignancy include weight loss and fever. If pulmonary metastasis has occurred, symptoms of lung involvement, such as dyspnoea, cough, shortness of breath and pain in the chest, may be evident.

Diagnostic Evaluation

In a child suspected of having Wilms tumour, special emphasis is placed on the history and physical examination for the presence of congenital anomalies (e.g. aniridia, developmental delay, hypospadias, cryptorchidism); a family history of cancer; and signs of malignancy, such as weight loss, enlarged liver and spleen, indications of anaemia and lymphadenopathy. The diagnostic workup includes: abdominal imaging studies (abdominal x-ray, ultrasound, CT or MRI of the abdomen); CT of the chest to look for lung metastases; and Doppler ultrasound of the inferior vena cava. Laboratory studies should include a FBC (polycythaemia is sometimes present if the tumour secretes excess erythropoietin), biochemical studies and urinalysis. Studies to assess intravascular extension of the tumour and tumour rupture also are essential.

Staging and Prognosis

There are two main staging systems for Wilms tumour, one used by the Children's Oncology Group and the other by the European group SIOP. In the Children's Oncology Group system, disease staging (ranging from stage I to V) is determined by results of imaging studies and pathological findings at nephrectomy (Box 29.5), with stage I being localised to one kidney and stage V indicating bilateral involvement by tumour. The histology of the tumour cells is also classified into two groups: favourable histology (FH) and anaplastic (unfavourable) histology; the anaplastic group is subdivided into diffuse and focal (Fernandez et al 2016). The best outcomes are associated with FH; diffuse anaplastic tumours have the worst outcomes.

Five-year survival rates for Wilms tumour with FH are above 90% (Ballentine & NZCCR Working Group 2017, Youlden & Aitken 2019). In addition to histology, prognosis depends on stage of disease at diagnosis, molecular features of the tumour and age, with older age conferring a worse prognosis.

Therapeutic Management

The standard of care is combined treatment with surgery and chemotherapy; radiation therapy may be used, based on clinical stage and tumour histology. In unilateral disease nephrectomy and lymph node sampling are performed; a transabdominal or thoracoabdominal incision is used for greatest visibility of the kidney. Great care is taken to keep the encapsulated tumour intact because intraoperative spill can seed cancer cells throughout the abdomen, lymph channel and bloodstream. If imaging studies do not indicate bilateral kidney involvement, exploration of the contralateral kidney is not necessary during the operative procedure (National Institutes of Health 2017).

BOX 29.5 Children's Oncology Group Staging of Wilms Tumour

Stage I—Tumour is limited to one kidney and completely resected without rupture or previous biopsy. All sampled lymph nodes negative for tumour.
Stage II—Tumour extends beyond kidney but is completely resected; lymph nodes do not contain tumour cells.
Stage III—There is postoperative residual tumour confined to abdomen. Lymph nodes in abdomen or pelvis contain tumour cells.
Stage IV—Haematogenous metastases with disease spread to the lung, liver, bone, brain or distant lymph nodes.
Stage V—Bilateral renal involvement is present at diagnosis.

The child may be treated with chemotherapy preoperatively under some circumstances (e.g. tumour is bilateral or child has a single kidney) after biopsy confirmation of the diagnosis. Preoperative chemotherapy reduces the size and vascular supply of the tumour, thereby making tumour removal easier (National Institutes of Health 2017). Standard chemotherapy regimens for Wilms tumour include some or all of the following: vincristine, dactinomycin, doxorubicin, cyclophosphamide and etoposide. Postoperative radiation therapy is indicated for children with tumours classified as stage II focal or diffuse anaplastic histology, stage III and IV (National Institutes of Health 2017). Options for stage V tumours may include preoperative chemotherapy and surgery, and/or renal transplantation.

Nursing Care Management

The nursing care of the child with Wilms tumour is similar to that of other cancers treated with surgery and chemotherapy, and possibly radiation therapy. However, some significant differences are discussed for each phase of nursing intervention.

Preoperative Care. As with many other cancers, the diagnosis of Wilms tumour is a shock. Frequently the child has no physical indication of the seriousness of the disorder other than a palpable abdominal mass. Because the parents usually discover the mass, the nurse needs to take into account their feelings regarding the diagnosis. Whereas some parents are grateful for detecting the tumour so it can be treated, others feel guilty for not finding it sooner or feel angry towards the healthcare professional, believing it was missed on earlier examinations.

The preoperative period is one of swift diagnostic workup. Typically, surgery is scheduled within 24 to 48 hours of admission. The nurse is faced with the challenge of preparing the child and parents for all laboratory and operative procedures. Explanations should be simple and repeated, with attention to what the child will experience. In addition to usual preoperative observations, monitor blood pressure because hypertension from excess renin production is a possibility.

There are several special preoperative concerns, the most important of which is not to palpate the tumour unless absolutely necessary because manipulation of the mass may cause dissemination of cancer cells to adjacent and distant sites.

Because chemotherapy and radiation therapy (if used) are usually begun immediately after surgery, parents need an explanation of what to expect, such as major benefits and side effects, although the timing of the information should be considered to avoid overwhelming the family. Ideally the nurse should be present during conferences between the medical practitioner and parents to answer questions as they arise afterwards.

Postoperative Care. Despite the extensive surgical intervention necessary in many children with Wilms tumour, the recovery period is usually rapid. The major nursing responsibilities are those after any abdominal surgery. Because of the risk for intestinal obstruction from vincristine-induced ileus, radiation-induced oedema and post-surgical adhesion formation, the nurse monitors gastrointestinal activity, such as bowel movements, bowel sounds, distension and vomiting. Other considerations are frequent evaluation of blood pressure and observation for signs of infection, especially during chemotherapy.

Support the Family. The postoperative period is frequently difficult for parents. The shock of seeing their child immediately after surgery may be the first realisation of the seriousness of the diagnosis. From surgery, the stage and pathology of the tumour are determined. The medical practitioner discusses this information with the parents. The nurse's presence during this conversation is important to provide additional support and assess the parents' understanding of this information.

Older children need an opportunity to deal with their feelings concerning the many procedures to which they have been subjected in rapid succession. Therapeutic play can be beneficial in helping children of any age understand what they have undergone and express their feelings.

Rhabdomyosarcoma

Sarcomas, including rhabdomyosarcoma (*rhabdo* means striated), are tumours arising from mesenchymal cells, which normally develop into muscle and other tissues (Wexler et al 2016). Approximately 23 cases per million children are diagnosed each year in Australia and New Zealand (Ballentine & NZCCR Working Group 2017, Youlden & Aitken 2019).

Rhabdomyosarcomas originate from undifferentiated mesenchymal cells in muscles, tendons, bursae and fascia, or in fibrous, connective, lymphatic or vascular tissue. The most common primary sites are the head and neck (especially the orbit), the genitourinary tract and the extremities, but these tumours can occur in other sites as well. Rhabdomyosarcoma is classified into histological subtypes (Box 29.6): embryonal, alveolar and pleomorphic. More than half are embryonal. The embryonal and alveolar subtypes are most common in children and have distinct genetic alterations in the tumour cells. At the molecular level, these genetic alterations appear to involve both muscle differentiation pathways and cell proliferation pathways (Wexler et al 2016). Rhabdomyosarcoma is associated with several genetic conditions (e.g. Li-Fraumeni cancer susceptibility syndrome, neurofibromatosis type 1).

Clinical Manifestations

The initial signs and symptoms are related to the site of the tumour and compression of adjacent organs (Table 29.5). Some tumour locations, such as the orbit, manifest early in the course of the illness. Other tumours, such as those of the retroperitoneal area, only produce symptoms when they are relatively big and cause organ compression. Unfortunately, many of the signs and symptoms attributable to rhabdomyosarcoma are vague and frequently suggest a common childhood illness, such as 'earache' or 'runny nose'. Often it is not possible to identify the site of the primary tumour.

Diagnostic Evaluation

Diagnosis begins with a careful history and physical examination, imaging studies and baseline laboratory studies. An extensive evaluation is then performed to determine the extent of disease. Metastatic evaluation includes chest x-ray and CT scan, CT/MRI for abdominal/pelvic tumours, MRI of the skull and brain for parameningeal tumours, imaging of regional lymph nodes, bilateral bone marrow aspirates and biopsies, and bone scan for selected patients. An excisional biopsy or surgical resection of the tumour, when possible, is done to confirm the diagnosis.

BOX 29.6 Subtypes of Rhabdomyosarcoma

Embryonal—Most common type; most frequently found in the head, neck, abdomen and genitourinary tract

Alveolar—Second most common type; most often seen in deep tissues of the extremities and trunk

Pleomorphic—Rare in children (adult form); most often occurs in soft parts of extremities and trunk

TABLE 29.5 Clinical Manifestations of Rhabdomyosarcoma According to Tumour Site

Location	Signs and Symptoms
Orbit	Rapidly developing unilateral proptosis Ecchymosis of conjunctiva Loss of extraocular movements (strabismus)
Nasopharynx	Stuffy nose (earliest sign) Nasal obstruction—dysphagia, nasal voice (obstruction of posterior nasal conches), serous otitis media (obstruction of eustachian tube) Pain (sore throat and ear) Epistaxis Palpable neck nodes Visible mass in oropharynx (late sign)
Paranasal sinuses	Nasal obstruction Local pain Discharge Sinusitis Swelling
Middle ear	Signs of chronic serous otitis media Pain Sanguinopurulent drainage Facial nerve palsy
Retroperitoneal area (usually a 'silent' tumour)	Abdominal mass Pain Signs of intestinal or genitourinary obstruction
Perineum	Visible superficial mass Bowel or bladder dysfunction (from tumour compression)

Staging and Prognosis

Careful staging is extremely important for planning treatment and determining the prognosis. Two staging systems are used in combination: a surgicopathological staging system (Box 29.7) and a modified tumour, node, metastasis (TNM) pretreatment staging system. A stage is assigned, based on primary site, tumour size and whether or not there is regional lymph node involvement or distant metastasis. A group is assigned based on the status of the surgical resection/biopsy, pathological assessment of the tumour margin and lymph node involvement before therapy. Then a risk group is assigned, based on stage, group and histology (National Institutes of Health 2017). Risk refers to the risk of disease recurrence.

Prognosis is related to age, with children ages 1 to 9 years having the best prognosis; primary tumour site, size and resectability; whether or not there is lymph node involvement or metastasis at diagnosis; and histological subtype. The alveolar histological subtype is associated with a worse outcome. Most rhabdomyosarcomas are curable with the use of contemporary multimodal therapy. More than 70% of patients with localised disease are expected to survive (Ballentine & NZCCR Working Group 2017, Youlden & Aitken 2019). If relapse occurs, the prognosis for long-term survival is poor.

BOX 29.7 Surgical-Pathological Staging of Rhabdomyosarcoma

Group I—Localised disease; tumour completely resected and regional nodes not involved
Group II—Localised disease; tumour completely removed; microscopic residual that may have spread into nearby lymph nodes
Group III—Incomplete resection with gross residual disease
Group IV—Metastatic disease present at diagnosis

Therapeutic Management

Rhabdomyosarcoma is treated with multimodality therapy that includes chemotherapy plus surgery or radiation therapy, or both modalities. The intensity and duration of chemotherapy are based on risk group. Some or all of the following chemotherapeutic drugs are used: vincristine, dactinomycin, cyclophosphamide and ifosfamide. Complete resection of the primary tumour before chemotherapy is advocated whenever possible, if it will not result in disfigurement, functional compromise or organ dysfunction. Otherwise, only an initial biopsy is performed. Radiation therapy is also based on risk group and tailored to the primary site and sites of metastatic disease.

Nursing Care Management

The nursing responsibilities in caring for a child with rhabdomyosarcoma are similar to those for other types of cancer, especially the other solid tumours for which surgery is employed. Specific objectives include: careful assessment for signs of tumour, especially during well-child examinations; preparation of the child and family for the multiple diagnostic tests; and supportive care during each stage of multimodal therapy. The reader is urged to review the Nursing Care Management section for cancer and Chapter 19 for emotional support of the family in the event of a poor prognosis.

Retinoblastoma

Retinoblastoma, so named because it arises from the retina, is the most common intraocular malignancy of childhood, with 20 cases per million children per year diagnosed (Ballentine & NZCCR Working Group 2017, Youlden & Aitken 2019). Retinoblastoma can be present at birth, can have single or multiple foci in one or both eyes and occurs in a heritable form. Of all cases of retinoblastoma, 60% are unilateral and non-hereditary (also called sporadic), 25% are bilateral and hereditary and 15% are unilateral and hereditary (Hurwitz et al 2016). Retinoblastoma occurs predominantly in very young children; most cases are diagnosed before 3 to 4 years of age. Children with hereditary retinoblastoma tend to be diagnosed at a younger age. In the hereditary form of retinoblastoma, germ-line mutation of the *RB1* gene is present. The mutation may have been inherited, occurred in a germ cell before conception or occurred in utero during embryogenesis (Hurwitz et al 2016). The two-hit model (discussed earlier in this chapter) was developed to explain hereditary and sporadic retinoblastoma. According to the model, as few as two events can lead to tumour formation; in the hereditary form, the 'first hit' occurs in the germ-line whereas both hits occur somatically in the sporadic form.

Clinical Manifestations

Retinoblastoma has few grossly obvious signs. Typically parents or relatives are the ones who first observe a whitish 'glow' in the pupil, known as the **cat's eye reflex**, or **leucocoria** (Fig 29.6), which prompts ophthalmoscopic examination. The reflex represents visualisation of the tumour as light momentarily falls on the mass. When a tumour arises in the macular region (area directly at the back of the retina when the eye is focused straight ahead), a white reflex may be visible when the tumour is small. It is best observed when a bright light is shining towards the child as the child looks forwards, which is why it may be discovered when a photograph with flash is taken.

When the tumour arises in the periphery of the retina, it must grow to a considerable size before light can strike it sufficiently to produce the cat's eye reflex. In this situation it is visible only when the child

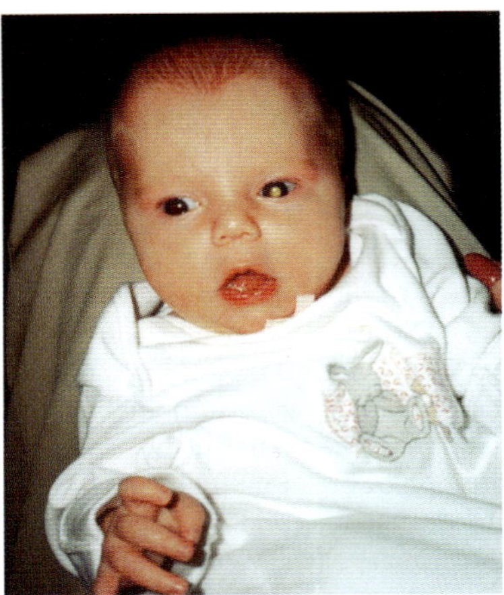

Fig 29.6 Cat's eye reflex. Whitish appearance of lens is produced as light falls on tumour mass in left eye.

BOX 29.8 International Classification for Intraocular Retinoblastoma

Group A—Small (3 mm or less) intraretinal tumours away from the optic disc and foveola
Group B—All remaining tumours that are larger than 3 mm and/or close to the optic disc or foveola but remain confined to the retina
Group C—Discrete local disease with minimal disease under the retina (subretinal seeding) or in the gelatinous material of the eye (vitreous seeding)
Group D—Large or poorly defined tumours with significant vitreous or subretinal seeding; retina may have become detached from the back of the eye
Group E—Tumour is very large, extending near the front of the eye, is bleeding or causing glaucoma, or has other features that indicate it is not possible to save the eye

looks sideways or if the observer stands at an oblique angle to the child's face as the child looks straight ahead. The fleeting nature of the reflex often results in a delayed diagnosis because healthcare professionals fail to appreciate the ominous significance of the parents' observation.

The next most common sign is strabismus resulting from poor fixation of the visually impaired eye, particularly if the tumour develops in the macula, the area of sharpest visual acuity. Blindness is usually a late sign, but it may not be obvious unless the parent consciously observes for behaviours indicating loss of sight, such as bumping into objects, slowed motor development or turning of the head to see objects lateral to the affected eye. Other late signs and symptoms include pain, orbital cellulitis and glaucoma.

Diagnostic Evaluation

A detailed family history and recording of eye signs and symptoms are essential. Children suspected of having retinoblastoma are referred to an ophthalmologist; the diagnosis usually is based on indirect ophthalmoscopy (under anaesthesia) and ultrasound, CT and MRI scans. Blood and tumour samples can be tested for *RB1* gene mutations.

Metastatic disease at the time of retinoblastoma diagnosis is rare. For patients with suspected metastatic disease, bone marrow aspirates and biopsies, bone scan and LP may be performed.

Staging and Prognosis

Staging of retinoblastomas is done under indirect ophthalmoscopy before surgery to accurately determine the tumour size (measured in disc diameters [DD]) and location (according to an imaginary line called the equator drawn on the midplane of the eye) (Hurwitz et al 2016).

Various classification systems have been used to stage or group retinoblastomas. The Reese-Ellsworth system classifies tumours according to five groups and is used to compare therapeutic results in patients treated with methods other than enucleation (i.e. radiation therapy). A revised classification system, the International Classification of Retinoblastoma, is based on the extent and location of the intraocular tumour; it better predicts globe salvage using contemporary treatments (Box 29.8). The overall 10-year survival rate is nearly 90% for unilateral and bilateral tumours (Hurwitz et al 2016). Retinoblastoma, like neuroblastoma, may spontaneously regress.

A major concern for long-term survivors is the development of SMNs. Children with bilateral disease (hereditary form) are more likely to develop subsequent cancers than are children with unilateral disease, and radiation therapy increases their risk.

Therapeutic Management

Treatment of retinoblastoma is complex. Enucleation may be used to treat advanced disease with optic nerve invasion in which vision cannot be salvaged. Radiation therapy can be used when there is vitreous seeding. Chemotherapy has been used to decrease the tumour size to allow treatment with local therapies such as plaque brachytherapy (surgical implantation of an iodine-125 applicator on the sclera until the maximum radiation dose has been delivered to the tumour), photocoagulation (use of a laser beam to destroy retinal blood vessels that supply nutrition to the tumour) and cryotherapy (freezing of the tumour, which destroys the microcirculation to the tumour and the cells themselves through microcrystal formation). Chemotherapy, along with radiation or high-dose chemotherapy with autologous stem cell rescue, is used to treat metastatic disease (Hurwitz et al 2016).

Nursing Care Management

Prepare the Family for Diagnostic and Therapeutic Procedures and Home Care. Because the tumour is usually diagnosed in infants or very young children, most of the preparation for diagnostic tests and treatment involves parents. Once the disease is staged, the medical practitioner confers with the parents regarding treatment. In most cases, enucleation can be avoided. In the event that enucleation is performed, the procedure and the benefits of a prosthesis are explained. Showing parents pictures of another child with an artificial eye may help with adjustment to the procedure (Fig 29.7). Although the loss of vision is distressing, most parents realise that there is no alternative. Emphasising that the unaffected eye retains normal vision and that the affected eye is probably already blind may be helpful in promoting acceptance of the imposed impairment.

After surgery the parents need to be prepared for the child's facial appearance. An eye patch is in place, and the child's face may be oedematous and ecchymotic. Parents often fear seeing the surgical site because they imagine a cavity in the skull. On the contrary, the lids are usually closed, and the area does not appear sunken because a surgically implanted sphere maintains the shape of the eyeball. The implant is covered with conjunctiva, and when the lids are open, the exposed area resembles the mucosal lining of the mouth. Once the child is fitted for a prosthesis, usually within 3 weeks, the facial appearance returns to normal.

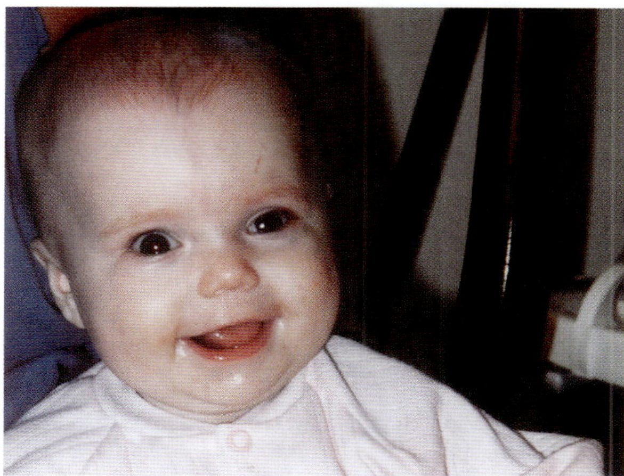

Fig 29.7 Infant with left prosthetic eye.

After an uneventful recovery from enucleation, plans can be made for discharge from the hospital, usually within 3 to 4 days postoperatively. Parents need instruction regarding care of the surgical site and preparation for any additional therapy. They should be given the opportunity to see the socket as soon after surgery as possible. A good time to do this without unduly pressuring them is during dressing changes. They should then be encouraged to participate in the dressing changes.

Care of the socket is minimal and easily accomplished. The wound itself is clean and has little or no drainage. If an antibiotic ointment is prescribed, it is applied in a thin line on the surface of the tissues of the socket. The dressing consists of an eye pad changed daily. Once the socket has healed completely, a dressing is no longer necessary, although there are several reasons for having the child continue to wear an eye patch. Infants and toddlers explore their environment with their hands, and without an eye patch in place, the socket is available to exploring fingers. Although there is little danger of the child injuring the socket, parents may feel more secure with the socket covered. This also helps prevent infection.

The ocularist, who fits and manufactures the prosthesis, gives initial instructions for care of the device. Once in place, the prosthesis need not be removed unless cleaning is necessary, in which case it is taken out by gently pulling down on the lower lid, which frees the lower edge of the prosthesis, and applying pressure to the upper lid. The prosthesis is cleaned by placing it in hot water and soaking it for several minutes. Reinsertion is easier if the prosthesis remains wet. To reinsert the prosthesis, the lids are separated; and with the prosthesis held in the correct position (it should be marked to indicate the nasal side), it is pushed up under the upper lid, allowing the lower lid to cover its lower edge.

Safety is a major concern to prevent damage to the unaffected eye. Safety measures should be practised at all times, and children should avoid rough contact sports or wear protective eyewear.

Support the Family. The diagnosis of retinoblastoma presents some special concerns in addition to those raised by any type of cancer. Families with a history of retinoblastoma may feel guilt for transmitting the mutation to their offspring, especially if they knowingly 'played the odds' in conceiving an affected child. Conversely, when parents are aware of the probability and have an affected child, early treatment results in such favourable outcomes that parental adjustment may be rapid. In families with no history of retinoblastoma, the diagnosis is a shock, frequently complicated by guilt for not having discovered it sooner. Because parents frequently are the first to observe the cat's eye reflex, they may be angry at themselves or others, especially healthcare professionals, if a more thorough examination was delayed. The nurse should consider each of these variables while offering supportive care to the family.

Other concerns also relate to the hereditary aspects of the disease. Of great importance to parents is the risk of retinoblastoma in their subsequent offspring and in the offspring of the surviving affected child. With improving prognoses for these children, genetic counselling is assuming greater importance. (See Chapter 3 for a discussion of the nurse's role in genetic counselling.)

Encourage these families to seek regular follow-up care for the affected child for early identification of possible SMNs. Offspring of unaffected parents and survivors should undergo regular ophthalmoscopy to detect retinoblastoma at its earliest stage.

Germ Cell Tumours

Germ cell tumours (GCTs) account for approximately 3% of cancers in children diagnosed each year in Australia and New Zealand (Ballentine & NZCCR Working Group 2017, Youlden & Aitken 2019). They can arise in gonadal and extragonadal sites and are broadly classified as teratomas (mature and immature) or malignant GCTs. GCTs can appear in various body sites, including the testicles (e.g. yolk sac tumour, teratoma), ovaries (e.g. teratoma, germinoma, yolk sac tumour), sacrococcyx, mediastinum and retroperitoneum (Frazier et al 2016). In general, most children with teratomas and localised gonadal tumours that are surgically resected can be observed without the need for further therapy. For patients with more advanced disease, the use of chemotherapy has produced excellent results.

Liver Tumours

Primary liver tumours are rare in childhood; they are divided into two main histological subtypes, hepatoblastoma and hepatocellular carcinoma, with hepatoblastoma being most common. Surgical resection is the treatment of choice for liver tumours, usually performed after the administration of chemotherapy to increase the likelihood of complete resection (Meyers et al 2016). Liver transplantation may be used in unresectable tumours. Survival rates for patients with hepatoblastoma can be as high as 90% with current therapies (Aronson & Meyers 2016).

THE CHILDHOOD CANCER SURVIVOR

Survival rates for children with cancer have greatly improved over the past decades, so that long-term survival is expected for more than 80% of children with access to contemporary therapy for cancer (Ballentine & NZCCR Working Group 2017, Youlden & Aitken 2019). Curative therapy can also produce adverse health outcomes, referred to as late effects, which may become apparent months to years after cancer treatment is completed. Survivorship research has demonstrated that 60% to 90% of adult survivors of childhood cancer develop chronic health conditions; of these, 20% to 80% experience severe or life-threatening complications (Landier et al 2016). Late effects are related to therapeutic exposures (chemotherapy, surgery, radiation therapy, SCT) and are also influenced by host factors such as genetic predisposition, age at diagnosis/treatment, comorbid health conditions and health habits (National Institutes of Health 2017).

Table 29.6 describes systemic late effects caused by cancer treatment that require careful nursing assessment. All survivors should have risk-based medical follow-up that includes a survivorship care plan for lifelong screening, surveillance and health promotion.

TABLE 29.6 Late Effects of Cancer Treatment

Systemic Effects and Clinical Manifestations	Associated Mode of Treatment
CENTRAL NERVOUS SYSTEM	
Leucoencephalopathy (syndrome ranging from lethargy, dementia and seizures to quadriplegia and death)	Methotrexate, intrathecal chemotherapy or CNS irradiation
Mineralising microangiopathy (headaches, focal seizures, incoordination, gait abnormalities)	Methotrexate or CNS irradiation
Peripheral neuropathy (footdrop, tingling sensation in hands and/or feet, incoordination)	Vincristine
Cognitive deficits (decline with intelligence, memory, attention, non-language skills)	Intrathecal chemotherapy or cranial irradiation (especially before 3 years old)
CARDIOVASCULAR	
Cardiomyopathy (tachycardia, tachypnoea, dyspnoea, shortness of breath, oedema, palpitations)	Anthracyclines (doxorubicin and daunorubicin) or irradiation to heart High-dose cyclophosphamide
Pericardial damage (pleural effusion, cardiomegaly)	Mediastinal irradiation
RESPIRATORY	
Pneumonitis (dyspnoea, non-productive cough, fever) Pulmonary fibrosis (dyspnoea, restrictive ventilation, decreased exercise tolerance)	Lung irradiation, alkylating agents, possibly bleomycin, vinblastine, cisplatin
GASTROINTESTINAL	
Chronic enteritis (colic, abdominal pain, vomiting, diarrhoea, obstipation, bleeding)	Abdominal irradiation, methotrexate, cytarabine
Hepatic fibrosis (jaundice, hepatomegaly)	Methotrexate, mercaptopurine
URINARY	
Haemorrhagic cystitis (microscopic haematuria to gross haemorrhage)	Cyclophosphamide; ifosfamide; irradiation
Bladder fibrosis (decreased bladder capacity, ureteral reflux) Tubular necrosis (decreased creatinine clearance)	Cisplatin
ENDOCRINE	
Thyroid dysfunction (see Chapter 31)	Irradiation to thyroid, pituitary gland, testes, ovaries
REPRODUCTIVE	
Possible gonadal damage, both sexes (delayed puberty, amenorrhoea, decreased sperm counts, increased follicle-stimulating and luteinising hormones, decreased testosterone or oestrogen)	Alkylating agents Irradiation to pituitary gland, testes, ovaries
SKELETAL	
Growth retardation (short stature)	Irradiation, long-term steroids
Spinal deformities, scoliosis, kyphosis, asymmetrical growth, pathological fractures	Irradiation
IMMUNE	
Asplenia (overwhelming infection, fever)	Splenectomy
SENSORY ORGANS	
Cataracts (opacity over pupil)	Cranial irradiation, high-dose steroids
Hearing (decreased hearing, especially with high-frequency loss)	Cisplatin
NEUROCOGNITIVE EFFECTS	
Reduced intelligence quotient (IQ) scores	Cranial irradiation, antimetabolite chemotherapy; high-dose steroids
Slow processing speed; inattention; memory impairment; and deficits in visual spatial skills and psychomotor speed	Cranial irradiation although chemotherapy alone may be linked to subtle deficits
ADDITIONAL EFFECTS	
Dental Problems Increased caries, periodontal disease, hypoplastic teeth, hypodontia (delayed or absent tooth development)	Irradiation to maxilla and mandible
Second Malignancies Bone and soft tissue tumours Leukaemia (ALL or AML)	Irradiation, alkylating agents

ALL, acute lymphoblastic leukaemia; *AML*, acute myeloid leukaemia; *CNS*, central nervous system.

Childhood cancer survivors have an elevated risk for disease and treatment-related morbidity and mortality that persists long after disease cure (Landier et al 2016). Survivorship research has contributed to better characterisation of late effects, as well as to modification of treatment regimens to minimise the risk of late effects. As therapeutic options evolve, nurses will need to stay current with ongoing research to determine best practices for continued improvement in both the duration and the quality of survival after childhood cancer.

REFERENCES

Allen, C. E., Kamdar, K. Y., Bollard, C. M., et al. (2016). Malignant non-Hodgkin lymphomas in children. In P. A. Pizzo & D. G. Poplack (Eds.), Principles and practices of pediatric oncology (7th ed.). Philadelphia: Lippincott.

Andrews, J., Galel, S. A., Wong, W., et al. (2016). Hematologic supportive care for children with cancer. In P. A. Pizzo & D. G. Poplack (Eds.), Principles and practice of pediatric oncology (7th ed.). Philadelphia: Lippincott.

Arceci, R. J., & Meshinchi, S. (2016). Acute myeloid leukaemia and myelodysplastic syndromes. In P. A. Pizzo & D. G. Poplack (Eds.), Principles and practice of pediatric oncology (7th ed.). Philadelphia: Lippincott.

Ardura, M. I., & Koh, A. Y. (2016). Infectious complications in pediatric cancer patients. In P. A. Pizzo & D. G. Poplack (Eds.), Principles and practice of pediatric oncology (7th ed.). Philadelphia: Lippincott.

Aronson, D. C., & Meyers, R. L. (2016). Malignant tumors of the liver in children. Seminars in Pediatric Surgery, 25(5), 265–275.

Australian Technical Advisory Group on Immunisation (ATAGI). (2018). Australian Immunisation Handbook, Australian Government Department of Health, Canberra. http://immunisationhandbook.health.gov.au

Australian and New Zealand Children's Haematology Oncology Group (ANZCHOG). (2020). *The Challenges of Childhood Cancer.* Victoria. https://anzchog.org/childhood-cancer/the-challenges-of-childhood-cancer/

Ballentine, K. & NZCCR Working Group. (2017). The incidence of childhood cancer in New Zealand 2010-2014: A report from the New Zealand Children's Cancer Registry. Auckland: National Cancer Network.

Becze, E. (2017). Nursing considerations for adverse events from CAR T-cell therapy. ONS Voice, May 9. https://voice.ons.org/news-and-views/nursing-considerations-for-adverse-events-from-car-t-cell-therapy

Bhatia, S., Landier, W., Hageman. L., et al. (2015). Acute Lymphoblastic Leukemia: A Children's Oncology Group Study. Oncology, 1(3), 287–295.

Brodeur, G. M., Hogarty, M. D., Bagatell, R., et al. (2016). Neuroblastoma. In P. A. Pizzo & D. G. Poplack (Eds.), Principles and practice of pediatric oncology (7th ed.). Philadelphia: Lippincott.

Burgoyne, L. L., Billups, C. A., Jirón, J. L., Jr., et al. (2012). Phantom limb pain in young cancer related amputees: Recent experience at St Jude Children's Research Hospital. Clinical Journal of Pain, 28, 222–225.

Cancer Australia. (2020). About Children's Cancer [Online]. Australian Government. https://childrenscancer.canceraustralia.gov.au/about-childrens-cancer

Cancer Australia. (2021). Targeted Therapies. Australian Government. https://www.canceraustralia.gov.au/affected-cancer/treatment/targeted-therapy

Cancer Institute of New South Wales. (2019). Prevention of antineoplastic induced nausea and vomiting [Online]. Australia. https://www.eviq.org.au/clinical-resources/side-effect-and-toxicity-management/gastrointestinal/7-prevention-of-antineoplastic-induced-nausea-and#management-of-high-emetogenic-risk-90-risk-of-e

Ceppi, F., Beck-Popovic, M., Bourquin, J. P., et al. (2017). Opportunities and challenges in the immunological therapy of pediatric malignancy: a concise snapshot. European Journal of Pediatrics, 176(9), 1163–1172.

Chaveli-Lopez, B., & Bagan-Sebastian, J. V. (2016). Treatment of oral mucositis due to chemotherapy. Journal of Clinical and Experimental Dental Research, 8(2), e201–e209.

Children's Oncology Group (COG). (2019a). Informed Consent [Online]. https://www.childrensoncologygroup.org/index.php/informed-consent-311

Children's Oncology Group (COG). (2019b). Tests and Procedures [Online]. https://www.childrensoncologygroup.org/index.php/testsandprocedures

Children's Oncology Group (COG). (2019c). What is a Clinical Trial? [Online]. https://www.childrensoncologygroup.org/index.php/clinicaltrials-136

Clinical Oncology Society of Australia (COSA). (2018). COSA guidelines for the safe prescribing, dispensing and administration of systemic cancer therapy [Online]. Australia. https://wiki.cancer.org.au/australiawiki/images/2/29/Cancer_chemotherapy_medication_safety_guidelines.pdf

Department of Health. (2020a). How is cancer diagnosed? [Online]. Australia. https://childrenscancer.canceraustralia.gov.au/about-childrens-cancer/how-cancer-diagnosed

Department of Health. (2020b). National Cervical Screening Program [Online]. Australia. http://www.cancerscreening.gov.au/internet/screening/publishing.nsf/Content/about-the-new-test

Effinger, K. E., Migliorati, C. A., Hudson, M. M., et al. (2014). Oral and dental late effects in survivors of childhood cancer: A Children's Oncology Group report. Supportive Care in Cancer, 22(7), 2009–2019.

European Society for Paediatric Oncology (SIOP Europe). (2020). Clinical Trials in Paediatric Oncology. https://www.siope.eu/european-research-and-standards/clinical-trials-in-paediatric-oncology/

Fernandez, C. V., Geller, J. I., Ehrlich, P. F., et al. (2016). Renal tumors. In P. A. Pizzo & D. G. Poplack (Eds.), Principles and practice of pediatric oncology (7th ed.). Philadelphia: Lippincott.

Fielding, F., Sanford, T. M., & Davis, M. P. (2013). Achieving effective control in cancer pain: A review of current guidelines. International Journal of Palliative Nursing, 19, 584–591.

Foggo, V., & Cavenagh, J. (2015). Malignant causes of fever of unknown origin. Clinical Medicine (London), 15, 292–294.

Freedman, J. L., Rheingold, S. R., & Fisher, M. J. (2016). Oncologic emergencies. In P. A. Pizzo & D. G. Poplack (Eds.), Principles and practice of pediatric oncology (7th ed.). Philadelphia: Lippincott.

Frazier, A. L., Olson, T. A., Schneider, D. R., et al. (2016). Germ cell tumors. In P. A. Pizzo & D. G. Poplack (Eds.), Principles and practice of pediatric oncology (7th ed.). Philadelphia: Lippincott.

Gore, L., DeGregori, J., & Porter, C. C. (2013). Targeting developmental pathways in children with cancer: What price success? The Lancet Oncology, 14(2), e70–e78.

Gorlick, R., Janeway, K., & Marina, N. (2016). Osteosarcoma. In P. A. Pizzo & D. G. Poplack (Eds.), Principles and practice of pediatric oncology (7th ed.). Philadelphia: Lippincott.

Gottschalk, S., Naik, S., Hegde, M., et al. (2016). Hematopoietic stem cell transplantation in pediatric oncology. In P. A. Pizzo & D. G. Poplack (Eds.), Principles and practice of pediatric oncology (7th ed.). Philadelphia: Lippincott.

Gupta, S., & Bhatia, S. (2017). Optimizing medication adherence in children with cancer. Current Opinion in Pediatrics, 29, 41–45.

Hawkins, D. S., Bolling, T., Brennan, B. M. D., et al. (2016). Ewing sarcoma. In P. A. Pizzo & D. G. Poplack (Eds.), Principles and practice of pediatric oncology (7th ed.). Philadelphia: Lippincott.

Hockenberry, M. J., Kline, N. E., & Rodgers, C. (2016). Nursing support of the child with cancer. In P. A. Pizzo & D. G. Poplack (Eds.), Principles and practice of pediatric oncology (7th ed.). Philadelphia: Lippincott.

Hurwitz, R. L., Shields, C. L., Shields, J. A., et al. (2016). Retinoblastoma. In P. A. Pizzo & D. G. Poplack (Eds.), Principles and practice of pediatric oncology (7th ed.). Philadelphia: Lippincott.

Johnson, A. (2018). An Update: Genetic Mutations and Childhood Cancers. The Journal for Nurse Practitioners, 14, 230–237.

Karakukcu, M., & Unal, E. (2015). Stem cell mobilization and collection from pediatric patients and healthy children. Transfusion and Apheresis Science, 53, 17–22.

Knudson, A. G., Hethcote, H. W., & Brown, B. W. (1975). Mutation and childhood cancer: A probabilistic model for the incidence of retinoblastoma. Procedures of the National Academy of Sciences, 72(12), 5116–5120.

Landier, W., Armenian, S. H., Meadows, A. T., et al. (2016). Late effects of childhood cancer and its treatment. In P. A. Pizzo & D. G. Poplack (Eds.),

Principles and practice of pediatric oncology (7th ed.). Philadelphia: Lippincott.

Lawson, C. M., Daley, B. J., Sams, V. G., et al. (2013). Factors that impact patient outcome: Nutrition assessment. Journal of the American Society of Parenteral and Enteral Nutrition, 37(5 Suppl.), 30S–38S.

Leukaemia Foundation. (2019). Childhood AML treatment. https://www.leukaemia.org.au/blood-cancer-information/types-of-blood-cancer/childhood-blood-cancers/childhood-all/

Luo, Y., & Anderson, T. A. (2016). Phantom limb pain: A review. International Anesthiology Clinics, 54, 121–139.

Leukaemia Foundation. (2021). Childhood Acute Lymphoblastic Leukaemia. https://www.leukaemia.org.au/blood-cancer-information/types-of-blood-cancer/childhood-blood-cancers/childhood-all/

Lymphoma Australia. (2021a). Hodgkin Lymphoma. https://www.lymphoma.org.au/types-of-lymphoma/hodgkin-lymphoma/

Lymphoma Australia. (2021b). Non-Hodgkin Lymphoma. https://www.lymphoma.org.au/types-of-lymphoma/non-hodgkin-lymphoma/

McLean, T. W., & Kemper, K. J. (2016). Complementary and alternative medical therapies in pediatric oncology. In P. A. Pizzo & D. G. Poplack (Eds.), Principles and practices of pediatric oncology (7th ed.). Philadelphia: Lippincott.

Metzger, M., Krasin, M. J., Choi, J. K., et al. (2016). Hodgkin lymphoma. In P. A. Pizzo & D. G. Poplack (Eds.), Principles and practices of pediatric oncology (7th ed.). Philadelphia: Lippincott.

Meyers, R. L., Trobough-Lotrario, A. D., Malogolowkin, M. H., et al. (2016). Pediatric liver tumors. In P. A. Pizzo & D. G. Poplack (Eds.), Principles and practice of pediatric oncology (7th ed.). Philadelphia: Lippincott.

Ministry of Health. (2020). Immunisation Handbook. Wellington: Ministry of Health. https://www.health.govt.nz/our-work/immunisation-handbook-2020/

Murphy, K. (ed.). (2011). The Children's Oncology Group: Family Handbook for Children with Cancer, United States of America: The Children's Oncology Group.

National Institutes of Health (NIH), National Cancer Institute. (2017). Neuroblastoma treatment. https://www.cancer.gov/types/neuroblastoma/hp/neuroblastoma-treatment-pdq

Parsons, D. W., Pollack, I. F., Hass-Kogan, D. A., et al. (2016). Gliomas, ependymomas, and other nonembryonal tumors of the central nervous system. In P. A. Pizzo & D. G. Poplack (Eds.), Principles and practice of pediatric oncology (7th ed.). Philadelphia: Lippincott.

Patel, P., Robinson, P. D., Thackray, J., et al. (2017). Guideline for the prevention of acute chemotherapy-induced nausea and vomiting in pediatric cancer patients: A focused update. Pediatric Blood and Cancer, 64(10), 28453189.

PDQ Pediatric Treatment Editorial Board. (2021). Childhood Cancer Genomics (PDQ): Health Professional Version. Bethesda, United States of America: National Cancer Institute. https://www.cancer.gov/types/childhood-cancers/pediatric-genomics-hp-pdq

PDQ Pediatric Treatment Editorial Board. (2020). Unusual Cancers of Childhood Treatment (PDQ)-Patient Version [Online]. https://www.cancer.gov/types/childhood-cancers/patient/unusual-cancers-childhood-pdq

Plon, S. E., & Malkin, D. (2016). Childhood cancer and heredity. In P. A. Pizzo & D. G. Poplack (Eds.), Principles and practice of pediatric oncology (7th ed.). Philadelphia: Lippincott.

Poussaint, T. Y., Panigrahy, A., & Huisman, T. A. (2015). Pediatric brain tumors. Pediatric Radiology, 45(Suppl3), S443–S453.

Rabin, K. R., Gramatges, M. M., Margolin, J. F., et al. (2016). Acute lymphoblastic leukaemia. In P. A. Pizzo & D. G. Poplack (Eds.), Principles and practice of pediatric oncology (7th ed.). Philadelphia: Lippincott.

Sarvaria, A., Jawdat, D., Madrigal, J. A., et al. (2017). Umbilical cord blood natural killer cells, their characteristics, and potential clinical applications. Frontiers in Immunology, 23(8), 329.

Scheurer, M. E., Lupo, P. J., & Bondy, M. L. (2016). Epidemiology of childhood cancer. In P. A. Pizzo & D. G. Poplack (Eds.), Principles and practice of pediatric oncology (7th ed.). Philadelphia: Lippincott.

Ullrich, C. K., Sourkes, B. M., & Wolfe, J. (2016). Palliative care for the child with cancer. In P. A. Pizzo & D. G. Poplack (Eds.), Principles and practice of pediatric oncology (7th ed.). Philadelphia: Lippincott.

Wexler, L. H., Skapek, S. X., & Helman, L. J. (2016). Rhabdomyosarcoma. In P. A. Pizzo & D. G. Poplack (Eds.), Principles and practice of pediatric oncology (7th ed.). Philadelphia: Lippincott.

Youlden, D. & Aitken, J. (2019). Childhood Cancer in Australia 1983-2015. Brisbane, Australia: Cancer Council Queensland

Zero Childhood Cancer. (2020). Translational Research. http://www.zerochildhoodcancer.org.au/page/44/the-research-behind-zero-childhood-cancer

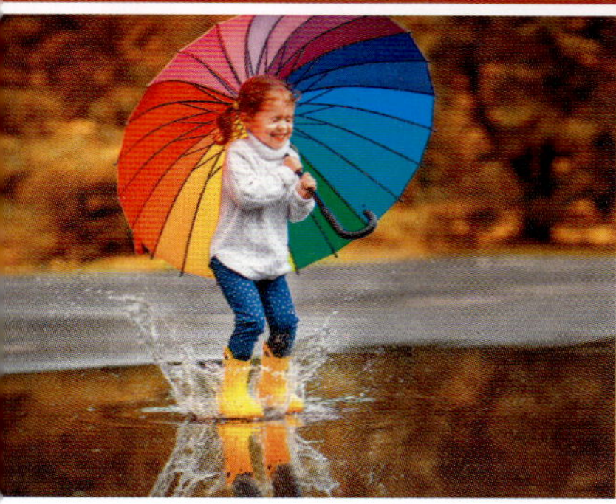

30

The Child with Cerebral Dysfunction

Emma Collins

LEARNING OUTCOMES

- Develop an understanding of intercranial regulation and effects on cerebral function.
- Develop an understanding of common problems children experience with cerebral dysfunction.
- Understand the complexities in assessment of children with cerebral dysfunction.
- Understand the importance of family-centred care and safety of children with cerebral dysfunction.

CEREBRAL STRUCTURE AND FUNCTION

The nervous system is made up of three intimately connected and functioning parts: the central nervous system (CNS), the peripheral nervous system and the autonomic nervous system. The CNS is composed of two cerebral hemispheres, the brainstem, the cerebellum and the spinal cord. The peripheral nervous system is composed of the cranial nerves (CNs) that arise from or travel to the brainstem and the spinal nerves that travel to or from the spinal cord. These nerves may be either motor (efferent) or sensory (afferent). The autonomic nervous system is composed of the sympathetic and parasympathetic systems, which provide automatic control of vital functions.

Development of the Neurological System

In contrast to other body tissues, which grow rapidly after birth, the nervous system grows proportionately more rapidly before birth. Two periods of rapid brain cell growth occur during fetal life. From 15 to 20 weeks of gestation there is a dramatic increase in the number of neurons. Another increase in growth rate begins at 30 weeks of gestation and extends to 1 year of age. This rapid growth during infancy continues during early childhood and slows to a more gradual rate during later childhood and adolescence. Brain volume is readily reflected in head circumference, which increases six times as much during the first year as during the second year of life. During the first 3 months of life infants will gain 6 cm in head circumference, 3 cm during the next 3 months and 1 cm per month from age 6 to 12 months. Fifty per cent of postnatal brain growth is achieved by age 1 year, 75% by age 3 and 90% by age 6. Cerebral blood flow (CBF) and oxygen consumption in childhood (up to age 6 years) is almost twice that of adults, which reflects an increased metabolic requirement consistent with growth and development.

The growth and final form of the brain depend on the development and multiplication of neurons. Creation of new cells occurs, in theory, only during the first 100 days of gestation. During the remainder of gestation, cells divide and multiply at the astonishing rate of 250,000 per minute. It is believed that no new nerve cells appear after the sixth month of fetal life. Postnatal growth consists of increasing the amount of cytoplasm around the nuclei of the 10 billion existing cells, increasing the number and intricacy of communications with other cells and advancing their peripheral axons to keep pace with expanding body dimensions.

The brain constitutes 12% of the body weight at birth. It doubles its weight in the first year, and by age 5 or 6 years its weight at birth has tripled. Thereafter, growth slows until in adulthood the brain is only about 2% of the total body weight. The surface configuration of the brain also changes with development. The early embryonic brain surface is smooth, but the sulci deepen with advancing development. This process continues throughout childhood. At birth the cortex is only about half of its adult thickness, although all the major surface features are present. There is little cortical control over body movements at birth, with movements guided principally by primitive reflexes. (See Chapter 7.) With advancing development and maturation, the brain, through association pathways, exercises increasing control over much of the reflex activity. This allows the growing child to perform progressively complex tasks that require coordinated movements. Persistence of primitive reflexes may suggest defective cortical development.

Cortical control is closely associated with the acquisition of a myelin coating on the nerves. Although nerve fibres are able to conduct impulses without this myelin sheath, the impulses travel at a slower rate and with more likelihood of diffusion. Myelinisation of the various nerve tracts in the CNS, which allows progressive neuromotor function, follows the cephalocaudal (head-to-toe) and proximodistal (near-to-far) sequence. It appears first with the fibres of the spinal cord and cranial nerves, then in the brainstem and corticospinal tracts.

Development of the nervous system proceeds on a continuum and generates the most complex structures within the embryo. The brain and spinal cord are among the first of the major organ systems to be recognised in the embryo and one of the last to finish significant development after birth. The rate of myelogenesis accelerates rapidly after birth. In general, the pathways concerned with sensation are myelinated early, before the motor pathways. The acquisition of motor skills depends on the maturation and myelination of the nervous system, and no amount of special training or practice will hasten the process. Most of an infant's advancing performance is a direct result of brain development indirectly influenced by environmental stimuli.

Central Nervous System

The bony skull forms the strongest covering and provides the primary protection to the brain. It is an expansible structure in the infant and young child due to incomplete ossification of the bones of the skull, but becomes rigid in the older child and adolescent. Blood is supplied to the dura mater by the middle meningeal artery, a branch of the external carotid artery. It enters the skull at a point inferior to the temporal bone, then branches over the surface of the dura, usually encased in a groove in the temporal and parietal bones after 2 years of age. Damage to this artery or to its branches is a common cause of an epidural haematoma.

Brain Coverings

Within the skull, three membranes (the meninges) cover and protect the brain: the dura mater, arachnoid membrane and pia mater (Fig 30.1). The tough outer membrane, the **dura mater**, is a double layer that serves as the outer meningeal layer and the inner periosteum of the cranial bones. These two layers are separated by the epidural space. The dura is closely attached to the skull in infancy, causing slower spread of blood in epidural haemorrhage. Because of this adherence, epidural haemorrhages are uncommon in the first 2 years of life.

Between these layers of dura inside the skull lie large venous sinuses. Sheets of the dura mater also extend downwards and inwards to form partitions within the cranium. Projecting downwards into the longitudinal fissure is a sheet of dura called the **falx cerebri**, which separates the cerebral hemispheres, and the **falx cerebelli**, which separates the cerebellar hemispheres. Another segment is a tentlike structure, the **tentorium**, which separates the cerebellum from the occipital lobe of the cerebrum. The large gap through which the brainstem passes is the tentorial hiatus.

The middle meningeal layer, the **arachnoid membrane**, is a delicate, avascular, weblike structure that loosely surrounds the brain. Between the arachnoid and the dura mater lies the subdural area, a potential space that normally contains only enough fluid to prevent adhesion between the two membranes. During cerebral trauma the fine blood vessels that bridge the subdural space are stretched and ruptured, causing venous blood to escape and spread freely, forming a subdural haemorrhage. The subdural space is small in children; therefore, small amounts of blood can increase intracranial haemorrhage significantly.

The innermost covering layer, the **pia mater**, is a delicate, transparent membrane that, unlike the other coverings, adheres closely to the outer surface of the brain, conforming to the folds (gyri) and furrows (sulci). Within the pial layer lie the arteries and veins of the brain. Between the pia mater and the arachnoid membrane is the subarachnoid space. Cerebrospinal fluid (CSF) fills the entire subarachnoid space surrounding the brain and spinal cord and acts as a protective cushion for the brain tissue. Fibrous filaments known as arachnoid trabeculae provide further protection and help anchor the brain. When the head receives a blow, these attachments allow the arachnoid to slide on the dura, preventing excessive movement.

The Brain

Each section of the brain plays a vital role in regulation and control of body function. Each hemisphere is artificially divided into lobes. Pressure on or damage to these lobes produces observable signs or symptoms directly related to the area of pathology. These signs provide clues to the location of the damage.

The two large cerebral hemispheres that occupy the anterior and medial fossae of the skull are separated in the upper part by the longitudinal fissure. This separation is complete anteriorly and posteriorly, but centrally the hemispheres are joined by the block of fibres known as the **corpus callosum**, the largest fibre bundle in the brain. These fibres interconnect cortical areas of the right and left hemispheres. Destruction of the corpus callosum causes hemispheric independence, or 'split brain'.

Situated deeply within each hemisphere and on each side of the midline are the basal ganglia (or cerebral nuclei), which serve as vital sorting areas for messages passing to and from the hemispheres. Connected to the hemispheres by thick bunches of nerve fibres is the brainstem, through which all nerve fibres traverse as they pass from the

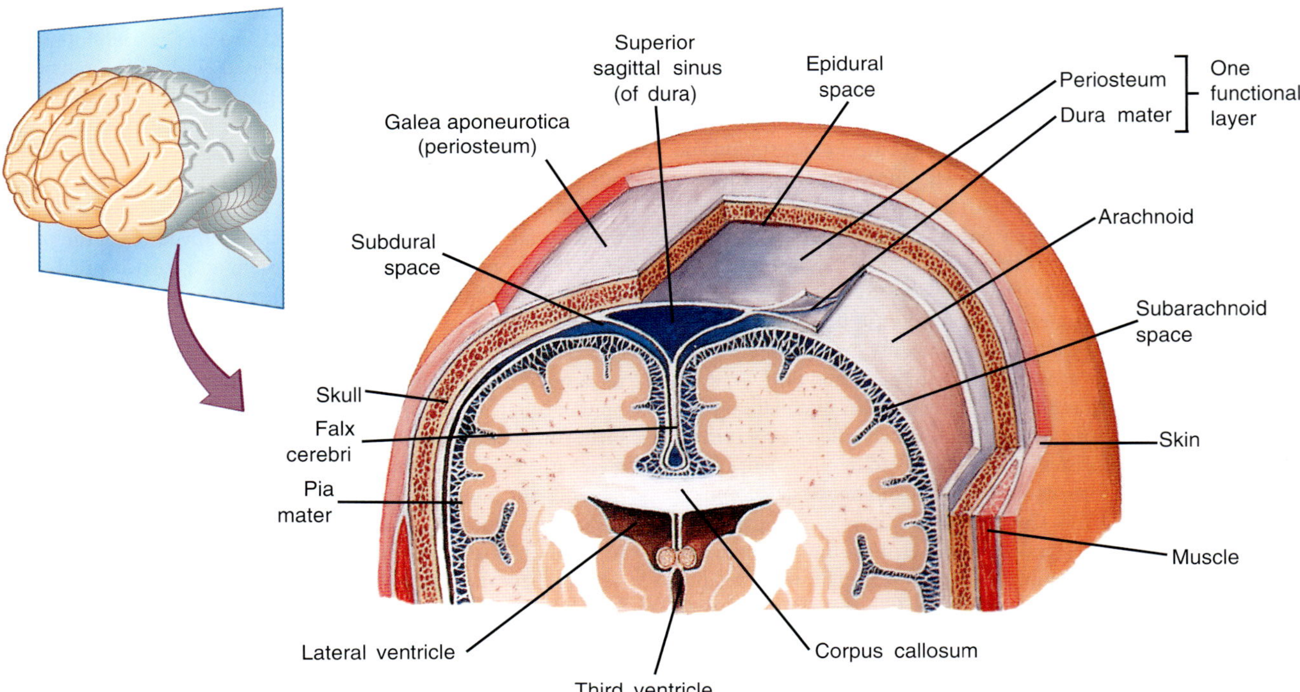

Fig 30.1 Coronal section of top of head showing meningeal layers. (Source: Patton, K. T., & Thibodeau, G. A. (2010). Anatomy and physiology (7th ed.). St Louis, MO: Mosby.)

hemispheres to the cerebellum and spinal cord. The brainstem extends from the base of the hemispheres through the foramen magnum, where it is continuous with the spinal cord. Within the cranium and behind the brainstem is the cerebellum. Any pressure exerted on the intracranial structures can cause compression of the brainstem and prolapse of the cerebellum through the foramen magnum.

Cerebral Blood Flow. The blood supply to the brain tissue is carried by the internal carotid arteries, which branch to supply the various brain segments. The volume of blood to the brain, which constitutes only 17% of the cardiac output, supplies the brain with 25% of the body's oxygen supply. The brain, an 'inactive' organ, uses 10 times the oxygen used by the body as a whole. Only the heart uses more oxygen per gram of tissue.

CBF is the result of two opposing forces: cerebral blood pressure (the difference between systemic arterial pressure and cerebral venous pressure) and cerebral vascular resistance. CBF remains constant at a cerebral blood pressure between 50 and 150 mmHg. Because cerebral venous pressure is usually very low and relatively constant, cerebral blood pressure is determined mainly by systemic arterial pressure.

Autoregulation. One of the most important factors in the control of CBF is autoregulation, the unique ability of cerebral arterial vessels to change their diameter in response to fluctuating cerebral perfusion pressure (CPP). The CPP is the mean arterial pressure (MAP) minus the intracranial pressure (ICP):

$$\text{CPP} = \text{MAP} - \text{ICP}$$

As a result, cerebral vessels maintain a constant blood flow during alterations in blood pressure and perfusion caused by body posture, increased ICP, decreased cardiac output or narrowing or occlusion in the major blood vessels of the neck. Autoregulation fails when the limits of cerebrovascular dilation are reached; at this point CBF decreases, causing clinical symptoms of ischaemia (nausea, fainting, dizziness, dim vision). Conversely, increased MAP leads to 'breakthrough of autoregulation', with increased CBF leading to microhaemorrhages and cerebral oedema. Autoregulation may be impaired locally or globally as a result of trauma or ischaemia.

Changes in arterial oxygen pressure (PaO_2) or arterial carbon dioxide pressure ($PaCO_2$) have a profound effect on autoregulation. Hypercapnia ($PaCO_2 > 45$ mmHg) or increased levels of lactic acid have a pronounced dilating effect on cerebral arterioles, which increases CBF and thus cerebral volume. Hypocapnia ($PaCO_2 < 35$ mmHg) constricts cerebral arterioles and decreases CBF. PaO_2 values between 70 and 100 mmHg have little effect on the cerebrovascular system. Profound hypoxia ($PaO_2 < 50$ mmHg) dramatically increases CBF. Consequently maintenance of the airway and effective hyperventilation are of primary importance in the initial management of the neurologically impaired patient. CPP is the most important physiological determinant because the brain relies on the delivery of oxygen and nutrients to function.

Oxygen. Metabolic requirements for oxygen by the brain are not affected by rest or sleep, but they are reduced by narcosis and coma and are altered by changes in temperature. CBF is not altered when body temperature is between 35°C and 40°C. Hyperthermia increases oxygen consumption by the brain. Hypothermia decreases oxygen consumption. The brain depends on a constant supply of oxygen-rich blood. Because the brain's need for oxygen is great in relation to the volume of blood supplied, the brain is capable of extracting more oxygen from each unit of circulating blood as needed.

Oxygen supply to the brain is compromised when the supply is inadequate as a result of impaired respiration, hypotension, increased ICP or vascular damage, spasm or compression. Neurons are highly susceptible to elevated $PaCO_2$ (a potent vasodilator). The metabolic damage to brain tissue caused by an inadequate supply of well-oxygenated blood can often exceed the effects of trauma. Respiratory acidosis resulting from increased $PaCO_2$ levels can produce symptoms indistinguishable from those of head injury.

Blood–Brain Barrier. The **blood–brain barrier (BBB)** is an anatomical–physiological feature of the brain that separates the brain parenchyma from the blood. Unlike capillaries in other parts of the body, cerebral capillaries have no fenestrations or pores. The tight junctions of the vascular endothelium are responsible for the selective nature of the BBB. The mature BBB allows facilitated diffusion of glucose and passive diffusion of water and carbon dioxide but is impermeable to protein and does not permit passage of many active substances. However, the BBB of the fetus and newborn is normally indiscriminately permeable, allowing protein and other large and small molecules to pass freely between the cerebral vessels and the brain. Conditions that cause cerebrovascular dilation (hypertension, hypercapnia, hypoxia, acidosis) disrupt the BBB. Hyperosmotic fluids, which cause shrinkage of vascular endothelium and widen the vascular junctions, also disrupt the BBB.

Increased Intracranial Pressure

The brain, tightly enclosed in the solid bony cranium, is well protected but highly vulnerable to pressure that may accumulate within the enclosure. Its total volume—brain (80%), CSF (10%) and blood (10%)—must remain approximately the same at all times. A change in the proportional volume of one of these components (e.g. increase or decrease in intracranial blood) must be accompanied by a compensatory change in another (e.g. decrease or increase in CSF). In this way the volume and pressure normally remain constant. Examples of compensatory changes are reduction in blood volume, decrease in production of CSF, increase in CSF absorption or shrinkage of brain mass by displacement of intracellular and extracellular fluid.

Children with open fontanels compensate for increased volume by skull expansion and widened sutures. However, at any age the capacity for spatial compensation is limited. An increase in ICP may be caused by tumours or other space-occupying lesions, accumulation of fluid within the ventricular system, bleeding or oedema of cerebral tissues. Once compensation is exhausted, any further increase in volume results in a rapid rise in ICP.

The early signs and symptoms of increased ICP are often subtle, such as headache, vomiting, personality changes, irritability and fatigue (Box 30.1). In older children subjective symptoms are headache, especially when arising after lying flat (e.g. on awakening in the morning) or when coughing, sneezing or bending over, and nausea and vomiting. The child may complain of double vision or blurred vision with movement of the head. Seizures may occur. In children whose cranial sutures have not closed, there is an increase in head circumference and tense or bulging fontanels. Cranial sutures may widen. Head circumference can enlarge until the child is 5 years of age if the condition progresses slowly. It is therefore essential that a head circumference measurement is completed regularly to see any pattern occurring. As pressure increases, the pupils become progressively sluggish in reaction and eventually become fixed and dilated. The level of consciousness progressively deteriorates from drowsiness to eventual coma. Problems related to increased ICP are discussed later in this chapter in relation to head injury and hydrocephalus. (See also Brain Tumours, Chapter 29.)

Physiological and biochemical changes within the cerebral vasculature serve to complicate the primary causes of increased ICP. Especially in cases of trauma, blood flow often initially increases as a result of venous congestion or vasomotor paralysis. If cerebral hypoxia is associated with the cerebral dysfunction, the compensatory vasodilation caused by oxygen deficiency will tend to increase the cerebral flow. However, blood flow is reduced as ICP progressively increases, with diminished blood supply to the brain tissues. The classic responses

BOX 30.1 Clinical Manifestations of Increased Intracranial Pressure in Infants and Children

Infants
- Tense, bulging fontanel
- Separated cranial sutures
- Irritability and restlessness
- Drowsiness
- Increased sleeping
- High-pitched cry
- Increased fronto-occipital circumference
- Distended scalp veins
- Poor feeding
- Crying when disturbed
- Setting-sun sign

Children
- Headache
- Nausea
- Forceful vomiting
- Diplopia, blurred vision
- Seizures
- Indifference, drowsiness
- Decline in school performance
- Diminished physical activity and motor performance
- Increased sleeping
- Inability to follow simple commands
- Lethargy

Late Signs in Infants and Children
- Bradycardia
- Decreased motor response to command
- Decreased sensory response to painful stimuli
- Alterations in pupil size and reactivity
- Extension or flexion posturing
- Cheyne-Stokes respirations
- Papillo-oedema
- Decreased consciousness
- Coma

observed in adults (widening pulse pressure, increased blood pressure) rarely occur in children or are very late signs. Periodic or irregular breathing is an ominous sign of brainstem (especially medullary) dysfunction that often precedes apnoea.

EVALUATION OF NEUROLOGICAL STATUS

Earlier chapters discuss methods to evaluate neurological function in relation to numerous aspects of child care. The neurological examination is an integral part of the health assessment (see Chapter 4) and newborn assessment (see Chapter 7). Chapter 34 discusses some of the tests used to differentiate neuromuscular disorders. The assessment tools and examinations in this chapter are primarily those used to assess intracranial integrity.

Assessment: General Aspects

Children younger than approximately 2 years of age require special evaluation because they are unable to respond to directions designed to elicit specific neurological responses. Early neurological responses in infants are primarily reflexive; these responses are gradually replaced by meaningful movement in the characteristic cephalocaudal direction of development. This evidence of progressive maturation reflects more extensive myelinisation and changes in neurochemical and electrophysiological properties.

Most information about infants and small children comes from observation of spontaneous and elicited reflex responses. It is also important to involve the family in your assessment. As infants and small children develop increasingly complex gross and fine motor skills and communication skills, more sophisticated techniques are used to assess acquisition of developmental milestones. Delay or deviation from expected milestones helps identify high-risk children. Persistence or reappearance of primitive reflexes indicates a pathological condition. In evaluating the infant or young child, it is important to obtain the history of the pregnancy, delivery, respiratory status at birth and neonatal health including any need for intensive care hospitalisation to determine the possible impact of intrauterine and extrauterine environmental influences known to affect the orderly maturation of the CNS. These influences include maternal infections, chemical exposure, trauma, medication, illicit drug use and metabolic insults.

History

A family history can sometimes offer clues regarding possible genetic disorders with neurological manifestations. A review of family members often identifies conditions that might otherwise be overlooked, especially increased number of miscarriages or siblings or relatives who died at an early age.

A health history provides valuable clues regarding the cause of neurological dysfunction. A history is assessed for injury with loss of consciousness, febrile illness, an encounter with an animal or insect, ingestion of neurotoxic substances, inhalation of chemicals, past illness and known diabetes mellitus or sickle cell disease. Sudden or progressive alterations in movement or mental abilities may provide clues for investigation. It is also important to ascertain the chronological course of the illness.

Physical Examination

Physical examination includes observation of the size and shape of the head (particularly in the infant and young child), spontaneous activity and postural reflex activity and sensory responses. Note whether the patient is lethargic, drowsy, stuporous, alert, active or irritable. The nurse also observes the overall tone, noting whether there is a normal flexed posture or one of extreme extension, opisthotonos or hypotonia. Symmetry of movement is also assessed.

Facial features may suggest a specific syndrome. A high-pitched, piercing cry in an infant is often associated with CNS disorders. An abnormal respiratory cycle, such as prolonged apnoea, ataxic breathing, paradoxical chest movement and hyperventilation, may be the result of a neurological problem.

Older children can be evaluated by the usual methods used in a neurological examination. In addition, an estimation of the level of development provides essential information about neurological function. This assessment is discussed throughout the book in relation to evaluation for specific disorders such as intellectual and developmental disabilities, failure to thrive, attention deficit/hyperactivity disorder, cerebral palsy, cerebral tumours and other physical or behavioural problems. Developmental screening tests can assess developmental progress in the young child.

Muscular activity and coordination, including ocular movements and gait, are valuable sources of information. Ocular movements, pupillary response, facial movements and mouth functions provide clues regarding CNS involvement or impingement. Testing reflexes, strength and coordination and for the presence and location of tremors, twitching, tics or other unusual movements is also an aspect of the neurological assessment (Box 30.2). Box 30.3 describes abnormalities of gait that indicate cerebral dysfunction.

Altered States of Consciousness

Consciousness implies awareness—the ability to respond to sensory stimuli and have subjective experiences. Consciousness has two aspects: alertness, an arousal-waking state that includes the ability to respond to stimuli, and cognition, which includes the ability to process stimuli and produce verbal and motor responses.

An **altered state of consciousness** usually refers to varying states of unconsciousness that may be momentary or may last for hours, days or indefinitely. Unconsciousness is depressed cerebral function—the inability to respond to sensory stimuli and have subjective experiences. Coma is defined as a state of unconsciousness from which the patient cannot be aroused, even with powerful stimuli.

BOX 30.2 Abnormal Involuntary Muscular Movements

Ataxia—Gross incoordination that may become worse with the eyes closed
Spasm—Involuntary contraction of a muscle
Spasticity—Prolonged and steady contraction of a muscle characterised by clonus (alternating relaxation and contraction of the muscle) and exaggerated reflexes
Rigidity—Inability to flex or extend a joint
Tremors—Constant small involuntary movements
Twitching—Spasmodic movements of short duration
Tic—Involuntary, compulsive, stereotyped movement of an associated group of muscles
Choreiform Movements—Quick, jerky, grossly uncoordinated, irregular movements that may disappear on relaxation
Athetosis—Slow, writhing, wormlike, constant, grossly uncoordinated movements that increase on voluntary activity and decrease on relaxation
Dystonia—Slow twisting movements of limbs or trunk
Associated Movements—Voluntary movement of one muscle accompanied by involuntary movement of another muscle
Mirroring Movements—Same as associated movements except with symmetrical muscle group

BOX 30.3 Abnormalities of Gait That Indicate Cerebral Dysfunction

Ataxia—Impaired ability to coordinate movements; staggering gait and postural imbalance.
Spastic Paraplegic Gait—Narrow-based gait with a tendency to walk on toes, along with flexion at knees and hips, and shuffling. Hips are adducted, and knees may strike each other with each step; in younger children a 'scissoring' position results when lower limbs cross because of increased adductor tone. Patients walk stiffly; take slow, deliberate steps; and have difficulty when attempting to walk on heels or run.
Spastic Hemiplegic Gait—Involved leg extended, circumducted, plantar flexion. The affected arm is flexed and adducted and does not swing.
Cerebellar Gait—Staggering, unsteadiness, wide-based gait; tendency to veer in one lateral direction; often accompanied by swaying of the trunk.
Extrapyramidal Gait—Rigidity, few automatic movements and bradykinesia (slowness of all movements) with associated bending of trunk and head, arms adducted at shoulders and flexed at elbows and wrists, fingers extended; festination (upper body moving forwards in advance of lower part), causing rapid steps and risk of falling.

The seat of consciousness, or 'alerting area', of the brain is in the reticular formation—the central core of the brainstem. The reticular formation extends from the midbrain to the medulla. The reticular activating system receives collaterals from and is stimulated by every major somatic and special sensory pathway in the brain. Disturbances of consciousness may occur when any part of the reticular, thalamic, hypothalamic and cortical circuits is sufficiently impaired. However, the effects may vary according to the areas involved. For example, small lesions of the reticular or hypothalamic regions produce a profound effect, whereas extensive impairment of the cortex is required to produce quantitatively similar results.

Aetiology

An altered state of consciousness may be the outcome of several processes that affect the CNS. Impaired neurological function can result from a direct or indirect cause. Some altered states, such as the diffuse changes observed in encephalitis, are directly related to cerebral insult. Others are the result of dysfunction in other organs or processes. For example, biochemical changes can impair neurological function without morphological findings, as in hypoglycaemia.

Level of Consciousness

Assessment of level of consciousness (LOC) remains the earliest indicator of improvement or deterioration in neurological status. LOC is determined by observations of the child's responses to the environment. Other diagnostic tests, such as motor activity, reflexes and vital signs, are more variable and do not necessarily directly parallel the depth of the comatose state. The most consistently used terms are described in Box 30.4.

Coma Assessment

Diminished alertness as a result of pathological conditions occurs on a continuum and is designated as the comatose state, which extends from somnolence at one end to deep coma at the other. To produce coma, one of the following must occur: (1) extensive, diffuse, bilateral cerebral hemispheric destruction (the brainstem may be intact); (2) a lesion in the diencephalon; or (3) destruction of the brainstem down to the level of the lower pons.

Several scales have been devised in an attempt to standardise the description and interpretation of the degree of depressed consciousness.

BOX 30.4 Levels of Consciousness

Full consciousness—Awake and alert, oriented to time, place and person; behaviour appropriate for age.
Confusion—Impaired decision-making.
Disorientation—Confusion regarding time, place and/or person; decreased level of consciousness.
Lethargy—Limited spontaneous movement, sluggish speech, drowsiness.
Obtundation—Arousable with stimulation.
Stupor—Remaining in a deep sleep, responsive only to vigorous and repeated stimulation.
Coma—No motor or verbal response to noxious (painful) stimuli.
Persistent Vegetative State (PVS)—Permanently lost function of the cerebral cortex. Eyes follow objects only by reflex or when attracted to the direction of loud sounds; all four limbs are spastic but can withdraw from painful stimuli; hands show reflexive grasping and groping; the face can grimace, some food may be swallowed and the child may groan or cry but utter no words.

Source: Modified from Seidel, H. M., Ball, J. W., Dains, J. E., et al (Eds.). (2006). Mosby's guide to physical examination (6th ed.). St Louis, MO: Mosby.

Some workplaces may also have specific scales. However, the most popular of these is the **Glasgow Coma Scale (GCS)**, which consists of a three-part assessment: eye opening, verbal response and motor response. The GCS was created to meet a clinical need to identify criteria for the consciousness level. For clinical purposes, the primary role of observation of the LOC is to detect a life-threatening complication such as cerebral oedema. The GCS requires observational skills and is readily reproducible between observers.

A paediatric version of the GCS recognises that expected verbal and motor responses must be related to the child's age (Fig 30.2). The paediatric coma scale does not assess verbal responses as such but records smiling, crying and interaction. It uses a 6-point motor scale that is inappropriate for children below the age of 6 months. In children under 5 years of age, speech is understood to be any sound at all, even crying. Young children demonstrate orientation by identifying their parents correctly or giving their own names.

The GCS in itself is not sufficient to determine depressed consciousness in all children. For example, because a child with quadriplegia cannot respond to commands physically, the child's GCS can be very

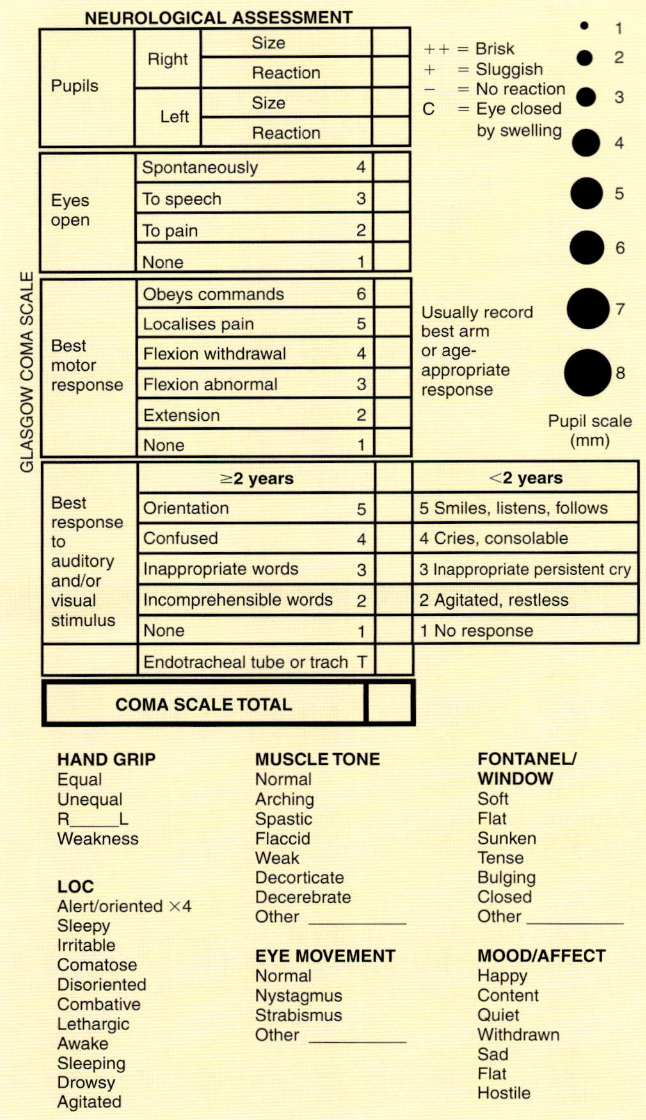

NEUROLOGICAL ASSESSMENT

GLASGOW COMA SCALE

Pupils			
Pupils	Right	Size	
		Reaction	
	Left	Size	
		Reaction	

++ = Brisk
+ = Sluggish
− = No reaction
C = Eye closed by swelling

Eyes open	Spontaneously	4	
	To speech	3	
	To pain	2	
	None	1	
Best motor response	Obeys commands	6	
	Localises pain	5	
	Flexion withdrawal	4	
	Flexion abnormal	3	
	Extension	2	
	None	1	

Usually record best arm or age-appropriate response

Pupil scale (mm): 1, 2, 3, 4, 5, 6, 7, 8

	≥2 years			<2 years
Best response to auditory and/or visual stimulus	Orientation	5		5 Smiles, listens, follows
	Confused	4		4 Cries, consolable
	Inappropriate words	3		3 Inappropriate persistent cry
	Incomprehensible words	2		2 Agitated, restless
	None	1		1 No response
	Endotracheal tube or trach	T		

COMA SCALE TOTAL	

HAND GRIP
Equal
Unequal
R_____L
Weakness

LOC
Alert/oriented ×4
Sleepy
Irritable
Comatose
Disoriented
Combative
Lethargic
Awake
Sleeping
Drowsy
Agitated

MUSCLE TONE
Normal
Arching
Spastic
Flaccid
Weak
Decorticate
Decerebrate
Other __________

EYE MOVEMENT
Normal
Nystagmus
Strabismus
Other __________

FONTANEL/ WINDOW
Soft
Flat
Sunken
Tense
Bulging
Closed
Other __________

MOOD/AFFECT
Happy
Content
Quiet
Withdrawn
Sad
Flat
Hostile

Fig 30.2 Paediatric coma scale.

low but the child may be cognitively intact. Nevertheless, the GCS provides a more objective method for evaluating the state of consciousness in most cases. Severely injured children (GCS $\leq$ 8) may have a consistent grading of motor response, verbal response and eye opening.

The GCS score performed during preadmission (i.e. assessment in the field), in the emergency department and throughout the inpatient admission is universally accepted as one criterion to determine the patient's prognosis (Braine & Cook 2017). GCS scores equal to or less than 5 are associated with poor outcome (Murphy et al 2017).

Irreversible Coma. There is no precise diagnosis for clinical death. Different tissues undergo permanent damage after varying periods of exposure to an ongoing insult; therefore, the brain (especially the cerebrum) has become the tissue of most importance in determining the time of death. The current concept of dying is a process that takes place over a finite interval of time rather than an event that occurs spontaneously. **Brain death** is a clinical diagnosis based the total cessation of brainstem and cortical brain function that causes irreversible widespread brain injury and coma. In children the most common causes are trauma, anoxic encephalopathy, infections and cerebral neoplasms. The pronouncement of brain death requires two conditions: (1) complete cessation of clinical evidence of brain function; and (2) irreversibility of the condition (Australian and New Zealand Intensive Care Society [ANZICS] 2019). It is essential to establish the absence of a reversible condition, especially a toxic and metabolic disorder, sedative-hypnotic drugs, paralytic agents, hypothermia, hypotension and surgically remediable conditions (Nakagawa et al 2012).

Organ transplantation has created a need to separate the process of death from the retrieval of viable tissues at a time when the brain is already dead. The clinical criteria for brain death must be met so that there is no error. It is essential that cultural considerations are adhered to and respected. At least two different attending medical practitioners should participate in the diagnosing of brain death in children (ANZICS 2019).

NURSING CARE GUIDELINES

Establishing Brain Death in Children

- Coma and apn ea must coexist. Child must exhibit complete loss of consciousness, vocalisation and volitional activity.
- Brainstem function must be absent, as defined by the following:
  - midposition or fully dilated pupils in both eyes that do not respond to light
  - absence of spontaneous eye movements and those induced by oculocephalic and caloric (oculovestibular) testing
  - absence of movement of bulbar musculature, including facial and oropharyngeal muscles
  - absence of the corneal, gag, cough, sucking and rooting reflexes
  - absence of respiratory movements when child is removed from ventilator; apnoea testing using standardised methods can be performed but is done after other criteria are met.
- Child must not be significantly hypothermic or hypotensive for age.
- Flaccid tone and absence of spontaneous or induced movements, including spinal cord events such as reflex withdrawal or spinal myoclonus, should exist.
- Examination should remain consistent with brain death throughout the observation and testing period.

Source: Data retrieved from Australia and New Zealand Intensive Care Society (ANZICS). (2019). The Statement on Death and Organ Donation. Edition 4. https://www .anzics.com.au/wp-content/uploads/2020/07/ANZICS-Statement-on-Death-and-Organ-Donation-Edition-4.pdf

Neurological Examination

The purpose of the neurological examination is to establish an accurate, objective baseline of neurological function. Therefore, it is essential that the neurological examination be documented in a descriptive and detailed fashion, thereby enhancing the ability to detect subtle changes in neurological status over time. Descriptions of behaviours should be simple, objective and easily interpreted; for example, 'Drowsy but awake and conversationally rational/oriented' or 'Sleepy but arousable with vigorous physical stimuli; pressure to nail base of right hand results in upper extremity flexion/lower extremity extension'.

Vital signs, observation of posture and movement (both spontaneous and elicited), eye examination, CN testing and reflex testing all provide valuable clues regarding the LOC, the site of involvement and the probable cause, but they do not necessarily parallel the depth of a comatose state.

Vital Signs

Pulse, respiration and blood pressure provide information regarding the adequacy of circulation and the possible underlying cause of altered consciousness. Autonomic activity is most intensively disturbed in deep coma and in brainstem lesions. Body temperature is often elevated; sometimes the elevation is extreme. High temperature is most often a sign of an acute infectious process or heatstroke, but it may be caused by ingestion of some drugs (especially salicylates, alcohol and barbiturates) or by intracranial bleeding, especially subarachnoid haemorrhage. Hypothalamic involvement may cause elevated or decreased temperature. Serious infection may produce hypothermia.

The pulse is variable and may be rapid, slow and bounding, or feeble. Blood pressure may be normal, elevated or very low. The Cushing reflex, or pressor response that causes a slowing of the pulse and an increase in blood pressure, is uncommon in children; when it does occur, it is a very late sign of increased ICP. Medications can also affect vital signs. For assessment purposes, actual changes in pulse and blood pressure are more important than the direction of the change.

Respirations are more often slow, deep and irregular. Slow and deep breathing often occurs in the heavy sleep caused by sedatives, after seizures or in cerebral infections. Slow, shallow breathing may result from sedatives or opioids. Hyperventilation (deep and rapid respirations) is usually the result of metabolic acidosis or abnormal stimulation of the respiratory centre in the medulla caused by salicylate poisoning, hepatic coma or Reye's syndrome. A pattern of alternating hyperventilation and breath-holding during wakefulness is common in Rett syndrome.

Breathing patterns have been described with a number of terms (e.g. *apneustic, cluster, ataxic, Cheyne-Stokes*). However, it is better to describe what is being observed rather than placing a label on it because the terms are often used and interpreted incorrectly. Periodic or irregular breathing is a sign of brainstem (especially medullary) dysfunction. This is an ominous sign that often precedes complete apnoea. The odour of the breath may provide additional clues (e.g. the fruity and acetone odour of ketosis, the foul odour of uraemia, the fetid odour of hepatic failure or the odour of alcohol).

Skin

The skin may offer clues to the cause of unconsciousness. The body surface should be examined for injury, needle marks, petechiae, bites and ticks. Evidence of toxic substances may be found on the hands, face, mouth and clothing—especially in small children.

Eyes

Assess pupil size and reactivity (Fig 30.3). Pupils either do or do not react to light. Pinpoint pupils are commonly observed in poisoning (e.g. opiate or barbiturate poisoning) or in brainstem dysfunction. Widely dilated and reactive pupils are often seen after seizures and may involve only one side. Widely dilated and fixed pupils suggest paralysis of CN III (oculomotor nerve) secondary to pressure from herniation of the brain through the tentorium. A unilateral fixed pupil usually suggests a lesion on the same side. Bilateral fixed pupils if present for more than 5 minutes usually imply brainstem damage. Dilated and non-reactive pupils also occur in hypothermia, anoxia, ischaemia, poisoning with atropine-like substances or prior instillation of

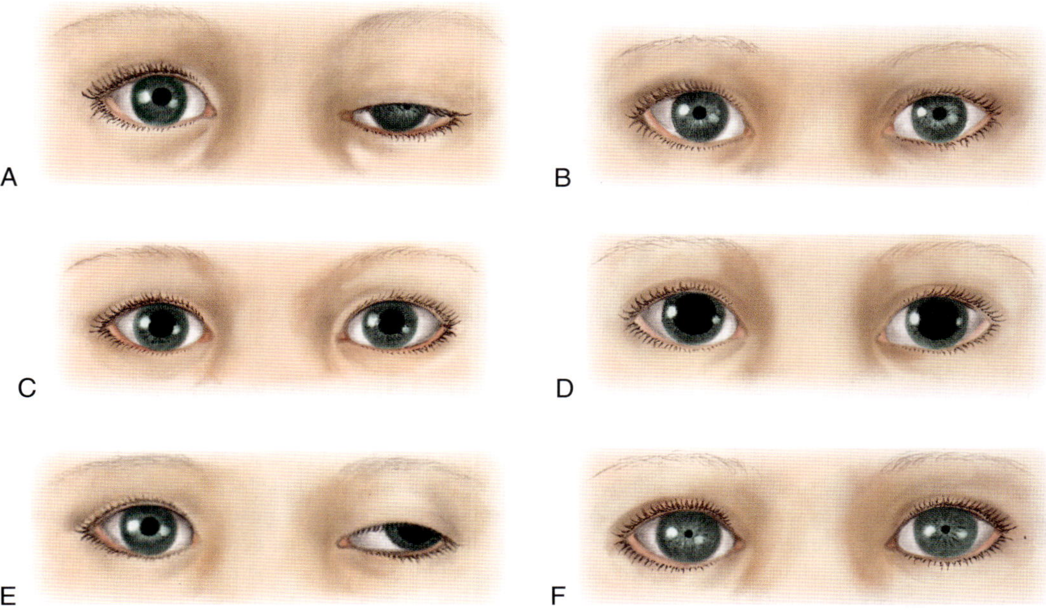

Fig 30.3 Variations in pupil size with altered states of consciousness. **(A)** Ipsilateral pupillary constriction with slight ptosis. **(B)** Bilateral small pupils. **(C)** Midposition, light fixed to all stimuli. **(D)** Bilateral dilated and fixed pupils. **(E)** Dilated pupils, left eye abducted with ptosis. **(F)** Pinpoint pupils.

mydriatic drugs. Some of the therapies used (e.g. barbiturates) can alter pupil size and reaction.

The description of eye movements should indicate whether one or both eyes are involved and how the reaction was elicited. Ask the parents if the child has strabismus which may cause the eyes to appear misaligned.

Blinking observed at rest or in response to a sudden loud noise or bright light implies that the pontine reticular formation is intact. The corneal reflex, blinking of the eyelids when the cornea is touched with a wisp of cotton, can test the integrity of the ophthalmic division of CN V (trigeminal nerve). Posttraumatic strabismus indicates CN VI (abducens nerve) damage.

Eye movements are assessed by the doll's head manoeuvre, in which the child's head is rotated quickly to one side and then to the other. When the brainstem centres for eye movement are intact, there is conjugate (paired or working together) movement of the eyes in the direction opposite the head rotation. Absence of this response suggests dysfunction of the brainstem or CN III. Downward or lateral deviation is often observed in association with pupillary dilation in dysfunction of CN III.

Funduscopic examination reveals additional clues. Because it takes 24 to 48 hours to develop, papillo-oedema (e.g. optic disc swelling, indistinct margins, haemorrhages, tortuosity of vessels, absence of venous pulsations), if it develops at all, will not be evident early in the course of unconsciousness. The presence of retinal haemorrhages in children is usually the result of accidental or inflicted trauma with intracranial bleeding (usually subarachnoid or subdural haemorrhage) but is sometimes caused by infection (Minns et al 2017).

Motor Function

Observation of spontaneous activity, posture and response to painful stimuli provides clues to the location and extent of cerebral dysfunction. Asymmetrical movements of the limbs or the absence of movement suggests paralysis. In haemiplegia the affected limb lies in external rotation and falls uncontrollably when lifted and allowed to drop. Observations should be described rather than labelled.

In the deeper comatose states the child has little or no spontaneous movement, and the musculature tends to be flaccid. There is considerable variability in motor behaviour in lesser degrees of coma. For example, the child may be relatively immobile or restless and hyperkinetic; muscle tone may be increased or decreased. Tremors, twitching and spasms of muscles are common observations. The patient may display purposeless plucking or tossing movements. Combative or negativistic behaviour is not uncommon. Hyperactivity is more common in acute febrile and toxic states than in cases of increased ICP. Seizures are common in children and may be present in coma as a result of any cause. Any repetitive movements and movements during seizures are described.

Posturing

Primitive postural reflexes emerge as cortical control over motor function is lost in brain dysfunction. These reflexes are evident in posturing and motor movements directly related to the area of the brain involved. Posturing reflects a balance between the lower exciting and the higher inhibiting influences. Strong muscles overcome weaker ones. Flexion posturing (Fig 30.4A) occurs with severe dysfunction of the cerebral cortex or with lesions to corticospinal tracts above the brainstem. Typical flexion posturing includes rigid flexion, with arms held tightly to the body; flexed elbows, wrists and fingers; plantar flexed feet; legs extended and internally rotated; and possibly fine tremors or intense stiffness. Extension posturing (Fig 30.4B) is a sign of dysfunction at the level of the midbrain or lesions to the brainstem.

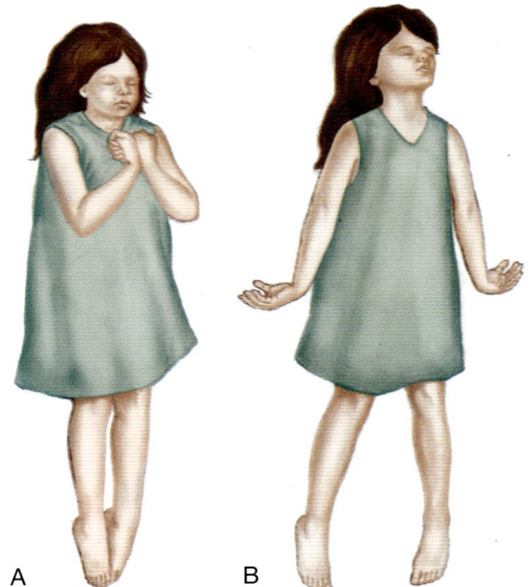

Fig 30.4 (**A**) Flexion posturing. (**B**) Extension posturing.

It is characterised by rigid extension and pronation of the arms and legs, flexed wrists and fingers, clenched jaw, extended neck and possibly an arched back. Unilateral extension posturing is often caused by tentorial herniation.

Posturing may not be evident when the child is quiet but can usually be elicited by applying painful stimuli such as a blunt object pressed on the base of the nail. Nurses should avoid applying thumb pressure to the supraorbital region of the frontal bone (risk of orbital damage). Noxious stimuli (e.g. suctioning), turning or touching will elicit a response. When the nurse is describing posturing, the stimulus needed to provoke the response is as important as the reaction.

Reflexes

Testing of certain reflexes, such as those present in an intact spinal cord, may be of limited value. In general, the corneal, pupillary, muscle-stretch, superficial and plantar reflexes tend to be absent in deep coma. The state of reflexes is variable in lighter grades of unconsciousness and depends on the underlying pathological process and the location of the lesion. The doll's eye reflex manoeuvre, described previously, reflects paralysis of CN III. The absence of corneal reflexes (CN V) and the presence of a tonic neck reflex are associated with severe brain damage. Babinski's reflex, in which the lateral portion of the bottom of the foot is stroked and causes the big toe to go up, may be of value if it is found to be present consistently in children older than 1 year. A positive Babinski's reflex is significant in the assessment of pyramidal tract lesions when it is unilateral and associated with other pyramidal signs. A fluctuating Babinski's reflex is often observed after seizures. (See Fig 7.7B.)

Special Diagnostic Procedures

Numerous diagnostic procedures are used for assessment of cerebral function. Laboratory tests that may help determine the cause of unconsciousness include blood glucose, urea nitrogen and electrolyte (pH, sodium, potassium, chloride, calcium and bicarbonate) tests; clotting studies, haematocrit and a full blood count; liver function tests; blood cultures if there is fever; and sometimes studies to detect lead or other toxic substances, such as drugs.

An electroencephalogram (EEG) may provide important information. For example, generalised random, slow activity may suggest suppressed cortical function, and localised slow activity may suggest a space-occupying lesion. A flat tracing is one of the criteria used as evidence of brain death. Examination of spinal fluid is carried out when toxic encephalopathy or infection is suspected. Lumbar puncture is delayed if intracranial haemorrhage is suspected, and is contraindicated in the presence of increased ICP because of the potential for brainstem herniation.

Auditory and visual evoked potentials are sometimes used in neurological evaluation of very young children. Brainstem auditory evoked potentials are useful for evaluating the continuity of brainstem auditory tracts and are particularly useful for detecting demyelinating disease and neoplasms of the brainstem and for distinguishing between brainstem and cortical lesions. For example, a normal evoked potential in a comatose patient suggests involvement of the cerebral hemispheres.

Highly sophisticated tests are carried out with specialised equipment. Two imaging techniques, computed tomography (CT) and magnetic resonance imaging (MRI), assist in diagnosis by scanning both soft tissues and solid matter. Most of these tests are listed in Table 30.1. Because these tests can be confronting to children, the nurse needs to prepare patients and their parents/guardians for the tests and provide support, distractions and reassurance during the tests. Consultation with a play specialist can also be helpful.

Children who are old enough to understand require careful explanation of the procedure, why it is being done, what they will experience and how they can help. School-age children usually appreciate a more detailed description of why contrast material is injected. Because children are often frightened of needles, they and their families need to be informed of any medication or contrast medium that will be administered intravenously. Special anxiety reduction strategies may be necessary for children who have blood-injury-injection (needle) phobia (McMurtry et al 2016). This phobia is the most inheritable of all phobias. The nurse should talk with parents to find out if they also have this phobia and will need help with anxiety management (Van Houtem et al 2013). When tests require venepuncture, the application of local anaesthetics can prevent pain and increase the chance of venepuncture success (Baxter et al 2013). Enlist the assistance of a play specialist who is invaluable at preparing children for procedures and a key part of the child health team.

The importance of lying still for tests needs to be stressed. Children unfamiliar with the machines can be shown a picture beforehand. Although radiographic examinations are not painful, the machinery often appears so frightening that the child protests because of anxiety. This is especially true of CT and MRI, both of which require that the child's head be placed within a special immobilising device. Chin and cheek pads are sometimes used to prevent the slightest head movement, and straps are applied to the body to prevent a slight change in body position. It is important to emphasise to the child that at no time is the procedure painful. There are many ways to help prepare a child for a CT or a MRI. This is usually a team approach done in partnership with the family. Many facilities have virtual reality experiences to prepare children for procedures such as this.

It is helpful for nurses to become acquainted with the equipment and the general environment in which the test will take place so they can better explain the procedure to children and their families at their level of understanding. Written material describing the procedure should be available for parents and may be appropriate to share with children. Equipment is often strange and ominous to children. They need constant reassurance from a trusted companion.

The nurse should not expect cooperation from a young child. Sedation may be required.

If a child does need to be sedated, they should be supported through the preparation and administration and assured that someone will remain with them (if this is possible). Children need continual support and reinforcement during procedures in which they remain conscious. Vital signs and physiological responses to the procedure are monitored throughout. Many diagnostic procedures performed on an outpatient basis require sedation, and children need recovery time and observation. The nurse should review written instructions with parents if the child is discharged after a procedure. Children who have undergone a procedure with a general anaesthetic require postanaesthesia care, including positioning to prevent aspiration of secretions and frequent assessment of vital signs, oxygen saturation and LOC. In addition, other neurological functions such as pupillary responses, motor strength and movement are tested at regular intervals. Any surgical wound resulting from the test is checked for bleeding, CSF leakage and other complications.

Consider children's emotional reactions to the procedure. They should be allowed and encouraged to express their feelings about the experience through verbal expression and therapeutic play. Parents also seek an explanation of the results of tests and procedures performed on their children. Nurses are in a unique position to provide support and education to parents regarding procedures.

THE CHILD WITH CEREBRAL COMPROMISE

Nursing Care of the Unconscious Child

The unconscious child requires nursing attendance with observation, recording and evaluation of changes in objective signs. These observations provide valuable information regarding the patient's progress and often serve as a guide to diagnosis and treatment. Therefore, careful and detailed observations are essential for the child's welfare. In addition, vital functions must be maintained and complications prevented through conscientious and meticulous nursing care. The outcome of unconsciousness is variable and ranges from early and complete recovery, to death within a few hours or days, or persistent and permanent unconsciousness, or recovery with varying degrees of residual mental or physical disability. The outcome and recovery of the unconscious child may depend on the level of nursing care and observational skills.

The nurse should direct emergency measures towards ensuring airway, breathing and circulation (ABC); stabilising the spine when indicated; treating shock; and reducing ICP (if present). Delayed treatment often leads to increased damage. Therapies for specific causes of unconsciousness begin as soon as emergency measures have been implemented; in many cases they occur concurrently. Because nursing care is closely related to the medical management, both are considered here.

Continual observation of the LOC, pupillary reaction and vital signs is essential to management of CNS disorders, and an integral part of nursing care. The frequency of observations depends on the cause of unconsciousness, the LOC and the progression of cerebral involvement. Intervals between observations may be as short as every 15 minutes or as long as every 2 hours. Significant alterations are reported immediately.

The temperature is measured every 2 to 4 hours, depending on the child's condition. An elevated temperature may occur in children with CNS dysfunction; therefore, a light covering may be sufficient. Vigorous efforts, such as tepid sponge baths or application of a hypothermia blanket, are needed to prevent brain damage if the temperature exceeds 40°C.

The LOC is assessed periodically, including pupillary size, equality and reaction to light. Signs of meningeal irritation, such as nuchal rigidity, need to be assessed. Assessment of LOC also includes response to vocal commands, spontaneous behaviour, resistance to care and

TABLE 30.1 Neurological Diagnostic Procedures

Test	Description	Purpose	Comments
Lumbar puncture (LP)	Spinal needle is inserted between L3 and L4 or L4 and L5 vertebral spaces into subarachnoid space; cerebrospinal fluid (CSF) pressure is measured, and sample is collected for examination.	Measures spinal fluid pressure Obtains CSF for laboratory analysis Injection of medication	Contraindicated in patients with increased ICP or infected skin over puncture site.
Subdural tap	Needle is inserted into anterior fontanel or coronal suture (midline to pupil).	Helps rule out subdural effusions Removes CSF to relieve pressure	Place infant in semierect position after subdural tap to minimise leakage from site; prevent child from crying if possible. Check site frequently for evidence of leakage.
Electroencephalography (EEG)	EEG records changes in electrical potential of brain. Electrodes are placed at various points to assess electrical function in a particular area. Impulses are recorded by electromagnetic pen or digitally.	Detects spikes, or bursts of electrical activity that indicate the potential for seizures Used to determine brain death	Patient should remain quiet during procedure; may require sedation. Minimise external stimuli during procedure.
Nuclear brain scan	Radioisotope is injected intravenously, then counted and recorded after fixed time intervals. Radioisotope accumulates in areas where blood–brain barrier is defective.	Identifies focal brain lesions (e.g. tumours, abscesses) Positive uptake of material with encephalitis and subdural haematoma Visualises CSF pathways	Requires intravenous (IV) access; patient may require sedation. In normal children or non-communicating hydrocephalus, no retrograde filling of ventricles occurs. Areas of concentrated uptake of material are termed *hot spots*.
Radiography	Skull films are taken from different views—lateral, posterolateral, axial (submentoventricular), half-axial.	Shows fractures, dislocations, spreading suture lines, craniostenosis Shows degenerative changes, bone erosion, calcifications	Simple, non-invasive procedure.
Computed tomography (CT) scan	Pinpoint x-ray beam is directed on horizontal or vertical plane to provide series of images that are fed into computer and assembled in image displayed on video screen. CT uses ionising radiation.	Visualises horizontal and vertical cross-section of brain in three planes (axial, coronal, sagittal) Distinguishes density of various intracranial tissues and structures—congenital abnormalities, haemorrhage, tumours, demyelinating and inflammatory processes, calcification	Requires IV access if contrast agent is used. Patient may require sedation.
Magnetic resonance imaging (MRI)	MRI produces radiofrequency emissions from elements (e.g. hydrogen, phosphorus) which are converted to visual images by computer.	Permits visualisation of morphological feature of target structures Permits tissue discrimination unavailable with many techniques	MRI is non-invasive procedure except when IV contrast agent is used. No exposure to radiation occurs. Patient may require sedation. MRI does not visualise bone detail or calcifications. No metal can be present in scanner.
Positron emission tomography (PET)	PET involves IV injection of positron-emitting radionucleotide; local concentrations are detected and transformed into visual display by computer.	Detects and measures blood volume and flow in brain, metabolic activity, biochemical changes within tissue	Requires lengthy period of immobility. Minimum exposure to radiation occurs. Patient may require sedation.

response to painful stimuli. Note any abnormal movements, changes in muscle tone or strength and body position. If a seizure occurs, describe the seizure, including the body areas involved from the beginning to the end of the seizure and the duration of seizure (see Box 30.9 later in this chapter).

Pain management for the unconscious child requires astute nursing observation and management and depends on the child's age and stage. Signs of pain include changes in behaviour (e.g. increased agitation and rigidity) and alterations in vital signs and perfusion (usually, an increased heart rate, respiratory rate and blood pressure and decreased oxygen saturation). Because these findings are not specific for pain, the nurse should be alert for their appearance during times of induced or suspected pain and for their disappearance after the inciting procedure or the administration of analgesia. A pain assessment record is used to document indications of pain and the effectiveness of interventions. The use of opioids, such as morphine, to relieve pain is controversial because they can mask signs of altered consciousness or depressed respirations. However, unrelieved pain activates the stress response, which can elevate ICP. To block the stress response, some practitioners advocate the use of analgesics, sedatives and, in some cases such as head injury, paralysing agents via continuous IV infusion. A commonly used combination is fentanyl, midazolam and vecuronium. If there are concerns about assessing the LOC or respiratory depression, naloxone can be used to reverse the opioid effects. Paracetamol and ibuprofen may also be effective analgesics for mild to moderate pain (Whittaker 2013). Regardless of the drugs used, adequate dosage and regular administration are essential to provide optimum pain relief.

Other measures to relieve discomfort include providing a quiet, dimly lit environment; limiting visitors; preventing any sudden, jarring movement, such as banging into the bed; limiting screen time; and preventing an increase in ICP. The latter is most effectively achieved by proper positioning and prevention of straining, such as during coughing, vomiting or defecating. Antiepileptic drugs, such as phenytoin or phenobarbitone, may be ordered for control of seizure activity.

Respiratory Management

Respiratory effectiveness is the primary concern in the care of the unconscious child, and establishment of an adequate airway is always the first priority. Carbon dioxide has a potent vasodilating effect and will increase CBF and ICP. Cerebral hypoxia at normal body temperature that lasts longer than 4 minutes often causes irreversible brain damage.

Children in lighter stages of coma may be able to cough and swallow, but those in deeper states of coma are unable to manage secretions, which tend to pool in the throat and pharynx. Dysfunction of CNs IX and X (glossopharyngeal and vagus nerves) places the child at risk of aspiration and cardiac arrest. Therefore, position the child with the head and body to the side to prevent aspiration of secretions, and empty the stomach to reduce the likelihood of vomiting. In infants, the blockage of air passages from secretions can happen in seconds. In addition, upper airway obstruction from laryngospasm is a common complication in comatose children.

An oral airway can be used for the child who is suffering a temporary loss of consciousness, such as after a contusion, seizure or anaesthesia. For children who remain unconscious for a longer time, a nasotracheal or orotracheal tube is inserted to maintain the open airway and facilitate removal of secretions. A tracheostomy is performed in cases in which laryngoscopy for introduction of an endotracheal tube would be difficult or dangerous or for a child who needs long-term ventilatory support. Suctioning is used only as needed to clear the airway, exerting care to prevent increasing ICP. Respiratory status is observed and evaluated regularly. Signs of respiratory distress may indicate a need for ventilator assistance.

Mechanical ventilation is usually indicated when the respiratory centre is involved. Blood gas analysis is performed regularly, and oxygen is administered when indicated. Moderately severe hypoxia and respiratory acidosis are often present, but they are not always evident from clinical manifestations. Hypoventilation often accompanies unconsciousness and may lead to respiratory alkalosis, or it may represent the body's attempt to compensate for metabolic acidosis. Therefore, blood gas and pH determinations are essential guides for electrolyte therapy. Chest physiotherapy is carried out on a regular basis, and the child's position is changed at least every 2 hours to prevent pulmonary complications. Regular oral hygiene is recommended to reduce the risk of ventilator-associated pneumonia (VAP) (Hua et al 2016).

Intracranial Pressure Monitoring

The selection of the type of ICP monitor should be guided by the clinical presentation and the therapeutic strategy chosen for each child. Indications for inserting an ICP monitor are: (1) GCS evaluation ≤ 8; (2) GCS evaluation > 8 with respiratory assistance; (3) deterioration of condition; and (4) subjective judgment regarding clinical appearance and response (Singhi & Tiwari 2009).

Four major types of ICP monitors are intraventricular catheter with or without fibroscopic sensors attached to a monitoring system, subarachnoid bolt (Richmond screw), epidural sensor and anterior fontanel pressure monitor. Transducers for both ventricular and subarachnoid monitoring should be set up without the use of a flush device. Direct ventricular pressure measurement remains the gold standard of ICP monitoring.

The catheter method involves introduction of a catheter into the lateral ventricle on the non-dominant side, if known, or placement in the subdural space. The catheter has the advantage of providing a means of extraventricular (or continuous) drainage of CSF to reduce pressure. A drainage bag attached to the system is kept at the level of the ventricles and can be lowered to decrease ICP. This device requires full penetration of the brain, requires skill and experience with placement and carries the risk of infection. Infection risks can be lowered by always using aseptic technique when handling the external ventricular drainage (EVD) system, manipulating the EVD as little as possible and sterile dressing changes only weekly or when the dressing is compromised, whichever occurs first (Hepburn-Smith et al 2016).

> **NURSING CARE CONSIDERATIONS**
>
> If the external ventricular drain is unclamped for CSF drainage, carefully monitor the level of the collection container. If the container is positioned too low, improper CSF decompression could lower ICP too rapidly, causing bleeding and pain.

With the bolt method the end of the bolt is placed into the subarachnoid space. The bolt cannot be adequately secured in a small child's pliant skull, although special modifications have been developed for children under 6 years of age. The placement of the bolt is not adjusted by anyone except the neurosurgeon who placed the device. The neurosurgeon is notified if a satisfactory waveform is not observed.

An epidural sensor can be placed between the dura and the skull through a burr hole and connected to a stopcock assembly and a transducer, which provides a readout of the pressure. Although less invasive, the epidural sensor may have inconsistent correlation of pressure readings. In infants a fontanel transducer can be used to detect impulses from a pressure sensor and convert them to electrical energy. The electrical energy is then converted to visible waves or numeric readings on an oscilloscope. ICP measurement from the anterior fontanel is non-invasive but may prove to be inaccurate if the equipment is poorly placed or inconsistently recalibrated. Intraparenchymal pressure monitoring devices (e.g. Camino) use fibreoptic technology and perform reliably.

ICP can be increased by direct instillation of solutions; therefore, antibiotics are administered systemically if a positive CSF culture is obtained. However, ICP monitoring rarely causes infection. CSF is a body fluid; therefore, implement standard precautions according to hospital policy.

Nurses caring for patients with intracranial monitoring devices must be acquainted with the system, assist with insertion, interpret the monitor readings and be able to distinguish between danger signals and mechanical dysfunction. Because systemic blood pressure, ICP and therefore CPP are normally lower in children, the child's age must be taken into account when deciding what constitutes abnormally high ICP or abnormally low CPP.

Several medical measures are available to treat increased ICP resulting from cerebral oedema. These include sedation, CSF drainage and osmotic diuretics. Osmotic diuretics may provide rapid relief of ICP in emergency situations. Although their effect is transient, lasting only about 6 hours, they can be lifesaving in emergencies. These substances are rapidly excreted by the kidneys and carry with them large quantities of sodium and water. Mannitol administered intravenously is the drug most commonly used for rapid reduction of ICP. The infusion is generally given slowly but may be pushed rapidly if there is herniation or impending herniation. Because of the profound diuretic effect of the drug, an indwelling catheter is inserted to ensure bladder emptying. $PaCO_2$ should be maintained at approximately 30 mmHg to produce vasoconstriction, which reduces CBF, thereby decreasing ICP. Recording and analysing the child's volume state, plasma sodium concentration and serum osmolarity can avert potential fluid and electrolyte problems. Administration of adrenocorticosteroids is not recommended for cerebral oedema secondary to head trauma.

Nursing Activities. In cases of high levels of increased ICP, nursing procedures tend to trigger reactive pressure waves in many children. For example, increased intrathoracic or abdominal pressure will be transmitted to the cranium. The goals of monitoring a child who is neurologically compromised include: maintaining CPP; controlling ICP, cerebral oedema and factors that increase cerebral metabolism (e.g. fever, seizures); and maintaining haemodynamic stability. Take particular care in positioning these patients to avoid neck vein compression that may further increase ICP by interfering with venous return.

NURSING CARE CONSIDERATIONS

Elevate the head of the bed 15 to 30 degrees, and position the child so that the head is maintained in midline to facilitate venous drainage and avoid jugular compression. Turning side to side is contraindicated because of the risk of jugular compression.

Sandbags or other support devices can help maintain correct head position. The child can be propped to one side or the other, and the use of a pressure-relieving or pressure-decreasing mattress decreases the chance of prolonged pressure to vulnerable skin areas. Frequent clinical assessment of the child cannot be replaced by an ICP monitoring device.

It is important to avoid activities that may increase ICP by causing pain or emotional stress. Clustering nursing activities together and minimising environmental stimuli by decreasing noxious procedures help control ICP. Range-of-motion exercises can be carried out gently but should not be performed vigorously. Any necessary disturbing procedures should be scheduled to take advantage of therapies that reduce ICP, such as osmotherapy and sedation. Make efforts to minimise or eliminate environmental noise, including managing the number of visitors. Assessment and intervention to relieve pain are important nursing functions to decrease ICP. Children with a raised ICP are usually cared for in a high dependency unit (HDU) or intensive care unit (ICU). Suctioning and percussion are often poorly tolerated; therefore, these procedures are contraindicated unless the child has concurrent respiratory problems. Hypoxia and the Valsalva manoeuvre associated with cough acutely elevate ICP. Vibration, which does not increase ICP, accomplishes excellent results and should be tried first if treatment is needed. If suctioning is necessary, it should be used judiciously and preceded by hyperventilation with 100% oxygen, which can be monitored during suctioning with a pulse oxygen sensor reading to determine oxygen saturation.

Nutrition and Hydration

In the unconscious child, fluids and calories are supplied initially by the IV route. The type of fluid administered depends on the patient's general condition. Children on the ketogenic diet and with certain metabolic disorders, such as pyruvate dehydrogenase deficiency, should receive normal saline rather than fluids containing glucose, which can cause seizures and worsen their condition. Fluid therapy requires careful monitoring and adjustment based on neurological signs and electrolyte determinations. Often, unconscious children cannot tolerate the same amounts of fluid as when they are healthy. Overhydration must be avoided to prevent fatal cerebral oedema. When cerebral oedema is a threat, fluids may be restricted to reduce the chance of fluid overload. Examine skin and mucous membranes for signs of dehydration. Adjustments to fluid administration are based on urinary output, serum electrolytes and osmolarity, blood pressure and arterial filling pressure. Observation for signs of altered fluid balance related to abnormal pituitary secretions is a part of nursing care.

Provide long-term nutrition in a balanced formula given by nasogastric or gastrostomy tube. The nasogastric tube is usually taped in place, with care taken to prevent pressure on the nares. Most children have continuous feedings. When bolus feedings are used, the tube is rinsed with water after each feeding. Tubes are replaced according to institutional policy. Irritation of the nasal mucosa is prevented by alternating nares each time the nasogastric tube is replaced.

Avoid overfeeding to prevent vomiting and the associated risk of aspiration. Stomach contents are aspirated with a syringe and measured before feeding to ascertain the amount remaining in the stomach. The removed contents may be refed. If the residual volume is excessive (depending on the child's size), consult the dietitian and medical practitioner regarding the composition and amount to determine whether changes are required to provide calories and nutrients in a smaller volume.

Altered Pituitary Secretion. An altered ability to handle fluid loads is attributed in part to the syndrome of inappropriate antidiuretic hormone (SIADH) and diabetes insipidus (DI) resulting from hypothalamic dysfunction. (See Chapter 31.) SIADH often accompanies CNS conditions such as head injury, meningitis, encephalitis, brain abscess, brain tumour and subarachnoid haemorrhage. In the child with SIADH, scant quantities of urine are excreted, electrolyte analysis reveals hyponatraemia and hypo-osmolality, and manifestations of over-hydration are evident. It is important to evaluate all parameters because the reduced urinary output might be erroneously interpreted as a sign of dehydration. The treatment of SIADH consists of fluid restriction until serum electrolytes and osmolality return to normal levels. If fluid restriction is not completely ineffective, medications such as sodium chloride and diuretics may be used.

DI may occur after intracranial trauma. In DI there is increased urinary volume and the accompanying danger of dehydration. See Table 30.2 for comparison of fluid changes in DI and SIADH. Adequate replacement of fluids is essential, and observation of electrolyte bal-

TABLE 30.2 Effects of Altered Pituitary Secretion

Measurement	Diabetes Insipidus	Syndrome of Inappropriate Antidiuretic Hormone Secretion
Urinary output	Increased	Decreased
Specific gravity	Decreased	Increased
Serum sodium	Increased (hypernatraemia)	Decreased (hyponatraemia)

ance is necessary to detect signs of hypernatraemia and hyperosmolality. Exogenous vasopressin may be administered.

Medications

The cause of unconsciousness determines specific drug therapies. Children with infectious processes are given antibiotics appropriate to the disease and the infecting organism. Corticosteroids are prescribed for inflammatory conditions and oedema. Cerebral oedema is an indication for osmotic diuretics. Antiepileptic medications are prescribed for seizure activity. Sedation in the combative child provides amnesic and anxiolytic properties in conjunction with a paralytic agent. This combination decreases ICP and allows treatment of cerebral oedema. Usual drugs include morphine and midazolam. Midazolam is attractive because of its short half-life.

Deep coma induced by the administration of barbiturates is controversial in the management of ICP. Barbiturates are currently reserved for the reduction of increased ICP when all else has failed. Barbiturates decrease the cerebral metabolic rate for oxygen and protect the brain during times of reduced CPP. Barbiturate coma requires extensive monitoring. EEG monitoring can assess depth of coma, record EEG background abnormalities that can help predict outcome and evaluate any seizure activity. Cardiovascular and respiratory support and ICP monitoring are needed to assess response to therapy. Paralysing agents such as vecuronium may be needed to aid in performing diagnostic tests, improving effectiveness of therapy and reducing the risks of secondary complications. Elevation of ICP or heart rate in patients who are being given paralysing agents or are under sedation may indicate the need for another dose of either or both medications or the need for pain medication.

Thermoregulation

Hyperthermia often accompanies cerebral dysfunction; if it is present, the nurse implements measures to reduce the temperature to prevent brain damage from hyperthermia and to reduce metabolic demands generated by the increased body temperature. Antipyretics are the method of choice for fever reduction; cooling devices are used for hyperthermia. Laboratory tests and other methods help determine the cause, if any, of the hyperthermia. Treatment with hypothermia and barbiturates increases the risk of iatrogenic complications.

Elimination

A urinary catheter may be inserted in the acute phase, but nappies may be used and weighed to record urinary output. The child who previously had bowel and bladder control is generally incontinent. If the child remains comatose for a long period, the indwelling catheter may be removed and periodic bladder emptying accomplished by intermittent catheterisation. Stool softeners are usually sufficient to maintain bowel function, but suppositories or enemas may be needed occasionally for adequate elimination and to prevent faecal impaction. The passage of liquid stool after a period of no bowel activity is usually a sign of impaction. To avoid this preventable problem, daily recording of bowel activity is essential.

Hygienic Care. Routine measures for cleansing and maintaining skin integrity are an integral part of nursing care of the unconscious child. Skinfolds require special attention to prevent excoriation. The child who is unable to move is prone to develop tissue breakdown and necrosis; therefore, the child is placed on a resilient appliance (e.g. air mattress) to prevent pressure on prominent areas of the body. The goal is prevention by regular change of position and inspection of vulnerable areas (e.g. the ankle, heels, trochanter, sacrum and shoulder). Unconscious children undergo numerous invasive procedures, and the skin sites used for these procedures require special assessment and intervention to promote healing and prevent infection. Keep bed linen and any clothing dry and free of wrinkles. Rubbing the back and extremities with lotion stimulates circulation and helps prevent drying of the skin. However, to prevent further tissue damage, do not massage reddened and non-blanching skin. If the child requires surgery or radiography, the nurse checks all dressings, bony sites, catheters and IV access lines before and after the procedure.

Oral care is performed at least twice daily because the mouth tends to become dry or coated with mucus. The teeth are carefully brushed with a soft toothbrush or cleaned with gauze saturated with saline. Lips are coated with ointment to protect them from drying, cracking or blistering.

The unconscious child is also prone to eye irritation. The corneal reflexes are absent; therefore, the eyes are easily irritated or damaged by linen, dust or other substances that may come in contact with them. Excessive dryness results from incomplete closure of the lids and/or decreased secretions, especially if the child is undergoing osmotherapy to reduce or prevent brain oedema.

Keep the child's hair combed and secure to prevent tangling. Keep the scalp clean with dry or wet shampoos as needed. The child's head may need to be shaved for tests or surgical procedures. It is important to consider any cultural practices in regard to hygiene. For example, many Māori families may want any hair that is shaved to be returned to them.

Positioning and Exercise. The unconscious child is positioned to minimise ICP and to prevent aspiration of saliva, nasogastric secretions and vomitus. The head of the bed is elevated, and the child is placed in a side-lying or semiprone position. A small, firm pillow is placed under the head, and the uppermost limbs are flexed and supported with pillows. The weight of the body should not rest on the dependent arm. In the semiprone position the child lies with the dependent arm at the side behind the body; the opposite side is supported on pillows, and the uppermost arm and leg are flexed and resting on the pillows. This position prevents undue pressure on the dependent extremities. The dependent position of the face encourages drainage of secretions and prevents the flaccid tongue from obstructing the airway.

Normal range-of-motion exercises help maintain function and prevent contractures of joints. Perform exercises gently to minimise increasing ICP and with full range of motion. Place a small rolled pad in the palms to help maintain proper positioning of fingers. Splinting may be needed to prevent severe contractures of the wrists, knees or ankles.

Stimulation

Sensory stimulation is as important in the care of the unconscious child as it is in the care of the alert child. For the temporarily unconscious or semiconscious child, sensory stimulation helps arouse the child to the conscious state and orient the child in terms of time and place. Auditory and tactile stimulation are especially valuable. Tactile stimulation is not appropriate for a child in whom it may elicit an undesirable response. However, for other children tactile contact often has a relaxing and calming effect. When the child's condition permits, holding or rocking the child is soothing and provides the body contact needed by young children.

Hearing is often intact in a state of coma. Hearing is the last sense to be lost and the first one to be regained; therefore, speak to the child as any other child. Conversation around the child should not include thoughtless or derogatory remarks. Soft music is often used to provide auditory stimulation. Singing the child's favourite songs or reading a favourite story is a strategy used to maintain the child's contact with a familiar world. Playing songs or favourite stories recorded in the parents' voices can provide a continuous source of familiar stimulation.

Family Support

Helping the parents of an unconscious child cope with the situation is especially difficult. They may demonstrate all the guilt, fear, hostility and anxiety of any parent of a seriously ill child. In addition, these parents face the uncertain outcome of the cerebral dysfunction. The fear of death, cognitive impairment or permanent physical disability is present. Nursing intervention with parents depends on the nature of the pathological condition, the parents' coping skills and the parent–child relationship before injury or illness.

Recovering from coma is a complex process and may be confusing for parents and family members, who are already anxious and overwhelmed. Understanding the stages of recovery may assist parents in coping with the situation. It is important to remember that comatose children may not complete all stages of the recovery process and that they may manifest characteristics of more than one stage at a time.

Level 1: No response—Child does not respond to stimuli but may be able to hear what is said in the room.

Level 2: Generalised response—Child responds to painful or unpleasant stimuli; responses may not be consistent and may be delayed.

Level 3: Localised response—Child responds purposefully to painful or unpleasant stimuli by trying to pull away; turns towards sounds; responds inconsistently to simple commands.

Level 4: Confused, agitated—Child becomes restless, aggressive, frustrated; exhibits abnormal behaviour; forgets answers to frequently asked questions.

Level 5: Confused, inappropriate—Child behaves more calmly; behaviour starts to normalise, but child may become frustrated; voice and face lack expression; follows simple commands; performs simple tasks.

Level 6: Confused, appropriate—Child is less frustrated and is able to concentrate for longer periods (up to 30 minutes); short-term memory is improving; responses to questions are more appropriate but may not be correct.

Level 7: Automatic, appropriate—Child's memory continues to improve, although details may not be clear; continues to have difficulty concentrating; decreased safety awareness and judgment.

Level 8: Purposeful—Child's basic thinking skills will have recovered to the maximum extent; incidental changes in social skills, memory and concentration may continue for months; child will fully understand what happened and may grieve over how things have changed. (Stages for recovery are based on the Rancho Levels of Cognitive Functioning, copyright Los Amigos Research and Educational Institute, 1990.)

Awakening from a coma is a gradual process; however, some children regain consciousness within a short time. If there is little or no residual effect, the child is discharged home fairly soon. The parents need the most intensive nursing intervention during the period of crisis and uncertainty. During the recovery phase the nurse gives them information, clarifies it as needed and encourages them to become involved in the child's care. Often the child's hospitalisation is brief; however, some children require extended hospitalisation for intensive therapy and rehabilitation. The parents of children who die require support and guidance to cope with the reality of the death and to resolve their grief.

Probably the most difficult situations are those that involve children who never regain consciousness. Unlike losing a child through death, these children lack finality, which often leaves the parents in a state of suspended grief. Like parents of dying children, parents of comatose children search for any signs of hope. Well-meaning friends and relatives relate instances of miraculous recoveries. The parents seek confirmation and support for such possibilities and assign erroneous meanings to any sign in the child that might be interpreted as evidence of recovery (e.g. reflexive muscle contractions).

At these times nurses need to respond with compassion and honesty. They can acknowledge that miraculous recoveries do occur but are rare. The important message is to maintain open communication with the family. It is also crucial to enlist the support of other services. Most services will have Aboriginal and Torres Strait Islander or Māori and Pacific Islander support workers to support families from a cultural perspective.

Like parents who lose a child through death, the parents of a child who is unconscious attempt to construct a representation of the child. They bring items that belong to the child, such as favourite toys or music. This may be interpreted as an attempt to provide stimulation for the child in the hope of eliciting a response, to let the hospital staff know the child as the unique individual he or she was and to reconstitute an image of the child 'lost' to them and for whom they mourn. The nurses' recognition and understanding of these behaviours and coping mechanisms is important to support the parents in their grief process.

In addition to the process of grieving for the 'lost' child, the parents may face difficult decisions. When the child's brain is so severely damaged that vital functions must be maintained by artificial means, the parents must make the final decision whether to remove the life-support systems and allow a natural death (Chen & Azueta 2017). After parents are provided with information about what allowing a natural death and removal from life-support mean, the parents may turn to both the provider and the nurses with their questions and concerns. Nurses play a critical role in assisting families in participating in their child's care to the greatest extent possible and in planning the child's death when that is the inevitable outcome of their neurological disorder (Bloomer et al 2016).

When the child has survived the cerebral insult but is physically and/or mentally limited, either minimally or severely, families must cope with and make decisions about the rehabilitation process and uncertain outcome. The family may need to make decisions whether to place their child in a chronic care facility or to care for their child at home. The drain on financial, emotional and social resources can be enormous.

For parents who choose to care for their child at home, planning begins early in the recovery process. Family members should become involved with the child's care as soon as they indicate an interest and ability to do so. They need education and support in learning to care for the child, regular follow-up observation and planning for home equipment, nursing and respite care. Parents need to understand that it is important to plan for periodic relief from the continuous care of the child.

Head Injury

Head injury is a pathological process involving the scalp, skull, meninges or brain as a result of mechanical force. Unintentional injuries are a health risk for children, with children less than 1 year of age having a significantly higher rate of severe head injury.

Aetiology

The most common causes of head injury in children are falls mainly from play equipment and trampolines, being struck by or striking an object with one's head and motor vehicle crashes. Neurological injury accounts for the highest mortality rate, with boys usually affected twice as often as girls. There are a number of head trauma strategies, including safety gates on stairs, restricting sleeping in the top bunk to children older than 6 years of age, seat belts and car seat use, and helmets during recreational activities such as biking and skateboarding. Furthermore, preventing child abuse is necessary and possible.

Many of the physical characteristics of children predispose them to craniocerebral trauma. For example, infants are often left unattended on beds, in high chairs and in other places from which they can fall. Because the head of an infant or toddler is proportionately large and heavy in relation to other body parts, it is the most likely to be injured. Incomplete motor development contributes to falls at young ages, and the natural curiosity and exuberance of children increase their risk for injury.

Pathophysiology

The pathology of brain injury is directly related to the force of impact. Intracranial contents (brain, blood, CSF) are damaged because the force is too great to be absorbed by the skull and musculoligamentous support of the head. Although nervous tissue is delicate, it usually requires a severe blow to cause significant damage.

A child's response to head injury is different to that of adults. The larger head size in proportion to body size and insufficient musculoskeletal support render the very young child particularly vulnerable to acceleration-deceleration injuries.

Primary head injuries are those that occur at the time of trauma and include skull fractures, contusions, intracranial haematomas and diffuse injuries. Subsequent complications include hypoxic brain injury, increased ICP and cerebral oedema. The predominant feature of a child's brain injury is the diffuse amount of swelling that occurs. Hypoxia and hypercapnia threaten the energy requirements of the brain and increase CBF. The added volume across the BBB along with the loss of autoregulation exacerbates cerebral oedema. Pressure inside the skull that is greater than arterial pressure results in inadequate perfusion. Because the cranium of very young children has the ability to expand and the thin skull is more compliant, they may tolerate increases in ICP better than older children and adults.

Physical forces act on the head through acceleration, deceleration or deformation. Acceleration or deceleration is more descriptive of the circumstances responsible for most head injuries. When the stationary head receives a blow, the sudden acceleration causes deformation of the skull and mass movement of the brain. Continued movement of the intracranial contents allows the brain to strike parts of the skull (e.g. the sharp edges of the sphenoid or the irregular surface of the anterior fossa) or the edges of the tentorium.

Although the brain volume remains unchanged, significant distortion and cavitation occur as the brain changes shape in response to the force transmitted from the impact to the skull. This deformation can cause bruising at the point of impact (coup) or at a distance as the brain collides with the unyielding surfaces opposite or far removed from the point of impact (contrecoup) (Fig 30.5). Thus a blow to the occipital region can cause severe injury to the frontal and temporal areas of the brain.

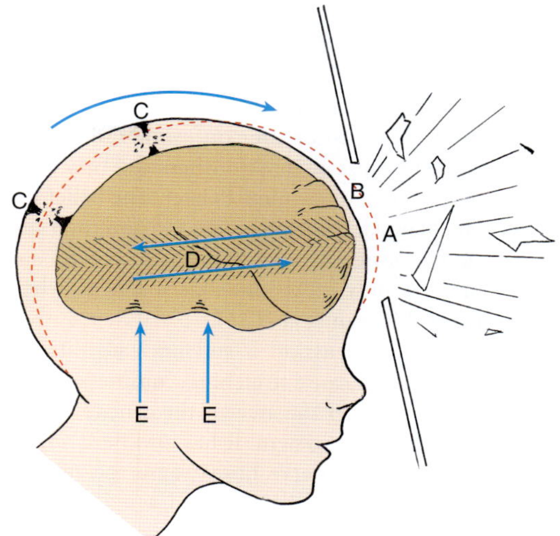

Fig 30.5 Mechanical distortion of cranium during closed head injury. (**A**) Preinjury contour of skull. (**B**) Immediate postinjury contour of skull. (**C**) Torn subdural vessels. (**D**) Shearing forces. (**E**) Trauma from contact with floor of cranium. (Source: Redrawn from Grubb, R. L., & Coxe, W. S. (1974). Central nervous system trauma: Cranial. In S. G. Eliasson, A. L. Presky, & W. B. Hardin (Eds.), Neurological pathophysiology. New York: Oxford University Press.)

When a moving head strikes a stationary surface, such as during a fall, sudden deceleration occurs and causes the greatest cerebral injury at the point of impact. Deceleration is responsible for most severe brainstem injuries.

Children with an acceleration-deceleration injury demonstrate diffuse generalised cerebral swelling produced by increased blood volume or by a redistribution of cerebral blood volume (cerebral hyperaemia) rather than by the increased water content (oedema).

Another effect of brain movement is shearing forces, which are caused by unequal movement or different rates of acceleration at various levels of the brain. A shearing force may tear small arteries that travel from the cerebral surfaces through the meninges to the dural sinuses and cause subdural haemorrhages. Shearing or stretching effects can also be transmitted to nerve fibres. Maximum stress from the shearing force occurs at the interface between structures of different density so that the grey matter (cell body) rapidly accelerates, whereas the white matter (axons) tends to lag behind. Although maximum shearing forces are at the cerebral surface and extend towards the centre of rotation within the brain, the most serious effects are often in the area of the brainstem. Severe compression of the skull can cause the brain to be forced through the tentorial opening and produce irreparable damage to the brainstem.

A GCS value of 8 or less in paediatric patients indicates severe injury and requires aggressive therapeutic management (Hartman & Cheifetz 2016). Three out of four children with a score of 3 or 4 will be severely disabled, be in a persistent vegetative state or die within a year of their injury (Fulkerson et al 2015). There are a number of studies that indicate the Simplified Motor Scale (SMS) is equivalent to the GCS in predictive power but the GCS is better for prognosticating death (Singh et al 2013).

Concussion. The most common and mildest traumatic brain injury is **concussion**, an alteration in mental status with or without loss of consciousness that occurs immediately after a head injury

(McCrea et al 2017). Direct head trauma and 'whiplash' seen with rapid acceleration and deceleration of the head are the most frequent causes in children. Sports-related activities are responsible for the majority of concussions (Mullally 2017).

The hallmarks of a concussion are confusion and amnesia. These are often not preceded by loss of consciousness and may occur immediately after the injury or several minutes later. The belief that loss of consciousness is the hallmark of concussion is a common misconception. A recent study among 182 adolescent athletes who sustained a concussion found that only 22% lost consciousness, whereas 34% experienced amnesia (Meehan et al 2013).

The pathogenesis of concussion is still unclear, but it may be a result of shearing forces that cause stretching, compression and tearing of nerve fibres, particularly in the area of the central brainstem, the seat of the reticular activating system. It has also been suggested that the anatomical alterations of nerve fibres cause the release of large quantities of acetylcholine into the CSF and a reduction in oxygen consumption with increased lactate production.

Contusion and Laceration. The terms *contusion* and *laceration* are used to describe visible bruising and tearing of cerebral tissue. Contusions represent petechial haemorrhages or localised bruising along the superficial aspects of the brain at the site of impact (coup injury) or a lesion remote from the site of direct trauma (contrecoup injury). In serious accidents there may be multiple sites of injury.

The major areas of the brain susceptible to contusion or laceration are the occipital, frontal and temporal lobes. In addition, the irregular surfaces of the anterior and middle fossae at the base of the skull are capable of producing bruises or lacerations on forceful impact. Contusions may cause focal disturbances in strength, sensation or visual awareness. The degree of brain damage in the contused areas varies according to the extent of vascular injury. Signs vary from mild, transient weakness of a limb to prolonged unconsciousness and paralysis. However, the signs and symptoms may be clinically indistinguishable from those of concussion.

Infants who are roughly shaken, referred to as shaken baby syndrome or abusive head trauma, can sustain profound neurological impairment, seizures, retinal haemorrhages (usually bilateral) and intracranial subarachnoid or subdural haemorrhages (Sieswerda-Hoogendoorn et al 2012).

Cerebral lacerations are generally associated with penetrating or depressed skull fractures. However, they may occur without fracture in small children. When brain tissue is actually torn, with bleeding into and around the tear, more severe and prolonged unconsciousness and paralysis usually occur, leaving permanent scarring and some degree of disability.

Fractures. Skull fractures result from a direct blow or injury to the skull and are often associated with intracranial injury. Many of the falls that resulted in a skull fracture in children younger than 2 years of age involved short distances of less than a metre, such as falls from a caregiver's arms (Burrows et al 2015).

The types of skull fractures that occur are linear, comminuted, depressed, open, basilar and growing fractures. As a rule, the faster the blow, the greater the likelihood of a depressed fracture; a low-velocity impact tends to produce a linear fracture.

Linear skull fractures are a single fracture line that starts at the point of maximum impact and spreads; however, they do not cross suture lines. Linear skull fractures constitute the majority of childhood skull fractures and typically occur in the parietal bone. Most linear skull fractures are associated with an overlying scalp haematoma, particularly in infants younger than 2 years of age and in the parietal or temporal region (Burns et al 2016). Scalp haematomas, in turn, are associated with the presence of intracranial injury whether there is a linear fracture or not (Burns et al 2016).

Comminuted fractures consist of multiple associated linear fractures. They usually result from intense impact, often from repeated blows against an object or ejection from a car at a high rate of speed. They may suggest child abuse.

Depressed fractures are those in which the bone is locally broken, usually into several irregular fragments that are pushed inwards. The greater the depression, the higher the risk of a tear in the dura or cortical laceration. Depressed skull fractures may be associated with direct underlying parenchymal damage and should be suspected when a child's head appears misshapen. Surgery may be needed to elevate the depressed bone fragment if there is an associated intracranial haematoma and if the depression is greater than 1 cm.

Basilar fractures involve the bones at the base of the skull in either the posterior or the anterior region. The bones involved are the ethmoid, sphenoid, temporal or occipital bones. These fractures usually result in a dural tear. Because of the proximity of the fracture line to structures surrounding the brainstem, a basal skull fracture is a serious head injury. Basilar fractures often involve frontal bone fractures. This can result in clinical features such as leakage of CSF from the nose (CSF rhinorrhoea) or ear (CSF otorrhoea), blood behind the tympanic membrane (haemotympanum), subcutaneous bleeding over the mastoid process that is located posterior to the ear and subcutaneous bleeding around the orbit (Bonfield et al 2014). Meningitis, although rare, is always a potential risk with CSF leakage.

Open fractures result in a communication between the skull and the scalp or the mucosa of the upper respiratory tract. The risk of CNS infection is increased with open fractures. Compound fractures consist of a skin laceration overlying the bone fracture. Open fractures that involve the paranasal sinuses or middle ear may lead to leakage of CSF (rhinorrhoea or otorrhoea). Prophylactic antibiotics are recommended to prevent osteomyelitis.

Growing skull fracture is an unusual complication of head trauma. The fracture is accompanied by an underlying tear in the dura or brain injury that fails to heal properly. A leptomeningeal cyst, dilated ventricles or herniated brain may result and cause growth of the original fracture. The majority of growing skull fractures occur before 30 months of age and occur in the parietal bone (Vezina et al 2017). Physical examination usually shows a swelling scalp and skull defect. Clinical neurological symptoms may be delayed for months to years after the initial skull fracture and include headache, seizures, hemiparesis and learning and intellectual disabilities (Vezina et al 2017).

Complications

The major complications of trauma to the head are haemorrhage, infection, oedema and herniation through the brainstem. Infection is always a hazard in open injuries. Oedema is related to tissue trauma. Vascular rupture may occur even in minor head injuries, causing haemorrhage between the skull and cerebral surfaces. Compression of the underlying brain produces effects that can be rapidly fatal or insidiously progressive.

Epidural Haematoma. Epidural (extradural) haematoma is a haemorrhage into the space between the dura and the skull. As the haematoma enlarges, the dura is stripped from the skull; this accumulation of blood results in a mass effect on the brain, forcing the underlying brain contents downwards as it expands (Fig 30.6A). Because bleeding is generally arterial, brain compression occurs rapidly. The lower incidence of epidural haematoma in childhood is attributed to the fact that the middle meningeal artery is not embedded in the skull's bone surface until approximately 2 years old. Therefore, a temporal bone fracture is less likely to lacerate the artery. However, occipital fractures are common with posterior fossa epidural haematomas (Sencer et al 2012).

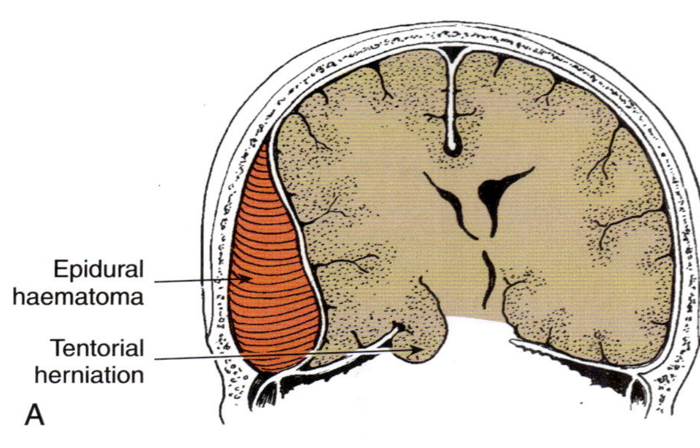

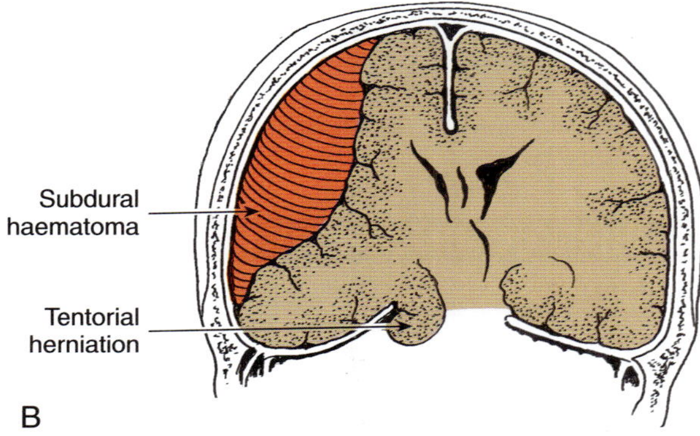

Fig 30.6 (**A**) Epidural (extradural) haematoma and compression of temporal lobe through tentorial herniation. (**B**) Subdural haematoma.

Epidural haematomas occur infrequently in infants and children, but they may occur after a low-velocity fall (Sencer et al 2012). Child abuse accounts for a significant number of cases of epidural haematomas in infants and children, whereas motor vehicle crashes account for most epidural haematomas in adolescents.

Because bleeding is generally arterial, brain compression occurs rapidly. Most often the expanding haematoma is located in the parietal and temporal regions (Teichert et al 2012), which forces the medial portion of the temporal lobe under the edge of the tentorium, where it places pressure on nerves and blood vessels. Pressure on the arterial supply and venous return to the reticular formation causes loss of consciousness; pressure on CN III produces dilation and (later) fixation of the ipsilateral pupil. Pressure on the fibres of the pyramidal tract is evidenced by contralateral weakness or paralysis and increased deep tendon reflexes. Extreme pressure may cause brain herniation and death. Expanding epidural haemorrhages may be better tolerated in young children with open sutures that allow for expansion of the skull. In addition, young children have larger subarachnoid and extracellular spaces, which provide space for the expanding haematoma without compression on the brain parenchyma.

The classic clinical picture of an epidural haemorrhage is a lucid interval of minutes to hours followed by rapidly altered mental status, then loss of consciousness or coma due to blood accumulation in the epidural space and compression of the brain. The child may be seen with varying degrees of impaired consciousness, depending on the severity of the traumatic injury. Common symptoms in a child with no neurological deficit are irritability, headache and vomiting. In infants less than 24 months of age common symptoms are scalp swelling, irritability and lethargy. They may also have seizures, reduced oral intake and increasing head circumference (Sellin et al 2017).

An epidural haematoma can be detected by an initial CT scan. If the severity of the child's symptoms is not recognised, herniation and death will result. **Cushing's triad** (systemic hypertension, bradycardia and respiratory depression) is a late sign of impending brainstem herniation.

NURSING CARE CONSIDERATIONS

Children with a subdural haematoma and retinal haemorrhages should be evaluated for the possibility of child abuse, especially shaken baby syndrome resulting in abusive head trauma.

Subdural Haematoma. A subdural haematoma is a haemorrhage between the dura and the arachnoid membrane that overlies the brain and the subarachnoid space. The haemorrhage may be from two sources: (1) tearing of the veins that bridge the subdural space; and (2) haemorrhage from the cortex of the brain caused by direct brain trauma (see Fig 30.6B). Subdural haematomas are much more common than epidural haematomas in infants and children.

Unlike epidural haemorrhage, which develops inwardly against the less resistant brain tissue, subdural haemorrhage tends to develop more slowly and spreads thinly and widely, crossing cranial sutures, until it is limited by the dural barriers: the falx and the tentorium. The small subdural space and the dura, which is firmly attached to the skull in this area, are highly vulnerable to increased ICP.

Subdural haematoma is fairly common in infants. Most often it is the result of assaults or violent shaking. The caregiver's response to infant crying, often perceived as inconsolable, is an important risk factor (Barr 2014). In neonates subdural haematoma can be a consequence of labour and delivery. Subdural haemorrhage can cause either acute or chronic subdural haematoma. Acute subdural haematoma may be associated with contusions or lacerations and develops within minutes or hours of injury. Chronic subdural haematoma is more common. The clinical course and manifestations vary depending on the damage sustained by the brain and the child's age.

Presenting signs of acute haematoma include irritability, vomiting, increased head circumference, bulging anterior fontanel (in the infant), lethargy, coma or seizures. In infants with open fontanels, large amounts of intracranial blood may accumulate, causing haemorrhagic shock or fever before there are any changes in the neurological examination (Squier & Mack 2009). Retinal haemorrhages and skull and skeletal fractures are suggestive of physical abuse. An infant who has an altered LOC and in whom the CT scan shows subarachnoid haemorrhage or subdural haematoma may have been physically abused. A child with a GCS of 12 or less or a decrease in GCS score by 2 or more points requires emergency consultation with the neurosurgeon (Huang et al 2016).

Closely observe older children for signs of neurological deterioration, including altered mental status, vomiting, lethargy and signs of increased ICP. Hemiparesis, hemiplegia and anisocoria (unequal pupils) are signs of brainstem compression and require emergency treatment targeted at decreasing ICP. The surgical management of subdural haematomas depends on the physical examination, size of the haematoma and presence of other abnormalities on the CT scan. Not all children require surgery or are candidates for surgery. Various surgical options to treat subdural haematomas include transfontanel percutaneous aspiration, subdural drains, placement of burr hole or craniotomy (Huang et al 2016).

Other Haemorrhagic Lesions. A subarachnoid haemorrhage is bleeding within the subarachnoid space, which is normally filled with CSF. Non-traumatic intracranial haemorrhages are rare in children. The most common causes of spontaneous intracranial haemorrhage in children are arteriovenous malformations and fistulas and brain tumours (Ding et al 2017). Sudden onset of a severe headache, headaches occurring out of sleep, first-time seizure and abnormal neurological examination are symptoms that require evaluation including neuroimaging (Blume 2017).

Cerebral Oedema. Some degree of brain oedema is expected after craniocerebral trauma and often accompanies any of the previously mentioned disorders. Cerebral oedema peaks at 24 to 72 hours after injury and may account for changes in a child's neurological status. Cerebral oedema associated with traumatic brain injury may be a result of two different mechanisms: cytotoxic oedema or vasogenic oedema. Cytotoxic oedema is a result of direct cell injury and is caused by intracellular swelling. In many cases the brain cells are irreversibly damaged. Vasogenic oedema is due to increased permeability of capillary endothelial cells, resulting in increased intracellular fluid. In vasogenic oedema the nerve cells are not primarily injured. Either mechanism can result in increased ICP as a result of increased intracranial volume and changes in CBF as a result of loss of autoregulation and/or hypercapnia or hypoxia. Children at risk for deterioration can be identified by abnormalities seen on non-contrast CT scans.

Sequelae of Traumatic Brain Injury. **Postconcussion syndrome** is a sequela to brain injury with or without loss of consciousness. Concussions usually resolve in 1 to 3 weeks without complications. Up to a third of children may have ongoing somatic, behavioural, cognitive and psychological symptoms including headaches, visual and balance problems, difficulty concentrating, irritability and changes in their sleep patterns (Morgan et al 2015). The pathophysiology of these symptoms is unclear. When these symptoms continue more than 4 weeks after the concussion the term *postconcussion syndrome* (PCS) is used (Zemek et al 2016). Risk factors for PCS in youth athletes include a personal or family history of mood disorders and other psychiatric illnesses and migraines (Morgan et al 2015). Previously concussion treatment guidelines recommended cognitive and physical rest as a path to recovery. Recent studies, though, have found that early participation in physical activity is significantly likely to prevent the development of PCS (Grool et al 2016).

Posttraumatic headaches, one of the most common symptoms after mild traumatic brain injury (TBI), may occur within 1 week to 3 months after a mild TBI. They occur in 25% to 75% of individuals and are most commonly classified as migraines (Kuczynski et al 2013). Posttraumatic headaches are treated based on the primary headache type, migraine or tension/chronic headache (Kacperski & Arthur 2016).

Posttraumatic seizures occur in a number of children who survive a head injury, often within 24 hours, but they can occur up to 1 week after the injury (Christensen 2012). In comparison to children with no brain injury, seizures are two times more likely to occur in children with mild TBI and seven times more likely to occur in children with severe head injury (Christensen 2012).

Hydrocephalus may develop after subarachnoid haemorrhage or infection. Normal-pressure hydrocephalus can be a complication of TBI. In infants, signs and symptoms include rapidly increasing head circumference, irritability, refusal to feed and sleepiness. The clinical signs and symptoms in children include changes in personality, developmental regression, ataxia and incontinence. These signs are also seen during posttraumatic amnesia, making early recognition of this syndrome difficult. Focal deficits, including optic atrophy, CN palsies, motor deficits, DI or aphasia, may be seen. The type of residual effect depends on the location and nature of the trauma.

Diagnostic Evaluation

A detailed health history, both past and present, is essential in evaluating the child with head trauma. Certain disorders such as drug allergies, haemophilia, diabetes mellitus or epilepsy may produce similar symptoms. Even a minor traumatic injury can aggravate a preexisting disease process, thereby producing neurological signs out of proportion to the injury.

After a minor injury, initial unconsciousness (if present) is brief. The child ordinarily exhibits a transient period of confusion, somnolence and listlessness; this period is most often accompanied by irritability, pallor and one episode of vomiting. A severe head injury requires immediate evaluation and treatment. Because head injuries are often accompanied by injuries in other areas (e.g. spine, viscera, extremities), the examination is performed with care to avoid further damage. Box 30.5 lists manifestations of head injury.

Initial Assessment. Priorities in the initial phase in the care of a child with a head injury include assessment of the ABC (airway, breathing, circulation); neurological examination focusing on mental status, papillary responses and motor responses; and assessment for spinal cord injury. The assessment is carried out quickly in relation to vital signs (see Nursing Care Considerations box).

NURSING CARE CONSIDERATIONS

Head Injury

1. Assess the child.
   - A—Airway
   - B—Breathing
   - C—Circulation
   - Neurological and thermoregulatory status
2. Stabilise the neck and spine immediately. Use jaw thrust to open airway, not chin lift.
3. Clean any abrasions with soap and water.
   - Apply clean dressing.
   - If the child is bleeding, apply ice to relieve pain and swelling.
4. Keep child nil by mouth (NBM) until instructed otherwise.
5. Assess pain but do not give analgesics or sedatives.
6. Check level of consciousness and pupillary reaction every 4 hours (including twice during the night) for 48 hours.
7. Seek medical attention for any of the following:
   - injury sustained at high speed (e.g. motor vehicle)
   - fall from a significant distance (height greater than that of the child)
   - injury sustained from great force (e.g. cricket bat)
   - injury sustained under suspicious circumstances
   - loss of consciousness
   - amnesia
   - discomfort (crying) more than 10 minutes after injury
   - headache that is severe, worsens, interferes with sleep or lasts more than 24 hours
   - vomiting three or more times or that begins or continues 4 to 6 hours after injury
   - swelling in front of or above earlobe or swelling that increases in size
   - fluid leak from ears or nose; blackened eyes
   - confusion or abnormal behaviour
   - difficulty arousing child from sleep
   - difficulty speaking
   - blurring of vision or diplopia
   - unsteady gait
   - difficulty using extremities; weakness or incoordination
   - neck pain or stiffness
   - pupils dilated, fixed or unequal
   - infant with bulging fontanel
   - seizures.

BOX 30.5 Clinical Manifestations of Acute Head Injury

Minor Injury
- May or may not lose consciousness
- Transient period of confusion
- Somnolence
- Listlessness
- Irritability
- Pallor
- Vomiting (one or more episodes)

Signs of Progression
- Altered mental status (e.g. difficulty arousing child)
- Mounting agitation
- Development of focal lateral neurological signs
- Marked changes in vital signs

Severe Injury
- Signs of increased intracranial pressure (see Box 30.1)
- Bulging fontanel (infant)
- Retinal haemorrhages
- Extraocular palsies (especially cranial nerve III)
- Hemiparesis
- Quadriplegia
- Elevated temperature
- Unsteady gait (older child)
- Papillo-oedema (older child)
- Retinal haemorrhages

Associated Signs
- Scalp trauma
- Other injuries (e.g. to extremities)

Ocular signs such as fixed, dilated and unequal pupils; fixed and constricted pupils; and pupils that are poorly reactive or unreactive to light and accommodation indicate increased ICP or brainstem involvement. It is important to remain with the patient who demonstrates fixed and dilated pupils because these are ominous signs often associated with impending respiratory arrest. Dilated, non-pulsating blood vessels indicate increased ICP before the appearance of papillo-oedema. Retinal haemorrhages often occur with acute head injuries, specifically with shaken baby syndrome.

Funduscopic examination should be performed routinely to detect retinal haemorrhages in a child with CNS trauma. Vestibulo-ocular symptoms such as diplopia, dizziness, motion sensitivity, eye-tracking and eye-focusing problems, photosensitivity and visual inattention may develop (Ellis et al 2015). Transient vision loss may occur after mild head trauma but may not be obvious in children unless this diagnosis is evaluated. Theories of possible causes are vasospasm or localised cerebral oedema.

Less urgent but important assessments include examination of the scalp for lacerations, widely separated sutures and the size and tension of fontanels, which indicate intracranial haemorrhage or rapidly developing cerebral oedema. Scalp lacerations may require surgical intervention. A significant amount of blood loss can occur from scalp lacerations. CT scan may be necessary to evaluate possible skull fractures and acute intracranial haemorrhage (Ryan et al 2016).

NURSING CARE CONSIDERATIONS

Bleeding from the nose or ears needs further evaluation, and a watery discharge from the nose (rhinorrhoea) that is positive for glucose (as tested with reagent strips) suggests leaking of CSF from a skull fracture.

A documented accurate assessment of clinical signs provides baseline information. Serial evaluations, preferably by a single observer, help detect changes in neurological status. Alterations in mental status, evidenced by increased difficulty in rousing the child, mounting agitation, development of focal neurological signs or marked changes in vital signs, usually indicate extension or progression of the basic pathological process.

Evaluation of reflexes provides information about cerebral and pyramidal involvement, although transient abnormalities of the primitive reflexes and Babinski's sign may be present in children with mild head trauma. Conscious, cooperative children are examined for cerebellar signs such as ataxia and dysmetria. Children may display unsteadiness, clumsiness or tremor with intentional movement after head injury. Temperature may be moderately elevated for 1 or 2 days after an initial mild hypothermia after injury. A persistent fever may indicate subarachnoid haemorrhage or infection.

Special Tests. After a thorough clinical examination, a variety of diagnostic tests are helpful in providing a more definitive diagnosis of the type and extent of the trauma. A haematocrit and urinalysis are typically done. Serum electrolytes and glucose may also be measured in children with severe head injuries; hyperglycaemia and disseminated intravascular coagulation are associated with a poor prognosis. The severity of a head injury may not be apparent on clinical examination of the child but detectable on a CT scan. Whenever the child has a history consistent with a serious head injury (as with an unrestrained occupant in a severe motor vehicle crash or a fall from greater than their own height), it is important to perform a scan even if the child initially appears alert and oriented. All children with head injuries who have any alteration of consciousness, headache, vomiting, skull fracture, seizure or predisposing medical condition should undergo a diagnostic evaluation that includes CT scanning.

MRI may be done to further assess cerebral oedema or other structural brain abnormalities. A neurodevelopmental assessment after early head injury may be useful in documenting cognitive impairment. Skull radiographs are of little benefit in diagnosing skull fractures. Other radiographic tests may be indicated, depending on the severity or cause of the trauma. Electroencephalography (EEG) is not helpful for diagnosis of a head injury but is useful for defining seizures and looking for subclinical seizures, which can impair consciousness (Gainza-Lein et al 2017). Lumbar puncture is rarely used for craniocerebral trauma and is contraindicated in the presence of increased ICP because of the possibility of herniation.

Therapeutic Management

The majority of children with mild TBI who have not lost consciousness can be cared for and observed at home after careful examination reveals no serious intracranial injury. The nurse should give parents both verbal and written instructions of signs and symptoms that warrant concern and the need for re-evaluation. These include persistent or worsening headaches, vomiting, change in mental status or behaviour, unsteady gait or seizure. The child should have a physical examination within 1 or 2 days after the injury. The manifestations of epidural haematoma in children do not generally appear until 24 hours or more after injury.

Maintaining contact with parents for continued observation and re-evaluation of the child, when indicated, facilitates early diagnosis and treatment of possible complications from head injury, such as haematoma, cerebral oedema and posttraumatic seizures. Children are generally hospitalised for 24 to 48 hours of observation if their family lives far from medical facilities or lacks transportation or a telephone, which would provide access to immediate help. Other circumstances, such as language or other communication barriers or even emotional trauma, may hinder learning and make it difficult for families to feel confident caring for their child at home.

Children with severe injuries, those who have lost consciousness for more than a few minutes and those with prolonged and continued seizures or other focal or diffuse neurological signs must be hospitalised until their condition is stable and their neurological signs have diminished. The child is maintained on NBM status or restricted to clear liquids (if able to take fluids by mouth) until it is determined that vomiting will not occur. IV fluids are indicated in the child who is comatose, displays dulled sensorium or is persistently vomiting.

The volume of IV fluid is carefully monitored to minimise the possibility of over-hydration in case of SIADH and cerebral oedema. However, damage to the hypothalamus or pituitary gland may produce DI with its accompanying hypertonicity and dehydration. Fluid balance is closely monitored by daily weight, strict intake and output measurement and serum osmolality (to detect early signs of water retention).

Sedating drugs are usually withheld in the acute phase. Headache is usually controlled with paracetamol; while opioids may be needed, they must be used with caution due to the role they play in the CNS. Antiepileptics are used for seizure control. Antibiotics are administered if there are lacerations or penetrating injuries. Prophylactic tetanus vaccine is given as appropriate. Cerebral oedema is managed as described for the unconscious child. Hyperthermia is controlled with tepid sponges or a hypothermia blanket.

Surgical Therapy. Approximately 10% to 30% of paediatric head traumas will result in skull fractures. Because of the greater capacity of a child's skull fracture to heal, conservative non-surgical management is often adequate. Children hit in the head or who have TBI as a result of a motor vehicle crash are more likely to require surgical intervention, especially if the frontal bones have been fractured (Bonfield et al 2014).

Scalp lacerations are sutured after careful examination of underlying bone. The use of topical anaesthesia such as EMLA or ALA (adrenaline/lignociane/amethocaine) and a procedural sedative such as midazolam provides non-invasive, effective anaesthesia for suturing, particularly when combined with biobehavioural techniques such as distraction.

Depressed fractures require surgical reduction and removal of bone fragments. Torn dura is also sutured. A skull fracture depressed more than the thickness of the skull or an intracranial haematoma that causes more than a 5-mm midline shift is an indication for surgery. Direct pressure should never be applied to a depressed skull fracture. Parents should be advised that hardware and wound infections may need further surgical intervention. Parents and other caregivers must be taught the importance of meticulous hand washing after surgical repair of a skull fracture.

Prognosis. The outcome of craniocerebral trauma depends on the extent of injury and complications. Neurological, cognitive, emotional and behavioural symptoms can result in significant impairment. They may not present until the child is older and preparing to reach certain developmental milestones (Babikian et al 2015). These symptoms can become chronic and include epilepsy, attention deficit/hyperactivity disorder and learning or psychiatric disorders. Children with learning and behaviour problems before their head trauma are more likely to suffer these consequences (Beauchamp & Anderson 2013). More than 90% of children with concussions or simple linear fractures recover without symptoms after the initial period.

Children may be more vulnerable than adults to long-term cognitive and behavioural dysfunction after diffuse brain injury. Contrary to what was previously thought about 'brain plasticity', evidence now indicates that children's brains may be especially vulnerable to early injury due to their ongoing maturation processes, which can be disrupted by head trauma (Babikian et al 2015). Parents of children who have suffered TBI should be advised to seek evaluation and treatment sooner rather than later if any of these symptoms present. TBI is recognised as a disability that may qualify a child for special education services.

True coma (i.e. not obeying commands, eyes closed and not speaking) usually does not last more than 2 weeks. A child's eventual outcome can range from brain death to a persistent vegetative state to complete recovery. However, even the best recovery may be associated with personality changes, including mood lability and loss of confidence, impaired short-term memory, headaches and subtle cognitive impairments. In general, 90% of the long-term neurological outcome has been achieved within 6 months to 1 year after the injury.

Nursing Care Management

The hospitalised child requires careful neurological assessment and evaluation repeated as frequently as every 15 minutes to establish a correct diagnosis, identify signs and symptoms of increased ICP, determine clinical management and prevent many complications. The goals of nursing management of the child with a head injury are to: maintain adequate ventilation, oxygenation and circulation; monitor and treat increased ICP; minimise cerebral oxygen requirements; and support the child and family during recovery. (See Quality Patient Outcomes box.)

QUALITY PATIENT OUTCOMES

Acute Head Injury

- Early recognition of signs and symptoms of increased intracranial pressure
- Adequate ventilation, oxygenation and circulation maintained
- Cerebral oxygen requirements minimised
- Sedation and analgesia provided while allowing for neurological assessment

The child is placed on bed rest, usually with the head of the bed elevated slightly and the head in midline position. Appropriate safety measures, such as side rails kept up and seizure precautions, are implemented. If the child is extremely restless, hard surfaces may be padded and restraints used to prevent further injury. Individualise care according to the child's specific needs.

A key nursing role is to provide analgesia for the child. Sedation needs to be administered with caution if the patient is already neurologically compromised. The conflict between the need to promote the child's comfort and relieve anxiety versus the need to assess for neurological changes presents a dilemma. Both goals can be achieved with close observation of the child's LOC and response to analgesics (using a pain assessment record) and effective communication with the provider. Decreasing restlessness after administration of an analgesic most likely reflects pain control rather than a decreasing LOC.

Children may be restless and irritable, but more often their reaction is to fall asleep when left undisturbed. A quiet environment can help reduce restlessness and irritability. Bright lights are irritating. This often makes checking the ocular responses more difficult and aggravating to the child.

Frequent examinations of vital signs, neurological signs and LOC are extremely important nursing observations. When possible, they should be performed by a single observer to better detect subtle changes that may indicate worsening of neurological status. Pupils are checked for size, symmetry, reaction to light and accommodation. Unless there is brainstem involvement, vital signs generally return to normal after the initial changes seen after injury.

The most important nursing observation is assessment of the child's LOC. In the progression of an injury, alterations in consciousness appear earlier than alterations of vital signs or focal neurological signs (see evaluation of responsiveness later in this chapter). Frequent examinations of alertness are fatiguing to the child; therefore, the child often desires to fall asleep, which may be confused with depressed consciousness. It is not uncommon to observe ocular divergence through the partially closed eyelids.

Observations of position and movement provide additional information. Note any abnormal posturing and whether it occurs continuously or intermittently. Questions nurses might ask include the following.

- Are the child's hand grips strong and equal in strength?
- Are there any signs of extension or flexion posturing?
- What is the child's response to auditory and physical stimulation?
- Is movement purposeful, random or absent?
- Are movement and sensation equal on both sides or restricted to one side only?

The child may report a headache or other discomfort. The child who is too young to describe a headache may be fussy and resist being handled. The child who suffers from vertigo often vigorously resists being moved from a position of comfort. Forcible movement causes the child to vomit and display spontaneous nystagmus. Seizures are relatively common in children at the time of head injury and may be of any type. Carefully observe any seizure activity and describe it in detail. Children in postictal states are more lethargic, with sluggish pupils.

Document drainage from any orifice. Bleeding from the ear suggests the possibility of a basal skull fracture. Clear nasal drainage is suggestive of an anterior basal skull fracture. Observe the amount and characteristics of the drainage.

Head trauma is often accompanied by other undetected injuries; therefore, any bruises, lacerations or evidence of internal injuries or fractures of the extremities are noted and reported. Associated injuries are evaluated and treated appropriately.

The child with a normal LOC is usually allowed clear liquids unless fluid is restricted. If the child has an IV infusion, it is maintained as prescribed. The diet is advanced to that appropriate for the child's age as soon as the condition permits. Intake and output are measured and recorded with attention to the development of constipation. Any incontinence of bowel or bladder is noted for the child who has been toilet trained.

Assessment for unusual behaviour can only be made in relation to the child's typical behaviour. For example, urinary incontinence during sleep would be of no consequence in a child who routinely wets the bed but would be highly significant for one who is always dry. Parents are invaluable resources in evaluating objective behaviours of their children. Information obtained from parents at or shortly after admission is essential in evaluating the child's behaviour (e.g. the ease with which the child is roused normally, the usual sleeping position, how much the child sleeps during the day, the child's motor activities [rolling over, sitting up, climbing], hearing and visual acuity, appetite and manner of eating [spoon, bottle, cup]). Documentation of the child's baseline developmental and behavioural level is crucial. There is less concern about a child who falls asleep several times during the day if this is consistent with the child's usual behaviour.

When the child is discharged, advise the parents of probable post-traumatic symptoms they may observe, such as behavioural changes, sleep disturbances, phobias and seizures. Parents should be taught seizure first aid. They should understand observations they need to make and when and how to contact the provider or health facility in case the child develops any unusual signs or symptoms. Emphasise the importance of follow-up evaluation.

Family Support. The emotional and educational support of the family presents a challenge. Witnessing the parents' grief and helplessness on seeing their child in an intensive care unit connected to monitoring equipment and in an altered state evokes empathy. The nurse can encourage the family to be involved in the child's care, to bring in familiar belongings or to make a recording of familiar voices and sounds. Parents may need a demonstration on how to touch or cuddle their child and may want to talk about their grief. The nurse listens attentively, reinforces what is being done to assist the child and directs parents towards signs and symptoms of recovery to instil hope without promises. Honesty and kindness, along with consistent and competent care, help families through this difficult time.

Rehabilitation. Rehabilitation and management of the child with permanent brain injury are essential aspects of care. Rehabilitation begins as soon as possible and usually involves the family and a rehabilitation team. The nurse makes a careful assessment of the child's capabilities and limitations and implements appropriate interventions to maximise the residual capacities. Brain Injury New Zealand (https://www.brain-injury.nz/) provides information and listings of rehabilitation services and support groups throughout the country.

The child with a disability resulting from head trauma requires functional assessment of his or her physical, cognitive, emotional and social levels. The child has experienced separation, pain, sensory deprivation and overload, changes in circadian cycle and fear of the unknown. Recovery and transition require new coping strategies at the same time that regressive and acting-out behaviours may start. Parents and children need honest communication for decision-making.

Paediatric rehabilitation focuses on the child's strengths and needs. The rehabilitation team should include physical medicine; rehabilitation nursing; nutritional counselling; physical, occupational and speech therapy; special education; and psychological, neuropsychological, child life and social services support.

Prevention. Preventive strategies are underused in almost all cases of accidental childhood injury. Head injuries occur in the most serious accidents—especially motor vehicle crashes, sports and falls.

Strides are being made in the prevention of secondary brain tissue damage after the initial head injury in children. This secondary injury is caused by altered cerebral blood flow that results in ischaemia, hypoxia and eventually the death of brain cells (Popernack et al 2015). Studies are ongoing in both humans and animals using therapeutic hypothermia, glucagon, blood pressure medications and antioxidants (Toth et al 2016). The roles of calcium, oxyradicals and prostaglandins are being investigated.

However, the greatest benefit lies in prevention of head injuries. Nurses can exert a valuable influence on behalf of children through education. Accidents occur that are preventable because unnecessary risks go unchecked. Inadequate supervision combined with a child's natural sense of curiosity and exploration can lead to lethal results. Nurses are in the unique position of influencing caregivers in terms of growth and development. The use of car seats; seat belts in prams and high chairs; and helmets for biking, skateboarding and other sports has been shown to reduce both the number and severity of head injuries in children (Ganti et al 2013, Gaw et al 2017).

Submersion Injury

Drowning is one of the major causes of unintentional injury-related death in children ages 1 to 19 years. In children ages 1 to 4 years it is the leading cause of unintentional injury-related death. The term *near-drowning* is no longer used; instead, the term *submersion injury* should be used up until the time of drowning-related death (Weiss 2010). In 2002 the World Congress on Drowning and the World Health Organization established a uniform definition: 'the process of respiratory impairment from submersion/immersion in liquid' and uniform classifications of death, no morbidity or morbidity (Weiss 2010).

Most cases of submersion injury are accidental, usually involving children who are helpless in water, such as inadequately attended children in or near swimming pools or infants in bathtubs; small children who fall into ponds, streams and dams, usually near home; occupants of leisure boats who fail to wear life jackets; children who have diving accidents; and children who are able to swim but overestimate their endurance. Accidental submersion injury occurs predominantly in males and toddlers (Fig 30.7). Aboriginal and Torres Strait Islander and Māori and Pacific Islander children tend to have a higher incidence of hospitalisation and mortality from submersion, as do children in remote areas of Australia (Australian Institute of Health and Welfare [AIHW] 2021, Moran et al 2017).

Pathophysiology

Physiologically most organ systems are affected, especially the pulmonary, cardiovascular and neurological systems. The major pulmonary changes that occur in submersion injury are directly related to the length of submersion (regardless of the type and amount of fluid aspirated), the victim's physiological response and the development and degree of immersion hypothermia. Cerebral hypoxia is a major component of morbidity and mortality in these individuals. Therefore, early and aggressive resuscitation is imperative.

Physiological factors in submersion injuries are hypothermia, aspiration and hypoxia. The temperature of the liquid plays an important role. Cold water decreases metabolic demands and activates the diving reflex, which causes blood to be shunted away from the periphery to vital organs (i.e. the brain and heart). Hypothermia occurs rapidly in infants and children, partly because of their large surface area relative to size and partly as a result of the cold water itself. Profound hypothermia is usually evidence of lengthy submersion. Prolonged submersion in cold liquids can impair cognition, coordination and muscle strength that ultimately results in loss of consciousness, decreased cardiac output and cardiac arrest (Caglar & Quan 2016). Submersion in cold water had previously been thought to be somewhat neuroprotective, but it is not (Quan et al 2014).

Submerged children struggle initially to stay above water, and often breath-holding leads to air hunger. Reflex inspiration eventually occurs, which leads to aspiration (Caglar & Quan 2016). Fluid is quickly absorbed in the pulmonary circulation, resulting in pulmonary oedema, atelectasis and airway spasm. Hypoxia is the primary problem because it results in global cell damage, with different cells tolerating variable lengths of anoxia. Neurons, especially cerebral cells, sustain irreversible damage after 4 to 6 minutes of submersion. The heart and lungs can survive up to 30 minutes. Regardless of the amount of water aspirated, the victim suffers arterial hypoxaemia (resulting from atelectasis and shunting of blood through the non-ventilated alveoli), combined respiratory acidosis (resulting from retained carbon dioxide) and metabolic acidosis (caused by build-up of acid metabolites because of anaerobic metabolism). Although electrolyte imbalances are contributing factors, they are not the major causes of morbidity and mortality. The pathological events are directly related to the duration of submersion. Approximately 10% of submersion injury victims die without aspirating fluid but succumb from acute asphyxia as a result of prolonged reflex laryngospasm.

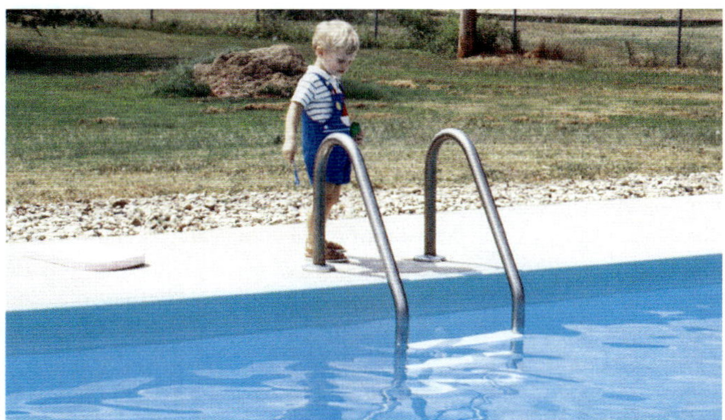

Fig 30.7 Water is fascinating for children; however, drowning is the second leading cause of accidental death in unsupervised situations.

Aspiration of fluid occurs in the majority of submersion injuries. The aspirated fluid results in pulmonary oedema, atelectasis, airway spasm and pneumonitis, which aggravates hypoxia. Submersion in salt water is associated with better outcomes than submersion in fresh water, although duration of the submersion is the main factor that predicts outcome (Quan et al 2016).

Clinical Manifestations

Clinical manifestations are directly related to the duration of loss of consciousness and neurological status after rescue and resuscitation.

Therapeutic Management

With rapid treatment some children can be saved. Resuscitative measures should begin at the scene, and the victim should be transported to the hospital with maximum ventilatory and circulatory support. In the hospital intensive pulmonary care is implemented and continued according to the patient's needs.

In general, management of the victim with a submersion injury is based on the degree of cerebral insult. The first priority is to restore oxygen delivery to the cells and prevent further hypoxic damage. A spontaneously breathing child does well in an oxygen-enriched atmosphere; the more severely affected child requires endotracheal intubation and mechanical ventilation. Blood gases and pH are monitored at frequent intervals as a guide to oxygen, fluid and electrolyte therapies. Rewarming the hypothermic patient is initiated. Seizures may occur due to hypoxia and cerebral oedema. Seizures result in increased cerebral oxygen consumption. Therefore, it is imperative to aggressively control seizure activity. In addition, blood glucose should be monitored; both hypoglycaemia and hyperglycaemia are harmful to the brain.

All children who have a submersion injury should be hospitalised for observation. Although some children do not appear to have sustained adverse effects from the event, respiratory compromise or cerebral oedema may occur within 24 hours after the incident. In the acute recovery period fever should be prevented although prophylactic antibiotics are not recommended. Aspiration pneumonia is a common complication that occurs approximately 48 to 72 hours after the episode. Bronchospasm, alveolar-capillary membrane damage, atelectasis, abscess formation and acute respiratory distress syndrome are other complications that occur after aspiration of fluid.

Prognosis. Children who have submersion injuries usually have a good outcome with no or mild neurological sequelae, no severe neurological disabilities and rarely morbidity (Caglar & Quan 2016). The best predictors of a good outcome are length of submersion less than 5 minutes and the presence of sinus rhythm, reactive pupils and neurological responsiveness at the scene. The worst outcomes are for children submerged for more than 10 minutes and unresponsive to advanced life support within 25 minutes. All children without spontaneous purposeful movement and normal brainstem function 24 hours after sustaining a submersion injury suffered severe neurological deficits or death (Caglar & Quan 2016).

Nursing Care Management

Nursing care depends on the child's condition. A child who survives may need intensive respiratory nursing care with attention to vital signs, mechanical ventilation or tracheostomy, blood gas determination, chest physiotherapy and IV infusion. Often the child has sustained a hypoxic insult and requires the same care as an unconscious child.

A difficult aspect in the care of the child who sustained a submersion injury is helping the parents cope with the grief, guilt and anger reactions. Given the magnitude of the event, parents need repeated assurance that everything possible is being done to treat their child.

If the child dies, the sudden, unexpected nature of the death and the particular circumstances of the accident, especially in terms of guilt for not preventing it, compound the grief. The parents of the child who survives face the anxiety of not knowing the final outcome—to what extent will their child recover? This situation generates such intense feelings of loneliness and guilt that it is important for families to know they are not alone. They should be reminded frequently that there are people to assist them through this crisis. Additional sources of support that can be recommended include psychiatric and social work consultants, community services and religious support. Self-help groups are excellent if available in the community.

Nurses often have difficulty relating to the parents if obvious neglect has precipitated the accident and subsequent problems; therefore, it is important for those who care for these children and their families to assess their own feelings about the situation, in addition to assessing the family's coping abilities and resources. Caring for victims of a submersion injury and their families requires the nurse to be sensitive to the needs of the child and the family and to recognise his or her own reactions and emotions.

Prevention. Most submersion injuries are preventable. The most common cause of submersion injury in infants and young children is inadequate adult supervision, including a momentary lapse of supervision. Parents are often unaware that they must be within arm's reach and constantly supervising without being distracted (Caglar & Quan 2016). Children with known risk factors such as epilepsy and autism require eyes-on surveillance. All parents and swimming pool owners should be familiar with basic cardiopulmonary resuscitation (CPR) because rapid, basic CPR is one of the keys to improving outcomes (Tobin et al 2017). Water safety and survival training should be required for all school-age children. Pool covers and fencing on all sides and the presence of lifeguards can prevent accidents.

Nurses can be active advocates in their communities. Nurses are also in a position to emphasise the importance of adequate adult supervision when children are around any body of water and should include the necessity of the adult not engaging in distracting activities.

THE CHILD WITH CEREBRAL MALFORMATION

Hydrocephalus

Hydrocephalus is a condition caused by an imbalance in the production and absorption of CSF in the ventricular system. The causes of hydrocephalus are varied and include either congenital (e.g. myelomeningocele, intrauterine viral infection [cytomegalovirus, toxoplasmosis], aqueduct stenosis) or acquired conditions such as intraventricular haemorrhage, tumour, CSF infection or head injury. The result is either: (1) impaired absorption of CSF fluid within the subarachnoid space, obliteration of the subarachnoid cisterns or malfunction of the arachnoid villi (non-obstructive or communicating hydrocephalus); or (2) obstruction to the flow of CSF through the ventricular system (obstructive or non-communicating hydrocephalus) (Kinsman & Johnston 2016).

Any imbalance of secretion and absorption causes an increased accumulation of CSF in the ventricles, which become dilated (ventriculomegaly) and compress the brain tissue against the surrounding rigid bony cranium. When this occurs before fusion of the cranial sutures, it causes enlargement of the skull and dilation of the ventricles. In children younger than 12 years old, previously closed sutures, especially the sagittal suture, may become diastatic or opened. After 12 years old, the sutures are fused and will not open.

Pathophysiology

To appreciate the condition, an understanding of the dynamics of CSF and the relationship between the various structures that make up the ventricular and subarachnoid spaces is necessary (Fig 30.8). The two mechanisms by which CSF is formed are secretion by the choroid plexuses and lymphatic-like drainage by the extracellular fluid of the brain. CSF circulates throughout the ventricular system and is then absorbed within the subarachnoid spaces by a mechanism that is not entirely clear.

Ventricular Circulation. The fluid flows from the lateral ventricles through the foramen of Monro to the third ventricle, where it combines with fluid secreted into the third ventricle. From there CSF flows through the aqueduct of Sylvius into the fourth ventricle, where more fluid is formed; it then leaves the fourth ventricle by way of the lateral foramen of Luschka and the midline foramen of Magendie and flows into the cisterna magna. From the cisterna magna, CSF flows to the cerebral and cerebellar subarachnoid spaces where it is absorbed. A large portion is absorbed through the arachnoid villi, but the sinuses, veins, brain substance and dura also participate in absorption.

The terms *communicating* and *non-communicating hydrocephalus* traditionally referred to obstructive and non-obstructive types of hydrocephalus. Because other diagnostic methods are now used, the terms may be used only as a reference point in the diagnosis. Hydrocephalus can also be classified according to the cause as either congenital or acquired hydrocephalus.

Aetiology

Rarely, a tumour of the choroid plexus causes increased CSF secretion. Most cases of hydrocephalus are a result of developmental malformations. Although the defect usually is apparent in early infancy, it may become evident at any time from the prenatal period to late childhood or early adulthood. Other causes include neoplasms, CNS infections (e.g. meningitis, encephalitis) and trauma (e.g. shaken baby syndrome). An obstruction to the normal flow can occur at any point in the CSF pathway to produce increased pressure and dilation of the pathways proximal to the site of obstruction.

Developmental defects (e.g. Chiari's malformation [see following discussion], aqueductal stenosis, aqueductal gliosis and atresia of the foramina of Luschka and Magendie [Dandy-Walker cyst]) account for most cases of hydrocephalus from birth to 2 years of age. Dandy-Walker cyst involves dilation of the fourth ventricle, partial or complete absence of the cerebellar vermis and enlargement of the posterior fossa resulting in hydrocephalus in about 80% of children with Dandy-Walker cyst (Shankar et al 2016).

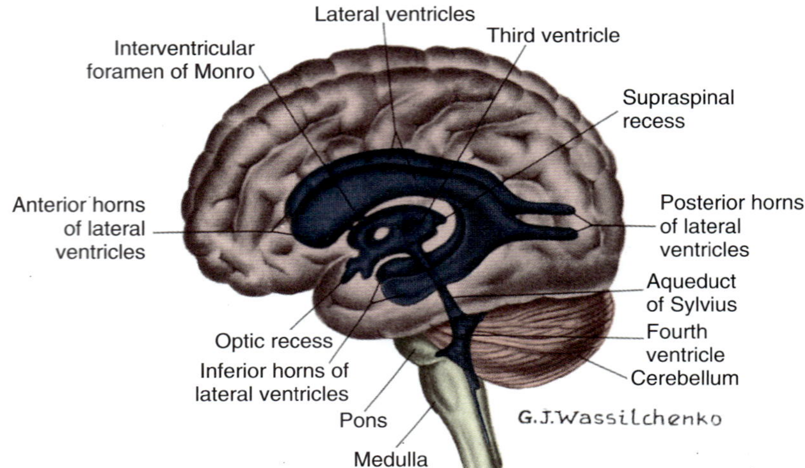

Fig 30.8 Cerebral ventricular system. (Source: Thompson, J. M., McFarland, G., Hirsch, J. E., et al. (2002). Mosby's clinical nursing (5th ed.). St Louis, MO: Mosby.)

Hydrocephalus is so often associated with myelomeningocele that all such infants should be observed for its development. In the remainder of cases there is a history of intrauterine infection (e.g. toxoplasmosis, cytomegalovirus), haemorrhage (e.g. posthaemorrhagic hydrocephalus in preterm infants) and neonatal meningoencephalitis (bacterial or viral). In older children hydrocephalus is most often a result of intracranial masses (e.g. vascular anomalies, cysts and tumours), preexisting developmental defects, intracranial infections, trauma or haemorrhage.

Chiari's Malformations I and II. Chiari's malformations are structural defects in the base of the skull and cerebellum. They occur when the lower cerebellum extends below the foramen magnum and into the upper spinal canal (Chiari's I) or when the lower cerebellum and brain stem protrude into the spinal canal through an enlarged foramen magnum (Chiari's II). Chiari's I malformation does not usually cause hydrocephalus. It is usually asymptomatic until adolescence when it can cause headaches, neck pain, frequent urination and lower limb progressive spasticity (Kinsman & Johnston 2016). Type II Chiari's malformation is seen almost exclusively with myelomeningocele, and results in obstruction of CSF flow causing the hydrocephalus.

Clinical Manifestations

The three factors that influence the clinical picture in hydrocephalus are the acuity of onset, timing of onset and associated structural malformations. In infancy, before closure of the cranial sutures, head enlargement (increasing occipitofrontal circumference [OFC]) is the predominant sign. The signs and symptoms in early to late childhood are caused by increased ICP. Specific manifestations are related to the location of the lesion.

Infancy. In infants with hydrocephalus, the head grows at an abnormal rate, although the first signs may be bulging fontanels with or without head enlargement (Fig 30.9). The anterior fontanel is tense, often bulging and non-pulsatile. Scalp veins are dilated, especially when the infant cries. With the increase in intracranial volume, the bones of the skull become thin and the sutures become palpably separated to produce the cracked-pot sound (**Macewen's sign**) on percussion of the skull. In severe cases there may be frontal protrusion, or **frontal bossing**, with depressed eyes, and the eyes may be rotated downwards, producing a **setting-sun sign**, in which the sclera may be visible above the iris. Pupils are sluggish, with unequal response to light.

The infant is irritable and lethargic, feeds poorly and may display changes in level of consciousness, opisthotonos (often extreme) and

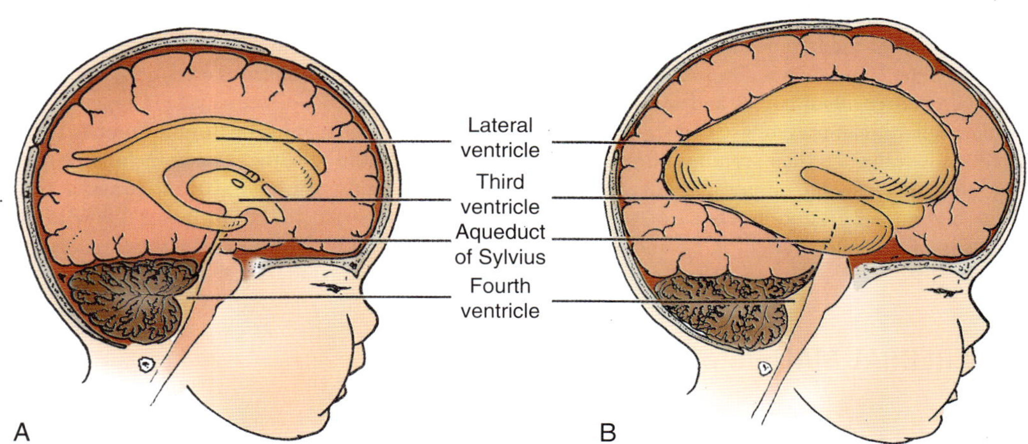

Fig 30.9 Hydrocephalus: a block in flow of cerebrospinal fluid. (**A**) Patent cerebrospinal fluid circulation. (**B**) Enlarged lateral and third ventricles caused by obstruction of circulation—stenosis of aqueduct of Sylvius.

lower extremity spasticity. The infant cries when picked up or rocked and quiets when allowed to lie still. Early infantile reflexes may persist and normally expected responses may not appear, indicating failure in the development of normal cortical inhibition.

Infants with Chiari's malformations may exhibit behaviours that reflect cranial nerve dysfunction as a result of brainstem compression, including swallowing difficulties, stridor, apnoea, aspiration, respiratory difficulties and arm weakness.

The preterm infant with posthaemorrhagic hydrocephalus may not exhibit any clinical signs and symptoms other than a gradual increase in head circumference. Alternatively, the nurse may note subtle seizure activity and alternating levels of consciousness. Ventricular size can be assessed by ultrasonography or CT scanning in preterm infants at high risk for intraventricular haemorrhage.

If hydrocephalus is allowed to progress, development of lower brainstem functions is disrupted, as manifested by difficulty in sucking and feeding and a shrill, brief, high-pitched cry. Eventually the skull becomes enlarged, and the cortex is destroyed. If the hydrocephalus is rapidly progressive, symptoms may include emesis, somnolence, seizures and cardiopulmonary distress.

Childhood. The signs and symptoms in early to late childhood are caused by increased ICP, and specific manifestations are related to the location of the focal lesion. Most commonly resulting from posterior fossa neoplasms and aqueduct stenosis, the clinical manifestations are primarily those associated with space-occupying lesions (i.e. headache on awakening with improvement after emesis, papillo-oedema, strabismus and extrapyramidal tract signs such as ataxia). As with infants, the child is irritable, lethargic, apathetic, confused and often incoherent. In one of the congenital defects with later onset (by age 3 months), the Dandy-Walker cyst, characteristic manifestations are a bulging occiput, nystagmus, ataxia and cranial nerve palsies.

Manifestations of Chiari's malformation in children over 3 years of age are related to spinal cord dysfunction rather than brainstem compression as observed in infants. Scoliosis proximal to the level of the myelomeningocele (usually associated with Chiari's malformation) and development of upper extremity spasticity, which may progress to weakness and atrophy, are common. Cranial nerve deficits are rare.

Diagnostic Evaluation

Antenatal diagnosis of fetal ventriculomegaly, which is associated with postnatal hydrocephalus, is possible with fetal ultrasonography as early as 14 to 15 weeks of gestation, often followed by fetal MRI (Pisapia et al 2017). There are ongoing trials in carefully selected pregnant women of fetal surgery for prevention of in utero brain damage from in utero hydrocephalus. Initial results were not promising, but recently outcomes have improved (Elbabaa et al 2017). Delivery is not currently recommended until fetal lung maturity has been achieved.

In infancy the diagnosis of hydrocephalus is based on head circumference that crosses one or more percentile lines on the head measurement chart within a period of 2 to 4 weeks and on associated neurological signs that are progressive. However, other diagnostic studies are needed to localise the site of CSF obstruction. Routine daily head circumference measurements are carried out in infants with myelomeningocele, haemorrhage or intrauterine viral or CNS infections. In evaluation of a preterm infant, specially adapted head circumference charts are consulted to distinguish abnormal head growth from rapid but normal head growth.

The primary diagnostic tools for detecting hydrocephalus in older infants and children are CT and MRI. Mild sedation or general anaesthesia is usually required for children under age 8 or with neurodevelopmental disabilities because the child must remain absolutely still for an accurate study. Diagnostic evaluation of children who have symptoms of hydrocephalus after infancy is similar to that employed in those with a suspected intracranial tumour.

Problems in differential diagnosis are related to the child whose head circumference is greater than the 95th percentile but whose head growth parallels the normal growth curve. It is sometimes valuable to measure the parental OFC to detect a possible normal familial characteristic (benign familial megalencephaly). (See Table 30.1 for diagnostic tests for neurological evaluation.)

Therapeutic Management

The treatment of hydrocephalus is directed towards relief of ventricular pressure, treatment of the cause of the ventriculomegaly, treatment of associated complications and management of problems related to the effect of the disorder on psychomotor development. The treatment is, with few exceptions, surgical.

Surgical Treatment. Improved neurosurgical techniques have established surgical treatment as the therapy of choice in almost all cases of hydrocephalus. This is accomplished by direct removal of an obstruction, such as resection of a neoplasm, cyst or haematoma, or, in rare instances of fluid overproduction, by choroid plexus extirpation (plexectomy or electric coagulation). However, most children require a shunt procedure that provides primary drainage of the CSF from the ventricles to an extracranial compartment, usually the peritoneum.

Most shunt systems consist of a ventricular catheter, a flush pump, a unidirectional flow valve and a distal catheter. All are radio-opaque for easy visualisation after placement, and all are tested for accuracy before insertion. A reservoir is frequently added to allow direct access to the ventricular system for administration of medications and removal of fluid. In all models the valves are designed to open at a predetermined intraventricular pressure and close when the pressure falls below that level, thus preventing backflow of fluid. Most shunts now in use have differential pressure and adjustable programmable valves with capability for changing the pressures with an external magnet, thus avoiding additional surgery.

The standard procedure for many years has been the **ventriculoperitoneal (VP) shunt**, especially in neonates and young infants (Fig 30.10). There is greater allowance for excess tubing, which minimises the number of revisions needed as the child grows. Because it requires repeated lengthening, the ventriculoatrial (VA) shunt (ventricle to right atrium) is reserved for older children who have attained

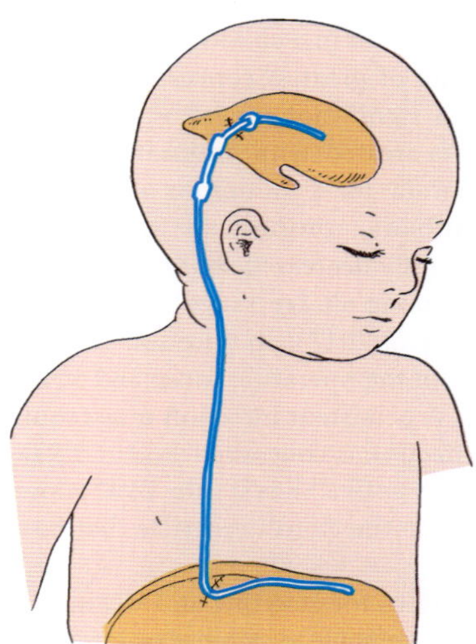

Fig 30.10 Ventriculoperitoneal shunt. Catheter is threaded beneath skin.

most of their somatic growth and children with abdominal pathological conditions. The VA shunt is contraindicated in children with cardiopulmonary disease or elevated CSF protein.

The initial shunt is placed when indicated on the basis of individual assessment. The timing of revisions varies widely. In most instances revisions are performed when physical signs indicate shunt malfunction (i.e. signs of elevated ICP). Sometimes revisions are planned for specific times during development. The initial success rate is relatively high. However, shunts are associated with complications that interfere with continued shunt function or that threaten the child's life.

Endoscopic third ventriculostomy (ETV) is a procedure that has potential for allowing greater independence from VA or VP shunting in children with obstructive hydrocephalus. ETV involves creating a small opening in the floor of the third ventricle, allowing CSF to flow freely through the previously blocked ventricle. Studies to date have not demonstrated improved short-term outcomes with ETV compared with VP shunting (Kulkarni et al 2016). Long-term outcomes need to be studied. VP shunts have a risk of infection and shunt failure whereas ETV does not; however, for the foreseeable future placement of a VP shunt for treatment of hydrocephalus remains a frequent neurosurgical procedure (Venable et al 2016).

Complications. The major complications of VP shunts are infection and malfunction. All shunts are subject to mechanical difficulties, such as kinking, plugging or separation and migration of tubing. Malfunction is most often caused by mechanical obstruction either within the ventricles from particulate matter (tissue or exudate) or at the distal end from thrombosis or displacement as a result of growth. Functional obstruction of a shunt's antisiphon device remains a common complication. About 22% of shunt failures are reported within the first 90 days, the majority of these within the first month (Venable et al 2016). The child with a shunt obstruction often is seen in an emergency visit with clinical manifestations of increased ICP, such as nausea, vomiting, irritability and a bulging fontanel, that is frequently accompanied by worsening neurological status.

One of the most common and serious complications, shunt infection, can occur at any time, but the period of greatest risk is within the first month after placement (Månsson et al 2017). Within 2 years shunt infection rates are reported to be approximately 5% to 10% (Månsson et al 2017). Infections include sepsis, bacterial endocarditis, wound infection, shunt nephritis, meningitis and ventriculitis and may be a result of intercurrent infections at the time of shunt placement. Brain abscess associated with colonic perforation and infection with a gram-negative enteric organism suggests an ascending shunt infection in a child who has a VP shunt. Meningitis and ventriculitis are of greatest concern because any complicating CNS infection is a significant predictor of future intellectual disability. Infection is treated with antibiotics administered intravenously or intrathecally for a minimum of 7 to 10 days. The use of perioperative antibiotic prophylaxis or antibiotic-impregnated shunts has significantly decreased shunt infection rates, particularly acute infections, among all age ranges of patients and all types of shunts (Månsson et al 2017). In addition measures to reduce the number of people in the operating room and strictly enforced hand washing can help. A persistent infection may require removal of the shunt until the infection is controlled, and an EVD, or external ventriculostomy, is used until CSF is sterile. EVD allows removal of CSF from a tube placed in the child's ventricle that flows by gravity into a collection device.

The primary reasons for inserting an EVD include unstable status, increased ICP that is difficult to stabilise or infection from an existing VP shunt. The EVD may drain CSF intermittently or continuously according to need. The EVD is a closed system made up of transparent pliable tubing that should be labelled, a collection bag and, at times, a drip chamber between the tubing and the collection bag. The EVD is placed at the level of the child's external auditory meatus with the head at a 20- to 30-degree elevation, depending on medical practitioner preference. Elevating the EVD above this level decreases the flow of CSF, and placing the device below the level of the external meatus increases the flow. Ambulation or sitting up in bed or a chair usually requires that the tubing be clamped to prevent imbalance in CSF drainage. In addition, the EVD is a closed sterile system. Aseptic technique should be used during any manipulation or maintenance of the EVD system, such as in relation to emptying the device or changing the scalp dressing (Hepburn-Smith et al 2016). Accurate and frequent documentation of the incision site, amount, colour and consistency of drainage into the device and the child's vital and neurological signs are an important part of the nursing care.

Another serious shunt-related complication is subdural haematoma caused by too-rapid reduction of ICP and, in some cases, tentorial herniation as a result of imbalance in CSF drainage. These complications can be averted by careful assessment of ICP before insertion of the shunt and use of correct valvular pressure. Other complications that may occur include peritonitis, abdominal abscesses, perforation of abdominal organs by catheter or trocar (at the time of insertion), fistulas, hernias and ileus. Some children require shunt lengthening as body growth occurs. This procedure usually involves replacing the distal catheter below the valve.

Prognosis. The prognosis of children with treated hydrocephalus depends largely on the cause of the dilated ventricles before shunt placement and the amount of irreversible brain damage before shunting (Kinsman & Johnston 2016). Those children with isolated aqueductal stenosis usually function cognitively like their typically developing peers (Kahle et al 2016). The neurological disorders seen in children after shunting for hydrocephalus are most often due to the underlying cause of the hydrocephalus rather than the hydrocephalus itself (Paulsen et al 2015).

Survivors have a high incidence of intellectual disability and learning disorders, including challenges with memory, processing and visuospatial skills requiring special education services. Tumours, meningitis and intraventricular haemorrhage are the conditions most closely associated with hydrocephalus accompanied by intellectual disability (Paulsen et al 2015). Children with myelomeningocele or intraventricular haemorrhage often have motor disabilities. As with all paediatric neurological conditions, social and behaviour problems are common, including attention deficit/hyperactivity disorder. Up to a third of children with hydrocephalus will have epilepsy (Kahle et al 2016).

Surgically treated hydrocephalus in patients with little or no evidence of irreversible brain damage has a survival rate of about 80%, with most deaths occurring within the first year of treatment (Paulsen et al 2015). Those with poor outcomes included children shunted for posthaemorrhagic hydrocephalus or meningitis. Most children who require shunting must depend on the shunt for the remainder of their life.

Nursing Care Management

The infant with suspected or confirmed hydrocephalus is observed carefully for signs of increasing ventricular size and increasing ICP. In infants the head is measured daily at the point of largest measurement. (See Chapter 4 for technique.) To avoid the likelihood of wide discrepancies, the point at which the measurements are taken is indicated on the head with a marking pen. Fontanels and suture lines are palpated for size, signs of bulging, tenseness and separation. Irritability, lethargy, seizure activity and altered vital signs and feeding behaviour may indicate an advancing pathological condition.

In older children, who are usually admitted to the hospital for elective or emergency shunt revision, the most valuable indicators of increasing ICP are an alteration in the child's level of consciousness, complaint of headache and changes in interaction with the environment. Changes are identified by observing and comparing present behaviour with customary behaviour, sleep patterns, developmental capabilities and habits obtained through a detailed history and a baseline assessment. This baseline information serves as a guide for postoperative assessment and evaluation of shunt function.

The nurse is responsible for preparing the child for diagnostic tests such as MRI or a CT scan and for assisting with procedures such as a ventricular tap, which is often performed to relieve excessive pressure and to obtain CSF during the preoperative period. Sedation is required because the child must remain absolutely still during diagnostic testing. A variety of drugs are available for sedation. (See Chapter 22 for preparing children for procedures.) If surgery is anticipated, IV infusions should not be placed in a scalp vein.

Postoperative Care. In addition to routine postoperative care and observation, the infant or child is positioned carefully on the unoperated side to prevent pressure on the shunt valve. The child remains flat to help avert complications resulting from too-rapid reduction of intracranial fluid. The surgeon indicates the position to be maintained and the extent of activity allowed.

The nurse continues observation for signs of increased ICP that indicate obstruction of the shunt. Neurological assessment includes pupil dilation (pressure causes compression or stretching of the oculomotor nerve, producing dilation on the same side as the pressure) and blood pressure (hypoxia to the brainstem causes variability in these vital signs). The nurse also observes for abdominal distension and constipation because CSF may cause peritonitis or a postoperative ileus as a complication of distal catheter placement.

Because infection is the greatest hazard of the postoperative period, nurses are continually on the alert for the usual manifestations of CSF infection, including elevated temperature, poor feeding, vomiting, decreased responsiveness and seizure activity. There may be signs of local inflammation at the operative sites and along the shunt tract. Antibiotics are administered by the IV route as ordered, and the nurse may need to assist with intraventricular instillation. Inspect the incision site for leakage, and test any suspected drainage for glucose, an indication of CSF.

Family Support. Specific needs and concerns of parents during periods of hospitalisation are related to the reason for the child's hospitalisation (e.g. shunt revision, infection, diagnosis) and the diagnostic and surgical procedures to which the child must be subjected. Parents may have little understanding of anatomy; therefore, they need further explanation and reinforcement of information that was given to them by the medical practitioner, neurosurgeon and nurse practitioners, including information about what to expect. They are especially frightened of any procedure that involves the brain. The fear of disability or brain damage is real and pervasive. Nurses can calm their anxiety with explanations of the rationale underlying the various nursing and medical activities such as positioning or testing and by simply being available and willing to listen to their concerns.

To prepare for the child's discharge and home care, instruct the parents on how to recognise signs that indicate shunt malfunction or infection. Active children may have injuries, such as a fall, that can damage the shunt, and the tubing may pull out of the distal insertion site or become disconnected during normal growth. Contact sports such as Australian rules football, rugby, boxing and wrestling are usually prohibited if a person has a VP shunt; other sports such as swimming, soccer and athletics are acceptable and even encouraged for the child's physical and emotional health. Families should consult with their child's neurosurgeon or neurosurgery nurse practitioner about activities after discharge as providers vary in their recommendations. Helmets must be worn for riding bikes, skateboards and scooters. It is also important for the nurse to encourage families to enrol infants and toddlers with hydrocephalus into an early childhood development program to monitor their development and quickly address any signs that they are not keeping up with their typically developing peers.

The management of hydrocephalus in a child is a demanding task for both the family and health professionals. Helping the family cope with the child's difficulties is an important nursing responsibility. Children with hydrocephalus have lifelong special healthcare needs. The nurse can provide optimum primary healthcare, including teaching families hand hygiene and hand washing, advice on immunisations, treatments for common infectious conditions or child care and school precautions. The overall aim is to establish realistic goals and an appropriate educational program that will assist the child in achieving the maximum potential. Families can be referred to community agencies for support and guidance.

INTRACRANIAL INFECTIONS

The nervous system is subject to infection by the same organisms that affect other organs of the body. However, the nervous system is limited in the ways in which it responds to injury. Laboratory studies are needed to identify the causative agent. The inflammatory process can affect the meninges (meningitis) or brain (encephalitis).

Meningitis can be caused by a variety of organisms, but the three main types are: (1) bacterial, or pyogenic, caused by pus-forming bacteria, especially meningococci and pneumococci organisms; (2) viral, or aseptic, caused by a wide variety of viral agents; and (3) tuberculous, caused by the tuberculin bacillus. The majority of children with acute febrile encephalopathy have either bacterial meningitis or viral meningitis as the underlying cause.

Bacterial Meningitis

Bacterial meningitis is an acute inflammation of the meninges and CSF. The advent of antimicrobial therapy has had a marked effect on the course and prognosis. Today, *H. influenzae* type b infection has been virtually eradicated among young children in areas where the Hib vaccine is administered routinely. Since the introduction of widespread vaccination for *S. pneumoniae,* the incidence of pneumococcal meningitis in children has decreased, but it remains the most common cause of meningitis in children ages 3 months to 11 years. It is also the most likely to result in death (Heckenberg et al 2014).

Aetiology

A variety of bacterial agents can cause bacterial meningitis. Since the introduction of vaccinations against most common causes of community-acquired pathogens, the incidence of bacterial meningitis has declined precipitously. It is now most common in children under 1 year of age (Marcdante & Kliegman 2016). The leading causes of neonatal meningitis are group B streptococcus (GBS) and *Escherichia coli* (Ku et al 2015).

Meningococcal meningitis is the only type readily transmitted by droplet infection from nasopharyngeal secretions and so has the potential to occur in outbreaks (Vetter et al 2016).

Maternal factors, such as premature rupture of fetal membranes and maternal infection during the last week of pregnancy, are major causes of neonatal meningitis. It is a devastating disease with significant morbidity and mortality. Children who survive neonatal meningitis are 10 times more likely to have moderate to severe disabilities than those who have not had meningitis (Ku et al 2015). The incidence of early-onset GBS meningitis has been reduced by more than 70% with the adoption of antenatal screening and administration of intrapartum prophylactic antibiotics (Ku et al 2015).

Risk factors for children developing meningitis include lack of immunisation to the specific pathogen; recent exposure to someone with invasive *Neisseria meningitidis* or *H. influenzae* type b disease; penetrating head trauma; cochlear implant devices; and anatomical defects such as midline facial defects, inner ear fistulas or recent placement of a ventricular shunt (Swanson 2015).

Pathophysiology

The most common route of infection is vascular dissemination from a focus of infection elsewhere. For example, organisms from the nasopharynx invade the underlying blood vessels, cross the BBB and multiply in the CSF. Invasion by direct extension from infections in the paranasal and mastoid sinuses is less common. Organisms also gain entry by direct implantation after penetrating wounds, skull fractures that provide an opening into the skin or sinuses, lumbar puncture or surgical procedures, anatomical abnormalities such as spina bifida or foreign bodies such as an internal ventricular shunt or an external ventricular device. Once implanted, the organisms spread into the CSF, by which the infection spreads throughout the subarachnoid space.

The infective process is like that seen in any bacterial infection: inflammation, exudation, white blood cell accumulation and varying degrees of tissue damage. The brain becomes hyperaemic and oedematous, and the entire surface of the brain is covered by a layer of purulent exudate that varies with the type of organism. For example, meningococcal exudate is most marked over the parietal, occipital and cerebellar regions; the thick, fibrinous exudate of pneumococcal infection is confined chiefly to the surface of the brain, particularly the anterior lobes; and the exudate of streptococcal infections is similar to that of pneumococcal infections, but thinner. As infection extends to the ventricles, thick pus, fibrin or adhesions may occlude the narrow passages and obstruct the flow of CSF.

Clinical Manifestations

The clinical manifestations of acute bacterial meningitis depend to a large extent on the child's age. The type of organism, the effectiveness of therapy for antecedent illness and whether it occurs as an isolated entity or as a complication of another illness or injury also influence the clinical manifestation (Box 30.6).

Children and Adolescents. The onset of illness may be abrupt and rapid, or develop progressively over one or several days, and may be preceded by a febrile illness. Most children with meningitis are seen with fever, chills, headache and vomiting that are associated with or quickly followed by alterations in sensorium; however, some may present only with lethargy and irritability (Weinberg & Thompson-Stone 2018). The child is extremely irritable and agitated and may develop seizures, photophobia, confusion, hallucinations, aggressive behaviour, drowsiness, stupor or coma.

The child resists flexion of the neck (nuchal rigidity). Kernig's and Brudzinski's signs are positive. Reflex responses are variable, although they show hyperactivity. The skin may be cold and cyanotic with poor peripheral perfusion.

BOX 30.6 Clinical Manifestations of Bacterial Meningitis

Children and Adolescents

- Usually abrupt onset
- Fever
- Chills
- Headache
- Vomiting
- Alterations in sensorium
- Seizures (often the initial sign)
- Irritability
- Agitation
- May develop the following:
  - photophobia
  - delirium
  - hallucinations
  - aggressive behaviour
  - drowsiness
  - stupor
  - coma
- Nuchal rigidity; may progress to opisthotonos
- Positive Kernig's and Brudzinski's signs
- Hyperactivity but variable reflex responses
- Signs and symptoms peculiar to individual organisms:
  - petechial or purpuric rashes (meningococcal infection), especially when associated with a shock-like state
  - joint involvement (meningococcal or *Haemophilus influenzae* infection)
  - chronically draining ear (pneumococcal meningitis)

Infants and Young Children

- Classic picture (above) rarely seen in children between 3 months and 2 years of age
- Fever
- Poor feeding
- Vomiting
- Marked irritability
- Frequent seizures (often accompanied by a high-pitched cry)
- Bulging fontanel
- Nuchal rigidity possible
- Brudzinski's and Kernig's signs not helpful in diagnosis
- Difficult to elicit and evaluate in this age group
- Subdural empyema (*H. influenzae* infection)

Neonates

Specific Signs

- Child well at birth but within a few days begins to look and behave poorly
- Refuses feedings
- Poor sucking ability
- Vomiting or diarrhoea
- Poor tone
- Lack of movement
- Weak cry
- Full, tense and bulging fontanel may appear late in course of illness
- Neck usually supple

Non-specific Signs That May Be Present

- Hypothermia or fever (depending on the infant's maturity)
- Jaundice
- Irritability
- Drowsiness
- Seizures
- Respiratory irregularities or apnoea
- Cyanosis
- Weight loss

Other signs and symptoms may appear that are specific to individual organisms. Petechial or purpuric rashes occur in 50% of cases and indicate a meningococcal infection (meningococcaemia), especially when the eruption is associated with a septic shock–like state. Joint involvement is seen in meningococcal and *H. influenzae* infection. A chronically draining ear commonly accompanies pneumococcal meningitis. *E. coli* infection may be associated with a congenital dermal sinus that communicates with the subarachnoid space.

Infants and Young Children. Between 3 months and 2 years of age the illness is characterised by fever or hypothermia, poor feeding, vomiting, marked irritability, restlessness, seizures and a bulging or tense fontanel, which are often accompanied by a high-pitched cry.

Neonates. Meningitis in newborn and premature infants is extremely difficult to diagnose. The vague and non-specific manifestations, which are characteristic of all neonatal sepsis, bear little resemblance to the findings in older children. These infants are usually well at birth but within a few days begin to appear ill. They refuse feedings, have poor sucking ability and may vomit or have diarrhoea. They display poor muscle tone and lack of movement and have a poor cry. Other non-specific signs that may be present include hypothermia or fever (depending on the infant's maturity), jaundice, irritability, drowsiness, seizures, respiratory irregularities or apnoea, cyanosis and weight loss. The full, tense and bulging fontanel may or may not be present until late in the course of the illness, and the neck is usually supple. Untreated, the infant's condition will decline to cardiovascular collapse, seizures and apnoea. Even with improved antibiotics and more rapid diagnosis, the prognosis of neonatal meningitis has not improved in decades; this is likely to be due to the virulence of the infectious pathogen (Gordon et al 2017).

Complications. The incidence of complications from acute bacterial meningitis has been significantly reduced with early diagnosis and vigorous antimicrobial therapy. If infection extends to the ventricles, thick pus, fibrin or adhesions may occlude the narrow passages, thereby obstructing the flow of CSF and causing obstructive hydrocephalus. Subdural effusions often occur, and thrombosis may occur in meningeal veins or venous sinuses. Destructive changes may take place in the cerebral cortex, and brain abscesses may form by direct extension of the infection or by vascular dissemination. Extension of the infection to the areas of the cranial nerves or compression necrosis from increased pressure may cause deafness, blindness or weakness or paralysis of facial or other muscles of the head and neck.

One of the most dramatic and serious complications usually associated with meningococcal infections is meningococcal sepsis, or meningococcaemia. When the onset is severe, sudden and rapid, it is known as the Waterhouse-Friderichsen syndrome. The syndrome is characterised by overwhelming septic shock, disseminated intravascular coagulation, massive bilateral adrenal haemorrhage and purpura (Fig 30.11). Meningococcaemia requires immediate emergency treatment, hospitalisation and intensive care because of the serious sequelae that can quickly develop (Weinberg & Thompson-Stone 2018).

Other acute complications of meningitis include SIADH (see Chapter 31), subdural effusions, seizures, cerebral oedema and herniation and hydrocephalus. Obstruction to the flow of CSF occurs during the acute phase of illness by clumping of purulent material in the drainage channels and during the chronic phase by adhesive arachnoiditis or fibrotic obstruction through any of the ventricular foramina. Postmeningitic complications in neonates include ventriculitis, which results in cystic, walled-off areas of the brain with fluid accumulation and pressure.

Extension of the inflammation to cranial nerves or compression and destruction of the nerves from ICP can produce permanent impairment of vision or hearing and other nerve palsies. CN VIII damage is usually followed by permanent deafness, the most common permanent neurological sequela of bacterial meningitis (Weinberg & Thompson-Stone 2018). Other long-term complications include cerebral palsy, cognitive impairments, learning disorders, attention deficit/hyperactivity disorder and seizures.

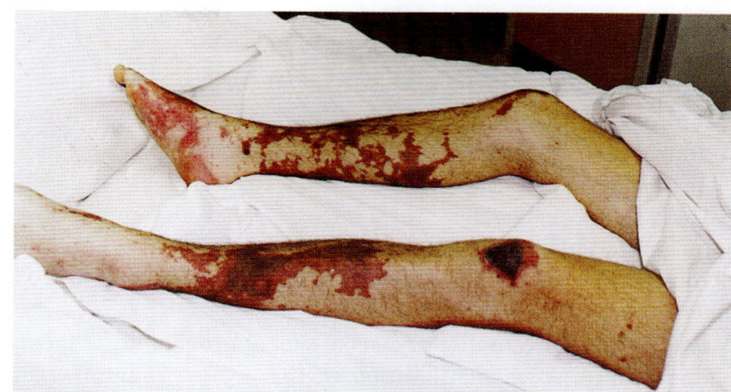

Fig 30.11 Purpura of the lower extremities of child suffering from meningococcaemia.

Hemiparesis and tetraparesis may result from damage caused by arteritis or thrombosis or other mechanisms. Behavioural changes occur in some children. Evidence indicates that psychometric and behavioural defects may be a significant concomitant sign of meningitis in childhood, although it is difficult to determine the degree to which meningitis affects the intelligence of young children. Meningitis in the neonatal period is more likely to cause lifelong impairments, including moderate to severe developmental delay, blindness, deafness and epilepsy (Swanson 2015).

Diagnostic Evaluation

A lumbar puncture is the definitive diagnostic test. The fluid pressure is measured, and samples are obtained for culture, Gram stain, blood cell count and determination of glucose and protein levels. The findings are usually diagnostic. Culture and sensitivity are needed to identify the causative organism. Spinal fluid pressure is usually elevated, but interpretation is often difficult when the child is crying. Sedation can alleviate the child's pain and fear associated with this procedure. If there is evidence or suspicion of increased ICP, a CT scan of the head may be warranted before the procedure (Weinberg & Thompson-Stone 2018).

The patient generally has an elevated white blood cell count, often predominantly polymorphonuclear leucocytes. The glucose level is reduced, generally in proportion to the duration and severity of the infection. The relationship between the CSF glucose and serum glucose levels is important in evaluating the glucose content of CSF; therefore, a serum glucose sample is drawn approximately 30 minutes before the lumbar puncture. Protein concentration is usually increased.

Blood culture is advisable for all children suspected of having meningitis if antibiotics are started before obtaining CSF. Blood culture will occasionally be positive when CSF culture is negative. Nose and throat cultures may provide helpful information in some cases.

Therapeutic Management

Acute bacterial meningitis is a medical emergency that requires early recognition and immediate therapy to prevent death and avoid residual disabilities. The initial therapeutic management includes the following:

- isolation precautions
- initiation of antimicrobial therapy
- maintenance of hydration

- maintenance of ventilation
- reduction of increased ICP
- management of systemic shock
- control of seizures
- control of temperature
- treatment of complications.

The child is usually moved to an intensive care unit for close observation. An IV infusion is started to facilitate administration of antimicrobial agents, fluids, antiepileptic drugs and blood, if needed. The child is placed in respiratory isolation.

Drugs. Until the causative organism is identified, empirical therapy is administered. After identification of the organism, antimicrobial agents are adjusted accordingly.

Non-specific Measures. Maintaining hydration is a prime concern. The patient's condition determines whether IV fluids are needed and the type and amount of fluid. The optimum hydration involves correction of any fluid deficits and electrolyte abnormalities, followed by fluid restriction until normal serum sodium levels and no signs of increased ICP are present. If needed, measures to decrease ICP are implemented (see earlier in the chapter); however, long-term fluid restriction is not the standard of care because a lack of fluid volume can reduce blood pressure and CPP, causing CNS ischaemia (Prober et al 2016a).

Complications, such as subdural effusion in infants and disseminated intravascular coagulation syndrome, are treated appropriately. Shock is managed by restoration of circulating blood volume and maintenance of electrolyte balance. Seizures can occur during the first few days of treatment. These are controlled with the appropriate antiepileptic drug.

Hearing loss is common. The patient should undergo auditory evaluation shortly after discharge so that audiology and speech and communication therapies can begin as soon as possible.

Prognosis. Less than 10% of cases of bacterial meningitis are fatal; the highest mortality rate is seen in pneumococcal meningitis and in infants under the age of 6 months (Prober et al 2016a). Prognosis is dependent in large part on the length of time between onset of illness and initiation of antibiotic therapy, rapidity of diagnosis after onset, type of organism, prolonged or complicated seizures, low CSF glucose concentration and adequacy of therapy. Up to half of those who recover from meningitis will have some neurodevelopmental sequelae ranging from mild behavioural and learning problems to profound hearing impairment, intractable epilepsy and significant intellectual disability (Prober et al 2016a).

The sequelae of bacterial meningitis occur most often when the disease occurs in the first 2 months of life and least often in children with meningococcal meningitis. The residual deficits in infants are primarily a result of communicating hydrocephalus and the greater effects of cerebritis on the immature brain. In older children the residual effects are related to the inflammatory process itself or result from vasculitis associated with the disease. Bacterial meningitis continues to cause substantial morbidity in infants and children.

Prevention. Vaccination is the foundation of prevention of CNS infections. Vaccines are available in Australia and New Zealand for pneumococci (types A, B, C, Y), W-135 meningococci and *H. influenzae* type b.

Nursing Care Management

Nurses should take the necessary precautions to protect themselves and others from possible infection. Teach parents proper hand washing technique and remind them as needed.

Keep the room as quiet as possible and environmental stimuli at a minimum as most children with meningitis are sensitive to noise, bright lights and other external stimuli. Help the family limit the number and frequency of visitors until the child is and feels better. Most children are more comfortable without a pillow under their head but with the head of the bed slightly elevated. Use pillows alongside a child in a side-lying position and between the child's knees for comfort in cases of nuchal rigidity. Avoid actions that cause pain or increase discomfort, such as lifting the child's head. Evaluating the child for pain and implementing appropriate relief measures are important ongoing interventions. Measures are used to ensure safety because the child is often restless, disoriented and subject to seizures. Prevention of falls is essential.

The nursing care of the child with meningitis is determined by the child's symptoms and treatment (see Box 30.6). Observation of vital signs, neurological signs, LOC, urinary output and other pertinent data is carried out at frequent intervals. The child who is unconscious is managed as described previously, and all children are observed carefully for signs of the complications just described, especially increased ICP, shock and respiratory distress. Frequent assessment of the open fontanels is needed in the infant because subdural effusions and obstructive hydrocephalus can develop as a complication of meningitis.

Administration of fluids and nourishment is determined by the child's status. The child who is not alert and oriented is given nothing by mouth. Other children are allowed clear liquids initially and, if tolerated, progress to a diet suitable for their age. Careful monitoring and recording of intake and output are needed to determine deviations that might indicate impending shock or increasing fluid accumulation, such as cerebral oedema or subdural effusion.

QUALITY PATIENT OUTCOMES

Bacterial Meningitis

- Early recognition of signs and symptoms of meningitis
- Antibiotics administered as soon as diagnosis is established
- Cerebral oedema prevented
- Exposure prevented by early isolation
- Side effects managed
- Neurological sequelae prevented

Family Support. The sudden nature of the illness makes emotional support of the child and parents extremely important. Parents are upset and concerned about their child's condition and often feel guilty for not having suspected the seriousness of the illness sooner. They need reassurance that the natural onset of meningitis is sudden and that they acted responsibly in seeking medical assistance when they did. The nurse encourages the parents to openly discuss their feelings to minimise blame and guilt. Some parents will benefit from referral to a hospital chaplain, social worker, psychologist or psychiatrist. The nurse keeps parents informed of the child's progress and of all procedures, results and treatments. In the event that the child's condition worsens, they need the same psychological care as other parents facing the possible death of their child. (See Chapter 19.)

Non-bacterial (Aseptic) Meningitis

The term *aseptic meningitis* refers to the onset of meningeal symptoms, fever and pleocytosis without bacterial growth from CSF cultures. Aseptic meningitis is caused by many different viruses, including arbovirus, enterovirus, herpes simplex virus, cytomegalovirus and human immunodeficiency virus. Enterovirus is the most common cause of aseptic meningitis (Prober et al 2016b). The onset may be abrupt or gradual, and many of the presenting signs and symptoms are the same

TABLE 30.3 Variation of Cerebrospinal Fluid Analysis in Bacterial and Viral Meningitis

Manifestations	Bacterial*	Viral
White blood cell count	Elevated; increased neutrophils	Slightly elevated; increased lymphocytes
Protein content	Elevated	Normal or slightly increased
Glucose content	Decreased	Normal
Gram stain; bacteria culture	Positive	Negative
Colour	Turbid or cloudy	Clear or slightly cloudy
Opening pressure	Elevated	Normal

*Results may vary in the neonate.

as bacterial meningitis, including headache, fever, photophobia and nuchal rigidity.

Diagnosis is based on clinical features and CSF findings. Table 30.3 lists variations in CSF values in bacterial and viral meningitis. It is important to differentiate this usually self-limiting disorder from the more serious forms of meningitis.

Treatment is primarily symptomatic, such as paracetamol for headache and muscle pain, maintenance of hydration and positioning for comfort. Until a definitive diagnosis is made, antimicrobial agents may be administered and isolation enforced as a precaution against the possibility that the disease might be of bacterial origin. Nursing care is similar to the care of the child with bacterial meningitis. The course of aseptic meningitis is usually much shorter and typically without significant complications.

Brain Abscess

Intracerebral abscesses form when pyogenic organisms gain access to neural tissue by way of the bloodstream from foci of infection or from direct inoculation of organisms from infections, penetrating trauma or surgical procedures. Chronic ear infection, mastoiditis, sinusitis and congenital heart disease are the most common predisposing factors for children with brain abscesses. The majority (70%) of brain abscesses are caused by aerobic and anaerobic streptococci (Prober & Mathew 2016). In neonates *Citrobacter* is most common, and fungi are more common in immunocompromised children (Prober & Mathew 2016).

The most common sites of intracerebral abscesses are the parietal, temporal and frontal lobes. Early signs of the disease are vague; however, the most common symptom is a severe headache. As the inflammatory process proceeds, symptoms intensify and include vomiting, lethargy, fever, seizures, papillo-oedema, focal neurological signs (hemiparesis) and progression to coma (Prober & Mathew 2016). Because mortality rates from brain abscesses may exceed 20%, prompt diagnosis and treatment are critical (Prober & Mathew 2016). Successful management consists of surgical drainage and antibiotic therapy. Surgical drainage is necessary if the mass is greater than 2 cm in diameter or there are signs of increased ICP. Where possible, the source of the infection is eradicated. Children may experience epilepsy, hemiparesis, cranial nerve abnormalities and behaviour/learning problems as long-term complications (Prober & Mathew 2016).

Encephalitis

Encephalitis is an inflammatory process of the CNS that is caused by a variety of organisms, including bacteria, spirochaetes, fungi, protozoa, helminths and viruses. Most infections are associated with viruses, and this discussion is limited to those agents.

Aetiology

Encephalitis can occur as a result of direct invasion of the CNS by a virus or postinfectious involvement of the CNS after a viral disease. Enteroviruses are the most common aetiology (Prober et al 2016b); however, the specific type of encephalitis may often not be identified.

Autoimmune encephalitis syndromes are a recently recognised cause of new-onset neurological deficits in children (Longoni et al 2016). In some children antibodies are identified, and there is a small group (< 20%) whose aetiology is a tumour, particularly ovarian teratoma, but the majority of children will not have either of these conditions (Dubey et al 2015). Diagnosis is usually based on clinical symptoms, which can be neurological, psychiatric or both (Scheer & John 2016). Neurological symptoms include seizures, encephalopathy and movement disorders (Dale et al 2017). Behavioural changes, hallucinations, anxiety and aggression are some of the more commonly seen psychiatric manifestations (Scheer & John 2016).

Herpes simplex encephalitis is an uncommon disease, but 30% of cases involve children. The initial clinical findings are non-specific (e.g. fever, altered mental status), but most cases evolve to demonstrate focal neurological signs and symptoms. Children may experience focal seizures. The CSF is abnormal in most cases. Because of a rise in the number of children with herpes simplex encephalitis, suspected cases require prompt attention, especially because the diagnosis can be difficult. CSF polymerase chain reaction (PCR) testing can confirm the clinical diagnosis rapidly. The early use of IV aciclovir reduces mortality and morbidity rates. Empiric therapy with aciclovir is given before precise virological diagnosis has been established.

The multiplicity of causes of viral encephalitis makes diagnosis difficult. Most are those involved with arthropod vectors (e.g. togaviruses and bunyaviruses) and those associated with haemorrhagic fevers (e.g. arenaviruses, filoviruses and hantaviruses).

Clinical Manifestations

The clinical features of encephalitis are similar regardless of the agent involved. Manifestations can range from a mild benign form that resembles aseptic meningitis, lasts a few days and is followed by rapid and complete recovery, to a rapidly progressing encephalitis with severe CNS involvement. The onset may be sudden or may be gradual with malaise, fever, headache, dizziness, apathy, nuchal rigidity, nausea and vomiting, ataxia, tremors, hyperactivity and speech difficulties. In severe cases the patient has high fever, stupor, seizures, disorientation, spasticity and coma that may proceed to death. Ocular palsies and paralysis also may occur.

Diagnostic Evaluation

The diagnosis is made on the basis of clinical findings and, where possible, identification of the specific virus. Early in the course of encephalitis, CT scan results may be normal. Later, haemorrhagic areas in the fronto-temporal region may be seen. Arboviruses are rarely detected in the blood or spinal fluid, but viruses of herpes, mumps, measles and enteroviruses may be found in the CSF. Serological testing may be required. The first blood sample should be drawn as soon as possible after onset, with the second sample drawn 2 or 3 weeks later.

Therapeutic Management

Patients suspected of having encephalitis are hospitalised promptly for observation, including ICP monitoring. In autoimmune encephalitis rapid initiation of immunotherapy, including corticosteroids, plasmapheresis and IV immunoglobulin, improves outcomes. Herpes simplex virus encephalitis is the only viral encephalitis that has specific treatment available. In other cases, treatment is primarily supportive and includes conscientious nursing care, control of cerebral manifestations and adequate nutrition and hydration, with observations and management as for other cerebral disorders.

Prognosis. Viral encephalitis can cause devastating neurological injury. The prognosis for the child with encephalitis depends on the child's age, the type of encephalitis and residual neurological damage. Very young children (less than 2 years of age) with viral encephalitis have an increased risk of neurological disability, including learning difficulties and epilepsy. About 80% of autoimmune encephalitis patients make a full or nearly full recovery (Longoni et al 2016).

Follow-up care with periodic re-evaluation and rehabilitation is important for patients who develop residual effects of encephalitis.

Nursing Care Management

Nursing care of the child with encephalitis is the same as for any unconscious child and for the child with meningitis. Additional nursing interventions include observation for deterioration in consciousness. Isolation of the child is not necessary; however, always use good hand washing technique. A main focus of nursing management is the control of rapidly rising ICP. Neurological monitoring, administration of medications and support of the child and parents are the major aspects of care.

SEIZURES AND EPILEPSY

A seizure is a 'transient occurrence of signs and/or symptoms due to abnormal excessive and synchronous neuronal activity in the brain' (Fisher et al 2014). Seizures are the most common paediatric neurological disorder. About 4% to 10% of children will have at least one seizure in the first 16 years of life (Mikati & Hani 2016). The manifestation of seizures depends on the region of the brain in which they originate and may include unconsciousness or altered consciousness, involuntary movements and changes in perception, behaviours, sensations and/or posture. Seizures are a symptom of an underlying disease process. They are individual events. Potential causes include infections, intracranial lesions or haemorrhage, metabolic disorders, trauma, brain malformations, genetic disorders or toxic ingestion.

Epilepsy is defined as two or more unprovoked seizures more than 24 hours apart and can be caused by a variety of pathological processes in the brain. A single seizure is not classified as epilepsy and is generally not treated with long-term antiepileptic drugs. Some seizures may result from an acute medical or neurological illness and cease after the illness is treated. In other cases, children may have one or more seizures without the cause ever being found.

When a child has had a seizure, it is important to classify the seizure, according to the International League Against Epilepsy (ILAE) Classification of the Epilepsies. Optimal treatment and prognosis require an accurate diagnosis and a determination of the cause whenever possible.

Epilepsy

The clinical definition of epilepsy was recently updated by the International League Against Epilepsy (ILAE):

> *Epilepsy is a disease of the brain defined by the following conditions: (1) at least two unprovoked seizures occurring more than 24 hours apart OR (2) one unprovoked seizure and a probability of further seizures similar to the general recurrence risk (at least 60%) after two unprovoked seizures occurring over the next 10 years.*
>
> ***(Fisher et al 2014)***

Seizures are a symptom of an underlying disease process. A single seizure event should be classified as epilepsy only if it meets criteria in number 2. Single seizures in children are generally not treated with long-term antiepileptic drugs. Some seizures may result from an acute medical or neurological illness and cease once the illness is treated. In other cases, children may have a single seizure without the cause ever being known.

Aetiology

Seizures in children have many different causes (Box 30.7). Seizures had been classified according to type and aetiology. The International League Against Epilepsy 2017 classification of seizures focuses on location of onset rather than aetiology: focal (formerly known as partial), generalised or unknown and unclassified (Fisher et al 2017). Focal

BOX 30.7 Aetiology of Seizures in Children

Non-recurrent (Acute)

- Febrile episodes
- Intracranial infection
- Intracranial haemorrhage
- Space-occupying lesions (cyst, tumour)
- Acute cerebral oedema
- Anoxia
- Toxins
- Drugs
- *Shigella* and *Salmonella* organisms
- Metabolic alterations:
  - Hypocalcaemia
  - Hypoglycaemia
  - Hyponatraemia or hypernatraemia
  - Hypomagnesaemia
  - Alkalosis
  - Disorders of amino acid metabolism
  - Deficiency states
  - Hyperbilirubinaemia

Recurrent (Chronic)

- Idiopathic epilepsy
- Epilepsy secondary to the following:
  - trauma
  - haemorrhage
  - anoxia
  - infections
  - toxins
  - degenerative phenomena
  - congenital defects
  - parasitic brain disease
  - hypoglycaemia injury
- Epilepsy—sensory stimulus
- Epilepsy-stimulating states:
  - narcolepsy and catalepsy
  - psychogenic
  - tetany from hypocalcaemia, alkalosis
- Hypoglycaemic states:
  - hyperinsulinism
  - hypopituitarism
  - adrenocortical insufficiency
  - hepatic disorders
- Uraemia
- Allergy
- Cardiovascular dysfunction or syncopal episodes
- Migraine

seizures are divided into those with preserved awareness and those with impaired awareness and those with or without motor manifestations. Generalised form onset seizures are also divided by their motor symptoms: tonic for the stiffening movements, clonic for the rhythmic jerking that may accompany tonic stiffening and absence for non-motor seizures. Unknown-onset seizures are classified using the same motor criteria as generalised seizures.

The causes of seizures in children are many. Acute reactive seizures are caused by an acute condition such as electrolyte imbalance, acute stroke, head trauma, meningitis or encephalitis. These seizures may continue and become epilepsy depending on the ability to treat the underlying condition. New-onset seizures may be the initial presentation of a child with a brain malformation. More than 100 genes have been found to cause epilepsy syndromes in children (Mikati & Hani 2016). Many, but not all, of these genetic orders cause intellectual disability in addition to epilepsy. The proportion of seizures and epilepsy for which we have no identifiable cause becomes smaller each year as neuroimaging and genetic testing improve. Those children who do not have an identifiable cause for their seizures and epilepsy have a better prognosis for eventual resolution of their epilepsy.

Incidence

Epilepsy and seizures are the most common neurological condition of children (Russ et al 2012). Epilepsy affects people of all ages, but particularly the very young and the elderly. Approximately 1 in every 10 children experience one or more seizures in the first 17 years of life (Russ et al 2012). The onset of epilepsy in children is highest during the first few months of life. The causative factors associated with childhood seizures are often linked to the child's age. In infants the most common causes are congenital brain malformations and genetic disorders, including metabolic disorders. Infections and epilepsy of unknown aetiology are common causes of seizures in childhood. Children with intellectual disability, cerebral palsy and/or autism spectrum disorder are more likely to have epilepsy than their typically developing peers.

Pathophysiology

Regardless of the aetiological factor or type of seizure, the basic mechanism is the same. Abnormal electrical discharges: (1) may arise from the simultaneous activation of neurons in both hemispheres of the brain (generalised seizures); (2) may be restricted to one area of the cerebral cortex, producing manifestations characteristic of that particular anatomical focus; or (3) may begin in a localised area of the cortex as a focal seizure and spread to other portions of the brain and, if sufficiently extensive, produce generalised seizure activity.

A seizure occurs when there is sudden excessive excitation and loss of inhibition within neuronal circuits, allowing the circuits to amplify their discharges simultaneously. These discharges occur in response to the activity of sodium, potassium, calcium and chloride ion channels. Normally these discharges are restrained by inhibitory mechanisms. In response to physiological stimuli, such as brain injury or infection, genetic abnormalities, severe hypoglycaemia, electrolyte imbalance, sleep deprivation and toxic exposures, these abnormal neuronal discharges can spread to nearby cortex and subcortical structures. Primary generalised seizures begin with abnormal discharges in both hemispheres, which can involve connections between the thalamus and neocortex. On the basis of these characteristic neuronal discharges (manifested as stereotypical symptoms observed and reported during seizures and/or as recorded by the EEG), seizures are designated as focal, generalised and unclassified epileptic seizures.

Seizure Classification and Clinical Manifestations

There are many different types of seizures, and each has unique clinical manifestations (Box 30.8). Seizures are classified into two major categories: (1) focal seizures (previously referred to as partial seizures), which have a local onset and involve a relatively small location in the brain; and (2) generalised seizures, which involve both hemispheres of the brain and are without local onset.

Focal Seizures (formerly known as Partial Seizures). Focal seizures may arise from any area of the cerebral cortex, but the frontal, temporal and parietal lobes are most often affected and are characterised by localised motor symptoms; somatosensory, psychic or autonomic symptoms; or a combination of these. The abnormal EEG discharges begin unilaterally and are evident as focal spikes or sharp waves. Focal seizures are subdivided into three types.

1. **Focal seizures without impaired awareness** (formerly simple partial seizures)—Sensory symptoms that occur in one part of the brain and cause no alteration of consciousness, often referred to as aura. Sometimes accompanied by motor movements.
2. **Focal seizures with impaired awareness** (formerly complex partial seizures)—Sensory and/or motor symptoms that result in a change or loss of consciousness.
3. **Focal to bilateral tonic–clonic seizures** (formerly simple or complex seizures secondarily generalised)—Focal seizures with or without awareness that evolve into generalised seizures, usually a tonic–clonic event.

Focal seizures exhibit manifestations related to where they occur in the brain. A clear description of the seizure (**ictal state**) by an eyewitness is a valuable aid in localising the brain area involved. Asking the child if he or she could hear, remember and respond during the event is also helpful for localisation. The initial event may provide the best clue for assessing the type of seizure and its localisation. Correctly localising the area of the brain involved with the seizure event is crucial for diagnostic and therapeutic reasons because many antiepileptic drugs are specific for each type of seizure.

In addition to the initial event, the circumstances that precipitated the episode are important. Identifying and eliminating triggering factors may be the only treatment needed. The **postictal state** (the period after a seizure) may be varied. The child may be drowsy, be uncoordinated, have transient aphasia or confusion and display some sensory or motor impairment. Document neurological changes. Weakness, hypotonia or inactivity of a body part may indicate an epileptogenic focus in the corresponding contralateral cortical region.

Focal seizures without impaired awareness. Focal seizures with motor signs originate from the primary motor cortex, located in the temporal lobe, which is the area of the brain that controls muscle movement. They are the most frequent type of focal seizure. The simplest form of focal seizures with motor signs is **clonus**, the rhythmic alternating contraction and relaxation of muscle groups.

Eye movements provide clues to the focus or origin of the seizure. Discharge in the cortex of one hemisphere tends to cause the eyes to deviate to the opposite side. Bilateral discharges tend to cause the eyes to move upwards or stare straight ahead. While deviated the eyes may rhythmically twitch.

Focal seizures with sensory symptoms are usually described as numbness, tingling or pins and needles. This may be the only symptom of a seizure, or it may spread to involve an adjacent sensory cortex or motor cortex. Auditory seizures may manifest as sounds becoming painfully loud, humming, buzzing or hissing. Visual seizures typically manifest as micropsia, macropsia or flashes of light or colours. Focal seizures with autonomic symptoms may consist of feelings of nausea or epigastric rising. Flushing or pallor, sweating or pupil dilation can be observed. Focal seizures with psychic symptoms may include speech

BOX 30.8 Classification and Clinical Manifestations of Partial and Generalised Seizures

Partial Seizures

Simple Partial Seizures with Motor Signs

- Characterised by the following:
  - Localised motor symptoms
  - Somatosensory, psychic, autonomic symptoms
  - Abnormal discharges remaining unilateral
- Manifestations
  - Aversive seizure (most common motor seizure in children)—Eye or eyes and head turn away from the side of the focus; awareness of movement or loss of consciousness
  - Rolandic (Sylvan) seizure—Tonic–clonic movements involving the face, salivation, arrested speech; most common during sleep
  - Jacksonian march (rare in children)—Orderly, sequential progression of clonic movements beginning in a foot, hand or face and moving, or 'marching', to adjacent body parts

Simple Partial Seizures with Sensory Signs

- Characterised by various sensations, including:
  - Numbness, tingling, prickling, paraesthesia or pain originating in one area (e.g. face or extremities) and spreading to other parts of the body
  - Visual sensations or formed images
  - Motor phenomena such as posturing or hypertonia

Focal Seizures with Impaired Awareness

- Observed more often in children from 3 years through adolescence
- Characterised by the following:
  - Period of altered behaviour
  - Amnesia for event (no recollection of behaviour)
  - Inability to respond to environment
  - Impaired consciousness during event
  - Drowsiness or sleep usually following seizure
  - Confusion and amnesia possibly prolonged
  - Complex sensory phenomena (aura)—Most frequent sensation is strange feeling in the pit of the stomach that rises towards the throat and is often accompanied by odd or unpleasant odours or tastes, complex auditory or visual hallucinations, ill-defined feelings of elation or strangeness (e.g. déjà vu, a feeling of familiarity in a strange environment), strong feelings of fear and anxiety, distorted sense of time and self, and in small children emission of a cry or attempt to run for help
- Patterns of motor behaviour:
  - Stereotypical
  - Similar with each subsequent seizure
  - May suddenly cease activity, appear dazed, stare into space, become confused and apathetic, and become limp or stiff or display some form of posturing
  - May be confused
  - May perform purposeless, complicated activities in a repetitive manner (automatisms), such as walking, running, kicking, laughing or speaking incoherently, most often followed by postictal confusion or sleep; may exhibit oropharyngeal activities, such as smacking, chewing, drooling, swallowing and nausea or abdominal pain followed by stiffness, a fall and postictal sleep; rarely manifests actions such as rage or temper tantrums; aggressive acts uncommon during seizure

Generalised Seizures

Tonic–Clonic Seizures (formerly known as Grand Mal)

- Most common and most dramatic of all seizure manifestations
- Occur without warning
- Tonic phase lasts approximately 10 to 20 seconds
- Manifestations:
  - Eyes roll upwards
  - Immediate loss of consciousness
  - If standing, falls to floor or ground
  - Stiffens in generalised, symmetrical tonic contraction of entire body musculature
  - Arms usually flexed
  - Legs, head and neck extended
  - May utter a peculiar piercing cry
  - Apnoeic, may become cyanotic
  - Increased salivation and loss of swallowing reflex
- Clonic phase: lasts about 30 seconds but can vary from only a few seconds to half an hour or longer
- Manifestations:
  - Violent jerking movements as the trunk and extremities undergo rhythmic contraction and relaxation
  - May foam at the mouth
  - May be incontinent of urine and faeces
- As event ends, movements less intense, occurring at longer intervals, then ceasing entirely
- ***Status Epilepticus***—Series of seizures at intervals too brief to allow the child to regain consciousness between the time one event ends and the next begins
  - Requires emergency intervention
  - Can lead to exhaustion, respiratory failure and death
- ***Postictal State:***
  - Appears to relax
  - May remain semiconscious and difficult to arouse
  - May awaken in a few minutes
  - Remains confused for several hours
  - Poor coordination
  - Mild impairment of fine motor movements
  - May have visual and speech difficulties
  - May vomit or complain of severe headache
  - When left alone, usually sleeps for several hours
  - On awakening is fully conscious
  - Usually feels tired and complains of sore muscles and headache
  - No recollection of entire event

Absence Seizures (formerly called Petit Mal)

- Characterised by the following:
  - Onset usually between 4 and 12 years of age
  - More common in girls than in boys
  - Usually cease at puberty
  - Brief loss of consciousness
  - Minimum or no alteration in muscle tone
  - May go unrecognised because of little change in child's behaviour
  - Abrupt onset; suddenly develops 20 or more attacks daily
  - Event often mistaken for inattentiveness or daydreaming
  - Events possibly precipitated by hyperventilation, hypoglycaemia, stresses (emotional and physiological), fatigue or sleeplessness
- Manifestations:
  - Brief loss of consciousness
  - Appear without warning or aura
  - Usually last about 5 to 10 seconds
  - Slight loss of muscle tone may cause child to drop objects
  - Ability to maintain postural control; seldom falls

BOX 30.8 Classification and Clinical Manifestations of Partial and Generalised Seizures—cont'd

- Minor movements such as lip smacking, twitching of eyelids or face or slight hand movements
- Not accompanied by incontinence
- Amnesia for episode
- May need to reorient self to previous activity

Atonic and Akinetic Seizures (also known as Drop Attacks)

- Characterised by the following:
  - Onset usually between 2 and 5 years of age
  - Sudden, momentary loss of muscle tone and postural control
  - Events recurring frequently during the day, particularly in the morning hours and shortly after awakening
- Manifestations:
  - Loss of tone causing child to fall to the floor violently; unable to break fall by putting out hand; may incur a serious injury to the face, head or shoulder
  - Loss of consciousness only momentary

Myoclonic Seizures

- May be isolated as benign essential myoclonus
- Characterised by the following:
  - Sudden, brief contractures of a muscle or group of muscles
  - Occur singly or repetitively
  - No postictal state
  - May or may not be symmetrical
  - May or may not include loss of consciousness

arrest or vocalisations, the sensation that an experience has occurred before (déjà vu), fear, displeasure, anger or irritability. The affective symptoms associated with focal seizures last only a few minutes and are unprovoked.

Focal seizures with impaired awareness. During the period of impaired consciousness the child may look vacant, dazed or frightened and be unable to respond when spoken to or to follow instructions and will not react when touched. Focal seizures with impaired awareness are the most common type of seizures. Focal seizures are observed in children of all ages and are the most common type in infants. These seizures may begin with an **aura**—a sensation or sensory phenomenon that precedes the seizure activity. Common sensations include a strange feeling at the bottom of the stomach that rises towards the throat, odd or unpleasant odours or taste, complex auditory or visual hallucinations or ill-defined feelings of strangeness (e.g. déjà vu). Small children may emit a cry as a manifestation of an aura. Strong feelings of fear and anxiety and a disturbed sense of time can be associated with an aura. The aura is part of the seizure event and is associated with EEG changes.

Another feature of a focal seizure may be **automatisms** (repetitive involuntary activities without purpose, carried out in a dreamy state). The predominant observations may be oropharyngeal activities such as: lip smacking, chewing, drooling, swallowing or picking at clothing or bed linens; ambulatory activities such as wandering or running; and verbal manifestations such as repeating words ('please, please', or 'help, help'). These automatisms may appear to be antisocial behaviours, such as removing clothes in public or attempting to open the door of a moving car. The child may begin walking or running and unknowingly run out into traffic or into obstacles. It is important to realise that the child's consciousness is impaired and that these actions are not deliberate. It is sometimes difficult to determine whether such behaviour is related to the seizure activity or to a behavioural deviation. If the behaviour results from seizure activity, all attempts to control such behaviour by physical restraint, with counselling or with behaviour plans will be ineffective. The child may suddenly cease activity, appear dazed, stare into space, become confused or apathetic, become limp or stiff or display some form of posturing. Because the seizure starts in the same part of the brain each time, the child will do the same thing during every event. The term *psychomotor seizure* was formerly used because of the frequent association of psychic symptoms and motor automatisms with focal seizures.

If the seizure involves areas of the brain that control motor function, the child exhibits movements such as jerking of the hands and arms. Focal seizures generally last only a few minutes. After the seizure the postictal period occurs, with signs of confusion and lack of recollection of the ictal period. Depending on the area of the brain involved during the episode, the child may sleep for a time.

Focal seizures that generalise. Focal seizures may spread and become generalised, usually into a tonic–clonic seizure. In such cases the focal seizure is considered the primary seizure event, and the generalised seizure is considered the secondary one. Thus it would be stated that the tonic–clonic seizure was not generalised at the onset but was a focal seizure that became a bilateral tonic–clonic or secondarily generalised seizure.

Generalised Seizures. Generalised seizures without a focal onset indicate that the initial involvement is from both hemispheres. Loss of consciousness and impairment of motor function occur from the outset. Unlike focal seizures that become generalised, there is no aura. Seizures can occur at any time, day or night. The interval between events may be minutes, hours, weeks or even years.

Tonic–clonic seizures. The generalised tonic–clonic seizure, formerly known as *grand mal*, is the most dramatic of all seizure manifestations of childhood. The seizure usually occurs without warning and consists of two distinct phases: tonic and clonic. In the tonic phase the child stiffens, the eyes roll upwards and the child loses consciousness. If standing, the child falls to the ground. The musculature stiffens in a generalised and symmetrical tonic contraction of the entire body. The arms usually flex, and the legs, head and neck extend. The mouth snaps shut, and the tongue may be bitten. The thoracic and abdominal muscles contract and sometimes produce a 'tonic cry' as air is forced over the vocal cords. Parents often misinterpret this as an expression of pain. The average tonic phase lasts 10 to 30 seconds, during which the child's respirations become slow and shallow and the child may become cyanotic. Autonomic phenomena that may be observed include increased blood pressure, increased heart rate, flushing and increased salivation.

In the clonic phase the tonic rigidity is replaced by intense jerking movements as the trunk and extremities undergo rhythmic contraction and relaxation. During this time the child cannot control oral secretions and may be incontinent of urine and faeces. As the seizure ends, the movements become less intense and occur at less frequent intervals until they cease entirely. The average clonic phase lasts 30 to 50 seconds.

In the postictal phase the child may remain semiconscious and difficult to arouse. The postictal phase can last 30 minutes to several hours (Mikati & Hani 2016). The child may remain confused or sleep.

He or she may have mild impairment of fine motor movements, have visual and speech difficulties and may vomit or complain of headache. On awakening, he or she is fully conscious but usually feels tired and may complain of sore muscles and a headache. The child has no recollection of the event.

Absence seizures. Absence seizures, formerly called *petit mal*, are generalised seizures. They have a sudden onset and are characterised by a brief loss of awareness, a blank stare and automatisms. Absence seizures are divided into typical and atypical. These seizures almost always first appear during childhood, usually between the ages of 5 to 8, and often stop spontaneously in the teenage years (Mikati & Hani 2016).

The onset of typical absence seizures is abrupt, with the child suddenly experiencing 20 or more events daily. Characteristically the brief loss of consciousness appears without warning and usually lasts 5 to 10 seconds. The child has a motionless blank stare that may be confused with inattentiveness or daydreaming. Slight loss of muscle tone may cause the child to drop objects, but he or she seldom falls. There may be automatisms such as lip smacking, twitching of the eyelids or face or fumbling with the clothes. The sudden arrest of activity and consciousness is not accompanied by incontinence. Although the child will not recall the episode, when the seizure ends, the child may be aware and able to report that he or she has missed things that happened. There is no postictal sleepiness. Most children can immediately resume previous activities but may be momentarily confused. Atypical absence seizures are accompanied by head nods and sudden myoclonic jerks. Atypical absence seizures, unlike typical absence seizures, can be difficult to treat (Mikati & Hani 2016).

Hyperventilation and photic stimulation are potent precipitators of absence seizures (Mikati & Hani 2016). If the child is involved in a group activity, such as classroom reading or discussion, he or she may need help to catch up with the group after the seizure. Frequent episodes can result in slowed intellectual processes and deterioration in schoolwork and behaviour. This is often the first indication of the problem. Absence seizures can be distinguished from daydreaming and attention deficit/hyperactivity disorder by attempting to physically interrupt the episode by touching the face and eyelashes. Children who are daydreaming will respond to touch, whereas those who are having an absence seizure cannot. The abnormal EEG pattern in absence epilepsy is diagnostic and distinguishes absence seizures from focal seizures.

Atonic seizures. Atonic seizures are a sudden, momentary and total loss of muscle tone. The onset is usually between 2 and 5 years of age. During a mild seizure the child may simply experience several sudden brief head drops. During a more severe episode the child suddenly falls to the ground, loses consciousness briefly and after a few seconds gets up as if nothing happened. Because of the sudden loss of tone, the child is unable to break the fall by putting out a hand, and can suffer injuries to the head, teeth and face. Therefore, if a child has frequent atonic seizures, wearing a helmet with a face guard when the child is up and walking around should be considered.

Myoclonic seizures. Myoclonic seizures are characterised by sudden, brief, shock-like movements of a muscle or group of muscles (Holmes 2018). The seizures may involve only the face and trunk or one or more extremities. They may occur singly or repetitively. The seizures may or may not be symmetrical. Myoclonic seizures often occur in combination with other seizure types. Myoclonic seizures should not be confused with myoclonic jerks that can occur normally in the course of falling asleep.

The myoclonic seizure can be confused with the exaggerated startle reflex often seen in children with severe developmental delays. The startle reflex occurs immediately after a stimulus such as a loud noise. The child will stiffly and rapidly extend all four extremities, sometimes with a cry, and then quickly return to his or her usual posture. An EEG with video recording can distinguish between the two events.

Tonic seizures. Tonic seizures are characterised by a sudden onset of increased tone. The child falls if standing. The child may involuntarily cry out because of contraction of the respiratory and abdominal muscles. Tonic seizures are longer than myoclonic seizures, with an average duration of 10 seconds. Postictal confusion, tiredness and headache are common.

Clonic seizures. Clonic seizures are characterised by loss of consciousness and decreased tone followed by jerking movements of the extremities. These movements may be more predominant in one extremity. The duration is typically from one to several minutes and may be followed by a rapid recovery or may have a period of postictal confusion.

Unknown-onset Epileptic Seizures. Unknown-onset epileptic seizures are seizures that lack sufficient information to classify. For example, the location of the onset of epileptic spasms, a type of seizure found predominantly in children under 2 years old, is often unknown. In addition to the seizures listed in the ILAE Classification of Epilepsies, several types of epileptic syndromes display a group of signs and symptoms that collectively characterise or indicate a particular condition. Several syndromes associated with epilepsy occur in infants and children. Two of these are West's syndrome and Lennox-Gastaut syndrome (LGS).

West's syndrome. Infantile spasms are the most common epilepsy of infancy. It has a peak onset between 4 and 8 months of life and rarely occurs after 2 years of age (Singhal et al 2018). The aetiology can be genetic, metabolic or structural but is unknown in about one-third of affected children. The pathophysiology is poorly understood. An abnormal EEG with hypsarrhythmia is pathognomonic. Nearly all children with infantile spasms have some degree of cognitive impairment (Singhal et al 2018).

Flexor spasms consist of brief contractions of the neck, trunk, arms and legs. The arms may either adduct or abduct, with the arms flexed at the elbow. Extensor spasms consist predominantly of extensor contractions resulting in abrupt extension of the neck and trunk with extensor adduction or abduction of the arms and legs. Eye deviation or nystagmus often occurs with infantile spasms. Infantile spasms may occur as a single event or in clusters, with as many as 150 seizures within a cluster. The infant often cries or is irritable during or after a cluster of spasms.

Adrenocorticotropic hormone (ACTH), an injectable hormonal treatment, is the first-line treatment recommended for infantile spasms. The use of high- versus low-dose therapy is controversial. Because of potential significant adverse side effects (e.g. immunosuppression, weight gain, hypertension, inconsolable crying and irritability) short-term therapy followed by a taper is recommended (Shumiloff et al 2013). ACTH is more likely to provide short-term resolution of infantile spasms, but longer-term resolution is no different when prednisolone (oral hormonal treatment) is used (Jones, Snead et al 2015). Due to the cost and difficulty obtaining ACTH, prednisone is considered to be a reasonable option by many neurologists.

Vigabatrin is usually the choice of treatment for infantile spasms in tuberous sclerosis (Hancock et al 2013). There is evidence that it works as well as hormonal treatment in the rare children with infantile spasms and normal development (Jones, Go et al 2015). Long-term use can damage the retinas, causing clinically asymptomatic peripheral visual field cuts. The risk of this visual field cut must be balanced with the benefit of controlling infantile spasms. New evidence suggests that combining vigabatrin with hormonal treatment is more effective than either treatment alone (O'Callaghan et al 2017).

The most recent Cochrane review of 18 randomised controlled studies found no single treatment proved to be more efficacious than any other in the treatment of infantile spasms; hormonal treatments resolve spasms more often than vigabatrin, but the hormonal treatments may cause more long-term side effects (Hancock et al 2013). Use of the ketogenic diet and other antiepileptic drugs as adjunctive therapy is increasing.

The diagnosis of infantile spasms is devastating for many families. Nurses play an important role in supporting these families while at the same time teaching them how to give injections, monitor blood pressure and blood glucose, avoid exposure to illness and adhere to all recommended appointments and procedures after discharge.

Lennox-Gastaut syndrome. Between 20% and 50% of infants who have infantile spasms eventually develop LGS (German & Maria 2018). LGS is diagnosed on three criteria: (1) the presence of multiple seizure types (atonic, myoclonic, tonic and atypical absence); (2) intellectual disability; and (3) slow spike wave discharges on EEG (Tenney & Glauser 2018). Onset of LGS is between 1 and 8 years of age. Children with LGS typically have multiple seizures daily. Tonic seizures are the most common. There are many causes of LGS; about one-third of children with LGS have no known cause. Causes include brain malformations and injury, neurocutaneous disorders, brain infections and genetic disorders. In addition to cognitive impairments, many of these children develop other problems, including hyperactivity, aggressive behaviour or autism spectrum disorder.

Treatment is challenging. Most children require more than one antiepileptic drug and even then many will continue to have some seizures. Drugs are chosen according to the types of seizures. In addition, the ketogenic diet or implantation of a vagus nerve stimulator may be efficacious for some of these children. The prognosis of LGS is typically poor. Additional family support is often required to maintain the child at home.

Diagnostic Evaluation

Establishing a diagnosis is critical for establishing a prognosis and planning appropriate treatment. The process of diagnosis in a child suspected of having epilepsy includes first determining whether the events thought to be seizures are epileptic seizures or non-epileptic events and then identifying the underlying cause, if possible. The assessment and diagnosis rely heavily on a thorough history, skilled observation and several diagnostic tests.

It is especially important to differentiate seizures from other brief alterations in consciousness or behaviour. Clinical entities that mimic seizures include staring, migraine headaches, toxic effects of drugs, syncope (fainting), breath-holding spells in infants and young children, movement disorders (tics, tremor, chorea), prolonged QT syndrome and other cardiac arrhythmias, sleep disturbances (sleepwalking, night terrors), psychogenic seizures, rage attacks and transient ischaemic attacks (rare in children). The toxic effects of maternal drug use and withdrawal from these drugs should be considered in the differential diagnosis of new-onset seizure activity in a newborn.

A detailed description of the seizure should be obtained from the caregiver(s) who witnessed it. Ask questions about the child's behaviour during the event, especially at the onset, and the time at which the seizure occurred (e.g. early morning, while awake or during sleep). Any factors that may have precipitated the seizure are important, including fever, infection, head trauma, anxiety, fatigue, sleep deprivation, menstrual cycle, alcohol and activity (e.g. hyperventilation or exposure to strong stimuli such as bright flashing light or loud noises). Record any sensory phenomena that the child can describe and if the child was able to hear during the seizure. The duration and progression of the seizure (if any) and the postictal feelings and behaviour (e.g. confusion, inability to speak, amnesia, headache and sleep) should also be noted. For children who have epilepsy, document how often they have seizures: daily, weekly or monthly. Knowing the age at which the child had his or her first seizure is important. It is important to determine whether more than one seizure type exists. It is often more informative to ask the parents to show you what the seizure looked like rather than relying on their verbal description. Demonstrating a seizure often reveals features, such as head turning, that would otherwise go unrecognised. Some seizures are overlooked by parents. For example, some parents may not identify brief head nods or brief single jerks as seizures unless specifically asked if their child has these symptoms.

A thorough medical history must be obtained, beginning with conception. Questions to consider include the following: Was the mother's pregnancy complicated by illness and drug use, either prescription or recreational? How old was the baby when discharged from the hospital after birth? Has the child had any overnight hospitalisations or surgeries? A complete history is designed to uncover possible risk factors for the development of seizures or epilepsy.

The family history should include whether other family members ever had a seizure of any kind, cognitive impairments, cerebral palsy, autism or other neurological disorders. Ask if there is a family history of sudden, unexpected deaths. A family history can offer clues to other paroxysmal disorders, such as migraine headaches, breath-holding spells, febrile seizures or neurological diseases.

A complete physical and neurological examination, including developmental assessment of language, learning, behaviour and motor abilities, may provide clues to the cause of the seizures. A number of laboratory and neuroimaging tests may be ordered depending on the child's age, whether it is a new-onset seizure, characteristics of the seizure and the history. Laboratory studies that may prove valuable include a white blood cell count (for signs of infection) and blood glucose measurements that may indicate hypoglycaemic episodes. Serum electrolytes, blood urea nitrogen, calcium, serum amino acids, lactate, ammonia and urine organic acids may indicate metabolic disturbances. Blood for chromosomal analysis may also be tested if a genetic aetiology is suspected. A toxicology screen should be performed if alcohol or drug ingestion or withdrawal is suspected. Lumbar puncture can confirm a suspected diagnosis of meningitis. CT may be done to detect a cerebral haemorrhage, infarctions, brain tumours and gross malformations. MRI provides greater anatomical detail and is used to detect developmental malformations, tumours and cortical dysplasias.

Most children with seizures will have an EEG. The EEG is the most useful tool for evaluating the child's risk of recurrent seizures, helping determine the type of seizure the child had and diagnosing the type of epilepsy. The EEG confirms the presence of abnormal electrical discharges and provides information on the seizure type and the location of onset. The EEG is carried out under varying conditions: with the child asleep, awake, awake with provocative stimulation (flashing lights, noise) and hyperventilation. Stimulation may elicit abnormal electrical activity that is recorded on the EEG. Various seizure types produce characteristic EEG patterns; for example, a three-per-second spike and wave pattern is observed in absence epilepsy and a slow spike and wave pattern in LGS.

A normal EEG does not rule out seizures. The EEG is only a surface recording, lasts approximately 1 hour and therefore may show normal interictal activity. If there is concern about whether a child has seizures or the seizure type cannot be determined, a long-term video EEG may be done to record the child during wakefulness and sleep. The full-body image is recorded on video, with selected EEG channels displayed on the same screen for simultaneous recording and viewing. Amplitude-integrated electroencephalography (aEEG) monitoring is increasingly available in neonatal and paediatric intensive care units. This is a method of continuous monitoring of brain activity using recordings from a handful of leads compared with the 24 leads of standard EEGs. aEEG is useful for diagnosing seizures when standard EEG or a neurophysiologist to interpret it is unavailable. Although the EEG is valuable, it should not be used alone to determine the type of seizure. Rather, the EEG interpretation with a thorough clinical description of the child's behaviour during the seizure will inform the correct classification of the seizure and the appropriate treatment choice.

Therapeutic Management

The goal of treatment of seizure disorders is to control the seizures or to reduce their frequency and severity, discover and correct the cause when possible and help the child live as normal a life as possible. Discovering and, when possible, correcting the underlying cause of the seizures can lead to complete control of all seizures. If the seizure activity is a manifestation of an infectious, traumatic or metabolic process, seizure therapy is instituted as part of the general therapeutic regimen. Management of epilepsy has four treatment options: drug therapy, the ketogenic diet, vagus nerve stimulation and epilepsy surgery.

Drug Therapy. It is known that persons predisposed to epilepsy have seizures when their basal level of neuronal excitability exceeds a critical point; no event occurs if the excitability is maintained below this threshold. The administration of antiepileptic drugs serves to raise this threshold and prevent seizures. Consequently, the primary therapy for epilepsy is the administration of the appropriate antiepileptic drug or combination of drugs in a dosage that provides the desired effect without causing adverse side effects or toxicity. Antiepileptic drugs are believed to exert their effect primarily by reducing the responsiveness of neurons to the sudden, high-frequency nerve impulses that arise in the epileptogenic focus. Thus the seizure is effectively suppressed; however, the abnormal brain waves may or may not be altered. The chance of total control of seizures depends on the underlying cause of the seizures. Children with epilepsy without any underlying pathology such as brain malformations or genetic disorders and with normal development have the best prognosis.

The initiation of anticonvulsant therapy is based on several factors, including the child's age, type of seizure, risk of recurrence and other comorbid or predisposing medical issues. For children who develop recurrent seizures or epilepsy, treatment is begun with a single drug known to be effective for the child's seizure type and have the lowest risk of adverse side effects. The dosage is gradually increased until the seizures are controlled. If a child develops intolerable side effects, the medication is stopped and another one tried. If the drug at maximum doses reduces but does not stop all seizures, a second drug is added in gradually increasing doses. When seizures are controlled, the first drug may be tapered to reduce the potential adverse effects and drug interactions of polytherapy. Monotherapy remains the treatment of choice for epilepsy, but a combination of medications may be a viable alternative for children who do not have total seizure control with only one medication (Mikati & Hani 2016).

If complete seizure control is maintained on an antiepileptic drug for 2 years, it may be safe to slowly discontinue the drug for patients with no risk factors. Risk factors for recurrence of seizures include history of status epilepticus, older age at onset, duration of treatment before seizure control is achieved, presence of a neurological dysfunction (e.g. motor or cognitive impairment) and abnormal EEG findings when the medication is stopped (Lee et al 2017). Recurrence occurs most often within the first year of discontinuation (Braun & Schmidt 2014). When seizure medications are discontinued, the dosage is decreased gradually over weeks or months. Sudden withdrawal of a drug is not recommended because it can cause seizures, which may be longer and more intense than previously, to recur.

Potential complications of drug therapy. The side effects of continued use of antiepileptic medications are often distressing to the child and family. Most side effects are transient and dose related, but drug reactions warrant immediate attention. A serious potential adverse side effect of antiepileptic medication is allergic drug rash. The rash can start with hives and is usually very pruritic. Allergic drug rashes from antiepileptic drugs can spread quickly and become severe, life-threatening events. The drug should be stopped with any signs of a rash. A medical practitioner or nurse practitioner should evaluate the child within 24 hours or sooner if the child develops oedema or respiratory problems. Treatment includes antihistamines, adrenaline, glucocorticosteroids, anabolic steroids and/or airway management, depending on the severity of the reaction (Blaszczyk et al 2015).

Sleepiness, changes in mood or behaviour, vision changes and ataxia are some of the potential side effects of antiepileptic medications. These are very distressing to both children and families. They often disappear over time or when drug dosages are reduced. Blood cell counts, urinalysis and liver function tests are obtained at regular intervals in children receiving some older antiepileptic medications that can affect organ function.

Knowledge of drug-to-drug interactions, including other medications such as antibiotics, is critical in caring for the child with epilepsy. Knowledge of potential adverse effects is also imperative. Severe, potentially life-threatening side effects can occur with specific antiepileptic medications. Therefore, critical thinking and careful monitoring are necessary in providing optimum care to the child with epilepsy.

Ketogenic Diet. The **ketogenic diet** is a high-fat, very-low-carbohydrate and adequate-protein diet that has shown effectiveness for treatment of epilepsy (Martin et al 2016). It is also the first-line treatment for certain metabolic disorders, including pyruvate dehydrogenase deficiency, glucose transporter type I deficiency and glutaric aciduria type I. Consumption of the ketogenic diet forces the body to shift from using glucose as the primary energy source to using fat, and the individual develops a state of ketosis. The diet is rigorous. All foods and liquids the child consumes must be carefully weighed and measured. There is a liquid formula available for children who cannot take solid food. The diet is deficient in vitamins and minerals; therefore, vitamin and mineral supplementation is necessary. Potential adverse side effects of the diet include constipation, hypoglycaemia during initiation of the diet, acidosis and lethargy. Less common but more serious side effects include urinary tract infections, kidney stones and insufficient weight gain (Luat et al 2016).

The ketogenic diet (and its variations) has been shown to be an effective and tolerable treatment for medically refractory epilepsy with seizure control comparable to or better than that obtained with antiepileptic medications in some children (Martin et al 2016).

Vagus Nerve Stimulation. Vagus nerve stimulation (VNS) was developed as palliative treatment for patients with seizures not controlled by drugs and who are not candidates for diet or surgical therapy

(Moshe et al 2015). The results in children have been mixed, with a usually modest reduction in seizures (Dhamne et al 2018). A programmable signal generator is implanted subcutaneously in the chest. Electrodes tunnelled underneath the skin deliver electrical impulses to the left vagus nerve (CN X). The device is programmed non-invasively to deliver a precise pattern of stimulation to the left vagus nerve. The patient or caregiver can activate the device using a magnet at the onset of a seizure. No long-term adverse effects have been reported with VNS, but dysphonia, throat or neck pain and cough can occur during stimulation.

Surgical Therapy. When seizures are caused by a haematoma, vascular malformation, tumour or other cerebral lesion, surgical removal is usually recommended. Epilepsy surgery is the most effective treatment for children with medically refractory epilepsy due to focal cortical dysplasia and mesial temporal sclerosis. About 80% of these patients will be seizure-free 4 years after surgery (Moosa & Gupta 2014).

Epilepsy surgery does not always eliminate the need for antiepileptic drug therapy. The goal is to improve seizure control without worsening or producing serious deficits. Some children will see improvements in their cognition, behaviour and quality of life (Ryvlin et al 2014). Types of surgeries include focal resection of the epileptogenic focus, functional hemispherectomy and corpus callosotomy, which severs the connection between the hemispheres.

Status Epilepticus. **Status epilepticus** is a continuous seizure that lasts more than 30 minutes or a series of seizures from which the child does not regain a premorbid level of consciousness (Fernandez et al 2018). The term *impending status epilepticus* is used for a continuous seizure or series of seizures lasting between 5 and 30 minutes with the designation that treatment should begin within 5 minutes (Fernandez et al 2018).

The initial treatment is directed towards support of vital functions, measuring blood glucose, administrating oxygen and gaining IV access, immediately followed by IV administration of antiepileptic agents. Simultaneously with life-support measures and emergency medications, the underlying cause of the status epilepticus is identified and corrected (Fernandez et al 2018).

Buccal or intranasal midazolam and rectal diazepam are simple, effective and safe treatments for home or prehospital management of prolonged seizures and impending status epilepticus (Brigo et al 2015). Time to cessation of the seizure with midazolam was 4 minutes shorter than with rectal diazepam (Brigo et al 2015). Respiratory depression is a potential side effect of these medications when more than two doses are given (Abend & Loddenkemper 2014); however, respiratory depression is not a side effect of rectal diazepam when it is administered as recommended (Shorvon 2011). Intranasal midazolam is safe and effective for stopping seizures but also is easier to administer than rectal diazepam (Glauser et al 2016).

For in-hospital management of status epilepticus is the first-line drug of choice (Glauser et al 2016). If IV access has not been established, rectal diazepam or intramuscular, intranasal or buccal midazolam should be given. It appears that the exact medication chosen is less important than choosing the one that can be administered fastest (Fernandez et al 2018). The child must be closely monitored during administration to detect early alterations in vital signs that may indicate impending respiratory depression. When a benzodiazepine (diazepam or lorazepam) is ineffective, IV phenytoin followed by phenobarbitone is given as the next line of treatment. This combination of therapy places the child at high risk for apnoea, and therefore respiratory support is generally necessary. Children may also receive other antiepileptic medications, including IV valproate or levetiracetam.

Nursing care of a child with status epilepticus includes monitoring vital signs as well as blood pressure and body temperature. During the first 30 to 45 minutes of the seizure the blood pressure may be elevated. Thereafter the blood pressure typically returns to normal but may be decreased depending on the medications being administered for seizure control. Hyperthermia requiring treatment may occur as a result of increased motor activity.

Status epilepticus is a medical emergency that requires immediate intervention to prevent possible brain injury or death. Diagnosis and correction of the underlying cause of the status epilepticus is essential.

Prognosis

Only about half of children who experience a first seizure will have additional seizures (El-Radhi 2015). Children who have cognitive impairments and/or cerebral palsy are at highest risk for developing epilepsy. Prognosis for eventual remission of childhood epilepsy depends on the aetiology and epilepsy syndrome diagnosis. Some syndromes almost always remit whereas others almost never do (Camfield & Camfield 2015). **Intractable seizures** are failure to control seizures after two appropriately selected antiepileptic medications are trialled (Wassenaar et al 2013). **Refractory seizures** are usually defined as the persistence of seizures despite adequate trials of three antiepileptic medications, alone or in combination (Téllez-Zenteno et al 2014).

Most deaths in children with epilepsy are due to factors associated with a child's coexisting neurological conditions and poorly controlled seizures (Berg & Rychlik 2015). Deaths from epilepsy in children who have no other neurological conditions occur at the same rate as childhood deaths from other causes, with the exception of drowning (Franklin et al 2017).

Nursing Care Management

An important nursing responsibility is to observe the seizure episode and accurately document the events. Record and note any alterations in behaviour preceding the seizure and the characteristics of the episode, such as sensory-hallucinatory phenomena (e.g. an aura), motor effects (e.g. eye movements, muscular contractions), alterations in consciousness and postictal state (Box 30.9). The nurse should describe only what is observed, rather than trying to label a seizure type. Note the time that the seizure began and the duration of the seizure.

Generalised seizures and other types with clear manifestations are easy to detect, but absence seizures may present more difficulties. They are easily misinterpreted as inattention. Any unusual behaviour, even seemingly inconsequential, such as a momentary interruption of activity, staring or mental blankness, should be described. The more detailed these descriptions, the more valuable they are for assessment (see Nursing Care Plan and Quality Patient Outcomes boxes).

QUALITY PATIENT OUTCOMES

Seizures

- Aetiology of seizure determined
- Seizures controlled or reduced in frequency and severity
- Family and child receive education to manage seizures
- Child adhering to treatment
- Side effects of treatment minimised

The child must be protected from injury during the seizure. Nursing observations made during the event provide valuable information for diagnosis and management of the disorder (see Nursing Care Considerations box).

NURSING CARE CONSIDERATIONS

Seizures

Tonic–clonic Seizure

During the Seizure

- Remain calm.
- Time the seizure episode.
- If child is standing or seated, ease child down to the floor.
- Place pillow or folded blanket under child's head.
- Loosen restrictive clothing.
- Remove eyeglasses.
- Clear area of any hazards or hard objects.
- Allow seizure to end without interference.
- If vomiting occurs, turn child to one side.
- Do *not:*
  - attempt to restrain child or use force
  - put anything in child's mouth
  - give any food or liquids.

After the Seizure

- Time postictal period.
- Check for breathing. Check position of head and tongue.
- Reposition if head is hyperextended.
- If breathing is not present, commence airway support, bag and mask and call medical emergency team.
- Keep child on side.
- Remain with child.
- Do not give food or liquids until child is fully alert and swallowing reflex has returned.
- Look for medical identification, and determine what factors occurred before onset of seizure that may have been triggering factors.
- Check head and body for possible injuries.
- Check inside of mouth to see if tongue or lips have been bitten.
- Ensure privacy for the patient especially if patient has become incontinent.

Focal Seizure with Impaired Consciousness

During the Seizure

- Do not restrain the child's movements.
- Remove harmful objects from area.
- Redirect to safe area.
- Do not agitate; instead, talk in calm, reassuring manner.
- Do not expect child to follow instructions.
- Watch to see if seizure generalises.

After the Seizure

- Stay with child and reassure until fully conscious.

Call for Emergency Support if

- child stops breathing
- there is evidence of injury or child is diabetic or pregnant
- seizure lasts for more than 5 minutes (unless seizures typically last longer than 5 minutes) and written medical order is present
- status epilepticus occurs
- pupils are not equal after seizure
- child vomits continuously 30 minutes after seizure has ended (sign of possible acute problem)
- child cannot be awakened and is unresponsive to pain after seizure has ended
- seizure occurs in water
- this is child's first seizure.

Source: Data from First Aid for Seizures, Epilepsy New Zealand. http://epilepsy.org.nz/viewobj/first_aid_for_seizures__2__updates_30_10_151.pdf?file-name=first-aid-for-seizures--2--updates-30-10-151.pdf&objID=170

Seizure precautions are required for children who are known to have seizures or who are under observation for seizures. The extent of these measures depends on the type and frequency of the seizure (Box 30.10).

Long-term Care. Care of the child with epilepsy involves physical care and instruction regarding the importance of adherence to the treatment plan. Probably more significant is support and education regarding the potential for the development of psychosocial, educational and emotional problems in children with epilepsy and their families. Few diseases generate as much anxiety among family, friends and school personnel as epilepsy (Jones & Reilly 2016). Fears and misconceptions about the disease and its treatment are common. Nursing care is directed towards educating the child and family about epilepsy and helping them develop strategies to cope with the psychological and sociological problems related to epilepsy.

Children with epilepsy are prescribed antiepileptic medications, which are administered at regular intervals to maintain adequate levels in the blood. The nurse can help the parents plan the administration of the medication at convenient times, usually breakfast and dinner or bedtime, to make taking the medication as easy as possible. It is important to talk with the family about the importance of giving the antiepileptic medication as scheduled to prevent recurrent seizures. Using a pill box can prevent accidentally missing doses. The seizure threshold may be lowered during any illness but particularly with fever. Therefore, parents should be aware that if their child has an illness he or she may be at increased risk for seizures. Parents should contact their health professional if their child misses medications due to vomiting.

Buccal and intranasal midazolam are useful adjunctive home treatments for children at risk for prolonged seizures or clusters of seizures and can minimise the need for hospitalisation while enhancing parental confidence.

Usually antiepileptic medications are continued until the child has been seizure free for 2 years (Lee et al 2017). The medication is then slowly tapered over a period of weeks to decrease the chances of precipitating a seizure.

Nurses should educate the child and parents about the possible adverse reactions to the medications used to treat seizures. Parents must understand the rare but potentially serious side effect of allergic reaction to the medication. They must immediately report rashes to the child's healthcare provider. More common but less serious potential side effects include excessive sleepiness, changes in appetite and worsening behaviour and mood. Parents should be encouraged to share their observations with their child's healthcare provider. Parents should understand that the child needs periodic physical assessment. Depending on the medication prescribed, some children will need regular testing of their full blood count and liver functions. Possible adverse effects on the haematopoietic system, liver and kidneys may be reflected in symptoms such as fever, sore throat, enlarged lymph nodes, jaundice and bleeding (e.g. abnormally easy bruising, petechiae, ecchymosis and epistaxis). The most common cause of status epilepticus in children taking antiepileptic medications is missed medication.

Triggering Factors. Careful and detailed documentation of seizures over time may indicate a pattern of seizures. About half of people

BOX 30.9 General Observations of the Child During a Seizure

Observations During Seizure

General Description

- Order of events (before, during and after)
- Duration of seizure
  - Tonic–clonic—from first signs of event until jerking stops
  - Absence—from loss of consciousness until consciousness is regained
  - Focal seizures with impaired awareness—from first sign of unresponsiveness, motor activity, automatisms until there are signs of responsiveness to environment

Onset

- Time of onset
- Significant precipitating events—missed medication dosage, illness, stress, sleep deprivation, menses

Behaviour

- Change in facial expression
- Cry or other sound
- Stereotypical or automatous movements
- Random activity (wandering)
- Position of eyes, head, body, extremities
- Unilateral or bilateral posturing of one or more extremities

Movement

- Change of position, if any
- Site of commencement—hand, thumb, mouth, generalised
- Tonic phase—length, parts of body involved
- Clonic phase—twitching or jerking movements, parts of body involved, sequence of parts involved, generalised, change in character of movements
- Lack of movement or muscle tone of body part or entire body

Face

- Colour change—pallor, cyanosis, flushing
- Perspiration
- Mouth—position, deviating to one side, teeth clenched, tongue bitten, frothing at mouth
- Lack of expression
- Asymmetrical expression

Eyes

- Position—straight ahead, deviation upwards or outwards, conjugate or divergent gaze
- Pupils—change in size, equality, reaction to light

Respiratory Effort

- Presence and length of apnoea

Other

- Incontinence

Postictal Observations

- Duration of postictal period
- State of consciousness
- Orientation
- Arousability
- Motor ability
  - Any change in motor function
  - Ability to move all extremities
  - Paresis or weakness
- Speech
- Sensations
  - Complaint of discomfort or pain
  - Any sensory impairment
  - Recollection of preseizure sensations or aura

BOX 30.10 Seizure Precautions

- The extent of precautions depends on type, severity and frequency of seizures. Precautions may include the following:
  - Side rails raised when child is sleeping or resting
  - Side rails and other hard objects padded
  - Waterproof mattress or pad on bed or cot
- Appropriate precautions during potentially hazardous activities may include the following:
  - Swimming with a companion
  - Showers preferred; bathing only with close supervision
  - Use of protective helmet and padding during bicycle riding, skateboarding and riding a scooter
  - Supervision during use of hazardous machinery or equipment
- Have child carry or wear medical identification.
- Alert other caregivers to need for any special precautions.
- Child may not drive or operate hazardous machinery or equipment unless seizure-free for designated period (varies by state).

12 years old and older with epilepsy can recognise at least one trigger for their seizures (Wassenaar et al 2014). When this occurs, the child, nurse or responsible adult can intervene to make changes in the lifestyle or environment that may prevent seizures or decrease their frequency. Often the necessary changes are simple but can make an enormous difference in the lives of the child and family.

The most precipitating factors for seizures in children include physical and psychological stress, sleep deprivation, fever and illness (Novakova et al 2013). Other precipitating factors include flickering lights, menstrual cycle, stimulant recreational drugs and alcohol (Wassenaar et al 2014). Some individuals have pattern-sensitive or photosensitive epilepsy, that is, seizures precipitated by changes in dark/light patterns, such as those that occur with a flash on a camera, motor vehicle headlights, reflections of light on snow or water, sunlight filtered through leafy trees or rotating blades on a fan. Most of these individuals have absence, myoclonic or generalised tonic–clonic seizures. A small minority of children have seizures while playing video games. Only these children need to be restricted from playing video games.

Family Support. Parental attitudes and management of a child with a seizure disorder vary. Whether the seizures result from illness, injury or unknown cause, the parents may feel guilt, anxiety and even humiliation. They want to know if the seizures will affect their child's ability to learn and develop. Seizures commonly accompany other manifestations of severe brain damage from disease or injury, but children with seizures, like any population of healthy children, display a wide range of intelligence.

Parents also wonder how the illness will affect their child's future. The answer to this question depends on the cause of the seizures and other comorbid conditions. In many cases parents can be reassured that the illness will not shorten their child's life and that their child can attend school, marry and have children. Educational materials and support groups may prove beneficial for families such as those available from Epilepsy New Zealand (http://epilepsy.org.nz/) or Australia's Epilepsy Foundation (https://epilepsyfoundation.org.au/).

The adolescent period may prove to be a trying time for the child with epilepsy. Limits imposed on the young person's activities at a time when freedom and independence are desired may bring the disability into sharp focus.

Epilepsy should not be a severe impairment to most youngsters. The nurse can help provide positive outcomes for the child and family by assuming the role of patient advocate, helping educate the public about the condition and working to make opportunities available to persons with the disorder.

Febrile Seizures

A febrile seizure is a seizure associated with a febrile illness in the absence of a CNS infection. By definition, children who have a febrile seizure cannot have a history of afebrile seizures, must have a temperature of at least 38°C and must be between the age of 6 and 60 months (Mikati & Hani 2016). Febrile seizures are the most common type of seizure, affecting 2% to 4% of children (Weiss et al 2016).

There is evidence for both genetic and environmental causes of febrile seizures. Children with a family history of febrile seizures are at increased risk for both a single febrile seizure (10% to 46%) and recurrent febrile seizures (Saghazadeh et al 2014). In some families the predisposition to febrile seizures is inherited as an autosomal dominant trait. In most families, though, the predisposition involves multiple genes that have not yet been found (Mikati & Hani 2016). Environmental factors include viral illness and age under 18 months old (Mewasingh 2014).

Most febrile seizures have stopped by the time the child is taken to a medical facility and require no treatment. There is no benefit of antiepileptic prophylaxis in these children; patients who were started on medication are exposed to several potential adverse side effects (Offringa et al 2017). Parents may be given a prescription to take home for a benzodiazepine for as-needed acute treatment of prolonged recurrent febrile seizures. The child whose seizure does not stop within 10 minutes of administration of acute treatment will need treatment for febrile status epilepticus with IV administration of both short-acting and long-acting antiepileptic medications.

Antipyretic therapy during febrile illness offers symptomatic relief for fever-associated symptoms but appears to be ineffective in preventing seizures (Patel et al 2015). Parental education and emotional support are important interventions. Parents need reassurance regarding the benign nature of febrile seizures. Several large studies show no difference in intelligence, memory, behaviour or academic performance in children with febrile seizures compared with either population or sibling controls (Weiss et al 2016).

Parents need education on what to do during a seizure, that is, turn the child on his or her side, never put anything in the child's mouth and time the seizure. Attempts to lower the temperature will not prevent a seizure. Tepid sponge baths are not recommended for several reasons: they are ineffective in significantly lowering the temperature, the shivering effect further increases metabolic output and cooling causes discomfort to the child. Parental education and emotional support are important interventions, and information may need to be repeated, depending on the parents' anxiety and education level.

Long-term antiepileptic therapy is usually not required for children with simple febrile seizures. Children whose initial simple febrile seizure becomes febrile status epilepticus have an increased risk of subsequent febrile status epilepticus. Risk of recurrence of a simple febrile seizure is about 30% (Hesdorffer et al 2016). The risk of developing epilepsy after having simple febrile seizures is less than 3%, whereas the risk increases to 12% to 22% if the child has had prolonged febrile seizures and febrile status epilepticus. The risk of developing epilepsy for children with simple febrile seizures is increased if they have a family history of seizures (Seinfeld et al 2016).

HEADACHE

Headaches are a common complaint of children. They can be either primary or secondary. Primary headaches are classified as migraine, tension-type headache, trigeminal autonomic cephalalgias and other primary headache disorders by the International Headache Society (2018). A secondary headache is caused from another condition and should resolve once the underlying cause is treated. Headaches can be the result of a variety of conditions, including TBI, brain tumour, brain infections, cerebrovascular disorders, withdrawal from or exposure to substances, vision problems, hunger, psychiatric disorders and medication overuse.

Assessment

It is important to determine the pattern of the headache—acute, acute recurrent, chronic progressive or chronic non-progressive (Langdon & DiSabella 2017). Other assessment information includes the presence of seizures, ataxia, lethargy, weakness, nausea or vomiting or any personality changes. Factors related to early development and past illnesses and a family history of headaches may also be pertinent. A 'headache diary', which includes times of onset and termination of headaches, intensity, associated events and actions taken and their effects, can be helpful for the patient and provider.

Clues to aetiology may be found in the family history, including information about the home or social situation (e.g. divorce, separation, alcoholism, school avoidance). Box 30.11 lists specific questions that often elicit needed information. Thorough physical and neurological examinations are performed. An abnormal neurological examination or unusual neurological symptoms indicate the need for further diagnostic tests (e.g. CT, MRI or EEG) (Hershey et al 2016).

NURSING CARE CONSIDERATIONS

During the health history and neurological assessment, the following abnormal signs require immediate follow-up for children.

- The headache progresses in frequency and severity over a brief period (2 to 3 weeks).
- It awakens the child from sleep (may also be migraine).
- It occurs in early morning.
- It is worse on arising.
- It is characterised by persistent occipital or frontal pain.
- It is accompanied by unexplained vomiting.
- It is associated with a change in gait, personality or behaviour.
- It is exacerbated by Valsalva manoeuvre (intensified by lowering head and straining, such as during a bowel movement, coughing or sneezing).

Tension-type headaches are common in children. They are typically frontal, the pain is described as a pressing or tightness and non-throbbing in character and they are not typically accompanied by nausea or vomiting.

Management of tension-type headaches begins with headache hygiene or prevention (Gofshteyn & Stephenson 2016). This includes adequate sleep, appropriate hydration and regular meals and exercise. If headaches continue after the child is following a headache hygiene plan, ibuprofen is usually the most effective pharmacological intervention. To prevent medication overuse headache, children with headaches should take no more than three doses of these medications per week (Kacperski et al 2016). Biofeedback, cognitive-behavioural

BOX 30.11 Questions for Evaluating Headaches

1. Do you have more than one type of headache?
2. How did the headache begin? Trauma? Infection?
3. How long has it been present?
4. Are the symptoms getting worse or staying the same?
5. How often do they occur?
6. How long do they last?
7. Do they occur at any special time or when certain things happen?
8. Do you have warning signs?
9. Where does it hurt?
10. How does the pain feel? Pounding? Sharp?
11. Do you feel sick in other ways during the headache? Abdominal pain? Nausea, vomiting?
12. Do you stop what you are doing during the headache?
13. Do you have any other health problems?
14. Are you taking any medicines regularly?
15. Are there some things you do that make the headache worse or better?
16. Does any one medicine make the headache better?
17. Does any one else in your family have headaches?
18. What do you think is causing your headaches?

Source: Modified from Rothner, A. D. (1993). Management of headaches in children and adolescents. Journal of Pain and Symptom Management, 8(2), 81–86.

therapy and relaxation techniques may be useful non-pharmacological interventions in children with recurrent tension-type headaches (Langdon & DiSabella 2017).

Migraine Headache

Migraine is in the top five common childhood diseases. Migraines can have their onset in very young children, including infants where they may manifest as colic. The onset tends to be earlier in boys than girls until puberty when girls have a twofold increase over boys in migraines. This is thought to be due to the effects of oestrogen (Langdon & DiSabella 2017).

The exact pathophysiology of migraines is not completely known. Genetics, neurotransmitters and neurophysiological mechanisms appear to be involved in varying degrees (Puledda et al 2017). Familial hemiplegic migraine has an identified autosomal dominant genetic cause. A number of other genes have been identified in diseases that are often accompanied by migraine (Sutherland & Griffiths 2017). Previously, it was thought that migraine headaches were caused by dilation of cerebral blood vessels; however, this is no longer thought to be correct. There is much attention on the specific vulnerability factors of the individual that leads to neuron dysfunction and the generation of the acute attack.

Revisions in the classification of migraine headaches introduced some new terms and eliminated, renamed or reclassified others. Migraine headaches are now classified as migraine without aura and migraine with aura; the latter category includes the following subtypes: auras and prodrome, familial hemiplegic migraine, sporadic hemiplegic migraine and basilar-type migraine (Box 30.12) (International Headache Society 2018).

Migraines are paroxysmal. The symptoms vary depending on age. Typical symptoms include nausea, vomiting and abdominal pain, which are relieved by sleep. Toddlers may be seen with episodic pallor, decreased activity and vomiting. In children the onset may be bifrontal, temporal and bilateral or unilateral. As children and adolescents advance in age, many will develop phonophobia and/or photophobia. Compared with adults, migraine headaches in children are generally

BOX 30.12 Migraine Patterns

Migraine with Aura

- Aura may be visual (most common); hemiparetic (tingling and numbness of lips, lower face; second most common); hemiparetic; hemiplegic; or aphasic
- Aura duration less than 1 hour and completely resolves. Followed by throbbing, unilateral or bilateral headache coupled with nausea, vomiting, photophobia and phonophobia.

Migraine without Aura

- Prodrome that consists of pallor, alteration in personality or change in appetite or thirst
- Unilateral or bilateral headache coupled with nausea and/or vomiting, photophobia and phonophobia
- Pulsating quality
- Moderate or severe pain intensity

Sporadic Hemiplegic Migraine

- Migraine with aura
- Motor weakness
- No first- or second-degree relative who also has migraine with aura and motor weakness

Basilar-type Migraine

- Recurrent attacks
- Headache typically occipital
- Symptoms may include dysarthria, vertigo, diplopia, vomiting and altered consciousness

shorter in duration. If the child falls asleep during the headache, the amount of time the child is asleep is counted as part of the duration (Hershey et al 2016). A family history of migraine is elicited in up to 90% of children with migraine; 28% of all children who have migraines experience a headache before age 15 years (Hershey et al 2016).

Like tension-type headaches, migraine management begins with headache hygiene. Keeping a headache diary can help with identifying triggers so they can be avoided. If these measures fail to prevent migraines, both abortive and prophylactic treatment may be needed. At the onset of the headache, the child should rest or sleep in a quiet, dark room when feasible. Migraine therapy, if administered early in the course of the headache, may provide rapid relief. Ibuprofen appears to be the safest and most effective treatment if given early (Patniyot & Gelfand 2016).

The outlook for a child with migraine is good, but the child and parents should be informed that predisposition to the headaches may be lifelong. Severe headaches can adversely affect the child's routine activities of daily living, including family relations and school. Many children and families will benefit from psychotherapy.

REFERENCES

Abend, N. S., & Loddenkemper, T. (2014). Pediatric status epilepticus management. Current Opinion in Pediatrics, 26(6), 668–674.

Australian and New Zealand Intensive Care Society (ANZICS). (2019). The ANZICS Statement of death and organ donation. https://www.anzics.com.au/wp-content/uploads/2020/07/ANZICS-Statement-on-Death-and-Organ-Donation-Edition-4.pdf

Australian Institute of Health and Welfare. (2021). Injury in Australia: drowning and submersion. https://www.aihw.gov.au/reports/injury/drowning-and-submersion

Babikian, T., Merkley, T., Savage, R. C., et al. (2015). Chronic aspects of pediatric traumatic brain injury: Review of the literature. Journal of Neurotrauma, 32(23), 1849–1860.
Barr, R. G. (2014). Crying as a trigger for abusive head trauma: A key to prevention. Pediatric Radiology, 44(Suppl4), S559–S564.
Baxter, A. L., Ewing, P. H., Young, G. B., et al. (2013). EMLA application exceeding two hours improves pediatric emergency department venipuncture success. Advanced Emergency Nursing Journal, 35(1), 67–75.
Beauchamp, M. H., & Anderson, V. (2013). Cognitive and psychopathological sequelae of pediatric traumatic brain injury. Handbook of Clinical Neurology, 112, 913–920.
Berg, A. T., & Rychlik, K. (2015). The course of childhood-onset epilepsy over the first two decades: A prospective, longitudinal study. Epilepsia, 56(1), 40–48.
Blaszczyk, B., Laso , W., & Czuczwar, S. J. (2015). Antiepileptic drugs and adverse skin reactions: An update. Pharmacological Reports, 67(3), 426–434.
Bloomer, M. J., Endacott, R., Copnell, B., et al. (2016). 'Something normal in a very, very abnormal environment' – Nursing work to honour the life of dying infants and children in neonatal and paediatric intensive care in Australia. Intensive and Critical Care Nursing, 33, 5–11.
Blume, H. K. (2017). Childhood headache: A brief review. Pediatric Annals, 46(4), e155–e165.
Bonfield, C. M., Naran, S., Adetayo, O. A., et al. (2014). Pediatric skull fractures: The need for surgical intervention, characteristics, complications, and outcomes. Journal of Neurosurgery. Pediatrics, 14(2), 205–211.
Braine, M. E., & Cook, N. (2017). The Glasgow Coma Scale and evidence-informed practice: A critical review of where we are and where we need to be. Journal of Clinical Nursing, 26(1–2), 280–293.
Braun, K. P., & Schmidt, D. (2014). Stopping antiepileptic drugs in seizure-free patients. Current Opinion in Neurology, 27(2), 219–226.
Brigo, F., Nardone, R., Tezzon, F., et al. (2015). Nonintravenous midazolam versus intravenous or rectal diazepam for the treatment of early status epilepticus: A systematic review with meta-analysis. Epilepsy and Behavior: E&B, 49, 325–336.
Burns, E., Grool, A. M., Klassen, T. P., et al. (2016). Scalp hematoma characteristics associated with intracranial injury in pediatric minor head injury. Academic Emergency Medicine: Official Journal of the Society for Academic Emergency Medicine, 23(5), 576–583.
Burrows, P., Trefan, L., Houston, R., et al. (2015). Head injury from falls in children younger than 6 years of age. Archives of Disease in Childhood, 100(11), 1032–1037.
Caglar, D., & Quan, L. (2016). Drowning and submersion injury. In R. Kliegman, B. Stanton, J. St. Geme, et al. (Eds.), Nelson textbook of pediatrics (20th ed.). Philadelphia PA: Elsevier/Saunders.
Camfield, P., & Camfield, C. (2015). Incidence, prevalence and aetiology of seizures and epilepsy in children. Epileptic Disorders: International Epilepsy Journal with Videotape, 17(2), 117–123.
Chen, D., & Azueta, D. (2017). Clarity of Confusion? Variability in uses of 'Allow Natural Death' in State POLSI forms. Journal of Palliative Medicine, 20(7), 695–696.
Christensen, J. (2012). Traumatic brain injury: Risks of epilepsy and implications for medicolegal assessment. Epilepsia, 53(Suppl. 4), 43–47.
Dale, R. C., Gorman, M. P., & Lim, M. (2017). Autoimmune encephalitis in children: Clinical phenomenology, therapeutics, and emerging challenges. Current Opinion in Neurology, 30(3), 334–344.
Dhamne, S. C., Kaye, H. L., & Rotenberg, A. (2018). Neuromodulation in epilepsy. In K. F. Swaiman, S. Ashwal, D. M. Ferriero, et al. (Eds.), Swaiman's pediatric neurology: Principles and practice (6th ed.). Philadelphia, PA: Elsevier.
Ding, D., Starke, R. M., Kano, H., et al. (2017). International multicenter cohort study of pediatric brain arteriovenous malformations. Part 1: Predictors of hemorrhagic presentation. Journal of Neurosurgery. Pediatrics, 19(2), 127–135.
Dubey, D., Sawhney, A., Greenberg, B., et al. (2015). The spectrum of autoimmune encephalopathies. Journal of Neuroimmunology, 287, 93–97.
Elbabaa, S. K., Gildehaus, A. M., & Pierson, M. J. (2017). First 60 fetal in-utero myelomeningocele repairs at Saint Louis Fetal Care Institute in the post-MOMS trial era: Hydrocephalus treatment outcomes (endoscopic third ventriculostomy versus ventriculo-peritoneal shunt). Child's Nervous System, 33(7), 1157–1168.
Ellis, M. J., Cordingley, D., Vis, S., et al. (2015). Vestibulo-ocular dysfunction in pediatric sports-related concussion. Journal of Neurosurgery. Pediatrics, 16(3), 248–255.
El-Radhi, A. S. (2015). Management of seizures in children. The British Journal of Nursing, 24(3), 152–155.
Fernandez, I. S., Abend, N. S., & Loddenkemper, T. (2018). Status epilepticus. In K. F. Swaiman, S. Ashwal, D. M. Ferriero, et al. (Eds.), Swaiman's pediatric neurology: Principles and practice (6th ed.). Philadelphia, PA: Elsevier.
Fisher, R. S., Acevedo, C., Arzimanoglou, A., et al. (2014). ILAE official report: A practical clinical definition of epilepsy. Epilepsia, 55(4), 475–482.
Fisher, R. S., Cross, J. H., French, J. A., et al. (2017). Operational classification of seizure types by the International League Against Epilepsy: Position paper of the ILAE commission for classification and terminology. Epilepsia, 58(4), 522–530.
Franklin, R. C., Pearn, J. H., & Peden, A. E. (2017). Drowning fatalities in childhood: The role of pre-existing medical conditions. Archives of Disease in Childhood, 102(10), 888–893.
Fulkerson, D. H., White, I. K., Rees, J. M., et al. (2015). Analysis of long-term (median 10.5 years) outcomes in children presenting with traumatic brain injury and an initial Glasgow Coma Scale score of 3 or 4. Journal of Neurosurgery. Pediatrics, 16(4), 410–419.
Gainza-Lein, M., Sanchez-Fernández, I., & Loddenkemper, T. (2017). Use of EEG in critically ill children and neonates in the United States of America. Journal of Neurology, 264(6), 1165–1173.
Ganti, L., Bodhit, A. N., Daneshvar, Y., et al. (2013). Impact of helmet use in traumatic brain injuries associated with recreational vehicles. Advances in Preventive Medicine, 2013, 450195.
Gaw, C. E., Chounthirath, T., & Smith, G. A. (2017). Nursery product-related injuries treated in United States emergency departments. Pediatrics, 139(4), e20162503.
Germain, B., & Maria, B. L. (2018). Epileptic encephalopathies: Clinical aspects, molecular features and pathogenesis, therapeutic targets and translational opportunities, and future research directions. Journal of Child Neurology, 33(1), 7–40.
Glauser, T., Shinnar, S., Gloss, D., et al. (2016). Evidence-based guideline: Treatment of convulsive status epilepticus in children and adults: Report of the guideline committee of the American Epilepsy Society. Epilepsy Currents, 16(1), 48–61.
Gofshteyn, J. S., & Stephenson, D. J. (2016). Diagnosis and management of childhood headache. Current Problems in Pediatric and Adolescent Health Care, 46(2), 36–51.
Gordon, S. M., Srinivasan, L., & Harris, M. C. (2017). Neonatal meningitis: Overcoming challenges in diagnosis, prognosis, and treatment with omics. Frontiers in Pediatrics, 5, 139.
Grool, A. M., Aglipay, M., Momoli, F., et al. (2016). Association between early participation in physical activity following acute concussion and persistent postconcussive symptoms in children and adolescents. The Journal of the American Medical Association, 316(23), 2504–2514.
Hancock, E. C., Osborne, J. P., & Edwards, S. W. (2013). Treatment of infantile spasms. Cochrane Database of Systematic Review, (6), CD001770.
Hartman, M. E., & Cheifetz, I. M. (2016). Pediatric emergencies and resuscitation. In R. M. Kliegman, B. F. Stanton, J. W. St Geme, et al. (Eds.), Nelson textbook of pediatrics (20th ed.). Philadelphia, PA: Elsevier/Saunders.
Heckenberg, S. G., Brouwer, M. C., & van de Beek, D. (2014). Bacterial meningitis. Handbook of Clinical Neurology, 121, 1361–1375.
Hepburn-Smith, M., Dynkevich, I., Spektor, M., et al. (2016). Establishment of an external ventricular drain best practice guideline: The quest for a comprehensive, universal standard for external ventricular drain care. The Journal of Neuroscience Nursing: Journal of the American Association of Neuroscience Nurses, 48(1), 54–65.
Hershey, A. D., Kabbouche, M. A., & O'Brien, H. L. (2016). Headaches. In R. M. Kliegman, B. F. Stanton, J. W. St Geme, et al. (Eds.), Nelson textbook of pediatrics (20th ed.). Philadelphia, PA: Elsevier/Saunders.
Hesdorffer, D. C., Shinnar, S., Lax, D. N., et al. (2016). Risk factors for subsequent febrile seizures in the FEBSTAT study. Epilepsia, 57(7), 1042–1047.

Holmes, G. L. (2018). Generalised seizures. In K. F. Swaiman, S. Ashwal, D. M. Ferriero, et al. (Eds.), Swaiman's pediatric neurology: Principles and practice (6th ed.). Philadelphia, PA: Elsevier.

Hua, F., Xie, H., Worthington, H. V., et al. (2016). Oral hygiene care for critically ill patients to prevent ventilator-associated pneumonia. Cochrane Database of Systematic Review, (10), CD008367.

Huang, K. T., Bi, W. L., Abd-El-Barr, M., et al. (2016). The neurocritical and neurosurgical care of subdural hematomas. Neurocritical Care, 24(2), 294–307.

International Headache Society. (2018). The international classification of headache disorders 3rd edition. https://www.ichd-3.org/.

Jones, K., Go, C., & Boyd, J. (2015). Vigabatrin as first-line treatment for infantile spasms not related to tuberous sclerosis complex. Pediatric Neurology, 53(2), 141–145.

Jones, C., & Reilly, C. (2016). Parental anxiety in childhood epilepsy: A systematic review. Epilepsia, 57(4), 529–537.

Jones, K., Snead, O. C., III, & Boyd, J. (2015). Adrenocorticotropic hormone versus prednisolone in the treatment of infantile spasms post vigabatrin failure. Journal of Child Neurology, 30(5), 595–600.

Kacperski, J., & Arthur, T. (2016). Management of post-traumatic headaches in children and adolescents. Headache, 56(1), 36–48.

Kacperski, J., Kabbouche, M. A., O'Brien, H. L., et al. (2016). The optimal management of headaches in children and adolescents. Therapeutic Advances in Neurological Disorders, 9(1), 53–68.

Kahle, K. T., Kulkarni, A. V., Limbrick, D. D., et al. (2016). Hydrocephalus in children. Lancet, 387(10020), 788–799.

Kinsman, S. L., & Johnston, M. V. (2016). Hydrocephalus. In R. M. Kliegman, B. F. Stanton, J. W. St Geme, et al. (Eds.), Nelson textbook of pediatrics (20th ed.). Philadelphia, PA: Elsevier/Saunders.

Ku, L. C., Boggess, K. A., & Cohen-Wolkowiez, M. (2015). Bacterial meningitis in infants. Clinics in Perinatology, 42(1), 29–45.

Kuczynski, A., Crawford, S., Bodell, L., et al. (2013). Characteristics of post-traumatic headaches in children following mild traumatic brain injury and their response to treatment: A prospective cohort. Developmental Medicine and Child Neurology, 55(7), 636–641.

Kulkarni, A. V., Sgouros, S., Constantini, S., et al. (2016). International infant hydrocephalus study: Initial results of a prospective, multicenter comparison of endoscopic third ventriculostomy (ETV) and shunt for infant hydrocephalus. Child's Nervous System, 32(6), 1039–1048.

Langdon, R., & DiSabella, M. T. (2017). Pediatric headache: An overview. Current Problems in Pediatric and Adolescent Health Care, 47(3), 44–56.

Lee, I. C., Li, S. Y., & Chen, Y. J. (2017). Seizure recurrence in children after stopping antiepileptic medication: 5-year follow-up. Pediatrics and Neonatology, 58(4), 338–343.

Longoni, G., Levy, D. M., & Yeh, E. A. (2016). The changing landscape of childhood inflammatory central nervous system disorders. The Journal of Pediatrics, 179, 24–32.

Luat, A. F., Coyle, L., & Kamat, D. (2016). The ketogenic diet: A practical guide for pediatricians. Pediatric Annals, 45(12), e446–e450.

Månsson, P. K., Johansson, S., Ziebell, M., et al. (2017). Forty years of shunt surgery at Rigshospitalet, Denmark: A retrospective study comparing past and present rates and causes of revision and infection. BMJ Open, 7(1), e013389.

Marcdante, K., & Kliegman, R. M. (2016). Meningitis. In R. Kliegman, B. Stanton, J. St. Geme, et al. (Eds.), Nelson textbook of pediatrics (20th ed.). Philadelphia, PA: Elsevier/Saunders.

Martin, H. A. (2017). The power of lidocaine, adrenaline (epinephrine), and tetracaine (LET) and a child life specialist when suturing lacerations in children. Journal of Emergency Nursing, 43(2), 169–170.

Martin, K., Jackson, C. F., Levy, R. G., et al. (2016). Ketogenic diet and other dietary treatments for epilepsy. Cochrane Database of Systematic Review, (2), CD001903.

McCrea, M. A., Nelson, L. D., & Guskiewicz, K. (2017). Diagnosis and management of acute concussion. Physical Medicine and Rehabilitation Clinics of North America, 28(2), 271–286.

McMurtry, C. M., Taddio, A., Noel, M., et al. (2016). Exposure-based interventions for the management of individuals with high levels of needle fear across the lifespan: A clinical practice guideline and call for further research. Cognitive Behaviour Therapy, 45(3), 217–235.

Meehan, W. P., Mannix, R. C., Stracciolini, A., et al. (2013). Symptom severity predicts prolonged recovery after sport-related concussion, but age and amnesia do not. The Journal of Pediatrics, 163(3), 721–725.

Mewasingh, L. D. (2014). Febrile seizures. BMJ Clinical Evidence, 2014, 0324.

Mikati, M. A., & Hani, A. J. (2016). Seizures in childhood. In R. M. Kliegman, B. F. Stanton, J. W. St Geme, et al. (Eds.), Nelson textbook of pediatrics (20th ed.). Philadelphia, PA: Elsevier/Saunders.

Minns, R. A., Jones, P. A., Tandon, A., et al. (2017). Raised intracranial pressure and retinal haemorrhages in childhood encephalopathies. Developmental Medicine and Child Neurology, 59(6), 597–604.

Moosa, A. N., & Gupta, A. (2014). Outcome after epilepsy surgery for cortical dysplasia in children. Child's Nervous System, 20(11), 1905–1911.

Moran, K., Webber, J., & Stanley, T. (2017). The 4Rs of Aquatic Rescue: educating the public about safety and risks of bystander rescue. International Journal of Injury Control & Safety Promotion, 24(3), 396–405. https://doi-org.op.idm.oclc.org/10.1080/17457300.2016.1224904

Morgan, C. D., Zuckerman, S. L., Lee, Y. M., et al. (2015). Predictors of postconcussion syndrome after sports-related concussion in young athletes: A matched case-control study. Journal of Neurosurgery. Pediatrics, 15(6), 589–598.

Moshe, S. L., Perucca, E., Ryvlin, P., et al. (2015). Epilepsy: New advances. Lancet, 385(9971), 884–898.

Mullally, W. J. (2017). Concussion. The American Journal of Medicine, 130(8), 885–892.

Murphy, S., Thomas, N. J., Gertz, S. J., et al. (2017). Tripartite stratification of the Glasgow Coma Scale in children with severe traumatic brain injury and mortality: An analysis from a multi-center comparative effectiveness study. Journal of Neurotrauma, 34(14), 2220–2229.

Novakova, B., Harris, P. R., Ponnusamy, A., et al. (2013). The role of stress as a trigger for epileptic seizures: A narrative review of evidence from human and animal studies. Epilepsia, 54(11), 1866–1876.

Nakagawa, T. A., Ashwal, S., Mathur, M., et al. (2012). Guidelines for the determination of brain death in infants and children: An update of the 1987 task force recommendations. Annals of Neurology, 71(4), 573–585.

O'Callaghan, F. J., Edwards, S. W., Alber, F. D., et al. (2017). Safety and effectiveness of hormonal treatment versus hormonal treatment with vigabatrin for infantile spasms (ICISS): A randomised, multicentre, open-label trial. The Lancet. Neurology, 16(1), 33–42.

Offringa, M., Newton, R., Cozijnsen, M. A., et al. (2017). Prophylactic drug management for febrile seizures in children. Cochrane Database of Systematic Review, (2), CD003031.

Patel, N., Ram, D., Swiderska, N., et al. (2015). Febrile seizures. BMJ (Clinical Research Ed.), 351, 1–7.

Patniyot, I. R., & Gelfand, A. A. (2016). Acute treatment therapies for pediatric migraine: A qualitative systematic review. Headache, 56(1), 49–70.

Paulsen, A. H., Lundar, T., & Lindegaard, K. F. (2015). Pediatric hydrocephalus: 40-year outcomes in 128 hydrocephalic patients treated with shunts during childhood. Assessment of surgical outcome, work participation, and health-related quality of life. Journal of Neurosurgery. Pediatrics, 16(6), 633–641.

Pisapia, J. M., Sinha, S., Zarnow, D. M., et al. (2017). Fetal ventriculomegaly: Diagnosis, treatment, and future directions. Child's Nervous System, 33(7), 1113–1123.

Popernack, M. L., Gray, N., & Reuter-Rice, K. (2015). Moderate-to-severe traumatic brain injury in children: Complications and rehabilitation strategies. Journal of Pediatric Health Care, 29(3), e1–e7.

Prober, C. G., & Mathew, R. (2016). Brain abscess. In R. M. Kliegman, B. F. Stanton, J. W. St Geme, et al. (Eds.), Nelson textbook of pediatrics (20th ed.). Philadelphia, PA: Elsevier/Saunders.

Prober, C. G., Srinivas, N. S., & Mathew, R. (2016a). Acute bacterial meningitis. In R. Kliegman, B. Stanton, J. St. Geme, et al. (Eds.), Nelson textbook of pediatrics (20th ed.). Philadelphia, PA: Elsevier/Saunders.

Prober, C. G., Srinivas, N. S., & Mathew, R. (2016b). Central nervous system infections. In R. M. Kliegman, B. F. Stanton, J. W. St Geme, et al. (Eds.), Nelson textbook of pediatrics (20th ed.). Philadelphia, PA: Elsevier/Saunders.

Puledda, F., Messina, R., & Goadsby, P. J. (2017). An update on migraine: Current understanding and future directions. Journal of Neurology, 264(9), 2031–2039.

Quan, L., Bierens, J. J., Lis, R., et al. (2016). Predicting outcome of drowning at the scene: A systematic review and meta-analyses. Resuscitation, 104, 63–75.

Quan, L., Mack, C. D., & Schiff, M. A. (2014). Association of water temperature and submersion duration and drowning outcome. Resuscitation, 85(6), 790–794.

Russ, S. A., Larson, K., & Halfon, N. (2012). A national profile of childhood epilepsy and seizure disorder. Pediatrics, 129(2), 256–264.

Ryan, M. E., Jaju, A., Ciolino, J. D., et al. (2016). Rapid MRI evaluation of acute intracranial haemorrhage in pediatric head trauma. Neuroradiology, 58(8), 793–799.

Ryvlin, P., Cross, J. H., & Rheims, S. (2014). Epilepsy surgery in children and adults. The Lancet. Neurology, 13(11), 1114–1126.

Saghazadeh, A., Mastrangelo, M., & Rezaei, N. (2014). Genetic background of febrile seizures. Reviews in the Neurosciences, 25(1), 129–161.

Scheer, S., & John, R. M. (2016). Anti–N-Methyl-D-Aspartate receptor encephalitis in children and adolescents. Journal of Pediatric Health Care, 30(4), 347–358.

Seinfeld, S. A., Pellock, J. M., Kjeldsen, M. J., et al. (2016). Epilepsy after febrile seizures: Twins suggest genetic influence. Pediatric Neurology, 55, 14–16.

Sellin, J. N., Moreno, A., Ryan, S. L., et al. (2017). Children presenting in delayed fashion after minor head trauma with scalp swelling: Do they require further workup? Child's Nervous System, 33(4), 647–652.

Sencer, A., Aras, Y., Akcakaya, M. O., et al. (2012). Posterior fossa epidural hematomas in children: Clinical experience with 40 cases. Journal of Neurosurgery. Pediatrics, 9(2), 139–143.

Shankar, P., Zamora, C., & Castillo, M. (2016). Congenital malformations of the brain and spine. Handbook of Clinical Neurology, 136, 1121–1137.

Shumiloff, N. A., Lam, W. M., & Manasco, K. B. (2013). Adrenocorticotropic hormone for the treatment of West Syndrome in children. The Annals of Pharmacotherapy, 47(5), 744–754.

Shorvon, S. D. (2011). The etiologic classification of epilepsy. Epilepsia, 52(6), 1052–1057.

Sieswerda-Hoogendoorn, T., Boos, S., Spivak, B., et al. (2012). Abusive head trauma part I: Clinical aspects. European Journal of Pediatrics, 171, 415–423.

Singh, B., Murad, M. H., Prokop, L. J., et al. (2013). Meta-analysis of Glasgow Coma Scale and simplified motor score in predicting traumatic brain injury outcomes. Brain Injury: [BI], 27(3), 293–300.

Singhal, N. S., Harini, C., & Sullivan, J. (2018). Epileptic spasms and myoclonic seizures. In K. F. Swaiman, S. Ashwal, D. M. Ferriero, et al. (Eds.), Swaiman's pediatric neurology: Principles and practice (6th ed.). Philadelphia, PA: Elsevier.

Singhi, S. C., & Tiwari, L. (2009). Management of intracranial hypertension. Indian Journal of Pediatrics, 76(5), 519–529.

Squier, W., & Mack, J. (2009). The neuropathology of infant subdural haemorrhage. Forensic Science International, 187(1–3), 6–13.

Swanson, D. (2015). Meningitis. Pediatrics in Review, 36(12), 514–524.

Sutherland, H. G., & Griffiths, L. R. (2017). Genetics of migraine: Insights into the molecular basis of migraine disorders. Headache, 57(4), 537–569.

Teichert, J. H., Rosales, P. R., Jr., Lopes, P. B., et al. (2012). Extradural hematoma in children: Case series of 33 patients. Pediatric Neurosurgery, 48(4), 216–220.

Téllez-Zenteno, J. F., Hernández-Ronquillo, L., Buckley, S., et al. (2014). A validation of the new definition of drug-resistant epilepsy by the International League Against Epilepsy. Epilepsia, 55(6), 829–834.

Tenney, J. R., & Glauser, T. (2018). Electroclinical syndromes: Childhood onset. In K. F. Swaiman, S. Ashwal, D. M. Ferriero, et al. (Eds.), Swaiman's pediatric neurology: Principles and practice (6th ed.). Philadelphia, PA: Elsevier.

Tobin, J. M., Ramos, W. D., Pu Y., et al. (2017). Bystander CPR is associated with neurologically favourable survival in cardiac arrest following drowning. Resuscitation, 115, 39–43.

Toth, P., Szarka, N., Farkas, E., et al. (2016). Traumatic brain injury-induced autoregulatory dysfunction and spreading depression-related neurovascular uncoupling: Pathomechanisms, perspectives, and therapeutic implications. American Journal of Physiology, Heart and Circulatory Physiology, 311(5), H1118–H1131.

Van Houtem, C. M., Laine, M. L., Boomsma, D. I., et al. (2013). A review and meta-analysis of the heritability of specific phobia subtypes and corresponding fears. Journal of Anxiety Disorders, 27(4), 379–388.

Venable, G. T., Rossi, N. B., & Morgan Jones, G. (2016). The preventable shunt revision rate: A potential quality metric for pediatric shunt surgery. Journal of Neurosurgery. Pediatrics, 18(1), 7–15.

Vetter, V., Baxter, R., Denizer, G., et al. (2016). Routinely vaccinating adolescents against meningococcus: Targeting transmission & disease. Expert Review of Vaccines, 15(5), 641–658.

Vezina, N., Al-Halabi, B., Shash, H., et al. (2017). A review of techniques used in the management of growing skull fractures. The Journal of Craniofacial Surgery, 28(3), 604–609.

Wassenaar, M., Kasteleijn-Nolst Trenite, D. G., de Haan, G. J., et al. (2014). Seizure precipitants in a community-based epilepsy cohort. Journal of Neurology, 261(4), 717–724.

Wassenaar, M., Leijten, F. S., Egberts, T. C., et al. (2013). Prognostic factors for medically intractable epilepsy: A systematic review. Epilepsy Research, 106(3), 301–310.

Weinberg, G. A., & Thompson-Stone, R. (2018). Bacterial infections of the nervous system. In K. F. Swaiman, S. Ashwal, D. M. Ferriero, et al. (Eds.), Swaiman's pediatric neurology: Principles and practice (6th ed.). Philadelphia, PA: Elsevier.

Weiss, J. (2010). Prevention of drowning. Pediatrics, 126, e253–e262.

Weiss, E. F., Masur, D., & Shinnar, S. (2016). Cognitive functioning one month and one year following febrile status epilepticus. Epilepsy & Behavior, 64, 283–288.

Whittaker, M. R. (2013). Opioid use and the risk of respiratory depression and death in the pediatric population. The Journal of Pediatric Pharmacology and Therapeutics, 18(4), 269–276.

Zemek, R., Barrowman, N., Freedman, S. B., et al. (2016). Clinical risk score for persistent postconcussion symptoms among children with acute concussion in the ED. The Journal of the American Medical Association, 315(10), 1014–1025.

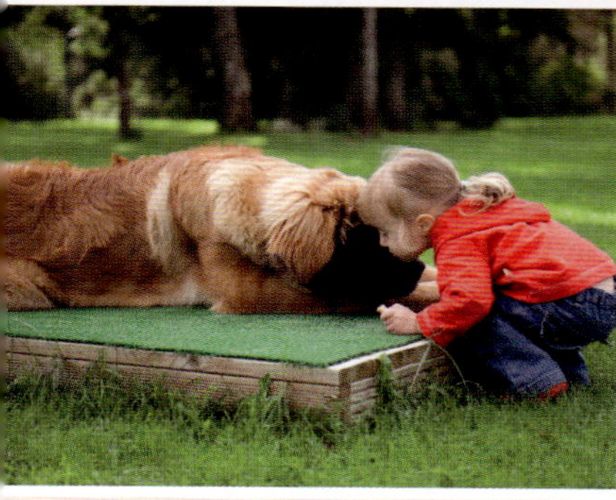

31

The Child with Endocrine Dysfunction

Lisa Speedie

LEARNING OUTCOMES

- Describe the endocrine system and begin to describe metabolic disorders
- Discuss family-centred care for the child and family for those with endocrine disorders
- Plan and implement nursing care for the child and family with endocrine and metabolic disorders

THE ENDOCRINE SYSTEM

The endocrine system controls and regulates metabolism; this includes energy production, growth, fluid and electrolyte balance, response to stress and sexual reproduction (Wheeler et al 2014). This system has three components: (1) the cell, which sends a chemical message using a hormone; (2) the target cells, or organs, which receive the chemical message; and (3) the environment through which the chemical is transported (e.g. blood, lymph, extracellular fluids) from the site of synthesis to the sites of cellular action.

The endocrine glands, which are distributed throughout the body, are listed in Box 31.1; also listed are several additional structures sometimes considered endocrine glands, although they are not usually included.

Hormones

A **hormone** is a complex chemical substance produced and secreted into body fluids by a cell or group of cells that exerts a physiological controlling effect on other cells (Garibaldi & Chemaitilly 2016). Local hormones create their effect near the point of secretion. For example, secretin, a digestive hormone made by cells lining the duodenum, stimulates the pancreas. General hormones are released by endocrine glands into the bloodstream, where they are carried to responsive tissues (Fig 31.1). Some of these hormones (such as thyroid hormone [TH] and growth hormone [GH]) affect most cells of the body, whereas others (such as the tropic hormones) produce their effects on specific tissues, called **target tissues**. These responsive, or target, tissues may be another endocrine gland, an organ or tissue (Gardner et al 2011). For example, pituitary hormones stimulate the adrenal glands and the thyroid gland to secrete adrenocorticotropic hormone (ACTH) and thyroid-stimulating hormone (TSH), respectively.

Control of Hormone Secretion

Regulation of hormonal secretion is often based on negative feedback. As a rule, endocrine glands have a tendency to oversecrete particular hormones. However, once the hormone's physiological effect has been achieved, this information is transmitted to the producing gland, either directly or indirectly, to inhibit further secretion. If the gland undersecretes, the inhibition is stopped and the gland increases production of the hormone again. As a result, the hormone is secreted according to the amount needed. This is the primary function of the tropic hormones.

The anterior pituitary gland, located below the hypothalamus, is often referred to as the master gland. It is primarily responsible for stimulation and inhibition of tropic hormones. Tropic (which literally means 'turning') hormones secreted by the anterior pituitary regulate the secretion of hormones from various target organs (Fig 31.2). As blood concentrations of the target hormones reach normal levels, a negative message is sent to the anterior pituitary to inhibit release of the tropic hormone. For example, TSH responds to low levels of circulating TH. As blood levels of TH reach normal concentrations, a negative feedback message is sent to the anterior pituitary, resulting in diminished release of TSH.

The pituitary gland is controlled by either hormonal or neuronal signals from the hypothalamus. Two types of substances are secreted from the hypothalamus: (1) releasing hormones and (2) inhibitory hormones. Both are secreted within the hypothalamus and transported by way of the pituitary portal system to the anterior pituitary, where they stimulate the secretion of tropic hormones. An example of this is the secretion of corticotropin-releasing factor (CRF) by the hypothalamus. CRF stimulates the pituitary to secrete ACTH. In this instance the anterior pituitary is the target of the hypothalamus. ACTH then stimulates the adrenals to secrete glucocorticoids, which have multiple target sites throughout the body. Pituitary hormones that lack feedback control from the product of a target tissue (e.g. GH, prolactin and melanocyte-stimulating hormone) require hypothalamic inhibitors and stimulators for their control.

Neuroendocrine Interrelationships

Two regulatory systems maintain haemostasis: the endocrine and the autonomic nervous systems (collectively known as the neuroendocrine system) (Wheeler et al 2014, Aslan & Cheung 2014). The autonomic nervous system consists of the sympathetic and parasympathetic systems that control non-voluntary functions—specifically that of smooth muscle, myocardium and glands. The parasympathetic system primarily regulates the digestive processes, whereas the sympathetic system functions to maintain homeostasis during times of stress.

The higher autonomic centres, located in the hypothalamus and limbic system, help control the functioning of both autonomic systems. Both sympathetic and parasympathetic nerve fibres secrete

BOX 31.1 Endocrine Glands

Pituitary gland (hypophysis cerebri)—A pea-sized gland that lies within a deep bony depression at the base of the cranium (the sella turcica) and is attached to the hypothalamus on the undersurface of the brain by a slender infundibulum, or pituitary stalk

Thyroid gland—Two large lateral lobes and a connecting portion, the isthmus, situated on the anterior aspect of the neck just below the larynx

Parathyroid glands—Four or five (more or less) small round bodies attached to the posterior surfaces of the lateral lobes of the thyroid gland

Adrenal glands—Pyramid-shaped glands situated on top of the kidneys, fitting like caps over these organs

Ovaries—Glands located in the female pelvis on each side of the uterus at the fimbriated end of the fallopian tubes

Testes—Oval-shaped glands situated within the male scrotum

Islets of Langerhans—Small clusters of endocrine cells within the pancreas situated between the acinar or exocrine-secreting portions of the gland

Structures Sometimes Considered Endocrine Glands

Pineal body (epiphysis cerebri)—A gland located in the cranial cavity behind the midbrain and third ventricle, the functions of which are largely speculative

Thymus—A gland situated behind the sternum and below the thyroid gland; plays an important role in immunity but only during fetal life and early childhood

Gastrointestinal glands—Mucosal lining of the gastrointestinal tract containing cells that produce hormones which play important roles in controlling and coordinating secretory and motor activities of digestion

Placenta—A body that secretes ovarian hormones and chorionic gonadotropin during gestation; only a temporary endocrine gland

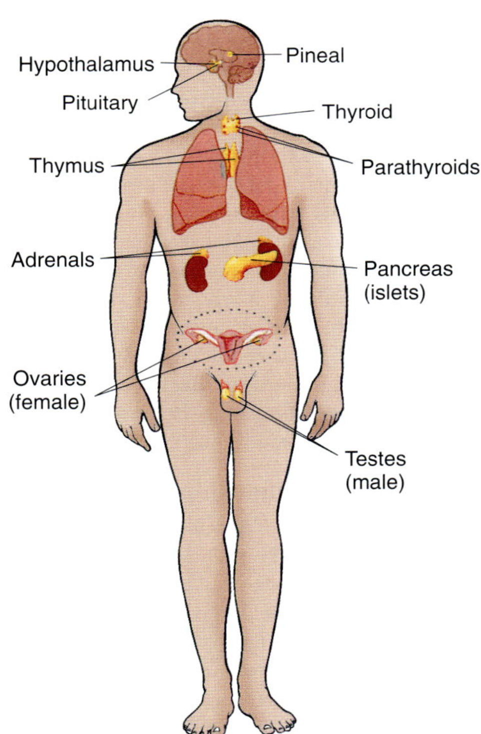

Fig 31.1 Location of the endocrine glands and structures sometimes considered endocrine glands. (Source: Thibodeau, G. A., & Patton, K. T. (2008). Structure and function of the body (13th ed.). St Louis, MO: Mosby.)

neurotransmitting substances: acetylcholine, released by cholinergical fibres, and noradrenaline, released by adrenergical fibres. Release of noradrenaline into the plasma produces the same effects as secretion of this substance by the adrenal medulla. Thus the interrelatedness between the two systems is demonstrated.

The neuroendocrine system acts by synthesising and releasing various chemical substances that regulate body functions. Information is carried by means of neural impulses in the autonomic system and by the blood in the endocrine system. In general, neural responses are more rapid and localised, whereas endocrine responses are more lasting and widespread. The two systems function synergistically because neural impulses transmitted to the central nervous system (CNS) stimulate the hypothalamus to manufacture and release several releasing or inhibiting factors.

Because of the interdependent relationship of these glands, a malfunction in one gland produces effects elsewhere. Endocrine dysfunction may result from an intrinsic defect in the target gland or from a diminished or elevated level of tropic hormones. Endocrine problems occur when there is hypofunction or hyperfunction of the glands. Primary hypofunction is usually associated with a more profound deficiency of the target gland hormone because little or no hormone is secreted. In secondary dysfunction the target glands secrete some of their hormones but in smaller amounts and less rapidly.

DISORDERS OF PITUITARY FUNCTION

The pituitary gland is divided into two lobes: the anterior pituitary (adenohypophysis) and the posterior pituitary (neurohypophysis). It is regulated by hormones secreted from the hypothalamus. The anterior pituitary is responsible for secreting GH, TSH, ACTH, follicle-stimulating hormone (FSH), luteinising hormone (LH) and prolactin. The posterior pituitary secretes antidiuretic hormone and oxytocin (Belfiore & LeRoith 2018).

Deficiencies of the anterior pituitary hormones may be due to organic defects or have an idiopathic aetiology. Clinical manifestations depend on the hormones involved and the age of the patient. If the tropic hormones are involved, the resulting disorder reflects the altered stimulus of the target gland. For example, if TSH is deficient, the thyroid gland does not secrete TH and the child displays clinical signs of hypothyroidism.

An overproduction of the anterior pituitary hormones can result in gigantism (caused by excess GH production during childhood), hyperthyroidism, hypercortisolism (Cushing's syndrome) and precocious puberty from excessive gonadotropins (LH and FSH). Overproduction may be caused by hyperplasia of the pituitary cells—which may eventually progress to a tumour (adenoma)—or a primary hypothalamic defect that results in an excess of the hormone's releasing factor. Although the initial clinical manifestations are a result of pituitary oversecretion, eventually pituitary insufficiency occurs and the signs of panhypopituitarism become evident. **Panhypopituitarism** is defined clinically as the loss of all anterior pituitary hormones, leaving only posterior pituitary function intact (Belfiore & LeRoith 2018).

Hypopituitarism

Hypopituitarism is the diminished secretion of one or more pituitary hormones. The consequences of the condition depend on the degree of dysfunction. It often leads to the following:

- gonadotropin deficiency (decrease in LH or FSH), where children show absence or regression of secondary sexual characteristics
- GH deficiency, where children display stunted somatic growth
- TSH deficiency, which produces hypothyroidism
- corticotropin deficiency, which results in manifestations of adrenal hypofunction.

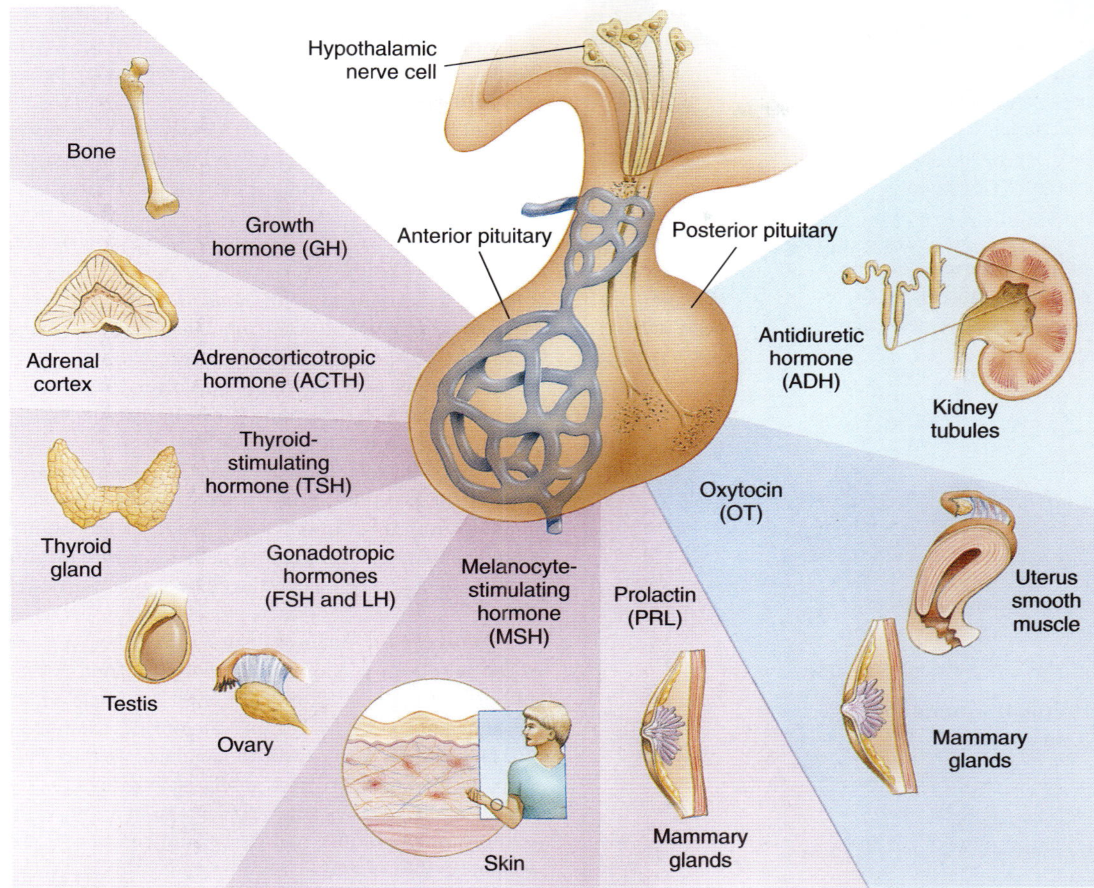

Fig 31.2 Principal anterior and posterior pituitary hormones and their target organs. (Source: Thibodeau, G. A., & Patton, K. T. (2008). Structure and function of the body (13th ed.). St Louis, MO: Mosby.)

Hypopituitarism can result from any of the conditions listed in Box 31.2. The most common organic cause of pituitary undersecretion is a tumour in the pituitary or hypothalamic region. Craniopharyngiomas are tumours known to invade these regions of the brain and cause panhypopituitarism (Box 31.3). A child may experience decreased growth velocity for some time before developing any symptoms or signs of increased intracranial pressure, local compression or the destructive effects of a tumour.

BOX 31.2 Causes of Hypopituitarism

- Aplasia or hypoplasia
- Developmental defects
- Idiopathic—Sporadic; genetic
- Destructive lesions
- Trauma—Perinatal; child abuse; basal skull fracture
- Irradiation—Central nervous system, eye, middle ear
- Autoimmune hypophysitis
- Surgery—Removal of pharyngeal pituitary, ablation of craniopharyngioma or other tumour
- Vascular—Aneurysm, infarct
- Functional deficiency
- Psychosocial dwarfism
- Anorexia nervosa

Congenital hypopituitarism can be seen in newborn infants and run in families, suggesting a genetic cause; however, the majority of cases have no genetic association (Schoenmakers et al 2015). Neonates may have symptoms of hypoglycaemia and seizure activity (Schoenmakers et al 2015). A child with combined GH deficiency and hypothyroidism should be screened for congenital pituitary defects and genetic mutations (Pine-Twaddell et al 2013, Belfiore & LeRoith 2018).

Idiopathic hypopituitarism, or idiopathic pituitary growth failure, is usually related to GH deficiency, which inhibits somatic growth in all cells of the body (Amin et al 2015).

Isolated GH deficiency without other associated pituitary hormone deficiencies or a known organic cause is also seen in children (Stanley 2012). **Growth failure** is defined as an absolute height of less than −2 standard deviations for age, or a linear growth velocity consistently less than −1 standard deviation for age. When this occurs without the presence of hypothyroidism, systemic disease or malnutrition, an abnormality of the GH–insulinlike growth factor (IGF) axis should be considered (Grimberg et al 2016).

Not all children with short stature have GH deficiency. In most instances the cause of short stature is considered idiopathic. Idiopathic short stature (ISS) is defined as a condition in which the height of an individual is more than two standard deviations below the mean height for their age, sex and population group, without evidence of systemic, endocrine, nutritional or chromosomal abnormalities (Argente 2016). Children with ISS fall into one of three groups: those

BOX 31.3 Clinical Manifestations of Panhypopituitarism

Growth Hormone
- Short stature but proportional height and weight
- Delayed epiphyseal closure
- Growth restriction
- Premature ageing common in later life
- Increased insulin sensitivity

Thyroid-stimulating Hormone
- Short stature with infantile proportions
- Dry, coarse skin; yellow discolouration, pallor
- Cold intolerance
- Constipation
- Somnolence
- Bradycardia
- Dyspnoea on exertion
- Delayed dentition, loss of teeth

Gonadotropins
- Absence of sexual maturation or loss of secondary sexual characteristics
- Atrophy of genitalia, prostate gland, breasts
- Amenorrhoea without menopausal symptoms
- Decreased spermatogenesis

Adrenocorticotropic Hormone
- Severe anorexia, weight loss
- Hypoglycaemia
- Hypotension
- Hyponatraemia, hyperkalaemia
- Adrenal apoplexy, especially in response to stress
- Circulatory collapse

Antidiuretic Hormone
- Polyuria
- Polydipsia
- Dehydration

Melanocyte-stimulating Hormone
- Decreased pigmentation

with familial short stature, those with constitutional delay of growth and puberty and those with an as yet unidentified cause of short stature. Familial short stature refers to healthy children who have ancestors with adult height in the lower percentiles and whose height during childhood is appropriate for genetic background (Fig 31.3). Constitutional delay of growth and puberty refers to individuals with delayed linear growth and delayed skeletal and sexual maturation for age (Amin et al 2015). GH therapy in children with ISS continues to be debated frequently by paediatric endocrinologists (Murray et al 2016).

Clinical Manifestations

Children with GH deficiency often grow normally during the first year and then follow a slowed growth curve that is below the third percentile. In children with a partial GH deficiency, the growth malformation is less marked than in children with complete GH deficiency. Height may be stunted more than weight because, with good nutrition, these children can become overweight or even obese. Their well-nourished appearance is an important diagnostic clue to differentiation from other disorders such as faltering growth. Skeletal proportions are normal for the age, but these children appear younger than their chronological age. Later in life, premature ageing is common. Bone age is delayed but is closely related to height age; the degree of growth delay depends on the duration and extent of the hormonal deficiency. Because of the underdeveloped jaw, teeth may be overcrowded and malpositioned.

Children with isolated GH deficiency have normal intelligence. However, emotional problems are common, especially as they near puberty, when their smallness becomes increasingly apparent in comparison with their peers.

Diagnostic Evaluation

Only a small number of children with delayed growth or short stature have hypopituitary dysfunction. Diagnostic evaluation is aimed at isolating organic causes, which, in addition to GH deficiency, may include brain tumour, hypothyroidism, oversecretion of cortisol, gonadal aplasia, chronic illness, nutritional inadequacy, Russell-Silver dwarfism or hypochondroplasia.

A complete diagnostic evaluation should include a family history, a history of the child's growth patterns and previous health status, a physical examination and a psychosocial evaluation. Specific radiographic imaging, including magnetic resonance imaging (MRI), endocrine studies and genetic testing, may also be warranted (Wheeler et al 2014).

Family History. A family history is of utmost importance in relating short stature to genetic background. The mid-parental height is an important prognosticator of the child's ultimate adult height. Normal adult height should fall within 5 cm of mid-parental height (Ferguson 2011). Children with constitutional delays frequently are the products of parents who experienced similar slow growth patterns and delayed sexual maturation. A small percentage of those with GH deficiency demonstrate an autosomal recessive inheritance pattern. Height and weight of siblings should be compared with the child's growth patterns at comparable age periods.

Child's History. The child's history should include a thorough prenatal history to rule out maternal disorders that may have influenced growth, such as malnutrition. Compare birth height and weight with gestational age. Children with hypopituitarism are usually of normal size and normal gestational age at birth.

Investigate the child's health history for evidence of chronic illness that may have influenced growth patterns, although a chronic illness, such as congenital heart disease, malabsorptive disorders, severe anaemia or neurological impairments, is usually identified long before the growth problem becomes a concern. Signs and symptoms suggesting a tumour, such as visual disturbances, headache and signs of increasing intracranial pressure, are important. With lesions involving the hypothalamus, the history may also reveal somnolence, thermodysregulation, epilepsy and polyphagia, resulting in obesity. Because a craniopharyngioma can affect the secretion of any of the pituitary hormones, assessment for hypothyroidism, hypoadrenalism and hypoaldosteronism should also be included.

Whenever possible, evaluate the child's growth patterns since birth, especially growth velocity, and compare them with standard measurements. The age of onset of short stature provides a significant diagnostic clue. When the clinician evaluates the results of plotting height and weight, upward or downward changes in height velocity in children older than 3 years may indicate a growth abnormality (Cheetham & Davies 2014).

Physical Examination. Accurate measurement of height (using a calibrated stadiometer) and weight and comparison with standard growth charts are essential. Multiple height measures reflect a more accurate assessment of abnormal growth patterns (Cheetham & Davies 2014). Other measurements may include crown-to-pubis and

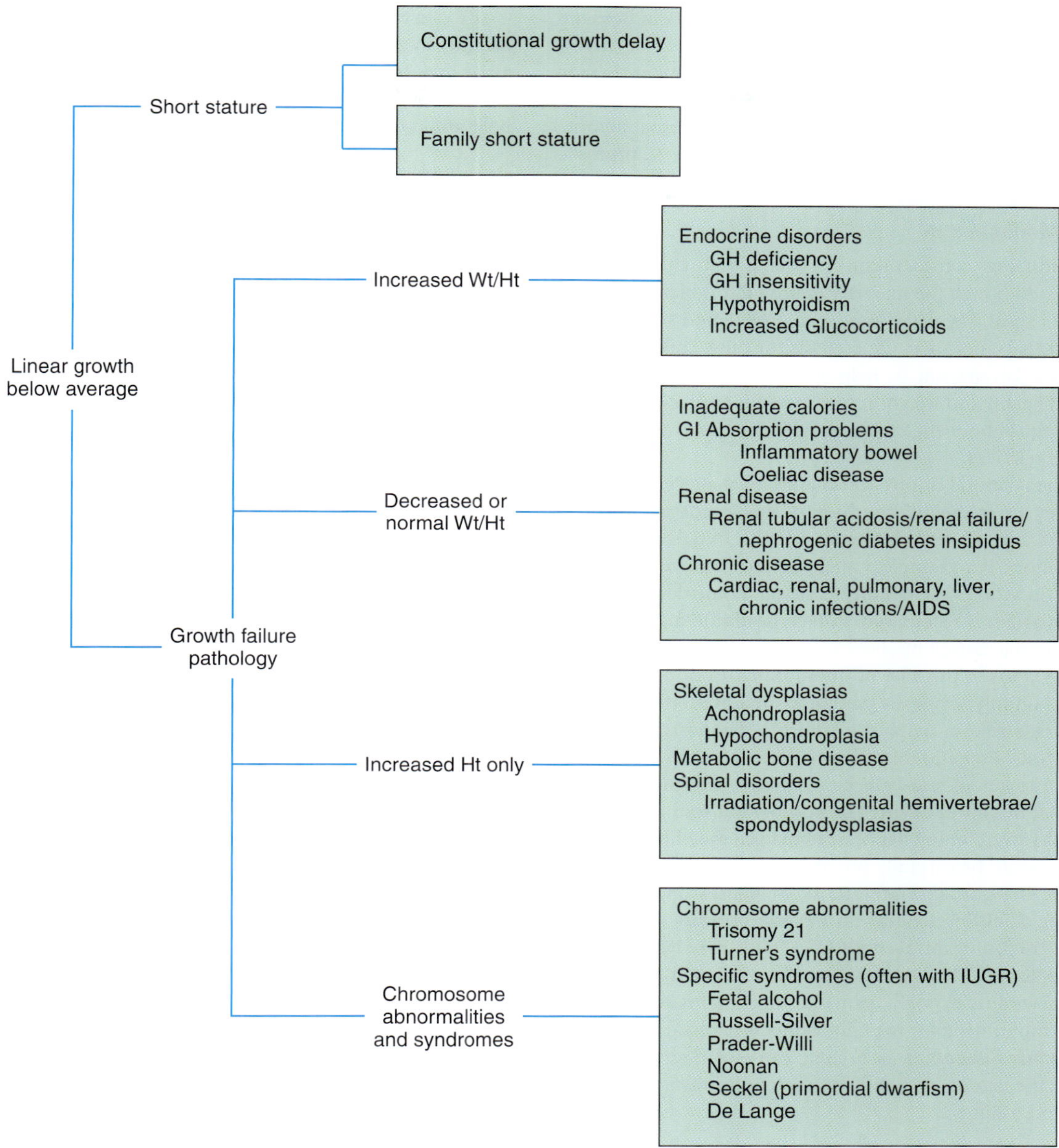

Fig 31.3 Causes of short stature. *AIDS*, acquired immunodeficiency syndrome; *GI*, gastrointestinal; *GH*, growth hormone; *IUGR*, intrauterine growth restriction; *Wt/Ht*, weight-to-height ratio. (Source: Vogiatzi, M. G., & Copeland, K. C. (1998). The short child. Pediatrics in Review, 19(3), 92–99.)

pubis-to-heel length to compare body proportions. Sexual development should be assessed and compared with age-appropriate development. Observation of general appearance yields valuable clues, especially signs of premature ageing and infantile facial features.

Radiographic Surveys. A skeletal survey in children less than 3 years of age and radiographic examination of the hand-wrist for centres of ossification (bone age) in older children are important in evaluating growth. Epiphyseal maturation is delayed in GH deficiency but consistent with height. This is in contrast with gonadal dysplasia, such as Turner's syndrome, in which bone age is near normal.

Endocrine Studies. Definitive diagnosis of GH deficiency is based on absent or subnormal reserves of pituitary GH. Measuring serum IGF-1 and IGF binding protein 3 (IGFBP3) levels may assist in the decision to pursue further testing for GH deficiency. It is recommended that GH stimulation tests be reserved for children with low serum IGF-1 and IGFBP-3 levels and poor growth who do not have other endocrine or non-endocrine causes for short stature (Wheeler et al 2014, Erdöl & Sağlam 2017). However, although the IGF-1 test is useful in detecting severe GH insensitivity, it may not be accurate in detecting less severe cases of idiopathic short stature (Erdöl & Sağlam 2017).

Therapeutic Management

Treatment of GH deficiency caused by organic lesions is directed towards correction of the underlying disease process (e.g. surgical removal or irradiation of a tumour). GH therapy in children with ISS continues to be debated frequently by paediatric endocrinologists (Erdöl & Sağlam 2017).

The child, family and healthcare team make the decision jointly to stop GH therapy. Growth rates of less than 2.5 cm per year and a bone age of more than 14 years in girls and more than 16 years in boys are often used as criteria to stop GH therapy (Parks & Felner 2016). Children with other hormone deficiencies require replacement therapy to correct the specific disorders. This may involve administration of thyroid extract, cortisone, testosterone or oestrogens and progesterone. The sex hormones are usually begun during adolescence to promote normal sexual maturation.

Nursing Care Management

The principal nursing consideration is identifying children with growth problems. Although the majority of growth problems are not a result of organic causes, any delay in normal growth and sexual development poses special emotional adjustments for these children.

The nurse is a key person in helping establish a diagnosis. For example, if serial height and weight records are not available, the nurse can question parents about the child's growth compared with that of siblings, peers or relatives.

Because the behavioural or physical changes that suggest a tumour are insidious, they are frequently overlooked. It is important to correlate the onset of any positive findings with the initial evidence of growth abnormalities. For example, visual problems and headaches are not uncommon in school-age children and can coincidentally occur after a growth problem is recognised. In fact, headache may represent the emotional trauma caused by short stature rather than be a symptom of a tumour. Pursue this line of questioning cautiously to avoid alarming parents unduly about the possibility of a brain tumour.

Part of a nurse's role in helping establish a diagnosis is assisting with diagnostic tests. Preparation of the child and family is especially important if a number of tests are being performed and the child requires particular attention during GH stimulation testing. Children also have difficulty overcoming hypoglycaemia generated by tests with insulin, so they should be carefully observed for signs of hypoglycaemia. Those receiving glucagon are at risk of nausea and vomiting. Patients receiving clonidine require close blood pressure monitoring. Nursing administration of intravenous (IV) fluids may be required if hypotension is detected. The use of arginine is often well tolerated by children, but it may cause hypoglycaemia in some infants and toddlers. Therefore, close monitoring for hypoglycaemia is necessary.

Child and Family Support. If an organic cause of the problem has been confirmed, the parents and child need an opportunity to express their thoughts and feelings.

Pituitary Hyperfunction

Excess GH before closure of the epiphyseal shafts results in proportional overgrowth of the long bones until the individual reaches a height of 2.4 m or more. Vertical growth is accompanied by rapid and increased development of muscles and viscera. Weight is increased but is usually in proportion to height. Proportional enlargement of head circumference also occurs and may result in delayed closure of the fontanels in young children. Children with a pituitary-secreting tumour may also demonstrate signs of increasing intracranial pressure, especially headache.

If oversecretion of GH occurs after epiphyseal closure, growth is in the transverse direction, producing a condition known as **acromegaly**. Typical facial features include the following:

- overgrowth of the head, lips, nose, tongue, jaw and paranasal and mastoid sinuses
- separation and malocclusion of the teeth in the enlarged jaw
- disproportion of the face to the cerebral division of the skull
- increased facial hair; thickened, deeply creased skin
- increased tendency towards hyperglycaemia and diabetes mellitus (DM).

Excessive secretion of GH by a pituitary adenoma causes most cases of acromegaly. Acromegaly can develop slowly, with patients being diagnosed as much as 10 years after their symptoms first appear. Left untreated, these patients have a higher mortality rate due to potential cardiovascular, metabolic and pulmonary complications (Pivonello et al 2017).

Diagnostic Evaluation

Diagnosis is based on a history of excessive growth during childhood and evidence of increased levels of IGF-1 concentration. If this is elevated, a specialised GH test will be done to assess for excess secretion (Erdöl & Sağlam 2017, Belfiore & LeRoith 2018). MRI may reveal a tumour in an enlarged sella turcica, normal bone age, enlargement of bones (such as the paranasal sinuses) and evidence of joint changes. Endocrine studies to confirm excess of other hormones, specifically thyroid, cortisol and sex hormones, should also be included in the differential diagnosis.

Therapeutic Management

If a lesion is present, surgical treatment by cryosurgery or hypophysectomy is performed to remove the tumour when possible. Transsphenoid surgery (TSS) is the most common surgical treatment for pituitary adenoma. External radiation (XRT) or radioactive implants may be used to destroy GH-secreting tissue. Medical therapy using drugs that can suppress GH may be used in conjunction with TSS and/or XRT to treat this disease (Maffezzoni et al 2016). Depending on the extent of surgical excision and degree of pituitary insufficiency, hormone replacement with thyroid extract, cortisone and sex hormones may be necessary.

Nursing Care Management

The primary nursing consideration is early identification of children with excessive growth rates. Although medical treatment of acromegaly will not reduce a patient's height, it will prevent further excess growth. Nurses in health assessment settings who are frequently involved in growth screening should refer children who demonstrate excessive linear growth for a medical evaluation. They should also observe for signs of a tumour, especially headache, and evidence of concurrent hormonal excesses, particularly the gonadotropins, which cause sexual precocity.

Precocious Puberty

Manifestations of sexual development before age 9 years in boys or age 8 years in girls have traditionally been considered precocious development, and these children were recommended for further evaluation (Brito et al 2016), but guidelines on this have been debated.

Normally the hypothalamic-releasing factors stimulate secretion of the gonadotropic hormone from the anterior pituitary at the time of puberty. In the male, interstitial cell–stimulating hormone stimulates Leydig cells of the testes to secrete testosterone. In the female FSH and LH stimulate the ovarian follicles to secrete oestrogens. This sequence of events is known as the **hypothalamic–pituitary–gonadal axis.** If for some reason the cycle undergoes premature activation, the child displays evidence of advanced or precocious puberty. Sex hormones affect bone growth, and premature exposure may cause short stature. Box 31.4 lists the causes of precocious puberty.

Isosexual precocious puberty is more common among girls than boys. Approximately 50% of children with precocious puberty have central precocious puberty (CPP), in which pubertal development is activated by the hypothalamic gonadotropin-releasing hormone (GnRH). This produces early maturation and development of the gonads, with secretion of sex hormones, development of secondary sexual characteristics and sometimes production of mature sperm

BOX 31.4 Precocious Puberty

Central Precocious Puberty
- Idiopathic, with or without hypothalamic hamartoma
- Secondary
  - Congenital anomalies
  - Postinflammatory: encephalitis, meningitis, abscess, granulomatous disease
  - Radiotherapy
  - Trauma
  - Neoplasms
- After effective treatment of long-standing pseudosexual precocity

Peripheral Precocious Puberty
- Familial male-limited precocious puberty
- Albright's syndrome
- Gonadal or extragonadal tumours
- Adrenal
  - Congenital adrenal hyperplasia
  - Adenoma, carcinoma
  - Glucocorticoid resistance
- Exogenous sex hormones
- Primary hypothyroidism

Incomplete Precocious Puberty
- Premature thelarche
- Premature menarche
- Premature pubarche or adrenarche

Source: Modified from Root, A. W. (2000). Precocious puberty. Pediatrics in Review, 21(1), 10–19.

and ova (Garibaldi & Chemaitilly 2016). CPP occurs more frequently in girls and is usually idiopathic, with 95% demonstrating no causative factor (Brito et al 2016). A CNS insult or structural abnormality occurs in more than 75% of boys with CPP (Garibaldi & Chemaitilly 2016).

Peripheral precocious puberty (PPP) refers to early puberty resulting from hormone stimulation other than the hypothalamic GnRH–stimulated pituitary gonadotropin release. Clinical findings normally associated with puberty may be seen as variations in normal sexual development (Brito et al 2016). They appear without other signs of puberty and are probably caused by unusual end-organ sensitivity to prepubertal levels of oestrogen or androgen. Included are premature thelarche (development of breasts in prepubertal girls), premature pubarche (premature adrenarche, early development of sexual hair) and premature menarche (isolated menses without other evidence of sexual development).

Therapeutic Management

Children with evidence of precocious puberty should be evaluated by a paediatric endocrinologist. In every case, an MRI of the brain should be performed to assess for hypothalamic brain tumour (Brito et al 2016). When there is no organic cause for CPP, patients will be monitored closely for growth. In 50% of cases, precocious pubertal development regresses or stops advancing without any treatment. CPP can be managed with monthly injections of a synthetic analogue of luteinising hormone–releasing hormone, which decreases the pituitary secretion of LH and FSH (Garibaldi & Chemaitilly 2016).

After initiation of treatment, breast development regresses or does not advance, and growth returns to normal rates, enhancing predicted height. Treatment is discontinued at a chronologically appropriate time, allowing pubertal changes to resume. Despite the early sexual development, maturation of the gonads and the appearance of secondary sexual characteristics proceed in the usual order. The most difficult time for the child is usually the school years before adolescence. After puberty, physical differences from peers are no longer present. Some patients, however, do not attain adult targeted height during therapy. The use of GH to improve adult height is being investigated with children with precocious puberty and advanced bone age (Garibaldi & Chemaitilly 2016).

Nursing Care Management

Psychological support and guidance of the child and family are the most important aspects of management. Parents and children need anticipatory guidance, support and information resources and reassurance. GnRH agonists are associated with side effects such as headache, emotional lability and vasodilation causing hot flushes (Harrington & Palmert 2016). Nurses are essential in providing medical education to the patient and family. Dress and activities for the physically precocious child should be appropriate to the chronological age. Sexual interest is not usually advanced beyond the child's chronological age, and parents need to understand that the child's mental age is congruent with the chronological age.

Although the child's sexual behaviour may be appropriate for the chronological age, the nurse should emphasise to parents that the child may be fertile. Usually no form of contraception is necessary unless the child is sexually active. In this situation proper counselling is important because hormonal forms of birth control, such as oestrogen pills, prematurely initiate epiphyseal closure, resulting in stunted linear growth.

Diabetes Insipidus

The principal disorder of posterior pituitary hypofunction is diabetes insipidus (DI). Also known as neurogenic DI, central diabetes insipidus results from the undersecretion of antidiuretic hormone (ADH), also known as vasopressin. This disease results in the production of large volumes of urine (polyuria), which leads to a state of uncontrolled diuresis (Belfiore & LeRoith 2018). Central DI is not to be confused with nephrogenic DI, a rare hereditary disorder affecting primarily males and caused by unresponsiveness of the renal tubules to the hormone. (See Chapter 24.)

Neurogenic DI may result from a number of different causes. Primary causes are familial or idiopathic; approximately 20% to 50% of the total cases are idiopathic (Belfiore & LeRoith 2018). More than 55 genetic mutations have been identified, which result in a deficiency of vasopressin and cause familial central DI (Belfiore & LeRoith 2018, Erdöl & Sağlam 2017). Secondary causes include trauma (accidental or surgical), tumours, granulomatous disease, Langerhans cell histiocytosis (LCH), autoimmune disease, infections (meningitis or encephalitis), cranial malformations and vascular anomalies (aneurysm). Certain drugs, such as alcohol or phenytoin (diphenylhydantoin), can cause a transient polyuria. DI may be an early sign of an evolving cerebral process (Belfiore & LeRoith 2018, Erdöl & Sağlam 2017).

Clinical Manifestations

The cardinal signs of DI are polyuria and polydipsia. In the older child, signs can include excessive urination accompanied by insatiable thirst so intense that the child does little more than go to the toilet and drink fluids. Frequently the first sign is enuresis. In the infant the initial symptom is irritability that is relieved with feedings of water but not milk. The infant is also prone to severe dehydration, electrolyte imbalance, hyperthermia, azotaemia and potential circulatory collapse. Other symptoms such as vomiting, constipation, fever, irritability, sleep issues, faltering growth and other growth problems may be seen.

Diagnostic Evaluation

Important points of assessment to be considered are in relation to hydration status and fluid balance, taking particular note of urine output, noting presence of intercurrent illness, such as urinary tract infection (UTI). Past history of DI with a similar episode should be documented in detail and any change in weight as marker of fluid status. Baseline investigations including urea and electrolytes, full ward uranalysis and paired serum and urine osmolality should be attended to.

Therapeutic Management

Rehydration. Rehydration is first-line treatment; the child should be closely monitored throughout the rehydration and a strict fluid balance attended. Rehydration therapy should be commenced after completing assessments and determining the level of dehydration and ongoing losses. For further therapeutic management, refer to your paediatric facility for the most current clinical guidelines. Many of the major paediatric hospitals have specific clinical guidelines that can be applied (The Royal Children's Hospital Melbourne [RCHM] n.d.).

Nursing Care Management

The initial objective is identification of the disorder. Because an early sign may be sudden enuresis in a child who is toilet trained, excessive thirst with bedwetting is an indication for further investigation. Another clue is persistent irritability and crying in an infant that is relieved only by bottle-feedings of water. After head trauma or certain neurosurgical procedures, the development of DI can be anticipated; therefore, closely monitor these patients.

Assessment includes measurement of body weight, serum electrolytes, blood urea nitrogen (BUN), haematocrit and urine specific gravity taken before surgery and every other day after the procedure. Fluid intake and output should be carefully measured and recorded. Alert patients are able to adjust intake to urine losses, but unconscious or very young patients require closer fluid observation. In children who are not toilet trained, collection of urine specimens may require application of a urine-collecting device.

For emergency purposes, these children should wear medical alert identification. School personnel need to be aware of the problem so they can grant children unrestricted use of the bathroom. Failure to permit this may result in embarrassing accidents that often result in a child's unwillingness to attend school. Medication may need to be kept at school depending on dosing schedules.

Syndrome of Inappropriate Antidiuretic Hormone

Oversecretion of the posterior pituitary antidiuretic hormone (ADH) causes the disorder known as syndrome of inappropriate antidiuretic hormone (SIADH). This disorder occurs with increased frequency in a variety of conditions that disrupt CNS function such as infection, tumour or surgery. It can also be the side effect of a variety of medications. SIADH is the most common cause of hyponatraemia in hospitalised patients (Cuesta et al 2016).

Excess ADH causes free water to be reabsorbed from the kidneys. As increased free water circulates, serum osmolality goes down and urine osmolality inappropriately increases. Clinical signs of SIADH are directly related to fluid retention and hyponatraemia. When hyponatraemia occurs acutely, swelling of the brain occurs (Giuliani & Peri 2014). When serum sodium levels are diminished to 120 mEq/L, affected children may display anorexia, nausea, vomiting, stomach cramps, irritability and personality changes. With progressive hyponatraemia, more serious neurological signs, such as stupor and seizures, may occur.

Fluid restriction is the immediate management of choice. Subsequent management depends on the cause and severity. Fluids may be restricted in anticipation of SIADH development postoperatively. Some children may be treated with oral sodium replacement. Severe SIADH may require hypertonic saline infusion that is only given in the hospital setting under close supervision (Cuesta et al 2016).

Nursing Care Management

The recognition of SIADH symptoms is the primary nursing goal. Close attention to measurements of intake and output, weight and monitoring for the development of neurological symptoms is essential, especially in patients at risk in the intensive care setting.

Seizure precautions are implemented in children at high risk for SIADH. The child and family need education and support regarding the rationale for fluid restrictions. The rare child with chronic SIADH is placed on long-term ADH-antagonising medication. The patient and family will need instruction regarding medication administration.

DISORDERS OF THYROID FUNCTION

The thyroid gland secretes two types of hormones: thyroid hormone (TH) and calcitonin. TH is made up of the hormones thyroxine (T_4) and triiodothyronine (T_3). The anterior pituitary hormone TSH controls the secretion of TH. TSH is regulated by the hypothalamic hormone thyrotropin-releasing factor (TRF) as a negative feedback response. Hypothyroidism or hyperthyroidism may result from a defect in the thyroid or from a disturbance in the secretion of TSH or TRF. Because the functions of T_3 and T_4 are qualitatively the same, the term *thyroid hormone* (TH) is used throughout the discussion (Box 31.5).

The synthesis of TH depends on available sources of dietary iodine and tyrosine. The thyroid is the only endocrine gland capable of storing excess amounts of hormones for release. During circulation T_4 and T_3 are bound to carrier proteins (thyroxine-binding globulin). They must be unbound before they are able to exert their metabolic effect.

The main physiological action of TH is to regulate metabolism and control the processes of growth and tissue differentiation, as outlined in Box 31.5. Unlike GH, TH is involved in many more diverse activities that influence the growth and development of body tissues. Therefore, a deficiency of TH exerts a more profound effect on growth than that seen in GH deficiency.

Calcitonin helps maintain blood calcium levels by decreasing the calcium concentration. It inhibits skeletal demineralisation and promotes calcium deposition in the bone. This effect is the opposite of parathyroid hormone (PTH).

Juvenile Hypothyroidism

Hypothyroidism is one of the most common endocrine problems of childhood. It may be either congenital or acquired and represents a deficiency in secretion of TH (Parks & Felner 2016). Hypothyroidism from dietary insufficiency of iodine is now rare in Australia and New Zealand because iodised salt is a readily available source of the nutrient.

Beyond infancy, a number of defects may cause primary hypothyroidism. For example, a congenital hypoplastic thyroid gland may provide sufficient amounts of TH during the first year or two but be inadequate when rapid body growth increases demands on the gland. A partial or complete thyroidectomy for cancer or thyrotoxicosis can leave insufficient thyroid tissue to furnish hormones for body requirements. Radiotherapy for Hodgkin's disease or other malignancies may lead to hypothyroidism (Metzger et al 2016). Infectious processes may cause hypothyroidism. It can also occur when dietary iodine is deficient.

BOX 31.5 Physiological Effects of Thyroid Hormone

- Regulates metabolic rate of all cells; protein, fat and carbohydrate catabolism; and nitrogen excretion
- Regulates body heat production and heat-dissipating mechanisms
- Regulates protein synthesis and catabolism, amino acid incorporation into protein and transcription of messenger ribonucleic acid
- Increases gluconeogenesis and peripheral utilisation of glucose
- Maintains appetite and secretion of gastrointestinal substances
- Maintains calcium mobilisation
- Stimulates cholesterol synthesis and hepatic mechanisms that remove cholesterol from the circulation; stimulates lipid turnover and free fatty acid release
- Regulates hepatic conversion of carotene to vitamin A
- Maintains growth hormone secretion, skeletal maturation and tissue differentiation
- Is necessary for muscle tone and vigour and normal skin constituents
- Maintains cardiac rate, force and output
- Affects respiratory rate, depth of oxygen utilisation and carbon dioxide formation
- Affects central nervous system development and cerebration during first 2 to 3 years
- Affects milk production during lactation and menstrual cycle fertility
- Maintains sensitivity to insulin and insulin degradation
- Affects red cell production
- Affects cortisol secretion, probably by directly affecting the adrenal glands and by increasing adrenocorticotropic hormone secretion

Thyromegaly (enlarged thyroid gland) and growth deceleration are seen in children with hypothyroidism. Growth and development are less impaired when hypothyroidism is acquired at a later age. Because brain growth is nearly complete by 2 to 3 years of age, intellectual disability and neurological sequelae are not associated with juvenile hypothyroidism. Clinical manifestations may include dry skin, puffiness around the eyes, sparse hair, constipation, sleepiness, lethargy and mental decline. Growth failure, delayed puberty and excessive weight gain can also be seen.

Therapy is TH replacement, the same as for hypothyroidism in the infant. In children with severe symptoms, the restoration of thyroid function is achieved more gradually with administration of increasing amounts of l-thyroxine over a period of 4 to 8 weeks. This is done to avoid symptoms of hyperthyroidism. Researchers have found that children treated early continue to have mild delays in reading, comprehension and arithmetic but should catch up over time (Pardo Campos et al 2017). Adolescents may demonstrate problems with memory, attention and visuospatial processing.

Nursing Care Management

Growth deceleration in a child whose growth has previously been normal should alert the observer to the possibility of hypothyroidism. Treatment is daily oral TH replacement. The importance of daily compliance and the need for periodic monitoring of serum thyroid levels should be stressed to patients and their families.

Goitre

A goitre is an enlargement or hypertrophy of the thyroid gland. It may occur with deficient (hypothyroid), excessive (hyperthyroid) or normal (euthyroid) TH secretion. It can be congenital or acquired. Congenital disease usually occurs as a result of maternal administration of antithyroid drugs or iodides during pregnancy. Acquired disease can result from increased secretion of pituitary TSH in response to decreased circulating levels of TH or from infiltrative neoplastic or inflammatory processes. In areas where dietary iodine (essential for TH production) is deficient, goitre can be endemic.

Enlargement of the thyroid gland may be mild and noticeable only when there is an increased demand for TH (e.g. during periods of rapid growth). Where iodine deficiency is severe, a large percentage of the population display goitres. Enlargement of the thyroid at birth can be sufficient to cause severe respiratory distress. Sporadic goitre is usually caused by lymphocytic thyroiditis, and intrinsic biochemical defects in synthesis of the hormones are associated with goitres. TH replacement is necessary to treat the hypothyroidism and reverse the TSH effect on the gland.

Nursing Care Management

Large goitres are identified by their obvious appearance. Smaller nodules may be evident only on palpation. Nurses in ambulatory settings need to be aware of the possibility of goitres and report such findings. Benign enlargement of the thyroid gland may occur during adolescence and should not be confused with pathological states. Nodules are rarely caused by a cancerous tumour but always require evaluation. Include questions regarding exposure to radiation in the assessment.

Chronic Lymphocytic Thyroiditis

Chronic lymphocytic thyroiditis (also known as Hashimoto's disease) is the most common cause of thyroid disease in children and adolescents and accounts for the largest percentage of juvenile hypothyroidism (Hanley et al 2016). It accounts for many of the enlarged thyroid glands formerly designated as thyroid hyperplasia of adolescence or adolescent goitre. Although lymphocytic thyroiditis can occur during the first 3 years of life, it occurs more frequently after age 6, with peak incidence occurring during adolescence. Some children may have subclinical hypothyroidism, but the presence of a goitre and elevated thyroglobulin antibody with progressive increase in both thyroid peroxidase antibody and TSH are predictive factors for development of overt hypothyroidism (Hanley 2016).

Pathophysiology

There is a strong genetic predisposition to the development of lymphocytic thyroiditis. In families this disease is closely related to other thyroid disorders (e.g. Graves' disease, idiopathic hypothyroidism, idiopathic myxoedema) and autoimmune disorders (e.g. pernicious anaemia, Addison's disease, type 1 DM and hypoparathyroidism).

Thyroid cell damage and death are autoimmune mediated by T-cells and cytokines. Lymphocytes infiltrate the thyroid gland and cause inflammation. Eventually, thyroid cells are replaced with fibrous tissue. Several antithyroid antibodies have been recognised in patients with thyroiditis and these antibodies are the best marker to determine a diagnosis (Caturegli et al 2014). The identification of genes involved in this disease has led to improved diagnostic testing and may lead to new treatments in the future (Tomer 2014).

Clinical Manifestations

Enlargement of the thyroid gland is often noted during routine examination. Parents may notice it when the youngster swallows. In most children the entire gland is enlarged symmetrically (but may be asymmetric) and is firm, freely movable and non-tender. There may signs of moderate tracheal compression (sense of fullness, hoarseness and dysphagia). However, it is extremely rare for a non-toxic diffuse goitre to enlarge enough to cause tracheal compression. Most children are euthyroid, but some display symptoms of hypothyroidism. Others have signs suggestive of hyperthyroidism, such as nervousness, irritability, tachycardia, increased sweating or hyperactivity.

Diagnostic Evaluation

Thyroid function tests are usually normal, although TSH levels may be slightly or moderately elevated. With progressive disease the T_4 decreases, followed by a decrease in T_3 levels and an increase in TSH. A variety of abnormalities in radioactive iodine uptake may be noted. The majority of children have serum antibody titres to thyroid antigens, but fewer children have a positive red blood cell haemgglutination test result. When both tests are used, almost all children with thyroid autoimmunity are detected. However, levels in children are lower than in adults; therefore, repeated measurements may be needed in questionable cases because titres may increase later in the disease.

Therapeutic Management

In many cases the goitre is transient and asymptomatic and regresses spontaneously within a year or two. Therapy of a non-toxic diffuse goitre is usually simple, uncomplicated and effective. Oral administration of TH decreases the size of the gland significantly and provides the feedback needed to suppress TSH stimulation, and the hyperplastic thyroid gland gradually regresses in size. Surgery is contraindicated in this disorder. Evaluate untreated patients periodically.

Nursing Care Management

Nursing care consists of identifying the youngster with thyroid enlargement, reassuring the child that the condition is probably only temporary and reinforcing instructions for thyroid therapy.

Hyperthyroidism

Graves' disease (GD) is the most common cause of hyperthyroidism in children. This disease runs in families and is autoimmune. Most cases of GD in children occur in adolescence, with a peak incidence at 12 to 14 years of age. Transient GD may be present at birth in children of thyrotoxic mothers. The incidence is higher in girls than in boys (Leger & Carel 2013, Erdöl & Sağlam 2017).

The hyperthyroidism of GD is caused by the generation of autoantibodies to the TSH receptor. This leads to excess secretion of TH. Currently, there is no cure for GD.

Clinical Manifestations

Signs and symptoms of hyperthyroidism develop gradually, with an interval between onset and diagnosis of approximately 6 to 12 months. Clinical features include irritability, hyperactivity, short attention span, tremors, insomnia and emotional lability. Gradual weight loss despite a voracious appetite occurs in half the cases. Linear growth and bone age are usually accelerated. Muscle weakness often occurs. Hyperactivity of the gastrointestinal tract may cause vomiting and frequent stooling. Cardiac manifestations can include rapid pulse at rest, widened pulse pressure, systolic murmur and cardiomegaly. Dyspnoea may occur during slight exertion, such as climbing stairs. The skin is warm, flushed and moist. Heat intolerance may be severe and is accompanied by diaphoresis. The hair is unusually fine and unable to hold a wave.

Exophthalmos (protruding eyeballs), observed in many children, is accompanied by a wide-eyed staring expression, increased blinking, lid lag, lack of convergence and absence of wrinkling of the forehead when looking upwards. If exophthalmos progresses, the eyelid may not completely cover the cornea. Visual disturbances may include blurred vision and loss of visual acuity. Eye disease associated with hyperthyroidism can develop before or after the clinical diagnosis.

Diagnostic Evaluation

The diagnosis of GD is established on the basis of increased levels of T_4 and T_3. TSH is suppressed to unmeasurable levels. Other tests are rarely indicated.

Therapeutic Management

Therapy for hyperthyroidism is controversial, but the end goal is the same: to decrease circulating TH. The three available treatments for children are antithyroid drugs, subtotal thyroidectomy and ablation with radioiodine (^{131}I iodide, RAI) (Hanley 2016). Each therapy has advantages and disadvantages.

When affected children exhibit signs and symptoms of hyperthyroidism (e.g. increased weight loss, pulse pressure and blood pressure), their activity should be limited to schoolwork only. Vigorous exercise is restricted until thyroid levels are decreased to normal or near-normal values.

Drug Therapy. Antithyroid drug (ATD) therapy interferes with the biosynthesis of TH. Generally, some improvement is noted within the first 2 weeks, with evidence of decreased nervousness, less fatigue, increased strength, a lowered pulse and weight gain. In many children an initial treatment course of 1 to 2 years is followed by a complete remission of the disorder. Others require 2 to 4 years before remission is achieved (Australian Paediatric Endocrine Group 2016).

ATD disadvantages include drug reactions (e.g. rash, hives, joint pain, nausea, vomiting) and chronic dependency on the drug. Remission is not achieved in many patients, and alternative treatments are required. The most serious side effect of ATDs is agranulocytosis (severe leucopenia), which generally occurs within the initial weeks or months of therapy. It is usually accompanied by a sore throat and fever. Treatment involves immediate discontinuation of the drug and the administration of antibiotics and glucocorticoids until symptoms resolve.

Thyroidectomy. Surgical treatment involves surgical ablation of the thyroid (thyroidectomy). Although this approach has the advantage of being a long-lasting form of therapy, it has a number of serious disadvantages. Hypothyroidism occurs along with the need for thyroxine therapy. Infrequently, recurrent laryngeal nerve palsy, permanent hypoparathyroidism, keloid formation and surgical morbidity and mortality do occur. Surgery in most centres is reserved for children who fail ATD therapy or who are prone to recurrence.

Radioiodine Therapy. Radioiodine may be a therapy of choice in young patients with GD who relapse after medical treatment (Hanley 2016). Low-dose RAI is administered to children to treat hyperthyroidism without resulting in hypothyroidism. The relapse rate is high in this case and may require multiple doses throughout life. RAI should be avoided in very young children due to the increased risk of cancer. More research on RAI in children is needed due to concerns over its potential long-term side effects, including thyroid cancer, hyperparathyroidism and high mortality rates (Australian Paediatric Endocrine Group 2016).

Thyrotoxicosis. Thyrotoxicosis (thyroid 'crisis' or thyroid 'storm') may occur from sudden release of TH. Although thyrotoxicosis is unusual in children, it can be life-threatening. Clinical signs of thyroid storm are acute onset of severe irritability and restlessness, vomiting, diarrhoea, hyperthermia, hypertension, severe tachycardia and prostration. There may be rapid progression to delirium, coma and death. A crisis may be precipitated by acute infection, surgical emergency or discontinuation of antithyroid therapy. In addition to ATD therapy, the administration of beta blockers is used to control symptoms until normal thyroid function is achieved (Leger & Carel 2013). Therapy is usually required for 2 to 3 weeks.

Nursing Care Management

Because the clinical manifestations of GD often appear gradually, the goitre and ophthalmic changes may not be noticed. Excessive activity may be attributed to behavioural problems. Nurses need to be alert to signs that suggest this disorder. Weight loss despite an excellent appetite, inattention, hyperactivity, unexplained fatigue, sleepiness and difficulty with fine motor skills may be seen. Exophthalmos, infrequent blinking and impairment of convergence are common presenting signs (Huang & LaFranchi 2016).

Surgical Care. If surgery is anticipated, iodine is administered for a few weeks before the procedure. Compliance with iodine therapy is essential to avoid the danger of thyroid crisis after sudden discontinuation.

Psychological preparation of children for thyroidectomy is similar to that for any other surgical procedure. (See Chapter 22.) However, the fear of having one's throat cut is unique to thyroidectomy. The nurse should explain that the throat is not cut, only the skin, to remove the gland. Children should be prepared for the dressing around the neck and the possibility of an endotracheal or 'breathing' tube after surgery.

Postoperative care involves positioning with the neck slightly flexed to avoid strain on the sutures and observation for bleeding and complications. The children learn to support the neck in this position when they sit up. Damage to the laryngeal nerve is evidenced by severe stridor or hoarseness, although some hoarseness is expected. **Laryngospasm**, a spasmodic contraction of the larynx, can be a life-threatening complication of thyroidectomy. Signs of laryngospasm are stridor, hoarseness and a feeling of tightness in the throat. Place a tracheostomy set near the bed for emergency use. The nurse should observe for signs of hypoparathyroidism, which causes hypocalcaemia, in the immediate postoperative period.

NURSING CARE CONSIDERATIONS

The earliest indication of hypoparathyroidism may be anxiety and mental depression, followed by paraesthesia and evidence of heightened neuromuscular excitability, such as the following:

- **Chvostek's sign**—Facial muscle spasm elicited by tapping the facial nerve in the region of the parotid gland
- **Trousseau's sign**—Carpal spasm elicited by pressure applied to nerves of the upper arm
- **Tetany**—Carpopedal spasm (sharp flexion of wrist and ankle joints), muscle twitching, cramps, seizures and stridor

DISORDERS OF PARATHYROID FUNCTION

The parathyroid glands secrete parathyroid hormone (PTH). Along with vitamin D and calcitonin, PTH regulates the homeostasis of serum calcium concentrations (Belfiore & LeRoith 2018). The effect of PTH on calcium is the opposite to that of calcitonin. Box 31.6 lists the principal effects of PTH on its target sites.

PTH and vitamin D work together to maintain serum calcium levels within a narrow normal range and mineralisation of bone. Secretion of PTH is controlled by a negative feedback system involving the serum calcium ion concentration. Low ionised calcium levels stimulate PTH secretion, causing absorption of calcium by the target tissues; high ionised calcium concentrations suppress PTH.

Hypoparathyroidism

Hypoparathyroidism is a spectrum of disorders that result in deficient PTH. Congenital hypoparathyroidism may be caused by a specific defect in the synthesis or cellular processing of PTH or by aplasia or hypoplasia of the gland (Belfiore & LeRoith 2018).

Hypoparathyroidism can occur secondary to other causes. Postoperative hypoparathyroidism may follow thyroidectomy with acute

BOX 31.6 Physiological Effects of Parathyroid Hormone

Bones—Increases osteoclastic activity, causing phosphate-producing bone demineralisation
Kidneys—Increases absorption of calcium and excretion of phosphate
Gastrointestinal tract—Promotes calcium absorption

or gradual onset. It may be transient or permanent. Two forms of transient hypoparathyroidism may be present in the newborn, both of which are the result of a relative PTH deficiency. One type is caused by maternal hyperparathyroidism. A more common form appears almost exclusively in infants fed a milk formula with a high phosphate-to-calcium ratio.

Clinical Manifestations

Symptoms vary from none to significant morbidity if treatment is not initiated. Mild deficiency may be identified through laboratory studies. Muscle cramps are an early symptom, progressing to numbness, stiffness and tingling in the hands and feet. A positive Chvostek's or Trousseau's sign or laryngeal spasms may be present. Convulsions with loss of consciousness may occur. These episodes may be preceded by abdominal discomfort, tonic rigidity, head retraction and cyanosis. Headaches and vomiting with increased intracranial pressure and papillo-oedema may occur and may suggest a brain tumour (Doyle 2016a).

Children with long-standing hypoparathyroidism often have dry, scaly, coarse skin and horizontal lines in the nails. Mucocutaneous eruptions caused by *Candida* organisms are common (Doyle 2016a). Dental and enamel hypoplasia often occurs. Cataracts develop in patients with untreated disease.

Diagnostic Evaluation

The diagnosis of hypoparathyroidism is made on the basis of clinical manifestations associated with decreased serum calcium and increased serum phosphorus. Levels of plasma PTH are low in idiopathic hypoparathyroidism but high in pseudohypoparathyroidism. End-organ responsiveness is tested by the administration of PTH with measurement of urinary cyclic adenosine monophosphate. Kidney function tests are included in the differential diagnosis to rule out kidney disease. Although bone radiographs are usually normal, they may demonstrate increased bone density and suppressed growth.

Therapeutic Management

The objective of treatment is to maintain normal serum calcium and phosphate levels with minimum complications. Acute or severe tetany is corrected immediately by IV administration of calcium gluconate and follow-up doses as necessary to achieve normal calcium levels. When diagnosis is confirmed, vitamin D therapy is begun.

Nursing Care Management

The initial objective is recognition of hypocalcaemia. Unexplained convulsions, irritability (especially to external stimuli), gastrointestinal symptoms (e.g. diarrhoea, vomiting, cramping) and positive signs of tetany should lead the nurse to suspect this disorder. Initial nursing care includes institution of seizure and safety precautions and observation for signs of laryngospasm such as stridor, hoarseness and a feeling of tightness in the throat. A tracheostomy set and injectable calcium gluconate should be located near the bedside for emergency use.

Because vitamin D toxicity can be a serious consequence of therapy, parents should watch for signs that include weakness, fatigue, lassitude, headache, nausea, vomiting and diarrhoea. Polyuria, polydipsia and nocturia are signs of early renal impairment.

Hyperparathyroidism

Hyperparathyroidism is rare in childhood but can be primary or secondary. The most common cause of primary hyperparathyroidism is adenoma of the gland (Doyle 2016b). Primary hyperparathyroidism is rarely seen in children, but when it occurs, it is often due to a single parathyroid adenoma (Pashtan et al 2013, Belfiore & LeRoith 2018). The most common causes of secondary hyperparathyroidism are chronic renal disease, renal osteodystrophy and congenital anomalies of the urinary tract. The common symptom of hyperparathyroidism is hypercalcaemia. Box 31.7 lists the manifestations of hyperparathyroidism.

Diagnostic Evaluation

Blood studies to identify elevated calcium and decreased phosphorus levels are routinely performed. Measurement of PTH, as well as several tests to isolate the cause of the hypercalcaemia, such as renal function studies, should be included. If parathyroid adenoma is suspected, imaging using ultrasound and a sestamibi nuclear subtraction study are recommended (Belfiore & LeRoith 2018).

Therapeutic Management

Treatment depends on the cause of hyperparathyroidism. The treatment of primary hyperparathyroidism is initially medication, but if this has no effect, surgical removal of the tumour or radioactive iodine is used (Huang & LaFranci 2016). Parathyroidectomy may cause recurrent laryngeal nerve damage, voice impairment and hypoparathyroidism (Huang & LaFranci 2016). Treatment of secondary hyperparathyroidism is directed at the underlying contributing cause, which subsequently restores the serum calcium balance.

Nursing Care Management

The initial nursing objective is recognition of hyperparathyroidism. Because secondary hyperparathyroidism is a consequence of chronic renal failure, the nurse is always alert to signs that suggest this complication, especially bone pain and fractures. Because urinary symptoms are the earliest indication, assessment of other body systems for evidence of high calcium levels is indicated when polyuria and polydipsia coexist. Clues to the possibility of hyperparathyroidism include: change in behaviour, especially inactivity; unexplained gastrointestinal symptoms; and cardiac irregularities.

If parathyroidectomy is anticipated, care is similar to that discussed for the child with hyperthyroidism. Because hypocalcaemia is a potential complication, observing for signs of tetany, instituting seizure precautions and having calcium gluconate available for emergency use are part of the nursing care.

BOX 31.7 Clinical Manifestations of Hyperparathyroidism

Gastrointestinal—Nausea, vomiting, abdominal discomfort and constipation

Central nervous system—Delusions, confusion, hallucinations, impaired memory, lack of interest and initiative, depression and varying levels of consciousness

Neuromuscular—Weakness, easy fatiguability, muscle atrophy (especially proximal muscles of the lower limbs), twitching of the tongue and paraesthesias in extremities

Skeletal—Vague bone pain, subperiosteal resorption of phalanges, spontaneous fractures and absence of lamina dura around the teeth

Renal—Polyuria and polydipsia, renal colic and hypertension

DISORDERS OF ADRENAL FUNCTION

Adrenal Hormones

The adrenal glands consist of two distinct portions: the cortex, or outer section; and the medulla, or inner core. The adrenal cortex secretes hormones, called steroids, that are essential to life. The adrenal medulla, the inner core, produces the catecholamines adrenaline and noradrenaline. These three chemicals are also produced by the sympathetic nervous system, so if the adrenal supply fails, the body will continue to function.

Adrenal Cortex

The cortex secretes three groups of hormones that are classified according to their biological activity: (1) glucocorticoids (cortisol, corticosterone); (2) mineralocorticoids (aldosterone); and (3) sex steroids (androgens, oestrogens and progestins). The glucocorticoids and mineralocorticoids affect metabolism and stress. The sex steroids influence sexual development but are not essential because the gonads secrete the major supply of these hormones.

Glucocorticoids. The most important glucocorticoids in humans are cortisol and corticosterone, the principal effects of which are listed in Box 31.8. Normally the hypothalamus secretes CRF, which causes the pituitary gland to produce ACTH, which stimulates the adrenal glands to produce glucocorticoids (primarily cortisol). Cortisol is the switch that controls this feedback. When blood levels of cortisol are low, the system turns on. When blood levels of cortisol rise, the system turns off.

In times of stress the anterior pituitary is stimulated by CRF from the hypothalamus, which causes the release of increased amounts of ACTH. Stressful stimuli capable of provoking this response include: trauma; anaesthesia; surgical intervention; sepsis; acute anoxia; hypothermia; hypoglycaemia; and emotional states, especially panic, anxiety or anger.

Mineralocorticoids. The most important mineralocorticoid is aldosterone. Like cortisol, it promotes sodium retention and potassium excretion in the renal tubules. Aldosterone is significantly more potent than that of the glucocorticoids in maintaining extracellular fluid volume, acid–base balance and normal potassium levels.

Aldosterone synthesis is regulated primarily by the renin-angiotensin system of the kidney. The juxtaglomerular cells of the kidney respond to decreased arterial pressure or blood volume and to

BOX 31.8 Physiological Effects of Glucocorticoids

- Stimulation of gluconeogenesis by the liver (a hyperglycaemic effect)
- Increased protein catabolism with resulting reduction in protein stores (except in the liver)
- Increased mobilisation and utilisation of fatty acids for energy
- Increased storage of adipose tissue in certain sites
- Decreased inflammatory and allergic reactions
- Regulation of fluid and electrolytes by promoting sodium retention and potassium excretion by the kidneys and by water diuresis through direct antagonistic action against antidiuretic hormone
- Increased gastric acid and pepsin production
- Suppression of lymphocytes, eosinophils and basophils, but elevation of neutrophils, erythrocytes and thrombocytes

decreased sodium concentrations by secreting the enzyme renin into the blood. Renin in turn converts angiotensinogen to angiotensin I and then to angiotensin II. Increased levels of angiotensin stimulate the adrenal cortex to secrete aldosterone, which preserves sodium, thereby retaining water. The renin-angiotensin mechanism also results in increased blood pressure.

Sex Steroids. Except for the first few days of life, the sex hormones are normally secreted in only minimum amounts until adolescence, at which time they play a role in pubertal changes. Their actions are the same as those of the gonadal hormones on internal and external sexual structures and skeletal growth.

Adrenal Medulla

The adrenal medulla secretes the catecholamines adrenaline and noradrenaline. Both hormones have essentially the same effects on different organs as those caused by direct sympathetic stimulation, except the hormonal effects last several times longer. Their major actions are listed in Box 31.9.

Although the catecholamines evoke similar responses from target sites, there are some important differences. Adrenaline has a greater effect on cardiac activity than noradrenaline, but it causes only weak constriction of the blood vessels of muscles in comparison with the effect of noradrenaline. As a result, noradrenaline elevates blood pressure, whereas adrenaline increases cardiac output. Another important difference is their effect on metabolism. Adrenaline increases the metabolic rate to a much greater extent than noradrenaline. These differences in action have been attributed to the catecholamines' effects on alpha- or beta-adrenergic receptors. Noradrenaline can only affect those effector cells that contain alpha receptors, which are mostly excitatory (constriction and contraction). Adrenaline, however, can affect both alpha and beta receptors, and beta receptors are mostly inhibitory (dilation and relaxation). Control of secretion of catecholamines, primarily in response to physiological or emotional stress, is through the hypothalamus. Also, stimulation of the sympathetic nervous system results in the release of adrenaline and noradrenaline from the sympathetic nerves and adrenal medulla. Both systems support each other, and one can be substituted for the other. For this reason no condition is attributable to hypofunction of the adrenal medulla. Even in bilateral adrenalectomy, catecholamine replacement is not necessary because the sympathetic release of these chemicals is sufficient to meet all the physiological functions required to cope with stressful events.

Phaeochromocytoma is a rare tumour characterised by secretion of catecholamines. The tumour most commonly arises from the chromaffin cells of the adrenal medulla but may occur wherever these cells are found, such as along the paraganglia of the aorta or thoracolumbar sympathetic chain. In children, they are frequently bilateral or multiple and are generally benign. Often there is a familial transmission of the condition as an autosomal dominant trait (White 2016a).

The clinical manifestations of phaeochromocytoma are caused by an increased production of catecholamines, producing hypertension, tachycardia, headache, decreased gastrointestinal activity and resulting constipation, increased metabolism with anorexia, weight loss, hyperglycaemia, polyuria, polydipsia, hyperventilation, nervousness, heat intolerance and diaphoresis. In severe cases, signs of congestive heart failure are evident.

BOX 31.9 Physiological Effects of Catecholamine Secretion

- Increased cardiac activity
- Vasoconstriction of blood vessels (elevation of blood pressure)
- Increased rate and depth of respirations
- Bronchial dilation
- Inhibition of gastrointestinal activity
- Increased muscular contraction
- Pupillary dilation
- Increased metabolic rate
- Heightened sensory awareness
- Diaphoresis

Acute Adrenocortical Insufficiency

The acute form of adrenocortical insufficiency (adrenal crisis) may have a number of causes during childhood. Although a rare disorder, some of the more common aetiological factors include haemorrhage into the gland from trauma, which may be caused by a prolonged, difficult labour and rapidly progressing infections, such as meningococcaemia, which result in haemorrhage and necrosis (Waterhouse-Friderichsen syndrome). Abrupt withdrawal of exogenous sources of cortisone or failure to increase endogenous supplies during stressor congenital adrenogenital hyperplasia of the salt-losing type can also cause adrenal crisis.

Clinical Manifestations

Early symptoms of adrenocortical insufficiency include increased irritability, headache, diffuse abdominal pain, weakness, nausea and vomiting and diarrhoea. Generalised haemorrhagic manifestations are present in Waterhouse-Friderichsen syndrome. Abnormal serum electrolyte levels include hyponatraemia and hyperkalaemia. Fever increases as the condition worsens and is accompanied by signs of CNS involvement, such as nuchal rigidity, convulsions, stupor and coma. The child is in a shocklike state with: a weak, rapid pulse; decreased blood pressure; shallow respirations; cold, clammy skin; and cyanosis. Circulatory collapse is the terminal event.

In the newborn, adrenal crisis is accompanied by extreme hyperpyrexia (high temperature), tachypnoea, cyanosis and seizures. Usually there is no evidence of infection or purpura. However, haemorrhage into the adrenal gland may be evident as a palpable retroperitoneal mass.

Diagnostic Evaluation

There is no rapid, definitive test for confirmation of acute adrenocortical insufficiency. Samples for measurement of plasma cortisol and ACTH levels should be sent for analysis, but this is too time consuming to be practical for initial diagnosis. Therefore, diagnosis is usually made based on clinical presentation, especially when haemorrhagic manifestations and signs of circulatory collapse despite adequate antibiotic therapy accompany a fulminating sepsis. Improvement with cortisol therapy confirms the diagnosis.

Therapeutic Management

Treatment involves replacement of cortisol, replacement of body fluids to combat dehydration and hypovolaemia, administration of glucose solutions to correct hypoglycaemia and specific antibiotic therapy in the presence of infection. Initially, IV hydrocortisone is administered. Normal saline containing 5% glucose is given parenterally to replace lost fluid, electrolytes and glucose. If haemorrhage has been severe, whole blood may be replaced. In the event that these measures do not reverse the circulatory collapse, vasopressors are used for immediate vasoconstriction and elevation of blood pressure.

After the child's condition has been stabilised, oral doses of cortisone, fluids and salt are given, similar to the regimen used for chronic adrenal insufficiency. To maintain sodium retention, aldosterone is replaced by synthetic salt-retaining steroids.

Nursing Care Management

Because of the abrupt onset and potentially fatal outcome of this condition, prompt recognition is essential. Vital signs and blood pressure are taken every 15 minutes. Seizure precautions are instituted. The nurse should monitor the child's response to fluid and cortisol replacement. Rapid administration of fluids can precipitate cardiac failure and overdosage with cortisol may cause hypotension and a sudden fall in temperature.

When the acute phase is over and the hypovolaemia has been corrected, the child is given oral fluids in small quantities. Rapid ingestion of oral fluids may induce vomiting, which increases dehydration. Therefore the nurse should plan a gradual schedule for reintroducing liquids. (See Quality Patient Outcomes box.)

QUALITY PATIENT OUTCOMES

Acute Adrenocortical Insufficiency

- Early recognition of signs and symptoms of acute adrenal crisis
- Hypokalaemia or hyperkalaemia prevented
- Fluid balance maintained
- Sufficient cortisol replacement

The sudden, severe nature of this disorder necessitates a great deal of emotional support for the child and family. The child may be placed in an intensive care unit where the surroundings are strange and frightening. Despite the need for emergency intervention, the nurse must be sensitive to the family's psychological needs and prepare them for each procedure.

Chronic Adrenocortical Insufficiency (Addison's disease)

Chronic adrenocortical insufficiency is rare in children. Causes include infection, a destructive lesion of the adrenal gland and autoimmune processes, but the cause may also be idiopathic. Because 90% of adrenal tissue must be non-functional before signs of insufficiency are manifested, onset of symptoms is often gradual. However, during periods of stress, when demands for additional cortisol are increased, symptoms of acute insufficiency may appear in a previously well child (Box 31.10).

Definitive diagnosis is based on measurements of functional cortisol reserve. The fasting serum cortisol and urinary 17-hydroxycorticosteroid levels are low and fail to rise, and plasma ACTH levels are elevated with corticotropin (ACTH) stimulation, the definitive test for the disease.

BOX 31.10 Clinical Manifestations of Acute and Chronic Adrenocortical Insufficiency

Clinical Manifestations of Acute Adrenocortical Insufficiency

Early Symptoms

- Increased irritability
- Headache
- Diffuse abdominal pain
- Weakness
- Nausea and vomiting
- Diarrhoea
- Generalised haemorrhagic manifestations (Waterhouse-Friderichsen syndrome)
- Fever (increases as condition worsens)
- Central nervous system signs:
  - nuchal rigidity
  - seizures
  - stupor
  - coma
- Shock-like state
- Weak, rapid pulse
- Decreased blood pressure
- Shallow respirations
- Cold, clammy skin
- Cyanosis
- Circulatory collapse (terminal event)

Newborn

- Hyperpyrexia
- Tachypnoea
- Cyanosis
- Seizures
- Gland evident as palpable retroperitoneal mass (haemorrhagic)

Clinical Manifestations of Chronic Adrenocortical Insufficiency

- Neurological symptoms
- Muscular weakness
- Mental fatigue
- Irritability, apathy and negativism
- Increased sleeping, listlessness
- Pigmentary changes
- Previous scars
- Palmar creases
- Mucous membranes
- Hair
- Hyperpigmentation over pressure points (elbows, knees or waist)
- Less frequently, vitiligo (loss of pigmentation)
- Gastrointestinal symptoms
- Dehydration
- Anorexia
- Weight loss
- Circulatory symptoms
- Hypotension
- Small heart size
- Dizziness
- Syncopal (fainting) attacks
- Hypoglycaemia
- Headache
- Hunger
- Weakness
- Trembling
- Sweating

Other Signs (Seen in Some Children)

- Recurrent, unexplained seizures
- Intense craving for salt
- Acute abdominal pain
- Electrolyte imbalances

Therapeutic Management

Treatment involves replacement of glucocorticoids (cortisol) and mineralocorticoids (aldosterone). Some children are able to be maintained solely on oral supplements of cortisol (cortisone or hydrocortisone preparations) with a liberal intake of salt. During stressful situations (e.g. fever, infection, emotional upset or surgery), the dosage must be tripled to accommodate the body's increased need for glucocorticoids. Failure to meet this requirement will precipitate an acute crisis. Overdosage produces appearance of cushingoid signs.

Children with more severe states of chronic adrenal insufficiency require mineralocorticoid replacement to maintain fluid and electrolyte balance.

Nursing Care Management

After the disorder is diagnosed, parents need guidance concerning drug therapy. They must be aware of the continuous need for cortisol replacement. Sudden termination of the drug because of inadequate supplies or inability to ingest the oral form because of vomiting places the child in danger of an acute adrenal crisis. Parents should always have a spare supply of medication.

Cushing's Syndrome

Cushing's syndrome is a characteristic group of manifestations caused by excessive circulating free cortisol (Table 31.1).

Cushing's syndrome is uncommon in children. When seen, it is often caused by excessive or prolonged steroid therapy that produces a cushingoid appearance (Fig 31.4). This condition is reversible after the steroids are gradually discontinued. Abrupt withdrawal will precipitate acute adrenal insufficiency. Gradual withdrawal of exogenous supplies is necessary to allow the anterior pituitary an opportunity to secrete increasing amounts of ACTH to stimulate the adrenals to produce cortisol.

Clinical Manifestations

Because the actions of cortisol are widespread, clinical manifestations are equally profound and diverse. The symptoms that produce changes in physical appearance occur early in the disorder and are of considerable concern to school-age and older children (Fig 31.5). The physiological disturbances, such as hyperglycaemia, susceptibility to infection, hypertension and hypokalaemia, may have life-threatening consequences unless recognised early and treated successfully. Children with short stature may be responding to increased cortisol levels, resulting in Cushing's syndrome. Cortisol inhibits the action of GH.

Diagnostic Evaluation

Several tests are helpful in confirming Cushing's syndrome. Serum cortisol levels should be measured at midnight and in the morning along with corticotropin hormone, urinary free cortisol, fasting blood glucose levels for hyperglycaemia, serum electrolyte levels for hypokalaemia and alkalosis, and 24-hour urinary levels of elevated 17-hydroxycorticoids and 17-ketosteroids (Lowitz & Keil 2015). Imaging of the pituitary and adrenal glands to assess for tumours, bone density studies for evidence of osteoporosis and skull radiographs to determine enlargement of the sella turcica may also aid in the diagnosis. Another procedure used to establish a more definitive diagnosis is the dexamethasone (cortisone) suppression test (Ceccato & Boscaro 2016). Administration of an exogenous supply of cortisone normally suppresses ACTH production. However, in individuals with Cushing's syndrome, cortisol levels remain elevated. This test is helpful in differentiating between children who are obese and those who appear to have cushingoid features.

TABLE 31.1 Clinical Manifestations of Cushing's Syndrome

Signs and Symptoms	Physiological Cause
Centripetal fat distribution Truncal obesity Supraclavicular fat pads Fat pads on neck and back (buffalo hump) Rounded or 'moon' face	Increased appetite and deposition of fat
Muscular wasting Thin extremities Pendulous abdomen Muscle weakness Thin skin and subcutaneous tissue Poor wound healing	Increased protein catabolism resulting in negative nitrogen balance
Increased frequency of infection Decreased inflammatory response	Decreased production and circulating levels of antibodies by lysis of fixed plasma cells and lymphocytes
Excessive bruising Petechial haemorrhages	Capillary weakness resulting from loss of protein
Facial plethora ('red cheeks') Reddish purple abdominal striae	Thin skin allowing capillary blood to be visible; increased colour from polycythaemia
Hypertension—arteriosclerosis	Increased salt and water retention (hypervolaemia)
Hypokalaemia Alkalosis	Increased excretion of potassium and hydrogen ions
Osteoporosis Compression fractures of vertebrae Kyphosis Backache	Increased glomerular filtration rate and excretion of calcium and decreased absorption of calcium from intestinal tract
Stunted linear growth (short stature) Delayed bone age	Increased levels of cortisol interfering with action of growth hormone
Hypercalciuria—renal calculi	Excessive amount of calcium in urine
Psychoses Irritability Insomnia Euphoria Depression Frank psychoses	Cause unknown
Peptic ulcer	Increased production of hydrochloric acid and pepsin and decreased gastric mucus production
Glycosuria	Increased gluconeogenesis by liver and decreased rate of glucose utilisation by cells
Latent or overt diabetes	Overstimulation of islets of Langerhans
Virilisation Hirsutism (excessive body hair) Acne Deepening of voice Clitoral enlargement Tendency towards male physique in female Amenorrhoea Impotence	Excess production of androgens

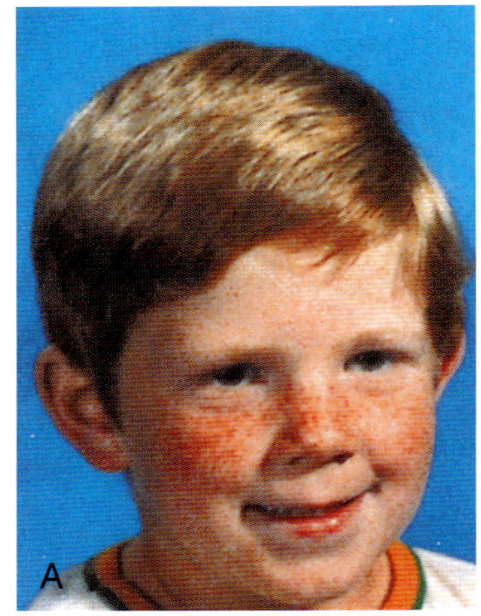

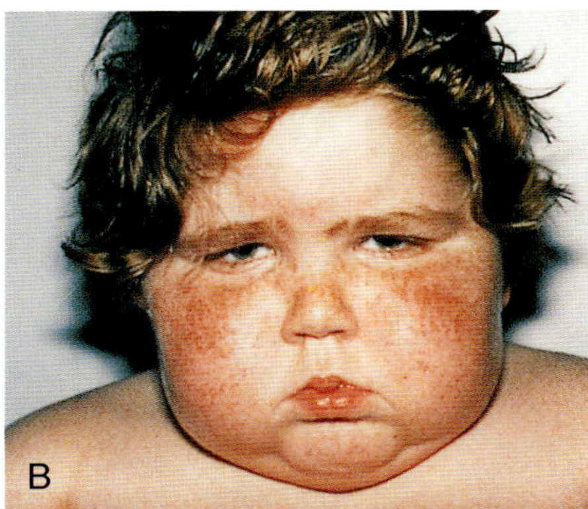

Fig 31.4 (**A**) Boy before development of Cushing's syndrome. (**B**) Same boy 4 months after onset of Cushing's syndrome. (Source: Zitelli, B. J., & Davis, H. W. (2007). Atlas of pediatric physical diagnosis (5th ed.). St Louis, MO: Mosby.)

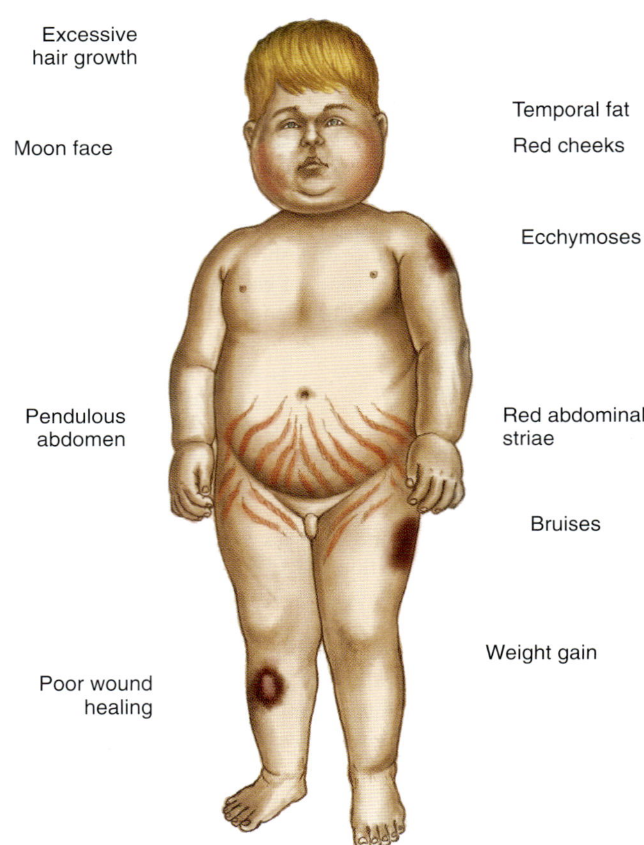

Fig 31.5 Characteristics of Cushing's syndrome.

NURSING CARE CONSIDERATIONS

Postoperative complications of adrenalectomy are related to the sudden withdrawal of cortisol. Observe for shock-like symptoms (e.g. hypotension, hyperpyrexia).

Therapeutic Management

Treatment depends on the cause. In most cases, surgical intervention involves bilateral adrenalectomy and postoperative replacement of the cortical hormones (the therapy for this is the same as that outlined for chronic adrenocortical insufficiency). If a pituitary tumour is found, surgical extirpation or irradiation may be chosen. In either of these instances, treatment of panhypopituitarism with replacement of GH, TH, ADH, gonadotropins and steroids may be necessary for an indefinite period (Lau et al 2015).

Nursing Care Management

Nursing care also depends on the cause. When cushingoid features are caused by steroid therapy, the effects may be lessened with administration of the drug early in the morning and on an alternate-day basis. Giving the drug early in the day maintains the normal diurnal pattern of cortisol secretion. If given during the evening, it is more likely to produce symptoms because endogenous cortisol levels are already low, and the additional supply exerts more pronounced effects. An alternate-day schedule allows the anterior pituitary an opportunity to maintain more normal hypothalamic–pituitary–adrenal control mechanisms.

If an organic cause is found, nursing care is related to the treatment regimen. Although a bilateral adrenalectomy permanently solves one condition, it reciprocally produces another syndrome.

Anorexia and nausea and vomiting are common and may be improved with the use of nasogastric decompression. Muscle and joint pain may be severe, requiring use of analgesics. The psychological depression can be profound and may not improve for months. Parents should be aware of the physiological reasons behind these symptoms in order to be supportive of the child.

Congenital Adrenal Hyperplasia

Congenital adrenal hyperplasia (CAH) is a family of disorders caused by decreased enzyme activity required for cortisol production in the adrenal cortex. The adrenal gland produces excessive amounts of cortisol precursors and androgens to compensate. There are seven types of biochemical defects with the most common defect being 21-hydroxylase deficiency, which constitutes more than 90% of all cases of CAH (El-Maouche et al 2017). This deficiency is an autosomal recessive disorder that results in improper steroid hormone synthesis (Mendes et al 2015).

Clinical Manifestations

Excessive androgens cause masculinisation of the urogenital system at approximately the tenth week of fetal development. The most pronounced abnormalities occur in girls, who are born with varying degrees of ambiguous genitalia. Masculinisation of external genitalia causes the clitoris to enlarge so that it appears as a small phallus. Fusion of the labia produces a saclike structure resembling the scrotum without testes. However, no abnormal changes occur in the internal sexual organs, although the vaginal orifice is usually closed by the fused labia. The label *ambiguous genitalia* should be applied to any infant with hypospadias or micropenis and no palpable gonads, and a diagnostic evaluation for CAH should be contemplated (Wheeler et al 2014).

Increased pigmentation of skin creases and genitalia caused by increased ACTH may be a subtle sign of adrenal insufficiency. A salt-wasting crisis frequently occurs, usually within the first few weeks of life (White 2016b). Infants fail to gain weight, and hyponatraemia and hyperkalaemia may be significant. Cardiac arrest can occur.

Untreated CAH results in early sexual maturation, with enlargement of the external sexual organs; development of axillary, pubic and facial hair; deepening of the voice; acne; and a marked increase in musculature with changes towards an adult male physique. However, in contrast to precocious puberty, breasts do not develop in girls, and they remain amenorrhoeic and infertile. In boys, the testes remain small and spermatogenesis does not occur. In both sexes, linear growth is accelerated and epiphyseal closure is premature, resulting in short stature by the end of puberty.

Diagnostic Evaluation

Clinical diagnosis is initially based on congenital abnormalities that lead to difficulty in assigning sex to the newborn and on signs and symptoms of adrenal insufficiency.

Therapeutic Management

After diagnosis is confirmed, medical management includes administration of glucocorticoids to suppress the abnormally high secretions of ACTH and adrenal androgens. If cortisone is begun early enough, it is very effective. Cortisone depresses the secretion of ACTH by the anterior pituitary, which in turn inhibits the secretion of adrenocorticosteroids, which stems the progressive virilisation. The signs and symptoms of masculinisation in girls gradually disappear, and excessive early linear growth is slowed. Puberty occurs normally at the appropriate age.

Gender assignment and surgical intervention in the newborn with ambiguous genitalia is complex and controversial. It is a significant stress for families, who need support and education from a multidisciplinary team of experienced specialists. Factors that influence gender assignment include genetic diagnosis, genital appearance, surgical options, fertility, and family and cultural preferences. Early reconstructive surgery should be considered only in the case of severe virilisation (El-Maouche et al 2017). Emphasis is on functional rather than cosmetic outcomes, and surgery can often be delayed. Reports concerning sexual satisfaction after partial clitoridectomy indicate that the capacity for orgasm and sexual gratification is not necessarily impaired. Male infants may require phallic reconstruction by an experienced surgeon.

Unfortunately, not all children with CAH are diagnosed at birth and raised in accordance with their genetic sex. Particularly in the case of affected females, masculinisation of the external genitalia may have led to sex assignment as a male. In males, diagnosis is usually delayed until early childhood, when signs of virilism appear. In these situations, it is advisable to continue rearing the child as a male in accordance with assigned sex and phenotype. Hormone replacement may be required to permit linear growth and to initiate male pubertal changes. Surgery is usually indicated to remove the female organs and reconstruct the phallus for satisfactory sexual relations. These individuals are not fertile.

Nursing Care Management

Of major importance is recognition of ambiguous genitalia and diagnostic confirmation in newborns. Parents need assistance in understanding and accepting the condition and time to grieve for the loss of perfection in their newborn child.

In general, rearing a genetically female child as a girl is preferred because of the success of surgical intervention and the satisfactory results with hormones in reversing virilism and providing a prospect of normal puberty and the ability to conceive. This is in contrast to the choice of rearing the child as a boy, in which case the child is sterile and may never be able to function satisfactorily in heterosexual relationships. If the parents persist in their decision to assign a male sex to a genetically female child, a psychological consultation should be requested to explore their motivations and ensure their understanding of the future consequences for the child.

Nursing care management regarding cortisol and aldosterone replacement is the same as that discussed for chronic adrenocortical insufficiency. Because infants are especially prone to dehydration and salt-losing crises, parents need to be aware of signs of dehydration and the urgency of immediate medical intervention to stabilise the child's condition. Parents should have injectable hydrocortisone available and know how to prepare and administer the intramuscular injection.

Parents should be referred for genetic counselling before they conceive another child because CAH is an autosomal recessive disorder. Prenatal diagnosis and treatment are available.

NURSING CARE CONSIDERATIONS

Advise parents that there is no physical harm in treating for suspected adrenal insufficiency that is not present, but the consequence of not treating acute adrenal insufficiency can be fatal.

Hyperaldosteronism

Excessive secretion of aldosterone may be caused by an adrenal tumour or, in some types of adrenogenital syndromes, result from enzymatic deficiency. The signs and symptoms are caused by increased sodium levels, water retention and potassium loss. Hypervolaemia causes hypertension and resultant headaches. Hypokalaemia results in muscular weakness, paraesthesia, episodes of paralysis and tetany, and may be responsible for polyuria and consequent polydipsia.

The clinical diagnosis is suspected when there are findings of hypertension, hypokalaemia and polyuria that fail to respond to ADH administration. Renin and angiotensin titres are abnormally low. Urinary levels of 17-hydroxycorticosteroids and 17-ketosteroids are normal in primary hyperaldosteronism caused by an aldosterone-secreting tumour but are usually abnormal in adrenogenital syndrome.

Therapeutic Management

Temporary treatment of the disorder involves replacement of potassium and administration of spironolactone (Aldactone), a diuretic that blocks the effects of aldosterone, thereby promoting excretion of sodium and water, while preserving potassium. Definitive treatment is similar to that for chronic adrenocortical insufficiency.

Nursing Care Management

An important nursing consideration is recognition of the syndrome, particularly in children with high blood pressure. Other clues include bedwetting, excessive thirst and unexplained weakness. After the diagnosis, nursing care is related to the treatment regimen. If diuretics are used, they should be administered in the morning to avoid accidents during the night. Children need unrestricted bathroom privileges at school. Potassium supplements should be mixed with fruit juice such as grape juice to increase their acceptability, and potassium-rich foods should be encouraged. Parents need to be aware of the signs of hypokalaemia and hyperkalaemia. After an adrenalectomy, nursing care is similar to that for chronic adrenocortical insufficiency.

Phaeochromocytoma

Phaeochromocytoma is a rare tumour characterised by secretion of catecholamines. The tumour most commonly arises from the chromaffin cells of the adrenal medulla but may occur wherever these cells are found, such as along the paraganglia of the aorta or thoracolumbar sympathetic chain. In children, they are frequently bilateral or multiple and are generally benign. Often there is a familial transmission of the condition as an autosomal dominant trait (White 2016a).

Clinical Manifestations

The clinical manifestations of phaeochromocytoma are caused by an increased production of catecholamines, producing hypertension, tachycardia, headache, decreased gastrointestinal activity with resulting constipation, increased metabolism with anorexia, weight loss, hyperglycaemia, polyuria, polydipsia, hyperventilation, nervousness, heat intolerance and diaphoresis. In severe cases, signs of congestive heart failure are evident.

Diagnostic Evaluation

The clinical manifestations mimic those of other disorders, such as hyperthyroidism or DM. Tests specific to these conditions may be performed as part of the differential diagnosis. In a small number of instances a palpable tumour suggests the diagnosis. Usually the tumour is identified by CT scan or MRI. Definitive tests include 24-hour measurement of urinary levels of the catecholamine metabolites (Young 2016).

Therapeutic Management

Definitive treatment consists of surgical removal of the tumour. In children, the tumours may be bilateral, requiring a bilateral adrenalectomy and lifelong glucocorticoid and mineralocorticoid therapy. The major complications that can occur during surgery are severe hypertension, tachyarrhythmias and hypotension. The first two are caused by excessive release of catecholamines during manipulation of the tumour, and the latter results from catecholamine withdrawal and hypovolaemic shock.

Preoperative medication to inhibit the effects of catecholamines is begun 1 to 3 weeks before surgery to prevent these complications. The major group of drugs used is the alpha-adrenergic blocking agents with or without beta-adrenergic blocking agents. To control catecholamine release after alpha-adrenergic blockage has been achieved, the child is given beta-adrenergic blocking agents.

Success of therapy is judged by lowering of blood pressure to normal, absence of hypertensive attacks (e.g. flushing or blanching, fainting, headache, palpitations, tachycardia, nausea and vomiting, profuse sweating), heat tolerance, decrease in perspiration and disappearance of hyperglycaemia.

Nursing Care Management

An initial nursing objective is identification of children with this disorder. Children with hypertension and hypertensive attacks should be assessed for phaeochromocytoma. Because of behavioural changes (nervousness, excitability, overactivity and even psychosis), increased cardiac and respiratory activity may appear to be related to an acute anxiety attack. Therefore a careful history of the onset of symptoms and association with stressful events is helpful in distinguishing between an organic and a psychological cause for the symptoms.

Preoperative nursing care involves frequent monitoring of vital signs and observation for evidence of hypertensive attacks and congestive heart failure. Therapeutic effects are evidenced by normal vital signs and absence of glycosuria. Note daily blood glucose levels, urine acetone and any signs of hyperglycaemia and report immediately.

NURSING CARE CONSIDERATIONS

Do not palpate the mass. Preoperative palpation of the mass releases catecholamines, which can stimulate severe hypertension and tachyarrhythmias.

The environment is made conducive to rest and free of emotional stress. This requires adequate preparation during hospital admission and before surgery. Parents are encouraged to room-in with their child and to participate in care. Play activities need to be tailored to the child's energy level without being overly strenuous or challenging because these can increase metabolic rate and promote frustration and anxiety.

After surgery, the child is observed for signs of shock from removal of excess catecholamines. If a bilateral adrenalectomy was performed, the nursing interventions are those discussed for chronic adrenocortical insufficiency.

DISORDERS OF PANCREATIC HORMONE SECRETION

Diabetes Mellitus

DM is a chronic disorder of metabolism characterised by hyperglycaemia and insulin resistance. It is the most common metabolic disease, resulting in metabolic adjustment or physiological change in almost all areas of the body.

In 2017 more than 6500 Australian children aged 0 to 14 years had type 1 diabetes. This equates to 141 cases per 100,000 population. Aboriginal and Torres Strait Islander children were less likely than non-Indigenous children to have type 1 diabetes (89 compared with 137 cases per 100,000). There was no obvious difference in the rate between boys and girls. What was noticeable was the increase with age, from 29 cases per 100,000 in 0 to 4 year olds to 256 cases per 100,000 in 10 to 14 year olds (AIHW 2020).

New Zealand has much lower numbers than Australia with approximately 2000 children and young people in New Zealand having type 1 diabetes in 2015, with the numbers showing males having slightly higher numbers than females (Ministry of Health 2015).

Type 1 diabetes is characterised by destruction of the pancreatic beta cells, which produce insulin; this usually leads to absolute insulin deficiency (Fig 31.6). Type 1 diabetes has two forms. Immune-mediated DM results from an autoimmune destruction of the beta cells; it typically starts in children or young adults who are slim, but it can arise in adults of any age. Idiopathic type 1 refers to rare forms of the disease that have no known cause.

Type 2 diabetes usually arises because of insulin resistance in which the body fails to use insulin properly combined with relative (rather than absolute) insulin deficiency. People with type 2 can range from predominantly insulin resistant with relative insulin deficiency to predominantly deficient in insulin secretion with some insulin resistance. It typically occurs in those who are older than 45 years of age, are

PATHOPHYSIOLOGY REVIEW

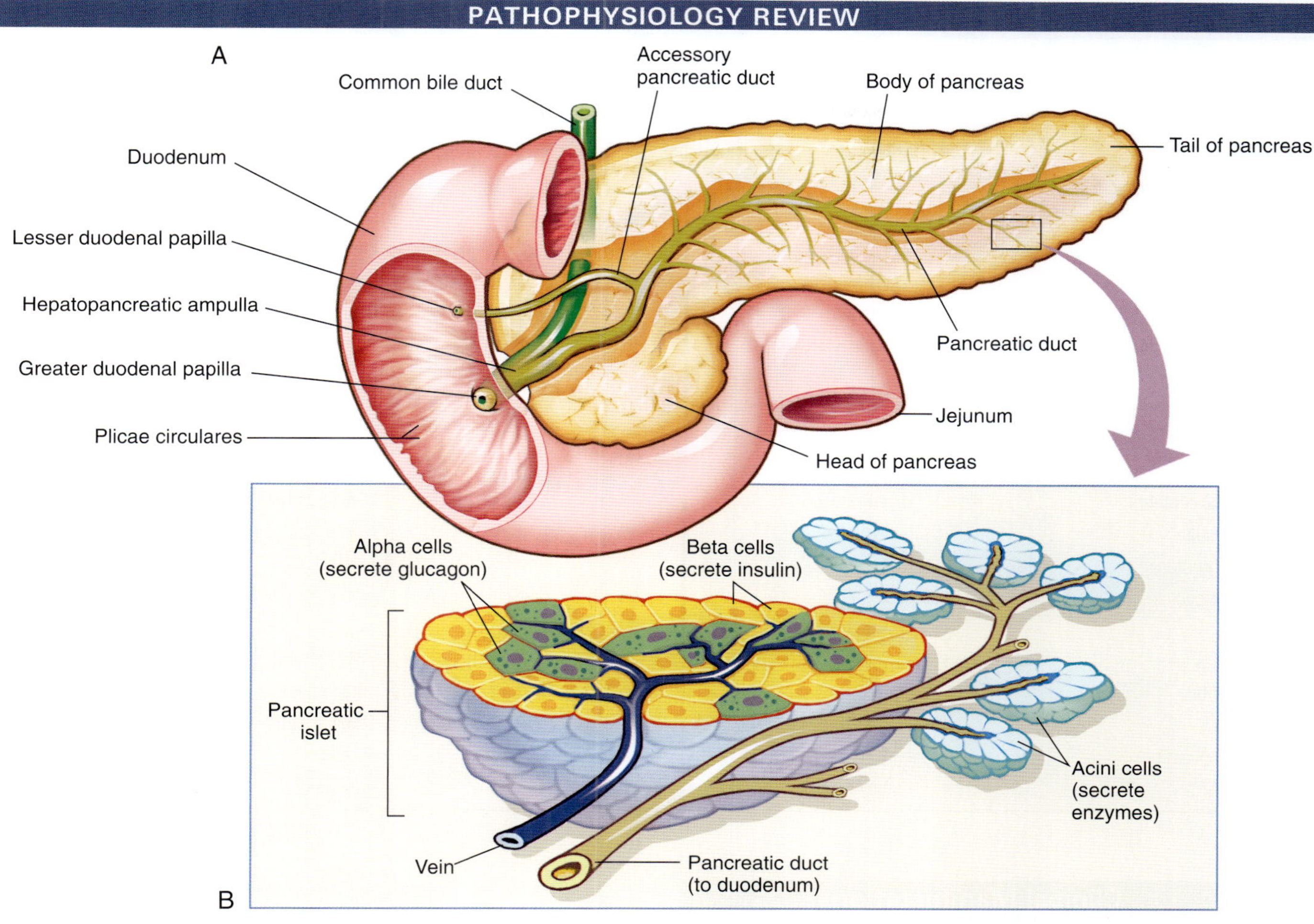

Fig 31.6 The pancreas. (**A**) The main and accessory ducts. (**B**) Glandular cells of the pancreatic islets. (Source: Patton, K. T., & Thibodeau, G. A. (2010). Anatomy and physiology (7th ed.). St Louis, MO: Mosby.)

overweight and sedentary and have a family history of diabetes (Table 31.2).

The symptomatology of diabetes is more readily recognisable in children than in adults, so it is surprising that the diagnosis may sometimes be missed or delayed. Diabetes is a great imitator; influenza, gastroenteritis and appendicitis are the conditions most often diagnosed when it turns out that the disease is really diabetes (Box 31.11).

Pathophysiology

Insulin is needed to support the metabolism of carbohydrates, fats, and proteins, primarily by facilitating the entry of these substances into the cells. Insulin is needed for the entry of glucose into the muscle and fat cells, prevention of mobilisation of fats from fat cells and storage of glucose as glycogen in the cells of liver and muscle. Insulin is not needed for the entry of glucose into nerve cells or vascular tissue. The chemical composition and molecular structure of insulin are such that it fits into receptor sites on the cell membrane. Here it initiates a sequence of poorly defined chemical reactions that alter the cell membrane to facilitate the entry of glucose into the cell and stimulate enzymatic systems outside the cell that metabolise the glucose for energy production.

With a deficiency of insulin, glucose is unable to enter the cells, and its concentration in the bloodstream increases. The increased concentration of glucose (hyperglycaemia) produces an osmotic gradient that causes the movement of body fluid from the intracellular space to the interstitial space and then to the extracellular space and into the glomerular filtrate to 'dilute' the hyperosmolar filtrate. Normally, the renal tubular capacity to transport glucose is adequate to reabsorb all the glucose in the glomerular filtrate. When the glucose concentration in the glomerular filtrate exceeds the renal threshold (180 mg/dL), glucose spills into the urine (glycosuria) along with an osmotic diversion of water (polyuria), a cardinal sign of diabetes. The urinary fluid losses cause the excessive thirst (polydipsia) observed in diabetes. This water 'washout' results in a depletion of other essential chemicals, especially potassium.

Protein is also wasted during insulin deficiency. Because glucose is unable to enter the cells, protein is broken down and converted to glucose by the liver (glucogenesis); this glucose then contributes to the hyperglycaemia. These mechanisms are similar to those seen in starvation when substrate (glucose) is absent. The body is actually in a state of starvation during insulin deficiency. Without the use of carbohydrates for energy, fat and protein stores are depleted as the body attempts to meet its energy needs. The hunger mechanism is triggered, but increased food intake (polyphagia) enhances the problem by further elevating blood glucose (Fig 31.7).

Ketoacidosis. When insulin is absent or insulin sensitivity is altered, glucose is unavailable for cellular metabolism, and the body chooses alternative sources of energy, principally fat. Consequently,

TABLE 31.2 Characteristics of Types 1 and 2 Diabetes Mellitus

Characteristic	Type 1	Type 2
Age at onset	< 20 years	Increasingly occurring in younger children
Type of onset	Abrupt	Gradual
Sex ratio	Affects males slightly more than females	Females outnumber males
Percentage of diabetic population	5%–8%	85%–90%
Heredity:		
• Family history	Sometimes	Frequently
• Human leucocyte antigen	Associations	No association
• Twin concordance	25%–50%	90%–100%
• Ethnic distribution	Primarily whites	Increased incidence in American Indians, Hispanics, African Americans
Presenting symptoms	Three Ps common—polyuria, polydipsia, polyphagia	May be related to long-term complications
Nutritional status	Underweight	Overweight
Insulin (natural):		
• Pancreatic content	Usually none	> 50% normal
• Serum insulin	Low to absent	High or low
• Primary resistance	Minimum	Marked
Islet cell antibodies	80%–85%	< 5%
Therapy:		
• Insulin	Always	20%–30% of patients
• Oral agents	Ineffective	Often effective
• Diet only	Ineffective	Often effective
Chronic complications	> 80%	Variable
Ketoacidosis	Common	Infrequent

BOX 31.11 Clinical Manifestations of Type 1 Diabetes Mellitus

- Polyphagia
- Polyuria
- Polydipsia
- Weight loss
- Enuresis or nocturia
- Irritability; 'not himself' or 'not herself'
- Shortened attention span
- Lowered frustration tolerance
- Dry skin
- Blurred vision
- Poor wound healing
- Fatigue
- Flushed skin
- Headache
- Frequent infections
- Hyperglycaemia
  - Elevated blood glucose levels
  - Glucosuria
- Diabetic ketosis
  - Ketones and glucose in urine
  - Dehydration in some cases
- Diabetic ketoacidosis
  - Dehydration
  - Electrolyte imbalance
  - Acidosis
  - Deep, rapid breathing (Kussmaul respirations)

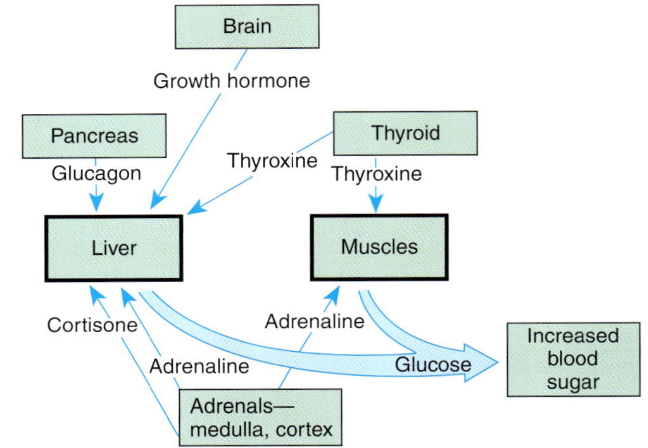

Fig 31.7 Body systems respond to hypoglycaemia in various ways to increase blood glucose level.

fats break down into fatty acids, and glycerol in the fat cells is converted by the liver to ketone bodies (e.g. beta-hydroxybutyric acid, acetoacetic acid, acetone). Any excess is eliminated in the urine (ketonuria) or the lungs (acetone breath). The ketone bodies in the blood (ketonaemia) are strong acids that lower serum pH, producing ketoacidosis.

Ketones are organic acids that readily produce excessive quantities of free hydrogen ions, causing a fall in plasma pH. Then chemical buffers in the plasma, principally bicarbonate, combine with the hydrogen ions to form carbonic acid, which readily dissociates into water and carbon dioxide. The respiratory system attempts to eliminate the excess carbon dioxide by increased depth and rate—**Kussmaul respirations**, or the hyperventilation characteristic of metabolic acidosis. The ketones are buffered by sodium and potassium in the plasma. The kidneys attempt to compensate for the increased pH by increasing tubular secretion of hydrogen and ammonium ions in exchange for fixed base, thus depleting the base buffer concentration.

With cellular death, potassium is released from the cells (intracellular fluid) into the bloodstream (extracellular fluid) and excreted by the kidneys, where the loss is accelerated by osmotic diuresis. The total body potassium is then decreased even though the serum potassium level may be elevated as a result of the decreased fluid volume in which it circulates. Alteration in serum and tissue potassium can lead to cardiac arrest.

If these conditions are not reversed by insulin therapy in combination with correction of the fluid deficiency and electrolyte imbalance, progressive deterioration occurs, with dehydration, electrolyte imbalance, acidosis, coma and death. **Diabetic ketoacidosis (DKA)** should be diagnosed promptly in a seriously ill patient and therapy instituted in an intensive care unit.

Long-term Complications. Long-term complications of diabetes involve both the microvasculature and the macrovasculature. The principal microvascular complications are nephropathy, retinopathy and neuropathy. Microvascular disease develops during the first 30 years of diabetes, beginning in the first 10 to 15 years after puberty, with renal involvement evidenced by proteinuria and clinically apparent retinopathy.

Macrovascular disease develops after 25 years of diabetes and creates the predominant problems in patients with type 2 DM. The process appears to be one of glycosylation, wherein proteins from the blood become deposited in the walls of small vessels (e.g. glomeruli), where they become trapped by 'sticky' glucose compounds (glycosyl radicals). The buildup of these substances over time causes narrowing of the vessels, with subsequent interference with microcirculation to the affected areas (Svoren & Jospe 2016).

With poor diabetic control, vascular changes can appear as early as 2½ to 3 years after diagnosis; however, with good to excellent control, changes can be postponed for 20 or more years. Intensive insulin therapy appears to delay the onset and slow the progression of retinopathy, nephropathy and neuropathy. However, children who have type 2 DM have a higher risk of long-term cardiovascular disease, including hypertension, stroke and myocardial infarction, than individuals who develop type 2 DM in adulthood (Reinehr 2013).

Other complications have been observed in children with type 1 DM. Hyperglycaemia appears to influence thyroid function, and altered function is frequently observed at the time of diagnosis and in poorly controlled diabetes. Limited mobility of small joints of the hand occurs in 30% of 7- to 18-year-old children with type 1 DM and appears to be related to changes in the skin and soft tissues surrounding the joint as a result of glycosylation.

Diagnostic Evaluation

Three groups of children who are candidates for diabetes are: (1) children who have glycosuria, polyuria and a history of weight loss or failure to gain despite a voracious appetite; (2) those with transient or persistent glycosuria; and (3) those who display manifestations of metabolic acidosis, with or without stupor or coma. In every case, diabetes must be considered if there is glycosuria, with or without ketonuria, and unexplained hyperglycaemia.

Glycosuria by itself is not diagnostic of diabetes. Other sugars, such as galactose, can produce a positive result with certain test strips, and a mild degree of glycosuria can be caused by other conditions, such as infection, trauma, emotional or physical stress, hyperalimentation and some renal or endocrine diseases.

DM is diagnosed based on any of the following four abnormal glucose metabolites: (1) 8-hour fasting blood glucose level of 126 mg/dL or more; (2) a random blood glucose value of 200 mg/dL or more accompanied by classic signs of diabetes; (3) an oral glucose tolerance test (OGTT) finding of 200 mg/dL or more in the 2-hour sample; or (4) haemoglobin A_{1C} of 6.5% or more (Laffel & Svoren 2015). Postprandial blood glucose determinations and the traditional OGTTs have yielded low detection rates in children and are not usually necessary for establishing a diagnosis. Serum insulin levels may be normal or moderately elevated at the onset of diabetes; delayed insulin response to glucose indicates impaired glucose tolerance.

Ketoacidosis must be differentiated from other causes of acidosis or coma, including hypoglycaemia, uraemia, gastroenteritis with metabolic acidosis, salicylate intoxication encephalitis and other intracranial lesions. DKA is a state of relative insulin insufficiency and may include the presence of hyperglycaemia (blood glucose level $\geq$ 200 mg/dL), acidosis (pH $<$ 7.30 and bicarbonate $<$ 15 mmol/L), glycosuria and ketonuria (Svoren & Jospe 2016).

Therapeutic Management

The management of the child with type 1 DM consists of a multidisciplinary approach involving the family; the child (when appropriate); and professionals, including a paediatric endocrinologist, diabetes nurse educator, nutritionist and exercise physiologist. Often psychological support from a mental health professional is also needed. Communication among the team members is essential and extends to other individuals in the child's life, such as grandparents, relatives, school and sports coach.

Insulin Therapy. Consultation about the individual insulin regimen should be made by the paediatric diabetes team in discussion with the family and child. Initial treatment will usually consist of a quick-acting insulin within 2 hours prior to a meal. Standard insulin regimens for newly diagnosed patients will comprise of either twice-daily mixture of short-acting and intermediate-acting insulins or multiple daily injections. The option of multiple daily injection regimens offer greater flexibility within daily living to fit around mealtimes, school, sport and leisure activities; however, the child needs to be old enough to have the ability and skills to self-administer the insulin using a pen device without parental supervision (RCHM n.d.).

Methods of administration. Daily insulin is administered subcutaneously by twice-daily injections, by multiple-dose injections or by means of an insulin infusion pump.

Monitoring. Daily monitoring of blood glucose levels is an essential aspect of appropriate DM management. Plasma blood glucose and haemoglobin A_{1C} vary according to age (Table 31.3). Plasma blood glucose and haemoglobin A_{1C} goal ranges are found in Table 31.4.

Blood glucose. Self-monitoring of blood glucose (SMBG) has improved diabetes management and is used successfully by children from the onset of their diabetes. By testing their own blood, children are able to change their insulin regimen to maintain their glucose level in the euglycaemic (normal) range of 80 to 120 mg/dL. Diabetes management depends to a great extent on SMBG. In general, children tolerate the testing well.

Glycosylated haemoglobin. The measurement of glycosylated haemoglobin (haemoglobin A_{1C}) levels is a satisfactory method for assessing control of the diabetes. As red blood cells circulate in the bloodstream, glucose molecules gradually attach to the haemoglobin A molecules and remain there for the lifetime of the red blood cell, approximately 120 days. The attachment is not reversible; therefore, this glycosylated haemoglobin reflects the average blood

TABLE 31.3 Plasma Blood Glucose and Haemoglobin A_{1C} Goals for Type 1 Diabetes Mellitus by Age-group

Age	Value* Before Meals (mg/dL)	Value* at Bedtime/Overnight (mg/dL)	Haemoglobin A_{1C} (%)	Implications
Toddlers and preschoolers (< 6 years)	100–180	110–200	≤ 8.5% (but ≥ 7.5%)	High risk and vulnerability to hypoglycaemia
School age (6–12 years)	90–180	100–180	< 8%	Risks of hypoglycaemia and relatively low risk of complications before puberty
Adolescents (> 12 years) and young adults	90–130	90–150	< 7.5%	Risk of hypoglycaemia Developmental and psychological issues

*Plasma blood glucose goal range.
Source: Modified from American Diabetes Association. (2005). Standards of medical care in diabetes. Diabetes Care, 28(Suppl), S4–S36.

TABLE 31.4 Comparison of Haemoglobin Blood Glucose Levels to Haemoglobin A_{1C}

Haemoglobin A_{1C} levels	Haemoglobin A_{1C} (%)	Mean Blood Glucose (mg/dL)	Mean Blood Glucose (mmol/L)
Severely elevated	14	360	20
	13	330	18.3
	12	300	16.7
	11	270	15
Elevated	10	240	13.3
	9	210	11.7
Slightly elevated	8	180	10
	7	150	8.3
Normal	6	120	6.7
	5	90	5
	4	60	3.3

Source: The Royal Children's Hospital. (n.d.) Diabetes mellitus. Clinical Practice Guidelines. https://www.rch.org.au/clinicalguide/guideline_index/Diabetes_mellitus/.

glucose levels over the previous 2 to 3 months. The test is a satisfactory method for assessing control, detecting incorrect testing, monitoring the effectiveness of changes in treatment, defining patients' goals and detecting non-adherence. Non-diabetic haemoglobin A_{1C} values are generally between 4% and 6% but can vary by laboratory. Diabetes control for children depends on age, with haemoglobin A_{1C} levels of 6.0% to 7.5% as good control, levels of 7.6% to 9.9% as fair control and levels of 10% or higher as poor control (Svoren & Jospe 2016).

Urine. Urine testing for glucose is no longer used for diabetes management. There is poor correlation between simultaneous glycosuria and blood glucose concentrations. However, urine testing can be carried out to detect evidence of ketonuria.

NURSING CARE CONSIDERATIONS

It is recommended that urine be tested for ketones every 3 hours during an illness or whenever the blood glucose level is over 240 mg/dL when illness is not present.

Nutrition. Essentially, the nutritional needs of children with diabetes are no different from those of healthy children. Children with diabetes need no special foods or supplements. They need sufficient calories to balance daily expenditure for energy and to satisfy the requirement for growth and development. Unlike children without diabetes, whose insulin is secreted in response to food intake, insulin injected subcutaneously has a relatively predictable time of onset, peak effect, duration of action and absorption rate depending on the type of insulin used. Consequently, the timing of food consumption must be regulated to correspond to the timing and action of the insulin prescribed.

Meals and snacks must be eaten according to peak insulin action, and the total number of calories and proportions of basic nutrients must be consistent from day to day. The constant release of insulin into the circulation makes the child prone to hypoglycaemia between the three daily meals unless a snack is provided between meals and at bedtime. The distribution of calories should be calculated to fit the activity pattern of each child.

Exercise. Exercise is encouraged and never restricted unless indicated by other health conditions. Exercise lowers blood glucose levels, depending on the intensity and duration of the activity. Consequently, exercise should be included as part of diabetes management, and the type and amount of exercise should be planned around the child's interests and capabilities. However, in most instances, children's activities are unplanned, and the resulting decrease in blood glucose can be compensated for by providing extra snacks before (and if the exercise is prolonged, during) the activity. In addition to a feeling of wellbeing, regular exercise aids in utilisation of food and often results in a reduction of insulin requirements.

Hypoglycaemia. Occasional episodes of hypoglycaemia are an integral part of insulin therapy, and an objective of diabetes management is to achieve the best possible glycaemic control while minimising the frequency and severity of hypoglycaemia. Even with good control, a child may frequently experience mild symptoms of hypoglycaemia. If the signs and symptoms are recognised early and promptly relieved by appropriate therapy, the child's activity should be interrupted for no more than a few minutes.

The signs and symptoms of hypoglycaemia are caused by both increased adrenergic activity and impaired brain function. The increased adrenergic nervous system activity plus increased secretion of catecholamines produces tachycardia, tremors, sweating, irritability, aggression and hunger (Svoren & Jospe 2016). Drowsiness, personality changes, mental confusion, loss of coordination, seizures and coma are more severe responses and reflect

TABLE 31.5 Comparison of Manifestations of Hypoglycaemia and Hyperglycaemia

Variable	Hypoglycaemia	Hyperglycaemia
Onset	Rapid (minutes)	Gradual (days)
Mood	Labile, irritable, nervous, weepy	Lethargic
Mental status	Difficulty concentrating, speaking, focusing, coordinating Nightmares	Dulled sensorium Confusion
Inward feeling	Shaky feeling	Thirst
	Hunger	Weakness
	Headache	Nausea and vomiting
	Dizziness	Abdominal pain
Skin	Pallor	Flushed
	Sweating	Signs of dehydration
Mucous membranes	Normal	Dry, crusty
Respirations	Shallow, normal	Deep, rapid (Kussmaul)
Pulse	Tachycardia, palpitations	Less rapid, weak
Breath odour	Normal	Fruity, acetone
Neurological	Tremors	Diminished reflexes Paraesthesia
Ominous signs	Late: Hyperreflexia, dilated pupils, seizure	Acidosis, coma
	Shock, coma	
Blood:		
• Glucose	Low: < 60 mg/dL	High: ≥ 250 mg/dL
• Ketones	Negative	High, large
• Osmolarity	Normal	High
• pH	Normal	Low (≤ 7.25)
• Haematocrit	Normal	High
• Bicarbonate	Normal	< 20 mEq/L
Urine:		
• Output	Normal	Polyuria (early) to oliguria (late)
• Glucose	Negative	Enuresis, nocturia
• Ketones	Negative or trace	High
Visual	Diplopia	Blurred vision

CNS glucose deprivation and the body's attempts to elevate the serum glucose levels.

It is often difficult to distinguish between hyperglycaemia and a hypoglycaemic reaction (Table 31.5). Because the symptoms are similar and usually begin with changes in behaviour, the simplest way to differentiate between the two is to test the blood glucose level. The blood glucose level is low in hypoglycaemia, but in hyperglycaemia the glucose level is significantly elevated. Urinary ketones may be present after hypoglycaemia as a result of starvation ketone production. In doubtful situations, it is safer to give the child some simple carbohydrate. This will help alleviate the symptoms in the case of hypoglycaemia but will do little harm if the child is hyperglycaemic.

Children are usually able to detect the onset of hypoglycaemia, but some are too young to implement treatment. Parents should become adept at recognising the onset of symptoms—for example, a change in a child's behaviour, such as tearfulness or euphoria. In the majority of cases, 10 to 15 g of simple carbohydrate, such as 1 tablespoon of table sugar, will elevate the blood glucose level and alleviate the symptoms. The simpler the carbohydrate, the more rapidly it will be absorbed (200 mL of milk equals 15 g of carbohydrate). The rapidly releasing sugar is followed by a complex carbohydrate, such as a slice of bread, and by a protein, such as peanut butter or milk.

For a mild reaction, milk or fruit juice is a good food to use in children. Milk supplies them with lactose or milk sugar, as well as a more prolonged action from the protein and fat (aids in decreased absorption). Other glucose sources include carbonated drinks (not sugarless), sherbet, gelatine or jelly beans/lollies. All children with diabetes should carry with them glucose tabs, sugar cubes or sugar-containing lollies, such as jellybeans.

Glucagon is sometimes prescribed for home treatment of hypoglycaemia. It is available as an emergency kit that must be mixed at the time of use and is administered intramuscularly or subcutaneously. Glucagon functions by releasing stored glycogen from the liver and requires about 15 to 20 minutes to elevate the blood glucose level.

When in doubt, it is best to assume hypoglycaemia and treat, but overtreatment could result in hyperglycaemia. The treatment may be repeated in 10 to 15 minutes if the initial response is not satisfactory. Rest and the addition of food should be part of the plan.

Morning hyperglycaemia. The management of elevated morning blood glucose levels depends on whether the increase is a true dawn phenomenon, insulin waning or a rebound hyperglycaemia (the **Somogyi effect**). Insulin waning is a progressive rise in blood glucose levels from bedtime to morning. It is treated by increasing the nocturnal insulin dose. The true dawn phenomenon shows relatively normal blood glucose level until about 3 am, when the level begins to rise. The Somogyi effect may occur at any time but often entails an elevated blood glucose level at bedtime and a drop at 2 am, with a rebound rise following. The treatment for this phenomenon is decreasing the nocturnal insulin dose to prevent the 2 am hypoglycaemia. The rebound rise in the blood glucose level is a result of counterregulatory hormones (adrenaline, GH and corticosteroids), which are stimulated by hypoglycaemia. More frequent blood monitoring (especially at times of anticipated peak insulin action) usually identifies these conditions. Trace amounts of urinary ketones aid in identifying undetected hypoglycaemia.

Illness Management. Illness alters diabetes management, and maintaining control is usually related to the seriousness of the illness. In a well-controlled child, an illness will run its course as it does in an unaffected child.

The goals during an illness are to restore euglycaemia, treat urinary ketones and maintain hydration. Monitor blood glucose levels and urinary ketones every 3 hours. Some hyperglycaemia and ketonuria are expected in most illnesses, even with diminished food intake, and are an indication for increased insulin. Insulin should never be omitted during an illness, although dosage requirements may increase, decrease or remain unchanged depending on the severity of the illness and the child's appetite. Often the child needs supplemental insulin between usual dose times. If the child vomits more than once, if blood glucose levels remain above 240 mg/dL or if urinary ketones remain high, notify the healthcare practitioner. Simple carbohydrates may be substituted for carbohydrate-containing exchanges in the meal plan. Although insulin and diet are important tools in sick-day care, fluids are the most important intervention. Fluids must be encouraged to prevent dehydration and to flush out ketones.

Therapeutic Management of Diabetic Ketoacidosis

DKA, the most complete state of insulin deficiency, is a life-threatening situation. Management consists of rapid assessment, adequate insulin to reduce the elevated blood glucose level, fluids to overcome dehydration and electrolyte replacement (especially potassium).

DKA constitutes an emergency situation, thus a child is admitted to an intensive care facility for management. The priority is to obtain a venous access for administration of fluids, electrolytes and insulin. The child should be weighed, measured and placed on a cardiac monitor. Blood glucose and ketone levels are determined at the bedside, and samples are obtained for laboratory measurement of glucose, electrolytes, BUN, arterial pH, PO_2, PCO_2, haemoglobin, haematocrit, white blood cell count and differential, calcium and phosphorus.

Oxygen may be administered to patients who are cyanotic and in whom arterial oxygen is less than 80%. Gastric suction is applied to unconscious children to avoid the possibility of pulmonary aspiration. Antibiotics may be administered to febrile children after appropriate specimens are obtained for culture. A Foley catheter may or may not be inserted for urine samples and measurement. Unless the child is unconscious, a collection bag is usually sufficient for accurate assessments.

Fluid and Electrolyte Therapy. All patients with DKA experience dehydration (10% of total body weight in severe ketoacidosis) because of the osmotic diuresis, accompanied by depletion of electrolytes, sodium, potassium, chloride, phosphate and magnesium. Serum pH and bicarbonate reflect the degree of acidosis. Prompt and adequate fluid therapy restores tissue perfusion and suppresses the elevated levels of stress hormones.

The initial hydrating solution is 0.9% saline solution. Traditionally, deficits have been replaced at a rate of 50% over the first 8 to 12 hours and the remaining 50% over the next 16 to 24 hours. Current trends suggest more cautious fluid management to reduce the risk of cerebral oedema. Therefore the fluid deficit should be replaced evenly over a period of 36 to 48 hours (Hamilton et al 2017).

NURSING CARE CONSIDERATIONS

Potassium must never be given until the serum potassium level is known to be normal or low and urinary voiding is observed. All maintenance IV fluids should include 30 to 40 mEq/L of potassium unless the potassium concentration is elevated or urinary output is absent. Never give potassium as a rapid IV bolus, or cardiac arrest may result.

Serum potassium levels may be normal on admission, but after fluid and insulin administration, the rapid return of potassium to the cells can seriously deplete serum levels, with the attendant risk of cardiac arrhythmias. As soon as the child has established renal function (is voiding at least 25 mL/hr) and insulin has been given, vigorous potassium replacement is implemented. The cardiac monitor is used as a guide to therapy, and configuration of T waves should be observed every 30 to 60 minutes to determine changes that might indicate alterations in potassium concentration (widening of the Q-T interval and the appearance of a U wave after a flattened T wave indicate hypokalaemia; an elevated and spreading T wave and shortening of the Q-T interval indicate hyperkalaemia).

Insulin should not be given until after urinary ketones and a blood glucose level have been obtained. Continuous IV regular insulin is given at a dosage of 0.1 U/kg/hr. Insulin therapy should be started after the initial rehydration bolus because serum glucose levels fall rapidly after volume expansion. Blood glucose levels should decrease by 50 to 100 mg/dL/hr. When blood glucose levels fall to 250 to 300 mg/dL, glucose is added to the IV solution. The goal is to maintain blood glucose levels between 120 and 240 mg/dL by adding 5% to 10% glucose. Sodium bicarbonate is used conservatively; it is used for pH less than 7.0, severe hyperkalaemia or cardiac instability. Because sodium bicarbonate has been associated with an increased risk for cerebral oedema, children receiving this substance must be carefully monitored for changes in level of consciousness.

When the critical period is over, the task of regulating the insulin dosage in relation to diet and activity is started. Children should be actively involved in their own care and are given responsibility according to their ability and the guidance of the nurse.

NURSING CARE CONSIDERATIONS

Because insulin can chemically bind to plastic tubing and in-line filters, thereby reducing the amount of medication reaching the systemic circulation, an insulin mixture is run through the tubing to saturate the insulin-binding sites before the infusion is started.

Nursing Care Management

Children with DM may be admitted to the hospital at the time of their initial diagnosis; during illness or surgery; or for episodes of ketoacidosis, which may be precipitated by any of a variety of factors. Many children are able to keep the disease under control with periodic assessment and adjustment of insulin, diet and activity as needed under the supervision of a practitioner. Under most circumstances, these children can be managed well at home and require hospitalisation only for serious illnesses or upsets.

Hospital Management. Children with DKA require intensive nursing care. Observe and record vital signs frequently. Hypotension caused by the contracted blood volume of the dehydrated state may cause decreased peripheral blood flow, which can be particularly hazardous to the heart, lungs and kidneys. An elevated temperature may indicate infection and should be reported so that treatment can be implemented immediately.

Maintain careful and accurate records, including vital signs (pulse, respiration, temperature and blood pressure), weight, IV fluids, electrolytes, insulin, blood glucose level and intake and output. Use a urine collection device or retention catheter to obtain the urine measurements, which include volume, specific gravity and glucose and ketone values. The volume relative to the glucose content is important because 5% glucose in a 300-mL sample is a significantly greater amount than a similar reading from a 75-mL sample. A diabetic flow sheet maintained at the bedside provides an ongoing record of the vital signs, urine and blood tests, amount of insulin given and intake and output. Assess and record the level of consciousness at frequent intervals. The comatose child generally regains consciousness fairly soon after initiation of therapy but is managed like any unconscious child until then.

Child and Family Education. Children and their families vary in educational background and the capacity to learn and understand the various aspects of the therapeutic program. Some families respond best to simple explanations and directions, whereas others expect thorough, in-depth information about the physiological processes and responses associated with the disease and its therapy. All the principles of teaching and learning are applied in the educational process; therefore, before beginning, the nurse must determine the optimum time, place, method and content to be taught. Self-management, the ultimate goal for children with diabetes, is more likely to occur when children understand the disease and the care it requires. Properly educated and motivated, most families should be able to follow a program of regulated control satisfactorily.

Medical Identification. One of the first things the nurse should call to the parents' attention is the need for the child to wear some means of medical identification. Usually recommended is the Medic-Alert identification.

Insulin. Families need to understand the treatment method and the insulin prescribed, including the effective duration, onset and peak action. They also need to know the characteristics of the various types of insulins, the proper mixing and dilution of insulins, even when they present in pen devices.

Injection Procedure. Learning to give insulin injections is a source of anxiety for both parents and children. It is helpful for the learner to know that this important aspect of care will become as routine as brushing the teeth.

Continuous subcutaneous insulin infusion. Some children are considered candidates for use of a portable insulin pump, and even some young children with unsatisfactory metabolic control can benefit from its use.

Monitoring. Nurses should also be prepared to teach and supervise blood glucose monitoring. SMBG is associated with few complications, and although it does not necessarily lead to improved metabolic control, it provides a more accurate assessment of blood glucose levels than can be obtained with the historical urine testing.

Urine testing. Testing for urinary ketones is recommended during times of illness and when blood glucose values are elevated. Information on a specific ketone-testing product should include correct procedure, storage and product expiration. Families need a clear understanding of home management of ketones (fluids and additional insulin as directed by the healthcare team).

Hyperglycaemia. Severe hyperglycaemia is most often caused by illness, growth, emotional upset or missed insulin doses. Emotional stress from school examinations or physical response to immunisations are examples of causes of hyperglycaemia. With careful glucose monitoring, any elevation can be managed by adjustment of insulin or food intake.

Signs of Hypoglycaemia. Hypoglycaemia is caused by imbalances of food intake, insulin and activity. Ideally, hypoglycaemia should be prevented, and parents need to be prepared to prevent, recognise and treat the problem. They should be familiar with the signs of hypoglycaemia and instructed in treatment, including care of the child with seizures. (See Chapter 30.) Hypoglycaemia can be managed effectively with the main implementation being intramuscular injection of glucagon if the child is unconscious.

Hygiene. All aspects of personal hygiene should be emphasised for children with diabetes. Children should be cautioned against wearing shoes without socks, wearing sandals and walking barefoot. Correct nail and extremity care tailored to the individual child (with the guidance of a podiatrist) can begin health practices that last a lifetime. Eyes should be checked once a year unless the child wears glasses and then as directed by the ophthalmologist. Regular dental care is emphasised, and cuts and scratches should be treated with plain soap and water unless otherwise indicated. Nappy rash in infants and candidal infections in teens may indicate poor diabetes control.

Exercise. Exercise is an important component of the treatment plan. If the child is more active at one time of the day than at another time, food or insulin can be altered to meet that activity pattern. Food should be increased in the summer, when children tend to be more active. Decreased activity on return to school may require a decrease in food intake or increase in insulin dosage. Children who are active in team sports need a snack about a half hour before the anticipated activity.

Food intake will usually need to be repeated for prolonged activity periods, often as frequently as every 45 minutes to 1 hour.

NURSING CARE CONSIDERATIONS

Ketonuria in the presence of hyperglycaemia is an early sign of ketoacidosis and a contraindication to exercise.

Record Keeping. Home records are an invaluable aid to diabetes self-management. The nurse and family devise a method to chart insulin administered, blood glucose values, urine ketone results and other factors and events that affect diabetes control.

Self-management. Self-management is the key to close control. Being able to make changes when they are needed rather than waiting until the next contact with healthcare professionals is important for self-management and gives the individual and family the feeling that they have control over the disease. As children grow and assume more responsibility for self-management, they develop confidence in their ability to manage their disease and confidence in themselves as persons. They learn to respond to the disease and to make more accurate interpretations and changes in treatment when they become adults.

REFERENCES

Amin, N., Mushtaq, T., & Alvi, S. (2015). Fifteen-minute consultation: the child with short stature. Archives of Disease in Childhood: Education and Practice, 100(4), 180–184.

Argente, J. (2016). Challenges in the management of short stature. Hormone Research in Paediatrics, 85(1), 2–10.

Australian Paediatric Endocrine Group. (2016). Hormones and Me. Disorders of the thyroid gland in children and adolescents. Merck Australia. https://d192ha6kdpe15x.cloudfront.net/apeg/assets/uploads/2016/03/Thyroid-Disorders-of-Childhood-And-Adolescence-Web-Version.pdf

Australian Institute of Health and Welfare. (2020). Australia's children. Children with diabetes, key findings. 3 April. https://www.aihw.gov.au/reports/children-youth/australias-children/contents/health/children-diabetes

Aslan, I. & Cheung, C. (2014). Early and late endocrine effects in pediatric central nervous system diseases. Journal of Pediatric Rehabilitation Medicine, 7(4), 281–294.

Belfiore, A. & LeRoith, D. (2018). Principles of Endocrinology and Hormone Action. 1st ed. Champaign, IL: Springer International Publishing.

Brito, V. N., Spinola-Castro, A. M., Kochi, C., et al. (2016). Central precocious puberty: revisiting the diagnosis and therapeutic management. Archives of Endocrinology and Metabolism, 60(2), 163–172.

Caturegli, P., De Remiqis, A., & Rose, N. R. (2014). Hashimoto thyroiditis: clinical and diagnostic criteria. Autoimmunity Reviews, 13(4–5), 391–397.

Ceccato, F., & Boscaro, M. (2016). Cushing's syndrome: screening and diagnosis. High Blood Pressure and Cardiovascular Prevention, 23(3), 209–215.

Cheetham, T., & Davies, J. H. (2014). Investigation and management of short stature. Archives of Disease in Childhood, 99(8), 767–771.

Cuesta, M., Garrahy, A., & Thompson, C. J. (2016). SIAD: practical recommendations for diagnosis and management. Journal of Endocrinological Investigation, 39(9), 991–1001.

Doyle, D. A. (2016a). Hypoparathyroidism. In R. M. Kliegman, B. Stanton, J. W. St Geme, et al. (Eds.), Nelson textbook of pediatrics (20th ed.). Philadelphia: Saunders.

Doyle, D. A. (2016b). Hyperparathyroidism. In R. M. Kliegman, B. Stanton, J. W. St Geme, et al. (Eds.), Nelson textbook of pediatrics (20th ed.). Philadelphia: Saunders.

El-Maouche, D., Arlt, W., & Merke, D. P. (2017). Congenital adrenal hyperplasia. Lancet, 390(10108), 2194–2210.

Erdöl, Ş., & Sağlam, H. (2016). Endocrine Dysfunctions in Patients with Inherited Metabolic Diseases. Journal of Clinical Research in Pediatric Endocrinology, 8(3), 330–333.

Ferguson, L. A. (2011). Growth hormone use in children: necessary or designer therapy? Journal of Pediatric Health Care, 25(11), 24–30.

Gardner, D. G., Anderson, M., & Nissenson, R. A. (2011). Hormones and hormone action. In D. G. Gardner & D. Shoback (Eds.), Basic and clinical endocrinology (9th ed.). New York: Lange Medical Books/ McGraw-Hill.

Garibaldi, L. R., & Chemaitilly, W. (2016). Disorders of pubertal development. In R. M. Kliegman, B. Stanton, J. W. St Geme, et al. (Eds.), Nelson textbook of pediatrics (20th ed.). Philadelphia: Saunders.

Giuliani, C., & Peri, A. (2014). Effects of hyponatremia on the brain. Journal of Clinical Medicine, 3(4), 1163–1677.

Grimberg, A., Divall, S. A., Polychronakos, C., et al. (2016). Guidelines for growth hormone deficiency and insulin-like growth factor-1 treatment in children and adolescents: growth hormone deficiency, idiopathic short stature, and primary insulin-like growth factor-1 deficiency. Hormone Research in Paediatrics, 86(6), 361–397.

Hamilton, H., Knudsen, G., Vaina, C. L., et al. (2017). Children and young people with diabetes: recognition and management. British Journal of Nursing, 26(6), 340–347.

Hanley, P., Lord, K., & Bauer, A. J. (2016). Thyroid disorders in children and adolescents: a review. Pediatrcs, 170(10), 1008–1019.

Harrington, J., & Palmert, M. R. (2016). Treatment of precocious puberty. In T. W. Post (Ed.), UpToDate. Waltham, MA.

Huang, S. A., & LaFranci, S. H. (2016). Hyperthyroidism. In R. M. Kliegman, B. Stanton, J. W. St Geme, et al. (Eds.), Nelson textbook of pediatrics (20th ed.). Philadelphia: Saunders.

Laffel, L., & Svoren, B. (2015). Epidemiology, presentation, and diagnosis of type 2 diabetes mellitus in children and adolescents. http://www.uptodate.com/contents/epidemiology-presentation-and-diagnosis-of-type-2-diabetes-mellitus-in-children-and-adolescents.

Lau, D., Rutledge, C., & Aghi, M. K. (2015). Cushing's disease: current medical therapies and molecular insights guiding future therapies. Neurosurgical Focus, 38(2), E11.

Leger, J., & Carel, J. C. (2013). Hyperthyroidism in childhood: causes, when and how to treat. Journal of Clinical Research in Pediatric Endocrinology, 5(Suppl. 1), 50–56.

Lowitz, J., & Keil, M. F. (2015). Cushing syndrome: establishing a timely diagnosis. Journal of Pediatric Nursing, 30(3), 528–530.

Maffezzoni, F., Frara, S., Doga, M., et al. (2016). New medical therapies of acromegaly. Growth Hormone and IGF Research, 30–31, 58–63.

Mendes, C., Vaz Matos, I., Ribeiro, L., et al. (2015). Congenital adrenal hyperplasia due to 21-hydroxylase deficiency: genotype-phenotype correlation. Acta Medica Portuguesa, 28(1), 56–62.

Metzger, M. L., Krasin, M. J., Choi, J. K., et al. (2016). Hodgkin lymphoma. In P. A. Pizzo & D. G. Poplack (Eds.), Principles and theories of pediatric oncology (7th ed.). Philadelphia: Lippincott Williams & Wilkins.

Murray, P. G., Dattani, M. T., & Clayton, P. E. (2016). Controversies in the diagnosis and management of growth hormone deficiency in childhood and adolescence. Archives of Disease in Childhood, 101(1), 96–100.

Ministry of Health. (2015). Living Well with Diabetes: A plan for people at high risk of or living with diabetes 2015–2020. Wellington: Ministry of Health. https://www.health.govt.nz/system/files/documents/publications/living-well-with-diabetes-oct15.pdf

Pardo Campos, M. L., Musso, M., Keselman, A., et al. (2017). Cognitive profiles of patients with early detected and treated congenital hypothyroidism. Archivos Argentinos de Pediatria, 11591, 12–17.

Parks, J. S., & Felner, E. I. (2016). Hypopituitarism. In R. M. Kliegman, B. Stanton, J. W. St Geme, et al. (Eds.), Nelson textbook of pediatrics (20th ed.). Philadelphia: Saunders.

Pashtan, I., Grogan, R. H., Kaplan, S. P., et al. (2013). Primary hyperparathyroidism in adolescents: the same but different. Pediatric Surgery International, 29(3), 275–279.

Pine-Twaddell, E., Romero, C., & Radovick, S. (2013). Vertical transmission of hypopituitarism: critical importance of appropriate interpretation of thyroid function tests and levothyroxine therapy during pregnancy. Thyroid, 23(7), 892–897.

Pivonello, R., Auriemma, R. S., Grasso, L. F., et al. (2017). Complications of acromegaly: cardiovascular, respiratory, and metabolic comorbidities. Pituitary, 20(1), 42–62.

Reinehr, T. (2013). Type 2 diabetes mellitus in children and adolescents. World Journal of Diabetes, 4(6), 270–281.

Schoenmakers, N., Alatzoglou, K. S., Chatterjee, V. K., et al. (2015). Recent advances in central congenital hypothyroidism. The Journal of Endocrinology, 227(3), R51–R71.

Stanley, T. (2012). Diagnosis of growth hormone deficiency in childhood. Current Opinion in Endocrinology, Diabetes and Obesity, 19, 47–52.

Svoren, B., & Jospe, N. (2016). Diabetes mellitus in children. In R. M. Kliegman, B. Stanton, J. W. St Geme, et al. (Eds.), Nelson textbook of pediatrics (20th ed.). Philadelphia: Saunders.

Tomer, Y. (2014). Mechanisms of autoimmune thyroid diseases: from genetics to epigenetics. Annual Review of Pathology: Mechanisms and Disease, 9, 147–156.

The Royal Children's Hospital (RCHM). (n.d.). Diabetes insipidus. Management. Clinical Practice Guidelines. https://www.rch.org.au/clinicalguide/guideline_index/Diabetes_insipidus/

Wheeler, D., Wong, H., Shanley, T., et al. (2014). Pediatric Critical Care Medicine: Volume 3: Gastroenterological, Endocrine, Renal, Hematologic, Oncologic and Immune Systems. 2nd ed. London: Springer London, Limited.

White, P. C. (2016a). Pheochromocytoma. In R. M. Kliegman, B. Stanton, J. W. St Geme, et al. (Eds.), Nelson textbook of pediatrics (20th ed.). Philadelphia: Saunders.

White, P. C. (2016b). Congenital adrenal hyperplasia and related disorders. In R. M. Kliegman, B. Stanton, J. W. St Geme, et al. (Eds.), Nelson textbook of pediatrics (20th ed.). Philadelphia: Saunders.

Young, W. F. (2016). Pheochromocytoma in children. In T. W. Post (Ed.), UpToDate. Waltham, MA.

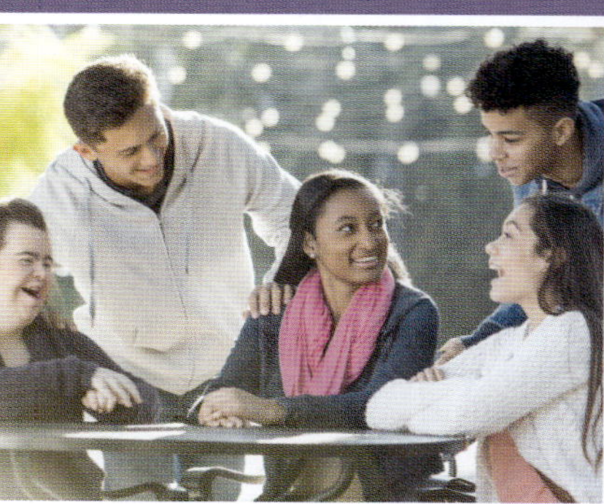

32 The Child with Integumentary Dysfunction

Ibi Patane

LEARNING OBJECTIVES

- Identify the principles of skin assessment
- Develop an understand of the principles of wound healing
- Develop an understand of common presentation and the treatment of skin integrity issues in the paediatric population

INTEGUMENTARY DYSFUNCTION

Skin Lesions

Lesions of the skin result from a variety of aetiological factors. Skin lesions originate from: (1) contact with injurious agents, such as infective organisms, toxic chemicals and physical trauma; (2) hereditary factors; (3) external factors, such as allergens; or (4) systemic diseases, such as varicella, lupus erythematosus and nutritional deficiency diseases. Responses are highly individualised in children. An agent that is harmless to one individual may be damaging to another, and a single agent may produce varying degrees of responses in different individuals.

Another factor in the aetiology of skin manifestations is the child's age. For example, infants and young children are subject to 'birthmark' malformations and atopic dermatitis that appear early in life. The school-age child is susceptible to tinea (ringworm) of the scalp and impetigo (school sores), and acne is a characteristic skin disorder of puberty. Children's typical social environments also make them susceptible to skin disorders. Exposure to smoke and children with food allergies, particularly peanut allergy, have also been associated with higher rates of atopic dermatitis and eczema. Contact dermatitis, such as to plants or chemicals (sunscreen, nickel, cosmetics), is seen only when the noxious agent is found in the environment. Similarly, insect bites are associated with seasonal activities during the summer and autumn months.

Skin of Younger Children

The major skin layers arise from different embryological origins. Early in the embryonic period, a single layer of epithelium forms from the ectoderm while simultaneously the corium develops from the mesenchyme. In infants and small children, the epidermis is loosely bound to the dermis. This poor adherence causes the layers to separate easily during an inflammatory process to form blisters. This is especially true in preterm infants, who have a propensity to blister formation and separation of the skin with minor trauma such as the removal of adhesive tape. In contrast, the skin of older children is thinner, and the cells of all the strata are more compressed.

Pathophysiology of Dermatitis

More than half of the dermatological problems in children are various forms of dermatitis. This implies a sequence of inflammatory changes in the skin that are grossly and microscopically similar but diverse in course and causation. Acute responses produce intercellular and intracellular oedema, the formation of intradermal vesicles and an initial infiltration of inflammatory cells into the epidermis. In the dermis, there is oedema, vascular dilation and early perivascular cellular infiltration. The location and manner of these reactions produce the lesions characteristic of each disorder. The changes are usually reversible, and the skin ordinarily recovers without blemish unless complicating factors such as ulceration from the primary irritant, scratching and infection are introduced or underlying vascular disease develops. In chronic conditions, permanent effects are seen that vary according to the disorder, the general condition of the affected individual and the available therapy.

Diagnostic Evaluation

Although the history and subjective symptoms of skin lesions are explored first, the obvious objective characteristics of the lesions are often noted simultaneously. Many skin lesions are diagnosed after careful inspection.

History and Symptoms

Many cutaneous lesions are associated with local symptoms. The most common local symptom is itching (**pruritus**), which varies in frequency and intensity. Pain or tenderness often accompanies some skin lesions. Other skin sensations such as burning, prickling, stinging or crawling are also described. Alterations in local feeling include absence of sensation (**anaesthesia**); excessive sensitivity (**hyperaesthesia**); diminished sensation (**hypoaesthesia**); or abnormal sensation, such as burning or prickling (**paraesthesia**). These symptoms may remain localised or migrate. They may also be constant or intermittent and may be aggravated by a specific activity, such as exposure to sunlight.

It is important to determine whether the child has an allergic condition such as asthma or history of a previous skin disease. Atopic dermatitis, often associated with allergies, frequently begins in infancy. Important questions for the parent include: when the lesion or symptom first appeared; whether it occurred with ingestion of a food or other substance, including any medication; and whether the condition was related to activity such as contact with plants, insects or chemicals. Finally, enquire if other children in the home or classroom have similar symptoms and if the child's parents or siblings have a history of atopy or allergic skin conditions.

Objective Findings

The skin lesions' distribution, size, location and morphology provide significant information. Skin lesions assume distinct characteristics that are related to the pathological process. The following are some terms.

- **Erythema**—A reddened area caused by increased amounts of oxygenated blood in the dermal vasculature
- **Ecchymoses (bruises)**—Localised red or purple discolourations caused by extravasation of blood into dermis and subcutaneous tissues
- **Petechiae**—Pinpoint, tiny and sharp circumscribed spots in the superficial layers of the epidermis
- **Primary lesions**—Skin changes produced by a causative factor; common primary lesions in paediatric skin disorders are macules, papules and vesicles
- **Secondary lesions**—Changes that result from alteration in the primary lesions, such as those caused by rubbing, scratching, medication or involution and healing
- **Distribution pattern**—The pattern in which lesions are distributed over the body, whether local or generalised, and the specific areas associated with the lesions
- **Configuration and arrangement**—The size, shape and arrangement of a lesion or groups of lesions (e.g. **discrete**, **clustered**, **diffuse** or **confluent**)

Extrinsic causes usually result from physical, chemical or allergic irritants or from an infectious agent such as bacteria, fungi, viruses or animal parasites. Intrinsic causes such as a specific infection (e.g. measles or chickenpox), drug sensitisation or other allergic phenomena can produce skin manifestations.

Laboratory Studies

When it is suspected that a skin problem might be related to a systemic disease, such as one of the collagen diseases or an immunodeficiency disease, studies are needed to rule out these possibilities. Diagnostic techniques include microscopic examination, cultures, skin scrapings or biopsy, cyto-diagnosis, patch testing and Wood light examination. Allergic skin testing and other laboratory tests such as blood count and sedimentation rate are used when indicated.

Wounds

Wounds are structural or physiological disruptions of the skin that activate normal or abnormal tissue repair responses. Wounds are classified as acute or chronic. **Acute wounds** are those that heal uneventfully within 2 to 3 weeks. **Chronic wounds** are those that do not heal in the expected timeframe or are associated with complications. Cofactors that disrupt or delay wound healing include compromised perfusion, malnutrition and infection. Wounds are classified in the same manner as burns: superficial, partial thickness, full-thickness and complex wounds that include muscle and/or bone. Some types of acute wounds are the following.

- **Abrasion**—Removal of the superficial layers of skin by rubbing or scraping
- **Avulsion**—Forcible pulling out or extraction of tissue
- **Laceration**—Torn or jagged wound; accidental cut wound
- **Incision**—Division of the skin made with a sharp object; cut
- **Penetrating wound**—Disruption of the skin surface that extends into underlying tissue or into a body cavity
- **Puncture**—Wound with a relatively small opening compared with the depth

Epidermal Injuries

Abrasions are the most common epidermal wounds in children, usually in the form of a skinned knee or elbow. In most injuries, the margins of the abraded area are superficial, involving only the outer layers of epidermis, although the central portion may extend into the dermis. Initially the defect is filled by a blood clot and necrotic debris, which subsequently dehydrate to form a scab. Epithelial tissue is composed of labile cells, which are constantly destroyed and replaced throughout the life span. Injury to these tissues results in **regeneration** (i.e. rapid replacement by similar cells).

Injury to Deeper Tissues

Tissues composed of **permanent cells** such as muscle and nerve cells are unable to regenerate. These tissues repair themselves by substituting fibrous connective tissue for the injured tissue. This fibrous tissue, or **scar**, serves as a patch to preserve or restore the continuity of the tissue. Wounds involving permanent cells include surgical incisions, lacerations, ulcers, evulsions and full-thickness burns. Injured cells of glandular organs and bones, composed of stable cells, multiply less vigorously and heal more slowly. With some wounds an overgrowth of nerve endings may occur, resulting in **allodynia**, or the sensation of pain from normally non-painful stimuli, such as light touch.

General Therapeutic Management

The human body intrinsically attempts to heal itself; therefore, treatment is directed towards eliminating or ameliorating factors that interfere with normal healing processes. Some disorders may demand aggressive therapy, but by and large the major aim of any treatment is to prevent further damage, eliminate the cause, prevent complications and provide relief from discomfort while tissues undergo healing. When possible, eliminate factors that contribute to the dermatitis and prolong the course of the disease. The most common offenders in paediatrics are environmental factors, including soaps (bubble baths and shampoos) and lotions; garments that are made of synthetic materials, have a rough texture (wool) or are tight-fitting; prolonged exposure to damp undergarments or swimsuits; and natural elements (plants and insects, dirt, sand, heat, cold, moisture and wind). Dermatitis can also be aggravated by home remedies, poor nutrition, exposure to smoke, scratching or physical irritation of the site and medications.

Dressings. No one dressing meets the needs of all wounds. The traditional dry gauze dressing should not be used on open wounds because it allows the wound surface to dry, does little to prevent bacterial invasion and adheres to the dried scab so that removal disturbs the newly regenerating epithelial cells. In most instances, traditional gauze dressings have been replaced by dressings that promote moist wound healing. Moist wound healing increases the rate of collagen synthesis and re-epithelialisation and decreases pain and inflammation. It also creates an environment for autolytic debridement of necrotic tissue, which creates a clean wound bed and enhances granulation. However, a balance must be achieved between creating a moist wound bed and maintaining a dry peri-wound area that protects the skin and wound from maceration. The dressing type and frequency of dressing changes help achieve this balance. The frequency of dressing changes is based on the presence of infection, the type of dressing, the location of the wound and the amount of drainage. Dressings should always be changed when they are loose or soiled. They should be changed more frequently in areas where contamination is likely (e.g. the sacral area, the buttocks, the tracheal area) or when wound infection is suspected or present.

Occlusive dressings can be classified according to their degree of permeability. The term *occlusive* is synonymous with impermeable, *semi-occlusive* is synonymous with semi-permeable and *non-occlusive* is synonymous with permeable. The use of silver-impregnated dressings for the treatment of wound care has re-emerged. Although several studies suggest that silver decreases the bacteria and bioburden in the wound and improves short-term healing of wounds and ulcers, the long-term effects remain unclear. It is known that silver can be highly toxic and harmful. In a recent study of children with scald injuries, the use of silver-based dressings and antibiotic creams produced poorer outcomes compared with bio-synthetic dressings which provided significantly increased healing time and the added advantage of not requiring daily dressings (Raymond et al 2018) which is significant in the paediatric context to reduce trauma.

Topical Therapy. A variety of agents and methods are available for treatment of dermatological problems. In selecting a therapeutic program, the practitioner considers: (1) the active ingredient of the agent; (2) the vehicle or base; (3) the cosmetic effect; (4) the cost; (5) instructions for the agent's use; and (6) the family preference. Practitioners aim to avoid overtreatment, particularly in young children. For example, when the dermatitis is acute, short-term topical medications such as steroids are used to reduce irritation, inflammation and spread of the disorder, then quickly tapered to mild or less frequent dosages to prevent side effects or long-term consequences.

Baths are especially useful in the treatment of widespread dermatitis because they evenly distribute the soothing antipruritic and anti-inflammatory solution, usually an oatmeal or mineral oil preparation. The temperature of the bathwater should be tepid, and the treatment usually lasts 15 to 30 minutes. Bleach baths (45 mL household bleach to 40 L bath water) twice a week has shown a significant reduction in the severity of atopic dermatitis in an Australian study (Page et al 2016). As with any paediatric treatment, therapeutic baths are always more interesting for the child when toys are available in the bath for water play.

Topical agents are applied to skin lesions to ease discomfort, prevent further injury and facilitate healing. The emollient action of ointments and allergen-free lotions provides a soothing film over the skin surface that reduces external stimuli. Regardless of the type of preparation used, parents need detailed information on the medication being applied, how to apply it and how long the preparation should remain on the skin or under an occlusive dressing.

Topical corticosteroid therapy. Glucocorticoids are the therapeutic agents used most frequently for skin disorders. Their local anti-inflammatory effects are merely palliative, so the medication is applied until the condition undergoes a remission or the causative agent is eliminated. Corticosteroids are applied directly to the affected area, are essentially non-sensitising and have only minor side effects. As with the use of any steroids, their use in large amounts may mask signs of infection, and symptoms may be exacerbated after termination of the drug. Families are cautioned that the medication cannot be used for all skin disorders. The concentrations available without prescription are not adequate for stubborn skin conditions (e.g. psoriasis, eczema) and may further aggravate inflammation caused by fungus or bacteria. When appropriate, it is important to counsel parents to apply only a thin film and to massage it into the skin because most parents and children apply more topical hydrocortisone than necessary for effective treatment. Parents and children should also be advised to use the application for no more than 5 to 7 days because these agents may cause depigmentation and other changes in the skin with extended use.

Other topical therapies. Other topical treatments include chemical cautery (especially useful for warts), cryosurgery, electrodesiccation (chiefly used for warts, granulomas and naevi), ultraviolet (UV) light therapy (primarily used in psoriasis and acne), laser therapy (especially for birthmarks) and special acne therapies such as dermabrasion and chemical peels. **Topical immunomodulators** are effective in reducing the itching of atopic dermatitis (eczema) and preventing flare-ups in children resistant to first-line treatment options. A large European multicentre study (Castellsague et al 2018) confirmed the association between increased risk of lymphoma and the use of these medications in children, so their use is no longer recommended in children.

Systemic Therapy. Systemic drugs may be used as an adjunct to topical therapy in some dermatological disorders. The drugs most frequently used are corticosteroids, antibiotics and antifungal agents. Corticosteroids are valuable in the treatment of severe skin disorders because of their capacity to inhibit inflammatory and allergic reactions. The dosage is carefully adjusted and gradually tapered to the minimum dosage that is effective and tolerated. Prolonged use of systematic corticosteroids may temporarily suppress the child's growth.

Antibiotics are used in cases of severe, chronic or widespread skin infections. However, because these drugs tend to produce hypersensitivity in some patients, they are used with caution. Oral antifungal agents are the only effective means for treating systemic fungal infections and tinea capitis.

Nursing Care Management

To help establish a diagnosis, it is important for nurses to accurately describe any deviation in the character of the skin, using both inspection and palpation. Note the colour, shape, size, character and distribution of the lesions or wounds. Describe the individual lesions using the accepted terminology, understanding that there may be more than one type of wound, lesion or rash. Assess wounds for depth of tissue damage, evidence of healing and signs of infection (e.g. drainage, warmth and odour).

To confirm or amplify the assessment findings made by inspection, gently palpate the skin to detect characteristics such as temperature, moisture, texture, elasticity and the presence of oedema. Indicate whether the findings are restricted to the area of the lesion(s) or are generalised.

A detailed history of the child's presenting illness, condition or wound and the description (or appearance) of symptoms provide additional information. Besides asking about past medical history and noting the allergy and medication list of the patient, a careful nursing history may provide clues that will assist in determining an uncertain diagnosis. During the interview process, the nurse should ask the following questions:

- How long has this been occurring?
- Is the child scratching the area?
- Is the child restless or irritable?
- Does the child favour or avoid using a certain body part?
- Has the child had a fever or other illnesses recently?
- Has the child been around chemicals, grasslands/bush, gardens or garden mulch?
- Has the child travelled recently or visited someone's home for the first time?

- Has the child recently eaten a new food?
- Do any classmates, playmates or siblings have similar lesions or illnesses?
- What has been done to treat the symptoms so far? Have any medications or home remedies been used?

Therapeutic treatments of skin disorders are typically aimed at providing comfort measures: rest, protection from infection or spread of the condition and relief of discomfort. Specific treatments, such as a definitive medication or physical treatment or technique, may be prescribed for chronic conditions or wounds. Only a few skin disorders are contagious, so it is usually not necessary to isolate the affected child unless there is a danger that the child may acquire a secondary infection (e.g. the child who is receiving large doses of corticosteroids or other immunosuppressant drugs or the child with an immunological deficiency disorder). However, when the skin manifestation is a viral exanthem such as chickenpox, infectious skin condition such as impetigo or an easily spread vector such as lice, the recommendation is to prevent exposing other susceptible children until the disorder is almost healed or the treatment is complete. The relevant health department guidelines should be accessed to ascertain exclusion from school/day care and relevant treatment.

Wound Care. Parents can generally manage small skin wounds at home. Instruct parents to wash their hands and then wash the wound gently with mild soap and water. Topical antibiotics and non-adherent dressings are usually applied to the wound while it is in the primary healing stage. Caution parents to avoid povidone-iodine, alcohol and hydrogen peroxide because these products are toxic to wounds. Wounds covering a very large area (> 15% of the body) need medical attention with the child undergoing conscious sedation and analgesia.

NURSING CARE CONSIDERATIONS

Do not put anything in a wound that you would not put in the eye. The safest solution is 0.9% sodium chloride (normal saline).

Open wounds are typically covered with a non-adherent dressing, such as a commercial adhesive bandage, although larger wounds may benefit from the use of occlusive dressings.

The location of the wound dictates careful physical assessment. For example, wounds over bony areas may contain bone chips, and clear fluid seeping from severe head wounds may indicate cerebrospinal fluid. For severe wounds that cannot be completely evaluated immediately and lacerations that require suturing, apply a clean pressure dressing over the affected area and transfer the child for emergency medical care. Puncture wounds should initially be irrigated with sterile 0.9% sodium chloride and then soaked in a basin of warm soapy water for several minutes before applying a clean dressing.

Relief of Symptoms. Most of the therapeutic regimens are intended to promote wound healing, prevent infection and provide relief of pruritus, the most common subjective complaint. Preventing scratching is of primary importance. Itching is believed to often result from stimulation of C fibres at the dermo-epidermal junction and the release of histamine and endopeptidases. These fibres are similar to but distinct from pain fibres and may be stimulated with a single scratch. Cooling the affected area and increasing the skin pH with an alkaline-containing compress, such as a baking soda or tepid bath, reduce the child's external stimuli and the urge to scratch.

Wet compresses or dressings cool the skin by evaporation, relieve itching and inflammation and cleanse the area by loosening and removing crusts and debris. Plain water can be applied on Kerlix gauze (rolls of pre-washed gauze with a crinkle-weave pattern); plain gauze; or (preferably) soft cotton cloths such as freshly laundered towels, bed sheets or pillowcases.

Pain and discomfort are usually managed with non-pharmacological measures such as positioning and rest, distraction techniques and individual preferences of comfort. Occlusive dressings applied over wounds reduce pain similar to cool or tepid compresses. Doses of mild analgesics such as paracetamol or ibuprofen, prescribed based on the patient's weight, may be recommended. Severe pain requires prescribed analgesic medication, often narcotics, and careful nursing assessment for infection or an underlying cause of discomfort. For severe wounds and burns, prescribed analgesic medications should be administered before each dressing change, debridement procedure or cleansing, allowing adequate time for the medicine to take therapeutic effect.

Wound healing may be facilitated by recombinant growth factor or a vacuum-assisted closure device. These therapies may be employed when wounds are large and in a location that creates challenges for therapy (e.g. sacral or groin wound) or when the child has associated conditions such as malnutrition or a comprised immune system, putting 'normal' wound healing at risk. Recombinant growth factors are human platelet–derived growth factors that are engineered outside the body. They foster the formation of new granulation tissue by stimulating the migration of fibroblasts, macrophages, smooth muscle cells and capillary endothelial cells to the wound site.

The vacuum-assisted closure (VAC) device uses a technique that involves placing a foam dressing into the wound, covering it with an occlusive dressing and applying gentle, continuous suction. The negative pressure of the suction is applied from the foam dressing to the wound surfaces. The mechanical force removes excess fluids from the wound, stimulates formation of granulation tissue, restores capillary flow and fosters closure of the wound. VAC has been used to prepare wounds for a skin graft and to treat complicated wounds such as some surgical wounds, burns and pressure ulcers (de Jesus et al 2018). The safety and efficacy of the VAC technique for infants and children for various conditions has been documented in recent studies (de Jesus et al 2018, Khurram et al 2019) but consideration must be given to protection of the more fragile paediatric tissue, fluid losses, pain and negative pressure levels used (de Jesus et al 2018).

Home Care and Family Support

Care of a child with a dermatological condition always involves the family, but few situations require hospitalisation, and most care is delivered at home. Because the family members must carry out the treatment plan, their cooperation is essential. The family may also need assistance in adapting equipment available for home therapy.

INFECTIONS OF THE SKIN

Bacterial Infections

Normally, the skin harbours a variety of bacterial flora, including the major pathogenic varieties of staphylococci and streptococci. The degree of pathogenicity of the organism depends on its invasiveness and toxicity, the integrity of the skin (the host's barrier) and the host's immune and cellular defences. Children with congenital or acquired immunodeficiency disorders (e.g. acquired immunodeficiency syndrome [AIDS]), children receiving immunosuppressant therapy and those with a malignancy such as leukaemia or lymphoma are at risk for developing bacterial infections.

Because of the characteristic 'walling-off' process of the inflammatory reaction (abscess formation), staphylococci are more difficult to treat, and the local infected area is associated with an increase in bacteria all over the skin surface that serves as a source of continuing infection. Since the early 2000s, the number of methicillin-resistant *Staphylococcus aureus* (MRSA) community-acquired infections rose dramatically until reaching a peak in 2010 and then steadily declining (Alzomor et al 2017). These factors underline the importance of careful hand washing and cleanliness when caring for infected children and their lesions to prevent the spread of infection and as an essential prophylactic measure when caring for infants and small children. Common bacterial skin disorders are outlined in Table 32.1 (see also Figs 32.1 and 32.2).

NURSING CARE CONSIDERATIONS

Impetigo is a particular problem for remote Aboriginal and Torres Strait Islander communities in Australia, and it is estimated that more than 80% of children have sores before reaching the age of 1 year. The risk of developing impetigo is 7 to 12 times higher when scabies (also endemic) is present. Infections in these populations are frequently undertreated and can lead to serious invasive bacterial infections, such as post-streptococcal glomerulonephritis explaining the high levels of renal disease also seen (Aung et al 2018).

TABLE 32.1 Bacterial Infections

Disorder and Organism	Manifestations	Management	Comments
Impetigo contagiosa—*Staphylococcus* (see Fig 32.1)	Begins as a reddish macule Becomes vesicular Ruptures easily, leaving superficial, moist erosion Tends to spread peripherally in sharply marginated irregular outlines Exudate dries to form heavy, honey-coloured crusts Pruritus common Systemic effects—Minimal or asymptomatic	Topical bactericidal ointment mupirocin Oral or parenteral antibiotics (penicillin) in severe or extensive lesions Vancomycin for methicillin-resistant *Staphylococcus aureus* (MRSA)	Tends to heal without scarring unless secondary infection Autoinoculable and contagious Common in toddlers and preschoolers May be superimposed on eczema
Pyoderma—*Staphylococcus, Streptococcus*	Deeper extension of infection into dermis Tissue reaction more severe Systemic effects—Fever, lymphangiitis, sepsis, liver disease, heart disease	Soap and water cleansing Topical antiseptic, such as chlorhexidine Mupirocin Antibiotics depending on causative organism: Cefalexin, intramuscular benzathine benzylpenicillin Bathing with antibacterial soap as prescribed Do not share washcloths or towels	Autoinoculable and contagious May heal with or without scarring
Folliculitis (pimple), furuncle (boil), carbuncle (multiple boils)—*Staphylococcus aureus,* methicillin-resistant *S. aureus* (MRSA)	Folliculitis—Infection of hair follicle Furuncle—Larger lesion with more redness and swelling at a single follicle Carbuncle—More extensive lesion with widespread inflammation and 'pointing' at several follicular orifices Systemic effects—Malaise if severe	Skin cleanliness Local warm, moist compresses Topical application of antibiotic agents Systemic antibiotics in severe cases Incision and drainage of severe lesions, followed by wound irrigations with antibiotics or suitable drain implantation MRSA infections: • Bleach baths (45 mL household bleach to 40 L bath water) • No sharing of towels or washcloths, changing of clothes and underwear daily, and washing them in hot water • Disposal of razors after one use • Application of mupirocin to nares bid for 2–4 weeks	Autoinoculable and contagious Furuncle and carbuncle tend to heal with scar formation Lesions should never be squeezed
Cellulitis—*Streptococcus, Staphylococcus, Haemophilus influenzae* (see Fig 32.2)	Inflammation of skin and subcutaneous tissues with intense redness, swelling and firm infiltration Lymphangiitis 'streaking' frequently seen Involvement of regional lymph nodes common May progress to abscess formation Systemic effects—Fever, malaise	Oral or parenteral antibiotics Rest and immobilisation of both affected area and child	Hospitalisation may be necessary for child with systemic symptoms Otitis media may be associated with facial cellulites
Staphylococcal scalded skin syndrome—*S. aureus*	Macular erythema with 'sandpaper' texture of involved skin Epidermis becomes wrinkled (in days or less), and large bullae appear Localised bullous impetigo in older child	Systemic antibiotics Gentle cleansing with saline	Infants subject to fluid loss; impaired body temperature regulation; and secondary infection, such as pneumonia, cellulitis and septicaemia Heals without scarring

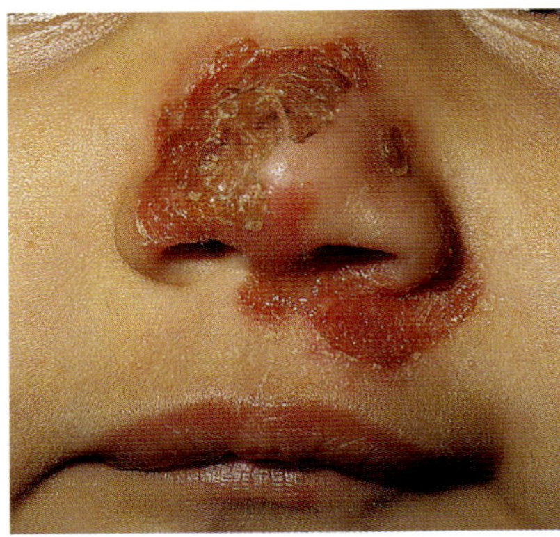

Fig 32.1 Impetigo contagiosa. (Source: Weston, W. L., & Lane, A. T. (2007). Color textbook of pediatric dermatology (4th ed.). St Louis, MO: Mosby.)

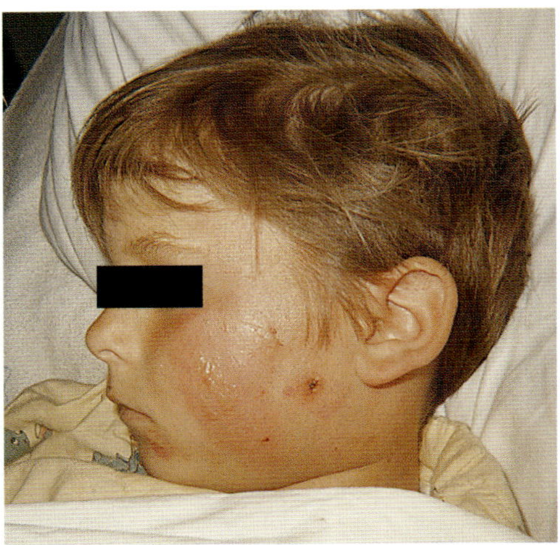

Fig 32.2 Cellulitis of cheek from a puncture wound. (Source: Weston, W. L., & Lane, A. T. (2007). Color textbook of pediatric dermatology (4th ed.). St Louis, MO: Mosby.)

Nursing Care Management. The major nursing functions related to bacterial skin infections are to prevent the spread of infection and to prevent complications. Impetigo contagiosa and MRSA infection can easily spread by self-inoculation; therefore, caution the child against touching the involved area. Hand washing is mandatory before and after contact with an affected child. Also emphasise hand washing to both the child and the family. Many children with atopic dermatitis are colonised with MRSA (Chopra et al 2017). For many bacterial infections and MRSA infection in particular, the child should be provided with washcloths and towels separate from those of other family members. The child's clothes should be changed daily and washed in hot water.

Children and parents are often tempted to squeeze follicular lesions. They must be warned that squeezing will not hasten the resolution of the infection and that there is a risk of making the lesion worse or spreading the infection. No attempt should be made to puncture the surface of the pustule with a needle or sharp instrument. A child with a stye may waken with the eyelids of the affected eye sealed shut with exudate. The child or the parents are instructed to gently wipe the eyelid from the inner to the outer edge with warm water and a clean washcloth until the exudate is removed.

The child with limited cellulitis of an extremity is usually managed at home on a regimen of oral antibiotics and warm compresses. The parents are taught the procedures and instructed in administration of the medication. Children with more extensive cellulitis, especially around a joint with lymphadenitis or on the face, are usually admitted to the hospital for parenteral antibiotics with continued treatment at home.

Viral Infections

Viruses are intracellular parasites that produce their effect by using the intracellular substances of the host cells. Composed of only a deoxyribonucleic acid (DNA) or ribonucleic acid (RNA) core enclosed in an antigenic protein shell, viruses are unable to provide for their own metabolic needs or to reproduce themselves. After a virus penetrates a cell of the host organism, it sheds the outer shell and disappears within the cell, where the nucleic acid core stimulates the host cell to form more virus material from its intracellular substance. In a viral infection, the epidermal cells react with inflammation and vesiculation (as in herpes simplex) or by proliferating to form growths (warts).

Many of the communicable viral diseases of childhood are associated with rashes, and each rash is characteristic. The type of lesion and the configuration of rubeola, rubella and chickenpox are described in Table 6.1. Other common viral disorders of the skin are outlined in Table 32.2.

Dermatophytoses (Fungal Infections)

The dermatophytoses (ringworm) are infections caused by a group of closely related filamentous fungi that invade primarily the stratum corneum, hair and nails. These are superficial infections by organisms that live on, not in, the skin. Dermatophytoses are designated by the Latin word *tinea,* with further designation relating to the area of the body where they are found (e.g. tinea capitis [ringworm of the scalp]). Table 32.3 outlines common dermatophytoses (see also Fig 32.3).

Dermatophyte infections are most often transmitted from one person to another or from infected animals to humans. Because the keratin is desquamated constantly, the fungus must multiply at a rate that equals the rate of keratin production to maintain itself; otherwise the infection would be shed with the discarded skin cells. Diagnosis is made from microscopic examination of scrapings taken from the advancing periphery of the lesion, which almost always produces a scale.

Nursing Care Management

When teaching families how to care for ringworm, the nurse should emphasise good health and hygiene. Because of the infectious nature of the disease, affected children should not exchange grooming items, headgear, scarves or other articles of apparel that have been in proximity to the infected area with other children. Because the infection can be acquired by animal-to-human transmission, all household pets should be examined for the disorder. Other sources of infection are seats in change rooms, seats in public transportation vehicles, helmets, communal showers and gym mats. The child may return to school/day care the day after the therapy is initiated, but the lesions must be covered.

For tinea capitis, both 2% ketoconazole and 1% selenium sulfide shampoos may reduce colony counts of dermatophytes. These shampoos can be used in combination with oral therapy to reduce the transmission of disease to others. The shampoo should be applied to the scalp for 5 to 10 minutes no more than once to twice weekly.

TABLE 32.2 Viral infections

Infection	Manifestations	Management	Comments
Verruca (warts) Cause—Human papillomavirus (various types)	Usually well-circumscribed, grey or brown, elevated, firm papules with a roughened, finely papillomatous texture Occur anywhere but usually appear on exposed areas such as fingers, hands, face and soles May be single or multiple Asymptomatic	Not uniformly successful Local destructive therapy, individualised according to location, type and number—surgical removal, electrocautery, curettage, cryotherapy (liquid nitrogen), caustic solutions (lactic acid and salicylic acid in flexible collodion, retinoic acid, salicylic acid plasters), laser ablation	Common in children Tend to disappear spontaneously Course unpredictable Most destructive techniques tend to leave scars Autoinoculable Repeated irritation will cause to enlarge
Verruca plantaris (plantar wart)	Located on plantar surface of feet and, because of pressure, are practically flat; may be surrounded by a collar of hyperkeratosis	Caustic chemical solution applied to wart and wear foam insole with hole cut to relieve pressure on wart; soak 20 minutes after 2–3 days; repeat until wart comes out	Destructive techniques tend to leave scars, which may cause problems with walking
Herpes simplex virus Type I (cold sore, fever blister) Type II (genital)	Grouped, burning and itching vesicles on inflammatory base, usually on or near mucocutaneous junctions (lips, nose, genitalia, buttocks) Vesicles dry, forming a crust followed by exfoliation and spontaneous healing in 8–10 days May be accompanied by regional lymphadenopathy	Avoidance of secondary infection Saline solution compresses during weeping stages Oral antiviral (aciclovir [Zovirax]) for initial infection or to reduce severity in recurrence; may also be given prophylactically for recurrent Valaciclovir (Valtrex), an oral antiviral, used for episodic treatment of recurrent genital herpes; reduces pain, stops viral shedding and has a more convenient administration schedule than aciclovir; primarily recommended for immunocompromised patients	Heal without scarring unless secondary infection Type I cold sores prevented by using sunscreens protecting against ultraviolet A and ultraviolet B light to prevent lip blisters Aggravated by corticosteroids Positive psychological effect from treatment May be fatal in children with depressed immunity
Varicella-zoster virus (herpes zoster; shingles)	Caused by same virus that causes varicella (chickenpox) Virus has affinity for posterior root ganglia, posterior horn of spinal cord and skin; crops of vesicles usually confined to dermatome following along course of affected nerve Usually preceded by neuralgic pain (rare in children), hyperaesthesias or itching May be accompanied by constitutional symptoms	Symptomatic Analgesics for pain Drying lotions sometimes helpful Ophthalmic variety: systemic corticotropin (adrenocorticotropic hormone) or corticosteroids Aciclovir or valaciclovir Preventive vaccine is available for persons > 50 years old	Pain in children usually minimal Postherpetic pain does not occur in children Chickenpox may follow exposure; isolate affected child from other children in a hospital or school May occur in children with depressed immunity; can be fatal
Molluscum contagiosum Cause—Pox virus	Flesh-coloured papules (1–20) with a central caseous plug (umbilicated) that occur on trunk, face and extremities; may be transmitted by sexual contact Usually asymptomatic	Cases in well children resolve spontaneously in about 18 months Treatment reserved for cosmetic purposes; alleviate discomfort; reduce autoinoculation; prevent secondary infection Numerous chemical removing agents including podophyllin; imiquimod cream These are painful treatments: use local anaesthesia Curettage, electrodessication or cryotherapy	Common in school-age children Spread by skin-to-skin contact, including autoinoculation and fomite-to-skin contact Outbreaks in day care centres have been reported

Systemic Mycotic (Fungal) Infections

Mycotic (systemic or deep fungal) infections have the capacity to invade the viscera, as well as the skin. The most common infections are the lung diseases, which are usually acquired by inhalation of fungal spores. These fungi produce a variable spectrum of disease, and some are common in certain geographic areas. They are not transmitted from person to person but appear to reside in the soil, from which their spores are airborne. The cutaneous lesions caused by deep fungal infections are granulomatous and appear as ulcers, plaques, nodules, fungating masses and abscesses. The course of deep fungal diseases is chronic with slow progression that favours sensitisation (Table 32.4).

SKIN DISORDERS RELATED TO CHEMICAL OR PHYSICAL CONTACTS

Contact Dermatitis

Contact dermatitis is an inflammatory reaction of the skin to chemical substances, natural or synthetic, that evoke a hypersensitivity response or direct irritation. The initial reaction occurs in an exposed region,

TABLE 32.3 **Dermatophytoses (Fungal Infections)**

Disease and Organism	Manifestations	Management	Comments
Tinea capitis—*Trichophyton tonsurans, Microsporum audouinii, Microsporum canis* (see Fig 32.3A)	Lesions in scalp but may extend to hairline or neck Characteristic configuration of scaly, circumscribed patches or patchy, scaling areas of alopecia Generally asymptomatic but severe, deep inflammatory reaction may occur that manifests as boggy, encrusted lesions (kerions) Pruritic Diagnosis: Microscopic examination of scales	Oral griseofulvin or terbinafine Selenium sulfide shampoos, used twice a week, may decrease infection and fungal shedding (Chen et al 2017)	Person-to-person transmission Animal-to-person transmission Rarely, permanent loss of hair *M. audouinii* transmitted from one human being to another directly or from personal items; *M. canis* usually contracted from household pets, especially cats Atopic individuals more susceptible
Tinea corporis—*Trichophyton rubrum, Trichophyton mentagrophytes, M. canis,* Epidermophyton (see Fig 32.3B)	Generally round or oval, erythematous scaling patch that spreads peripherally and clears centrally; may involve nails (tinea unguium) Diagnosis—Direct microscopic examination of scales Usually unilateral	Oral griseofulvin Local application of antifungal preparation applied 2.5 cm beyond periphery of lesion twice daily; application for 10 days. Oral antifungal needed if response limited (Nazarko 2017).	Usually of animal origin from infected pets but may occur from human transmission, soil or fomites Majority of infections in children caused by *M. canis* and *M. audouinii* Tinea gladiatorum is commonly seen in wrestlers
Tinea cruris ('jock itch')—*Epidermophyton floccosum, T. rubrum, T. mentagrophytes*	Skin response similar to tinea corporis Localised to medial proximal aspect of thigh and crural fold; may involve scrotum in males Pruritic Diagnosis—Same as for tinea corporis	Local application of topical antifungal twice daily for 2–4 weeks	Rare in preadolescent children Health education regarding transmission via person-to-person (direct or indirect) Occurs in close association with tinea pedis and tinea unguium
Tinea pedis ('athlete's foot')—*T. rubrum, Trichophyton interdigitale, E. floccosum* Tinea unguium: Nail infection	On intertriginous areas between toes or on plantar surface of feet Lesions vary: Maceration and fissuring between toes Patches with pinhead-sized vesicles on plantar surface Pruritic Diagnosis—Direct microscopic examination of scrapings	Local applications of topical antifungal cream/powder. Elimination of conditions of heat and perspiration by use of clean, light socks and well-ventilated shoes; avoidance of occlusive shoes (Sasagawa 2019)	Most frequent in adolescents and adults; rare in children, but occurrence increases with wearing of plastic shoes Common in locations such as showers, change rooms and swimming pools where fungi proliferate
Candidiasis (moniliasis)—*Candida albicans*	Grows in chronically moist areas Inflamed areas with white exudate, scaly plaques and easy bleeding Pruritic Diagnosis—Characteristic appearance; microscopic identification of scrapings; candidaemia diagnosed from cultures (blood, cerebrospinal fluid, bone marrow); tissue biopsy Chronic or recurrent often seen with HIV infection and immunocompromised child	Oral thrush: good oral hygiene accompanied by topical antifungal and systemic antifungal for persistent cases or patients who are immuno-compromised (Millsop & Fazel 2017) Genital thrush: topical antifungal, antibiotics if secondary infection (Cohen 2017, Folster-Holst 2018)	Common form of nappy rash (see Fig 32.8) Oral form common in infants (see Chapter 8) Vaginal form in females Disseminated disease in very-low-birth-weight infants and immunosuppressed children

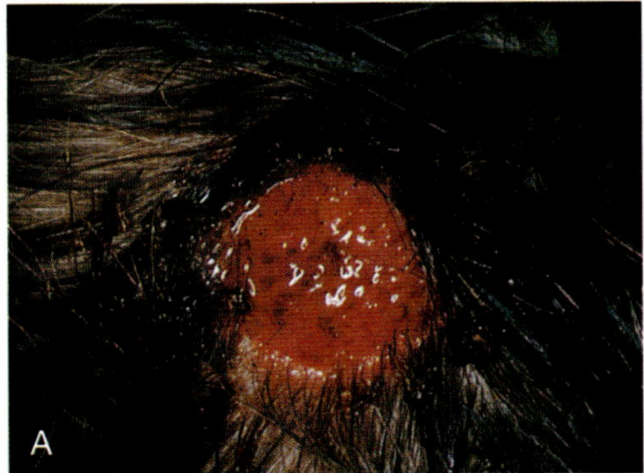

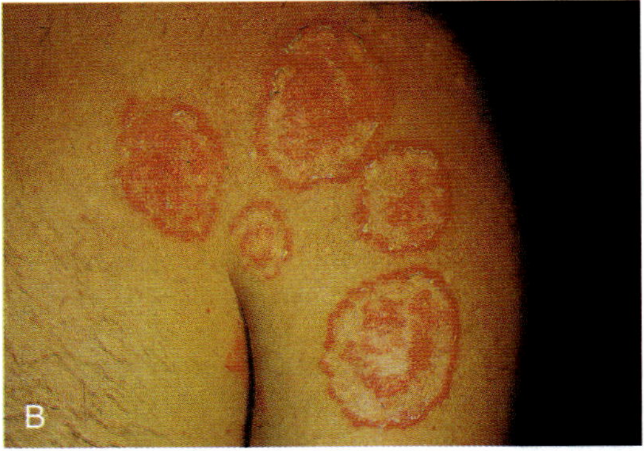

Fig 32.3 (**A**) Tinea capitis. (**B**) Tinea corporis. Both infections are caused by *Microsporum canis*, the 'kitten' or 'puppy' fungus. (Source: Habif, T. P. (2004). Clinical dermatology: A color guide to diagnosis and therapy (4th ed.). St Louis, MO: Mosby.)

TABLE 32.4 Systemic mycoses

Disorder and Organism	Skin Manifestations	Systemic Manifestations	Management	Comments
Cryptococcosis—*Cryptococcus neoformans* (*Torula histolytica*)	Usually on face; acneiform, firm, nodular, painless eruption	CNS manifestations—Headache, dizziness, stiff neck and signs of increased intracranial pressure Low-grade fever, mild cough, lung infiltration	IV amphotericin B (liposomal) may be administered intrathecal for CNS involvement Excision and drainage of local lesions	Acquired by inhalation of contaminate soil (bird faeces) Has occurred in northern Australia and Papua New Guinea Increased incidence in persons with defects in T-lymphocyte–mediated immunity (HIV, leukaemia, systemic lupus, AIDS or organ transplant) No person-to-person transmission
Histoplasmosis—*Histoplasma capsulatum*	Not distinctive or uniform but most appear as punched-out or granulomatous ulcers Erythema nodosum in adolescents	General systemic symptoms may include pallor, diarrhoea, vomiting, irregular spiking temperature, hepatosplenomegaly and pulmonary symptoms Any tissue of body may be involved with related symptoms	IV amphotericin B (liposomal) for severe cases Itraconazole for mild to moderate infections	Organism cultured from soil, especially where contaminated with fowl droppings Fungus enters through skin or mucous membranes of mouth and respiratory tract Occurs worldwide including a limited number of cases in parts of Australia Disseminated diseases most common in infants and children younger than 2 years

most commonly the face and neck, backs of the hands, forearms, male genitalia and lower legs. There is characteristically a sharp demarcation between inflamed and normal skin that ranges from a faint, transient erythema to massive bullae on an erythematous swollen base. Itching is a constant symptom.

The cause may be a primary irritant or a sensitising agent. A **primary irritant** is one that irritates any skin. A **sensitising agent** produces an irritation on those individuals who have encountered the irritant or something chemically related to it, have undergone an immunological change and have become sensitised. Prior exposure is not necessarily a factor in the reaction. A sensitiser irritates in relatively low concentrations only persons who are allergic to it.

The major goal in treatment is to prevent further exposure of the skin to the offending substance and testing may be required to ascertain the offending allergen. Provided there is no further irritation, the skin's normal recuperative powers will often produce healing without treatment. If required, treatment will be tailored to the restoration of the skin and symptomatic treatment after removal and avoidance of the allergen (Pelletier et al 2016).

The most frequent offenders are plant (chrysanthemums, primula, tomato plants, grevillea and English ivy in Australia/New Zealand), animal (wool, feathers and furs) and metal irritants (nickel found in jewellery, belt buckles and the fasteners on sleep suits and denim). In infants, contact dermatitis occurs on the convex surfaces of the nappy area. Other agents that produce contact dermatitis include vegetable irritants (oleoresins, oils and turpentine), synthetic fabrics (e.g. shoe components), dyes, cosmetics, perfumes and soaps (including bubble baths).

Nursing Care Management

Nurses frequently detect evidence of contact dermatitis during routine physical assessments. Skin manifestations in specific areas suggest limited contact, such as around the eyes (mascara), areas of the body covered by clothing but not protected by undergarments (wool) or areas of the body not covered by clothing (ultraviolet [UV] injury). Generalised involvement is more likely to be caused by bubble bath, laundry soap, body soap or lotion. Often nurses can determine the offending agent and counsel families regarding management. If the lesions persist, are extensive or show evidence of infection, medical evaluation is indicated.

Allergic Contact Dermatitis from Plants

In Australia and New Zealand, common plants causing contact dermatitis are chrysanthemums, primula, tomato plants, grevillea, English ivy and occasionally rhus trees. This contact produces a weepy itch rash, usually a few days after contact with the allergen. The rash will appear on the areas where direct exposure occurred (Australasian Society of Clinical Immunology and Allergy [ASCIA] 2019). Treatment relies on identification and avoidance of the allergen, will be symptomatic and, as with any contact dermatitis, is aimed at restoring skin integrity (Pelletier et al 2016).

Drug Reactions

Although drugs can adversely affect any organ of the body, reactions to medications are seen more often in the skin than in any other organ. The reaction may be a result of toxicity related to drug concentration, individual intolerance to the therapeutic dosage of the drug or an allergic or idiosyncratic response. The manifestations may be associated with side effects or secondary effects of a drug, either of which are unrelated to its primary pharmacological actions.

Nursing Care Management

The most effective means of management is prevention, documentation and assessment. Frequent offenders in drug reactions are penicillin and sulfonamides, and nurses must be alert to this possibility. However, even commonplace drugs such as aspirin and phenobarbital (phenobarbitone), chemical agents in some foods, flavouring agents and preservatives are capable of producing an undesired response. A careful nursing assessment (observation, inspection and palpation) of the skin is paramount for any child receiving medication, especially intravenously. Noting the child's behaviour and frequency of scratching is also critical.

SKIN DISORDERS RELATED TO ANIMAL CONTACTS

Arthropod Bites and Stings

Arthropods include insects and arachnids, such as mosquitoes, mites, ticks, spiders and scorpions. All scorpions in Australia are relatively harmless and while they may bite and cause a painful irritation, their venom is non-fatal. Although all spiders produce venom that is injected via fangs, some are unable to pierce the skin and others produce venom that is insufficiently toxic to be harmful. There are several spiders in Australia that produce venom that can be harmful and/or fatal. The funnel-web spider can inject venom deadly enough to require immediate attention. Children bitten by these arachnids must receive medical attention as soon as possible. Redback and mouse spiders are also offending creatures; their manifestations and management are outlined in Table 32.5. White-tailed spiders have been maligned for causing necrotic injuries, but this is now proven to be untrue and their bites cause little more than local irritation.

When a hymenopteran (bees in particular) stings, its barbed stinger penetrates the skin. As long as the stinger remains in the skin, the muscles push the stinger deeper and the venom is pumped into the wound. The best approach is to remove the stinger as quickly as possible and to get away from the vicinity of other insects to prevent further injury. Children who have become sensitised to hymenopteran bites may demonstrate a severe systemic response that can be life-threatening. One sting can produce generalised urticaria, respiratory difficulty (from laryngeal oedema), hypotension and death. Intramuscular administration of adrenaline provides immediate relief and must be available for emergency use.

Scabies

Scabies is an endemic infestation caused by the scabies mite, *Sarcoptes scabiei*. Lesions are created as the impregnated female burrows into the stratum corneum of the epidermis (never into living tissue) to deposit her eggs and faeces. The inflammatory response causes intense pruritus that leads to punctate discrete excoriations secondary to the itching (Box 32.1). Maculopapular lesions are characteristically distributed in intertriginous areas: interdigital surfaces, the axillary-cubital area, popliteal folds and the inguinal region. The observer must look for discrete papules, burrows or vesicles (Fig 32.4). Scabies is transmitted primarily through prolonged close personal contact, and it affects persons regardless of age, sex, personal hygiene and socioeconomic status.

NURSING CARE CONSIDERATIONS

In Australia, scabies is endemic in many Aboriginal and Torres Strait Islander populations and it is estimated that about 70% of infants are infected by the age of 1 year (Kearns et al 2015). Overcrowding and the tropical climate contributes to the scabies burden.

Skin lesions can lead to cellulitis or abscesses (Thomas et al 2017). Secondary infections are caused by scratching and contribute to high rates of pyoderma causing complications of acute post-streptococcal glomerulonephritis, contributing to high rates of chronic kidney disease and sepsis. Rheumatic fever and rheumatic heart disease occur in this population at the highest rate in the world, causing limited life span and reduced mortality (Thomas et al 2017). Crusted scabies can develop, which is a rare, severe manifestation where the scabies infestation is in the millions of mites, resulting in lichenification and yellow-green crusts. This is a disfiguring disease which can lead to sepsis and death (Hardy et al 2017) and the rate of crusted scabies in Aboriginal and Torres Strait Islander populations is one of the highest in the world.

Nursing Care Management

The treatment of scabies is the application of a scabicide. The drug of choice in children and infants older than 2 months of age is

TABLE 32.5 Skin Lesions Caused By Arthropods

Mechanism and Characteristic	Manifestations	Management
INSECT BITES—FLIES, ANTS, MOSQUITOES, FLEAS		
Mechanism—Foreign protein in insects' saliva introduced when skin is penetrated for a blood meal Distribution: Almost everywhere—Fleas, mosquitoes, ants Suburbs and rural areas—Bees Urban areas—Hornets, wasps, yellow jackets	Hypersensitivity reaction Papular urticaria Firm papules; may be capped by vesicles or excoriated Little or no reaction in non-sensitised person	Treatment: Use antipruritic agents and baths Administer antihistamines Treat secondary infection Prevention: Avoid contact Remove focus, such as untreated furniture, mattresses, carpets and pets, where insects may live Apply insect repellent or wear protective clothing when exposure is anticipated
HYMENOPTERANS—BEES, WASPS, FIRE ANTS		
Mechanism: Injection of venom through stinging apparatus Venom contains histamine; allergenic proteins; and often a spreading factor, hyaluronidase Severe reactions caused by hypersensitivity or multiple stings Fire ants are rare in Australia and are the focus of a large eradication program	Local reaction—Small red area, wheal, itching and heat Systemic reactions—May be mild to severe, including generalised oedema, pain, nausea and vomiting, confusion, respiratory impairment and shock	Treatment: Carefully scrape off stinger or pull out stinger as quickly as possible Cleanse with soap and water Apply cool compresses Apply common household product (e.g. lemon juice) Administer antihistamines Severe reactions—Administer adrenaline, corticosteroids; treat for shock Prevention: Teach child to wear shoes; to avoid wearing bright clothing, flowery prints, shiny jewellery or perfumed grooming products (cologne, scented hairspray), which might attract the insect; and to avoid places where the insect may be contacted Hypersensitive children should wear medical identification to indicate allergy and therapy needed; family should keep emergency medication and be taught its administration

TABLE 32.5 Skin Lesions Caused By Arthropods—cont'd

Mechanism and Characteristic	Manifestations	Management
AUSTRALIAN SPIDERS		
Funnel web spider (*Atrax robustus* species) The most venomous spider in the world. Shiny, dark brown large spider Live in dark, moist places.	Autonomic and neuromuscular excess, hypoxia, pulmonary oedema, hypotension and cardiogenic shock. Requires immediate medical treatment with anticholinergic medication and transfer to a medical facility for antivenom	Treatment: Pressure immobilisation bandage Immediate medical treatment with anticholinergic medication Transfer to a medical facility for antivenom Ongoing treatment includes: • antivenom • dobutamine • noradrenaline • high-dose insulin • pain relief • sedation May require ventilation Prevention: Teach children to avoid possible nesting sites
Mouse spider (*Missulena* species) Medium to large spider with large fangs, less aggressive than the funnel-web spider. Live in burrows in soil	Most cases cause local neurotoxic effects or minor systemic effects like numbness, swelling or local pain Severe effects rare.	Treatment: Initial first aid is pressure bandage with immobilisation As the mouse spider is similar in appearance to the funnel-web spider, observation in hospital should occur for 4 hours after the bite Prevention: Teach children to avoid possible nesting sites
Redback spider Females are 1 cm and males < 5 mm A black spider, the female has an hourglass red shape of their back Often found in backyards and homes Females are responsible for causing harm Note: *The Katipo spider in New Zealand is closely related to the redback and the advice and treatment are the same*	Rarely cause significant envenoming Pain at the site of the bite may increase in the days after the bite, often lasting for days Generalised symptoms such as headache, fatigue, nausea/vomiting may manifest Systemic effects rare	Treatment: Adequate analgesia Clean the wound Apply ice to the bite Symptomatic treatment Do not use pressure immobilisation bandage Antivenom rarely required but can induce pain relief Resuscitation not required Prevention: Check children's play areas; these spiders like heat and open areas and avoid damp areas or water
White-tailed spider Sized 12–18 mm with a dark reddish grey colour and a cylindrical body Like to dwell in homes and in fabrics like towels and sheets	May cause local irritation and swelling; at worst a red lesion persisting for 5–12 days Rumoured to cause necrotic arachnidism but this is unfounded	Treatment: Clean the site Treat with ice pack Prevention: Shake out linen before use
TICKS		
Mechanism—In process of sucking blood, head and mouth parts are buried in skin Characteristics: Feed on blood of mammals Significant in humans because of pathological organism carried May be vectors of various infectious diseases, such as Queensland tick typhus, Flinders Island spotted fever, tick paralysis No evidence for spread of Lyme disease in Australia Must attach and feed for 1–2 hours to transmit disease Usual habitat is wooded area	Tick usually attached to skin with head embedded Firm, discrete, intensely pruritic nodules at site of attachment May cause urticaria or persistent localised oedema	Treatment: Grasp tick with tweezers (forceps) as close as possible to point of attachment Pull straight up with steady, even pressure; if using bare hands, use a tissue to touch tick during removal; wash hands thoroughly with soap and water Remove any remaining part (e.g. head) with sterile needle Cleanse wounds with soap and disinfectant Prevention—Teach children to avoid areas where prevalent Inspect skin (especially scalp) after being in wooded areas Use insecticide repellent prior to entering infested areas.

BOX 32.1 Clinical Manifestations of Scabies

Lesion
- **Children**—Minute greyish brown, threadlike (mite burrows), pruritic
  - Black dot at end of burrow (mite)
- **Infants**—Eczematous eruption, pruritic

Distribution
- **Generally in intertriginous areas**—Interdigital, axillary-cubital, popliteal, inguinal
- **Children older than 2 years of age**—Primarily hands and wrists
- **Children younger than 2 years**—Primarily feet and ankles

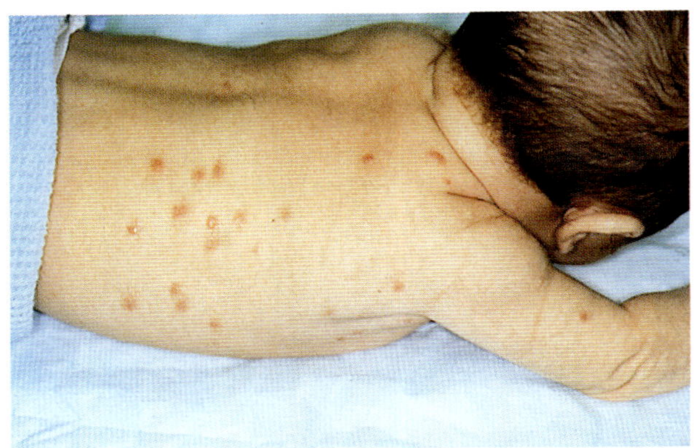

Fig 32.4 Scabies. (Source: McCance, K., & Huether, S. (2010). Pathophysiology: The biological basis for disease in adults and children (6th ed.). St Louis, MO: Mosby/Elsevier.)

permethrin 5% cream. First-line treatment choice is crotamiton (Eurax) for infants younger than 2 months, permethrin 5% (Lyclear) for infants older than 2 months. If this is not available then second-line treatment would be benzl benzoate (Ascabiol) for children older than 6 months (Hardy et al 2017). Alternative drugs are 10% crotamiton (cream or lotion).

Ivermectin, an oral medication, may be used to treat scabies in patients with secondary excoriations for whom topical scabicides are irritating and not well tolerated or whose infestation is refractory. However, the safety and efficacy of ivermectin for children weighing less than 15 kg has not been established (Thomas et al 2017, Hardy et al 2017). Thomas and colleagues (2017) conducted research into using tea tree oil formulated into a cream which is promising as it is better tolerated, improves compliance and the scabies mites are developing resistance to current treatments.

Because of the length of time between infestation and physical symptoms (30 to 60 days), all persons who were in close contact with the affected child need treatment. This may include siblings, boyfriends or girlfriends, babysitters, grandparents and immediate family members. The objective is to treat as thoroughly as possible the first time. Enough medication for the entire family should be prescribed.

Crusted scabies requires hospital admission, isolation and intensive treatment with both topical and oral formulations (Hardy et al 2017).

BOX 32.2 Clinical Manifestations of Pediculosis

- Pruritus (caused by crawling insects and insect saliva on skin)
- Nits observable on hair shaft (see Fig 32.5)

Distribution
- Occipital area
- Behind ears
- Nape of neck
- Eyebrows and eyelashes (occasionally) (caused by pubic lice)

Pediculosis Capitis

Pediculosis capitis (head lice) is an infestation of the scalp by *Pediculus humanus capitis,* a common parasite in school-age children. These lice infestations create embarrassment and concern in the family and community. They can also cause a child to be ridiculed by other children. An important nursing role is education about pediculosis. Nurses should emphasise that anyone can get pediculosis; it has no respect for age, socioeconomic level or cleanliness.

The adult louse lives only about 48 hours when away from a human host, and the life span of the average female is 1 month. The female lays her eggs at night at the junction of a hair shaft and close to the skin because the eggs need a warm environment. The **nits**, or eggs, hatch in approximately 7 to 10 days. Itching, caused by the crawling insect and saliva on the skin, is usually the only symptom. The louse is a blood-sucking organism that requires approximately five meals a day. Common areas involved are the occipital area, behind the ears and the nape of the neck (Box 32.2).

Diagnostic Evaluation

Diagnosis is made by observation of the white eggs (nits) firmly attached to the hair shafts (Fig 32.5). Lice are small and greyish-tan, have no wings and are visible to the naked eye. Observation of the white eggs (nits) firmly attached to the hair shafts confirms the diagnosis. The nits, or eggs, appear as tiny whitish oval specks adhering to the hair shaft about 6 mm from the scalp. The adherent nature of the nits distinguishes them from dandruff, which falls off readily. Empty nit cases, indicating hatched lice, are translucent rather than white and are located more than 6 mm from the scalp. Because of their brief life span and mobility, adult lice are more difficult to locate. Nits must be differentiated from dandruff, lint, hair spray and other items of similar size and shape. Scratch marks or inflammatory papules, caused by secondary infection, are also found on the scalp in the vulnerable areas.

Therapeutic Management

Treatment consists of the application of hair conditioner or pediculicides and manual removal of nit cases. The product of choice for infants and children should contain permethrin, which kills adult lice and nits. There are several products that can be obtained from the chemist without prescription and are effective and safe but hair conditioner has been found to be as effective and is less toxic, better tolerated and cheaper (Queensland Government 2019). Most experts advise a second treatment at 7 to 10 days to ensure a cure. However, malathion is not recommended for children younger than 2 years of age.

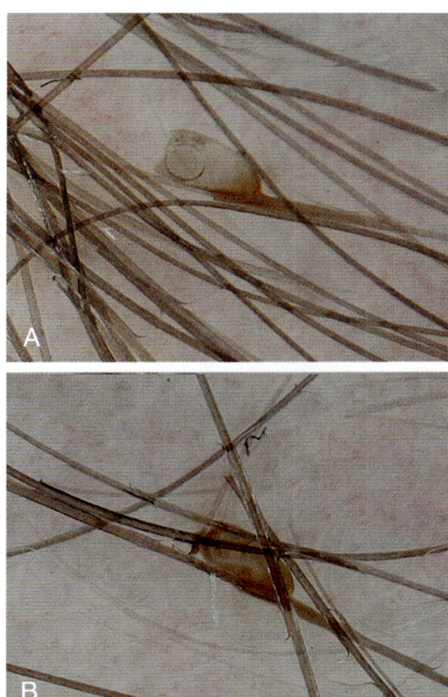

Fig 32.5 (**A**) Empty nit case. (**B**) Viable nits. (Source: Stefani, A. D., Hofmann-Wellenhof, R., & Zalaudek, I. (2006). Dermoscopy for diagnosis and treatment monitoring of pediculosis capitis. Journal of the American Academy of Dermatology, 54(5), 909–911.)

Nursing Care Management

An important nursing role is educating the parents about pediculosis. Nurses should emphasise that *anyone* can get pediculosis; it has no respect for age, gender, socioeconomic level or cleanliness. Lice do not jump or fly, but they can be transmitted from one person to another on personal items. Children are cautioned against sharing combs, hair ornaments, hats, caps, scarves, coats and other items used on or near the hair although spread by these means is now thought to be rare (Queensland Government 2019).

If evidence of infestation is found, it is important to treat the child.

> **NURSING CARE CONSIDERATIONS**
>
> Current advice is as follows.
>
> 1. Treat with hair conditioner, which stuns the lice and assists removal. The conditioner is applied generously through the hair which is then combed out and washed. This needs to be repeated after 7 to 10 days (Queensland Government 2019). Head lice are becoming immune to chemical treatments which can be expensive and toxic, so this is the recommended current treatment.
> 2. Treat with pediculicide according to the directions on the label of the pediculicide (Queensland Government 2019). Parents are advised to read the directions carefully before beginning treatment.

Live lice survive for up to 48 hours away from the host, but nits are shed into the environment and are capable of hatching in 7 to 10 days; retreatment is required. Therefore, measures must be taken to prevent further infestation. It is no longer recommended as necessary to wash all linen that has been in contact with the affected child due to the short life span of the live lice away from the scalp/hair environment, but control measures such as tying up long hair and avoiding play with head-to-head contact is recommended, along with regular checks and treatment of all children in a school/day care setting where head lice are detected (Queensland Government 2019).

Rickettsial Diseases

The organisms responsible for a number of disorders are transmitted to human beings via arthropods. Mammals become infected only through the bites of infected lice, fleas, ticks and mites, all of which serve as both infectors and reservoirs. Rickettsiae are intracellular parasites, similar in size to bacteria that inhabit the alimentary tract of a wide range of natural hosts. Rickettsial diseases are more common in temperate and tropical climates where humans live in association with arthropods. Infection in humans is incidental (except epidemic typhus) and not necessary for the survival of the rickettsial species. However, after the organism invades a human, it causes a disease that varies in intensity from a benign, self-limiting illness to a disease that is fulminating and fatal.

In Australia, tick bites can result in several conditions: Queensland tick typhus, Flinders Island spotted fever, Australian spotted fever and Q fever. The Australian paralysis tick can cause a paralysis syndrome with involvement of the cranial nerves, ataxia and ascending, flaccid paralysis. This generally affects animals but could affect a small child if bitten (Graves & Stenos 2017). Tick bites generally cause firm papules, erythema with intense itching due to the substances found in the ticks' saliva; later reactions can be nodules due to retained mouth parts of the tick (Haddad et al 2018).

Nursing Care Management

The major emphasis of nursing care should be educating parents to protect their children from exposure to ticks. Children should avoid tick-infested areas or wear light-coloured clothing so that ticks can be spotted easily, tuck pant legs into socks and wear a long-sleeved shirt tucked into pants when in wooded areas. Parents and children need to perform regular tick checks when they are in infested areas (with special attention to the scalp, neck, armpits and groin areas). Parents should also be alert for signs of the skin lesion, especially if their children have been in tick-infested areas.

Parents should also be educated regarding tick removal in the event of a tick bite. The tick should be grasped firmly with tweezers and pulled straight out. The application of insecticide, nail polish or petrolatum jelly is not recommended and does not appear to have an effect on tick withdrawal as has been hypothesised. Concerns about tick engorgement or tick remains left in the person's body (such as the tick head) is uncommon; there is no need for medical examination of the tick itself. After the tick is removed, wash the bite area with an iodine scrub, rubbing alcohol or plain soap and water.

Insect repellents containing diethyltoluamide (DEET) and permethrin can protect against ticks, but parents should use these chemicals cautiously. Although there have been reports of serious neurological complications in children resulting from frequent and excessive application of DEET repellents, the risk is low when they are used properly. Products with DEET should be applied sparingly according to label instructions and not applied to a child's face, hands or any areas of irritated skin. Permethrin-treated clothing has also been shown to be effective in repelling ticks (Haddad et el 2018). After the child returns indoors, treated skin should be washed with soap and water.

Animal Bites

Animal bites are common in childhood. The present discussion is directed primarily towards dog bites because most animal bites to children are caused by dogs. Cat bites are less frequent, although cat scratches are extremely common (see Cat-Scratch Disease, later in this chapter).

Most injuries caused by dogs or cats are to the upper extremities. Small children are likely to be bitten or scratched on the head, face and neck because they tend to put their heads near the animal's head and flail their arms rather than protecting their heads. Most dogs involved are owned by the family of the victim or by a neighbour. Injuries vary in intensity from small puncture wounds to complete evulsion of tissue that is associated with significant crush injury. Animal bites are potentially serious because of the likelihood of significant infection.

Therapeutic Management

General wound care consists of rinsing the wound with copious amounts of saline or lactated Ringer's solution under pressure via a large syringe and of washing the surrounding skin with mild soap. A clean pressure dressing is applied, and the extremity is elevated if the wound is bleeding. Medical evaluation is advised because of the danger of tetanus. Bites from wild animals, such as bats and rodents, are potentially dangerous.

Prophylactic antibiotics are indicated for puncture wounds and wounds in areas that may prove to be cosmetically or functionally impaired if infected. Extensive lacerations are debrided and loosely sutured to allow drainage in the event of infection. Tetanus toxoid is administered according to standard guidelines (see Immunisations, Chapter 6). Injuries to poorly vascularised areas, such as the hands, are more likely to become infected than those in more vascularised areas, such as the face; puncture wounds are more likely to become infected than lacerations.

Nursing Care Management

The most important aspect related to animal bites is prevention. Children should understand animal behaviour and develop respect for animals. Parents should monitor their children's behaviour with dogs and cats and instruct them not to tease or surprise dogs, invade their territory, interfere with their feeding or sleeping, take their toys, approach strange animals or interact with sick or injured animals or animals with young. Parents who are considering getting a pet, especially a dog, for themselves or their children should select a dog that has a high level of sociability with children and is unlikely to be a danger to them.

Human Bites

Children often acquire lacerations from the teeth of other humans in rough play, during fights or as victims of child abuse. Some young children bite others out of frustration or anger. Because human dental plaque and gingiva harbour pathogenic organisms, all human bites should receive attention. Delayed treatment increases the risk of infection.

The wound is washed vigorously with soap and water, and a pressure dressing is applied to stop bleeding. Ice applications minimise discomfort and swelling. Increased pain or redness at the wound site is an indication that the child should receive medical attention for antibiotic therapy. Tetanus toxoid is needed if the child is insufficiently immunised. Wounds larger than 6 mm should receive medical attention.

Cat-scratch Disease

Cat-scratch disease is the most common cause of regional lymphadenitis in children and adolescents. It usually follows the scratch or bite of an animal (a cat or kitten in 99% of cases) and is caused by *Bartonella henselae*, a gram-negative bacterium (Nelson et al 2016).

The usual manifestations are a painless, non-pruritic erythematous papule at the site of inoculation, followed by regional lymphadenitis. The lymph nodes most commonly involved are axillary, epitrochlear, cervical, submandibular, inguinal and preauricular. The disease may persist for several months before gradual resolution. In some children, especially those who are immunocompromised, the adenitis may progress to suppuration. Some children may develop serious complications that include encephalitis, hepatitis and Parinaud's oculoglandular syndrome. This syndrome is characterised by granulomatous lesions on the palpebral conjunctiva associated with swelling of the ipsilateral preauricular nodes.

Children should be cautioned about playing with aggressive kittens that bite or scratch. Wounds should be washed with soap and water. Analgesics may be given if there is discomfort. Treatment is supportive, with antibiotic therapy where indicated. Most children can continue normal activities during the disease. Flea control will reduce the transmission and spread of the infection between cats (Nelson 2016). The animals are not ill during the time they transmit the disease, and most authorities do not recommend disposal of a cherished pet.

Flying Fox (Bat) Bites

Flying foxes are known to spread lyssa virus. In 1996 a version of this virus was identified in Australia—Australian bat lyssavirus (ABLV). This virus only affects about 1% of flying foxes and is more likely to affect ill or injured flying foxes. Therefore, children should be cautioned against handling flying foxes and any bites must be treated appropriately to prevent serious infection of lyssavirus, which leads to paralysis, convulsions, delirium and death. It is important to seek urgent medical attention in the case of a flying fox bite as treatment prior to becoming ill is imperative (Queensland Government 2020).

MISCELLANEOUS SKIN DISORDERS

A number of miscellaneous skin lesions occur in children. Some occur as a result of congenital disorders and are inherited as an autosomal dominant trait (Table 32.6). **Ichthyoses** are a heterogeneous group of disorders characterised by scaling that create challenging problems in treatment. These disorders are not discussed in detail here because of their wide variability.

SKIN DISORDERS ASSOCIATED WITH SPECIFIC AGE GROUPS

Several common dermatological conditions are confined to children in specific age groups. These conditions include nappy rash and atopic and seborrhoeic dermatitis, which occurs predominantly in infants, and acne, which is most common in adolescence.

Nappy Rash

Nappy rash is common in infants and one of several acute inflammatory skin disorders caused either directly or indirectly by wearing nappies. The peak age of occurrence is 9 to 12 months of age, and the incidence is greater in bottle-fed infants than in breastfed infants.

Pathophysiology and Clinical Manifestations

Nappy rash is caused by prolonged and repetitive contact with an irritant (e.g. urine, faeces, soaps, detergents, ointments, friction). Although the irritant in the majority of cases is urine and faeces, a combination of factors contributes to irritation.

TABLE 32.6 **Miscellaneous Skin Disorders**

Disease and Causative Agent	Local Manifestations	Management	Comments
Urticaria—Usually lallergic response to drugs or infection	Development of wheals Vary in size and configuration and tend to appear quickly, spread irregularly, and fade within a few hours May be constant or intermittent, sparse or profuse, small or large, discrete or confluent May be acute, chronic or recurrent in acute attacks	Topical soothing and antipruritic applications Antihistamines Cortisone in severe cases Severe involvement may require adrenaline	Known aetiological agents should be avoided May be accompanied by malaise, fever, lymphadenopathy Severe cases may involve mucous membranes, internal organs and joints Obstruction to air passages constitutes medical emergency
Intertrigo—Mechanical trauma and aggravating factors of excessive heat, moisture and sweat retention	Red, inflamed, moist, partially denuded, marginated areas, the shape of which is determined by location Appears where opposing skin surfaces rub together, such as intergluteal folds, groin, neck and axilla Excessive moisture and obesity are often factors	Maintenance of cleanliness and dryness of affected areas Skinfolds kept separated with a generous supply of non-medicated powder Expose to air and light Remove excess clothing	A form of nappy irritation Prevent recurrence by keeping susceptible areas clean and dry Frequently associated with overheating from too much clothing Common in tracheostomy patients with short necks and copious secretions
Psoriasis—Cause unknown; hereditary predisposition; may be triggered by stress	Round, thick, dry, reddish patches covered with coarse, silvery scales over trunk and extremities; first lesions commonly appear in scalp; facial lesions more common in children than in adults Affected cells proliferate at a much more rapid rate than normal cells	Tar preparations in combination with ultraviolet B light or natural sunlight Topical corticosteroids Topical vitamin D analogue calcipotriol Saline solutions followed by a tar shampoo to remove scales Keratolytic agents (salicylic acid) Acitretin Emollients may provide relief	Uncommon in children younger than 6 years Affected patients are otherwise healthy Coal tar acts synergistically with ultraviolet light Keratolytic agents enhance absorption of corticosteroids Humidifiers may help in winter
Alopecia			
Alopecia areata	Sudden onset of asymptomatic, non-inflammatory, round, bald patches in hairy parts of body	Psychological support	Family history in 10% to 26% of cases Some concern regarding drug therapy safety
Traumatic alopecia	Traction alopecia around scalp margins from tight hair styles (e.g. plaits, ponytails, corn rows)	Counselling regarding hair styling, use of hair cosmetics, hot combs, rollers	More prevalent in African American children and adolescents Prolonged traction can produce fibrosis of hair root and permanent loss
Trichotillomania	Compulsive hair pulling	Determine and treat cause	Chronic hair pulling may require psychological therapy
Tinea capitis	See Table 32.2	See Table 32.2	See Table 32.2
Erythema multiforme (Stevens-Johnson syndrome)—Cause unknown; associated with ingestion of some drugs; often follows upper respiratory tract infection	Erythematous papular rash Lesions enlarge by peripheral expansion, develop central vesicle Involves most skin surfaces except scalp May extend to mucous membranes, especially oral, ocular and urethral	Symptomatic and supportive Maintenance of adequate intake of fluids (oral or intravenous), calories and protein Moist wound care, hydrogels. Appropriate treatment of complications Diligent monitoring of urine volume and specific gravity, haemoglobin and haematocrit, serum electrolyte levels, total body weight	Rash often preceded by fever and malaise Complications include renal failure and severe eye disease Respiratory involvement in a number of cases Self-limiting, but recovery may extend for weeks; skin lesions may subside without scarring; mucous membrane lesions may persist for months Recurrence rate, 20%; mortality rate as high as 10% High mutation rate
Neurofibromatosis—Inherited disorder; autosomal dominant inheritance pattern	Café-au-lait spots, pigmented naevi, axillary freckling Slow-growing cutaneous and subcutaneous neurofibromas	Symptomatic treatment of associated manifestations (e.g. speech defects, seizures, skeletal defects [scoliosis, kyphosis], learning disabilities) Surgical removal of troublesome tumours	Refer to support groups. Family needs to know about genetic implications

Prolonged contact of the skin with nappy wetness produces higher friction, greater abrasion damage, increased trans-epidermal permeability and increased microbial counts. Healthy skin is less resistant to potential irritants (Fig 32.6).

Nursing Care Management

Nursing interventions are aimed at altering the three factors that produce dermatitis: wetness, pH and faecal irritants. The most significant factor amenable to intervention is the moist environment created in the nappy area. Changing the nappy as soon as it becomes wet eliminates a large part of the problem, and removing the nappy to expose healthy skin to air facilitates drying. The use of a hair dryer or heat lamp is not recommended because these devices can cause burns.

Atopic Dermatitis (Eczema)

Atopic dermatitis (AD), also referred to as eczema, refers to a descriptive category of dermatological diseases and not to a specific aetiology. AD is a chronic relapsing inflammatory skin disorder that results in itching and lesions (Fig 32.7; Saini & Pansare 2019). It occurs in 20% to 30% of children (Saini & Pansare 2019). AD manifests in three forms based on the child's age and the distribution of lesions.

1. **Infantile (infantile eczema)**—Usually begins at 2 to 6 months of age; generally undergoes spontaneous remission by 3 years of age
2. **Childhood**—May follow the infantile form; occurs at 2 to 3 years of age; 90% of children have manifestations by age 5 years
3. **Preadolescent and adolescent**—Begins at about 12 years of age; may continue into the early adult years or indefinitely

The diagnosis of AD is based on a combination of history and morphological findings (Box 32.3). Although symptoms can vary among individuals, one symptom that is common is pruritus. Itching can be mild, moderate or severe, and can intensify the inflammation and erythema associated with the lesions; itching can become so severe that the lesions bleed. Lesions gradually disappear when the scratching is stopped.

Although the cause is not fully understood, AD is believed to have genetic and environmental factors. The majority of children with infantile AD have a family history of eczema, asthma, food allergies or allergic rhinitis, which strongly supports a genetic predisposition. The cause is unknown but appears to be related to abnormal function of the skin, including alterations in perspiration, peripheral vascular function, heat tolerance and immune dysregulation (Saini & Pansare 2019). Manifestations of the chronic disease improve in humid climates and get worse in the autumn and winter, when homes are heated and environmental humidity is lower. The disorder can be controlled but not cured. A recent study of 250 patients with AD showed that the severity of AD significantly affected their quality of life, with more severe disease resulting in a lower quality of life (Holm et al 2016). Furthermore, the study reported a lower quality of life among females and among patients with eczema on their face (Holm et al 2016).

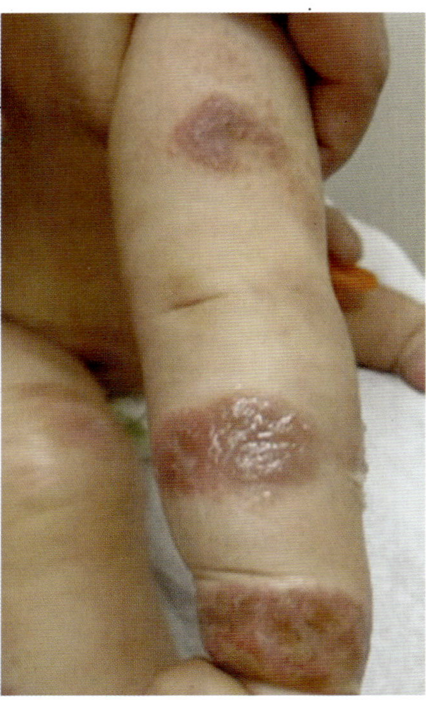

Fig 32.7 Atopic dermatitis. (Source: Gupta, D. (2015). Atopic dermatitis. Medical Clinics of North America, 99(6), 1269–1285.)

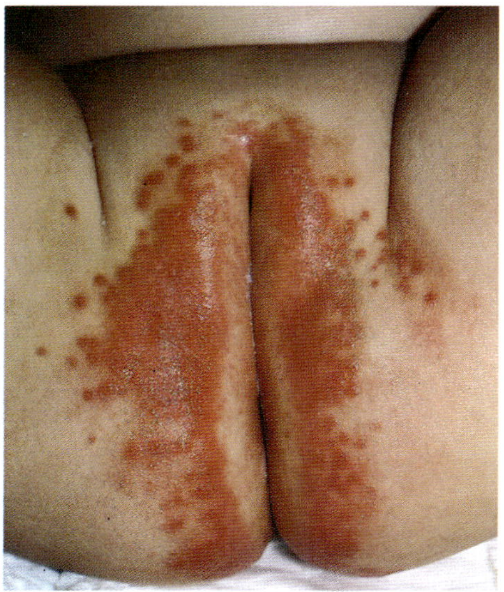

Fig 32.6 Candidiasis of nappy area. Note the beefy red central erythema with satellite pustules. (Source: Paller, A. S., & Mancini, A. J. (2011). Hurwitz clinical pediatric dermatology (4th ed.). St Louis, MO: Saunders Elsevier.)

Therapeutic Management

The major goals of management are to: (1) hydrate the skin; (2) relieve pruritus; (3) reduce flare-ups or inflammation; and (4) prevent and control secondary infection. The general measures for managing AD focus on reducing pruritus and other aspects of the disease. Management strategies include: avoiding exposure to skin irritants or allergens; avoiding overheating; and administrating medications such as antihistamines, topical immunomodulators, topical steroids and (sometimes) mild sedatives as indicated. Phototherapy, biological agents and probiotic therapy may also be used for severe cases (Saini & Pansare 2019).

Enhancing skin hydration and preventing dry, flaky skin are accomplished in a number of ways, depending on the child's skin characteristics and individual needs. A tepid bath with a mild soap (Dove or Neutrogena), no soap or an emulsifying oil followed immediately by application of an emollient (within 3 minutes) assists in trapping moisture and preventing its loss. Bubble baths and harsh soaps should be avoided. The bath may need to be repeated once or twice daily, depending on the child's status; excessive bathing without emollient application only dries out the skin. Some lotions are not effective, and emollients should be chosen carefully to prevent excessive skin drying.

BOX 32.3 Clinical Manifestations of Atopic Dermatitis

Distribution of Lesions

- **Infantile form**—Generalised, especially face, scalp, neck and extensor surfaces of extremities
- **Childhood form**—Flexural areas (antecubital and popliteal fossae, neck), wrists, ankles and feet
- **Preadolescent and adolescent form**—Face, sides of neck, hands, feet, face and antecubital and popliteal fossae (to a lesser extent)

Appearance of Lesions

Infantile Form

- Erythema
- Vesicles
- Papules
- Weeping
- Oozing
- Crusting
- Scaling
- Often symmetrical

Childhood Form

- Symmetrical involvement
- Clusters of small erythematous or flesh-coloured papules or minimally scaling patches
- Dry and may be hyperpigmented
- Lichenification (thickened skin with accentuation of creases)
- Keratosis pilaris (follicular hyperkeratosis) common

Adolescent or Adult Form

- Same as childhood manifestations
- Dry, thick lesions (lichenified plaques) common
- Confluent papules

Other Physical Manifestations

- Intense itching
- Unaffected skin dry and rough
- May exhibit one or more of the following:
  - lymphadenopathy, especially near affected sites
  - increased palmar creases (many cases)
  - atopic pleats (extra line or groove of lower eyelid)
  - prone to cold hands
  - pityriasis alba (small, poorly defined areas of hypopigmentation)
  - facial pallor (especially around nose, mouth and ears)
  - bluish discolouration beneath eyes ('allergic shiners')
  - increased susceptibility to unusual cutaneous infections (especially viral)

Soap free skin cleaners such as Cetaphil are acceptable lotions for skin hydration. A night-time bath followed by emollient application and dressing in soft cotton pyjamas or use of wet wraps may help alleviate most night-time pruritus.

Oral antihistamine drugs (such as Polaramine) usually relieve moderate or severe pruritus. Non-sedating antihistamines such as loratadine (Claratyne) or fexofenadine (Telfast) may be preferred for daytime pruritus relief. Because pruritus increases at night, a mildly sedating antihistamine may be needed.

Occasional flare-ups require the use of topical steroids to diminish inflammation. Low-, moderate- or high-potency topical corticosteroids are prescribed, depending on the degree of involvement, the area of the body to be treated, the child's age, the potential for local side effects (striae, skin atrophy and pigment changes) and the type of vehicle to be used (e.g. cream, lotion, ointment). Patients receiving topical corticosteroid therapy for chronic conditions should be evaluated for risk factors for suboptimal linear growth and reduced bone density. Topical immunomodulators, a non-steroidal treatment for AD, are best used at the beginning of a 'flare-up' just as the skin becomes red and itches. Second-line management for children with AD includes immunomodulator medications such as pimecrolimus (Langan et al 2020). Pimecrolimus is a short term medication only and only approved for the use in children 3 months and above (Langan et al 2020).

If secondary skin infections occur in children with AD, these infections are managed with appropriate systemic antibiotics. Obtaining cultures from affected areas and the child's nares is helpful to ensure appropriate therapy (Page et al 2016).

Nursing Care Management

Assessment of the child with AD includes a family history for evidence of atopy, a history of previous involvement and any environmental or dietary factors associated with the present and previous exacerbations. The skin lesions are examined for type, distribution and evidence of secondary infection. Parents are interviewed regarding the child's behaviour, especially in relation to scratching, irritability and sleeping patterns. Exploration of the family's feelings and methods of coping is also important.

Wet wraps and compresses are applied and medications for pruritus or infection are administered as directed. The family is given explicit instructions on the preparation and use of soaks, special baths and topical medications, including the order of application if more than one is prescribed. It is important to emphasise that one thick application of topical medication is *not* equivalent to several thin applications and that excessive use of an agent (particularly steroids) can be hazardous. If children have difficulty remaining still for a 10- or 15-minute soak, bath or dressing application, these can be carried out at naptime or when the child is engrossed in watching television, listening to a story or playing with bath toys. For more severe cases, wet wraps which are the application of wet dressings using tubular elastic bandages that are worn at night-time have been shown to alleviate the itching and severity of the condition. More information on the use and application of wet wraps or wet dressings can be found through the Royal Children's Hospital Melbourne website Kid's Health Info (Eczema).

Diet modification may prevent skin exacerbations. When a hypoallergenic diet is prescribed, parents need help to understand the reason for the diet and the guidelines for avoiding hyperallergenic foods. Because hypoallergenic diets take time before visible effects are apparent, parents need reassurance that results may not be seen immediately. If airborne allergens make eczema worse, the family is counselled about 'allergy proofing' the home (see Asthma, Chapter 26).

Family Support. Parents are assured that the lesions will not produce scarring (unless secondarily infected) and that the disease is not contagious. However, the child may have repeated exacerbations and remissions. Spontaneous and permanent remission takes place at approximately 2 to 3 years of age in most children with the infantile disorder.

During acute phases, emotional stress can become intense for the family. They need time to discuss negative feelings and to be reassured that these feelings are normal. Stress tends to aggravate the severity of the condition. Therefore, efforts to relieve as much anxiety as possible in both the parents and the child have a beneficial emotional and physical effect.

Seborrhoeic Dermatitis

Seborrhoeic dermatitis is a chronic, recurrent, inflammatory reaction of the skin. It occurs most commonly on the scalp (cradle cap) but may involve the eyelids (blepharitis), external ear canal (otitis externa), nasolabial folds and inguinal region. The cause is unknown, although it is more common in early infancy, when sebum production is increased. The lesions are characteristically thick, adherent, yellowish, scaly, oily patches that may or may not be mildly pruritic. Unlike AD, seborrhoeic dermatitis is not associated with a positive family history for allergy and is common in infants shortly after birth and in adolescents after puberty. Diagnosis is made primarily on the basis of the appearance and the location of the crusts or scales.

Nursing Care Management

Cradle cap may be prevented with adequate scalp hygiene. Frequently, parents omit shampooing the infant's hair for fear of damaging the 'soft spots', or fontanels. The nurse should discuss how to shampoo the infant's hair and emphasise that the fontanel is similar to skin anywhere else on the body—it does not puncture or tear with mild pressure.

Acne

Acne vulgaris is the most common skin problem treated by doctors during adolescence. Acne is caused by testosterone, a hormone present in boys and girls that increases during puberty. It stimulates the sebaceous glands of the skin to enlarge, or produce oil, and plug the pores. Comedogenesis (formation of comedones) results in a non-inflammatory lesion that may be either an open comedone ('blackhead') or a closed comedone ('whitehead').

Acne affects more than 90% of Australian teenagers (Gebauer 2018). Although the disorder can appear before the age of 10 years, the peak incidence occurs in middle to late adolescence (age 16 to 17 years in girls and 17 to 18 years in boys). It is more common in boys than in girls. After this age period, the disease usually decreases in severity, but it may persist into adulthood. The degree to which an individual is affected may range from nothing more than a few isolated comedones to a severe inflammatory reaction. Although the disease is self-limiting and not life-threatening, it has great significance to adolescents who can suffer higher levels of anxiety, depression and low self-esteem (Zaenglin 2018) and can cause permanent scarring (Gebauer 2018). Health professionals should not underestimate the impact that acne has on teenagers.

Numerous factors affect the development and course of acne. Its distribution in families and a high degree of concordance in identical twins suggest hereditary factors (Zaenglein 2018). Premenstrual flare-ups of acne occur in nearly 70% of adolescent girls, suggesting a hormonal cause. Studies do not indicate a clear association between stress and acne, but adolescents commonly cite stress as a cause for acne outbreaks. Cosmetics containing lanolin, petrolatum, vegetable oils, lauryl alcohol, butyl stearate and oleic acid can increase comedone production. Exposure to oils in cooking grease can be a precursor in adolescents who work over fast-food restaurant hot oils. There may be an association with the intake of dairy products and high glycaemic index foods that may potentiate hormonal and inflammatory factors that contribute to acne severity. In patients with known insulin resistance there has been demonstrated improvement in acne with a low-glycaemic diet; however, in others results are less convincing with link of dietary influences including milk and dairy products unclear (Fiedler et al 2017, Zaenglein 2018).

Pathophysiology

Four pathophysiological factors have the greatest influence on acne development: (1) excessive sebum production; (2) alterations in follicular growth; (3) differentiation with colonisation of *Propionibacterium acnes*; and (4) an accompanying immune response and inflammation (Bhat et al 2017). Acne severity is proportional to the sebum secretion rate, which is genetically determined and increases at the time of adrenocortical maturation. Inflammation occurs with the proliferation of *P. acnes,* which draws in neutrophils, causing inflammatory papules, pustules, nodules and cysts (Fig 32.8). Acne can be categorised as comedonal, inflammatory or both and can be classified as mild, moderate or severe based on the number and type of comedones, extent of affected skin and systemic involvement (Zaenglein 2018).

Therapeutic Management

Successful management of acne depends on a cooperative effort among the healthcare provider, adolescent and parents. Unlike many other dermatological conditions, acne lesions resolve slowly and improvement may not be apparent for at least 6 weeks. Individual comedones can take several weeks to months to resolve, and papules and pustules usually resolve in about 1 week. The multifactorial causes of acne necessitate a combined approach for successful treatment. Treatment consists of general measures of care and specific treatments determined by the type of lesions involved.

General Measures. The practitioner provides the adolescent with an overall explanation of the disease process, emphasising the patient's involvement. Improvement of the adolescent's overall health status is part of the general management. Adequate rest, moderate exercise, a well-balanced diet, reduction of emotional stress and elimination of any foci of infection are all part of general health promotion.

Cleansing. Dirt or oil on the surface of the skin does not cause acne. Gentle cleansing with a mild cleanser once or twice daily is usually sufficient. Antibacterial soaps are ineffective and may cause dryness when used in combination with topical acne medications. For some adolescents, hygiene of the hair and scalp appears to be related to the clinical activity of the acne. Acne on the forehead may improve with brushing the hair away from the forehead and more frequent shampooing. Heavy cleaning and poor quality, cheaper soaps can exacerbate the problem (Gebauer 2017).

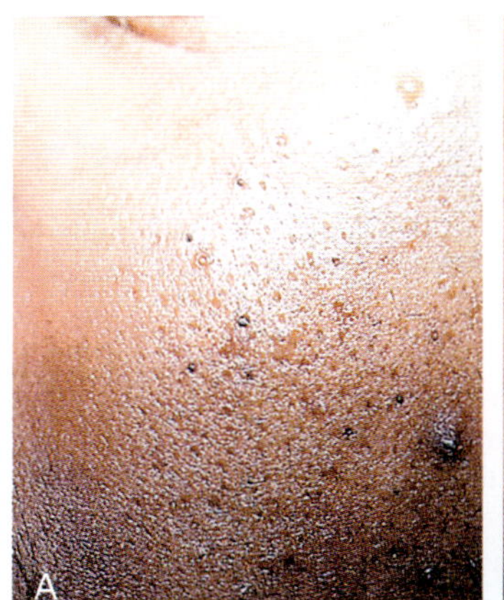

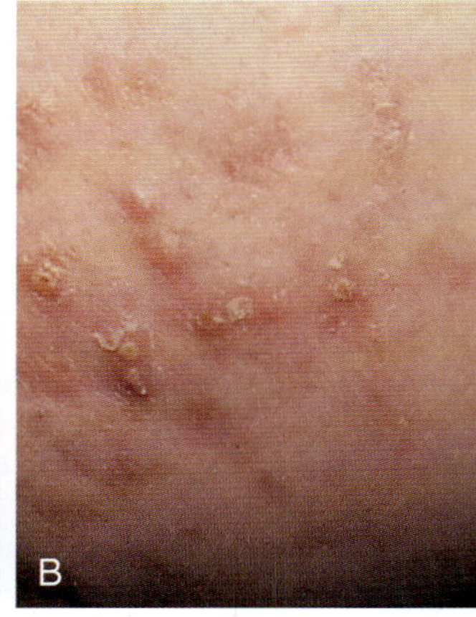

Fig 32.8 Acne vulgaris. (**A**) Acne vulgaris. (**B**) Comedones with a few inflammatory pustules. (Source: Zitelli, B. J., McIntire, S. C., & Nowalk, A. J. (2012). Zitelli and Davis' atlas of pediatric physical diagnosis (6th ed.). St Louis, MO: Saunders.)

Medications. Treatment success depends on commitment from the adolescent. Before prescribing treatment, the practitioner should determine the adolescent's level of comfort and readiness to begin treatment. The adolescent should be reminded that clinical improvement may take weeks to months. Early intervention, most often with topical medications, may prevent the development of more severe acne.

Tretinoin (ReTrieve Cream, Stieva-A) is often used to treat acne vulgaris where papules and/or pustules are predominate. The cream is applied to the lesions nightly for up to at least 6-8 weeks with the aim to decrease when the acne responds satisfactorily to treatment. The cream can cause significant and ongoing side effects during use and is not suitable for all children/adolescents. Transient stinging, overwhelming feeling of warmth to the area of use, peeling, erythema and changes to pigmentation can be experienced. Photosensitivity can developed, reversible elevation of liver enzymes and bilirubin. On the rare occasion allergy and contact dermatitis is experienced. Tretinoin should be used solely on its own and it is not recommended as montherapy for deep cystic nodular acne or severe pustular acne. If the acne does not improve within 6–8 weeks of use further assessment with general practitioner or dermatologist should be followed up before continuing use.

Topical **benzoyl peroxide** is an antibacterial agent that inhibits the growth of *P. acnes* organisms. It is effective against both inflammatory and non-inflammatory acne and is an effective first-line agent. This medication is available as a cream, gel or wash. Benzoyl peroxide and salicylic acid are the most effective acne treatment kits available over the counter. The patient should be informed that the medication may have a bleaching effect on sheets, bedclothes and towels. The adolescent can be reassured that skin bleaching will not occur. Accommodation to the medication can be gained with a gradual increase in the strength and frequency of application.

When inflammatory lesions accompany the comedones, a **topical antibacterial agent** may be prescribed. These agents are used to prevent new lesions and to treat pre-existing acne. Dapsone gel has demonstrated efficacy in treatment of inflammatory acne (Zaenglein 2018). Retinoid in combination with antimicrobials also improves the penetration of these topical agents and is the only means to address three of the pathogenic causes of acne: keratinisation, *P. acnes* and inflammation. Side effects of the topical medications include erythema, dryness and burning; using the medications every other day will decrease the adverse effects.

Systemic antibiotic therapy is initiated when moderate to severe acne does not respond to topical treatments. The foundation for using systemic antibiotics in acne treatment has been the elimination of the inflammatory effects of *P. acnes* by suppressing the bacteria and should be used in combination with topical retinoids and benzoyl peroxide but use of oral antibiotics should be limited to 3- to 4-month courses due to increasing microbial resistance. Adolescent girls with mild to moderate acne may respond well to topical treatment and the addition of an **oral contraceptive pill (OCP)** (Gebauer 2018). OCPs reduce the endogenous androgen production and decrease the bioavailability of the woman's circulating androgens. Both of these actions result in decreased acne.

Isotretinoin, 13-*cis*-retinoic acid (Oratane, Roaccutane), is a potent and effective oral agent that is reserved for severe cystic acne that has not responded to other treatments. Isotretinoin is the only agent available that affects factors involved in the development of acne. However, treatment with isotretinoin should be managed *only* by a dermatologist. Adolescents with multiple, active, deep dermal or subcutaneous cystic and nodular acne lesions are treated for 20 weeks. Multiple side effects can occur, including dry skin and mucous membranes, nasal irritation, dry eyes, decreased night vision, photosensitivity, arthralgia, headaches, mood changes, aggressive or violent behaviours, depression and suicidal ideation. Adolescents taking this drug should be monitored for depression, depressive symptoms and suicidal ideation (Oliveira et al 2018). The drug should be given only at the recommended doses for no longer than the recommended duration. The most significant side effects of this drug are the teratogenic effects. Isotretinoin is absolutely contraindicated in pregnant women. Sexually active young women must use an effective contraceptive method during treatment and for 1 month after treatment. Patients receiving isotretinoin should also be monitored for elevated cholesterol and triglyceride levels. Significant elevation may require discontinuation of the medication.

Nursing Care Management

Because acne is so common and its appearance may seem so mild, the healthcare provider may underestimate the relative importance of the disease to the adolescent. The nurse should assess the individual adolescent's level of distress, current management and perceived success of any regimen before initiating a referral. If adolescents do not perceive the acne to be a problem, they may lack motivation to follow the treatment plan.

The nurse can provide ongoing support for the adolescent when a treatment plan is initiated. Discuss the use of medications and basic skin care information in detail with the adolescent. Written instructions should accompany the verbal discussion. Information to dispel myths regarding the use of abrasive cleansing products can prevent unnecessary costs and trauma to the skin. Adolescents need education about the factors that aggravate and damage the skin, such as too vigorous scrubbing. In addition, picking, squeezing and manual expression with fingernails break down the ductal walls of lesions and cause the acne to worsen.

COLD INJURY

In cold injuries the nature of the heat-regulating mechanisms of the body are such that the inner portion of the body, or core, produces heat and the periphery, or outer area, conserves or dissipates heat. When the body attempts to conserve heat, the outer tissues are subjected to low temperatures and local trauma may result.

Chilblain, redness and swelling of the skin, occurs when extremities, usually the hands, are exposed intermittently to temperatures of 1.1°C to 15.5°C. The response may vary but is characterised by intense vasodilation that increases the temperature of involved tissues above that of unaffected tissue and produces oedematous, reddish blue patches that itch and burn. As warming takes place, the sensations become more intense, but ordinarily they subside in a few days.

Frostbite is the term used to describe tissue damage caused when excessive heat loss to local tissues allows ice crystals to form in tissues. The frostbitten part appears white or blanched, feels solid and is without sensation. Rapid rewarming is associated with less tissue necrosis than slow thawing. It restores blood flow and shortens the period of cellular damage. Rewarming produces a flush (sometimes deep purple) and a return of sensation, which is extremely painful. Large blisters may appear in 24 to 48 hours after rewarming and begin to reabsorb within 5 to 10 days followed by the formation of a hard black eschar. Superficial injury often heals without incident. Rewarming is accomplished by immersing the part in well-agitated water at 37.8°C to 42.2°C. Discomfort is managed with analgesics and sedatives. Care of blistered skin is similar to that described for burns. It is seldom possible to estimate the extent of tissue loss until new skin layers are revealed after the eschar layer separates.

REFERENCES

Alzomor, O., Alfawaz, T., & Alshahrani, D. (2017). Invasive community-acquired methicillin-resistant Staphylococcus aureus (CA-MRSA) infection in children: case series and literature review. International Journal of Pediatrics & Adolescent Medicine, 4(3), 119–123. https://www.sciencedirect.com/science/article/pii/S2352646717300595?via%3Dihub

Aung, P., Cuningham, W., Hwang, K., et al. (2018). Scabies and risk of skin sores in remote Australian Aboriginal communities: A self-controlled case series study. PLoS Neglected Tropical Diseases, 12(7), e0006668.

Australasian Society of Clinical Immunology and Allergy (ASCIA). (2019). Contact dermatitis. Plants may also cause allergic contact dermatitis. https://www.allergy.org.au/patients/skin-allergy/contact-dermatitis

Bhat, Y. J., Latief, I., & Hassan, I. (2017). Update on etiopathogenesis and treatment of acne. Indian Journal of Dermatology, Venereology and Leprology, 83(3), 298–306.

Castellsague, J., Kuiper, J., Pottegård, A., et al. (2018). A cohort study on the risk of lymphoma and skin cancer in users of topical tacrolimus, pimecrolimus, and corticosteroids (Joint European Longitudinal Lymphoma and Skin Cancer Evaluation – JOELLE study). Clinical Epidemiology, 10, 299–310.

Chopra, R., Vakharia, P., Sacotte, R., et al. (2017). Efficacy of bleach baths in reducing severity of atopic dermatitis: A systematic review and meta-analysis. Annals of Allergy, Asthma & Immunology, 119(5), 435–440.

de Jesus, L., Martins, A., Oliveira, P., et al. (2018). Negative pressure wound therapy in pediatric surgery: How and when to use. Journal of Pediatric Surgery, 53(4), 585–591.

Fiedler, F., Stangl, G. I., Fiedler, E., et al. (2017). Acne and nutrition: A systematic review. Acta Dermato-Venereologica, 97(1), 7–9.

Gebauer, K. (2017). Acne in adolescents. Australian Family Physician, 46(12), 892–895.

Graves, S., & Stenos, J. (2017). Tick-borne infectious diseases in Australia. Medical Journal of Australia, 206(7), 320–324.

Haddad, V., Haddad, M., Santos, M., et al. (2018). Skin manifestations of tick bites in humans. Anais Brasileiros de Dermatologia, 93(2), 251–255.

Hardy, M., Engelmann, D. & Steer, A. (2017). Scabies: A clinical update. *Focus:* The Royal Australian College of General Practitioners, 46(5), 264–268. https://www.racgp.org.au/download/Documents/AFP/2017/May/AFP-MAY-Focus-Steer.pdf

Holm, J. G., Agner, T., Clausen, M. L., et al. (2016). Quality of life and disease severity in patients with atopic dermatitis. Journal of the European Academy of Dermatology and Venereology, 30(1), 1760–1767.

Kearns, T., Speare, R., Cheng, A., et al. (2015). Impact of an ivermectin mass drug administration on scabies prevalence in a remote Australian Aboriginal community. PLoS Neglected Tropical Diseases, 9(10). doi:10.1371/journal.pntd.0004151

Khurram, M., Sarfraz A., & Yaseen, M. (2019). Vacuum-assisted wound closure therapy in pediatric lower limb trauma. The International Journal of Lower Extremity Wounds, 18(3), 317–322.

Langan, S., Irvine, A. & Weidinger, S. (2020). Atopic dermatitis. The Lancet (British edition), 396(10247), 345–360.

Nelson, C., Saha, S. & Mead, P. (2016). Cat-scratch disease in the United States, 2005-2013. Emerging Infectious Diseases, 22(10), 1741–1746.

Oliveira, J. M., Sobreira, G., Velosa, J., et al. (2018). Association of isotretinoin with depression and suicide: A review of current literature. Journal of Cutaneous Medicine and Surgery, 22(1), 58–64.

Page, S. S., Weston, S., & Loh, R. (2016). Atopic dermatitis in children. Australian Family Physician, 45(5), 293–296.

Pelletier, J., Perez, C. & Jacob, S. (2016). Contact Dermatitis in Pediatrics. Pediatric Annals, 45(8), e287–e292.

Queensland Government. (2019). Head lice. 26 April. http://conditions.health.qld.gov.au/HealthCondition/condition/14/165/351/Head-Lice

Queensland Government. (2020). Australian Bat Lyssavirus. 27 August. http://conditions.health.qld.gov.au/HealthCondition/condition/14/217/10/australian-bat-lyssavirus

Raymond, S., Zecevic, A., Larson, S., et al. (2018). Delayed Healing Associated with Silver Sulfadiazine Use for Partial Thickness Scald Burns in Children. The American Surgeon, 84(6), 836–840.

Saini, S. & Pansare, M. (2019). New insights and treatments in atopic dermatitis. Pediatric Clinics of North America, 66(5), 1021–1033.

Thomas. J., Christenson, J., Walker, E., et al. (2017). Scabies—An ancient itch that is still rampant today. Journal of Clinical Pharmacy and Therapeutics, 42(6), 793–799, https://doi.org/10.1111/jcpt.12631

Zaenglein, A. (2018). Acne vulgaris. 'The New England Journal of Medicine, 379(14), 1343–1352. https://pubmed.ncbi.nlm.nih.gov/30281982/

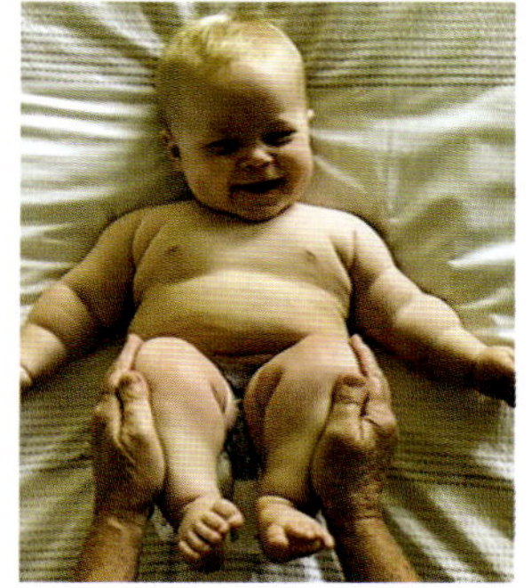

33

The Child with Musculoskeletal or Articular Dysfunction

Patience Moyo

LEARNING OUTCOMES

- Discuss the pathophysiology of various musculoskeletal or articular dysfunctions that are prevalent among children.
- Discuss the clinical manifestations of various musculoskeletal or articular dysfunctions that are common among children.
- Describe the nursing care/management of a child with a musculoskeletal or articular dysfunction.
- Describe the support mechanisms for the children's family/carer during the management of musculoskeletal or articular dysfunctions.
- Discuss the potential complications of musculoskeletal or articular dysfunctions in children and identify the strategies that are necessary to prevent the identified complications.

THE CHILD AND TRAUMA

Trauma Management

Epidemiology of Trauma

Trauma is a leading cause of death in children older than age 1 year (see Chapter 1) and an important cause of disability during childhood and adolescence. In many ways, childhood trauma differs little from trauma in adults. However, the child's developmental stage affects many aspects of injury, including the type of injury incurred and the physiological response to injury.

Unintentional injuries are the leading cause of death in children 0 to 14 years of age in Australia. In this age group, 88% of all deaths are noted to come from unintentional injuries, with motor vehicle crashes accounting for the largest percentage of deaths (Kidsafe WA 2018).

Childhood Characteristics

Certain developmental characteristics of children at various ages render them more susceptible to injury. For example, the large head of infants and toddlers predisposes them to head injury, especially in falls or motor vehicle injuries. Also, the relatively large spleen and liver and the broad costal arch make these structures prone to direct trauma. Because of their light weight and small size, infants and small children are easily thrown around in a moving vehicle. Their natural curiosity and their propensity for using large muscles lure them to attempt potentially hazardous activities.

Later, in school-age children and adolescents, whose bone growth outstrips muscle growth, difficulty controlling movement can contribute to physical injury. This is also a time when many children attempt to engage in activities beyond their physical capabilities to keep up with more agile companions and to meet the expectations of adults and older siblings. They are also vulnerable to a 'dare'. Risk-taking compounded by a feeling of invulnerability is also characteristic of adolescence. Children of school age and early adolescence may also be encouraged to continue engaging in sports activities after suffering a contusion or injury and are therefore subject to repetitive injuries.

Unintentional or Accidental Injury

Among the leading causes of morbidity in children are medical problems resulting from traumatic injury that occurs at home or school, in a motor vehicle or in association with recreational activities. Children's everyday activities include vigorous play that may involve such things as climbing, falling, running into immovable objects and receiving blows to any part of the body. All of these activities make them prone to injury. School-age children and adolescents are vulnerable to multiple and severe trauma because they are mobile on bikes, motorcycles and/or vehicles; they are also active in sports. Speed and congested surroundings often increase the chance of injury.

Young children and adolescents usually do not calculate risks as they learn to manipulate their environment and achieve developmental goals. Therefore, accidents are a part of many childhood experiences. Fortunately, when children fall or are hit, their body's resilience protects them from serious damage to soft tissue, the musculoskeletal system or other body organs. Their bones are more flexible with less density than those of adults and therefore do not offer the rigid resistance to external forces making it more likely for a child to sustain a fracture.

Child Abuse or Non-accidental Injury

Unfortunately, careless handling of an infant or child (in some instances intentional physical abuse) is not uncommon. A multitude of different types of bone and soft tissue injury are inflicted on children by adults, and smaller children who are unable to protect themselves are most vulnerable.

A traumatic incident that produces physical injury to an infant or child may be the outcome of an accident that was no one's fault, or it may be associated with child abuse. A well-documented history and a careful examination are essential to determine the cause of the injury. Emergency department (ED) and paediatric health professionals should be alert to situations in which the child's injuries are not congruent with the parent's description of the incident; the child's behaviours, such as fearful mannerisms or lack of crying, are not the expected ones; or radiographs show multiple healed fractures. Accounts of injury inconsistent with developmental abilities can alert the provider to possible abuse as well. For example, a 6-month-old infant cannot 'climb out of the cot and break her leg'. Reporting these incidents will aid in securing help for the child and family. Mandatory reporting is a requirement as governed by the various state/territory child protection legislation such as the *Child and Young Persons (Care and Protection) Act 1998* (NSW) or the *Child & Young People Act 2008* (ACT). (See Nursing Care Considerations box.)

NURSING CARE CONSIDERATIONS

Distinguishing Unintentional From Intentional Fractures

Distinguishing abusive (non-accidental) from unintentional fractures can be challenging. The history, location of the injury, radiographs and associated injuries must be carefully considered. Details of the history to consider include delay in seeking medical care and an inappropriate clinical history or the report of a change in the child's health, behaviour or activity level but no report of injury. The history should be collected from the carer or person accompanying the child as well as from the child when relevant and safe to do so. It is important that the child's actual words are recorded. Open-ended questions must be used to avoid questions that insinuate that a particular individual is responsible for the injuries. Statements made by the child during the physical examination should be recorded verbatim.

Studies have shown that children less than 2 years of age and those that were born prematurely or have comorbid medical conditions are more likely to suffer a non-accidental injury. In addition, risk of abuse is increased if parents feel isolated, perceive an absence of support or lack a connection to the community. The average age for children who presented with non-accidental fractures was 9.7 months (Stephens & Oates 2014). The most common fractures in non-accidental injury involved the skull, and most of these fractures occurred in children between 4 to 12 years of age (Stephens & Oates 2014).

Although not diagnostic of an intentional injury, the location of a fracture can raise suspicions about the actual cause. In an infant, midshaft or metaphyseal humerus fractures and radius-ulna, tibia-fibula and femur fractures are not common and raise suspicion about the likelihood of abuse. Rib fractures, scapular fractures, bilateral fractures, complex skull fractures and vertebral fractures or subluxations are also suspicious. In contrast, in children older than 1 year of age, supracondylar humerus fractures and fractures of the clavicle, distal extremity and femur are most frequently related to an unintentional or accidental injury.

In children of all ages, radiographic evidence of previous fractures at different stages of healing may indicate repeated trauma and raise concern about intentional injuries. The presence of bruises, burns and additional soft tissue injuries in children may also prompt further evaluation to determine whether the child has been subjected to intentional harm. One mnemonic used to prompt consideration of the possibility of intentional physical abuse is the five Bs:

Bumps
Bruises
Breaks
Burns
anything that happens in the **B**athroom.

There are some guidelines which have been developed to help healthcare professionals to identify non-accidental injuries such as the New South Wales Health Suspected Child Abuse and Neglect (SCAN) Medical Protocol (Appendix 1) available via the following link: https://www1.health.nsw.gov.au/pds/ActivePDSDocuments/GL2014_012.pdf

Prevention of Injury

Increasingly, healthcare providers are recognising the importance of injury prevention efforts in preserving the health and wellbeing of children. Nurses have an important role to play in these efforts.

Leading causes of non-fatal injury to children include falls, being struck by or against an object, motor vehicle or transportation-related accidents, overexertion, bites or stings and being cut or pierced. Falls are the leading cause of non-fatal injury among children ages 0 to 14 years. Being struck by or against a person or object is the leading cause of non-fatal injury in older children 15 to 19 years of age. Foreign body causes occur in young children, especially those between 0 and 4 years of age, whereas sports injuries or overexertion occur in school-age children and adolescents (Centers for Disease Control and Prevention 2015).

Unintentional, preventable injury is the primary cause of paediatric mortality and a significant contributor to morbidity, including permanent disability. Both morbidity and mortality rates could be reduced dramatically by improved efforts at injury prevention. Studies have indicated a general lack of public awareness regarding risks, causes and prevention of injury to children. Studies also show that injury prevention counselling is effective both in reducing hazards in the home and in increasing car seat use. Nurses can be active in legislative efforts, public awareness campaigns, group classes on injury prevention and individual prevention counselling with children and families.

Nurses in ED and outpatient clinic settings can provide instructions related to injury prevention on an individual basis as developmentally appropriate.

Accident prevention among adolescents presents a unique challenge to all healthcare workers. For accident prevention to be effective, adolescents must perceive the specific interventions as having an impact on their lives. Adolescents are concerned with body image and often feel indestructible unless their own life or the life of a close friend is touched by a catastrophic debilitating injury or death. With increased emphasis in society on having fun and enjoying life to its fullest (today) regardless of the consequences (tomorrow), it is difficult for adolescents to understand the need to follow the rules laid down by authority figures.

Concern is also increasing about injuries to older school-age children and adolescents from the use of motorcycles (for which many states have no laws on minimum age for riders), skateboards, scooters and motor vehicles. Activities involving such vehicles and equipment, although safe in and of themselves when conducted according to safety guidelines (of the manufacturer), may be dangerous for children and adolescents who are unable to appreciate the risks involved, not only to self, but to others as well. Adolescents are known for taking risks, and the approval of their peers often compounds risk-taking behaviours in games such as car surfing and breath-holding games. Parents may not be aware that their teens are partaking in such games which are present in the online environment and a frank discussion between parents and adolescents may be required. Nurses who work with adolescents and their families need to be aware of such games and be ready to discuss the effects of risk-taking with teens.

Emergency Management

The Nursing Care Considerations box outlines guidelines for care of the child at the scene of an injury. After level of consciousness is assessed, the concerns are for airway, breathing and circulation (ABC), after which other injuries are managed as indicated by the assessment. When spinal trauma is a possibility, open the airway using the modified jaw thrust manoeuvre, which is accomplished by grasping the angles of the victim's lower jaw and lifting with both hands, one on each side, and displacing the mandible upwards and outwards (without head tilt or chin lift). Otherwise a head tilt–chin lift manoeuvre is effective in opening the victim's airway.

NURSING CARE CONSIDERATIONS

Trauma

Before entering trauma area, observe for potential threats or dangers to rescuers and bystanders. Be aware of potential for further injuries to the child.

Observe scene for signs and mechanism of injury (e.g. head-on motor vehicle injury), which helps determine proper course of action for treating the child's injuries.

Do not move child before arrival of the medical emergency team (MET) unless the child is in danger of further injury. If it is necessary to move the child, follow appropriate steps to prevent further injury (e.g. stabilise cervical spine to avoid exacerbation of spinal injury during movement).

Primary Assessment and Intervention

A primary survey should be conducted following the mnemonic DRSABCDE (Danger, Response, Send for help, Airway, Breathing, Circulation, Disability and Exposure). Any life-threatening problem(s) noted during any stage should be treated first or escalated immediately prior to moving onto the next step of the assessment.

Assess level of consciousness. Use the AVPU method.

A—Child is **a**lert.
V—Child responds to **v**erbal stimulus.
P—Child responds to **p**ainful stimulus.
U—Child is **u**nresponsive to any stimulus.

Open airway, using the appropriate method.

- In a child with head, trunk or multisystem trauma, modified jaw thrust is preferred method.
- At this point, cervical spine should be manually immobilised and held in alignment with rest of spinal column and should not be released until MET personnel have immobilised the child with appropriate equipment.

Activate the rapid response system or MET call if the child appears to be pubertal or older or if you witnessed sudden collapse. If the child has not reached puberty, perform 2 minutes of cardiopulmonary resuscitation (CPR) (as per assessment); then activate the rapid response system or MET call and call for an automatic external defibrillator (AED).

If no response to stimulation and no pulse is detected, begin chest compressions. Compress at a rate of at least 100 to 120 compressions per minute.*

After 15 compressions administer 2 breaths—each breath is administered over 1 second. Avoid overventilating.*

Continue chest compressions and ventilations until person shows signs of responsiveness, breathing or MET arrives.

If an AED with paediatric capability is available, apply the paediatric pads, turn on the AED and follow the AED directions. Avoid interrupting chest compressions for more than 10 seconds.*

A pulse check may be made if 5 cycles of 15 compressions and 2 breaths have been administered.*

- Palpate carotid artery in children 1 year or older.
- Palpate brachial artery in infants younger than 1 year.

If pulse present, assess for breathing. If necessary, begin rescue breathing.*

Observe for haemorrhage. If the child has severe life-threatening bleeding, control of bleeding should be prioritised over management of airway and breathing problems (Australian Resuscitation Council [ARC] 2017, p. 1).

Prior to controlling bleeding, there is need to don appropriate personal protective equipment (PPE) as per standard precautions (e.g. gloves, goggles).

Control bleeding with a gloved or protected hand.

1. Apply direct firm pressure to wound site using hand(s) or pad.
2. Elevate wound site.
3. Apply pressure to appropriate arterial pressure point.

If competent, apply an arterial tourniquet above the bleeding point only as a last resort if there is life-threatening bleeding which is not controlled by firm pressure application to the wound (ANZCOR Guideline 9.1.1 2017, p. 1). Once a tourniquet is applied, it should not be loosened. If a tourniquet is not available, ineffective or cannot be applied, then apply a haemostatic dressing. It is important to also consider having the child lie down and be still and immobilise the limb to restrict movement to aid in controlling bleeding as appropriate (ANZCOR Guideline 9.1.1 2017, p. 1) .

Assess for further injury.

Do not remove objects protruding from child's body but rather apply pressure around the object.

Check for evidence of decreased motor or sensory function in extremities.

- Infant and young child—Observe spontaneous movement in extremities.
- Older child—Ask if able to wiggle extremities.

Evaluate pain—Present, absent; severe, mild.

- Attempt to alleviate with non-pharmacological techniques.
- Encourage use of analgesics when emergency personnel arrive.

Assess pulses in extremity distal to injury.

- Check colour and temperature of extremities.

Manage any injuries appropriately (e.g. splint fractures)

Maintain body heat.

Identify child.

Obtain information regarding the injury from witnesses, if any.

*Further reading: For detailed instructions for performing CPR, see The Australian Resuscitation Guidelines at: https://resus.org.au/guidelines/

Spinal cord injury is always suspected in a patient with any injuries above the shoulders (e.g. head, trunk or multisystem trauma). Only in a fully equipped trauma centre with radiography and other diagnostic testing such as computed tomography (CT) or magnetic resonance imaging (MRI) can spinal cord injury be ruled out or diagnosed. Therefore, the patient is treated as if the spinal cord injury were present, until cleared for spinal precautions by a medical officer. Immobilise the cervical spine by maintaining the head in a neutral position and not allowing movement of the head or body in any direction. Padding of approximately 2.5 cm may be required under a child's shoulders for those below the age of 8 years (ARC 2016, p. 4).

NURSING CARE CONSIDERATIONS

In any situation in which spinal cord injury is suspected or is a possibility, the child should be calmed, reassured and told not to move. *No one should be allowed to move the child unless the entire spine is stabilised.* A rigid cervical collar is used to immobilise the cervical spine, and the child is placed supine on a rigid immobilisation board. Infants and small children are removed from a vehicle in their car seats; no attempt should be made to take them out of their seats unless medically necessary.

Assessment of the child involves observation from head to toe because infants and young children are unable to communicate except by crying and other behaviours. Therefore, pinpointing areas of pain is difficult. To check for any motor or sensory dysfunction in the extremities, the nurse should note any spontaneous movement, which provides the best clue in infants and young children. Older children are able to follow directions to wiggle toes or fingers, demonstrate a grasp, 'push down on the pedal' or lift legs off the floor or stretcher. It is important to determine whether the child has any existing health problems that might have implications for the circumstances of the injury and for therapeutic management. Ask any witnesses for details about the incident to aid in assessment of the child's emotional responses.

In the prehospital setting, the nurse's role consists of contacting MET and providing basic life support until MET personnel arrive on the scene. The nurse's role is limited to basic life support because the nurse has no standing orders or protocols under which to work in the prehospital setting (see Nursing Care Considerations box). Call the MET as soon as possible so that the patient can receive advanced life support before and during transport. A paediatric trauma triage system with personnel designated to care for an injured child is essential to provide excellent trauma patient care.

Attempting to transport a child by vehicle wastes valuable time in obtaining help. Transportation by the MET is recommended. Services in most large communities can institute advanced life support immediately or en route to a medical facility.

NURSING CARE CONSIDERATIONS

It is imperative that the MET be called to respond as soon as possible. Family, friends or strangers should *not* transport the trauma victim.

Systematic Assessment

Several factors can affect a child's response to trauma. An undetected congenital anomaly can contribute to a complicated injury. Acute gastric distension occurs frequently in children because of the crying and screaming that accompany an injury. The temperature of young children is unstable because of their large surface area in relation to body mass, and temperature maintenance is critical in trauma management. Children also experience rapid metabolic changes. When they are ill, children are really ill, but as they recover, they change very rapidly. In addition, children have a small volume of blood in absolute terms. Whereas blood volume is 60% of total body weight in the adult, it is 70% to 85% in the child.

The first priority on admission to an emergency facility is rapid assessment of ABC status. Because the overwhelming majority of childhood injuries are the result of blunt-impact trauma, multiple organ involvement is a common finding. Therefore, it is essential to perform a systematic assessment of the trauma victim.

The secondary survey is a systematic head-to-toe search for any additional injuries not originally addressed in the primary survey. However, children are often an exception to the head-to-toe approach. It may be preferable to complete the secondary survey on the injured child in a toe-to-head direction. This approach may allow the rescuer to gain the child's trust as the survey progresses and the rescuer moves gradually into the child's personal space. Throughout the assessment, the nurse observes for areas of deformity, oedema, ecchymosis, bleeding, haematoma, paralysis or pain.

THE IMMOBILISED CHILD

Immobilisation

One of the most difficult aspects of illness is the immobility it often imposes on a child. Children's natural tendency to be mobile influences all elements of growth and development—physical, social, psychological and emotional. Impaired physical mobility related to disability or imposed activity restrictions presents a definite challenge to children, their families and their caregivers.

Causes of Immobilisation

For some children immobilisation may be due to a disability. For those children without disabilities, illness or injury is the usual reason for immobilisation or restriction of activities. When children are ill, they are content to remain quiet, and most of them instinctively reduce their activity. It is children who are forced to remain inactive because of physical limitations or therapy who display the multiple effects of restricted movement.

The most frequent reasons for immobility are congenital defects (e.g. spina bifida); neuromuscular conditions (e.g. cerebral palsy, muscular dystrophy, spinal muscular atrophy); the need for prolonged mechanical ventilation and sedation; and infections or injuries that impair the integumentary system (e.g. severe burns), the musculoskeletal system (e.g. complex fractures or osteomyelitis) or the neurological system (e.g. spinal cord injury, Guillain-Barré syndrome or traumatic brain injury and coma). Sometimes therapies such as traction or surgery are responsible for prolonged immobilisation, although the trend is towards early mobilisation, early discharge and outpatient care.

Physiological Effects of Immobilisation

Many clinical studies, including space program research, have documented predictable consequences that occur after immobilisation and the absence of gravitational force. Functional and metabolic responses to restricted movement occur in most of the body systems. Each has a direct influence on the child's growth and development because homeostatic mechanisms thrive on normal use and need feedback to maintain dynamic equilibrium. Inactivity leads to a decrease in the functional capabilities of the whole body as dramatically as the lack of physical exercise leads to muscle weakness.

Immobilisation from illness, injury or a sedentary lifestyle can limit function and potentially delay a child from meeting age-appropriate milestones. Most of the pathological changes that take place during immobilisation arise from decreased muscle strength and mass, decreased metabolism and bone demineralisation. The three are closely interrelated, with one change leading to or affecting another. Some results of immobilisation are primary and produce a direct effect; other pathophysiological consequences occur frequently but seem to be more indirect and are therefore secondary effects. Many pathophysiological changes affect more than one body system, with the primary or secondary effect being demonstrated in multiple systems.

The major effects of immobilisation (Fig 33.1) are related directly or indirectly to decreased muscle activity, which produces numerous primary changes in both muscular and bone structures, along with secondary alterations in the cardiovascular, respiratory, metabolic and renal systems. The major consequences are as follows:

- significant loss of muscle strength, endurance and muscle mass (atrophy)
- bone demineralisation leading to osteoporosis
- loss of joint mobility and contracture.

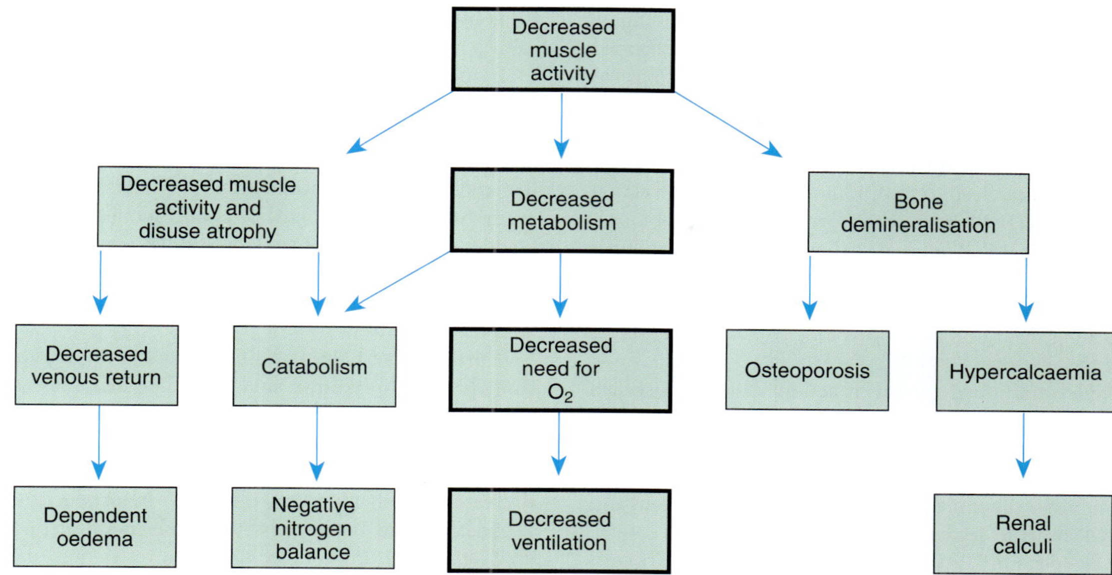

Fig 33.1 Physiological effects of immobilisation.

The larger the portion of the body immobilised and the longer the immobilisation, the greater the hazards of immobility.

Muscular System. Inactive muscle loses strength at the rate of 3% per day, and several weeks or months are sometimes required for function to be regained when there is no primary neuromuscular deficit. Stretching can occur as muscle loses its tone or as excessive strain is put on weakened muscle (e.g. stretching by tight bed covers or poor body position that produces foot drop as experienced by some children with disability). The disuse leads to tissue breakdown and muscle **atrophy**. The chief intracellular muscle enzyme, creatine, is released into the serum as the muscle atrophies; therefore, serum levels provide an indication of the amount of muscle mass undergoing degeneration. Muscle inactivity also affects the cardiovascular system by decreasing venous return and cardiac output. In general, muscle atrophy causes decreased strength and endurance.

In children who have limited mobility, such as children who are unconscious or partially or fully paralysed, joint mobility becomes restricted. In the absence of normal structural stretching, collagen fibres generated within the joint become fibrotic and further limit movement. This tissue fibrosis creates shortening of the muscles and contracture of the joint. Any decrease in circulation to the joint caused by oedema, inflammation or restrictive positioning contributes to further fibrotic changes. The problem rapidly becomes cyclic as the contracture leads to muscle fatigue and pain, which causes the child to protect the site, thus leading to more fibrosis. This process is further exaggerated because body flexor muscles are stronger than extensor muscles, and unless range of motion is re-established within 3 to 7 days, contractures will develop. Passive or active range-of-motion exercises and proper positioning can help prevent joint stiffness and contractures. Frequent disabling contractures are hip flexion, knee flexion, plantar flexion of the feet and shoulder stiffness.

Skeletal System. The daily stresses on bone created by motion and weight bearing maintain the balance between bone formation (osteoblastic activity) and bone resorption (osteoclastic activity). When these stresses are diminished, bone formation ceases while bone destruction continues leading to a disruption in the state of equilibrium. Bone calcium becomes severely depleted, and secretion of phosphorus and nitrogen is increased. This demineralisation of the bone (osteopenia) makes the skeletal structures prone to pathological fractures and increases calcium ion concentration in the blood (hypercalcaemia).

Cardiovascular System. Immobility has three major cardiovascular consequences: orthostatic intolerance, increased workload of the heart and thrombus formation. During movement, muscle contraction causes pressure on peripheral veins, which in turn causes the venous valves to close and thus assists in return of the blood to the heart when the individual is in an upright position. In the absence of this assistance, blood tends to pool in the dependent areas, reducing the blood supply to the trunk and brain. In addition, direct reflex stimulation to the splanchnic and peripheral vessels causes them to constrict when a person is upright. Impairment of this neurovascular orthostatic reflex activity from lack of motion causes further interference with venous return. The individual displays signs of excessive autonomic activity (e.g. pallor, sweating and restlessness, which are frequently followed by fainting). The child with a spinal cord injury has unique problems with orthostatic intolerance, which is discussed in Chapter 34.

NURSING CARE CONSIDERATIONS

Carefully evaluate: sudden chest pain and dyspnoea; sudden onset of shortness of breath; air hunger; or pain, redness and swelling in the lower extremities; skin warm to touch and limb cramps; and changes in the colour of skin (red/blue colour), which sometimes indicates deep vein thrombosis.

Changes in vascular resistance caused by the horizontal position and immobility alter the distribution of blood within the body. The reduction in gravity pressure to the extremities causes much of the total blood volume to be redistributed from lower extremities to other parts of the body. Consequently, there is an increase in the venous return and the volume of blood to be handled by the heart, which is reflected in elevated blood pressure. As a result, cardiac output and stroke volume are increased, and a progressive increase in heart rate occurs. When immobilisation extends over time, there is a compensatory decrease in blood volume and a decrease in heart rate and blood pressure.

Without muscle contraction, venous stasis and increased intravascular pressure in the extremities often lead to dependent oedema. If undue pressure is exerted on the major veins by positioning or mechanical devices, the likelihood of interstitial oedema is increased. Oedematous tissue, especially tissue located over an area that receives much of the body's weight, is prone to skin breakdown.

Circulatory stasis combined with hypercoagulability of the blood, which results from factors such as damage to the endothelium of blood vessels (Virchow triad), can lead to thrombus and embolus formation. **Deep vein thrombosis** (DVT) involves the formation of a thrombus in a deep vein such as the iliac and femoral veins and can cause significant morbidity if it remains undetected and untreated. DVT may develop with prolonged venous stasis in conditions such as obesity, chronic heart failure, prolonged surgical procedure, long trips without exercise or prolonged immobilisation.

The state of deconditioned cardiac function, caused by skeletal muscle inactivity, can produce a variety of secondary problems in other systems. However, the major clinical manifestation is increased pulse and heart rate in response to an active exercise program. After prolonged immobility, the child should build up activity tolerance slowly to allow the heart to regain optimum capabilities.

Respiratory System. Initially the effects of immobilisation are compensatory or adaptive. The basal metabolic rate is decreased because with reduced expenditure of energy the cells require less oxygen and produce less carbon dioxide. Lessened demand for oxygen–carbon dioxide exchange causes the respirations to become slower and more shallow. In children, chest expansion may be limited by: the child's position (e.g. supine); abdominal distension caused by accumulation of faeces, gas or fluid; and by mechanical restriction such as from a brace or constricting binder. Pain (e.g. chest tube in place) may also limit deep breathing and adequate chest expansion. More effort is required to expand the lungs in the supine position. Reduced muscle power and coordination secondary to altered innervation can also hinder respiratory movement.

Prolonged immobility also reduces the normal movement of secretions from the tracheobronchial tree, particularly in the presence of impaired muscle function and without positional changes that normally facilitate removal of secretions. A weak and ineffectual cough reflex contributes to stasis of secretions and the possibility of airway obstruction in the smaller airways of children. Shallow respirations and obstruction of the airway with thick mucus are factors in the development of secondary complications such as atelectasis and pneumonia.

Gastrointestinal System. Prolonged immobility produces a state of negative nitrogen balance resulting from the increased catabolic activity related to muscle atrophy. This and the reduced energy requirements contribute to a diminished appetite and a resulting decrease in ingestion of nutrients (anorexia). Eating and feeding become more difficult with immobility, and the risk of aspiration is increased. Associated psychological factors further influence intake.

The process of elimination depends on the integration of smooth and skeletal muscle activity and on visceral reflex patterns. Immobility may interfere with these mechanisms, as well as with the gravitational effect on stool passing through the intestines. Slowing of stool in the colon causes the faeces to become hard (**faecal impaction**), and the bowel wall is not stimulated to further its peristaltic movement down the tract to the rectum. Weakened muscles used in defecation (diaphragmatic and abdominal muscles) are unable to produce the intraabdominal pressure needed for elimination. Sometimes embarrassment in using a bedpan or bedside commode may be the cause of not responding to the urge to defecate.

Renal System. The urinary system is designed to function in an upright posture. When the gravitational force is altered by the reclining position, the peristaltic contractions of the ureters are insufficient to overcome gravitational resistance. Consequently, there may be stasis of urine in the renal pelvis, and any particulate matter that settles in the calyces may serve as nuclei for calculi formation or as foci for infection.

In the horizontal position the individual has difficulty relaxing the perineal musculature and external sphincter sufficiently to initiate the integrated reflex micturition mechanism, which involves the external sphincter, the internal sphincter and the detrusor muscle of the bladder wall. If adequate intraabdominal pressure is exerted, voiding can occur, but if the individual does not respond to the sensation to void, bladder distension leads to stasis and its complications add to embarrassing overflow incontinence. In time, reflux and back pressure may impair renal function, and urinary tract infection is always a hazard with urine retention.

Normally the kidney is able to handle the increased metabolites from protein breakdown and bone demineralisation. However, the increased level of calcium excreted may predispose the person to calculus formation. Formation of **renal calculi** (kidney stones) is further favoured by urinary stasis, infection and alkaline urine caused by the decreased production of the acid by-products of metabolism. Haematuria may be the only clue to the condition.

Metabolism. Immobility or severe restriction of activity is often accompanied by decreased or inappropriate nutritional intake, which frequently leads to a decreased basal metabolic rate, a negative nitrogen balance associated with catabolism and a high serum calcium level.

All body systems are influenced by a decrease in metabolism. The altered energy level leads to further fatigue and lack of motivation for moving. Immobilised persons often feel sluggish and have a poor appetite, particularly for protein foods. The protein breakdown in the body related to a loss of muscle and other tissues is more apt to be severe after injury or surgery. Protein breakdown produces nitrogenous wastes, and on the fifth or sixth day of catabolic protein metabolism, an increase in urinary nitrogen level develops that contributes to anaemia and delayed healing.

Another metabolic problem is **hypercalcaemia** associated with bone catabolism. Completely immobilised children or adolescents are especially prone to hypercalcaemia. Symptoms, which include nausea and vomiting, polydipsia, polyuria and lethargy, usually appear 4 to 8 weeks after immobilisation. In quadriplegia, symptoms may occur within 10 days and last for as long as 6 months. The accelerated rate of bone metabolism in children makes the bone demineralisation a greater hazard. Larger amounts of calcium are released into the blood than the kidney can excrete, and calcium continues to accumulate in serum. High levels of serum calcium decrease neuronal permeability, which can lead to a depression of the central and peripheral nervous systems. Symptoms are a result of the depressed nervous system, and include smooth and skeletal muscle fatigue, diminished reflexes and atony of the gastrointestinal tract.

A child with bone demineralisation may not develop hypercalcaemia, but the excess amount of calcium that the kidneys are required to excrete may produce a negative calcium balance, with more calcium than citric acid lost in the urine. This imbalance causes the urine to become alkaline, with the potential danger of renal calculi, especially if there is an accompanying retention of urine.

Integumentary System. The following factors play a major role in skin breakdown: moisture, friction, shear and pressure (see also Chapter 22, Maintaining Healthy Skin). Circulation to the skin is reduced during inactivity and may be further impeded by dependent oedema. Circulation is especially compromised in places where the bone surface is near the skin, such as areas over the sacrum, occiput, trochanter and heel, and continued impairment causes rapid necrosis with ulcer formation. Friction and mechanical irritation from appliances such as straps, rods and tubing and the friction of bedclothes during turning or other movement can produce skin breakdown.

Healing capacity is also impaired by poor circulation, negative nitrogen balance and anaemia. Immobilisation often makes it difficult to carry out adequate cleansing and hygienic measures, which may also contribute to tissue breakdown in areas that are difficult to reach.

Cellular breakdown caused by prolonged pressure has several characteristics. Normally when pressure is applied to the skin, the skin appears pale but becomes very red, or hyperaemic, after the pressure is removed. This reactive hyperaemia should disappear within 5 to 15 minutes. Prolonged redness (> 30 minutes) indicates that a pressure area is developing and treatment should begin. Other manifestations of tissue ischaemia include an increase in temperature in the area, blistering, swelling and dark purple or black areas. The pressure area may be limited to the skin and subcutaneous layers or may be deeper and more extensive. The skin changes observed may represent the top of a cone-shaped area with widespread tissue destruction, beneath which tissue rapidly ulcerates and creates a large pressure ulcer that sometimes extends to the bone. Figure 33.2 illustrates the sequence of events in tissue breakdown.

Neurosensory System. Studies indicate that immobilisation does not produce neurosensory consequences directly; however, two occurrences—loss of innervation and sensory and perceptual deprivation—are common.

Peripheral nerves, in contrast to skeletal muscles, do not degenerate with disuse, but loss of innervation takes place if nerves are damaged by pressure or if their blood supply is disrupted. Improper body positioning, improperly applied casts or restraints or fluid build-up within a compartment (compartment syndrome) can place excessive pressure on nerves and blood vessels that can lead to ischaemia and nerve degeneration. Frequent sites of nerve compression phenomenon are the peroneal nerve, where pressure results in **foot drop**, and the radial nerve, where pressure leads to **wrist drop**. These complications significantly interfere with attempts to regain functional use of the extremities, but they can be prevented by conscientious nursing assessment and intervention. Preventing pressure on vulnerable areas and avoiding extreme positions of flexion and extension that apply inappropriate pressure on nerves and blood vessels reduce the likelihood of compression injury. Periodic plantarflexion and dorsiflexion of the feet and hands by passive or active range of motion will stimulate circulation and keep nerves from becoming pinched. Numbness, tingling, change in sensation and loss of motion are symptoms of neurological impairment and should be evaluated immediately.

Psychological Effects of Immobilisation

For children, one of the most difficult aspects of illness is immobilisation. Throughout childhood, physical activity is an integral part of daily life and is essential for physical growth and development. It also serves children as an instrument for communication and expression and as a means for learning about and understanding their world. Activity helps them deal with a variety of feelings and impulses and provides a mechanism by which they can exert control over inner tensions. Children respond to anxiety with increased activity. Removal of this power deprives them of necessary input and a natural outlet for their feelings and fantasies. Through movement children also gain sensory input, which provides an essential element for developing and maintaining body image.

Active children have many opportunities for input from a wide variety of settings. When they are immobilised by disease or as a part of a treatment regimen, they experience diminished environmental stimuli with a loss of tactile, vestibular and proprioceptive input and an altered perception of themselves and their environment. Sudden or gradual immobilisation narrows the amount and variety of environmental stimuli they receive by means of all their senses: touch, sight, hearing, taste, smell and proprioception. This sensory deprivation frequently leads to feelings of isolation, boredom and being forgotten, especially by peers. Nursing interventions involving the use of diversion activities, schoolwork, structured television viewing and computer games can assist the child in maintaining usual activities.

The struggle for independence is thwarted by imposed immobility. For toddlers, exploration and imitative behaviours are essential to

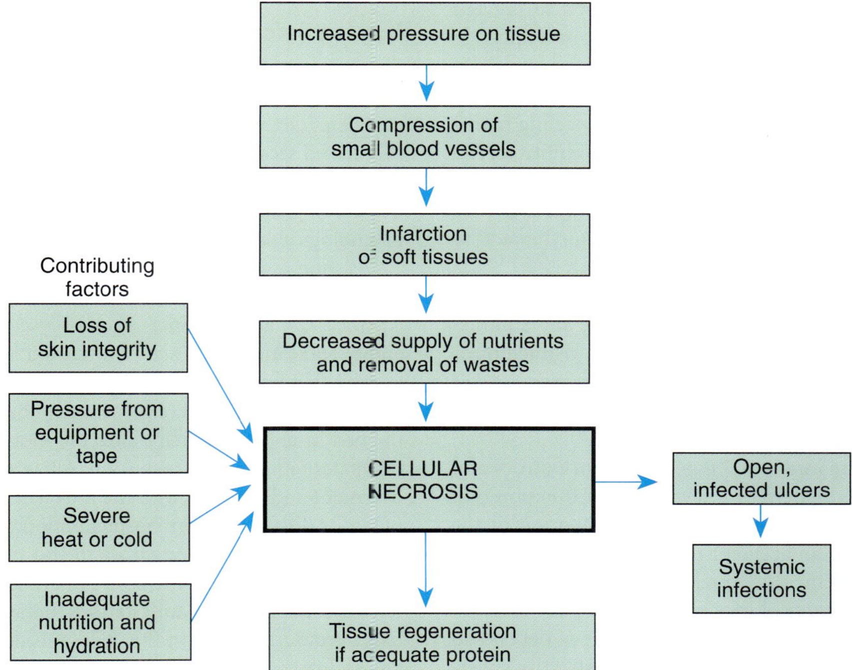

Fig 33.2 Sequence of events in tissue breakdown.

BOX 33.1 Behavioural Changes in Immobilised Children

Higher-than-normal level of anxiety leads to the following:
- restlessness
- difficulty with problem-solving
- inability to concentrate on activities
- depression
- regression
- egocentrism.

Monotony leads to the following:
- sluggish intellectual responses
- sluggish psychomotor responses
- decreased communication skills
- increased fantasising
- hallucinations
- disorientation
- dependence
- acting-out behaviour
- depression.

developing a sense of autonomy; preschooler's expression of initiative is evidenced by their penchant for vigorous physical activity; school-age children's development is strongly influenced by physical achievement and competition; and adolescents rely on mobility to achieve independence. The quest for mastery at every stage of development is related to mobility.

Behavioural changes occur when children experience prolonged sensory deprivation. Some of these behaviours are indications of a higher-than-normal level of anxiety (Box 33.1). Children are likely to become depressed over their loss of ability to function or the marked changes in body image. Significant others often notice regressive behaviour and a greater reliance on them for tasks the children are able to perform. Children seek attention by reverting to earlier developmental behaviours, such as wanting to be fed, bed-wetting and baby talk. In many ways, immobilised children are realistically dependent on others; therefore, intelligent and sensitive care is required to prevent major developmental regressions during the period of immobility.

Limbs that are immobilised by casts, traction or paralysis transmit less sensory data than typical. Sensory impairment may be a concomitant problem of the involved part. Numbness or loss of feeling markedly alters proprioception. Children who have limited ability to feel others touching them not only experience less tactile stimulation in a physical sense but are also deprived of warm, loving feelings that arise from being touched. The loss of feeling from touch can further add to their sense of being isolated and unwanted.

Children often react to immobility with active protest, anger and aggressive behaviour, or they may become quiet, passive and submissive. Often children believe that the immobilisation is a justified punishment for misbehaviour. Children should be allowed to express their anger, but this expression should be within the limits of safety to their self-esteem and not damaging to the integrity of others.

The most difficult situations are those involving major injuries and diseases that produce a disfigurement or a severe loss of function that directly affects a child's self-image, such as burns, amputation or the sudden, catastrophic effects of an accident that leave a healthy, active child disabled. Children have difficulty expressing feelings of anger and hostility when they are at the mercy of the environment. They dare not speak out against or defy authority figures on which they depend so completely. Consequently, their aggression may be masked by cheerfulness or rigidity. When they are unable to express their anger, the aggression is often displayed inappropriately through regressive behaviour and outbursts of crying or temper tantrums over insignificant irritations. Adolescents and older school-age children should vary their daily routine to fit their needs for independence; allowing this age group to stay up late at night and sleep in during the daytime (within reasonable limits to accommodate treatment needs) may help decrease struggles over other inconsequential matters and at the same time allow a daily pattern of life. Encourage parents to continue setting limits and not abandon disciplinary measures with children who are confined to bed due to trauma or illness.

Effects of Immobilisation on Families

Even brief periods of child immobilisation may disrupt the functioning of a family, and a child's catastrophic illness or disability may severely tax their resources and coping abilities. The need for instruction concerning medical and nursing care, community resources to contact and emotional support are paramount. Many families have unmet needs, operate from crisis to crisis and are unable to use outside help appropriately. For these families, the new situation can be disruptive; therefore, a multidisciplinary team must help the family members identify unmet needs and solve problems. The following are commonly occurring problems.

- Financial strains may decrease or totally eliminate the family's resources.
- Attention is focused, at least temporarily, on the affected member; therefore, other members of the family, especially siblings, may feel that they are being neglected or that their needs may not be met.
- The family may have difficulty accepting the child's altered body condition.
- Individual family members may be unable to express their feelings and may have difficulty coping with the crisis.
- Parents often experience guilt over their child's condition and need for immobilisation. Their perception of failing to protect the child forms the basis for their difficulty coping.

The family's needs often must be met through the services of a multidisciplinary team and nurses play a key role in anticipating the services the family will need and coordinating appropriate care.

Nursing Care Management

Physical assessment of the child who is immobilised for any number of reasons (e.g. injury or illness) includes a focus not only on the injured part (e.g. fracture) but also on the functioning of other systems that may be affected secondarily: the circulatory, renal, respiratory, muscular and gastrointestinal systems. With long-term immobilisation, there may also be neurological impairment and changes in metabolism. In addition, the psychological impact of immobilisation should be assessed.

As soon as possible, the child should wear street clothes and resume school and preinjury hobbies. Play is the most useful tool of nursing (see Chapter 22), and activities should be selected on the basis of interest, ability and limitations. Activities should include some form of physical activity that encourages the use of uninvolved muscles and joints. Any activity that is tolerated (e.g. turning in bed or changing the position of the bed in the room) helps alter the monotony of immobilisation and dissipates tension and frustration. Allow a parent and/or sibling to stay overnight and room-in with the hospitalised child to prevent the effects of family disruption from hospitalisation. Make every effort to minimise family disruption resulting from the hospitalisation.

Nursing assessment includes gathering psychosocial data, in addition to assessing physical manifestations, because long-term immobilisation has a profound effect on the child and the family. Nursing approaches are evaluated frequently and continued, discontinued or modified to meet the changing problems and goals. Table 33.1 summarises

TABLE 33.1 Summary of Physical Effects of Immobilisation with Nursing Interventions*

Primary Effects	Secondary Effects	Nursing Considerations
		MUSCULAR SYSTEM
Decreased muscle strength, tone and endurance	Decreased venous return and decreased cardiac output	Use antiembolism stockings or intermittent compression devices to promote venous return (monitor circulatory and neurovascular status of extremities when such devices are used).
	Decreased metabolism and need for oxygen	Plan play activities to use uninvolved extremities.
	Decreased exercise tolerance	Place in upright posture when possible.
	Bone demineralisation	Perform passive range-of-motion exercises.
Disuse atrophy and loss of muscle mass	Catabolism Loss of strength	Have patient perform range-of-motion, active, passive and stretching exercises.
Loss of joint mobility	Contractures, ankylosis of joints	Maintain correct body alignment. Use joint splints as indicated to prevent further deformity. Maintain range of motion.
Weak back muscles	Secondary spinal deformities	Maintain body alignment.
Weak abdominal muscles	Impaired respiration	See nursing considerations for respiratory system.
		SKELETAL SYSTEM
Bone demineralisation—osteoporosis, hypercalcaemia	Negative bone calcium uptake Pathological fractures Calcium deposits Extraosseous bone formation, especially at hip, knee, elbow and shoulder Renal calculi	With paralysis use upright posture on tilt table. Handle extremities carefully when turning and positioning. Administer calcium-mobilising drugs (diphosphonates) and normal saline infusions as ordered. Ensure adequate intake of fluid; monitor output. Acidify urine. Promptly treat urinary tract infections.
Negative bone calcium uptake	Life-threatening electrolyte imbalance	Monitor serum calcium levels. Provide electrolyte replacement as indicated.
		METABOLISM
Decreased metabolic rate	Slowing of all systems Decreased food intake	Mobilise as soon as possible. Have patient perform active and passive resistance and deep-breathing exercises. Ensure adequate food intake. Provide a high-protein diet.
Negative nitrogen balance	Decline in nutritional state	Encourage small, frequent feedings with protein and preferred foods.
	Impaired healing	Monitor for and prevent pressure areas.
Hypercalcaemia	Electrolyte imbalance	See nursing consideration for skeletal system.
Decreased production of stress hormones	Decreased physical and emotional coping capacity	Identify causes of stress. Implement appropriate interventions to lower physical and psychosocial stresses.
		CARDIOVASCULAR SYSTEM
Decreased efficiency of orthostatic neurovascular reflexes	Inability to adapt readily to upright position (orthostatic intolerance) Pooling of blood in extremities in upright posture	Monitor peripheral pulses and skin temperature changes. Use antiembolism stockings or intermittent compression devices to decrease pooling when upright.
Diminished vasopressor mechanism	Orthostatic intolerance with syncope, hypertension, decreased cerebral blood flow, tachycardia	Provide abdominal support. In severe cases use antigravitational pants. Position horizontally.
Altered distribution of blood volume	Increased cardiac workload Decreased exercise tolerance	Monitor hydration, blood pressure and urinary output.
Venous stasis	Pulmonary emboli or thrombi	Encourage and assist with frequent position changes. Elevate extremities without knee flexion. Ensure adequate fluid intake. Have patient perform active or passive exercises or movement as needed. Prescribe routine wearing of antiembolism stockings or intermittent compression devices. Monitor for signs of pulmonary embolism—sudden dyspnoea, chest pain, respiratory arrest. Promptly intervene to maintain adequate oxygenation if signs and symptoms of pulmonary emboli are noted.

Continued

TABLE 33.1 **Summary of Physical Effects of Immobilisation with Nursing Interventions—cont'd**

Primary Effects	Secondary Effects	Nursing Considerations
		Measure circumference of extremities periodically. Give anticoagulant drugs as prescribed.
Dependent oedema	Tissue breakdown and susceptibility to infection	Administer skin care. Turn every 2–4 hours. Monitor skin colour, temperature and integrity. Use pressure-reduction surface as necessary to prevent skin breakdown.
		RESPIRATORY SYSTEM
Decreased need for oxygen	Altered oxygen–carbon dioxide exchange and metabolism	Promote exercise as tolerated. Encourage deep-breathing exercises.
Decreased chest expansion and diminished vital capacity	Diminished oxygen intake Dyspnoea and inadequate arterial oxygen saturation; acidosis	Position for optimum chest expansion. Semi-Fowler's position may assist in lung expansion if patient can tolerate. Use prone positioning without pressure on abdomen to allow gravity to aid in diaphragmatic excursion. Ensure that patient maintains proper alignment when sitting to prevent pressure on respiratory mechanism.
Poor abdominal tone and distension	Interference with diaphragmatic excursion	Avoid restriction of chest and abdominal musculature. Supply torso support to promote chest expansion.
Mechanical or biochemical secretion retention	Hypostatic pneumonia Bacterial and viral pneumonia Atelectasis	Change position frequently. Use incentive spirometer. Monitor breath sounds. Encourage deep-breathing exercises. Implement airway clearance techniques as necessary.
Loss of respiratory muscle strength	Poor cough	Encourage coughing and deep breathing. Support chest wall by splinting with pillow when patient coughs. Use incentive spirometer. Observe for signs of respiratory distress with pulse oximetry or blood gas measurement as necessary.
	Upper respiratory tract infection	Prevent contact with infected persons. Provide adequate hydration. Administer immunisations as necessary (pneumococcal, meningococcal).
		GASTROINTESTINAL SYSTEM
Distension caused by poor abdominal muscle tone	Interference with respiratory movements	Monitor bowel sounds. Encourage small, frequent feedings.
	Difficulty in feeding in prone position	Have patient sit in upright position in bedside chair if possible.
No specific primary effect	Possible constipation caused by gravitational effect on faeces through ascending colon or weakened smooth muscle tone	Carry out bowel training program with hydration, stool softeners, increased fibre intake and mild laxatives if necessary.
	Anorexia	Stimulate appetite with favoured foods.
		URINARY SYSTEM
Alteration of gravitational force	Difficulty in voiding in prone position	Position as upright as possible to void.
Impaired ureteral peristalsis	Urinary retention in calyces and bladder infection Renal calculi	Hydrate to ensure adequate urinary output for age. Stimulate bladder emptying with warm running water as necessary. Catheterise only for severe urinary retention. Administer antibiotics as indicated.
		INTEGUMENTARY SYSTEM
Altered tissue integrity	Decreased circulation and pressure leading to tissue injury	Turn and reposition at least every 2–4 hours. Frequently inspect total skin surface. Eliminate mechanical factors causing pressure, friction, moisture or irritation. Place on pressure-relief mattress.
	Difficulty with personal hygiene	Assess ability to perform self-care and assist with bathing, grooming and toileting as needed. Encourage self-care to potential ability. Ensure adequate intake of protein, vitamins and minerals.

*Individualise care according to the child's needs; interventions may vary in different institutions.

the physical effects of immobilisation and appropriate nursing care management. With the increased trend towards early mobilisation, early discharge and home healthcare, many children are discharged home after a few days of hospitalisation. Follow-up treatment may take place in the home or at an outpatient ambulatory facility.

The Child in a Cast

Children may be placed into a cast for different reasons, including treatment of a fracture or after a surgery to maintain alignment. In many situations, the joints above and below the site of injury are immobilised to eliminate the possibility of movement that might cause displacement at the site. Three major types of casts are used for immobilisation: upper extremity to immobilise the wrist or elbow; lower extremity to immobilise the ankle or knee; and spica to immobilise the hip and knee (Fig 33.3). Fig 33.4 shows a full spica cast with a hip abduction and Fig 33.5 shows a full spica cast with water proofing to assist with nursing care.

The Cast

Casts are constructed from gauze bandages impregnated with plaster of Paris or, more commonly, synthetic lighter-weight and water-resistant materials (e.g. waterproof liners, fibreglass and polyurethane resin). Both types of casting material produce heat from a chemical reaction activated by water immediately after application. The lightweight casts are used more often for casting in children and are available in a variety of colours. Plaster casts are usually reserved for situations that require moulding closely to the body part.

Cast Application. The child's developmental age should be considered before the cast is applied. For preschoolers who fear bodily harm and fantasise the loss of an extremity, use a plastic doll or stuffed animal to explain the procedure beforehand. Toddlers and preschoolers do not have easily defined body boundaries; if an extremity is wrapped in a bandage, splint or cast, to the young child the extremity ceases to function or exist. During the application of the cast, use

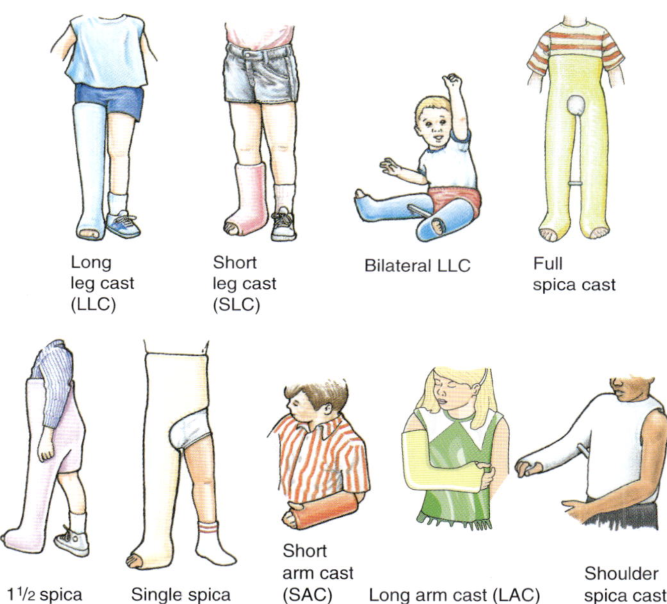

Fig 33.3 Types of casts.

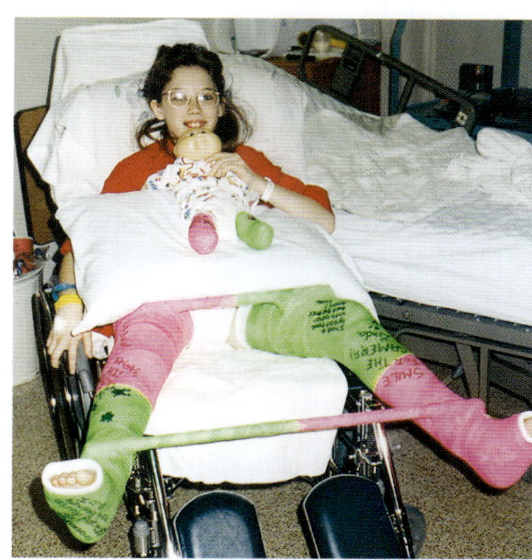

Fig 33.4 Spica cast with hip abductor. Note casts on doll as well.

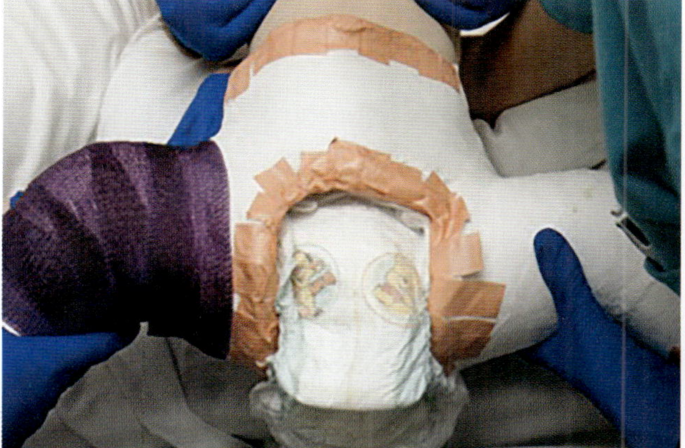

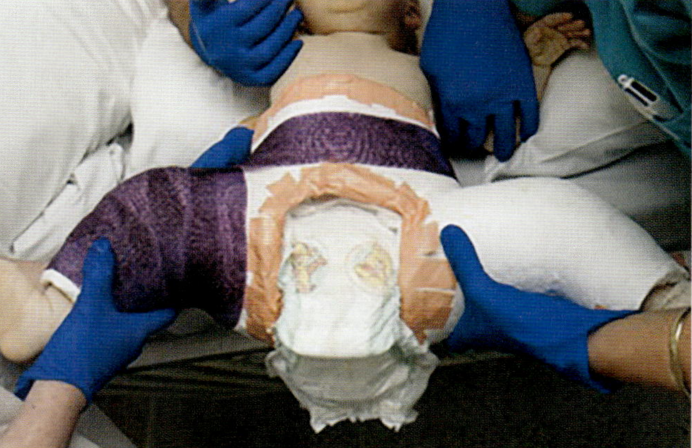

Fig 33.5 Hip spica cast—placement of nappy and waterproof taping to edges for care of young child. (Source: The Royal Children's Hospital Melbourne (RCHM). (2018). Hip spica nursing care. Clinical Guidelines (Nursing). February. https://www.rch.org.au/rchcpg/hospital_clinical_guideline_index/Hip_spica_nursing_care/)

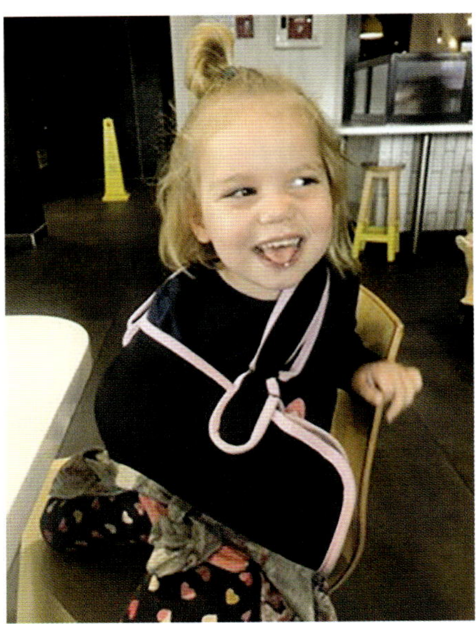

Fig 33.6 Young children come to regard a cast or sling as part of their body. (Source: L. Kendrick.)

various distraction methods, including discussing favourite pets or activities at school and blowing bubbles.

It is important to note that there are some local clinical guidelines/policy directives to follow for the application of the cast and these must be adhered to so as to prevent any further harm to the child. Many children adapt quickly to a cast and sling in their everyday life (Fig 33.6).

NURSING CARE CONSIDERATIONS

Most often, a plaster cast may be applied initially until the swelling is reduced, then apply a fibreglass cast. It is important for the plaster casts to be kept dry to prevent being weakened when wet. Heated fans or dryers are not used because they cause the cast to dry on the outside and remain wet beneath. They may also cause burns from heat conduction by the cast to the underlying tissue.

Cast Removal. Cutting the cast to remove it or to relieve tightness is frequently a frightening experience for children.

Preparation for the procedure helps reduce anxiety, especially if the nurse has established a trusting relationship with the child. Many young children come to regard the cast as part of themselves, which intensifies their fear of removal. They need continual reassurance that all is going well and that their behaviour is accepted.

If the cast has been in place for a lengthy period of time, decreased muscle mass may be noted. The child and family should be reassured that resuming exercise and routine activities will gradually return function and appearance (provided there was no significant trauma beforehand).

NURSING CARE CONSIDERATIONS

Immediately report any abnormal neurovascular observations that include the five Ps of ischaemia: pain, especially with passive range of motion; pallor; pulselessness (an ominous and late sign); paraesthesia; and paralysis.

During the first few hours after a cast is applied, the chief concern is that the extremity may continue to swell to the extent that the cast becomes a tourniquet, shutting off circulation and producing neurovascular complications (compartment syndrome). One measure to reduce the likelihood of this problem is to elevate the body part and thereby increase venous return. If oedema is excessive, casts are bivalved (i.e. cut to make anterior and posterior halves that are held together with an elastic bandage). The cast and the involved extremity are observed frequently to assess neurovascular integrity and detect any signs of compromise. Permanent muscle and tissue damage can occur within a few hours.

Appropriate cast care guidelines for the child's parents and caregivers are necessary before discharge. Instructions are also given for checking for signs and symptoms that indicate the cast is too tight (see Family-Centred Care box). Parents should also be told to take the child to their healthcare professional if the cast becomes too loose because a loose cast no longer serves its purpose.

FAMILY-CENTRED CARE

Cast Care

- Keep the casted part of the body elevated on pillows or similar support for the first day or as directed by the healthcare professional.
- Expose the plaster cast to air until dry.
- A wet plaster cast should be lifted and supported with the palms of the hands only in order to avoid indenting with the fingers and creating pressure points.
- Observe the fingers or toes for any evidence of swelling or discolouration (darker or lighter than a comparable extremity) and contact the healthcare professional immediately if noted.
- Check movement and sensation of the visible fingers or toes frequently and contact the healthcare professional regarding any changes noted.
- Encourage frequent rest for a few days, and elevate the injured arm or leg while resting.
- Do not allow the affected limb to hang in a dependent position for more than 30 minutes (to prevent swelling and circulatory stasis).
- Keep an injured arm or hand elevated (e.g. in a sling) most of the time; supporting it on pillows at chest level is helpful.
- Elevate an injured leg when the child is sitting and avoid standing for too long.
- Keep plaster casts dry at all times to prevent them being weakened when wet.
- Do not allow the child to put anything inside the cast.
- Keep small items that might be placed inside the cast away from young children.
- Examine the skin at the cast edges to detect irritation or breakdown. Pad the cast accordingly.
- Instruct the child and parents to avoid placing the cast in water (e.g. tub, shower, swimming pool).
- If the patient is incontinent, protect the cast with waterproof tape and plastic. Use nappies, pull-ups or other guards.

The Child in Traction

With the increased emphasis on outpatient care of acute and chronic illnesses to cut healthcare costs, developmental and social considerations, immobilisation problems and advanced surgical techniques, traction is used with decreasing frequency. Most skeletal traction is applied in children after a severe or complex injury to allow physiological stability, align bone fragments and permit closer evaluation of the injured site. New technology has developed orthopaedic fixation devices that allow for partial or full mobility, thus preventing long-term immobilisation and its consequences. In many cases, surgical intervention may be carried out within a matter of hours to days; therefore, skeletal traction devices described herein may be used infrequently in paediatrics.

Purposes of Traction

The primary purposes of traction are as follows.

1. To realign bone fragments
2. To provide rest for an extremity
3. To help prevent or improve contracture deformity
4. To correct a joint deformity
5. To treat a dislocation
6. To allow preoperative or postoperative positioning and alignment
7. To provide immobilisation of specific areas of the body
8. To reduce muscle spasms

The three primary purposes of traction for reduction of fractures are as follows:

1. To fatigue the involved muscle and reduce muscle spasm so that bones can be realigned
2. To position the distal and proximal bone ends in the desired realignment to promote satisfactory bone healing
3. To immobilise the fracture site until realignment has been achieved and sufficient healing has taken place to permit casting or splinting

When two forces of given direction and magnitude act on an object at the same point simultaneously from opposite directions, the object either changes its state of rest or motion or remains in equilibrium. The use of traction in the management of fractures is the direct application of such forces to reduce or realign the bone at the fracture site. The three essential components of traction management are traction, counter traction and friction. **Traction** (forward force) is produced by attaching weight to the distal bone fragment. Body weight provides **counter traction** (backward force), and the patient's contact with the bed constitutes the **frictional** force (Fig 33.7). These forces are used to align the distal and proximal bone fragments by adjusting the line of pull upwards or downwards and by adducting or abducting the extremity. To attain equilibrium, the amount of forward force is adjusted by adding weight to or subtracting weight from the traction. Counter traction can be increased by elevating the foot of the bed to create a greater gravitational pull to the backward force.

The all-or-none law, characteristic of muscle contractility, applies to muscle relaxation as well. The muscle is fatigued by applying constant stress to the muscle so that the build-up of lactic acid will produce muscle relaxation. When muscles are stretched, muscle spasm ceases, which permits the realignment of the bone ends. The continuous maintenance of traction is important during this phase because releasing the traction allows the muscle to contract normally and again cause malpositioning of the bone ends.

The realignment of bone fragments is a gradual process that is achieved more rapidly in infants, who have limited muscle tone compared with muscular teenagers. The desired vector force, bone alignment and callus formation are checked periodically by radiographic examination. The traction pull to some degree immobilises the fracture site; however, adjunct immobilising devices such as splints or casts are sometimes used with skeletal traction. Immobilisation with traction is maintained until the bone ends are in satisfactory realignment, after which a less confining type of immobilisation—a cast, pins or external stabilisation device—is applied. In injuries in which there is severe soft tissue swelling or vascular and nerve damage, it is customary to use traction until these complications have been resolved and it is safe to apply a cast.

Types of Traction

The pull needed for traction can be applied to the distal bone fragment in several ways. The main types of traction include manual, skin and skeletal traction (Box 33.2). The type of traction applied is determined primarily by the child's age, the condition of the soft tissues and the type and degree of displacement of the fracture. Fractures most commonly treated by application of traction are those involving the femur and vertebrae.

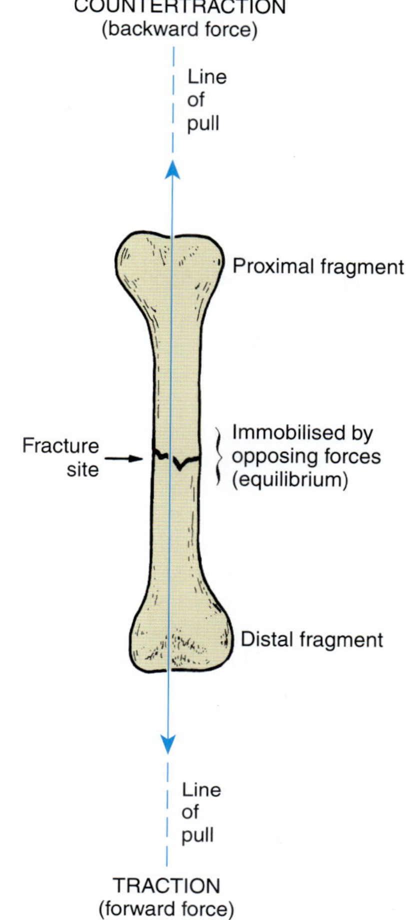

Fig 33.7 Application of traction for maintaining equilibrium.

BOX 33.2 Types of Traction

Manual Traction—Applied to the body part by the hands placed distal to the fracture site. Manual traction may be provided during application of a cast but more commonly when a closed reduction is performed.

Skin Traction—Applied directly to the skin surface and indirectly to the skeletal structures. The pulling mechanism is attached to the skin with adhesive material or an elastic bandage. Both types are applied over soft, foam-backed traction straps to distribute the traction pull.

Skeletal Traction—Applied directly to the skeletal structure by a pin, wire or tongs inserted into or through the diameter of the bone distal to the fracture.

A common site for a femoral fracture is the middle third of the shaft (see Fig 33.21A later in this chapter). With such a fracture there may be significant overriding but minimal displacement. In a fracture of the lower third of the femoral shaft, the pull of the gastrocnemius muscle causes the distal fragment to become downwardly displaced. Femur fractures in young children can often be reduced followed by

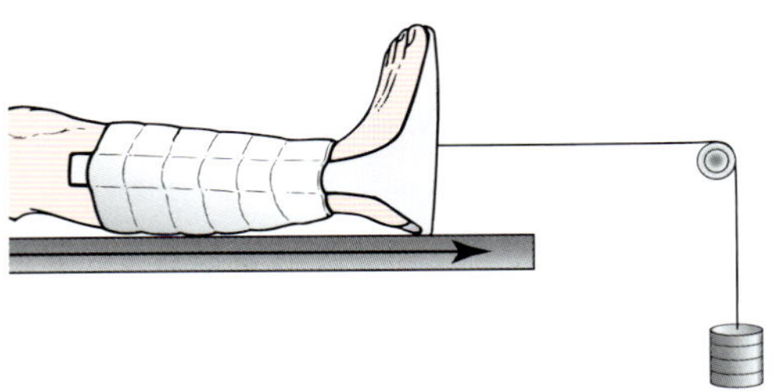

Fig 33.8 Buck extension traction.

application of a hip spica cast. When traction is necessary, several types may be used based on the initial assessment.

Buck extension traction is a type of skin traction applied with the legs in an extended position (Fig 33.8). Buck extension traction is used primarily for short-term immobilisation, such as preoperative management of a child with a dislocated hip, or for correction of contractures or bone deformities, such as in Legg-Calvé-Perthes disease.

A common skeletal traction is 90-degree–90-degree traction (90-90 traction). The lower leg is supported by a boot cast or a calf sling, and a skeletal Steinmann pin or Kirschner wire is placed in the distal fragment of the femur. This type of traction results in a 90-degree angle at both the hip and the knee. It achieves the desired line of pull for reducing the fracture and provides adequate immobilisation of the fracture site. The use of 90-90 traction also supports the lower extremity in a desired position with good venous return. From a nursing standpoint, this type of traction facilitates position changes, toileting and prevention of complications related to traction.

Balanced suspension traction may be used with or without skin or skeletal traction. Unless it is combined with another type of traction, balanced suspension merely holds the leg in a desired flexed position to relax the hip and hamstring muscles and does not exert any traction directly on a body part.

The cervical area is a vulnerable site for flexion or extension injuries to muscles, vertebrae or the spinal cord. Cervical muscle trauma without other complications is treated with a cervical soft or hard collar to relieve the weight of the head on the fracture site. When a child's cervical vertebra is displaced or fractured, it may be necessary to reduce and immobilise the site with cervical skeletal traction. The spinal cord runs through the intravertebral canal, and dislocation or fracture of the vertebrae can also cause spinal cord injury. Nursing assessment of neurological function is essential to prevent further injury during the application and use of cervical skeletal traction.

Most cervical traction is accomplished with the use of a halo brace or halo vest (Fig 33.9A). This device consists of a steel halo attached to the outer skull by four screws; several rigid bars connect the halo to a vest that is worn around the chest. This provides greater mobility of the rest of the body, while limiting cervical spinal motion completely. Gardner-Wells tongs may also be used to immobilise the cervical spine (Fig 33.9B). With cervical traction, the neck muscles fatigue with constant traction pull and the vertebral bodies gradually separate so the spinal cord is no longer pinched between the vertebrae. Immobilisation until fracture healing or surgical fixation can occur is an essential goal of cervical traction. If immobilisation is needed in a young child, a special cervical spine cast (Minerva cast) may be applied.

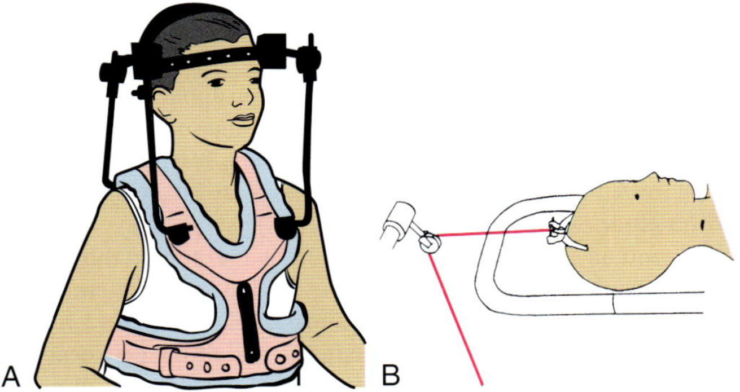

Fig 33.9 (**A**) Halo vest. (**B**) Cervical traction with Gardner-Wells tong.

Nursing Care Management

To assess the child in traction, it is essential to know the purpose or reason for application of traction and understand the basic principles of its use. Routine assessment of both the child and the traction apparatus is required. Many of the nursing problems associated with traction in a child are related to immobility. However, a number of physical needs related to traction require attention and vigilance.

In addition to routine skin observation and care, the child in skeletal traction will need special skin care at the pin site according to hospital policy or provider preference. Pin sites should be frequently assessed and cleaned to prevent infection; after the first 48 to 72 hours, pin site care may be performed once daily with normal saline swabs unless directed otherwise by the orthopaedic medical officer (The Sydney Children's Hospital Network 2014). Before the child's discharge, parents and caregivers are taught pin site care, including how to observe for infection or pin instability, using a return demonstration method. A pressure-reduction device, such as a foam overlay or an alternating-pressure mattress, reduces the chance of skin breakdown.

When the child is first placed in traction, increased discomfort is common as a result of the traction pull fatiguing the muscle. Orthopaedic conditions are associated with a higher-than-average number of painful events and a higher percentage of bodily symptoms than other common conditions. Analgesics (including opioids) and muscle relaxants help during this phase of care and should be administered liberally with close attention paid to possible adverse effects.

Distraction

Unlike traction, which helps bones realign and fuse properly, distraction is the process of separating opposing bone to encourage generation of new bone in the created space. An osteotomy is performed to allow for distraction and either an external or an internal device is utilised. Distraction can be used when limbs are of unequal lengths or if there is an angular deformity of a limb.

Monolateral, Taylor spatial frame and Ilizarov external fixators are common external fixation devices. The Ilizarov external fixator uses a system of wires, rings and telescoping rods that permits limb lengthening to occur by manual distraction (Fig 33.10). In addition to lengthening bones, the device can be used to correct angular or rotational deformities or to immobilise fractures. The device is attached surgically by securing a series of external full or half rings to the bone with wires. External telescoping rods connect the rings to each other. Manual distraction is accomplished by manipulating the rods to increase the distance between the rings. A special osteotomy or corticotomy involves cutting only the cortex of the bone, while preserving its blood supply, bone marrow, endosteum and periosteum. Capillary blood flow to the transected area is essential for proper bone growth. The bone may be lengthened approximately 1 mm per day or about 2.5 cm per month.

The use of motorised internal fixation devices is a relatively new treatment for correcting limb length discrepancies. Intramedullary nails are placed within the bone and an electrical or magnetic remote is utilised to control the distraction of the bone. This technique is typically performed in adolescents or skeletally mature individuals.

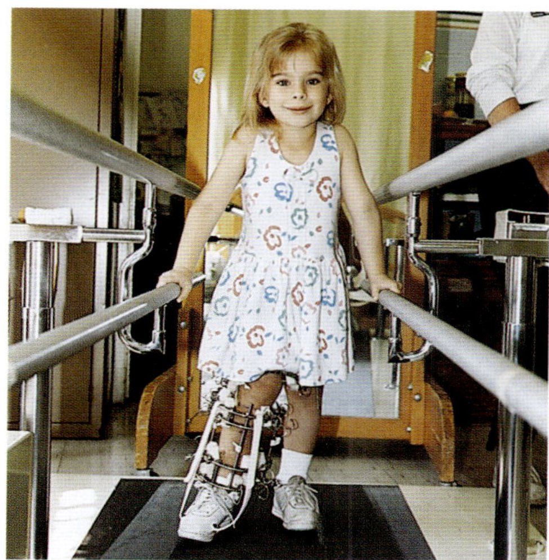

Fig 33.10 Child with Ilizarov external fixator (on right leg) during physical therapy on parallel bars.

Nursing Care Management

Successful use of external fixation depends on the child's and family's cooperation; therefore, before surgery, they must be fully informed about the appearance of the device, the way it accomplishes bone growth, required alterations in activities and home and follow-up care. Children are involved in learning to adjust the device to accomplish distraction. Children and parents should be instructed in pin care, including observation for infection and loosening of pins. Close monitoring of neurovascular status and changes of the involved extremity are also important.

Children who participate actively in their care report less discomfort. Because the device may be external, the child and family need to be prepared for the reactions of others. Partial weight bearing is allowed, and the child needs to learn to walk with crutches. Alterations in activity include modifications at school and in physical education. Full weight bearing is not allowed until the distraction is completed and bone consolidation has occurred. Follow-up care is essential to maintain appropriate distraction until the desired limb length is achieved. The device is removed surgically after the bone has consolidated; the child may need to use crutches or have a cast for 4 to 6 weeks after removal of the device to reduce the risk of fracture.

Amputation

A child may be born with the congenital absence of a body part, experience a traumatic loss of an extremity or require a surgical amputation for a pathological condition such as osteosarcoma. With today's surgical technology and the quick thinking of bystanders who save a traumatically amputated body part, some children have had fingers and arms sewn back on with varying degrees of functional use regained.

Surgical amputation or the surgical repair of a permanently severed limb focuses on constructing an adequately nourished residual limb. For lower extremities the presence of a smooth, healthy, padded stump, free of nerve endings, is important for prosthesis fitting and subsequent ambulation. In some situations in which there is no vascular or neurological deficit, a cast is applied to the stump immediately after the procedure, and a pylon, metal extension and artificial foot are attached so that the patient can walk on the temporary prosthesis within a few hours.

Nursing Care Management

Extremity stump shaping is done postoperatively with special elastic bandaging using a figure eight compression bandage, which applies pressure in a conical fashion. This technique decreases stump oedema, controls haemorrhage and aids in developing desired contours so that the child will bear weight on the posterior aspect of the skin flap rather than on the end of the stump. Postoperative complications for which the nurse should be vigilant include haemorrhage and infection of the operative site.

Postoperatively, the stump may be elevated for the first 24 hours, but after this time the extremity should not be left in this position because contractures in the proximal joint will develop and seriously hamper ambulation. Monitoring proper body alignment further decreases the risk of flexion contractures. Children who undergo amputation of a lower extremity should be turned not only from side to side but also from front to back. As the child progresses, encourage him or her to lie prone at least three times a day, increasing the time prone to tolerance of an hour at a time.

For children who have had an amputation, phantom limb pain is an expected experience because the nerve-brain connections are still present. Phantom pain is real pain and should be treated appropriately with analgesics and other pain-relieving measures. Gradually these sensations fade, although in many amputees they persist for years. Preoperative discussion of this phenomenon helps a child understand these feelings and not hide the experience from others. Limb pain, especially pain that increases with ambulation, should be evaluated for the possibility of a neuroma at the free nerve endings in the stump or a poorly fitting prosthesis. Chronic pain may also be related to weakness or joint instability, injury to the nerve or fibrosis of soft tissues. Pain in the contralateral extremity may result from asymmetric weight bearing.

Mobilisation Devices

Orthotics and Prosthetics

Developments in the fields of **orthotics** (fabrication and fitting of braces) and **prosthetics** (fabrication and fitting of artificial limbs) have resulted in lighter and better-fitting devices and thus greater patient compliance in using them. Orthoses are often used to prevent deformity, increase the energy efficiency of gait and control alignment. Braces that facilitate walking can sometimes stabilise paralysed or markedly weakened extremities. Special joint hinges permit the hip, knee and ankle to flex while sitting, whereas the leg is held rigid during ambulation. Well-fitted orthoses promote ambulation, whereas ill-fitting braces throw off the child's balance and frequently cause muscle stress and tissue breakdown. An orthosis must fit each body curvature to avoid undue pressure on tissues and imbalance between muscle groups. Bony prominences where a brace has contact, such as along the spine, chin, iliac crests, ankles and feet, are observed closely for pressure or irritation and are padded as necessary. In the growing child, braces need frequent adjustment and replacement if long-term use is necessary.

Types of orthoses are described based on the joints controlled by the orthosis. The ankle-foot orthosis (AFO) is used to prevent foot drop due to bed rest, trauma to the foot or paralysis of the muscles in the foot; to prevent heelcord tightening; or to support the foot in proper position for standing and walking. Shorter styles of bracing for the foot include a supramalleolar orthosis (SMO) and foot orthosis. The child will have custom made orthoses to encompass the foot, ankle and leg. A cast will be made initially (Fig 33.11) before a final AFO is fitted (Fig 33.12).

The knee-ankle-foot orthosis (KAFO) is used to prevent buckling of the knee, to support the extremity when there is paralysis or

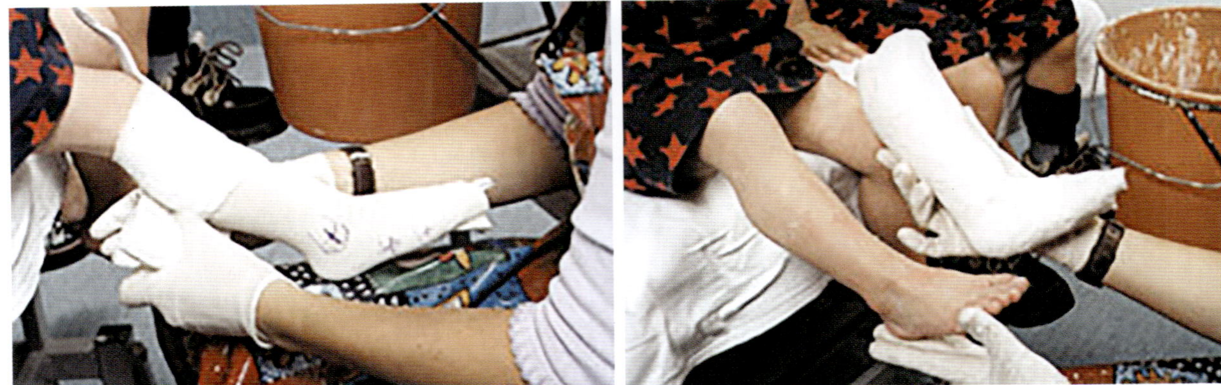

Fig 33.11 Custom-made orthoses to encompass the foot; ankle and leg will be made first. (Source: RCHM. (n.d.). Ankle-Foot Orthoses AFOs. Orthotic and Prosthetic Unit. https://www.rch.org.au/orthotic/info_for_parents/AnkleFoot_Orthoses_AFOs/)

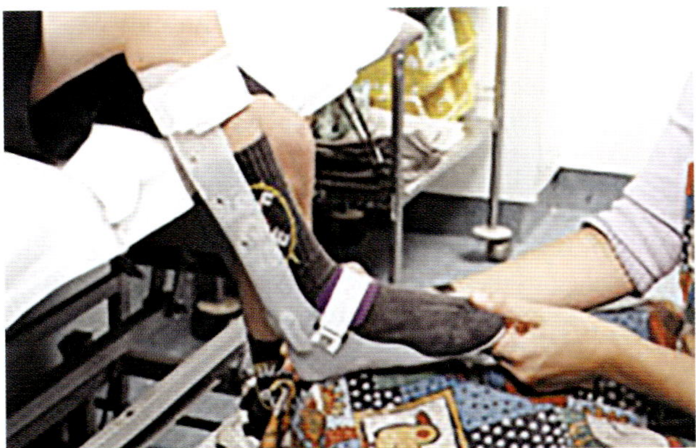

Fig 33.12 Fitting of the final AFO. (Source: RCHM. (n.d.). Ankle-Foot Orthoses AFOs. Orthotic and Prosthetic Unit. https://www.rch.org.au/orthotic/info_for_parents/AnkleFoot_Orthoses_AFOs/)

marked weakness of the quadriceps muscle or to protect the limb when the bone structure is weak. The hip-knee-ankle-foot orthosis (HKAFO) is used to provide various types of control for the knee and ankle joints as described earlier, as well as the hip (e.g. flail lower limb and paralysis). The reciprocal gait orthosis (RGO) is a type of HKAFO that has a mechanism allowing children with significant paraplegia to walk in a reciprocal fashion on a flat surface. RGOs are used in children with spinal cord injury, sacral agenesis and spina bifida.

The thoracolumbosacral orthosis (TLSO) and cervical thoracolumbosacral orthosis (CTLSO) are custom moulded and fit snugly around the trunk of the body to exert pressure on the ribs and back to support the spine in a straight position.

When prostheses are prescribed, the provider considers many factors: level of amputation, age, weight, activity, agility and skin condition. Each prosthesis is custom made or fabricated of various plastic and foam materials. Development of myoelectric devices, use of new cosmetic materials in terminal gloves and feet, and socket construction using computer-aided design and computer-aided manufacturing are but a few of the recent changes with positive effects for patients who require prostheses.

Nursing Care Management

Meticulous skin care under a brace is necessary. Protective clothing should be worn under braces to protect the skin from friction and pressure. Assessment of all areas that make contact with the brace every 1 to 2 hours for the first few days after application is recommended. If any area is reddened, the brace should be removed for at least 30 minutes. If the redness does not disappear, the nurse should notify the provider or orthotist (see Family-Centred Care box).

FAMILY-CENTRED CARE

Orthoses

Care of Skin

- If the child has decreased sensation in the legs, check the skin condition more frequently than every 4 hours.
- If the child complains of a burning sensation under the brace, remove the brace promptly and observe the skin for any reddened areas. If the child complains of burning several times, contact the provider or orthoptist/prosthetist.
- If a small blister or open area develops, cover it with a sterile bandage and check the skin more often. Do not put alcohol on open areas. The child should avoid wearing the device until the skin heals.
- Sometimes open areas are slow to heal. If no sign of healing occurs after 3 days, contact the provider or orthoptist/prosthetist.
- Lotions and creams will soften the skin and should be used only if the skin is dry.

Care of Orthoses

- Clean the plastic sections of the brace with soap and water and dry them thoroughly.
- Check all screws or fasteners periodically to make certain they are tight.
- If the brace is broken, out of alignment or causing skin problems, notify the orthotist.

Before a prosthesis is applied, the condition of the skin must be assessed, with special note taken of areas of redness or breaks in the integrity of the skin. Prevention of skin breakdown is best accomplished through good hygiene of the residual limb, proper fitting of the artificial limb and prosthetic training (see Family-Centred Care box).

Crutches, Canes and Walkers

Crutches, canes and walkers are used when children need support for balance while walking, are not allowed to bear weight or can place only part of their body weight on an extremity, such as with a lower leg injury. There are many types of crutches, and the selection depends on

FAMILY-CENTRED CARE

Prostheses

Care of Residual Limb

- Wash with mild, non-perfumed soap, rinse and dry thoroughly daily.
- Check skin for redness, blisters, sensitive areas or signs of infection.

Care of Prosthesis

- Routinely wash the socket with water and mild soap, rinse and dry thoroughly.
- Check straps and rubber bands with each application.
- Check joints to ensure that they operate smoothly.
- Replace worn or broken parts (heels, soles, straps) as needed.
- Use 100% cotton stump socks to absorb perspiration, prevent skin friction and provide comfort.
- Change socks daily, and wash and dry following instructions provided by prosthetist.

the child's individual needs. In children with limited hand and arm strength or function, the use of trough crutches allows the weight to be assumed by the elbow. For small children who have not yet learned to walk or those who are unsteady, front or reverse walkers are typically used (Fig 33.13).

Children must be properly fitted with a crutch, cane or walker to prevent both poor posture and crutch pressure on the axilla during ambulation. A physiotherapist usually measures the child and teaches crutch, cane or walker use; however, nurses in some areas such as the ED do teach children crutch walking.

Wheelchairs

Wheelchairs are used temporarily or permanently as a means of transportation. A wheelchair for temporary use should fit the child and contain any adaptations needed, such as an elevating leg rests or reclining back. The child learns how to transfer in and out of the chair and how to move it safely. Prescribing a wheelchair for permanent use is the joint responsibility of the provider and therapist after an assessment of home and surroundings. A wheelchair should be neither too small nor too large and preferably should be adaptable as the child grows (Fig 33.14).

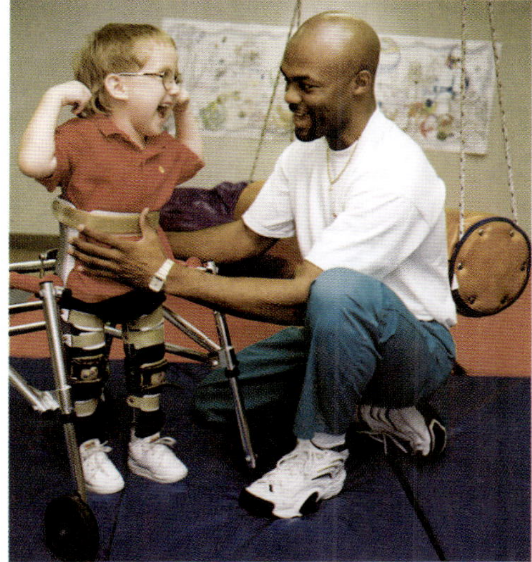

Fig 33.13 Young child with rear-rolling walker. (Source: Courtesy Texas Children's Hospital, Houston.)

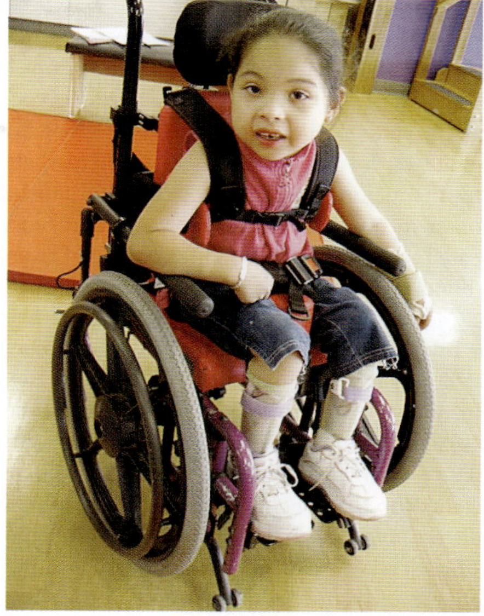

Fig 33.14 Child in wheelchair, which should be scaled appropriately to child's size. Note AFOs and left wrist splint to prevent contractures. (Source: Courtesy Texas Children's Hospital, Houston.)

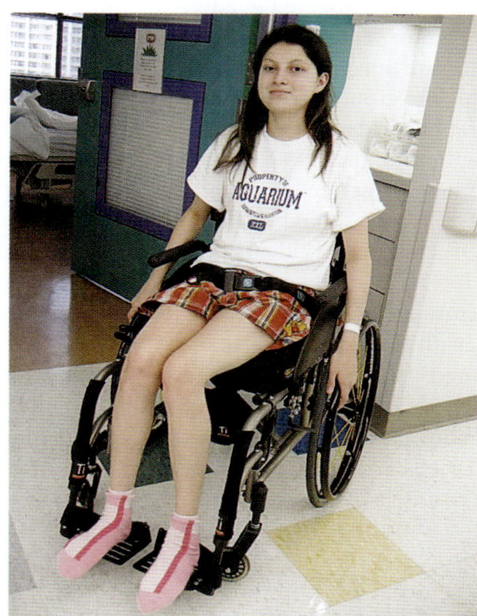

Fig 33.15 A wheelchair allows adolescent mobility and independence. (Source: Courtesy Texas Children's Hospital, Houston.)

Children with lower extremity paraplegia require upper arm strengthening exercises and instruction on transfer techniques before wheelchair mobilisation (Fig 33.15). Often a tilt table is used to overcome the problem of orthostatic intolerance before the child is able to tolerate wheelchair sitting.

Various motorised chairs are available for children with marked upper extremity weakness, and mouth- or cheek-operated models are available for children who do not have the use of upper extremities so they can operate the wheelchairs independently. Very small children who have permanent paralysis of the lower extremities are provided with specially designed units that allow independent mobility.

THE CHILD WITH A FRACTURE

The process of **ossification**, the gradual conversion of precursor substances (i.e. cartilage) to bony structures, begins in the embryo and continues until the child is 18 to 21 years of age. In long bones this process progresses outwards from the **diaphysis**, the hard, shaft-like portion that constitutes the major part of the bone. Within this hard, compact shaft is the hollow medullary canal composed of the bone marrow. The **epiphyses**, located at the ends of long bones, consist of layers of cartilage, subchondral bone and sponge-like cancellous bone. Situated between the diaphysis and the epiphysis is the **physis** (**growth plate**), which plays a major role in the longitudinal growth of the developing child (Fig 33.16). The **periosteum**, or thin, tough membrane covering all bones, contains blood vessels that nourish the living bone. Damage to this thin membrane can be a major problem in bone growth and healing.

Bones fracture when the resistance of the bone against the stress being exerted yields to the stress force. Fractures are a common injury at any age but are more likely to occur in children and the elderly. Because childhood is a time of rapid bone growth, the patterns of fractures, problems of diagnosis and methods of treatment are different in children compared with adults. An adult's bones are strong and require a violent traumatic force to fracture, which is accompanied by massive injury to surrounding soft tissues. In children the bones are more easily injured, and fractures may result from minor falls or twists and are less likely to be accompanied by soft tissue damage. Features of children's fractures not observed in adults are listed in Box 33.3.

Aside from motor vehicle crashes or falls from heights, true injuries causing fracture are uncommon in infancy; therefore, bony injuries in children of this age group warrant further investigation. In any small child, radiographic evidence of fractures at various stages of healing, with few exceptions, indicates a non-accidental injury or child abuse. Any investigation of fractures in infants and young children, particularly multiple fractures, should include the suspicion of osteogenesis imperfecta (OI) after non-accidental injury has been ruled out.

A distal forearm (radius, ulna or both) fracture is the most common fracture in children. The clavicle is also a common fracture in childhood, with approximately half of clavicle fractures occurring in children younger than 10 years of age. A common mechanism of injury is a fall with an outstretched hand or direct trauma to the bone (Fig 33.17). In neonates, fractures of the clavicle may occur with a large newborn and a small maternal pelvis. Hip fractures are uncommon in children and require a great deal of force to produce. A femoral neck fracture may be sustained in children 6 or 7 years of age as a result of pedestrian–motor vehicle crashes because in these children the hip is at the same level as a motor vehicle bumper. In older children, the femur is the most likely target; in adolescents knee injuries are common with this type of accident.

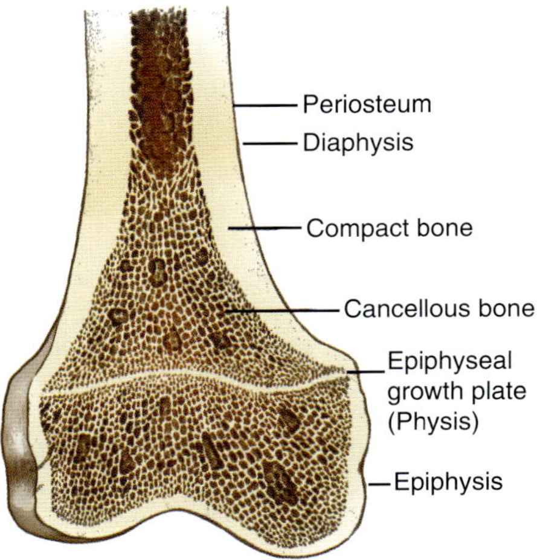

Fig 33.16 Diagram of bone showing relationships of compact and cancellous bone, epiphysis, physis and diaphysis.

BOX 33.3 Features of Fractures in Children

- The growth plate, a thick, elastic portion of bone where growth takes place, serves to absorb shock and protect joint surfaces from injury and is the means by which the limb is able to grow and to straighten itself. Growth is stimulated by a fracture in the diaphysis, whereas damage to the growth plate can cause shortening and often a progressive angular deformity.
- The periosteum of a child's bone is thicker and stronger and has more active osteogenic potential than that of an adult's bone.
- The pliable bones of the growing child are more porous than those of the adult, which allows them to bend, buckle and break in a 'greenstick' manner. The greater porosity increases the flexibility of the bone and dissipates and absorbs a significant amount of the force on impact.
- Healing is more rapid in children, and the rapidity is inversely related to the child's age. The younger the child, the more rapid the healing process. Non-union of bone fragments is uncommon except in severe injuries in children.
- Stiffness is unusual and, unlike in adults, an uninjured joint in a child can be immobilised for a long period without producing stiffness that lasts longer than a few minutes. Injured joints do become stiff, however, and the current trend is towards early mobilisation and active range-of-motion exercises as preventive measures.
- Children only complain when something is wrong. Unreasonable crying, restlessness and calling for the parents are usually indications that something is amiss and requires investigation.

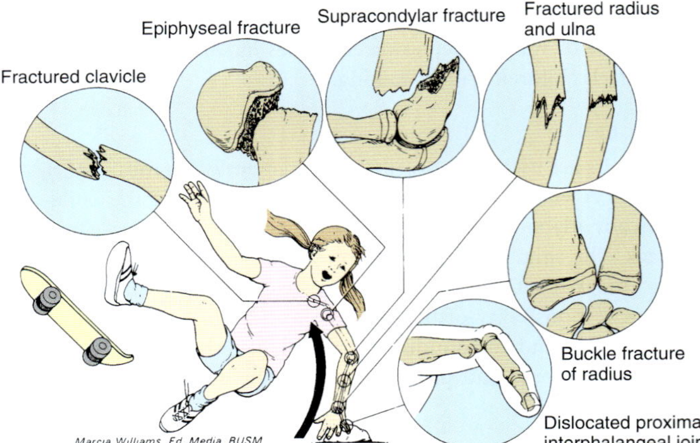

Fig 33.17 Trauma resulting from progression of force in fall on outstretched hand.

Types of Fractures. A fractured bone consists of fragments: the fragment closest to the midline or trunk, called the proximal fragment, and the fragment furthest from the midline, or the distal fragment. When fracture fragments are separated, the fracture is **complete**; when fragments remain attached, the fracture is said to be **incomplete**. The fracture line can be any of the following.

- Transverse—Crosswise, at right angles to the long axis of the bone
- Oblique—Slanting but straight, between a horizontal and a perpendicular direction
- Spiral—Slanting and circular, twisting around the bone shaft

The twisting of an extremity while the bone is breaking results in a **spiral** fracture. If the fracture injury does not produce a break in the

BOX 33.4 Types of Fracture in Children

Plastic deformation—Occurs when the bone is bent but not broken. A child's flexible bone can be bent 45 degrees or more before breaking. However, if bent, the bone will straighten slowly but not completely to produce some deformity but without the angulation seen when the bone breaks. Bends occur most commonly in the ulna and fibula, often in association with fractures of the radius and tibia.

Buckle, or Torus, Fracture—Produced by compression of the porous bone; appears as a raised or bulging projection at the fracture site. These fractures occur in the most porous portion of the bone near the metaphysis (the portion of the bone shaft adjacent to the epiphysis) and are more common in young children.

Greenstick Fracture—Occurs when a bone is angulated beyond the limits of bending. The compressed side bends, and the tension side fails, causing an incomplete fracture similar to the break observed when a green stick is broken.

Complete Fracture—Divides the bone fragments. These fragments often remain attached by a periosteal hinge, which can aid or hinder reduction.

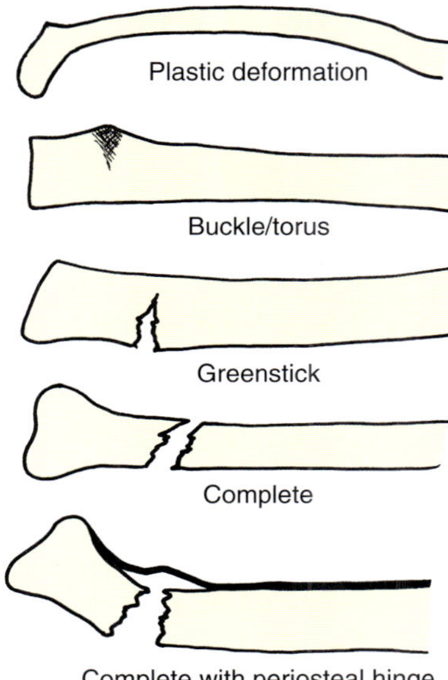

Fig 33.18 Common types of fracture in children. Note that there are subclassifications of complete fractures based on characteristics of the fracture line.

skin, it is a **simple**, or closed, fracture. Open, or **compound**, fractures are those with an open wound through which the bone protrudes. If the bone fragments cause damage to other organs or tissues (e.g. the lung or bladder), the injury is said to be **complicated**. When small fragments of bone are broken from the fractured shaft and lie in the surrounding tissue, the fracture is called **comminuted**. This type of fracture is rare in children. The types of fracture that occur most often in children are shown in Box 33.4 and Fig 33.18.

Growth Plate or Physeal Injuries. The weakest point of long bones is the cartilage growth plate or the physis. Consequently, this is a frequent site of injury during childhood trauma. The Salter-Harris classification is typically used to describe growth plate injuries, as indicated in Fig 33.19. Detection of physeal injuries is sometimes difficult but critical in determining whether bone growth will be affected. Close monitoring and early treatment, if indicated, are essential to prevent longitudinal or angular growth deformities (or both).

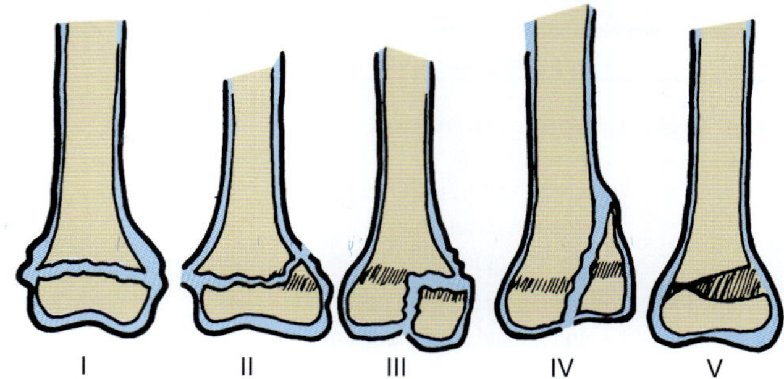

Fig 33.19 Types of physeal injuries developed by orthopaedists R. B. Salter and W. R. Harris: type I, separation or slip of growth plate without fracture of the bone; type II, separation of growth plate and breaking off of section of metaphysis; type III, fracture of physis extending through the epiphysis into the joint surface; type IV, fracture of growth plate, epiphysis and metaphysis; type V, crushing, comminuted fracture of the physis.

Bone Healing and Remodelling

Immediately after a fracture occurs, the muscles contract and physiologically splint the injured area. This phenomenon accounts for the muscle tightness observed over a fracture site and the deformity that is produced as the muscles pull the bone ends out of alignment. This muscle response must be overcome by traction or complete muscle relaxation (i.e. anaesthesia) in order for the distal bone fragment to be realigned to the proximal bone fragment.

Bone healing follows a patterned sequence. Fig 33.20 shows three broad overlapping phases: inflammatory, restorative and remodelling. Bone healing can be described more definitively in terms of five stages (Table 33.2). When the bone breaks, the envelope of subcutaneous tissue, muscle and periosteal tissue surrounding the site is torn; blood vessels rupture; and a haematoma forms. The ends of the fractured bone segments, deprived of circulation, die as far back as the nearest collateral circulation. Necrotic tissue accumulates, and an inflammatory response takes place at the site, with its characteristic vasodilation, plasma exudation and oedema. The organisation and reabsorption of the haematoma proceeds, and the restorative phase begins with the reestablishment of local circulation. Repair requires an adequate blood supply and immobilisation of the fracture fragments.

When there is a break in the continuity of bone, the periosteal and intraosseous osteoblasts are stimulated to maximum activity. New osteoblasts are formed in immense numbers almost immediately after the injury and begin building a bridge, as evidenced by a bulging growth of osteoblastic tissue and new bone matrix between the fractured bone fragments. This is followed by deposition of calcium salts to form callus, which provides stability (Fig 33.21B).

Bone healing is characteristically rapid in children because of the thickened periosteum and generous blood supply. In the young child, for example, there is frequently a solid union of the femoral shaft in

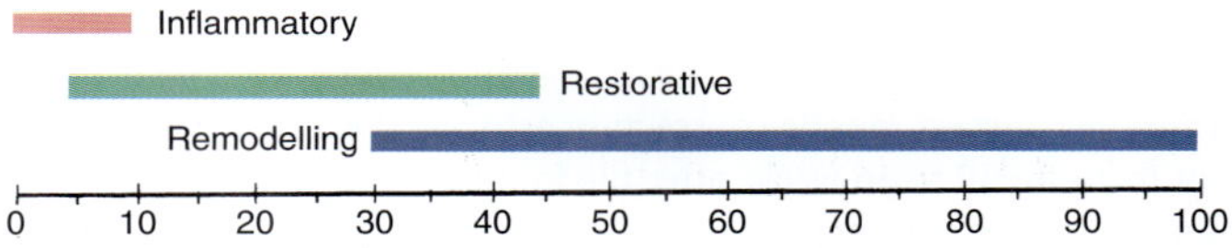

Fig 33.20 Approximate time spent in inflammatory, restorative and remodelling phases of bone healing. Scale indicates percentage of healing time.

TABLE 33.2 Stages of Bone Healing

Time*	Physiological Events
Stage 1: Haematoma Formation	
Impact	Fracture occurs. Injury to soft tissue envelops site. Periosteal tissue tears. Vessels rupture.
3–5 minutes	Bleeding occurs from bone and tissues into area between and around bone fragments.
First 24 hours	Haematoma forms and clots; fibrin assists in clotting periosteal membrane to aid in repair. Clot provides fibrin network for cellular invasion. Granulation tissue forms by fibroblasts and new capillaries. Osteoblastic activity stimulated.
Stage 2: Cellular Proliferation	
After 24 hours	Blood supply increases, bringing available calcium, phosphate and fibroblasts. Cells proliferate at ends of bone fragments and differentiate into cartilage and connective tissue.
Next few days	Haematoma becomes granulation tissue, which develops into a framework for bone-forming substances. Fibroblasts convert to osteoblasts (cells that form bone marrow).
2–3 days	*Halisteresis* (softening of bone ends) occurs for 3 to 6 mm; bone cells are resorbed.
Stage 3: Callus Formation	
6–10 days	Fibroblasts form in granulation tissue; form bone in areas adjacent to surface of bone shaft; form cartilage at surfaces more distal to blood supply. *Provisional callus* develops, bridging fracture ends; holds bone together but will not support body weight.
14–21 days	*True callus* develops, seen on radiographs; more than needed is formed, but with remodelling, excess callus is resorbed. Cartilage differentiates to bone tissue.
Stage 4: Ossification	
3–10 weeks	Callus forms into bone, which grows beneath periosteum of fragments; fuses (knits together) fracture defect. Also called *union stage*.
Stage 5: Consolidation and Remodelling	
After 9 months	Bone marrow cavity is restored. Compact bone forms according to stress patterns. Remodelling occurs according to Wolff's law. Fracture line is always visible on radiographs.

*Healing time is more rapid in infants and in cancellous (spongy) bone; may be delayed if complications occur.

3 to 4 weeks, whereas in the adult, callus sufficient to avoid deformities from the constant muscle contraction associated with movement may not form for 10 to 16 weeks after the injury. The approximate healing times for a femoral shaft fracture are as follows.

- Neonatal period—2 to 3 weeks
- Early childhood—4 weeks

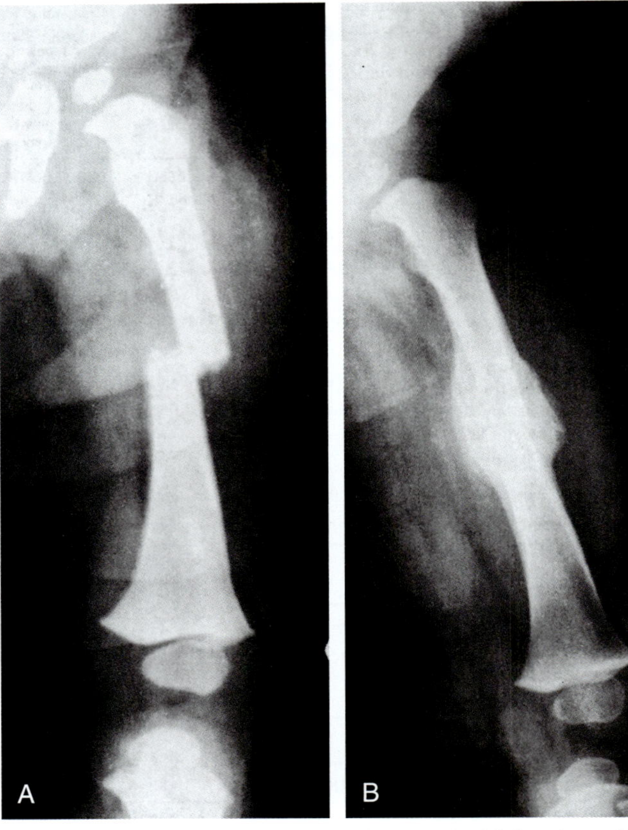

Fig 33.21 Fractured femur. Most femur fractures in childhood are of the spiral type shown here. Note comparison of (**A**) original x-ray film and (**B**) 6-month post fracture film showing callus formation.

- Later childhood—6 to 8 weeks
- Adolescence—8 to 12 weeks

Remodelling is a unique process that occurs in the healing of long bone fractures in growing children. When a bone remodels, the irregularities produced by the fracture become distinct because hollows are filled in and angles are rounded off in the healing process, which gives the bone a straighter, more typical appearance. The build-up of new bone or callus restores a portion of the normal bone structure in most cases despite observable malalignment. The younger the child and the closer the proximity of the fracture to the growth plate, the greater the degree of remodelling that is able to take place. Various factors such as the type and location of the fracture, the child's age and the amount of fragment angulation or rotation influence the degree of correction in alignment that can be obtained by remodelling.

The position of the bone fragments in relation to one another influences the rapidity of healing and the residual deformity. For example, a gap between fragments delays (or prevents) healing (Fig 33.22A). Healing is prompt and complete with end-to-end apposition (Fig 33.22B), but the fracture can stimulate accelerated growth of the neighbouring physis, causing bony overgrowth and increased length of the extremity. Angulation deformity caused by an incomplete fracture (Fig 33.22C) may remodel in the young child, but the degree of residual deformity depends on the relationship of the angulation of the bone fragments to the angle of the joint. This requires careful evaluation and reduction to prevent permanent deformity.

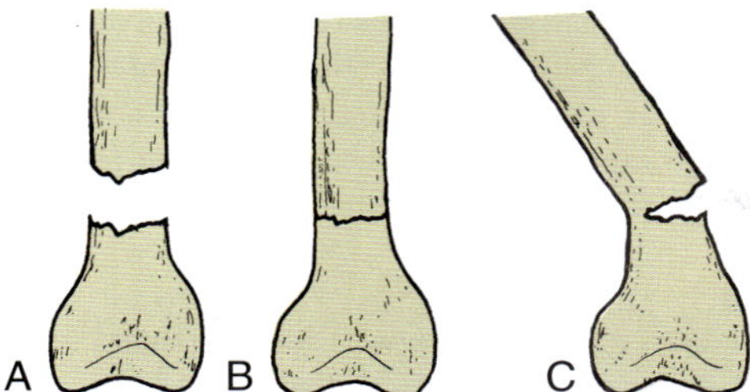

Fig 33.22 Relationships of fracture fragments. (**A**) Gap between fragments. (**B**) End-to-end apposition. (**C**) Angulation of incomplete fracture.

Wolff's law is applied in treating children with orthopaedic problems. Paraphrased, it states that bone will grow in the direction in which stress is placed on it. Examples of the use of this law are the hip spica cast with an abduction bar for treating developmental dysplasia of the hip and application of casts or traction at a selected angle to influence the direction of bone healing.

Bone healing in any age group is greatly influenced by the injured person's general health. The child with a fracture requires adequate nutrition for optimum bone healing. When nutritional intake is insufficient, vitamin and mineral supplementation may be necessary. Consumption of carbonated soft drinks should be limited or completely eliminated as the phosphoric acid in these drinks may interfere with calcium absorption.

Diagnostic Evaluation

A history of the injury or events leading up to the injury is helpful but often may be lacking for childhood injuries. Infants and toddlers are unable to clearly communicate the details of what occurred. Older children may not be reliable informants or volunteer information (even under direct questioning) if the injury occurred during questionable activities. In cases of child abuse, parents or caregivers may deliberately give false information to protect themselves or family members. Whenever possible, it is helpful to get information from someone who witnessed the injury.

Children demonstrate the usual signs of injury: generalised swelling, pain or tenderness and diminished functional use of the affected part. There may be bruising or severe muscular rigidity which are also frequent signs in adults. More often, the fracture is remarkably stable because of the usually intact periosteum. The child may even be able to use an affected arm or walk on a fractured leg.

Although neurological and vascular damage is much less frequent in children than in adult patients, the integrity of these structures must be thoroughly assessed. This is often difficult in infants and young children, who are unable to cooperate. Vascular injury is most likely to occur with supracondylar fractures of the humerus and femur. Femoral and popliteal vessels and the sciatic nerve are prone to trauma in femoral fractures. Humeral fractures may cause damage to the medial, ulnar or radial nerves and to the brachial artery.

Radiographic examination is the most useful diagnostic tool for assessing skeletal trauma. The calcium deposits in bone make the entire structure radio-opaque. However, during normal growth and development, much of the skeleton of infants and young children is composed of radiolucent growth cartilage that does not appear on radiographs. Radiographs are sometimes less reliable than gross deformity and point tenderness in predicting extremity fractures. Healthcare providers may also obtain a film of the uninjured limb for a direct comparison to help identify minor alterations in alignment. Radiographic films are also taken after fracture reduction and during the healing process to confirm satisfactory progress.

NURSING CARE CONSIDERATIONS

A fracture should be strongly suspected in a small child who refuses to walk or crawl. However, the fact that a child walks on a suspected fractured extremity does not rule out a fracture. Be on the watch for any signs of compartment syndrome (to be discussed in more detail in the fracture complication section); report any excessive pain which is one of the earliest signs of compartment syndrome (The Sydney Children's Hospitals Network 2019). It is also important to consider other differential diagnoses such as osteomyelitis, septic arthritis or malignancy (The Sydney Children's Hospitals Network 2019).

Therapeutic Management

The goals of fracture management are as follows:

- re-establish alignment and length of the bony fragments (reduction)
- retain alignment and length (immobilisation)
- restore function to the injured parts
- prevent further injury and deformity.

The majority of children's fractures heal well, and non-union is rare. Fractures are splinted (see Research Focus box) or casted to immobilise and protect the injured extremity. Children with displaced fractures may have a surgical reduction and fixation (internal or external) rather than being immobilised by traction. Box 33.5 describes factors that determine the type of reduction method for fractures. Some injuries may require immediate medical attention. These include open fractures, compartment syndrome with and without fracture, fractures associated with vascular or nerve injuries and joint dislocations that cannot be reduced.

RESEARCH FOCUS

Removable Splints

Handoll and colleagues (2018) conducted an integrated review of randomised controlled trials and quasi randomised trials comparing the management of displaced distal radial fractures in children and noted that there was evidence of maximum return to previous function for all those who had correct initial diagnosis with whatever treatment was instituted. They went on to add that the results concluded the need to move away from managing the injuries with casts and hence the use of the removable splints was considered to be ideal.

Nursing Care Management

Nurses often conduct the initial assessment of a child with a suspected fracture (see Nursing Care Considerations box). The child and parents may be frightened and upset, and the child is often in pain. Therefore, if the child is alert and there is no sign of haemorrhage, the initial nursing interventions are directed at calming and reassuring the child and parents so that a more thorough assessment can be easily accomplished.

BOX 33.5 Factors in Determining the Reduction Method for Fractures

- Age of child
- Degree of displacement
- Amount of overriding (bone)
- Degree of oedema
- Condition of skin and soft tissue
- Sensation and circulation distal to fracture

NURSING CARE CONSIDERATIONS

Fracture

Assess the extent of injury—five Ps:

- **P**ain and point of tenderness
- **P**ulselessness—distal to the fracture site (late and ominous sign)
- **P**allor
- **P**araesthesia—sensation distal to the fracture site
- **P**aralysis—movement distal to the fracture site.

Determine the mechanism of injury.

Provide adequate analgesia in line with the local policy guidelines.

Move the injured part as little as possible.

Cover open wounds with sterile or clean dressing.

Immobilise the limb, including the joints above and below the fracture site; do not attempt to reduce the fracture or push protruding bone under the skin.

- Soft splint (with pillow or folded towel)
- Rigid splint (rolled newspaper or magazine)
- Uninjured leg can serve as splint for leg fracture if no splint is available

Reassess neurovascular status and continue to monitor hourly until stable in line with the neurovascular assessment practice guidelines.

Apply manual traction if circulatory compromise is present.

Elevate the injured limb if possible using a sling or pillow as appropriate.

Apply cold to the injured area (no longer than 20 minutes with each application).

Call emergency medical services.

Fracture Complications

Circulatory Impairment

If the trauma or immobilising device restricts blood flow in veins or arteries of the affected extremity, bone healing will be seriously impaired. Careful assessment of the pulses, capillary refill, skin colour and temperature is an important nursing responsibility. In the upper extremity, brachial, radial, ulnar and digital pulses are felt. In the leg, femoral, popliteal, posterior tibial and dorsalis pedis pulses are checked. After injury, swelling of tissues occurs more rapidly in the child than in the adult.

Closely associated with an inadequate blood supply is a low haematocrit value, which can result from the initial blood loss or surgically induced anaemia. Although the blood flow may be adequate, a lowered amount of haemoglobin will not provide a sufficient supply of oxygen for tissue repair.

Nerve Compression Syndromes

Nerve damage can occur at the time of injury, develop in the process of realignment or arise as a complication of use of an immobilising apparatus. The syndromes are classified according to the anatomical area affected and can involve the median nerve (carpal tunnel syndrome), ulnar nerve (at wrist or elbow), radial nerve, posterior tibial nerve (tarsal tunnel syndrome), common peroneal nerve or sciatic nerve. Peroneal nerve damage can result in foot drop, and radial nerve impairment produces wrist drop. Both these disabilities can significantly interfere with activities of daily living.

Sensory testing with touch and pinprick and evaluation of motor strength by asking the child to move the unaffected joint distal to the injury are common means of determining neurological involvement. Subjective symptoms are pain or discomfort, muscular weakness, a burning sensation, limitation of motion and altered sensation. Because the fear of pain limits the child's cooperation, play can be the nurse's most valuable tool.

Treatment is alleviation of pressure on the nerve. The healthcare provider determines whether correcting the alignment will alleviate pressure on the nerve or whether surgical intervention is necessary. At times, sensory or motor changes indicate ischaemia, and the treatment is correction of the vascular disturbance.

Acute Compartment Syndromes

A compartment is a group of muscles surrounded by tough, inelastic fascial tissue. **Acute compartment syndrome (ACS)** occurs when pressure within this closed space increases and compromises circulation to the muscles and nerves within the space. Muscles and nerves of both upper and lower extremities are enclosed within such compartments. The most frequent causes of compartment syndrome are tight dressings or casts, skin traction, haemorrhage, trauma, burns and surgery. Other causes include an increase in compartment contents (e.g. haemorrhage, venous obstruction, infiltrated IV infusion, exudate) and externally applied pressure, such as lying on the affected limb.

NURSING CARE CONSIDERATIONS

Assessing for compartment syndrome includes monitoring for the five Ps of ischaemia (pain, pallor, pulselessness, paraesthesia and paralysis).

Signs and symptoms of compartment syndrome reflect a deficit in or deterioration of neuromuscular status in the anatomical area surrounding the involved structures. Clinical manifestations of compartment syndrome may occur as early as 30 minutes after the ischaemia develops and can be difficult to recognise in small children or in those who have a head injury. A palpable peripheral pulse and brisk capillary refill may be present despite increasing compartmental pressure. Tenseness may be noted on palpation of the area. The neuromuscular symptoms of compartment syndrome are severe pain that is out of proportion to the injury or pain not controlled by analgesia which worsens with limb movement (although pain is not always a manifestation), pallor or cyanosis, oedema, absence of pulses in the extremity (usually a late sign), loss of sensation, firm, tense shiny skin and motor weakness. Sensory deficit in the affected limb is reported to be the most reliable physical finding of compartment syndrome (Agency for Clinical Innovation [ACI] 2018a, Mencio et al 2015).

Unrelieved, the occlusive hypoxic process can cause some contracture if ischaemia lasts as little as 6 hours. A great deal of muscle damage occurs after 12 to 24 hours; 48 hours of ischaemia produces severe deformity, with muscle fibrosis and contractures in 5 to 10 days. If not treated, the contracture leads to severe deformity and paralysis.

If you suspect compartment syndrome, reassess the neurovascular status with another registered nurse/junior medical officer and notify the orthopaedic registrar/consultant immediately (ACI 2018a).

The immediate treatment is to remove any mechanically obstructive materials, such as tight bandages, and extend the joint to free blood vessels. The limb needs to be elevated to the heart level; any elevation beyond this level will result in decreased perfusion to the limb altogether (ACI 2018b). If tolerated, apply ice as appropriate (ACI 2018b). Monitor the neurovascular signs half hourly until the patient is reviewed (ACI 2018b). The patient should be kept nil by mouth in case of a surgical intervention being required. Provide adequate analgesia. If the symptoms do not improve within a few hours, arteriography is done in anticipation of a possible need for surgical intervention (**fasciotomy**) to decrease arterial spasms and to improve the blood supply by separation of the fascial sheaths of the involved muscles. Because early detection is important in preventing permanent damage to tissues, in certain high-risk situations specialists may recommend continuous monitoring of compartment pressures by way of a small, slit-tip catheter; Wick catheter; or needle inserted into the compartment.

Volkmann contracture (ischaemic muscular atrophy) is a serious, persistent flexion contraction of the forearm and hand caused by massive infarction of muscle. Pressure caused by a cast or tight bandage or by swelling from the injury in the area of the elbow begins with arterial occlusion and then progresses to muscle anoxia and reflex vasospasms. Finally, the lack of blood supply leads to muscle necrosis and replacement with fibrous tissue, which produces paralysis and a claw-like hand contracture. Any fracture that requires excessive traction can be complicated by Volkmann contracture; however, it occurs most often in the elbow.

Physeal Damage

Growth of bone originates from the physis or growth plate, and damage to this structure can result in unequal lengths of the extremities or angular deformity. This is most concerning in the lower extremities. Surgical intervention may be required if the limb length inequality becomes large enough. This may involve slowing the growth on the longer leg with a procedure called an epiphysiodesis or lengthening the bones in the shorter or affected extremity. Angular deformities may develop if a physeal bar or bony bridge forms across the growth plate. If less than 50% of the physis is involved a surgical procedure to resect the bar may be performed.

Non-union

Bone healing and callus formation can span and repair only a limited space between bone fragments. When bone fragments cannot be maintained in correct alignment for repair due to inadequate reduction or poor immobilisation, bone healing is impaired. The factors most likely to interfere with bone healing and to cause delayed union or non-union, based on the physiological needs for bone healing, are listed in Box 33.6.

The haematoma, which becomes the matrix for bone deposition in the break, must be free of infection or bits of adipose or connective tissue. Nutrients and bone-forming cells brought to the area by way of the bloodstream provide the vital ingredients for repair.

Sometimes artificial means are employed to facilitate bone healing. Bone grafting becomes necessary when bone non-union occurs. The donor site is usually the tibia or the iliac crest. Bleeding of bone ends may need to be artificially stimulated, and at times holes are drilled near the bone ends in an attempt to increase circulation. Postsurgical immobilisation of the recipient area is crucial to the success of the graft.

BOX 33.6 Factors that Interfere with Bone Healing

- Separation of bone fragments at fracture site
- Interposition of tissue between bone fragments
- Loss of bone tissue, especially from necrosis
- Infection
- Poor nutrition
- Interruption of blood supply
- Diseases that influence calcium metabolism (e.g. vitamin D deficiency)
- Bone cancer
- Administration of corticosteroids

Malunion

Malunion is fracture union with increased angulation or deformity at the fracture site. It can be detected at any stage in the healing process or after complete healing. Unsatisfactory reduction is the usual reason for malunion. A cast or splint that allows fracture movement is also likely to result in malunion. Periodic radiographic examinations help detect this complication and prevent it from becoming a major long-term problem.

Excessive deformity can be corrected during the healing process through realignment and re-immobilisation. However, attempts at correction may cause delayed union or non-union; therefore, the degree of deformity is carefully evaluated in light of these complications. The probability that sufficient spontaneous alignment will occur with growth and continuation of the healing process also is considered. Correction of the malunion when healing is near completion or completed requires surgical intervention.

Infection

Osteomyelitis, infection of the bone, is often secondary to a bloodstream infection but is a potential risk with open fractures, pressure ulcers or when bone surgery has been performed. Any bacterial organism can cause this infectious process; however, *Staphylococcus aureus* is the pathogen most frequently identified (Lewis et al 2017, The Royal Children's Hospital Melbourne [RCHM] n.d.).

Kidney Stones

Although uncommon in children, development of renal calculi is a potential risk whenever the child has a limb that is non–weight bearing for a long time, especially if the circumstances also produce urinary stasis. Measures to prevent the formation of renal calculi include maintaining optimal hydration, mobilising the child as much as possible and checking closely the amount and characteristics of urinary output. Any urinary tract infection should be treated promptly with appropriate antimicrobials and urine acidification because the nucleus of a calculus is often composed of bacterial debris or calcium and the build-up of stone is precipitated by alkaline urine. An associated problem, hypercalcaemia, was reviewed in the section on problems of the immobilised child.

Pulmonary Emboli

Blood, air or fat emboli can be a hazard to the child with a fracture. As post injury bleeding and clotting occur, a small piece of the clot has the potential to travel to vital organs, such as the lung, heart or brain, and produce a life-threatening vascular obstruction and ischaemia. Generally the pulmonary system is the most frequent site of emboli deposition, but it may not occur until 6 to 8 weeks after the injury.

Fat emboli are the greatest threat in an individual with multiple fractures, particularly fractures of the long bones such as the femur. Fat droplets from the marrow are transferred to the general circulation by the venous-arterial route, where they can be transported to the lung or brain. This type of embolism occurs within the first 24 hours, generally in the second 12 hours after the injury occurs. Adolescents are those usually affected in the paediatric age groups.

Intermittent compression devices are used to prevent venous pooling in the lower extremities when prolonged immobilisation is required. These devices are inflatable sleeves that allow cyclic emptying and filling of leg veins; the devices are used in children with spinal cord injury once mobilisation is initiated to decrease the effects of orthostatic intolerance. Anticoagulant drug therapy, passive and active range of motion and early mobilisation are also used to decrease venous stasis and prevent thrombus development.

NURSING CARE CONSIDERATIONS

Pulmonary embolism should be suspected in a child with a history of recent surgery, major trauma or prolonged immobilisation who suddenly develops chest pain and dyspnoea. The severe dyspnoea must be treated immediately by elevating the head when possible and administering oxygen by mask or nasal cannula; an IV line should be established. This is a medical emergency.

INJURIES AND HEALTH PROBLEMS RELATED TO SPORTS PARTICIPATION

Adolescents probably spend more time and energy practising and participating in sports activities than members of any other age group. Sports and game participation contributes significantly to growth and development, the education process and good health. It provides exercise for growing muscles, interaction with peers and a socially acceptable means of enjoying stimulation and conflict.

Every sport has some potential for injury to the participant—whether the young person participates in serious competition or purely for enjoyment. Serious injury is not limited to the athlete who competes in rough contact sports; a large number of severe or fatal injuries occur to those who engage in milder physical activity but are not physically prepared for it. For example, a person's body build may not be suited to the sport, muscles and support systems (respiratory and cardiovascular) may not have been sufficiently conditioned to withstand the rigors of the physical stress or the child or adolescent may not possess the insight and judgment to recognise when an activity is beyond his or her capabilities. Rapidly growing bones, muscles, joints and tendons are especially vulnerable to unusual strain.

Preparation for Sports

Among adolescents of the same age, the degree of physical maturation varies greatly, and many of the physical characteristics important in sports are related to hormone production. Consequently, physical strength, coordination, endurance and size vary considerably among children and adolescents who wish to compete against one another. Sports competition between young people who differ markedly in strength and agility is unfair and hazardous. Matching of candidates for sports should be based on physical maturity, height, weight and physical fitness and skills, particularly in sports involving rigorous body contact.

Categorising sports and activities according to the probability of collision and strenuousness can help estimate the risk of one sustaining an injury. Collision or contact sports for males and females such as football, basketball, hockey and soccer tend to have the highest injury rates, followed by other contact sports (Fig 33.23). In addition, Sports Medicine Australia (2017) has published safety guidelines that provide criteria for determining inclusion or exclusion of the young athlete based on common medical and surgical conditions and relative risks in various sports categories. This serves as a useful guideline for the health professional in counselling youth regarding sports activities (Sports Medicine Australia 2017).

Sports Medicine Australia (2017) encourages sports participation by young persons and encourages adults close to sports activities to be aware of the early warning signs of fatigue, dehydration and injury. Athletes should seek assistance when an injury is suspected and not 'work through' injuries caused by overuse (e.g. shin splints, stress fractures, tendonitis and apophysitis). Children and adolescents should be aware of not 'working through' non-contact, repetitive sports also as this may also have long-term impacts on growth (Sports Medicine Australia 2017) (Fig 30.24).

The role of healthcare professionals, specifically nurses, in relation to sports injuries focuses on prevention, treatment and rehabilitation. Of these areas, prevention is perhaps the most important. Children should use appropriate protective equipment that is properly maintained and fitted. The sports environment should make maximum provision for safety and availability of first aid and medical services.

Types of Injury

The injuries sustained in sports or recreational activities can involve any part of the body and range from relatively minor cuts, bruises and abrasions to severe closed head injuries such as concussion or totally incapacitating central nervous system injuries or death.

Some sports are particularly dangerous for children and adolescents. Snowmobiling, snowboarding, use of all-terrain vehicles (ATVs), skateboarding, motorcycle riding, bicycle riding and using trampolines

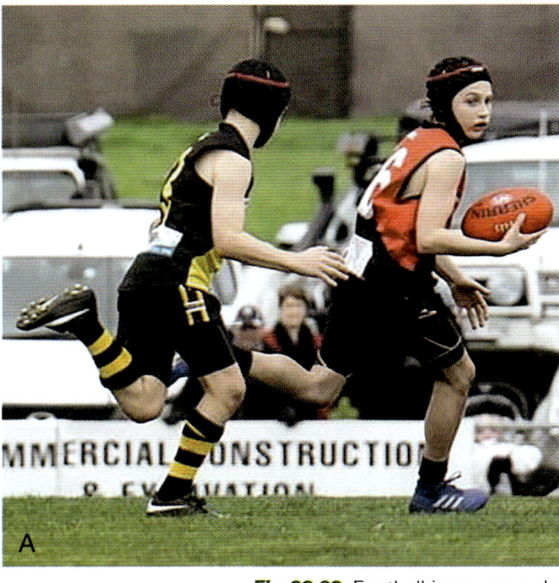

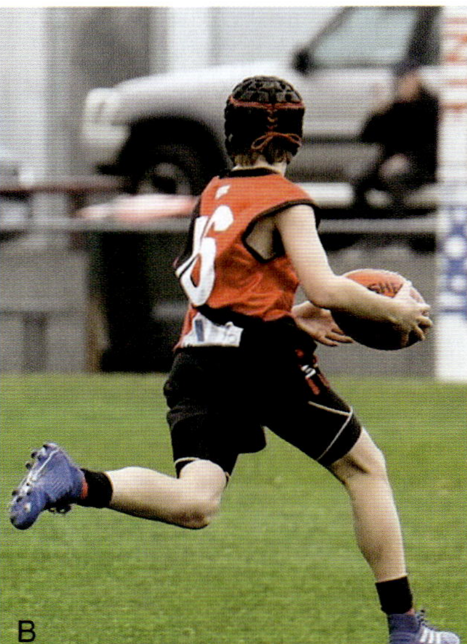

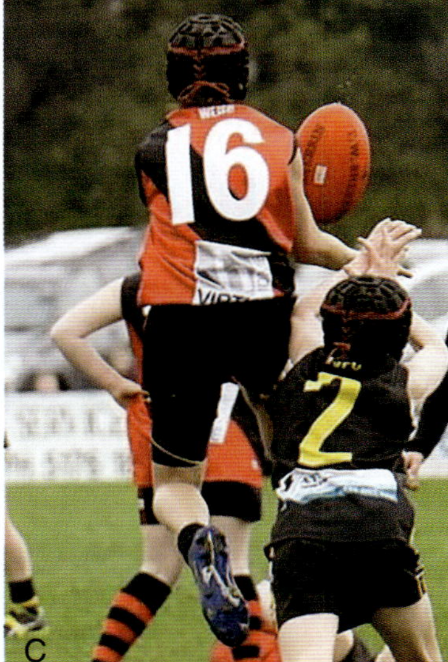

Fig 33.23 Football is an example of a strenuous collision sport with a high risk of serious injury.

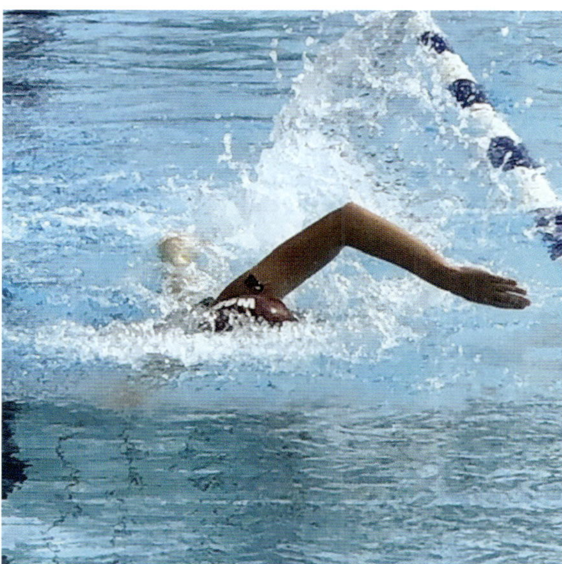

Fig 33.24 Competitive swimming is an example of strenuous and repetitive non-contact sport with high risk of serious injury where children and adolescents may 'work through it' and cause further damage.

are examples of sports and recreational activities that can lead to significant injuries in connection with inappropriate use, failure to wear protective equipment or participation by children who are underage. The Australian Institute of Health and Welfare (AIHW 2017) reported high rates of sport-related concussion related to Australian Rules football for the years 2012–13. Ankle injuries are the most common competitive sports–related injuries, with significant numbers occurring in the 15 to 24 years age group predominantly in soccer and football (AIHW 2017). Recent attention has focused on the management and prevention of concussion injuries among adolescent as well as adult athletes.

A variety of injuries can result when an external force is applied that causes severe stress on tissue, muscle and skeletal structures (Fig 33.25). The body structures attempt to absorb the force, but when they are unable to do so, injuries occur. Two general types of injury are recognised. The first is **acute trauma**, which is defined as a sudden, acute injury from a major force. Among such injuries are fractures of long bones and the axial skeleton; sprains of joint ligaments; strains of muscle tendon units; and contusions, including those of muscle tendon units and overlying soft tissue. The second type is repetitive **overuse injuries**, or microtrauma, which result from repetitive injury to tissue over a long period. Overuse injuries include stress fractures, bursitis, tendonitis, apophysitis and at times injuries of the joint surface.

Contusions

Contusions are a common sports injury and are often considered to be 'part of the game'. A contusion is damage to the soft tissue, subcutaneous structures and muscle. The tearing of these tissues and small blood vessels and the ensuing inflammatory response lead to haemorrhage, oedema and associated pain when the child or adolescent attempts to move the injured part. The escape of blood into the tissues is observed as ecchymosis, a black-and-blue discolouration.

The most serious contusions are those involving the quadriceps; they are common in strenuous, collision-type sports and usually result from being kicked or kneed in the thigh. Large contusions cause gross

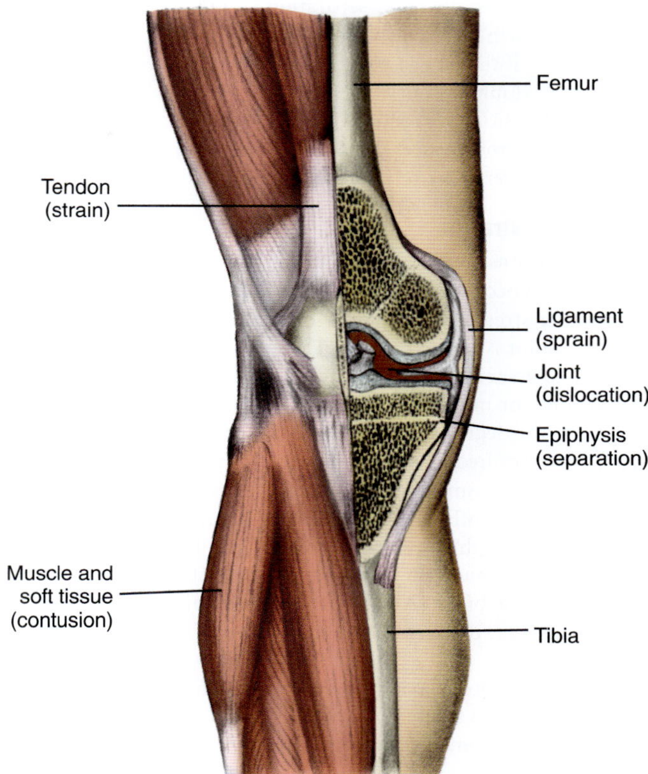

Fig 33.25 Sites of injury to bones, joints and soft tissues.

swelling, pain and disability and usually receive immediate attention from healthcare personnel. The less spectacular, smaller injuries may go unnoticed, so continued participation is allowed. They can become disabling after rest, however, because of pain and muscle spasm. The young athlete is frequently instructed to 'work it out' or disregard the pain. *Myositis ossificans* may occur from deep contusions to the biceps or quadriceps muscles; this condition may result in a restriction of flexibility of the affected limb.

Immediate treatment of a contusion consists of application of cold as in the treatment of sprains described later. Return to participation is allowed when the strength and range of motion of the affected extremity are equal to those of the opposite extremity.

Dislocations

Long bones are held in approximation to one another at the joint by ligaments. Joints can be tight or loose, and loose joints are more likely to be dislocated. A dislocation occurs when the force of stress on the ligament is great enough to disrupt the normal position of the opposing bone ends or the bone end and its socket. The predominant symptom is pain that increases with attempted passive or active movement of the extremity. In dislocations there may be an obvious deformity and inability to move the joint. Simple dislocations should be reduced as soon as possible with the child under mild sedation and often local anaesthesia. Increased swelling, which makes reduction difficult and increases the risk of neurovascular problems, can complicate an unreduced dislocation. Treatment depends on the location and severity of the injury.

Dislocations are less common in children than in those who are skeletally mature, but some types are specific to the younger age groups. Before final closure of the physis (growth plate), injuries to the joints are more likely to cause separation of the epiphysis from the metaphysis (growth plate injury) than dislocation.

Dislocation of the patella occurs spontaneously in some children; in others it is a result of injury. The patella is typically dislocated laterally. Most dislocations are reduced either spontaneously or by a companion before a provider sees the child. Therapy is immobilisation for 3 to 4 weeks. Surgery may be indicated to treat recurrent dislocations.

Sprains and Strains

Sprains and strains are the most common high school sports-related injury. A sprain occurs when trauma to a joint is so severe that a ligament is either stretched or partially or completely torn by the force created as a joint is twisted or wrenched. This is often accompanied by damage to associated blood vessels, muscles, tendons and nerves. As a guideline for management and prognosis, sprains are classified according to the degree of injury (Box 33.7). Because of the number of ligaments required to maintain knee stability, the knee is one of the joints most commonly injured in sports. It is also the largest joint and consequently is more prone to injury. Ankle sprains in children, even though considered to be mild injuries, were noted to take longer to heal and also to have a high chance of contributing to chronic ankle instability (AIHW 2017). These injuries are common in individuals who participate in sports, especially in the paediatric age group.

The presence of joint laxity is the most valid indicator of the severity of a sprain. With a severe injury the athlete complains that the joint 'feels loose' or as if 'something is coming apart' and may describe hearing a 'snap', 'pop' or 'tearing'. Pain is seldom the principal subjective symptom. There is a rapid onset with swelling, often diffuse, accompanied by immediate disability and appreciable reluctance to use the injured joint.

A strain is a microscopic tear to the musculotendinous unit and has features in common with sprains. The area is painful to the touch and is swollen. The severity is evaluated as grade I, II or III, as for sprains, except that the degree of laxity does not apply. Even with severe grade III injuries, complaints of laxity are rare. Most strains happen over time rather than suddenly, and the rapidity of the appearance provides clues regarding severity. In general the more rapidly the strain occurs, the more severe the injury. When the strain involves the muscular portion, there is more bleeding, often palpable soon after injury and before oedema obscures the haematoma.

Therapeutic Management

The first 6 to 12 hours is the most critical period for virtually all soft tissue injuries. Basic principles for managing sprains and other soft tissue injuries are summarised in the mnemonics RICE and ICES.

BOX 33.7 Classification of Sprains

Grade I—Mild injury; involves overstretching or microscopic tearing but without haemorrhage or increased instability of the involved joint. Swelling may develop later.

Grade II—Moderate injury; involves partial, overt tearing of the ligament with at least some ligamentous continuity remaining; usually immediate pain and swelling with decreased function.

Grade III—Severe injury; total loss of ligamentous continuity (i.e. disruption of one or more ligaments or the musculotendinous unit). Pain is immediate but subsides because none of the pain fibres is being stretched. Swelling may be minimal because haemorrhage extravasates outside of the area into soft tissues.

R—Rest
I—Ice
C—Compression
E—Elevation

I—Ice
C—Compression
E—Elevation
S—Support

There is still controversy over whether heat or ice should be used during the rehabilitative phase of management. Regardless of the method used, it should be accompanied by appropriate exercise, depending on the severity of the injury, and carried out under the direction of a competent professional experienced in the care of sports injuries.

Ice has a rapid cooling effect on tissues that reduces pain and the magnitude of the stretch reflex by decreasing muscle spindle response, afferent nerve discharge and the afferent loop response (monosynaptic reflex). Secondary effects are achieved by vasoconstriction, decrease in muscle nerve velocity and increase in muscle viscosity. Also, the decreased temperature slows metabolism, which reduces tissue oxygen requirements. Oedema formation is reduced when fewer histamine-like substances are released. Nine to 15 minutes of ice exposure produces deep-tissue vasodilation without increased metabolism. However, the effects last up to 7 hours. Ice therapy should be intermittent, and ice should never be applied for more than 30 minutes at a time to prevent tissue damage.

Elevating the extremity uses gravity to facilitate venous return and reduce oedema formation in the damaged area. The point of injury must be kept at least 10 cm above the level of the heart for therapy to be effective (Fig 33.26). Allowing the extremity to be dependent causes excessive fluid accumulation in the area of injury, which delays healing and causes painful swelling.

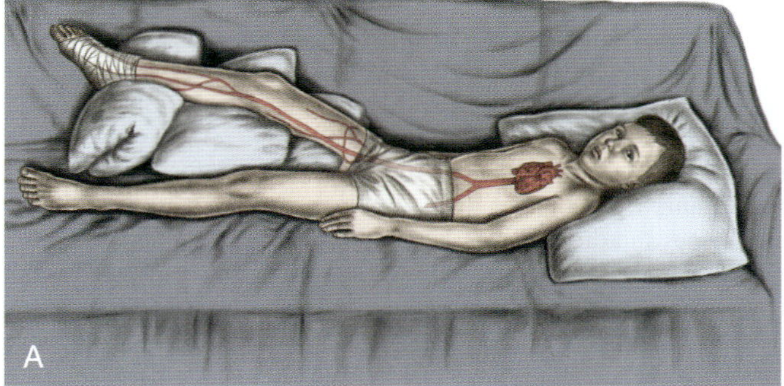

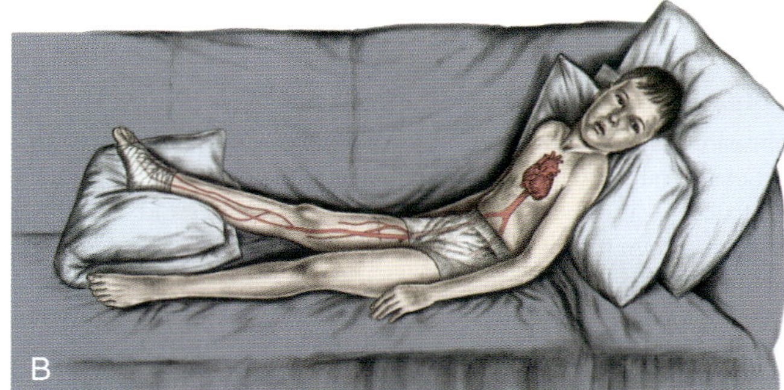

Fig 33.26 Correct and incorrect methods for elevating a lower extremity. (**A**) Correct method: lower leg elevated on pillows; ankle above heart level. (**B**) Incorrect positioning: ankle below level of heart.

Overuse Injury

To excel in sports, the young athlete is forced to train longer, harder and earlier in life than previously. The rewards are an increased level of fitness, better performance, faster times and the satisfaction of attaining a personal goal. With the increase in the number of children participating in a wide variety of sports year-round, more **overuse injuries** are being seen in the paediatric age group. More paediatric athletes are also specialising in one sport and participating year-round. It is recommended for the paediatric athletes to take a break from their usual sport for at least 2 to 3 months per year to reduce the risk of overuse injuries (Kidsafe WA 2018).

The risk of overuse injury is always present and can be related to several factors: training errors, muscle-tendon imbalance, anatomical malalignment (e.g. femoral anteversion, excessive lumbar lordosis, tibial torsion), incorrect footwear or playing surface, an associated disease state and growth (growth cartilage is less resistant to microtrauma). Chronic pain in athletes is often associated with overuse injury, which can occur at any level of athletic participation. The common feature in overuse injuries is the repetitive microtrauma that occurs to a particular anatomical structure. Performing the same movements time and time again can cause several types of injury: (1) frictional, or rubbing of one structure against another; (2) tractional, or repeated pull on a ligament or tendon; and (3) cyclic, or repetitive loading of impact forces (stress fractures). The end result is inflammation of the involved structure with complaints of pain, tenderness, swelling and disability.

Stress Fractures

Given the intensity and duration of sports training, many young athletes suffer stress fractures, especially after a recent increase in training regimens. These fractures occur as a result of repeated muscle contraction and occur most often in sports involving repetitive weight bearing such as running, gymnastics and basketball. They occur less often in swimming (in the upper extremities). Tibial stress fractures are most common.

The most common symptom of stress fracture is a sharp, persistent, progressive pain or a deep, persistent dull ache located over the bone. Sometimes there is pain on impact (heel strike), but the most important clinical sign is pain over the involved bony surface. Diagnosis is based on clinical observation. Plain radiographs are rarely diagnostic of stress fractures during the initial few weeks because callus formation is not yet evident. An MRI may more closely delineate a soft tissue injury/inflammation.

Therapeutic Management

Inflammation is common to all overuse syndromes; therefore, management involves rest or alteration of activities, physical therapies and medication. Rest is the primary therapy, usually interpreted as reduced activity and the use of alternative exercise—not bed rest or immobilisation with casting. The main purpose is to alleviate the repetitive stress that initiated the symptoms. It is important to keep the child or adolescent mobile, and training can be continued. Alternative exercise is selected that maintains conditioning without aggravating the injury. For example, pool running (treading water in the deep end of a pool) uses the same movements as running but without the weight bearing. Bicycling, swimming and rowing are viable alternatives.

Other modalities include cryotherapy and cold whirlpool baths, and sometimes taping, bracing, splinting and other orthoses are employed, depending on the injury. Medications such as non-steroidal anti-inflammatory drugs (NSAIDs) are sometimes prescribed to reduce inflammation and pain. Topical medications are of questionable value.

Exercise-induced Heat Stress

Infants, children and adolescents are at greater risk for heat-related illness than adults (AIHW 2017). Several characteristics of infants and children render them more vulnerable to heat stress. The greater ratio of surface area to body mass in infants and young children leads to increased transfer of heat between the body and the environment. Although infants do not exercise they may become overheated through environmental exposure (e.g. being left in a closed car). Children produce more metabolic heat for body mass during exercise and have a reduced capacity to convey heat from the body core to the skin. Also, children do not have the sweating capacity of adults and take longer to become acclimatised to hot conditions. Young children may not feel the need to drink a sufficient amount of fluid during extended exercise.

Heat cramps are caused by sodium depletion, which in turn potentiates the effects of calcium on skeletal muscle. They most often occur as a result of strenuous exercise in a hot environment. Cramps most frequently involve the leg muscles. Vital signs are usually normal, but the core temperature may be elevated. The child sweats profusely, but mentation is normal. Treatment consists of rest and replacement of fluid and electrolytes. Ingestion of dilute sports drinks or electrolyte replacement liquids is helpful.

Heat exhaustion, or heat stress, is a condition that usually occurs during vigorous exercise in a hot environment. It results from excessive loss of fluids, especially in poorly acclimatised and dehydrated children. The onset may be gradual, with initial complaints that include thirst, headache, fatigue, dizziness, anxiety or nausea and vomiting. The child usually has a clear sensorium but may be somewhat disoriented. The temperature can be normal or mildly elevated; sweating is profuse. Tachycardia, hypotension (usually postural) and syncope may be observed secondary to intravascular volume depletion. Treatment is to move the child to a cool environment, provide rest and replace fluid volume. The child with a clear sensorium can receive oral replacement fluids, but often IV fluids are required due to vomiting. External cooling methods are not necessary.

Heatstroke represents a failure of normal thermoregulatory mechanisms. Heatstroke usually occurs during or immediately after physical activity, especially in the unacclimatised adolescent who is exercising vigorously. The onset is rapid, with initial symptoms of headache, weakness and disorientation. Central nervous system manifestations may be agitation, confusion and lethargy. Loss of consciousness may occur without warning and may be accompanied by nuchal rigidity, posturing and convulsions. Sweating may not be present. The temperature is typically higher than 40°C, and there is severe volume depletion. Immediate care is relocation to a cool environment, removal of clothing, application of cool water (wet towels or immersion) and use of fans. The child should be transported to the nearest hospital immediately.

Acute care includes rapid cooling until core temperature reaches 38.9°C to prevent overcooling. Antipyretics are not used because they are metabolised by the liver, which is already not functioning properly. Renal and liver failure are common sequelae to heatstroke. Treatment includes careful monitoring of temperature and other vital signs, supportive care such as supplemental oxygen administration and cautious fluid and electrolyte replacement. Prevention remains the best treatment for hyperthermia. If the temperature is elevated, time in the sun should be decreased. Activity should be stopped if the humidity is elevated as well. The athlete should drink plenty of fluids, preferably with low sugar content.

Health Concerns Associated with Sports

Nutrition

Some athletes are motivated to enhance their performance by any and all means available. They are eager to learn about nutrition, and many are influenced by misconceptions, fads and superstitions regarding certain foods. Physical performance is affected by energy and body composition. The young athlete must maintain a diet that provides sufficient nutrients and energy to meet metabolic needs for optimum functioning. Physical training increases the need for energy and for more nutrients that convert food energy into chemical energy for physical performance.

There is no evidence to indicate that food supplements, extra vitamins, sports bars or high-protein diets are needed to meet the demands of heavy physical exercise or improve physical performance in children or adolescents. In addition, there are no scientific data, other than anecdotal reports, supporting the benefits of such supplements in increasing physical performance (Burke & Peeling 2018). Athletes should be given accurate information regarding the lack of proven safety for such supplements. Young athletes need considerably more calories than the recommended dietary allowance (RDA). When the basic requirements for growth and activity are met by a balanced diet of protein, grains and cereals, fruits and vegetables and dairy products, the additional calories needed for the extra exertion can be selected as desired. The athlete can obtain these extra calories by eating additional helpings from any of the basic four food groups, but many of the additional calories are provided by complex carbohydrates found in foods such as vegetables, pastas and bread.

The recommended dietary energy intake for adolescents involved in sports is a caloric intake from carbohydrates which matches the exercise demands, protein intake of 1.3 to 1.8 g/kg/day and 20% to 35% from fat (Sports Dietitians Australia 2019). It should be noted, however, that energy requirements vary depending on the sport and the children or adolescent's age and body build. Adolescent athletes need additional iron and calcium intake from appropriate food sources to meet growth and developmental needs and to replace amounts lost in competition.

Water and Electrolytes. Considerable water is lost from the body through perspiration, urination and evaporation from the respiratory tract. Water losses, especially from the skin, increase as the duration and intensity of exercise increase and as the environmental temperature rises. Although thirst is experienced early in dehydration, it is unreliable as an indicator of fluid deficit. Water is recommended as *the best drink* for most athletes. Very little water is exchanged in the stomach, and it must reach the intestines for absorption. The best fluids for rapid gastric emptying are cold, have low osmolality and have a large volume. Fluids should never be restricted during activity. Drinking carbonated beverages is discouraged. Fluids containing 6% to 8% carbohydrates appear to have a faster gastric emptying time than water and may be tolerated by adolescent athletes (Kleinman & Greer 2014).

Small amounts of electrolytes, especially sodium and chloride, are lost during exercise. Because sweat is quite dilute relative to plasma, excessive perspiration can result in excessive loss of water and an increase in plasma concentrations of sodium chloride. Therefore, it is more important to replace water than sodium and chloride. Children should be well hydrated before beginning strenuous exercise or sports, especially in warm climates or environments. Athletes should hydrate with water regardless of thirst during strenuous exercise or activity. Periodic drinking breaks are encouraged, and adults or other team members should be alert to the child who has complaints such as headache, cramping, nausea or vertigo. The use of salt tablets or table salt is unnecessary and may actually be harmful. Athletes usually derive sufficient salt replacement from the diet. Energy drinks are not recommended in children and adolescents participating in sports activities as these may lead to increased caloric intake which would lead to increased weight gain and consequential obesity (Dezbrow et al 2014).

Minerals. The basic diet does not satisfy the iron requirement of 10% to 15% of female athletes, most of whom are teenage girls who tend to become iron depleted after menarche. Young boys who are experiencing rapid adolescent growth and who have irregular and inadequate diets also are at risk of iron depletion. These children may need iron supplements; however, Dezbrow and colleagues (2014) do not recommend iron supplementation in athletes whose iron stores are adequate. Athletes who are participating in weight-restrictive sports or who are otherwise restricting dietary intake may need supplemental iron. There is currently no evidence that iron supplementation in healthy individuals enhances sports performance (Dezbrow et al 2014) Consideration for iron supplementation should only be done if medically indicated under the guidance of a medical practitioner (Dezbrow et al 2014).

Adequate calcium intake during puberty is essential to promote mineralisation of the growing skeleton. The recommended dietary reference intake (DRI) for calcium in adolescents ages 14 to 18 years is 1300 mg/day and the national reverence value for Vitamin D for children of all ages is 5 microgram/day, yet few adolescents meet this goal. Calcium plays a vital role in nerve transmission, muscle contraction and blood coagulation. Female athletes who engage in intensive training may develop amenorrhoea, with subsequent decreased bone mineral density, osteopenia and osteoporosis. Although the last two conditions may not occur immediately, stress fractures and impaired muscle contractions may be seen with low calcium intake. The best sources of additional calcium for athletes are non-fat dairy products. A well-balanced diet can provide the necessary calcium intake if adolescent athletes are made aware of the requirements and of the long-term consequences of poor nutrition.

Weight. Control of body weight by restricting water or food intake or increasing sweat loss is dangerous. Weight loss should not exceed 1.5% of total body weight per week (Kleinman & Greer 2014). Young athletes need appropriate information about nutrition to dispel the allure of fads and fallacies about diet and performance. A sports nutritionist should be consulted for determining an optimal diet based on amount of energy expenditure and energy requirements. The optimum diet for an athlete is one that contains the essential food groups and that is adjusted to the energy requirements of the sport in which the child or adolescent is engaged. Such a dietary plan should provide adequate nutrition for top physical efficiency and performance, maintenance of physical fitness and desirable body weight and optimum function of all organ systems.

Considerations for the Female Athlete

The syndrome known as **female athlete triad** was initially defined in 1997 as amenorrhoea, osteoporosis and low caloric intake or disordered eating. The definition has evolved to become more inclusive and represent the spectrum of this disorder ranging from health to disease. The three components of female athlete triad have been renamed to menstrual function, bone mineral density and energy availability; female athletes may present with any or all of these components (Brown et al 2017). The triad was originally described in athletes in sports for which thinness was desired (e.g. gymnasts, ballet dancers, figure skaters and long-distance runners) but is now recognised in virtually all sports. The phenomenon has been attributed to a complex interplay of physical, genetic, hormonal, nutritional, psychological and environmental factors that include the stress of competition, decreased protein consumption and altered lean-to-fat body ratio.

Menstrual irregularities can be common in adolescent girls but have been found to be more common in athletes. Adolescent athletes with amenorrhoea have a lower bone mineral density and are more likely to sustain a musculoskeletal injury than their peers. In addition, amenorrhoea or oligomenorrhoea has been associated with cardiovascular risk factors such as endothelial dysfunction. Low oestrogen levels and nutritional intake lead to a deficit in bone mineral density. The majority or nearly 90% of bone mass is reached by late adolescence. Girls with diminished oestrogen secretion in delayed menarche will reach late adolescence with low bone density and will be subject to stress fractures and osteoporosis.

Energy availability is defined as the amount of energy left in the body after exercise training; a spectrum of eating disorders is commonly seen, ranging from poor eating habits to eating disorders (Brown et al 2017). Disordered eating is less severe and more subtle than eating disorders such as anorexia and bulimia. Disordered eating includes food restrictions, rigid food patterns, fasting, vomiting and the use of diet pills and laxatives. The goal is to achieve a specific body image that is seen as desirable for the sport and is influenced by others such as coaches, teammates or peers. Disordered eating results in poor protein intake, low fat intake and inadequate caloric intake. Adolescent females should increase calcium intake to four to six servings per day of low-fat dairy products (recommendation for 1300 mg of calcium and the national reverence value for Vitamin D for children of all ages is 5 microgram/day) (Dezbrow et al 2014). In addition, they should consume adequate protein and calories to meet the energy and metabolic needs of exercise. Trainers and coaches also need to be aware of the potentially long-term results of intensive, prolonged exercise in pubertal girls.

Treatment may be long term and often involves development of an appropriate nutritional plan with a multidisciplinary team approach. However, education alone may not provide adequate incentive to change behaviour, and psychological health interventions may be required.

Substance Misuse by Athletes

Young athletes may use various performance-enhancing substances in an attempt to augment their athletic performance. Athletes believe that these substances, also known as *ergogenic aids*, increase strength and endurance, delay the onset of fatigue, increase the ability to concentrate and decrease sensitivity to pain. Examples of substances athletes use include psychomotor stimulants (e.g. amphetamines), anabolic-androgenic steroids (AAS), ephedra, androstenedione (andro), dehydroepiandrosterone (DHEA), creatine, guarana, ginseng, amino acid and protein supplements and excess amounts of vitamins (e.g. nicotinic acid (niacin), vitamin A, vitamin B_6).

Because many of these substances are considered natural, people willingly use them without further investigating potential hazards. The belief is that anything 'natural', even if consumed in excess of the DRI, must be perfectly fine for the body because it will be rapidly metabolised and excreted without causing harm. This is not necessarily true for all substances, however, and parents, coaches, trainers, athletes and healthcare workers should be knowledgeable about the effects of such substances. Rather than prohibiting their use, a better approach, especially for adolescents, is to provide open, informed discussion on the availability of appropriate substitutes that exist in foods that are indeed healthy to consume yet provide beneficial effects for athletic performance. Schools may include such discussions in existing curricula for their athletes and encourage participation in these educational programs.

Amphetamines and related drugs, such as methylphenidate (Ritalin), as well as caffeine, ephedra or other stimulants, may be taken to provide a sense of increased alertness and relief of fatigue; however, obscuring fatigue may permit participants to exceed their limits and precipitate a sudden collapse.

Creatine is reported to be the most commonly used performance-enhancing substance among athletes; it is a naturally occurring compound that supplies energy to muscles, builds muscle mass, increases recovery after strenuous exercise and improves strength. Other misused drugs include stimulants intended for bronchodilation, decongestants, agents for weight gain or loss, physiological agents used to enhance oxygen-carrying capacity and nutritional supplements taken in doses greater than required.

Anabolic steroids are a source of concern to health professionals. Black market supplies of anabolic steroids are of poor quality and potency. The user develops larger-appearing muscles and increased body weight and body water, but reports on the side effects of these drugs outweigh any benefits for performance during athletic competition. Although the psychological effect may be beneficial, many valid studies have failed to demonstrate any safety and improvement in performance (Jagim et al 2018).

Adolescents and young adults rely on poor sources of information about the potential hazards of steroid use (e.g. friends, television, muscle magazines) and are generally poorly informed about their potential negative side effects. Healthcare professionals need to be aware of the clinical manifestations of steroid use. Health hazards outweigh any potential gain that the drug might provide.

Sudden Death

A death associated with sports produces renewed anxiety in both parents and healthcare professionals. The term *sudden* or *instantaneous death* is applied to death that occurs within minutes of the onset of the cause of death or within 24 hours of the episode. *Sudden cardiac arrest* is also a term used to describe the athlete who experiences a sudden death. The incidence of sudden death among children involved in sports has been estimated to be 1.0 per 100,000 per year (Providência et al 2017). Genetically inherited cardiomyopathies are identified as the most common cause of sudden death in young athletes (Sports Medicine and Fitness 2017). Most studies show that causes of sudden cardiac death are due to hypertrophic cardiomyopathy (Sports Medicine and Fitness 2016). Overall survival rates for young athletes experiencing sudden cardiac arrest during an athletic event improve if the event occurs in later adolescence towards improved survival in the latter years of the study (Providência et al 2017).

Causes of sudden death are related to three main risk factors: (1) sports with a high inherent risk for sports-related sudden death; (2) recognised or unknown underlying medical problems in child participants; and (3) the sports environment (e.g. the rules, equipment, practice fields or areas of sport participation and ambient temperature of the geographic area). Some experts advocate screening all youth athletes with a 12-lead electrocardiogram to detect disorders such as Brugada syndrome, long QT syndrome, hypertrophic cardiomyopathy and dilated cardiomyopathy, but this remains somewhat controversial. A comprehensive health history and physical examination may be helpful in identifying children and adolescents with risk factors for further diagnostic investigation and it is recommended to institute an 'athlete-centred model of care' which considers the factors such as clinical disease severity, family history, personal and social factors and exercise factors and implications (adverse clinical outcomes; e.g. cardiac arrest, psychological trauma and legalities) (Sweeting & Semsarian 2018). Chapter 19 discusses the impact of sudden death on the family and relevant nursing interventions.

Sports. Sports associated with the greatest risk of sudden death are those involving collision and frequent body contact. Examples of collision sports are football, rugby and boxing. There is a high potential for serious injury or fatality in sports such as mountain or rock climbing and hang-gliding. Sports that involve high-velocity objects, such as baseball and hockey, may result in death from serious head or chest injuries. Riding vehicles such as motorbikes, mountain bikes, ATVs and snowboards can also be considered high-risk sports.

Medical Conditions. The most frequent medical causes of sudden death during sports activity are cardiac abnormalities, especially idiopathic hypertrophic subaortic stenosis (hypertrophic cardiomyopathy). Manifestations suggestive of hypertrophic cardiomyopathy include a typical triad of severe chest pain, dizziness and dyspnoea. Unfortunately some affected individuals never display signs of disease until they collapse during a sports event. A history of sudden death of a relative or relatives in the second or third decade of life often offers a clue to recognition. Well-trained athletes often display evidence of hypertrophic cardiomyopathy, the so-called athlete's heart, but the condition is not pathological.

Congenital coronary artery malformation is the second most common cause of sudden death in athletes. Additional causes include valvular heart disease, atherosclerotic coronary artery disease, dilated cardiomyopathy, Marfan syndrome and myocarditis. Children with systemic hypertension, some types of cardiac arrhythmias such as prolonged QT syndrome and some forms of heart block will face restrictions in the type and amount of exercise they can tolerate safely. Commotio cordis is a common cause of sudden death in athletes without previous history of heart disease. This occurs after a blunt, non-penetrating blow to the chest, which produces ventricular fibrillation. Commotio cordis is more common in children and adolescents, with a mean age at occurrence of 13 years, and the blow may not be perceived as being that unusual or significant enough to produce such drastic results.

Appropriate use of an automatic external defibrillator (AED) by civilian bystanders or healthcare workers may save the life of an athlete who experiences a life-threatening cardiac emergency. A school-based AED program provides a high survival rate for student athletes and non-athletes who experience sudden cardiac arrest (Sweeting & Semsarian 2018).

Environmental Causes. Environmental factors that are potential causes of sudden death include playing conditions, clothing, equipment, rules used by officials governing a sport and outdoor temperature. Heatstroke and hypothermia are the most serious environment-related causes of death in athletes (Sports Medicine and Fitness 2016).

Nurse's Role in Children's Sports

Nurses may become involved in children's sports activities in preparation and evaluation of children for activities, provision of anticipatory guidance and counselling about athletic competition and nutrition, prevention of injuries, treatment of injuries and rehabilitation after injuries. Selecting an appropriate sport for both recreation and competition is a joint effort of the child or adolescent, parents and health professionals. Children are introduced to sports as part of family activities and school physical education programs, and both parents and children are influenced by media exposure to a variety of sports. Children are highly influenced by the popularity of and exposure afforded athletics in the school setting, especially in high school.

The best approach to counselling children and parents regarding sports participation is to encourage activities that are most likely to provide pleasure and physical benefits throughout childhood and into adulthood. Caution parents against overprogramming children to allow ample time for other activities and associations. Burnout among children and adolescents who continuously participate in sports is increasing. Children and adolescents are encouraged to take periodic breaks from such activities to allow physical healing, refresh the mind and work on strength and conditioning (Kidsafe WA 2018).

MUSCULOSKELETAL DYSFUNCTION

Torticollis

Torticollis, or wry neck, which can be either congenital or acquired, is a condition of limited neck motion. The condition is characterised by the neck being in a flexed position and the head drawn or tilted laterally to the affected side, while the chin is pointed towards the opposite side. Congenital muscular torticollis often occurs as a result of abnormal positioning in utero, causing a contracture of the sternocleidomastoid muscle. Torticollis is a manifestation rather than a disease entity and may be associated with a number of conditions, including congenital abnormality of the cervical spine or a traumatic lesion of the sternocleidomastoid muscle.

In early infancy a firm, non-tender mass may be felt in the mid-portion of the sternocleidomastoid muscle. The mass regresses and is replaced by fibrous tissue. If the condition remains untreated, permanent limitation of neck movement results. Plagiocephaly and facial asymmetry often occur as a result of the contractured sternocleidomastoid muscle. Children may have other associated musculoskeletal conditions, including foot deformities or developmental dysplasia of the hips; a thorough physical examination should be performed for all infants.

Treatment of simple torticollis consists of gentle stretching exercises. A physiotherapist typically establishes the treatment regimen to be followed by the family with the goal of achieving full, symmetrical cervical range of motion. If stretching exercises are unsuccessful, surgical release of the sternocleidomastoid muscle may be needed. Increasingly, surgical correction by age 12 to 18 months is recommended to prevent muscle contracture and further progression of plagiocephaly. Other causes of torticollis occur in infancy or may develop at a later age but are not discussed in this text.

Nursing Care Management

Nurses should be alert to the possibility of torticollis in infants with limited head movement. After diagnosis, the nurse should supervise the family in performing stretching exercises and ensure proper technique. The nurse should also suggest that the child be positioned in a way that encourages turning the head and neck in the direction of limited range of motion; for example, placing interesting toys or activities towards one side.

Kyphosis and Lordosis

The spine, which consists of numerous segments, can acquire deformation curves of three types: kyphosis, lordosis and scoliosis (Fig 33.27). Kyphosis is the lateral convex angulation in the curvature of the thoracic spine (see Fig 33.27B). If it is increased (greater than 45 degrees), it may occur secondary to disease processes such as tuberculosis, chronic arthritis, osteodystrophy or compression fractures of the thoracic spine. Postural kyphosis is a common type of kyphosis in which the deformity is flexible and there are no radiographic vertebral body abnormalities or changes. Children, especially during the time when skeletal growth outpaces growth of muscle, are prone to postural roundback deformity. This is particularly common in self-conscious adolescent girls who assume a round-shouldered slouching posture in an attempt to hide their developing breasts and increasing height. No intervention is necessary other than education.

Scheuermann kyphosis is a thoracic curve of greater than 45 degrees, with wedging of more than 5 degrees of at least three adjacent vertebral bodies and vertebral irregularity. Onset occurs typically during the prepubertal growth spurt at approximately 10 to 12 years of age and is seen more frequently in males than females. Young adolescents often present with pain along with the visible kyphosis. The deformity has a degree of rigidity and lack of spine extension flexibility. Treatment for Scheuermann disease includes physical therapy working on increasing spine flexibility and strength as well as addressing potential lumbar hyperlordosis and hamstring or hip flexor tightness. Use of a spine brace may be indicated in children who are still

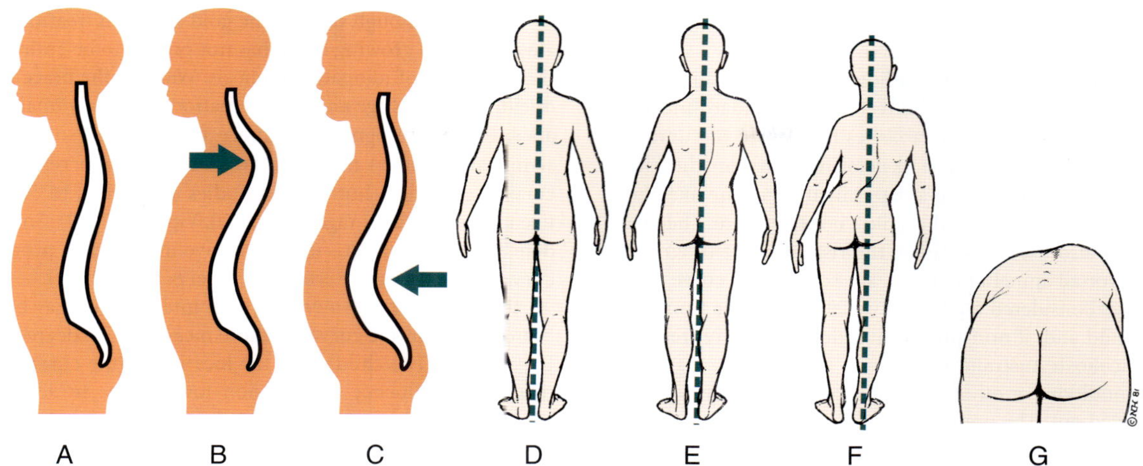

Fig 33.27 Defects of spinal column. (A) Normal spine. (B) Kyphosis. (C) Lordosis. (D) Normal spine in balance. (E) Mild scoliosis in balance. (F) Severe scoliosis not in balance. (G) Rib hump and flank asymmetry seen in flexion caused by rotary component.

growing. Surgical correction may be considered for severe, painful or progressive deforming curves.

Lordosis is the lateral inward curve of the cervical and lumbar spine (see Fig 33.27C). Hyperlordosis may be a secondary complication of a disease process, the result of trauma or idiopathic. Hyperlordosis is a normal observation in toddlers, and in older children it is often seen in association with flexion contractures of the hip, obesity, congenital dislocated hip and slipped capital femoral epiphysis.

Spondylolysis is a fracture sustained at the pars interarticularis. Spondylolisthesis is the forward slipping of one vertebral body on another. It most often involves L5 moving forwards over S1. The condition may be asymptomatic, or it may cause lower back pain or neurological compromise more typically seen with spondylolisthesis than spondylolysis. Treatment is usually non-surgical; however, spinal fusion may be indicated in cases of severe, progressive slip.

Idiopathic Scoliosis

Scoliosis is a complex spinal deformity in three planes, usually involving lateral curvature, spinal rotation causing rib asymmetry and, when in the thoracic spine, often thoracic hypokyphosis (see Fig 33.27E–G and Fig 33.28). Scoliosis is the most common spinal deformity and is classified according to age of onset: *congenital* occurs in fetal development; *infantile* occurs at birth up to 3 years of age; *juvenile* occurs in children 3 to 10 years of age; and *adolescent* occurs at 10 years of age or older. Scoliosis may be caused by a number of conditions and may occur alone or in association with other diseases, particularly neuromuscular conditions (neuromuscular scoliosis). In most cases, however, there is no apparent cause, hence the name *idiopathic scoliosis.* The following discussion involves the adolescent type, which is often called adolescent idiopathic scoliosis. There appears to be a genetic component to the aetiology of idiopathic scoliosis; however, the exact relationship has yet to be established.

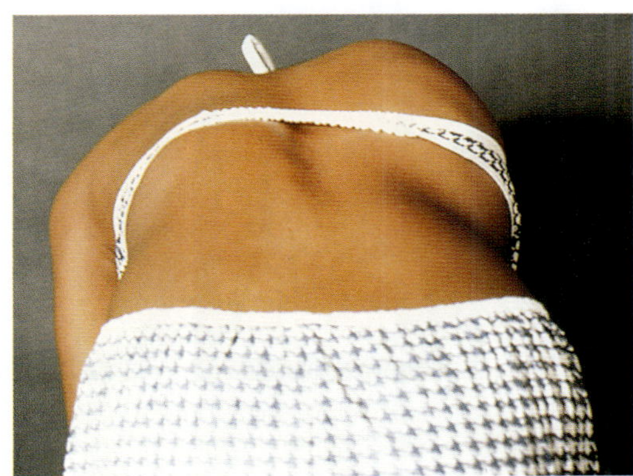

Fig 33.28 Moderate thoracic idiopathic adolescent scoliosis. Forward flexion reveals a mild rib hump deformity.

Clinical Manifestations

Idiopathic scoliosis is most commonly identified during the preadolescent growth spurt. Parents frequently bring a child for follow-up on an abnormal school scoliosis screening or because of ill-fitting clothes, such as poorly fitting jeans. Scoliosis Australia (2021) published a policy favouring scoliosis screening for preadolescents and adolescents in the school, medical practitioner's office or nurses' clinic which is available at: https://www.scoliosis-australia.org/policies-programs/policy-re-screening/. Self-assessment using the National Self-Detection Program for Scoliosis Fact Sheet and early treatment of minor curvatures by family doctors is recommended (Scoliosis Australia 2021). Girls should be screened at ages 10 and 12 years, whereas boys should be screened once either at age 13 or 14 years. In New Zealand, a smartphone application to detect scoliosis called ScoliScreen was developed; it is easy and free to use (see https://app.scoliscreen.com/).

The benefits of early detection, referral and medical treatment are considered to be significant, but the persons performing the screenings must be educated in the detection of spinal deformity (Scoliosis Australia 2021).

Diagnostic Evaluation

The standing child, wearing only shorts/briefs and viewed from behind, may exhibit asymmetry of shoulder height, scapular or flank shape or hip height or may demonstrate pelvic obliquity. Cutaneous changes may also be observed. When the child bends forwards at the waist so that the trunk is parallel with the floor and the arms hang free (the Adams position), asymmetry of ribs and flanks may also be appreciated (see Fig 33.27G and Fig 33.28). A scoliometer is used in the initial screening to measure truncal rotation (as does the Adams test). Often a primary curve and a compensatory curve will place the head in alignment with the gluteal cleft. With an uncompensated curve, however, the head and hips are not aligned.

Definitive diagnosis is made by radiographs of the child in the standing position and use of the Cobb technique (standard measurement of angle curvature), which establishes the degree of curvature. The Risser scale is used to evaluate skeletal maturity on the radiographs. This scale assists in making a determination of the likely progression of the spinal curvature as the child's bones mature. The sexual maturity rating is also used to evaluate the risk of curve progression in adolescents. Not all spinal curvatures are scoliosis. A curve of less than 10 degrees is considered a postural variation. Curves from 10 to 25 degrees are mild and, if non-progressive, do not require treatment (Hresko 2013, Scoliosis Australia 2021).

Intraspinal conditions or other disease processes that may cause scoliosis must be ruled out. The presence of pain, sacral dimpling or hairy patches, cutaneous vascular changes, absent or abnormal reflexes, bowel or bladder incontinence or left thoracic curve may indicate an intraspinal abnormality such as syringomyelia, diastematomyelia or tethered cord syndrome. An MRI scan is usually obtained for evaluation.

Therapeutic Management

Current management options include observation with regular clinical and radiographic evaluation, orthotic intervention (bracing) and surgical spinal fusion (Fig 33.29). Treatment decisions are based on the magnitude, location and type of curve; the age and skeletal maturity of the child or adolescent; and any underlying or contributing disease process.

Bracing and Exercise. For moderate curves (25 to 45 degrees) in the growing child and adolescent, bracing may be the treatment of choice. Historically bracing has not been shown to be curative; the goal is to slow the progression of the curvature to allow skeletal growth and maturity. The two most common types of TLSOs are the Boston and Wilmington braces, which are customised underarm orthoses made of plastic with corrective external forces using lateral pads to help prevent progression (Fig 33.30).

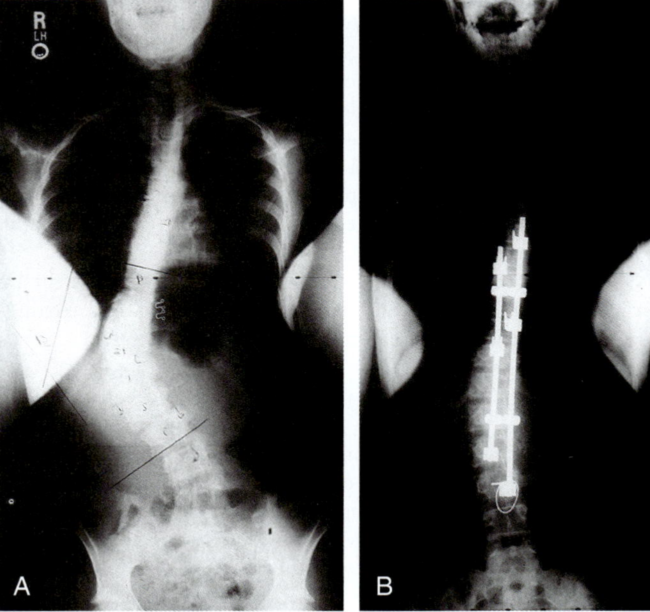

Fig 33.29 Radiographs showing severe scoliosis before surgical correction (**A**) and after surgical correction of scoliosis, including internal fixation (**B**).

Bracing, although used as the gold standard treatment for moderate curves in a growing child, has not proved to be entirely effective in the treatment of idiopathic scoliosis. Wearing the brace is challenging due to the child's age and preoccupation with body image and appearance. Experts recognise that brace treatment in some children with significant scoliosis may help avoid surgical intervention by slowing curve progression, but further studies are needed to clarify the effectiveness of bracing (Yagci et al 2020, Yip et al 2018). Some recent evidence suggests that bracing is effective in slowing a progressive spinal curvature in moderate scoliosis (Yagci & Yakut 2019).

Operative Management. Surgical intervention may be required for correction of severe curves or those measuring 45 degrees or more (see Fig 33.29A). The child's age, the location of the curvature and curve magnitude influence the decision for surgery. In addition, thoracic curves with a magnitude greater than 50 degrees and lumbar curves greater than 30 degrees are more likely to progress after skeletal maturity (Gregory 2020, Newton et al 2014). Any progressive or severe curve that does not respond to more conservative bracing measures requires surgical correction. Neuromuscular, dysplastic and congenital curves, which eventually progress, are best treated with early surgical stabilisation. Difficulties with balance or seating, respiratory excursion or pain are also considered.

There are a number of surgical techniques for severe scoliosis. One surgical intervention consists of realignment and straightening of the spine with internal fixation and instrumentation combined with bony fusion (**arthrodesis**). Posterior and/or anterior surgical approaches may be implemented. The goals of spinal fusion surgery are to improve the curvatures on the sagittal and coronal planes to provide a solid, pain-free fusion in a well-balanced torso (balanced shoulders and pelvis), with maximum mobility of the remaining spinal segments.

Spinal fusion can lead to decreased spinal mobility in the long term. Other methods of surgical treatment are therefore being explored, including vertebral body stapling and anterior tethering. These types of surgical techniques do not require a fusion and may alter spinal growth by inhibiting growth of the anterior vertebral growth plate while still allowing for continued posterior growth thereby improving the spinal curvature or deformity (Cahill et al 2017).

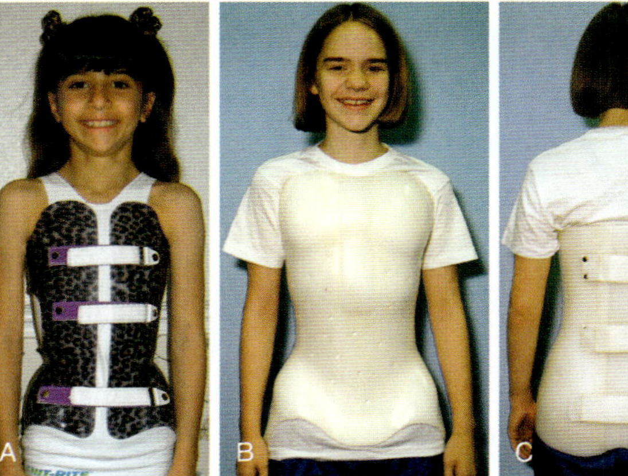

Fig 33.30 (**A**) Standard thoracolumbosacral orthosis (TLSO) brace for idiopathic scoliosis. Note the colour and design incorporated into the brace to make it more acceptable to children and adolescents. (**B**) and (**C**) Variation of a standard TLSO brace that fastens in the back to provide needed support for the spinal curvature.

Nursing Care Management

Treatment for scoliosis extends over a significant portion of the affected child's period of growth. In adolescents this period is the one in which their identity, both physical and psychological, is formed. The identification of scoliosis as a 'deformity', in combination with unattractive appliances and a significant surgical procedure, can have a negative effect on the already fragile adolescent body image. The adolescent and family require excellent nursing care to meet not only physical needs but also psychological needs associated with the diagnosis, surgery, postoperative recovery and eventual rehabilitation.

Although adolescents are encouraged to participate in most peer activities, necessary therapeutic modifications are likely to make them feel different and isolated. Nursing care of the adolescent who is facing scoliosis surgery, potential social isolation, pain and uncertainty, not to mention misunderstood emotions and body image issues, must be evaluated from the adolescent's perspective to be successful in meeting the individual's needs.

Preoperative Care. The preoperative workup usually involves a radiographic series, including bending or traction spine films, possible pulmonary function studies and serological laboratory studies (including prothrombin, partial thromboplastin and bleeding times; blood count; electrolyte levels; urinalysis and urine culture; and blood levels of any medications).

Surgery for spinal fusion is complex, and often adolescents who require the procedure due to idiopathic scoliosis are not familiar with medical terms or procedures. Preoperative teaching is critical for the adolescent to be able to cooperate and participate in his or her treatment and recovery. Because the surgery is extensive, the patient is taught how to manage his or her own patient-controlled analgesia (PCA) pump; how to log-roll; and the use and function of other equipment, such as a chest tube (for anterior spinal fusion) and Foley urinary catheter. Meeting with a peer and his or her family members who have undergone a similar surgery may also be of value.

Postoperative Care. After surgery, patients are monitored in an acute care setting and log-rolled when changing position to prevent damage to the fusion and instrumentation. In some cases an immobilisation brace or cast is used postoperatively depending on the type of surgical intervention. Skin care is important, and pressure-relieving mattresses or beds may be needed to prevent pressure wounds. (See Maintaining Healthy Skin, Chapter 22.)

In addition to the usual postoperative assessments of wound, circulation and vital signs, the neurological status of the patient's extremities requires special attention. Prompt recognition of any neurological impairment is imperative because delayed paralysis may develop that requires surgical intervention. Common postoperative problems after spinal fusion include neurological injury or spinal cord injury, hypotension from acute blood loss, wound infection, syndrome of inappropriate antidiuretic hormone, atelectasis, pneumothorax, ileus, delayed neurological injury and implanted hardware complications (Swann et al 2016). Superior mesenteric artery syndrome may occur several days after spinal surgery; this involves duodenal compression by the aorta and superior mesenteric artery and may result in acute partial or complete duodenal obstruction. Clinical manifestations include epigastric pain, belching, nausea and copious vomiting; symptoms are aggravated in the supine position and often relieved with the patient in a left lateral decubitus or prone position.

The adolescent usually has considerable pain for the first few days after surgery and requires frequent administration of pain medication, preferably opioids administered intravenously on a regular schedule. For children able to understand the concept, PCA is recommended. In most cases the patient begins walking as soon as possible. Depending on the instrumentation used and the surgical approach, most patients are walking by the second or third postoperative day and are discharged by 5 to 7 days. In addition to pain management, the patient is evaluated for skin integrity, adequate urinary output, fluid and electrolyte balance and ileus. Discharge planning should include a timetable for follow-up with the provider and resumption of regular activities.

Encourage the family to become involved in the patient's care to facilitate the transition from hospital to home management. An organisation that provides education and services to both families and professionals is Scoliosis Australia.

Skeletal Limb Deficiency

Congenital limb deficiencies are characterised by underdevelopment of skeletal elements of the extremities. The range of malformation or deficiency can extend from minor defects of the digit to serious abnormalities such as amelia (absence of an entire extremity) or hemimelia (partial absence of an extremity), which includes phocomelia, an interposed deficiency of long bones with relatively good development of hands and feet attached at or near the shoulder or the hip. Most reduction deficiencies involve anomalies in the development of the limb, but prenatal destruction of the limb can occur, such as full or partial amputation of a limb in utero from constriction by an amniotic band (amniotic band syndrome). Neonates with congenital limb deficiencies often have associated malformations and should be thoroughly assessed for cardiovascular, central nervous system, renal and digestive abnormalities (Wilson 2014).

Pathophysiology

Limb deficiencies can be attributed to both genetic and environmental causes and originate at any stage of limb development. Formation of limbs may be suppressed at the time of limb bud formation, or there may be interference in later stages of differentiation and growth. A family history of a deficiency increases the risk of a similar deficiency in a child demonstrating the inheritable or genetic nature of limb deficiencies. Prenatal environmental insults have been implicated in a number of cases, such as the well-publicised thalidomide tragedy in the late 1950s and early 1960s, which demonstrated a clear relationship between the time of exposure of the pregnant woman to the antiemetic drug and the presence and type of limb deformity in the newborn. There are still drugs that may have similar teratogenic effects in the first trimester of pregnancy; medication administration during this time period should be carefully evaluated by the provider (Stanger et al 2017).

Therapeutic Management

The child with a limb deficiency should be fitted with prosthetic devices, and the devices should be applied at the earliest possible stage of development in an attempt to match the infant's motor readiness. This favours natural progression of prosthetic use. For example, an infant with an upper extremity deficiency is fitted with a simple passive device between 3 and 6 months of age, when limb exploration is active, sitting is beginning (with the extremities needed for support) and bilateral hand activities are encouraged. Lower limb prostheses are applied when the infant is ready to pull to a standing position.

In preparation for prosthetic devices, surgical modification may be necessary to ensure the most favourable use of the device because severe deformity can interfere with its effective use. Phocomelic digits are preserved for controlling switches of externally powered appliances in the upper extremities. Digits (in both the upper and the lower extremities) provide the child with surfaces for tactile exploration and stimulation. Prostheses are replaced to accommodate the child's growth and increasing capabilities.

Nursing Care Management

Prosthetic application, training and habilitation are most successfully carried out in a centre that specialises in meeting the special needs of these children, especially very young children and those with multiple amputations. Management involves a prosthetist, who specialises in the development, fitting and maintenance of prosthetic limbs, and other healthcare providers such as physical and occupational therapists. Parents need support and are encouraged to assist the child in making age-appropriate adjustments to the environment. Although these children need assistance, overprotection may produce overdependence, with later maladjustment to school and other situations.

Developmental Dysplasia of the Hip

The broad term **developmental dysplasia of the hip (DDH)** describes a spectrum of disorders related to abnormal development of the hip that may occur at any time during fetal life, infancy and childhood. A change in terminology from *congenital hip dysplasia* and *congenital dislocation of the hip* to DDH more properly reflects the varying onset and types of hip abnormalities in which there is a shallow acetabulum and femoral head subluxation or dislocation.

The incidence of hip instability is approximately 7 per 1000 live births, and approximately 17% to 23% of infants with DDH are born with a breech intrauterine position. Girls are more commonly affected than boys, and there is a positive family history in approximately 120/1000 of affected individuals. Additional risk factors for DDH include firstborn child, oligohydramnios, hip asymmetry and other musculoskeletal conditions including torticollis and metatarsus adductus or foot deformities (Weinstein 2014a). Tight swaddling and carrying babies with hips flexed is also noted to contribute to DDH (Williams 2018).

Pathophysiology

The cause of DDH is unknown, but certain factors such as female gender, first pregnancy, family history, breech intrauterine position, high birth weight, joint laxity and postnatal positioning are believed to affect the risk of DDH. Predisposing factors associated with DDH may be divided into three broad categories: physiological factors, including maternal hormone secretion and intrauterine positioning; mechanical factors, which involve breech presentation, multiple fetuses, oligohydramnios and large infant size, as well as continued maintenance of the hips in adduction and extension that with time can cause dislocation and genetic factors, which include a higher incidence of DDH in siblings of affected infants and even greater incidence of recurrence if a sibling and one parent were affected.

Recently it has been recommended that infants' hips be placed in slight flexion and abduction during swaddling. Further, it was recommended that infants' knees be maintained in slight flexion and that forced or prolonged passive hip extension in the first months of life be avoided. These recommendations were made based on evidence that demonstrated a significant relationship between tight swaddling and hip dysplasia and are aimed at decreasing the incidence of DDH in infants (Williams 2018).

DDH can be categorised into two major groups: idiopathic, in which the infant is neurologically intact, and teratologic, which involves a neuromuscular defect such as arthrogryposis or myelomeningocele. The teratological forms usually occur in utero and are much less common.

Three degrees of DDH are illustrated in Figure 33.31 and are outlined here.

1. Acetabular dysplasia—This is the mildest form of DDH, in which there is a delay in acetabular development evidenced by osseous hypoplasia of the acetabular roof that is oblique and shallow. The femoral head remains in the acetabulum with no subluxation or dislocation.
2. Subluxation—The largest percentage of DDH, subluxation implies incomplete dislocation. The femoral head remains in contact with the acetabulum, but a stretched capsule and ligamentum teres cause the head of the femur to be partially displaced. Pressure on the cartilaginous acetabulum inhibits ossification and produces a flattening of the socket.
3. Dislocation—This is the most severe form of DDH. The femoral head loses contact with the acetabulum and is displaced posteriorly and superiorly.

Diagnostic Evaluation

The diagnosis of DDH should be made in the newborn period if possible because treatment initiated before 2 months of age achieves the highest rate of success. In the newborn period, hip dysplasia usually appears as hip joint laxity. Subluxation and the tendency to dislocate can be demonstrated by the Ortolani and Barlow tests (Fig 33.32D). Before attending to the assessment, all nurses and midwives should review their facility's policies as to who can attend to the assessment and if it is within their scope of practice.

With the infant quiet and relaxed in the supine position on a firm surface with the legs facing the examiner, the hips and knees are flexed (not forced) at right angles. The examiner places the middle finger of each hand over the greater trochanter and the thumbs on the inner side of the thigh at a point opposite the lesser trochanter. The knees are

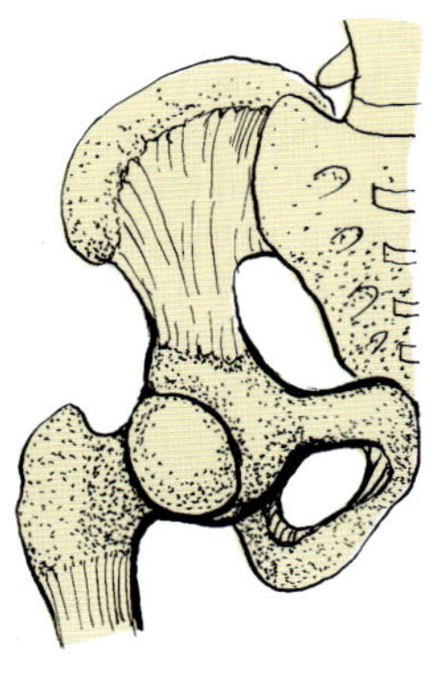
Normal

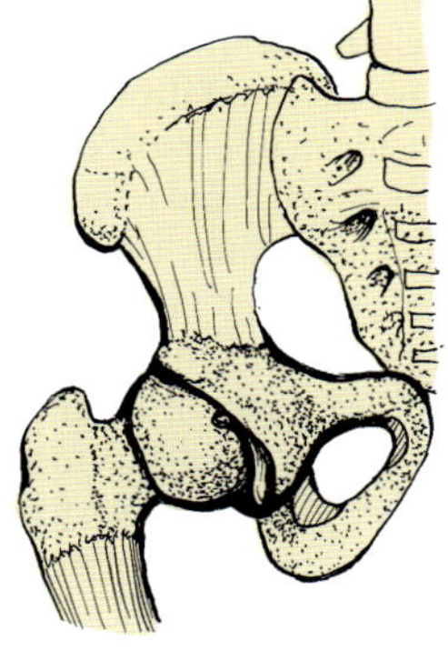
Dysplasia

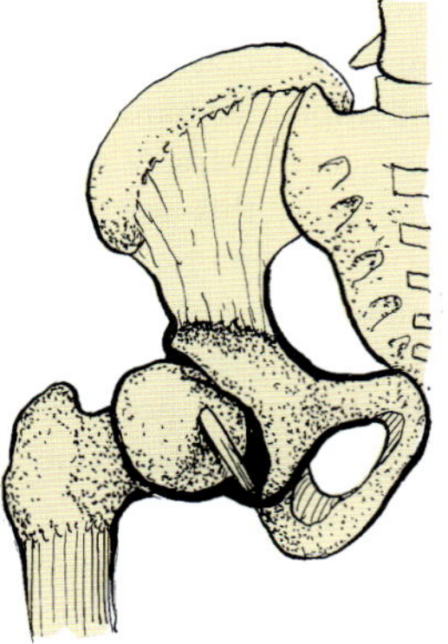
Subluxation

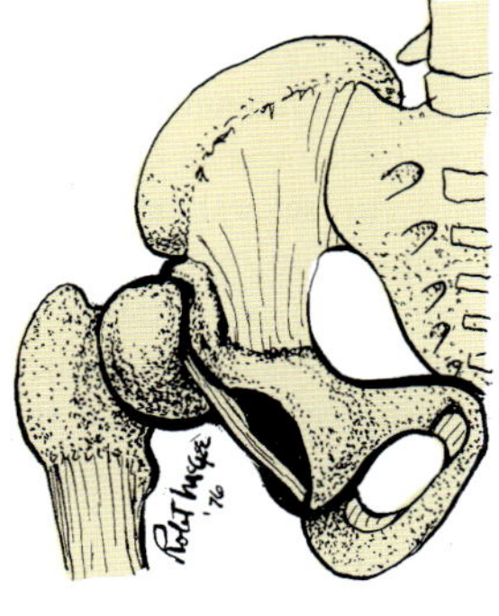
Dislocation

Fig 33.31 Configuration and relationship of structures in developmental dysplasia of the hip.

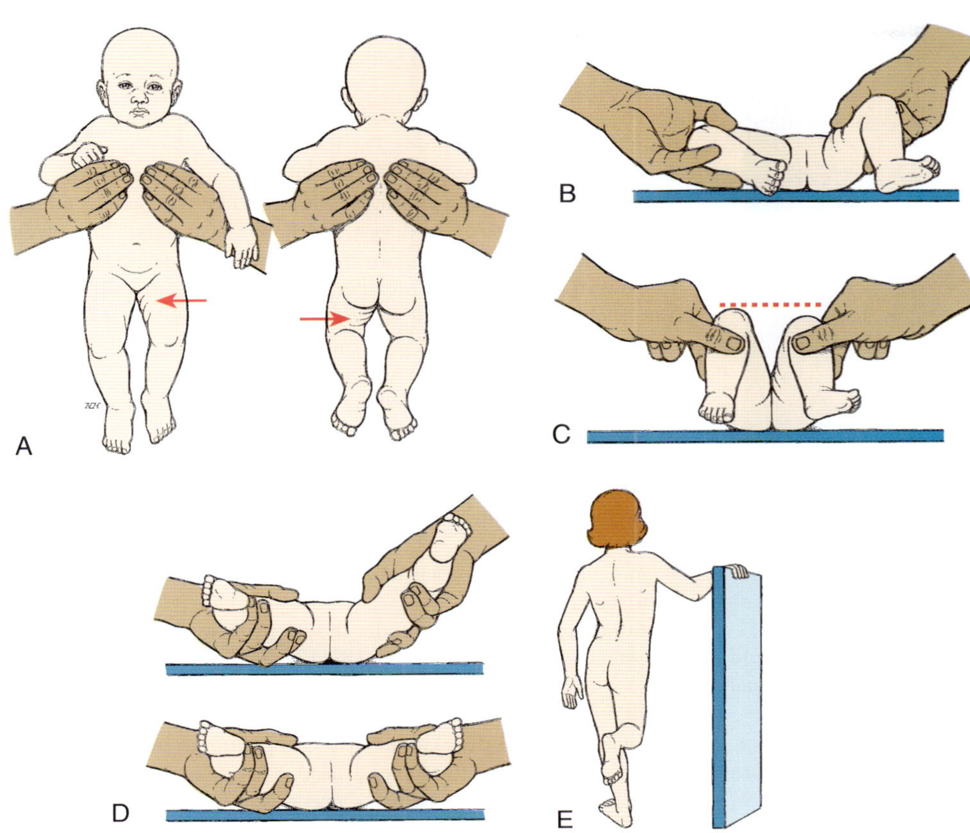

Fig 33.32 Signs of developmental dysplasia of hip. **(A)** Asymmetry of gluteal and thigh folds. **(B)** Limited hip abduction, as seen in flexion. **(C)** Apparent shortening of femur, as indicated by level of knees in flexion. **(D)** Ortolani test. **(E)** Positive Trendelenburg sign (if child is weight bearing).

carried to midabduction and each hip joint is submitted, one at a time, first to forward pressure exerted behind the trochanter and then to backward pressure exerted from the thumbs in front as the opposite joint is held steady. If the femoral head can be felt to slip forwards into the acetabulum on pressure from behind, it is dislocated (Ortolani test). If with hip flexion and adduction, the femoral head is felt to slip out over the posterior lip of the acetabulum, the hip is said to be dislocatable or 'unstable' (Barlow test). Sometimes an audible 'clunk' can be heard on exit or entry of the femur out of or into the acetabulum. The audible clunk is not pathological and occurs as a result of breaking surface tension across the hip joint, knee rotation, snapping of gluteal tendons or patellofemoral motion.

NURSING CARE CONSIDERATIONS

The Barlow and Ortolani manoeuvres should be performed only by an experienced clinician, nursing, midwifery and medical, to prevent an injury to the infant's hips.

The Ortolani and Barlow manoeuvres are most reliable from birth to 4 weeks of age. Adduction contractures develop at about 6 to 10 weeks of age, and the Ortolani sign disappears. After this time, the most sensitive test is limited hip abduction (Fig 33.32B). Other signs are shortening of the thigh on the affected side (Galeazzi sign) (Fig 33.32C), asymmetrical thigh and gluteal folds (Fig 33.32A) and broadening of the perineum (in bilateral hip dislocations).

In the older infant and child, the affected leg appears shorter than the other. In both unilateral and bilateral dislocations the greater trochanter is prominent and appears above a line from the anterosuperior iliac spine to the tuberosity of the ischium. There may be telescoping or piston mobility, meaning that the head of the femur can be felt to move up and down in the buttock when the extended thigh is pushed first towards the child's head and then pulled distally. Instability of the hip on weight bearing produces a characteristic waddling gait and marked lumbar lordosis in bilateral hip dislocations. When the child stands first on one foot and then on the other (holding onto a chair, rail or someone's hand), bearing weight on the affected hip, the pelvis tilts downwards on the normal side instead of upwards as it would with normal stability (positive Trendelenburg sign) (Fig 33.32E).

Radiographic examination in early infancy is not reliable because ossification of the femoral head does not normally take place until 4 to 6 months of life. However, the cartilaginous femoral head can be visualised directly by ultrasonography. Universal newborn screening with ultrasonography has been proposed; however, numerous studies reveal that this approach has a high rate of false-positive results and subsequent overtreatment. Therefore, ultrasonography is considered an adjunct to the physical examination and recommended for young infants with known risk factors. In infants older than 6 months of age and in children, pelvis radiographs are obtained to confirm the diagnosis. Some local paediatric clinical guidelines for screening and early detection of DDH which healthcare staff can refer to are at: https://www.rch.org.au/kidsinfo/fact_sheets/Denis_Browne_Bar_for_DDH/.

Therapeutic Management

Treatment is begun as soon as the condition is recognised because early intervention is more favourable to the restoration of normal bony architecture and function. The longer treatment is delayed, the more severe the deformity, the more difficult the treatment and the less favourable the prognosis. The treatment varies with the child's age and

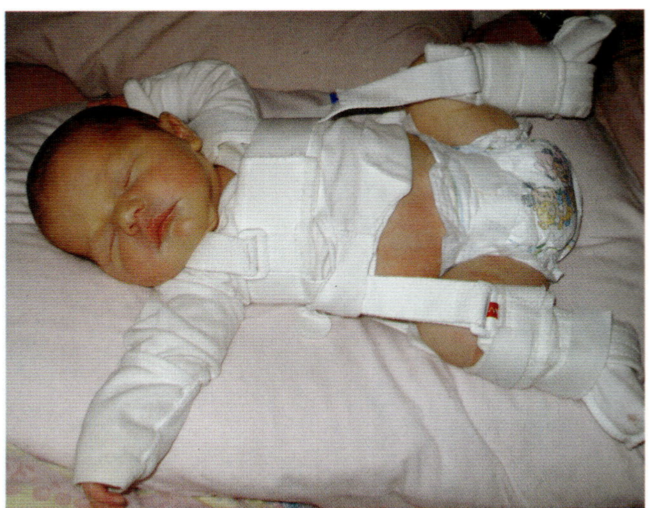

Fig 33.33 Child in Pavlik harness. (Source: Courtesy Amanda Politte, St Louis, MO.)

the extent of the dysplasia. The goal of treatment is to obtain and maintain a safe, congruent position of the hip joint to promote normal hip joint development.

Newborn to 6 Months. The hip joint is maintained, by dynamic splinting, in a safe position with the proximal femur centred in the acetabulum in a degree of flexion. A variety of abduction devices are available; of these, the Pavlik harness is the most widely used, and with time, motion and gravity, the hip works into a more abducted, reduced position (Fig 33.33). The harness does not rigidly immobilise the hip but acts to prevent hip extension and adduction. The Pavlik harness is worn continuously until the hip is stable on both clinical and ultrasound examination, usually within 6 to 12 weeks (or for as long as recommended by the doctor). It is highly effective when the device is well constructed, follow-up care is adequate and the parents follow instructions in its use. If young infants' hips fail to locate with the Pavlik harness, then surgical closed reduction and spica casting may be warranted.

Ages 6 to 24 Months. In this age group, the Pavlik harness has a low success rate. Therefore, surgical treatment with a closed reduction is recommended, and the child is placed in a spica cast for approximately 12 weeks. If the hip is not reducible, a surgical open reduction may be necessary. A hip abduction orthosis may be used after spica casting in order to maintain the hip in an appropriate, stable position and further promote hip development.

Older Child. Correction of the hip deformity in the older child is inherently more difficult than in the preceding age groups because secondary adaptive changes and other aetiological factors (such as juvenile arthritis or cerebral palsy) complicate the condition. Operative reduction, which may involve preoperative traction, tenotomy of contracted muscles and pelvic osteotomy procedures designed to construct an acetabular roof, often combined with proximal femoral osteotomy, is usually required. After cast removal, range-of-motion exercises help restore movement. Other rehabilitation measures may include muscle strengthening, a period of crutch or walker use and gait training.

Nursing Care Management

Nurses are in a unique position to detect DDH in the newborn. During the infant assessment process and routine nurturing activities, the nurse inspects the hips and extremities for any deviations from normal. These observations are reported to the attending provider for further examination. The ambulatory child who displays a limp or waddling gait is also referred for evaluation. Non-ambulatory children with cerebral palsy or spina bifida should be assessed for evidence of hip problems as well.

The primary nursing goal is teaching parents to apply and maintain the reduction device or brace. The Pavlik harness allows for easy handling of the infant and usually produces less apprehension in the parent than heavy braces and casts. It is important that parents understand the correct use of the device, which may or may not allow for its removal during bathing. Removing the harness is determined individually on the basis of the provider's recommendations, the degree of hip instability and the family's level of understanding. Parents should be instructed not to adjust the harness.

Skin care is an important aspect of the care of an infant in a Pavlik harness. The following instructions for preventing skin breakdown are stressed.

- Check frequently (at least two to three times per day) for red areas under the straps and at skin folds.
- Gently massage healthy skin under the straps once a day to stimulate circulation.
- In general, avoid lotions and powders because they can cake and irritate the skin.
- Always place the nappy under the straps; frequent nappy changes are required to prevent soiling the harness.

Legg-Calvé-Perthes Disease

Legg-Calvé-Perthes disease is a self-limiting disorder in which there is avascular necrosis of the femoral head. The disease affects children ages 2 to 12 years, but most cases occur as an isolated event in boys between 4 and 8 years of age. The male-to-female ratio is 4 or 5 to 1. In approximately 10% of cases, the involvement is bilateral; most of the affected children have a skeletal age significantly below their chronological age (Weinstein 2014b).

Pathophysiology

The cause of the disease is unknown, but a temporary disturbance of circulation to the femoral capital epiphysis produces an ischaemic aseptic necrosis of the femoral head. During middle childhood, circulation to the femoral epiphysis is more tenuous than at other ages, being supplied almost entirely by the lateral retinacular vessels. Activity causes microfractures of the soft ischaemic epiphysis, which tends to induce synovitis, stiffness and hip adductor contracture.

The pathological events seem to take place in four stages (Box 33.8). The entire disease process may encompass as few as 18 months or continue for several years. The reformed femoral head may be severely altered or minimally affected.

BOX 33.8 Radiographic Stages of Legg-Calvé-Perthes Disease

Stage I—Aseptic necrosis or infarction of the femoral capital epiphysis with degenerative changes producing flattening of the upper surface of the femoral head (the avascular stage)

Stage II—Capital bone resorption and revascularisation with fragmentation (vascular resorption of the epiphysis) that gives a mottled appearance on radiographs (the fragmentation, or revascularisation, stage)

Stage III—New bone formation, which is represented on radiographs as calcification and ossification or increased density in the areas of radiolucency; this filling-in process appears to take place from the periphery of the head centrally (the reparative stage)

Stage IV—Gradual reformation of the head of the femur without radiolucency and, it is hoped, to a spherical form (the regenerative stage)

Clinical Manifestations and Diagnostic Evaluation

The onset of Legg-Calvé-Perthes disease is usually insidious, and the history may reveal only intermittent appearance of a limp on the affected side or a symptom complex, including hip soreness, ache or stiffness, which can be constant or intermittent. The parents may report seeing the child limping, and the limp may become more pronounced with increased activity. The pain may be experienced in the hip, along the entire thigh or in the vicinity of the knee joint. The pain and limp are often more evident on arising and at the end of a long day of activities. The pain is usually accompanied by joint dysfunction and limited range of motion at the hip. There may be a vague history of trauma but not necessarily. The diagnosis is established by characteristic radiographic findings and, occasionally, by MRI.

Therapeutic Management

Because deformity occurs early in the disease process, the aims of treatment are to eliminate hip irritability; restore and maintain adequate hip range of motion; prevent capital femoral epiphyseal collapse, extrusion or subluxation; and preserve as well-rounded femoral head as possible at time of healing. Treatment varies according to the child's age at the time of diagnosis and the appearance of the femoral head and position within the acetabulum.

The initial therapy is rest or activity restrictions and limited weight bearing, which helps reduce inflammation and irritability of the hip. The use of NSAIDs can provide relief of pain or discomfort; physical therapy or range-of-motion exercises help restore hip motion. In some cases, traction is applied to stretch tight adductor muscles and improve containment of the femoral head. Abduction braces or casting may also be used for containment. If non-surgical or conservative management is unsuccessful, surgical reconstruction or containment procedures such as a pelvic or proximal femoral osteotomy may be necessary.

The disease is self-limiting, but the ultimate outcome of therapy depends on early and efficient treatment and the child's age at the onset of the disorder. Children 5 years and younger, whose epiphyses are more cartilaginous, tend to have the best prognosis or outcome. Children over 9 years old have a significant risk for degenerative arthritis, especially if they have femoral head deformity at the time of diagnosis. The later the diagnosis is made, the more femoral head damage will have occurred before treatment is implemented.

Nursing Care Management

Because these children are largely cared for on an outpatient basis, the major emphasis of nursing care is on teaching the family the required care and management. The family needs to comprehend the diagnosis and the importance of compliance with the prescribed regimen to achieve the desired outcome. The child and the family may rely on the nurse to help them understand and adjust to therapeutic measures.

One of the most difficult aspects associated with the disorder is the need to cope with a normally active child who feels well but must remain relatively inactive. It is important to emphasise that children should continue to attend school and engage in activities that can be adapted to the prescribed regimen. Suitable activities must be devised to meet the needs of the child in the process of developing a sense of initiative or industry.

Slipped Capital Femoral Epiphysis

Slipped capital femoral epiphysis (SCFE) refers to the spontaneous displacement of the proximal femoral epiphysis in relationship to the femoral neck and shaft. In most cases, the femoral head stays within the acetabulum while the femoral neck and shaft moves anteriorly and rotates externally relative to the femoral epiphysis. It develops most frequently shortly before or during accelerated growth and the onset of puberty (children between the ages of 10 and 16 years; median age 13 years for boys and 12 years for girls) and is commonly observed in boys and obese children. SCFE has a reported prevalence of 2 to 13 in 100,000 globally, with bilateral involvement occurring in up to 60% of cases (Wills 2017, Kay & Kim 2014).

Pathophysiology

Most cases of SCFE are idiopathic, although it can be associated with endocrine disorders such as hypothyroidism, growth hormone therapy, renal osteodystrophy due to secondary hyperparathyroidism, and previous radiation therapy to the femoral head. The cause of idiopathic SCFE is multifactorial, with a variety of mechanical factors playing a part, including obesity, physeal architecture and orientation and pubertal hormone changes that affect physeal strength. Although obesity stresses the physeal plate, SCFE can also occur in children who are not obese.

Clinical Manifestations and Diagnostic Evaluation

SCFE is suspected when an adolescent or preadolescent displays clinical signs of a limp or complains of intermittent or continuous pain in the hip, groin, thigh or knee. Onset may be acute, chronic or acute-on-chronic. The child or adolescent often lies stiff with the lower extremity flexed, abducted and externally rotated because of the pain; any attempts to move the limb are met with significant resistance. The limp of a child with SCFE often reveals a Trendelenburg gait with an external foot progression angle on the affected side. In an unstable SCFE, the child is unable to bear weight because of severe pain.

Physical examination reveals range-of-motion restrictions of both hip flexion and hip extension as well as limited internal rotation. The affected hip falls into obligate external rotation as it is flexed. The diagnosis is confirmed by anteroposterior and frog-leg or cross-table lateral radiographs that reveal a change in the position of the femoral neck relative to the proximal femoral epiphysis. With a more severe or progressive slip, displacement may lead to an uncovered upper portion of the femoral neck adjacent to the physis. The growth plate appears widened and irregularities may be seen at the metaphysis. Lateral view radiographs are more sensitive at detecting a mild SCFE.

Therapeutic Management

The treatment goals of SCFE are to prevent further slipping at the proximal femur until physeal closure, avoid further complications such as avascular necrosis and maintain adequate hip function. Once the diagnosis is established, the child should be non-weight bearing to prevent further slippage. SCFE is an emergency and requires early diagnosis and treatment to increase the likelihood of an acceptable outcome.

Surgical treatment is necessary and varies with the degree of displacement or slippage. Current recommended treatment is with in situ fixation or pinning, which involves the placement of a single pin or alternatively multiple pins or screws through the femoral neck into the proximal femoral epiphysis to prevent further slippage. Most surgeons prefer to take the child to surgery within 24 hours of the onset of acute symptoms and avoid further risk of avascular necrosis. Postsurgical care includes non-weight bearing or limited weight bearing with crutches until acceptable painless range of motion is achieved. Activities may be limited for a length of time. Fixation or pins remain in place at least until the physis is closed and often are not removed.

Nursing Care Management

Nursing care involves preparing the child and family for the surgical procedure and recovery. Postoperative care involves haemodynamic stabilisation, pain management and assessment for complications. The adolescent is taught the proper use of crutches and the importance of avoiding any weight bearing on the affected hip. Self-care and performance of activities of daily living to capability are encouraged to promote confidence and decrease a sense of helplessness.

Metatarsus Adductus

Metatarsus adductus is the most common congenital foot deformity. The deformity is characterised by medial adduction of the toes and forefoot, frequently in association with inversion and convexity of the lateral border of the foot (kidney shaped). In most instances, it is a result of abnormal intrauterine positioning, particularly in a firstborn child, and is usually detected at birth. Metatarsus adductus can be divided into three categories: type I, in which the forefoot is flexible and corrects easily into abduction with manipulation; type II, in which the forefoot is only partially flexible and corrects only to neutral position with active manipulation; and type III, in which the forefoot is rigid and will not stretch to a neutral position with manipulation. Unlike a clubfoot, with which it is often confused, the angulation occurs at the tarsometatarsal joint, while the heel and ankle remain in a neutral position. Ankle range of motion is normal. The deformity often causes a pigeon-toed or intoeing gait in the child. A thorough hip examination should be performed for all infants with metatarsus adductus, as an increased risk of hip dysplasia is associated with foot deformities.

Management depends on the flexibility of the deformity. The majority of cases spontaneously correct with no treatment over the first 4 years of life. Interventions such as stretching and bracing or corrective shoes have not been shown to be effective. However, the parents can perform gentle forefoot abduction stretching. For partly flexible or rigid deformities, serial manipulation and casting can be considered to correct the defect, after which a corrective shoe or orthosis may be used to help prevent a recurrence; risk of recurrence is reported to be as high as 37%. Surgical correction is rarely required for the condition, as even those with residual deformity tend to not have long-term functional disability. Surgery may be considered in children over 4 to 6 years of age who have considerable pain on ambulation or difficulties with shoe wear as a result of the deformity (Claytor & Bazner-Chandler 2017, Mosca 2014).

Nursing Care Management

The nursing role primarily involves identifying the defect so that early education and instruction to the parents can be initiated. The nurse teaches the parents how to hold the heel firmly and to stretch only the forefoot; otherwise, undue force on the heel may produce a valgus deformity. If casting or an orthosis is needed, the nurse instructs the parents in cast care and care of the brace.

Congenital Talipes Equinovarus (Clubfoot)

Congenital talipes equinovarus, also referred to as clubfoot, is a complex deformity of the ankle and foot that includes forefoot adduction, cavus, hindfoot varus and ankle equinus (Fig 33.34). Congenital talipes equinovarus involves bone deformity and malposition with soft tissue contracture. It may occur as an isolated deformity or in association with other conditions or syndromes, such as spina bifida, arthrogryposis, constriction band or chromosomal abnormalities.

The incidence of congenital talipes equinovarus in the general population is approximately 1.5 per 1000 live births, with 3.5 per 1000 live births among the Indigenous population more than the Caucasian population at 1.1 per 1000 live births (Ansar et al 2018). Boys are affected twice as often as girls. Bilateral clubfeet occur in 50% of the cases and unilaterally mostly seen to occur on the right side (Ansar et al 2018). The precise aetiology of congenital talipes equinovarus is unclear but is likely to be a result of multiple mechanisms. However, there is a strong genetic or familial tendency. Other possible theories as to the cause of congenital talipes equinovarus include arrested or abnormal fetal development or abnormal positioning and restricted movement in utero, although the evidence is inconclusive (Mosca 2014).

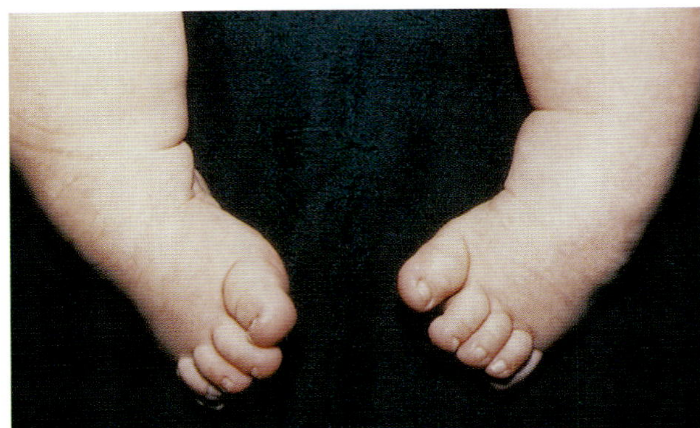

Fig 33.34 Bilateral congenital talipes equinovarus (congenital clubfoot).

Diagnostic Evaluation

A congenital talipes equinovarus deformity is readily apparent at birth if it has not been detected prenatally through ultrasonography. Once it is detected, a careful yet comprehensive physical assessment of the affected foot (or feet) should be completed to allow for appropriate decision-making regarding treatment plans and prognosis. The affected foot (or feet) is usually smaller and shorter, with an empty heel pad and a midfoot plantar crease. When the deformity is unilateral, the affected limb may be shorter and calf atrophy is present. Generally, imaging such as radiographs or ultrasonography is not necessary for diagnosis. A thorough hip examination should be performed for all infants with a clubfoot; an increased risk of hip dysplasia is associated with clubfoot deformities.

Therapeutic Management

The goal of treatment for congenital talipes equinovarus is to achieve a painless, plantigrade and stable foot. Once the diagnosis is established, treatment is ideally initiated in the newborn period and involves three stages: (1) correction of the deformity; (2) maintenance of the correction until normal muscle balance is regained; and (3) follow-up observation to avert possible recurrence of the deformity. Some feet respond to treatment readily; some respond only to prolonged, vigorous and sustained efforts; and the improvement in others remains disappointing even with maximum effort. Parents should realise that outcomes are not always predictable and depend on the severity of the deformity, age of the child at initial intervention, compliance with treatment protocols and development of bones, muscles and nerves.

The common approach to congenital talipes equinovarus management and treatment is the Ponseti method (Ponseti 1996). Serial casting is begun within the first month of life. Weekly gentle manipulation and stretching of the foot along with placement of serial long-leg casts allow for gradual repositioning of the foot (Fig 33.35). The extremity or extremities are casted until maximum correction is achieved, usually within 5 to 8 weeks. The majority of the time, a percutaneous heelcord tenotomy is performed at the end of casting to correct the equinus deformity. After the tenotomy, a long-leg cast is applied and left in place for 3 weeks. After the completion of casting, a Denis Browne bar with Ponseti sandals placed in abduction are fitted to maintain the correction and prevent recurrence. The foot abduction brace is used at night-time for 3 to 5 years. Inability to achieve an

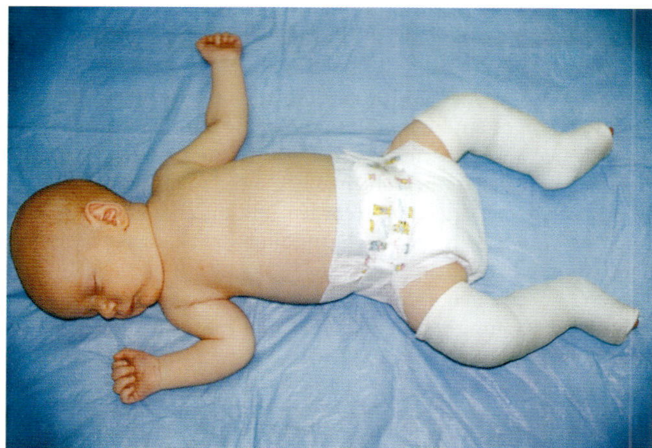

Fig 33.35 Feet casted for correction of bilateral clubfeet.

acceptable foot alignment and ankle range of motion after casting and tenotomy indicates the need for additional surgical intervention.

Nursing Care Management

Nursing care of the child with congenital talipes equinovarus is the same as for any child who has a cast. Because the child will spend considerable time in a corrective device, nursing care plans include both long- and short-term goals. Careful observation of the skin and circulation is particularly important in young infants because of their rapid growth rate.

Because treatment and follow-up care are handled in the orthopaedic clinic or outpatient department, parent education and support are important in the nursing care of these children. Parents need to understand the diagnosis, the overall treatment program, the importance of regular cast changes and the role they play in the long-term effectiveness of the therapy. Nursing responsibilities include reinforcing and clarifying the orthopaedic provider's explanations and instructions, teaching parents about care of the cast or bracing (including vigilant observation for potential problems) and encouraging parents to facilitate normal development within the limitations imposed by the deformity or therapy.

ORTHOPAEDIC INFECTIONS

Osteomyelitis

Osteomyelitis, an infectious process involving the bone, may occur at any age but most frequently is seen in children 10 years of age or younger. *Staphylococcus aureus* is the most common causative organism. Neonates are also likely to have osteomyelitis caused by group B streptococci. Since the advent of *Haemophilus influenzae* type b immunisation in the late 1980s, *H. influenzae* has become a less common causative pathogen. *Kingella kingae* and methicillin-resistant *S. aureus* (MRSA), however, are emerging as potential causative organisms in musculoskeletal infections (Tande et al 2020, Stans 2014).

Acute haematogenous osteomyelitis results when a blood-borne bacterium causes an infection in the bone. Common foci include infected lesions, upper respiratory tract infections, otitis media, tonsillitis, abscessed teeth, pyelonephritis and infected burns. Exogenous osteomyelitis is acquired from direct inoculation of the bone from a puncture wound, open fracture, surgical contamination or adjacent tissue infection. Subacute osteomyelitis has a longer course and may be caused by less virulent microbes with a walled-off abscess or Brodie abscess, typically in the proximal or distal tibia. Chronic osteomyelitis is a progression of acute osteomyelitis and is characterised by the presence of dead bone, bone loss and drainage and sinus tracts. Generally healthy bone is not likely to become infected. Factors that contribute to infection include inoculation with a large number of organisms, presence of a foreign body, bone injury, high virulence of an organism, immunosuppression and malnutrition. Certain types and locations of bone are also more vulnerable to infection. The limbs most commonly affected include the foot, femur, tibia and pelvis.

PATHOPHYSIOLOGY REVIEW

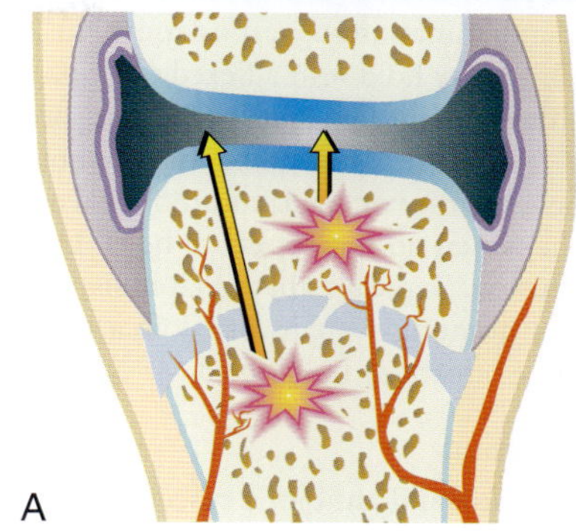

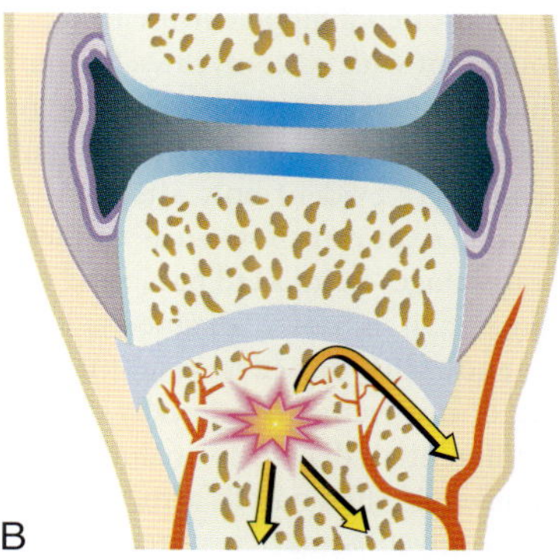

Fig 33.36 Pathogenesis of acute osteomyelitis differs with age. (**A**) In infants younger than 1 year, the epiphysis is nourished by penetrating arteries through the physis, allowing development of the condition within the epiphysis. (**B**) In children up to 15 years of age, the infection is restricted to below the physis because of interruption of the vessels.

Pathophysiology

In acute osteomyelitis, bacteria adhere to bone, causing a suppurative infection with inflammatory cells, oedema, vascular congestion and small-vessel thrombosis; the result is bone destruction, abscess formation and dead bone (sequestrum). Infection within the bone can rupture through the cortex into the subperiosteal space, stripping loose periosteum and forming an abscess. As dead bone is resorbed, new bone is formed along the live bone and infection borders. This surrounding sheath of live bone is called an involucrum. Sinus tracts from perforations in the involucrum may drain pus through soft tissue to the skin.

The pathology of osteomyelitis is different in infants, children older than 1 year of age and adults. In infants blood vessels cross the growth plate into the epiphysis and joint space, which allows infection to spread into the joint. In children the infection is contained by the growth plate, and joint infection is less likely (unless the infection is intracapsular) (Fig 33.36).

Clinical Manifestations

In children severe pain, fever, irritability and tenderness with or without local signs of inflammation suggest osteomyelitis. The extremity is tender, and the child may hold it in a flexed position and resist movement. In infants these symptoms may be minimal or absent, and pain may be difficult to localise. The infant may demonstrate pain with movement of the extremity or hold it immobile. Fever is uncommon in infants, and they often do not appear to be ill. Infants may have an adjacent joint effusion. Typically the metaphysis of long bones—the tibia, femur and/or humerus—are involved. In a small portion of children more than one bone may be affected.

Diagnostic Evaluation

Organism identification and antibiotic susceptibility testing are essential for effective therapy. Obtain cultures of aspirated subperiosteal pus along with cultures of blood, joint fluid and infected skin samples. Bone biopsy may be indicated if blood culture results and radiographic findings are not consistent with osteomyelitis. Supporting evidence for osteomyelitis includes leucocytosis, elevated erythrocyte sedimentation rate and elevated C-reactive protein. Radiographic signs, except for soft tissue swelling, are evident only after 2 to 3 weeks. A three-phase technetium bone scan can show areas of increased blood flow, such as occurs in early stages in infected bone, and is useful in locating multiple sites; however, it is not a diagnostic test. CT can detect bone destruction, and MRI provides anatomical details useful in delineating the area of involvement, especially if surgical intervention is planned. The differential diagnosis includes trauma, malignant lesions, leukaemia, juvenile rheumatoid arthritis and acute rheumatic fever. Sometimes osteomyelitis may be unrecognised if it occurs as a complication of a severe toxic and debilitating disease.

Therapeutic Management

Surgical management with aspiration and drainage of the bone or joint affected should be performed as soon as possible. Specimen cultures are obtained during the procedure to help identify the specific organism responsible for the infection. Aspiration also assists in determining whether there is an abscess or septic joint that requires surgical drainage.

After culture specimens are obtained, empiric therapy is started with IV antibiotics covering the most likely organisms. When the infective agent is identified, administration of the appropriate antibiotic is initiated and continued for at least 4 weeks, but the length of therapy is determined by the duration of the symptoms, the response to treatment and the sensitivity of the organism. In selected cases oral antibiotic therapy may follow a shorter IV course. Due to the prolonged duration of high-dose antibiotic therapy, it is important to monitor for haematological, renal, hepatic, ototoxic and other potential side effects.

Nursing Care Management

During the acute phase of illness, any movement of the affected limb causes discomfort to the child, so the child is positioned comfortably with the affected limb supported. Moving and turning are carried out carefully and gently to minimise discomfort. The child may require pain medication (see Chapter 5) or sedation. Take vital signs and record them frequently, and implement measures to reduce a significant temperature elevation.

Antibiotic therapy requires careful observation and monitoring of the IV equipment and site. Because more than one antibiotic is usually administered, the compatibility of the drugs must be determined and care taken to avoid mixing incompatible drugs. The stability of the drugs and their toxic nature are also considered when determining the rate of administration. The infusion device must be well situated in the vein to ensure that the drug does not infiltrate into surrounding tissues, where it may produce tissue damage.

The wound is managed according to the provider's directions. Administration of antibiotic solution directly into the wound is most efficiently accomplished using a regular infusion set-up that is prepared and regulated in the same manner as for any IV infusion. Intake and output are measured and recorded, and the character of both the wound and drainage is noted. The amount and character of drainage on the wound dressing are also noted.

As the infection subsides, physical therapy is instituted to ensure restoration of optimum function. The child is usually discharged on a regimen of antibiotics (either IV or oral), and progress is monitored closely.

Septic Arthritis

Septic (suppurative) arthritis is a bacterial infection in the joint. It usually results from haematogenous spread or from direct extension of an adjacent cellulitis or osteomyelitis. Direct inoculation from trauma accounts for 15% to 20% of septic arthritis cases. The most common causative organism is *S. aureus*. Community-acquired MRSA is commonly a cause of septic arthritis. In addition to *S. aureus*, pathogens seen in neonates include group B and A *Streptococcus*, *Escherichia coli* and *Streptococcus pneumoniae*. In children 2 months to 5 years of age, *S. aureus*, *Streptococcus pyogenes*, *S. pneumoniae* and *K. kingae* are the primary organisms causing infection, whereas children older than 5 years are more likely to be infected by *S. aureus* and *S. pyogenes*; sexually active adolescents may be infected by *N. gonorrhoeae* (Kerin 2017, Montgomery & Epps 2017).

Knees, hips, ankles and elbows are the most commonly affected joints. Clinical manifestations include severe joint pain, swelling, warmth of overlying tissue and occasionally erythema. The child is resistant to any joint movement. Features of systemic illness such as fever, malaise, headache, nausea, vomiting and irritability may also be present.

Therapeutic and Nursing Care Management

The affected joint is aspirated and the specimen evaluated by Gram stain, culture and determination of leucocyte count. In addition, blood cultures and full blood counts with differential, erythrocyte sedimentation rate and C-reactive protein levels should be monitored. Surgical decompression of the joint along with irrigation and debridement is recommended. Early radiographic findings are limited to soft tissue swelling but may reveal a foreign body, and such films always provide a baseline for comparison. MRI and CT scans provide more detailed images of inflammation, cartilage loss, joint narrowing, erosions and marrow involvement.

IV antibiotic therapy is based on Gram stain results and clinical presentation. The benefits of serial aspiration to demonstrate sterility of synovial fluid and reduce pressure or pain are controversial. Pain management is an important aspect of nursing care, particularly with involvement of a large joint such as the hip. Surgical intervention may also be required if there was a penetrating wound or a foreign object was possibly involved. Physical therapy may be initiated to maintain range of motion and prevent contractures, similar to the nursing care for osteomyelitis.

Skeletal Tuberculosis

In children, tuberculous infection of the bones and joints is acquired by lymphohaematogenous spread at the time of primary infection. Occasionally it is from chronic pulmonary tuberculosis. Skeletal tuberculous infection is not common but should be considered in communities with high tuberculosis case rates. The infection is most likely to involve the vertebrae, causing a paravertebral abscess formation. If the spine infection is progressive, it results in destruction of the vertebral bodies and results in hyperkyphosis deformity. Symptoms are insidious. The child may report persistent or intermittent pain. Other findings include joint swelling and stiffness; fever and weight loss are not common. Tuberculous arthritis can also affect single joints such as a knee or hip and tends to cause severe destruction of adjacent bone. Infection in the fingers causes spina ventosa, a tuberculous dactylitis.

As with pulmonary tuberculosis, the index case should be located. A family and environmental history needs to be obtained and skin tests performed. (See also Tuberculosis, Chapter 26.) Results of tuberculin skin tests are positive for the majority of children with tuberculous arthritis; however, the results are not diagnostic, and the clinical and laboratory features do not differentiate tubercular arthritis from a non-tuberculous septic arthritis. Diagnosis requires isolation of *Mycobacterium tuberculosis* from the site. Patients with the susceptible organism start treatment with combined antituberculosis chemotherapy (isoniazid, rifampicin and pyrazinamide); directly observed therapy is preferred and should be continued for 1 year.

Nursing care depends on the site and extent of infection. Tuberculous spondylitis and hip infection may require immobilisation and additional surgical management. Nursing care is the same as for osteomyelitis, with the addition of isolation requirements.

SKELETAL AND ARTICULAR DYSFUNCTION

Osteogenesis Imperfecta

Osteogenesis imperfecta (OI) is the most common osteoporosis syndrome in children, characterised by excessive fractures and bone deformity; most affected children have moderate to severe growth restriction. There are at least 11 types of OI, accounting for significant disease variability. Clinical features include: varying degrees of bone fragility, deformity and fracture; blue sclerae; hearing loss; and dentinogenesis imperfecta (hypoplastic discoloured teeth). The inheritance pattern is autosomal dominant in the majority of cases, although forms demonstrate autosomal recessive inheritance.

Most types of OI have defects in the *COL1A1* or *COL1A2* genes, which code for polypeptide chains in type 1 procollagen, a precursor of type 1 collagen, a major structural component of bone. The error results in faulty bone mineralisation, abnormal bone architecture and increased susceptibility to fracture. Recently genetic studies have found OI types caused by genetic mutations not associated with defective collagen production (Arshad & Bishop 2021, Marini & Blissett 2013). Additional autosomal recessive genetic types of OI have been described and include *CRTAP, PPIB, SERPINH1, LEPRE1, PLOD2, FKBP10, LRP5* and *SP7* (Arshad & Bishop 2021, Laron & Pandya 2013).

Classifications for OI are based on clinical features and patterns of inheritance (Box 33.9). Clinically, type I is the most common, with wide variability of bone fragility; some affected family members have significant deformity and disability, whereas others lead agile, active lives. Type II variants are the most severe and are considered lethal in infancy. Type III OI is characterised by multiple fractures, bone deformity and severe disability; affected individuals rarely live to 30 years of age. Type IV is similar to type I with blue or white sclerae. Another variant, or type V, has been described in which those affected have a hyperplastic callus, a radiodense metaphyseal band and calcification of the interosseous membrane of the forearm; no collagen mutations are noted in this group (Tauer et al 2019, Marini 2016). A type VI has been described with a characteristic mineralisation defect, which does not respond to pamidronate therapy as types I to V do (Land et al 2007).

BOX 33.9 Classification of Osteogenesis Imperfecta*

Type I[†]

- **A**—Mild bone fragility; blue sclerae; normal teeth; hearing loss (occurs between ages 20 and 30 years); autosomal dominant inheritance
- **B**—Same as A except dentinogenesis imperfecta instead of normal teeth
- **C**—Same as B but no bone fragility

Type II—Lethal; stillborn or die in early infancy; severe bone fragility, multiple fractures at birth; 10% of cases of OI; autosomal recessive inheritance

Type III—Severe bone fragility leading to severe progressive deformities; normal sclerae; marked growth failure; most autosomal recessive inheritance; few autosomal dominant inheritance

Type IV

- **A**—Mild to moderate bone fragility; normal sclerae; normal teeth; short ; variable deformity; autosomal dominant inheritance
- **B**—Same as A except dentinogenesis imperfecta instead of normal teeth; approximately 6% of cases of OI

Type V—Clinically similar to type IV; hyperplastic callus; ossification of interosseous membranes between tibia/fibula and radius/ulna; collagen mutation negative

Type VI—Clinically similar to type IV; rare; sclerae and dentition normal; moderate to severe bone fragility; diagnosis by bone biopsy because of similarities to other types

Types VII and VIII (recessive form)—Clinically overlap types II and III but have white sclerae, rhizomelia and small to normal head circumference; severe osteochondroplasia and short stature in survivors. Type VII is associated with *CRTAP* gene and Type VIII is associated with the *LEPRE1* genetic mutation (Marini *2016).

*Two-thirds of cases are type I.
†This classification is based on that proposed by Sillence and colleagues (1979), which originally included OI types I through IV. Additional types have been described but are not included herein.
OI, osteogenesis imperfecta.

However, a small group of children with OI VI responded favourably to denosumab, a RANK ligand inhibitor (Semler et al 2012, Trejo & Rauch 2016). Children affected with this type have no dental involvement and normal sclerae; a bone biopsy is the only way to establish a diagnosis because of the similarities to other types. Types VII and VIII overlap types II and III in relation to clinical features, but those who survive these types have white sclerae, a normal-to-small head circumference, short stature and rhizomelia (Marini 2016).

Therapeutic Management

The treatment for OI has historically been primarily supportive, although patients and families are optimistic about new research advances. Bone marrow transplant for severe OI was first reported in 1999 with positive results; however, this is still considered an experimental treatment, and long-term follow-up of such children has not been published. The long-term effectiveness of bone marrow transplant for OI in comparison to the complications of the treatment have yet to be fully explored (Arshad & Bishop 2021).

Therapeutic management should focus on decreasing the number of fractures, decreasing pain, increasing growth, improving bone metabolism and optimising function. Bisphosphonate therapy with pamidronate or alendronate to promote increased bone density and prevent fractures has become standard therapy for many children with OI. Bisphosphonate therapy reportedly is more beneficial for increasing vertebral bone density but is considered less effective for long bones (Marini 2016). Others report effectiveness of pamidronate in children with moderate to severe OI (Arshad & Bishop 2021). Trejo and Rauch

(2016) suggest that data are inadequate to recommend the use of bisphosphonate therapy in children with OI for sole treatment of bone mineral density reduction.

The rehabilitative approach to management is directed to preventing positional contractures and deformities, muscle weakness and osteoporosis and malalignment of lower extremity joints, prohibiting weight bearing. Lightweight braces and splints help support limbs, prevent fractures and aid in ambulation. Physical therapy helps prevent disuse osteoporosis and strengthens muscles, which in turn improves bone density. Surgery is sometimes used to help treat the manifestations of the disease. Surgical techniques are used to correct deformities that interfere with bracing, standing or walking. For the child with recurrent fractures, inserting an intramedullary rod provides stability to bones.

Nursing Care Management

Infants and children with this disorder require careful handling to prevent fractures. They must be supported when they are being turned, positioned, moved and held. Even changing a nappy may cause a fracture in severely affected infants. These children should never be held by the ankles when the nappy is being changed but should be gently lifted by the buttocks or supported with pillows; however, nurses should not be afraid to touch or handle the infant or child with OI. Such children need compassionate handling and care as much as any other patient. Parents who care for such children on a regular basis can often share tips for handling the child without causing fractures.

It is recommended that blood pressure be obtained with a manual cuff to prevent fractures. In addition nurses should be aware that such children, although smaller in stature than same-age children, have normal intelligence and should receive adequate information and instructions regarding their care. Involving parents in the daily care of the child is essential (Madonia 2012). Children receiving bisphosphonate therapy should be closely monitored for respiratory infections and should receive appropriate immunisations for the prevention of childhood communicable diseases. Live virus vaccines may not be recommended in children on bisphosphonate therapy, and an infectious disease specialist should be consulted. Skin care for children with OI is essential; infants with OI may need frequent repositioning of the head to prevent posterior occipital flattening or other cranial moulding. Oral and dental care should be performed on a regular basis and with extreme care due to bone and tooth fragility (Madonia 2012). Parents of the child undergoing bone marrow transplant need adequate written information and instructions regarding special care in regard to the various chemotherapeutic drugs required (Madonia 2012). (See also Bone Marrow Transplantation, Chapter 29.)

Children with current fractures or healing fractures should be screened for OI; the assumption that abuse or neglect is the cause of fractures in children must be carefully evaluated by a multidisciplinary team. A detailed history, no evidence of associated soft tissue injury and the presence of other symptoms related to OI help determine the diagnosis.

Both parents and the affected child need education regarding the child's limitations and guidelines in planning suitable activities that promote optimum development and protect the child from harm. Realistic occupational planning and genetic counselling are part of the long-term goals of care.

Juvenile Idiopathic Arthritis

Juvenile idiopathic arthritis (JIA) refers to chronic childhood arthritis. A group of heterogeneous chronic autoimmune diseases, JIA causes inflammation in the synovium, joints and surrounding tissue. The cause of JIA is unknown. Some theories speculate that the disorder arises when an infectious agent activates an autoimmune inflammatory process in a genetically predisposed child. Although a genetic susceptibility to JIA is known, such as human leucocyte antigen (HLA) polymorphisms, the *PTPN22* gene and the *IL2RA/CD 25* gene, the genetic contribution is complicated and still not well understood (John & Brady 2017). The reported incidence of chronic childhood arthritis is approximately 1 per 1000 children (Arthritis Australia 2017). JIA starts before age 16 years with two peak onsets: between 1 and 3 and between 8 and 10 years of age. There is a female predominance of 2:1.

Pathophysiology

The disease process is characterised by chronic synovial inflammation causing joint effusion and eventual erosion, destruction and fibrosis of the articular cartilage. Adhesions between joint surfaces and ankylosis of joints occur if the process persists.

Clinical Manifestations

Whether single or multiple joints are involved, stiffness, swelling and loss of motion develop in the affected joints. The swelling results from soft tissue oedema, joint effusion and synovial thickening. The affected joints may be warm and tender to the touch, but it is not uncommon for pain not to be reported. Erythema is not typical, and a warm, painful red joint is always suspect for infection. The limited motion early in the disease is a result of muscle spasm and joint inflammation; later it is caused by ankylosis or soft tissue contracture. Morning stiffness of the joint(s) is characteristic and present on arising in the morning or after inactivity. Functional change may be an obvious limp or subtle modifications of joint motion that protect the involved joint, such as fisting to avoid wrist extension with pressure. In severe, long-standing cases growth is significantly restricted. Corticosteroid therapy can be a contributing factor. There may be growth disturbances, either overgrowth or undergrowth, adjacent to the inflamed joints (e.g. altered leg length after knee involvement) and micrognathia (receding chin) from temporomandibular arthritis.

Classification. The International League of Associations for Rheumatology classification of JIA, developed in 1997, revised and published in 1998 and revised again in 2001, lists seven disease categories, each with its own set of criteria and exclusions: systemic arthritis, oligoarthritis, rheumatoid factor (RF)–negative polyarthritis, RF-positive polyarthritis, psoriatic arthritis, enthesitis-related arthritis and undifferentiated arthritis (John & Brady 2017) (Box 33.10).

Course and Prognosis

The outcome of JIA is variable and unpredictable. Even in severe forms, JIA is rarely life-threatening and is significantly different from adult rheumatoid arthritis. Features that distinguish JIA from adult disease include: onset before 16 years of age; a negative rheumatoid factor (in 90% of cases); classic symptoms of systemic arthritis, including quotidian fever, rash and pericarditis; development of uveitis (inflammation of the iris and ciliary body) as a complication (in 8% to 20% of cases); and a tendency for the arthritis to become inactive.

Juvenile arthritis affects 1 in 1000 children (AIHW 2019). Children with juvenile arthritis can experience short- and long-term life-limiting symptoms, and it lowers their quality of life with disability and pain, impacting on physical and social wellbeing (AIHW 2019). Their arthritis can cause significant joint deformity and functional disability requiring medication, physical therapy and perhaps future joint

BOX 33.10 International League of Associations for Rheumatology Classification of Juvenile Idiopathic Arthritis

Systemic Arthritis

Definition—Arthritis in one or more joints with or preceded by fever for at least 2 weeks' duration that is documented to be daily for at least 3 days, and accompanied by one or more of the following: evanescent (non-fixed) erythematous rash, generalised lymph node enlargement, hepatomegaly and/or splenomegaly, serositis.

Exclusions—a, b, c, d*

Oligoarthritis

Definition—Arthritis affecting one to four joints during the first 6 months of disease. Two subcategories are recognised: (1) persistent oligoarthritis, which never extends over four affected joints during disease course; and (2) extended oligoarthritis, which affects more than four joints after 6 months of disease.

Exclusions—a, b, c, d, e*

Polyarthritis (Rheumatoid Factor Negative)

Definition—Arthritis affecting five or more joints during the first 6 months of the disease and a negative rheumatoid factor.

Exclusions—a, b, c, e*

Polyarthritis (Rheumatoid Factor Positive)

Definition—Arthritis affecting five or more joints during the first 6 months of disease and two or more positive rheumatoid factor tests at least 3 months apart during the first 6 months of disease.

Exclusions—a, b, c, e*

Psoriatic Arthritis

Definition—Arthritis and psoriasis, or arthritis and at least two of the following: (1) dactylitis; (2) nail pitting or onycholysis; and (3) psoriasis in a first-degree relative.

Exclusions—b, c, d, e*

Enthesitis-related Arthritis

Definition—Arthritis and enthesitis (inflammation at a tendon insertion site), or arthritis or enthesitis with at least two of the following: (1) presence or history of sacroiliac joint tenderness and/or inflammatory lumbosacral pain; (2) presence of HLA-B27 antigen; (3) onset of arthritis in a male over 6 years of age; (4) symptomatic anterior uveitis; and (5) a history of ankylosing spondylitis, enthesitis-related arthritis, sacroiliitis with inflammatory bowel disease, Reiter syndrome or acute anterior uveitis in a first-degree relative.

Exclusions—a, d, e*

Undifferentiated Arthritis

Definition—Arthritis that fulfils criteria in no category or in two or more of the above categories.

*Exclusions: (a) Psoriasis or a history of psoriasis in the patient or first-degree relative; (b) arthritis in an HLA-B27–positive male beginning after the sixth birthday; (c) ankylosing spondylitis, enthesitis-related arthritis, sacroiliitis with inflammatory bowel disease, Reiter syndrome, or symptomatic anterior uveitis, or a history of one of these disorders in a first-degree relative; (d) the presence of immunoglobulin M rheumatoid factor on at least two occasions at least 3 months apart; (e) the presence of systemic juvenile idiopathic arthritis in the patient (Petty et al 2004).

HLA, human leucocyte antigen.

replacement. Chronic and acute uveitis is an extraarticular complication of JIA that may cause permanent vision loss if undiagnosed and not aggressively treated. Although many children have minimal arthritis, it can produce severe physical, functional and emotional impairment.

Diagnostic Evaluation

JIA is a diagnosis of exclusion; there are no definitive tests. Criteria include onset before 16 years, arthritis in one or more joints for 6 weeks or longer and exclusion of other causes (John & Brady 2017). Laboratory test results may provide supporting evidence of disease. An elevated sedimentation rate or C-reactive protein may or may not be present. Leucocytosis is frequently present during flares of systemic disease. Tests for RF give positive results in only 10% of the children with JIA. The presence of antinuclear antibodies is common in JIA, but they are not specific for arthritis; however, their presence helps identify children with pauciarticular disease, who are at greater risk for uveitis.

Therapeutic Management

There is no cure for JIA. The major goals of therapy are to control pain, preserve joint range of motion and function, minimise the effects of inflammation such as joint deformity and promote normal growth and development. Achievement of these goals requires a family-centred approach with collaboration among the child, family and healthcare team. The team includes: the primary care practitioner; paediatric rheumatologist; social worker; occupational therapists; physiotherapist; and a community of friends, relatives and teachers. The treatment plan is individualised, but it can be complicated and intrusive, including medications, physical and occupational therapy, slit-lamp eye examinations, splints, comfort measures, dietary management, modification of school activities and psychosocial support.

Chronic uveitis can cause permanent vision loss, glaucoma and cataracts. Slit-lamp ophthalmological examinations at regular intervals are required to diagnose chronic anterior uveitis (iridocyclitis), inflammation of the anterior segments of the eye, iris and ciliary body. The majority of affected children have a relatively good visual prognosis if the inflammation is detected and treated early; however, most cases are asymptomatic. Consequently, routine slit-lamp examinations are critical. The children at greatest risk for development of uveitis have pauciarticular disease and a positive antinuclear antibody (John & Brady 2017). Infections, injuries and surgical procedures often precipitate a flare-up of the arthritis; therefore, prompt recognition and treatment of infections are necessary.

Medications. Treatment guidelines are divided into four groups: children with: (1) four or fewer affected joints; (2) five or more affected joints; (3) systemic arthritis with active systemic features; and (4) systemic arthritis with active arthritis. Each path provides recommendations for stepwise escalation of medication therapy (Beukelman et al 2011). All tracks consider poor prognostic indicators, such as: erosions on radiographs; arthritis of the hip, cervical spine, ankle or wrist; and a positive rheumatoid factor. Additionally, each track takes into account disease activity levels that include elevated acute phase reactants and global assessments of both the provider and the patient/parent.

A variety of antirheumatic drugs are available. NSAIDs are used alone or in combination with other drugs, depending on the amount of disease activity and poor prognostic features. Common NSAIDs include ibuprofen, naproxen, diclofenac, indomethacin and meloxicam. NSAIDs offer an immediate analgesic effect, but the anti-inflammatory effect requires larger doses and more time to achieve. Patient and family education regarding potential gastrointestinal, renal and hepatic side effects and reduced clotting is essential. Parents should monitor the child for abdominal pain and blood in the stool. Naproxen has the potential side effect of skin fragility; patients need to use sunscreen and report unusual skin lesions.

Additional medication is required in most children with arthritis. The agents used are **disease-modifying antirheumatic drugs (DMARDs)** and include the non-biological drugs methotrexate and sulfasalazine. The decision to use DMARDs at initiation of therapy or later in the escalation of therapy is guided by the amount of disease activity and poor prognostic features. Families may be overwhelmed by the potential adverse effects, including liver disease, bone marrow suppression, gastrointestinal disturbance, teratogenic effects and the alarming but unconfirmed risk of carcinogenesis. Methotrexate is effective, however, and the potential benefits outweigh the potential risks. Methotrexate therapy has also improved uveitis in children with uveitis resistant to steroid treatment. Laboratory monitoring of liver enzyme levels and blood counts is crucial. A daily folic acid supplement can help reduce the occurrence of oral ulcers. Taking methotrexate at bedtime may help reduce nausea.

Frank discussion about sexual activity and birth defects is critical. Sexually active teenagers need effective contraception and documented menstrual periods, as well as pregnancy tests if periods are not regular. As a precaution, pregnant caregivers and those trying to conceive need to avoid contact with methotrexate.

Alcohol consumption is another sensitive topic that needs to be discussed honestly because it increases the risk of hepatotoxicity. Patients should avoid additional over-the-counter NSAIDs and to take paracetamol for episodes of fever. Parents should always discuss methotrexate drug interactions with providers prescribing medications for interval illness. During some illnesses, especially varicella, methotrexate should be discontinued because it can suppress the immune response. Sulfasalazine may be selected in children with axial arthritis, a positive test result for HLA-B27 or symptoms of inflammatory bowel disease, given this drug's success in these select groups of patients.

Biological DMARDs. Biological DMARDs are initiated when there is significant disease activity and/or poor prognostic indicators after unsuccessful treatment with methotrexate. Tumour necrosis factor alpha (TNF-alpha) inhibitors are the most frequently used biological DMARDs and include etanercept, infliximab and adalimumab. Etanercept blocks the binding of TNF-alpha with cell surface receptors, and adalimumab and infliximab are monoclonal antibody TNF-alpha blocking agents. All three reduce the proinflammatory response that promotes arthritis. TNF-alpha inhibitors are seen to be effective and well tolerated (Chang & Girgis 2017).

Although TNF-alpha inhibitors have been found safe and effective, parents need to inform providers of any unusual symptoms in the child given the relatively limited experience with these drugs and the potential for long-term side effects (Chang & Girgis 2017). The potential for malignancy, particularly lymphoma, is continuing to be monitored in children on TNF blockers. Increased infection risk is the most common adverse effect. Parents should withhold TNF-alpha inhibitors during a concurrent infection and promptly report symptoms of infection to their provider for assessment and treatment. A negative tuberculin skin test should be obtained before starting a biological DMARD; yearly follow-up skin testing has been suggested.

Glucocorticoids. Glucocorticoids are potent anti-inflammatory agents; however, systemic steroids will not cure arthritis, and the significant adverse effects of long-term steroid use are undesirable. Steroids are administered when there is high disease activity or poor prognostic features. Prednisone is given orally in a burst and taper or at the lowest effective dosage. Use of an alternate-day schedule may help reduce side effects. High-dose IV steroids may provide sustained improvement for children with severe arthritis and pericarditis associated with systemic disease. Intraarticular injections of long-acting steroids have proven effective in treating limited arthritis with minimal adverse effects and frequently provided sustained control and, in some, a remission. Children may require procedural sedation or general anaesthesia, which affects risk-benefit considerations, but it is critical to have a cooperative patient for good procedure outcome.

Physical Management. Programs of physical therapy are individualised for each child and are designed to reach the ultimate goal of preserving function and preventing deformity. Physical therapy is directed towards specific joints and focuses on strengthening muscles, mobilising restricted joints and preventing or correcting deformities. Occupational therapists assume responsibility for evaluating and improving performance of activities of daily living.

General treatment and maintenance programs vary. Physical therapists may be involved several times per week, or their visits may be limited to monthly evaluations to review the home program for compliance, effectiveness and need. Muscle strength is frequently lost around the involved joints, and inactivity leads to generalised weakness. However, performance of the normal activities of daily living and the child's natural tendency to be active are usually sufficient to maintain muscle strength and joint mobility. Unless there is a specific risk of injury related to arthritis, the child should not be restricted from regular play, dance, exercise programs and even individual and team sports. Activity modifications may be needed to accommodate joint limitations, but exercise should be encouraged; a sedentary lifestyle contributes to a deconditioned state, which further limits physical activity and ultimately influences the child's quality of life.

Exercising in a pool is excellent because it allows freedom of movement with support. When joints are inflamed, heavy resistance aggravates the pain. At such times, simple isometric or tensing exercises that do not involve joint movement are generally tolerated. Range-of-motion exercises are an important aspect of therapy and are continued after evidence of disease has disappeared in order to detect any signs of recurrence.

Providers may recommend night-time splinting to help minimise pain and prevent or reduce flexion deformity. Vigilance is required to detect loss of motion, and vigorous attention must be given to specialised passive stretching, positioning and resting splints to prevent deformity.

Surgery. The benefits of synovectomy, an established therapeutic procedure in adults, are questionable in children with arthritis. Synovectomy is used primarily in pauciarticular disease when all other therapy has been unsuccessful. In cases of synovitis, intraarticular steroid injection is an alternative to synovectomy and may be tried once or twice before surgery is performed. Joint replacement is proving to be successful in older children who are fully grown.

Nursing Care Management

Nursing care of children with JIA involves assessment of their general health, the status of involved joints and their emotional responses to all of the ramifications of the disease: pain, physical restrictions, therapies and self-concept, especially in preadolescents and adolescents.

The effects of the disease are manifested in every aspect of the child's life, including physical activities, social experiences and personality development. Children's adjustment to the stresses and demands of the disease and the level of functioning they achieve are related largely to the reaction and support they receive from their family and the healthcare professionals involved in their care and management.

Relieve Pain. Multiple factors influence the pain of arthritis: disease severity, functional status, individual pain threshold, family variables and psychological adjustment. Although complete pain relief is desirable, it is probably unrealistic. The aim is to provide as much relief as possible with anti-inflammatory medication and other therapies to help children tolerate the pain and complete the activities of daily living. At present, opioid administration is not a routine therapy for the chronic pain of arthritis. Non-pharmacological modalities such as relaxation may be helpful.

Promote General Strength

Diet and exercise. The general health of children with arthritis and their siblings must be considered but may be overlooked as parents and health personnel concentrate on the disease. Maintenance of a well-balanced diet and assessment of nutritional status are integral parts of health supervision. A daily children's complete multivitamin with iron is a reasonable dietary supplement, but there is no 'arthritis diet' or foods to avoid that are specifically associated with arthritis. Unfortunately children with arthritis have not been spared the nationwide obesity epidemic. After assessing the child growth chart, make a referral to a dietitian for children who are underweight or overweight due to malnutrition. Excessive weight causes additional strain on inflamed joints. Joint pain during or after exercise impedes active play, which perpetuates the vicious cycle of inactivity and weight gain. Encourage daily physical exercise, starting with a gradual program of walking and slowly advancing to more active play as tolerated. When school is out, parents and children should devise a family plan for exercise that includes a variety of options such as games, sports, dance, yoga, swimming, bike riding and walking. This builds good habits for an active lifestyle for the entire family.

Sleep and rest. Children with JIA report sleep pattern disturbances which contribute to anxiety and depression resulting in reduced quality of life (Fair et al 2019). Restorative sleep is essential. Children should get 8 to 10 hours of night-time sleep. Daytime naps are discouraged, especially because inactivity provokes stiffness and prolonged naps can interfere with sleepiness at bedtime. Fatigue should be handled with rest rather than sleep. Thirty to 60 minutes of relaxation—viewing television, reading, playing video games, using the computer or listening to music—is refuelling and less likely to disrupt night-time sleep than a nap.

Encourage School Attendance. School-aged children should attend school, even on days when there is joint pain. Staying home will not improve arthritis. If joint pain and stiffness prevent school attendance, the rheumatologist should be notified and the child assessed. The rheumatology team can make recommendations to the school to maximise attendance and participation.

Facilitate Compliance. For any medical or physical plan of therapy to be effective, the family must agree to it and understand the benefits of treatment and the problems associated with non-compliance. Review a simple written list of exercise benefits and complications of joint immobility. At the outset, elicit barriers to a plan from the child and parents. If a child cannot swallow pills or refuses injections, the given modality is not acceptable. If parents know they cannot monitor or enforce a complicated medication and physical therapy schedule, the plan needs to be simplified to honestly reflect the actual care that is being provided. If joint range-of-motion exercises are too painful and emotionally difficult for parents to implement despite use of pre-therapy analgesics and comfort measures, then physiotherapy home visits or outpatient physiotherapy sessions need to be considered.

Encourage Comfort Measures and Activities of Daily Living. Application of heat has been beneficial to children with arthritis. Moist heat is best for relieving pain and stiffness, and the most efficient and practical method is via the bathtub. Sometimes a daily whirlpool bath or hot packs may be used as needed for temporary relief of acute swelling and pain.

The child. Changes in personality may accompany JIA, as with any chronic illness. These changes may be temporary, such as demanding, irritable behaviour, or they may be persistent, such as passive hostility, uncommunicativeness and manipulativeness. Families need confirmation that adjusting to a chronic illness is difficult. Consider and encourage support referrals to social workers, counsellors and psychologists. (See Chapter 19.)

The family. Parents and patients need to hear that nurses promote independence. The child's participation in extracurricular activities, including play with friends, scouting, youth groups, dancing and sports, is recommended. Nurses also support assigning children family chores and allowing older children to hold a part-time job, which fosters self-reliance. Attendance at one of the several juvenile arthritis camps available to children with JIA is a confidence-boosting experience they will never forget.

Most of the reactions, problems and concerns of families of a child with JIA are those of any parents of a child with a chronic illness or disability. The impact of the diagnosis is felt most acutely by the parents, who demonstrate anxiety, guilt and all the manifestations of the grief process. The concerns and needs of these families are discussed extensively in Chapter 19, and the reader is directed to this chapter for additional guidance in planning care.

Systemic Lupus Erythematosus

Systemic lupus erythematosus (SLE) is a chronic multisystem autoimmune disease of the blood vessels and connective tissue, which is estimated to affect more than 20,000 people in Australia and New Zealand (Australian Society of Clinical Immunology and Allergy [ASCIA] 2019). It typically manifests between the ages of 10 and 19 years, and onset before 5 years of age is unusual. There is a 4:3 female/male predominance in the first 10 years of life, which increases to 4:1 in the second decade.

Its course and symptoms are variable and unpredictable, with mild to life-threatening complications. SLE in children tends to be more severe at onset and has a more aggressive clinical course than adult-onset disease (John & Brady 2017). Other types of lupus erythematosus include chronic cutaneous lupus erythematosus (discoid lupus erythematosus), drug-induced lupus erythematosus, subacute cutaneous lupus erythematosus and neonatal lupus erythematosus. Neonatal lupus erythematosus occurs when maternal autoantibodies cross the placenta and cause transient lupus-like symptoms in the newborn, with the potential lethal complication of heart block. The remaining discussion focuses on SLE.

Aetiology

The cause of SLE is not known. It appears to result from a complex interaction of genetics with an unidentified trigger that causes the disease to activate. Suspected triggers include exposure to ultraviolet light, oestrogen, pregnancy, infections and drugs. Complement deficiencies C1q, C4 and C1s are associated with an increased risk of developing SLE. The major histocompatibility complex (MHC) Class II and III alleles are associated with an increased risk for developing SLE. There is a racial difference, with non-Caucasian children at increased risk of developing SLE.

Pathophysiology

SLE is the result of an abnormal immune response causing production of abnormal antibodies and formation of immune complexes. These immune complexes are deposited in tissues, causing inflammation and inciting other proinflammatory mediators that result in tissue injury and damage. Immune complex deposition in the glomerulus of the kidney causes lupus nephritis, a life-threatening complication of SLE. Almost any tissue in the body can be damaged by this abnormal inflammatory response, including the brain, heart, lungs, liver, gastrointestinal tract, spleen, joint tissues, muscles and skin.

Clinical Manifestations

The onset of SLE can be insidious, with intermittent constitutional symptoms such as fever, fatigue, weight loss and arthralgia. However, rapid involvement of vital organs, primarily the kidneys, can herald an accelerated course with potentially fatal outcome. Reports suggest that survival rates in children with SLE have significantly improved; 5-year survival rates are over 90% and 15 year survival rates are 85% (Gilek-Seibert 2020). Box 33.11 lists the manifestations related to the various tissues involved.

Rash is a common feature in SLE. The erythematous malar 'butterfly' rash that spares the nasolabial fold is a suggestive feature but not pathognomonic. Maculopapular rashes are frequent and can occur anywhere but typically are found on sun-exposed skin. Nails and hair can be involved, with red, cracked cuticles; periungual telangiectasia; and patchy or diffuse alopecia. Raynaud's phenomenon, or spasm of the blood vessels, causes cool hands and feet with pain and a characteristic tricolour (purple- or blue-white-red) change. Raynaud's phenomenon usually appears as a response to cold exposure and can cause significant tissue damage. In addition to colour changes in the extremities, vascular necrosis and digital ulceration can occur. Arthritis and tenosynovitis are common in SLE. The arthritis is usually painful and typically of short duration; joint deformity is unusual.

Renal involvement is a serious complication caused primarily by deposition of circulating immune complexes in the glomerular basement membrane with cellular infiltrates. Lupus nephritis is usually asymptomatic; consequently, monitoring of urine and renal function is required to detect disease. Kidney biopsy is required for lupus nephritis classification. There are six classes, depending on the type and extent of the renal lesion. Specific treatment is based on the class of nephritis. Although outcomes have improved for children with renal disease, the course is difficult to predict. Most children improve, although some remain the same or progress to renal failure, requiring dialysis and transplantation.

Neuropsychiatric lupus is another serious complication found in approximately 25% of paediatric SLE patients. Central nervous system involvement is seen within the first year of SLE diagnosis (Kivity et al 2015). Symptoms can vary from manifestations as subtle as inability to concentrate to frank psychosis and seizure. Headaches are common with variable severity. Assess school performance and emotional stability at each visit as possible indicators of central nervous system involvement.

Cardiovascular disease results in significant mortality and morbidity in lupus. The immune dysregulation of SLE directly contributes to premature atherosclerosis. Children with SLE have an increased rate of dyslipidaemia complicated by the secondary effects of corticosteroids (Szabó et al 2017). Treatment includes exercise and dietary changes to promote a healthy weight, cardiovascular fitness and management of hypertension. Studies are currently under way to assess the usefulness of statins in paediatric lupus for future evidence-based treatment of premature atherosclerosis in SLE.

Diagnostic Evaluation

SLE is a clinical diagnosis supported by specific abnormal results on laboratory tests. The American College of Rheumatology criteria for the classification of SLE in adults has a sensitivity of 96% and a specificity of 96% if 4 of the 11 criteria are present (Box 33.12). The SLE workup includes an extensive history taking and physical examination with enquiry about school performance and behaviour change. Initial laboratory tests include: full blood count with differential; comprehensive metabolic chemistry panel; microscopic urinalysis; rapid plasma reagin test; quantitative determination of immunoglobulin levels; and tests for antinuclear antibodies, anti-deoxyribonucleic acid antibodies, complement 3 (C3), complement 4 (C4), lupus anticoagulant and antiphospholipid antibodies.

A diagnosis of lupus should not be made without consideration of all medications being taken and their side effects. Some commonly used drugs such as minocycline, procainamide, hydralazine and chlorpromazine can cause lupus-like symptoms. Minocycline, a common acne treatment, may not be considered important by the teenager and omitted from the history, so an accurate recent past and present medication history is essential for treatment. Drug-induced lupus resolves with time after the triggering medication has been discontinued.

BOX 33.11 Manifestations of Systemic Lupus Erythematosus

Constitutional—Fever, fatigue, weight loss, anorexia
Cutaneous—Erythematosus butterfly rash over bridge of nose and across cheeks, discoid rash, photosensitivity, mucocutaneous ulceration, alopecia, periungual telangiectasias
Musculoskeletal—Arthritis, arthralgia, myositis, myalgia, tenosynovitis
Neurological—Headache, seizure, forgetfulness, behaviour change, change in school performance, psychosis, chorea, stroke, cranial and peripheral neuropathy, pseudotumour cerebri
Pulmonary and Cardiac—Pleuritis, basilar pneumonitis, atelectasis, pericarditis, myocarditis and endocarditis
Renal—Glomerulonephritis, nephrotic syndrome, hypertension
Gastrointestinal—Abdominal pain, nausea, vomiting, blood in stool, abdominal crisis, oesophageal dysfunction, colitis
Hepatic, Splenic and Nodal—Hepatomegaly, splenomegaly, lymphadenopathy
Haematological—Anaemia, cytopenia
Ophthalmological—Cotton wool spots, papillo-oedema, retinopathy
Vascular—Raynaud's phenomenon, thrombophlebitis, livedo reticularis

BOX 33.12 Classification Criteria for Systemic Lupus Erythematosus

Malar Rash—Fixed malar erythema
Discoid Rash—Patchy erythematous lesions
Photosensitivity—Rash with sunlight exposure
Oronasal Ulcers—Painless ulcers in mouth and nose
Arthritis—Swelling, tenderness or effusion in two or more peripheral joints (non-erosive)
Serositis—Pleuritis, pericarditis
Renal Disorder—Proteinuria, casts in urine
Neurological Disorder—Psychosis, seizures
Haematological Disorder—Haemolytic anaemia, thrombocytopenia, leucopenia, lymphopenia
Immunological Disorder—Anti–double-stranded deoxyribonucleic acid, anti-Sm, antiphospholipid antibodies; lupus anticoagulant; false-positive result on syphilis test (rapid plasma reagin)
Antinuclear Antibodies—Presence of antinuclear antibody by immunofluorescence or an equivalent assay

*The presence of four criteria is required for classification as systemic lupus erythematosus.

Therapeutic Management

There is no cure for SLE; the management goal is to reverse or minimise disease activity with appropriate medications while helping the child and family cope with the complications of the disease and treatment.

Medications. Since the 1950s, corticosteroids have been the mainstay of SLE therapy. They are effective anti-inflammatory and immunosuppressive agents. Unfortunately, the use of steroids is hampered by side effects, which include growth delay, decreased resistance to infection, osteoporosis, weight gain, hypertension, development of cushingoid features and cataracts, and diabetes risks. Generally, a dosage sufficient to control symptoms is prescribed, and then the dosage is tapered to the lowest level possible to achieve an acceptable balance between disease activity and steroid side effects. For severe disease, IV pulse (high-dose) steroids are given on an intermittent schedule, which may allow reduction in the daily steroid dose with better compliance and fewer cushingoid features. Topical steroids are used for cutaneous lesions, but prolonged therapy thins the skin; consequently, facial application needs to be brief or with medication of lower concentration. A medical identification tag should be worn by children undergoing chronic steroid therapy so that administration of stress steroids can be considered in emergency situations.

Other medications used include NSAIDs such as naproxen and ibuprofen for pain associated with arthritis, arthralgia and myalgia. Nurses need to instruct patients to take NSAIDs with food to help prevent gastrointestinal side effects. Methotrexate may be used in patients with stubborn arthritis that has not responded to NSAIDs and hydroxychloroquine and allows a lower dose of glucocorticoids to be used. Azathioprine, another steroid sparer, has been useful in treatment of SLE thrombocytopenia. Both methotrexate and azathioprine have significant potential adverse effects, including potential for increased infection, malignancy risks, liver and lung toxicity, and birth defects. Well-documented discussions of these risks with patients and parents are required.

Cyclophosphamide, a potent immunosuppressive chemotherapy agent, used in combination with corticosteroids, is effective in treating proliferative lupus nephritis and neuropsychiatric lupus. A detailed cyclophosphamide education session should be held for patient and family to clearly describe potential benefits and risks, including infertility and future malignancy.

Mycophenolate mofetil, a purine inhibitor, has been used with success in adult lupus nephritis and is currently being used as a steroid-sparing agent in active paediatric lupus and as maintenance therapy after standard cyclophosphamide treatment for lupus nephritis. It is also being evaluated as an alternative to standard treatment of lupus nephritis to cyclophosphamide (Mok 2016). Mycophenolate mofetil is an attractive alternative, if successful, because it is less toxic and better tolerated than cyclophosphamide; however, it is not without potential side effects, including increased infection risk, liver toxicity and birth defects. Sexually active females need to be on effective contraception.

New biological treatments are being developed that focus on the immune dysregulation in SLE, cancer and other autoimmune diseases. Belimumab is an IgG1-lambda monoclonal antibody that reduces the activity of B cell–mediated immunity and the autoimmune response by blocking receptors on B lymphocytes. It has been approved in adults with SLE and may be used off-label in select paediatric lupus, while paediatric studies are ongoing (John & Brady 2017). Rituximab is a monoclonal antibody that eliminates CD20-positive B cells without affecting early B cells or plasma cells. This results in decreased antibody formation and has been used off-label in paediatric lupus patients who have not responded to standard therapy (Kallash et al 2019). Individuals with neuropsychiatric involvement may require antidepressants, antineuropathy and antiepileptic drugs (Kivity et al 2015).

General Measures

In addition to medication, treatment includes general measures such as patient and family education, rest and exercise, proper diet, sun avoidance and social support. SLE is complex and requires ongoing patient education. Families and patients need up-to-date, understandable information so they can become informed decision makers and participate in disease management. Nurses are duty bound to discuss with families any information they bring to appointments from the internet, friends and family. As healthcare providers critically evaluate disease information with families, families learn the skills needed to become self-advocates. Families also want to hear about the impact of SLE on growth and development, childbearing, schooling and career choice. The message should be optimistic and clear, with few exceptions: 'Prepare for the future; you will attend school, graduate, have children and work'.

There is no specific SLE diet, but a balanced diet that does not exceed calorie expenditure is essential for maintaining appropriate weight on corticosteroid therapy. A low-salt diet may be required if the patient becomes nephrotic or hypertensive. A low-fat diet is indicated in children with dyslipidaemia. Maximising peak bone mass in adolescent SLE is essential, especially because both SLE and its treatment with glucocorticoids increase the risk of osteoporosis. A diet rich in calcium and vitamin D is essential to prevent osteoporosis. If dietary calcium is not sufficient, calcium and vitamin D supplements need to be recommended. Consultation with a registered dietitian will help the family develop an individualised diet that meshes with their lifestyle.

The benefits of a regular exercise program include weight maintenance, cardiovascular fitness and osteoporosis prevention, all of which help minimise SLE complications and corticosteroid side effects. Unfortunately, many children stop participation in sports after diagnosis. Current evidence recommends exercise as adjunct therapy which is effective in controlling pain and fatigue (Sheikh et al 2019).

Social support from family, friends, teachers, counsellors and professional social workers and therapists can help the child and family through difficult times and promote adaptation to an illness that is not going to go away. Destructive coping mechanisms need to be identified and replaced with behaviours that enhance adaptation and healthy outcomes. Organisations that can help children and families learn about and adjust to the disease are Arthritis Australia and Arthritis New Zealand*.

Nursing Care Management

Fostering adaptation and self-advocacy is the primary nursing goal. Patient and family acceptance and understanding of this life-threatening and therapeutically intrusive disease are big challenges for any nurse. Patient education is started at diagnosis and continued at every opportunity; repetition is good. Encourage family members to call with questions and concerns. Advise patients to write down their questions so they are prepared during the appointment.

With older children, sexual activity and contraception must be discussed; birth defects are associated with mycophenolate and methotrexate. Additionally, pregnancy is a potential trigger for disease flare. Honest discussion about healthy, responsible reproductive choices with

*Arthritis Australia: https://arthritisaustralia.com.au/types-of-arthritis/lupus-systemic-lupus-erythematosus/; Arthritis New Zealand: https://www.arthritis.org.nz/forms-of-arthritis/lupus/

both the teenager and the parents is important for establishing communication. The parents and teenager should know that the teenager can come to the nurse with reproductive concerns. Because oestrogen can trigger disease flare, low-dose oestrogen or progestin-only oral contraceptives are preferred. Some teenagers choose the compliance-friendly Depo-Provera (medroxyprogesterone) 3-month injections. Again, frank discussion about risks and benefits is essential.

Prevention of infection includes hand washing (especially at school) and preprocedure antibiotic coverage for routine events such as dental cleaning. Immunisation vaccinations should be maintained in SLE, except live vaccines should be withheld in patients on immunosuppressive therapy.

Teaching patients how to find ways to adapt positively to SLE with normal growth and development as the goal will give them self-advocacy skills. Nurses should apply the principles of adjusting to a chronic illness that are discussed in Chapter 19.

REFERENCES

Agency for Clinical Innovation (ACI). (2018a). Acute Compartment Syndrome. Musculoskeletal Network: Factsheet. November. https://www.aci.health.nsw.gov.au/__data/assets/pdf_file/0007/458188/ACI_0133-MSK-compartment-syndrome-consumer-fsheet.PDF

Agency for Clinical Innovation (ACI). (2018b). Musculoskeletal Network. Neurovascular Assessment guide. November. https://www.aci.health.nsw.gov.au/__data/assets/pdf_file/0004/458185/ACI_0147-MSK-compartment-guide_V4.pdf

Ansar A., Rahman A.E., Romero, L., et al. (2018). Systematic review and meta-analysis of global birth prevalence of clubfoot: a study protocol. BMJ Open, 8, e019246. https://doi.org/10.1136/bmjopen-2017-019246

Arshad, F. & Bishop, N. (2021). Osteogenesis imperfecta in children. Bone, 12 March, 115914.

Arthritis Australia. (2017). Juvenile idiopathic arthritis (children). https://arthritisaustralia.com.au/types-of-arthritis/jia/

Australian Institute of Health and Welfare (AIHW). (2019). Juvenile Arthritis. What is Juvenile Arthritis? https://www.aihw.gov.au/reports/chronic-musculoskeletal-conditions/juvenile-arthritis/contents/what-is-juvenile-arthritis-1

Australian Institute of Health and Welfare (AIHW): Kreisfeld R, Harrison JE, & Tovell A. (2017). Hospital care for Australian sports injury, 2012–13. Injury research and statistics series no. 105. Cat. no. INJCAT 181. Canberra: AIHW. https://www.aihw.gov.au/getmedia/080b164c-eaa2-4f7c-b438-015797a9474e/aihw-injcat-181.pdf.aspx?inline=true

Australian Resuscitation Council (ARC). (2016). Guidelines & New Zealand Resuscitation Council. First Aid Guidelines – Trauma. ANZCOR Guideline 9.1.6 – Management of Suspected Spinal Injury. January, p. 4.

Australian Resuscitation Council (ARC). (2017). Guidelines & New Zealand Resuscitation Council. First Aid Guidelines – Trauma. ANZCOR Guideline 9.1.1 – Frist Aid for Management of Bleeding. July, p. 1.

Australian Society of Clinical Immunology and Allergy (ASCIA). (2019). Systemic Lupus Erythematosus (SLE). https://www.allergy.org.au/images/pcc/ASCIA_PCC_Systemic_Lupus_Erythematosus_2019.pdf

Beukelman, T., Patkar, N. M., Saag, K. G., et al. (2011). 2011 American College of Rheumatology recommendations for the treatment of juvenile idiopathic arthritis: Initiation and safety monitoring of therapeutic agents for the treatment of arthritis and systemic features. Arthritis Care & Research, 63(4), 465–482.

Brown, K. A., Dewoolkar, A. V., Baker, N., et al. (2017). The female athlete triad: special considerations for adolescent female athletes. Translational Pediatrics, 6(3), 144–149. https://doi.org/10.21037/tp.2017.04.04

Burke, L. M., & Peeling, P. (2018). Methodologies for Investigating Performance Changes with Supplement Use. International Journal of Sport Nutrition and Exercise Metabolism, 28, 159–169. https://doi.org/10.1123/ijsnem.2017-0325

Cahill, P. J., Auriemma, M., Dakwar, E., et al. (2017). Factors predictive of outcomes in vertebral body stapling for idiopathic scoliosis. Science Direct: Spine Deformity, 6(1), 28–37. https://doi.org/10.1016/j.jspd.2017.03.004

Centers for Disease Control and Prevention. (2015). Web-based injury statistics query and reporting system (WISQARS). Centers for Disease Control and Prevention National Center for Injury Prevention and Control. http://www.cdc.gov/injury/wisqars/index.html

Chang, J., & Girgis, L. (2017). Clinical use of anti-TNF-α biological agents: A guide for GPs. Australian Family Physician, 36(12), 1035–1038. https://www.racgp.org.au/afpbackissues/2007/200712/200712Chang.pdf

Claytor, C. M., & Bazner-Chandler, J. (2017). Musculoskeletal Disorders. In Burns, C.E., Dunn, A.M., Brady, et al. (2017). Pediatric Primary Care (6th ed.). St Louis, Missouri: Elsevier.

Dezbrow, B., Burke, L. M., Fallon, K., et al. (2014). Sports Dietitians Australia Position Statement: Sports Nutrition for the Adolescent Athlete. International Journal of Sport Nutrition and Exercise Metabolism, 24, 570–584. http://dx.doi.org/10.1123/ijsnem.2014-0031

Fair, D. C., Rodriguez, M., Knight, A. M., et al. (2019). Depression and anxiety in patients with juvenile idiopathic arthritis: Current insights and impact on quality of life, a systematic review. Dove Press Journal: Open Access Rheumatology: Research and Reviews, 11, 237–252. https://doi.org/10.2147/OARRR.S174408

Gilek-Seibert, K. (2020). Systemic Lupus Erythematosus. In Ferri, F.F. Ferri's Clinical Advisor 2020. Philadelphia: Elsevier.

Gregory, E. (2020). Scoliosis. In Ferri, F.F. Ferri's clinical advisor 2020. Elsevier: Philadelphia.

Handoll, H. H., Elliott, J., Iheozor-Ejiofor, Z., et al. (2018). Interventions for treating wrist fractures in children. Cochrane Database System Review, (12), CD012470. https://doi.org/10.1002/14651858.CD012470.pub2

Hresko, M. T. (2013). Idiopathic scoliosis in adolescents. New England Journal of Medicine, 368(9), 834–841.

Jagim, A. R., Stecker, R. A., Harty, P. S. et al. (2018). Safety of Creatine Supplementation in Active Adolescents and Youth: A Brief Review. Frontiers in Nutrition, 115(5). https://doi.org/10.3389/fnut.2018.00115

John, R. M. & Brady, M. A,. (2017). Atopic, Rheumatic, and Immunodeficiency Disorders. In Burns, C.E., Dunn, A.M., Brady, M.A., et al. (2017). Pediatric Primary Care (6th ed.). Missouri: Elsevier.

Kay, R. M., & Kim, Y. J. (2014). Slipped capital femoral epiphysis. In S. L. Weinstein & J. M. Flynn (Eds.), Lovell and Winter's Pediatric Orthopaedics. Philadelphia, PA: Lippincott Williams & Wilkins.

Kerin, K. D. (2017). Infectious Arthritis. In Buttaro, T.M., Trybulski, J., Polgar-Bailey, P. & Sanberg-Cook, J. (2017). Primary Care: A collaborative practice (5th ed.). Missouri: Elsevier.

Kidsafe WA. (2018). Childhood Injury Bulletin Research Report: Sporting Injuries. https://www.kidsafewa.com.au/professionals/wa-childhood-injury-bulletins-reports/

Kivity, S., Agmon-Levin, N., Zandman-Goddard, G., et al. (2015). Neuropsychiatric lupus: a mosaic of clinical presentations. Bio Med Central Medicine, 13(43), 1–11. https://doi.org/10.1186/s12916-015-0269-8

Kleinman, R. E., & Greer, F. R. (2014). Pediatric nutrition. Elk Grove Village, IL: American Academy of Pediatrics.

Land, C., Rauch, F., Travers, R., et al. (2007). Osteogenesis imperfecta type VI in childhood and adolescence: Effects of cyclical intravenous pamidronate treatment. Bone, 40(3), 638–644.

Laron, D., & Pandya, N. K. (2013). Advances in the orthopedic management of osteogenesis imperfect. Orthopaedic Clinics of North America, 44(4), 565–573.

Lewis, S. L. Hagler, D., Bucher, L., et al. (2017). Osteomyelitis. In Lewis, S.L., Bucher, L., Heitkemper, M.M. & Harding, M.M. (Eds.) Clinical Companion to Medical-Surgical Nursing, (10th ed). Elsevier.

Kallash, M., Smoyer, W. E., & Mahan, J. D. (2019). Rituximab Use in the Management of Childhood Nephrotic Syndrome. Frontiers in Pediatrics, 7(178), 1–10. https://doi.org/10.3389/fped.2019.00178

Madonia, L. (2012). Osteogenesis imperfecta and bone narrow transplant. Journal of Pediatric Oncology Nursing, 29(1), 37–44.
Marini, J. C. (2016). Osteogenesis imperfecta. In R. M. Kliegman, B. F. Stanton, J. W. St Geme, et al. (Eds.), Nelson textbook of pediatrics (20th ed.). Philadelphia, PA: Saunders.
Marini, J. C., & Blissett, A. R. (2013). New genes in bone development: What's new in osteogenesis imperfecta. Journal of Clinical Endocrinology and Metabolism, 98(8), 3095–3103.
Mencio, G. A., Swiontkowski, M. F., & Green, N. E. (2015). Green's skeletal trauma in children. Philadelphia, PA: Elsevier/Saunders.
Mok, C. C. (2016). Con: Cyclophosphamide for the treatment of lupus nephritis. Nephrology Dialysis Transplantation, 31(7), 1053–1057. https://doi.org/10.1093/ndt/gfw068
Montgomery, N. I., & Epps, H. R. (2017). Pediatric septic arthritis. Orthopaedic Clinics of North America, 48(2), 209–216.
Mosca, V. S. (2014). The foot. In S. L. Weinstein & J. M. Flynn (Eds.), Lovell and Winter's Pediatric Orthopaedics. Philadelphia, PA: Lippincott Williams & Wilkins.
Newton, P. O., Wenger, D. R., & Yaszay, B. (2014). Idiopathic scoliosis. In S. L. Weinstein & J. M. Flynn (Eds.), Lovell and Winter's Pediatric Orthopaedics. Philadelphia, PA: Lippincott Williams & Wilkins.
Petty, R. E., Southwood, T. R., Manners, P., et al. (2004). International League of Associations for Rheumatology classification of juvenile idiopathic arthritis: Second revision, Edmonton, 2001. The Journal of Rheumatology, 31(2), 390–392.
Ponseti, I. V. (1996). Congenital clubfoot: Fundamentals of treatment. Oxford: Oxford University Press.
Providência, R., Teixeira, C., Oliver Segal, O., et al. (2017). Is it time to loosen the restrictions on athletes with cardiac disorders competing in sport? British Journal of Sports Medicine, 51(14). http://dx.doi.org/10.1136/bjsports-2016-097002
Rauch, F., Munns, C. F., Land, C., et al. (2009). Risedronate in the treatment of mild pediatric osteogenesis imperfecta: A randomized placebo-controlled study. Journal of Bone and Mineral Research: The Official Journal of the American Society for Bone and Mineral Research, 24(7), 1282–1289.
Scoliosis Australia. (2021). Adolescent idiopathic scoliosis. https://www.scoliosis-australia.org/about-scoliosis/adolescent-idiopathic-scoliosis/
Semler, O., Netzer, C., Hoyer-Kuhn, H., et al. (2012). First use of the RANKL antibody denosumab in osteogenesis imperfect type VI. Journal of Musculoskeletal and Neuronal Interactions, 12(3), 183–188.
Sheikh, S. Z., Kaufman, K., Gordon, B.-B., et al. (2019). Evaluation of the self-directed format of walk with ease in patients with systemic lupus erythematosus: the Walk-SLE Pilot Study. Lupus, 28(6), 764–770. https://doi.org/10.1177/0961203319846387
Sillence, D. O., Senn, A., & Danks, D. M. (1979). Genetic heterogeneity in osteogenesis imperfecta. Journal of Medical Genetics, 16(2), 101–116.
Sports Dietitians Australia. (2019). Nutrition for the adolescent athlete. Fact sheet. https://www.sportsdietitians.com.au/wp-content/uploads/2019/08/Adolescent-Nutrition.pdf
Sports Medicine Australia. (2017). Safety guidelines for children and young people in sport and recreation. https://sma.org.au/sma-site-content/uploads/2017/08/childrensafetyguidelines-fulldoc.pdf
Stanger, M., Coulter, C., & Giavedoni, B. (2017). Limb deficiencies and amputations. In Palisano, R.J., Orlin, M.N. & Schreiber, J. (2017). Campbell's Physical Therapy for Children (5th ed). Missouri: Elsevier.
Stans, A. A. (2014). Musculoskeletal infection. In S. L. Weinstein & J. M. Flynn (Eds.), Lovell and Winter's Pediatric Orthopaedics. Philadelphia, PA: Lippincott Williams & Wilkins.
Stephens, S., & Oates, K. (2014). The placement of children following non-accidental head injuries: Are they protected from further harm? Child Abuse Review, 24, 67–76. https://doi.org/10.1002/car.2335
Swann, M. C., Hoes, K. S., Aoun, S. G., et al. (2016). Postoperative complications of spine surgery. Best Practice & Research Clinical Anaesthesiology, 30(1), 103–120. https://doi.org/10.1016/j.bpa.2016.01.002
Sweeting, J., & Semsarian, C. (2018). Sudden cardiac death in athletes. Heart, Lung and Circulation, 27(9), 1072–1077. https://doi.org/10.1016/j.hlc.2018.03.026
Szabó, M. Z., Szodoray, P., & Kiss, E. (2017). Dyslipidemia in systemic lupus erythematosus. Immunologic Research, 65(2), 543–550. https://doi.org/10.1007/s12026-016-8892-9
Tande, A. J., Steckelberg, J. M., Osmon, D. R., et al. (2020). Osteomyelitis. In Bennett, J.E., Dolin, R. & Blaser, M.J. (2020) Mandell, Douglas & Bennett's Principles and Practice of Infectious Diseases, 9th (ed). Philadelphia: Elsevier.
Tauer, J., Robinson, M., & Rauch, F. (2019). Osteogenesis imperfecta: new perspectives from clinical and translational research: new developments in osteogenesis imperfecta. JBMR Plus, 3(8), e10174. https://asbmr.onlinelibrary.wiley.com/doi/pdfdirect/10.1002/jbm4.10174
The Royal Children's Hospital Melbourne (RCHM). (n.d.). Osteomyelitis and septic arthritis. https://www.rch.org.au/clinicalguide/guideline_index/Osteomyelitis_and_septic_arthritis/
The Sydney Children's Hospital Network. (2014). Guideline: Orthopaedic traction: care and management. Orthopaedic traction: care and management. Practice Guideline. Guideline No: 2014-9099 v5.p.5. https://www.schn.health.nsw.gov.au/_policies/pdf/2014-9099.pdf
The Sydney Children's Hospital Network. (2019). Fracture management. Practice Guideline. Guideline No: 2014-9097 v4. p.4–14. https://www.schn.health.nsw.gov.au/_policies/pdf/2014-9097.pdf
Trejo, P., & Rauch, F. (2016). Osteogenesis imperfecta in children and adolescents—new developments in diagnosis and treatment. Osteoporosis International, 27(12), 3427–3437.
Weinstein, S. L. (2014a). Developmental hip dysplasia and dislocation. In S. L. Weinstein & J. M. Flynn (Eds.), Lovell and Winter's Pediatric Orthopaedics. Philadelphia, PA: Lippincott Williams & Wilkins.
Weinstein, S. L. (2014b). Legg-Calvé-Perthes syndrome. In S. L. Weinstein & J. M. Flynn (Eds.), Lovell and Winter's Pediatric Orthopaedics. Philadelphia, PA: Lippincott Williams & Wilkins.
Williams, N. (2018). Improving early detection of developmental dysplasia of the hip through general practitioner assessment and surveillance. Australian Journal of General Practice, 47(9), 615–619. https://doi.org/10.31128/AJGP-03-18-4524
Willock, J., Habiballah, L., Long, D., et al. (2016). A comparison of the performance of the Braden Q and the Glamorgan paediatric pressure ulcer risk assessment scales in general and intensive care paediatric and neonatal units. Journal of Tissue Viability, 25(2), 119–126. https://doi.org/10.1016/j.jtv.2016.03.001
Wilson, D. (2014). Musculoskeletal or Articular Dysfunction. In Perry, S.E., Hockenberry, M.J., Lowdermilk, D.L. & Wilson, D. Maternal child nursing care (6th ed). Canada: Elsevier.
Wills, J. M. (2017). Orthopedic Conditions. In Palisano, R.J., Orlin, M.N. & Schreiber, J. Campbell's Physical Therapy for Children, (5th ed.). Canada: Elsevier.
Yagci, G., Karatel, M., & Yakut, Y. (2020). Body awareness and its relation to quality of life in individuals with idiopathic scoliosis. Perceptual and Motor Skills, 127(5), 841–857.
Yip, B., Li, X., Leung, C., et al. (2018). Trial Protocol: The use of mindfulness-based intervention for improving bracing compliance for adolescent idiopathic scoliosis patients: protocol for a randomised, controlled trial. Journal of Physiotherapy, 64(3), 193. https://www.sciencedirect.com/science/article/pii/S1836955318300420?via%3Dihub

34

The Child with Neuromuscular or Muscular Dysfunction

Andrea Middleton

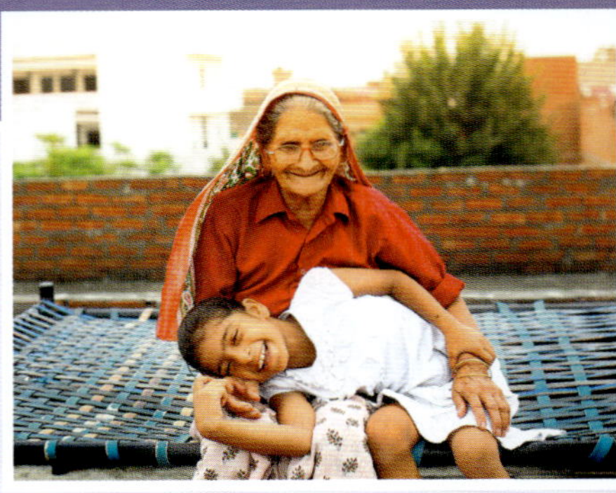

LEARNING OUTCOMES

- Develop an understanding of neuromuscular or muscular dysfunction.
- Develop an understanding of common problems children experience with neuromuscular or muscular dysfunction.
- Understand the complexities in assessment of children with neuromuscular or muscular dysfunction.
- Understand the importance of family-centred care and safety of children with neuromuscular or muscular dysfunction.

NEUROMUSCULAR DYSFUNCTION

Weakness or abnormal skeletal muscle function may represent a defect in the muscle itself or reflect a pathological disorder at some point along the neural pathway from the cortex of the brain to the neuromuscular junction. Identifying the source of muscular dysfunction includes not only the testing of muscle function but also the systematic elimination of possible disorders of neural structures on which muscle function depends for its stimulus. In a few disorders muscle disease may be accompanied by a neurological disorder.

Some clinical features are shared by muscle disease (myopathy), which differs in many ways from muscular dysfunction resulting from disorders of neuronal structures—brain, cranial nerve nuclei, long nerve tracts, anterior horn cells of the spinal cord and peripheral nerves. Motor function is accomplished by means of the simple reflex arcs or by way of impulses transmitted from the cerebral cortex and other centres in the brain through the various nerve pathways of the central nervous system (CNS). The upper motor neurons consist of cells that lie in the cerebral cortex and fibres that traverse the brainstem and spinal cord to terminate at their synapses with the anterior horn cells. The lower motor neurons consist of the anterior horn cells, axons and peripheral nerve branches. The motor unit consists of the lower motor neuron, the neuromuscular (or myoneural) junction and the muscle fibres it supplies (Fig 34.1). The upper motor neuronal pathways from the cerebrum to the lower motor neuron are described as: (1) pyramidal—those whose fibres extend from the cortex, come together in the medulla, cross from one side to the other, then extend down the cord to synapse with anterior horn motor neurons; and (2) extrapyramidal—a complex network of motor neurons that comprise relays between motor areas of the cortex, basal ganglia, thalamus, cerebellum and brainstem.

Classification and Diagnosis

The site of pathological disturbance determines the type of muscular dysfunction. In general, upper motor neuron lesions produce weakness associated with spasticity, increased deep tendon reflexes and abnormal superficial reflexes. The primary disorder of upper motor neuron dysfunction is cerebral palsy (CP). Lower motor neuron lesions interrupt the reflex arc, causing weakness and atrophy of the skeletal muscles involved with associated hypotonia or flaccidity, which eventually progress to atrophy with varying degrees of contracture deformity. A disorder of the extrapyramidal pathway and the cerebellum rarely produces muscle weakness.

Lower motor neuron involvement is usually symmetrical (except that of poliomyelitis and single peripheral nerve disease), whereas disorders of the pyramidal tract are more often asymmetrical. Muscle wasting is characteristic of lower motor neuron lesions and more marked than in diseases of muscles. Deep tendon reflexes are briskly active in upper motor neuron disease, are diminished or absent in lower motor neuron disease and depend on the progress of muscle degeneration in the myopathies.

These disorders can also be categorised according to onset: those in which there is acute onset of flaccid paralysis and those with more gradual onset and progressive degeneration. In most instances the sudden appearance of flaccid paralysis in a previously healthy child is due to an infectious process. Neurotoxins (e.g. botulism, tick paralysis or heavy metal poisoning), pressure on the spinal cord from tumours or abscesses and spinal cord injury (SCI) are less likely causes. Hereditary factors and metabolic disease are more often responsible for muscular weakness and atrophy of gradual onset.

Classification

The most useful classification of neuromuscular disorders is one that defines the site of origin of the pathological lesion: the anterior horn cells of the spinal cord, the peripheral nerves, the neuromuscular junction and the muscles.

Diseases of Anterior Horn Cells. Diseases and disorders that affect the anterior horn cells are the result of destruction or atrophy of the anterior horn of the spinal column along with the inability to transfer impulses from sensory neurons to motor neurons. Enteroviruses, which have a worldwide distribution, are prominent aetiological agents that selectively affect anterior horn cells. Inherited disorders, primarily the spinal muscular atrophies, cause degeneration of the anterior horn cells.

Neuropathies. Disorders affecting peripheral nerves may be mononeuropathies, which involve a single nerve and the muscles it innervates, or polyneuropathies, which involve multiple nerves and the muscles they supply. Neuropathies are caused by a number of hereditary diseases, traumatic injuries, infections, poisons and (secondarily)

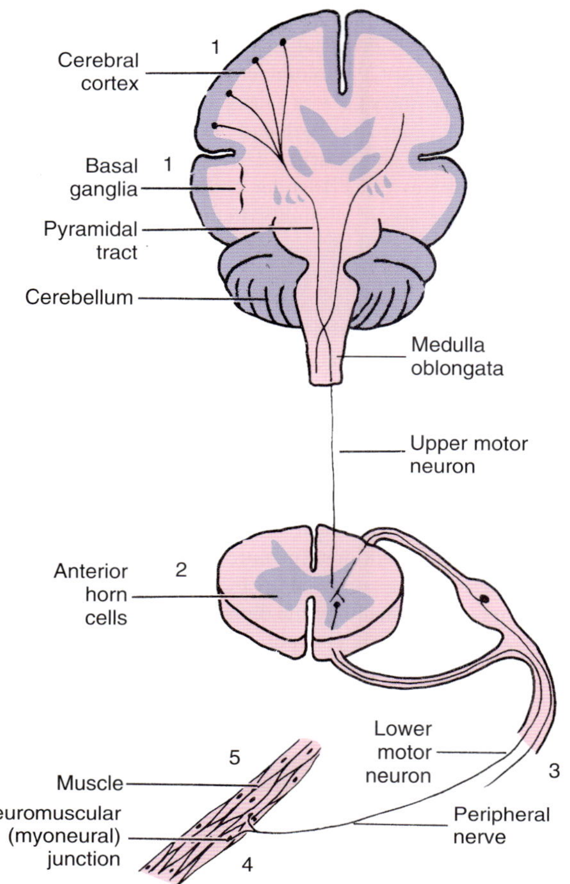

Fig 34.1 Site of origin for neuromuscular disorders. 1, Cerebral palsy; 2, poliomyelitis, spinal muscular atrophy; 3, mononeuropathies, polyneuropathies; 4, neurotoxic disorders; 5, muscular dystrophies.

some metabolic diseases. Polyneuropathy can be restricted to specific areas (as in diabetes mellitus). Some hereditary diseases involve skeletal muscles extensively. The distal limbs (feet and hands) are usually affected first, with gait disturbance and footdrop being early manifestations. The involvement gradually progresses proximally as the disorder becomes more severe.

In some polyneuropathies there is segmented or patchy loss of the myelin sheath of nerve fibres; in others the primary process appears to be progressive degeneration of nerve fibres. Examples of acute and chronic polyneuropathies are Guillain-Barré syndrome (infectious polyneuritis) and Charcot-Marie Tooth disease (peroneal muscular atrophy), respectively.

Neuromuscular Junction Disease. Disorders involving a neurohumoral deficiency interfere with transmission of nerve impulses to muscles at the neuromuscular junction. Normally nerve impulses are transmitted to skeletal muscles across the neuromuscular junction by acetylcholine. This is accomplished in three steps: (1) acetylcholine is released from vesicles in the terminal nerve endings; (2) it then diffuses across the junction and contacts receptor sites in the muscle membrane, stimulating the muscle to contract; and (3) it is removed by the action of cholinesterase. Interference at any of these three steps will block transmission of nerve impulses and prevent muscular contraction.

Several toxic substances act at the neuromuscular junction to inhibit nerve impulses to the skeletal muscles. Examples of toxins that prevent the release of acetylcholine are those that produce the paralysis of botulism and tick paralysis. Action at receptor sites is also blocked by the drug curare. Paralysis resulting from inhibition of cholinesterase release is caused by poisoning with organic phosphate insecticides.

Diseases of Muscles. Diseases of skeletal muscles can be inflammatory (such as polymyositis), the result of endocrine dysfunction (such as hypothyroidism and hyperthyroidism) or the result of congenital defects (e.g. absence of muscle, periodic paralysis and the various muscular dystrophies [MDs] and myotonias). Inflammation occurs in a number of infectious illnesses such as trichinosis, toxoplasmosis and those caused by the enteroviruses (coxsackieviruses and echoviruses).

Diagnostic Tools

Several general diagnostic tools aid in differentiating diseases with similar manifestations. In addition, a number of more definitive tests are used to establish a specific diagnosis. The neurological examination is a basic test that helps assess the extent of motor and sensory function.

The electromyogram (EMG) measures the electrical potentials generated in individual muscles. A small metal disc is placed on the skin overlying the muscle to be tested, or a sterile needle electrode is inserted directly into the muscle. The electrical activity generated in the skeletal muscles is measured at rest, with slight voluntary contraction and with maximum contraction. The electrical activity is amplified and displayed on a cathode ray oscilloscope. Needle electrodes are sensitive enough to pick up the activity of a single muscle fibre; thus this is usually the method of choice. However, the procedure is traumatic for children. It is often not useful because it requires cooperation. A topical anaesthetic should be considered to decrease pain. Nerve conduction velocity, or the velocity of electrical impulse conduction along motor or sensory nerves, is often measured in conjunction with the EMG. Certain diseases affect the peripheral nerves, prolonging the conduction time from the point of stimulation of the nerve to the muscle and increasing the duration of the evoked potential of the muscle.

Muscle biopsy may be used to confirm and classify muscle disorders. The vastus lateralis is the most commonly sampled muscle. Procedural sedation may be required. Serum enzyme measurements are helpful in diagnosing and monitoring the course of muscular disease, but these are used as adjuncts in the diagnosis of most neuromuscular diseases. The intracellular enzyme creatine (phosphokinase) kinase (CK) is present in muscle tissues, including cardiac muscle, and the brain. It is released in large amounts in some muscular diseases, such as MD. CK is not elevated in neurogenic disease. Genetic testing is becoming increasingly valuable in the diagnosis of many neuromuscular conditions and may make muscle biopsies less necessary. Because of the increasing complexities of choosing appropriate genetic tests, genetic counselling may be appropriate.

Cerebral Palsy

Cerebral palsy (CP) has been defined as a disorder of posture and movement from static brain injury perinatally or postnatally, which limits activity (Ferris 2015, Newman 2017, Patterson et al 2017). In addition to motor disorders, the condition often involves disturbances of sensation, perception, communication, cognition and behaviour; secondary musculoskeletal problems; and epilepsy (Newman 2017). The aetiology, clinical features and course vary and are characterised by abnormal muscle tone and coordination as the primary disturbances. CP is the most common permanent physical disability of childhood, and the incidence is reported to range from 1.5 to over 4 per 1000 live births internationally (Starship 2019). The 2018

Australian Cerebral Palsy Register summary report identified a decline in the prevalence of CP, which may be reflected in the improved survival of extremely low birth weight (ELBW) and very low birth weight (VLBW) infants (AusACPDM 2018). The New Zealand CP register was established in 2015 and is yet to publish data.

Aetiology

A variety of prenatal, perinatal and postnatal factors contribute to the development of CP, singly or multifactorially (Box 34.1). The human brain undergoes development during the prenatal period and up to 2 years of age. A brain insult or injury occurring during this period may result in CP.

Although the prevalent traditional hypothesis has been that CP results from perinatal problems, especially birth asphyxia, it is now believed that CP results more often from existing prenatal brain abnormalities. However, the exact cause of these abnormalities remains elusive. It has been estimated that as many as 70% to 80% of the cases of CP are caused by unknown prenatal factors (Krigger 2006, MacLennan et al 2015).

In general, infants exposed to maternal and perinatal infections are at increased risk for the development of CP as a result of the effects on the developing brain. Although CP occurs in term births, preterm birth of ELBW and VLBW infants continues to be the single most important risk factor for CP. Still, in some cases no identifiable cause is determined. Periventricular leucomalacia and intracerebral haemorrhage in low birth weight infants are significant risk factors in the development of CP. Perinatal ischaemic stroke is also associated with a later diagnosis of CP (Golomb et al 2007).

In some children their CP was caused by a brain injury that happened more than 28 days after birth and before 2 years of age (e.g. due to stroke, infection or an accident). There were proportionally more Aboriginal and Torres Strait Islander children in this group. These children had more severe disability than other children with CP (AusACPDM 2018).

Pathophysiology

It is difficult to establish a precise location of neurological lesions on the basis of aetiology or clinical signs because there is no characteristic pathological picture. In some cases, there are gross malformations of the brain. In others, there may be evidence of vascular occlusion, atrophy, loss of neurons and laminar degeneration that produce narrower gyri, wider sulci and low brain weight. Anoxia appears to play the most significant role in the pathological state of brain damage, which is often secondary to other causative mechanisms.

There are a few exceptions. In some cases, the manifestations or aetiology is related to anatomical areas. For example, CP associated with preterm birth is usually spastic diplegia caused by hypoxic infarction or haemorrhage with periventricular leucomalacia in the area adjacent to the lateral ventricles. The athetoid (extrapyramidal) type of CP is most likely to be associated with birth asphyxia but can also be

BOX 34.1 Aetiological Risk Factors for Cerebral Palsy

Prenatal

Maternal

1. Diabetes mellitus or hyperthyroidism
2. Exposure to radiation or toxins
3. Malnutrition
4. Seizure disorder or cognitive impairment
5. Infections
6. Incompetent cervix
7. Bleeding
8. Polyhydramnios
9. Genetic abnormalities
10. Previous child with development disabilities
11. Previous premature birth
12. Previous fetal loss
13. Medication use (e.g. thyroid, oestrogen, progesterone)
14. Inflammatory response
15. Severe proteinuria

Gestational

1. Chromosome abnormalities
2. Genetic syndromes
3. Teratogens
4. Rh incompatibility
5. Infections
6. Congenital malformations
7. Fetal development abnormalities
8. Problems in placental functioning
9. Inflammatory response

Labour and Delivery

1. Premature delivery
2. Prolonged rupture of membranes
3. Prolonged fetal heart rate depression
4. Abnormal presentation
5. Long labour
6. Pre-eclampsia
7. Asphyxia

Perinatal

1. Prematurity and associated problems
2. Sepsis and/or central nervous system infection
3. Seizures
4. Intraventricular haemorrhage
5. Periventricular leucomalacia
6. Meconium aspiration
7. Number of days on mechanical ventilation
8. Persistent pulmonary hypertension
9. Intrauterine growth restriction
10. Low birth weight
11. Perinatal stroke
12. Unknown

Childhood or Postnatal

1. Brain injury
2. Meningitis or encephalitis
3. Toxins
4. Traumatic brain injury
5. Infections
6. Stroke

Unknown

1. Unknown prenatal factors that contribute to the development of CP; possibly as many as 70% to 80% of CP (Krigger 2006)

CP, cerebral palsy.
Source: From Jackson, P. L., Vessey, J. A., & Schapiro, N. A. (Eds.). (2010). Primary care of the child with a chronic illness (5th ed.). St Louis, MO: Mosby.

caused by kernicterus and metabolic genetic disorders such as mitochondrial disorders and glutaric aciduria (Johnston 2016, Keys & Chaves-Carballo 2013). Hemiplegic (hemiparetic) CP is often associated with a focal cerebral infarction (stroke) secondary to an intrauterine or perinatal thromboembolism, usually a result of maternal thrombosis or hereditary clotting disorder (Johnston 2016). Cerebellar hypoplasia and sometimes severe neonatal hypoglycaemia are related to ataxic CP. Generalised cortical and cerebral atrophy often cause severe quadriparesis with cognitive impairment and microcephaly.

Clinical Classification

The Gross Motor Functional Classification System (GMFCS) (Sehrawat et al 2014), Functional Mobility Scale (FMS) (Sehrawat et al 2014, Eliasson 2006), Manual Ability Classification Scale (MACS) and Communication Functional Classification Scale (CFCS) (Hidecker 2011) have been used by several authors to guide care of children with CP.

CP has four primary types of movement disorders: spastic, dyskinetic, ataxic and mixed (Box 34.2) (Nehring 2010). The most common clinical type, spastic CP (Cerebral Palsy Alliance 2018), represents an upper motor neuron muscular weakness. The reflex arc is intact, and the characteristic physical signs are increased stretch reflexes, increased muscle tone and (often) weakness. Early neurological manifestations are usually generalised hypotonia or decreased tone that lasts for a few weeks or may extend for months or even as long as a year.

Clinical Manifestations

The alert observer may suspect CP when a child demonstrates some of the groups of manifestations in Box 34.3.

Delayed Gross Motor Development. Delayed gross motor development is a universal manifestation of CP. The child shows a delay in all motor accomplishments, and the discrepancy between motor ability and expected achievement tends to increase with successive developmental milestones as growth advances. It is especially significant if other developmental behaviours, such as language and personal-social achievement, are normal. Delayed development of the ability to balance may also slow the progression of milestones.

Abnormal Motor Performance. Neuromotor dysfunction is particularly evident in motor performance. An early sign is preferential unilateral hand use that may be apparent at approximately 6 months of age. Hand dominance does not normally develop until the preschool years. Abnormal crawling with propulsion by hand movements only and with lower extremities and hips hiked along, much like a 'bunny hop', occurs in diplegia. Children with hemiplegia have an asymmetrical crawl, using the unaffected arm and leg to propel themselves on either the buttocks or the abdomen. Spasticity may cause the child to stand or walk on the toes. Uncoordinated or involuntary movements are characteristic of dyskinetic CP, and facial grimacing and writhing movements of the tongue, fingers and toes are signs of athetosis. Other significant signs of motor dysfunction are poor sucking and feeding difficulties, with persistent tongue thrust. Head staggering, tremor on reaching and truncal ataxia are also common. Hand preference in the first 2 years of life is reported to be a sign of hemiplegic CP (Berker & Yalçin 2008).

Alterations of Muscle Tone. Increased or decreased resistance to passive movements is a sign of abnormal muscle tone. The child may exhibit opisthotonic postures (exaggerated arching of the back) and may feel stiff on handling or dressing. Also, there is difficulty in changing nappies because of spasticity of the hip adductor muscles and lower extremities. When pulled to a sitting position, the child may extend the entire body and be rigid and unbending at the hip and knee joints. This is an early sign of spasticity.

BOX 34.2 Clinical Classification of Cerebral Palsy

Spastic (Pyramidal)

- Characterised by persistent primitive reflexes, positive Babinski's reflex, ankle clonus, exaggerated stretch reflexes, eventual development of contractures
- Seventy per cent to 80% of all cases of CP
- **Diplegia**—All extremities affected; lower more than upper (30% to 40% of spastic CP)
- **Tetraplegia**—All four extremities involved: legs and trunk, mouth, pharynx and tongue (10% to 15% of spastic CP)
- **Triplegia**—Three limbs involved
- **Monoplegia**—Only one limb involved
- **Hemiplegia**—Motor dysfunction on one side of the body; upper extremity more affected than lower (20% to 30% of spastic CP)
- Hypertonicity with poor control of posture, balance and coordinated motion
- Impairment of fine and gross motor skills

Dyskinetic (Non-spastic, Extrapyramidal)

- **Athetoid**—Chorea (involuntary, irregular, jerking movements); characterised by slow, wormlike, writhing movements that usually involve the extremities, trunk, neck, facial muscles and tongue
- **Dystonic**—Slow, twisting movements of the trunk or extremities; abnormal posture
- Involvement of the pharyngeal, laryngeal and oral muscles causing drooling and dysarthria (imperfect speech articulation)

Ataxic (Non-spastic, Extrapyramidal)

- Wide-based gait
- Rapid, repetitive movements performed poorly
- Disintegration of movements of the upper extremities when the child reaches for objects

Mixed Type

- Combination of spastic CP and dyskinetic CP
- May be labelled *mixed* when no specific motor pattern is dominant; however, this term is losing favour to more precise descriptions of motor function and affected area of brain involved

Source: Data from Nehring, W. (2010). Cerebral palsy. In P. J. Allen, J. A. Vessey, & N. A. Schapiro (Eds.), Primary care of the child with a chronic condition (5th ed.). St Louis, MO: Mosby; Jones, M. W., Morgan, E., Shelton, J. E., et al. (2007). Cerebral palsy: Introduction and diagnosis, part 1. Journal of Pediatric Health Care, 21(3), 146–152.

Abnormal Posture. Children with spastic CP assume abnormal postures at rest or when their position is changed. From an early age, a child lying in a prone position will maintain the hips higher than the trunk with the legs and arms flexed or drawn under the body. In the supine position spasticity is evident by scissoring (legs in crossed position; knees, hips and ankles stiff) and extension of the legs, with the feet plantar flexed. This posture is exaggerated when the child is suspended vertically or when others try to make the child bear weight. Depending on the degree of impairment, spasticity may be mild or severe. A persistent infantile resting and sleeping posture (i.e. arms abducted at shoulders, elbows flexed and hands fisted) is a sign of spasticity when it remains constant after 4 to 5 months of age. The hemiparetic child may rest with the affected arm adducted and held against the torso, with the elbow pronated and slightly flexed and the hand closed.

Reflex Abnormalities. Persistence of primitive reflexes is one of the earliest clues to CP (e.g. obligatory tonic neck reflex at any age or nonobligatory persistence beyond 6 months of age, and the persistence or

BOX 34.3 Clinical Manifestations of Cerebral Palsy (at Time of Diagnosis)

Delayed Gross Motor Development
- A universal manifestation
- Delay in all motor accomplishments
- Increases as growth advances
- Delays more obvious as growth advances

Abnormal Motor Performance
- Very early preferential unilateral hand preference
- Abnormal and asymmetrical crawl
- Standing or walking on toes
- Uncoordinated or involuntary movements
- Poor sucking
- Feeding difficulties
- Persistent tongue thrust

Alterations of Muscle Tone
- Increased or decreased resistance to passive movements
- Opisthotonic posturing (arching of back)
- Feels stiff on handling or dressing
- Difficulty in changing nappies
- Rigid and unbending at the hip and knee joints when pulled to sitting position (early sign)

Abnormal Postures
- Maintains hips higher than trunk in prone position with legs and arms flexed or drawn under the body
- Scissoring and extension of legs with feet plantar flexed in supine position
- Persistent infantile resting and sleeping position
- Arms abducted at shoulders
- Elbows flexed
- Hands fisted

Reflex Abnormalities
- Persistence of primitive infantile reflexes
- Obligatory tonic neck reflex at any age
- Non-persistence beyond 6 months of age
- Persistence or hyperactivity of the Moro, plantar and palmar grasp reflexes
- Hyperreflexia, ankle clonus and stretch reflexes elicited in many muscle groups on fast, passive movements

Associated Disabilities
- Altered learning and reasoning
- Seizures
- Impaired behavioural and interpersonal relationships
- Sensory impairment (vision, hearing)

Source: From Nehring, W. M. (2010). Cerebral palsy. In P. J. Allen, J. A. Vessey, & N. A. Schapiro (Eds.), Primary care of the child with a chronic condition (5th ed.). St Louis, MO: Mosby; Adapted from Jones, M. W., Morgan, E., & Shelton, J. E. (2007). Primary care of the child with cerebral palsy: A review of systems (part II). Journal of Pediatric Health Care, 21(4), 226–237.

even hyperactivity of the Moro, plantar and palmar grasp reflexes). Hyperreflexia, ankle clonus and stretch reflexes can be elicited from many muscle groups on fast passive movements (e.g. resistance to passive abduction when the hips are suddenly separated [adductor catch]).

Associated Disabilities and Problems. Some of the disabilities associated with CP are visual impairment, hearing impairment, behavioural problems, communication and speech difficulties, seizures and intellectual impairment. Additional sensory deficits such as hypersensitivity, hyposensitivity and balance difficulties may occur in children with CP (Nehring 2010).

Intellectual impairment is a concern, although children with CP have a wide range of intelligence, and 50% to 60% are within normal limits. Speech difficulties are often interpreted as a sign of cognitive impairment. Assessing the intelligence of a child with CP is often difficult because of the motor and sensory deficits. Tests carried out periodically over time should determine the degree of intelligence. Many persons with CP who have severely limiting physical involvement actually have the least intellectual impairment. As a group, children with athetosis and ataxia are intellectually superior to those with other types of CP. The incidence of severe or profound impairment is highest in rigid and atonic CP. Improved communication devices (e.g. communication jacket, computerised communication) have revealed that some people with quadriplegic spastic CP have normal intelligence.

The manifestations of attention-deficit/hyperactivity disorder may occur in children with CP. The primary presenting symptoms are poor attention span, marked distractibility, hyperactive behaviour and defects of integration. (See Chapter 16.) Seizures are more likely to accompany postnatally acquired hemiplegia. They are an unusual finding in ataxia and diplegia. The most common types of seizures are generalised tonic-clonic seizures and minor motor types (Nehring 2010).

Poor control of oral musculature may contribute to a number of problems. Abnormal posture and motor performance and alterations in muscle tone affect chewing, swallowing and talking. Occupational and speech-language therapy interventions may be necessary to assist some children with feeding and speech. Coughing and choking, especially while eating, may predispose the child with CP to aspiration, which may not be readily apparent. Respiratory problems may result from and coexist with feeding difficulties in children with CP; respiratory symptoms observed during feedings include apnoea, dyspnoea, tachypnoea, coughing and choking and hypoxaemia (Nehring 2010). Many children with CP may also have gastro-oesophageal reflux.

Motor impairment associated with CP contributes to other problems. Children with CP who are non-ambulatory have an increased risk of developing orthopaedic complications such as unilateral or bilateral hip dislocations, scoliosis and joint contractures resulting from unbalanced muscle tone.

A variety of factors, including decreased mobility, decreased fluid intake, a fear of toileting, poor positioning on the toilet and lack of fibre intake, may be responsible for constipation (Nehring 2010). Stool softeners, laxatives and a bowel management program may be required to prevent chronic constipation.

Increased incidence of dental caries results from improper dental hygiene, congenital enamel defects (hypoplasia of primary teeth), high carbohydrate intake and retention, dietary imbalance with poor nutritional intake, inadequate fluoride and difficulty in mouth closure and drooling. Spastic or clonic movements can cause gagging or biting down on the toothbrush, thus interfering with cleaning techniques. Oral hypersensitivity is also common, which causes the child to resist dental hygiene. Malocclusion can occur in as many as 90% of these children. Gingivitis is secondary to inadequate dental hygiene and may be further complicated by the use of antiepileptic drugs (AEDs) such as phenytoin (Nehring 2010).

Skin breakdown may occur with prolonged positioning, especially with underweight children with bony prominences and those who are unable to reposition themselves or who may have insensate areas of skin.

Nystagmus and amblyopia are common and may require surgery, corrective lenses or both. Hearing impairment is also common in children with CP. Some loss is caused by sensorineural involvement. Affected infants may spend increased amounts of time lying flat. This predisposes them to otitis media, which may result in conductive hearing loss.

Diagnostic Evaluation

Infants at risk according to known aetiological factors associated with CP warrant careful assessment during early infancy to identify the signs of muscular dysfunction as early as possible. The neurological examination and history are the primary modalities for diagnosis. Neuroimaging of the child with suspected brain abnormality and CP is now recommended for diagnostic assessment, with MRI being a strong predictor of CP when performed at term (corrected age); general movements assessment also had a strong predictive value in children over 2 years of age and under 5 years of age (Bosanquet et al 2013). MRI has the capability of early identification of infants at risk for CP (George et al 2017). MRI was useful in predicting language development in people with certain brain lesions (Choi et al 2017). Metabolic and genetic testing is recommended if no structural abnormality is identified by neuroimaging; laboratory tests are no longer recommended in the diagnostic process for CP.

Early recognition is made more difficult by the lack of reliable neonatal neurological signs. However, the nurse should monitor infants with known aetiological risk factors and evaluate them closely in the first 2 years of life. Because cortical control of movement does not occur until later in infancy, motor impairment associated with voluntary control is usually not apparent until after 2 to 4 months of age at the earliest. More often the diagnosis cannot be confirmed until the age of 1 or 2 years because motor tone abnormalities may be indicative of another neuromuscular condition. In addition, some children who show signs consistent with CP before 2 years do not demonstrate such signs after 2 years (Nehring 2010). However, there is no consensus regarding an age cut-off for the onset of symptoms.

Establishing a diagnosis may be easier with the persistence of primitive reflexes: either the asymmetrical tonic neck reflex or persistent Moro reflex (beyond 4 months of age), and the crossed extensor reflex. The tonic neck reflex normally disappears between 4 and 6 months of age. An obligatory response is considered abnormal. This is elicited by turning the infant's head to one side and holding it there for 20 seconds. When a crying infant is unable to move from the asymmetrical posturing of the tonic neck reflex, it is considered obligatory and an abnormal response. The crossed extensor reflex, which normally disappears by 4 months, is elicited by applying a noxious stimulus to the sole of one foot with the knee extended. Normally the contralateral foot responds with extensor, abduction and then adduction movements. The possibility of CP is suggested if these reflexes occur after 4 months.

A thorough knowledge of normal variations of motor development is required for detecting abnormal progress, and a careful history is necessary to detect possible aetiological factors. Observe the child's spontaneous movements and behaviour, including posture; attitude; and muscle size, function and tone. Because children with CP often have sensory deficits, it is appropriate to evaluate the child for hearing and vision deficits.

Therapeutic Management: General Concepts

The goals of therapy for children with CP are early recognition and promotion of an optimum developmental course to enable affected children to attain their potential within the limits of their dysfunction. The disorder is permanent, and therapy is chiefly symptomatic and preventive.

The beneficial influences of a rehabilitation program on both child and family are based on recognising the disability as early as possible and implementing treatment. Parents are essential to a treatment program. Consider their goals and desires, their cooperation and their confidence in all aspects of management. With early diagnosis parents can begin to provide the sensorimotor experiences essential to cognitive development because CNS structures depend on stimulation and use to attain and maintain their functional integrity.

The broad aims of therapy are to: (1) establish locomotion, communication and self-help skills; (2) gain optimum appearance and integration of motor functions; (3) correct associated defects as early and effectively as possible; (4) provide educational opportunities adapted to the individual child's needs and capabilities; and (5) promote socialisation experiences with other affected and unaffected children. Each child is evaluated and managed on an individual basis. The plan of therapy may involve a variety of settings, facilities and specially trained persons. The scope of the child's needs requires multidisciplinary planning and care coordination among professionals and the child's family (Box 34.4). The outcome for the child and family with CP is normalisation and promotion of self-care activities that empower the child and family to achieve maximum potential.

Mobilising Devices. Many children with CP wear ankle-foot orthoses (AFOs) (braces) and a variety of orthotics. Orthotics are moulded to fit the feet and are worn inside the shoes. Devices are often used to help prevent or reduce deformity, increase the energy efficiency of gait and control alignment. Some of the more commonly used mobility devices include wheeled scooter boards that allow children to propel themselves while the abdomen or total body is supported and the legs are positioned with wedges to prevent scissoring. Wheeled go-carts provide good sitting balance and serve as an early 'wheelchair' experience for young children. Strollers can be equipped with custom seats for dependent mobilisation. Special devices for independent mobilisation that may or may not allow the upper extremities to remain free are particularly valuable for children with lower extremity involvement (Fig 34.2). A number of wheelchairs can be customised to meet the needs and preferences of older children.

Surgery. Surgical intervention is usually reserved for the child who does not respond to the more conservative measures such as orthotics, but it is also indicated for the child whose spasticity causes progressive deformities. Orthopaedic surgery may be required to correct contracture or spastic deformities, to provide stability for an uncontrollable joint, to address bone malalignment (e.g. lever arm dysfunction) and to provide balanced muscle power. This includes tendon-lengthening procedures (especially heel-cord lengthening), release of spastic wrist flexor muscles and correction of hip and adductor muscle spasticity or contracture to improve locomotion. Orthopaedic specialists with special interest in CP will implement hip observation protocols for children considered at risk for hip abnormalities. Hip surveillance and surgical salvage choices are individual for each person with CP. There is not one procedure that fits all. Orthopaedic surgery is generally not performed until after the child is 6 years of age (Nehring 2010). Surgery is used primarily to improve function rather than for cosmetic purposes and is followed by physical therapy. Surgery may also be performed to improve caloric intake, correct gastro-oesophageal reflux disease, prevent aspiration and correct associated dental problems (Nehring 2010).

Neurosurgical procedures are used only in selected cases. Selective dorsal rhizotomy has provided marked improvement in some children with CP (Nordmark et al 2008). After selective dorsal rhizotomy, gait was improved in children with CP (Rumberg et al 2016). However, achieving the benefits from the surgery requires intensive physical therapy and family commitment. Because the procedure results in flaccid muscles, the child must relearn to sit, stand and walk.

BOX 34.4 Therapeutic Interventions for Cerebral Palsy

Interdisciplinary developmental and physical assessment with recommendations may include the following.

Physical Therapy

Orthotic Devices

- Braces
- Splints
- Casting
- Moulded orthoses

Adaptive Equipment

- Scooters, bicycles and tricycles
- Wheelchairs
- Boards
- Standing devices

Functional (Neuromuscular) Electrical Stimulation (in Combination with Dynamic Splinting)

Occupational Therapy

Adaptive Equipment

- Utensils for functional use (e.g. eating, writing)
- Switches
- Computers

Speech-language Therapy

- Oral-motor skills
- Adaptive communication techniques

Special Education

- Early intervention programs
- Specialised learning programs and support services in school
- Socialisation to promote self-concept development

Surgical Intervention

- Orthopaedic (e.g. tendon transfers, muscle lengthening, spinal deformities)
- Neurological (e.g. neurectomies)
- Selective dorsal rhizotomy
- Feeding (e.g. gastrostomy)
- Dental

Medication Therapy

- Medications to treat the following:
  - Spasticity
  - Pain
  - Secondary conditions (e.g. seizure disorder, chronic constipation, urinary tract infections, gastro-oesophageal reflux)
- Primary care for health supervision and acute childhood illnesses

Behavioural Therapy

Care Coordination

- Care coordination of specialised services and community resources in collaboration with the child's family

Source: Modified from Nehring, W. M. (2010). Cerebral palsy. In P. J. Allen, J. A. Vessey, & N. A. Schapiro (Eds.), Primary care of the child with a chronic condition (5th ed.). St Louis, MO: Mosby.

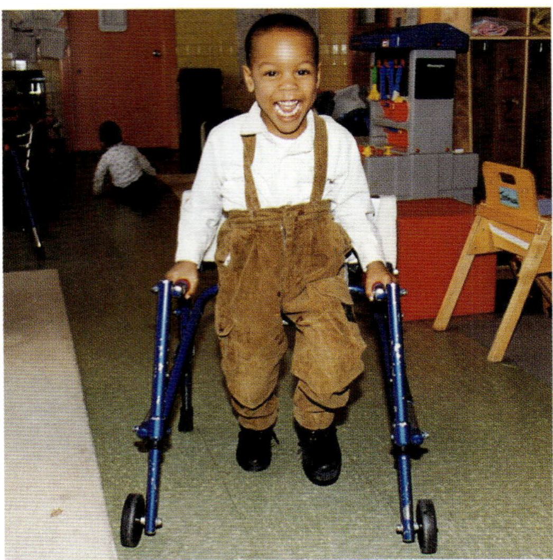

Fig 34.2 Child ambulating with use of assistive device.

Medication. Intense pain may occur with muscle spasms in patients with CP. Children with CP may also experience pain as a result of painful procedures such as injection with botulinum toxin type A (botox), surgical procedures intended to reduce contracture deformities, abdominal pain related to position and gastro-oesophageal reflux and pain associated with physical therapy. Therefore, pain management is an important aspect of the care of the child with CP.

Botox is used to reduce spasticity in targeted muscles of the upper and lower extremities (Lukban et al 2009). Botox is injected into a selected muscle (commonly the quadriceps, gastrocnemius or medial hamstrings), where it acts to inhibit the release of acetylcholine into a specific muscle group, thereby preventing muscle movement. When it is administered early in the course of the illness, this may prevent affected muscle contractures, particularly in lower extremities, thus avoiding surgical procedures with possible adverse effects. The goal is to allow stretching of the muscle; as it relaxes, it permits ambulation with an AFO. The major reported adverse effects of botox injection include pain at the injection site and a temporary weakness (Lukban et al 2009). Prime candidates for botox injections are children with spasticity confined to the lower extremities. The onset of action occurs within 24 to 72 hours, with a peak effect observed at 2 weeks and a duration of action of 3 to 6 months.

The neurosurgical and pharmacological approach to managing the spasticity associated with CP involves the implantation of a pump to infuse baclofen directly into the intrathecal space surrounding the spinal cord to provide relief of spasticity. High doses of oral baclofen are associated with significant side effects, including drowsiness and confusion, yet are often unable to provide adequate relief of spasticity. Direct infusion of baclofen into the intrathecal space provides relief without as many side effects (Motta et al 2011). Intrathecal baclofen is especially helpful in improving comfort (Morton et al 2011).

Patients may be screened before pump placement by the infusion of a 'test dose' of intrathecal baclofen delivered via a lumbar puncture. Close monitoring for side effects (e.g. hypotonia, somnolence, seizures, nausea, vomiting, headache and catheter- or pump-related problems) and relief of spasticity occurs for several hours after the infusion. If a positive effect occurs, the patient is considered a candidate for pump placement.

The pump is placed in the subcutaneous space of the midabdomen; it is about the size of a hockey puck. An intrathecal catheter is tunnelled from the lumbar area to the abdomen and connected to the pump. The pump is filled with baclofen and programmed to provide a set dose using a telemetry wand and a computer. The patient remains hospitalised for several days to adjust the dosage and ensure proper healing. Outpatient visits to refill the pump and make dosage adjustments occur about every 4 to 6 weeks, depending on the patient's response to the treatment. Benefits of intrathecal baclofen include fewer systemic side effects, dosage titration for maximising effects and reversibility of therapy with removal of the pump if so desired. Abrupt withdrawal of intrathecal baclofen, especially at high doses, may result in adverse effects such as rebound spasticity, pruritus, hyperthermia, rhabdomyolysis, disseminated intravascular coagulation, multiorgan failure and death; in some cases intrathecal baclofen withdrawal may mimic sepsis. Treatment of withdrawal centres on re-establishing the medication dosage, with improvements observed within 1 to 2 hours. Hospitalisation and surgery may be required for withdrawal as a result of pump or catheter failure.

Technical Aids. A wide variety of technical aids are available to improve the functioning of children with CP. These include electromechanical toys that employ the concept of biofeedback and operate from a head unit. The toy is manipulated only when the head and trunk are in correct alignment. Computerised toys and games can also enhance eye–hand coordination.

Computers combined with voice synthesisers help children with speech difficulties to 'speak'. Smart phones and tablets with speech applications are appropriate for some children. These and other devices print messages onto screen monitors and paper. These devices have made it apparent that some children have been erroneously considered to be cognitively impaired. Computers have also increased the possibilities for increased mobility via wheelchairs and specially designed mobilisation devices.

Sensors can be activated and deactivated using a head-stick, a voluntary muscle such as the tongue or any other voluntary muscle movement over which the child has control. The application of this technology makes it possible for older persons with CP to eventually function in their own apartments and can be extended into the workplace.

Associated problems. Children with CP often have sensory deficits, which require the attention of appropriate specialists. Speech-language therapy involves the services of a speech-language pathologist (SLP) who may also assist with feeding problems. Dental care is especially important for children with CP and often is overlooked. Regular visits to the dentist and dental prophylaxis, including brushing, fluoride and flossing (after several teeth are present), should begin as soon as the teeth erupt. This is especially important for children given phenytoin, who often develop gum hyperplasia. Additional problems common among children with CP include constipation caused by neurological deficits and lack of exercise; poor bladder control and urinary retention; chronic respiratory tract infections and aspiration pneumonia, which occur as a result of gastro-oesophageal reflux, abnormal muscle tone, immobility and altered positioning; and skin problems as a result of altered positioning, poor nutrition and immobility. Hip dislocation occurs often in children with CP. Latex allergy has also been reported in children with CP (Nehring 2010).

Therapeutic Management: Therapies and Education

Physical Therapy. Physical therapy is one of the most commonly used treatment modalities in children with CP. In general, physical therapy is directed towards good skeletal alignment for the child with spasticity; training in purposeful acts, even in the face of involuntary motion, for the child with athetosis; and gait training and maximum development of proprioceptive sense for the child with ataxia.

An active therapy program involves the family, the physical therapist (PT), the occupational therapist (OT) and other members of the healthcare team. Developing a treatment program that can be carried out at home is of utmost importance. The major approach uses traditional types of therapeutic exercises that consist of stretching; passive, active and resistive movements applied to specific muscle groups or joints to maintain or increase range of motion; strength; or endurance. Neuromuscular electrical stimulation combined with dynamic splinting may benefit some children (Wright et al 2012). No therapeutic approach is able to achieve spectacular changes in the ultimate outcome of motor disability. Early efforts focus on alleviating abnormal postures by positioning and range-of-motion exercises. Passive range-of-motion exercises, stretching and elongation exercises are valuable at any age, even when the child is too young to cooperate. Some active extension can be performed when the child is old enough to cooperate, with passive motion applied to complete joint extension. Prevention of contracture deformity is a prime function of physical therapy. Seating, mobility, strength and endurance are other key goals.

Functional and Adaptive Training (Occupational Therapy). Training in manual skills and activities of daily living (ADLs) proceeds along developmental lines and according to the child's functional level. Sitting, balancing, crawling and walking are encouraged at appropriate ages and are accompanied by stimulation of protective extension and equilibrium reactions. Hand activities are started early to improve motor function and provide the child with sensory experiences and information about the environment. As the child progresses from simple feeding and self-care activities, training is extended to include other tasks (e.g. cooking or use of keyboard or computer mouse) that are within the child's developmental and functional capabilities.

Incorporating play into the therapeutic program often requires great ingenuity and inventiveness from those involved in the child's care. Objects and toys are chosen to provide needed sensory input using a variety of shapes, forms and textures. Nurses can help parents integrate therapy into play activities in natural ways.

Children with CP may need considerable help (and patience) in learning to feed and dress themselves and care for personal hygiene needs. A feeding program may be developed by an OT in conjunction with an SLP. Children should be fed in the normal eating position. When they have difficulty sucking and swallowing, it is tempting to hold them in a semireclining posture to make use of gravity flow. However, this method does not promote active swallowing, and the neck hyperextension may even interfere with swallowing. A more flexed sitting position, with the arms brought forwards to decrease the tendency towards back and neck extension, is more natural during bottle- or spoon-feeding and encourages active swallowing.

Because jaw control is compromised, more normal control can be achieved if the feeder provides stability for the oral mechanism from the side or front of the face. When directed from the front, the middle finger of the non-feeding hand is placed posterior to the bony portion of the chin, the thumb is placed below the bottom lip and the index finger is placed parallel to the child's mandible (Fig 34.3). Manual jaw control from the side assists with head control, correction of neck and trunk hyperextension and jaw stabilisation. The middle finger of the non-feeding hand is placed posterior to the bony portion of the chin, the index finger is placed on the chin below the lower lip and the thumb is placed obliquely across the cheek to provide lateral jaw stability (Fig 34.4).

In all ADLs it is important to capitalise on the child's assets and compensate for liabilities. The level of expected independence is related to both gross and fine motor manipulation. Even when complete independence in a specific activity is not realistic, the child

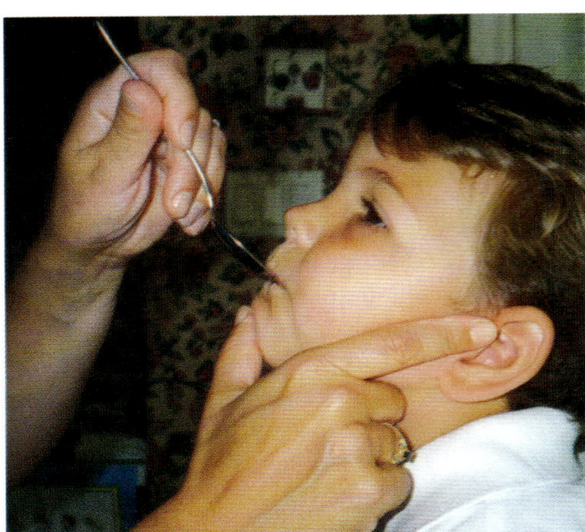

Fig 34.3 Manual jaw control provided anteriorly.

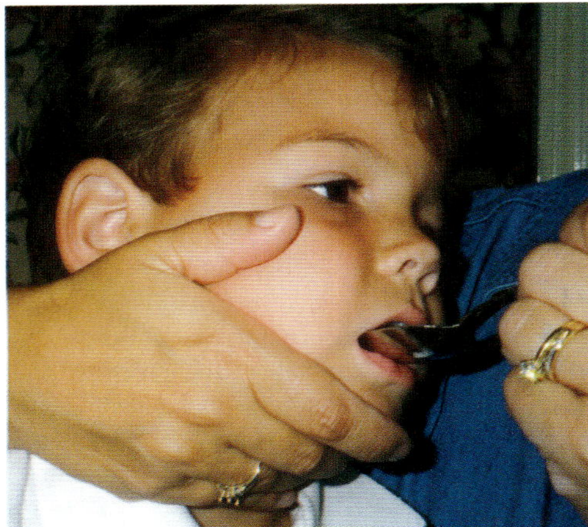

Fig 34.4 Manual jaw control provided from the side.

should learn any part of the task that he or she can master. However, motor function is not the sole purpose of learning to be as independent as possible. Any accomplishment promotes self-reliance and self-esteem for healthier personality development.

Speech Therapy. Speech training under the supervision of an SLP begins early, before the child learns poor habits of communication. Parents and others can help by following the directions of the speech therapist and by talking to the child slowly while using pictures or handling objects about which the adult is speaking. Feeding techniques such as forcing the child to use the lips and tongue in eating facilitate speech. An example of this technique is placing food at the side of the tongue, first one side and then the other, and making the child use the lips to take food from a spoon rather than placing it directly on the tongue. If severe dysarthria prevents articulate speech and the child has reasonable intelligence, the child learns non-verbal communication (e.g. sign language). (See Chapter 20.)

Education. As in all aspects of care, educational requirements are determined by the child's needs and potential. This includes the severity of the child's disease and the presence and degree of associated conditions that affect learning and participation, such as learning impairment, abnormal actions or behaviours, impaired vision or hearing and seizures. Children with mild to moderate cognitive involvement are generally able to participate, for varying amounts of time, in regular classes. Integration of these children into regular classrooms should be the initial goal. Teachers' assistants often work one-on-one with children in both settings. Prevocational and vocational counselling and guidance are arranged at adolescence. Education is geared towards the child's assets at any phase or in any setting. Nurses should be aware of early intervention programs and provisions for special education and related services for children and should support parents in their efforts to obtain appropriate educational services for the child. Bourke-Taylor and colleagues (2018) emphasised the importance of collaboration among team members of school-age children with CP in schools, in the community, in healthcare and across the life span for best outcomes.

Prognosis. The prognosis for the child with CP depends largely on the type and severity of the condition. Children with mild to moderate involvement (85%) have the capability of achieving ambulation between the ages of 2 and 7 years (Berker & Yalçin 2008). If the child does not achieve independent ambulation by this time, chances are poor for ambulation and independence.

Children with CP may have difficulty with hearing, spatial perception, speech and learning (Cerebral Palsy Society 2021). Many children with severe spastic tetraplegic CP have normal intelligence. Growth is affected in children with spastic tetraplegia, and many children remain below the 5th percentile for age and sex. Vocational rehabilitation and higher education are possible for adults with CP. Children with severe CP, difficulty with movement and feeding problems often succumb to respiratory tract infection in childhood. The few survival rate studies on children or adults with CP show that survival is influenced by existing comorbidities (Nehring 2010). In general, the more medically fragile children are least likely to survive to adulthood (Westbom et al 2011).

Nursing Care Management

Assessment. Nursing assessment includes risk identification of infants with aetiological factors that are associated with CP. Ongoing assessment of infants for abnormal muscle tone, inability to achieve developmental milestones and persistence of neonatal reflexes alert the nurse to investigate further.

Reinforce Therapeutic Plan and Assist in Normalisation. Because children are being treated at an earlier age, parents are participating at an earlier stage in treatment programs for their disabled child. They learn the proper handling and home care of young children with CP and need carefully programmed steps so that their expanded parental role can be melded into the established relationship. Close work with other multidisciplinary team members is essential. Nurses reinforce the therapeutic plan and assist the family in devising and modifying equipment and activities to continue the therapy program in the home.

Some children have difficulty keeping their head upright. Because of this, they can neither explore much of their environment nor process the information. Parents need to be complimented on their efforts to provide a stimulating environment for these children. These infants are at risk for delayed development in holding up their heads, righting their shoulders and trunks for stable posture, sitting, pulling, standing and crawling. Most parents of children with impaired movements benefit from support and practical suggestions for feeding, moving, holding and encouraging the infant to explore hands and feet and to play. Helping parents incorporate therapeutic suggestions into typical daily activities is an important normalising strategy.

Although practical advice is important, the nurse, OT or PT should offer suggestions at a pace that can be absorbed by the parents. Encourage the parents to define their concerns, acknowledge the concerns as genuine and ask the parents what approaches they have tried and for how long. In this way the nurse is able to find out what works, what does not work and what the parents would like to try next. Give the parents positive feedback for their observations of the infant, the progress they note and how they differentiate the child's needs.

Address Health Maintenance Needs. Because children with CP expend so much energy in their efforts to accomplish ADLs, more frequent rest periods should be arranged to avoid the fatigue that may aggravate their limited capabilities. Meeting the child's nutritional needs may be a challenge because of gastro-oesophageal reflux, feeding and swallowing difficulties, chronic constipation and subsequent anorexia and absence or diminished ability to independently feed himself or herself (Jones et al 2007). As a result of being ELBW or VLBW in combination with these feeding problems, children with CP are at risk for failure to thrive, and the nurse must ensure an adequate caloric intake. Children with spasticity expend more energy and often require more energy intake than same-age counterparts to maintain adequate growth. Nutritional supplements such as high-calorie milk products (e.g. Pediasure) may be necessary to provide adequate caloric intake after the child has reached 1 year of age. Additional nutritional concerns include providing adequate intake of fruits and fibre to enhance gastrointestinal (GI) motility, routinely monitoring child's growth on a standardised growth chart and avoiding overfeeding and obesity (Jones et al 2007).

Routine assessment of skin status is imperative in children with CP who are limited in movement or who must remain in assistive devices such as a wheelchair for a prolonged period. The overall nutritional status may also be a risk factor for skin breakdown. Care must be taken to ensure that adequate objective skin assessments are routinely performed. If skin breakdown does occur, consult a skin and wound specialist for treatment and further prevention.

Gastrostomy feedings may be necessary to supplement regular feedings and ensure adequate weight gain, particularly in children at risk for growth failure and chronic malnutrition, those with severe CP and subsequent oral feeding difficulties and children whose wellbeing is affected by illness and decreased fluid or medication intake (Rogers 2004). Oral feedings may be continued to maintain oral-motor skills. Weight gain is perceived as an important measure of adequate oral feeding efficiency (Rogers 2004).

Parents may need assistance and advice with medication administration through a gastrostomy tube to prevent clogging. Pills may be crushed and mixed with small amounts of water but not other liquids, such as formula or elixir medications, because these may act together to form a sludge that can interfere with gastrostomy tube function. When crushed pills or tablets are administered, flush the feeding tube with more water after instilling the dissolved pill in water. The pharmacist can provide information regarding crushed pills and tablets and elixirs, which should not be mixed together when administered via gastrostomy or nasogastric tube. A skin-level gastrostomy is particularly suited for the child with CP.

Safety precautions are implemented, such as having children wear protective helmets if they are subject to falls or capable of injuring their heads on hard objects. Because the child with CP is at risk for altered proprioception and subsequent falls, parents should adapt the home and play environment to the child's particular needs to prevent bodily harm. Transportation of the child with motor problems and restricted mobility may be especially challenging for the family and child. Attention must be given to the child's safety when riding in a motor vehicle; an approved safety restraint should be used at all times.

Appropriate immunisations should be administered to prevent childhood illnesses and protect against respiratory tract infections such as influenza. Depending on the level of involvement, dental problems may be more common in children with CP, which creates a need for meticulous attention to all aspects of dental care.

Support the Family. The nursing interventions that are probably most valuable to the family are support and help in coping with the emotional aspects of a chronic disorder, many of which are discussed in Chapter 19. Initially the parents need information and support in understanding the implications of the diagnosis and all the feelings it engenders. Later they need clarification regarding what they can expect from the child and from healthcare professionals. Educating families in the principles of family-centred care and parent–professional collaboration is essential. The family also may require help modifying the home environment for care of the child. Transportation to the practitioner's office and other healthcare agencies often requires special considerations.

Care management for the child and family with CP is an important nursing role. In many cases the family assumes complete care of the child and becomes quite adept at caring for her or his individual needs. The home health nurse or case manager has an important role in the support and encouragement of families who assume the primary care of a child with CP. Having a child with CP implies numerous problems of daily management, with changes in family life, and the nurse needs to stress principles of normalisation.

The nurse can support the parents by acknowledging and addressing their concerns and frustrations and by noting and appreciating their problem-solving skills and their approaches to helping the child. Siblings of a child with a disability are also affected and may respond with overt or less evident behavioural problems. The family needs a relationship with nurses who can provide continued contact, support and encouragement through the long process of rehabilitation.

Parents can also find help and support from parent groups, where they can share experiences, accomplishments, problems and concerns while deriving comfort and practical information. For example, parents can understand from others what it is like to have a child with CP.

Care of the Hospitalised Child. CP is not a condition that requires hospitalisation; therefore, when children with CP are hospitalised, they are usually admitted for an associated illness or for corrective surgery. To facilitate the care and management of hospitalised children with CP, the therapy program should be continued (insofar as their condition allows) while they are hospitalised. This should be incorporated into the multidisciplinary care plan, with every effort expended to make certain the ground that has been so laboriously gained is not lost. Encouraging the parent to room-in and actively participate in the child's care facilitates a continuation of the home therapy program and helps the child adjust to an unfamiliar environment. However, it is equally important to remember that a hospitalisation may be the first time a parent can defer care to a nurse and not be the primary caregiver. This respite may be crucial to the parent's wellbeing. Respect the parent's preference in this regard.

DEFECTS OF NEURAL TUBE CLOSURE

Abnormalities that derive from the embryonic neural tube (**neural tube defects [NTDs]**) constitute the largest group of congenital anomalies with multifactorial inheritance. Normally the spinal cord and cauda equina are encased in a protective sheath of bone and meninges (Fig 34.5A). Failure of neural tube closure produces defects of varying degrees (Box 34.5). They may involve the entire length of the neural tube or may be restricted to a small area.

Aetiology

Two of the defects, anencephaly and spina bifida (SB), occur in association with each other more often than would be expected by chance,

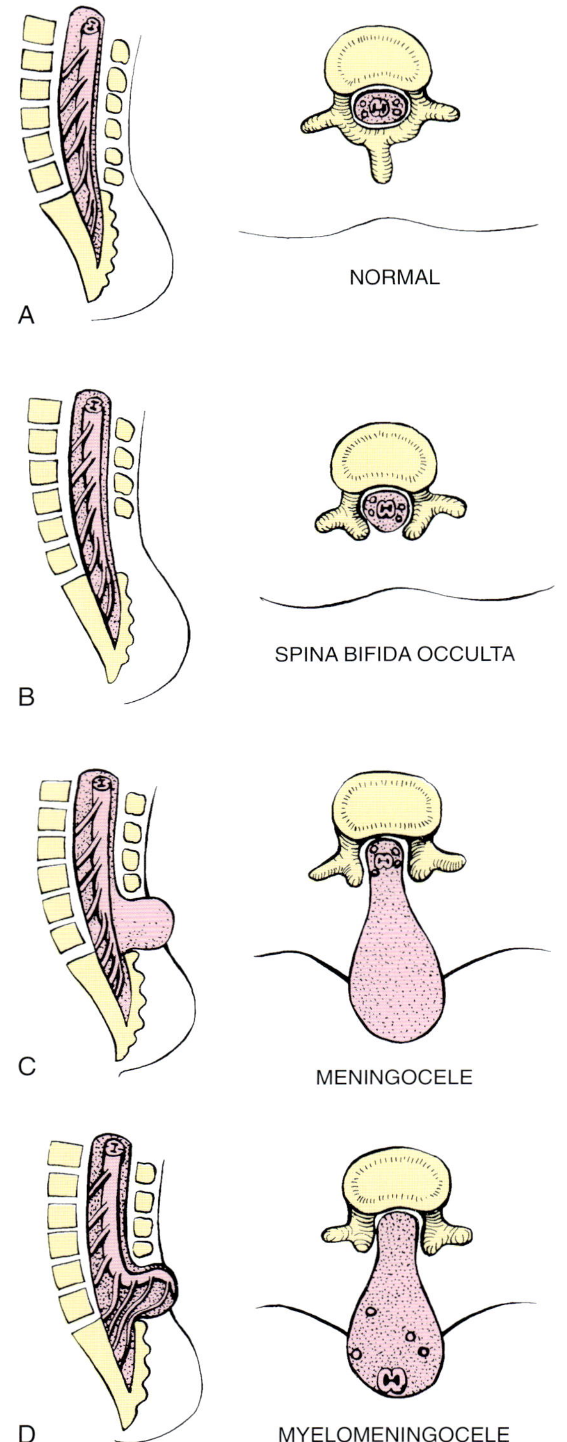

Fig 34.5 (**A**) through (**D**), Midline defects of osseous spine with varying degrees of neural herniations.

suggesting a common origin. The CNS defects may alternate in siblings, which also tends to support the theory of a common origin.

The decline in NTDs in the late 1990s has been attributed in large part to the addition of folic acid to cereal grain products (Department of Health 2010). Population-based studies have also witnessed a substantial decrease in NTDs since food fortification with folic acid and folic acid supplementation recommendations were made (Collins et al 2011). Increased use of prenatal diagnostic techniques and termination of pregnancies have also affected the overall incidence of NTDs.

BOX 34.5 Neural Tube Defects

Cranioschisis—A skull defect through which various tissues protrude
Exencephaly—Brain totally exposed or extruded through an associated skull defect; fetus usually aborted
Anencephaly—Congenital malformation in which both cerebral hemispheres are absent.
Encephalocele—Herniation of brain and meninges through a defect in the skull producing a fluid-filled sac
Rachischisis or Spina Bifida—Fissure in the spinal column that leaves the meninges and spinal cord exposed
Meningocele—Hernial protrusion of a saclike cyst of meninges filled with spinal fluid (see Fig 34.5C)
Myelomeningocele (meningomyelocele)—Hernial protrusion of a saclike cyst containing meninges, spinal fluid and a portion of the spinal cord with its nerves (see Fig 34.5D)

Most authorities believe that the primary defect in NTDs is a failure of neural tube closure during the embryo's early development (between the third and fourth week). However, evidence also implicates a multifactorial origin, including drugs, radiation, maternal malnutrition, chemicals and possibly a genetic mutation in folate pathways in some cases, which may result in abnormal development (Kinsman & Johnston 2015).

Additional factors predisposing the infant to NTDs include maternal obesity, previous NTD pregnancy, Hispanic ancestry, low folic acid intake, gestational diabetes, hot tub or sauna use, low maternal vitamin B_{12} status and the use of antiepileptic drugs (e.g. valproic acid) in pregnancy (Agopian et al 2013). The degree of neurological dysfunction depends on where the sac protrudes through the vertebrae, the anatomical level of the defect and the amount of nerve tissue involved (Fig 34.6). Most myelomeningoceles involve the lumbar or lumbosacral area.

It is recommended that women take at least 0.5 mg of folic acid for at least the month before a planned pregnancy and for the first 3 months of pregnancy to reduce the risk of NTDs and SB (Royal Australian and New Zealand College of Obstetricians and Gynaecologists [RANZCOG] 2019).

The following discussion of NTDs is limited to the two most common types: (1) anencephaly, a defect incompatible with life; and (2) SB, in particular myelomeningocele, an abnormality that causes significant disability.

Anencephaly

Anencephaly, the most serious NTD, is a congenital malformation in which both cerebral hemispheres are absent. If the child with exencephaly (where brain protrudes from the skull) survives, degeneration of the brain to a spongiform mass occurs, with no bony covering. The condition is incompatible with life, and many affected infants are stillborn. For those who survive, no specific treatment is available. The infants have a portion of the brainstem and are able to maintain vital functions (such as temperature regulation and cardiac and respiratory function) for a few hours to several weeks but eventually die of respiratory failure.

Traditionally these infants have been provided comfort measures, but with no effort at resuscitation. Ethical and moral questions are encountered regarding treatment and withdrawal of support systems (e.g. feedings) if the newborn survives the first few days of life, as well as use of the organs for donor transplants. During this time the family requires emotional support and counselling to cope with the birth of an infant with a fatal defect. Referral to neonatal palliative care or hospice should be made as soon as possible (see Palliative Care in Childhood Terminal Illness, Chapter 19).

Spina Bifida and Myelodysplasia

Myelodysplasia refers broadly to any malformation of the spinal canal and cord. Midline defects involving failure of the osseous (bony) spine to close are called **spina bifida**, the most common defect of the CNS. SB is categorised into two types: SB occulta and SB cystica.

SB occulta refers to a defect that is not visible externally. It occurs most commonly in the lumbosacral area (L5 and S1) (Fig 34.5B). Routine radiographic examinations indicate that the disorder may occur in as many as 10% to 30% of the general population. However, it may not be apparent unless there are associated cutaneous manifestations or neuromuscular disturbances. Superficial cutaneous indications include a skin depression or dimple (which may also mark the outlet of a dermal sinus tract that extends to the subarachnoid space); port-wine angiomatous naevi; dark tufts of hair; and soft, subcutaneous lipomas. These signs may be absent, appear singly or be present in combination.

If associated neurological involvement is present, the defect is known as occult spinal dysraphism. Fibrous bands and adhesions, an intraspinal **lipoma** (fatty tumour) or subcutaneous lipoma (lipomyelomeningocele), a dermoid or epidermoid cyst, diastematomyelia (spinal cord split in two) or a tethered cord can distort the spinal cord or roots. The usual cause is abnormal adhesion, or tethering, to a bony or fixed structure, resulting in traction on the spinal cord and cauda equina. (See Figs 34.7 and 34.8 for areas innervated by specific spinal nerves.)

Neuromuscular disturbances usually consist of progressive or static changes in gait with foot weakness, foot deformity or bowel and bladder sphincter disturbances. Some manifestations may not be evident until the child walks or is toilet trained.

Plain radiography is employed to disclose the precise bony defect in the symptomatic lesion and to establish the diagnosis in the suspected, non-symptomatic occult variety. MRI is the most sensitive tool for evaluating the defect. CT, ultrasonography and myelography are also used to differentiate between SB occulta and other spinal disorders.

SB cystica refers to a visible defect with an external saclike protrusion. The two major forms of SB cystica are meningocele, which encases meninges and spinal fluid but no neural elements (Fig 34.5C), and myelomeningocele (or meningomyelocele), which contains meninges, spinal fluid and nerves (Fig 34.5D). Neurological deficit is not associated with meningocele but occurs in varying, often serious, degrees in myelomeningocele.

Myelomeningocele (Meningomyelocele)

Myelomeningocele (MMC) develops during the first 28 days of pregnancy when the neural tube fails to close and fuse at some point along its length. It may be detected prenatally or at birth, accounts for 90% of spinal cord lesions and may be located at any point along the spinal column. Usually the sac is encased in a fine membrane that is prone to tears through which cerebrospinal fluid (CSF) leaks. In other instances the sac may be covered by dura, meninges or skin, in which case there is rapid and spontaneous epithelialisation. The largest number (75%) of myelomeningoceles occur in the lumbar or lumbosacral area (see Fig 34.6). The location and magnitude of the defect determine the nature and extent of neurological impairment. When the defect is below the second lumbar vertebra, the nerves of the cauda equina are involved, giving rise to symptoms such as flaccid, areflexic partial paralysis of the lower extremities and varying degrees of sensory deficit. Unlike an SCI, the degree of deficit is not necessarily uniform on both sides but may vary between extremities, depending on the compromise to specific nerves from malformation or tethering.

The anomaly most frequently associated with myelomeningocele is **hydrocephalus**; approximately 80% to 85% of children with SB develop hydrocephalus (Burke et al 2011, Kinsman & Johnston 2015). Although present at birth, hydrocephalus may not be apparent until shortly thereafter, or after the primary closure of the opening on the back. Careful monitoring of head circumference, fontanel tension and ventricular size by head ultrasonography can indicate its

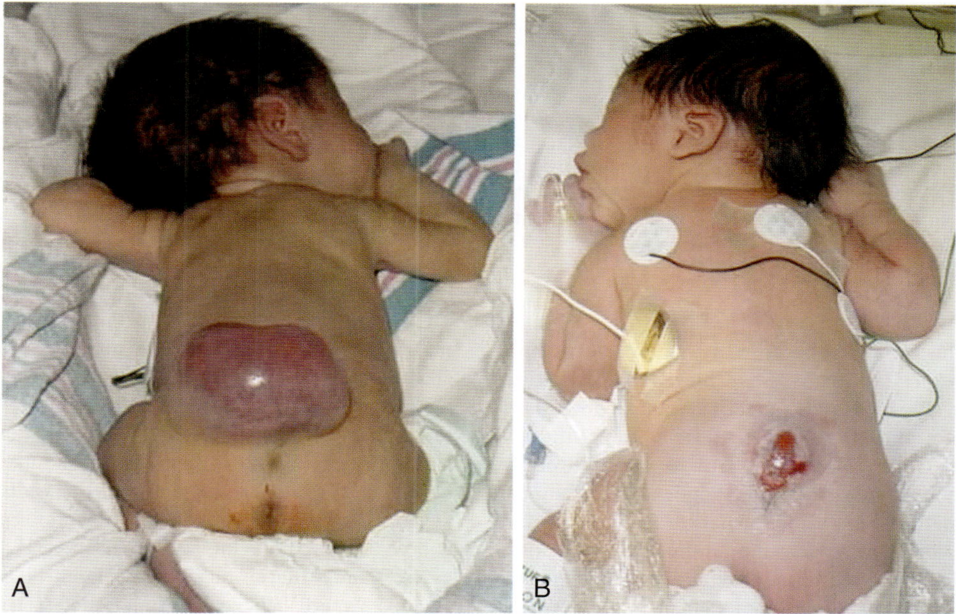

Fig 34.6 (**A**) Myelomeningocele with intact sac. (**B**) Myelomeningocele with ruptured sac. (Source: Courtesy Dr Robert C. Dauser, Neurosurgery, Baylor College of Medicine, Houston, TX.)

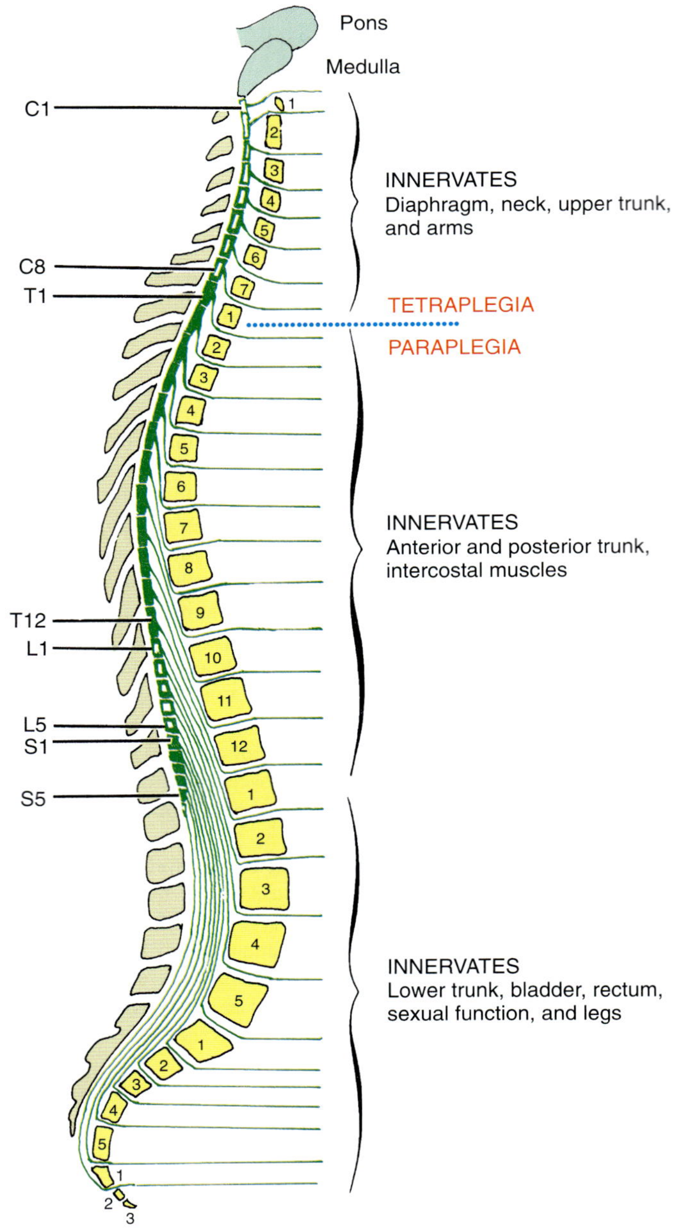

Fig 34.7 Relationships of spinal cord segments and spinal nerves to vertebral bodies. Cervical nerves exit through intervertebral foramina above their respective vertebral bodies (seven cervical vertebrae and eight cervical nerves). Spinal cord ends at L1–L2 vertebral level.

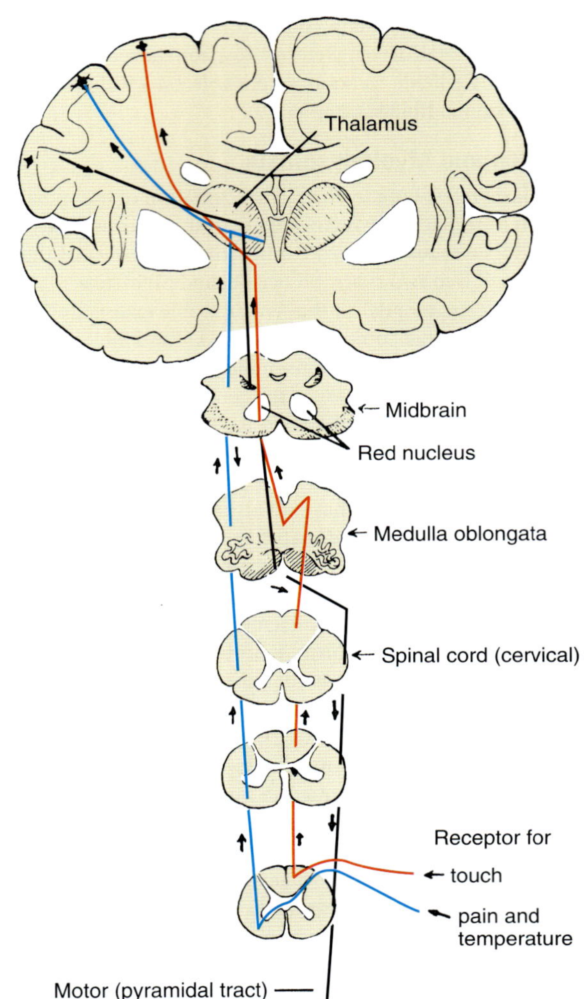

Fig 34.8 Main motor and sensory pathways. Perception of touch, passive motion, position and vibration is transmitted through posterior tract in spinal cord through medial lemniscus in brainstem to thalamus and through internal capsule to cortex (pathway is represented by *solid red line*). Pain and temperature sensations are transmitted through anterolateral tract and lateral lemniscus to thalamus, then through internal capsule to cortex (*blue line*). Motor impulses are transmitted by pyramidal tract, descending from cerebral cortex, crossing in medulla to opposite side and continuing to anterior horns of spinal cord (*black line*). (Source: Conway, B. L. (1978). Carini and Owens' neurological and neurosurgical nursing (7th ed.). St Louis, MO: Mosby.)

presence. Hydrocephalus can occur because the NTD itself disrupts the flow of CSF (see p. 841). In many cases **Chiari's malformation** (type II) is responsible. Type II Chiari's malformation (a downward herniation of the brain into the brainstem) is present, though asymptomatic, in many children with SB. It can, however, adversely affect respiratory function, causing episodic apnoea. Other clinical symptoms of problematic Chiari's malformation include stridor, hoarse cry from vocal cord paralysis, feeding difficulties, aspiration pneumonia and, in older children, upper extremity spasticity. The appearance of such symptoms should not be taken for granted; immediate referral is required to prevent further neurological deterioration.

Pathophysiology

The pathophysiology of SB is best understood when related to the normal formative stages of the nervous system. At approximately 20 days of gestation, a decided depression, the neural groove, appears in the dorsal ectoderm of the embryo. During the fourth week of gestation, the groove deepens rapidly and its elevated margins develop laterally and fuse dorsally to form the neural tube. Neural tube formation begins in the cervical region near the centre of the embryo and advances in both directions—caudally and cephalically—until by the end of the fourth week of gestation, the ends of the neural tube, the anterior and posterior neuropores, close.

Most experts believe the primary defect in neural tube malformations is a failure of neural tube closure. However, some evidence indicates that the defects are a result of splitting of the already closed neural tube as a result of an abnormal increase in CSF pressure during the first trimester.

The degree of neurological dysfunction depends on where the sac protrudes through the vertebrae, the anatomical level of the defect and the amount of nerve tissue involved. One classification designates the level of functional mobility in relationship to the anatomical level of the defect. For example, children with a high lumbar-thoracic defect may be able to walk short distances using long leg braces and by early adolescence must use a wheelchair for mobility; children with a low lumbar defect can walk with short leg braces and forearm crutches (Liptak & Dosa 2010). This classification system, however, does not describe genitourinary and bowel function. About 80% of patients with myelomeningocele develop a type II Chiari's malformation (Kinsman & Johnston 2015). There is some evidence that prolonged exposure of the MMC sac to amniotic fluid predisposes to the development of hindbrain herniation and type II Chiari's malformation (Adzick 2013).

Clinical Manifestations

The manifestations of SB vary widely according to the degree of the spinal defect. The defect is readily apparent on inspection. The degree of neurological dysfunction is directly related to the anatomical level of the defect and thus the nerves involved. Sensory disturbances usually parallel motor dysfunction. The upper level of sensory and motor impairment can be determined by observation of the infant's response to a pinprick over the legs and trunk. The infant responds to the sensory stimulus with limb movement, arousal and crying. When withdrawal activity is used to determine the lowest level of spinal cord function, the response to pinprick should begin above the lesion.

Defective nerve supply to the bladder affects both sphincter and detrusor tone, which often causes constant dribbling of urine or produces overflow incontinence. This can often be mistaken for normal voiding patterns in the newborn. Some infants with SB, however, are able to void in a stream and achieve complete bladder emptying with each void.

Frequently the infant has poor anal sphincter tone and poor anal skin reflex, which result in lack of bowel control and sometimes rectal prolapse. Avoid taking rectal temperatures in affected infants. Because bowel sphincter function is frequently affected, the thermometer can cause irritation and rectal prolapse. If the defect is below the third sacral vertebra, the infant has no motor impairment but may have saddle anaesthesia with bladder and anal sphincter paralysis.

Sometimes the denervation to the muscles of the lower extremities produces joint deformities in utero. These are primarily flexion or extension contractures, talipes valgus or varus contractures, kyphosis, lumbosacral scoliosis and hip dislocations. The extent and severity of these associated orthopaedic deformities again depend on the degree of nerve involvement. Most flexion deformities result from the pull of stronger, fully innervated muscles acting without the counterpull of their non-functioning paralysed antagonists. Box 34.6 provides a summary of clinical manifestations of SB cystica and occulta.

Diagnostic Evaluation

The diagnosis of SB is made on the basis of clinical manifestations (see Box 34.6) and examination of the meningeal sac (see Fig 34.6A). Diagnostic measures used to evaluate the brain and spinal cord include MRI, ultrasonography and CT. A neurological evaluation will determine the extent of involvement of bowel and bladder function, as well as lower extremity neuromuscular involvement. Flaccid paralysis of the lower extremities is a common finding with absent deep tendon reflexes.

BOX 34.6 Clinical Manifestations of Spina Bifida

Spina Bifida Cystica

- Sensory disturbances usually parallel to motor dysfunction
- Below second lumbar vertebra:
  - flaccid, partial paralysis of lower extremities
  - varying degrees of sensory deficit
  - overflow incontinence with constant dribbling of urine
  - lack of bowel control
  - rectal prolapse (sometimes)
- Below third sacral vertebra:
  - no motor impairment
  - bladder and anal sphincter paralysis
- Joint deformities (sometimes produced in utero):
  - talipes valgus or varus (foot) contractures
  - kyphosis
  - lumbosacral scoliosis
  - hip dislocation

Spina Bifida Occulta

- Frequently no observable manifestations
- May be associated with one or more cutaneous manifestations:
  - skin depression or dimple
  - port-wine angiomatous naevi
  - dark tufts of hair
  - soft, subcutaneous lipomas
- May be neuromuscular disturbances:
  - progressive disturbance of gait with foot weakness
  - bowel and bladder sphincter disturbances

Prenatal Detection. It is possible to determine the presence of some major open NTDs prenatally. Ultrasonographic scanning of the uterus and elevated maternal concentrations of α-fetoprotein (AFP, or MS-AFP), a fetal-specific γ-1-globulin, in amniotic fluid may indicate anencephaly or myelomeningocele. The optimum time for performing these diagnostic tests is between 16 and 18 weeks of gestation before AFP concentrations normally diminish and in sufficient time to permit a therapeutic abortion. It is recommended that such diagnostic procedures and genetic counselling be considered for all mothers who have borne an affected child, and testing is offered to all pregnant women (RANZCOG 2018). Chorionic villus sampling is also a method for prenatal diagnosis of NTDs; however, it carries certain risks (skeletal limb depletion) and is not recommended before 10 weeks of gestation (Simpson et al 2012).

Therapeutic Management

Management of the child who has a myelomeningocele requires a multidisciplinary team approach involving the specialties of neurology, neurosurgery, paediatrics, urology, orthopaedics, rehabilitation, physical therapy, occupational therapy and social services, as well as intensive nursing care in a variety of specialty areas. The collaborative efforts of these specialists focus on the following:

- the myelomeningocele and the problems associated with the defect—hydrocephalus, paralysis, orthopaedic deformities (e.g. developmental dysplasia of the hip, clubfoot) and genitourinary abnormalities
- possible acquired problems that may or may not be associated, such as type II Chiari's malformation, meningitis, seizures, hypoxia, tethered cord and haemorrhage
- other abnormalities, such as cardiac or GI malformations.

Initial Care. Care of the newborn involves preventing infection; performing a neurological assessment, including observation for associated anomalies; and dealing with the impact of the anomaly on the family. Although meningoceles are repaired early, especially if the sac is in danger of rupturing, the philosophy regarding skin closure of myelomeningocele varies. Most authorities believe that early closure, within the first 24 to 72 hours, offers the most favourable outcome. Surgical closure within the first 24 hours is recommended if the sac is leaking CSF (Kinsman & Johnston 2015). Early closure, preferably in the first 12 to 18 hours, not only prevents local infection and trauma to the exposed tissues but also avoids stretching other nerve roots (which may occur as the meningeal sac expands during the first hours after birth), thus preventing further motor impairment. Broad-spectrum antibiotics are initiated, and neurotoxic substances such as povidone-iodine are avoided at the malformation.

Associated problems are assessed and managed by appropriate surgical and supportive measures. Shunt procedures provide relief from imminent or progressive hydrocephalus (see Chapter 30). When diagnosed, ventriculitis, meningitis and urinary tract infection are treated with vigorous antibiotic therapy and supportive measures. Surgical intervention for type II Chiari's malformation is indicated only when the child is symptomatic (i.e. high-pitched crowing cry, stridor, respiratory difficulties, apnoea, failure to thrive, gastro-oesophageal reflux, oral-motor difficulties, upper extremity spasticity).

Improved surgical techniques do not alter the major physical disability and deformity or chronic urinary tract infections that affect the quality of life for these children. Superimposed on these physical problems are the disorder's effects on family life and finances and on school and hospital services.

Musculoskeletal Considerations. According to most orthopaedists, musculoskeletal problems that will affect later locomotion should be evaluated early and treatment, where indicated, instituted without delay. Neurological assessment determines the neurosegmental level of the lesion, spasticity and progressive paralysis, potential for deformity and functional expectations. Orthopaedic and musculoskeletal management includes preventing joint contractures, correcting the existing deformity, preventing or minimising effects of motor and sensory deficits, preventing skin breakdown and obtaining the best possible function of affected lower extremities. Common musculoskeletal problems requiring attention in SB include deformities of the knees, hips, feet and spine; fractures and insensate skin further complicate orthopaedic care. Other problems that may occur later include kyphosis and scoliosis (Lazzaretti & Pearson 2010, Liptak & Dosa 2010). About 50% of infants born with myelomeningocele will have clubfoot (Sandler 2010). Because children with MMC often have decreased sensitivity in lower extremities, preventive skin care is important. A high percentage (60%) of children seen in a wound clinic for skin breakdown had myelomeningocele at birth (Samaniego 2003). The most common wound sites were the foot and ankle, with the buttocks being the second most common site. Pressure wounds are more common in patients who use wheelchairs for mobility (Ottolini et al 2013).

The status of the neurological deficit remains the most important factor in determining the child's ultimate functional abilities; however, many children with lumbar and sacral myelomeningocele are able to achieve functional ambulation (Kinsman & Johnston 2015). With technological advances, a variety of lightweight orthoses, including braces, special 'walking' devices and custom-built wheelchairs, are available to provide mobility to children with spinal cord lesions (see also Chapter 30). Early in infancy, intervention with passive range-of-motion exercises, positioning and stretching exercises may help decrease the incidence of muscle contractures. Corrective surgical procedures, when indicated, are best initiated at an early age so that the child will not lag significantly behind age-mates in developmental progress. The degree of lower extremity function guides decisions about whether orthopaedic surgery will be needed.

Physical therapy and musculoskeletal management of children with myelomeningocele are continual processes to achieve optimum function and ambulation when possible. Problems such as type II Chiari's malformation, hydrocephalus and a tethered spinal cord can complicate expectations. A common complication is tethered cord syndrome in which there is a presumed traction injury to the distal spinal cord with subtle and progressive loss of neural function; this may occur any time but is more common during periods of rapid growth and can be precipitated by ventricular shunt failure (Burke et al 2011).

Management of Genitourinary Function. Myelomeningocele is one of the most common causes of neuropathic (neurogenic) bladder dysfunction among children. Neurological deficits can affect the innervation of the bladder, impairing the ability to store and empty urine. As many as 90% of children with SB will experience some form of voiding dysfunction. A child with a neuropathic bladder will require care across the life span. The goals of urological treatment should be individualised to the child's developmental stage. In infants the goal of treatment is to preserve renal function. In older children the goal is to preserve renal function and achieve optimum urinary continence. Urinary incontinence is a chronic, often debilitating problem for the child. In addition, the neuropathic bladder may produce **urinary system distress**, characterised by symptomatic urinary tract infections, ureterohydronephrosis, vesicoureteral reflux or renal insufficiency. The characteristics of bladder dysfunction in children vary according to the level of the neurological lesion and the influence of bony growth and development of the spine. In addition, the presence of type II Chiari's malformation and subsequent hydrocephalus has the potential to affect bladder function, although spinal influences predominate.

During infancy, urinary incontinence is normally physiological, but urinary system distress may occur. Ongoing urological monitoring is essential. Evidence is growing that early intervention, based on evaluation during the neonatal period and before complications occur, improves bladder function, reduces the subsequent risk of urinary system distress and reduces the need for reconstructive surgery of the lower urinary tract. Ultrasonography of the bladder and ureters and routine urinalysis (and urine cultures when indicated) are used to detect urinary system distress before renal function is compromised. In addition, urodynamic testing is used to identify bladder dysfunction that predisposes the child to urinary system distress (Gray & Moore 2009, Snodgrass & Gargollo 2010). These conditions include high-pressure detrusor hyperreflexia (reflex contractions of the detrusor muscle) with vesicosphincter dyssynergia (incoordination of detrusor and sphincter muscles), low bladder wall compliance (poor distensibility of the bladder wall causing increased intravesical pressures during urine filling and storage) or detrusor areflexia (absence of detrusor contractions caused by the spinal defect).

Infants may have one of several predominant neuropathic bladder disorders. Detrusor contractions associated with vesicosphincter dyssynergia are particularly common. Some infants are able to empty the bladder efficiently despite incoordination between the sphincter mechanism and detrusor, but the majority experience chronic residual urine, urinary tract infections or more serious types of urinary system distress. A minority of infants have poor detrusor contraction strength or detrusor areflexia. This condition is particularly damaging to the urinary system when it coexists with low bladder wall compliance and an elevated detrusor leak point pressure. Low bladder wall compliance occurs when collagen or fibrosis causes stiffening of the bladder wall. This stiffened bladder wall raises intravesical pressures, obstructing the bladder, ureters and, ultimately, the nephron. The impact of low bladder wall compliance is directly related to the influence of the bladder outlet. Among children with myelodysplasia, the urethral muscles are typically weakened, and collagen replaces much of the muscle tissue. As a result, the sphincter is fixed, so it neither closes efficiently to prevent urinary leakage nor opens well enough to allow urinary flow with a detrusor contraction. When the magnitude of the pressure required to drive urine across the abnormal sphincter is greater than 40 cmH_2O (the detrusor leak point pressure) and the compliance of the bladder wall is low (< 10 cmH_2O), the risk of urinary system distress is high.

In contrast, a small number of infants experience effective detrusor contractions without vesicosphincter dyssynergia. Effective bladder evacuation is likely among this group, and the incidence of urinary system distress during the first year of life is low.

As the child grows, detrusor hyperreflexia is often replaced by deficient detrusor contraction strength and **stress urinary incontinence (SUI)** (leakage produced by physical exertion). The bladder wall is often poorly compliant (producing chronically elevated intravesical pressures), and the bladder outlet, while incompetent, obstructs the outflow of urine. When the detrusor leak point pressure exceeds 40 cmH_2O, the child is predisposed to chronic urinary leakage and urinary distress symptoms, including recurrent urinary tract infections and reflux. When the detrusor leak point pressure is lower than 40 cmH_2O, urinary leakage is more severe, although the risk of urinary system distress is lessened. Thus the child with more severe urinary incontinence is less predisposed than the 'drier' child to serious urinary tract infections.

Infants with myelomeningocele and a neurogenic bladder who are not at risk for urinary system distress are managed by nappy containment and watchful waiting. The infant empties the bladder into a nappy, the urine is routinely monitored for infection and the upper urinary tracts are monitored for evidence of urinary system distress (dilation of the ureters, renal pelvises or collecting systems) via serial ultrasonography.

In contrast, children with evidence of urinary system distress, or those considered at risk based on early urodynamic testing, undergo **clean intermittent catheterisation (CIC)**, typically in combination with an antispasmodic medication such as oxybutynin or propantheline (De Jong et al 2008, Gray & Moore 2009). Anticholinergic medications are prescribed because they reduce detrusor muscle tone and reduce bladder pressures both during urine filling and storage and during micturition. CIC is not intended to prevent spontaneous voiding. Instead, it ensures routine, regular bladder evacuation, further preventing deleterious elevation of intravesical pressures. Usually, the parents learn to catheterise the infant every 4 hours during the day and once each night. Follow-up evaluation, consisting of serial ultrasonography and urinalysis, is completed every 3 to 6 months as indicated.

Infants with significant urinary system distress and neuropathic bladder dysfunction at birth sometimes require temporary urinary diversion to ensure adequate urine outflow and prevent further damage to the upper urinary tracts. A vesicostomy is a relatively simple procedure wherein the anterior bladder wall is brought to the abdominal wall, creating a small stoma for urinary drainage. Urine is contained via a nappy, but using two nappies or use of a larger nappy that can be placed higher on the abdomen is necessary for adequate urine containment. Meticulous skin care is necessary because the perineal skin is exposed to continuous urinary leakage.

Among older children the quest for continence typically begins with a CIC program. The parents learn the procedure and teach the child to self-catheterise as soon as possible, usually by 6 years of age (Gray & Moore 2009). The child with detrusor hyperreflexia and dyssynergia often responds well to antispasmodic medications and CIC. In contrast, the child with poor bladder wall compliance and SUI often requires a combination of antispasmodic medications to reduce intravesical filling pressures and a sympathetic agonist (such as imipramine, pseudoephedrine or phenylpropanolamine) to enhance sphincter competence. Unfortunately, the combination of medications and CIC is typically only partially effective, and more aggressive interventions are often required to render the neuropathic bladder both continent and free from its predisposition towards producing urinary system distress. It is important that a careful history is taken by the provider to identify other problems that may be contributing to persistent incontinence. Factors that can affect bladder continence include caffeinated drinks, constipation or lack of access to bathrooms (Metcalfe 2017).

When the child cannot attain continence by conservative measures, surgery is considered. Augmentation enterocystoplasty (or gastrocystoplasty) is a surgical procedure that increases bladder capacity, reverses or halts the negative effects of the poorly compliant bladder wall and reduces harmfully high bladder pressures caused by detrusor hyperreflexia with vesicosphincter dyssynergia. A detubularised segment of large or small bowel or a wedge of the fundus of the stomach has been used to successfully augment bladder capacity. The choice of segment varies according to the surgeon's preference and the status of the patient's urinary and GI systems. Large and small bowel segments produce significant volumes of mucus that may clog catheters used for CIC. Augmentation with the stomach produces less mucus, and its acidic secretions may reduce the urinary system's predisposition to infection. The bladder must be irrigated to decrease mucus within the bladder; this also decreases the possible complications of infection, stones and bladder perforation.

Even though augmentation of the bladder may improve or resolve urinary leakage related to detrusor hyperreflexia or urinary system distress caused by low bladder wall compliance, the SUI produced by the abnormal sphincter mechanism typically persists. Several surgical procedures help correct this intrinsic sphincter deficiency. The Mitrofanoff procedure uses the appendix to provide an alternative route for intermittent catheterisation. The appendix is removed from the colon and used to create a continent conduit between the abdominal wall and the bladder. The resulting stoma is relatively small and produces minimum mucus. The ureter may be used as an alternative to the appendix for some children. If the appendix is insufficient, a segment of tapered intestine, ileum or colon may be used to create a conduit (Monti tube) (Gray & Moore 2009). CIC through the easily accessible abdominal route fosters greater independence in children, especially in those unable to transfer from wheelchair to toilet to perform CIC.

When intrinsic sphincter deficiency produces only mild stress urinary leakage, the construction of a Mitrofanoff route alone may be sufficient to achieve continence between catheterisation episodes. However, when SUI is more severe, a suburethral sling or suburethral collagen injection is used to alleviate intrinsic sphincter deficiency.

The suburethral sling is a slip of fascia or synthetic material that is placed below the proximal third of the urethra. The sling may be placed in a fashion that uses only slight tension to obstruct the urethra and prevent SUI. The sling may be used for both boys and girls, and the procedure can be completed at the same time as the augmentation enterocystoplasty is constructed. After augmentation enterocystoplasty and placement of a suburethral sling, the patient can expect to evacuate the bladder by CIC of the appendiceal Mitrofanoff route (appendicovesicostomy) or the urethra if a Mitrofanoff route has not been constructed.

Because of advances in neurogenic bladder management, adolescents and young adults with myelomeningocele and neurogenic bladder have been followed for up to 30 years without evidence of deterioration in renal function. Nevertheless, urinary and faecal incontinence are common, and these conditions lead to significant, and sometimes devastating, problems with growth and developmental tasks, including establishing independence and social and intimate relationships. This observation underscores the need to aggressively manage both continence and the threat of urinary system distress from an early age and to establish an expectation of social continence critical to providing these patients with the skills they need to thrive as adolescents and adults. Newborns with SB and normal urodynamics require close follow-up care during the first several years of life to prevent deterioration in urodynamic status as a result of neurological deterioration.

Bowel Control. Some degree of faecal continence can be achieved in most children with myelomeningocele with diet modification, regular toilet habits and prevention of constipation and impaction. It is frequently a lengthy process. Dietary fibre supplements (recommended age of child in years + 5 g/day), laxatives, suppositories or enemas aid in producing regular evacuation. Older children and adolescents seeking more independence may attain bowel continence and higher quality of life after undergoing an **antegrade continence enema** (ACE) procedure (Doolin 2006). In a procedure similar to the Mitrofanoff, the appendix or ileum is used to create a catheterisable channel with attachment of the proximal end to the colon. The distal end of the channel exits through a small abdominal stoma. Every 1 or 2 days, a catheter is passed through the stoma, allowing enema solution to be instilled directly into the colon. After administration of the enema solution, the child sits on the toilet for 30 to 60 minutes as stool is flushed out through the rectum. The frequency of enemas and volume of solution used to completely evacuate the bowel vary among individuals.

Prognosis

The early prognosis for the child with myelomeningocele depends on the neurological deficit present at birth, including motor ability, bladder innervation and associated neurological anomalies. Early surgical repair of the spinal defect, antibiotic therapy to reduce the incidence of meningitis and ventriculitis, prevention of urinary system dysfunction and early detection and correction of hydrocephalus have significantly increased the survival rate and quality of life in such children. Mortality rates are reported to be 10% to 15%, with many deaths occurring before the age of 4 years (Kinsman & Johnston 2015). Many young adults with SB achieve partial independent living and gainful employment. Reports of survival rates vary, and many include adults who were born before medical advances and surgical techniques seen in the past 25 years. Coordinated care for adults with SB is essential; however, multidisciplinary adult care is often inadequate (Lazzaretti & Pearson 2010). One of the factors associated with early death among adults with MMC is hydrocephalus and shunt failure (Mourtzinos & Stoffel 2010). This chronic condition has an array of associated complications, including hydrocephalus and shunt malfunctions, tethered cord syndrome, scoliosis, type II Chiari's malformation development, bowel and bladder management issues, latex allergy and epilepsy. However, based on current medical knowledge and ethical considerations, aggressive early management is favoured for the child with myelomeningocele.

Nursing Care Management

The basic needs of the infant with a myelomeningocele are essentially the same as for any newborn infant. (See Chapter 8.) Special needs related to the defect and potential complications are discussed in the following section. As the child matures, the problems increase and involve all aspects of daily living; therefore, care is directly related to the child's rehabilitation at each stage of development.

Assessment. At the time of delivery an examination is performed to assess the intactness of the membranous cyst. During transport to the nursery, make every effort to prevent trauma to this protective covering. In addition to the routine assessment of the newborn (see Chapter 7), assess the infant for the level of neurological involvement. Note movement of extremities or skin response, especially an anal reflex that might provide clues to the degree of motor or sensory impairment.

Care of the Myelomeningocele Sac. The infant is usually placed in a humidicrib so that temperature can be maintained without clothing or covers that might irritate the CNS lesion. Before surgical closure, the myelomeningocele is kept from drying by the application of a sterile, moist, non-adherent dressing. The moistening solution is usually sterile normal saline. Dressings are changed frequently (every 2 to 4 hours), and the sac is inspected closely for leaks, abrasions, irritation and signs of infection. The sac must be cleansed carefully if it becomes soiled or contaminated. Sometimes the sac ruptures during delivery or transport, and any opening in the sac greatly increases the risk of infection to the CNS (Fig 34.6B).

Positioning. One of the most important and challenging aspects of early care of the infant with myelomeningocele is positioning. Before surgery the infant remains in the prone position to minimise tension on the sac and the risk of trauma. The prone position allows for optimum positioning of the legs, especially in cases of associated hip dysplasia.

The infant's head is turned to one side for feeding. Fortunately, most defects are repaired early, and the infant can be held for feeding and routine care soon after surgery. Physical therapy consultation may be necessary for difficult positioning problems. SLP consultation may be needed for difficulty with oral-motor skills that may indicate complications caused by a Chiari's malformation.

General Care. Changing the infant's nappy may be contraindicated until the defect has been repaired and healing is well advanced or epithelialisation has taken place. The padding beneath the nappy area is changed as needed to keep the skin dry and free of irritation. When the nurse detects urinary retention (the bladder is still an abdominal organ in early infancy), CIC is employed. Because the bowel sphincter is frequently affected, there may be continual passage of stool, often misinterpreted as diarrhoea, which is a constant irritant to the skin and a source of infection to the spinal lesion.

Areas of sensory and motor impairment are subject to skin breakdown and therefore require meticulous care. The infant may be placed on a pressure-reducing mattress or a mattress to prevent pressure on the knees and ankles.

Gentle range-of-motion exercises are carried out to prevent contractures, and stretching of contractures is performed when indicated. However, these exercises may be restricted to the foot, ankle and knee joint. When the hip joints are unstable, stretching against tight hip flexors or adductor muscles, which act much like bowstrings, may aggravate a tendency towards subluxation. A physical therapy consultation is often necessary to develop a multidisciplinary plan to prevent long-term complications.

Some infants with unrepaired myelomeningocele are unable to be held in the arms and cuddled as unaffected infants are, so their need for tactile stimulation is met by caressing, stroking and other comfort measures. To facilitate handling and reduce parental anxiety, the infant can recline on a pillow placed in the parent's lap.

Ophthalmic complications may occur in children with SB and hydrocephalus. The appearance of a squint, other ocular motility or papillo-oedema usually denotes hydrocephalus and is reported.

Ophthalmological follow-up care, particularly in children with shunts, is generally included in the multidisciplinary care plan.

Postoperative Care. Postoperative care for the infant with myelomeningocele involves the same basic care as for any postsurgical infant: monitoring vital signs, weight and intake and output; maintaining body temperature; assessing and relieving pain; providing nourishment; and observing for signs of infection. The wound is managed according to the surgeon's directions, and general care is continued as preoperatively.

The prone position is maintained after operative closure, although many neurosurgeons allow a side-lying or partial side-lying position unless it aggravates a coexisting hip dysplasia or permits undesirable hip flexion. This offers an opportunity for position changes, which reduces the risk of pressure sores and facilitates feeding. Once the effects of anaesthesia have subsided and the infant is alert, feedings may resume unless there are other anomalies or associated complications.

Nursing assessments are carried out for implementation of comfort measures in the postoperative period. The infant can be held upright against the body, taking care to avoid pressure on the operative site. In the case of an unusually large defect, skin grafting may be required for wound closure; the infant must then be kept prone postoperatively with as little movement as possible to prevent tension on the skin graft.

The nurse can assist in determining the extent of neuromuscular involvement. Note movement of the extremities or skin response, especially an anal reflex, that might provide clues to the degree of motor or sensory status. Measure head circumference daily and examine the fontanels for signs of tension or bulging. The nurse is also alert to early signs of infection, such as elevated or decreased temperature (axillary), irritability and lethargy, and to signs of increased intracranial pressure. Urinary catheterisation may be needed for urine retention. Although it may not have been a problem preoperatively, swelling around the operative site may cause transient urine retention, which resolves in 2 to 5 days.

Family Support and Home Care. As soon as the parents are able to cope with the infant's condition, encourage them to become involved in care. They need to learn how to continue at home the care that has been initiated in the hospital: positioning, feeding, skin care and range-of-motion exercises when appropriate. Parents also need to learn CIC technique when prescribed. The family needs to know the signs of complications and how to reach assistance when needed.

As the child grows and develops, parents need guidance to encourage and stimulate the infant to accomplish age-appropriate developmental tasks within the limits imposed by the disabilities. Upper limb movement can be stimulated early by placing the infant on the floor in a prone position with toys within reach. Activities that encourage body consciousness, such as rolling over and pulling to a sitting position, are encouraged at the appropriate times. The parents may need help to modify appliances and activities normally expected of a growing child. A standing table, frame or parapodium is helpful for a variety of activities, and it is best for the child to begin supported weight bearing and standing as close as possible to the expected time for standing to occur.

It is important for the family to understand the nature of sensory deficit in a child with a spinal defect. The child will be insensitive to pressure or other sources of tissue injury. Therefore, the family must be alert to hot or cold items that could cause thermal injury to tissues and remember to inspect the skin regularly for signs of pressure, especially over bony prominences. Because of sensory impairment, the child is unaware of bladder discomfort. Therefore, signs of urinary tract infections may go unnoticed. Urinary tract infection is often considered when the child becomes ill.

The long-range planning with and support of the parents and newborn begin in the hospital and extend throughout childhood and even into young adulthood. The life expectancy of children with SB extends well into adulthood; therefore, planning should involve long-term goals and plans for optimum function as an adult. Long-range planning goals should include a discussion of achievement of functional mobility, urinary continence and as much bowel continence as physically possible. Discussion about aspects of adulthood such as having a mate, sexual relationships and bearing and rearing children is important and should not be overlooked (Rowe & Jadhav 2008). The unique service needs of adolescents with SB as they attempt to gain independence from family and establish a life of their own have not been adequately addressed in the literature (Sawyer & Macnee 2010). Betz and colleagues (2010) interviewed young people with SB making the transition to adulthood. Some common themes that emerged among these young people were challenges in preparation for self-management, limited social relationships, awareness of their cognitive challenges and the cost of independence.

Nurses assume an important role as a central member of the health team. As a coordinator, the nurse reviews information with the family, takes responsibility for family teaching and acts as a liaison between inpatient and outpatient services. The child may require numerous hospitalisations over the years, and each one will be a source of stress to which the younger child is especially vulnerable.

Changes in functional ability, particularly in the lower extremities, bowel or bladder, may indicate the presence of a tethered cord, one that is bound low or restricted in an abnormal position by scar tissue. These symptoms usually occur after a growth spurt and can best be detected with MRI. Tethering can be repaired surgically but, unfortunately, may recur.

Rehabilitation involves solving not only problems of self-help and locomotion but also the most distressing problem of incontinence, which threatens the child's social acceptability. Assistance in preparing the child and the school regarding the special needs of children with disabilities helps the parents provide a better initial adjustment to broader social experiences.

Hypotonia

Decreased muscle tone may be observed in the neonatal period and is one of the most common presenting symptoms in neuromuscular disorders. Hypotonia in neonates born before 37 weeks may be due to neuromuscular immaturity or perinatal maternal medications. (See also Chapter 9.) Monitor such infants over time for neuromuscular tone and make further evaluation if physiological immaturity is not determined to be a contributing factor. Hypotonia may also indicate a variety of systemic conditions. Common causes are cerebral trauma or perinatal hypoxia, but most neuromuscular disorders with hypotonia as the presenting symptom, especially Down syndrome and spinal muscular atrophy, are genetically determined. Additional conditions that may present in the neonatal period include inborn errors of metabolism such as glycogen storage disease; congenital and metabolic myopathies; cerebral dysgenesis such as lissencephaly; and congenital muscular dystrophies.

Clinical Manifestations

Hypotonia is marked by diminished muscle tone and weakness in both spontaneous and passive motion and reflex testing. The affected infant, when placed in a supine position, assumes a characteristic 'frog-leg posture' or lies in some other unusual position at rest. Normally the neonate or infant who is held in horizontal suspension (i.e. with the examiner's hand supporting the infant under the chest) responds by slightly raising the head with the back relatively straight, the arms flexed and slightly abducted and the knees partly flexed. The hypotonic infant droops over the supporting hand with head and extremities hanging loosely, resembling an inverted U. The muscles feel atrophied when palpated, and there is marked head lag when the infant is pulled to a sitting position. Poor sucking may be noted. *Floppy infant syndrome* was the term traditionally used to describe infants with hypotonia.

Diagnostic evaluation

The infant with hypotonia presents a diagnostic challenge. The child's and family's history and the physical examination offer important clues to the general category of causes, such as central or motor neuron disorders. Laboratory diagnosis may include a CK level specific for skeletal muscle. Molecular deoxyribonucleic acid (DNA) analysis may eliminate the need for additional invasive tests when a definitive diagnosis is made for a hereditary myopathy or neuropathy (Sarnat 2015a). Nerve conduction velocity, electromyography (EMG) and muscle biopsy may be used in diagnostic testing. Accurate diagnosis is essential for appropriate treatment, genetic implications and family counselling.

Therapeutic and Nursing Care Management

The management of an infant with hypotonia is determined by the cause of the hypotonia. It is a nursing responsibility to record and report findings that suggest hypotonia in an infant so that further evaluation can be carried out and therapeutic measures implemented if indicated.

Spinal Muscular Atrophy Type 1 (Werdnig-Hoffmann disease)

Spinal muscular atrophy (SMA) type 1 (Werdnig-Hoffmann disease) is a disorder characterised by progressive weakness and wasting of skeletal muscles caused by degeneration of anterior horn cells. It is inherited as an autosomal recessive trait and is the most common paralytic form of the **floppy infant syndrome (congenital hypotonia)**. The sites of the pathological condition are the anterior horn cells of the spinal cord and the motor nuclei of the brainstem, but the primary effect is atrophy of skeletal muscles.

Clinical Manifestations

The age of onset is variable, but the earlier the onset, the more disseminated and severe the motor weakness. The disorder may be manifested early—often at birth—and almost always before 2 years of age; death may occur as a result of respiratory failure by age 2 years (Iannaccone & Burghes 2002).

The manifestations (Box 34.7) and prognosis are categorised according to the age of onset, severity of weakness and clinical course; some children may fluctuate between exhibiting symptoms of types 1 and 2 or types 2 and 3 in regard to clinical function (Sarnat 2015a). Some experts also categorise SMA according to the highest level of motor function; type 1 includes 'non-sitters', type 2 includes 'sitters' and type 3 includes 'walkers' (Iannaccone 2007). A severe rare fetal form of SMA, classified as type 0, is reported to be quite lethal in the perinatal period; motor neuron degeneration may be noted as early as midgestation in type 0 (Sarnat 2015a). Type 4 may present between 20 and 30 years of age and may be referred to as proximal adult-type SMA (Prior 2010).

BOX 34.7 Clinical Manifestations of Spinal Muscular Atrophy

Type 1 (Werdnig-Hoffmann Disease)

- Clinical manifestations within first few weeks or months of life
- Onset within 6 months of life
- Inactivity the most prominent feature
- Infant lying in a frog-leg position with legs externally rotated, abducted and flexed at knees
- Generalised weakness
- Absent deep tendon reflexes
- Limited movements of shoulder and arm muscles
- Active movement usually limited to fingers and toes
- Diaphragmatic breathing with sternal retractions (diaphragmatic paralysis may occur)
- Abnormal tongue movements (at rest)
- Weak cry and cough
- Poor suck reflex
- Fatigues quickly during feedings (if breastfed, may lose weight before noticeable)
- Failure to thrive (nutritional)
- Alert facies
- Normal sensation and intellect
- Affected infants not able to sit alone, roll over or walk
- Early death possible from respiratory failure or infection

Type 2 (Intermediate Spinal Muscular Atrophy)

- Onset before age 18 months
  - **Early**—Weakness confined to arms and legs
  - **Later**—Becomes generalised
- Legs usually involved to greater extent than arms
- Prominent pectus excavatum
- Movements absent during complete relaxation or sleep
- Some infants able to sit if placed in position, but few can ambulate
- For most, life span varies from 7 months to 7 years, although many have normal life expectancy

Type 3 (Kugelberg-Welander Syndrome; Mild Spinal Muscular Atrophy)

- Onset of symptoms after 18 months of age
- Normal head control and ability to sit unassisted by 6–8 months of age
- Thigh and hip muscles weak
- Scoliosis common
- Failure to walk a common presentation
- In those who manage to walk:
  - Waddling gait
  - Genu recurvatum
  - Protuberant abdomen
  - Ambulation becoming increasingly difficult
  - Permanent use of wheelchair by second decade
- Deep tendon reflexes may be present early but disappear

Type IV (Adult Spinal Muscular Atrophy)

- Rare, adult-onset spinal muscular atrophy usually in second or third decade of life; muscle weakness is first symptom

Diagnostic Evaluation

The diagnosis is based on the molecular genetic marker for the *SMN* (survival motor neuron) gene, which is located on chromosome *5q13*. Prenatal diagnosis may be made by genetic analysis of circulating fetal cells in maternal blood or circulating fetal cells in amniotic fluid. The risk for subsequent affected offspring in carriers of the mutant gene or in families with known cases of SMA may also be evaluated genetically. Further diagnostic studies include muscle electromyography (EMG), which demonstrates a denervation pattern, and muscle biopsy;

however, the genetic analysis has become the gold standard for diagnosis of the condition (Sarnat 2015a).

Therapeutic Management

There is no cure for the disease, and treatment is symptomatic and supportive, primarily preventing joint contractures and treating orthopaedic problems, the most serious of which is scoliosis. Hip subluxation and dislocation may also occur. Many children benefit from powered wheelchairs, lifts, special pressure-adjustable mattresses and accessible environmental controls. Muscle and joint contractures require careful attention and care to prevent further complications. Nutritional growth failure may occur in infants and toddlers as a result of poor feeding; supplemental gastrostomy feedings may be required to maintain adequate nutritional status and maintain weight gain. The use of lower extremity orthoses may assist with ambulation, but eventually the child may be required to use a wheelchair permanently as muscle atrophy progresses. Restrictive lung disease is the most serious complication of SMA (Iannaccone 2007). Upper respiratory tract infections often occur and are treated with antibiotic therapy; they are the cause of death in many children. Rapid eye movement (REM)–related sleep-disordered breathing is common in children with SMA type 1; this progresses to sleep-disordered breathing during REM and non-REM sleep followed by respiratory failure, which often requires nocturnal non-invasive mechanical ventilation (Schroth 2009). Non-invasive ventilation methods such as bilevel positive airway pressure (BiPAP) have decreased the morbidity and increased the survival rate of children with SMA types 1 and 2. Children with SMA type 1 who undergo tracheotomy and invasive ventilation often remain ventilator dependent for the rest of their lives; some families choose to withdraw support when invasive ventilation becomes necessary (Mercuri et al 2012). Palliative care is an important aspect of care for families of children with SMA type 1. A decreased ability to cough and clear secretions may be managed with airway clearance therapies such as the cough assist machine and manual cough assistance. Guidelines for the standardisation of respiratory care for patients with SMA have been published elsewhere (Schroth 2009).

In addition to non-invasive respiratory support, some infants and children may benefit from tracheostomy and mechanical ventilation. If untreated, some infants may die of respiratory complications in infancy.

Associated medical conditions in survivors include gastro-oesophageal reflux, scoliosis, early-onset puberty, hip dysplasia and recurrent oral candidiasis (Bach 2007). A referral to paediatric palliative care may help the families of children with SMA make decisions about the benefits and burdens of treatment options.

A new therapy to treat SMA is an antisense oligonucleotide (ASO) called Spinraza (nusinersen) that consists of small strings of synthetic nucleotides that selectively bind ribonucleic acid (RNA). It was designed to treat infants with SMA. In recent studies, treated infants experienced a statistically significant improvement in motor milestones compared with those not treated. The medication is given by intrathecal injection. This allows it to be delivered directly to the CSF around the spinal cord, where motor neurons degenerate in SMA patients due to insufficient levels of SMN protein. Spinraza is designed to alter the splicing of SMN2 to increase the production of full-length SMN protein. Although not a cure, it is showing promise of improving motor skills in infants with SMA (Finkel et al 2016).

Nursing Care Management

An infant or a small child with progressive muscle weakness requires nursing care similar to that of an immobilised patient. However, the underlying goal of treatment should be to assist the child and family in dealing with the illness while progressing towards a life of normalisation within the child's capabilities. Special attention should be directed to preventing muscle and joint contractures, promoting independence in performance of ADLs and becoming incorporated into the mainstream of school when possible. In addition, parents need support and resources to be able to provide for the child and remain an intact family. Because children with neuromuscular disease have abnormal breathing patterns that often contribute to early death, it is important to assess adequate oxygenation, especially during the sleep phase when shallow breathing occurs and hypoxaemia may develop. Home pulse oximetry may be used to assess the child during sleep and provide non-invasive mechanical ventilation as necessary (Bush et al 2005, Young et al 2007). Supportive care also includes management of orthoses and other orthopaedic equipment as required. Because children with SMA are intellectually normal, verbal, tactile and auditory stimulation are important aspects of developmental care. Supporting them so they can see the activities around them and transporting them in appropriate equipment (e.g. wagon, power wheelchair) for a change of environment provide stimulation and a broader scope of contacts.

Children who are able to sit require proper support and attention to alignment to prevent deformities and other complications. Children who survive beyond infancy need attention to educational needs and opportunities for social interaction with other children. Parents who have not sought genetic counselling should be encouraged to do so to evaluate further risk potential.

Juvenile Spinal Muscular Atrophy (Kugelberg-Welander disease)

Spinal muscular atrophy type 3 (Kugelberg-Welander disease) is a result of anterior horn cell and motor nerve degeneration. The disease is characterised by a pattern of muscular weakness similar to that of infantile SMA (see Box 34.7). Several modes of inheritance have been reported for the disease: autosomal recessive, autosomal dominant and X-linked recessive.

The onset occurs from younger than 1 year of age into adulthood, with symptoms resembling group 3 infantile SMA. Proximal muscle weakness (especially of the lower limbs) and muscular atrophy are the predominant features. The disease runs a slowly progressive course. Some children lose the ability to walk 8 to 9 years after the onset of symptoms, but many can still walk after 30 years or more. One source notes that approximately half of all children with SMA type 3 lose ambulation by age 14 years and may require a wheelchair when falls are more frequent (Mercuri 2012). Many affected persons have a normal life expectancy.

Therapeutic and Nursing Care Management

Promising results from ongoing clinical trials suggest treatments that increase SMN protein might provide clinical benefit to patients with SMA (Chiriboga et al 2016). However, the management is primarily symptomatic and supportive and is related to maintaining mobility as long as possible, preventing complications such as skin breakdown, optimising and maintaining respiratory function and providing support to the child and family. The discussion of family support in the section for Duchenne muscular dystrophy is also applicable to families of children with SMA.

Guillain-Barré Syndrome

Guillain-Barré syndrome (GBS), also known as *infectious polyneuritis*, is an uncommon acute demyelinating polyneuropathy with a progressive, usually ascending, flaccid paralysis. The hallmark of GBS is acute peripheral motor weakness. The paralysis usually occurs approximately 10 days after a non-specific viral infection; GBS has also been reported after administration of certain vaccines (e.g. rabies, influenza, polio and meningococcal) (Sarnat 2015b). Several subtypes of GBS include acute inflammatory demyelinating neuropathy, acute motor axonal neuropathy, acute motor sensory axonal neuropathy and Miller Fisher syndrome. Children are less often affected than adults; among children, those between ages 4 and 10 years have higher susceptibility. The male-to-female ratio is reported to be 1.5 to 1. Two peak periods with an increased incidence of GBS have been identified: late adolescence and young adulthood.

Chronic inflammatory demyelinating polyradiculoneuropathies (CIDPs) are chronic types of GBS that recur intermittently or do not improve over a period of months to years (Sarnat 2015b). The following discussion focuses on GBS.

Congenital GBS is rare, yet may occur in the neonatal period, and consists of hypotonia, weakness and decreased or absent reflexes. Maternal neuromuscular disease may or may not be present. Diagnosis is established by the same criteria as in older children, but the symptoms gradually subside over the first few months of life and disappear by 12 months (Sarnat 2015b).

Pathophysiology

GBS is an immune-mediated disease often associated with a number of viral or bacterial infections or the administration of certain vaccines. It has been associated with infectious mononucleosis, measles, mumps, *Campylobacter jejuni* (gastroenteritis), cytomegalovirus, *Borrelia burgdorferi* (Lyme disease), Epstein-Barr virus, *Helicobacter pylori* and *Mycoplasma* and *Pneumocystis* infections. Onset of GBS symptoms usually occurs within 10 days of the primary infection. Pathological changes in spinal and cranial nerves consist of inflammation and oedema with rapid, segmented demyelination and compression of nerve roots within the dural sheath. Nerve conduction is impaired, producing ascending partial or complete paralysis of muscles innervated by the involved nerves. GBS has three phases.

1. Acute—Phase starts when symptoms begin and continues until new symptoms stop appearing or deterioration ceases; it may last as long as 4 weeks.
2. Plateau—Symptoms remain constant without further deterioration; it may last from days to weeks.
3. Recovery—Patient begins to improve and progress to optimal recovery; it usually lasts a few weeks to months, depending on the deficits incurred by the illness.

Clinical Manifestations

A mild influenza-like illness or sore throat usually precedes the paralytic manifestations of GBS. The onset can be rapid, reaching peak activity within 24 hours, or there may be a gradual progression of symptoms over days or weeks. Neurological symptoms initially involve muscle tenderness that sometimes is accompanied by paraesthesia and cramps. Proximal muscle weakness progressing to paralysis usually occurs before distal weakness, and there is a tendency towards symmetrical involvement. In most patients paralysis ascends from the lower extremities, often involving the muscles of the trunk and upper extremities and those supplied by cranial nerves. The seventh cranial (facial) nerve is often affected.

Tendon reflexes are depressed or absent, and paralysis is flaccid. Paralysis may involve facial, extraocular, labial, lingual, pharyngeal and laryngeal muscles. Evidence of intercostal and phrenic nerve involvement includes breathlessness in vocalisations and shallow, irregular respirations. There may be variable degrees of sensory impairment. Most patients complain of muscle tenderness or sensitivity to slight pressure. Lower limb pain and back pain are common in children with GBS. Urinary incontinence or retention and constipation are often present. Abdominal pain and fatigue have also been reported in children with GBS (Lyons 2008).

Autonomic nervous system disturbances may occur in children and adolescents with severe muscle involvement and respiratory muscle paralysis. These include orthostatic hypotension; hypertension; and vagal responses such as bradycardia, asystole and heart block (Laskowski-Jones 2007).

Diagnostic Evaluation

Diagnosis is based on the paralytic manifestations, CSF analysis and EMG. Motor nerve conduction velocities are greatly reduced. Sensory nerve conduction time is often slowed. CSF analysis reveals an elevated protein concentration, and fewer than 10 WBCs/mm^3 and normal glucose level (Sarnat 2015b). Other laboratory studies are usually noncontributory. The symmetrical nature of the paralysis helps differentiate this disorder from spinal paralytic poliomyelitis, which usually affects sporadic muscles.

Therapeutic Management

Treatment of GBS is primarily supportive. In the acute phase, patients are hospitalised because respiratory and pharyngeal involvement may require assisted ventilation, sometimes with a temporary tracheostomy. Treatment modalities include aggressive ventilatory support in the event of respiratory compromise, intravenous (IV) administration of immunoglobulin (IVIg) and sometimes steroids; plasmapheresis and immunosuppressive drugs may also be used. Plasmapheresis has been shown to decrease the length of recovery in patients with severe GBS; however, it is expensive, and side effects include hypotension, fever, bleeding disorders, chills, urticaria and bradycardia. Further evidence reports equal benefits to treatment of GBS with IVIg administration or plasmapheresis; both sped up recovery time in studies reviewed (Hughes & Cornblath 2005). There is evidence, however, of significant improvement in children with high-dose IVIg therapy (versus supportive treatment alone) (Hughes et al 2012). IVIg is now recommended as the primary treatment of GBS when administered within 2 weeks of disease onset (Hughes 2008). Corticosteroids alone do not decrease the symptoms or shorten the duration of the disease.

Additional medications that may be administered during the acute phase include a low molecular weight heparin to prevent deep vein thrombosis (DVT), a mild laxative or stool softener to prevent constipation and pain medication such as paracetamol. Chronic neuropathic pain after GBS may be treated with gabapentin, which is reported to be more effective than carbamazepine (Sarnat 2015b).

Rehabilitation after the acute phase may involve physical therapy, occupational therapy and speech therapy. Additional consideration should be given to problems of general weakness and retraining for toileting and feeding (Lyons 2008).

Prognosis. Better outcomes are associated with younger age, no requirement for mechanical respiratory assistance, slower progression of disease, normal peripheral nerve function on EMG and treatment with either IVIg or plasmapheresis. Recovery usually begins within 2 to 3 weeks, and most patients regain full muscle strength. The recovery of muscle strength progresses in the reverse order of onset of paralysis, with lower extremity strength being the last to recover. Poor prognosis with subsequent residual effects in children is reportedly associated with cranial nerve involvement, extensive disability at time of presentation and intubation.

Most deaths associated with GBS are caused by respiratory failure; therefore, early diagnosis and access to respiratory support are especially important. The rate of recovery is usually related to the degree of involvement and may extend from a few weeks to months. The greater the degree of paralysis, the longer the recovery phase.

Nursing Care Management

Nursing care is primarily supportive and is the same as that required for children with immobilisation and respiratory compromise. The emphasis of care is on close observation to assess the extent of paralysis and on prevention of complications, including aspiration, ventilator-associated pneumonia (VAP), atelectasis, DVT, pressure ulcer, fear and anxiety, autonomic dysfunction and pain.

During the acute phase of the disease, the nurse should carefully observe the child's condition for possible difficulty in swallowing and respiratory involvement. Vital signs are monitored frequently, as well as neurological signs and level of consciousness. For children who develop difficulty breathing, the care is the same as that for any child with respiratory distress requiring mechanical ventilation.

A key to recovery in the child with GBS is the prevention of muscle and joint contractures, so passive range-of-motion exercises must be carried out routinely to maintain vital function. Although the child may have a generalised paralysis, cognitive function remains intact; therefore, it is important for nursing care to involve communication with the child or adolescent regarding procedures and treatments that may be frightening, especially if mechanical ventilation is required. Encourage parents to talk to the child and make eye and physical contact and to reassure the child during this phase of the illness.

Pain management is crucial in the care of children with GBS. Although neuromuscular impairment may make pain perception more difficult to evaluate accurately, objective pain scales should be used. Gabapentin and carbamazepine may be used to manage neuropathic pain in patients with GBS.

Physical therapy may be limited to passive range-of-motion exercises during the evolving phase of the disease. Later, as the disease stabilises and recovery begins, an active physical therapy program is implemented to prevent contracture deformities and facilitate muscle recovery. This may include active exercise, gait training and bracing.

Throughout the course of the illness, child and parent support are paramount. The usual rapidity of the paralysis and the long recovery period greatly tax the emotional reserves of all family members. The parents and child benefit from repeated reassurance that recovery is occurring and from realistic information regarding the possibility of permanent disability. In the event of a residual disability, the family needs assistance in accepting and adjusting to the loss of function.

Spinal Cord Injuries

SCIs with major neurological involvement are not a common cause of physical disability in children. However, many children with these injuries are admitted to major medical centres, and because of the increased survival rate as a result of improved management, nurses have an important role in the care of children with SCI.

The principles of management and nursing care of the child with a spinal cord lesion apply regardless of cause. In addition to care related to the immobilised child, as discussed in Chapter 33, children with damage to the spinal cord present additional problems—specifically, complications related to the neuropathology of the central and autonomic nervous systems. The extent of paralysis is determined by both neurological and clinical assessment. Although the majority of children with SCI are paraplegic, some are tetraplegic (quadriplegic). Some children with tetraplegia are able to move only their face and neck muscles, whereas others are able to lift and bend their arms but are unable to perform fine hand movements. Almost every physiological system is disrupted in a child with high-level tetraplegia. Not only are the central and peripheral nerves impaired, but there is also autonomic nervous system dysfunction. Vital structures such as blood vessels, lungs, bladder and bowel are affected. Therefore, an understanding of neuromuscular physiology is essential to effectively care for the child with damage or injury to the spinal cord.

Essential Neuromuscular Physiology

The spinal cord extends from the medulla oblongata to the lower border of the first lumbar vertebra and contains millions of nerve fibres. However, because of its protected location, a considerable amount of direct trauma is required to cause injury. Posteriorly the cord is protected by the spinous processes, which are stabilised by related ligaments and muscles. It is further protected by the spinal fluid, which surrounds it and absorbs some of the shock.

Spinal Nerves. The 31 nerves of the spinal cord are divided into five segments (Fig 34.7). The cervical cord segments lie within the first seven vertebrae. The remaining cord segments—thoracic (12), lumbar (5), sacral (5) and coccygeal (1)—extend from the first thoracic vertebra to the lower level of the first lumbar vertebra. Therefore, the cord constituents do not anatomically match by number the 33 associated vertebrae. However, nerves that arise from the spinal cord exit from the spinal column at the numerically corresponding vertebrae. In describing injuries to the spinal cord, the highest point at which there is normal function is referred to in relation to the vertebra; for example, an intact cord at the sixth cervical vertebra is designated a C6 injury.

Certain areas of the curved vertebral column are less stable and more prone to damage from severe flexion and twisting. These sites are the cervical area and the junction of the thoracic and lumbar regions. The cervical vertebrae are fractured most often, and this high level of injury causes extensive paralysis and many associated neurological problems (Table 34.1). Also, traumatic tearing or embolic occlusion of the arteries supplying these areas can markedly jeopardise the cord tissue. Impaired blood supply often produces severe neurological deficit, which can extend to complete loss of cord function at the level of injury.

Cell bodies of interneurons and motor neurons within the spinal cord are identified as H-shaped grey matter surrounded by columns of white myelinated nerve fibres. Each column serves as a route for a specific type of impulse, such as touch, vibration, pain and temperature (Fig 34.8). Nerve pathways in the spinal cord transmit sensory and motor impulses between peripheral receptors and the brain, conduct impulses through the reflex arc and convey sympathetic and parasympathetic nerve impulses from the brain to peripheral structures.

Sensory transmission begins when peripheral receptors pick up a wide variety of stimuli and transfer the impulses, by means of peripheral nerves, to the spinal nerves, where they make ganglionic connections and enter the cord posteriorly. At this point the impulses travel in two directions: across the interneuron connection and then to the motor neurons (reflex arc), or up the spinal cord to predetermined areas of the brain. Motor impulses are transmitted from the cerebral cortex to the medulla (where nerve tracts cross) and proceed down descending motor pathways to the desired level within the spinal cord. Here they connect with the anterior horn cells and are transmitted to the muscle fibres by means of the lower motor neurons to complete a meaningful movement.

A network of nerves that serves the major muscle groups constitutes a plexus. Total involvement of any one of these plexuses seriously impairs function to the areas it innervates. Box 34.8 describes the three major plexuses.

TABLE 34.1 Functional Significance of Spinal Cord Lesions

Highest Intact Cord Segment	Muscle Innervation	Functional Capacity	Functional Goals
TETRAPLEGIA			
C1–C3	None below chin, including phrenic nerve to diaphragm	No voluntary control below chin Respiratory paralysis complete May cause bradycardia or tachycardia, vomiting	Mechanical ventilation; can be taught glossopharyngeal breathing to be used for short periods Electric wheelchair Adaptive equipment for special tasks in bed or wheelchair using mouth stick
C4	Intact sternocleidomastoid, trapezius, upper cervical paraspinal muscle	No voluntary function of upper extremities, trunk or lower extremities All neck movements Mechanical ventilation dependent	Electric wheelchair Externally powered devices and adaptive equipment for special tasks in bed or wheelchair with mouth stick, such as turning pages, using computer Totally dependent for activities of daily living
C5	Partial deltoid, biceps, major muscles of rotator cuffs at shoulders Diaphragm	Abduction, flexion and extension of arm Flexion and extension of forearm Unable to roll over or attain sitting position Abdominal respiration Poor respiratory reserve	Electric wheelchair Requires attendant to assist in moving and transfer to wheelchair Adaptive devices for self-feeding, grooming, using computer Vocational potential with adaptive devices
C6	Pectoralis major, serratus anterior, latissimus dorsi muscles Complete deltoid and brachioradialis muscles Partial triceps muscle	Significant increase in function over that with lesion at C5 level Adduction and medial rotation of arm Wrist extension Good elbow flexion	Cuff strapped to hand to permit use of implements for self-care and other activities Able to assist in dressing and transfer Hand rim extension to permit independence in wheelchair
C7	Triceps and finger flexion and extensor muscle Shoulder depressor muscles Still nerve disruption to intercostal muscles	With elbow stabilised in extension and intact shoulder depressor muscles, able to lift body weight Grasp and release still weak; dexterity lacking	Almost complete independence within limitations of wheelchair Requires some assistance in transfer and lower extremity dressing Hand splints helpful Can roll over in bed, sit up in bed and eat independently Homebound employment possible; outside work usually not feasible
PARAPLEGIA			
T1–T10	Full innervation of upper extremity muscles	Full use of upper extremities, including intrinsic muscles of hand Trunk balance poor—may have difficulty lifting trunk sufficiently to put on lower extremity clothing Considerable energy expenditure to put on long leg braces with extensive attachments	Completely wheelchair dependent Trunk balance benefits from training Able to drive motor vehicle with hand controls May be braced for standing May hold job away from home Can manage adapted public transportation
T10–L2	Full abdominal and upper back muscle control	Good trunk balance Good respiratory reserve Can accomplish moderate hip hiking using external oblique and latissimus dorsi muscles	Ambulation with bilateral long braces using four-point or swing-through crutch gait Usually able to negotiate kerbs Some able to use regular public transportation Few vocational limitations as long as does not require much walking or standing
L3–L4	Quadriceps muscle Partial gluteus and hamstring muscles	May have lumbar lordosis Floppy ankles	Ambulates well, often with short leg braces with or without cane Difficulty in getting out of wheelchair May never require wheelchair

BOX 34.8 The Three Major Plexuses

1. **Cervical Plexus (C1–C4)**—Innervates the neck and diaphragm
2. **Brachial Plexus (C4–T1)**—Supplies the shoulders, chest and arms
3. **Lumbosacral Plexus (L1–S4)**—Transmits impulses to the lower trunk and legs

Upper versus Lower Motor Neurons. Upper motor neurons extend from cerebral centres to cells in the spinal column; lower motor neurons consist of anterior horn cells and spinal and peripheral nerves. Motor fibres of the reflex arc are lower motor neurons. This is an important point because relative dominance of the CNS over reflex arcs suppresses some reflex responses. When the higher centres no longer exert an influence in SCI, spastic responses are observed in muscles innervated by the intact lower motor neurons. Most SCIs involve upper motor neurons; children born with spinal cord defects have primarily lower motor neuron deficits (see Fig 34.7). Box 34.9 outlines manifestations of upper and lower motor neuron syndromes.

Effect on Sensory and Motor Tracts. Voluntary muscle control is lost after complete transection of the cord. In partial transection, function is altered to varying degrees depending on the areas innervated by involved nerves. The crossing of motor tracts at various levels makes it possible for an injured person to have motor paralysis in one leg but retain pain and temperature sensation in that leg, while the opposite leg retains its motor function but loses pain and temperature sensation.

Although a transected cord injury leads to sensory loss, it is not uncommon for the injured person to experience pain. For example, smooth or skeletal muscle spasms, destruction of the myelin sheath (impulses cross to adjacent nerves) and scar formation or irritation of nerve endings may cause pain. Pain suffered by a person with tetraplegia or paraplegia is often intensified because of loss of sensation in other parts. Severe and prolonged pain should be medically evaluated for a treatable pathological condition.

Effect on Autonomic System. Sympathetic and parasympathetic systems receive both excitatory and inhibitory stimuli from autonomic centres in the cerebral cortex, limbic system and hypothalamus. The stimuli are transmitted by means of a feedback mechanism within the ascending fibres of the cord that normally controls descending input. Axons of the many CNS neurons synapse with autonomic preganglionic fibres and thus are able to alter their patterned responses. Box 34.10 describes the most significant effects of autonomic disruption.

BOX 34.9 Differences in Clinical Manifestations Between Upper and Lower Motor Neuron Syndromes

Upper Motor Neuron Syndrome

- Spastic paralysis in muscle groups below lesion (intact reflex arcs below lesion)
- Hyperreflexia with tendon reflexes exaggerated, Babinski's reflex present
- No wasting of muscle mass because of increased muscle tone
- Flexion contractures and spasms of muscle groups below lesion level common
- No skin or tissue changes

Lower Motor Neuron Syndrome

- Flaccid paralysis caused by muscle atonia (reflex arcs permanently damaged)
- Reflex with associated muscle response absent
- Marked atrophy of atonic muscle
- Fasciculations (local twitching of muscle groups) common
- No flexor spasms
- Loss of hair
- Skin and tissue changes
- Cornified nails

BOX 34.10 Significant Effects of Autonomic Disruption

- Decreased muscle tone and impairment of vasoconstrictive effects of sympathetic innervation cause venous pooling; diminished venous return to the heart; decreased cardiac output; and hypotension, especially orthostatic hypotension (orthostatic intolerance).
- Thermoregulatory disruption in the hypothalamus and skin receptors causes blood vessels to remain dilated during the initial stage, an inability to sweat in response to increased environmental temperature and a possible rapid elevation in body temperature.
- Voluntary bowel and bladder functions are lost because of damage to nerve fibres that innervate these organs.
- Altered sexual function (lack of erection, ejaculation and orgasm) results from interference with numerous autonomic nerve fibres and plexuses.

Aetiology

The most common cause of serious spinal cord damage in children is trauma involving motor vehicle crashes (MVC) (including motor bikes and all-terrain vehicles), sports injuries (especially from diving, trampoline activities, gymnastics and football), birth trauma and non-accidental trauma.

Congenital defects of the spine such as myelomeningocele also may in some cases produce the effects of SCI (see p. 981).

Transverse myelitis (inflammation of the spinal cord) may be caused by illness and has also been reported to develop from inadvertent intraarterial administration of long-acting penicillin injected into the buttocks. Damage can be extensive enough to result in paraplegia or even lower limb amputation.

In MVCs, most SCIs in children are a result of indirect trauma caused by sudden hyperflexion or hyperextension of the neck, often combined with a rotational force. Trauma to the spinal cord without evidence of vertebral fracture or dislocation (**SCI without radiographic abnormality**, or SCIWORA) is particularly likely to occur in an MVC when proper safety restraints are not used. An unrestrained child becomes a projectile during sudden deceleration and is subject to injury from contact with a variety of objects inside and outside the vehicle. Individuals who use only a lap seat belt restraint are at greater risk for SCI than those who use a combination lap and shoulder restraint. High cervical spine injuries have been reported in children younger than 2 years who are improperly restrained in forward-facing car seats. Infants who are improperly restrained in an infant car seat may experience cervical trauma in a car crash. Small children may also be severely injured by front seat air bags being deployed.

Falling from heights occurs less often in children than in adults, but vertebral compression from blows to the head or buttocks can occur in water sports (diving and surfing), falls from horses or other athletic activities. Birth injuries may occur in breech births from traction force on the spinal cord during birth of the head and shoulders. When shaken, infants commonly sustain cervical cord damage, as well as subdural haematoma and retinal haemorrhage; cognitive impairment and death may occur subsequent to the traumatic event. Infants have weak neck muscles, and during vigorous shaking, their large and heavy heads rapidly wobble back and forth.

Because of the marked mobility of the neck, fracture or **subluxation** (partial dislocation) is the most common immediate cause of SCI, particularly in the lower cervical region. Although unusual in adults, SCI without fracture is common in children, whose spines are suppler, weaker and more mobile than those of adults. Therefore, the force is more easily dissipated over a larger number of segments. In infants and small children younger than 5 years, upper cervical spine fractures and spinal compression are more common, but adolescents tend to have lower cervical and thoracolumbar fracture dislocations (Pruitt & McMahon 2015, Rekate 2015). Children who suffer SCI before puberty are reported to experience a higher incidence of musculoskeletal complications such as scoliosis and hip dislocation (Vogel et al 2012).

Pathophysiology

The severity of the force, the mechanisms of the injury and the degree of the individual's muscular relaxation at the time of the injury greatly influence the extent of the trauma. SCIs are classified as either *complete* or *incomplete.* In a complete injury, there is no motor or sensory function more than three segments below the neurological level of the injury (Mathison et al 2008). Incomplete lesions have several typical characteristics (Mathison et al 2008).

- Central cord syndrome—Central grey matter destruction and preservation of peripheral tracts; tetraplegia with sacral sparing common; some motor recovery gained.
- Anterior cord syndrome—Complete motor and sensory loss with trunk and lower extremity proprioception and sensation of pressure.
- Posterior cord syndrome—Loss of sensation, pain and proprioception with normal cord function, including motor function; able to move extremities but have difficulty controlling such movements.
- Brown-Séquard syndrome—Unilateral cord lesion with a motor deficit on the opposite side of the body from the primary insult; absence of pain and temperature sensation on the opposite side from the injury.
- Spinal cord concussion—Transient loss of neural function below the level of the acute spinal cord lesion, resulting in flaccid paralysis and loss of tendon, autonomic and cutaneous reflex activity; may last hours to weeks.

The American Spinal Injury Association (ASIA) (Kirshblum et al 2011) International Standards for Neurological Classification of Spinal Cord Injury worksheet was recently revised and published in the cited reference. The ASIA Impairment Scale (Box 34.11) combines motor and sensory function and is used to determine the severity of impairment from the injury (complete or incomplete). It may also be used to measure neurological changes and functional goals for rehabilitation (Mathison et al 2008).

The injury sustained can affect any of the spinal nerves, and the higher the injury, the more extensive the damage. The child can be left with complete or partial paralysis of the lower extremities (**paraplegia**) or with damage at a higher level and without functional use of any of the four extremities (**tetraplegia**). A high cervical cord injury that affects the phrenic nerve paralyses the diaphragm and leaves the child dependent on mechanical ventilation.

A mild but equally frightening form of cord trauma is **spinal cord compression**, a temporary neural dysfunction without visible damage to the cord. Complete tetraplegia can result but initially may not be differentiated from serious cord injury.

Clinical Manifestations

It is often difficult to determine the extent and severity of damage at first. Immediate loss of function is caused by both anatomical and impaired physiological function, and improved function may not be evident for weeks or even months. Manifestation of the initial response to acute SCI is flaccid paralysis below the level of the damage. This stage is often referred to as **spinal shock syndrome** and is caused by the sudden disruption of central and autonomic pathways. Local effects of cord oedema and ischaemia produce a physiological transection with or without an anatomical severance. Most children with an SCI experience some spinal shock. Manifestations include the absence of reflexes at or below the cord lesion, with flaccidity or limpness of the involved muscles, loss of sensation and motor function and autonomic dysfunction (i.e. symptoms of hypotension, low or high body temperature, loss of bladder and bowel control and autonomic dysreflexia). It is estimated that 25% to 50% of children with SCI will have a delay in the onset of neurological abnormalities ranging from 30 minutes to 4 days (Vogel et al 2012).

Autonomic paralysis also affects thermoregulatory functions. Afferent impulses from temperature receptors in the skin are not integrated; therefore, the patient is subject to temperature increases or decreases in response to alterations in environmental temperature. Hyperthermia can result from excessive ambient temperature, such as too many covers.

Except in the situations previously mentioned, flaccid paralysis is replaced by spinal reflex activity and increasing spasticity or, in incomplete lesions, greater or lesser degree of neurological recovery.

The paralytic nature of autonomic function is replaced by **autonomic dysreflexia**, especially when the lesions are above the midthoracic level. This autonomic phenomenon is caused by visceral distension or irritation, particularly of the bowel or bladder. Sensory impulses are triggered and travel to the cord lesion, where they are blocked, which causes activation of sympathetic reflex action with disturbed central inhibitory control. Excessive sympathetic activity is manifested by a flushing face, sweating forehead, pupillary constriction, marked hypertension, headache and bradycardia. The precipitating stimulus may be merely a full bladder or rectum or other internal or external sensory input. It can be a catastrophic event unless the irritation is relieved.

Additional clinical findings of SCI may include numbness, tingling or burning; priapism; weakness; and loss of bowel and bladder control (Hayes & Arriola 2005).

BOX 34.11 American Spinal Injury Association Impairment Scale

A—Complete: No motor or sensory function is preserved in the sacral segments S4–S5.

B—Sensory Incomplete: Sensory but not motor function is preserved below the neurological level and includes the sacral segments S4–S5, or deep anal pressure, AND no motor function is preserved more than three levels below the motor level on either side of the body.

C—Motor Incomplete: Motor function is preserved below the neurological level,* and more than half of key muscle functions below the single neurologic level of injury have a muscle grade less than 3.

D—Motor Incomplete: Motor function is preserved below the neurological level,* and at least half (or more) of key muscles below the neurological level have a muscle grade of 3 or more.

E—Normal: If sensation and motor function as tested with the International Standards for Neurological Classification of Spinal Cord Injury (ISNCSCI) are graded as normal in all segments, and the patient had prior deficits, then the AIS grade is E. Someone without an initial SCI does not receive an AIS grade.

*For further details and instructions see the online page at http://www.asia-spinalinjury.org/elearning/ISNCSCI_Exam_Sheet_r4.pdf.
Source: Used with permission, American Spinal Injury Association, 2011.

Neurogenic shock occurs as a result of a disruption in the descending sympathetic pathways with loss of vasomotor tone and sympathetic innervations to the cardiovascular system (Hayes & Arriola 2005). Hypotension, bradycardia and peripheral vasodilation occur as a result of neurogenic shock.

Children with suspected SCI may have suffered multiple injuries (e.g. MVC); therefore, multiple clinical manifestations may occur that may mask those of an SCI.

In the final stage neurological signs are stabilised in terms of loss and recovery of function. The major emphasis is on rehabilitation. A problem unique to injury in childhood is progressive spinal deformity usually not seen in adults or in adolescents near the end of the growth period. Scoliosis develops in the majority of children with high thoracic and cervical lesions and is almost certain to occur in children with tetraplegia whose injury occurred in infancy or early childhood.

Diagnostic Evaluation

A history of the injury provides valuable clues regarding the possible type of damage incurred and directions for further assessment without the risk of additional damage. A complete neurological examination determines whether damage was incurred and, if so, the level and extent of any nerve impairment. A neurological unit of the CNS is considered normal if reflex arcs are functioning, sensory tracts are intact when each dermatome is examined separately and voluntary motor response demonstrates an ability to move a body part against gravity on command.

Testing a reflex arc is accomplished by stimulating the peripheral receptors at a specific site, such as eliciting the patellar reflex. Symmetrical testing is performed to determine unilateral or bilateral neurological deficit. A sufficient number of reflexes are examined to test motor function thoroughly. The blunt end of a safety pin is used to assess pressure sensitivity, and the sharp point is used to elicit pain. Hot and cold water, a tuning fork and cotton may also be used to determinxe specific sensory loss (e.g. temperature, vibration and light touch).

The ASIA dermatome classification worksheet is used to determine the extent of neurological damage (Fig 34.9). Body surface zones, or **dermatomes**, accurately correspond to the spinal cord segment receiving the sensory input from the peripheral nerves in that zone. Systematically pinpricking the body surface in each zone determines intactness of sensory pathways. Fig 34.9 illustrates the zones and the spinal cord segments they represent. The examiner tests for each specific sensory fibre in the dermatome areas in which neurological deficit is suspected.

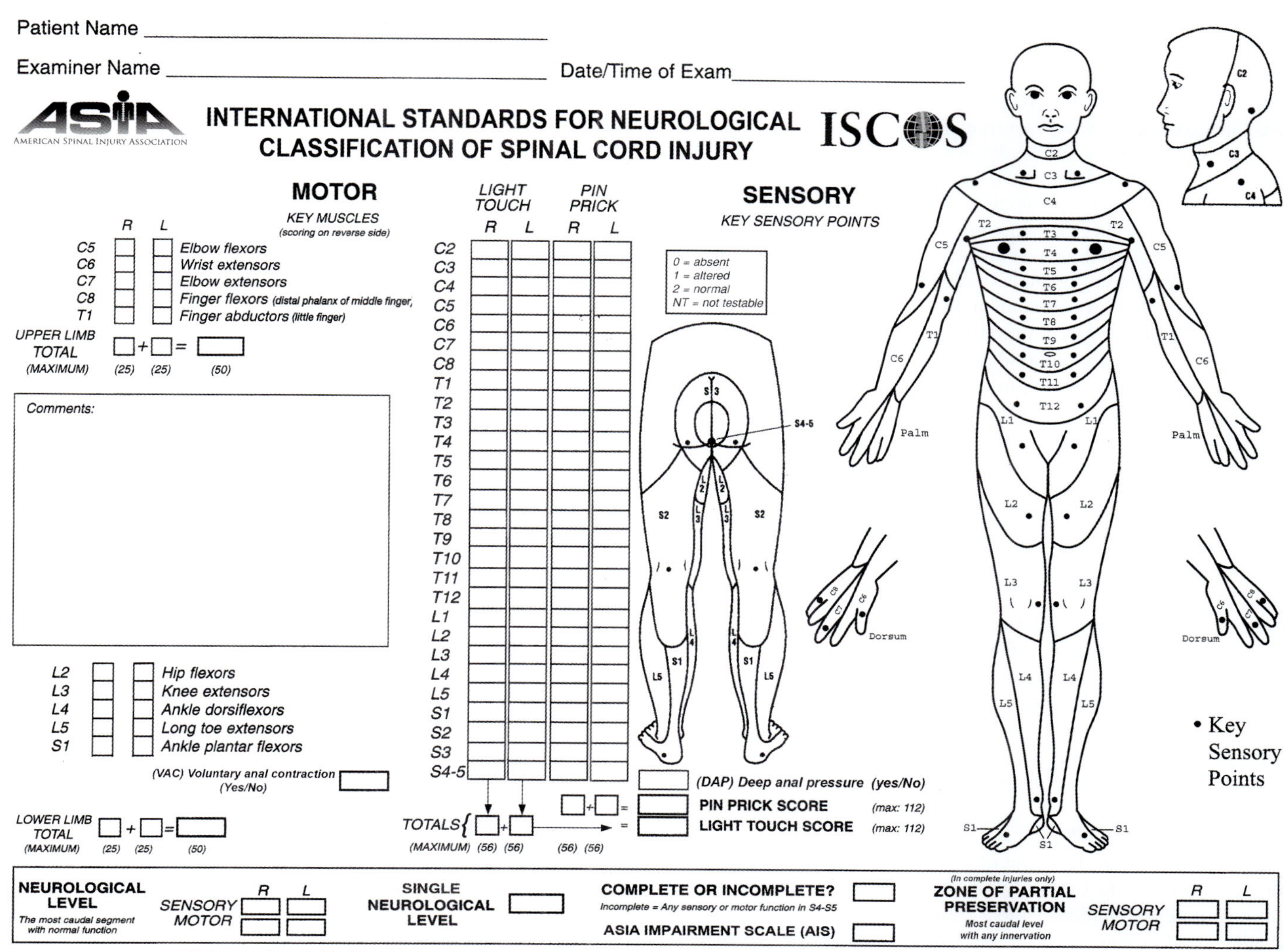

Patient Name ______

Examiner Name ______ Date/Time of Exam ______

ASIA — American Spinal Injury Association

INTERNATIONAL STANDARDS FOR NEUROLOGICAL CLASSIFICATION OF SPINAL CORD INJURY — ISCOS

MOTOR — KEY MUSCLES (scoring on reverse side)

	R	L	
C5			Elbow flexors
C6			Wrist extensors
C7			Elbow extensors
C8			Finger flexors (distal phalanx of middle finger)
T1			Finger abductors (little finger)

UPPER LIMB TOTAL (MAXIMUM) ☐ + ☐ = ☐ (25) (25) (50)

Comments:

	R	L	
L2			Hip flexors
L3			Knee extensors
L4			Ankle dorsiflexors
L5			Long toe extensors
S1			Ankle plantar flexors

(VAC) Voluntary anal contraction (Yes/No) ☐

LOWER LIMB TOTAL (MAXIMUM) ☐ + ☐ = ☐ (25) (25) (50)

	LIGHT TOUCH R	LIGHT TOUCH L	PIN PRICK R	PIN PRICK L
C2				
C3				
C4				
C5				
C6				
C7				
C8				
T1				
T2				
T3				
T4				
T5				
T6				
T7				
T8				
T9				
T10				
T11				
T12				
L1				
L2				
L3				
L4				
L5				
S1				
S2				
S3				
S4-5				

TOTALS { ☐ + ☐ ☐ + ☐ = ☐
(MAXIMUM) (56) (56) (56) (56)

SENSORY — KEY SENSORY POINTS

0 = absent
1 = altered
2 = normal
NT = not testable

(DAP) Deep anal pressure (yes/No) ☐

PIN PRICK SCORE (max: 112)

LIGHT TOUCH SCORE (max: 112)

NEUROLOGICAL LEVEL (The most caudal segment with normal function)	R	L	SINGLE NEUROLOGICAL LEVEL	COMPLETE OR INCOMPLETE? (Incomplete = Any sensory or motor function in S4-S5)	ZONE OF PARTIAL PRESERVATION (In complete injuries only) (Most caudal level with any innervation)	R	L
SENSORY					SENSORY		
MOTOR				ASIA IMPAIRMENT SCALE (AIS)	MOTOR		

This form may be copied freely but should not be altered without permission from the American Spinal Injury Association.

REV 04/11

Fig 34.9 ASIA classification of spinal cord injury. (Source: Used with permission, American Spinal Injury Association, 2011. http://asia-spinalinjury.org/?s=ASIA+spinal+cord+injury+classification)

Matching cord level to vertebra is more difficult in infants and young children than it is in older children and adults because the sacral and several lower lumbar cord segments lie at a lower position, especially during the first 2 years of life. The spinal anatomy approaches adult configuration by the time the child reaches age 7 or 8 years; by late adolescence the conus medullaris has usually reached the level of L1.

Motor system evaluation includes observing gait if the child is able to walk; noting balance maintenance with the child's eyes open and closed; and noting the ability to lift, flex and extend the arms and legs. Testing muscle strength with and without resistance and against gravity provides clues to the specific nature and degree of motor dysfunction. The number of muscles in any muscle group that remain completely intact in the upper extremities makes a marked difference in the individual's ability to provide self-care, especially at high injury levels. Hip movement is necessary for ambulation with braces and crutches.

The degree to which supportive aids are needed for ambulation is determined by the strength, stability and movement of the pelvis, trunk, hip flexor muscles and quadriceps muscles. A general guideline for determining the capacity for self-help is that a person with paraplegia who has function down to and including the quadriceps muscle or muscle function below the L3 level will have little difficulty in learning to walk with or without braces and crutches. It is especially vital that children with lumbar levels of injury be taught to walk functionally so that they are weight bearing at least part of the time; this minimises the risk of osteoporosis and hypercalcaemia. The functional significance of the spinal cord lesion level is given in Table 34.1.

If a CNS pathological disorder is detected, a body system assessment is performed to determine the degree of autonomic impairment. Because the cord and CNS directly influence the function of the autonomic nerves, the specific sympathetically related organ systems are examined for skeletal muscle and vascular tone and body temperature regulation. For example, bladder and GI functions have sympathetic and parasympathetic innervation and local reflexes.

CT and MRI scans are important for localising the lesion, but the nature of the spine in childhood often creates difficulty in interpretation. Guidelines for diagnostic imaging of children with suspected SCI have been published elsewhere (Rozelle et al 2013). Small children often have no radiographic evidence of vertebral or spinal injury despite significant injuries ranging from complete transection with major haemorrhage to minor haemorrhage, oedema or normal neural findings. This condition, SCIWORA, is reported to occur in approximately 64% of children 5 years of age or younger and in 19% to 32% of older children with SCIs (Launay et al 2005, Mathison et al 2008, Vogel et al 2012). The younger the child, the more likely for SCIWORA to occur—up to 72% of children 5 and under (Schottler et al 2012). SCIWORA is also a common finding in very young children who are victims of abuse (primarily shaken baby syndrome) because of the elasticity and incomplete ossification of the vertebrae. SCIWORA is more common in children under the age of 8 years, and injury to the cervical spine is common. Diagnostic scans must be taken carefully and with sufficient help to prevent further damage to the spine.

Therapeutic Management

Initial care begins at the scene of the accident or crash with proper immobilisation of the cervical, thoracic and lumbar spine. Immobilisation should take into account the age and size of the child; smaller children have a larger head size, which may make effective immobilisation on a rigid board difficult (Rozelle et al 2013). Because of the complexity of these injuries, it is usually recommended that these persons be transported to a spinal injury centre for care by specially trained healthcare personnel as soon as possible after the injury for appropriate diagnostic evaluation and intervention.

The initial management of the child with a suspected SCI should begin with an assessment of the ABCs: **A**irway, **B**reathing and **C**irculation. The airway should be opened using the jaw-thrust technique to minimise damage to the cervical spine. The child is monitored for cardiovascular instability, and measures are taken to support systemic blood pressure and maintain optimal cardiac output. Because MVCs and other trauma in children may involve internal organ damage and potential bleeding, abdominal distension and other signs are acted on immediately to prevent further systemic shock. After the child is stabilised and transported to a regional trauma centre, a thorough evaluation of neurological status and any other associated trauma is carried out by the multidisciplinary team. In the emergency department, spinal immobilisation should be maintained until a thorough neurological assessment has been completed and SCI is ruled out; in children, this typically involves a CT scan and possibly an MRI. Additional interventions are discussed in the Nursing Care Management section. Assessment of neurological status using the Glasgow Coma Scale (see Chapter 30) is important; a helpful assessment is represented in the mnemonic AVPU: **A**lert; responds to **V**erbal stimuli; responds to **P**ainful stimuli; and **U**nresponsive. A secondary assessment tool in the emergency department follows the mnemonic AMPLE: **A**llergies, **M**edications, **P**ast medical history, **L**ast meal or fluids and **E**nvironment and Events leading to the incident (Avarello & Cantor 2007).

IV methylprednisolone may be started within the first 12 hours after the injury to decrease inflammation and minimise further injury; however, its use in small children is controversial. Studies of methylprednisolone administration in adults with SCI have shown mixed results, with experts recommending against its use in acute SCI (Hurlbert et al 2013).

In children with upper motor neuron involvement, the spasticity that develops may require administration of an antispasmodic medication such as diazepam. Baclofen is considered the drug of choice for reducing muscle spasticity (Vogel et al 2012). Gabapentin may be used to treat neuropathic pain (Hayes & Arriola 2005). Botulinum toxin type A and α_2-adrenergic agonists may be used in older children with SCI to decrease muscle spasticity.

A number of progressive rehabilitation modalities have been developed in recent years that have the potential for increasing the quality of life for children with SCI. One treatment is functional electrical stimulation (FES), also referred to as *functional neuromuscular stimulation* or *neuromuscular electrical stimulation*. With this treatment, an electrical stimulator is surgically implanted under the skin in the abdomen and electrode leads are tunnelled to paralysed leg muscles, enabling the child to sit, stand and walk with the aid of crutches, a walker or other orthoses. The stimulator can also be used to elicit a voluntary grasp and release with the hand. Before the latter can be accomplished, a number of surgical tendon transfers may be required for elbow extension, wrist extension and finger and thumb flexion. In addition, FES has therapeutic benefits, which include increased muscle strength, improved gait function and increased cardiovascular fitness (Thrasher & Popovic 2008). Tendon transfers have been shown to be successful in enhancing hand and arm function, increasing pinch force and facilitating independence in ADLs (Hosalkar et al 2009). Restoration of hand and arm function enables children with SCI to perform self-catheterisation and achieve greater independence in personal hygiene.

Exercise is considered an integral part of SCI rehabilitation; exercise may enhance neuroplasticity and decrease further muscle atrophy.

Examples of exercise modalities in SCI patients include upper body strength training and hand cycling (Hosalkar et al 2009).

Administration of pharmacological agents such as clonidine hydrochloride may improve ambulation in patients with partial SCIs, and exercise therapy through interactive locomotor training has helped some individuals with SCI regain ambulatory function.

A number of orthoses or ambulation aids such as crutches may still be necessary to achieve upright mobility, yet as robotic technology advances, so do the chances for improved mobilisation in children with SCI. Mechanical or robotic orthoses may be used in conjunction with FES to enable ambulation in persons with SCI (To et al 2005). Gait training may be achieved with a number of different modalities, including a stationary cycle; however, no specific method has proved superior to the others. FES has also been effective in reducing complications from bladder and bowel incontinence and in assisting males in achieving penile erection. Ambulation is an important part of rehabilitation in SCI; retrospective studies found that ambulation was dependent on age at injury and extent of neurological injury (as measured by ASIA motor scales). Age (younger) and lesser neurological impairment are key predictors for ambulation (Vogel et al 2012). A knee-ankle-foot orthosis and reciprocating-gait orthosis may also be used to assist with early rehabilitation and ambulation (Vogel et al 2012). Additional detailed information regarding ambulation and orthotics for children have been published elsewhere (Calhoun et al 2013).

Surgical interventions for SCI include early cord decompression (decompression laminectomy) and cervical or thoracic fusion. Crutchfield, Vinke or Gardner-Wells tongs and skeletal traction may be used for early cervical vertebral stabilisation. A halo vest or Minerva jacket may be suited for ambulation after the acute phase. (See also Cervical Traction, Chapter 33.) After cervical spinal fusion, a hard cervical collar or sterno-occipital-mandibular immobiliser brace may be worn until the fusion is solidified. When SCI occurs in young children and preteens, scoliosis develops over time and often requires surgical consideration (Parent et al 2011).

Prognosis. The ultimate outlook for spinal cord function after injury depends on the completeness of the cord transection, site of injury, complicating damage to the neuronal tissue and success of treatment regimens aimed at recovery of lost muscle movement and ability. Healing of the injury and the return of neurological function are related to two factors.

1. Although individual nerve fibres do regenerate, they do not necessarily reconnect or make synaptic connections with the distal portion of the severed fibres; the chance of numerous fibres reconnecting is highly unlikely.
2. The damage resulting from cord ischaemia produces necrosis in the grey and white matter of the cord tissue, which does not regenerate if the axon cylinder is not intact.

In children the prognosis for recovery is considered better than in adults because children have rapid healing of bone and ligaments and increased potential for nervous system regeneration. Paraplegia is more common in children under 12 years, whereas older children and adolescents tend to have incomplete injuries (Mathison 2008). Shavelle and colleagues (2007) reported an increased likelihood of mortality among children less than 16 years of age who suffered an SCI in comparison to adults with similar injuries. Children with incomplete injuries (and who are not ventilator dependent) had a projected 83% chance of normal life expectancy, whereas those with high-level cervical injuries who are not ventilator dependent had a 50% chance of having a normal life expectancy. One study found that adults who had an SCI as children (less than 18 years of age at time of incident) had comparable or greater degrees of education in comparison to the general population of the same age (Vogel et al 2011). The same study found lower employment rates for adults with paediatric-onset SCI, lower rates of independent living and independent driving and lower rates of marriage in this select population.

In general, recovery of motor function in children with thoracic lesions is variable. Cervical injuries are also variable in the extent of damage. Incomplete lesions produce hemiplegia, whereas complete transection implies some involvement of all extremities—from partial use of the upper extremities to complete paralysis, including the need for some type of assisted ventilation. Lumbar injury may involve partial or complete loss of function in the lower extremities and bladder. With rapidly advancing surgical technology, use of computers in medicine and newer treatment modalities such as FES, there are increasing hope and evidence that functional mobility and independence can be restored in children with SCI.

Nursing Care Management

The nursing care of the child affected by SCI is complex and challenging. A multidisciplinary SCI team is equipped to manage the acute phase of the injury, and some members, including the nurse, may follow the patient to eventual recovery. Nursing management is concerned with ensuring adequate initial stabilisation of the entire spinal column with a rigid cervical collar with supportive blocks on a rigid backboard. The traumatic event causing the injury may or may not be recalled if the child lost consciousness; such events are extremely frightening to the child. The young child may also be frightened by the immobilisation process and the inability to move extremities; therefore, it is important to reassure and comfort the child during this process.

During the acute phase of the injury it is imperative that airway patency be ensured, complications prevented and function maintained. Evaluate the extent of the neurological damage early to establish a baseline for neurological function. Continual assessment of sensory and motor function should occur to prevent further deterioration of neurological status as a result of spinal cord oedema. The ASIA Impairment Scale can be used to assess neurological function on a routine basis during the patient's recovery. Once the patient is admitted, further evaluation of their ability to perform ADLs and need for assistance during recovery can be made with the Functional Independence Measure scale.

Nursing care during the acute phase should also focus on frequent monitoring of neurological signs to determine any changes in neurological function that require further intervention (e.g. level of consciousness using the Glasgow Coma Scale). In addition to airway maintenance, the nurse monitors for changes in haemodynamic status that may require immediate medical attention. Neurogenic shock consists of hypotension, bradycardia and vasodilation. Inotropic medications may be required to maintain adequate perfusion. Renal function is closely monitored by measuring urinary output and fluids administered. The child with a head injury may experience elevated intracranial pressure; therefore, changes in neurological status are reported to the practitioner. Fluid restriction may be required if intracranial pressure is elevated, so fluid intake should be closely monitored.

The nursing care of the child with an SCI is, in most respects, the same as that of any immobilised child (see The Immobilised Child, Chapter 33). Additional aspects of care that should be addressed on an individual basis include hypercalcaemia in adolescent boys, DVT, latex sensitisation, pain, hypothermia and hyperthermia, spasticity, autonomic dysreflexia and sleep-disordered breathing (Vogel et al 2012).

Respiratory Care. The child with a high-level cervical injury (C3 and above) requires continuous ventilatory assistance. In most instances a tracheostomy is the method of choice for greater ease in clearing secretions and for less trauma to tissues during long-term ventilatory dependence. Patient-triggered synchronous intermittent mandatory ventilation (SIMV–assist/control mode) may be required to maintain adequate oxygenation. In an acute care centre, respiratory therapy personnel are often responsible for establishing and maintaining the equipment, but the nurse must understand how it works and recognise mechanical malfunction and deviations from the prescribed rate and volume. In case of malfunction the nurse must be prepared to maintain respirations manually with a self-inflating bag-valve-mask device. In many home care situations the family is responsible for the care of ventilatory assistance devices; therefore, adequate family training and availability of the nurse (or durable medical equipment representative) for questions related to the equipment and evaluation of the child's breathing are essential. For some children, breathing pacemaker devices (phrenic nerve stimulators) are implanted to stimulate the phrenic nerve and produce diaphragmatic contractions and lung expansion without assisted ventilation.

Children with lesions below the C4 level are seldom ventilator dependent, but pulmonary vital capacity is significantly reduced. Position them for optimum chest expansion, and use a variety of breathing exercises and assistive devices to stimulate deep breathing. Chest physiotherapy is performed as needed to mobilise secretions, and flow-by oxygen may be needed occasionally. Regular monitoring of breath sounds to assess for adequate ventilation in all lung fields is part of routine care.

The cough reflex may be markedly diminished, which, combined with weak intercostal muscles, may mean the child has difficulty with secretions. Increasing the elastic qualities of the lung by breathing exercises, mechanical cough assist techniques and incentive spirometry helps the child achieve a productive cough. (See discussion of airway management and airway clearance devices under Muscular Dystrophies: Therapeutic Management.)

Cardiovascular Care. Children with SCI may experience cardiovascular instability as a result of loss of vagal tone, vagal stimulation during procedures such as oral suctioning or insertion of a nasogastric tube, turning and endotracheal suctioning. Close monitoring of heart rate and blood pressure is essential to detect any signs of decreased cardiac output. Pneumothorax may occur, resulting in a mediastinal shift and decreased cardiac output. Autonomic dysreflexia may occur and result in decreased cardiac output (see discussion later).

The child with loss of muscle tone and prolonged immobility may be at high risk for the development of DVT. In addition, major reparative surgery for associated injuries and spinal decompression place the child at risk for thrombus formation. DVT is prevented with the use of pneumatic compression devices and low molecular weight heparin during the acute phase of care. Fluid and electrolyte balance may be impaired as a result of trauma and associated injuries or decreased fluid intake during the recovery period. Fluid intake should be closely monitored, especially with regard to the development of pulmonary oedema and intracranial pressure. The child may require nasogastric tube feedings due to anorexia and immobility.

Temperature Regulation. Temperature is often poorly regulated in children with SCI; therefore, body temperature must be monitored closely for fluctuations. In small children hypothermia may occur relative to large body surface and inability to mount an appropriate metabolic response to the initial injury, so close attention should be given to preserving body temperature. Response to environmental temperature changes may be slow or absent, and the ability to dissipate heat through the process of shivering may be compromised.

During the spinal shock stage the dilated capillaries conducting body heat to the subcutaneous tissues cause heat loss. Without the capacity to sweat, the body retains heat in hot weather. An elevated temperature that cannot be corrected by environmental measures should be evaluated to rule out urinary or upper respiratory tract infection. However, excessive perspiration observed in sentient areas usually indicates an elevated ambient temperature.

Skin Care. Children with SCI have unique needs in relation to skin care. Because of decreased sensation and impaired mobility, they depend on others to assess and assist in the management of intact skin. Skin care practices are the same as those for any child who is immobilised. A skin score scale such as the Braden Q Scale can objectively evaluate risks for skin breakdown and skin conditions (Noonan et al 2011). Keep an alternating-pressure mattress or other pressure relief/reduction device underneath the child, and inspect the skin thoroughly at least twice a day for signs of pressure, especially over bony prominences. Prevention of skin breakdown is much easier than treatment. A number of factors contribute to the risk of skin breakdown in these children: decreased sensation, inadequate nutrition, muscle spasticity, impaired peripheral circulation, diaphoresis, mechanical shearing from assistive devices and improper positioning.

The areas most likely to be affected are the sacrum, scapulae, heels and occiput when the child is supine; the trochanters and the lateral aspect of the ankles, heels and knees when the child is in a side-lying position; and the ischial tuberosities when the child is sitting. The pressure wound may begin in deeper tissues and be visible on the surface only at a later stage. Therefore, areas that feel firm, irregular or warm or that appear to be only slightly reddened require careful evaluation. Keeping the skin clean and dry is particularly important in these children, especially those who are incontinent of urine or stool or those who have significant diaphoresis. When there is any evidence of skin breakdown, treatment to prevent further breakdown is implemented promptly. When orthotic devices such as AFOs and braces are used, skin care and vigilance for pressure areas are also important in the prevention of pressure ulcers. Prolonged use of wheelchairs without special sacral protection may also lead to skin ulceration.

The child who is heavily sedated or who is being given muscle paralytics should receive appropriate eye care to prevent corneal damage (e.g. artificial tears, ointment and impermeable eye shield). Additional nursing care may involve the administration of histamine blockers and proton pump inhibitors to prevent stress ulcers by reducing the secretion of hydrochloric acid.

Physical Therapy. An important consideration for the child with SCI is achievement of mobility and ambulation. A developmental approach should be considered in the rehabilitation phase (Calhoun et al 2013). Range-of-motion, passive and active exercises are carried out under the guidance of a personal trainer.

Unless there are contraindications, exercises during the period of immobilisation are aimed at maintaining and increasing the strength of the child's intact musculature. Upper extremity strengthening is especially important to the paraplegic child, who must rely on these muscle groups for turning, transferring, dressing, parallel bar walking, gait training and other activities. Children are usually eager to use their muscles and respond to interesting and innovative activities.

Neurogenic Bladder. When the bladder is denervated, as in the acute stage of spinal shock syndrome or after lower motor neuron damage, the bladder wall is flaccid. Lack of muscle tone inhibits the bladder's ability to respond to changes in passive pressure, causing overdistension. Therefore, it is important to prevent distension by periodic emptying, even though there may be dribbling between emptyings.

In contrast, an upper motor neuron lesion causes increased bladder tone and contractions that often include the urinary sphincter. Thus although the bladder empties periodically by reflex action, complete emptying is prevented, resulting in urinary retention and ureteral reflux.

In school-age children and adolescents, achieving bladder and bowel continence is a significant developmental issue related to self-esteem and perception of self in relation to peers. Therefore, it is imperative to consider options that best meet the child's physiological and emotional needs.

Surgical options for children with neurogenic bladder include the creation of a urinary stoma, made possible by removing the appendix and creating a urinary diversion from the bladder to the exterior, usually the umbilicus, thus making self-catheterisation more private, especially with the recovery of hand and elbow movement (with tendon transfers). Other options include surgical bladder augmentation to increase capacity and FES to restore micturition on command without a urinary catheter (Merenda & Hickey 2005).

Emptying the bladder by clean intermittent catheterisation (CIC) is also an option for children with SCI; older children who are functionally capable can learn to perform self-catheterisation. Encourage the child to adhere to a schedule for CIC and to maintain a regular pattern of fluid intake throughout the day; they should avoid large intakes of fluid without considering the need for more frequent CIC. Caffeinated beverages and other caffeinated foods are used sparingly to avoid bladder overdistension with increased urine formation (Francis 2007). Latex catheters should be avoided to prevent the development of latex allergy (if it is not already present). Bladder-training programs usually begin with intermittent bladder emptying at regular intervals that are gradually increased.

Urinary tract infections are common due to urinary stasis. A regular schedule of CIC may help prevent such infections. Encourage the child to increase fluid intake by approximately 240 mL/day and use CIC every 3 to 4 hours.

Maintenance of bladder dynamics and control of urinary tract infections are of utmost importance. Pyelonephritis and renal failure are the most significant causes of death in long-standing paraplegia.

Bowel Training. The loss of bowel function is considered to be one of the most stressful events when quality-of-life issues are considered in persons with SCI; however, successful bowel training is easier to institute than bladder management. The aim is to control defecation until an appropriate time and place are found. Merenda and Hickey (2005) propose four components in a successful bowel management program: desired stool consistency (i.e. a soft stool), a regular evacuation pattern, upright positioning for planned evacuation and motivation and commitment from the child and family.

A diet with sufficient fibre (age in years plus 5 g is recommended) for adequate stool bulk and insertion of a glycerin or bisacodyl (Dulcolax) suppository at a convenient time, either morning or evening, are often all that are necessary to induce a bowel movement within a short time. The probability of an accident between times diminishes once the bowel is completely evacuated. The key to adequate bowel training is to maintain consistency in the time of day for evacuation.

Autonomic Dysreflexia. Children with high-level lesions are susceptible to the development of autonomic dysreflexia, which requires prompt action to prevent encephalopathy and shock. Clinical manifestations of autonomic dysreflexia include an increase in systemic blood pressure, headache, bradycardia, profuse diaphoresis, cardiac arrhythmias, flushing, piloerection, blurred vision, nasal congestion, anxiety, spots on the visual field or absent or minimum symptoms. A quick assessment may rule out other causes, such as orthostatic intolerance. After that, vital signs, including blood pressure, are taken while the bladder is checked for distension (the usual precipitating cause). The bladder is drained slowly; if this does not relieve symptoms, any tight clothing is loosened and the bowel is checked for the pressure of impacted faeces.

Other potential causes of autonomic dysreflexia in SCI children include bowel impaction and abdominal distension, pressure ulcers, tight clothing, burns, DVT, menses, trauma, fractures, pregnancy, labour, surgery or invasive procedures, any painful stimulus and hyperthermia (Vogel et al 2012). If removal of the causative agent is unsuccessful in controlling the syndrome, IV administration of an antihypertensive drug is indicated, followed by oral maintenance doses. Antispasmodics may also be administered.

Remobilisation. As soon as the condition warrants, the child is moved from a reclining to an upright position. Cardiovascular deconditioning and impaired autonomic responses below the level of injury will cause pooling of blood in the extremities (because of peripheral vasodilation); a drop in blood pressure; and a feeling of light-headedness, dizziness or fainting on sudden assumption of an upright posture, often referred to as **orthostatic intolerance**. Therefore, an upright position must be accomplished gradually by first placing the child (who is secured by passive restraint) on a head-up tilt table. The table is slowly elevated from a horizontal to a 30-degree semireclining position. This is performed twice daily for 20 to 30 minutes, with the angle gradually increased until 90 degrees vertical is reached.

During the procedure the vital signs are monitored, and the child's behaviour is observed for subjective symptoms of syncope. The pooling of blood is reduced by using elastic antiembolism stockings and sequential pneumatic compression devices, which consist of inflatable sleeves that fit on the legs and compress the leg muscles for cyclic emptying and filling of leg veins. The process of achieving an upright posture may require several weeks. After tolerance is achieved, the child will be ready to begin using a wheelchair. Getting the child up should be accomplished slowly by gradually elevating the bed over 20 to 30 minutes before placing the child in the wheelchair and then gradually lowering the legs after the child has been in the chair a short time.

All adaptive devices help children increase their mobility, function and endurance. The child with some lower extremity function progresses to parallel bars and then to a walker. The child with tetraplegia learns to use a wheelchair—among the most valuable aids available to the child with an SCI. The wheelchair should be selected carefully in relation to where it will be used, the architectural barriers and the child's functional capacity. For children with severe upper extremity paralysis, a variety of motorised wheelchairs are used; however, the more complex they are, the greater their cost, weight and tendency to break down. Wheelchair tolerance is gained over time and is accompanied by measures to prevent orthostatic hypotension and pressure sores.

A variety of orthoses and other appliances can be adapted for use by many children. The primary purpose of lower extremity bracing in the child with an SCI is for ambulation, although correction of deformities may be attempted. However, the efficacy is limited because of the tendency to develop pressure lesions over insensate areas. The higher the lesion, the more support required, with the accompanying difficulties of getting into the orthosis and the greater energy expended in using the appliance. The energy required in walking with crutches and braces is two to four times greater than that required for normal walking.

Children, with their natural and overwhelming desire for mobility, usually attain or even surpass the maximum expectation in ambulation. However, as they approach adulthood, the increasing weight and energy cost usually cause them to resort to predominant use of the wheelchair for mobility and the pursuit of more intellectual and vocational interests. Wheelchair mobility has the advantages of requiring no more energy than normal walking and allowing the person with paraplegia to maintain the speed of other pedestrians on level ground.

Physical Rehabilitation. The process of physical rehabilitation usually begins once the child is medically stable and associated problems have been managed. The major aims of physical rehabilitation are to prepare the child and family to achieve normalisation and resume life at home and in the community. Additional goals of rehabilitation in children with SCI are to promote independence in mobility and self-care skills, academic achievement, independent living and employment.

Members of the multidisciplinary rehabilitation team cooperate with one another and the family to identify the child's needs and to plan realistic interventions. Integration of activities is coordinated by one team member, most often a specialist in physical medicine and rehabilitation. Members of the team attempt to achieve their collaborative goals through mutual trust, good communication, professional respect and sincere interest in the child and family. Training in the rehabilitation centre promotes maximum achievement commensurate with each child's physical capacities (Fig 34.10). Instruction for home routine is stressed and includes all the precautions and management implemented in the acute care centre (e.g. skin care, nutrition, bladder and bowel training, gait training) and an exercise program.

Inpatient physical rehabilitation of children with tetraplegia takes approximately 2 to 4 months; children with paraplegia can achieve these goals in 1 to 3 months but require constant vigilance to avoid complications. Emotional adjustments take longer, especially in older children and adolescents. In most children the outlook is favourable unless the life-threatening consequences of urinary pathological condition are severe or the emotional adjustment is poor.

Psychosocial Rehabilitation. Early-acquired or congenital disability is usually more readily accepted by children than paralysis that appears later in childhood. Rehabilitation efforts should include not only the child's emotional responses but also those of the persons closest to the child. Intensive education is important so that family members understand the nature of the disability, the therapeutic regimen and complications and are able to provide the physical and emotional support the child needs.

As with any disability, treat children as normally as possible and encourage them in developmental tasks at the age at which they would typically be expected to acquire abilities and perform activities. However, the goals must be realistic, and children should not be forced beyond their capabilities. Vogel and colleagues (2012) emphasise the need for children and adolescents with SCI to assume responsibility for their own care. When this is not physically possible, they should direct others in their care. Encouraging self-care is important in the emotional and physical rehabilitation of the child or adolescent with SCI.

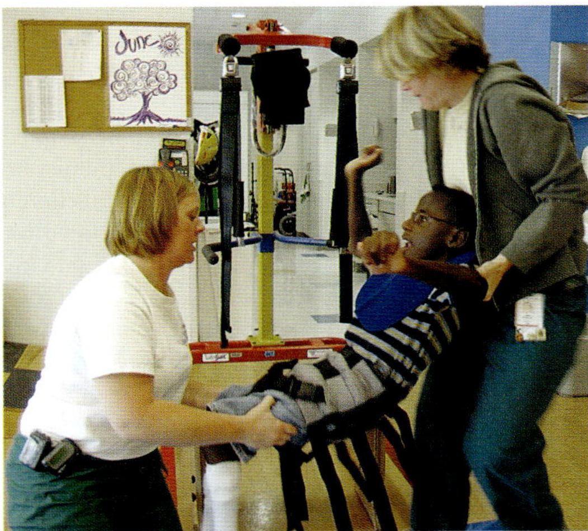

Fig 34.10 Training in a rehabilitation facility can promote achievement and encourage the child to strive to reach his maximum physical abilities. (Source: Courtesy of E. Jacob, Texas Children's Hospital, Houston.)

Severe depression can be emotionally and intellectually immobilising, but it indicates that the child is no longer hiding behind denial. In rehabilitation it is desirable for the child to begin to express negative feelings towards the situation because these feelings, redirected by efforts of the rehabilitation team, are the ones that will motivate the child towards learning a new way of life. Anxiety and depression in young children and adolescents with SCI are associated with a poorer quality of life (Anderson et al 2009).

The needs of young children and adolescents who are permanently disabled must be re-evaluated periodically by the total rehabilitation team, including the children and their families. Vocational rehabilitation is important for helping these adolescents find meaningful work activities and enrol in formal educational programs as desired.

Sexuality. Issues related to loss of sexual function also apply to adolescents with debilitating neuromuscular diseases such as Duchenne's muscular dystrophy (DMD) and SMA. The problems of self-image are particularly significant when children with SCI reach puberty, especially if the disability was acquired during early adolescence. Sexual development and awareness and changing perceptions of body image are prominent aspects of adolescence; a loss that affects these areas is often devastating. Development of secondary sexual characteristics does not seem to be altered by SCIs, and it is now believed that with comprehensive rehabilitation, motivated young people can look forward to successful participation in marital and family activities.

In females, if the injury occurs after the onset of menstruation, there is usually a temporary cessation and irregularity in menstrual flow, but menstruation resumes in the majority of cases. Ovulation and conception are possible, but only about 50% of females experience vaginal or clitoral orgasms, although they can learn to use other erogenous zones for a sexual experience. This is important to emphasise in sex education because many females have the misconception that they are unable to conceive because they lack sensation. FES may help some women with SCI achieve orgasm. Education is important because the pregnant paraplegic or tetraplegic patient may be unaware that she is in labour, and those with a high-level injury are subject to autonomic dysreflexia during labour.

More attention has been focused on rehabilitating male sexual function (erection and ejaculation) than female sexual function until the last two decades. A number of pharmacological (prostaglandin E_1) and mechanical devices (e.g. penile implants, vacuum pump devices) now make it possible for males to participate in sexual intercourse and produce offspring, provided that fertility has not been affected by associated complications. Penile injections with vasoactive substances (prostaglandin E_1) are reported to be effective in 90% of men (DeForge et al 2006). However, sildenafil (Viagra) is now considered the treatment of choice for the sexually active male. Adolescents with SCI should be counselled regarding condom use and the symptoms of latex allergy.

As soon as adolescent males become aware of their functional loss, they will be concerned about sexual capacities, regardless of the type of sexual activities experienced before the SCI. The healthcare professional should take the initiative in discussing sexuality with adolescents and their families. Parents of younger children may want to know about their children's sexual and reproductive potential. As their interest and understanding increase, adolescents need to know the specifics of physiology, the prognosis and sexual techniques related to their

TABLE 34.2 **Characteristics of Major Muscular Dystrophies**

Primary Myopathy and Inheritance Pattern	Age of Onset	Initial Manifestations	Progression	Therapy
Duchenne's X-linked recessive, sporadic	Early childhood; ages 3–5 years	Lordosis Waddling gait Frequent falls Toe walking Difficulty in rising from floor and climbing stairs Fat deposits replace wasted gastrocnemius muscles	Rapid Ultimately involves all voluntary muscles Death usually occurs at ages 15–30 years	Supportive Physical therapy to prevent disuse atrophy of unaffected muscles
Becker X-linked recessive, sporadic	> 7 years of age	Same as Duchenne's	Much slower progression than Duchenne's	Same as Duchenne's
Myotonic Autosomal dominant	Early infancy, except for severe congenital form	Facial wasting and hypotonia	Progressive muscle wasting into adolescence and adulthood; affects multiple organs	Treatment of cardiac, ocular, endocrine and gastrointestinal complications
Limb-girdle Autosomal recessive (usually, but 16 genetic forms are recognised and some are autosomal dominant)	Late childhood or adolescence; > 8 years of age	Weakness of proximal muscles of both pelvic and shoulder girdles	Variable but usually slow Most become incapacitated within 20 years of onset; in some, disability may remain slight	Supportive Physical therapy to prevent disuse atrophy of unaffected muscles
Facioscapulohumeral (Landouzy-Dejerine) Autosomal dominant	Early adolescence; > 8 years of age	Lack of facial mobility Difficulty raising arms over head Forward slope of shoulders	Very slow May be intervals with no progression Considerable disability in time, but life span unaffected	Supportive

particular problems. The practitioner should provide them with information about what can be expected regarding erection, ejaculation and other sexual experiences.

A knowledgeable rehabilitation team is valuable to adolescents as they experience concerns regarding loss as a sexual being. This is especially true in paraplegia or tetraplegia. Most sexual counselling for adolescents with SCI focuses on developing the idea that sex means different things to different people. Most rehabilitation teams have an active counselling program to help adolescents learn intimacy and how to function sexually within their limitations. Through individual and group counselling they gain new attitudes concerning sexuality and experiences exclusive or inclusive of intercourse. Guidelines for sexual and reproductive healthcare of persons with SCI are published elsewhere (Consortium for Spinal Cord Medicine 2010).

Transition to Adulthood. With the ultimate goal of making an effective transition to adulthood, adolescents with SCI often face challenges similar to others with chronic and debilitating conditions. Issues such as housing, education, personal assistance care, transportation, medical care and specialised medical care must be addressed in a coordinated transition program (Vogel et al 2012). The concepts of care coordination for children and adolescents requiring home care also apply to adolescents making the transition to adulthood because different healthcare services may be needed or requirements may change for benefits for those no longer dependent on parents.

MUSCULAR DYSFUNCTION

Muscular Dystrophies

The MDs constitute the largest and most important single group of muscle diseases of childhood (Table 34.2). They have a genetic origin in which there is gradual, progressive degeneration of muscle fibres, and they are characterised by progressive weakness and wasting of symmetrical groups of skeletal muscles, with increasing disability and deformity. In all forms of MD there is insidious loss of strength, but each differs in regard to the muscle groups affected, age of onset, rate of progression and inheritance patterns.

The basic defect in MD is still being clarified but appears to be caused by a metabolic disturbance unrelated to the nervous system. Initial sites of muscle involvement are illustrated in Fig 34.11.

Treatment of the MDs consists mainly of providing supportive measures (including physical therapy; orthopaedic procedures to minimise deformity; and ventilatory support, including airway clearance techniques) and assisting the affected child in meeting the demands of daily living.

Facioscapulohumeral (Landouzy-Dejerine) muscular dystrophy is inherited as an autosomal dominant disorder with onset in early adolescence. It is characterised by difficulty in raising the arms over the head, lack of facial mobility and a forward slope of the shoulders. The progression is slow, and the life span is usually unaffected.

Limb-girdle muscular dystrophy (LGMD) is a heterogenous group of disorders with autosomal dominant and recessive inheritance whose clinical manifestations often appear in later childhood, adolescence or early adulthood with variable but usually slow progression (Quan 2011). All types of LGMD are characterised by weakness of proximal muscles of the pelvic and shoulder girdles. Other forms of MD include myotonic dystrophy, scapulohumeral MD (Emery-Dreifuss MD), fascioscapulohumeral MD (Landouzy-Dejerine disease) and congenital MD; these forms consist of subtypes of MD.

Duchenne's muscular dystrophy is discussed in the following section.

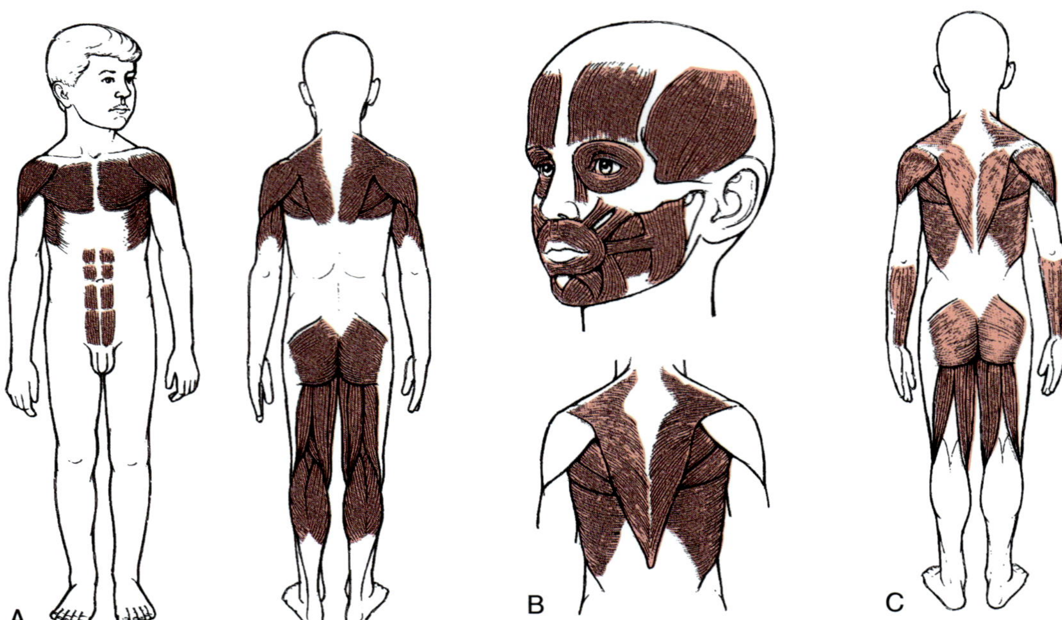

Fig 34.11 Initial muscle groups involved in muscular dystrophies. (**A**) Pseudohypertrophic (Duchenne's). (**B**) Facioscapulohumeral. (**C**) Limb-girdle.

Duchenne's Muscular Dystrophy

DMD is the most severe and most common MD of childhood. It is inherited as an X-linked recessive trait, and the single-gene defect is located on the short arm of the X chromosome. DMD has a high mutation rate, with a negative family history in approximately 65% to 75% of all cases; therefore, genetic counselling is an important aspect of the care of the family. Approximately 30% of DMD patients are new mutations and the mother is not the carrier (Sarnat 2015c).

As in all X-linked disorders, males are affected almost exclusively. The female carrier may have an elevated serum CK, but muscle weakness is usually not a problem; however, about 10% of female carriers develop cardiomyopathy (Manzur, Kinali et al 2008). In rare instances a female may be identified with DMD disease yet with muscular weakness that is milder than in boys (Sarnat 2015c).

At the genetic level, both DMD and Becker MD result from mutations of the gene that encodes dystrophin, a protein product in skeletal muscle. Dystrophin is absent from the muscle of children with DMD and is reduced or abnormal in children with Becker MD. The absence of dystrophin leads to a number of problems in muscle, including muscle fibre degeneration. A deficiency of dystrophin isoforms in brain tissue causes cognitive and intellectual impairment (Manzur, Kinali et al 2008). Children with Becker MD have a later onset of symptoms, which are usually not as severe as those seen in DMD. There is a strong correlation between the clinical severity of these disorders and the type of genetic mutation and dystrophin protein alterations. Survival has increased with newer ventilation technologies, and median age is reported as high as 27 years in those being ventilated; types of ventilation used were not described in the report (Rall & Grimm 2012).

Clinical Manifestations

Most children with DMD reach the appropriate developmental milestones early in life, although they may have mild, subtle delays. Evidence of muscle weakness usually appears during the third to seventh year, although there may have been a history of delay in motor development, particularly walking. Difficulties in running, riding a bicycle and climbing stairs are usually the first symptoms noted. Later, abnormal gait on a level surface becomes apparent. In the early years, rapid developmental gains may mask the progression of the disease. Questioning the parents may reveal that the child has difficulty in rising from a sitting or supine position. Occasionally the parents notice enlarged calves.

Typically, affected boys have a waddling gait and lordosis, fall frequently and develop a characteristic manner of rising from a squatting or sitting position on the floor (Gower sign) (Fig 34.12). Lordosis occurs as a result of weakened pelvic muscles, and the waddling gait is a result of weakness in the gluteus medius and maximus muscles (Battista 2010). Muscles, especially in the calves, thighs and upper arms, become enlarged from fatty infiltration and feel unusually firm or woody on palpation. The term *pseudohypertrophy* is derived from this muscular enlargement. Profound muscular atrophy occurs in the later stages; contractures and deformities involving large and small joints are common complications as the disease progresses. Ambulation usually becomes impossible by 12 years of age. The loss of mobilisation further increases the spectrum of complications, which may include osteoporosis, fractures, constipation, skin breakdown and psychosocial and behavioural problems. Atrophy of facial, oropharyngeal and respiratory muscles does not occur until the advanced stage of the disease. Ultimately the disease process involves the diaphragm and auxiliary muscles of respiration, and cardiomegaly is common.

Mild to moderate cognitive impairment is commonly associated with MD. The mean intelligence quotient (IQ) is approximately 20 points below normal, and frank mental deficit is present in 20% to 30% of these children. Verbal IQ is markedly low in males with DMD, and emotional disturbance is more common than in other children with disabilities; however, children with DMD should be involved in early learning programs and eventually moved into regular classrooms as much as possible.

Complications. The major complications of MD include contractures, scoliosis, disuse atrophy, infections, obesity and respiratory and cardiopulmonary problems. Contracture deformities of the hips, knees and ankles occur from early selective muscle involvement and often

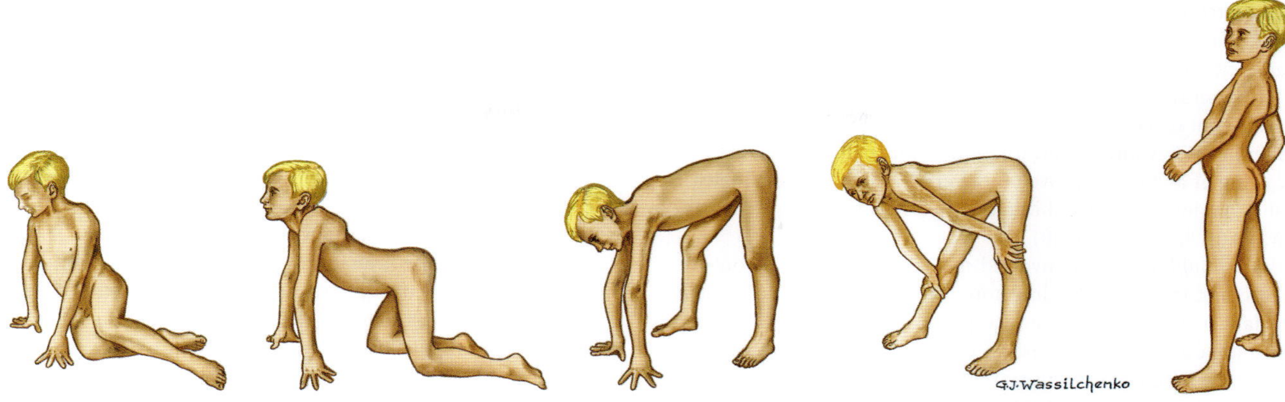

Fig 34.12 Child with Duchenne's muscular dystrophy attains standing posture by kneeling, then gradually pushing their torso upright (with knees straight) by 'walking' their hands up their legs (Gower sign). Note marked lordosis in upright position.

exaggerate the weakness. Passive range-of-motion exercises, stretching and active exercises under the supervision of a personal trainer are effective in treating reducible contractures. Non-reducible contractures require wedge casting or surgical reduction. Scoliosis caused by muscle imbalance is common in children who lose ambulatory capability and tends to progress even when the child becomes dependent on a wheelchair. Bracing with an orthosis may be required, but in many cases spinal fusion surgery is performed to prevent complications associated with cardiac and pulmonary restriction.

Atrophy of disuse from prolonged inactivity occurs readily when children are immobilised or confined to bed with illness, injury or surgery. To minimise this complication, physical therapy should begin if bed rest extends beyond a few days. To maintain muscle strength, a daily goal for well children with moderate disability should be at least 3 hours of ambulation.

Pulmonary infections become increasingly frequent as the dystrophic process produces a progressive decrease in pulmonary vital capacity as a result of weakness of the primary, secondary and associated muscles of respiration. Consequently, even minor upper respiratory tract infections may become serious in these children. The eventual cause of death is usually respiratory tract infection or cardiac failure; however, much progress has been made in providing ventilatory methods to prolong and maintain quality of life. Prompt and vigorous antibiotic therapy, supplemented by postural drainage and aggressive airway clearance methods, is effective. Because of the respiratory musculature weakness, these children are unable to cough effectively and secretions collect easily.

Obesity is a common complication that contributes to premature loss of ambulation. Children who have restricted opportunities for physical activity and who suffer from boredom easily consume calories in excess of their needs. This may be compounded by overfeeding by well-meaning family and friends. Proper dietary intake and a diversified recreational program help reduce the likelihood of obesity and enable children to maintain ambulation and functional independence for a longer time.

Cardiac manifestations are usually late events but may occur in ambulatory children. The most significant of these, cardiac failure, is difficult to correct in advanced cases, but treatment with digoxin and diuretics is often beneficial in the early stages of the disease.

Diagnostic Evaluation

MD is suspected on the basis of clinical manifestations (see Box 34.12) and confirmed by molecular genetic detection of deficient dystrophin by DNA analysis from peripheral blood or in muscle tissue obtained by biopsy. The diagnosis of DMD is primarily established by blood polymerase chain reaction (PCR) for the dystrophin gene mutation (Sarnat 2015c). Diagnostic techniques such as multiplex PCR have made it possible to diagnose 98% of the DMD mutations. Prenatal diagnosis is also possible as early as 12 weeks of gestation. However, ethical questions exist regarding diagnosing a condition in the fetus when no treatment exists.

BOX 34.12 Characteristics of Duchenne's Muscular Dystrophy

- Early onset, usually between 3 and 5 years of age
- Progressive muscular weakness, wasting and contractures
- Calf muscle hypertrophy in most patients
- Loss of independent ambulation by 9–12 years of age
- Slowly progressive, generalised weakness during adolescence
- Relentless progression until death from respiratory or cardiac failure

Serum enzyme measurement, muscle biopsy and EMG may also be used in establishing the diagnosis. Serum CK levels are extremely high in the first 2 years of life, before the onset of clinical weakness. If the child demonstrates the usual characteristics, has a positive family history for DMD and the PCR is positive, the muscle biopsy may be deferred.

Muscle biopsy reveals degeneration of muscle fibres, with fibrosis and fatty tissue replacement. EMG readings show a decrease in amplitude and duration of motor unit potentials.

Therapeutic Management. Currently no curative treatment exists for childhood MD. Increased muscle bulk and muscle power have been reported after a course of corticosteroids. Several clinical trials demonstrated increased muscle strength and improved performance and pulmonary function, with significant decrease in the progression of weakness, when prednisone was administered for 6 months to 2 years (Manzur, Kuntzer et al 2008). Corticosteroid administration also prolonged ambulation, preserved respiratory function and decreased the incidence of scoliosis and cardiomyopathy (Manzur, Kinali et al 2008). Major side effects in these studies included weight gain and a cushingoid facial appearance.

Maintaining optimum function in all muscles for as long as possible is the primary goal; secondary is the prevention of contractures. In general, children who remain as active as possible are able to avoid wheelchair use for a longer time. Maintenance of function often includes stretching exercises, strength and muscle training, breathing exercises and use of incentive spirometry to increase and maintain vital lung capacity, airway clearance, range-of-motion exercises, surgery to release contracture deformities, bracing and performance of ADLs. Knee-ankle-foot orthoses have been shown to prolong ambulation for 18 to 24 months beyond the termination of independent ambulation. Serial casting of ankles has proven more effective than surgical release of Achilles tendons in many children with DMD to prevent contractures (Manzur, Kinali et al 2008).

Parents should always be involved in making decisions about the child's care, and teaching regarding home safety and prevention of falls is important as well. Also encourage parents to have the child keep follow-up appointments for medical care and physical and occupational therapy. Because respiratory tract infections are most troublesome in these children, encourage regular influenza and pneumococcal vaccines and avoidance of contact with persons with respiratory tract infections as much as possible. Baseline pulmonary function testing, electrocardiograms and echocardiograms are also recommended.

Eventually, respiratory and cardiac problems become the central focus of the debilitating illness. Referral to palliative care may help the family evaluate the benefits and burdens of various treatments. The child and parents should be involved in discussion of long-term ventilation options. Cardiac and respiratory assessment during wake-sleep cycles is imperative. Children with neuromuscular disease eventually develop abnormal breathing patterns, particularly during REM sleep, and hypoxia occurs as a result of inadequate oxygenation. The sleep-disordered breathing of DMD results in symptoms such as frequent night awakenings, morning headache and daytime sleepiness. Polysomnography should be performed once daytime symptoms of sleep-disordered breathing occur. Non-invasive positive pressure ventilation should be considered in such children to prevent further hypoventilation and cardiorespiratory deterioration (Culebras 2008). Respiratory care for children with neuromuscular conditions such as SMA and DMD may involve the use of non-invasive ventilation with BiPAP on a temporary or full-time basis, mechanically assisted coughing (MAC), or tracheostomy and relief of airway obstruction with coughing and suctioning devices; the tracheostomy, however, is associated with more complications (Simonds 2006, Young et al 2007).

Several devices are available for children with neuromuscular disease to assist in clearing the airway when the cough reflex is ineffective or diminished. The *mechanical cough in-exsufflator* (MIE) (also referred to as cough assist) has been found to be safe and effective in the daily management of respiratory function (Kravitz 2009). The MIE delivers positive inspiratory pressures at a set rate, followed by negative pressure exsufflation coordinated with the patient's own breathing rhythm. The exsufflation is designed to mimic a cough reflex so mucus can be effectively cleared. Airway suctioning after exsufflation is accomplished as necessary to clear the airways. In children the MIE device may be connected directly to a tracheostomy or used with a mouthpiece or face mask.

Survival in individuals with DMD may be prolonged several years with the use of non-invasive ventilation and airway clearance devices such as cough assist as alternatives to tracheotomy and airway suctioning (Simonds 2006).

Genetic counselling is recommended for parents, sisters and maternal aunts and their daughters. (See Chapter 3.) Long-term care, end-of-life care and palliative care options are issues that the healthcare team must discuss with the child and family affected by MD (Finder 2009). Professional counselling is necessary in some cases to allow frank discussion of these issues, and referrals should be made as appropriate.

Nursing Care Management

The care and management of a child with MD involve the combined efforts of a multidisciplinary healthcare team. Nurses can help clarify the roles of these healthcare professionals to family and others. The major emphasis of nursing care is to assist the child and family in coping with the progressive, incapacitating and fatal nature of the disease; to help design a program that will afford a greater degree of independence and reduce the predictable and preventable disabilities associated with the disorder; and to help the child and family deal constructively with the limitations the disease imposes on their daily lives. Because of advances in technology, children with MD may live into early adulthood; therefore, the goals of care should also involve decisions regarding quality of life, achievement of independence and transition to adulthood.

Working closely with other team members, nurses assist the family in developing the child's self-help skills to give the child the satisfaction of being as independent as possible for as long as possible. It is tempting for parents to overprotect their affected children. Children derive pleasure and build self-esteem from performing actions that visibly please their parents. Therefore, parents must be helped to develop a balance between limiting the child's activity because of muscular weakness and allowing the child to accomplish things alone. This requires continual evaluation of the child's capabilities, which are often difficult to assess. Most children with MD instinctively recognise the need to be as independent as possible and strive to do so.

Practical difficulties faced by families are the physical limitations of housing, transportation and mobility. Housing accommodations must be made so the child who uses a wheelchair can be mobile in the home setting. Transportation in a car restraint seat adapted for the child with weakened neck and back musculature will be necessary, and eventually a wheelchair-accessible vehicle will be required. Discuss diet, nutritional needs and nutrition modification according to the needs of the individual child and family. Nutritional needs decrease the more a child uses a wheelchair, and dietary modifications should be made in conjunction with a paediatric dietitian to ensure the child is receiving an adequate amount of the necessary nutrients to maintain bone health and prevent constipation.

Parents' social activities may be restricted, and the family's activities must be continually modified to meet the needs of the affected child. (See Chapter 21.) When the child becomes increasingly incapacitated, the family may consider home care to provide the care needed. The nurse as case manager can assist the family in making this difficult transition. Unless the child is severely incapacitated, he or she should also be involved in the decisions regarding such care. Nurses can assist with decision-making by exploring all available options and resources and supporting the child and family in the decision.

Each child's therapy program is tailored to individual needs and capabilities, and family members should be active participants. Parents often need assistance with the physical therapy program and education regarding a home regimen of exercises and activity. Many parents erroneously believe that by exerting sufficient effort, the child can overcome the weakness and prevent progression of the disease process. They should also be advised to notify the nurse or other designated person when the child becomes even temporarily bedridden so that the exercise program can be modified and continued during this time.

Children with MD tend to become socially isolated as their physical condition deteriorates to the point that they can no longer keep up with friends and classmates. Their physical capabilities diminish, and their dependency increases at the age at which most children are expanding their range of interests and relationships. To gain peer associations, they often learn and employ behaviours that bring them the rewards of other children's company. These friends are often children who have been rejected by more able-bodied classmates.

Older boys with MD may also need psychiatric or psychological counselling to deal with issues such as depression, anger and quality of life. Parents need encouragement to become involved in support groups because there is evidence that adequate social support from family, community and other parents is crucial to appropriate coping in families with children with chronic illness.

Nurses are especially valuable healthcare professionals as they come to know the family and the family's challenges. Nurses can be alert to the problems and needs of the families and make necessary referrals when supplementary services are indicated.

REFERENCES

Adzick, N. S. (2013). Fetal surgery for spina bifida: past, present, future. Seminars in Pediatric Surgery, 22(1), 10–17.

Agopian, A. J., Tinker, S. C., Lupo, P. J., et al. (2013). Proportion of neural tube defects attributable to known risk factors. Birth Defects Research. Part A, Clinical and Molecular Teratology, 97(1), 42–46.

Anderson, C. J., Kelly, E. M., Klaas, S. J., et al. (2009). Anxiety and depression in children and adolescents with spinal cord injuries. Developmental Medicine and Child Neurology, 51(10), 826–832.

Avarello, J. T., & Cantor, R. M. (2007). Pediatric major trauma: an approach to evaluation and management. Emergency Medicine Clinics of North America, 25(3), 803–836.

Australasian Academy of Cerebral Palsy and Developmental Medicine (AusACPDM). (2018). Australian Cerebral Palsy Register. https://www.ausacpdm.org.au/resources/australian-cerebral-palsy-register/

Bach, J. R. (2007). Medical considerations of long-term survival of Werdnig-Hoffmann disease. American Journal of Physical Medicine and Rehabilitation, 86(5), 349–355.

Battista, V. (2010). Muscular dystrophy, Duchenne. In P. L. Jackson, J. A. Vessey, & N. A. Schapiro (Eds.), Primary care of the child with a chronic illness (5th ed.). St Louis: Mosby.

Berker, A. N., & Yalçin, M. S. (2008). Cerebral palsy: orthopedic aspects and rehabilitation. Pediatric Clinics of North America, 55(5), 1209–1225.

Betz, C., Linroth, R., Butler, C., et al. (2010). Spina bifida: what we learned from consumers. Pediatric Clinics of North America, 57(4), 935–944.

Bosanquet, M., Copeland, L., Ware, R., et al. (2013). A systematic review of tests to predict cerebral palsy in young children. Developmental Medicine and Child Neurology, 55(5), 418–426.

Bourke-Taylor, H. M., Cotter, C., Lalor, A., et al. (2018). School success and participation for students with cerebral palsy: a qualitative study exploring multiple perspectives. Disability and Rehabilitation, 40(18), 2163–2171.

Burke, R., Liptak, G. S., & Council on Children with Disabilities. (2011). Providing a primary care medical home for children and youth with spina bifida. Pediatrics, 128(6), e1645–e1658.

Bush, A., Fraser, J., & Jardine, E. (2005). Respiratory management of the infant with type 1 spinal muscular atrophy. Archives of Disease in Childhood, 90(7), 709–711.

Calhoun, C. L., Schottler, J., & Vogel, L. C. (2013). Recommendations for mobility in children with spinal cord injury. Topics in Spinal Cord Injury Rehabilitation, 19(2), 142–151.

Cerebral Palsy Alliance. (2018). Types of cerebral palsy. https://cerebralpalsy.org.au/our-research/about-cerebral-palsy/what-is-cerebral-palsy/types-of-cerebral-palsy/

Cerebral Palsy Society (2021). Effects of cerebral palsy. https://cerebralpalsy.org.nz/cerebral-palsy/what-is-cerebral-palsy/effects-of-cerebral-palsy/

Chiriboga, C. A., Swoboda, K. J., Darras, B. T., et al. (2016). Results from a phase 1 study of nusinersen (ISIS-SMN Rx) in children with spinal muscular atrophy. Neurology, 86(10), 890–897.

Choi, J. Y., Choi, Y. S., & Park, E. S. (2017). Language development and brain magnetic resonance imaging characteristics in preschool children with cerebral palsy. Journal of Speech, Language, and Hearing Research, 60(5), 1330–1338.

Collins, J. S., Atkinson, K. K., Dean, J. H., et al. (2011). Long-term maintenance of neural tube defects prevention in a high-prevalence state. The Journal of Pediatrics, 159(1), 143–149.

Consortium for Spinal Cord Medicine. (2010). Sexuality and reproductive health in adults with spinal cord injury: a clinical practice guideline for health-care professionals. The Journal of Spinal Cord Medicine, 33(3), 281–336.

Culebras, A. (2008). Sleep-disordered breathing in neuromuscular disease. Sleep Medicine Clinics, 3(3), 377–386.

DeForge, D., Blackmer, J., Garritty, C., et al. (2006). Male erectile dysfunction following spinal cord injury: a systematic review. Spinal Cord, 44(8), 465–473.

De Jong, T. P., Chrzan, R., Klijn, A. J., et al. (2008). Treatment of the neurogenic bladder in spina bifida. Pediatric Nephrology (Berlin, Germany), 23(6), 889–896.

Department of Health. (2010). Folate facts. https://www1.health.gov.au/internet/main/publishing.nsf/Content/health-pubhlth-strateg-folate-fofacts.htm

Doolin, E. (2006). Bowel management for patients with myelodysplasia. The Surgical Clinics of North America, 86(2), 505–514.

Eliasson, A. C., Krumlinde-Sundholm, L., & Rösblad, B. (2006). The Manual Ability Classification System (MACS) for children with cerebral palsy: scale development and evidence of validity and reliability. Developmental Medicine and Child Neurology, 48(7), 549–554.

Ferris, F. (2015). Cerebral Palsy. In R. M. Kliegman, B. F. Stanton, J. W. St Geme, et al. (Eds.), Nelson textbook of pediatrics (20th ed.). Philadelphia: Saunders.

Finder, J. D. (2009). A 2009 perspective on the 2004 American Thoracic Society statement, 'Respiratory care of the patient with Duchenne muscular dystrophy'. Pediatrics, 123(Suppl. 4), S239–S241.

Finkel, R. S., Chiriboga, C. A., Vajsar, J., et al. (2016). Treatment of infantile-onset spinal muscular atrophy with nusinersen: a phase 2, open-label, dose escalation study. Lancet, 388, 3017–3026.

Francis, R. (2007). Physiology and management of bladder and bowel continence following spinal cord injury. Ostomy/Wound Management, 53(12), 18–27.

George, J. M., Fiori, S., Fripp, J., et al. (2017). Validation of an MRI brain injury and growth scoring system in very preterm infants scanned at 29- to 35-week postmenstrual age. American Journal of Neuroradiology, 38(7), 1435–1442.

Golomb, M. R., Saha, C., Garg, B. P., et al. (2007). Association of cerebral palsy with other disabilities in children with perinatal arterial ischemic stroke. Pediatric Neurology, 37(4), 245–249.

Gray, M., & Moore, K. N. (2009). Urologic disorders: adult and pediatric care. St Louis: Mosby.

Hayes, J. S., & Arriola, T. (2005). Pediatric spinal injuries. Pediatric Nursing, 31(6), 464–467.

Hidecker, M. J., Paneth, N., Rosenbaum, P. L., et al. (2011). Developing and validating the Communication Function Classification System for individuals with cerebral palsy. Developmental Medicine and Child Neurology, 53(8), 704–710.

Hosalkar, H., Pandya, N. K., Hsu, J., et al. (2009). Specialty update: what's new in orthopaedic rehabilitation. The Journal of Bone and Joint Surgery. American Volume, 91(9), 2296–2310.

Hughes, R. (2008). The role of IVIG in autoimmune neuropathies: the latest evidence. Journal of Neurology, 255(Suppl. 3), 7–11.

Hughes, R. A., & Cornblath, D. R. (2005). Guillain-Barré syndrome. Lancet, 366(9497), 1653–1666.

Hughes, R., Swan, A., & Van Doorn, P. (2012). Intravenous immunoglobulin for Guillain-Barré Syndrome. Cochrane Database of Systematic Review, (7), CD002063.

Hurlbert, R. J., Hadley, M. N., Walters, B. C., et al. (2013). Pharmacological therapy for acute spinal cord injury. Neurosurgery, 72(3 Suppl.), 93–105.

Iannaccone, S. T. (2007). Modern management of spinal muscular atrophy. Journal of Child Neurology, 22(8), 974–978.

Iannaccone, S. T., & Burghes, A. (2002). Spinal muscular atrophies. Advances in Neurology, 88, 83–98.

Johnston, B. (2016). Early Intervention in Children with Developmental Disabilities. BMH Medical Journal, 3(1), 1–4.

Jones, M. W., Morgan, E., & Shelton, J. E. (2007). Primary care of the child with cerebral palsy: a review of systems (part II). Journal of Pediatric Health Care, 21(4), 226–237.

Keys, D. E., & Chaves-Carballo, E. (2013). Brain safari sick children sick brains and other maladies. California: Bookstand Publishing.

Kinsman, S., & Johnston, M. (2015). Myelomeningocele. In R. M. Kliegman, B. F. Stanton, J. W. St Geme, et al. (Eds.), Nelson textbook of pediatrics (20th ed.). Philadelphia: Saunders/Elsevier.

Kirshblum, S. C., Waring, W., Biering-Sorensen, F., et al. (2011). Reference for the 2011 revision of the international standards for neurological classification of spinal cord injury. The Journal of Spinal Cord Medicine, 34(6), 547–554.

Kravitz, R. M. (2009). Airway clearance in Duchenne muscular dystrophy. Pediatrics, 123(Suppl. 4), S231–S235.

Krigger, K. W. (2006). Cerebral palsy: an overview. American Family Physician, 73(1), 91–100, 101–102.

Laskowski-Jones, L. (2007). Peripheral nerve and spinal cord problems. In S. L. Lewis, M. M. Heitkemper, S. R. Dirksen, et al. (Eds.), Medical-surgical nursing: assessment and management of clinical problems (7th ed.). St Louis: Mosby/Elsevier.

Launay, F., Leet, A. I., & Sponseller, P. D. (2005). Pediatric spinal cord injury without radiographic abnormality: a meta-analysis. Clinical Orthopaedics and Related Research, 433, 166–170.

Lazzaretti, C. C., & Pearson, C. (2010). Myelodysplasia. In P. J. Allen, J. A. Vessey, & N. A. Schapiro (Eds.), Primary care of the child with a chronic condition (5th ed.). St Louis: Mosby.

Liptak, G. S., & Dosa, N. P. (2010). Myelomeningocele. Pediatrics in Review, 31(11), 443–450.

Lukban, M. B., Rosales, R. L., & Dressler, D. (2009). Effectiveness of botulinum toxin A for upper and lower limb spasticity in children with cerebral palsy: a summary of evidence. Journal of Neural Transmission, 116(3), 319–331.

Lyons, R. (2008). Elusive belly pain and Guillain-Barré syndrome. Journal of Pediatric Health Care, 22(5), 310–314.

MacLennan, A. H., Thompson, S. C., & Gecz, J. (2015). Cerebral palsy: causes, pathways, and the role of genetic variants. American Journal of Obstetrics and Gynecology, 213(6), 779–788. http://www.ajog.org/article/S0002-9378(15)00510-4/fulltext?cc=y=.

Manzur, A. Y., Kinali, M., & Muntoni, F. (2008). Update on the management of Duchenne muscular dystrophy. Archives of Disease in Childhood, 93(11), 986–990.

Manzur, A. Y., Kuntzer, T., Pike, M., et al. (2008). Glucocorticoid corticosteroids for Duchenne muscular dystrophy. Cochrane Database of Systematic Review, (1), CD003725.

Mathison, D. J., Kadom, N., & Krug, S. E. (2008). Spinal cord injury in the pediatric patient. Clinical Pediatric Emergency Medicine, 9(2), 106–123.

Mercuri, E., Bertini, E., & Iannaconne, S. T. (2012). Childhood spinal muscular atrophy: controversies and challenges. The Lancet. Neurology, 11(5), 443–452.

Merenda, L. A., & Hickey, K. (2005). Key elements of a bladder and bowel management for children with spinal cord injuries. SCI Nursing: A Publication of the American Association of Spinal Cord Injury Nurses, 22(1), 8–14.

Metcalfe, P. D. (2017). Neuropathic bladder: investigation and treatment through their lifetime. Canadian Urological Association Journal, 11(1–2Suppl1), S81–S86.

Morton, R., Gray, N., & Vloeberghs, M. (2011). Controlled study of the effects of continuous intrathecal baclofen infusion in non-ambulant children with cerebral palsy. Developmental Medicine and Child Neurology, 53, 736–741.

Motta, F., Antonello, C., & Stignani, C. (2011). Intrathecal baclofen and motor function in cerebral palsy. Developmental Medicine and Child Neurology, 53, 443–448.

Mourtzinos, A., & Stoffel, J. T. (2010). Management of goals for the spina bifida neurogenic bladder: a review from infancy to adulthood. The Urologic Clinics of North America, 37(4), 527–535.

Nehring, W. M. (2010). Cerebral palsy. In P. L. Jackson, J. A. Vessey, & N. A. Schapiro (Eds.), Primary care of the child with a chronic illness (5th ed.). St Louis: Mosby.

Newman, T. (2017). What's to know about Cerebral Palsy? http://www.medicalnewstoday.com/articles/152712.php.

Noonan, C., Quigley, S., & Curley, M. (2011). Using the Braden Q scale to predict pressure ulcer risk in pediatric patients. Journal of Pediatric Nursing, 26(6), 566–575.

Nordmark, E., Josenby, A. L., Lagergren, J., et al. (2008). Long-term outcomes 5 years after selective dorsal rhizotomy. BMC Pediatrics, 8, 54.

Ottolini, K., Harris, A. B., Amling, J. K., et al. (2013). Wound care challenges in children and adults with spina bifida: an open-cohort study. Journal of Pediatric Rehabilitation Medicine, 6(1), 1–10.

Parent, S., Mac-Thiong, J. M., Roy-Beaudry, M., et al. (2011). Spinal cord injury in the pediatric population: a systematic review of the literature. Journal of Neurotrauma, 28(8), 1515–1524.

Patterson, M. C., Bridgemohan, C., & Armsby, C. (2017): Clinical features and classification of cerebral palsy. https://www.uptodate.com/contents/clinical-features-and-classification-of-cerebral-palsy

Prior, T. (2010). Spinal muscular atrophy: newborn and carrier screening. Obstetrics and Gynecology Clinics of North America, 37(1), 23–26.

Pruitt, D. W., & McMahon, M. A. (2015). Spinal cord injury and autonomic crisis management. In R. M. Kliegman, B. F. Stanton, J. W. St Geme, et al. (Eds.), Nelson textbook of pediatrics (20th ed.). Philadelphia: Saunders/Elsevier.

Quan, D. (2011). Muscular dystrophies and neurologic diseases that present as myopathy. Rheumatic Diseases Clinics of North America, 37(2), 233–244.

Rall, S., & Grimm, T. (2012). Survival in Duchenne muscular dystrophy. Acta Myologica: Myopathies and Cardiomyopathies, 31(2), 117–120.

Rekate, H. L. (2015). Spinal cord injuries in children. In R. M. Kliegman, B. F. Stanton, J. W. St Geme, et al. (Eds.), Nelson textbook of pediatrics (20th ed.). Philadelphia: Saunders/Elsevier.

Rogers, B. (2004). Feeding method and health outcomes of children with cerebral palsy. The Journal of Pediatrics, 145(2 Suppl.), S28–S32.

Rowe, D. E., & Jadhav, A. L. (2008). Care of the adolescent with spina bifida. Pediatric Clinics of North America, 55(6), 1359–1374.

Royal Australian and New Zealand College of Obstetricians and Gynaecologists (RANZCOG). (2019). Planning for pregnancy. https://ranzcog.edu.au/womens-health/patient-information-resources/planning-for-pregnancy

Royal Australian and New Zealand College of Obstetricians and Gynaecologists (RANZCOG). (2018). Prenatal screening and diagnostic testing for fetal chromosomal and genetic conditions. https://ranzcog.edu.au/RANZCOG_SITE/media/RANZCOG-MEDIA/Women%27s%20Health/Statement%20and%20guidelines/Clinical-Obstetrics/Prenatal-screening_1.pdf?ext=.pdf

Rozelle, C. J., Arabi, B., Dhall, S. S., et al. (2013). Management of pediatric cervical spine and spinal cord injuries. Neurosurgery, 72(3 Suppl.), 205–226.

Rumberg, F., Bakir, M. S., Taylor, W. R., et al. (2016). The effects of selective dorsal rhizotomy on balance and symmetry of gait in children with cerebral palsy. PLoS ONE, 11(4), e0152930.

Samaniego, I. A. (2003). A sore spot in pediatrics: risk factors for pressure ulcers. Pediatric Nursing, 29(4), 278–282.

Sandler, A. D. (2010). Children with spina bifida: key clinical issues. Pediatric Clinics of North America, 57(4), 879–892.

Sarnat, H. B. (2015a). Spinal muscular atrophies. In R. M. Kliegman, B. F. Stanton, J. St Geme, et al. (Eds.), Nelson textbook of pediatrics (20th ed.). Philadelphia: Saunders.

Sarnat, H. B. (2015b). Guillain-Barré syndrome. In R. M. Kliegman, B. F. Stanton, J. St Geme, et al. (Eds.), Nelson textbook of pediatrics (20th ed.). Philadelphia: Saunders.

Sarnat, H. B. (2015c). Muscular dystrophies. In R. M. Kliegman, B. F. Stanton, J. W. St Geme, et al. (Eds.), Nelson textbook of pediatrics (20th ed.). Philadelphia: Saunders.

Sawyer, S., & Macnee, S. (2010). Transition to adult healthcare for adolescents with spina bifida: research issues. Developmental Disabilities Research Reviews, 16(1), 60–65.

Schottler, J., Vogel, L., & Sturm, P. (2012). Spinal cord injuries in young children: a review of children injured at 5 years of age and younger. Developmental Medicine and Child Neurology, 54, 1138–1143.

Schroth, M. K. (2009). Special considerations in the respiratory management of spinal muscular atrophy. Pediatrics, 123(Suppl. 4), S245–S249.

Sehrawat, N., Marwaha, M., Bansal, K., et al. (2014). Cerebral palsy: a dental update. International Journal of Clinical Pediatric Dentistry, 7(2), 109–118.

Shavelle, R. M., DeVivo, M. J., Paculdo, D. R., et al. (2007). Long-term survival after childhood spinal cord injury. The Journal of Spinal Cord Medicine, 30(Suppl. 1), S48–S54.

Simonds, A. K. (2006). Recent advances in respiratory care for neuromuscular disease. Chest, 130(6), 1879–1886.

Simpson, J. L., Richards, D. S., & Otaño, L. (2012). Prenatal genetic diagnosis. In S. G. Gabbe, J. R. Niebyl, J. L. Simpson, et al. (Eds.), Obstetrics: normal and problem pregnancies (6th ed.). Philadelphia: Saunders.

Snodgrass, W., & Gargollo, P. (2010). Urologic care of the neurogenic bladder in children. The Urologic Clinics of North America, 37(2), 207–214.

Starship. (2019). New Zealand Cerebral Palsy Register. https://www.starship.org.nz/health-professionals/cerebral-palsy-research/

Thrasher, T. A., & Popovic, M. R. (2008). Functional electrical stimulation of walking: function, exercise and rehabilitation. Annales de Readaptation et de Medecine Physique: Revue Scientifique de la Societe Francaise de Reeducation Fonctionnelle de Readaptation et de Medecine Physique, 51(6), 452–460.

To, C. S., Kirsch, R. F., Kobetic, R., et al. (2005). Simulation of a functional neuromuscular stimulation powered mechanical gait orthosis with coordinated joint locking. IEEE Transactions on Neural Systems and Rehabilitation Engineering: A Publication of the IEEE Engineering in Medicine and Biology Society, 13(2), 227–235.

Vogel, L. C., Betz, R. R., & Mulcahey, M. J. (2012). Spinal cord injuries in children and adolescents. In Verhaagen, J., & MacDonald, J. W., Eds. Handbook of Clinical Neurology, 109(3), 131–148.

Vogel, L. C., Chlan, K. M., Zebracki, K., et al. (2011). Long-term outcomes of adults with pediatric-onset spinal cord injuries as a function of neurologic impairment. The Journal of Spinal Cord Medicine, 34(1), 60–66.

Westbom, L., Bergstrand, L., Wagner, P., et al. (2011). Survival at 19 years of age in a total population of children and young people with cerebral palsy. Developmental Medicine and Child Neurology, 53, 806–814.

Wright, P., Durham, S., Ewins, D., et al. (2012). Neuromuscular electrical stimulation for children with cerebral palsy: a review. Archives of Disease in Childhood, 97(4), 364–371.

Young, H. K., Lowe, A., & Fitzgerald, D. A. (2007). Outcome of noninvasive ventilation in children with neuromuscular disease. Neurology, 68(3), 198–201.

INDEX

Page numbers followed by 'b' indicate boxes; 'f', figures; 't', tables.

A

abdomen, physical examination, 153
  auscultation, 89
  inspection, 88–89, 89f
  palpation, 89, 89b
  structures, 88, 88f
abdominal pain, 101
abnormal uterine bleeding (AUB), 403–405, 404b
absence seizures, 854
absent testis, 585
abusive head trauma, 329
accidental injury, 1
Accident Compensation Corporation (ACC), 2–3
Achilles reflex, 93, 94f
acidosis, chronic kidney disease (CKD), 581
acne, 908–909, 908f
acne vulgaris, 908, 908f
acquired immunity, 123b
acquired immunodeficiency syndrome (AIDS), 27, 778–780
acrocentric chromosomes, 28–29
acrocyanosis, 154
acromegaly, pituitary function, 870
active immunity, 123b
acute appendicitis, 609–610, 609b
acute compartment syndrome (ACS), 932–933
acute diarrhoea, 594–595, 598b, 599–600t
acute epiglottitis, 653–655
acute glomerulonephritis (AGN)
  aetiology, 568
  clinical manifestations, 568–569
  diagnostic evaluation, 569
  hypertension, 569
  pathophysiology, 568
  poststreptococcal glomerulonephritis *vs.* nephrotic syndrome, 568, 568t
  systemic disease process, 567–568, 567t
  therapeutic management, 569–570
acute hepatitis, 622–624, 622t
  clinical manifestations, 623–624
  diagnostic evaluation, 624
  hepatitis A virus (HAV), 622–623
  hepatitis B virus (HBV), 623
  hepatitis C virus (HCV), 623
  hepatitis D virus (HDV), 623
  hepatitis E virus (HEV), 623
  nursing care management, 624
  pathophysiology, 623
  therapeutic management, 624
acute infections, 653, 653f
acute kidney injury (AKI), 575–578
  aetiology, 575–576
  clinical manifestations, 576
  diagnostic evaluation, 576
  laboratory findings, 577t
  nursing care management, 578
  pathophysiology, 576
  therapeutic management, 576–578
    complications, 578
    diuretic/high-output, phase, 578
    fluid and calories, 577
    hyperkalaemia, 577–578
    hypertension, 578
    prognosis, 578
acute laryngitis, 655
acute *laryngotracheobronchitis* (LTB), 655–656, 656f
acute lung injury (ALI), 670–672
acute lymphoblastic leukaemia (ALL)
  clinical manifestations, 798–799

acute lymphoblastic leukaemia *(Continued)*
  clinical staging and prognosis, 798, 798t
  diagnostic evaluation, 799
  treatment, 799
acute myeloid leukaemia (AML), 799–800, 800f
acute otitis externa (AOE), 653
acute poststreptococcal glomerulonephritis (APSGN), 568
acute respiratory distress syndrome (ARDS), 670–672, 671f
acute spasmodic laryngitis, 656
acute streptococcal pharyngitis, 645–646, 645t, 646t
acute viral nasopharyngitis, 644–645, 645b
Addison's disease
  clinical manifestations, 878, 878b
  nursing care management, 879
  therapeutic management, 879
ADHD. *See* attention deficit/hyperactivity disorder (ADHD)
adolescence. *See also* growth and development promotion, adolescence
  Aboriginal and Torres Strait Islander children, 396
  abortion, 410–411, 410b
  alcohol use, 394
  chronic/complex diseases, 431
  depression and suicide, 394
  dietary habits and eating disorders, 393, 393f
  female reproductive system
    abnormal uterine bleeding (AUB), 403–405, 404b
    endometriosis, 402–403, 403f
    gynaecological examination, 401
    menstrual disorders, 401–402
    premenstrual dysphoric disorder (PMDD), 403
    sexually transmitted bacterial infections, 406–408
    sexually transmitted infections (STIs), 405–406, 406b
    sexually transmitted protozoa infections, 406
    sexually transmitted viral infections, 408–409
    vaginal infections, 405
    vulvar pain, 405
  health and wellbeing, 396
  health promotion, 391–392
  health screening, 392
  hypertension, 395
  infectious diseases and immunisation, 395
  intentional and unintentional injury, 392–393
  LGBTIQ+, 397
  male reproductive system
    epididymitis, 400–401
    gynaecomastia, 401
    penile conditions, 400
    testicular torsion, 401
    varicocele, 400
  nursing care management, 397
  physical activity, 393, 393f
  physical, sexual and emotional abuse, 394
  pregnancy
    complications, 409–410
    fathers, 410
    incidence, 409
    medical concerns, 409
    mother–infant relationships, 410
    nursing care management, 410
  psychosocial adjustment, 392
  rural, 397
  school and learning problems, 394–395
  self-assessed health status, 396–397
  sexual behaviour, 393–394
  sexually transmitted infections (STIs), 393–394
  sleep deprivation and insomnia, 396
  tobacco use, 394
  unintended pregnancy, 393–394

adoption, 15
adrenal cortex, 876–877
adrenal function
  acute adrenocortical insufficiency, 877–878
  adrenal hormones, 876–877
  CAH, 880–881
  chronic adrenocortical insufficiency, 878–879, 878b
  Cushing's syndrome, 879–880, 879t, 880f
  hyperaldosteronism, 881–882
  phaeochromocytoma, 882
adrenal hormones
  cortex, 876–877
  medulla, 877
adrenal medulla, 877
adrenocortical insufficiency
  acute
    clinical manifestations, 877, 878b
    diagnostic evaluation, 877
    nursing care management, 878
    therapeutic management, 877
  chronic
    clinical manifestations, 878, 878b
    nursing care management, 879
    therapeutic management, 879
adrenocorticotropic hormone (ACTH), 854
AGA. *See* appropriate for gestational age (AGA)
aggression, preschooler, 318–319
AGN. *See* acute glomerulonephritis (AGN)
AHMAC. *See* Australian Health Ministers' Advisory Council (AHMAC)
AIDS. *See* acquired immunodeficiency syndrome (AIDS)
air leak syndromes
  clinical manifestations, 218
  nursing care management, 218
  pulmonary interstitial emphysema (PIE), 218
  therapeutic management, 218
AKI. *See* acute kidney injury (AKI)
alcohol use, adolescence, 394
allele, 25–27b
allergic contact dermatitis, 899
allergic rhinitis, 675–697
alopecia, 795
alpha-fetoprotein (AFP), 25–27b
Alport's syndrome (AS), 574
ambiguous genitalia, 587
amenorrhoea, 401–402
amniocentesis, 25–27b
amphetamines, 939
anabolic steroids, 939
anaemia, 224
  burn, 544
  chronic kidney disease (CKD), 579, 580b, 581
  impaired/decreased red blood cells production
    aplastic anaemia (AA), 771, 771b
    blood clotting, 772f
    haemophilia, 772–775, 773t
    haemostasis, 771–772
    immune thrombocytopenia, 775–776
    von Willebrand disease (vWD), 775
  increased destruction, red blood cells, 763–771
  increased red blood cells destruction
    beta-thalassaemia (β-thalassaemia/Cooley's anaemia), 768–771, 769b, 769f
    hereditary spherocytosis (HS), 763
    sickle cell anaemia (SCA), 763–768, 764f, 765b, 767b, 768f
  nutritional deficiencies, 760–763
    iron deficiency anaemia (IDA), 760–763, 760b, 762t

analgesia
  administration, 110, 111–112b
  co-analgesic drugs, 109
  epidural, 112
  equipment needs, 115b
  timing, 110
  transmucosal and transdermal, 112, 112f
anencephaly, 970–971
aneuploidy, 25–27b, 29
Angelman's syndrome, 39
ankle-foot orthosis (AFO), 925
anorchism, 585
anorectal malformations (ARMs), 633–634, 633b, 633f
antegrade continence enema (ACE), 976
anthropometry, 63–64
antibody, 123b
anticipatory grief, 208
anticipatory guidance
  infant, 269–270
  preschooler, 322–323
  school-age children, 358
  toddlerhood, 308
antidiuretic hormone (ADH), 526
antidotes, poisoning, 328
antigens, 123b, 185
antisense oligonucleotide (ASO), 979
antithyroid drug (ATD) therapy, 874
antitoxin, 123b
anus, physical assessment, 91, 154
anxiety disorders, 377–378
AOE. *See* acute otitis externa (AOE)
AOP. *See* apnoea of prematurity (AOP)
Apert syndrome, 173b
Apgar scoring system, 140, 140t
aphthous stomatitis, 134
aplastic anaemia (AA), 771, 771b
apnoea, 152–153, 211
apnoea of prematurity (AOP)
  causes of, 212b
  classification, 211
  clinical manifestations, 211
  nursing care management, 212
  pathophysiology, 211
  therapeutic management, 211–212
apoptosis, 784
appetite, 360–361
appropriate for gestational age (AGA), 143
APSGN. *See* acute poststreptococcal glomerulonephritis (APSGN)
arachnoid membrane, 820
ARMs. *See* anorectal malformations (ARMs)
arterial oxygen pressure (PaO_2), 821
arthropods, 900, 900–901t
ASD. *See* autism spectrum disorder (ASD)
aseptic meningitis, 848–849, 849t
aspiration pneumonia, 668–669, 668b
association, 25–27b, 28
asthma, 677–687, 678b, 678f, 679f, 680f, 682f, 684t, 688f
atonic seizures, 854
atopic dermatitis (eczema) (AD)
  child's age, 906
  clinical manifestations, 906, 907b
  nursing care management, 907–908
  therapeutic management, 906–907
atresia, 627
attention deficit/hyperactivity disorder (ADHD)
  aetiology, 370
  clinical manifestations, 370
  diagnostic evaluation, 370–371
  nursing care management, 371–372
  symptoms, 369
  therapeutic management, 371
attenuate, 123b
AUB. *See* abnormal uterine bleeding (AUB)
aura, focal seizures, 853
Australian Health Ministers' Advisory Council (AHMAC), 9
Australia's children reports, 2b
Australia's health system, 2
authoritarian, 14
authoritative parenting, 14
autism spectrum disorders (ASDs), 105
  aetiology, 463
  clinical manifestations, 463
  definition, 462–463
  diagnostic evaluation, 463
  nursing care management, 463–464
  prognosis, 463
autologous transplantation, 791
automatisms, focal seizures, 853
autonomic dysreflexia, 984
autosomal dominant inheritance, 33–34, 33f, 34f, 35–37t
autosomal recessive inheritance, 34, 37f
autosome aneuploidies, 29–31, 30t
autosomes, 25–27b, 28
azotaemia, 526–527

B
BA. *See* biliary atresia (BA)
Babinski's reflex, 154, 154f, 155t, 826
bacterial infections, 894–896, 895t
bacterial meningitis
  aetiology, 845–846
  clinical manifestations, 846–847, 846b, 847f
  diagnostic evaluation, 847
  nursing care management, 848
  pathophysiology, 846
  therapeutic management, 847–848
bacterial tracheitis, 657
bacterial vaginosis (BV), 405
balanced translocation carriers, 32
balanitis, 584
Ballard Scale (BS), 143, 144f
basal metabolic rate (BMR), 522
basilar fractures, 834
BAT. *See* brown adipose tissue (BAT)
bathing, infection and injury prevention, 157
behavioural assessment, 141–142
  cry, 141–142
  Newborn Behavioural Observations (NBO) assessment, 141
  sleep-wake states, 141, 142t
  state modulation, 141
behavioural components
  anorexia nervosa (AN), 413–416, 414b
    signs of, 416b
  anxiety disorders, 377–378
  attention deficit/hyperactivity disorder (ADHD)
    aetiology, 370
    clinical manifestations, 370
    diagnostic evaluation, 370–371
    nursing care management, 371–372
    symptoms, 369
    therapeutic management, 371
  bulimia nervosa (BN), 413–416
  childhood depression, 376–377, 377b
  childhood schizophrenia, 377
  conduct disorders, 378–379, 378t
  functional abdominal pain (FAP), 375–376
  Gilles de la Tourette's syndrome (GTS), 372–373
  learning disabilities, 372
  posttraumatic stress disorder (PTSD), 373–374
  school phobia, 374–375
  tic disorders, 372, 372b
behaviour modification, 363
behaviour therapy, 364–365
benzoyl peroxide, 909
beta-thalassaemia (β-thalassaemia/Cooley's anaemia), 768–771, 769b, 769f
bicycle-associated injuries, 6
bilateral cleft lip, 175, 176f
bile, 593
biliary atresia (BA), 624–626, 625f
bilirubin encephalopathy, 180–181
bilirubin-induced neurological dysfunction, 180–181
binocularity, 241–242
biological development
  adolescence
    breasts development, 384f
    genital development, 385f
    in girls, 384f
    gonadotropin-releasing hormone (GnRH), 382–383, 383f
    physiological changes, 386
    pubertal sexual maturation, 383–386
    puberty, 382, 386
    pubic hair growth, 385f
    reproductive hormones, 383
    Tanner stages, 383b
  infant
    fine motor development, 245, 245f
    gross motor behaviour, 245
    head control, 245–246, 246f
    locomotion, 247, 248f
    maturation of systems, 242–245
    proportional changes, 241, 242b, 242f
    rolling over, 246
    sensory changes, 241–242, 242b, 243b, 243f
    sitting, 246–247, 247f
    skills, 241
  preschooler
    gross and fine motor behaviour, 310–311, 311f
    physical growth rate, 310
  school-age children, 337–340
    maturation of systems, 337–338
    physical changes, 337, 338f
    preadolescence, 338
    prepubescence, 338
    puberty, 338
  toddler, 290–292
    gross and fine motor development, 291–292
    maturation of systems, 291
    proportional changes, 290, 291f
    sensory changes, 290–291
biological therapy, children's cancer, 790–791
bipolar disorder, 376
birth injuries
  fractures
    crepitus, 170
    intracranial pressure (ICP), 170
    nursing care management, 170–171
  head injury, 168–169
    caput succedaneum, 168, 170f
    cephalhaematoma, 169, 170f
    skull fractures, 168
    subgaleal haemorrhage, 169, 170f
  maternal factors, 168
  nerve injuries
    brachial palsy, 171, 171f
    facial paralysis, 171, 171f
    nursing care management, 172
    phrenic nerve paralysis, 171
  soft tissue injury, 168, 169b
  types, 168, 169b
birthmarks, 179–180, 180f
birth weight, 143, 145f
bladder exstrophy, 586–587, 586f
blindness and low vision
  aetiology, 458–460
  definition and classification, 458
  eye injuries, 460b
  nursing care management, 460–462
  types, 459–460b
blood–brain barrier (BBB), 821
blood clotting, 772f
blood pressure (BP), 72, 74f
  physical assessment, 145, 151f

blood specimens, 498–500
from arterial vessels, 499–500
capillary methods, 500, 500f
from central venous catheters, 498–499
from peripheral veins, 499
blood transfusion therapy, 759–760, 759t
blood urea nitrogen (BUN), 543
BMR. *See* basal metabolic rate (BMR)
body fluids distribution, 524–526t. *See also* electrolyte balance
basal metabolic rate (BMR), 522
extracellular fluid (ECF), 520
intracellular fluid (ICF), 520
total body water (TBW), 520, 522, 522f
water balance
fluid movement mechanisms, 520–522
in infants, 522–523
internal control mechanisms, 522b
pathophysiology, 520–521, 521f
requirements, 522t
body mass index (BMI), 360
bonding and attachment behaviours, 142, 142b
bone marrow aspiration/biopsy, 496, 786
bone tumours
clinical manifestations, 809
diagnostic evaluation, 809
Ewing's sarcoma, 810–811
osteosarcoma, 809–810
prognosis, 809
bottle-feeding, infection and injury prevention, 160
Bowen's family systems theory, 11
bowleg/genu varum, 91–92, 92f
BP. *See* blood pressure (BP)
brachial palsy, 171, 171f
bradycardia, 152–153
brain abscess, 849
brain coverings, 820, 820f
brain neuromatrix, 98
brain tumours
clinical manifestations, 803, 805t
diagnostic evaluation, 803–804
location, 803, 804f
nursing care management
assessment, 806–807
comfort measures, 807
diagnostic and operative procedures, 806
family support, 807
fluid regulation, 807
optimum functioning, 807–808
positioning, 807
postoperative complications, 806
signs and symptoms, 805–806
therapeutic management, 804
breastfeeding
drug-exposed infants, 232
infection and injury prevention, 159–160, 159t, 160b, 161–162t, 162f
premature infants, 203
sepsis, 221
brief resolved unexplained event (BRUE), 287–288
broader influences, child health
economy and poverty, 20–21
ethnicity, 20
mass media, 19–20
media effects, 20, 21t
parental education, 21–22
positive media, 20, 20b
race, 20
refugee and immigration, 22
religion/spiritual identity, 22–23, 22f, 23b
social media, 19–20
bronchiolitis, 657–659, 659b
bronchitis, 657
brown adipose tissue (BAT), 138
BRUE. *See* brief resolved unexplained event (BRUE)
BS. *See* Ballard Scale (BS)
Buck extension traction, 924, 924f
bullous impetigo, 179
bullying, 343
BUN. *See* blood urea nitrogen (BUN)
burns, 101–102
epidemiology and aetiology, 538–539
major burns management, 546–548, 546b
minor burns management, 546
nursing care management, 550–553
prevention, 553
skin grafts
adherent allograft, 549f
mesh graft, 550f
requirements, 550b
sheet graft, 550f
split-thickness removal, 550f
types, 549b
therapeutic management, 545–550
wound characteristics
complications, 544–545
injury depth, 540, 540f, 541f
injury extent, 539, 539f
injury severity, 540–541, 542f
pathophysiology, 541–545
systemic responses, 543–544, 543f
zones, 543b, 543f
wound management, 548–550, 548b, 548f
BV. *See* bacterial vaginosis (BV)

C
CAH. *See* congenital adrenal hyperplasia (CAH)
calcitonin, 872
cancer pain, 102, 102t, 116–117
candidiasis, 178, 405
caput succedaneum, 168, 170f
cardiac catheterisation
congenital heart defects, 723–724, 724f
congenital heart disease, 708
altered haemodynamics, 708, 709f
clinical consequences of, 708
nursing care, 724–730
congestive heart failure, 709–723, 710f
altered haemodynamics, 709
clinical manifestations, 710–711, 711b
nursing care management, 712–714
skin-to-skin cuddles, 713f
diagnostic, 706–707, 707t
electrophysiological studies, 707
hypoxaemia, 714
altered haemodynamics, 714
aortic stenosis, 719f
atrial septal defect, 717f
atrioventricular canal defect, 717f
clinical manifestations, 714–715, 714f
coarctation of the aorta, 719f
diagnostic evaluation, 715
great vessels transposition, 722f
mixed defects, 720–722b
nursing care management, 723
obstructive defects, 718b
pulmonary blood flow, 719–720b
pulmonary stenosis, 719f
shunt procedures, 723t
Tetralogy of Fallot, 720f
therapeutic management, 715–723, 715f, 716–717b
tricuspid atresia, 720f
ventricular septal defect, 717f
interventional, 707
cardiogenic shock, 531
cardiovascular system
burn shock, 543
complications, 223–225
caregiver–child interaction, 331–332
carrier, 25–27b
catecholamine secretion, 877, 877b
cat-scratch disease, 904
cat's eye reflex/leucocoria, 813, 814f
cavernous venous haemangiomas, 179
CCHD. *See* critical congenital heart disease (CCHD)
CDI. *See* Children's Depression Inventory (CDI)
cell-mediated immunity, 778
central nervous system (CNS)
cerebral dysfunction, 819–821, 820f
children's cancer
brain tumours. *See* bone tumours
neuroblastoma, 808–809
central nervous system depressants, 417
central nervous system stimulants, 418
centromere, 25–27b
cephalhaematoma, 169, 170f
cephalocaudal-proximodistal laws, 139
cephalopelvic disproportion, 168
cerebral blood flow (CBF), 821
cerebral dysfunction
cerebral structure and function
central nervous system, 819–821
intracranial pressure, 821–822, 822b
neurological system, 819
headaches
assessment, 860–861, 861b
migraine, 861, 861b
head injury
aetiology, 833
complications, 834–836
diagnostic evaluation, 836–837, 836b, 837b
nursing care management, 838–839, 838b
pathophysiology, 833–834, 833f
therapeutic management, 837–838
hydrocephalus
aetiology, 841–842
clinical manifestations, 842–843, 842f
diagnostic evaluation, 843
nursing care management, 844–845
pathophysiology, 841, 842f
therapeutic management, 843–844
intracranial infections
bacterial meningitis, 845–848
brain abscess, 849
encephalitis, 849–850
non-bacterial (aseptic) meningitis, 848–849, 849t
neurological status
altered state of consciousness, 823–824
diagnostic procedures, 826–827, 828t
history, 822
neurological examination, 825–826
physical examination, 822–823, 823b
seizures and epilepsy
aetiology, 850–851, 850b
clinical manifestations, 851, 852–853b
definition, 850
diagnostic evaluation, 855–856
febrile seizure, 860
focal seizures, 851–853
generalised seizures, 853–854
incidence, 851
LGS, 855
nursing care management, 857–860, 857b, 858b, 859b
pathophysiology, 851
prognosis, 857
therapeutic management, 856–857
unknown-onset epileptic seizures, 854–855
submersion injury
accidental submersion injury, 840, 840f
clinical manifestations, 840
drowning, 839–840
nursing care management, 841
pathophysiology, 840
therapeutic management, 840–841
unconscious child
elimination, 831
family support, 832

cerebral dysfunction *(Continued)*
intracranial pressure monitoring, 829–830
LOC, 827–828
medications, 831
nutrition and hydration, 830–831, 831t
pain management, 828–829
respiratory management, 829
stimulation, 831–832
thermoregulation, 831
cerebral hypoperfusion, 72
cerebral malformation. *See* hydrocephalus
cerebral oedema, 836
cerebral palsy (CP)
aetiology, 962, 962b
clinical classification, 963, 963b
clinical features, 961–962
clinical manifestations, 963–965, 964b
diagnostic evaluation, 965
nursing care management, 968–969
pathophysiology, 962–963
therapeutic management, 966b
associated problems, 967
education, 968
functional and adaptive training, 967–968, 968f
medication, 966–967
mobilising devices, 965, 966f
physical therapy, 967
prognosis, 968
rehabilitation program, 965
speech therapy, 968
surgery, 965
technical aids, 967
cervical thoracolumbosacral orthosis (CTLSO), 926
cervical traction, 924, 924f
CGN. *See* chronic glomerulonephritis (CGN)
chemotherapy
administering and handling chemotherapeutic agents, 789–790, 790f
adrenal and gonadal hormones, 789
alkylating agents, 789
central venous lines, 789, 789f
role of, 787–788
venous access devices, 788
chest, physical examination, 83–84, 83f, 84f, 152
Chiari's malformation, 842
myelomeningocele, 971–972
chickenpox, 128, 131f
chilblain, 909
child abuse/non-accidental injury, 911–912
childhood depression, 376–377, 377b
childhood health problems
childhood mortality, 7
infant mortality, 6–7, 7f
injuries, 4–6, 6f
low birth weight (LBW), 4
mental health problems, 6
obesity, 4, 5f
type 2 diabetes, 4
very low birth weight (VLBW), 4
childhood schizophrenia, 377
child maltreatment
abusive head trauma, 329
caregiver–child interaction, 331–332
clinical manifestations, 333b
discharge plan, 335
history and interview, 332
Munchausen syndrome by proxy (MSBP), 329–330
neglect, 329
nursing care management, 334
physical abuse, 329–330
factors predisposing to, 330
physical assessment, 332–334
poison prevention, 329b
prevention, 335
child maltreatment *(Continued)*
sexual abuse
abusers and victims characteristics, 330–331
initiation and perpetuation, 331
nursing care of, 331
types, 330
warning signs of, 331b
social problems, 328–329
child neglect, 329
children's cancer
aetiology, 784
blood and lymph systems
acute lymphoblastic leukaemia, 798–799
acute myeloid leukaemia, 799–800, 800f
Hodgkin's lymphoma, 801–802
non-Hodgkin's lymphoma, 802–803, 803b
nursing care management, 800–801
bone tumours
clinical manifestations, 809
diagnostic evaluation, 809
Ewing's sarcoma, 810–811
osteosarcoma, 809–810
prognosis, 809
challenges, 783
clinical trials, 786–787
complications of therapy, 791–792
diagnostic evaluation
history, 784–785
laboratory tests, 786
pathological and molecular evaluation, 786
physical examination, 785
procedures and imaging, 786
symptoms, 785
tests and procedures, 785
epidemiology, 783
nervous system tumours
brain tumours. *See* bone tumours
neuroblastoma, 808–809
nursing care management
altered nutrition, 794–795
anaemia, 794
completion of therapy, 797–798
family education, 797
haematopoietic stem cell transplantation, 796
haemorrhage, 793–794
haemorrhagic cystitis, 795
health promotion, 797
infection, 793
mucosal ulceration, 795
nausea and vomiting, 794
neurological problems, 795
pain management, 796–797
preparation, 796
quality patient outcomes, 792b
signs and symptoms, 792–793, 792b
steroid effects, 795–796
risk factors, 784, 785t
solid tumours
GCTs, 815
liver tumours, 815
retinoblastoma, 813–815
rhabdomyosarcoma, 812–813, 813t
Wilms tumour, 811–812
survival rates, 815–817, 816t
treatment modalities
biological therapy, 790–791
chemotherapy, 787–790
haematopoietic stem cell transplant, 791
surgery, 787, 788t
Children's Depression Inventory (CDI), 107
Children's Headline Indicators (CHIs), 1, 2b
child wellbeing, 9
chimeric antigen receptor (CAR) T-cell therapy, 790–791
CHIs. *See* Children's Headline Indicators (CHIs)
Chlamydia, 406–407
choanal atresia, 675
chorionic villi sampling (CVS), 25–27b
chromosome, 25–27b
aberrations, 25–27b
abnormalities, 784
acrocentric, 25–27b
deletion, 31–32
instability syndromes, 33
metacentric, 25–27b
submetacentric, 25–27b
chromosome breakage, 31
reciprocal translocation, 32
translocation, 32
chronic/complex diseases
adjustment, 427
children care
chronic conditions, 423, 424t
family-centred care, 424
family healthcare provider communication, 424
normalisation, 424–425
shared decision-making, 424, 425b
siblings, 423
therapeutic relationships, 424
child with
coping mechanisms, 428
developmental aspects, 428, 428f, 429–430t
hopefulness, 428
family of child
anticipated parental stress, 425b
concurrent stresses, 426–427
coping mechanisms, 427
goal, 425
parental differences, 425–426
parental empowerment, 427
parental roles, 425
parents tasks, 425, 425b
siblings, 426, 426b
single-parent families, 426
nursing care of, 428–432
activities of daily living, 431
adolescence, 431
assessment, 428
diagnosis, 428
early childhood, 431
family's coping methods, 428–430, 430b
normal development promotion, 431
primary healthcare, 431
safe transportation, 431
school age, 431
reintegration and acknowledgment, 427
shock and denial, 427
support system, 427
chronic diarrhoea, 595, 601b
chronic glomerulonephritis (CGN), 570
chronic kidney disease (CKD), 578–581
aetiology, 579
anaemia, 579, 580b
bone demineralisation, 579, 579b
clinical manifestations, 580
diagnostic evaluation, 580
growth disturbance, 579–580, 580b
nursing care management, 581
pathophysiology, 579–580
progressive deterioration, 578–579
therapeutic management, 580–581
chronic lung disease
mild, 219
nursing care management, 220
pathophysiology, 219
prognosis, 220
therapeutic management, 219–220
chronic lymphocytic thyroiditis, 873–874
chronic non-specific diarrhoea (CNSD), 595
cigarette smoking, 233–234
circulatory system, extrauterine life, newborn, 137–138

circumcision, infection and injury prevention, 158
cirrhosis, 626–627
CKD. *See* chronic kidney disease (CKD)
clean intermittent catheterisation (CIC), 975
cleft lip/cleft palate (CL/CP), 174–178
  aetiology, 174
  diagnostic evaluation, 175, 176f
  feeding, 177
  long-term problems, 176–177
  nursing care management, 177–178
  pathophysiology, 174–175, 175f
  preoperative care, 177–178
  surgical correction, 175–176
  variations, 175f
clinical nurse specialist (CNS), 8
cloacal exstrophy, 586–587
clonus, 851
CMA. *See* cow's milk allergy (CMA)
CNS. *See* clinical nurse specialist (CNS)
CNSD. *See* chronic non-specific diarrhoea (CNSD)
COAG. *See* council of Australian Governments (COAG)
cocaine, 417
cocooning, 123b
coeliac disease (gluten-sensitive enteropathy), 619–620, 619b
cognitive development
  adolescence
    formal operational thought, 386–387
    self conceptions, 387
    social cognition, 387
  infant
    affect, 250
    imitation, 250
    mental representation, 250
    object permanence, 250
    primary circular reactions, 250
    reflexes, 250
    secondary circular reactions, 250
    sensorimotor phase, 249–250, 249f, 249t
    separation event, 249–250
    zone of proximal development, 250
  school-age children
    concrete operations, 340
    conservation, 340, 341f
  toddler
    causal relationship, 293
    domestic mimicry, 294, 294f
    mental symbolisation, 294–295
    object permanence, 294
    preoperational phase, 294
    preoperational thinking, 294, 295b
    sensorimotor phase, 292–293, 293t
    spatial relationships, 294
    tertiary circular reactions, 293
cognitive disability (CD)
  aetiology, 448–449
  diagnosis and classification, 448
  incidence, 448
  nursing care of
    child and family education, 449–452, 450f
    Down syndrome, 452, 453b, 453f
    fragile X syndrome (FXS), 454–455, 454b
cognitive therapy, 378
cold injury, 909
colic (paroxysmal abdominal pain)
  aetiology, 281
  characteristics, 281
  nursing care management, 282
  sleep problems, 282, 283t
  therapeutic management, 282
collagen, 558
coma assessment, 823–824, 824f
combination vaccine, 123b
commercially prepared formulas, infection and injury prevention, 160–162
comminuted fractures, 834
communicable diseases
  child and family support, 134
  of childhood, 128, 129–131t
    chickenpox, 128, 131f
    erythema infectiosum, 128, 131f
    exanthem subitum, 128, 131f
    measles, 128, 132f
    rubella, 128, 132f
    scarlet fever, 128, 133f
  comfortness, 133
  complications, 132–133
  conjunctivitis
    clinical manifestations, 134, 134b
    nursing care management, 134
    therapeutic management, 134
  incidence, 128
  nursing care management, 128–134
  primary prevention, 128
  prodromal symptoms, 128
  stomatitis
    aphthous stomatitis, 134
    herpetic gingivostomatitis (HGS), 135, 135f
    nursing care management, 135
    therapeutic management, 135
communication
  autism spectrum disorders (ASDs)
    aetiology, 463
    clinical manifestations, 463
    definition, 462–463
    diagnostic evaluation, 463
    nursing care management, 463–464
    prognosis, 463
  with children
    adolescence, 55, 55b
    egocentric, 54, 54f
    infancy, 53–54
    interpreters, 53b
    school-age years, 54
  computer privacy and applications, 50
  and interviewing, 50
  with parents
    anticipatory guidance, 52
    blocks, 52, 53b
    directing the focus, 51–52
    empathy, 52
    information overload, 52
    interpreter, 52–53, 53b
    listening and cultural awareness, 52
    nurse's relationship, 51
    silence, 52
    to talk, 51
  patient teaching, 50
  privacy and confidentiality, 50, 51f
  techniques
    play, 55–57
    verbal and non-verbal, 56–57b
  telehealth and counselling, 50–51
  telephone triage, 50–51, 51b
compensated shock, 532–533
complementary and alternative medicine (CAM), 797
compound heterozygous, 34
concordant, 25–27b
concussion, head injury, 833–834
conduct disorders, 378–379, 378t
conduction, stable body temperature, 156
congenital, 25–27b
  anomalies, 27–28
congenital adrenal hyperplasia (CAH), 588
  clinical manifestations, 880–881
  diagnostic evaluation, 881
  nursing care management, 881
  therapeutic management, 881
  types, 880
congenital aganglionic megacolon, 606–607, 606f, 607b
congenital diaphragmatic hernia (CDH), 673–675
congenital heart disease, 708
  altered haemodynamics, 708, 709f
  clinical consequences of, 708
  nursing care, 724–730
congenital hypopituitarism, 867
congenital lactase deficiency, 279
congenital nephrotic syndrome–Finnish type, 571
congenital talipes equinovarus/clubfoot
  diagnostic evaluation, 948
  incidence, 948
  nursing care management, 949
  therapeutic management, 948–949, 949f
congestive heart failure, 709–723, 710f
  altered haemodynamics, 709
  clinical manifestations, 710–711, 711b
  nursing care management, 712–714
  skin-to-skin cuddles, 713f
conjugate vaccine, 123b
conjunctivitis
  clinical manifestations, 134, 134b
  nursing care management, 134
  therapeutic management, 134
constipation
  childhood, 602
  encopresis, 602
  functional, 602
  idiopathic, 602
  infancy, 602
  newborn period, 602
  nursing care management, 602–603
  obstipation, 602
  therapeutic management, 602
contact dermatitis, 897–899
contiguous gene syndromes, 32
continence disorders
  encopresis, 368–369
    aetiology, 368
    clinical manifestations, 368–369, 369b
    nursing care management, 369
    therapeutic management, 369
    type, 368
  enuresis, 366–369
    aetiology and pathophysiology, 367
    clinical manifestations, 367
    diagnostic evaluation, 367
    nursing care management, 368
    therapeutic management, 367–368
    type, 366
continuous venovenous haemofiltration (CVVH), 583
contraception, 411, 412–413t
contusion, head injury, 834
convection, stable body temperature, 156
Cooley's anaemia, 768–771, 769b, 769f
coronavirus (Covid-19), 9, 122, 125–126, 493, 650
  immunisations, 125–126
corpus callosum, 820
cortical necrosis, 576
corticosteroids, 831
co-sleeping, children, 324b
Council of Australian Governments (COAG), 9
cow's milk allergy (CMA), 278–279, 278b
cranial deformities
  abnormal skull configurations, 172–173, 172f
  bossing, 172–173
  cleft lip/cleft palate (CL/CP), 174–178
    aetiology, 174
    diagnostic evaluation, 175, 176f
    feeding, 177
    long-term problems, 176–177
    nursing care management, 177–178
    pathophysiology, 174–175, 175f
    preoperative care, 177–178
    surgical correction, 175–176
    variations, 175f
  craniofacial abnormalities, 174

cranial deformities *(Continued)*
craniosynostosis, 173–174
with abnormal bone growth, 173b
defined, 173
nursing care management, 174
therapeutic management, 173
Pierre Robin sequence (PRS), 174
primary (genetic) microcephaly, 173
secondary (non-genetic) microcephaly, 173
Zika virus (ZIKV), 173
craniofacial abnormalities, 174
craniosynostosis, 173–174
with abnormal bone growth, 173b
defined, 173
nursing care management, 174
therapeutic management, 173
craniotabes, 151
crawling, 247
crawl reflex, 155t, 156f
creatine, 939
creeping, 247
critical congenital heart disease (CCHD), 150–151
crossing-over, 25–27b
croup syndromes, 654t
acute epiglottitis, 653–655
acute infections, 653, 653f
acute laryngitis, 655
acute *laryngotracheobronchitis* (LTB), 655–656, 656f
acute spasmodic laryngitis, 656
bacterial tracheitis, 657
Crouzon syndrome, 173b
cry, behavioural assessment, 141–142
cryptorchidism, 585
cultural diffusion, 19
cultural safety, 18
Cushing's syndrome
characteristics, 879, 880f
clinical manifestations, 879, 879t
development, 879, 880f
diagnostic evaluation, 879
nursing care management, 880
therapeutic management, 880
cyberbullying, 343
cystic fibrosis (CF), 687–696, 690f
cytogenetic diagnostic techniques, 44
cytogenetics, 25–27b

D

dance reflex, 155t, 156f
deafness and hearing
aetiology, 455
clinical manifestations, 457b
definition and classification, 455, 456t
hearing aids, 456f
lip-reading, 457
nursing care management, 456–458
pathology, 455
sign language, 457
socialisation, 457
speech-language therapy, 457
symptom severity, 455
therapeutic management, 455–456
deep tendon reflexes, 93, 93f
deformations, 25–27b, 27–28
dehydration
antidiuretic hormone (ADH), 526
azotaemia, 526–527
clinical manifestations, 527t
degree of, 526–527
evaluation, 527t
hypertonic, 526
hypotonic, 523–526
isotonic, 523
oliguria, 526–527
paediatric, 527b
parenteral fluid therapy, 528–529
dehydration *(Continued)*
shock, 526–527
skin elasticity, 528f
therapeutic management, 528–529
types, 523–526
deletion, 25–27b
de novo mutation, 33–34
dental decay
diagnostic evaluation, 365–366
nursing care management, 366
pathophysiology, 365
therapeutic management, 366
dental disorders
dental decay
diagnostic evaluation, 365–366
nursing care management, 366
pathophysiology, 365
therapeutic management, 366
trauma, 366
dental health
during infancy, 264
school-age children
brushing, 355
health education, 355
secondary teeth eruption, 354, 355f
toddlerhood, 304, 305f
depressed fractures, 834
depression
adolescence, 394
life-threatening illness, 445
dermatological problems, newborn
birthmarks, 179–180, 180f
bullous impetigo, 179
candidiasis, 178
erythema toxicum neonatorum, 178
herpes simplex virus (HSV), 178–179
oral candidiasis, 178, 178f
dermatophytoses, 896, 898f, 898t
detrusor, 558
developmental dysplasia of the hip (DDH)
diagnostic evaluation, 944–945, 945f
incidence, 944
pathophysiology, 944, 944f
therapeutic management, 945–946, 946f
developmental lactase deficiency, 279
dextrocardia, 153
DHBs. *See* district health boards (DHBs)
diabetes insipidus (DI), 830–831, 871–872
diabetes mellitus (DM)
diagnostic evaluation, 885
nursing care management, 888–889
pathophysiology, 883–885, 884f
therapeutic management
diabetic ketoacidosis, 888
exercise, 886
hypoglycaemia, 886–887, 887t
illness management, 887
insulin therapy, 885
monitoring, 885–886, 886t
nutrition, 886
type 1 diabetes, 882, 883f, 884b, 884t
type 2 diabetes, 882–883, 884t
diabetic ketoacidosis (DKA), 885
therapeutic management, 888
dialysis, 581
diarrhoea
acute diarrhoea, 594–595, 598b, 599–600t
aetiology, 595
causes, 594
chronic diarrhoea, 595, 601b
chronic non-specific diarrhoea (CNSD), 595
diagnostic evaluation, 597–598
fluid and electrolyte loss, 598b
fluid replacement, 601b
intractable diarrhoea of infancy, 595
nursing care management, 602
diarrhoea *(Continued)*
pathophysiology, 595–597
predispose, 601b
therapeutic management, 598–601
types, 594–595
diet
chronic kidney disease (CKD), 580–581
obesity, 363
diphtheria, immunisations, 123–124
diploid, 25–27b
diploid cells, 28–29
discipline
school-age children
dishonest behaviour, 348–349
parent–child relationships, 348
disease-modifying antirheumatic drugs (DMARDs), 954
disjunction phenomenon, 29
disorders of sex development (DSD)
family support, 588
obstructive uropathy, 588–590, 588f
pathophysiology, 587–588
therapeutic management, 588
disruptions, 27–28
disseminated intravascular coagulation (DIC), 792
distal tubular acidosis (Type I), 573–574
distributive shock, 531
district health boards (DHBs), 2–3
DNA, 25–27b
DNA, nuclear (nDNA), 25–27b
dominant, 25–27b
Down syndrome, 453f
aetiology, 452
clinical manifestations, 453b
diagnostic evaluation, 452
nursing care management, 452–454
prognosis, 452
therapeutic management, 452
drug-exposed infants
breastfeeding, 232
cigarette smoking, 233–234
clinical manifestations, 231
fetal alcohol spectrum disorder (FASD), 232–233
intrauterine drug and alcohol exposure, 230–231
marijuana exposure, 232
maternal infections, 234–236t, 234–236
methadone exposure, 232
methamphetamine exposure, 232
Neonatal Abstinence Scoring System, 231–232
neonatal abstinence syndrome (NAS), 231
nursing care management, 231–232, 234, 236
opiate exposure, 232
therapeutic management, 231
withdrawal signs, 231b
DSD. *See* disorders of sex development (DSD)
dual-earner families, 17–18
Duchenne's muscular dystrophy (DMD)
clinical manifestations, 992–993, 993f
diagnostic evaluation, 993–994, 993b
nursing care management, 994–995
X-linked disorders, 992
dura mater, cerebral dysfunction, 820
Duvall's developmental stages, 12, 13b
dying and death, 440–441, 441–442b, 441f
dysmaturity, high-risk conditions
postterm infants, 211
premature infants
aetiology, 210–211
characteristics, 211
nursing care management, 211
therapeutic management, 211
dysmenorrhoea, 402
dysplasias, 28
dyspnoea, 874
dyssomnias, 282

E

early childhood caries (ECC), 304, 305f
early-onset sepsis (EOS), 221
ears, physical examination, 152
  auditory testing, 81, 81t
  external structures, 79, 79f
  internal structures, 79–81, 80f, 81f
eating disorders
  adolescence, 393, 393f
  clinical manifestations, 414–415
  complications, 415
  diagnostic evaluation, 415
  epidemiology, 414
  nursing care management, 416
  pathophysiology, 414
  therapeutic management, 415–416
EBP. *See* evidence-based practice (EBP)
economy and poverty, child health, 20–21
ectopic pregnancy, 409
Edwards' syndrome, 31
electroencephalography (EEG), 229
electrolyte balance, 524–526t
  dehydration
    antidiuretic hormone (ADH), 526
    azotaemia, 526–527
    clinical manifestations, 527t
    degree of, 526–527
    evaluation, 527t
    hypertonic, 526
    hypotonic, 523–526
    isotonic, 523
    oliguria, 526–527
    paediatric, 527b
    parenteral fluid therapy, 528–529
    shock, 526–527
    skin elasticity, 528f
    therapeutic management, 528–529
    types, 523–526
  extracellular fluid (ECF), 523
  oedema, 529–530
  water intoxication, 529
electronic continuous thermometers, 72
electronic intermittent thermometers, 72
elevated temperatures
  symptoms, 490
  therapeutic management, 490–491
    family teaching and home care, 491
    fever, 490–491, 491b
    hyperthermia, 491
embryogenesis, 27–28
emotional abuse, 329
  adolescence, 394
emotional neglect, 329
encephalitis
  aetiology, 849
  clinical manifestations, 849
  diagnostic evaluation, 849
  nursing care management, 850
  therapeutic management, 849–850
encopresis, 368–369, 602
  aetiology, 368
  clinical manifestations, 368–369, 369b
  nursing care management, 369
  therapeutic management, 369
  type, 368
endocrine dysfunction
  adrenal function
    acute adrenocortical insufficiency, 877–878
    adrenal hormones, 876–877
    CAH, 880–881
    chronic adrenocortical insufficiency, 878–879, 878b
    Cushing's syndrome, 879–880, 879t, 880f
    hyperaldosteronism, 881–882
    phaeochromocytoma, 882
  components, 865
  hormone, 865, 866f
endocrine dysfunction *(Continued)*
  neuroendocrine interrelationships, 865–866
  pancreatic hormone secretion. *See* pancreatic hormone secretion
  parathyroid hormone
    hyperparathyroidism, 876, 876b
    hypoparathyroidism, 875–876
    physiological effects, 875b
  pituitary function. *See* pituitary function
  structures, 865, 866b
  thyroid function
    chronic lymphocytic thyroiditis, 873–874
    goitre, 873
    hyperthyroidism, 874–875
    juvenile hypothyroidism, 872–873
    thyroid hormone, 872, 873b
    types, 872
endocrine system, extrauterine life, newborn, 139
end of life, nursing care of, 437–440, 438b, 439t, 440b, 440f
endometriosis, 402–403, 403f
end-tidal carbon dioxide monitoring ($ETCO_2$), 640
enema, 516
en face position, parent–infant bonding (attachment), 163, 163f
enterohepatic circulation, 182
enterohepatic shunting, 182
enuresis, 366–369
  aetiology and pathophysiology, 367
  clinical manifestations, 367
  diagnostic evaluation, 367
  nursing care management, 368
  therapeutic management, 367–368
  type, 366
environmental tobacco exposure, 673
EOS. *See* early-onset sepsis (EOS)
epididymitis, 400–401
epidural haematoma, 834–835, 835f
epigenetics, 784
epilepsy. *See* seizures
epispadias, 586–587
epithelial pearls, 153
Epstein pearls, 152
Erb's palsy, 171, 171f
erythema infectiosum, 128, 131f
erythema toxicum neonatorum, 178
erythroblastosis fetalis, 185
erythropoietin, 243
escharotomy, 543, 543f
ethical decision-making, 8
ethnicity, 20
euploidy, 29
eutectic mixture of local anaesthetics (EMLA), 796
evaporation, stable body temperature, 156
evidence-based practice (EBP), 8–9
Ewing's sarcoma
  nursing care management, 811
  therapeutic management, 810
exanthem subitum, 128, 131f
exercise, 683–684
exercise-associated amenorrhoea, 402
exercise-induced bronchospasm (EIB), 683–684
exercise-induced heat stress, 937
exophthalmos, 874
exposure therapy, 378
extracellular fluid (ECF), 520, 523
extrauterine life, newborn
  immediate adjustments
    circulatory system, 137–138
    respiratory system, 137
  physiological status
    endocrine system, 139
    fluid and electrolyte balance, 138
    gastrointestinal system, 138, 139b
    haematopoietic system, 138
    hearing, 140
extrauterine life, newborn *(Continued)*
    against infection, 139
    integumentary system, 139
    musculoskeletal system, 139
    neurological system, 139
    renal system, 138
    smell, 140
    taste, 140
    thermoregulation, 138
    touch, 140
    vision, 140
extremities
  physical assessment, 91–92, 92f, 154, 154f, 155t
  venepuncture/injection, 494–495, 495f
eyes
  infection and injury prevention, 156
  physical examination
    accommodation, 77
    bulbar conjunctiva, 76
    colour vision, 79
    cornea, 77
    external structures, 76, 77f
    fovea centralis, 77
    fundus, 77, 77f
    internal structures, 77
    lacrimal punctum, 76
    macula, 77
    meibomian/sebaceous glands, 76
    ocular alignment, 77–78, 78f
    optic disc, 77
    palpebral conjunctivae, 76
    palpebral fissures, 76
    peripheral vision, 78–79
    PERRLA, 77
    sclera, 76
    vision testing, 77–79
    visual acuity testing, 78

F

facial paralysis, 171, 171f
facioscapulohumeral (Landouzy-Déjerine) muscular dystrophy, 991
failure to thrive (FTT), 279, 281b
faltering growth
  diagnostic evaluation, 280
  failure to thrive (FTT), 279, 281b
  growth measurements, 280
  inadequate caloric intake, 280
  nursing care management, 281
  prognosis, 280
  therapeutic management, 280
falx cerebelli, 820
falx cerebri, 820
familial nephritis (Alport's syndrome), 574
family
  affinal, 11
  and application, 11, 12t
  assessment, 61, 61–62b
  consanguineous, 11
  definition, 11
  developmental theory, 12–13, 13b
  family of origin, 11
  health history, 60
  hereditary disorders
    genetic evaluation and counselling, 47
    genetic testing, 45–46
    nurses role, 47–48, 48b
    prenatal testing, 46–47, 46b
  household, 11
  nursing interventions, 13
  parents communication
    anticipatory guidance, 52
    blocks, 52, 53b
    directing the focus, 51–52
    empathy, 52
    information overload, 52

family (Continued)
interpreter, 52–53, 53b
listening and cultural awareness, 52
nurse's relationship, 51
silence, 52
to talk, 51
roles and relationships, 13–14
parental roles, 14
role learning, 14
sociocultural influences, 18
strengths and functioning style, 13, 13b
stress theory, 12
structure, 60–61
systems theory
adaptability, 11
boundary, 11
components, 11
feedback, 11
general systems theory, 11
theory, 11
family-centred care, 7–8, 208–209
chronic/complex diseases, 424
hospitalisation stressors, 467–469
beneficial effects, 469
loss of control, 469
parental reactions, 469–470, 470b
post-hospital behaviours, 469, 469b
risk factors, 469, 469b
separation anxiety, 467–468, 468b
sibling reactions, 470
nursing care of
complementary medicine practices, 472b
discharge and home care preparation, 476–477
hospitalisation preparation, 470, 471–472b
nursing interventions, 472–475, 473f, 474b
parent participation, 476
play functions, in hospital, 474b
special hospital situations
ambulatory/outpatient setting, 477
emergency admission, 478–479, 478b
intensive care unit (ICU), 479, 479b, 479f
isolation, 477
family developmental theory, 12–13, 13b
family education, children's cancer, 797
family stress theory, 12
family systems theory
adaptability, 11
boundary, 11
components, 11
feedback, 11
general systems theory, 11
FAS. *See* fetal alcohol syndrome (FAS)
fasciotomy, 543, 543f
FASD. *See* fetal alcohol spectrum disorder (FASD)
fatty liver disease, 362
FDI. *See* Functional Disability Inventory (FDI)
fears, school-age children, 350
febrile seizure, 860
feeding
cleft lip/cleft palate (CL/CP), 177
family teaching and home care, 516
gastrostomy feeding, 514–515, 514f, 515f
gavage, 202–203, 512–514, 514f
infection and injury prevention, 160
nasoduodenal and nasojejunal tubes, 515
nipple-feeding, 203
non-nutritive sucking, 511
oral, 203
resistance, 203, 204b
sick child, 489–490, 490b
tolerance, 202
total parenteral nutrition (TPN), 515–516
female athlete triad, 938–939
female genitalia, physical assessment, 153
female reproductive system
abnormal uterine bleeding (AUB), 403–405, 404b
endometriosis, 402–403, 403f
gynaecological examination, 401
menstrual disorders, 401–402
premenstrual dysphoric disorder (PMDD), 403
sexually transmitted bacterial infections, 406–408
sexually transmitted infections (STIs), 405–406, 406b
sexually transmitted protozoa infections, 406
sexually transmitted viral infections, 408–409
vaginal infections, 405
vulvar pain, 405
femoral hernia, 89, 89f, 632
femoral venepuncture, 494, 495f
fetal alcohol spectrum disorder (FASD), 232–233
fetal alcohol syndrome (FAS), 232–233, 233b
fever, 490–491, 491b
fine motor development, 245, 245f
FISH analysis, 25–27b
flea bite dermatitis, 178
flow cytometry method, 786
fluid and electrolyte disturbances, nursing responsibilities
anaphylaxis, 536–537, 536b, 537b
assessment, 530–531
clinical observations, 530–531
extrauterine life, newborn, 138
history, 530
septic shock, 535–536, 535b, 535t
shock
aetiology, 531
clinical manifestations, 532–533, 532t
diagnostic evaluation, 533
family support, 534–535
nursing care management, 534
pathophysiology, 532
therapeutic management, 533–534
types, 531b
toxic shock syndrome (TSS), 538
fluid balance
aerosol therapy, 511
complications, 510
family teaching and home care, 511
gastrostomy administration, 511
infusion pumps, 509–510
intake and output measurement, 507
maintenance, 510
nasogastric administration, 511, 512–513b, 513–514b
optic, otic and nasal administration, 511, 511f
orogastric administration, 511
parenteral fluid therapy, 507–508, 508f
peripheral intravenous line, 508–509, 508f, 509f
removal, 510
rectal administration, 510–511
safety catheters and needleless systems, 509
fluorescence in situ hybridisation (FISH), 786
focal seizures, 851–853
food sensitivity, 276–279
allergens, 276
allergies, 276
anaphylaxis, 278b
atopy, 277
challenge testing, 279
Cow's milk allergy (CMA), 278–279, 278b
diagnosis and therapeutic management, 277–278
hyperallergenic foods and sources, 276, 277b
immediate GI hypersensitivity, 277
intolerance, 276
lactose intolerance, 279
nursing care management, 278
sensitisation, 276
foreign body ingestion, 605–606
and aspiration, 666–668, 667f
foreign body, nose, 668
foster care, 18
fractures, birth injuries
crepitus, 170
intracranial pressure (ICP), 170
nursing care management, 170–171
fragile X syndrome (FXS), 32–33
cause, 454
clinical manifestations, 454, 454b
inheritance pattern, 454
nursing care management, 454–455
prognosis, 454
therapeutic management, 454
frenulum, upper lip, 152
frostbite, 909
FTT. *See* failure to thrive (FTT)
functional abdominal pain (FAP), 375–376
Functional Disability Inventory (FDI), 107

G

GABHS infection. *See* group A β-haemolytic streptococci (GABHS) infection
gag reflex, 152
galactosaemia
clinical features, 43–44
galactokinase deficiency, 44
incidence, 43
laboratory tests, 44
mild bariants, 44
nursing care management, 44
prognosis, 44
screening considerations, 44
treatment, 44
gamete (germ cell), 25–27b
gametes, 28–29
gametogenesis, 25–27b
gastrointestinal (GI) bleeding, 620–622
gastrointestinal (GI) dysfunction
absorption, 593–594, 594f
acute gastroenteritis, 604b
assessment, 594
clinical manifestations, 594, 595b
constipation
childhood, 602
encopresis, 602
functional, 602
idiopathic, 602
infancy, 602
newborn period, 602
nursing care management, 602–603
obstipation, 602
therapeutic management, 602
development of, 592
diagnostic procedures, 594, 596–597t
diarrhoea
acute diarrhoea, 594–595, 598b, 599–600t
aetiology, 595
causes, 594
chronic diarrhoea, 595, 601b
chronic non-specific diarrhoea (CNSD), 595
diagnostic evaluation, 597–598
fluid and electrolyte loss, 598b
fluid replacement, 601b
intractable diarrhoea of infancy, 595
nursing care management, 602
pathophysiology, 595–597
predispose, 601b
therapeutic management, 598–601
types, 594–595
digestion, 592–593
foreign body ingestion, 605–606
functions, 593b
haematemesis, 622b
hepatic disorders
acute hepatitis, 622–624, 622t
biliary atresia (BA), 624–626, 625f
cirrhosis, 626–627

gastrointestinal (GI) dysfunction *(Continued)*
hernias
anorectal malformations (ARMs), 633–634, 633b, 633f
femoral hernia, 632
inguinal hernia, 631–632, 632f
umbilical hernia, 631, 631f
inflammatory conditions
acute appendicitis, 609–610, 609b
inflammatory bowel disease (IBD), 611–614, 612f, 612t
Meckel's diverticulum, 610–611, 611b
peptic ulcer disease (PUD), 614–616, 615b, 615f
malabsorption syndromes
absorptive defects, 619
anatomical defects, 619
coeliac disease (gluten-sensitive enteropathy), 619–620, 619b
complication, 618–619
digestive defects, 619
gastrointestinal (GI) bleeding, 620–622
short bowel syndrome (SBS), 620
motility disorders
gastro-oesophageal reflux (GOR), 607–608, 608b
Hirschsprung's disease (HD), 606–607, 606f, 607b
irritable bowel syndrome (IBS), 608–609
obstructive disorders
hypertrophic pyloric stenosis (HPS), 616–617, 616f, 617b
intussusception, 617–618, 618b, 618f
malrotation and volvulus, 618
mechanical (paralytic) intestinal obstruction, 616b
pica, 605
structural defects
abdominal wall defects, 629–631
atresia, 627
oesophageal atresia (OA), 627–629, 627f
tracheo-oesophageal fistula (TOF), 627–629, 627f
vomiting, 603–605, 603t
gastrointestinal system
burn, 543–544
extrauterine life, newborn, 138, 139b
gastro-oesophageal reflux (GOR), 607–608, 608b
gastroschisis, 630–631, 630f
gastrostomy feeding, 514–515, 514f, 515f
gavage feeding, 512–514, 514f
gender identity, 296
gene, 25–27b
generalised seizures, 853–854
genetic counselling, 25–27b
genetic disorders, 28–33
autosome aneuploidies, 29–31, 30t
autosomes, 28
numerical chromosome abnormalities, 28–29, 29f, 30f
polygenic disorders, 28
sex chromosome aneuploidies, 31
single-gene disorders, 28
structural chromosome abnormalities, 31–33, 32f
genetic/genomic nursing competencies
acquired immunodeficiency syndrome (AIDS), 27
Angelman's syndrome, 39
congenital anomalies, 27–28
evidence, 27
expansion mutation, 39
genes, 25–27, 28t
genetic disorders, 28–33
autosome aneuploidies, 29–31, 30t
autosomes, 28
numerical chromosome abnormalities, 28–29, 29f, 30f
polygenic disorders, 28
sex chromosome aneuploidies, 31
single-gene disorders, 28
structural chromosome abnormalities, 31–33, 32f
genomic imprinting, 39
hereditary cancer predisposition genes, 40–41
carcinogenesis process, 40
genetic/genomic nursing competencies *(Continued)*
mismatch repair genes, 40–41
oncogenes, 40
tumour suppressor genes, 40
locus heterogeneity, 38
messenger RNA (mRNA), 25–27
mitochondrial disorders, 39–40, 40t
new mutation, 25–27
pharmacogenomics, 27
point mutations, 38
premutation, 39
single-gene disorders
allele, 33
autosomal dominant inheritance, 33–34, 33f, 34f, 35–37t
autosomal recessive inheritance, 34, 37f
Mendelian-inherited genetic disorders, 34, 35–37t
reduced/incomplete penetrance, 33
sex-linked inheritance patterns, 34–37
sex-linked traits, 37, 38f
variable expressivity, 33
X-linked dominant inheritance, 37, 39f
X-linked recessive inheritance, 37, 38f
uniparental disomy, 39
variable expression, 38–39
genetics, 25–27b
genetic testing, hereditary disorders, 45–46
genitalia, physical examination
in adolescents, 89–90
female, 91, 91f
male, 90–91, 90f
genitourinary tract
defects
bladder exstrophy, 586–587, 586f
cloacal exstrophy, 586–587
cryptorchidism, 585
epispadias, 586–587
hydrocele, 584–585
hypospadias, 586, 586f
phimosis, 584
disorders
urinary tract infection (UTI), 563–566
vesicoureteral reflux (VUR), 563–566
genome, 25–27b
genomics, 25–27b
genotype, 25–27b
germ cells, 28–29
germ cell tumours (GCTs), 815
germ-line mutations, 784
gestational age, 143
appropriate for gestational age (AGA), 143
Ballard Scale (BS), 143, 144f
birth weight, 143, 145f
large for gestational age (LGA), 143
New Ballard Scale (NBS), 143
small-for-gestational-age (SGA), 143
tests used, 145b
GI dysfunction. *See* gastrointestinal (GI) dysfunction
Gilles de la Tourette's syndrome (GTS), 372–373
glandular fever (infectious mononucleosis), 648–649
Glasgow Coma Scale (GCS), 823–824
glomerular disease
acute glomerulonephritis (AGN), 567–570
chronic glomerulonephritis (CGN), 570
nephrotic syndrome, 570–573
glomerular filtration, 556–557
glucocorticoids, 876, 876b
glucose-6-phosphate dehydrogenase (G6PD) deficiency, 45
glycosylated haemoglobin, 885–886
goitre, 873
gonadotropin-releasing hormone (GnRH), 382–383, 383f
gonorrhoea, 407
GOR. *See* gastro-oesophageal reflux (GOR)
granulocyte colony-stimulating factor (G-CSF), 793
grasp reflex, 154, 154f, 155t
Graves' disease (GD)
clinical manifestations, 874
diagnostic evaluation, 874
nursing care management, 874–875
therapeutic management, 874
grieving family care, 441–444, 443–444t
gross motor behaviour, 245
Gross Motor Functional Classification System (GMFCS), 963
group A β-haemolytic streptococci (GABHS) infection, 645, 645t, 646t
growing skull fracture, 834
growth and development promotion, adolescence, 382t
biological development
breasts development, 384f
genital development, 385f
in girls, 384f
gonadotropin-releasing hormone (GnRH), 382–383, 383f
physiological changes, 386
pubertal sexual maturation, 383–386
puberty, 382, 386
pubic hair growth, 385f
reproductive hormones, 383
Tanner stages, 383b
cognitive development
formal operational thought, 386–387
self conceptions, 387
social cognition, 387
moral development, 387
phases, 381
psychosocial development
autonomy development, 388
gender, 389
identity development, 388
intimacy, 390
self-identity, 389–390
sexuality, 388–390
sexual orientation, 388–389
social environments
cyberbullying, 391
families, 390
peer groups, 390, 390f
schools, 390–391
social media, 391
spiritual development, 387–388
value autonomy, 387
growth and development promotion, infant
biological development
fine motor development, 245, 245f
gross motor behaviour, 245
head control, 245–246, 246f
locomotion, 247, 248f
maturation of systems, 242–245
proportional changes, 241, 242b, 242f
rolling over, 246
sensory changes, 241–242, 242b, 243b, 243f
sitting, 246–247, 247f
skills, 241
body image development, 250–251, 250f
cognitive development
affect, 250
imitation, 250
mental representation, 250
object permanence, 250
primary circular reactions, 250
reflexes, 250
secondary circular reactions, 250
sensorimotor phase, 249–250, 249f, 249t
separation event, 249–250
zone of proximal development, 250
gender identity development, 251
psychosocial development
breastfeeding, 249
primary narcissism, 247–248

growth and development promotion, infant *(Continued)*
sense of trust, 247–249
social development, 254–258t
attachment, 251–252
child care arrangements, 259–260
language development, 252
personal-social behaviour, 252–253
play, 253
prolonged separation effects, 251–252
separation anxiety, 252, 253–259
shaken baby syndrome, 259
soother use, 260–261
spoiled child syndrome, 259
stranger fear, 252, 252f, 253–259
teething, 261, 261f
thumb sucking, 260–261
temperament, 253
growth and development promotion, preschooler, 315–316t
aggression, 318–319
biological development
gross and fine motor behaviour, 310–311, 311f
physical growth rate, 310
body image development, 313
cognitive development, preoperational phase, 312, 312f
fears, 319–320
kindergarten experience, 317
moral development, 312
psychosocial development
oedipal stage, 311
sense of initiative, 311
sex education, 317–318
sexuality development, 313
social development
language, 313
personal-social behaviour, 314
play, 314, 317f
screen time, 314–317
speech problems, 319
spiritual development, 312
stress, 319, 320b
temperament, 317
growth and development promotion, school-age children, 346–347t
biological development, 337–340
maturation of systems, 337–338
physical changes, 337, 338f
preadolescence, 338
prepubescence, 338
puberty, 338
body image development, 345
cognitive development
concrete operations, 340
conservation, 340, 341f
language development, 342
moral development, 341–342
psychosocial development
inferiority, 339
latency period, 338
sense of industry, 338–339, 339f
self-concept development, 345–347
self-esteem, 345–347
sex education, 347–348
nurse's role, 348
sexuality development, 347–348
social development, 342–344
bullying, 343
cyberbullying, 343
ego mastery, 345
peer groups, 342–343
play, 344–345, 345f
quiet games and activities, 344–345, 345f
relationships with families, 343–344
rules and rituals, 344
social relationships and cooperation, 342–343, 343f
temperament, 339–340
growth and development promotion, toddler, 299–300t
biological development, 290–292
gross and fine motor development, 291–292
maturation of systems, 291
proportional changes, 290, 291f
sensory changes, 290–291
body image development, 295–296
cognitive development
causal relationship, 293
domestic mimicry, 294, 294f
mental symbolisation, 294–295
object permanence, 294
preoperational phase, 294
preoperational thinking, 294, 295b
sensorimotor phase, 292–293, 293t
spatial relationships, 294
tertiary circular reactions, 293
gender identity, 296
moral development, 295
psychosocial development, 292
regression, 302
sense of autonomy, 292
social development
individuation, 296
language development, 296–297
personal-social behaviour, 297
play, 297–298, 298f
rapprochement, 296
separation, 296
transitional objects, 296, 297f
spiritual development, 295
stress, 302
temperament, 298
temper tantrums, 301–302
toilet training, 298–301
growth measurements, physical examination
arm circumference, 71
growth charts, 68–69, 69f
head circumference, 71, 71f
height, 69–70, 70f
length, 69, 70f
parameters, 68
skinfold thickness, 70–71
weight, 70, 71f
GTS. *See* Gilles de la Tourette's syndrome (GTS)
Guillain-Barré syndrome (GBS)
clinical manifestations, 980
diagnostic evaluation, 980
nursing care management, 981
pathophysiology, 980
therapeutic management, 980–981
gynaecomastia, 401

H

haemangiomas of infancy, 179
haematemesis, 622b
haematological complications, 223–225
haematological system
assessment, 756
full blood count, 755t
haemoglobin, 754
Henoch-Schönlein purpura (HSP), 776–777
immunological deficiency disorders, 777–780
macrophages, 752
neutropenia, 776
phagocytosis, 752
platelets, 755–756
red blood cell disorders
anaemia, 756–759, 757f, 758b. *See also* anaemia
blood transfusion therapy, 759–760, 759t
red blood cells (erythrocytes), 752–753, 753f
white blood cells (leucocytes), 754–755
haematopoietic stem cell transplant (SCT), 791
haematopoietic system
extrauterine life, newborn, 138
haematuria, 574
haemodialysis, 581–582
haemolytic disease of the newborn (HDN), 186f
blood incompatibility
ABO incompatibility, 187, 187t
agglutination, 185
antigens, 185
Rh incompatibility isoimmunisation, 185–187
clinical manifestations, 187
diagnostic evaluation, 187
nursing care management, 188
therapeutic management
ABO incompatibility, 188
exchange transfusion, 188
intrauterine transfusion, 188
prognosis, 188
Rh isoimmunisation prevention, 187–188
haemophilia, 772–775, 773t
haemophilus influenzae type B, immunisations, 124
haemorrhagic cystitis, 795
haemorrhagic disease of the newborn, 192
haemostasis, 771–772
HAIs. *See* healthcare-associated infections (HAIs)
haploid, 25–27b
haploid cells, 28–29
Hashimoto's disease, 873–874
HAV. *See* hepatitis A virus (HAV)
HBV. *See* hepatitis B virus (HBV)
HCV. *See* hepatitis C virus (HCV)
HDN. *See* haemolytic disease of the newborn (HDN)
HDV. *See* hepatitis D virus (HDV)
headaches, 101
assessment, 860–861, 861b
migraine, 861, 861b
head and neck, physical assessment, 76, 151, 152f
head control, 245–246, 246f
head injury
aetiology, 833
birth injuries, 168–169
caput succedaneum, 168, 170f
cephalhaematoma, 169, 170f
skull fractures, 168
subgaleal haemorrhage, 169, 170f
complications
cerebral oedema, 836
epidural haematoma, 834–835, 835f
haemorrhagic lesions, 835–836
subdural haematoma, 835, 835f
traumatic brain injury, 836
diagnostic evaluation, 836–837, 836b, 837b
nursing care management, 838–839, 838b
pathophysiology, 833–834, 833f
therapeutic management, 837–838
health behaviours, school-age children, 350
healthcare-associated infections (HAIs), 121
health history
birth history, 58–59
chief complaint, 57
current medications, 59
dietary history, 59
direct, 57
family assessment, 61, 61–62b
family health history, 60
family structure, 60–61
growth and development, 59
habits, 59–60, 59b
immunisations, 59
indirect, 57
informant, 57
information identification, 57
paediatric, 57, 58b
pain, 59b
present illness, 58–59
previous illnesses, injuries and surgeries, 59
psychosocial history, 61–62
review of systems, 62–63, 62–63b
sexual history, 60, 60b

health promotion, children's cancer, 797
hearing. *See also* ears
  extrauterine life, newborn, 140
  major developmental characteristics, 243b
heart, physical examination, 153
  heart murmurs, 87, 88t, 145
  heart sound direction, 87, 87f, 88t
  position of, 86, 86f
  pulse location, 86, 87f
heart transplantation, 748–749
  nursing care management, 749
heel punctures, infection and injury prevention, 157b
hemizygote, 25–27b
Henoch-Schönlein purpura (HSP), 776–777
hepatic disorders
  acute hepatitis, 622–624, 622t
  biliary atresia (BA), 624–626, 625f
  cirrhosis, 626–627
hepatitis, 409
hepatitis A virus (HAV), 622–623
  immunisations, 123
hepatitis B vaccine administration, infection and injury prevention, 156
hepatitis B virus (HBV), 623
  immunisations, 122
hepatitis C virus (HCV), 623
hepatitis D virus (HDV), 623
hepatitis E virus (HEV), 623
herd immunity, 123b
hereditary cancer predisposition genes, 40–41
  carcinogenesis process, 40
  mismatch repair genes, 40–41
  oncogenes, 40
  tumour suppressor genes, 40
hereditary disorders
  genetic evaluation and counselling, 47
  genetic testing, 45–46
  nurses role, 47–48, 48b
  prenatal testing, 46–47, 46b
hereditary spherocytosis (HS), 763
hernias
  anorectal malformations (ARMs), 633–634, 633b, 633f
  femoral hernia, 632
  inguinal hernia, 631–632, 632f
  umbilical hernia, 631, 631f
herpes simplex virus (HSV), 178–179, 408–409, 662
herpetic gingivostomatitis (HGS), 135, 135f
heteroplasmy, 40
heterozygote, 25–27b
heterozygous carrier, 34
HEV. *See* hepatitis E virus (HEV)
HGS. *See* herpetic gingivostomatitis (HGS)
HIE. *See* hypoxic-ischaemic encephalopathy (HIE)
high-risk newborns
  classification, 196–197, 198b
  identification, 196–197
  intensive care facilities, 197–198
    family-centred care, 197
    organisation of services, 198
    transport unit, 198
  late-premature infant, 196, 197t
  nursing care of
    arousal states, 206t
    assessment, 198–199, 198–199b
    auditory environment, 208
    behavioural states, 206
    breastfeeding, 203
    complications, 198
    discharge planning and home care, 209–210
    facilitated tucking, 207
    feeding resistance, 203, 204b
    gavage feeding, 202–203
    growth maintenance, 201–202
    hydration, 201
    individualised developmental care, 204–206
    infection prevention, 201
high-risk newborns *(Continued)*
    kangaroo care, 207
    medications administration, 203–204
    monitoring physiological data, 199–210
    neonatal loss, 210
    neurodevelopmental impairment, 204
    nipple-feeding, 203
    nutritional needs, 202
    oral feeding, 203
    parent–infant relationships, 208–209, 209f
    pathology examinations, 199
    pulse oximetry, 199
    rapid eye movement (REM), 206
    respiratory support, 200
    safety measures, 199
    sensory system, 207
    siblings, 209
    skin care, 203
    state organisation, 206
    support groups, 209
    synactive theory of infant development, 204, 205t
    therapeutic handling, 207, 207b
    therapeutic positioning, 207–208, 208b
    thermoregulation, 200–201, 200f
    visual environment, 208
hip-knee-ankle-foot orthosis (HKAFO), 925–926
Hirschsprung's disease (HD), 606–607, 606f, 607b
HIV. *See* human immunodeficiency virus (HIV)
Hodgkin's lymphoma
  clinical manifestations, 802
  clinical staging and prognosis, 801, 801b
  diagnostic evaluation, 802
  histological types, 801
  lymphadenopathy and organ involvement, 801, 801f
  nursing care management, 802
  therapeutic management, 802
homologous, 25–27b
homozygote, 25–27b
hormone, endocrine system, 865, 866f
HPV. *See* human papillomavirus (HPV)
HSV. *See* herpes simplex virus (HSV)
Human Genome project, 25–27b
human immunodeficiency virus (HIV), 409
  infection, 778–780
  prevention, 406
human leucocyte antigens (HLAs), 777, 791
human milk, infection and injury prevention, 158–159
human papillomavirus (HPV), 408
  immunisations, 122, 125
human parvovirus B19, 132
hyaline membrane, 213
hydrocarbon aspiration pneumonia, 668–669
hydrocele, 153, 584–585
hydrocephalus, 836
  aetiology, 841–842
  clinical manifestations, 842–843, 842f
  diagnostic evaluation, 843
  nursing care management, 844–845
  pathophysiology, 841, 842f
  therapeutic management
    complications, 844
    prognosis, 844
    surgical treatment, 843–844, 843f
hydronephrosis, 588
hydrops fetalis, 185–187
hydroureteronephrosis, 588
5-Hydroxytryptamine-3 (5-HT_3), 794
hyperaldosteronism
  clinical diagnosis, 881
  nursing care management, 881–882
  signs and symptoms, 881
  therapeutic management, 881
hyperbilirubinaemia, 180–185
  clinical manifestations, 182
  diagnostic evaluation, 182–183, 183f
hyperbilirubinaemia *(Continued)*
  jaundice/icterus, 180
    in breastfeeding infants, 182, 184
    physiological, 182
  neonatal, 184b
  nursing care management, 184–185
  pathophysiology, 180–182
    late-preterm infants risk, 181–182
    prodromal symptoms, 182
    unconjugated bilirubin, 180–182, 181t
  phototherapy, 184
    and parent–infant interaction, 185b
  prognosis, 184
  therapeutic management, 183–184
hypercalcaemia, 916
hyperglycaemia
  glucose intolerance, 190
  nursing care management, 190–191
hyperkalaemia, 577–578
hyperleucocytosis, 792
hyperparathyroidism, 876, 876b
hypertension
  acute kidney injury (AKI), 578
  adolescence, 395
  chronic kidney disease (CKD), 581
hyperthermia, 491
hyperthyroidism
  clinical manifestations, 874
  diagnostic evaluation, 874
  nursing care management, 874–875
  therapeutic management, 874
hypertonic dehydration, 526
hypertrophic pyloric stenosis (HPS), 616–617, 616f, 617b
hypervitaminosis, 273–274
hypocalcaemia, 191
hypoglycaemia, 230, 886–887, 887t
  at-risk assessments, 188
  clinical manifestations, 189
  diagnostic evaluation, 189
  nursing care management, 189, 190f
  pathophysiology, 188–189
  therapeutic management, 189
hypogonadotropic amenorrhoea, 402
hypoparathyroidism, 875–876
hypopituitarism
  cause of, 867, 867b, 869f
  clinical manifestations, 868, 868b
  condition, 866
  congenital hypopituitarism, 867
  diagnostic evaluation, 868–869
  growth failure, 867
  idiopathic hypopituitarism, 867
  nursing care management, 870
  therapeutic management, 869–870
hypospadias, 586, 586f
hypotensive (decompensated) shock, 533
hypothalamic–pituitary–gonadal axis, 870
hypothalamus, 865
hypotonia, 154
  clinical manifestations, 977–978
  definition, 977
  diagnostic evaluation, 978
  therapeutic and nursing care management, 978
hypotonic dehydration, 523–526
hypovolaemic shock, 531
hypoxaemia, 714
  altered haemodynamics, 714
  aortic stenosis, 719f
  atrial septal defect, 717f
  atrioventricular canal defect, 717f
  clinical manifestations, 714–715, 714f
  coarctation of the aorta, 719f
  diagnostic evaluation, 715
  great vessels transposition, 722f
  mixed defects, 720–722b
  nursing care management, 723

hypoxaemia (Continued)
obstructive defects, 718b
pulmonary blood flow, 719–720b
pulmonary stenosis, 719f
shunt procedures, 723t
Tetralogy of Fallot, 720f
therapeutic management, 715–723, 715f, 716–717b
tricuspid atresia, 720f
ventricular septal defect, 717f
hypoxic-ischaemic encephalopathy (HIE), 226

I
IBD. *See* inflammatory bowel disease (IBD)
IBS. *See* irritable bowel syndrome (IBS)
ICH. *See* intracranial haemorrhage (ICH)
ichthyoses, 904
ictal state, 851
idiopathic hypopituitarism, 867
idiopathic scoliosis
clinical manifestations, 941
diagnostic evaluation, 941–942
nursing care management, 943
therapeutic management, 942, 942f
thoracic idiopathic adolescent scoliosis, 941, 941f
idiopathic thrombocytopenic purpura (ITP), 775–776
IDMs. *See* infants of diabetic mothers (IDMs)
IEMs. *See* inborn errors of metabolism (IEMs)
Ig. *See* immunoglobulin (Ig)
ileus, 609
immobilised child
causes of, 914
families effects, 918
nursing care management, 918–921, 919–920t
physiological effects
cardiovascular system, 915–916
gastrointestinal system, 916
integumentary system, 916–917
metabolism, 916
muscular system, 915
neurosensory system, 917
primary/secondary effect, 914, 915f
renal system, 916
respiratory system, 916
skeletal system, 915
psychological effects, 917–918, 918b
immune thrombocytopenia, 775–776
immunisations, 122–128, 123b, 126b
administration, 127–128
adolescence, 395
COVID-19, 125–126
diphtheria, 123–124
haemophilus influenzae type B, 124
hepatitis A virus (HAV), 123
hepatitis B virus (HBV), 122
human papillomavirus, 125
influenza, 125
measles, mumps and rubella (MMR), 124
meningococcal disease, 125
order of injections, 128b
pertussis, 124
pneumococcal disease, 124–125
polio, 124
reactions, 126
rotavirus, 125
schedule for, 122
tetanus, 123
varicella, 124
immunity, 123b
immunoglobulin (Ig), 123b
immunological deficiency disorders, 777–780
imprinting, 25–27b
inactivated poliovirus (IPV), 124
inborn errors of metabolism (IEMs)
cytogenetic diagnostic techniques, 44
galactosaemia
clinical features, 43–44
inborn errors of metabolism (Continued)
galactokinase deficiency, 44
incidence, 43
laboratory tests, 44
mild bariants, 44
nursing care management, 44
prognosis, 44
screening considerations, 44
treatment, 44
metabolic pathways, 41, 41f
mode of inheritance, 41
molecular diagnostic techniques, 44
phenylketonuria (PKU)
clinical manifestations, 43
diagnostic evaluation, 43
incidence, 42
nursing care management, 43
pathophysiology, 42, 42f
prognosis, 43
therapeutic management, 43
predisposition genetic testing, 45
prenatal diagnosis, 41–42
therapeutic management
environmental modification, 45
phenotype modification, 45
infant feeding, infection and injury prevention, 158
infantile haemangiomas, 179, 180f
infants of diabetic mothers (IDMs)
clinical manifestations, 230, 230f
hypoglycaemia, 230
incidence, 229–230
nursing care management, 230
severity, 230
therapeutic management, 230
infection control
airborne precautions, 121
contact precautions, 121–122
contraindications and precautions, 126–127
droplet precautions, 121
healthcare-associated infections (HAIs), 121
immunisations, 122–128, 126b
administration, 127–128
COVID-19, 125–126
diphtheria, 123–124
haemophilus influenzae type B, 124
hepatitis A virus (HAV), 123
hepatitis B virus (HBV), 122
human papillomavirus, 125
influenza, 125
measles, mumps and rubella (MMR), 124
meningococcal disease, 125
order of injections, 128b
pertussis, 124
pneumococcal disease, 124–125
polio, 124
reactions, 126
rotavirus, 125
schedule for, 122
tetanus, 123
varicella, 124
standard precautions, 121
transmission-based precautions, 121
infectious processes, high-risk newborns
necrotising enterocolitis (NEC)
clinical manifestations, 223
diagnostic evaluation, 223
nursing care management, 223
pathophysiology, 222–223
therapeutic management, 223
sepsis, 220–222
bacterial infection, 220–221
breastfeeding, 221
clinical manifestations, 221–222, 222b
diagnostic evaluation, 222
mortality rate, 221
nursing care management, 222
infectious processes, high-risk newborns (Continued)
pathophysiology, 221
prognosis, 222
sources of, 221
therapeutic management, 222
infective endocarditis (IE)
clinical manifestations, 730
diagnostic evaluation, 731
nursing care management, 731
pathophysiology, 730
therapeutic management, 731
inflammatory bowel disease (IBD), 611–614, 612f, 612t
aetiology, 611
clinical manifestations, 612t
clinical signs and symptoms, 612
diagnostic evaluation, 612–613
nursing care management, 613–614
pathophysiology, 611
therapeutic management, 613
ulcerative colitis/Crohn's disease, 612f
inflammatory conditions
acute appendicitis, 609–610, 609b
inflammatory bowel disease (IBD), 611–614, 612f, 612t
Meckel's diverticulum, 610–611, 611b
peptic ulcer disease (PUD), 614–616, 615b, 615f
influenza, 649
immunisations, 125
informed consent
conditions, 481
eligibility for, 482
requirements, 481–482
infrared thermometers, 72
inguinal hernia, 89, 89f, 631–632, 632f
injury prevention
falls, 358
during infancy, 264–269, 265–266b, 267–268t
nurse's role, 268–269, 269b, 358
preschooler, 322
at school, 358
school-age children, 355–358, 356t
bicycle injury, 357
motor vehicle injury, 357
risk-taking behaviour, 357
toddlerhood
accidental poisoning, 307, 307f
aspiration and suffocation, 307–308
bodily harm, 308
burns, 306, 306f
causes of, 304–305
drowning, 306
falls, 307
land transport injuries, 305–306
insomnia, 396
insulin, 883
integumentary dysfunction
acne, 908–909, 908f
animal contacts
animal bites, 903–904
arthropod bites and stings, 900, 900–901t
cat-scratch disease, 904
flying foxes, 904
human bites, 904
pediculosis capitis, 902–903, 903f
rickettsial diseases, 903
scabies, 900–902, 902b, 902f
atopic dermatitis (eczema)
child's age, 906
clinical manifestations, 906, 907b
nursing care management, 907–908
therapeutic management, 906–907
chemical/physical contacts
allergic contact dermatitis, 899
contact dermatitis, 897–899
drug reactions, 899
cold injury, 909
congenital disorders, 905t

integumentary dysfunction *(Continued)*
ichthyoses, 904
nappy rash, 904–906, 906f
seborrhoeic dermatitis, 908
skin infections
bacterial infections, 894–896, 895t
dermatophytoses, 896, 898f, 898t
systemic mycotic infections, 897, 899t
viral infections, 896, 897t
skin lesions
aetiology, 891
diagnostic evaluation, 891
history and symptoms, 891–892
laboratory studies, 892
objective findings, 892
origin, 891
pathophysiology of dermatitis, 891
younger children, 891
wounds
acute wounds, 892
chronic wounds, 892
deeper tissues, 892
epidermal injuries, 892
home care and family support, 894
nursing care management, 893–894
therapeutic management, 892–893
integumentary system, extrauterine life, newborn, 139
intellectual disability, 448
intelligence quotient (IQ) test score, 448
intensive care facilities, 197–198
family-centred care, 197
organisation of services, 198
transport unit, 198
intercostal retractions, 152
intermittent compression devices, 933
intestinal parasitic diseases
causes, 135
nursing care management, 135–136
prevention, 136b
threadworm, 135, 135b
intracellular fluid (ICF), 520
intracerebellar haemorrhage, 228
intracranial haemorrhage (ICH)
intracerebellar haemorrhage, 228
nursing care management, 228
subarachnoid haemorrhage, 227
subdural haemorrhage, 227
intracranial pressure (ICP) monitoring
signs and symptoms, 821, 822b
unconscious child, 829–830
intractable diarrhoea of infancy, 595
intractable seizures, 857
intravenous immunoglobulin (IVIg), 123b
intraventricular haemorrhage (IVH)
clinical manifestations, 227
diagnostic evaluation, 227
nursing care management, 227
pathophysiology, 226–227
therapeutic management, 227
intussusception, 617–618, 618b, 618f
IPV. *See* inactivated poliovirus (IPV)
irritable bowel syndrome (IBS), 608–609
isotonic dehydration, 523
isotretinoin, 13-*cis*-retinoic acid, 909
IVH. *See* intraventricular haemorrhage (IVH)

J
jaundice/icterus, 180
in breastfeeding infants, 182, 184
physiological, 182
jitteriness, 228–229
joint legal custody, 16
joint physical custody, 16
joints, physical examination, 92
juvenile hypothyroidism, 872–873
juvenile idiopathic arthritis (JIA)
musculoskeletal/articular dysfunction, 952–955
clinical manifestations, 952, 953b
course and prognosis, 952–953
diagnostic evaluation, 953
nursing care management, 954–955
pathophysiology, 952
therapeutic management, 953–954
juvenile spinal muscular atrophy, 979

K
kangaroo care, 207
karyotype, 25–27b, 28–29
Kawasaki disease (KD), 734–737
clinical manifestations, 734–735, 735b
pathophysiology, 734
therapeutic management, 736
kernicterus, 180–181
ketoacidosis, 883–885
ketogenic diet, 363, 856
ketones, 884–885
kidney transplantation
donor tissue selection, 583
immune response suppression, 583
nursing care management, 584
patient education, 584
procedure, 583
prognosis, 584
rejection, 583–584
kindergarten experience, 317
kinship care, 17–18
Klinefelter's syndrome, 31, 31f
knee-ankle-foot orthosis (KAFO), 925–926
knee-jerk reflex, 93, 93f
knock-knee/genu valgum, 92, 92f
Kugelberg-Welander disease, 979
Kussmaul respirations, 884–885
kwashiorkor, 274–275

L
laceration, head injury, 834
large for gestational age (LGA), 143
laryngospasm, 875
late-onset lactase deficiency, 279
late-onset sepsis, 221
late-premature infant, 196, 197t
LBW. *See* low birth weight (LBW)
LCPUFAs. *See* long-chain polyunsaturated fatty acids (LCPUFAs)
learning disabilities, 372
lecithin/sphingomyelin (L/S) ratio, 215
Legg-Calvé-Perthes disease
clinical manifestations, 947
diagnostic evaluation, 947
nursing care management, 947
pathophysiology, 946
therapeutic management, 947
Lennox-Gastaut syndrome (LGS), 855
leukaemia
acute lymphoblastic leukaemia, 798–799
clinical manifestations, 798–799
clinical staging and prognosis, 798, 798t
diagnostic evaluation, 799
treatment, 799
level of consciousness (LOC), 823, 823b, 827–828
LGA. *See* large for gestational age (LGA)
life-threatening illness, 444–446
Li-Fraumeni syndrome, 784
limb-girdle muscular dystrophy (LGMD), 991
lingual frenulum, 152
lipoid pneumonia, 669
lip-reading, 457
liver tumours, 815
locus, 25–27b
long-chain polyunsaturated fatty acids (LCPUFAs), 160
low birth weight (LBW), 4
LP. *See* lumbar puncture (LP)
lumbar puncture (LP), 495–496, 495f, 786
lung distensibility, 213
lungs, physical examination, 152–153
auscultation, 85–86, 86b
lobes location, 84–85, 85f
lymph nodes, physical examination, 76, 76f
lymphocytes, 139
lymphokines, 778
lymphomas
Hodgkin's lymphoma, 801–802, 801f
non-Hodgkin's lymphoma, 802–803, 803b

M
Macewen's sign, 842
macrominerals, 274
major histocompatibility complex (MHC), 777
malabsorption syndromes
absorptive defects, 619
anatomical defects, 619
coeliac disease (gluten-sensitive enteropathy), 619–620, 619b
complication, 618–619
digestive defects, 619
gastrointestinal (GI) bleeding, 620–622
short bowel syndrome (SBS), 620
male genitalia, physical assessment, 153–154
male reproductive system
epididymitis, 400–401
gynaecomastia, 401
penile conditions, 400
testicular torsion, 401
varicocele, 400
malformation, 25–27b, 28
major, 25–27b
minor, 25–27b
malignant hyperthermia (MH), 486
marasmus, 274–275
marijuana exposure, 232
MAS. *See* meconium aspiration syndrome (MAS)
mass media, 19–20
maternal attachment, 163
maternal conditions
drug-exposed infants
breastfeeding, 232
cigarette smoking, 233–234
clinical manifestations, 231
fetal alcohol spectrum disorder (FASD), 232–233
intrauterine drug and alcohol exposure, 230–231
marijuana exposure, 232
maternal infections, 234–236t, 234–236
methadone exposure, 232
methamphetamine exposure, 232
Neonatal Abstinence Scoring System, 231–232
neonatal abstinence syndrome (NAS), 231
nursing care management, 231–232, 234, 236
opiate exposure, 232
therapeutic management, 231
withdrawal signs, 231b
infants of diabetic mothers (IDMs)
clinical manifestations, 230, 230f
hypoglycaemia, 230
incidence, 229–230
nursing care management, 230
severity, 230
therapeutic management, 230
MBS. *See* Medicare Benefits Schedule (MBS)
McBurney's point, 609
MCNS. *See* minimal change nephrotic syndrome (MCNS)
measles, 128, 132f
measles, mumps and rubella (MMR), 124
Meckel's diverticulum, 610–611, 611b

meconium aspiration syndrome (MAS), 217f
clinical manifestations, 217
diagnostic evaluation, 217–218
nursing care management, 218
pathophysiology, 217
therapeutic management, 218
Medicare Benefits Schedule (MBS), 2
medication administration
dosage check, 501
drug dosage, 500–501
identification, 501
intramuscular administration, 502–505, 503t, 504–505b, 504f
intravenous administration, 505–507
central venous catheters, 505–507, 506f
intraosseous infusion, 507
peripheral intermittent infusion device, 505
oral administration, 501–502
parenteral administration, 501
subcutaneous and intradermal administration, 505
meiosis, 25–27b
mendelian inheritance, 25–27b
mendelian-inherited genetic disorders, 34, 35–37t
meningococcal disease, immunisations, 125
meningomyelocele, 971–977
menstrual disorders, 401–402
metabolic acidosis, burn, 544
metacentric chromosomes, 28–29
meta-iodobenzylguanidine (MIBG) scan, 786
metatarsus adductus, 948
methadone exposure, 232
methamphetamine exposure, 232
methylation, 37
MH. *See* malignant hyperthermia (MH)
microcephaly, 173
microdeletion, 25–27b
microminerals/trace elements, 274
migraine headache, 861, 861b
migrating motor complex (MMC), 138
milia, 139
mineralocorticoid, 876–877
minimal change nephrotic syndrome (MCNS), 570–571
minimum residual disease (MRD) testing, 786
mitochondrial (mtDNA), 25–27b
mitochondrial disorders, 39–40, 40t
mitochondrion, 25–27b
mitosis, 25–27b
mitotic non-disjunction, 29, 29f, 30f
MMC. *See* migrating motor complex (MMC)
mobilisation devices
crutches, canes and walkers, 926–927, 927f
nursing care management, 926–927
orthotics and prosthetics, 925–926, 926f
wheelchairs, 927, 927f
molecular diagnostic techniques, 44
monosomy, 25–27b, 29
monovalent vaccine, 123b
morning hyperglycaemia, 887
Moro reflex, 155t, 156f
mosaic Down syndrome, 30–31
mosaicism, 25–27b, 29
motility disorders
gastro-oesophageal reflux (GOR), 607–608, 608b
Hirschsprung's disease (HD), 606–607, 606f, 607b
irritable bowel syndrome (IBS), 608–609
motor vehicle injuries, 264–268, 270f
moulding therapy, 286
mourning, 444
mouth and throat, physical examination
buccal mucosa, 82
child positioning, 82, 82f
internal structures, 82–83, 83f
mucosal ulceration, 795
multifactorial, 25–27b
Munchausen syndrome by proxy (MSBP), 329–330
muscles, physical examination, 92
muscular dystrophies (MD)
characteristics, 991, 991t
DMD
clinical manifestations, 992–993, 993f
diagnostic evaluation, 993–994, 993b
nursing care management, 994–995
X-linked disorders, 992
facioscapulohumeral (Landouzy-Déjerine) muscular dystrophy, 991
LGMD, 991
muscle involvement, 992f
musculoskeletal and abnormal growth acceleration, obesity, 362–363
musculoskeletal/articular dysfunction
amputation, 925
casting
application, 921–922, 922f
family-centred care, 922b
nursing care, 922b
removal, 922
spica cast, 921, 921f
types of, 921, 921f
congenital talipes equinovarus
diagnostic evaluation, 948
incidence, 948
nursing care management, 949
therapeutic management, 948–949, 949f
DDH
diagnostic evaluation, 944–945, 945f
incidence, 944
pathophysiology, 944, 944f
therapeutic management, 945–946, 946f
distraction, 924–925, 925f
fracture
ACS, 932–933
bone healing and remodelling, 929–931, 929f, 930f, 930t, 931f
circulatory impairment, 932
compact and cancellous bone, epiphysis, physis and diaphysis, 928, 928f
diagnostic evaluation, 931
distal forearm, 928, 928f
features, 928, 928b
growth plate/physeal injuries, 929, 929f
infection, 933
kidney stones, 933
malunion, 933
nerve compression syndromes, 932
non-union, 933, 933b
nursing care management, 931–932, 932b
ossification, 928
physeal damage, 933
pulmonary emboli, 933–934
therapeutic management, 931, 931b
types of, 928–929, 929b, 929f
idiopathic scoliosis
clinical manifestations, 941
diagnostic evaluation, 941–942
nursing care management, 943
therapeutic management, 942, 942f
thoracic idiopathic adolescent scoliosis, 941, 941f
immobilisation
causes of, 914
families effects, 918
nursing care management, 918–921, 919–920t
physiological effects, 914–917, 915f, 917f
psychological effects, 917–918, 918b
JIA
clinical manifestations, 952, 953b
course and prognosis, 952–953
diagnostic evaluation, 953
nursing care management, 954–955
pathophysiology, 952
therapeutic management, 953–954
musculoskeletal/articular dysfunction *(Continued)*
kyphosis and lordosis, 940–941, 941f
Legg-Calvé-Perthes disease
clinical manifestations, 947
diagnostic evaluation, 947
nursing care management, 947
pathophysiology, 946
therapeutic management, 947
metatarsus adductus, 948
mobilisation devices
crutches, canes and walkers, 926–927, 927f
nursing care management, 926–927
orthotics and prosthetics, 925–926, 926f
wheelchairs, 927, 927f
orthopaedic infections
osteomyelitis, 949–950, 949f
septic arthritis, 950
tuberculosis, 950–951
osteogenesis imperfecta
classification, 951, 951b
nursing care management, 952
therapeutic management, 951–952
types, 951
SCFE, 947–948
skeletal limb deficiency, 943–944
SLE
aetiology, 955
clinical manifestations, 956, 956b
course and symptoms, 955
diagnostic evaluation, 956, 956b
general measures, 957
nursing care management, 957–958
pathophysiology, 955–956
therapeutic management, 957
sports participation
contusions, 935
dislocations, 935–936
overuse injury, 937
preparation, 934, 934f, 935f
sprains and strains, 936, 936b, 936f
types of, 934–935, 935f
torticollis, 940
traction
nursing care management, 924
purposes of, 923, 923f
types of, 923–924, 923b, 924f
trauma management
characteristics, 911
child abuse/non-accidental injury, 911–912
emergency management, 912–914, 913b
epidemiology, 911
prevention, 912
systematic assessment, 914
unintentional/accidental injury, 911, 912b
musculoskeletal pain, 101
musculoskeletal system, extrauterine life, newborn, 139
mutation, 25–27b
myelodysplasia, 971
myelomeningocele (MMC)
Chiari's malformation, 971–972
clinical manifestations, 973
diagnostic evaluation, 973
intact sac, 971, 971f
nursing care management, 976–977
pathophysiology, 972–973
prognosis, 976
therapeutic management
bowel control, 976
genitourinary function, 974–976
initial care, 974
multidisciplinary team approach, 973
musculoskeletal considerations, 974
myoclonic seizures, 854
Myositis ossificans, 935
myringotomy, 652

N

NAFLD. *See* non-alcoholic fatty liver disease (NAFLD)
nappy rash
  clinical manifestations, 904–906, 906f
  nursing care management, 905
  pathophysiology, 904–906, 905f
narcotics, 417
NAS. *See* neonatal abstinence syndrome (NAS)
Nasoduodenal and nasojejunal tubes, 515
National Federation Reform Council (NFRC), 9
national Health Strategies for Children, 9
natural immunity, 123b
NBO assessment. *See* Newborn Behavioural Observations (NBO) assessment
NBS. *See* New Ballard Scale (NBS)
NEC. *See* necrotising enterocolitis (NEC)
necrotising enterocolitis (NEC)
  clinical manifestations, 223
  diagnostic evaluation, 223
  nursing care management, 223
  pathophysiology, 222–223
  therapeutic management, 223
needlestick pain, 100, 115b
Neonatal Abstinence Scoring System, 231–232
neonatal abstinence syndrome (NAS), 231
neonatal haemorrhagic stroke (NHS), 228
neonatal/perinatal stroke, 228
neonatal seizures
  causes of, 228b
  classifications, 229t
  clinical manifestations, 228–229
  diagnostic evaluation, 229
  jitteriness, 228–229
  nursing care management, 229
  pathophysiology, 228
  spasms, 229
  therapeutic management, 229
  tremor, 229
nephrogenic diabetes insipidus (NDI), 574
nephrotic syndrome
  classification, 572b
  clinical manifestations, 571–572
  congenital nephrotic syndrome–Finnish type, 571
  diagnostic evaluation, 572
  minimal change nephrotic syndrome (MCNS), 570–571
  nursing care management, 573
  pathophysiology, 571, 571f
  secondary nephrotic syndrome, 571
  therapeutic management, 572
  types, 570–571
nerve compression syndromes, 932
nerve injuries
  brachial palsy, 171, 171f
  facial paralysis, 171, 171f
  nursing care management, 172
  phrenic nerve paralysis, 171
neural tube defects (NTDs), 970b
  aetiology, 969–970
  anencephaly, 970–971
  Guillain-Barré syndrome, 979–981
  hypotonia, 977–978
  juvenile spinal muscular atrophy, 979
  myelomeningocele, 971–977
  spina bifida and myelodysplasia, 971, 973b
  spinal cord and cauda equina, 970f
  spinal cord injuries
    aetiology, 983–984
    autonomic system, 983, 983b
    clinical manifestations, 984–985
    diagnostic evaluation, 985–986, 985f
    nursing care management, 987–991, 990f
    pathophysiology, 984, 984b
    principles, 981
    sensory and motor tracts, 983
    spinal nerves, 981, 982t
neural tube defects *(Continued)*
    therapeutic management, 986–987
    upper *vs.* lower motor neurons, 983, 983b
  spinal muscular atrophy type 1, 978–979, 978b
neuroblastoma
  clinical manifestations, 808
  diagnostic evaluation, 808
  nursing care management, 809
  staging and prognosis, 808–809, 808b
  therapeutic management, 809
neuroendocrine system, 865–866
  burn, 544
neurogenic shock, 985
neurological assessment, physical examination, 92–93
  cerebellar function, 92, 93b
  cranial nerves, 93, 94f, 95t, 96f
  reflexes, 92–93, 93f
neurological disturbance, 225–229
  intracranial haemorrhage (ICH)
    intracerebellar haemorrhage, 228
    nursing care management, 228
    subarachnoid haemorrhage, 227
    subdural haemorrhage, 227
  intraventricular haemorrhage (IVH)
    clinical manifestations, 227
    diagnostic evaluation, 227
    nursing care management, 227
    pathophysiology, 226–227
    therapeutic management, 227
  neonatal/perinatal stroke, 228
  neonatal seizures
    causes of, 228b
    classifications, 229t
    clinical manifestations, 228–229
    diagnostic evaluation, 229
    jitteriness, 228–229
    nursing care management, 229
    pathophysiology, 228
    spasms, 229
    therapeutic management, 229
    tremor, 229
  perinatal hypoxic-ischaemic brain injury
    causes, 225–226
    clinical manifestations, 226
    hypoxic-ischaemic encephalopathy (HIE), 226
    nursing care management, 226
    therapeutic hypothermia, 226, 226f
neurological status
  altered state of consciousness
    aetiology, 823
    coma assessment, 823–824, 824f
    LOC, 823, 823b
  diagnostic procedures, 826–827
  history, 822
  neurological examination
    eyes, 825–826, 825f
    motor function, 826
    posturing, 826, 826f
    reflexes, 826
    skin, 825
    vital signs, 825
  physical examination, 822–823, 823b
neurological system
  cerebral dysfunction, 819
  extrauterine life, newborn, 139
  physical assessment, 154–155
neuromuscular/muscular dysfunction
  cerebral palsy
    aetiology, 962, 962b
    clinical classification, 963, 963b
    clinical features, 961–962
    clinical manifestations, 963–965, 964b
    diagnostic evaluation, 965
    nursing care management, 968–969
    pathophysiology, 962–963
    therapeutic management, 965–968, 966b, 968f
neuromuscular/muscular dysfunction *(Continued)*
  classification, 960–961
  clinical features, 960
  diagnostic tools, 961
  muscular dystrophies
    characteristics, 991, 991t
    DMD. *See* Duchenne's muscular dystrophy (DMD)
    facioscapulohumeral (Landouzy-Déjerine) muscular dystrophy, 991
    LGMD, 991
    muscle involvement, 992f
  NTDs. *See* neural tube defects (NTDs)
  site of origin, 960, 961f
neuropathic pain syndromes, 101
neutropenia, 776
New Ballard Scale (NBS), 143
newborn and family, nursing and midwifery care
  Apgar scoring system, 140, 140t
  behavioural assessment, 141–142
    cry, 141–142
    Newborn Behavioural Observations (NBO) assessment, 141
    sleep-wake states, 141, 142t
    state modulation, 141
  bonding and attachment behaviours, 142, 142b
  discharge and home care, 165, 165b
  gestational age, 143
    appropriate for gestational age (AGA), 143
    Ballard Scale (BS), 143, 144f
    birth weight, 143, 145f
    large for gestational age (LGA), 143
    New Ballard Scale (NBS), 143
    small-for-gestational-age (SGA), 143
    tests used, 145b
  infection and injury prevention
    acculturation, 158b
    bathing, 157
    bottle-feeding, 160
    breastfeeding, 159–160, 159t, 160b, 161–162t, 162f
    circumcision, 158
    commercially prepared formulas, 160–162
    eye care, 156
    feeding schedules, 160
    heel punctures, 157b
    hepatitis B vaccine administration, 156
    human milk, 158–159
    identification, 156
    infant feeding, 158
    newborn screening, 156–157
    umbilicus, 157
    universal newborn hearing screening, 157
    vitamin K administration, 156
  parent–infant bonding (attachment)
    en face position, 163, 163f
    infant behaviour, 162–163
    maternal attachment, 163
    multiple births and subsequent children, 165
    neonates complexity, 162
    paternal engrossment, 163–164, 164f
    siblings, 164, 164f
  patent airway, 155–156
  periods of reactivity, 141, 141t
  physical assessment, 140, 143, 146t
    abdomen, 153
    axilla temperature measurements, 143
    back and anus, 154
    blood pressure (BP), 145, 151f
    chest, 152
    critical congenital heart disease (CCHD), 150–151
    ears, 152
    extremities, 154, 154f, 155t
    eyes, 151–152
    female genitalia, 153
    flexion position, neonate, 151, 151f
    head, 151, 152f
    heart, 153

newborn and family, nursing and midwifery care *(Continued)*
- lungs, 152–153
- male genitalia, 153–154
- measurements of, 143, 150f
- mouth and throat, 152
- neck, 152
- neurological system, 154–155
- nose, 152
- skin, 151
- sutures and fontanels location, 150f
- temporal artery thermometers (TATs), 145
- vital signs, 143–151

stable body temperature
- conduction, 156
- convection, 156
- evaporation, 156
- radiation, 156

Newborn Behavioural Observations (NBO) assessment, 141
newborn rash, 178
newborn screening, infection and injury prevention, 156–157
New Zealand's Health System, 2–3
NFRC. *See* National Federation Reform Council (NFRC)
NHS. *See* neonatal haemorrhagic stroke (NHS)
NICU Network Neurobehavioral Scale (NNNS), 232
non-alcoholic fatty liver disease (NAFLD), 362
non-bacterial (aseptic) meningitis, 848–849, 849t
non-disjunction chromosome distribution, 25–27b, 29
non-Hodgkin's lymphoma, 802–803, 803b
non-shivering thermogenesis (NST), 138
noradrenaline, 877
normothermia, 71–72
nose, physical examination, 152
- external structures, 81–82, 82f
- internal structures, 82

NST. *See* non-shivering thermogenesis (NST)
nuchal cord, 168
nucleotides, 160
nutrition
- assessment
  - anthropometry, 63–64
  - biochemical tests, 64
  - clinical examination, 63–64, 65–67t
  - dietary intake, 63
  - evaluation of, 64
  - food diary, 63
  - 24-hour recall, 63
- in children
  - mineral imbalances, 274
  - nursing care management, 274
  - obesity, 272–273
  - vitamin imbalances, 273–274
- faltering growth
  - diagnostic evaluation, 280
  - failure to thrive (FTT), 279, 281b
  - growth measurements, 280
  - inadequate caloric intake, 280
  - nursing care management, 281
  - prognosis, 280
  - therapeutic management, 280
- food sensitivity, 276–279
  - allergens, 276
  - allergies, 276
  - anaphylaxis, 278b
  - atopy, 277
  - challenge testing, 279
  - cow's milk allergy (CMA), 278–279, 278b
  - diagnosis and therapeutic management, 277–278
  - hyperallergenic foods and sources, 276, 277b
  - immediate GI hypersensitivity, 277
  - intolerance, 276
  - lactose intolerance, 279
  - nursing care management, 278
  - sensitisation, 276

nutrition *(Continued)*
- during infancy, 261–263
  - first 6 months, 262–263
  - second 6 months, 263
  - solid foods, 263
  - weaning, 263
- preschooler, 320, 321f
- school-age children, 351–352
- severe acute malnutrition (protein–energy malnutrition)
  - factor causing, 274–275
  - nursing care management, 275–276
  - therapeutic management, 275
- toddlerhood
  - feeding, 302, 303t
  - finger foods, 303f
  - nursing care management, 303
  - nutritional counselling, 303
  - physiological anorexia, 302

O

obesity, 4, 5f
- aetiology and pathophysiology, 360–361
  - anorexigenic substances, 360–361
  - appetite, 360–361
  - caloric equilibrium, 361
  - community and institutional contributors, 361
  - diseases, 360
  - energy balance, 360
  - genetic factors, 360
  - low metabolism, 361
  - orexigenic substances, 360–361
  - personal and interpersonal factors, 361
- in children
  - assessment and management, 272–273
  - causes of, 272
  - incidence, 272
- complications, 362–363
- diagnostic evaluation, 361–362
- family involvement, 365
- nursing care management, 364–365
- prevention, 364b, 365
- prognosis, 365
- stages, 364b
- therapeutic management, 363–364

obstructive disorders
- hypertrophic pyloric stenosis (HPS), 616–617, 616f, 617b
- intussusception, 617–618, 618b, 618f
- malrotation and volvulus, 618
- mechanical (paralytic) intestinal obstruction, 616b

obstructive shock, 531
obstructive sleep apnoea, 696–697
obstructive uropathy, 588f
- clinical manifestations, 589
- diagnostic evaluation, 589
- hydronephrosis, 588
- hydroureteronephrosis, 588
- nursing care management, 589–590
- pathophysiology, 589
- ureterocele, 588

occlusive dressings, 893
oedema, 529–530
oesophageal atresia (OA), 627–629, 627f
oligohydramnios, 588–589
oliguria, 526–527
OM. *See* otitis media (OM)
omphalitis, 153
omphalocele, 629–630, 630f
oncogenes, 25–27b, 784
ondansetron, 794
open fractures, 834
opiate exposure, 232
opioids, 109, 109–110b
oral candidiasis, 178, 178f
oral contraceptive pill (OCP), 909
oral healthcare, preschooler, 322

oral rehydration solutions (ORSs), 528, 598
oral rehydration therapy (ORT), 598
orthopaedic infections
- osteomyelitis
  - clinical manifestations, 950
  - definition, 949
  - diagnostic evaluation, 950
  - nursing care management, 950
  - pathophysiology, 949, 949f
  - therapeutic management, 950
- septic arthritis, 950
- tuberculosis, 950–951

orthostatic hypotension (OH), 72
orthotics, 925–926, 926b, 926f
osteodystrophy, 581
osteogenesis imperfecta (OI)
- classification, 951, 951b
- nursing care management, 952
- therapeutic management, 951–952
- types, 951

osteomyelitis, 933
- clinical manifestations, 950
- definition, 949
- diagnostic evaluation, 950
- nursing care management, 950
- pathophysiology, 949, 949f
- therapeutic management, 950

osteosarcoma
- nursing care management, 810
- therapeutic management, 809–810

ostomies, 516
otitis media (OM), 650–653, 650b, 651b, 651f
overweight, 360
oxygen, 821

P

paediatric nursing
- childhood health problems
  - childhood mortality, 7
  - infant mortality, 6–7, 7f
  - injuries, 4–6, 6f
  - low birth weight (LBW), 4
  - mental health problems, 6
  - obesity, 4, 5f
  - type 2 diabetes, 4
  - very low birth weight (VLBW), 4
- child wellbeing, 9
- clinical nurse specialist (CNS), 8
- coordination and collaboration, 8
- ethical decision-making, 8
- evidence-based practice (EBP), 8–9
- family-centred care, 7–8
- healthcare for, 1–3
  - accidental injury, 1
  - Australia's children reports, 2b
  - Australia's health system, 2
  - Children's Headline Indicators (CHIs), 1, 2b
  - immunisation rates, 1
  - New Zealand's Health System, 2–3
  - private healthcare policies, 3
- health promotion, 3–4
  - development, 3
  - health indicators, 3
  - nutrition, 3–4
  - oral health, 4
- National Health Strategies for Children, 9
- philosophy of care, 7–8
- therapeutic relationship, 8

paediatric procedures
- compliance
  - behavioural strategies, 488
  - methods, 487–488
  - organisational strategies, 488
  - treatment strategies, 488
- diagnostic and therapeutic procedures, 482–484
  - family education, 484, 484b

paediatric procedures *(Continued)*
performance of, 483–484
physical preparation, 483
postprocedural support, 484
psychological preparation, 482–483, 483t
informed consent
conditions, 481
eligibility for, 482
requirements, 481–482
surgical procedures, 484–487
intraoperative care, 485
postoperative care, 485–487, 486t, 487b
preoperative care, 484–485, 485t
pain
acute
invasive procedures, 98–100
needlestick pain, 100, 115b
postoperative pain, 100
assessment tools, 103
autism spectrum disorder (ASD), 105
biobehavioural strategies, 113–114b
brain neuromatrix, 98
children's cancer, 796–797
chronic
abdominal pain, 101
common sites, 100
headaches, 101
musculoskeletal pain, 101
neuropathic pain syndromes, 101
treatment, 116
chronic and recurrent pain assessment, 105–108
Children's Depression Inventory (CDI), 107
Functional Disability Inventory (FDI), 107
pain diaries, 107
Pediatric Pain Questionnaire (PPQ), 105–107
sleep disruption, 107–108
cognitively impaired children, 104
definition, 97, 98t
measurement tools, 103
mixed-pain conditions
burn pain, 101–102
cancer pain, 102, 102t, 116–117
sickle cell pain (SCD), 102–103, 117
model, 97–98, 99f
observational pain measures, 103–104, 103t, 104f
paediatric intensive care unit, 104
positron emission tomography, 97–98
post anaesthesia, 104
preterm infants/neonates, 98, 100b, 104, 105t
prevalence, 97
prevention and treatment
analgesia equipment needs, 115b
analgesia timing, 110
analgesic administration, 110, 111–112b
biobehavioural interventions, 108–109, 108b, 109f
co-analgesic drugs, 109
end-of-life care, 117
epidural analgesia, 112
medication dose, 109–110
non-opioids, 109
obese and overweight children, 116
opioids, 109, 109–110b
patient-controlled analgesia (PCA), 110–112
pharmacological management, 109–117
program goals, 108b
sedation levels, 115, 115b
side effects, 112–114, 113b
transmucosal and transdermal analgesia, 112, 112f
tricyclic antidepressants, 117b
self-report pain rating scales, 104–105, 106–107t
syndromes, 98
palliative care, childhood terminal illness, 432–437, 432b, 433b, 434t, 435b
pancreatic hormone secretion, diabetes mellitus
diagnostic evaluation, 885
nursing care management, 888–889
pathophysiology, 883–885, 884f
therapeutic management, 885–887, 886t, 887t
type 1 diabetes, 882, 883f, 884b, 884t
type 2 diabetes, 882–883, 884t
panhypopituitarism, 866, 868b
parachute reflex, 241, 242f
parasomnias, 282
parathyroid hormone (PTH)
hyperparathyroidism, 876
hypoparathyroidism, 875–876
physiological effects, 875b
PARDS severity classification, 670t
parental education, 21–22
parent–infant bonding (attachment)
en face position, 163, 163f
infant behaviour, 162–163
maternal attachment, 163
multiple births and subsequent children, 165
neonates complexity, 162
paternal engrossment, 163–164, 164f
premature infants, 208–209, 209f
siblings, 164, 164f
parenting
adoption, 15
after separation, 16
authoritarian, 14
authoritative, 14
cross-racial and international adoption, 15
discipline, 14
dual-earner families, 17–18
feelings and behaviours, 16, 17b
foster care, 18
joint legal custody, 16
joint physical custody, 16
kinship care, 17–18
limit setting, 14
misbehaviour, 15
permissive, 14
reconstituted families, 17
relationship breakdown, 15–16, 16f
single, 16–17
situations, 15–18
styles, 14
passive immunity, 123b
Patau's syndrome, 31
patellar reflex, 93, 93f
patent ductus arteriosus (PDA)
clinical manifestations, 224
incidence, 223–224
nursing care management, 224
therapeutic management, 224
paternal engrossment, 163–164, 164f
patient-controlled analgesia (PCA), 110–112
PBS. *See* Pharmaceutical Benefits Scheme (PBS)
PDA. *See* patent ductus arteriosus (PDA)
Pediatric Pain Questionnaire (PPQ), 105–107
pediculosis capitis
diagnostic evaluation, 902, 903f
nursing care management, 903
therapeutic management, 902
pedigree chart (family tree, genogram), 25–27b
peer cultures, 19, 19f
pelvic inflammatory disease (PID), 407–408
pelvis and ureters, renal dysfunction, 558
penetrance, 25–27b
peptic ulcer disease (PUD), 614–616, 615b, 615f
perinatal environmental factors
chemical agents, 192–193
radiation, 193
perinatal hypoxic-ischaemic brain injury
causes, 225–226
clinical manifestations, 226
perinatal hypoxic-ischaemic brain injury *(Continued)*
hypoxic-ischaemic encephalopathy (HIE), 226
nursing care management, 226
therapeutic hypothermia, 226, 226f
periodic breathing, 152–153
peripheral blood stem cell transplant (PBSCT), 791
peripherally inserted central catheters (PICCs), 506
peristalsis, 558
peritoneal dialysis, 582–583
peritonitis, 609
permanent cells, 892
persistent cloaca, 633
persistent depressive disorder, 376
persistent pulmonary hypertension of the newborn (PPHN)
nursing care management, 219
primary, 219
pulmonary vasculature, 218–219
therapeutic management, 219
pertussis, immunisations, 124
pertussis (whooping cough), 663
PHACE syndrome haemangiomas, 180
phaeochromocytoma, 882
phagocytes, 139
Pharmaceutical Benefits Scheme (PBS), 2
pharmacogenomics, 27
phenotype, 25–27b
phenylketonuria (PKU)
clinical manifestations, 43
diagnostic evaluation, 43
incidence, 42
nursing care management, 43
pathophysiology, 42, 42f
prognosis, 43
therapeutic management, 43
phimosis, 584
phlegmon, 609
phototherapy, 184
and parent–infant interaction, 185b
phrenic nerve paralysis, 171
physeal damage, 933
physical abuse, 329–330
adolescence, 394
factors predisposing to, 330
physical activity, school-age children
exercise, 353
organised athletics goals, 353b
physical fitness, 353
skills acquisition, 353–354, 354f
television, video games and the internet, 354, 355b
physical examination
abdomen
auscultation, 89
inspection, 88–89, 89f
palpation, 89, 89b
structures, 88, 88f
age-specific approaches, 67, 68t
anus, 91
chest, 83–84, 83f, 84f
child preparation, 64–67, 67b, 69f
developmental assessment, 93
ears
auditory testing, 81, 81t
external structures, 79, 79f
internal structures, 79–81, 80f, 81f
extremities, 91–92, 92f
eyes
accommodation, 77
bulbar conjunctiva, 76
colour vision, 79
cornea, 77
external structures, 76, 77f
fovea centralis, 77
fundus, 77, 77f
internal structures, 77

physical examination *(Continued)*
lacrimal punctum, 76
macula, 77
meibomian/sebaceous glands, 76
ocular alignment, 77–78, 78f
optic disc, 77
palpebral conjunctivae, 76
palpebral fissures, 76
peripheral vision, 78–79
PERRLA, 77
sclera, 76
vision testing, 77–79
visual acuity testing, 78
general appearance, 72–74
genitalia
in adolescents, 89–90
female, 91, 91f
male, 90–91, 90f
growth measurements
arm circumference, 71
growth charts, 68–69, 69f
head circumference, 71, 71f
height, 69–70, 70f
length, 69, 70f
parameters, 68
skinfold thickness, 70–71
weight, 70, 71f
head and neck, 76
heart
heart murmurs, 87, 88t
heart sound direction, 87, 87f, 88t
position of, 86, 86f
pulse location, 86, 87f
joints, 92
lungs
auscultation, 85–86, 86b
lobes location, 84–85, 85f
lymph nodes, 76, 76f
mouth and throat
buccal mucosa, 82
child positioning, 82, 82f
internal structures, 82–83, 83f
muscles, 92
neurological assessment, 92–93
cerebellar function, 92, 93b
cranial nerves, 93, 94f, 95t, 96f
reflexes, 92–93, 93f
nose
external structures, 81–82, 82f
internal structures, 82
paper-doll technique, 67, 69f
physiological measurements
apical impulse, 72
bladder width, 72
blood pressure, 72, 74f
core temperature, 71–72, 73t
cuff bladder length, 72
cuff size, 72, 74f
electronic continuous thermometers, 72
electronic intermittent thermometers, 72
elements, 71
infrared thermometers, 72
normothermia, 71–72
orthostatic hypotension (OH), 72
pulse grading, 72, 74t
respiration, 72
sequence of, 64
skin
accessory structures, 75, 75f
colour changes, 74–75, 75t
tissue turgor, 75
spine, 91
physical neglect, 329
phytates/oxalates, 274
pia mater, cerebral dysfunction, 820
pica, 605
PID. *See* pelvic inflammatory disease (PID)
PIE. *See* pulmonary interstitial emphysema (PIE)
Pierre Robin sequence (PRS), 173b, 174, 675
pilonidal sinus, 154
pincer grasp, 245, 245f
pituitary function
anterior pituitary hormones, 866
diabetes insipidus, 871–872
hypopituitarism
cause of, 867, 867b, 869f
clinical manifestations, 868, 868b
condition, 866
congenital hypopituitarism, 867
diagnostic evaluation, 868–869
growth failure, 867
idiopathic hypopituitarism, 867
nursing care management, 870
therapeutic management, 869–870
pituitary hyperfunction, 870
precocious puberty, 870–871, 871b
SIADH, 872
pituitary gland, 865
pituitary hyperfunction, 870
PKU. *See* phenylketonuria (PKU)
PMDD. *See* premenstrual dysphoric disorder (PMDD)
pneumococcal disease, immunisations, 124–125
Pneumocystis pneumonia, 793
pneumonia
atypical, 660
bacterial, 660–662
community-acquired pneumonia, 662f
neonatal, 662
signs of, 661b
types, 659–660, 660b
viral, 660
pneumothorax, 218, 663b, 663f
point of maximum intensity (PMI), 153
poisoning
children, 324–328, 325–326b
acute single-dose paracetamol poisoning, 328f
assessment, 328
developmental characteristics, 325
emergency treatment, 325–328
gastric decontamination, 328
recurrence prevention, 328
prevention, 329b
polio, immunisations, 124
polycythaemia, 224
polygenic disorders, 25–27b, 28
polyploidy, 25–27b
polyvalent vaccine, 123b
positional plagiocephaly (PP), 286f
diagnostic evaluation, 286
mild facial asymmetry, 286
nursing care management, 286–287
therapeutic management, 286
positive media, 20, 20b
postconcussion syndrome (PCS), 836
postictal state, 851
posttraumatic headaches, 836
posttraumatic seizures, 836
posttraumatic stress disorder (PTSD), 373–374
powder inhalation, 669
PP. *See* positional plagiocephaly (PP)
precocious puberty, 870–871, 871b
premature infants
nursing care of
arousal states, 206t
auditory environment, 208
behavioural states, 206
breastfeeding, 203
discharge planning and home care, 209–210
feeding resistance, 203, 204b
gavage feeding, 202–203
premature infants *(Continued)*
kangaroo care, 207
neurodevelopmental impairment, 204
nipple-feeding, 203
nutritional needs, 202
oral feeding, 203
parent–infant relationships, 208–209, 209f
pulse oximetry, 199
rapid eye movement (REM), 206
siblings, 209
skin care, 203
synactive theory of infant development, 204, 205t
respiratory function, 211–220
premenstrual dysphoric disorder (PMDD), 403
prenatal testing, hereditary disorders, 46–47, 46b
primary irritant, 899
primary lactase deficiency, 279
primary narcissism, psychosocial development, 247–248
private healthcare policies, 3
private health insurance, 2
proband (index case), 25–27b
probiotics, 202
procedures positioning
bone marrow aspiration/biopsy, 496
extremity venepuncture/injection, 494–495, 495f
femoral venepuncture, 494, 495f
lumbar puncture (LP), 495–496, 495f
prosthetics, 925–926, 926f, 927b
proteinuria, unexplained, 574–575
proximal tubular acidosis (Type II), 573
PRS. *See* Pierre Robin sequence (PRS)
pseudomenstruation, 153
psychological maltreatment, 329
psychosocial development
adolescence
autonomy development, 388
gender, 389
identity development, 388
intimacy, 390
self-identity, 389–390
sexuality, 388–390
sexual orientation, 388–389
infant
breastfeeding, 249
primary narcissism, 247–248
sense of trust, 247–249
preschooler
oedipal stage, 311
sense of initiative, 311
school-age children
inferiority, 339
latency period, 338
sense of industry, 338–339, 339f
toddler, 292
psychotic depression, 376
PTSD. *See* posttraumatic stress disorder (PTSD)
pubertal sexual maturation, 383–386
puberty, 382, 386
PUD. *See* peptic ulcer disease (PUD)
pulmonary emboli, 933–934
pulmonary hypertension (PH), 745–747, 746t
clinical manifestations, 746
diagnostic evaluation, 746
nursing care management, 746–747
pathophysiology, 746
therapeutic management, 746
pulmonary interstitial emphysema (PIE), 213, 218
pulmonary oedema, 213, 669–670
pulse oximetry, 199, 640
Punnett squares, 33, 34f

Q

quadriceps reflex, 93, 93f

R

race, 20
radiation, stable body temperature, 156
radiation therapy, children's cancer, 787, 788t
radioiodine, 874
rapid eye movement (REM), 206
RDS. *See* respiratory distress syndrome (RDS)
recessive, 25–27b
recombination, 25–27b
reconstituted families, 17
rectal atresia, 633
rectal stenosis, 633
refeeding syndrome, 275, 415
referred pain, 609
reflexes, 250. *See also individual reflex type*
refractory seizures, 857
refugee and immigration, 22
rehydration, pituitary function, 372
religion/spiritual identity, 22–23, 22f, 23b
REM. *See* rapid eye movement (REM)
renal dysfunction
  disorders of sex development (DSD)
    family support, 588
    obstructive uropathy, 588–590, 588f
    pathophysiology, 587–588
    therapeutic management, 588
  excretion, 556
  genitourinary tract defects
    bladder exstrophy, 586–587, 586f
    cloacal exstrophy, 586–587
    cryptorchidism, 585
    epispadias, 586–587
    hydrocele, 584–585
    hypospadias, 586, 586f
    phimosis, 584
  genitourinary tract disorders
    urinary tract infection (UTI), 563–566
    vesicoureteral reflux (VUR), 563–566
  glomerular disease
    acute glomerulonephritis (AGN), 567–570
    chronic glomerulonephritis (CGN), 570
    nephrotic syndrome, 570–573
  glomerular filtration, 556–557
  miscellaneous
    acute kidney injury (AKI), 575–578
    chronic kidney disease (CKD), 578–581
    familial nephritis (Alport's syndrome), 574
    renal failure, 575
    renal trauma, 575
    unexplained proteinuria, 574–575
  pathophysiology, 557, 557f
  pelvis and ureters, 558
  physiology, 556–558
  reabsorption, 556
  renal development and function, 558
  renal replacement therapy
    continuous venovenous haemofiltration (CVVH), 583
    dialysis, 581
    fluid and electrolyte movement, 581, 581b
    haemodialysis, 581–582
    peritoneal dialysis, 582–583
    transplantation, 583–584
  secretion, 556
  tubular disorders
    nephrogenic diabetes insipidus (NDI), 574
    renal tubular acidosis (RTA), 573–574
    tubular function, 573
  tubular function, 557
  urethrovesical unit, 558–563
    blood tests, 560, 563t
    clinical manifestations, 559, 559b
    collagen, 558
    detrusor, 558
    nursing care management, 563
    radiological tests, 560, 561–562t
renal dysfunction *(Continued)*
    urinary continence, 558
    urine tests, 560, 560–561t
renal failure, 575
renal replacement therapy
  continuous venovenous haemofiltration (CVVH), 583
  dialysis, 581
  fluid and electrolyte movement, 581, 581b
  haemodialysis, 581–582
  peritoneal dialysis, 582–583
  transplantation, 583–584
renal system
  burn, 543
  extrauterine life, newborn, 138
renal trauma, 575
renal tubular acidosis (RTA), 573–574
repositioning and physical therapy (RPPT), 286
reproduction
  adolescent abortion, 410–411, 410b
  adolescent pregnancy
    complications, 409–410
    fathers, 410
    incidence, 409
    medical concerns, 409
    mother–infant relationships, 410
    nursing care management, 410
  contraception, 411, 412–413t
  sexual assault (rape), 411
resiliency model, family stress, 12
respiratory distress syndrome (RDS)
  clinical manifestations, 213–214, 214f
  diagnostic evaluation, 214–215
  factors, 214t
  medical therapies, 216
  nursing care management, 216–217
  oxygen therapy, 215–216, 216f
  pathophysiology, 212–213, 212f, 213f
  positive pressure ventilation, 216
  prevention, 216
  surfactant, 212, 215
  therapeutic management, 215–216
respiratory dysfunction
  croup syndromes, 654t
    acute epiglottitis, 653–655
    acute infections, 653, 653f
    acute laryngitis, 655
    acute laryngotracheobronchitis (LTB), 655–656, 656f
    acute spasmodic laryngitis, 656
    bacterial tracheitis, 657
  diagnostic procedures
    blood gas determination, 640
    non-invasive monitoring, 640–641
    pulmonary function tests, 639–640
    radiology, 640
  function, 638
  infections
    aetiology and characteristics, 641
    clinical manifestations, 641
    nursing care of, 641–644, 642b, 643b
  long-term respiratory dysfunction
    allergic rhinitis, 675–697
    asthma, 677–687, 678b, 678f, 679f, 680f, 682f, 684t, 688f
    cystic fibrosis (CF), 687–696, 690f
    exercise, 683–684
    exercise-induced bronchospasm (EIB), 683–684
    obstructive sleep apnoea, 696–697
    puffer *vs.* puffer and spacer, 687f
  lower airways infections, 657t
    bronchiolitis, 657–659, 659b
    bronchitis, 657
    pneumonia. *See* pneumonia
    respiratory syncytial virus (RSV), 657–659, 658b
  non-infectious irritants
    acute lung injury (ALI), 670–672
respiratory dysfunction *(Continued)*
    acute respiratory distress syndrome (ARDS), 670–672, 671f
    aspiration pneumonia, 668–669, 668b
    environmental tobacco exposure 673
    foreign body ingestion and aspiration, 666–668, 667f
    foreign body, nose, 668
    PARDS severity classification, 670t
    pulmonary oedema, 669–670
    smoke inhalation injury, 672–673
  pertussis (whooping cough), 663
  physical assessment, 639
    chest pain, 639
    clubbing, 639
    colour changes of the skin, 639
    grunting, 639
    head bobbing, 639
    nasal flaring, 639
    noisy breathing, 639
    recession, 639
    respiration, 639
    stridor, 639
    wheezing, 639
  respiratory failure, 697, 698b
  structural defects
    choanal atresia, 675
    congenital diaphragmatic hernia (CDH), 673–675
    Pierre Robin sequence (PRS), 675
  tract defences, 638–639
  tract structure, 637–638
  tuberculosis, 663–666, 664b
  upper respiratory tract infections (URTI)
    acute otitis externa (AOE), 653
    acute streptococcal pharyngitis, 645–646, 645t, 646t
    acute viral nasopharyngitis, 644–645, 645b
    coronavirus (Covid-19), 650
    glandular fever (infectious mononucleosis), 648–649
    influenza, 649
    otitis media (OM), 650–653, 650b, 651b, 651f
    tonsillitis, 646–648, 646f
respiratory function, high-risk newborns
  air leak syndromes
    clinical manifestations, 218
    nursing care management, 218
    pulmonary interstitial emphysema (PIE), 218
    therapeutic management, 218
  apnoea of prematurity (AOP)
    causes of, 212b
    classification, 211
    clinical manifestations, 211
    nursing care management, 212
    pathophysiology, 211
    therapeutic management, 211–212
  chronic lung disease
    mild, 219
    nursing care management, 220
    pathophysiology, 219
    prognosis, 220
    therapeutic management, 219–220
  meconium aspiration syndrome (MAS), 217f
    clinical manifestations, 217
    diagnostic evaluation, 217–218
    nursing care management, 218
    pathophysiology, 217
    therapeutic management, 218
  persistent pulmonary hypertension of the newborn (PPHN)
    nursing care management, 219
    primary, 219
    pulmonary vasculature, 218–219
    therapeutic management, 219
  respiratory distress syndrome (RDS)
    clinical manifestations, 213–214, 214f
    diagnostic evaluation, 214–215

respiratory function, high-risk newborns *(Continued)*
factors, 214t
medical therapies, 216
nursing care management, 216–217
oxygen therapy, 215–216, 216f
pathophysiology, 212–213, 212f, 213f
positive pressure ventilation, 216
prevention, 216
surfactant, 212, 215
therapeutic management, 215–216
respiratory management, unconscious child, 829
respiratory secretion specimens, 500
respiratory syncytial virus (RSV), 657–659, 658b
retinoblastoma
clinical manifestations, 813–814
diagnostic evaluation, 814
nursing care management, 814–815, 815f
staging and prognosis, 814
therapeutic management, 814
two-hit model, 813
retinoblastoma gene (*Rb1*), 784
retinopathy of prematurity (ROP), 224–225, 225b
rhabdomyosarcoma
clinical manifestations, 812, 813t
diagnostic evaluation, 812
embryonal and alveolar subtypes, 812, 812b
nursing care management, 813
staging and prognosis, 813, 813b
therapeutic management, 813
rheumatic heart disease (RHD), 731–734
aetiology, 732
clinical manifestations, 732b
diagnostic evaluation, 733
nursing care management, 733–734
pathophysiology, 734
pathophysiology and clinical manifestations, 732–733
risk groups, 731, 732t
therapeutic management, 733
rickettsial diseases, nursing care management, 903
RNA, 25–27b
robertsonian translocations, 32, 32f
rooting reflex, 152
ROP. *See* retinopathy of prematurity (ROP)
rotavirus, 595
immunisations, 125
rubella, 128, 132f

S

safety
environmental factors, 492–493, 492f
falls prevention, 492–493
infants and children transport, 493–494
infection control, 493
mummy restraint/swaddle, 494, 495f
protective measures, 491
restraining methods, 494
toys, 492
SAM. *See* severe acute malnutrition (SAM)
Sarcoptes scabiei, 900
SBS. *See* short bowel syndrome (SBS)
scabies, 900–902, 902b, 902f
scarlet fever, 128, 133f, 645
SCD. *See* sickle cell disease (SCD)
school communities
community, 19
cultural diffusion, 19
peer cultures, 19, 19f
school health and school connectedness, 18–19
schools, 19
school health and school connectedness, 18–19
school phobia, 374–375
SCU. *See* severe childhood under-nutrition (SCU)
seasonal affective disorder, 376
seborrhoeic dermatitis, 908
secondary lactase deficiency, 279
seizures
cerebral dysfunction
aetiology, 850–851, 850b
clinical manifestations, 851, 852–853b
definition, 850
diagnostic evaluation, 855–856
febrile seizure, 860
focal seizures, 851–853
generalised seizures, 853–854
incidence, 851
LGS, 855
nursing care management, 857–860, 857b, 858b, 859b
pathophysiology, 851
prognosis, 857
therapeutic management, 856–857
unknown-onset epileptic seizures, 854–855
self-concept development, 345–347
self-esteem, 345–347
self-harm
aetiology, 418
definition, 418
diagnostic evaluation, 418
prevalence, 418
therapeutic management, 418
types, 418b
self-monitoring of blood glucose (SMBG), 885
sensitising irritant, 899
sensory loss
blindness and low vision
aetiology, 458–460
definition and classification, 458
eye injuries, 460b
nursing care management, 460–462
types, 459–460b
deafness and hearing
aetiology, 455
clinical manifestations, 457b
definition and classification, 455, 456t
hearing aids, 456f
lip-reading, 457
nursing care management, 456–458
pathology, 455
sign language, 457
socialisation, 457
speech-language therapy, 457
symptom severity, 455
therapeutic management, 455–456
sepsis, 220–222
bacterial infection, 220–221
breastfeeding, 221
clinical manifestations, 221–222, 222b
diagnostic evaluation, 222
mortality rate, 221
nursing care management, 222
pathophysiology, 221
prognosis, 222
sources of, 221
therapeutic management, 222
septic arthritis, 950
sequence, 28
setting-sun sign, 842
severe acute malnutrition (protein–energy malnutrition)
factor causing, 274–275
nursing care management, 275–276
therapeutic management, 275
severe acute malnutrition (SAM), 274–275
severe childhood under-nutrition (SCU), 274–275
sex chromosome aneuploidies, 31
sex education, 317–318, 347–348
nurse's role, 348
sex-linked inheritance patterns, 25–27b, 34–37
sex steroids, 877
sexual abuse
abusers and victims characteristics, 330–331
adolescence, 394
initiation and perpetuation, 331
nursing care of, 331
types, 330
warning signs of, 331b
sexual assault (rape), 411
sexuality development, school-age children, 347–348
sexually transmitted bacterial infections, 406–408
sexually transmitted infections (STIs), 393–394, 405–406, 406b
sexually transmitted protozoa infections, 406
sexually transmitted viral infections, 408–409
SGA. *See* small-for-gestational-age (SGA)
shock, 526–527
aetiology, 531
clinical manifestations, 532–533, 532t
diagnostic evaluation, 533
family support, 534–535
nursing care management, 534
pathophysiology, 532
therapeutic management, 533–534
types, 531b
short bowel syndrome (SBS), 620
siblings, 164, 164f
chronic/complex diseases, 426, 426b
premature infants, 209
sickle cell anaemia (SCA), 763–768, 764f, 765b, 767b, 768f
sickle cell disease (SCD), 273
sickle cell pain (SCD), 102–103, 117
SIDS. *See* sudden infant death syndrome (SIDS)
single-gene disorders, 28
allele, 33
autosomal dominant inheritance, 33–34, 33f, 34f, 35–37t
autosomal recessive inheritance, 34, 37f
Mendelian-inherited genetic disorders, 34, 35–37t
reduced/incomplete penetrance, 33
sex-linked inheritance patterns, 34–37
sex-linked traits, 37, 38f
variable expressivity, 33
X-linked dominant inheritance, 37, 39f
X-linked recessive inheritance, 37, 38f
sinus arrhythmia, 243
SIRS. *See* systemic inflammatory response syndrome (SIRS)
skeletal limb deficiency
nursing care management, 944
pathophysiology, 943
therapeutic management, 943
skin care, 488b
bathing, 489
epidermal stripping, 489
hair care, 489
healthy skin, 488–489
oral hygiene, 489
pressure ulcers, 488–489
shear, 489
skin elasticity, 528f
skin grafts
adherent allograft, 549f
mesh graft, 550f
requirements, 550b
sheet graft, 550f
split-thickness removal, 550f
types, 549b
skin infections
bacterial infections, 894–896, 895t
dermatophytoses, 896, 898f, 898t
systemic mycotic infections, 897, 899t
viral infections, 896, 897t
skin lesions, integumentary dysfunction
aetiology, 891
diagnostic evaluation, 891

skin lesions, integumentary dysfunction *(Continued)*
history and symptoms, 891–892
laboratory studies, 892
objective findings, 892
origin, 891
pathophysiology of dermatitis, 891
younger children, 891
skin, physical examination, 151
accessory structures, 75, 75f
colour changes, 74–75, 75t
tissue turgor, 75
skull fractures, 834
sleep and activity
during infancy, 263–264
preschooler, 320–322
school-age children, 352–353
toddlerhood, 303–304
sleep deprivation, 396
sleep disruption, 107–108
sleep problems, children, 324
sleep-wake states, 141, 142t
slipped capital femoral epiphysis (SCFE), 947–948
small-for-gestational-age (SGA), 143
smegma, 153
smell, extrauterine life, newborn, 140
smoke inhalation injury, 672–673
social development, 254–258t
attachment, 251–252
child care arrangements, 259–260
language development, 252
personal-social behaviour, 252–253
play, 253
preschooler
language, 313
personal-social behaviour, 314
play, 314, 317f
screen time, 314–317
prolonged separation effects, 251–252
school-age children, 342–344
bullying, 343
cyberbullying, 343
ego mastery, 345
peer groups, 342–343
play, 344–345, 345f
quiet games and activities, 344–345, 345f
relationships with families, 343–344
rules and rituals, 344
social relationships and cooperation, 342–343, 343f
separation anxiety, 252, 253–259
shaken baby syndrome, 259
soother use, 260–261
spoiled child syndrome, 259
stranger fear, 252, 252f, 253–259
teething, 261, 261f
thumb sucking, 260–261
toddler
individuation, 296
language development, 295–297
personal-social behaviour, 297
play, 297–298, 298f
rapprochement, 296
separation, 296
transitional objects, 296, 297f
social media, 19–20
soft tissue injury, 168, 169b
solid tumours
GCTs, 815
liver tumours, 815
retinoblastoma, 813–815
rhabdomyosarcoma, 812–813, 813t
Wilms tumour, 811–812
somatic cell, 25–27b
Somogyi effect, 887
specimens collection
blood specimens, 498–500
from arterial vessels, 499–500
specimens collection *(Continued)*
capillary methods, 500, 500f
from central venous catheters, 498–499
from peripheral veins, 499
respiratory secretion specimens, 500
stool specimens, 498
urine specimens, 496–498
bladder catheterisation, 496–498, 497t
collection bags, 496
lignocaine, 497–498b
twenty-four-hour collection, 496
speech-language therapy, 457
speech problems, preschooler, 319
spina bifida (SB), 971, 973b
spinal cord compression, 792
spinal cord injuries (SCIs)
aetiology, 983–984
autonomic system, 983, 983b
clinical manifestations, 984–985
diagnostic evaluation, 985–986, 985f
nursing care management
acute phase, 987
autonomic dysreflexia, 989
cardiovascular care, 988
neurogenic bladder, 988–989
physical rehabilitation, 990, 990f
physical therapy, 988
psychosocial rehabilitation, 990
remobilisation, 989–990
respiratory care, 987–988
sexuality, 990–991
skin care, 988
temperature regulation, 988
transition to adulthood, 991
pathophysiology, 984, 984b
principles, 981
sensory and motor tracts, 983
spinal nerves, 981, 982t
therapeutic management, 986–987
upper *vs.* lower motor neurons, 983, 983b
spinal cord injury, 913
spinal muscular atrophy (SMA) type 1
clinical manifestations, 978, 978b
diagnostic evaluation, 978–979
nursing care management, 979
therapeutic management, 979
spinal shock syndrome, 984
spine, physical examination, 91
spinraza, 979
spiritual development, 295
adolescence, 387–388
preschooler, 312
sporadic, 25–27b
sports participation
contusions, 935
dislocations, 935–936
exercise-induced heat stress, 937
female athlete triad, 938–939
nurse's role, 940
nutrition, 937–938
overuse injury, 937
preparation, 934, 934f, 935f
sprains and strains, 936, 936b, 936f
substance misuse, 939
sudden death, 939–940
types of, 934–935, 935f
status epilepticus, 857
stereopsis, 242
steroid effects, 795–796
STIs. *See* sexually transmitted infections (STIs)
stomatitis
aphthous stomatitis, 134
herpetic gingivostomatitis (HGS), 135, 135f
nursing care management, 135
therapeutic management, 135
stooling patterns, newborns, 138, 139b
stool specimens, 498
strawberry haemangioma, 179, 180f
stress
anticipated parental, 425b
concurrent, 426–427
fractures, 937
growth and development promotion, toddler, 302
life-threatening illness, 445–446
preschooler, 319, 320b
school-age children, 349–350, 351b
stress urinary incontinence (SUI), 975
structural chromosome abnormalities, 31–33, 32f
structural defects
abdominal wall defects, 629–631
atresia, 627
oesophageal atresia (OA), 627–629, 627f
tracheo-oesophageal fistula (TOF), 627–629, 627f
subarachnoid haemorrhage, 227
subdural haematoma, 835, 835f
subdural haemorrhage, 227
subgaleal haemorrhage, 169, 170f
submersion injury
accidental submersion injury, 840, 840f
clinical manifestations, 840
drowning, 839–840
nursing care management, 841
pathophysiology, 840
therapeutic management, 840–841
submetacentric chromosomes, 28–29
substance abuse
alcohol, 417
central nervous system depressants, 417
central nervous system stimulants, 418
cocaine, 417
drugs abuse, 416–417
illicit drugs, 416
mind-altering drugs, 418
motivation, 416
narcotics, 417
nursing care management, 418
tobacco
aetiology, 417
incidence, 417
nursing care management, 417
sucking reflex, 152
sudden death, 939–940
sudden infant death syndrome (SIDS)
aetiology, 282–283
definition, 282
epidemiology, 282, 284t
family care, 285
genetic predisposition, 282–283
nursing care management, 285
prevention, 282
protective factors, 284
risk factors
co-sleeping, 283
of infants, 284–285
maternal smoking, 283
prone sleeping, 283
soft bedding, 283–284
sudden unexpected death in infancy (SUDI), 6
suicide
adolescence, 394
aetiology, 419
attempt, 418
ideation, 418
mental health services, 420b
motivation, 419
nursing care management, 419–420
suicidal ideation, 418
suicide attempt, 418
therapeutic management, 419
warning signs of, 419b
superego, 311
superior vena cava syndrome (SVCS), 792

supramalleolar orthosis (SMO), 925
synactive theory of infant development, 204, 205t
syncope, 72
syndrome, 25–27b, 28
syndrome of inappropriate antidiuretic hormone (SIADH), 830, 831t
  pituitary function, 872
syphilis, 407
systemic antibiotic therapy, 909
systemic hypertension, 737–740
  aetiology, 737, 738b
  clinical manifestations, 737
  diagnostic evaluation, 738–739, 739t
  nursing care management, 740
  therapeutic management, 739–740
systemic inflammatory response syndrome (SIRS), 535, 535b
systemic lupus erythematosus (SLE)
  aetiology, 955
  clinical manifestations, 956, 956b
  course and symptoms, 955
  diagnostic evaluation, 956, 956b
  general measures, 957
  nursing care management, 957–958
  pathophysiology, 955–956
  therapeutic management, 957
systemic mycotic infections, 897, 899t

T

tachypnoea, 639
Tanner stages, 383b
targeted therapy, 786
taste, extrauterine life, newborn, 140
TATs. *See* temporal artery thermometers (TATs)
TBW. *See* total body water (TBW)
TCM. *See* transcutaneous monitoring (TCM)
telehealth and counselling, 50–51
telephone triage, 50–51, 51b
telomere, 25–27b
temper tantrums, 301–302
temporal artery thermometers (TATs), 145
tension pneumothorax, 218
tension-type headaches, 860–861
tentorium, cerebral dysfunction, 820
teratogen, 25–27b, 192
testicular torsion, 401
tetanus, immunisations, 123
thermoregulation
  extrauterine life, newborn, 138
  low-birth-weight (LBW) infant, 200
  non-shivering thermogenesis, 200
  plastic wrap, 200, 200f
  sterile cloth/disposable drapes, 201
  thermal stability, 200
thoracolumbosacral orthosis (TLSO), 926
thyroidectomy, 874
thyroid function
  chronic lymphocytic thyroiditis, 873–874
  goitre, 873
  hyperthyroidism
    clinical manifestations, 874
    diagnostic evaluation, 874
    nursing care management, 874–875
    therapeutic management, 874
  juvenile hypothyroidism, 872–873
  thyroid hormone, 872, 873b
  types, 872
thyroid hormone (TH). *See* thyroid function
thyroid-stimulating hormone (TSH), 865, 867f
thyrotoxicosis, 874
tic disorders, 372, 372b
tinea capitis, 896, 898f
tinea corporis, 896, 898f
tobacco
  adolescence, 394
  aetiology, 417
tobacco *(Continued)*
  incidence, 417
  nursing care management, 417
TOF. *See* tracheo-oesophageal fistula (TOF)
toilet training, toddler, 298–301
tonic–clonic seizures, 853–854
tonic neck reflex, 155t, 156f
tonsillitis, 646–648, 646f
tooth avulsion, 366
topical antibacterial agent, 909
topical corticosteroid therapy, 893
topical immunomodulators, 893
TORCHS complex, 234
torticollis, 171, 940
total body water (TBW), 520, 522, 522f
touch, extrauterine life, newborn, 140
toxic shock syndrome (TSS), 538
toxoid, 123b
TPN. *See* total parenteral nutrition (TPN)
tracheomalacia, 628
tracheo-oesophageal fistula (TOF), 627–629, 627f
transcription, 25–27b
transcutaneous monitoring (TCM), 640
translation, 25–27b
translocation, 25–27b
translocation Down syndrome, 30
transverse myelitis, 983
trauma management
  characteristics, 911
  child abuse/non-accidental injury, 911–912
  emergency management, 912–914, 913b
  epidemiology, 911
  prevention, 912
  systematic assessment, 914
  unintentional/accidental injury, 911, 912b
traumatic brain injury (TBI), 836
Treacher Collins syndrome, 173b
trichomoniasis, 406
tricyclic antidepressants, 117b
trisomy, 25–27b, 29, 30
trisomy 13, 31
trisomy 18, 31
trisomy 21, 29–31
tuberculosis, 950–951
tubular disorders
  nephrogenic diabetes insipidus (NDI), 574
  renal tubular acidosis (RTA), 573–574
  tubular function, 573
tubular necrosis, 576
tumour lysis syndrome, 791–792
tumour marker test, 786
tumour suppressor genes, 784
Turner's syndrome, 31
type 1 diabetes, 882, 883f, 884b, 884t
type 2 diabetes, 4, 882–883, 884t
  insulin resistance, 362

U

umbilical cord blood, 791
umbilical hernias, 88–89, 89f, 631, 631f
umbilicus, infection and injury prevention, 157
unconscious child
  elimination, 831
  family support, 832
  intracranial pressure monitoring, 829–830
  LOC, 827–828
  medications, 831
  nutrition and hydration, 830–831, 831t
  pain management, 828–829
  respiratory management, 829
  stimulation, 831–832
  thermoregulation, 831
unintentional/accidental injury, 911
uniparental disomy, 39
universal newborn hearing screening, infection and injury prevention, 157
unknown-onset epileptic seizures, 854–855
upper respiratory tract infections (URTI)
  acute otitis externa (AOE), 653
  acute streptococcal pharyngitis, 645–646, 645t, 646t
  acute viral nasopharyngitis, 644–645, 645b
  coronavirus (Covid-19), 650
  glandular fever (infectious mononucleosis), 648–649
  influenza, 649
  otitis media (OM), 650–653, 650b, 651b, 651f
  tonsillitis, 646–648, 646f
ureterocele, 588
urethrovesical unit, 558–563
  blood tests, 560, 563t
  clinical manifestations, 559, 559b
  collagen, 558
  detrusor, 558
  nursing care management, 563
  radiological tests, 560, 561–562t
  urinary continence, 558
  urine tests, 560, 560–561t
urinary continence, 558
urinary system distress, 974
urinary tract infection (UTI)
  aetiology, 563
  clinical manifestations, 563–564, 564b
  diagnostic evaluation, 564
  fluid requirements, 565b
  nursing care management, 565–566
  preventing measures, 566b
  side effects, 565t
  signs and symptoms, 563
  specimen collection, 564b
  therapeutic management, 565
urine specimens, 496–498
  bladder catheterisation, 496–498, 497t
  collection bags, 496
  lignocaine, 497–498b
  twenty-four-hour collection, 496
urine testing, diabetes mellitus, 886

V

vaccination, 123b
vaccine, 123b
vacuum-assisted closure (VAC) device, 894
vaginal infections, 405
vagus nerve stimulation (VNS), 856–857
varicella, immunisations, 124
varicella-zoster immunoglobulin (VariZIG), 133
varicella-zoster virus, 132
varicocele, 400
vaso-occlusive crisis (VOC) pain, 102–103
velocardiofacial syndrome, 33
ventriculoperitoneal (VP) shunt, 843–844, 843f
vermiform appendix, 609
vernix caseosa, 139, 244
vertigo, 72
very low birth weight (VLBW), 4
vesicants, 790
vesicoureteral reflux (VUR)
  grades, 566, 566f
  with infection, 566
  nursing care management, 567
  therapeutic management, 566–567
vigabatrin, 854–855
vincristine, 795
viral infections, 896, 897t
vision
  extrauterine life, newborn, 140
  major developmental characteristics, 242b
vitamin A deficiency, 273
vitamin D-resistant rickets, 273
vitamin K administration
  infection and injury prevention, 156

vitamin K–deficiency bleeding. *See* haemorrhagic disease of the newborn
VLBW. *See* very low birth weight (VLBW)
VOC pain. *See* vaso-occlusive crisis (VOC) pain
volutrauma, 216
vomiting, 603–605, 603t
von Willebrand disease (vWD), 775
vulvar pain, 405
VUR. *See* vesicoureteral reflux (VUR)

W

'walling-off' process, 894–895
water balance
  fluid movement mechanisms, 520–522
  in infants, 522–523
  internal control mechanisms, 522b
  pathophysiology, 520–521, 521f
  requirements, 522t
water intoxication, 529
Werdnig-Hoffmann disease, 978–979, 978b
West's syndrome, 854–855
Wilms tumour
  clinical manifestations, 811
  definition, 811
  diagnostic evaluation, 811
  nursing care management, 812
  staging and prognosis, 811, 811b
  therapeutic management, 811–812
Wiskott-Aldrich syndrome, 784
Wolff 's law, 931
wounds
  acute wounds, 892
  chronic wounds, 892
  deeper tissues, 892
  epidermal injuries, 892
  home care and family support, 894
wounds *(Continued)*
  nursing care management, 893–894
  therapeutic management
    dressing, 892–893
    systemic therapy, 893
    topical therapy, 893

X

X inactivation (lyonisation), 25–27b
X-linked dominant inheritance, 37, 39f
X-linked inheritance, 25–27b
X-linked recessive inheritance, 37, 38f

Z

Zika virus (ZIKV), 173
zygote, 25–27b